PATIENT TEACHING TABLES

Patient teaching information for . . .

BUILDING YOUR CRITICAL THINKING SKILLS

PHARMACOTHERAPEUTICS:

A Nursing Process Approach
Fourth Edition

PHARMACOTHERAPEUTICS:

A Nursing Process Approach
Fourth Edition

Merrily A. Kuhn, RNC, PhD
President, Educational Services, Inc.
Hamburg, New York
Associate Professor
Daemen College
Amherst, New York

 **F. A. DAVIS COMPANY · Philadelphia**

F. A. Davis Company
1915 Arch Street
Philadelphia, PA 19103

Printed in the United States of America

Last digit indicates print number: 10 9 8 7 6 5 4 3 2 1

Publisher, Nursing: Robert G. Martone
Cover Designer: Louis J. Forgione

As new scientific information becomes available through basic and clinical research, recommended treatments and drug therapies undergo changes. The author(s) and publisher have done everything possible to make this book accurate, up to date, and in accord with accepted standards at the time of publication. The authors, editors, and publisher are not responsible for errors or omissions or for consequences from application of the book, and make no warranty, expressed or implied, in regard to the contents of the book. Any practice described in this book should be applied by the reader in accordance with professional standards of care used in regard to the unique circumstances that may apply in each situation. The reader is advised always to check product information (package inserts) for changes and new information regarding dose and contraindications before administering any drug. Caution is especially urged when using new or infrequently ordered drugs.

Library of Congress Cataloging-in-Publication Data

Kuhn, Merrily A., 1945–
    Pharmacotherapeutics : a nursing process approach / Merrily A. Kuhn. — 4th ed.
      p. cm.
    Includes bibliographical references and index.
    ISBN 0-8036-0287-1
    1. Chemotherapy. 2. Pharmacology. 3. Nursing. I. Title.
    [DNLM: 1. Drug Therapy—nurses' instruction. 2. Pharmacology—nurses' instruction. 3. Nursing
    Process. WB 320 K96p 1997]
    RM262.M373 1997
    615.5'8—dc21
    DNLM/DLC
    for Library of Congress   97-7202
                                                                CIP

To my parents, Audrey M. and Norbert J. Kuhn
for their love and encouragement

To my husband, James A. Kulwicki
for his daily concern, devotion, and love

To Helen Ruggles
for her unending energy in typing and organizing the manuscript

To all my students

PREFACE

The ever-expanding role of pharmacology in the practice of nursing demands that students be provided not only with reliable and current pharmacologic information but also with an understanding of the nurse's role in applying the knowledge of drugs to patient care. The previous editions of *Pharmacotherapeutics: A Nursing Process Approach* revolutionized the way nursing students learned pharmacology by integrating the nursing process with pharmacologic content. The fourth edition continues the tradition, further enhancing the relationship between nursing and pharmacology.

The fourth edition is tailored to meet the needs of faculty and students in a demanding curriculum in which "the time is short and the learning long" due to the expansion of the nurse's role in pharmacotherapeutics, as well as the increase in new drug information, which needs to be learned. The book's innovative nursing-based approach has been refined, its text has been condensed, and its pharmacology has been updated. Several new features that allow the student to more rapidly acquire insights into fundamental pharmacologic principles and to develop a theoretical base for the skills involved in administering medications have been added: clinical alerts, specialty boxes on critical-thinking and home health care, and a critical pathway of care, to name a few. The result is a streamlined text that has been improved in its nursing and pharmacologic content as well as its design and pedagogic features.

STRUCTURE

The book consists of 68 chapters divided into 16 units. Unit I covers the nursing process as applied to drugs and drug administration, and also the fundamentals of drug therapy, including the safe administration of drugs. Unit II provides in-depth coverage on the three phases of drug action, drug interactions, and drug toxicity, including adverse reactions and poisoning. Unit III discusses pharmacotherapeutics for neonate/pediatric patients and geriatric patients, and ethnic/cultural considerations for drug therapy, including information on how drugs are handled by different ethnic groups and how patient compliance can be enhanced through understanding cultural beliefs. Unit IV contains chapters on drugs used in diagnostic testing, intravenous therapy, major body electrolytes, vitamins, minerals, and iron products, and enteral and parenteral nutritional agents (including exciting new research). Units V through XV present pharmacologic information using a body systems approach. Each unit begins with a chapter that discusses the anatomy and physiology of that particular system, followed by chapters in which appropriate drugs are discussed in detail. Drug groups are presented according to action, pharmacokinetics, uses, contraindications and precautions, adverse effects, and interactions, and then individual drugs are delineated in the same way. Important drugs in each major drug group also appear in accompanying drug tables, making the book useful as both a standard text and as a convenient drug reference. Each chapter in these units ends with a Using the Nursing Process section, which covers all steps of the nursing process. Entries in each step have been bulleted and condensed for easier reading. Unit XVI covers selected issues in pharmacotherapeutics—enzymes as therapeutic agents, using the nursing process with patients who abuse drugs, alcohol, and other substances (including smoking deterrents), and emergency situations, hypotension, and shock.

FEATURES

The book's pedagogic features make teaching and learning more straightforward.

CHAPTER OPENER

In addition to the Chapter Outline and Learning Objectives that open each chapter, a list of important terms introduced in that chapter is included. These key terms are not only italicized in the text for easy identification but are also defined within the text.

DRUG TABLES

The comprehensive drug tables that have been a major part of the previous editions have not only been greatly condensed, but have also been separated into smaller units. An important ongoing strength of the fourth edition is the division of the "Nursing Implications" column of the book's Drug Tables into Assessment, Intervention, and Evaluation sections that incorporate valuable patient teaching information. This ties the nursing process firmly and directly to the book's pharmacologic content for specific drugs and aids in planning and delivering nursing care to patients receiving medications. Also, page numbers for Drug Tables (as well as for Nursing Process and Patient Teaching Tables, and specialty boxes), are supplied inside the book's front and back covers and at the opening of each chapter in which they appear.

NURSING PROCESS TABLES

The Nursing Process Tables include assessment parameters, nursing actions with rationales, and desired outcomes/evaluation criteria. The tables provide guidelines that can be tailored to specific patients. At the end of each table are additional suggested nursing diagnoses.

PATIENT TEACHING TABLES

Patient teaching tables indicate how long the drug is to be taken, how it is to be administered, current drug-drug and drug-food interactions, what to do if a dose is omitted, how and when to stop medication, how (when necessary) to alter the dose, food and alcohol restrictions, common adverse effects, and proper storage. If they follow institutional guidelines, the patient teaching tables can be copied and given to a patient.

BUILDING YOUR CRITICAL-THINKING SKILLS BOX

The latest teaching concept of nursing education is the use of critical-thinking. Several critical-thinking situations are included in each section. The *Building Your Critical-Thinking Skills* box presents a patient scenario, followed by questions that teach the student how to use the critical-thinking process—focusing on an inquiry, analyzing and synthesizing the situation, posing a new supposition, and resolving the problem. The use of these critical-thinking exercises assists the nurse to follow a pattern when solving critical-thinking problems.

DELIVERING HOME HEALTH CARE BOX

As more patients are being discharged earlier, the health-care industry is moving toward more home health care. Several *Delivering Home Health Care* boxes—on such topics as pain medication, diabetic care, oxygen therapy, IV therapy in the home, and many more—are included to help bridge the gap between the hospital and home. These boxes include information on drug preparation and administration, including before, during, and after administration, emphasizing how home delivery is different from hospital care. Patient teaching for the home is also included.

CRITICAL PATHWAY OF CARE

Critical pathways of care establish a time-sequenced approach to organizing multidisciplinary interventions—diagnostic testing, medication administration, treatments, consultations, patient education, and discharge planning—to address collaborative, outcome-driven patient care. A critical pathway of care for the manic patient is included in Chapter 26 (Drugs Used To Treat Mood Disorders).

CHAPTER REVIEW QUESTIONS

Each chapter ends with four to seven questions that can be used to test the student's knowledge. The answers are found in Appendix A.

BIBLIOGRAPHY

A bibliography is provided for each chapter. These can be found in Appendix B.

INDEX

The fourth edition provides one comprehensive index, with generic drug names printed in a second color and drug classifications in boldface type. This will make locating a specific drug or drug classifications quick and easy.

CHAPTER UPDATES

There has been continuous refinement and updating of pharmacologic information since the third edition via annual Drug Information Updates provided each September. This content has been incorporated and expanded as needed in both the text and Drug Tables. Life span issues in pharmacology have been addressed in chapters on obstetric, neonatal/pediatric, and the older adult in drug therapy, and increased emphasis has been placed on pediatric dosage information when available. New material on ethnic/cultural considerations for patient teaching and strategies for compliance has been added to Chapter 9 (Ethnic/Cultural Considerations for Drug Therapy) to help meet the needs of multicultural clients. When available, information on how drugs are handled by different ethnic groups is included. Exciting new research has been added to the enteral and parenteral nutrition chapter (Chapter 14). The latest information on conscious sedation has been added to Skeletal Muscle Relaxants and Neuromuscular Blocking Agents (Chapter 22), including the nursing care associated with administering these medications. Drug therapy for Alzheimer's disease and multiple sclerosis is included in Chapter 23. A new chapter, *Pharmacotherapeutics and Principles of Psychobiology* (Chapter 24), has been added, which includes new research findings on brain function and neurotransmitters. The latest information on new drugs and drug groups has been added to Antihyperlipidemic Agents (Chapter 33), Antidiabetic Agents (Chapter 45), and Agents Used in the Management of HIV Infection and AIDS (Chapter 61).

ANCILLARIES

Ancillaries for the fourth edition of *Pharmacotherapeutics: A Nursing Process Approach* include an instructor's guide with 600 questions, a testbank diskette containing 800 questions for computer-generated exams, a transparency set, a computer disk to print out patient/family teaching guidelines for the major drug classes, and a yearly drug information update.

INSTRUCTOR'S GUIDE

The *Instructor's Guide* was carefully designed to save valuable course preparation time. Using a chapter-by-chapter approach, individual information elements (tables, figures, text sections) are evaluated from a teaching perspective, which emphasizes an integrated format, identifies key points for students, and suggests related interactive activities. A Focus Element feature can be used to spark small group discussions or to develop short quizzes. Includes 600 test questions.

TESTBANK

Perhaps the most exciting aspect of the *Instructor's Guide,* the testbank diskette (otherwise known as Cybertest), allow even the most computer-phobic instructor to quickly and confidently produce tests and exams. The software is self-guided, and putting together a test with associated answer key has never been so easy. Cybertest really *will* do it all for you, or you can select the exam questions yourself. You can modify questions to suit your particular course requirements and student needs, or even add your own questions and then save your customized course for future use! The computer disk contains 800 test questions in addition to the 600 questions covered with the Instructor's Guide.

TRANSPARENCY PACKAGE

A Transparency Package containing the illustrations most useful for presentation in a classroom setting has been prepared and is made available free of charge to instructors adopting the textbook for their students.

DRUG INFORMATION UPDATE

An annual Drug Information Update, which tracks new drugs, new information about drugs already in the text, and discontinued drugs helps keep the book as up to date as possible throughout its edition life. This Update is made available without charge to instructors each September. Photocopying of Update contents for distribution to students is encouraged.

COMPLIMENTARY PATIENT/FAMILY TEACHING COMPUTER DISK

The text now includes a complimentary electronic disk containing 56 patient teaching guidelines for the major drug classifications. These tables may be printed out, individualized, and distributed to patients upon discharge.

Merrily A. Kuhn, RNC, PhD

ACKNOWLEDGMENTS

Many people have helped to make this fourth edition a reality. To them I offer my special thanks:

To Helen Ruggles, who typed and modified this manuscript many times. She turned hand-written material of dubious legibility into letter-perfect typed copy. Helen also obtained permissions and kept tract of artwork and table preparation.

To Susan Doherty, who assisted with obtaining contracts and paying the bills during manuscript preparation.

To Ruth DeGeorge, Editorial Assistant, who kept track of the manuscript and reviewers.

To the contributors, who shared their expertise, generated many ideas, and rewrote their chapters as new concepts were incorporated into the manuscript.

To the many reviewers who, through their constructive criticisms, helped to bring this manuscript to completion.

To Art Oftner, Nursing Developmental Editor, for streamlining the design and content of the fourth edition.

To Herb Powell, Director of Production, and Bob Butler, Production Manager, who managed the production process.

Merrily A. Kuhn

CONTRIBUTORS

Christine M. Bellari, MS, RN
Assistant Professor of Nursing
Erie Community College-North
Williamsville, New York

Laurie L. Briceland, PharmD
Associate Professor
Albany College of Pharmacy
Albany, New York

Janet M. Brucker, MS, RN, CNRN
Assistant Director of Nursing
Texas Children's Hospital
Houston, Texas

Meredith A. Davison, PhD
School of Public Health
University of Illinois and Chicago
Chicago, Illinois

Marilynn E. Doenges, RN, BSN, MA, CA
Clinical Specialist
Adult Psychiatric/Mental Health Nursing
Private Practice
Instructor
Beth-El College of Nursing
Colorado Springs, Colorado

Barbara L. Herlihy, RN, PhD
Professor of Nursing
Incarnate Word College
San Antonio, Texas

Jeremiah T. Herlihy, PhD
Associate Professor of Physiology
University of Texas Health Science Center
at San Antonio
San Antonio, Texas

Frank Hicks, PhD, RN, CCRN
Assistant Professor
Loyola University Medical Center
Niehoff School of Nursing
Maywood, Illinois

Robert W. Hirnle, MS, RRT
Director, Respiratory Care Program
Highline College
Des Moines, Washington

Kenneth A. Kellick, PharmD
Clinical Pharmacy Coordinator
VAMC Buffalo
Clinical Instructor in Pharmacy
SUNY Buffalo
Buffalo, New York

Merrily A. Kuhn, RNC, PhD
President, Educational Services, Inc.
Hamburg, New York
Associate Professor
Daemen College
Amherst, New York

Carol Ann Maull, RN, PhD
Associate Professor
Daemen College
Amherst, New York

Patricia Robin McCartney, RNC, PhD
Clinical Assistant Professor
SUNY at Buffalo
Staff Nurse Labor & Delivery
Children's Hospital of Buffalo
Buffalo, New York

Mary Frances Moorhouse, RN, CCP, CCRN, CRRN
Nurse Consultant
TNT-RN Enterprises
Colorado Springs, Colorado

Anne Marie Moraca-Sawicki, RN, BSN, MSN
Clinical Nurse Specialist, Adult Health-Oncology
Surgical Nurse Coordinator/Administrative
Assistant for
Dr. Richard L. Sawicki
Niagara Falls, New York

Ellen O'Donnell, RN, CRNA
Staff Nurse
St. Luke's Roosevelt Hospital Center
Smithers Division
New York City, New York

Sandra L. Preston, PharmD
Albany Medical Center
Division of Clinical Pharmacology
Department of Medicine
Albany, New York

Brenda K. Shelton, MS, RN, CCRN, OCN
Critical Care Clinical Nurse Specialist
Johns Hopkins Oncology Center
Baltimore, Maryland

Mary C. Townsend, RN, MN, CS
Coordinator of Mental Health Nursing
Oklahoma City University
School of Nursing
Oklahoma City, Oklahoma

Kelly D. Wallin, MS, RN, C
Staff Development Specialist
Texas Children's Hospital
Houston, Texas

CONSULTANTS

Denise Arena, PhD
Clinical Pharmacist
Beth Israel
Deconess Medical Center
Boston, Massachusetts

Theresa Bracken, MS, RN
Mercy Care
1 Bethesda Drive
Hornell, New York

Kathryn A. Cartechine, MSN, RN
Assistant Professor of Nursing
Kent State University
Stark Regional Campus
Canton, Ohio

Mary Ann Daily, RN, DNS, CS
Cedar Crest College
Nursing Department
30th & Walnut Streets
Allentown, Pennsylvania

Barbara Herlihy, PhD
University of Incarnate Word College
4301 Broadway
San Antonio, Texas

Sister Grace Henke, SC, RN, MSN, EdD
Instructor
St. Vincent's Hospital
School of Nursing
27 Christopher Street
New York, New York

Rita Hickey, RN, BA, CCRN
Nursing Instructor
Southeastern Community College
South Campus
335 Messenger Road
Keokuk, Iowa

Frank D. Hicks, RN, PhD, CCRN
Assistant Professor
Medical–Surgical Nursing
Loyola University Medical Center
Niehoff School of Nursing
Maywood, Illinois

Mary Jo Kirkpatrick, RN, MSN
Mississippi University of Women
College Drive Shattuck Building
Columbus, Mississippi

Anita Andrews Kovalsky, RN, MN, EdD
Associate Professor of Nursing
Community College of Allegheny County
Boyce Campus
Monroeville, Pennsylvania

Lynne Kreutzer-Baraglia, RN, MS
Administrative Dean and Academic Faculty
Concordia University and West Suburban College of
    Nursing
Erie at Austin
Oak Park, Illinois

Lori Jane Duntz Lord, R, Ph
Staff Pharmacist
University of Connecticut School of Pharmacy
Storrs, Connecticut

Margaretta Lust, RN, MSN
Professor
Florida Community College at Jacksonville
Jacksonville, Florida

Karen Malloy, RN, MSN
Assistant Professor of Nursing
Howard County Junior College
Extension Campus
Kerrville, Texas

Margaret McKee, RN, MS
Instructor
Jennie Edmundson Hospital
School of Nursing
Council Bluffs, Iowa

Steven B. Meisel, PharmD
Assistant Director of Clinical Services
Pharmacy Department
Fairview-Southdale Hospital
Edina, Minnesota

Amy Ricupera, PhD
Clinical Pharmacist
Beth Israel
Deconess Medical Center
Boston, Massachusettes

Mary Jo Morrissey, RN, BSN
Instructor
University of South Alabama
Department of Nursing
1504 Springhill Avenue
Mobile, Alabama

Gail Ropelewski-Ryan, RN, BSN, MSN
Professor
Nurse Education, Health, Physical Education and
  Recreation
Corning Community College
1 Corning Drive
Corning, New York

Ann W. Oberle, RN, MN
Assistant Professor
Northwestern State University
College of Nursing
Shreveport, Louisiana

Valerie C. Scanlon, PhD
Professor
College of Mount St. Vincent
Riverdale, New York

Sandra Oglesby, RN, MS
Nursing Instructor
Cochise College
Main Campus
Douglas, Arizona

Debra Spring, RN, MS
Instructor
Hinds Community College
750 Chadwick
Jackson, Mississippi

CONTENTS

RESOLUTIONS TO BUILDING YOUR CRITICAL THINKING SKILLS BEGIN ON PAGE 1068

DRUG CLASS INDEX

UNIT 1

THE NURSING PROCESS AND FUNDAMENTALS OF DRUG THERAPY

UNIT OUTLINE

CHAPTER 1

Pharmacology and the Nurse's Role

Merrily A. Kuhn, RNC, PhD
Anne Marie Moraca-Sawicki, RN, BSN, MSN

CHAPTER OUTLINE

Pharmacology and Pharmacotherapeutics
Development of the Nurse's Role in Drug Administration
Historical Perspectives on Drug Standards
United States Drug Legislation
Canadian Drug Legislation
Patient Package Inserts
International Drug Control Efforts

KEY TERMS

Bioequivalence
Drug (medication)
Liability
Over-the-counter (OTC) medications
Patient package inserts (PPIs)
Pharmacology
Pharmacotherapeutics

LEARNING OBJECTIVES

After reading this chapter, the student will be able to:

1. List and define the three stages in the development of the science of therapeutics.
2. List the seven medication "rights."
3. Discuss drug laws and their impact on drug administration.
4. Explain the purpose of Drug Schedules and the ways in which drugs are classified into these categories.
5. Explain the process by which a new drug is developed and marketed.
6. Compare the United States and Canadian controlled-drug laws.

The problem of illness and disease is as old as mankind. Even before there were written historical records, people left behind evidence of attempts to intervene in the disease process. Throughout history there have always been those who nurtured or attended to the sick and injured, the earliest form of nursing. Three distinct stages in the historical development of the science of therapeutics have been identified: the mystical stage, the empirical stage, and the specific stage (Table 1–1).

Since the specific stage, advances in medicine and pharmacology and the creation of drug-related legislation and standards have dramatically changed the nurse's role. This chapter discusses the effects that the history, legislation, and standards associated with the therapeutic use of drugs have had, and continue to have, on the nursing

profession. General nursing responsibilities related to the administration of medications are also covered.

PHARMACOLOGY AND PHARMACOTHERAPEUTICS

Many people believe that there is a pill to cure every pain or symptom, and they are accustomed to consuming large numbers of drugs or medications on a daily basis. *Pharmacology* is the scientific study of all aspects of drugs, including their source, properties, uses, actions, and effects. Table 1–2 gives an overview of the history of pharmacology and highlights some important drug discoveries. A

Table 1–1. STAGES IN THE DEVELOPMENT OF THERAPEUTICS		
Development Stage	**Explanation**	**Examples of Treatments/Drugs Used**
Mystical stage	Oldest stage in the development of pharmacology, dates back to ancient man's earliest efforts to treat illness. This stage was steeped in religious and superstitious beliefs (magic).	Prayers, crude forms of surgery and exorcisms, unrefined medicinal herbs, and early drugs.
Empirical stage	Second stage in development of pharmacology. Based on clinical knowledge that a drug was effective, though the mechanisms of drug action were unknown. Modern medicine still uses empirical knowledge to some extent. This stage began about the time of man's ability to leave written records. Superstition/religion still played a large role in therapeutics.	Prayers/superstitious beliefs coupled with the use of medicinal herbs, spices, ritual baths. The use of effective pharmacologic drugs appeared. Some drugs still in use first appeared then. Some examples are castor oil, opium, and colchicine.
Specific stage	Beginning of modern era of pharmacology. It began in late Middle Ages. Based on rational principles and understanding of mechanisms of drug actions.	Refined botanical drug products as well as synthetic drugs were developed. Examples include insulins, vitamins, antineoplastics, anesthetics, antibiotics, immunizations, and tranquilizers.

drug or *medication* is a medicinal substance or agent given to produce a specific effect on the body. A drug can be derived from natural products (e.g., penicillins, which were first developed from molds) or from synthetics (e.g., antacids). Drugs can have various effects on the body ranging from very little effect, to therapeutic, to toxic, to fatal. By definition, a drug must have an effect. *Pharmacotherapeutics* is the treatment of all aspects of disease with medication to diagnose, treat, or cure. Medication can be prescribed by a physician, dentist, osteopath, podiatrist, and, in most states, a nurse practitioner or physician's assistant. Medications are prepared and dispensed in a pharmacy, usually by a licensed pharmacist. A pharmacist (druggist) is one who is licensed to prepare and sell or dispense drugs and compounds and to make up prescriptions. The pharmacist usually has a bachelor of science degree in pharmacy, but some may have more advanced degrees (PharmD). Pharmacists are a good source of information for the nurse because of their specialized education and around-the-clock availability in most hospitals. Pharmaceutical companies also employ pharmacists to answer questions that cannot be answered by the local pharmacist. Telephone numbers for drug companies are listed in the *Physicians' Desk Reference* (PDR), which is readily available in all hospitals and nursing homes.

The pharmacist may be assisted by a pharmacologist (a specialist in pharmacology). The pharmacologist has at least a master's degree, most often a PhD degree, with additional course work in pharmacology. The pharmacologist is primarily responsible for research in pharmaceutical companies, in patient populations, and in educational institutions.

DEVELOPMENT OF THE NURSE'S ROLE IN DRUG ADMINISTRATION

The administration of medicinal substances in an attempt to treat illness dates back to man's earliest days. Likewise, the presence of nurturing individuals to care for or nurse the ill predates recorded history. Although there was no organized, educated corps of nurses before Florence Nightingale opened the first nursing school in the 1860s, those who practiced nursing did administer medications. When Nightingale began her school, she advocated the selection of qualified, competent, well-trained nurses who could use a theoretical framework to practice the profession. She stressed that nurses needed to know the correct preparation, dosage, administration technique, desired effect, and side effects of the medications they administered.

In 1919, the National League for Nursing's Committee on Education published the earliest curriculum guidelines for nursing schools. This volume was called the *Standard Curriculum for Schools of Nursing* and included guidelines for two courses on medication administration. The introductory course, entitled "Drugs and Solutions," was meant to familiarize students with weights, measures, solutions, and symbols used in medication administration. The name of this course has had an enduring quality and has served at least in part as the title for several nursing texts on drug doses and calculations. The second medication course dealt with the study of drugs, their actions, administration, and reactions (adverse effects). The National League for Nursing has updated its curriculum standards for schools of nursing throughout the 20th century.

During the 1950s the administration of medications constituted a great part of the professional nurse's time. Patient teaching became an important nursing task, as the nurse was often responsible for teaching the patient to self-administer insulin and other medications. Nurses also became concerned with the legal aspects of medication administration much more than in the past. Nursing responsibilities also began to expand into new areas of medication administration. Gradually, nurses became responsible for venipuncture and for starting intravenous infusions, previously physician-only tasks.

The 1960s was an era of rights—civil rights, individual rights, patient rights. "Right" became a watchword of sorts, denoting ideas or tasks that were good, ideal, or imperative. During the 1960s the idea of the *Five Rights* of medication came into use. Two additional rights have been added in the 1980s and 1990s. These rights are ingrained into each student nurse's consciousness. The

Table 1–2. HISTORY OF PHARMACOLOGY

Historical Era	Discovery/Development/Characteristics
Pre-Christian Era	Medicine men or priests were responsible for the religious and medicinal aspects of the healing arts. Women practiced the day-to-day nurturing of and caring for the young, aged, and infirm.
	Earliest known written prescription (2100 BC) containing 15 formulas for cures recorded in a tablet by the ancient Sumerians.
	The Egyptian Ebers papyrus (1550 BC) records prescriptions for the treatment of skin ulcers, sores, and other conditions. Ancient Egyptians used castor oil, aloe, opium, colchicine, belladonna, and mandrake.
	The ancient Greeks built temples in which they practiced the healing arts. The temples became healing centers (hospitals).
	The Greek physician Hippocrates (born 460 BC), called the Father of Medicine because his influence has lasted through the ages, believed that disease was the result of natural causes that could be treated through the use of medicines derived from plant and animal products. He stressed principles such as observation (assessment), diagnosis, and treatment.
Early Post-Christian Era	The Greek physician Dioscorides (1st century AD) prepared a formulary arranged according to drug source (plant, animal, mineral) rather than by disease entity. For each drug, he described methods of identification (source), drug preparation and administration, and therapeutic indications.
	Another Greek physician, Galen (131–201 AD), erroneously believed that health was a perfect balance of four humors in the human system. However, he popularized the principle of polypharmacy and was the first to prepare rosewater ointment (cold cream).
	Christianity declared the official church of Rome (311 AD). The role of monasteries became increasingly significant to both medicine and learning as a whole. Monks collected and hand-copied works of pharmacy and medicine, preserving them.
	Arabian influence began in the 8th century as the Arabs spread across the Holy Land. They established hospitals and medical schools. As early as 800 AD the Muslims had evolved a separate profession of pharmacists who were respected members of a health care system. The Arabs originated alcohol, aromatic water, juleps, and syrups; introduced the use of decimal notation (which they acquired from India); and compiled great formularies, which were extensive and represented the first set of drug standards.
	The rise of the universities began in the 8th century with the founding of the University of Salerno.
	Popular medicines of the early post-Christian era were mistletoe, primrose, henbane, clover, wormwood, belladonna, and mandragora. Modern remedies dating from this era include the use of colchicine for gout, iron for anemia, and rhubarb for dysentery and liver complaints.
Late Middle Ages	Universities founded during this period included those in Paris (1110), Bologna (1113), Oxford (1167), Cambridge (1209), and Naples (1224).
	Christian Crusades, which began in 1095, affected the practice of pharmacy in Europe when Crusaders brought back Arabian science and pharmacy knowledge.
	By the 13th century, many spices, opium, and sugar (used almost exclusively for medicines) were being traded to Europe from other lands. During the same period, European pharmacies began to spring up as separate entities where medicines were compounded and dispensed.
	By the 14th and 15th centuries, many strides were being made in science and medicine. It was also during this time that epidemic disease, including leprosy and the bubonic plague (the Black Death), became prevalent.
	During the 15th century many medical schools were established in Europe, and the science of alchemy became popular.
	The invention of printing (1438) helped spread the knowledge of medicine and pharmacy.
16th Century	Valerius Cordus produced the first pharmacopeia to be printed and used in a community (1535).
	Paracelsus (1493–1541), son of a German physician and chemist, taught that diseases were actual entities that should be specifically treated with simple but specific compounds. His teachings marked the beginning of the specific stage in the development of the science of therapeutics.
17th Century	Many new drugs, including tincture of benzoin, ipecac, senna, alcoholic tincture of opium (laudanum), guaiacum, cinchona, and coca were introduced.
	The first London *Pharmacopeia,* published in 1618, contained 1028 simple drugs and 932 preparations and compounds.
18th Century	Patient care during this time was poor because "sisters" who cared for the ill and dispensed medications had no preparation or training and were often social outcasts, debtors, or criminals working off jail sentences. This era is often referred to as the dark age of nursing.
	Two extremely important advances in pharmacology introduced in the latter part of this century included the introduction of the infusion of digitalis for the treatment of heart disease by William Withering of England (1785) and the introduction of smallpox immunization by English physician Edward Jenner (1796).
19th Century	During this century chemistry became an individual, highly specialized science, and pharmaceutical chemistry became an important subdivision.
	The discovery of morphine (isolated by Serturner in 1815 in his German apothecary) was the first *active principle* (that portion of a chemical substance responsible for its therapeutic effect). Among other drugs discovered during this period were strychnine and atropine.
	Drs. Morton and Wells, dentists, demonstrated the successful use of ether as a general anesthetic (1846). Sir J. Y. Simpson used chloroform for anesthesia in 1847.
	In the 1850s salicylic and benzoic acids were synthesized.
	In this century it also became possible to administer drugs in more palatable forms, and manufacturing plants were established for the production of drugs, which led to greater accuracy of dosage.

Table 1–2. **HISTORY OF PHARMACOLOGY,** *Continued*	
Historical Era	**Discovery/Development/Characteristics**
19th Century, *Continued*	National pharmacopeias, including the French *Codex* published in 1818 and the *United States Pharmacopeia* (USP) published in 1820, were produced in an effort to maintain standards of drug preparations. The first national standard for Great Britain was published in 1864.
	In the 1860s, Florence Nightingale established the first school of nursing. She advocated the selection of qualified, competent, well-trained nurses who could use a theoretical framework to practice the profession.
20th Century	The German physician Paul Ehrlich introduced salvarsan for the treatment of syphilis (1907).
	Frederick Banting discovered insulin for the treatment of diabetes mellitus (1922).
	Dr. Alexander Fleming discovered penicillin while studying mold at the University of London (1929). Dr. Howard Florey at Oxford University is credited with the isolation of the penicillin molecule, its assay and dosage, as well as definite proof of its clinical usefulness. It was not until 1941 that the first patient was treated with penicillin.
	During the 1940s other antibiotics, as well as antihistamines, glucocorticoids, and antimalarials were developed.
	During the 1950s antihypertensives and oral contraceptives were developed. In 1955 Dr. Jonas Salk developed the poliomyelitis vaccine.
	The 1960s saw the development of antiviral agents, the Sabin vaccine (oral form of polio vaccine), and levodopa (for management of Parkinson's disease).
	During the 1970s the antineoplastic antibiotics Adriamycin and bleomycin and the histamine receptor antagonist cimetidine were introduced.
	The 1980s saw the introduction of new drugs as well as new classes of drugs, such as calcium channel blockers (used in the treatment of dysrhythmias, angina pectoris, and hypertension).

Seven Rights refer to (1) the right drug, (2) the right dose, (3) by the right route, (4) at the right time, (5) to the right patient, (6) the right of the patient to refuse medication, and (7) the right documentation.

By 1980 a new landmark had occurred in nursing practice. Legislation was passed in most states granting prescriptive authority to advanced-practice nurses. Nurse practitioners who prescribe medications are limited to medications in a drug formulary or must prescribe under the supervision of a physician, or both.

NEW HORIZONS IN DRUG THERAPY

The role of the professional nurse has evolved from the dependent role of "physician handmaiden" to a collaborative position in the health-care team. Once nursing practice was based on the medical model, but it is evolving a conceptual basis of practice of its own. The nursing process, itself a theoretical tool, is a part of every nurse's daily practice. The steps of the nursing process, as detailed in Chapter 2, form a cyclic and dynamic framework on which nurses can build to meet patient-care needs relative to the administration of medications. Nursing research continues to play an integral role in medication administration and in other areas of nursing practice.

Administering medications to patients remains one of the most important—and legally the most risk-filled—aspects of nursing practice today. Nurses are responsible not only for the medications they administer but also for the administration of medications they direct others to give. *Liability*, a legal term denoting responsibility for a failure to act that causes harm to another (e.g., failure to administer an anticonvulsant drug, which results in patient seizures and injury) or taking an action that fails to meet minimum standards of care, thereby causing harm to another (e.g., administering a 10-fold overdose as a result of misplacing the decimal point while calculating

dosage), is an important concept in the nurse's accountability for medication-related activities. Studies have shown that a frequent cause of malpractice suits is related to drug errors, many of which are easily preventable.

Patient education and health teaching continue to grow in importance as a result of much-needed concern for wellness maintenance and preventive-care measures. Television and radio commercials are responsible for the general public's medication orientation. The drug industry spends millions of dollars annually to promote the sale of over-the-counter as well as prescription drugs to consumers.

Certainly, medications have a place in the field of contemporary medicine; many conditions are controlled or cured with the help of medications. Other conditions, however, are best not treated with medications but rather with alternative forms of therapy: diet, stress reduction, and exercise, for example. The health team is primarily responsible for ensuring that the patient is adequately informed about the appropriate form of therapy, and the nurse often assumes the responsibility for this patient education because of the nurse's closer contact with the patient and family.

Pharmacologic comprehension is only one part of the nurse's responsibility. The nurse has ethical and legal responsibility to share with patients all information needed to assist them in achieving optimal health. Every prescribed therapy has advantages and disadvantages, and the health team—including nurse, physician, pharmacist, and therapy personnel—has a responsibility to share this information with patients and their families.

In the 1980s, concern over the spiraling costs of health care dramatically changed the method used by insurance companies to pay for health services. The resulting trend of discharging patients sooner has also increased the need for patient/family education in the administration of medications and observation for effectiveness and adverse effects. Nurses play an increasingly important role in patient/family teaching of medication-related matters, especially in motivating patient compliance. It is estimated that nearly half of patients do not take medications as directed.

Patients are extremely concerned about the costs of medications and health care. Those with the most limited financial resources are often the patients who require the most medications. During the 1980s the cost of prescription drugs increased by 268%. The average cost of a prescription in 1970 was $4; in 1980, $5.91; and in 1994, $42 (*Blue Cross News*, 1994). Although people over the age of 65 constitute approximately 12% of the population, they consume about 30% of all prescription drugs. The cost difference between a generic drug and a name-brand drug can be significant. (Generic and name-brand drugs are discussed in Chapter 3). For example, a patient taking Inderal, 40 mg 3 times a day, can expect to pay almost $30 for a 1-month supply. The generic, propranolol hydrochloride, costs only about $12.50 per month. The cost savings per year for the patient would be over $220. In 1984, the first year of the bioequivalence law, the Federal Trade Commission (FTC) estimated that the use of generic drugs saved consumers approximately $236 million.

HISTORICAL PERSPECTIVES ON DRUG STANDARDS

There was no legal control over the use or sale of any drugs until the early 1900s. This was of no particular significance because of the scarcity of effective drugs on the market. The drugs available were usually natural products prescribed and often supplied by the healer. The publication of the *United States Pharmacopeia* (USP) in 1820 was the first attempt to standardize drug purity. This widely recognized reference lists all approved medicines by the official name (generic); defines drugs as to source and physical and chemical properties; lists drug category, dosage, and method of storage; and provides tests for the purity and identity of an unknown compound. The USP is revised and updated every 5 years. Drugs are deleted when clinical use shows unacceptably high toxicity or when newer, more effective agents are developed. Originally, the USP restricted its coverage to single drugs. However, by the turn of the century, it was apparent that a reference was needed for mixtures and formulas. The *National Formulary* (NF) in 1888 became such a reference and was a supplement to the USP. The two books have been combined and are now called the USP-NF.

UNITED STATES DRUG LEGISLATION

The important drug laws are summarized in Table 1–3. The Federal Food, Drug and Cosmetic Act (FFDCA) of 1906 was the first federal law designed to protect the public by restricting the manufacture and distribution of drugs. This law designated the USP and NF as the official standards and empowered the federal government to enforce those standards. All drugs sold were required to

Table 1–3. SUMMARY OF UNITED STATES DRUG LAWS

Drug Legislation	Summary of Law
Federal Food, Drug and Cosmetic Act of 1906	First federal law designed to protect the public by restricting manufacture and sale of drugs. Set *USP* and NF as official standards and gave federal government authority to enforce standards. All drugs sold had to meet strength and purity standards.
Sherley Amendment of 1912	Added to FFDCA; prohibited use of fraudulent therapeutic claims by drug manufacturers.
Harrison Narcotic Act of 1914	First federal law aimed at curbing drug addiction and dependence. Established word *narcotic* as legal term.
Federal Food, Drug and Cosmetic Act of 1938	Made it mandatory for companies to perform toxicity tests on lab animals prior to seeking FDA approval to market any new drug. Labels and other literature must be included with all prescription drugs listing possible harmful effects. Requires medical devices to be safe and effective; cosmetics must be safe. FDA has power to prevent marketing or recall from market any drug it deems unsafe or not adequately tested.
Durham-Humphrey Amendment of 1952	First law to recognize class of drugs that could be sold OTC without a prescription. Two categories of drugs then existed: OTCs and prescription.
Drug Amendment of 1962 (Kefauver-Harris Act)	Required all drugs not only to be safe, but also to be proved effective before marketing. Also required all drugs marketed between 1938 and 1962 to be tested for effectiveness. There are five categories in addition to "effective" ("possibly effective," "probably effective," and so on). All drugs in classes other than "effective" must be so designated and upgraded to the "effective" rating or removed from the market within FDA-set time limits.
Controlled Substances Act of 1970	Strengthened law enforcement against drug abuse, increased research into drug abuse prevention and treatment, developed five schedules (categories) of drugs based on abuse potential and medical effectiveness. Schedule I drugs are those with highest abuse potential and are available only for research purposes. All controlled substances have set limits on the number of times a prescription can be refilled.
Drug Regulation and Reform Act of 1978	Allows a shorter period of time for new drug investigative efforts, thus speeding up ability to get new drugs to the public.
Drug Price Competition and Patent Term Restoration Act of 1984	Allows generic drug companies to market generic drugs by proving bioequivalence rather than duplicating original companies' clinical trials. Also grants longer patent protection on new drugs.

meet the strength and purity standards set down by the USP and NF. The FFDCA of 1906 was designed to protect the public from the "manufacture of adulterated or mis-branded or poisonous or deleterious foods, drugs, medicines, and liquors." It also required that any drug containing an opiate must state on the label the type and amount of narcotic. In 1912, the Sherley Amendment was added to the FFDCA. This amendment increased federal involvement in the manufacture and sale of drugs by prohibiting the use of fraudulent therapeutic claims.

For more than 20 years following the FFDCA, several legislative attempts to ensure drug safety met with little success until a tragedy in 1937 made it clear that drugs must be tested to ensure safety before being marketed. In 1937, an elixir of sulfanilamide was marketed by a manufacturer using diethylene glycol as a solvent for the then-new anti-infective sulfanilamide. Because the pharmacologic effects of the solvent were not tested in animals prior to marketing, its toxicity went undiscovered until reports of patient deaths came pouring in. More than 100 lives were lost in this unfortunate incident, and the public outcry resulted in new legislation to help guarantee greater safety in prescription drug products.

The resulting Federal Food, Drug and Cosmetic Act (FFDCA) of 1938 was passed, making it mandatory for manufacturers to perform toxicity tests in laboratory animals before seeking approval from the Food and Drug Administration (FDA) to market any new drug. This law empowered the FDA to keep a drug from the market and to order drug recalls if the agency decided that a drug's safety was not adequately tested or that it was too dangerous for the use for which it was intended.

An important focus of the 1938 FFDCA was the drug label. Specific requirements for all drug labels were outlined. All drug labels must contain the following:

1. No false or misleading statements.
2. The dose or frequency of use suggested.
3. The name and business address of the manufacturer, packer, or distributor.
4. A list of all habit-forming drugs in a product, as well as the statement, "Warning—May Be Habit Forming."
5. The kind, quantity, and proportion of certain specified ingredients, including alcohol, atropine, digitalis, and other agents that could be harmful to certain individuals.
6. Adequate directions for safe use and warnings against unsafe use by children, pregnant women, and persons with pathologic conditions.
7. During an experimental testing period, the statement, "Caution: New Drug—Limited by Federal Law to Investigational Use."

The FFDCA was amended in 1945 and expanded to require that certain drugs such as insulin and antibiotics must be from a batch certified before sale by the federal government. The FFDCA was further amended in 1952 by the Durham-Humphrey Amendment, which was the first law to recognize over-the-counter (OTC) drugs. This allowed certain drugs such as aspirin to be sold without a prescription.

OVER-THE-COUNTER DRUGS

Over-the-counter (OTC), nonlegend, and nonprescription are all adjectives describing drugs that an individual may purchase without a prescription. By definition, the FDA has found them to be safe for use without medical supervision.

OTC drugs became a legal classification through the passage of the Durham-Humphrey Amendment to the Federal Food, Drug and Cosmetic Act. This amendment required that each drug be classified as legend or nonlegend. Legend drugs must bear the statement, "Caution: Federal Law Prohibits Dispensing Without a Prescription," and are therefore not available for general purchase by the public. In 1962, the Kefauver-Harris Drug Amendments further required a pharmaceutical manufacturer to prove, prior to marketing, that a drug is effective for its intended indications. Before 1962, prior proof of safety was all that was necessary. This was required only for the prescription drugs; the nonprescription drugs (OTCs) had no such requirement.

In 1972, the FDA implemented a massive review of all OTC drug products to ensure that only those drugs that could be proved effective as well as safe are available for purchase. This review, which is still in progress, assesses the product ingredients for safety and effectiveness and evaluates the advertising claims and labeling. The process used in evaluating more than 300,000 nonprescription products identifies the active ingredients, broken down by therapeutic category, and then evaluates only these ingredients. By reviewing the product labels, the FDA identified only 700 active ingredients. This finding suggests that many products may contain the same ingredients.

Although the FDA review process is not complete, changes in OTC medications have occurred. Ingredients determined to be unsafe have been removed from the market (e.g., phenacetin). Some prescription ingredients have been evaluated as safe for self-medication in certain doses and changed to a nonprescription status (e.g., diphenhydramine and ibuprofen).

Over-the-counter products and drugs manufactured and marketed for self-medication are divided into groups based on the symptoms they are intended to treat. These drugs include analgesics and antipyretics, antihistamines, decongestants, antitussives and expectorants, local anesthetic agents for various sites, antacids, and laxatives. Each of these drug groups is discussed in the appropriate chapter elsewhere in this book.

SAFETY AND EFFICACY

From 1938 to 1962 the approval of new drugs was based solely upon proof of safety for use in humans. Senator Estes Kefauver of Tennessee tried to initiate an investigation into the drug industry when it became known that many drug companies were raking in huge profits and that some of the drug promotion was false and misleading. The senator's efforts were largely ignored until the thalidomide tragedy. Thalidomide is a hypnotic sedative that causes toxicity in humans. When the drug was marketed in Europe in the early 1960s, that toxicity was unforeseen, and use of thalidomide by European women in the early stages of pregnancy resulted in the birth of hundreds of deformed babies. The drug affects limb development, and many of the deformed babies were born with stunted limbs or no arms, or legs, or any limbs. A tragedy of this scale was avoided in the United States because thalidomide was not yet marketed here. However, babies were born in the United States with thalidomide-associated deformities when women who traveled abroad obtained the drug outside this country. Thalidomide is available in the U.S. today as an experimental treatment for cachecia and weight loss associated with cancer therapy and HIV. The same human immunosuppressive virus toxic effects are still present so birth control information must be taught to all women who are to receive the drug.

Again, public outcry over the tragedy spurred the legislature to action. The Kefauver-Harris Amendment was passed in 1962, and this law went into effect in 1963. This law requires that both safety and efficacy of a drug be proved before it is marketed. This act also required that all drugs marketed between 1938 and 1962 be evaluated for effectiveness.

To facilitate this tremendous task, the FDA signed a contract in 1966 with the National Academy of Sciences and its research arm, the National Research Council (NAS-NRC), to independently study all supporting data for therapeutic claims. This study was called the Drug Efficacy Study Implementation (DESI). According to the study, each drug would be rated for effectiveness and designated by one of the following categories: effective, probably effective, possibly effective, ineffective, ineffective as a fixed combination, and effective but (Table 1–4).

Thousands of drugs and therapeutic claims were studied, and the drugs rated "ineffective" were withdrawn from the market. Those drugs rated "possibly effective" or "probably effective" were withdrawn or reformulated. The drugs were allowed to remain on the market while claims were substantiated and scientific data collected. Drugs classified "probably effective" and "possibly effective" had to be upgraded to the "effective" category within a time limit set by the FDA or the drug would be withdrawn from the market. Drug ratings are required to be prominently displayed on the label. Substantial evidence of effectiveness must be in the form of adequate, well-controlled scientific and clinical investigations by qualified experts. Uncontrolled observations and testimonial-type endorsements are not acceptable scientific evidence. These categories are still in effect.

The two most recent drug laws concern the development of prescription drugs. The first deals with the development of new drugs and the second with the marketing of generic drugs. In 1978 the Drug Regulation and Reform Act was passed. This law allows for a shorter time for new drug investigative efforts, thereby speeding the release of new drugs to the public. The second law, The Drug Price Competition and Patent Term Restoration Act of 1984, has two major components: The first made it possible for generic-drug companies to market generic versions of drugs by proving bioequivalence rather than duplicating costly clinical trials undertaken when the drugs were introduced; the second granted longer patent protection (17 years) to innovator drug companies for the discovery of new drugs. *Bioequivalence* indicates that a drug in two or more similar dosage forms reaches the general circulation at the same relative rate and to the same relative extent.

CONTROLLED SUBSTANCES LAWS

The Harrison Narcotic Act of 1914 was the first federal law aimed at curbing drug addiction and dependence. It was also the first law concerned with narcotics to be passed by any nation, establishing the word "narcotic" as a legal term. This law regulated the importation, manufacture, sale, and use of opium, cocaine, marijuana, and all their compounds and derivatives, as well as other synthetic compounds capable of producing physical or psychologic dependence.

The most significant drug legislation of the modern era is the Comprehensive Drug Abuse Prevention and Control Act of 1970, also known as the Controlled Substances Act. This law was passed in an effort to control the rapidly increasing problem of drug abuse and misuse in the United States. The Controlled Substances Act went into effect May 1, 1971. In addition to providing increased research into drug abuse prevention and treatment of drug dependency, it also strengthened existing law enforcement and established drug schedules. In July 1983, the Drug Enforcement Administration (DEA) of the Department of Justice became the nation's sole legal drug enforcement agency. The DEA replaced the Bureau of Narcotics and Dangerous Drugs.

In an effort to better control drug distribution and assist with the campaign against drug abuse, a classification system was developed to categorize drugs according to their abuse potential. Controlled drugs are categorized into five different schedules, to which different regulations apply. Table 1–5 lists these controlled drugs in their appropriate schedules.

Schedule I

Drugs in Schedule I are available only for research (investigative) purposes. There is no other legal use for drugs in this schedule. Separate research registration and

---

Table 1–4. DRUG EFFECTIVENESS CATEGORIES

Effective: There is substantial evidence of effectiveness.

Probably effective: Additional evidence is required to rate the drug effective.

Possibly effective: Effectiveness might be shown eventually, but at the present time there is little evidence of efficacy.

Ineffective: There is no substantial evidence of effectiveness.

Ineffective as a fixed combination: Even though one or more components might be effective if used alone, the product is not acceptable in fixed-dosage combination for reasons of safety or because there is no evidence of contribution of each component to claimed effect.

Effective but: Although effective, there is an appropriate qualification or restriction imposed on the drug, which is still under consideration by the NAS-NRC and the FDA; the drug is effective for some recommended uses but not for all, thus requiring label changes.

Table 1–5. SCHEDULES OF CONTROLLED DRUGS IN THE UNITED STATES

SCHEDULE I: *All nonresearch use forbidden*

Narcotics

heroin, cocaine

Hallucinogens

LSD, MDA, STP, DMT, DET, mescaline, peyote, bufotenin, ibogaine, psilocybin, marijuana

SCHEDULE II: *No telephoned prescriptions, no refills*

Narcotics

Opium

Opium alkaloids and derived phenanthrene alkaloids: morphine, codeine, hydromorphone (Dilaudid), oxymorphone (Numorphan), oxycodone (14-hydroxydihydrocodeinone, a component of Percodan)

Designated synthetic drugs: meperidine (Demerol), alphaprodine (Nisentil), anileridine (Leritine), methadone, levorphanol (Levo-Dromoran), phenazocine (Prinadol)

Stimulants

Coca leaves and cocaine

Amphetamine

Dextroamphetamine

Methamphetamine

Phenmetrazine (Preludin)

Methylphenidate (Ritalin)

Depressants

Amobarbital

Pentobarbital

Secobarbital

Mixtures of above (Tuinal)

Phencyclidine (PCP)

Antiemetic: THC (tetrahydrocannabinol)—nabilone

SCHEDULE III: *Prescription must be rewritten after 6 months or 5 refills*

Narcotics

The following opiates in combination with one or more active non-narcotic ingredients, provided the amount does not exceed that shown:

Codeine and dihydrocodeine: Not to exceed 1800 mg/dL or 90 mg/tablet or other dose unit

Dihydrocodeinone (hydrocodone and in Hycodan): Not to exceed 300 mg/dL or 15 mg/tablet

Opium: 500 mg/dL, or 25 mg/5 mL, or other dosage unit (paregoric)

Narcotic antagonist

Nalorphine

Depressants

Schedule II barbiturates in mixtures with uncontrolled drugs or in suppository dose form

Butabarbital (Butisol)

Glutethimide (Doriden)

Methyprylon (Noludar)

Stimulants

Benzphetamine (Didrex)

Diethylpropion (Tenuate)

Mazindol (Sanorex)

Phendimetrazine

SCHEDULE IV: *Prescription must be rewritten after 6 months or 5 refills. Differs from Schedule III in penalties for illegal possession*

Narcotics

Pentazocine (Talwin)

Propoxyphene (Darvon)

Stimulants

Phentermine

Fenfluramine (Pondimin)

Depressants

Benzodiazepines: chlordiazepoxide (Librium); clonazepam (Klonopin); clorazepate (Tranxene); diazepam (Valium); flurazepam (Dalmane); halazepam (Paxipam); lorazepam (Ativan); oxazepam (Serax); prazepam (Verstran); quazepam; triazolam (Halcion)

Chloral hydrate

Ethchlorvynol (Placidyl)

Meprobamate

Mephobarbital (Mebaral)

Paraldehyde

Phenobarbital

SCHEDULE V: *As any other (non-narcotic) prescription drug; may also be dispensed without prescription unless additional state regulations apply*

Narcotics

Diphenoxylate (not more than 2.5 mg and not less than 0.025 mg of atropine per dosage unit, as in Lomotil)

The following drugs in combination with other active non-narcotic ingredients and provided the amount per 100 mL or 100 g does not exceed that shown: codeine: 200 mg; dihydrocodeine: 100 mg; ethylmorphine: 100 mg clearance from the FDA are required before any drug in Schedule I can be legally obtained. The only exception is the use of peyote by Native Americans in religious rituals. Examples of drugs in Schedule I are heroin, LSD, MDA, mescaline, and psilocybin.

Schedule II

Drugs in this class have accepted therapeutic uses but also have a high potential for abuse. They are known to be physically and/or psychologically addictive. Dependence on these drugs may readily develop if these drugs are taken for extended periods of time or are misused. Drugs in this class include amphetamines, cocaine, morphine, opium, and some barbiturates.

Prescriptions for substances in Schedule II may not be refilled; the prescriber must newly write each prescription. In the hospital setting, an order written with a dosage schedule and an as-needed (prn) notation, such as "Tuinal capsule at hs prn," is no longer valid after 72 hours. The physician must rewrite the order every 3 days if the patient is to continue to receive the medication. Hospital orders listing specific dosing schedules such as "Amobarbital 10 mg qid" are no longer valid after 7 days and must be reordered by the physician at that time. These above reordering regulations apply to all drugs in Schedule II. In emergency situations, the physician is allowed to prescribe a Schedule II substance over the telephone. The nurse obtaining such an order must record it in the patient's chart, and it must then be countersigned by the physician within 48 hours of the verbal order.

Schedule III

Drugs included in Schedule III have a lower abuse potential than those in either Schedule I or II, although they may also be abused. Examples of drugs in this class are codeine in combination with non-narcotic drugs, paregoric, butabarbital (Butisol), and some weaker stimulants such as mazindol. Telephone orders by physicians for drugs in Schedules III and IV are acceptable. Prescriptions for drugs in Schedules III and IV must be rewritten every 6 months or after five refills, whichever comes first.

Schedule IV

Schedule IV is similar to Schedule III except for the penalties for obtaining drugs in this class illegally (illegal possession of controlled substances). Examples of drugs included in this class are propoxyphene (Darvon), chlordiazepoxide (Librium), and diazepam (Valium). Schedule IV drugs are also subject to abuse and have become quite popular among drug abusers. Oftentimes, patients become psychologically addicted or habituated to drugs of this class (especially tranquilizers and sleeping pills) without realizing they have become dependent. ("Those aren't habit-forming; I take them all the time.")

Schedule V

According to federal law, the drugs listed in Schedule V have a low abuse potential, do not require a prescription, and may be sold over the counter. However, most states have stricter laws than the federal statutes and therefore do require a prescription for drugs in Schedule V. Those states that require prescriptions for these drugs follow the same regulations as for drugs in Schedules III and IV. In those states in which the federal law is observed (no prescription required), pharmacies are allowed to dispense only specific amounts of drugs within a specific time period. Both the drug and the time it was dispensed must be recorded in a ledger book signed by the pharmacist and the patient.

Drug Schedule Changes

Drugs may be moved from one schedule to another. For example, propoxyphene (Darvon) was listed as a Schedule V drug several years ago. However, because of an increase in the misuse and abuse of the drug, as well as its frequent involvement in overdoses it was moved to Schedule IV. Likewise, a drug can be moved from a more restrictive class to a less restrictive one, such as from Schedule I to Schedule II. This occurred in the case of THC (tetrahydrocannabinol). This substance was listed on Schedule I (investigational use only) for many years until a legitimate clinical use for it was recently discovered: Tetrahydrocannabinol (an active ingredient in marijuana) possesses antiemetic properties especially helpful for patients undergoing cancer chemotherapy.

Possession and Handling of Narcotics

It is unlawful for an individual to possess a controlled substance (illegal possession) unless it has been obtained by a valid prescription or order or unless its possession is pursuant to the course of professional practice. Whenever a nurse administers controlled substances such as narcotics from stock supplies, the date, time of administration, drug name and dose, prescriber's name, patient's name, and administering nurse's name must all be recorded in the narcotics log. Stock supplies of narcotics must be kept in locked medicine cabinets or carts, and nurses are responsible for accurate accounting of all narcotics dispensed on their units. The nurse coming on duty generally double-checks the drug count with the nurse whose shift is ending.

When narcotics are ordered for patients and are not used, they must be returned to their origination point, such as the hospital pharmacy. Likewise, if a dose of narcotic is contaminated, such as when a tablet accidentally falls on the floor, it is also returned to the pharmacy and marked as a contaminated dose. Some hospitals have narcotic return envelopes to return contaminated or refused doses of narcotics. Such doses are signed for on the narcotics log as "returned to pharmacy." The handling of controlled substances is a responsibility that should never be taken lightly. It is a crime for any individual to transfer a drug listed in Schedule II, III, or IV to anyone other than the patient for whom it was ordered. Violation of the Controlled Substances Act can result in a fine, imprisonment, or both. Any nurse who violates this act is also subject to loss of license and the right to practice nursing.

DEVELOPMENT OF NEW DRUGS

The development of a new drug begins with animal screenings to determine possible uses. New chemicals or drugs are first given to several species of animals in an effort to determine a database for pharmacologic use, adverse effects, and possible toxic effects. The dosage range is studied in various animals, and the minimum effective dose, effective dose, and toxic or lethal dose are determined. This type of testing can indicate possible drug actions and warn of probable dangers. Although this testing provides necessary background information, no animal model compares perfectly to the human model. Animal studies serve as a basis for the consideration of human studies. The FDA reviews the animal-study data for safety and effectiveness before it decides whether to approve the application for Investigational New Drug (IND).

Three phases of testing in human subjects occur once IND status is granted by the FDA. These studies must provide evidence of efficacy, safety, and risk-to-benefit ratio for the new drug intended for human use. The risk-to-benefit ratio concerns the risks of drug side effects or toxicity versus benefits to be obtained by taking the medication. For example, a potential antineoplastic drug or AIDS drug would be allowed more latitude of risk because the potential benefits of such drugs are worth the risk.

Phase 1 Clinical Studies

This stage of drug development focuses on small studies of healthy volunteers under the supervision of a clinical pharmacologist. The volunteers are given the new substance and the absorption, distribution, metabolism, and excretion of the drug are all monitored. All effects (e.g., adverse or toxic) of the substance upon the volunteers are recorded and provide information that is useful in determining the potential of future testing.

Phase 2 Clinical Studies

In this phase of study, a small, select group of volunteers helps to determine the potential use of the substance in actual disease and to determine more closely the proper dosing for achievement of therapeutic goals. Patients are again closely observed for any dangerous side effects or toxic effects. Data from long-term animal studies are also reviewed and compared with the human results. Animal studies are also observed to determine what effects, if any, the substance has upon fertility and reproduction. Refinement of dosage is generally achieved during this phase.

Phase 3 Clinical Studies

In this phase of study, large numbers of patients are treated with the substance to determine adverse effects, safety, and efficacy. Most of the risks associated with therapy are discovered at this stage. Double-blind studies, in which neither the patient nor the researcher knows if the drug or a placebo (inactive substance) is given, are often used, because this type of study reduces bias.

New Drug Application and Postmarket Surveillance

Once all three phases of study are complete, the data are reviewed and evaluated by the FDA. If it finds the drug to be safe and effective, then a New Drug Application (NDA) is granted to the innovator drug company. After the NDA is approved, a post-market surveillance begins. The drug company markets the drug and keeps careful records of the results of therapy on patients, who are provided by medical personnel. The drug company must advise the FDA of any adverse effects and updates regarding therapy. During the early years of use of a newly patented drug, the drug company is responsible for protecting the public by providing necessary updates. Sometimes a medication is discovered to be toxic in some patients, and this is discovered only in the post-market surveillance phase. Sometimes such effects are not readily observable in test populations but do become evident when a drug is marketed to large groups in which rare toxic effects are noted. Such was the case when the drug Omniflox was introduced. It was subsequently withdrawn from the market because of serious side effects.

COMMUNITY AND INSTITUTIONAL DRUG REGULATIONS

When the laws of a community or state or the regulations of an institution differ substantially from the federal laws governing pharmaceuticals, the stricter law generally applies. The most obvious examples are Schedule V drugs in the United States, which federal law says may be dispensed without a prescription. Many states, however, have enacted requirements that these drugs be dispensed by prescription only. Thus, in those states the stricter law, the one requiring the prescription, applies. The nurse should be familiar with all local, state, and federal laws concerning pharmaceuticals so as to practice within the regulations. Always check institutional policies when beginning a new job so that procedures are followed correctly.

CANADIAN DRUG LEGISLATION

Canadian drug laws developed in a fashion similar to that in the United States. The first Canadian drug legislation in 1875 prevented the sale of adulterated food, drink, and drugs.

The Drugs Directorate of Health Protection Branch, Department of Health and Welfare, is responsible for administering the Food and Drug Acts of Canada. These acts control the research and development of new drugs, drug advertising, product information, and the continuous monitoring of the safety of all drug products. The distribution of all potentially addictive drugs is also controlled by these acts.

The most recent Canadian drug legislation is the Narcotic Control Act of 1982. This law is similar in scope to the 1970 United States Comprehensive Drug Abuse Prevention and Control Act. As in the United States, the Canadian law designates classifications of drugs, with category of placement dependent on the abuse potential of the substances involved (Table 1–6). The Canadian drug schedule lists stimulants, barbiturates, and other drugs, such as anabolic steroids, subject to potential abuse in section G of their categorization.

In Canada, as in the United States, strict accounting of the dispensing of all narcotic and hypnotic drugs must be kept by nurses. Hospital-log records must contain the following information for each controlled drug administered: patient's name, prescriber's name, medication name, date and time of administration, name of administering nurse, and the number of remaining doses in the package. These hospital records are kept by the hospital pharmacy. In Canada, any nurse, physician, or pharmacist engaged in the illegal transportation or distribution

Table 1–6. SUMMARY OF CANADIAN DRUG CLASSIFICATIONS—PRESCRIPTION AND RESTRICTED

Classification	Description	Refills
Narcotic Drug (N) Schedule N drugs e.g., codeine, Demerol, Dilaudid, Leritine, Lomotil, morphine, Hycodan, Corutol-DH, Robidone, Tylenol #4, Percodan, Percocet, Tussionex, Novahistex-DH, Numorphan, methadone, heroin (hospitals only), Talwin C pd., Darvon-N 64a.	All straight narcotic drugs. All narcotic drugs for parenteral use. All narcotic compounds containing more than 1 narcotic drug. All narcotic compounds containing less than 2 other non-narcotic ingredients. All products containing hydrocodone, oxycodone, heroin, methadone, pentazocine, propoxyphene.	Refills not permitted. All reorders written or verbal, must be new prescriptions. Narcotics may be prescribed to be dispensed in divided portions, subject to professional discretion.
Narcotic Preparations (N) (oral prescription narcotics) Schedule N preparations e.g., AC with codeine 15, 30, or 60 mg, Cheracol, Cophylac Expectorant, Tylenol #2, #3, 692, Darvon-N compound.	All combinations containing only 1 narcotic drug and 2 or more non-narcotic medicinal ingredients in a recognized therapeutic dose not intended for parenteral use.	Refills not permitted. All reorders must be new written prescriptions. Narcotics may be prescribed to be dispensed in divided portions, subject to professional discretion.
Controlled Drugs (C) Schedule G Drugs e.g., Dexedrine, Mequelon, Nembutal, Seconal, Tuinal, Ritalin.	All straight controlled drugs. All combinations containing more than 1 controlled drug.	Refills not permitted, if original prescription is verbal. An original written or verbal prescription may be refilled if the prescriber has indicated in writing or verbally the number of times and dates for, or intervals between, refills.
Controlled Drug Preparations Schedule G preparations e.g., Carbrital, Mandrax.	All combinations containing only 1 controlled drug and 1 or more medicinal ingredients in a recognized therapeutic dose.	Same as above.
Controlled drugs in Schedule to Part G of Regulation (C) e.g., Amytal, Butisol, Daybarb, Donnatal, Mebaral, Plexonal, Tenuate, Ionamin, Amesec, Tedral, anabolic steroids.	Barbituric acid (except secobarbital and pentobarbital), butorphanol, chlorphentermine, diethylpropion, phentermine, thiobarbituric acid and their salts and derivatives. All combinations containing only 1 controlled drug listed above and 1 or more medicinal ingredients in a therapeutic dose.	An original written prescription may be refilled if prescriber has authorized in writing the number of refills and dates for, or intervals between, refills.
Schedule E and F Drugs (Pr) e.g., antibiotics, antidepressants, antipsychotics, steroids, oral contraceptives.	All drugs listed in Schedule F of Food and Drug Regulations. All drugs listed in Schedule E of the Health Disciplines Act.	An original written or verbal prescription may be refilled if the prescriber has authorized in writing or verbally the number of times it may be refilled.
Restricted Drugs Schedule H Drugs e.g., lysergic acid diethylamide (LSD), N, N-dimethyltryptamine (DMT).	Drugs with no recognized medicinal use and significant danger of physiologic and psychologic side effects; available only to institutions for research.	Not applicable.

NOTES: Table is adapted; for complete details refer to the official information.
Prescriptions must be held in sequence as to date and number and must be retained for not less than 6 years.
Drug names used are made for illustrative purposes only. Not a complete listing.
Legislation can change; keep abreast of changes in prescription requirements.
Table courtesy of Ontario College of Pharmacists, 230 St. George St., Toronto, Ontario, Canada, M5R 2N5. Revised July 1992.

of drugs may be held liable and subject to criminal prosecution and penalties.

PATIENT PACKAGE INSERTS

Patient package inserts (PPIs) remain a controversial topic. These information sheets with complete drug information for patient use had been proposed by the federal government for inclusion in all prescription drugs. However, their introduction was delayed because of opposition from most state regulatory agencies. The state agencies that oppose PPIs feel that the complex information contained in them would not be wisely used or would be misunderstood by the average patient and would, therefore, be more detrimental than helpful to the patient. This system has spawned efforts to increase patient education activities in hospitals. Some drug companies have developed "commercial PPIs" for use by the health-care worker in patient teaching. Patients are actively pursuing health information more than ever before. There has been explosive growth of consumer information drug books in recent years. The government is actively pursuing the requirement of standardized patient information sheets for each prescription filled because of the high cost of treating patients for preventable adverse drug effects.

INTERNATIONAL DRUG CONTROL EFFORTS

The first attempt to control drugs at the international level through legal means and treaties occurred in 1912 at the first Opium Conference, held at the Hague. At that time, international treaties were drawn up that legally obligated governments to do the following: (1) limit the manufacture and trade of opium to medicinal and scientific needs, (2) control the production and distribution of raw opium, and (3) establish a system of governmental licensing to control the manufacture and trade of drugs covered by the convention.

Government representatives in 1961 formed the Single Convention on Narcotic Drugs, which took effect in 1964. This act consolidated all existing treaties into one document for the control of all narcotic substances by the following: (1) outlawing the production, manufacture, trade, and use of narcotics for nonmedical purposes; (2) limiting the possession of all narcotic substances to authorized persons for medical and scientific purposes; (3) providing for international control of all opium transactions by the national monopolies (countries such as Turkey, which are designated to produce opium) and authorizing production only by licensed farmers in areas and on plots designated by these monopolies; and (4) requiring import certificates and export authorizations as a means of better control.

Obviously the task of enforcing such laws is monumental. An International Narcotics Control Board was established to enforce the international drug laws; however, it is not possible to completely stem the tide of illegal drug traffic. The illegal-drug industry has become a multibillion-dollar-a-year industry with equipment and techniques that are state of the art and often superior to the surveillance equipment of law enforcement officials. In recent years, the tremendous popularity of cocaine as a drug of abuse has multiplied the problem of illegal drug traffic 100-fold. As always, the opiates remain popular drugs of abuse. Drug enforcement officials cite the following staggering statistic in relation to their job: in one year an estimated 1400 tons of opium are circulated in the illegal-drug market, in contrast to the 800 tons handled through proper channels and that are sufficient for world medical needs.

International drug control efforts continue. Laws in this area continue to be modified as needed, and enforcement efforts are being stepped up on an international level. The United States has had several high-level meetings and has updated treaties in Central America to help reduce the tremendous traffic in illegal cocaine.

The bibliography for this chapter can be found in Appendix B, which begins on page 1054.

CHAPTER REVIEW QUESTIONS*

1. A major responsibility of the nursing profession is to:
   a. Discourage the use of over-the-counter medications.
   b. Teach consumers about the benefits and dangers of medications.
   c. Control the administration of medications in the hospital setting.
   d. Alter the consumer's values and beliefs concerning medication use.

2. The empirical stage of therapeutics was characterized by:
   a. A lack of detailed record keeping.
   b. Clinical evidence that a drug was effective.
   c. An understanding of drug action.
   d. All of the above.

3. The Federal Food, Drug, and Cosmetic Act (FFDCA) of 1906 contributed to medication safety by:
   a. Empowering state governments to enforce official drug standards.
   b. Requiring only narcotic drugs to comply with standards set by the USP and NF.
   c. Requiring synthetic drugs to list side effects on the label.
   d. Designating the USP and the NF as official drug standards.

4. Pharmacotherapeutics is defined as:
   a. Using pharmacists to dispense medications.
   b. Studying drug actions on a living system.
   c. Treating all aspects of disease with medications.
   d. Using a combination of therapies to treat disease.

*See Appendix A, which begins on page 1051, for answers.

CHAPTER 2

The Pharmacologic Application of the Nursing Process

Merrily A. Kuhn, RNC, PhD

CHAPTER OUTLINE

Assessment
Nursing Diagnosis
Evaluation

BOXES

Building Your Critical Thinking Skills, 21

KEY TERMS

Adverse effects
Critical thinking
Drug allergy
Idiosyncratic reaction

Nursing process
Placebo
Toxic effect

LEARNING OBJECTIVES

After reading this chapter, the student will be able to:

1. Apply the nursing process to solving problems in nursing practice related to pharmacology.
2. Explain how nursing diagnoses might lead to the formulation of a plan for intervention involving pharmacotherapeutics.
3. Discuss the components of a plan for nursing intervention in relation to pharmacologic needs of the patient.
4. Evaluate the sources from which data are accumulated for evaluation of the nursing process and explain how criteria are determined to measure success of a treatment program.
5. Identify patient factors and characteristics of patient factors that correlate with noncompliance.

The *nursing process* is the organized approach to problem solving and decision making that serves as the framework for the provision of nursing care. It consists of a series of five planned, logical steps—assessment, diagnosis, planning, intervention, and evaluation—that produce a definite result. The nursing process is open, cyclic, dynamic, and adaptive. It is cyclic because each reassessment reinitiates the process; dynamic because it involves constantly changing variables and relationships, making it ongoing rather than static; and adaptive because it changes for each patient and for each patient condition.

The nursing process begins with data collection, the assessment phase. From these data, the nurse determines priorities for the care to be given. Nursing outcomes and nursing diagnoses are developed to meet the established

priorities. The nurse then plans the nursing intervention necessary to implement the care. Care is given, and outcomes are subjected to evaluation. If the nursing care in any phase fails to meet patient needs, or if new needs are found, the nursing process recycles to the assessment phase and begins anew.

Many conceptual models of nursing practice use the nursing process directly or indirectly as their basis. The nursing process forms the operational basis of nursing case management, described by The American Nurses' Association as " . . . a health care delivery process whose goals are to provide quality health care, decrease fragmentation, enhance the client's quality of life and contains costs." Case management strives to organize client care through an episode of illness so that specific clinical and financial outcomes are achieved within an allotted time frame. This time frame is commonly determined by established protocols for length of stay.

Critical pathways of care (CPCs) serve as tools for documenting nursing care in a case management system. CPCs are based on expected rather than problem-based outcomes for goal achievement within a designated length of stay. They are altered or individualized only if the patient needs care that deviates from the established pathway. Generally, a critical pathway of care contains nursing diagnoses and categories of care, time dimensions, and goals and/or actions. For an example of this tool, see the Critical Pathway of Care for the Manic Patient in Chapter 26.

This chapter briefly reviews the five steps of the nursing process and discusses how they are applied during medication administration.

ASSESSMENT

Assessment, the first step of the nursing process, involves gathering information from and about each patient to identify the patient's disease history, current health problems, needs, problems, strengths, and weaknesses. A need can be for knowledge about the new drug just ordered. A problem may be the unwillingness to comply with the prescribed diabetic diet because the patient is now taking insulin. A strength may be a supportive family unit, whereas a weakness may be lack of motivation to take the medication. The nurse enters the data she or he gathers into the database, the body of accumulated information. The data base serves as a starting point for the nursing care the patient is to receive.

The data-gathering phase has two interrelated phases: (1) the verbal, or talking and listening, phase and (2) physical assessment, or hands-on, phase. The verbal interchange phase occurs first, with the taking of the health history from the patient when possible or the patient's spouse or another family member if needed. It is very important to obtain information from the patient about past and current use of medications, level of knowledge, and compliance. The physical assessment, or hands-on, phase further clarifies previously obtained information during performance of the physical examination.

VERBAL INTERCHANGE PHASE

During the verbal interchange phase, the nurse-interviewer listens attentively to what the patient and family are saying. The nurse also listens for whole thoughts and ideas, not merely for isolated facts. Facts themselves are not as important as the ideas that bind them together. For example, a diabetic patient tells you facts about how he watches his diet and injects his insulin daily, but the whole thought includes the idea that he does not accept his diabetes and is really not following his diet. At the conclusion of the interview, the nurse summarizes the data to ensure that the patient, family, and nurse all understand the same information.

When medications are to be administered, the nurse must ask the following questions during the assessment:

1. Does the patient have any allergies to food, animal dander, chemicals, medications, or anything else in his or her environment? If the patient response is positive to any of these factors, the nurse must elicit additional information. This includes a complete description by the patient of what happens when the patient comes in contact with or is exposed to any of the offending agents or irritants. Allergic reaction (anaphylaxis) may be manifested by rash, laryngeal edema, and/or cardiovascular collapse. Some side effects such as nausea, vomiting, dizziness, and drowsiness are often incorrectly termed allergic reactions. Cross-allergies are common; that is, a patient who is allergic to shellfish may be allergic to contrast media dyes used in diagnostic x-ray studies because the dyes contain iodine. A patient who is allergic to beef or pork may show similar allergies to insulin, heparin, or surfactant prepared from these animal sources.

2. What medications does the patient currently take? The nurse asks about prescription medicines, over-the-counter (OTC) medications, vitamins, medications provided by friends, folk medicines, and recreational drugs. Medications frequently interact with each other; therefore, it is important to know everything the patient is taking. For example, a patient taking aspirin may encounter bleeding problems when an anticoagulant such as warfarin is administered. (Drug interactions are discussed further in Chapter 5.)

3. Why is the patient taking prescription and/or OTC medications? Perhaps a certain medication proved helpful to a friend or represents a new health fad, such as the use of vitamins A, C, and E as antioxidants to reduce the incidence of heart disease. Often drugs are psychosomatically effective, that is, effective because the patient desires them to be, a *placebo* effect. The patient may take a medication that interferes with the desired action of other preparations, such as a pep pill taken with a tranquilizer or a sleeping pill. These medications may have been obtained from friends or from a physician not involved in treating the patient's present condition.

4. What is the condition of the patient's skin, particularly if the patient has been self-administering intramuscular medication or has been taking street drugs? The nurse assesses skin for color, because a patient taking street drugs may be jaundiced from hepatitis; for bruises, because a patient taking anticoagulants may have large hematomas on the skin; and for abscesses or infections, because a patient injecting insulin may not have good technique or may not be rotating sites properly.

5. What is the patient's daily use of tobacco, marijuana, or alcohol? For instance, a heavy cigarette smoker (more than one pack a day) may require larger doses of theophylline, a bronchodilator, and insulin than does a nonsmoker. When the patient stops smoking, he or she must notify the physician so that the med-

ication's toxic and therapeutic effects can be monitored closely and the dose adjusted as needed.

Marijuana potentiates the effects of many medications, particularly psychoactive agents and medications for pain or hypertension. Doses of these drugs may need to be modified.

Alcohol interferes with or potentiates the action of many medications. It is best that the patient refrain from drinking while taking antihypertensives, tranquilizers, and all central nervous system depressants; otherwise, the patient may become overly sedated or may become dizzy or faint, resulting in a fall.

6. How much coffee, tea, cola, and other caffeine-containing beverages does the patient drink daily? Caffeine interacts with various medications. For example, the xanthine bronchodilators (theophylline) are chemically related to caffeine. The patient must limit caffeine intake to a prescribed quantity to forestall toxic effects.

7. Does the patient have any medical problems that would affect the way drugs are metabolized (broken down) in the body? Such medical problems, which include renal, hepatic, gastrointestinal, and cardiac disease, might contraindicate the use of a certain medication or indicate that drug dosages need to be reduced.

HANDS-ON PHASE

The next phase of the assessment process is gathering of information from the patient's physical body. For example, the nurse might obtain baseline blood pressure before administering antihypertensives or obtain blood sugars before administering insulin. Once the data have been collected, the nurse proceeds to the second step of the nursing process, establishing a nursing diagnosis.

NURSING DIAGNOSIS

Nursing diagnoses identify the patient's actual or potential health status. The diagnostic statement is developed from the objective and subjective information obtained in the health-status database. Nursing diagnoses are specific to a particular patient and lead to the development of both short-term and long-term patient outcomes during the planning stage. They are the base on which all nursing care is organized and delivered.

Acceptable nursing diagnoses, approved by the North American Nursing Diagnosis Association (NANDA), are integrated throughout this book (see other publications for a complete list). The nursing diagnoses in the Nursing Process tables found in most chapters of this text include "related to" and "as evidenced by" statements. Table 2–1 offers several examples of nursing diagnoses the nurse could develop when administering medications. One of the most common nursing diagnoses, noncompliance, is a multifaceted problem in which any single cue, by itself, may not be significant in predicting noncompliance.

Table 2–1. EXAMPLES OF NURSING DIAGNOSES RELATED TO DRUG ADMINISTRATION

Knowledge deficit, related to insufficient instruction regarding new antihypertensive medication as evidenced by inability to recognize antihypertensives.

Noncompliance, related to inability to accept diagnosis and treatment regimen as evidenced by not taking medication as ordered.

Alterations in bowel activity, related to inappropriate administration of prescription cathartics as evidenced by diarrhea followed by constipation.

Impairment of skin integrity, related to poor insulin injection techniques and lack of site rotation as evidenced by destruction of skin and disruption of skin surfaces.

Anxiety, related to hair loss secondary to chemotherapy as evidenced by restlessness, facial tension, and insomnia.

Mother's anxiety, related to administration of insulin to 6-year-old son as evidence by increased extraneous body movements, hand trembling, and facial tension.

However, when a patient demonstrates a cluster of such cues, the nurse anticipates that the patient is a strong candidate to exhibit noncompliant behaviors (Table 2–2).

PLANNING

Planning is a systematic process in which short-term and long-term goals or expected patient outcomes are established, and the manner of implementation is determined. Many people may be involved with planning: one or more nurses, the client, family members or significant others, and other members of the health-care team. During the planning stage, the nurse designs strategies or interventions required to prevent, reduce, or eliminate the client health problems identified and validated during the diagnostic phase. The nurse must ensure that the patient has accepted this diagnosis and is willing to comply with the treatment plan. Research has shown that the patient who is unwilling to accept the diagnosis does not comply with the treatment regimen.

Planning involves establishing objectives that encompass the physical, psychologic, spiritual, and sociocultural/lifestyle needs of the patient and family. For example, a patient's physical need might be to learn to administer his or her bronchodilating medication via a metered-dose inhaler. A family's psychosocial need might be to respond appropriately to a newly diagnosed cancer requiring chemotherapy. Sociocultural/lifestyle needs might require changing a lifelong habit of eating "on the run" because of the new diagnosis of diabetes now requiring insulin injections.

During the planning stage, the nurse preparing to give medications must answer the following questions to proceed with medication administration:

1. What observations must be made relative to the effect of the medication? What is the action of the drug within the body? For example, is the pulse or blood pressure to change?

2. What route will be used to administer the medication? The patient's condition, including the ability to

Table 2–2. ASSESSMENT OF CUES PREDICTIVE OF NONCOMPLIANCE

Patient Factors to Be Assessed	Characteristics of Patient Factors That Correlate with Noncompliance	Method of Nursing Assessment
Feelings regarding illness	Subjectively believes illness is not as severe as perceived by health professionals	Ask "How would you describe the severity of your illness?"
Locus of control	Demonstrates cues of external locus of control, believes that powerful figures, luck, and/or fate are controlling life	Ask "What do you think caused this health problem?" "What do you think needs to be done to overcome this health problem?" "What are your goals for treatment?"
Beliefs regarding health status	Believes he or she is less susceptible to actual and potential illness than other people	Ask "How do you feel about the statement, 'I worry a lot about my health'?" Ask "Would you describe yourself as being healthy or unhealthy?"
Beliefs regarding the effectiveness of medical care	Believes medical care is not effective	Ask "How would you describe the effectiveness of your care?"
Feelings of satisfaction with treatment	Expresses dissatisfaction	Ask "How do you feel about your care?"
Feelings about prior care	Feels dissatisfied: "It was a waste of time and money"	Ask "How do you feel about your past care?"
Patient's perceptions of health-care plan	Perceives plans to be A. Difficult to follow B. Vague and ambiguous C. Disruptive to premorbid lifestyle	Ask "How do you feel about your plan of care?" "How does this plan affect your daily routine?"
Patient's perceptions of goals of treatment	A. Does not believe goals are relevant to him or her B. Believes self was not involved in setting goals C. Views goals as being vague or too difficult to achieve	Ask "How do you feel about the goals of the health-care plan?" "What are your goals for your treatment?" "How do you feel about this statement, 'The doctor wants me to come back even though it is not necessary'?"
Patient's perceptions of physician	A. Views as being unfriendly and uncaring B. Perceives as rejecting the patient's concerns and feelings C. Views as disagreeing with the patient's goals D. Communicates in an ambiguous manner. (This feeling may be intensified with the use of medical and technical jargon) E. Experiences feelings of disruption in the continuity of care by members of the health team F. Believes the physician does not show any interest in patient compliance	Ask "Describe your doctor." "How do you feel right after you see your doctor?"
Level of trust in physician and health-care system	Believes one should not trust physicians or hospitals	Ask "How much trust do you have in medical care?" "How do you feel about medical care?"
Intentions of compliance	Never intends to comply	Ask "How do you intend to take your medications?" "How do you feel about this statement, 'I try to do what my doctor tells me, without question'?"
Coping mechanisms	Uses denial* and repression, which result in not recognizing need for treatment or being unable to mobilize energies to cope	Assess for cues of denial, such as, "I'm not ill."
Level of self-esteem	Low	Assess for verbal cues, such as, "Don't bother with me, I'm not worth the effort," and nonverbal cues of disinterest in self.

Table 2–2. ASSESSMENT OF CUES PREDICTIVE OF NONCOMPLIANCE, *Continued*

Patient Factors to Be Assessed	Characteristics of Patient Factors That Correlate with Noncompliance	Method of Nursing Assessment
Reactions to illness	A. Reacts with anger, aggression, and demanding behaviors B. Exhibits low level of fear and anxiety, which decreases motivation to respond to danger C. Exhibits high level of fear and panic, which immobilizes attempts to cope with danger D. Exhibits depression, which limits abilities to learn and to cope	Assess for verbal and nonverbal cues of anxiety, fear, anger, depression, hopelessness, helplessness, worthlessness. Ask "How do you feel regarding your illness?"
Methods of compliance with prior treatment regimens	Exhibits noncompliance; states, "I never take medicines"	Ask "How often did you take your medicine for a past illness?"
Methods of compliance with concurrent medication regimens	Exhibits noncompliance	Ask "How often do you take your pills for concurrent illness?"
Reactions of mother of young children	A. Expresses feelings of being unable to get through the day with the children B. Has no situational supports to help care for the children	Ask "Who helps you with your children?" "How often do you have time for yourself?"
Financial status	A. Poverty level B. Unemployed C. Lacks medical insurance D. Believes medications are not worth what they cost	Check financial data on admissions form.
Status of family	A. Family is experiencing conflict and insecurity B. Lives alone	Assess for nonverbal cues of family disharmony. Ask "Who do you live with?" "When you want to talk about a problem, whom do you go to?"
Level of symptoms	A. Currently asymptomatic B. Feels he or she has returned to "normal"	Ask "What are the symptoms of your illness now?"
Side effects resulting from drugs	Noncompliances increases with A. Dizziness B. Fatigue C. Gastrointestinal distress D. Impotence E. Side effects that interfere with work abilities	Ask "What side effects are you experiencing now?" "How do they affect your work?" "How do they affect your daily activities?"

*The nurse must recognize that denial is considered adaptive during the initial stages of coping with a crisis. It is imperative that this mechanism be allowed unless it totally interferes with the progress of treatment.

take medication by mouth, and level of consciousness are important considerations. Will the route need to be altered because of nothing-by-mouth status that may be necessitated by surgery?

3. Are any precautions required to administer the medication, such as a side rail in the upright position when narcotics are administered?

4. Are any special considerations needed because of the patient's age, physical condition, or mental state? For example, a liquid preparation should not be ordered for a blind patient unless someone is available to measure the medication.

5. Are specific nursing measures required to adminis-

ter the medication safely? For example, the apical pulse is always taken before administering any digitalis preparation.

6. Does the patient or family have special learning needs relative to administering the medication at home, such as acquiring specific skills such as injection technique?

The goals or expected outcomes developed from the nursing diagnoses become, in turn, the outcome criteria. The outcome criteria provide the direction for the nursing intervention, provide a time span for the activities, serve as evaluation criteria, and aid in determining at what point the original problem has been resolved. Examples of patient goals or outcomes related to medication administration include the following:

- Before his or her discharge, the patient accurately describes why and how digoxin is taken.
- The patient identifies why he or she cannot eat or drink dairy products for at least 2 hours after taking tetracycline.
- The patient states why it is important to avoid alcohol when taking antifungal medications.
- The patient demonstrates proper injection technique.

After all feasible solutions are examined, the nursing-care plan is established. The nursing-care plan or client-care plan provides a detailed guide for patient care and focuses on the actions the nurse takes to address the patient's identified nursing diagnosis and to meet the stated goals.

INTERVENTION

During the intervention stage, the nursing care actually given is based on the nursing orders developed from the outcome criteria. A typical nursing order would be "Explain digitalis to the patient and give him or her time to ask questions; return in 1 hour and offer to repeat the explanation or discuss any further questions." Nursing care can involve discussing diet or drugs with the patient; performing procedures, such as changing a dressing or giving an injection; or providing psychological support to a patient receiving immunosuppressive drugs for a recent kidney transplant.

The nurse is involved not only with direct care of ill patients but also with health maintenance and disease prevention. Often, with good nursing care and teaching, chronic illness can be mitigated or controlled. For example, a patient with hypertension who controls weight and takes medications as prescribed may be able to avoid a critical cerebrovascular accident.

Nursing interventions may be dependent, independent, or collaborative. Dependent nursing actions are carried out on the order of a physician, such as the actual administration of the medication. Independent nursing actions are activities that the nurse initiates as a result of the nurse's own knowledge and skills, such as teaching a patient injection technique for the administration of insulin. Collaborative nursing actions are activities that are performed jointly with another member of the health team or as a joint decision by the nurse and another health-team member. An example of a collaborative intervention is the nurse and the respiratory therapist working together to teach the patient proper administration of medications with a hand-held inhaler and breathing exercises.

Critical thinking is central to nursing interventions. Every minute while caring for a patient, the nurse is analyzing, synthesizing, solving problems, setting priorities, and evaluating what is being done to and for the patient. Critical thinking is a high-level cognitive function that is reflective, reasonable, and focused on "why" and "how" instead of "what." See the Building Your Critical Thinking Skills box, which describes critical thinking and explains how it can improve nursing care. Throughout this text, this box presents situations with unresolved problems, followed by questions. Answering the questions will help the nurse or student to resolve the problem using critical thinking skills.

Patient Teaching

Health teaching is an important nursing function during the intervention stage. Often, the patient and significant others must not only acquire new knowledge and skills but also radically alter their behavior. Patients are unlikely to modify their behavior unless they thoroughly understand why it is necessary to do so and how they will benefit from change. Cultural and ethnic issues are also involved with teaching and compliance and are all discussed in detail in Chapter 9.

Health teaching also includes teaching the patient about adverse or toxic effects of a drug. An *adverse effect* is any undesired, unintended, and noxious effect of a drug occurring after a drug is administered for prophylactic, diagnostic, or therapeutic purposes. A *toxic effect* is an effect that can result in harm to the patient and must be treated by either stopping the drug or altering the dose. Adverse and toxic effects are described in more detail in Chapter 6. General information that patients need to be taught about their medications before discharge is discussed in detail in Chapter 3, and patient teaching for specific drug classes is found in tables throughout the text.

EVALUATION

During the evaluation stage, the nurse determines whether the previously established outcome criteria have been met and whether the nursing interventions can be terminated or must be reviewed or changed. Objective and subjective data are also evaluated. The nurse obtains objective data from a follow-up physical assessment or laboratory work. Subjective data, such as how the patient feels, how and whether the medication is being taken, and whether a prescribed diet is being followed, are obtained from the patient. If the desired effects of the medication cannot be observed in the patient, the nurse helps to determine why this is so. Several plausible reasons may exist: The patient may not be taking the medication as ordered, the medication may be ineffective for this patient at this time, or the medication may not have been ordered in a correct therapeutic dose for this patient. If the patient is not complying with the treatment regimen previously established, the nurse must ascertain the reason for the lack of compliance and determine what to do to achieve compliance (see Table 2–2). After this determination is made, the nurse, with the patient's help, rewrites the goals and objectives.

When the patient receives medications, the nurse has specific points to evaluate early in the intervention as well as during a later visit. The nurse evaluates the following:

1. Does the patient exhibit signs or symptoms that indicate the medication is effective (or ineffective)? A reduction of blood pressure when taking antihypertensives or diminution or absence of seizure activity when taking anticonvulsants is a sign that the medication is effective. If medications are ineffective, this is reported to the physician.

2. Is the patient experiencing any secondary effects? A secondary effect is any effect that is experienced other than the intended effect. Secondary effects include adverse effects, toxic effects, drug allergies, and idiosyncratic reactions. A *drug allergy* is a form of adverse drug reaction precipitated by interaction of the drug and the body's immune system. An *idiosyncratic reaction* is an unusual and unpredictable reaction to a drug occurring in a small portion of the total population, often associated with genetic defects. All these reactions are discussed in detail in Chapter 6. The nurse reports all suspected adverse drug reactions to the physician.

3. Is the patient experiencing the effects of drug interactions? Interactions may occur between two drugs (e.g., warfarin and aspirin) or between a drug and one or more foods (e.g., monoamine oxidase [MAO] inhibitors and red wine). Drug-drug and drug-food interactions can result in a toxic effect. For example, an interaction between warfarin and aspirin can cause severe bleeding, or an interaction between an MAO inhibitor and red wine can cause a hypertensive crisis. Drugs may also interfere with the results of laboratory tests. Drug interactions are discussed in detail in Chapter 5.

4. Does the patient comprehend all of the material previously taught about the medications?

5. Can the patient apply information when test situations are given?

6. Can the patient recognize each of his or her medications and differentiate among them?

7. Does the patient have all the knowledge or skill needed to administer the medications at home?

8. Is the patient taking the medication as ordered? The best way to elicit this information is to ask the patient, "How are you taking your medication?" The nurse should ascertain, or solicit, the following information: (1) Is the patient taking the medication as prescribed or only when he or she remembers? (2) Is the patient taking it at the correct times? and (3) Is the patient taking it in the correct way, with food or between meals, and using the correct technique, for example, injecting it intramuscularly or subcutaneously? Is the patient rotating sites correctly?

It is important for the nurse to understand (1) the expected action of the medication in the body, (2) how to assess and teach the patient about medication to ensure compliance, and (3) how to recognize when the medication is effective or not effective. By knowing and understanding this information, the nurse is able to use the nursing process in caring for the patient requiring medications.

The bibliography for this chapter can be found in Appendix B, which begins on page 1054.

CHAPTER REVIEW QUESTIONS*

1. What is the *first* condition that must be met for a patient to comply with the medication regimen?
   a. Adequate knowledge about the disease process.
   b. Examination of cultural beliefs.
   c. Acceptance of the diagnosis.
   d. Adequate family support.

2. Which of the following statements by Mr. Wilson may indicate noncompliance with his drug therapy prior to his hospitalization?
   a. "I'm responsible for my life and how I'm feeling."
   b. "I always get good treatment from my doctor."
   c. "These pills are costing me a lot of money."
   d. "My blood pressure isn't as bad as the doctor thinks."

3. Mr. Wilson tells the nurse that he was given a number of pamphlets on hypertension and his medications after his diagnosis. A significant factor that *may* be related to noncompliance in this case would be:
   a. Occupation.
   b. Readability level.
   c. Cultural background.
   d. Religious preference.

4. During the planning stage of the nursing process:
   a. The patient's actual and potential health problems are identified.
   b. Nursing actions are based on nursing orders.
   c. Objective and subjective data are evaluated.
   d. Goals are established that become the outcomes of nursing care.

*See Appendix A, which begins on page 1051, for answers.

BUILDING YOUR CRITICAL THINKING SKILLS

INTRODUCTION TO CRITICAL THINKING

Critical Thinking is often defined as thinking about your thinking. Thinking is not a static process, but rather a dynamic process that changes continually. In critical thinking, a conclusion is reached through a process of inquiry. The focus of the inquiry is the unresolved problem that needs to be analyzed creatively to arrive at a new solution. By recalling facts—for example, the patient's history or condition, adverse effects of medications, signs and symptoms of drug toxicity—and synthesizing this information with what you know about the problem, a new supposition can be developed. Final resolution to the problem is an intervention based on the new supposition. One of the biggest obstacles to critical thinking is getting into a rut. "This is the way we have always done. . . ." Being willing to ask questions, even from experts, expands one's awareness and solidifies new knowledge.

Critical thinking differentiates the professional from the technical nurse. The technical nurse operates machines, follows established routines, and gathers and records facts. The professional nurse uses critical thinking to analyze and interpret available information and then makes decisions and/or judgments to achieve the desired outcomes, rather than acting solely on orders or protocols. For example, the technical nurse titrates Nipride to the ordered blood pressure of 140/85. However, the professional nurse takes note of the patient's mental response—he is becoming combative and confused—and his urinary output, which is only 5 mL for the last 30 minutes. The professional nurse, using critical thinking, realizes that the ordered blood pressure is too low to maintain adequate cerebral and renal perfusion. The critically thinking professional nurse then calls the physician to obtain a higher base blood pressure.

CHAPTER 3

Administering Medications with Safety

Merrily A. Kuhn, RNC, PhD

CHAPTER OUTLINE

Medication Administration
Using the Nursing Process

KEY TERMS

Aerosol	Intrathecal
Anesthetic	Local effect
Antibiotics	Miosis
Anti-inflammatories	Mydriasis
Antiseptic	Nebulizer
Astringent	Ophthalmic route
Bactericidal	Otic route
Bacteriostatic	Parenteral
Buccal	Reference drug
Cleansing agent	Spray
Emollient	Sublingual
First-pass effect	Suppository
Foams	Systemic effect
Fungicides	Trade (brand or proprietary)
Gels	name
Generic	Transdermal
Intradermal	Troche

LEARNING OBJECTIVES

After reading this chapter, the student will be able to:

1. Formulate a specific plan to assess the patient receiving medications.
2. Plan the nursing intervention necessary to safely administer medications to any patient.
3. Evaluate the nursing intervention and the patient at various stages to ensure patient safety.

All patients receiving medications have the right to have the medications administered safely. The nurse assumes certain responsibilities and always follows the Seven Rights of Medication Administration, shown in Figure 3–1: (1) the right medication, (2) the right patient, (3) the right dose, (4) the right route, (5) the right time, (6) the right of the patient to refuse medication, and (7) the right documentation. The nurse also assumes the responsibility for teaching patients all they need to know to administer the medications safely at home. In selected chapters, a Delivering Home Health Care box details medication administration and other drug-related consid-

erations in the home setting. Ethnic and cultural considerations for drug administration are discussed in Chapter 9.

MEDICATION ADMINISTRATION

Aspects of medication administration discussed in this chapter include preparation and nursing care before, during, and after medication administration. For the actual

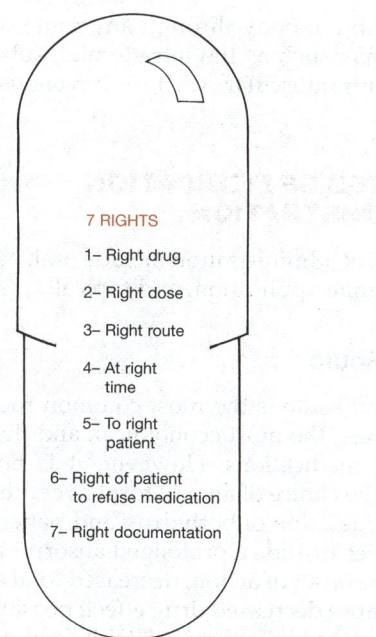

Figure 3–1. The Seven Medication Rights for administering drugs.

techniques of medication administration, please refer to a fundamentals text.

DRUG NAMES AND PREPARATIONS

Most medications today have four names: chemical, *generic* (nonproprietary), *trade* (brand or proprietary), and official. The chemical name is primarily used by chemists and represents the chemical formulation of a drug. The generic can be either handed down from antiquity (colchicine), acquired from biochemistry (nitroglycerin), or assigned by the United States Adopted Name (USAN) Council. A manufacturer is given a 17-year patent on a generic drug. Once the drug is patented, the manufacturer can recover part of the investment used in research and development by licensing other companies or itself to produce or sell the drug. The trade name is created by the manufacturer and is always capitalized. If the name is registered, the trademark symbol is found at the upper right of the name (e.g., Valium®).

Both generic and trade drugs are regulated by law with respect to the amount and purity of the drug. However, only a relatively small amount of a tablet or capsule is composed of active drug. The remainder is made up of nonmedicinal substances, which are not regulated. The ultimate formulation of the drug may affect the drug's action. Consumer groups have caused legislators to enact generic drug laws in many states. These laws require pharmacists to fill prescriptions with a generic form of a prescribed drug unless the prescriber writes ''DAW,'' which stands for ''dispense as written,'' (as shown in Figure 3–2). Generic drugs are often less expensive than trade drugs; therefore, the cost of medical care can be reduced by their use.

The official name, often the generic, is listed in an official compendium, *The United States Pharmacopeia–*

National Formulary (USP-NF). Canada does not designate a compendium as official.

The U.S. Food and Drug Administration (FDA) selects one formulation of a drug, usually the original of its kind, as a *reference drug*, which is the standard for all other drugs of its group. The FDA then uses this standard to test all other equivalent drugs for potency, efficacy, bioavailability, and other criteria (concepts are fully discussed in Chapter 4).

MEDICATION PREPARATIONS—LOCAL AND SYSTEMIC

Medications are administered to have either a local or a systemic effect. A *local effect* is one in which the effects of medications are confined to one area of the body. Antiseptics, anti-inflammatories, and some anesthetics are used locally. A *systemic effect* is obtained when the medication is absorbed and delivered to the body tissues by way of the vascular system. Some medications, although applied locally, such as nitroglycerin ointment, have a systemic effect due to their absorption through the skin.

Local Medications

Local medications affect only one part of the body and are generally applied to the skin (topically), the mucous membranes, or a joint cavity (by injection). When medications are applied topically, the skin usually acts as a barrier and does not allow them to be absorbed. The mucous membranes line all external cavities of the body, that is, the mouth, nose, eye, throat, rectum, vagina, and urethra, and are excellent surfaces for medication absorption because of the large number of capillaries directly beneath the surface. Injection of medication into a joint cavity is generally undertaken to reduce inflammation in the joint. Its effect is due to the presence of the large number of capillaries in the joint.

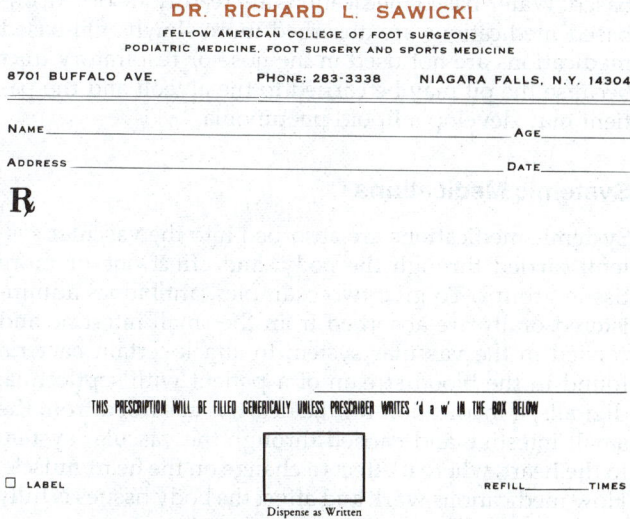

Figure 3–2. Sample prescription form currently in use in New York since July 1987. All prescriptions are filled generically unless the prescriber writes ''DAW'' in the box. (Courtesy of Dr. Richard L. Sawicki, Niagara Falls, NY.)

Local medications come in many forms, including aerosols, ointments, creams, pastes, powders, tinctures (medications mixed with alcohol), and lotions. Local medications can also be obtained as *gels, foams,* and *suppositories* for rectal, vaginal, and urethral application. The medication can also be administered through douche or irrigation into the vagina or through an enema or irrigation into the rectum. *Sprays, aerosols,* gases (including oxygen and carbon dioxide), and *nebulizers* are methods of introducing local or systemic medications, or both, into the respiratory system. Local medications in many different forms (gels, pastes, liquids) can be administered onto the surface of the mucous membranes and teeth to clean teeth or to freshen breath. Throat lozenges or *troches* are also used locally to produce relief for a sore mouth or throat. Many of these preparations are available over the counter (OTC).

Local medications are used for the following specific effects:

1. *Astringents* cause vasoconstriction and tissue contraction, which either decreases or arrests secretions, thereby toughening tissue.
2. *Emollients* soothe and soften and often reduce dryness of the skin.
3. *Cleansing agents* help to remove dirt, crusts, secretions, and debris from wherever applied.
4. *Anesthetics* produce a loss of feeling or sensation in a part of the body.
5. *Antiseptics* and *bacteriostatic* agents inhibit the growth or multiplication of bacteria.
6. *Antibiotics* and/or *bactericidal* agents—chemical compounds either produced by or obtained from certain living cells, especially yeasts and molds, or made from synthetic compounds—are antagonistic to other forms of life.
7. *Anti-inflammatories* reduce or counteract inflammation.
8. *Fungicides* are agents that destroy fungi.

Local medications can be water based (aqueous) or oil based. Water-based medications are readily absorbed; oil-based medications are absorbed more slowly. Oil-based medications are not used in the nose or respiratory tract because the oil may be carried to the alveoli and the patient may develop a lipoid pneumonia.

Systemic Medications

Systemic medications are absorbed into the vascular system, carried through the body, and affect one or more tissue groups. To give two examples, antibiotics administered orally are absorbed from the small intestine and carried in the vascular system to attack certain bacteria found in the blood stream of a patient with septicemia; digitalis, a medication for the heart, is absorbed from the small intestine and carried through the vascular system to the heart, where it effects a change on the heart muscle. How medications work and affect the body tissues is fully discussed in Chapter 4.

Systemic medications can be administered orally, topically, parenterally, or applied to mucous membranes. *Parenteral* is a term that refers to a medication's introduction into the body through any route other than gastrointestinal, such as the intradermal, subcutaneous (SC or SQ), intramuscular (IM), intravenous (IV), or rectal routes.

ROUTES OF MEDICATION ADMINISTRATION

Routes of administration include oral, parenteral, mucous membrane application, and topical.

Oral Route

The oral route is the most common route and is usually the safest, the most economical, and the easiest route for giving medications. However, it is not necessarily the best. The choice of an oral form over other forms involves a consideration of both drug and patient variables. Drug variables include a prolonged absorption time, which delays the onset of action; decreased total absorption, which may cause decreased drug effect; possible gastrointestinal upset; possible interaction with food and other medications; and possible prolonged effect. The patient variables include the patient's age; how quickly the pharmacologic action is needed; the patient's mental status, neurologic state, gastrointestinal function and mobility, and ability to swallow the medication (in some cases, liquid forms of the medication may be used); and very important, the physiologic integrity of the patient, such as his or her current illness and organ function. (These variables are discussed in more detail in Chapter 4.)

Oral medications are administered with sufficient amounts of water to ensure that they enter the stomach. The administration of water with an oral medication often enhances absorption; for example, the action of expectorants such as guaifenesin and iodide products may be enhanced by drinking six to eight glasses of water daily. Exceptions include some cough medicines that are given for a local soothing effect on the throat.

The oral route of administration has some disadvantages. Patients may object to the taste of the medication, or the medication may cause gastric upset, constipation, or diarrhea. Some medications may harm or stain the teeth. The medication may also be destroyed by gastrointestinal secretions and thus fail to produce its desired effects. Oral medications may also be inadvertently aspirated by the seriously ill, old, or young patient.

The nurse must know the correct time to administer oral medications. Some oral medications are best administered with food to enhance absorption or to decrease their gastric irritation, whereas others are given on an empty stomach. At times, medications can upset an empty stomach. Therefore, it may be necessary to modify the time schedule so that the medication can be administered at mealtime.

Oral medications are available in two forms: solid and liquid. The solid forms available include tablets, capsules, caplets, and powders. These forms are featured in Table 3–1. Tablets, capsules, and caplets are often stamped or embossed with the pharmaceutical company's name, drug name, and/or an identifying number and may occasionally be crushed and mixed in applesauce or other

Table 3–1. SOME COMMON MEDICATION DOSAGE FORMS

Route	Form	Description	Example
Oral	Tablet	Compressed powder or granulated drugs; breaks apart quickly in the stomach	Acetylsalicylic acid (aspirin)
Oral	Tablet (enteric coated)	Compressed powder or granulated drugs that are coated so that they dissolve slowly in the intestine	Ecotrin
Oral	Capsule	Gelatin covered; dissolves in either the stomach or the intestine	Propoxyphene (Darvon)
Oral	Caplet	Compressed powder or granulated drugs with smooth outer coating resembling a capsule, making it easier to swallow for some patients	Acetaminophen (Tylenol)*
Oral	Syrup	Solution with sugar, water, and flavoring; may pose problems for the diabetic patient	Robitussin
Oral	Elixir	Hydroalcoholic liquid flavored with volatile oil and slightly sweetened; may pose problems for the diabetic and alcoholic patients taking disulfiram (Antabuse)	Terpin hydrate
Oral	Emulsion	Mixture of oils and water	Agoral Plain
Oral	Gel and magma	Viscous suspension of mineral precipitates in water; shake well before use	Magnesium hydroxide (Milk of Magnesia)
Oral	Aromatic water	Aqueous solution with various oils	Saturated solution potassium iodide (SSKI)
Oral	Tincture	Extract of drugs in alcohol	Camphorated tincture of opium
Oral	Fluid extract	Concentrated liquid preparation of vegetable drugs	Fluid extract of belladonna
Oral	Extract	Concentrated preparation made by evaporating the hydroalcoholic solvent; may be more potent than active drug	Belladonna extract
Oral	Lozenge (troche)	Flattened disk intended to be held in the mouth until dissolved; often contains sweeteners, flavors, and color	Cepacol lozenges
Oral	Effervescent tablet	Large tablet that forms a bubbling solution	K-Lor
Rectal	Suppository	Solid dosage form inserted into body cavity where drug is released as the solid (cocoa butter, glycerin, gelatin) melts	Tigan
Topical	Powder	Topical product applied to dry the skin	Cornstarch
Topical	Lotion	Liquid preparation that may be soothing or medicinal	Calamine
Topical	Ointment	Fatty, soft substance for external use	White petrolatum jelly (Vaseline)
Topical	Transdermal disk (patch)	Medicated dressing applied to skin; releases its medication topically for systemic absorption	Nitroglycerin (Transderm-Nitro)
Parenteral	Powder	Mixed with sterile solution for parenteral administration	Penicillin G
Parenteral	Emulsion	Mixture of oil and water	Interlipid solutions
Parenteral	Solution	Liquid preparation containing dissolved compounds	D/ Electrolyte #2

*Many other forms available.

medium for patients who have difficulty swallowing or mixed in a bowl to be administered down a feeding tube. These products may be enteric coated, which delays the release of the medication until it reaches the small intestine. Enteric-coated medications are not administered concurrently with antacids, because the high pH of the antacid allows the enteric coating on the drug to break down in the stomach. Tablets and capsules may also be sustained-release, extended-release, long-acting, controlled-release, or prolonged-action products. These types of products are designed to release the drug over a long period to reduce the number of doses a patient must take each day. Unlike regular tablets or capsules, enteric-coated or sustained-release products are never crushed, because this destroys the sustained-release property.

The liquid forms include syrups, elixirs, emulsions, gels or magmas, tinctures, aromatic waters, fluid extracts, and extracts.

Parenteral Route

The parenteral route is used for medications entering the body through any route other than orally through the gas-

trointestinal system. All medication entering the body in this manner must be sterile and, because these drugs may enter the bloodstream readily, great care is always taken when administering them to patients. Parenteral medications are generally more expensive than their oral forms because of the greater cost of preparation. The administration of medications through the parenteral route takes specialized education. Only the physician, nurse, or other specially trained persons administer parenteral medication. The law regarding parenteral medication administration varies from state to state.

There are several parenteral routes that can be used, including the *intradermal* route, just under the surface of the skin; SC or SQ, into the subcutaneous tissue; IM, into the muscle tissue; and IV, into the vein. Parenteral medications are also given into a joint, the intra-articular route; into an artery, the intra-arterial route; into the spinal column, the intraspinal route; into the pleural space of the lung, the intrapleural route; and into the spinal or subarachnoid space, the *intrathecal* route. The drugs are administered from a sterile syringe and needle. The needles vary in diameter (gauge) from 14 to 26 gauge and in length from ⅜ inch to 3 inches. In selecting a needle, the

Table 3–2. INJECTION EQUIPMENT FOR PARENTERAL MEDICATION

| Type of Injection | Needle | | Syringe/Other Equipment | General Use |
	Gauge	Length		
Intradermal	26	⅜"	Tuberculin	Skin testing
Subcutaneous	25	½"	Tuberculin, insulin	For drugs that are destroyed by GI system, or rapid action is required
Intramuscular	20–23	1–3"	2–5 mL	For drugs that are destroyed by GI system, or rapid action is required
Intravenous fluid	20, 21	1–4"	Butterfly argyle, intercath connected to bottle or IV bag with tubing	When fast action is required
Blood	16, 18	1–4"	Bottle or bag with appropriate tubing	Replacement of blood products
Intra-articular	18, 19	2"	2–5 mL	Reduction of inflammation
Intraspinal	14–16	1–4"	2–5 mL	Anesthesia, pain relief
Intrapleural	14–16	4"	10–50 mL	Withdraw fluid/chemotherapy
Intrathecal	14–16	1–2"	2–5 mL	Chemotherapy

gauge and length are determined by the viscosity of the medication being administered and by the site of the medication deposit. Table 3–2 features injection equipment for parenteral medication and the general use of each route.

Many side effects can be experienced from parenteral administration. The medication may damage or stain the tissues, improper techniques may result in a local or systemic infection or in nerve injury at the injection site, the skin may slough at the injection site or become abscessed; or the patient may experience prolonged pain.

Mucous Membrane Application

Medications are often applied to the mucous membranes of the mouth and throat, the sublingual or buccal surfaces, the nose or other parts of the respiratory system (sprays, inhalants), the eye, the genitourinary system (vaginal douches, suppositories, creams, foams), and the gastrointestinal system (rectal suppositories or enemas). Medications applied to the mucous membranes of the nose, eye, and vagina are often given for their local effect, but systemic absorption can occur. A systemic effect may be desirable as, for example, when an aspirin suppository is given rectally for temperature control.

Sublingual Route When the *sublingual* route is used, the medication is placed under the tongue. Medications are quickly dissolved because of the dosage design, and because the tongue is a very vascular area, medications are quickly absorbed. In general, more medication is absorbed sublingually than through the oral route because the medication is not damaged by gastric secretions or metabolized by the liver through the *first-pass effect*, the combined inactivation of an orally administered medication in the liver. This concept is explained in a later chapter. The patient holds the sublingual medication under the tongue until it is dissolved and is instructed not to swallow the medication or drink any liquid while the medication remains under the tongue. Lingual sprays are also available; the same directions are given to the patient.

Buccal Route Several drugs are formulated to be applied to the mucous membranes of the mouth, that is, by the *buccal* route. Formulations for buccal adminstration include tablets and troches.

An example of a buccal tablet is nitroglycerin. Troches or lozenges are excellent forms for topical application of antibiotics, antifungals, and local anesthetics in the mouth. Swallowing these products would be undesirable because they would be destroyed in the gastrointestinal tract. The patient is instructed to keep these products against the buccal surface of the mouth until they are completely dissolved, usually 5 to 10 minutes, but a hard-candy base can be used to delay absorption. Patients should report any irritation to the mouth.

Inhalation Route Inhalants, usually sprays, are forced through the mouth or nose by a small amount of pressure into the lower respiratory tract. These medications require a pressure device such as a hand bulb, an atomizer, or a nebulizer to deliver the medication. Inhalants are often used for bronchodilation, that is, dilating the lower air passages to make it easier for the patient to exchange gases. Inhalants are local-acting medications and are generally not meant to be absorbed systemically, although with some drugs systemic absorption does occur and results in occasional side effects. It is important for the nurse to teach the patient the proper technique for inhaling these products. These techniques are discussed in greater depth in Chapter 40.

Vaginal Route Medications inserted into the vagina include foams, gels, creams, suppositories, compressed tablets, douches, troches, and irrigations. Medications such as contraceptives, anti-infectives, and anti-inflammatories are administered for their local action and are often inserted into the vagina with an applicator to ensure that the medication is well positioned. It is important that the nurse teach the patient about proper administration.

Rectal Route The rectum, an extremely vascular area with many small capillaries that enhance absorption, is used for administration of both local and systemic medications. Medication forms such as suppositories or enemas are administered for their local effect to treat hemorrhoids or constipation or for their systemic effect to treat respiratory conditions, to reduce temperature, and for many other effects. Suppositories, usually absorbed slowly, are designed to melt at body temperature, so they are best stored in the refrigerator or in a cool place. Most rectal suppositories are packaged in foil wrappers. Patients are taught that the foil is removed and the suppository lubricated with water or soluble gel before insertion.

Most patients identify the rectal route with an enema. Therefore, if medications such as bronchodilators, analgesics, or antipyretics are being administered, the patient should understand that the medication is not to be expelled. Systemic rectal medications may cause irritation, burning, and itching in the rectal area. When irritation arises, the medication may need to be discontinued.

Topical Administration

Topical medication can be applied to the skin (lotions, ointments, creams, patches), the eye (drops, ointments, irrigations), and the ear (drops or irrigation). Medications administered topically are often given for their local effect. However, some medications (nitroglycerin, estrogen) are applied topically but are absorbed and have systemic effect.

Dermal (Skin) Medications   The skin can be treated topically with many products to manage or treat local skin irritation or infections. These products are best applied to newly washed and dried skin in small amounts. Applications are made gently, by patting rather than by rubbing. When applying topical medication, wear gloves to avoid skin contact with the medication.

Transdermal Route   The *transdermal* route uses disks (patches) of medicated dressing applied to the skin that release their medication topically for systemic absorption, as shown in Figure 3–3. Several medications, such as nitroglycerin (treats acute chest pain), clonidine hydrochloride (Catapres, reduces blood pressure), nicotine (for smoking cessation), and estrogen (a female hormone), are available in this long-acting form. The adhesive-backed disks are applied to a nonhairy area and may be effective for up to 1 week. All disks can be worn safely during bathing or showering, and some of the disks remain effective even while swimming.

Ophthalmic Route   The *ophthalmic route* is used to administer medications into the left eye (OS), the right eye (OD), or both eyes (OU) to diagnose and treat eye disorders. Eye medications can dilate the pupil (*mydriasis*), constrict the pupil (*miosis*), or act as a local anesthetic, anti-inflammatory, or anti-infective. Patients need to receive sufficient teaching to administer these medications safely.

Otic Route   The *otic route* refers to medications that are administered into the ear canal. Formulations include powders, ointments, and drops. Drugs administered by this route include anti-infectives, anti-inflammatories, and local anesthetics. The ear canal can also be irrigated.

THE MEDICATION ORDER

Traditionally, the nurse receives the clearly and completely written medication order from the physician. When the nurse receives a medication order in the hospital, it includes the name of the medication, the dose, the route, and the number of times to be given daily. The order may be written in abbreviated form. Table 3–3 lists common abbrevations for medication orders. As an example, the physician orders Demerol 100 mg IM q 3 hr prn (when required). This means the patient receives Demerol 100 mg intramuscularly, when the patient requires, at least 3 hours apart. Another order might read penicillin G 400,000 units PO tid (three times daily). This means the patient receives penicillin G 400,000 units (usually one tablet) by mouth three times a day. Often several tid times can be chosen: 10 AM, 2 PM, and 6 PM; 8 AM, 4 PM, and midnight; 9 AM, 6 PM, and 1 AM; or 10 AM, 6 PM, and 2 AM. The nurse must know the drug's action to administer the medication at the correct times. The best time to administer penicillin G is 8 AM, 4 PM, and midnight; 9 AM, 6 PM, and 1 AM; or 10 AM, 6 PM, and 2 AM. Any of these regimens evenly spaces the dosage to maintain a constant serum level. The nurse is always able to alter the drug administration times for appropriate reasons. Antibiotics, antidysrhythmics, and bronchodilators are best given around the clock or at regular intervals to keep the medication at a therapeutic level in the blood for the entire 24 hours.

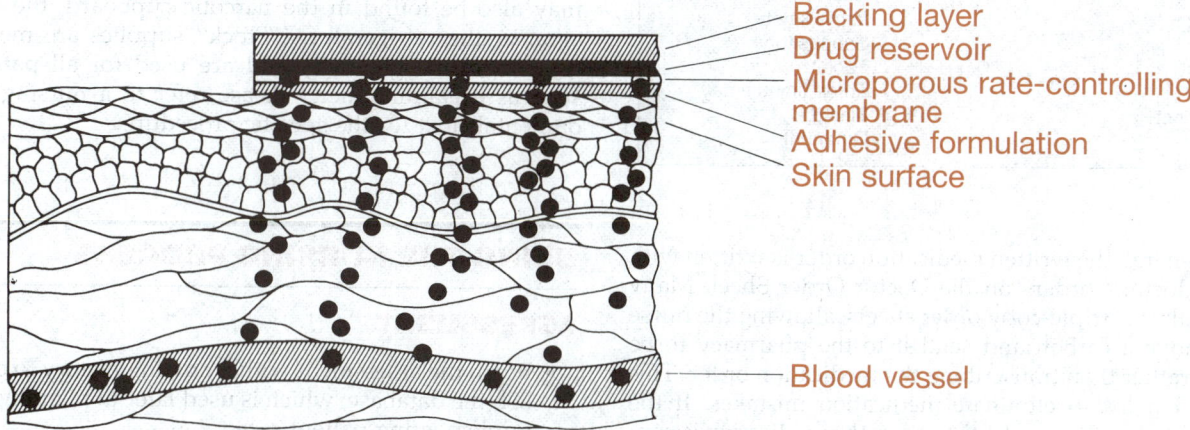

Backing layer
Drug reservoir
Microporous rate-controlling membrane
Adhesive formulation
Skin surface

Blood vessel

Figure 3–3. Typical structure of a transdermal patch, a unique way to deliver medicine to the body. Four separate layers are inside the Transderm® system. Applied like an adhesive bandage, the Transderm system provides a consistent and controlled amount of medication through the skin and directly into the bloodstream over an extended period of time. Transdermal delivery systems provide medication without interfering with the patient's daily activities or without the patient having to take pills several times a day. (Courtesy of CIBA-GEIGY Corporation, Summit, NJ.)

Table 3–3. COMMON ABBREVIATIONS FOR MEDICATION ORDERS

Abbreviation	Meaning
ac	Before meals
AD	Right ear
AS	Left ear
aq	Water
ag dest	Distilled water
AU	Both ears
aur	Ear
bid	Two times a day
c̄	With
caps	Capsule
comp	Compound
dil	Dilute
dr	Dram
elix	Elixir
fld	Fluid
gm or g	Gram
gr	Grain
gtt	A drop, drops
h or hr	Hour
hs	At bedtime
IM	Intramuscular
IU	International unit
IV	Intravenous
L	Liter
m	Minim
mcg (μg)	Microgram
mg	Milligram
ml, mL	Milliliter
noct	At night
OD	Right eye
OS	Left eye
OU	Both eyes
oz	Ounce
pc	After meals
PO	By mouth
prn	When required
U	Unit
qd	Every day
qh	Every hour
q 2 hr or q2h	Every 2 hours
q 3 hr or q3h	Every 3 hours
q 4 hr or q4h	Every 4 hours
qid	Four times a day
qs	As much as is required
s̄	Without
Sig or S	Write on label
s̄s̄	One-half
stat	Immediately
supp	Suppository
tab	Tablet
tid	Three times a day
tr or tinct	Tincture
ung	Ointment

administering each medication. Usually the pharmacy keeps a list of each patient's medications that is checked daily by the pharmacist, who then alerts the medical and nursing staff of possible drug interactions, duplications of medications, wrong doses, and other problems.

The nurse who is in doubt about a medication order, either because it is illegibly written or because it is of questionable dose or use, should never give the medication until verifying the order with the physician who wrote it. The nurse may also refuse to give the medication if the physician is known to be in error or, if, in the judgment of the nurse, the administration may result in harm to the patient. The abbreviations listed in Table 3–3 should be used cautiously. Many dosing mistakes are made because of improper interpretation of abbreviations as shown in Table 3–4.

The medication order can also be verbal, often given over the phone. All verbal orders are written in the patient's chart as they are received and are repeated back to the physician to ensure accuracy. In addition, the physician's full name, the date, and the time are written in the chart. The orders should be countersigned by the physician as soon as possible, most often within 24 hours in acute-care facilities. Some institutions also demand that the telephone order be tape-recorded.

The pharmacist dispenses the correct medication to the hospital units. The nurse is then responsible for checking for the correct dose, administering the drug, and instructing the patient about the use of the drug. The nurse's responsibilities also include observing the patient for both therapeutic and nontherapeutic drug effects. Any unusual responses are reported and recorded in the chart, and the next dose of the drug is withheld until the physician examines the patient.

THE MEDICATION AREA

Most hospitals and other institutions keep medications in a special location that is private and quiet. Often, the medications are stored in a room or on a special medication cart in which each patient has his or her own box or drawer that is stocked by the pharmacy, but medications may also be found in the narcotic cupboard, the stock area, or the refrigerator. ("Stock" supplies are medications available generally and are used for all patients, such as acetaminophen.) Please refer to a nursing fundamentals text for the specific procedure.

In general, the written medication order is written with other doctors' orders on the Doctor Order Sheet. Many hospitals use triple-copy order sheets, allowing the nurse to remove a carbon and send it to the pharmacy to be filled, rather than transcribing the medication order. This method helps to eliminate medication mistakes. If the nurse needs to transcribe the order, the medication is copied verbatim onto a pharmacy order form and sent to the pharmacy. The nurse prepares the medication card or sheet to administer the medication; however, the chart is the only authentic record and should be checked before

USING THE NURSING PROCESS

ASSESSMENT

- Begin the assessment with a nursing history to establish the database, which is used later in planning and implementing patient care.
- Obtain a medication history, including the use of prescription medications (specifically ask females about the use of birth control pills, as many women forget to mention them), over-the-counter medications, al-

Table 3–4. COMMONLY MISINTERPRETED ABBREVIATIONS

Order	Abbreviation or Problem	Intended Meaning	Misinterpretation	Correction
d/c meds: *Digoxin 0.25mg* *Lasix 40mg* *KCl 20mEq*	D/C	Discharge discontinue	Patients' medications have been prematurely discontinued when D/C, intended to mean "discharge," was misinterpreted as "discontinue," when followed by a list of drugs.	Write out "discharge" and "discontinue."
Vit B12 1 µg im Now *µg*		Microgram	When handwritten, this can easily be mistaken for "mg."	Use "mcg."
Diabinese 250mg t̄ 1d *t̄ 1D*		Once daily	Mistaken as "t.i.d."	Write it out.
Digoxin 0.25g q.d.	q.d.	Every day	The period after the "q" has sometimes been mistaken for an "i," and the drug has been given qid rather than daily.	Write it out.
Lasix 200 p. today	200	200 mg	Usual PO dose is 40–120 mg. This would have meant giving 15 tabs.	Do not write over orders.
Tylenol #3 qid prn	#3	#3 is specific dosage	Three tabs of Tylenol were administered.	Beware of ambiguous drug names.
100 ml of 5% D c̄ 100 ml HCl	HCl	KCl	KCl was misinterpreted for HCl because HCl is rarely used.	Question dose of KCl, which was too high.

cohol, and recreational drugs. If the patient is taking other medications, determine why they are being taken and what information the patient understands about those medications.

- Obtain an allergy history to prevent medication reactions. Many cross-allergies exist between medications as well as between foods and medications.
- Obtain a smoking history and intake of coffee, tea, and other caffeine beverages.
- Assess the patient's weight, because many medications are ordered based on the patient's current weight. It may be necessary to determine body surface area (BSA) to calculate proper dosage. BSA can be calculated using a nomogram, shown in Figure 3–4. Nomograms are also available for children and are discussed in Chapter 7.
- Assess the patient's skin, particularly noting color, bruises, needle marks, and infection. If these are present, injections are not performed in these areas.
- Help select the most appropriate route of administration for the specific medication as needed. Consider the patient's age and physical condition when determining the route. For example, a patient receiving digoxin 0.25 mg daily by mouth who is NPO (nothing by mouth) after surgery needs to receive digoxin by another route.
- Become familiar with the medication policies within the employment setting to determine when the physician must be notified to rewrite the order. Also assess the medication order for accuracy and completeness. If there is any doubt about the order, the physician is consulted first.

Nurses, after special education, are now able to prescribe and modify drug dosage and timing. These responsibilities are being used in all areas of patient care. Education remains a crucial factor in adequate preparation for this new role.

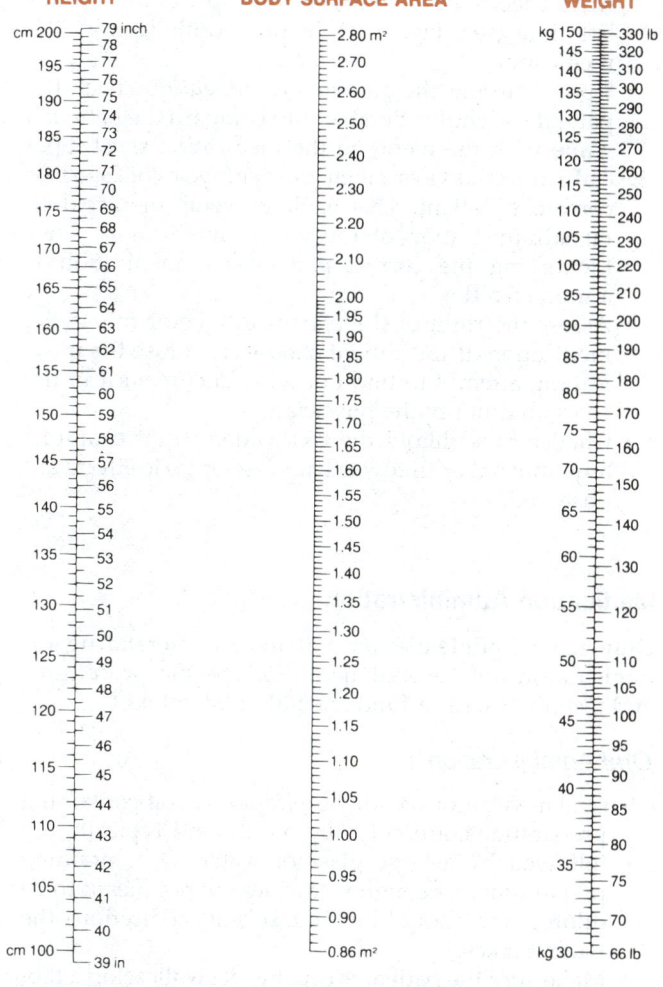

Figure 3–4. Body surface area of adults. Nomogram for determining body surface area from height and weight. (Documenta Geigy Scientific Tables, 8 ed. Vol. 1, 1981. Courtesy of CIBA-GEIGY Corporation, Summit, NJ.)

NURSING DIAGNOSIS

- Nursing diagnoses are established as the nurse prepares to administer medication to the patient. These nursing diagnoses may be established by the nurse when the locus of control is with the nurse, as in an acute-care situation, or by both the nurse and patient when the locus of control is shared. Typical examples of nursing diagnoses when administering medications include the following: Anxiety related to IM injection; Knowledge Deficit related to current need for IV therapy; Knowledge Deficit related to the use of transdermal nitroglycerin; and Risk for Injury related to medication administration. Additional nursing diagnoses that can be used during drug administration are reviewed throughout this text.

PLANNING AND INTERVENTION

- During the planning phase, the nurse plans to administer the medication safely to the patient and to advise the patient (and/or family) regarding information about the medication regimen. The nurse always checks the Seven Rights of Medication Administration (see Fig. 3–1) before administering the medication.
- Upon entering the patient's room, *always* check the patient's identification band to compare the patient's name with the name on the medication sheet. Special care is always taken to identify a confused or comatose patient. This habit prevents the accidental administration of the wrong medication. After identifying the correct patient, the medication is administered.
- Assess the right of the patient to take or refuse the medication. If the patient chooses to refuse the medication, attempt to find out why, document it in the chart, and notify the physician.
- Choose to withhold the medication if, for example, any unusual or untoward adverse or toxic effects are observed.

Medication Administration

Only general guidelines for oral and parenteral drug administration are covered here. For specific procedures and techniques, see a fundamental nursing text.

Oral Administration

- Oral medications, with the exception of oil-containing preparations, are taken by mouth and typically are followed by a large glass of water. Oil-containing preparations or cough medicines are not meant to be diluted and should be the last oral medications the patient takes.
- Make sure the patient is capable of swallowing a tablet or capsule before administering it.
- The patient should be sitting, standing, or lying on his or her side—not lying supine—when tablets or capsules are administered. When tablets or capsules are taken when the patient is supine, the medication often adheres to the esophageal mucosa and disintegrates, thus causing irritation of the esophageal mucosa or improper absorption.
- Crush tablets or open capsules and mix with a food or liquid if the patient has difficulty swallowing. Always check with the pharmacist before crushing tablets or opening capsules. Enteric-coated tablets cannot be crushed. Also, not all capsules can or should be opened.
- Make sure to measure the correct amount when administering liquid medications. In the home when a teaspoon or a tablespoon is the dosage amount ordered, patients are taught to use only accurate measuring devices, not their flatware, as measures.
- In patients, especially the young and old, who have difficulty taking liquids from a glass, administer the medication into the side of the patient's mouth with a syringe that has a Brody tip. The fluid can then be expelled into the mouth very slowly, allowing the patient sufficient time to swallow. A straw may also be used to give small quantities of medication.
- Insert oral medication through a feeding tube if necessary. If the patient has a nasogastric (NG) tube inserted, tablets may be crushed or capsules opened, mixed with a liquid, and, in most cases, administered through the NG tube. The NG tube is flushed before and after and clamped for 30 to 60 minutes after the medication is administered to allow the medication to pass into the small intestine.

Parenteral Administration

- Select the proper size syringe and needle (see Table 3–2). Medications are available in single-dose vials, multidose vials, ampules, or cartridges.
- If two medications are ordered at the same time, always check with a drug reference chart or the pharmacist to make sure the medications are physically compatible and/or will not cause a harmful drug-drug interaction before mixing them together. If unsure, it is always best to give the patient two injections rather than take the chance of mixing two incompatible drugs. Generally, narcotics and anticholinergics such as meperidine (Demerol) and atropine (standard preoperative medications) can be combined safely. In most instances, insulins can be safely mixed together in the same syringe, but time-dependent factors need to be considered. (More information on insulin can be found in Chapter 45.) Some medications (e.g., antibiotics) may be inactivated by other medications, so compatibility always must be ascertained.
- Institute universal precautions (e.g., wear gloves) when preparing to administer the drug to the patient.
- Select the medication, calculate the dose, and administer the medication. When administering medication to the very young or old, special techniques may be useful. Such techniques are reviewed in Chapter 7 (pediatric patients) and Chapter 8 (geriatric patients).

- Several strategies that may be helpful when planning to administer a pain-free parenteral injection (IM, SC) are as follows:
  1. Select a site away from skin lesions, abrasions, excoriations, lipodystrophies, or lipohypertrophies.
  2. Distract the patient by talking to him or her.
  3. Hold the needle steady.
  4. Inject the medication into or through a relaxed muscle.
  5. Insert and remove the needle quickly.
  6. Inject the medication slowly.
  7. Hold an alcohol pad firmly against the skin as the needle is removed from the site. This provides countertraction in the skin. The needle will then not pull the tissues and cause discomfort as it is removed.
  8. Rotate injection sites.
  9. Use a sharp needle free of burrs.
  10. Select the smallest gauge needle compatible with the medication to be injected.
  11. An ice cube may be applied to the site before injecting the medication in some selected situations.
  12. Apply direct pressure to the area.
  13. Massage the area to hasten absorption, except when administering iron dextran (InFED), heparin, or insulin.
  14. Use the Z-track technique, shown in Figure 3–5, which is the safest and most comfortable technique for giving IM injections, to patients between the ages of 8 and 60.

Intramuscular Injections   The patient must be positioned correctly for IM injections, depending on where the injection site. In addition, needle length may be an important consideration if the patient has considerable body fat.

- The patient should be sitting if an injection is to be administered in the arm (deltoid) or be lying down, either on the side or prone, if an injection is to be administered in the buttocks or legs. When using the leg for IM injections, it is best to use the lateral surface. If injections are received in the anterior surface of the leg, the medication may form a hard mass that

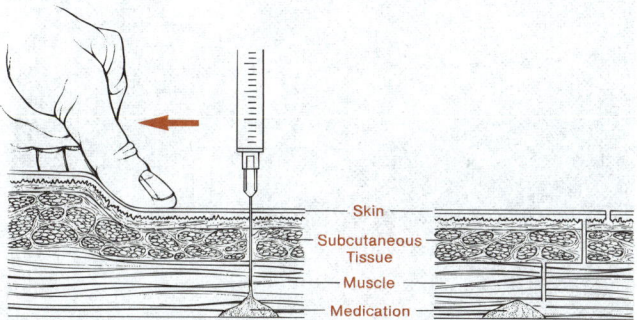

Figure 3–5. A Z-track intramuscular injection. The skin is pulled to one side for the injection. After the injection, when the skin returns to its normal position, the track is interrupted, keeping the medication from seeping back out.

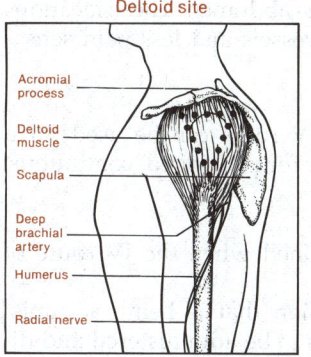 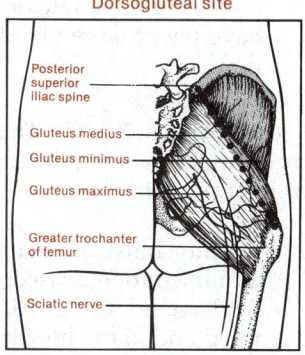

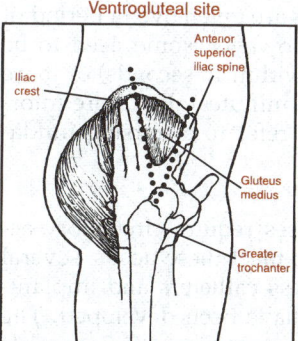 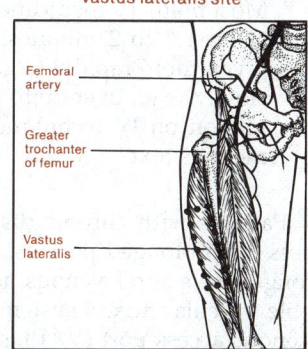

Figure 3–6. IM injection sites. (A) Deltoid site: The mid-deltoid area is located by forming a rectangle, the top of which is at the level of the lower edge of the acromion, and the bottom of which is at the level of the axilla; the sides are one-third and two-thirds of the way around the outer aspect of the patient's arm. (B) Dorsogluteal site: To avoid the sciatic nerve and accompanying blood vessels, an injection site is chosen above and lateral to a line drawn from the greater trochanter to the posterior superior iliac spine. (C) Ventrogluteal site: The nurse's palm is placed on the greater trochanter and the index finger is placed on the anterior superior iliac spine; the IM injection is made into the middle of the triangle formed by the nurse's fingers and the iliac crest. (D) Vastus lateralis site: The patient is supine or sitting for the injection. (*Source:* Deglin, JH and Vallerand, AH: Davis's Drug Guide for Nurses. FA Davis, Philadelphia, 1992, p. 1238, Appendix H, 3rd ed, with permission.)

becomes painful when the patient walks. Sites for IM injection are shown in Figure 3–6.

- Use a needle long enough to deposit the medication into the muscle. Injections intended for the muscle may in fact not reach the muscle but rather are deposited in fat. This is especially true for adult women, who have a thicker gluteal fat layer than men. (Children have less gluteal fat, so injections given to them usually go into the muscle.) Injections deposited in fat may be absorbed more slowly than those deposited in muscle.

Subcutaneous Injections   Because subcutaneous injections are not deep, some sites are more suitable than others.

- Subcutaneous injections are generally administered in the outer surface of the upper arm, the anterior portion of the thigh, or the abdomen. These locations have fewer large blood vessels and less pain sensation.

Intravenous Route The IV route can be used for a medication needed quickly or for prolonged, continuous, or intermittent infusion.

- Sterility must be maintained when the IV route of administration is used.
- Understand the medication that is being administered and know how it is to be administered and diluted.
- The medication is inserted directly into a vein and may be administered as a bolus, that is, a concentrated dose of medication given over a short period. Most bolus IV medications are given over a period of at least 1 to 2 minutes. However, some need to be given more rapidly (e.g., within 10 seconds) or more slowly (e.g., over 10 to 20 minutes). For more information on IV techniques, refer to a nursing fundamentals text.

Patients with chronic diseases require circulatory access for prolonged periods. To meet these needs, several long-term central venous access catheters and implantable vascular access systems have been developed. The venous access port (VAP), shown in Figure 3–7, consists of a radiopaque silicone catheter and an injection port with a self-sealing silicone-rubber system. The principal differences between the VAP systems are the size, shape, and composition (stainless steel/plastic) of the portal. Each manufacturer guarantees the septum for an indefinite number of punctures in the range of 1000 to 2000. The VAPs are implanted surgically. VAPs may be used for blood sampling, bolus injection, and continuous infusions. To access the port, the VAP is palpated; the port is entered with a special Huber needle, shown in Figure 3–8.

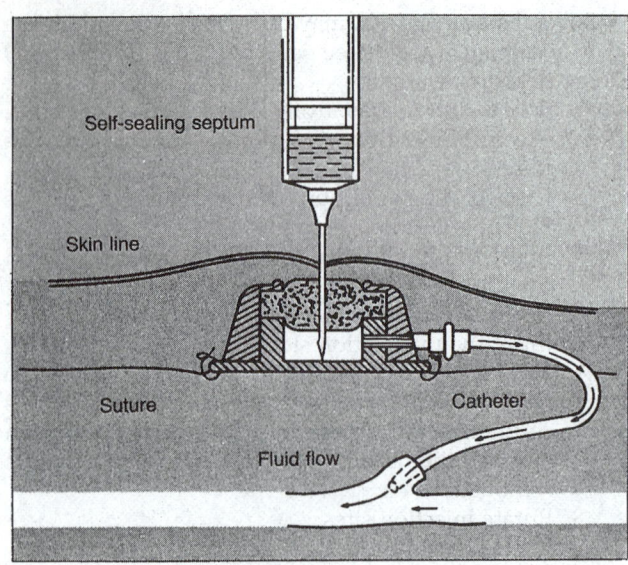

Figure 3–8. The Huber needle is pushed firmly through the skin and self-sealing septum until it hits the bottom of the portal chamber. (From Knox, LS: Implantable venous access devices. Critical Care Nurse 7 (1):71, 1987, with permission.)

Several long-term central venous access catheters are available. These catheters are placed under sterile technique into the right atrium of the heart by way of a large central vein, as shown in Figure 3–9. After tip placement, the catheter is tunneled subcutaneously for several inches to the desired exit site. A small Dacron cuff is attached to the catheter, promoting the ingrowth of fibrous tissue. The Dacron cuff assists in securing the catheter in place and reduces the potential of infection caused by the migration of bacteria in the subcutaneous tunnel. These special catheters are available with 1, 2, and 3 inner lumens.

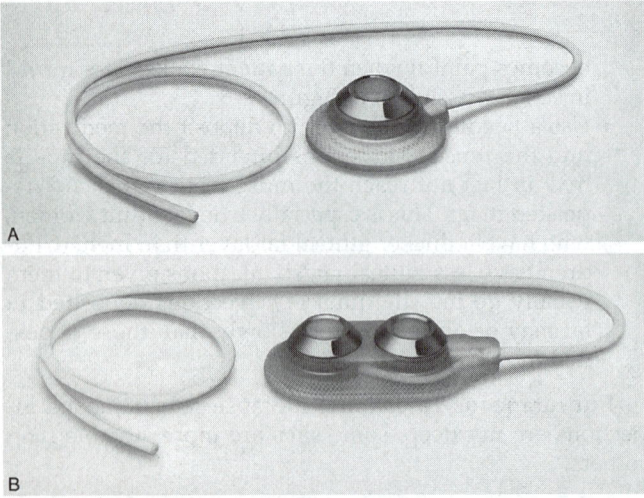

Figure 3–7. (A) VAP/Mediport II. (B) Mediport II DL. (Courtesy of Cormed, Inc., a subsidiary of Bard MedSystems Division, C. F. Bard, Inc., Medina, NY.)

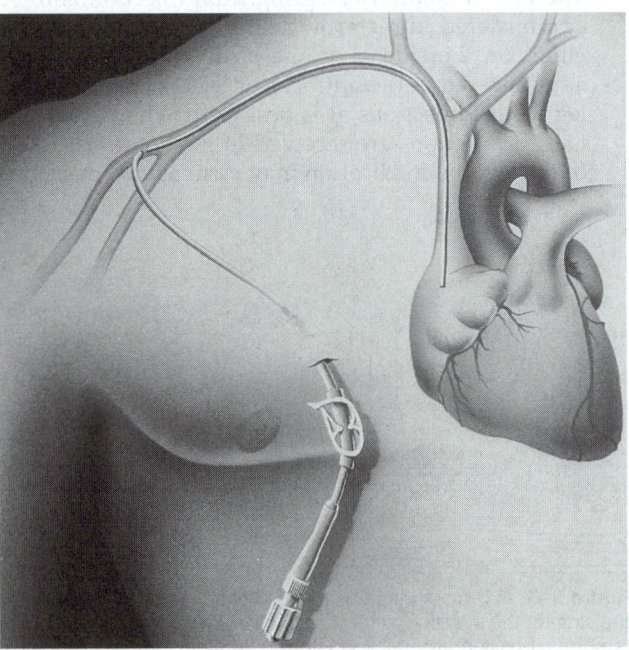

Figure 3–9. Corcath. (Courtesy of Cormed, Inc., a subsidiary of Bard MedSystems Division, C. F. Bard, Inc., Medina, NY.)

Their main advantage is that they do not need to be heparinized after each use. (A heparin flush is used once weekly.) Only a saline flush is needed to clear the catheter. These special implantable catheters are often used in chronically ill patients who are being cared for at home.

Nursing Responsibilities in Medication Administration

- Along with the Seven Rights of Medication Administration, additional points that must be remembered include the following:

1. When preparing medications, always give full, undivided attention to this task.
2. Wash hands prior to administering any medication.
3. Never leave the medication tray or cart unattended. If the nurse must leave the patient's room, the nurse always takes the unadministered medicines.
4. Develop a habit of verifying the medicine card, sheet, or Kardex with the original doctor's orders. This helps to ensure patient safety.
5. Daily, check the patient's allergy list to ensure that the patient is not receiving a medication to which he or she is allergic.
6. Check the discontinuation date on the medication sheet to ensure that medications are given only for the ordered period.
7. Make sure that hypnotics, narcotics, and antibiotics are either discontinued or reordered on their renewal date.
8. Sign out narcotics and hypnotics in the appropriate location at the time they are taken from the narcotic cabinet. Always verify the narcotic count before removing the medication.
9. Never administer medications that have been prepared by someone else. The only exception is medication prepared by the pharmacist.
10. Never administer medications from a bottle whose label is missing or illegible.
11. Never return an unused medication to a stock bottle.
12. When entering a patient's room, identify the patient by name and verify the name by checking the identification bracelet. Then compare the medication sheet with the identification bracelet.
13. Always assist the patient in taking the medication. Never leave the medication for the patient on the assumption that the patient will take it.
14. Always answer all questions the patient asks about the medication.
15. If the patient expresses doubt or concern about receiving a particular medication, always recheck the medication and the original order. Often patients are very familiar with their medications and their questions help prevent a drug error.
16. Follow oral medication with sufficient amounts of water, except when administering oil-based preparations and cough medications. Medications that taste particularly unpleasant may be diluted with juice or other diluents if no possible interaction might occur, or they can be followed with juice or other beverage. The best fluid to follow oral medication is 3½ ozs of cold, carbonated water.
17. Provide for patient privacy when administering a parenteral medication. Always wear gloves during the procedure.
18. Chart the medication administration after it has been given; never chart medications before their administration.
19. Keep all equipment—carts, trays, medicine cups, and water pitchers—meticulously clean. Clean and straighten the medicine preparation area when finished. Wash hands between patients when administering parenteral medications.

Preventing Medication Administration Errors Medication errors can be made by many people: the physician, the pharmacist, the nurse, and the patient.

- If an error is made or found, follow the formal reporting procedure used by the institution involved. Research on medication errors has determined that only approximately one error out of every ten is reported. Medication errors must be reported and documented as they are made. The patient's illness and recovery may be thwarted by poor reporting.
- Some common causes of medication error include the wrong patient, the wrong dose, omission of a dose, the wrong time, the wrong route, and the wrong medication. To prevent medication errors *always* observe the following:

1. Check ambiguous drug orders.
2. Check ambiguous drug names.
3. Beware of atypical drug names.
4. Never use the dropper of one medication to administer another medication.
5. Question the use of multiple tablets, ampules, or vials to provide a single dose.
6. Question unusually small and large doses.
7. Be suspicious of abrupt and excessive increases and decreases of medication.
8. Question the term "midnight" on an order to determine the date.
9. Refuse to interpret illegible handwriting.

Patient Teaching

- The nurse is also responsible for patient education concerning both medical and nursing regimens and all drug education. Patients have a right to know what is wrong with them, what and why products or treatments are prescribed, and what the anticipated results will be. Patient education leads to increased compliance with therapy.
- Patients must know specific information about the medications they are taking. Table 3–5 lists the kinds of medication-related information that generally must be included in teaching the patient prior to discharge. The Patient Teaching tables found throughout the text follow this format, with the information tailored specifically to each drug class. The nurse discusses this material with the patient and family. Ta-

---

Table 3–5. INFORMATION FOUND IN PATIENT TEACHING TABLES

1. General use
2. How long the drug is to be taken
3. How the drug is to be administered, including special preparation and time of administration
4. Interactions to be aware of, including drug-food, drug-drug, or prescription drug–OTC drug interactions
5. Food/alcohol reactions
6. What the patient should do if he or she forgets a dose
7. How the medication is to be stopped or what problems will develop if the medication is stopped abruptly
8. Information on altering the dose
9. Side effects to be aware of and those that need to be reported to the physician immediately
10. Storage instructions

---

bles may be duplicated and given to patients for handy reference at home.

Evaluation

- During the evaluation stage, the nurse evaluates the expected outcomes and goals, the evaluation criteria. Then the nurse evaluates the effectiveness of the medication. What was the desired action of the medication? And is that action being achieved? If not, what is the possible cause: a drug-drug or drug-food inter-

action, improper dosing, or lack of patient compliance? Is the patient experiencing any adverse or toxic effects?

- If parenteral medications have been administered, ascertain that injection sites have been rotated and evaluate for complications such as abscess formation, infections, phlebitis, allergic reactions, and infiltration of IV solution.
- Evaluate medications for interactions. In the 1970s, little was understood about drug interactions; today, entire books feature the subject, and new information accumulates daily. Any possible drug interactions must be anticipated. Always check with the physician or pharmacist if a problem is suspected. Chapter 5 discussed drug interactions in detail.
- Evaluate the patient for toxic reactions. Toxicology, which includes the study of adverse drug reactions, has become a science of its own in recent years. Chapter 6 discusses toxicology in detail.
- Evaluate patient teaching. Does the patient understand what was taught, and can the patient apply this information in everyday life?

The professional nurse is ultimately responsible for total patient care and safety. Only the nurse with a broad understanding of the medications being administered can confidently administer drugs with safety to patients.

The bibliography for this chapter can be found in Appendix B, which begins on page 1054.

CHAPTER REVIEW QUESTIONS*

1. Local medication preparations may be:
   a. Applied to the skin for rapid reabsorption.
   b. Injected into muscle tissue for altered absorption.
   c. Injected into a joint cavity.
   d. Administered safely to all patients.

2. Which statement is *true* regarding administration of medication by the oral route?
   a. Gastric upsets rarely occur.
   b. Inadvertent aspiration may occur in the seriously ill patient.
   c. Water given with the medication retards absorption.
   d. Oral administration is best for all patients.

3. Parenteral administration of medications includes all of the following routes *except*:
   a. Oral.
   b. Intra-articular.

   c. Subcutaneous.
   d. Intrathecal.

4. To prevent medication errors, the nurse will:
   a. Interpret illegible handwriting carefully.
   b. Question the use of multiple tablets to provide a single dose.
   c. Use the dropper of one medication to administer another.
   d. Decline to investigate atypical drug names.

5. One characteristic of generic medications is that they are often:
   a. Less expensive than brand name drugs.
   b. Not as potent as brand name drugs.
   c. More difficult to obtain from the pharmacist.
   d. Less regulated by law with respect to drug purity.

*See Appendix A, which begins on page 1051, for answers.

UNIT 2

BASIC PHARMACOLOGIC PRINCIPLES

UNIT OUTLINE

CHAPTER 4

Pharmaceutical, Pharmacokinetic, and Pharmacodynamic Phases of Drug Action

Merrily A. Kuhn, RNC, PhD

CHAPTER OUTLINE

The Pharmaceutical Phase
The Pharmacokinetic Phase
The Pharmacodynamic Phase
Pharmacokinetic and Pharmacodynamic Implications for
  the Nurse

KEY TERMS

Absorption
Active transport
Accumulation
Agonist
Antagonist
Bioavailability
Biologic half-life
Biotransformation
Clearance
Chronopharmacology
Desensitization
Diffusion
Dissolution
Distribution
Efficacy
Enterohepatic recirculation
Excretion
Facilitated diffusion
Filtration
Hepatic first-pass effect
Hyperactivity
  (supersensitivity)

Immunopharmacology
Induction
Ionized
Loading dose
Maintenance dose
Nonionized
Passive transport
Pharmaceutical phase or
  process
Pharmacodynamic phase
Pharmacokinetic phase
Placebo
Potency
Prodrug
Receptor
Selectivity
Solubility
Steady state
Teratogenic effects
Therapeutic index
Volume of distribution

LEARNING OBJECTIVES

After reading this chapter, the student will be able to:

1. Differentiate among the pharmaceutical, pharmacokinetic, and pharmacodynamic phases of medication action.

2. Assess factors that affect how a drug acts in the body.

3. Distinguish among the pharmacokinetic phases of absorption, distribution, biotransformation, and excretion.

4. Define biologic half-life, effective concentration, peak plasma levels, therapeutic blood level, and minimum and maximum effective levels.

Medications are administered to achieve a specific result or therapeutic effect in the body. Medications may *treat* (e.g., aspirin for arthritic pain), *cure* (e.g., antibiotics for pneumonia), or *control* (e.g., insulin for diabetes). After administration, a medication proceeds through three specific phases of drug action as it passes through the body: the pharmaceutical, pharmacokinetic, and pharmacodynamic, as shown in Figure 4–1.

THE PHARMACEUTICAL PHASE

The *pharmaceutical phase* describes that stage during which the medication enters the body in one form and changes into another form to be utilized. For example, a swallowed tablet or capsule is dissolved into solution by the gastrointestinal secretions and is then ready for absorption into the bloodstream. The ability of a drug to move into solution is called *dissolution*. Liquid medications such as syrups and elixirs are generally ready for absorption faster than capsules or tablets. When the medication is in a form the body can utilize, the next phase begins.

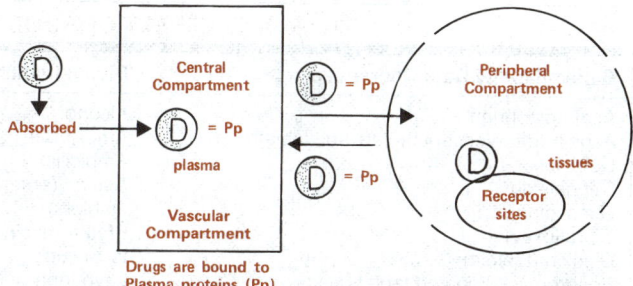

Figure 4–2. Drug distribution. The body has two compartments that hold medication: the central vascular compartment and the peripheral compartment. Drugs (D) are carried on plasma protein (Pp) in the vascular compartment. As the drug enters the peripheral compartment, the drug and plasma protein separate. The drug enters the peripheral compartment and the plasma protein remains in the vascular compartment.

THE PHARMACOKINETIC PHASE

The *pharmacokinetic phase* describes how the body works on drugs and consists of four major processes: absorption, distribution, biotransformation (metabolism), and excretion. In this phase the medication is absorbed into the systemic circulation, distributed to the tissues to act on appropriate cells, biotransformed (broken down or metabolized), and excreted from the body. Many basic principles of biochemistry and enzymology, along with principles of active and passive transport, are applied to understanding these four pharmacokinetic processes.

ABSORPTION

Absorption is the movement of drugs from their site of administration into the vascular bed (central compartment). The vascular bed, which contains the blood and plasma, is where drug molecules travel to reach their site(s) of action, as shown in Figure 4–2. Many factors—solubility, pharmaceutical processing, pH, presence or absence of food, drug concentration, circulation to the absorption site, the absorbing surface, and the route of administration—influence the absorption of drugs. These factors are important considerations in the selection of a drug's route of administration.

Factors Affecting the Rate and Extent of Absorption

Bioavailability For a medication to be absorbed, it must be available. The *bioavailability* of a medication depends on the solubility of the outer covering of a tablet or capsule, pharmaceutical processing of the drug, and the pH of the medication, all of which can enhance or retard the rate of dissolution of the drug. Bioavailability can be simply stated as the percentage of the medication absorbed. Dosage forms of a drug from different manufacturers (and even different lots of preparations from a single manufacturer) sometimes differ in their bioavailability. Bioavailability also depends on the presence or

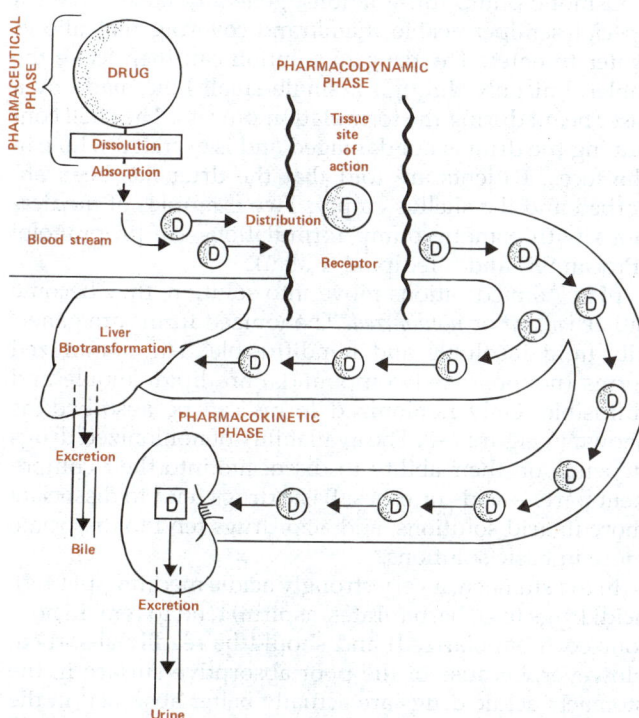

Figure 4–1. The phases of drug action. The pharmaceutical phase describes the stage during which the medication enters the body in one form and changes into another form in order to be utilized. Pharmacokinetic phase of a typical medication: The medication is absorbed into the bloodstream, distributed to its site of action, biotransformed in the liver, and then excreted by either the liver or the kidneys. The pharmacodynamic stage assesses the patient's response to drug therapy and assists in determining the proper dose and dosing schedule.

Table 4–1. EFFECT OF FOOD ON BIOAVAILABILITY OF DRUGS		
Bioavailability Rate Decreased	**Bioavailability Extent Decreased**	**Bioavailability Extent Increased**
Acetaminophen	Alcohol	Diazepam
Aspirin (effervescent tablets and tablets)	Amoxicillin	Dicumarol
Cefaclor	Ampicillin	Erythromycin ethyl succinate (coated
Cephalexin	Aspirin (enteric-coated tablets,	tablets, suspension)
Cimetidine	tablets)	Erythromycin stearate
Ciprofloxacin	Erythromycin	Griseofulvin
Digoxin (tablets)	Isoniazid	Hydralazine
Erythromycin (coated tablets and	Levodopa	Hydrochlorothiazide
tablets)	Nafcillin	Lithium citrate
Furosemide	Penicillin G	Metoprolol
Ibuprofen	Penicillin V (suspension, tablets)	Nitrofurantoin
Nitrofurantoin	Rifampin	Phenytoin
Phenobarbital	Tetracycline	Proprandol
		Spironolactone

This is only a partial listing.

absence of food within the gastrointestinal tract, which can increase or decrease a drug's absorption rate or extent. The *rate* is the speed at which a drug becomes available; *extent* refers to the amount of drug that is absorbed and therefore available. The drug may complex with food, making less drug available for absorption, or food can slow the rate of drug absorption by not allowing enough drug in contact with the intestinal wall. Bioavailability extent can also be increased with food as a result of the increased activity and the effect of food on pH within the intestinal system. Table 4–1 features several drugs for which bioavailability is affected by food.

Drug Solubility *Solubility* is the ability of a medication to dissolve and form a solution in body fluids, which allows the drug to be available for absorption into cells and tissues. The solubility of a medication affects the quantity available for absorption. Lipid-soluble products enter the vascular system more readily than other substances because most cell membranes contain a fatty acid layer. Also, only lipid-soluble substances can readily cross into the brain. Medications may react with each other (e.g., digitalis glycosides and antacids) or with substances within the body (e.g., antacids with phosphate) to form an insoluble precipitate that cannot be absorbed. The nurse must be aware of the possible reactions (discussed specifically in Chapter 5 and throughout this text) to avoid solubility problems. Medications in an aqueous solution are very quickly absorbed when given parenterally.

Pharmaceutical Processing Pharmaceutical processing can either enhance or delay absorption. The binders or excipients, such as alcohol, dextrose, starch, oils, or other chemicals, used to produce and stabilize a drug product ultimately affect the solubility of the drug. Alcohol-based products have enhanced absorption and availability, whereas oil-based products have delayed absorption and availability.

Pharmaceutical processing also includes the dosage form—liquids, tablets, or capsules. Liquids are available more readily because they are already in solution. Enteric-coated tablets are designed to be released only after they enter the relatively alkaline small intestine. Time-release (sustained-release) tablets are prepared so that only a part

of the medication enters solution at a time, producing a longer duration of action. Capsules, in general, are absorbed more readily than tablets. Once the capsule is destroyed, the powder or granules within have a greater surface area than a compressed tablet, thereby enhancing absorption.

Repeat-action tablets carry an initial dose in an outer shell and a second dose in an inner shell. The inner shell disintegrates later in the intestinal tract.

Osmotic pump formulations, generally tablets, have a special semipermeable membrane covering that allows water to enter. The drug in solution can then leave the tablet, but only through a single small hole made by a laser beam during the formulation process. The shell containing the drug is not damaged and is excreted whole in the feces. Patients are told that the drug has been absorbed and the shell is empty. Two examples of medications with osmotic pump formulations are propranolol (Procan SR) and nifedipine (Calan).

pH As medications move into solution, they become either *ionized* or *nonionized*. The ionized forms are generally lipid insoluble and nondiffusible. The nonionized forms (nonpolarized compounds) are lipid soluble and diffusible. Only nonionized forms can be absorbed, as shown in Figure 4–3. The availability of nonionized drugs depends on their ability to dissociate into their component parts—acids or bases. Basic drugs tend to dissociate more in acid solutions, and acid drugs tend to dissociate more in basic solutions.

In the stomach, a very strongly acidic medium (pH 1.4), acid drugs (e.g., barbiturates, aspirin) tend to remain nonionized (nonpolarized) and should be readily absorbed. However, because of the poor absorptive surface in the stomach, acidic drugs are actually better absorbed in the small intestine. By administering an antacid concurrently with an acidic drug, however, absorption can be enhanced. Basic drugs (e.g., quinidine, morphine) tend to remain ionized and, therefore, are not absorbed across the stomach.

In the intestines, where pH increases to 4.0 to 5.0, formerly ionized basic drugs (quinine, digitalis) reunite to form nonionized (nonpolarized) compounds, and their absorption is enhanced. Acid drugs return to their ionized

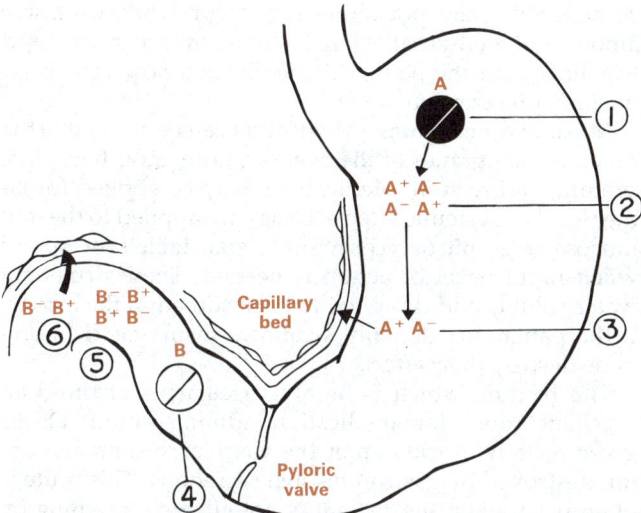

Figure 4–3. Steps in absorption of an oral tablet. (A = acid tablet, e.g., aspirin; B = basic tablet, e.g., quinidine). (1) An acid drug reaches the stomach, (2) becomes nonionized, and (3) is ready for absorption. (4) A basic drug enters the duodenum where pH increases to 6.0 to 8.0, (5) becomes nonionized, and (6) is absorbed.

form and should have reduced absorption. However, because of the increased surface area and increased absorption of the small intestine, the majority of acidic drugs are also absorbed in the small intestine.

Presence or Absence of Food The presence or absence of food in the gastrointestinal tract alters the rate of absorption of medications. The acidic contents of the stomach may increase the destruction of medications (e.g., penicillin G) because food slows the emptying time of the stomach and increases the time of the medication's contact with the digestive juices. Drugs especially susceptible to this destruction are given only parenterally. Food can also cause adsorption or adherence of the drug to food due to chemical or physical action, resulting in decreased absorption. Calcium-containing foods, for example, greatly reduce the absorption of the antibiotic tetracycline, allowing less drug to be available, resulting in inadequate systemic antibacterial action. In general, but not always, an empty stomach enhances absorption, whereas food delays absorption.

Concentration of the Drug The concentration of a drug influences its rate of absorption. The more concentrated a drug, the more rapidly it is absorbed from the area of high concentration in the gastrointestinal system to a low concentration in the blood.

Circulation to the Site of Absorption Blood flow in the administration and absorption sites affects the amount of drug absorbed. Reduced blood flow, as occurs in peripheral vascular disease or shock or with concurrent administration of vasoconstrictor drugs, reduces the absorption of a drug. Increased blood flow, as occurs with local massage, local application of heat, exercise, metabolic disease (hyperthyroidism), or concurrent administration of vasodilator drugs, enhances the absorption of a drug.

Absorbing Surface The absorbing surface, such as the intestinal mucosa, the skin, or the pulmonary alveolar ep-

ithelium, is the surface to which the drug is exposed for absorption. The larger the surface area, the more drug is absorbed. Scar tissue has a decreased absorbing area, so medications should not be administered near scars.

Route of Administration Each route of administration varies in how, where, at what rate, and to what extent it is absorbed.

Mechanisms of Absorption

Medications move through the body and into target cells through active and passive transport, as shown in Figure 4–4. All mechanisms enable the medication to penetrate the cell membrane to allow the medication to act within the cell.

Active transport requires energy and "carriers." The carrier is structurally or chemically specific and can carry only specific drugs. Active transport, generally a one-way transport process, moves substances against a concentration gradient (moving from areas of low concentration to high concentration). The carriers (proteins), form complexes with the drug molecule, moving the drug across the cell membrane before dissociating from the drug, leaving the drug free to act within the cell. Energy is consumed during active transport because of the work performed by the carrier.

Passive transport allows drug molecules to move into and out of cells with the concentration gradient (from high to low areas of concentration) without the expenditure of cellular energy. The concentration of medication

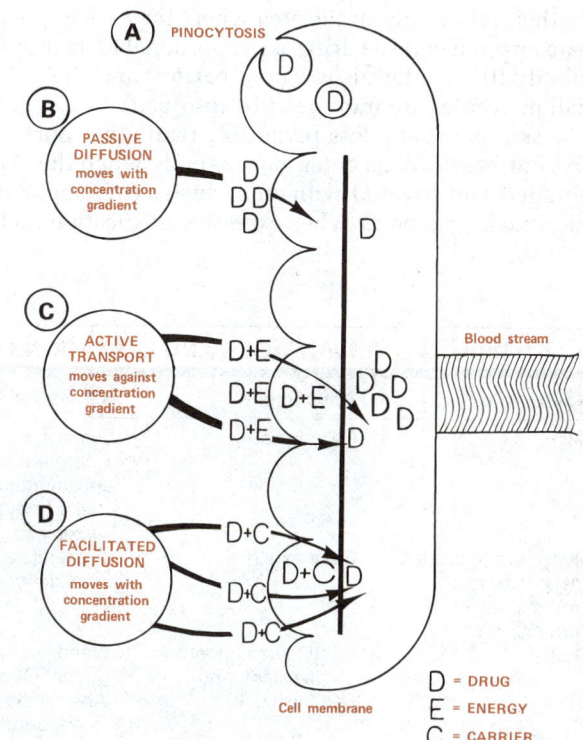

Figure 4–4. Movement of medications. Medications move across the cell membrane by passive diffusion (B)—moving *with* a concentration gradient; active transport (C)—moving *against* a concentration gradient so energy is required; facilitated diffusion (D)—moving *with* a concentration gradient but a *carrier* is needed.

is always highest in the original compartment. For example, a relatively high concentration of drug in the small intestine promotes the movement of the drug into the bloodstream. And, once distribution occurs, a high concentration of drug in the blood promotes the movement of the drug into extracellular fluids or into the cell. Passive diffusion is limited by the concentration of the drug at the membrane site and by the area of the membrane where diffusion occurs.

Several distinct processes are involved in passive transport: filtration, diffusion, and facilitated diffusion. *Filtration* is a process of moving particles through a barrier containing holes or spaces through which the liquid may pass, but which are too small to permit the solid particles to pass. In *diffusion*, molecules move from areas of high concentration to areas of low concentration. In *facilitated diffusion*, a carrier is needed to cross the cell membrane, but energy is not required because the drug does not move across a concentration gradient.

Routes of Absorption

The routes of absorption of medication include skin, mucous membranes, gastrointestinal (oral), parenteral, and inhalation. Table 4–2 features the advantages and limitations of each of these routes.

Skin Medications placed on the surface of the skin may be for systemic or local action. Topical systemically acting medications, such as nitroglycerin ointment or nicerate patches, are absorbed into the vascular system and eventually reach their target tissues. Locally acting medications, such as anti-infective ointments or emollients, have their effect only in the area where they are applied. The absorption of these drugs is proportional to their lipid solubility (the epidermis is a lipid barrier) and their size (small molecules are more readily absorbed).

The skin is usually less permeable than other ports of entry, but medications enter more rapidly when the skin is abraded and covered with an occlusive dressing. Systemic toxicity can occur when excessive medication is absorbed. Salicylate poisoning can occur when excessive amounts of methyl salicylate (oil of wintergreen) are used to relieve arthritic pain. This medication now requires a doctor's prescription.

Mucous Membranes Medication can be applied to the mucous membranes of the eye, ear, nose, mouth, vagina, urethra, and rectum. Medications may be applied for either local or systemic effects. Drugs are applied to the oral mucosa (e.g., nitroglycerin sublingual tablets or spray) when rapid onset of action is needed. These drugs are water soluble and designed to be absorbed in the mouth. If the patient accidentally swallows them, gastric secretions destroy their effects.

The rectum, which is highly vascular, is at times an excellent route for medication administration. Drugs given rectally quickly enter the vascular system and are not destroyed by gastrointestinal secretions. This route is often used when the patient is not allowed anything by mouth or when the medication can be destroyed by gastric secretions or can irritate the stomach or intestinal lining. Medications administered through this route include aspirin and morphine. Both medications may be irritating to the upper gastrointestinal tract if given by mouth, but cause fewer side effects when given rectally.

Gastrointestinal Route Most oral medications are absorbed from the small intestine. (Some exceptions are alcohol, alcohol-based drugs such as elixirs, and aspirin, which are absorbed across the stomach.) Dissolution, solubility, pharmaceutical processing, concentration of the drug, circulation to the site, and absorbing surface are all considered when administering oral medications. The presence or absence of food and antacids affects absorption.

Parenteral Route Parenteral medications are given through the intravenous, intramuscular, or subcutaneous route. Because they are more rapidly absorbed, they generally have an onset of action earlier than oral medications. The intravenous administration of medication provides immediate availability because it bypasses the absorption process. Injections given intramuscularly (IM)

Table 4–2. ADVANTAGES AND LIMITATIONS OF VARIOUS ROUTES FOR DRUG ADMINISTRATION			
Route	**Advantages**	**Limitations**	**Examples of Common Medications**
Skin	Easy to use	Intact epidermis generally not permeable. Inflammation or abrasion can lead to systemic absorption with toxic effects.	Local: Anesthetics, antibiotics, antiseptics, emollients, steroids Systemic: Antihistamines, vasodilators, hormones
Mucous membranes (eye, ear, nose, mouth, vagina, urethra, rectum)	Easy to use	Systemic absorption can occur readily from local drugs.	Local: Anesthetics, antibiotics, miotics, mydriatics Systemic: Antipyretics, bronchodilators, vasodilators
Oral	Easy to use, most convenient, and economical	Needs cooperative patient and an intact GI system. Absorption may be sporadic and undependable.	Local: Antacids, laxatives, antidiarrheals Systemic: Steroids, antibiotics, analgesics, cardiac medications, and many others
Parenteral	Generally prompt absorption	Sterile technique is required. Possibly results in pain and necrosis at site.	Local: Steroids into joints Systemic: Antibiotics, insulin, analgesics, and many others
Inhalation (respiratory tract)	Large surface area for rapid absorption	Poor ability to regulate dose. Many drugs cause irritation.	Local: Bronchodilators, mucolytics Systemic: Oxygen, anesthetics

or subcutaneously (SC) penetrate tissues, and thus absorption into the vascular system is not as rapid as the intravenous route. Patients with poor circulation or low blood pressure are given IM or SC medications cautiously because the absorption of the drugs may be delayed, thus delaying or even canceling their therapeutic effect. Patients receiving medications by this route may be unable to take the medication by mouth, or the medication itself (insulin, for example) may be destroyed by the gastrointestinal system, leaving the parenteral route the only one available.

Inhalation   Gases, volatile medications, and aerosols may be administered into the respiratory tract, either through regular inhalation (anesthetics) or with pressure assistance (bronchodilators). These medications take the form of fine mists that easily move across the alveolar membrane into the pulmonary capillary bed to have either a local effect in the lung or a systemic effect.

DISTRIBUTION

As the medication is absorbed into the bloodstream, several phases of *distribution* occur; these phases depend on cardiac output and regional blood flow. In the initial phase, medication is distributed to high blood-flow areas such as the heart, liver, kidney, and brain, usually within several minutes. During the second phase, which may take up to several hours, medication is distributed to areas of slower blood flow, such as the muscle, bone, middle ear, skin, and fat. When cardiac output is reduced, adequate tissue levels of medication are difficult to obtain. Superimposed on patterns of distribution of blood flow are factors that determine the rate at which drugs diffuse into tissues. These include the protein-binding capacity of the drug, the drug's solubility, the ratio of drug within body compartments, the manner in which the drug is stored in the body, the amount of drug in plasma, the drug's volume of distribution, and the ability of the drug to cross central nervous system and placental barriers.

Plasma Protein Binding

As the medication is absorbed into the vascular system, it is transported by protein molecules in the plasma, usually albumin, to its site of action, as shown in Figure 4–5. The plasma proteins are generally unable to exit from the vascular system because of their large molecular size; similarly, the units of medication that are attached to the proteins cannot exit unless they are freed from their binding sites. This drug-protein complex is termed "bound drug." Unattached drug that is available to produce an effect is termed "free drug." Only free or unbound drug is available to distribute out of blood vessels and act on body cells to elicit a pharmacologic response.

Plasma protein bindings range from very stable to very unstable. The stronger the binding, the slower the freeing of the medication, resulting in a longer duration of action, which may or may not be beneficial. As medication is biotransformed, more drug is usually released from the binding sites.

Because most medications are bound in the serum to albumin, the patient with hypoalbuminemia has diffi-

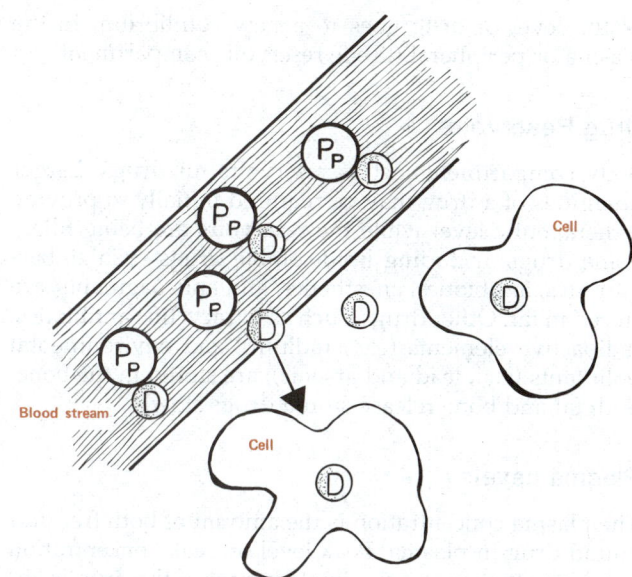

Figure 4–5. Medications (D) bind with plasma proteins (Pp) to be transported through the bloodstream. As the medication is freed from the plasma protein-binding site, it enters the tissues.

culty transporting medications. Many body hormones are also carried on protein. Because there is less protein to transport the drug molecules, excess free drug may result in an exaggerated pharmacologic effect that could prove dangerous to the patient.

Competition for Protein-Binding Sites   Occasionally, two or more medications compete for the same plasma protein-binding site. When this occurs, the drug with the strongest affinity for the binding site (i.e., a drug that is more than 85% to 90% protein bound) displaces the other drug. When this form of drug interaction occurs, the drug displaced may produce a toxic effect because a large concentration of the drug is now free in the central compartment. For example, when aspirin (antiarthritic) is given concurrently with warfarin (*Coumadin*, anticoagulant), aspirin displaces warfarin from the binding site, thereby increasing the free warfarin concentration in the central compartment, causing the patient to be at risk for bleeding.

Solubility

Distribution also depends on solubility. Lipid-soluble drugs readily move across the capillary endothelial membrane. Lipid-insoluble drugs permeate these membranes poorly and are therefore restricted in their distribution. For example, diazepam (Valium), a lipid-soluble drug, is distributed widely to adipose tissue and the brain, but lorazepam (Ativan), a water-soluble drug, is not well distributed to the brain.

Equilibrium

Equilibrium is achieved when a stable ratio of drug is found within all body compartments including the central and the peripheral compartments. The ratio does not have to be equal in each compartment but in fact may change as the level of drug goes to a new equilibrium in the plasma or peripheral (tissue reservoir) compartment.

Drug Reservoirs

Body compartments act as reservoirs for drugs. Larger quantities of a drug may be required initially to provide a therapeutic level while the reservoirs are being filled. Some drugs, including lipid-soluble drugs such as barbiturates, antibiotics, anesthetics, and anticoagulants, are stored in fat. Other drugs, such as tetracycline antibiotics, radioactive elements (e.g., radium), and environmental pollutants (e.g., lead and arsenic), are stored in the bone. Both fat and bone release stored drugs slowly.

Plasma Levels

The plasma concentration is the amount of both free and bound drug in plasma. Peak level or peak concentration is achieved when the maximal amount of the drug is absorbed into the plasma or in the target tissue. As the peak level is reached, maximal effect usually occurs. (The qualifier ''usually'' is necessary because peak level takes into account both bound and free drug, and all of the drug may not yet be active to cause maximal effect.)

Volume of Distribution

The *volume of distribution* (V_d) of a drug refers to the volume (blood, fat, and total body water) in which the drug would appear to be distributed during its steady state if the drug existed throughout that volume at the same concentration as in the plasma. Therefore, if a drug is highly concentrated in the tissues, its apparent V_d may be many times larger than that of total body water. The V_d ultimately determines the drug dosage.

A highly water-soluble drug has a small volume of distribution and a high blood concentration level. A highly fat-soluble drug has a large volume of distribution and a low blood concentration level. Factors that tend to keep a drug in circulation (high water solubility, high serum protein binding) result in a lower volume of distribution but a high blood level. Conversely, factors that promote the movement of a drug from the blood to other compartments (high lipid solubility, high degree of tissue binding) result in a higher volume of distribution and consequently a lower blood level.

Central Nervous System and Placental Barriers

The central nervous system (CNS), composed of the brain and spinal cord, has distribution barriers that discourage or prevent medications from entering. Only drugs that are very lipid soluble and not tightly bound to plasma proteins can cross the blood-brain barrier well and produce appreciable actions in the CNS. (Some examples are alcohol, atropine, scopolamine, general anesthetics, steroid hormones, sedative-hypnotics, and penicillin G.) Brain capillaries differ from their counterparts in most tissues by the tight junctions and absence of intercellular pores.

In addition, the unique arrangement of glial cells (astrocytes) around the blood vessels contributes to slow diffusion of medications into the CNS.

The blood-brain barrier is an important mechanism that protects the brain from chemical substances. The blood-brain barrier refers to an active transport system that pumps drug out of the brain after diffusion has allowed it to enter. However, for example, meningitis occurs, this transport system fails, and higher amounts of penicillin are allowed to remain in the brain.

The placenta is considered to be a lipid membrane that allows passage of substances by simple diffusion. Today it is believed that the fetus is generally exposed to the same drug concentrations as the mother. Placental transfer is responsible for the many untoward effects on the fetus that result from maternal use of drugs such as alcohol, cigarettes, narcotics, CNS depressants, and others. Some drugs (e.g., dilantin, streptomycin, cortisone) given during the first trimester of pregnancy may result in *teratogenic effects*, that is, they may cause physical defects in the developing fetus (see Chapter 48 for more information).

BIOTRANSFORMATION

Biotransformation or metabolism refers to the enzymatic alteration of a drug molecule. During biotransformation, some drugs are converted to inactive metabolites ready for excretion. However, a number of medications—*prodrugs*—become active only after this chemical reaction (e.g., the conversion of 6-mercaptopurine to 6-mercaptopurine ribonucleotide). Other medications are effective both before and after biotransformation (e.g., the conversion of phenylbutazone to oxyphenbutazone).

Most medications are biotransformed in the liver, but biotransformation can also occur in the renal tissue, lungs, blood plasma, and intestinal mucosa. Factors that affect biotransformation include the extent of plasma protein binding, drug storage in reservoirs, liver function, blood flow to the liver, presence of other substances that can either induce or inhibit liver function, and age.

Hepatic First-Pass Effect

Some medications absorbed into the vascular system from the portal system are metabolized almost completely by the liver on their first pass. This is called the *hepatic first-pass effect*. Medications administered parenterally bypass the hepatic system. Examples of drugs subject to the first-pass effect include amitriptyline (Elavil), lidocaine, and propranolol (Inderal). A drug such as lidocaine is not effective by the oral route and must be given parenterally. With propranolol (and other drugs mostly metabolized by the liver on the first pass), oral doses are much higher than parenteral doses: oral doses range from 40 to 160 mg; parenteral (IV) doses range from 1 to 2 mg.

Hepatic Enzymes

The liver has thousands of enzymes capable of catalyzing the transformation of active medication into inactive metabolites. Most medications are catalyzed by different enzymes, which catalyze or accelerate the reaction but are not destroyed by the reaction. In certain instances, such as those in which the patient has hepatitis, or liver degeneration, particular enzymes may exist in lowered concentration. In these cases, the medication may circulate for a longer time and trigger toxic reactions. At other times, the particular enzyme may increase in concentration (e.g., it may be triggered by another drug) and hasten the transformation of the medication into its inactive metabolite, thereby decreasing its effectiveness. For example, a person who smokes typically has an increase in several liver enzymes. If this patient receives the bronchodilator theophylline, the increase in the enzyme that helps to metabolize theophylline causes a lower theophylline plasma level. An increase in theophylline dosage may be necessary.

As mentioned previously, one drug may stimulate the production or synthesis of a liver enzyme that increases the biotransformation of a totally unrelated medication. This process is called *induction*. For example, barbiturates induce the synthesis of the liver enzyme that biotransforms warfarin. Thus, when barbiturates are given concurrently with warfarin, the dose of warfarin must be increased to achieve optimum effects. Many other examples of drug interactions are discussed in Chapter 5.

Cytochrome P-450 Enzyme System

The cytochrome P-450 enzyme system is the primary oxidative enzyme system within the liver. This system of enzymes is found in the microsomal fraction of the endoplasmic reticulum in hepatocytes. The microsomal enzymes within the liver also contribute to the biotransformation of fatty acids, steroid hormones, and conjugate bilirubin.

When the nurse administers medications to the very young or very old patient, the possibility of toxic drug complications must be considered. The young patient may not have a fully developed liver enzyme system, whereas the elderly or debilitated patient may have diminished function of the liver enzyme systems. These patients must be assessed carefully and continually for possible toxic drug effects associated with abnormal biotransformation.

EXCRETION

In the process of *excretion*, medications are eliminated from the body unchanged or as metabolites mostly through the renal system, but also in lesser amounts through the gastrointestinal and respiratory systems and through sweat, saliva, and breast milk. The rate of excretion varies with the concentration of the drug; as the drug concentration rises within the serum, excretion also rises. If excretion falls behind, serum levels rise, leading to a phenomenon called accumulation. *Accumulation* is the result of the gradual increase in the blood level of drugs. Without dosage adjustments, the increased level of the medication in the blood is likely to result in serious or toxic effects in the patient.

Clearance

Clearance is a measure of speed at which a drug leaves the body either through the kidney or the liver. A drug has a low clearance rate if it is removed from the body slowly or a high clearance rate if it is removed from the body rapidly. A drug with a high clearance often requires more frequent administration and higher doses than a drug with a low clearance. Clearance equals the volume of distribution divided by biologic half-life. Clearances are stated in milliliters per minute or liters per hour and sometimes normalized to weight. For example, aspirin has a clearance of 9.3 mL/min per kg. This means that 9.3 mL is eliminated each minute per kilogram of body weight. If renal function or clearance is reduced, the time needed to eliminate the aspirin is increased. Thus, it may be necessary to reduce the dose or increase the time between doses to prevent adverse or toxic effects.

Biologic Half-Life

The biotransformation and excretion of a medication determine the drug's *biologic half-life*, which is the amount of time required for elimination processes to reduce the original plasma concentration by 50%. For example, a 500-mg dose of a medication with a half-life of 3 hours is given: 250 mg remains in the body after 3 hours, 125 mg remains after 6 hours, 62.5 mg remains after 9 hours, and 31.25 mg remains after 12 hours, as shown in Figure 4–6. It takes approximately five half-lives for a single dose of a medication to be totally excreted.

The half-life of a drug ultimately determines how often the drug is to be administered. In general, drugs such as guanfacine (Tenex), with a half-life of 17 hours, can be

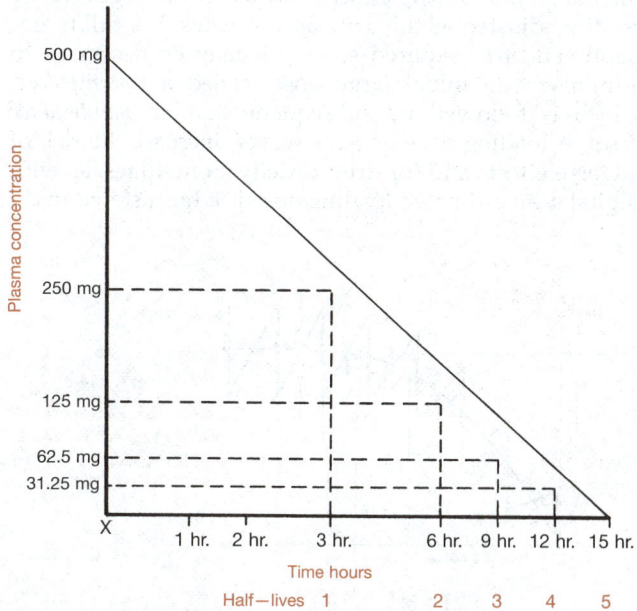

Figure 4–6. Linear medication curve. Shows the biologic half-life of a medication: A dose of 500 mg of the drug, which has a half-life of 3 hours, is given at point X. At 3 hours, 250 mg is excreted; at 6 hours, an additional 125 mg is excreted; at 9 hours, an additional 62.5 mg is excreted. This continues for approximately five half-lives.

given once daily. On the other hand, drugs such as methyldopa (Aldomet), with a half-life of only 1 hour, need to be given more often (2 to 4 times daily). The half-life is usually not dose dependent; therefore, doubling the dose will *not* double the half-life. Half-lives do not necessarily reflect duration of action.

The half-life for a given medication generally remains the same, within an individual patient, if all body systems are functioning normally. However, a patient's health status can affect a drug's half-life. For example, in the patient with renal or hepatic disease, a drug's half-life may increase. This results in the drug remaining in the body longer, which may cause accumulation, leading to possible toxicity. In some cases, drug dosages need to be reduced.

Steady State

With additional doses of a drug, a *steady state*, reached in approximately five half-lives, occurs when the rate of a drug's administration equals its rate of excretion. Figure 4–7 illustrates several dosing schedules to achieve a steady state. After five half-lives, all methods achieve a steady state, but the minimum and maximum plasma concentration differ markedly.

Loading Doses

The way a drug is first administered affects how quickly it reaches full therapeutic effect and steady state. When a drug is administered on a dosage schedule that is satisfactory for maintenance therapy, a partial effect occurs promptly, but full therapeutic effect does not occur for five half-lives. If the therapeutic situation is not acute, this dosage schedule may be preferred because it minimizes the risk of initial drug effects, and patient dosages can be readily adjusted as the drug accumulates. If a full therapeutic effect is required sooner, it may be necessary to administer an initial large dose, called a *loading dose*, which is followed by subsequent smaller *maintenance doses*. A loading dose does, however, increase the risk of adverse effects and/or drug toxicity. Sometimes, as with digitalis, an estimated loading dose is administered in divided fractions to permit at least some monitoring for efficacy and safety.

Renal Drug Excretion

The kidney usually removes the medication that is unbound and free in the plasma. Several factors directly affect the rate of excretion of medications from the kidney: the maturity of the kidney, kidney function (the absence or presence of disease), and circulatory function (the ability of the heart and blood vessels to deliver a blood supply to the kidney). The renal excretion of most drugs is closely correlated with creatinine clearance. However, other factors such as volume of distribution, drug metabolism, and protein binding must be considered.

Some medications, such as penicillin, are totally excreted on the first pass through the kidney. This accounts for the medication's short half-life. Other medications need several passes through the kidney to be totally excreted, because of passive tubular absorption. The excretion time of some medications may depend on urinary pH. When the tubular urine is made more acidic, for example, the excretion of weak acid medications is reduced, because the formation of the nonionized (nonpolar) molecules is favored and their reabsorption into the blood is increased. In a similar fashion, the excretion of weak bases is delayed in an alkaline urine because of increased recovery or reabsorption in the kidney and thus reduced excretion. By altering the urinary pH, it is possible to enhance or delay excretion of certain medications. However, with other treatment methods available today, changing the urinary pH is seldom an important part of the treatment regimen, although it may still be used.

If the kidneys are damaged, extracorporeal dialysis may be employed as a substitute. The artificial kidney is designed to perform the kidney's function, to remove wastes from the body. Any medication that is normally removed by the kidney can generally be removed through dialysis. Dialysis may be particularly helpful in treating cases of accidental or deliberate poisoning or drug overdose even if the kidney is functioning. Dialysis can achieve a rapid reduction of the toxic plasma level of the medication or poison.

Gastrointestinal Excretion

Medications excreted through the gastrointestinal system are mainly unabsorbed oral medications or metabolites of certain medications. Medications already absorbed can be excreted into the bile. However, drugs in bile can be reabsorbed in the intestine and recirculated again in a process called *enterohepatic recirculation*, shown in Figure 4–8. This recirculation of drug can prolong drug action. The administration of laxatives or cathartics can stimulate peristalsis and thus hasten drug elimination.

Pulmonary Excretion

Pulmonary excretion occurs most commonly with gases or volatile liquid general anesthetic agents. (See Chapter 21 for more information.) The pulmonary system also excretes limited amounts of alcohol. Alcohol is readily ab-

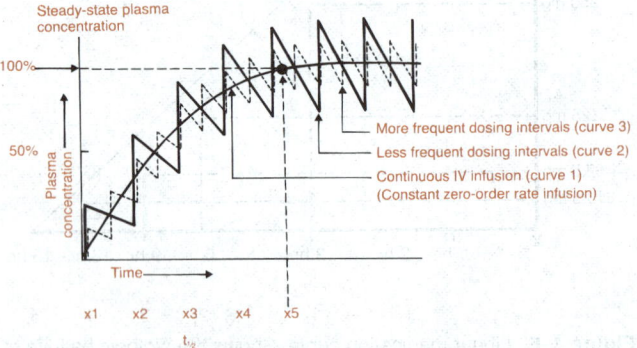

Figure 4–7. Dosing curve. Relationship between dosing at a continuous IV rate with a constant zero-order rate infusion and two different rates—more frequent and less frequent—and their minimum/maximum plasma concentrations. All three methods reach steady-state at the same time—in five half-lives.

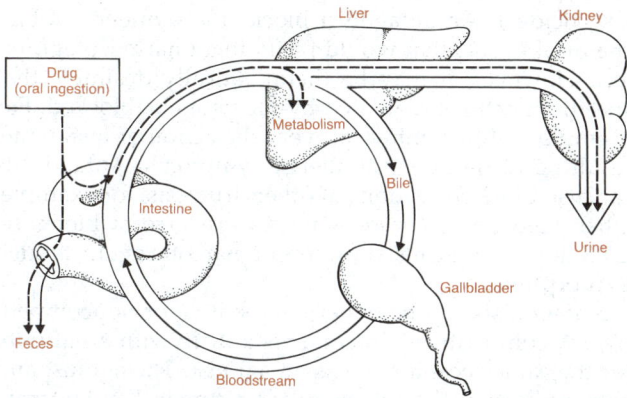

Figure 4–8. Enterohepatic recycling. A drug enters the GI system, is absorbed, and goes to the liver for metabolism. The active metabolites are secreted in bile, and the bile is then excreted into the gastrointestinal system. Eighty percent of bile is reabsorbed each day so the active metabolites recirculate for a long time. Some of the active drug or metabolites may go to the kidney for excretion.

sorbed through the stomach mucosa and, after entering the vascular system, is then partially excreted into the lungs and exhaled. A Breathalyzer test can be used quickly and inexpensively to calculate the percentage of alcohol consumed by an individual.

Other Routes of Excretion

The skin, although the largest organ in the body, eliminates a comparatively small amount of drugs. Several substances—arsenic, mercury, and polycyclic hydrocarbons—are all eliminated through the skin.

Excretion of drugs in sweat, saliva, and tears is relatively unimportant. Drugs excreted in saliva are usually swallowed, and their fate then follows other oral drugs. The hair, a modified epidermal structure, eliminates insignificant amounts of drug. However, hair samples may be examined in forensic medicine to help determine the cause of death. Traces of mercury have been found in Mozart's hair and may have contributed to his manic behavior during the preparation of his last major work, the *Requiem*.

THE PHARMACODYNAMIC PHASE

The *pharmacodynamic phase* describes the biochemical and physiologic action and effects of drugs in the body. This phase occurs when the medication reaches the target cell, tissue, or organ and a therapeutic effect results. Most medications are thought to work with a receptor at their site of action. The combination of the cell or structure with the drug is referred to as the *action*; what occurs as a result of the combination is the *effect* of the drug. Some medications have direct action on the tissues and cells to produce effects, whereas others may have a more indirect effect on the resultant activity. For example, the treatment of hypertension is accomplished with agents (e.g., hydralazine) that act directly on the blood vessels and in-

direct-acting agents (e.g., clonidine) that affect the brain centers for control of blood vessel tone.

MECHANISMS OF DRUG ACTION

Medications, once they reach their site of action, work through two major mechanisms. They may (1) alter the cell environment through physical or chemical processes or (2) alter cell function, mainly through drug-receptor interactions.

Physical and Chemical Mechanisms

Drugs can alter the environment of the cell through either physical or chemical processes that usually do not affect cell function. Physical processes include alteration of surface tension, lubrication, adsorption, osmosis, and ionizing radiation. Drugs also alter the cell environment through chemical processes such as inactivation, alteration of pH, alteration of body fluid chemistry, and chelation. Table 4–3 gives examples of each of these physical and chemical processes.

Drug-Receptor Interactions

Medications are thought to have an affinity for certain receptor sites. A *receptor* is the reactive site of a cell or tissue that can be occupied by a drug and result in a pharmacologic response. Receptors are most often cellular proteins or nucleic acids, but they can also be enzymes, carbohydrates, or lipids. A drug effect is produced because the interaction of the drug and the receptor alter

Table 4–3. PHYSICAL AND CHEMICAL PROCESSES THAT ALTER CELL ENVIRONMENT

Process	Example
Physical Process	
Alteration of surface tension	Stool softener reducing the surface tension of feces
Lubrication	Mineral oil facilitating the passage of feces
Absorption	Activated charcoal given orally to absorb harmful chemicals in the GI tract
Osmosis	Magnesium hydroxide (laxative) retaining water in the intestinal lumen
Ionizing radiation	Racioactive tracers used in diagnostic testing
Chemical Process	
Inactivation	Phosphate-binding antacids preventing the absorption of phosphate
Alteration in pH	Antacids given orally to neutralize gastric acidity
Alteration in body fluid chemistry	Ammonium chloride given intravenously to reverse metabolic alkalosis
Chelation	Dimercaprol combining with heavy metals (arsenic, mercury, lead) to form a complex that can be more readily excreted to prevent toxicity

cell function, which brings about biochemical and physiologic changes in the body (therapeutic response). A drug cannot, however, create a new function in a cell; the drug can only modify existing cell function. The stronger the affinity a drug has for a target receptor (i.e., a drug and its receptor with a compatible chemical shape), the more likely is the therapeutic response. Drug concentrations in cells or organs with no receptor sites have little effect.

Drugs can interact with a receptor to change cell function by altering cell membranes or cellular processes or by affecting specialized regions within the cell. The following are examples of how drug-receptor interactions change cell function: by altering transport mechanisms, permeability, or ion distribution; by depressing membrane function; or by supporting or inhibiting energy metabolism. Such interactions can also produce reactions that modify the synthesis, release, or inactivation of neurotransmitters, such as interactions produced by acetylcholine and norepinephrine.

Types of Receptors Receptors are believed to have evolved for the specific purpose of interacting with endogenous regulators, such as hormones and neurotransmitters. Many receptors and receptor subtypes have been identified, including adrenergic receptors (subtypes alpha$_1$, alpha$_2$, beta$_1$, beta$_2$ dopaminergic); cholinergic receptors (subtypes muscarinic$_1$, muscarinic$_2$ and nicotinic$_1$, nicotinic$_2$); histaminic receptors (subtypes H$_1$, H$_2$). A number of therapeutic agents have been developed that have selectivity for specific subtype receptors. With most of these drugs, therapeutic effects are enhanced, while unwanted effects are minimized.

Agonists, Antagonists, and Partial Agonists Endogenous regulators in the body that occupy receptors elicit either agonist action, which activates receptor functions, or antagonist action, which prevents receptor functions, as shown in Figure 4–9. Drugs also elicit agonist or antagonist action when occupying receptors. Some drugs elicit both types of action.

When a drug acts as an *agonist*, it complexes with and alters the functional properties of the receptor (e.g., terbutaline). As an *antagonist*, the drug inhibits or prevents the action of a natural agonist, either through competition for the receptor site (e.g., antihistamines) or interaction with other components of the effector mechanism (e.g.,

insecticides). An antagonist blocks the sequence of biochemical events that would result in a pharmacologic effect. However, it may be therapeutically desirable that specific functions regulated by receptors be blocked. For example, antihistamines prevent the action of histamine, resulting in the relief of allergy symptoms. Antagonists can also block the actions of other drugs, as, for example, when naloxone (*Narcan*) is used to reverse or block the CNS depression caused by certain narcotic agonists such as morphine.

Antagonists can be either competitive or noncompetitive. A competitive antagonist is a drug with an affinity for the same receptor site as an agonist. The agonist and antagonist (e.g., the anticoagulant dicumarol and vitamin K) both compete for the same receptor sites. The drug occupying the most receptor sites determines the type of reaction. A noncompetitive antagonist is a drug that prevents an agonist from producing any effect at a receptor site, usually by an irreversible-acting drug that fails to leave the receptor. Heavy metals such as lead, mercury, antimony, and arsenic are noncompetitive inhibitors.

Some drugs interact not only with a receptor to produce some pharmacologic response but also simultaneously antagonize the action of another agonist that interacts with the same receptor. Drugs such as pentazocine (Talwin) that act this way are called partial agonists or agonist-antagonists.

Reversible and Irreversible Interactions In most cases the interaction of the drug with a receptor is reversible; that is, the drug-receptor effect is terminated by the drug leaving the receptor. If the concentration of drug remains high in the vicinity of the receptor, the drug has an effect at the receptor. As the concentration of drug decreases, the receptors will no longer be filled and the drug effect is reversed.

Some drug-receptor interactions are irreversible. With certain substances, such as environmental pollutants, pesticides, and nerve gas, the drug-receptor combination alters both the drug and the receptor, so the drug-receptor becomes inseparable. In other reactions, the drug-receptor binding is very strong, and the drug remains on the receptor for a long time.

Drug-Enzyme Interactions Some drugs are thought to produce their effects through enzymatic action. A drug may so closely resemble the enzyme that the drug may combine with the normal enzyme substrate and allow the enzyme to be freed. A group of drugs called antimetabolites, which have enzymatic action, is discussed in Chapter 55.

Another effect of medications on enzymes is to produce an increase or decrease in the amount of the enzymes and, as a result, change cell or tissue response in the body. Because enzymes determine the rates of chemical reactions, their levels directly influence the biochemical activity of cells. The relaxation of the bronchioles in the lung is accomplished by enzyme stimulation of adenylcyclase by isoproterenol to produce more high-energy 3',5'-cyclic AMP, whereas aminophylline maintains this high-energy compound by inhibition of the enzyme phosphodiesterase, which breaks down 3',5'-cyclic AMP. The result of treatment with either medication is relief of bronchial constriction.

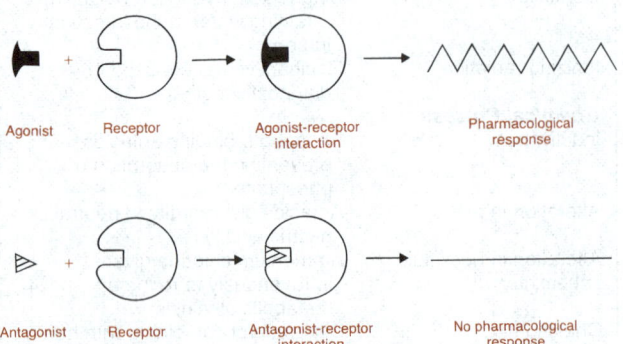

Agonist   Receptor   Agonist-receptor interaction   Pharmacological response

Antagonist   Receptor   Antagonist-receptor interaction   No pharmacological response

Figure 4–9. Agonist/antagonist effect. A drug acting as an agonist fits into a receptor, and a drug effect occurs. A drug acting as an antagonist can combine with a receptor, but does not quite fit, so no drug response occurs.

Other Drug-Receptor Interactions Drugs that interact with nucleic acids or other cellular components can be utilized in the treatment of tumors and cancer. For example, the ability of some drugs to halve the growth of cells enables these medications to slow or cause regression in the spread of the disease. The ability of the antibiotics to specifically disrupt the production of bacterial proteins, which usually destroys the bacteria, provides a safe and nonharmful treatment of infections in patients.

Clinical Implications of Drug-Receptor Interactions

If receptors are continually stimulated, their responsiveness may be decreased; this decrease is referred to as *desensitization* or down-regulation. This decrease in responsiveness may be due to an actual decrease in number or a change in the existing receptors or both. The end state of desensitization is termed *refractoriness*. As an example, desensitization may occur with repeated use of beta-adrenergic bronchodilators such as isoproterenol (Isuprel) for the treatment of asthma or nitroglycerin for the treatment of angina. With repeated use, the effectiveness of the drugs is reduced, thus requiring a larger dose or a change of medication. Nitroglycerin patches or ointment are used for only a 12-hour period and administered again after a 12-hour resting interval. This allows the receptors to return to normal.

When a receptor's activity is chronically activated or inhibited by a drug, a state of *hyperreactivity* or supersensitivity to a drug may occur. The receptors must then be allowed to return to normal. For example, hyperreactivity can occur following long-term use of an antagonistic drug like propranolol (Inderal). If the drug is rapidly withdrawn, the patient may experience an increased number of anginal attacks or a hypertensive episode, which were previously controlled with the drug. This is due to increased sensitivity of the beta-adrenergic receptors to epinephrine, which the propranolol was blocking.

DRUG EFFECT

The effects of medications can be immediate or delayed, desired (beneficial or therapeutic), or undesired (adverse or toxic). Drugs can also cause unusual effects—idiosyncratic effects—that occur in only a small percentage of individuals. The degree to which a drug produces a pharmacologic response or effect is partly determined by (1) the availability of receptor sites; (2) the location and function of receptors with which the drug interacts; (3) the kind of drug action (direct or indirect) on target cells, tissues, or organs; and (4) the concentration of the drug at the receptor sites. The effect of a drug results from its action and is dose related (over a limited range). A dose-effect relationship helps to determine the therapeutic range and the onset of action, peak concentration, and duration of action of a drug. When the dose-effect relationship is used to explain pharmacodynamic variables that affect the intensity of a drug's effect, a dose-response curve is graphed.

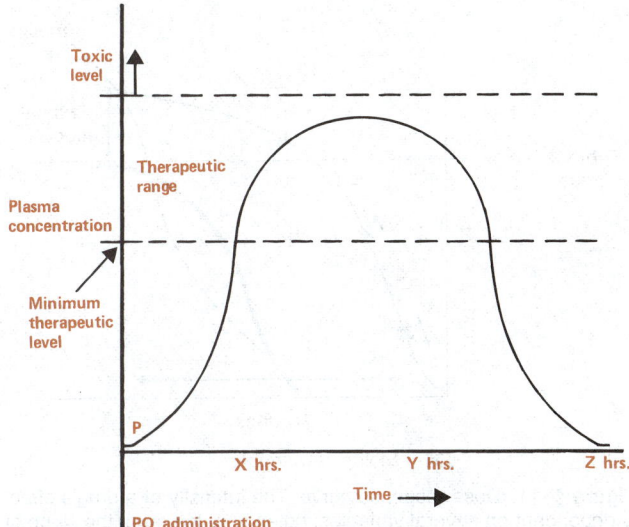

Figure 4–10. Concave time medication curve. A curve representing an oral drug administered at P time. The drug reaches its peak therapeutic level at Y hours. The concave curve represents the time arriving at (X hours) and time leaving (Z hours) the therapeutic drug level.

Dose-Effect Relationships

The dose-effect relationship is commonly derived from the drug's peak effect after a single dose of the medication. This effect can be graphically represented by a curve that may be linear (see Fig. 4–6) or may curve upward, downward, as shown in Figure 4–10, or sigmoidally. The sigmoid curve is the most common. Each curve has a time of onset of action when the drug is entering the central and peripheral compartments; a duration of action time, during which the therapeutic effect occurs; a peak concentration level, which is reached when the absorption rate equals the elimination rate; and the termination of action time, during which the drug is being eliminated. During this last phase, the next dose of the medication is administered to prevent the blood concentration level from dropping below what is desired.

Dose-Response Relationships

The intensity of a drug's effect depends on several response variables: biologic variables, potency, slope of the dose-response curve, and maximal efficacy, as shown in Figure 4–11. When medications are given, they are all subject to known and unknown sources of biologic variation. Known sources include the patient's body weight and composition, age, nutritional status, ethnic origin, genetic makeup, disease state, immunity status, psychology, environment, and body rhythms. Individual variations in drug response explain why each patient reacts differently to medications. This topic is discussed later in the chapter.

The *potency* of a drug is the relationship between the dose of the drug and the intensity of its effect. A drug is said to be potent when it possesses high intrinsic activity at low unit doses. Potency is influenced by absorption, distribution, biotransformation, excretion, and ability to

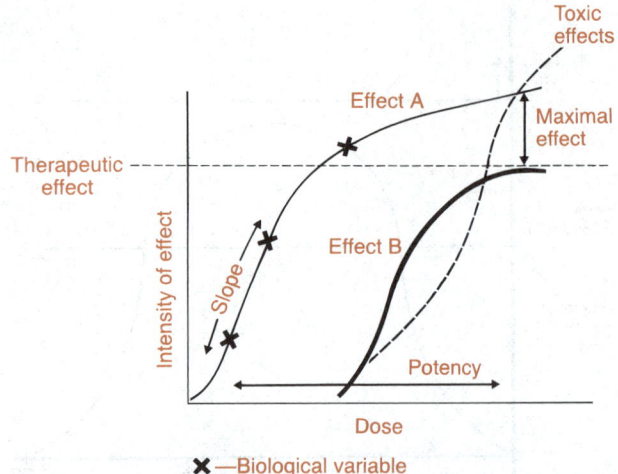

Figure 4–11. Dose-response curve. The intensity of a drug's effect is dependent on several variables: potency of the drug, the slope of the response curve, biological variables (X), and maximal effect (efficacy). A drug may have several effects (A and B). However, the appearance of adverse effects (broken line) may preclude using the drug to obtain effect B.

combine with receptors. Potency is taken into consideration when drug doses are established. With an extremely potent drug, the resulting miniscule doses can be difficult to measure and dispense; with a drug that has extremely low potency, high doses may need to be administered daily. When switching between different drugs, such as from morphine to hydromorphone (Dilaudid), relative potency (the ratio of equieffective doses) must be considered by the physician. For example, 10 mg morphine equals 1 mg hydromorphone. Therefore, hydromorphone is the more potent drug. However, it does not matter because both doses are equally effective.

The slope of the dose-response curve (see Fig. 4–11) demonstrates the ability of the drug to produce an effect. The steeper the slope, the more readily the drug binds with receptors and the quicker the drug effect.

The *efficacy* of a drug refers to its maximal effect. The efficacy of a drug is indicated on Figure 4–11 by a plateau. For example, aspirin effectively controls mild to moderate pain; morphine effectively controls pain at all levels. Thus, morphine is more efficacious in relieving intense pain than aspirin.

Selectivity

A medication is also described in terms of its selectivity (or spectrum of activity). *Selectivity* refers to the effects that the medication precipitates. Medications rarely produce a single effect; most produce multiple effects. However, one effect generally is elicited more readily than another. Drug selectivity is best described by summarizing the pattern and incidence of adverse and toxic effects produced by a therapeutic dose of the medication and by indicating the proportion of patients who, because they experienced these effects, had to lower the dosage or discontinue the medication. (A therapeutic dose is one that produces the desired effect; a nontherapeutic dose—too high or too low—does not.) A medication reference book

that lists all known adverse and toxic effects is of little use in determining selectivity. The best reference should at least indicate the most common and the least common adverse or toxic effects to assess and which effects to evaluate.

Therapeutic Index

The *therapeutic index* (margin of safety) describes the relative safety of a drug. A drug's therapeutic index is equal to the lethal dose (kills 50% of animals given the drug) divided by the effective dose (produces a specific therapeutic effect in 50% of animals given the drug). The closer the ratio is to 1, the greater the potential danger to the patient.

PHARMACOKINETIC AND PHARMACODYNAMIC IMPLICATIONS FOR THE NURSE

Nurses need a basic understanding of both pharmacokinetics and phamacodynamics to administer drugs safely and effectively. Knowledge of the pharmacokinetic principles used to establish the route, dosage, and timing of drug administration help the nurse avoid medication errors. In addition, the nurse may need to question physicians about their drug orders. For example, the nurse who knows that his or her patient has severe vomiting should ask the physician why oral medication was ordered for the patient when rectal or parenteral administration would be more beneficial. (The physician's order is questioned because vomiting decreases the gastrointestinal absorption of drugs.)

Knowledge of pharmacodynamics is applied when assessing patients for drug responses—both beneficial and harmful. The nurse also must know about the actions and effects of drugs to educate patients about their medications and to support, for example, a conviction that a patient is receiving inappropriate drug therapy. Because the pharmaceutical, pharmacokinetic, and pharmacodynamic phases are individualized, the nurse also must understand what factors will affect the patient's response to drug therapy.

MONITORING DRUG CONCENTRATION IN SERUM

To ensure that a therapeutic drug level is maintained and to guide therapy, serum monitoring of the drug level may be performed. The nurse performs an important role in collecting the information needed for the proper interpretation of serum concentration data, listed in Table 4–4.

To monitor serum levels, two blood levels are usually obtained: the peak level, usually drawn one-half hour after the medication is totally administered, and the trough level, usually drawn one-half hour before the next dose. The timing of both the peak and trough draws may vary, depending on the drug being monitored. If levels are not drawn at these specified times, but the physician assumes

Table 4–4. INFORMATION COLLECTED BY THE NURSE FOR PROPER INTERPRETATION OF DRUG SERUM LEVELS

Information	Reason for Importance
Drug, drug dose, and dosage regimen	Used to determine whether a steady state has been reached
Time at which blood sample was taken	Drug plasma concentrations vary between consecutive doses
Patient's weight and age	May affect the action of the drug
Patient's use of other medication	Drug interactions may affect the pharmacokinetics (absorption, distribution, biotransformation, excretion) of the drug being assayed
Patient's pathophysiologic condition	Disease states can affect the onset, peak, and duration of drug action because of alterations in pharmacokinetic factors (half-life, distribution, etc.)

they were, misinterpretation of the results occurs. Peak levels monitor possible toxic levels. Trough levels monitor whether the level remains within the therapeutic range.

Drug monitoring is of particular value in the following circumstances:

1. There is known to be considerable individual variation between the oral dose and plasma level obtained (e.g., aminophylline).
2. Therapeutic levels are close to toxic levels (e.g., lithium and gentamicin).
3. Toxicity is suspected.
4. Noncompliance is suspected.
5. Therapeutic effect must be maximized (as in sepsis).
6. Normal response to standard dosing does not occur.
7. A change in dosage or route of a drug's administration is made .
8. Long-term therapy is planned. (Levels may be drawn every 4 to 6 months.)
9. Long-term therapy has been used, and tolerance is suspected.
10. The drug is given for an episodic syndrome such as epilepsy or cardiac dysrhythmia.

When serum levels are available, the physician and/or clinical pharmacist determine the serum level best suited to each patient's overall needs. For example, gentamicin (peak 4 to 10 μg/mL, trough 1 to 3 μg/mL) therapy may be prescribed for a patient in several ways: Gentle therapy—peak 6 μg/mL, trough 1 μg/mL; moderate therapy—peak 8 μg/mL, trough 2 μg/mL; aggressive therapy—peak 10 μg/mL, trough 3 μg/mL.

When a peak or trough serum level is too high, the dose can be reduced or the time interval between doses increased. When a peak or trough serum level is too low, the dose can be increased or the time interval between the doses decreased. In addition, the physician examines other causes that could elevate or reduce these levels.

INDIVIDUAL PATIENT VARIATION IN DRUG RESPONSES

Each patient has a unique response to drug therapy. Individual variations occur because of differences in body weight and composition, age, diet and nutrition, ethnic origin, genetics, pathophysiology, immunity, psychology, environment, and body rhythms.

Body Weight and Composition

The average adult dose of aspirin is 10 grains (650 mg). Different reactions would be expected if this dose were given to a person weighing 100 lb and to one weighing 250 lb. The 100-lb person would receive a therapeutic effect, whereas the 250-lb person would have less than a therapeutic effect. Therefore, many medications are ordered based on body weight.

The average adult dose is calculated on the premise that it produces a specific effect in 50% of the population between ages 18 and 65 and weighing about 150 lb (70 kg). This means that very thin or obese individuals may have to receive adjusted doses to achieve the same result. Pediatric doses are calculated on body weight expressed as milligrams per kilogram (mg/kg) or on body surface area (BSA) expressed as milligrams per square meter (mg/m^2). A chart or nomogram plotting the weight in accordance with the height is used to determine the total BSA. (See Chapter 7 for more information on pediatric drug administration.)

A drug's therapeutic action and effect can also be influenced by body composition. A different proportion of fat to lean body mass can affect the distribution, tissue saturation at the site(s) of action, and elimination of a drug.

Age

The very young and the very old tend to react differently than the middle-aged person to medication. The immature liver or kidneys of the very young may delay drug metabolism and excretion. Delayed distribution, metabolism, and excretion are common in the elderly because of disease conditions or normal deterioration of body systems. Age may also affect the route chosen: an older person—when acutely ill and because of poor circulation in the extremities—is not given an intramuscular injection; instead, the medication is administered intravenously.

Diet and Nutrition

The obese and/or frail person have altered distribution. Dieting, with rapid loss of body fat, may release into the bloodstream highly fat-soluble drugs (barbiturates, anticoagulants) that have been stored in the body's fatty tissue.

Drug absorption can be increased or decreased by the presence of food in the gastrointestinal track. A diet high in fat leads to increased plasma fatty acids, which may bind albumin and displace protein-bound drugs. Metabolism of drugs may be increased by a high-protein, low-carbohydrate diet; foods such as cabbage or brussel sprouts; and charcoal-broiled foods. High-protein or high-fat diets may also decrease the biliary excretion of some drugs. High-fiber diets may increase excretion.

The frail and/or undernourished person may have hypoalbuminemia. This results in an increased serum level of protein-bound drugs, which may increase the risk of overdose.

Ethnic Origin

Clinical differences in the physiologic response to drugs among various ethnic groups are being found. (This topic is discussed in detail in Chapter 9.) For example, alcohol is metabolized by the enzyme alcohol dehydrogenase in Caucasians; in Asians, the enzyme that metabolizes alcohol is aldehydehydrogenase, which works faster and may result in circulatory flushing and palpitation. Caffeine is excreted faster in Caucasians than in Asians. Antihypertensives such as beta-adrenergic blockers are less effective in African-Americans (so higher doses or combination drug therapy is needed), but more effective in Chinese men (so that half as much is needed). Angiotensin-converting enzyme inhibitors are less effective in African-Americans than in Caucasians. Psychotropic medications like alprazolam (Xanax) are needed in smaller doses in Asians than in Caucasians. Haloperidol (Haldol) reaches a higher plasma level in Asians than in Caucasians. Because of these physiologic variations, the nurse needs to carefully assess patients from different areas of the world for drug effectiveness and side effects.

Genetics

Genetic makeup determines the rate at which a patient metabolizes and eliminates drugs. Patients who metabolize drugs more rapidly may need a higher dose or more frequent administration of a drug. Patients who metabolize drugs more slowly may need a lower dose or less frequent administration of a drug. Some patients have a genetically determined insufficiency that does not allow them to metabolize certain drugs, such as succinylcholine (a muscle relaxant). Patients with this insufficiency who are administered succinylcholine suffer prolonged muscle relaxation and possibly fatal respiratory arrest.

Pathophysiology

Patients who have various pathologic diseases, such as those of the liver, kidney, or heart, react differently to medications. If a medication must be given to a patient with underlying organ disease, the patient is assessed closely for further damage to the organ and for differences in response to various medications, such as longer duration of action or toxic effects. Often a drug reactivates an old problem. For example, a patient taking two aspirin tablets four times a day to treat an arthritis flare-up may aggravate an ulcer condition dormant for some years, with resultant severe burning stomach pain. Using enteric-coated or buffered aspirin or taking aspirin with food may eliminate or mitigate the untoward side effect of plain aspirin.

Immunity

The patient's immune system also affects how he or she responds to medication. *Immunopharmacology* is concerned with the underlying mechanisms by which endogenous and synthetic chemicals interact with the cells of the immune system. Research in this area has contributed to the development of antibodies that are frequently used today as specific probes for the quantitative and qualitative analysis of many different classes of chemicals.

Occasionally, when the patient receives a medication, the immune system is activated and produces antibodies to the foreign antigen (the medication). The next time this or a similar medication is taken, a systemic reaction may occur. As an example, a child is given penicillin for an ear infection. The ear infection is subsequently cured, and the child experiences no difficulties from the medication. Ten years later, the child develops pneumonia, and penicillin is again prescribed. This time, 30 minutes after the first dose of penicillin, the patient experiences generalized urticaria. This patient has developed antibodies against penicillin and must be told that he or she is allergic to penicillin. From now on, this patient should not receive penicillin or its related preparations and should carry a card identifying the allergy.

Psychology

The hopes, fears, and expectations of the individual often affect the action of a medication. If the patient is confident that an injection will relieve pain, it probably will; however, if the patient does not expect pain to lessen, it probably will not. Research indicates that the body produces natural substances called endorphins that help a person to control pain. If a person thinks the pain will be relieved, more endorphins are produced, ultimately relieving the pain. The body's release of endorphins may explain why placebos are effective. (A *placebo* is an inactive substance or preparation given to satisfy the patient's perceived need for drug therapy.)

Environment

The climate in which the patient lives may affect how he or she reacts to certain medications. This is a factor of reactivity rather than a true pharmacologic change. Extremes of temperature in the environment may affect the action and/or side effects of some drugs such as the phenothiazines, which may impair body temperature regulation.

Body Rhythms

Chronobiology (the study of body rhythms) has revealed countless patterns in the workings of the body. The adrenal glands produce most of the day's supply of the hormone cortisol in a few hours beginning around 4:00 AM, primarily to prepare the body for stresses that are to come. Skin cells divide more rapidly at night; bone marrow makes more blood cells from 6:00 PM to 10:00 PM. The activity of the immune system is also cyclic, with the majority of natural killer cells being produced in the early morning. A person who gets 3 hours less sleep per night than usual has a 50% decrease in the functioning of the immune system. For individuals living in synchronization with the world at large, body temperature peaks between 6 and 8 PM and bottoms between 4 and 6 AM.

Because drugs depend on enzymes and act on targets such as the skin, bone, or liver, chronobiologists suggest that body rhythms can have a profound effect on how drugs act. *Chronopharmacology* is a science that investigates drug effects as a function of biological timing and determines the best time to optimize dosing to enhance both effectiveness and tolerance of a drug. In fact, giving the same dose of the drug at a different time may be the same as giving a completely different dose. Today we know that more aspirin reaches the bloodstream if it is taken at 7:00 AM than if it is taken at 11:00 PM. A single dose of antacid taken at night is more effective than two or three doses taken during the day. Alcohol, the most

common of drugs, is more potent around midnight than the same amount consumed in the morning. Indomethacin (*Indocin*) used to treat arthritis is less likely to cause stomach pain or vertigo at bedtime. In a study with healthy males, the same dose of IV potassium produced a 40% higher plasma concentration when administered at midnight rather than at noontime. Perhaps the most dramatic effects of timing are seen in the use of the anticancer drugs doxorubicin and cisplatin. Doxorubicin can destroy the bone marrow and elevate the heart rate. It is best administered in the morning when bone marrow cells are not dividing as quickly. Cisplatin can cause irreversible kidney damage. It is best administered in the evening when the kidneys process large quantities of fluid and may actually absorb less platinum from cisplatin, producing less renal toxicity.

The bibliography for this chapter can be found in Appendix B, which begins on page 1054.

CHAPTER REVIEW QUESTIONS*

1. Which statement reflects the pharmacokinetic phase of drug administration?
   a. The immature drug-receptor interactions of the very young are usually irreversible.
   b. Medications enter the body in solid form and change into solution for absorption and utilization.
   c. Medication absorption, distribution to tissues, biotransformation, and elimination from the body are studied.
   d. A therapeutic effect occurs as the medication reaches the target cell.

2. During the phase of drug distribution:
   a. Most medications are bound in the serum to hormones.
   b. Reduced cardiac output increases tissue drug saturation and concentration.
   c. Tissues such as the bone and middle ear take longer for drug distribution.
   d. Substances pass the placental barrier by an active transport system.

3. Which statement is *true* regarding the half-life of medications?
   a. Doubling the dose doubles the medication half-life.
   b. Approximately six half-lives are required for a single dose of a medication to be completely excreted.

c. Patients with renal or hepatic disease usually have decreased drug half-lives.
   d. The half-life of a drug determines how often the drug is to be administered.

4. Regarding the absorption stage of the pharmacokinetic phase of drug administration:
   a. Medications injected directly by the intravenous route bypass the absorption process and are rapidly available for utilization by the body.
   b. Most oral medications are absorbed from the large intestine.
   c. The convoluted lining of the stomach enhances absorption into the central compartment.
   d. Tetracycline (an antibiotic) is better absorbed if given with an antacid.

5. During the pharmacodynamic phase of medication action:
   a. Medications are detoxified or broken down by the liver.
   b. Alterations in cell environment or cell function rarely occur.
   c. The biochemical and physiologic effects of the drug are studied.
   d. Medications are dissolved into absorbable, nonionized compounds.

*See Appendix A, which begins on page 1051, for answers.

CHAPTER 5

Drug Interactions

Merrily A. Kuhn, RNC, PhD

CHAPTER OUTLINE

Drug Incompatibilities
Drug Interaction Mechansims
Drug-Food Interactions
Patient-Related Factors That Affect Drug Interactions
Effects of Drugs on Laboratory Test Results
Legal Implications

KEY TERMS

Additive	In vitro
Antagonistic	Incompatibility
Antidote	Potentiation
Complexation	Sequestration
Drug interaction	Synergistic
In vivo	

LEARNING OBJECTIVES

After reading this chapter, the student will be able to:

1. Understand the differences between pharmacokinetic drug interactions, pharmacodynamic drug interactions, and combined drug toxicities.
2. Define the drug interaction terms additive, synergistic, potentiation, and antagonistic.
3. Identify selected drug-drug and drug-food interactions.
4. Describe the different levels at which drugs may interact.

Today, with over 1000 unique pharmacologic substances available, the potential exists for over 55 million individual, unique drug interactions. The number of significant drug interactions continues to grow and poses a potentially serious threat to the patient. Studies show that 5% to 10% of hospital admissions can be attributed to adverse drug interactions, most of which could have been prevented. Studies also show general surgical patients are at higher risk for drug interactions, with an incidence of 17% to 20% or more. For the benefit of the patient, all personnel involved with drug administration need a working knowledge of potential drug interactions.

A *drug interaction* "occurs whenever the diagnostic, preventive, therapeutic, or toxic action of a drug is modified in or on the body by another pharmacologically acting chemical substance, whether that be a prescription drug, an over-the-counter drug, or something in the diet or the environment." (Hayes, AH, Jr: How drugs affect drugs. Emerg Med (13):114–117, July 15, 1981). The interaction can be physical, chemical, or biologic. A drug interaction is the by-product of the administration of two or more drugs or a drug-food combination. Drugs can also affect the results of standard laboratory tests. Some drug interactions are intentional and beneficial to the patient; how-

ever, the majority are unintentional and potentially harmful. The potential sites of action for drug interactions within the body are featured in Figure 5–1.

DRUG INCOMPATIBILITIES

A drug *incompatibility* is not synonymous with a drug interaction. Drug incompatibilities are chemical or physical reactions that occur among two or more drugs and can occur during mixing outside the body (*in vitro*) or inside the body (*in vivo*).

CHEMICAL INCOMPATIBILITIES

Chemical incompatibilities between two drugs change the molecular structure of the drug(s) or solution(s), altering pharmacologic properties. A precipitate may form or a color change may occur. Chemical incompatibilities may be beneficial as when protamine sulfate (weak anticoagulant) is administered to stop the activity of heparin (anticoagulant). Together, these two drugs form an ionic bond that has *no* anticoagulant activity. Chemical incom-

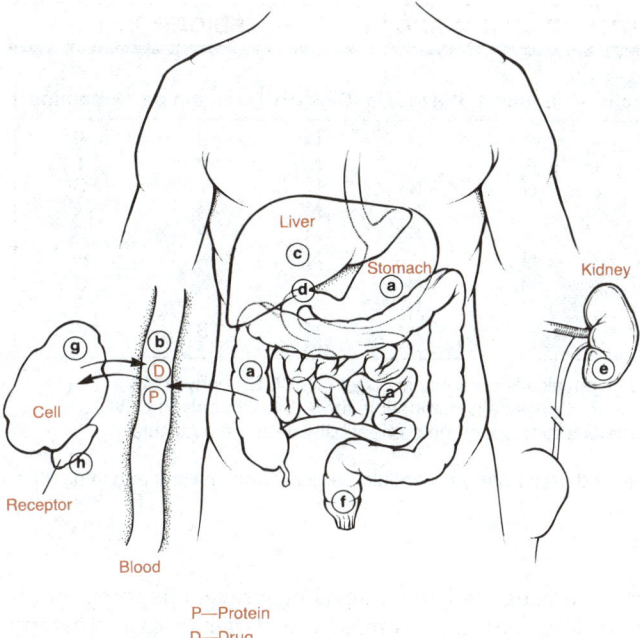

P—Protein
D—Drug

Figure 5–1. Drug interaction sites within the body. Drug interactions can occur in numerous sites within the body. (a) Absorption can be enhanced or reduced in the gut; (b) protein binding can be affected within the vasculature; (c) biotransformation can be affected in the liver; (d) excretion can be affected either through bile, (e) the kidney, or (f) in feces; (g) tissue binding of one drug may be affected by another; and finally, (h) drugs may have an effect through action on specific receptors.

patibilities may also be harmful. For example, when multivitamins and antibiotics are mixed in the same IV solution, the multivitamins change the solution's pH, thereby inactivating the antibiotic.

PHYSICAL INCOMPATIBILITIES

Physical incompatibilities occur when two drugs are loosely bound to each other, but still retain their original pharmacologic properties. The end result of a physical incompatibility is usually a precipitate. For example, mixing phenytoin (Dilantin, an anticonvulsant) with dextrose forms a precipitate in the IV bottle or tubing. Therefore, phenytoin is mixed only with saline solutions.

Incompatibilities are of prime concern in the preparation of large-volume parenterals that contain vitamin or electrolyte additives or both and in the preparation of preoperative medications in which two or more drugs are to be added in the same syringe. Some incompatibilities for IV medications are listed in Table 5–1.

It is essential that the nurse research incompatibility potentials before administering medication. Nurses can most easily obtain information on drug incompatibilities for large-volume parenterals from the reference guides available to pharmacists. Communication with the pharmacist helps the nurse avoid the potential inactivation or precipitation of two or more drugs mixed together in the same parenteral solution or syringe and decreases the risk of causing harm or discomfort to the patient.

DRUG INTERACTION MECHANISMS

In vivo drug interaction mechanisms can be divided into several general categories: (1) pharmacokinetic interactions, (2) pharmacodynamic interactions, and (3) combined toxicities.

Pharmacokinetic interactions comprise reactions in which the absorption, distribution, biotransformation, or excretion of one drug is affected by another drug. Pharmacodynamic interactions result from the combined pharmacologic effects of drugs. Such effects may be additive, synergistic, potentiated, or antagonistic. Action on the same receptor may or may not be involved. Combined toxicity results when two drugs with toxic effects on the same organ are combined for therapy. When used together, permanent damage to organs can occur.

PHARMACOKINETIC INTERACTIONS

Through research and clinical practice, the knowledge of pharmacokinetic interactions grows daily. The primary causes of these interactions and the resulting significance of concurrent drug administration is reviewed briefly.

The major mechanisms of pharmacokinetic interactions include interactions in which gastrointestinal absorption of a drug is affected, plasma protein binding is modified, drug metabolism is stimulated or inhibited. Details of these mechanisms are provided in Table 5–2.

Absorption

Medications given orally are absorbed through the gastrointestinal tract. Absorption depends on the function of the gastrointestinal tract itself. Normal tract function assumes normal motility and normal bacterial flora. Absorption of most medication depends on the time it is within either the stomach or the intestine. The faster the drug passes through the intestinal tract, the less drug is absorbed. For example, patients who abuse cathartics tend to have reduced absorption of oral medications. Other drugs, such as morphine and codeine, prolong emptying time within the small intestine, which may result in increased drug absorption. Conversely, anticholinergics increase gastric emptying time and therefore may decrease drug absorption.

Modification of gastrointestinal absorption can also occur secondary to physiochemical characteristics of the contents of the gastrointestinal tract itself. By altering pH, such as with antacids or histamine antagonist inhibitors, solubility and stability of medications may be affected, reducing or increasing drug absorption. When the pH is lowered, acidic drugs are absorbed more readily; when the pH is elevated, basic drugs are absorbed more readily. Antacids decrease the absorption of many drugs by complexing with them (e.g. digoxin and tetracycline products) or by altering the pH of the tract (e.g., aspirin and barbiturates).

Additional problems that can occur in the bowel include complexation and sequestration. *Complexation* occurs when nonabsorbable complexes are formed through

Table 5–1. PHYSICAL AND CHEMICAL COMPATIBILITY FOR MIXING AND INFUSING MEDICATIONS

	Aminophylline	Ampicillin	Bretylium	Calcium chloride	Cefazolin	Cimetidine	Diazepam	Digoxin	Dobutamine	Dopamine
Aminophylline		P	D	N	S	I	N	P	B	P
Ampicillin	P		N	N	S	A	N	N	N	I
Bretylium	D	N		C	C	N	N	D	I	C
Cefazolin	S	S	N	N		P	N	N	N	N
Cimetidine	I	A	N	N	P		N	M	P	P
Diazepam	N	N	N	N	N	N		N	N	N
Digoxin	P	N	D	P	N	M	N		N	N
Dobutamine	B	N	I	I	N	P	N	N		S
Dopamine	P	I	C	D	N	P	N	N	S	

C = physically and chemically compatible; P = physically compatible; D = physically compatible only in D5W; S = physically compatible only in 0.9% NaCl; A = physically compatible for 4–8 hours; B = physically compatible for 4–8 hours only in D5W; M = manufacturer claims medication should not be mixed with other medications but some compatibility data are available; I = incompatible; N = information on compatibility is not available.
This is only a portion of a chart. The most current compatibility chart obtained from pharmacy should be used when mixing and infusing IV drugs. Modified in 1996.

combinations of two or more drugs (e.g., antacids and either digoxin or tetracycline products) or drug and food combinations (e.g., cholestyramine and food containing vitamins A, D, K, B_{12}, or folic acid). *Sequestration* occurs when the drug is surrounded by a lipoid substance. For example, when the fat-soluble vitamins A, D, E, and K are combined with mineral oil, the mineral oil surrounds the vitamins and the vitamins cannot come in contact with the bowel surface and therefore cannot be absorbed.

The initial site of potential drug interactions, the intestine, is where the metals—aluminum, calcium, and magnesium—can tie up tetracycline and decrease its absorption. Antacids, milk, and dairy products, which contain

these metals, chelate tetracycline, prevent its complete absorption, and compromise the patient's drug therapy. How can this drug interaction be prevented in the patient using tetracycline four times a day and an antacid four times a day? The patient is instructed to take the tetracycline on an empty stomach 1 hour before each meal and 1 hour before bedtime. The antacid, which is most effective when taken after a meal, is administered 1 hour after each meal and at bedtime. When drugs interfere at the point of absorption, the administration times are staggered so that the doses of each drug are at least 1 to 2 hours apart. By staggering the administration times, the patient is not denied either medication.

Table 5–2. DRUG INTERACTIONS AFFECTING ABSORPTION, PROTEIN BINDING, BIOTRANSFORMATION, AND EXCRETION

Drug	Interacting Drug	Result/Effect	Probable Mechanism
Absorption			
Antacids	Isoniazid	Decreased isoniazid absorption	Decreased gastric emptying
Metoclopramide	Cimetidine	Decreased cimetidine absorption	Increased gastric emptying
Cimetidine	Ketoconazole	Decreased ketoconazole absorption	Increased gastric pH
Cholestyramine	Warfarin	Decreased warfarin effect	Complexation
Iron	Tetracycline	Decreased tetracycline absorption	Chelation
Protein Binding			
Warfarin	Clofibrate	Increased anticoagulant effect of warfarin	Warfarin displaced from binding sites
Methotrexate	Probenecid	Possible increased methotrexate toxicity	Methotrexate displaced from binding sites
Biotransformation			
Allopurinol	Theophylline	Increased pharmacologic effect of theophylline	Enzyme inhibition (allopurinol—enzyme inhibitor)
Phenobarbital	Diazepam	Decreased plasma concentration of diazepam	Enzyme induction (phenobarbital—enzyme inducer)
Phenytoin	Isoniazid	Reduced biotransformation of both drugs	Competition for same pathway
Renal Excretion			
Quinidine	Digoxin	Increased digoxin effect	Decreased tubular secretion
Diuretics	Lithium	Increased lithium toxicity	Increased tubular reabsorption
Antacids	Salicylates	Decreased salicylate effect	Increased urine pH
Tetracycline	Lithium	Increased lithium toxicity	Decreased renal excretion of lithium

Examples only, not a complete listing.

Drug absorption can also be affected by an alteration in the intestinal mucosa. If the mucosa is destroyed by disease or drugs (e.g., antineoplastics), absorption within the intestinal tract may be affected. Increased absorption may occur because destroyed mucosa leaves more vascular bed exposed, allowing more drug to be absorbed. Decreased absorption may occur because the mucosal layer of the intestine is destroyed and no longer functions properly.

Protein and Tissue Binding

Many drugs are extensively bound to plasma proteins. Drugs are pharmacologically inactive unless they are free from their binding sites on the protein. While protein bound, the drug can neither perform its intended therapeutic action nor be eliminated from the body. (See Chapter 4 for more information on protein binding.)

The percentage of protein-bound drug remains constant in each patient and generally does not pose any serious clinical problems. However, an increase in unbound or free drug in the plasma enhances not only the pharmacologic effect but also promotes the renal and/or hepatic elimination of the drug. In general, protein displacement drug interactions tend to be self-limiting, with generally only a transient increase in pharmacologic effect. However, the possibility of harm to the patient still exists because highly protein-bound drugs and their clinical effects can be influenced by other mechanisms. An illustration of this occurs with warfarin, an oral anticoagulant that is highly protein bound and whose therapeutic effect is a direct result of the amount of free drug in the blood. Phenylbutazone (Butazolidin, an anti-inflammatory drug) increases the anticoagulant effect of warfarin by displacing warfarin from its binding sites. Of greater importance, however, is that this agent inhibits the elimination of warfarin by the liver and prolongs its anticoagulant effect.

Drugs can also displace other drugs from tissue-binding sites with similar results as with protein-binding displacement. For example, quinidine (an antidysrhythmic) displaces digoxin from its binding sites in skeletal muscle. If quinidine and digoxin are given concurrently, the digoxin dosage usually must be reduced by 50% to prevent digitalis toxicity.

Drug interactions can also increase penetration of other drugs into tissue. Concurrent administration of acetazolamide (*Diamox*) and acetylsalicylic acid (aspirin) causes increased penetration of acetylsalicylic acid into the brain although the mechanism is unknown.

Biotransformation

The biotransformation (metabolism) of many drugs is mediated largely by the liver. Biotransformation is one determinant of drug concentration at a particular site of action where a drug exerts its pharmacologic effect. Therefore, any change in the activity of drug-metabolizing enzymes in the liver can affect drug action. Drugs that cause metabolic changes by affecting drug-metabolizing enzyme activity in the liver can be divided into several categories: drugs that increase enzyme activity through enzyme induction, drugs that inhibit enzyme activity, and drugs that compete for the same pathway. Enzyme induction involves the synthesis of new enzyme and takes place gradually in about 7 to 10 days. Enzyme inhibition usually takes place over 1 to 2 weeks (or sometimes longer), but may occur within 24 to 48 hours. Thus, the nurse needs to understand the likely time course of such interactions to monitor the patient appropriately.

Enzyme Induction There are literally hundreds of drugs or chemicals that can stimulate hepatic enzyme activity. Enzyme induction can be advantageous. For example, in the treatment of neonatal hyperbilirubinemia, phenobarbital accelerates the metabolism and thus the excretion of bilirubin. Enzyme induction, which speeds up the metabolism of a drug, may also be responsible for the patient's developing tolerance to certain drugs such as barbiturates. Because the same dose is metabolized more quickly, reduced effects are obtained from the drug.

Phenobarbital is considered the classic stimulator (inducer) of liver drug metabolism. It stimulates the liver to produce more microsomal enzymes, which in turn increases the biotransformation of a variety of drugs and decreases their plasma concentration. If phenobarbital or other well-known enzyme inducers such as rifampin and phenytoin are administered, the dose of the induced drug should be increased. The effect of phenobarbital on drug metabolism is usually seen within a few days; the maximum effect is seen within 2 to 3 weeks.

Alcohol also has an effect on drug biotransformation. It increases the metabolism and decreases the activity of drugs such as warfarin, isoniazid (INH, an antitubercular), and phenytoin (Dilantin). Tobacco and marijuana increase the metabolism of theophylline. Some drugs, such as phenobarbital and carbamazepine (Tegretol, an anticonvulsant), increase both the metabolism of other drugs and their own metabolism. With enzyme induction, the dose of the affected drug may have to be increased to maintain a therapeutic level.

Enzyme Inhibition In enzyme inhibition, one drug inhibits the metabolism of another drug by decreasing the activity of drug-metabolizing enzymes. This results in an increased pharmacologic effect of one or more of the drugs because plasma concentrations remain high. Cimetidine (Tagamet, an antiulcer agent), a well-known enzyme inhibitor, decreases the enzyme-metabolizing activity of several drugs, including lidocaine, phenytoin, propranolol, some benzodiazepines, and warfarin, which may lead to increased serum levels and possibly toxicity. Serum levels of these drugs may need to be monitored. Other enzyme inhibitors include allopurinol, oral anticoagulants, tricyclic antidepressants, erythromycin, and ciprofloxacin.

Competition For Same Pathway Occasionally, two (or more) drugs (e.g., phenytoin and isoniazid) given concurrently are biotransformed by the same enzyme. Because the drugs compete for the same enzyme, the rate of biotransformation for each drug is reduced, which results in an increased duration of action. With repeated doses of these drugs, toxic levels may occur.

Excretion

Interference with drug excretion can either delay or enhance drug effect. Excretion can be altered within the gastrointestinal tract by cathartics, food, narcotics, and stress; within the bilary tract by obstruction; or within the urinary system. Any stage of urinary function can be affected.

Some drugs are actively secreted by a similar process in the renal tubules. When such drugs are administered together, interference with the elimination of one or both drugs may occur. Examples of drugs that interact by this mechanism include penicillins, cephalosporins, salicylates, and thiazide diuretics.

Diuretics (except potassium-sparing diuretics) decrease renal clearance of lithium (Lithane), an antimanic drug, which can lead to lithium intoxication. Because lithium has a narrow therapeutic index (margin of safety), increased serum levels caused by this interaction can have serious consequences. When these agents are used together, frequent monitoring of lithium's serum level is necessary.

The use of probenecid (Benemid, an antigout drug) to block the renal secretion of penicillin is an example of an advantageous drug interaction. Instead of treating patients over several days with penicillin, one large dose of penicillin is administered with probenecid. Probenecid keeps the amount of penicillin in the body at higher levels for a longer period than could have been achieved by giving the penicillin alone.

Alteration of fluid and electrolyte balance can also modify the therapeutic effect and toxicities of other drugs. Hypokalemia—induced by many diuretics and corticosteroids—increases the likelihood of digitalis toxicity and can antagonize antidysrhythmic drugs. Drugs that induce sodium and water retention—phenylbutazone (Butazolidin, an anti-inflammatory drug) and corticosteroids—may negate the effect of antihypertensives or diuretics. Conversely, drugs that cause excessive diuresis—loop diuretics—may potentiate the hypotensive effects of antihypertensives and peripheral vasodilators.

PHARMACODYNAMIC INTERACTIONS

Pharmacodynamic interactions can occur when drugs with similar actions or similar adverse effects are administered together. The combined effect may be additive, synergistic, antagonistic, or potentiated. Table 5–3 features some examples of these interactions.

Additive

An *additive* effect occurs when two or more drugs having the same overt effect are combined and the result is the sum of the individual effects relative to the doses used. (If drug A has an effect of 1 and drug B has an effect of 1, the combination produces a 1 + 1 = 2 effect.) This additive effect may be harmful or beneficial. An example of a harmful additive effect is the increased incidence of gas-

Table 5–3. PHARMACODYNAMIC INTERACTIONS

Drug 1	+	Drug 2	Effects
Additive			
Beta-adrenergic blockers		Halothane	Hypotension
		Diltiazem and verapamil	Cardiac failure, AV conduction disturbances, and sinus bradycardia
		Diazoxide	Severe hypotension
Captopril		Most anesthetics	Hypotension
		Potassium supplements	Hyperkalemia
		Spironolactone	Hyperkalemia
Corticosteroids		Furosemide	Increased potassium loss
Furosemide		Aminoglycosides	Increased ototoxicity and nephrotoxicity
Smoking (marijuana)		Antidepressants (tricyclic)	Marked sinus tachycardia
Diazepam		Alcohol	Increased CNS depression
Digoxin		Methyldopa	Sinus bradycardia
Heparin		Alcohol	Increased bleeding
Nitroglycerin		Diazoxide	Severe hypotension
Nonsteroidal anti-inflammatory drugs		Alcohol	Increased GI bleeding
Synergistic			
Beta-adrenergic blockers		Ergot alkaloids	Severe peripheral vasoconstriction, possible gangrene
Lithium		Carbamazepine	Increased neurotoxicity
		Phenytoin	Increased lithium toxicity
Theophylline		Halothane	Increased ventricular dysrhythmias
Amphotericin B		Aminoglycosides	Increased nephrotoxicity
Potentiated			
Phenothiazides		Narcotics	Enhanced analgesic effect
Antagonistic			
Beta-adrenergic blockers		Sympathomimetics	Decreased antihypertensive effect, decreased bronchodilator effect

Source: Medical Letter Handbook of Adverse Drug Interactions. The Medical Letter, New Rochelle, N.Y., 1991. Modified in 1996. This is not a complete list.

trointestinal bleeding when alcohol is combined with a salicylate (aspirin and others). This drug interaction is additive because each agent alone can cause gastrointestinal bleeding. Combining two pain-relieving drugs such as aspirin and codeine is an example of a beneficial additive effect. The combination controls pain better than either drug alone.

Synergistic

A *synergistic* effect occurs when two or more drugs, with or without the same overt effect, are used together to yield a combined effect that has an outcome greater than the sum of the single drugs' active components alone. (If drug A has an effect of 1 and drug B has an effect of 1, the combination produces a 1 + 1 = 5 effect, rather than the 1 + 1 = 2 effect as expected.) This is exemplified by the prolonged hypnotic effect of chloral hydrate (a hypnotic) that occurs when it is combined with alcohol, which causes CNS depression. Unfortunately, the synergistic effect produced by this interaction can result in coma or death. On the positive side, a synergistic effect is obtained by combining various groups of antibiotics (e.g., penicillins or cephalosporins with aminoglycosides).

Another type of synergistic reaction occurs when two or more drugs produce a similar effect but do so by exerting actions at different sites or by different mechanisms. For example, the combination of a diuretic (which lowers blood volume) and a beta-adrenergic blocker (which dilates blood vessels to lower blood pressure) lowers blood pressure better than either drug could when administered alone.

Potentiation

Potentiation describes a particular type of synergistic effect—that is, a drug interaction in which only one of two drugs exerts the action that is made greater by the presence of the second drug. (If drug A has an effect of 1 and drug B has an effect of 1, the combination produces an effect that is two (or more) times the effect of drug B.) For example, when a phenothiazide is administered with a narcotic, the analgesic effect of the narcotic is enhanced (i.e., potentiated).

Antagonistic

Antagonistic reactions have the opposite effect of synergism and result in a combined effect that is less than either active component alone. In other words, adding a second drug may diminish or eliminate the effect of the first. (If drug A has an effect of 1 and drug B has an effect of 1, the combination produces a 1 + 1 = 0 effect.) For example, when protamine sulfate (an anticoagulant) is administered as an *antidote* to a patient experiencing bleeding secondary to the anticoagulant action of heparin, bleeding lessens or ceases. This effect occurs because protamine sulfate is a strong base that neutralizes acidic heparin by binding with it to form a stable compound with no anticoagulant effect.

COMBINED TOXICITY

Combining two or more drugs with the same or similar adverse or toxic effects on the same organ may result in an additive or synergistic toxic effect. For example, the combination of furosemide (Lasix, a diuretic) and an aminoglycoside antibiotic, both of which can cause ototoxicity, may cause a combined toxicity leading to eighth cranial nerve damage and deafness.

CLINICAL IMPLICATIONS OF DRUG-DRUG INTERACTIONS

Many drugs are capable of interacting. However, if two drugs are known to adversely interact, it does not mean that they can never be administered together. To prevent interactions, the dosages and/or the schedule of administration of the drugs is altered. The dosages of the drugs must be carefully balanced and adjusted to minimize interactions. The patient must be taught the importance of not missing a dose of either medication. Proper scheduling of drugs can also minimize or eliminate interactions.

Table 5–4. OVER-THE-COUNTER MEDICATIONS AND PRESCRIPTION DRUG INTERACTIONS

OTC Drug	Prescription Drug(s)	Interaction
Analgesics	Many	↑ Hepatotoxic effects
Acetasalicylic acid (ASA) or aspirin	Anticoagulants	↑ Bleeding
	Corticosteroids	↑ Gastric mucosa bleeding
	Anti-inflammatories	
	Oral antidiabetics	Potentiates effects of many drugs
	Barbiturates	
	Phenytoin	
Antacids	Many	Impairs absorption
Antidiarrheals	Many	Slows absorption
Antihistamines	CNS depressants	↑ CNS effects
	Tricyclic antidepressants	↑ Side effects
		Blurred vision
	Carbamazepine	Constipation
	Disopyramide	Dry mouth
Bronchodilators	Digitalis	↑ Toxic effects
	Thyroid drugs	
	Vasopressors	↑ Hypertensive effects
	Oral antidiabetics	↓ Effectiveness of antihypertensive
Decongestants	Antihypertensives	↓ Possibility of hypertension
Expectorants	Heparin	↑ Risk of hemorrhage
Vitamin B₆	Levodopa	↓ Effectiveness of levodopa
Vitamin B complex	Anticoagulants	↑ Bleeding
Vitamin C	Barbiturates	↓ Excretion
	Salicylates	
	Sulfonamides	
	Amphetamines	↑ Excretion
	Atropine	
	Quinidine	

This is only a partial list. Always consult current interaction sources before drug administration.

The patient needs to understand why the medications are taken at alternate times rather than together.

Patients also have to be taught about taking over-the-counter (OTC) products. Many OTC products, when combined with prescription drugs, cause interactions (Table 5–4). Patients are taught to always check with their pharmacist or physician before taking any OTC preparations.

DRUG-FOOD INTERACTIONS

Food is known to induce physiologic changes in the gastrointestinal tract that may decrease, increase, or delay the absorption of drugs; or the drug may take longer to reach peak blood levels after a dose.

FOODS DECREASING DRUG EFFECTIVENESS

Foods can act in various ways to decrease drug effectiveness. Foods can bind with drugs, allowing less to be absorbed; increase the hydrolysis of drugs in the intestine; or reduce the effect of absorbed drugs through various mechanisms.

Several drugs are known to bind with certain foods, thus decreasing their absorption. The erythromycins or fluoroquinolones readily bind with any food that is present; therefore, they are administered one hour before or two hours after food. Tetracyclines bind with milk, cheese products, and all antacids, forming an insoluble precipitate that is excreted rather than absorbed. Foods that are high in iron may also reduce the absorption of tetracycline. Tetracycline must be administered at least one hour before or two hours after a meal.

Calcium binds with chocolate, oxalic acid (in spinach), and phytic acid (in nuts, legumes, and cereal grains), reducing its absorption. Patients who are taking calcium for hypocalcemia must avoid chocolate and foods containing oxalic and phytic acids. Calcium also inhibits the absorption of tetracycline.

Bran can decrease the absorption of digoxin.

High-protein foods (eggs, meat, protein supplements) decrease the absorption of levodopa (Dopar) in the intestine. Proteins are metabolized to amino acids in the intestinal lumen, and levodopa, an amino acid derivative, competes with the amino acids for active transport across the intestinal wall. To minimize this reaction, protein intake is spread equally in three meals a day. More than 10 mg/day of vitamin B_6 also decreases levodopa's effectiveness. Patients taking levodopa are cautioned to avoid vitamin B_6 supplements (either alone or in multivitamin combinations).

Erythromycin is hydrolyzed more quickly in the intestine in the presence of acid foods like tomatoes, fruits, and vegetable and fruit juices. These foods should be limited when taking erythromycin.

Several food-drug combinations can actually reduce the effectiveness of absorbed drugs. Both natural licorice (contains glycyrrhizic acid) and tyramine-rich foods reduce the effectiveness of antihypertensives. Licorice is related to and acts like aldosterone: it enhances sodium retention and potassium excretion in the distal tubule of the kidney, thus elevating blood pressure. Tyramine-rich foods (aged or fermented foods, bananas, yogurt, and sour cream, to name just a few) enhance the release of norepinephrine from sympathetic axons, resulting in vasoconstriction and hypertension.

Patients taking theophylline are instructed not to eat charcoal-broiled meats. The combination of theophylline and charcoal-broiled meats can result in a decrease in theophylline's plasma half-life, increasing elimination and thus reducing effectiveness.

FOODS INCREASING DRUG EFFECTIVENESS

Food may promote the absorption of some drugs. Griseofulvin, (Grifulvin, an antifungal agent), is better absorbed when taken with meals containing fat; therefore, patients may be encouraged to increase the fat content of their diet. Other drugs, such as hydrochlorothiazide (HydroDiuril, a diuretic) and metoprolol (Lopressor, a beta-blocker) appear to be better absorbed after ingestion of food.

Monoamine oxidase (MAO) inhibitors, a specific class of antidepressant medications, increase levels of norepinephrine and serotonin in the central nervous system and potentiate the cardiovascular effects of substances such as tyramine. The combination of MAO inhibitors and foods containing tyramine can cause an acute hypertensive crisis, resulting in symptoms of severe occipital headache, palpitations, stiff neck, nausea, and vomiting. Thus, tyramine-containing foods are avoided during and for 2 to 3 weeks after MAO inhibitor therapy.

The effects of MAO inhibitors can also be enhanced by concurrent caffeine and monosodium glutamate (MSG), a flavor enhancer. Chinese food often contains large amounts of MSG, so patients are cautioned about eating Chinese food, especially in restaurants. It is now mandated in many states that a sign must be posted if MSG is used in food. Consuming large amounts of MSG without taking any medication can also cause symptoms of throbbing in the head, lightheadedness, tightness in the jaw, shoulders, and backache. These symptoms are related to arterial vasodilitation and reflex sympathetic stimulation.

PATIENT-RELATED FACTORS THAT AFFECT DRUG INTERACTIONS

Patient-related factors that may influence the response to drug interactions are chronic disease states, diet, environment, genetic makeup, and age.

Patients affected by chronic disease states may be predisposed to the adverse effects of drug interactions. This is a consideration in patients afflicted with endocrine diseases (e.g., diabetes and thyroid conditions), alcoholism, various diseases of the gastrointestinal tract, renal failure, and hepatic dysfunction.

Dietary excesses or insufficiencies may predispose some patients to untoward effects from certain drugs. Excesses of caffeine may have an antagonistic effect with central nervous system depressants. Sucrose, when taken in excess, may have a tendency to decrease sexual activity, particularly in patients taking large doses of aspirin. Excessive licorice intake may cause pseudoaldosteronism (hypoaldosteronism), which causes symptoms of aldosterone suppression. Vitamin C may increase the secretion of weakly basic drugs like atropine or quinidine and therefore inhibit their effects, or it may decrease the excretion of weak acids like barbiturates, aspirin, and sulfonamides and therefore potentiate their effects. Patients taking isoniazid should ingest limited amounts of foods with high histamine content, especially Swiss cheese and tuna fish. The combination causes severe headaches, redness and itching of the eyes and face, chills, palpitations, pulse-rate variations, and loose stools.

Various drugs can also precipitate dietary deficiencies. Long-term therapy with anticonvulsants can cause folate and vitamin D deficiencies manifested by muscle weakness, breathlessness, or bone pain. Increasing folate and vitamin D–rich foods in the diet may be helpful. Phenytoin and phenobarbital can also cause intestinal malabsorption of calcium and subsequent development of osteomalacia. Chronic aspirin ingestion can deplete folic acid and "pseudosenility" may occur in the elderly patient. D-Penicillamine (Cuprimine, an antiarthritic drug) chelates zinc and copper and may precipitate deficiencies of these elements.

Alcohol intake may also precipitate drug interactions. In the United States, approximately 104 million individuals consume alcohol regularly. Alcohol can cause interactions with many types of drugs, including antihypertensives, CNS depressants, antipsychotic agents, analgesics, anticoagulants, diuretics, cardiotonics, antidysrhythmics, and antidiabetic agents. The amount of alcohol consumed on a daily basis must be considered when these drugs are administered.

Environmental factors are considered in patients exposed to smoking, insecticides, and air pollution. For example, exposure to pesticides induces many drug-metabolizing enzymes, causing a decreased therapeutic effect in patients given drugs such as barbiturates, warfarin, or corticosteroids. In patients taking theophylline who also smoke, the clearance of theophylline is increased by approximately 30% to 40%, thus requiring a higher dose of the theophylline. These environmental influences are just beginning to be intensely investigated by researchers.

Another area of new research is the effect a patient's genetic makeup may have on drug disposition and adverse drug interactions.

Age can affect the patient's ability to handle potential drug interactions. Older patients, because of multiple chronic disease states, compromised kidney function, and possible dietary insufficiencies, must be closely monitored.

EFFECTS OF DRUGS ON LABORATORY TEST RESULTS

Many drugs can affect the results of standard laboratory tests. For example, amphotericin B (anti-infective), diuretics, and corticosteroids decrease serum potassium levels. Nicotine, estrogen, and adrenergic agents can increase serum cortisol (hormone) levels. Laboratory test results for creatinine levels are artificially elevated (i.e., actual creatinine level is lower than what tests record) in patients taking certain cephalosporins, leading to inadequate drug dosages if this information is not considered.

Some drugs produce false-positive results in urine glucose testing. These include cephalothin, isoniazid, levodopa, and probenicid.

LEGAL IMPLICATIONS

As the information on drug interactions grows, the legal responsibility of nurses also increases. Current legal guidelines suggest that the nurse is responsible for only published interactions that are well known. It is the nurse's responsibility to question all orders when there is a potential for interaction that may adversely affect the patient. The nurse must always assess the patient for symptoms of changing behavior or changing signs and symptoms and for any unusual or unexpected side or toxic effect that could indicate a drug interaction is occurring. The nurse has the legal right and responsibility to withhold further doses of the medication that is suspected of causing the problem until the physician can evaluate the patient.

The bibliography for this chapter can be found in Appendix B, which begins on page 1054.

CHAPTER REVIEW QUESTIONS*

1. A pharmacokinetic drug interaction:
   a. Occurs in the drug preparation phase of drug therapy.
   b. Produces the majority of drug incompatibility reactions.
   c. May have additive, synergistic, or antagonistic effects.
   d. Affects the absorption, distribution, biotransformation, and excretion of drugs.

2. A pharmacodynamic drug interaction:
   a. Occurs when liver function is compromised.
   b. Refers to a type of drug incompatibility.
   c. May have additive, synergistic, or antagonistic effects.
   d. Occurs when plasma protein binding is modified.

*See Appendix A, which begins on page 1051, for answers.

3. An antagonistic drug interaction occurs when:
   a. Drug absorption is decreased by the presence of food in the stomach.
   b. A second drug is added to diminish or eliminate the effect of the first.
   c. A second drug is added that has the same overt effect as the first.
   d. Drug distribution is enhanced by displacement of protein-bound drug.

4. Medications that increase or inhibit liver enzyme activity can affect drug action. Which of the following statements is *true* regarding biotransformation in the liver?
   a. Alcohol inhibits liver enzyme activity, resulting in increased activity of certain drugs.
   b. Phenobarbital stimulates liver enzyme activity, resulting in increased metabolism of certain drugs.
   c. Cimetidine (Tagamet) stimulates liver enzyme activity, resulting in increased effect of certain drugs.

d. Rifampin inhibits liver enzyme activity, resulting in decreased metabolism of certain drugs.

5. An additive drug interaction results when:
   a. Two drugs having the same overt effect are combined.
   b. One of two drugs exerts the action that is made greater by the presence of the second drug.
   c. Two drugs, not possessing the same overt effect, are used together to yield a combined effect.
   d. Two drugs produce a combined effect that is less than either active component alone.

6. A synergistic drug interaction occurs when the following drugs are administered together:
   a. Aspirin and codeine.
   b. Diazepam (Valium) and alcohol.
   c. Propranolol (Inderal) and epinephrine.
   d. Heparin and alcohol.

CHAPTER 6

Drug Toxicity, Adverse Drug Reactions, and Poisoning

Merrily A. Kuhn, RNC, PhD

CHAPTER OUTLINE

Adverse Drug Reactions
Poisoning by Drugs or Chemicals
Using the Nursing Process in Overdose/Poisoning

BOXES

Building Your Critical Thinking Skills, 71

KEY TERMS

Anaphylactic reaction	Bronchorrhea
Anaphylactoid reaction	Pharmacogenetics
Anaphylaxis	Photoallergic
Antibody	Photosensitivity
Antigen	Phototoxic
Antigenic	Interstitial nephritis
Atopic reaction	Teratogenic
Atopy	Toxicology

LEARNING OBJECTIVES

After reading this chapter, the student will be able to:

1. Differentiate among toxic, allergic, idiosyncratic, delayed, and teratogenic drug reactions.
2. Identify the four types of hypersensitivity reactions and their relationship to medication administration.
3. Understand drug-induced tissue and organ toxicities.
4. Identify selected drugs that cause toxic effects to the skin, liver, kidney, eye, ear, lung, and sexual organs.
5. Understand the principles of caring for a patient who has taken a poison or drug overdose.
6. Identify selected drugs removed from the body with dialysis, plasmapheresis, and hemoperfusion.

Toxicology is that aspect of pharmacology dealing with the adverse effects of drugs on living organisms. Toxicology is concerned not only with drugs used in therapy but also with many other chemicals that may be responsible for household, environmental, or industrial intoxication. Two federal agencies, the Food and Drug Administration (FDA) and the Environmental Protection Agency (EPA), ensure that the risk is low relative to the beneficial effect when an agent is used for its intended purpose in the general population. The FDA regulates drugs, cosmetics, and food additives in interstate commerce. The EPA regulates most other chemicals.

In general, when pharmacologic products are admin-istered, the benefit should outweigh the risk. However, the use of any pharmacologic product has certain risks, including the possibility of toxic reactions, especially with drug overdose.

ADVERSE DRUG REACTIONS

The terms "adverse reaction," "adverse effect," or "side effect" describe the potential unwanted effects that patients experience as a result of drug therapy. In this text, these terms are used interchangeably and collectively.

Adverse drug reactions (ADRs) range from those that are uncomfortable (but tolerated), such as nausea and dizziness, to those that are life threatening, such as seizures and cardiac arrest. ADRs may occur relatively soon after a drug is started, that is, within a minute (e.g., anaphylaxis), days (e.g., gastrointestinal bleeding), or weeks (e.g., renal failure). These are generally referred to as "acute" or short-term adverse effects. On the other hand, drug toxicities may be "delayed," that is, the toxicity may become manifest only months or years after a drug is started.

Assessment and evaluation of cumulative toxic effects are receiving increased attention because of chronic exposure to low concentrations of various natural and synthetic chemical substances in the environment. Numerous studies have investigated the incidence of adverse reactions. The incidence of adverse reactions ranges from 10% to 30% of hospitalized medical patients who then have a death rate of approximately 0.1% to 0.5%. In addition, 2% to 6% of hospital admissions are the result of adverse reactions. Adverse effects are more likely to occur in female patients, elderly patients, patients with impaired renal function, and patients taking many medications.

ADRs are classified into two major categories: type A reactions and type B reactions. Type A reactions produce 70% to 80% of all ADRs and are dose dependent and related to the pharmacologic effect of the drug. Type A reactions are often predictable and preventable. Type B reactions are immunologic or idiosyncratic reactions that are not dose dependent or an extension of the pharmacologic action of the drug. Type B reactions are usually not predictable or avoidable.

TYPE A REACTIONS

Type A reactions can be either primary or secondary.

Primary Reactions

The same pharmacologic mechanisms that account for a drug's efficacy account for many of its adverse effects, as most drug-induced adverse or toxic events are expected extensions of a drug's known pharmacologic properties. Examples include excessive drowsiness and lethargy from sedatives and hypnotics, increased bleeding tendencies from anticoagulants, excessive slowing of the heart from cardiac glycosides, and hypotension from antihypertensives. An overdose may also occur. For example, a drug may be accidentally taken by the patient as a result of poor patient teaching or understanding; or a medication may have been ordered for the patient without regard to hepatic or renal function or age considerations, resulting in an excessive dose. Most pharmacologic toxicities can be avoided by adjusting the dosage carefully to patient requirements and by vigilant monitoring on the part of the nurse.

Secondary Reactions

Some patients may develop undesirable secondary reactions including severe drowsiness and sleepiness from antihistamines, excessive tiredness and impotence from antihypertensives, and extreme agitation from theophylline bronchodilators. At times, reduction of the dose may be sufficient to lessen or stop these reactions, or the drug may need to be discontinued.

TYPE B REACTIONS

Type B reactions can be either allergic or idiosyncratic.

Allergic Reactions

Drug allergies or hypersensitivity reactions range from very mild (e.g., urticaria), with no need to discontinue the drug, to very severe and possibly life threatening (anaphylactic reaction). Patients reporting drug allergies need to be carefully evaluated because, in many instances, they are in fact experiencing adverse effects (e.g., nausea or vomiting).

Most drugs are made of relatively small molecules and have no *antigenic* activity, that is, they do not have the properties of an *antigen* (a substance that can provoke an immune response). Therefore, drugs must obtain antigenic properties and stimulate antibody production before they can produce an allergic reaction. An *antibody* is a serum protein that combines with and destroys antigens, (e.g., immunoglobulin). This is accomplished when a drug, acting as a hapten, combines with some body protein (carrier molecule) and forms a drug-protein complex. It is the drug-protein complex that has antigenic activity and invokes specific antibody formation, thereby sensitizing the body to the drug, as shown in Figure 6–1. The synthesis of antibodies usually occurs after a latent period of at least 1 to 2 weeks. When the individual is subsequently exposed to the chemical, an antigen-antibody interaction results in the typical manifestations of an allergy. Even extremely small quantities of the antigen can provoke a reaction.

Drug allergies may manifest themselves over a full spectrum of immediate and delayed reactions. For example, skin reactions may extend from mild rash to severe exfoliative dermatitis, and blood vessel reactions may extend from acute urticaria and angioedema to severe arteritis and localized degeneration.

Drug allergies are classified into four types: types I, II,

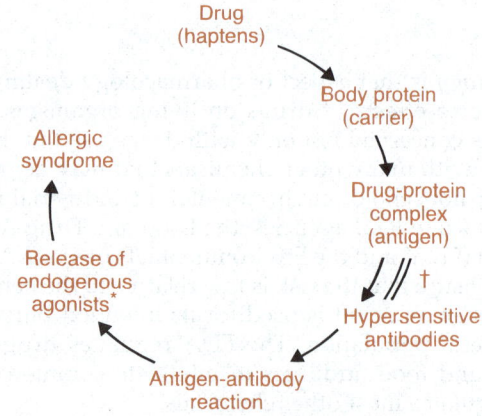

Figure 6–1. Drug allergic syndrome.

III, and IV. Each type is briefly described as to its etiology and pathology.

Type I (Anaphylactic or Atopic Reaction) A type I hypersensitivity reaction is a common type of drug allergy, but may also be activated by environmental pollens, foods, insect bites, and certain household cleaning agents. Two types of type I reactions can occur: (1) *anaphylaxis*, which refers to an acute reaction occurring in the skin and in the lung and cardiovascular systems and resulting in cardiovascular/respiratory collapse; and (2) *atopy*, which refers to a chronic reaction within the lung or in the skin that depends on the antigen, the frequency of contact or the route of contact, and the sensitivity of the organ system to the antigen. Both reactions share the same etiology and pathology.

On previous exposure to the agent (e.g., penicillin), IgE antibodies are formed that attach to basophils (fixed) and mast cells (circulating) found in profusion in connective tissue, the skin, and the mucous membranes. When the drug is administered again (challenging dose), the basophils and mast cells degranulate, liberating large doses of histamine and other humoral substances. These substances cause bronchoconstriction in the smooth muscles of the lung, peripheral vasodilatation, increased vascular permeability, and increased mucous production in the lung. If this reaction remains local, erythema and local edema occur. However, if the reaction becomes systemic, anaphylaxis occurs.

Anaphylactic reactions are a systemic reaction to the antigen that consequently affects many tissues and organs in the body. The release of histamine and other humoral substances results in contraction of smooth muscle and increased vascular permeability within the lung. Edema occurs around the eyes, on the skin, and in mucous membranes. Laryngeal edema often results in acute dyspnea. Hives or severe urticaria may appear on the skin surface. Within the vascular system the fluid shifts may result in hypotension and even cardiovascular collapse.

During an *anaphylactoid reaction*, the offending agent enters the body and works by nonimmunologic activating systems that cause degranulation of mast cells and basophils of the humoral system. Once the humoral system is activated, the same mediators are released and the clinical symptoms are indistinguishable from anaphylaxis.

Drugs that are capable of causing an anaphylactic or anaphylactoid reaction include penicillins, cephalosporins, tetracyclines, salicylates, iodides, blood products, diagnostic agents, venoms, hormones, thiazides, and others. Anaphylaxis is an acute medical emergency that is treated with epinephrine, antihistamines, bronchodilators, vasopressors, and other emergency procedures.

Atopic reactions from the inhalation of environmental antigens may cause bronchial asthma with resulting dyspnea and wheezing. Repeated exposure can result in hypertrophy of smooth muscle and can exaggerate bronchoconstriction.

Contact with irritants may cause atopic eczema resulting in urticaria, hives, and angioedema. These reactions are more common than anaphylaxis. The urticaria involves superficial capillaries, while the angioedema affects deeper skin capillaries. Drugs can also cause dermatologic manifestations (discussed in Chapter 65).

Type II (Cytotoxic Reaction) In a type II hypersensitivity reaction (cytotoxic reaction, immune complex syndromes, serum sickness), the foreign antigen adheres to the surface of the host's own cells (target cell). Antibodies are then formed by the host, which attach to the target cell. Generally, this reaction involves the activation of complement, a series of enzymatic proteins in normal serum that, in the presence of a specific sensitizer—often an antigen-antibody complex—destroy bacteria and other cells. When complement surrounds the target cells, destruction of the target cell occurs, either through phagocytosis or cell lysis. The ultimate effect on the host depends on the number and type of cells destroyed.

Drugs known to cause serum sickness include sulfonomides, penicillins, cephalosporins, salicylates, phenytoin (Dilantin), procainamide (Pronestyl), diphtheria and tetanus antitoxin, and others. Immediately after the drug is administered, the person develops antibodies of the IgG and IgM variety. Within several days to a week, the antibodies become so numerous that they begin to complex with red blood cells, platelets, and basophils. Histamine and other humoral substances are released, enter the bloodstream, and are soon deposited in many tissues. The patient then presents with fever, arthralgia, rash, splenomegaly, and lymph node enlargement. In severe reactions, hemolytic reactions, glomerulonephritis, thrombocytopenia, leukopenia, and vascular purpura may be seen. Usually, the reaction is self-limiting, and recovery occurs within several days to weeks after the drug is discontinued.

The exact mechanism of type II drug reactions is poorly understood. Several mechanisms have been suggested: hypersensitivity to the drug, contaminants or impurities in the drug, inflammation from the injection site, a direct pyrogenic effect, alteration of the thermoregulation center in the central nervous system, or biochemical defects within the patient.

Type III (Auto-Immune Reaction) A type III hypersensitivity reaction, also called an autoimmune reaction or a complex-mediated hypersensitivity reaction, is associated with a defect in the ability of the body to clear antigen-antibody complexes. These complexes then deposit on normal tissue and the antibody portion activates the complement cascade and thus the inflammatory response. Anaphylatoxins and neutrophils release necrotizing enzymes that produce local ischemia and necrosis as a consequence of complement activation. The mechanism is active in autoimmune diseases such as glomerulonephritis, rheumatoid arthritis, systemic lupus erythematosus, scleroderma, and many others. Drugs capable of causing a type III reaction include penicillins, phenytoin, and streptomycin.

Type IV (Cell-Mediated Hypersensitivity) A Type IV hypersensitivity reaction is mediated through T lymphocytes rather than antibodies and may be of two varieties: (1) a cell-mediated response or (2) a delayed hypersensitivity response. A cell-mediated response occurs as a result of T-cell contact with, and subsequent destruction of, the antigen. The T cell may also activate macrophages, which results in the lysis of other cells. Transplant rejection is, in part, a cell-mediated response.

Delayed hypersensitivity responses are due to the specific interaction of T cells with the antigen. The T cell–antigen reaction releases substances (macrophage migration inhibitory factor [MIF], macrophage activating factor [MAF], chemotactic factors, and others) that attract macrophages into the area. These factors also modulate the inflammatory response. The tuberculin skin test response is a good example of delayed hypersensitivity used to determine whether an individual has been sensitized to tuberculosis (TB). If the patient was previously exposed to TB, the skin test causes reddening and induration of the skin about 12 hours after intradermal injection. This reaction peaks within 24 to 72 hours. This response is elicited only when sensitized lymphocytes are present.

The two drugs that commonly cause a delayed hypersensitivity response are benzene and phenol, which are used primarily in topical preparations. Prior exposure is required. On the second or third exposure, by-products of these drugs penetrate the skin and combine with larger molecules in the skin, thus activating T lymphocytes. The T lymphocytes produce many chemical mediators, which, within 6 to 12 hours, cause the symptoms of contact dermatitis. The product should be completely washed from the skin and not used again.

Idiosyncratic Reactions

An idiosyncratic reaction is an unexpected, abnormal, or peculiar reaction to a drug occurring in a small portion of the total population and usually associated with a genetic defect. *Pharmacogenetics* deals with altered drug responses that are under hereditary control. For example, a patient who has decreased production of hepatic N-acetyltransferase and who takes procainamide (Pronestyl) has slower metabolism of procainamide and may develop toxic effects and symptoms of systemic lupus erythematosus; persons having a decreased production of glucose-6-phosphate dehydrogenase (about 10% of black males) develop a serious hemolytic anemia when they receive primaquine (antimalarial preparation); and, persons (in certain families whose genetic defect has yet to be discovered) receiving general anesthetics (such as halothane [*Fluothane*]) may develop malignant hyperthermia associated with high fever and skeletal muscle rigidity. The membranes within the muscle cells of this latter group release abnormal amounts of calcium ions when exposed to various chemicals, thus producing increased muscular heat.

Tests are available for detecting several drug idiosyncrasies. Red cell susceptibility to destruction by drugs can be determined by taking a small blood sample and checking the reaction of erythrocytes when a potent hemolysis-producing chemical is added. Patients suspected of developing malignant hyperthermia can have an assessment of their serum level of the enzyme creatinine phosphokinase. The nursing history is an important tool to determine which patients, based on their family history, may be prone to this reaction. Anytime the patient presents with an unusual or peculiar reaction, the suspected drug is always withheld until the physician has the opportunity to assess and evaluate the patient.

DELAYED TOXICITY

Most toxic effects occur at a predictable, usually short, time after administration. However, some reactions occur several days to several years after exposure. For example, aplastic anemia caused by chloramphenicol (Chloromycetin) may appear weeks after the drug is discontinued. Hepatotoxicity occuring after large doses of acetaminophen (Tylenol) is usually not apparent for 24 to 48 hours. Prolonged toxic effects, such as bronchogenic tumors, may occur many years after exposure to asbestos. Today it is speculated that women exposed to Agent Orange in Vietnam have an increased number of abortions and children born with birth defects, while men exposed have an increased number of malignancies. Delayed toxicity may also occur in the offspring, such as the increased incidence of cancer of the cervix in teenage daughters or testicular cancer in sons born to women who received diethylstilbestrol (DES) to reduce the symptoms of morning sickness during pregnancy.

Delayed toxicities obviously cannot be assessed or evaluated in a short period of time. Consequently, there is an urgent need for reliable, predictive, short-term tests for such toxicities.

DRUG-INDUCED TISSUE AND ORGAN TOXICITIES

Drugs can affect tissues, structures, and organs within the body either directly or indirectly. The organs most frequently affected include the skin, hematologic system, eye, kidney, liver, ear, lung, and sexual organs. Drugs can also mutate genetic codes in the body.

Dermatologic Reactions

The skin is the organ most commonly affected by allergic drug reactions. The majority of "drug rashes" consist of macules (flat red spots) or papules (raised red spots), which are highly pruritic. People who are prone to or already have skin problems are more likely to have an allergic skin reaction. Dermatologic reactions can also be life threatening and long lasting. Exfoliative dermatitis and erythema multiforme majus (Stevens-Johnson syndrome) are two very severe skin reactions that can occur secondary to the administration of sulfonamides and certain other drugs (see Chapter 65).

A unique form of dermatologic hypersensitivity is *photosensitivity* following exposure to sunlight. Two types of skin reaction occur: photoallergic and phototoxic. A *photoallergic* reaction often presents as a papular eruption on sun-exposed areas, similar in appearance to a contact dermatitis. It is thought to be associated with the photosensitizing drug forming an antigen by absorption of sunlight and the subsequent combination with a skin protein. A *phototoxic* reaction is characterized by a severe sunburn and is often not diagnosed as a hypersensitivity reaction. A phototoxic reaction is probably the result of a photosensitizing chemical absorbing ultraviolet radiation energy to such an extent that it becomes toxic to epidermal cells. A list of photosensitive drugs is provided in Chapter 65.

Blood Dyscrasias

Drugs can affect formed elements of the blood—erythrocytes, leukocytes, and thrombocytes—resulting in hemolytic or aplastic anemia, leukopenia, and thrombocytopenia. All of these conditions are very serious and could result in death if not diagnosed early. Any complaints of generalized weakness, fatigue, infection, or easy bruising are reported to the physician and the medication profile reviewed for potential drug-induced effects.

Hemolytic anemia can result secondary to a type II allergic reaction. A Coombs' test of the blood can detect the presence of the abnormal immunoglobulins both in the serum and attached to the red cell. Aplastic anemia is a very serious disorder that is fatal in over half of patients despite treatment efforts. Drugs known to cause aplastic anemia include chloramphenicol (Chloromycetin), phenylbutazone (Butazolidin), trimethadione (Tridione), and certain sulfonamides. Because most patients taking these drugs do not develop aplastic anemia, this reaction is thought to be idiosyncratic. Patients must have frequent blood counts performed to monitor for these anemias; if blood counts drop, the drug responsible is discontinued.

In leukopenia, the white cells, the primary defense mechanism for the body, are greatly reduced. Leukopenia can occur in a more specialized form, referred to as agranulocytosis, in which only the granulocytes are affected. When either condition is diagnosed, the drug responsible is discontinued immediately.

Thrombocytopenia—a reduction in platelets—develops occasionally. Drugs known to cause thrombocytopenia are quinidine, meprobamate (Equanil), chlorothiazide (Diuril), and some anti-infectives. Most patients recover quickly when the drug responsible is discontinued.

Ocular Toxicity

The eye, because of its delicate structure, is particularly subject to both direct and indirect injury by drugs. Patients may complain of blurring when taking anticholinergic products and of disturbances of color vision when taking digitalis products. These symptoms are generally mild and are reversible when the drugs are discontinued.

More serious complaints include changes in the cornea, lens, retina, and optic nerve. Before patients start on medications known to cause these changes, a complete eye examination is performed and then repeated periodically during therapy. If the patient notes changes in vision, the drug is discontinued immediately to prevent further damage (see Chapter 63).

Nephrotoxicity

The kidneys are subjected to injury from drugs or chemicals that are excreted through the kidney or that are carried by blood and flow through the kidney. The kidney is at risk because it has the highest blood supply per gram of any tissue in the body. This allows circulating agents to be delivered at 50 times the "usual" rate to tissues. The kidney also has the highest oxygen consumption and glucose production per gram. *Interstitial nephritis* or toxic nephropathy can occur secondary to various antibiotics, including the aminoglycosides, polymyxin B, and colistin (*Coly-Micin S*); analgesics such as salicylates; nonsteroidal anti-inflammatory drugs; anticancer drugs; heavy metals; and immune complex inducers such as penicillamine, captopril (Capoten), or gold salts. Patients should have baseline blood urea nitrogen and creatinine levels drawn prior to therapy and then periodically during therapy. The drug responsible is discontinued when these levels begin to rise. Nephrotoxicity secondary to medications is discussed more fully in Chapter 38.

Hepatotoxicity

Because of the liver's anatomic location and function, it is the first organ to receive medication once it is absorbed from the intestine. This makes the liver prone to both parenchyma (the mass of functioning liver cells) and bile channel injury. Any patient with depressed liver function may be more prone to liver injury, and liver necrosis can ensue. Reaction of the liver often results in hepatitis with increased enzyme levels, jaundice, and pruritus. Liver function studies are obtained prior to starting the patient on drugs known to cause liver injury and then are performed periodically during therapy (see Chapter 53). Drugs that may be hepatotoxic include methotrexate, halothane, gold salts, probenecid, and acetaminophen (overdose). These drugs may cause hepatotoxicity at normal doses, so close monitoring is needed.

Ototoxicity

Ototoxicity can result as a primary or secondary effect of medication. Toxic medications affecting the ear may affect both branches of the eighth cranial nerve—vestibular and auditory—resulting in dizziness, balance difficulties, and hearing loss. Ototoxicity often occurs in conjunction with nephrotoxicity because the medications that are not excreted by the kidney accumulate in other tissues (see Chapter 64). The drug class best known for causing ototoxic effects is the aminoglycosides.

Lung Toxicity

The lung may be negatively affected by drugs. Chemotherapeutic drugs (e.g., busulfan, bleomycin, and carmustine) and the antidysrhythmic drug amiodarone may precipitate pulmonary fibrosis. Frequent lung assessments including chest x-ray are performed to monitor for pulmonary changes.

Asthma may also be precipitated by drugs, particularly aspirin, anti-infectives (penicillins, streptomycin, tetracyclines, erythromycins, and chloramphenicol), and isoproterenol. Patients with underlying asthma are more prone to an acute attack when given these drugs. However, even patients with no known lung disease may be affected. Patients must be encouraged to report any changes in breathing pattern.

Sexual Dysfunction

Both male and female sexual function may be affected by medication. Toxic effects may range from a decreased sexual interest to impotence (see Chapter 47).

Mutagenic Effects

Several drugs (androgenic hormones, antineoplastic agents, caffeine, chlorpromazine, colchicine, estrogenic hormones, ether, and griseofulvin) can change the genetic composition of humans and are considered mutagenic. The largest genetic unit that can be involved in a mutation is a chromosome, while the smallest unit is a base pair present in the DNA molecule.

Today, we know that certain chemicals and drugs are capable of inducing carcinogenesis; they are called carcinogens. These products (environmental pollutants) are becoming a national health problem. Chemically induced carcinogenesis usually requires long exposure periods to carcinogens. Table 6–1 lists several substances recognized as being potentially carcinogenic.

TERATOGENIC REACTIONS

Administering certain drugs to pregnant women, particularly during the first trimester of pregnancy, can result in fetal deformities. These drugs are said to be *teratogenic*. The FDA has established five catergories indicating the potential for a drug to cause birth defects. Further information and the FDA listing are provided in Chapter 48. Whenever a drug is administered to a pregnant woman, the benefit-to-risk ratio must be assessed.

REPORTING ADVERSE DRUG REACTIONS

In both hospital and ambulatory settings, adverse drug reactions (ADRs) are underreported. The Joint Commission of Accreditation of Health Care Organizations (JCAHO) requires ADR reporting in hospitals. Each hospital should have a systematic process to monitor, report, and evaluate ADRs.

The FDA also has a spontaneous reporting system that is computerized. However, there is a very low rate of reporting. The purpose of the spontaneous reporting system is to collect, sort, and examine reports of clinically significant ADRs, evaluate the probability that the event was caused by the drug, seek trends to prevent further reactions, and provide guidelines for managing reactions. New drugs are usually studied for only 2 to 3 years with 2000 to 3000 patients. Therefore, uncommon or delayed reactions are unlikely to be identified prior to release of the drug. These reports may lead to actual withdrawal of the drug from the market or changes in product labeling.

POISONING BY DRUGS OR CHEMICALS

Poisons are described as chemical substances capable of causing harm to living substances even in small amounts. Even safe therapeutic products can become poisons if taken in large enough quantities.

Table 6–2 reviews the signs and symptoms of commonly overdosed drugs and toxic substances and reviews overdose management, including specific drugs used as antidotes. Typically, drugs such as aspirin and acetaminophen (Tylenol) are safe products. However, when taken accidentally or deliberately in large doses, death can result. Sedatives, hypnotics, and tranquilizers are all safe drugs when administered in therapeutic doses. However, these drugs can become toxic when combined with large amounts of ethanol (alcohol) or illegal drugs (cocaine, heroin, and so on). Only 37% of reported cases of poisoning are caused by a single agent. In 25% of cases, ethanol is one of the agents named and is the most common agent implicated in adult poisoning.

Children, if left unattended, often consume drugs prescribed for older siblings, parents, or grandparents. Most adult medications are toxic to small children. Household chemicals, such as cleaners and bleaches, or products found in the basement or garage, such as turpentine, petroleum distillates, gasoline, organophosphates (pesticides), and rat poisons, are also toxic.

Overdoses and poisonings are a common medical emergency. Poisoning is the fifth most common cause of accidental death in the United States. Recent epidemiologic data indicate that there are approximately 5 million cases of poisoning annually with over 13,000 deaths, with 1000 of these deaths in children under age 5. This number has been decreasing over several years. This decrease is probably due to the combined effort of the American Academy of Pediatrics (poisoning prevention) and the American Association of Poison Control Centers (centers located around the country).

The toxic activity of a poison depends on a number of variables, especially the amount of toxic substance and its metabolic route. Generally, the more substance is absorbed, the more toxic is the effect. Also, poisons injected into the bloodstream or inhaled have a more rapid onset of action. Poisons may have effects on almost all organs and tissues in the body, including the renal or hepatic

Table 6–1. SUBSTANCES POTENTIALLY CARCINOGENIC

Drugs	Other Substances
Androgens	Asbestos
Antineoplastics	Benzene
Busulfan	3.4-Benzopyrene
Clofibrate	Carbon tetrachloride
Corticosteroids	Chloroform
Cyclamates	Dioxane
Estrogens	Herbicides
Griseofulvin	Nitrosamines
Metronidazole	Pesticides
Nitrites	Tobacco smoke
Nitrofurans	TRIS (flame retardant)
Oral contraceptives	Trypan blue
Progestins	

Table 6–2. COMMONLY OVERDOSED DRUGS AND TOXIC AGENTS

Agent	Signs and Symptoms	Clinical Management	Specific Drugs for Management
Acetaminophen	Anorexia, nausea, vomiting, delayed onset of symptoms of jaundice, hypoglycemia, encephalopathy, and hepatic failure	Prevent further absorption of drug. Assess liver function for 3–5 days.	Acetylcysteine (Mucomyst)
Alcohol	Depressed sensorium, odor on breath, hypoglycemia, dehydration, visual disturbances, slowed respiration, flushing, fast pulse, ataxia; hallucinations, tremors, and convulsions (withdrawal effects)	Assess neurologic and metabolic systems; support cardiovascular and neurologic systems. Monitor liver function.	Glucose solution IV for dehydration; diazepam (Valium) for withdrawal symptoms.
Amphetamines	Toxic (paranoid) psychosis, hyperthermia, flushing, increased blood pressure, dilated pupils, auditory and visual hallucinations, seizures, tachycardia, needle marks in intravenous users, tachypnea	Prevent further reabsorption. Supportive treatment. Protect from further injury. Acidification of urine to increase elimination of drug.	Diazepam (Valium)
Anticholinergics (atropine, scopolamine)	Tachycardia, decreased secretions, urinary retention, dilated pupils, hallucinations, confusion, dry skin, fever, flushing	Assess cardiac activity.	Physostigmine
Antifreeze	Metabolic acidosis, hypocalcemia, renal failure	Prevent further reabsorption. Monitor blood alcohol and glucose levels. Include glucose in ethanol infusion.	Ethanol
Arsenic	Garlicky breath, vomiting, profuse diarrhea, abdominal colic, jaundice	Monitor blood pressure, respiratory status. Arsenic excreted by kidneys with BAL.	Dimercaprol (BAL)
Barbiturates	Tense vesicular skin lesions, coma, nystagmus, drowsiness, ataxia, slurred speech	Prevent further absorption. Supportive care; ventilate with oxygen if necessary. Dialyze if necessary.	Sodium bicarbonate to alkalinize the urine.
Carbon monoxide	Red skin, coal-gas odor, bullae, cyanosis	Monitor oxyhemoglobin.	Oxygen via hyperbaric chamber
Cocaine	Perforated nasal septum, dilated pupils, psychosis, delusions, hyperthermia, tachycardia	See amphetamines.	See amphetamines
Cyanide	Bitter-almond odor to breath, convulsion, coma, abnormal ECG	Prevent further reabsorption. Administer oxygen, monitor oxygen level, ventilate if necessary.	Sodium nitrate, amyl nitrite, sodium thiosulfate
Diazepam (Valium)	Euphoria (sometimes), ataxia, nystagmus, progressive CNS depression	See barbiturates.	See barbiturates
Digitalis products	Visual disturbances, delirium, abnormal ECG, nausea, vomiting, slowed pulse	Prevent further reabsorption. Monitor cardiac activity; treat arrhythmias.	Potassium, phenytoin (Dilantin), digoxin immune FAB (Digibind)
Gasoline	Distinctive odor, choking, pulmonary infiltrates, feeling of lightness, transitory visual hallucinations	Do not induce vomiting. Use gastric lavage to remove gasoline.	Calcium disodium edetate (EDTA) if gasoline is leaded
Heroin	Coma, decreased blood pressure, respiration, and pulse; miosis, needle marks	Assess respiratory and cardiovascular systems; support as necessary.	Naloxone (Narcan)

Continued on the following page

Table 6–2. COMMONLY OVERDOSED DRUGS AND TOXIC AGENTS, *Continued*

Agent	Signs and Symptoms	Clinical Management	Specific Drugs for Management
Hydrocarbons (cleaning fluids)	Pulmonary edema, lipid pneumonia, tinnitus, convulsions, diplopia, ventricular fibrillation	Prevent further reabsorption. Emesis or cathartics. Supportive care. Assess liver function.	Cathartics
Iron	Diarrhea, coma, bloody vomiting, radiopacity on radiograph, hypotension	Prevent further absorption. Urine turns red as iron is being excreted. Treatment discontinued when urine returns to normal.	Deferoxamine (Desferal)
Isopropyl alcohol	Severe gastritis, acetonemia with normoglycemia, acetone odor on breath, emesis	See alcohol.	See alcohol
Lead	Severe abdominal pain, increased blood pressure, milky vomitus, convulsions, muscle weakness, metallic taste, anorexia, encephalopathy, ataxia, paralysis, constipation	See arsenic.	Dimercaprol (BAL), penicillamine, calcium disodium edetate (EDTA)
LSD	Hallucinations, dilated pupils, mild tachycardia, bleeding disorder, confusion, agitation, sweating	See amphetamines.	See amphetamines.
Mercury	Stomatitis, gingivitis, colitis, nephrotic syndrome	Monitor renal function. Prevent further reabsorption.	D-penicillamine (Cuprimine)
Methadone (Dolophine)	Miosis; coma; lowered pulse, blood pressure, and respiration; transient response to narcotic antagonist naloxone	See heroin.	Naloxone (Narcan)
Mushrooms	Nausea, vomiting, hallucinations, delayed liver failure and renal failure	Prevent further absorption, emesis, lavage, supportive care; assess renal and hepatic systems.	Supportive therapy
Organophosphates	Miotic pupils, cramps, bronchorrhea, salivation, lacrimation, urination, defecation, sweating, skeletal muscle weakness, and paralysis	Prevent further reabsorption. Monitor respiratory rate; ventilate if necessary.	Atropine sulfate, pralidoxime (Protopam)
Phenothiazines	Postural hypotension, hypothermia, miosis, tremor, dystonic disorder, radiopacity on radiograph of abdomen, increased Q–T interval on ECG	Prevent further reabsorption. Monitor vital signs; expand volume if necessary to maintain blood pressure.	Diphenhydramine (Benadryl), adsorbents (activated charcoal, kaolin, pectin)
Salicylates	Hyperventilation, vomiting, fever, bleeding, acidosis, purpura	Prevent reabsorption by emesis or lavage. Dialysis or alkalinization of urine.	Adsorbents, sodium bicarbonate
Strychnine	Stiff neck, status epilepticus, cyanosis, opisthotonos	Prevent further reabsorption; supportive care. Avoid aural, visual, or tactile stimulation.	Supportive therapy
Tricyclic antidepressants	Paralytic ileus, supraventricular arrhythmias, convulsions, response to physostigmine, radiopacity on radiograph	Prevent further reabsorption. Monitor cardiac activity. Antiarrhythmics may be necessary.	Physostigmine, diazepam (Valium), adsorbents

systems, gastrointestinal system, hematologic system, and especially the central nervous system.

USING THE NURSING PROCESS IN OVERDOSE/POISONING

ASSESSMENT

The diagnosis of ADRs from overdose or poisoning is often difficult. Patients may arrive in the emergency department in mental states that range from alert to unconscious with seizures, with the unconscious state often difficult to differentiate from other disease states.

- Obtain a history as soon as possible from an alert patient. If a friend or relative accompanies an unconscious patient, a history is obtained, including the potential of poisoning and the possible products. The history should contain the following:
  - Date and time of overdose/poisoning
  - Reasons for overdose/poisoning
  - Circumstances surrounding overdose/poisoning
  - Last food/meal ingested (food and time)
  - Drug history
  - Drug abuse history
  - Disease history
  - Manifestations of overdose/poisoning and prior treatment
- Obtain laboratory toxicology screening from samples of blood, urine, and gastrointestinal contents to determine the causative agent as ordered. Quantitative determinations are needed for relatively few substances: acetaminophen, salicylates, diazepam (Valium), barbiturates, phencyclidine (PCP), cocaine, iron, lead, methyl alcohol, theophylline, lithium, and digitalis glycosides. For some of these, two plasma samples are obtained 1 or more hours apart, depending on the half-life of the drug involved, to determine if the concentration of the toxic substance is increasing or decreasing and thus to determine the needed therapy.
- Perform a thorough physical examination to obtain the following information:
  - Vital signs
  - Level of consciousness
  - Behavioral characteristics
  - Motor signs
  - Autonomic signs (diaphoresis, *bronchorrhea* [excessive discharge of mucus from the bronchi], bronchospasm, urinary retention, and so on)
  - Ancillary finding (pupil size, presence or absence of nystagmus, gag reflex, and status of oculocephalogyric reflex)

All of these gathered data are analyzed before the treatment is determined for optimal patient care.

NURSING DIAGNOSIS

Develop nursing diagnoses appropriate for the patient with a severe adverse drug reaction. Typical nursing diagnoses include the following: Risk for Poisoning, Altered Protection, Altered Thought Processes, Impaired Gas Exchange, and Altered Tissue Perfusion.

INTERVENTION

The primary goals of intervention are to work with the physician to do the following:

1. Institute supportive measures to maintain all vital functions such as patent airway and an IV access for fluid challenges or drug therapy.
2. Remove the toxic substance from the body; for example, wash chemicals from skin or remove from gastrointestinal system if possible through emesis (Chapter 51).
3. Administer antidote, if available (see Table 6–2).

- Provide supportive measures including cardiopulmonary resuscitation, ventilators, fluid recussitation, chelation, diuresis, cathartics, and other supportive drugs to control blood pressure or seizures. Volume depletion secondary to vomiting, diarrhea, and sweating is promptly corrected with normal saline or Ringer's solution, particularly in the young child or geriatric patient. Hypotension severe enough to require correction frequently necessitates monitoring of central venous or pulmonary artery pressures to determine fluid needs.

  Some severely poisoned patients may benefit from the use of artificial organs to enhance elimination of toxins from the blood. Hemodialysis, hemoperfusion, and plasmapheresis are considered state of the art in invasive detoxification.

  Hemodialysis exposes blood to a semipermeable membrane to remove low-molecular-weight toxins. Examples of drugs removed by dialysis include salicylates, isoniozid (INH), cephalosporins, and penicillins. Hemoperfusion percolates blood through absorbent columns to extract lipid- or protein-bound substances. Plasmapheresis is a modified phlebotomy procedure in which the cellular components of the blood are returned to the patient. The plasma and plasma proteins are replaced with fresh plasma or a suitable colloid. The use of this procedure in the treatment of severely intoxicated patients is of benefit, particularly for those strongly protein-bound toxins that are not well dialyzed or adsorbed. The ideal drug for removal by plasma exchange is one that is highly protein-bound, has a small volume of distribution, and has a prolonged half-life, such as loop diuretics, anticoagulants, anti-inflammatory drugs, and hypoglycemic agents.
- Protect self and others from contamination. It may be necessary to wear a gown, gloves, and a mask, and to discard contaminated supplies and clothing by double-bagging when dealing with poisons such as organophosphate pesticides (e.g., malathion or Diazinon).
- Provide psychologic support for families during this period of crisis. Nurses are often in a position to teach the patient or family how to avoid overdoses and poisonings and what steps to take if poisoning occurs. Poison control center numbers (there are over 600 in

the United States) are available in most telephone books around the country. All hospital emergency rooms have a listing of the closest centers. The Centers for Disease Control (CDC) in Atlanta, Georgia, is a source for hard-to-find data and rare antidotes.

Patient Teaching

- Teach poisoning prevention. Nurses can teach parents about storage of drugs and chemicals around the house. Parents are taught to make a room-by-room inventory of hazardous substances. Identify all harmful substances and make sure they are clearly identified for adult use and are out of the reach of children. All chemicals should be kept in their original, labeled containers with locked childproof caps. Chemicals are stored whenever possible in high, tightly shut or locked cabinets. When the container is empty, it is discarded. Household or garden chemicals are never mixed. When parents administer medications to children, they should not refer to the medication as candy. Do not trust child-resistant containers. No bottle top can be made so fail-safe that a child cannot find some way to get it off (Ekins, 1995).
- Teach families with young children to have activated charcoal and syrup of ipecac on hand. However, these products are not to be used unless the poison center or emergency department has suggested their use.
- Teach patients and families to read the directions carefully before they take a drug or use chemicals. Improper use may result in accidental poisoning. Do not combine chemical solutions. At least 60,000 people a year dial poison centers because they have inhaled dangerous fumes. The most common combinations are bleach and tile cleaner and bleach and ammonia. Always take a drug or use a chemical in a well-lighted area. Taking drugs in a dimly lit room increases the chance of error.
- Teach patients to take all of their prescription medications. If for any reason medications are left over, they should be destroyed—for example, by flushing them down the toilet. Tossing a bottle of pills in the garbage or even opening the bottle and tossing loose pills in the garbage increases the likelihood of accidental overdose/poisoning. Also, patients are taught to discard old medications. Do not save any for a "next time."
- Teach individuals what is proper first aid after a drug overdose/poisoning. Call poison centers or nearby hospitals or clinics immediately when a poisoning is suspected. The patient with the empty container of pills or chemicals is transported to the nearest emergency department. If transportation must be delayed, the nearest hospital is called to determine immediate first aid. First aid may be either to induce vomiting or to give milk, depending on the substance consumed.

EVALUATION

- Evaluate the patient's vital signs often during the acute overdose/poisoning episode. If the poisoning is severe, the patient is placed in an intensive care setting until the poisonous substance is eliminated or the acute symptoms are brought under control.
- Evaluate the effectiveness of the antidote.
- Evaluate the safety of the home environment, particularly when children have consumed poisonous substances. Work with parents to identify unsafe products. Teach them to store these products in a locked cabinet.

The bibliography for this chapter can be found in Appendix B, which begins on page 1054.

CHAPTER REVIEW QUESTIONS*

1. Toxicology is concerned with all of the following *except*:
   a. Drugs used in therapy.
   b. Environmental pollution.
   c. Industrial waste.
   d. Safety-related injuries.

2. Which of the following statements is *true* regarding the adverse effects of drug therapy?
   a. Pharmacologic products should be tested to ensure that there are no risks involved.
   b. Toxic effects will occur in all persons given sufficient dosage.
   c. Drug allergies and hypersensitivity reactions are effects that can be predicted.
   d. Adverse reactions to drugs usually take only minutes to manifest.

3. Adverse reactions are more likely to occur in:
   a. Male patients.
   b. Very young patients.

   c. Patients with nerve damage.
   d. Patients with renal dysfunction.

4. Which of the following is an example of primary drug reaction?
   a. Excessive drowsiness from antihistamines.
   b. Impotence from antihypertensives.
   c. Excessive lethargy from sedative.
   d. Extreme agitation from bronchodilators.

5. Which of the following is an example of secondary drug reaction?
   a. Impotence from antihypertensives.
   b. Increased bleeding tendencies from anticoagulants.
   c. Hypotension from antihypertensives.
   d. Drowsiness from hypnotics.

6. Atopic reactions may result from:
   a. Lysis of target cells.
   b. IgM antibodies attached to mast cells.
   c. Contact with lymphokine.
   d. IgA deficiency.

*See Appendix A, which begins on page 1051, for answers.

POISONING

Case Study 1: Isoniazid

An 8-year-old girl is admitted to the emergency room with persistent seizures. Her parents state the seizures started about 1 hour ago. History reveals the child's grandfather contracted pulmonary tuberculosis (TB). The child is currently taking prophylactic isoniazid (INH). The mother relates the child complained of numbness and tingling in the extremities for 2 or 3 days prior to onset of seizure activity. Multiple doses of intravenous diazepam (Valium) fail to control the seizures. The patient's temperature is normal.

1. What significance could her drug history have for her seizure activity?
2. Considering the side effects of isoniazid, what additional assessments should the nurse make?
3. What implications does isoniazid have for the administration of diazepam?
4. What is the best course of immediate action for this patient?
5. What teaching should be included in the nurse's discharge plan?

Case Study 2: Lead poisoning

A 50-year-old patient comes to the clinic with abdominal pain and weakness of one month's duration. The pain is fairly constant and cramping, but not associated with meals. His hemoglobin and hematocrit are normal. However, the patient relates a 4-pound weight loss and anorexia. Suspecting an ulcer, the nurse practitioner prescribes cimetidine (Tagamet) and requests that the patient return in 1 week. At the follow-up visit, the man states the pain is worse. Abdominal examination is unremarkable. However the patient's hemoglobin and hematocrit are now reduced, and he complains of weakness in his hands. Psychosocial assessment reveals the patient is an auto-mechanic and repairs radiators.

1. What data would indicate a need to revise the diagnosis of peptic ulcer?
2. Why is the patient's occupation important in determining the cause of his symptoms?
3. What is the most appropriate therapy for this man considering the revised diagnosis?
4. What teaching needs to be done with this patient?

BIOPSYCHOSOCIAL CONSIDERATIONS FOR DRUG THERAPY

Pharmacotherapeutics for the Neonate and the Pediatric Patient

Janet M. Brucker, MS, RN, CNRN
Kelly D. Wallin, MS, RN, C

CHAPTER OUTLINE

Pharmacokinetic Implications for the Pediatric Patient
Dose Calculations
Using the Nursing Process for the Pediatric Patient

TABLES
Nursing Process

KEY TERMS

Bilirubin
Hypertonic solution
Hypotonic solution
Isotonic solution
Kernicterus

LEARNING OBJECTIVES

After reading this chapter, the student will be able to:

1. Identify physiologic differences of neonates and children affecting the pharmacokinetic phases of drug administration.
2. Assess the neonate and pediatric patient to develop a database using principles of growth and development.
3. Plan nursing interventions that are appropriate for drug administration to the neonate and pediatric patient.
4. Evaluate the effectiveness of medications in patients of various ages.
5. Choose appropriate teaching strategies to gain pediatric patient compliance.

The neonatal-pediatric nurse faces the challenge of managing human responses within a changing tapestry of anatomic, physiologic, and psychosocial variations. With patients ranging in age from 24 weeks gestation (14 weeks premature) to 18 years and older, optimal nursing care and patient outcomes can be achieved only through an awareness of the developmental phenomena affecting the responses of infants and children to health problems.

From a pharmacotherapeutic perspective, developmental variations clearly indicate that a child should not be treated simply as a smaller version of an adult. There are differences between children of different ages in the ways in which they absorb, distribute, metabolize, and excrete drugs. Dosages and administration techniques vary among age groups—tiny amounts of medication to be administered amid diminutive physical characteristics such

as veins require ingenuity and versatility on the part of health care professionals. Children may respond to drugs much more quickly and dramatically than adults do. Compounding the challenge is the fact that, for most drugs, there exists little research-based information related to their safety and efficacy in children.

PHARMACOKINETIC IMPLICATIONS FOR THE PEDIATRIC PATIENT

Children's response to drugs varies dramatically between the neonatal, infant, younger childhood, and adolescent periods. Normal processes of growth and development bring about physiologic alterations in each of the pharmacokinetic processes of absorption, distribution, biotransformation (metabolism), and excretion. These alterations are taken into consideration when managing drug therapy for the infant and child.

DRUG ABSORPTION

Several maturational factors affect the absorption process. Gastric emptying is variable and therefore unreliable, especially in infancy. In neonates, a drug administered orally or via gastric tube normally remains in the stomach less than 3 hours, whereas in older infants and children, gastric emptying normally takes up to 6 hours. Therefore, a drug that is absorbed in the stomach normally has a therapeutic effect in neonates that is diminished in comparison to that seen in older infants given an equivalent dose for body weight. Consequently, there may be a more rapid and increased therapeutic response to intestinally absorbed drugs in neonates than in older children due to the drug reaching the intestine more quickly. Throughout the first week following birth, gastric acidity is increased; the acidity then decreases after one week and reaches adult normal levels by 6 to 9 months.

▼ CLINICAL ALERT

Gastric acidity is considered when administering drugs to the newborn, because many drugs are either deactivated or enhanced by a lower gastric pH. Other factors affecting absorption of orally administered drugs in the infant and child under 2 years of age include increased intestinal length compared to body length, rapid and unpredictable peristalsis, and frequent eating patterns coupled with a diet high in milk, which may inhibit gastric absorption.

Absorption of drugs administered topically and intramuscularly also varies with respect to age group. Certainly, the smaller the muscle size, the less volume capacity and absorptive surface exists for absorption of the intramuscular (IM) injection. In neonates, blood flow and tissue perfusion of muscles are immature, thereby increasing the obstacles to absorption of IM drugs. Topically applied medications may be absorbed in greater amounts in infants because of their thinner stratum corneum (the outer layer of skin), potentially resulting in systemic rather than localized responses. Because the skin of infants and children is more alkaline than acidic, they are more prone to skin infections (skin acidity acts as a bactericide). This alkalinity promotes more frequent use of topical medications to prevent or treat skin infections until skin pH normalizes after puberty.

DRUG DISTRIBUTION

Age also affects distribution to target tissues after the drugs are absorbed. Because children have a higher proportion of total body fluids for body weight than adults

(from 85% in the premature infant to 60% in the adult), they have a greater fluid volume in which the drug is distributed. This may result in decreased serum drug distribution due to dilution. In addition, a greater proportion of children's fluids are found in the extracellular space (60% of total body fluids in the premature infant compared to 40% in the adult). The younger the individual, the more rapidly extracellular fluid (ECF) is exchanged. Therefore, because most drugs are distributed primarily to the ECF in infants and children, the drug is eliminated rapidly. This, in combination with the higher volume of distribution in younger patients, may require increased dosages to maintain therapeutic drug levels. As the infant or child matures, these doses must then be adjusted.

Plasma protein levels also contribute to variations in drug distribution in infants and children. The lower serum albumin concentration in neonates offers fewer protein-binding sites for drugs, resulting in higher serum levels of unbound, active drug. Although the higher serum level may lead to increased clearance and subsequent decreased half-life, it may also result in increased toxicity. This is because the pharmacologic effect in the patient is achieved by the unbound drug particles. For example, when a total serum drug level of 10 mg/L is reported in a child (90% of which is protein bound, leaving an unbound active level of 1.0 mg/L), the same total serum level in a neonate consists of an active level of 3.0 mg/L. This occurs because neonates have less protein-binding capacity than older children. Because of the higher proportion of drug in the unbound state, neonates are at a higher risk for development of toxic side effects. To adjust for this maturational difference, the neonatal dosage of a particular drug may need to be decreased while the dosing frequency is increased.

Drug management may be further complicated by conditions such as hyperbilirubinemia, in which *bilirubin* (bile pigment produced by hemoglobin degeneration) competes with drugs for available protein-binding sites. If hyperbilirubinemia is present, drugs with weak binding power may lead to toxic unbound levels. Conversely, drugs with stronger binding power may displace bilirubin from binding sites and increase the risk of *kernicterus*, a condition in infants in which bilirubin infiltrates the brain and spinal cord. Close monitoring of neonates for therapeutic versus toxic responses to medications is clearly needed.

DRUG BIOTRANSFORMATION/ METABOLISM

The process of biotransformation (metabolism) also functions variably with age. Hepatic function is immature in neonates. Maturation is characterized by a sudden increase in metabolic rate at 2 to 3 weeks of age followed by a more gradual continued increase. The metabolic rate continues to increase until it peaks at 24 months, then decreases as the child matures. The relatively low metabolic rate of neonates can result in a drug's prolonged half-life and therapeutic effect. Consequently, doses and dosing frequencies should be adjusted accordingly until the metabolic "spurt" occurs a few weeks after birth. Failure to do so has been associated with the so-called gray baby syndrome, which is characterized by cardiovascular collapse and cyanosis associated with administration of certain drugs.

Metabolism of drugs is also affected by temperature regulation which, in infants and younger children, is unstable and subject to dramatic fluctuations. The increase or decrease in metabolic rate subsequent to temperature variations results in alterations in drug half-life and duration of therapeutic effect.

DRUG EXCRETION

Maturational features also affect the excretion of drugs. Full-term neonates have only 30% of the glomerular filtration rate and tubular secretion capacity of the adult. Premature infants have only 15% of the renal capacity of the adult kidney. Renal function increases until, at 6 to 12 months, it equals that of the adult. Of that increase, 50% occurs between birth and 3 weeks of age. Slower clearance through the kidneys may result in increased drug half-life by allowing accumulation of those drugs that are primarily dependent on renal excretion (like the penicillins and aminoglycosides). Generally, by the time infants reach 5 weeks of age, the standard pediatric doses may be given. However, ongoing measurement of serum concentrations of those drugs that have a propensity for toxicity is an important means of managing drug therapy in infants and children.

In conclusion, rapid physiologic changes that occur, especially in the first year of life, demand vigilance in assessing and managing the responses of neonates and pediatric patients to pharmacologic intervention.

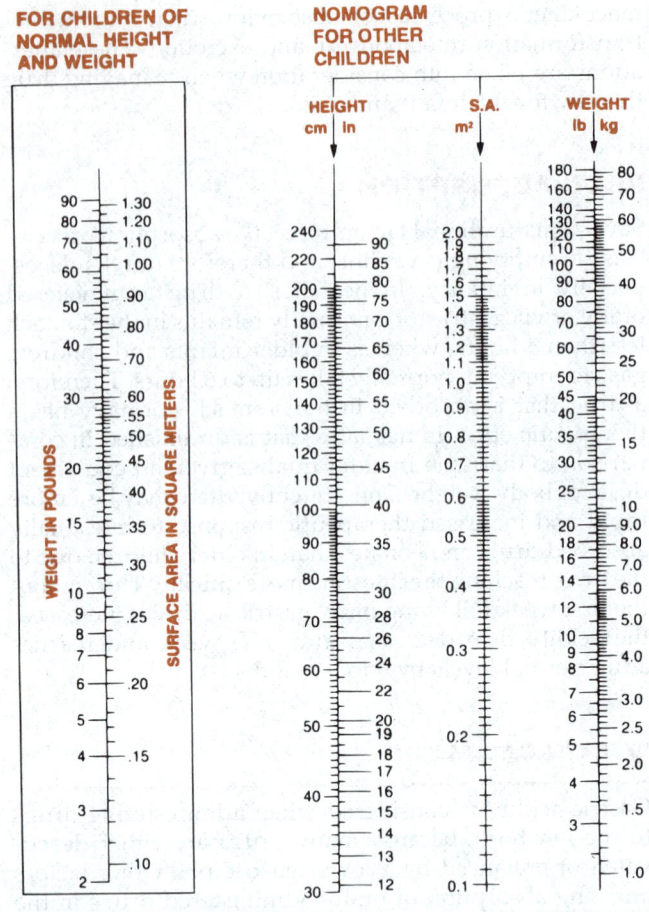

Figure 7–1. West's nomogram. Plot child's height and weight; draw a line between the two points. The point where the line intersects the surface-area line is the child's surface area.

DOSE CALCULATIONS

In light of the changing physiology of the neonate and pediatric patient, pediatric drug dosages are not as readily available in the medication manuals as are the dosages for adult patients. The dosage for each drug prescribed must be individually calculated at the time of prescription and must take into consideration the child's age and physiological characteristics. Several formulas are available that combine such factors as age, height, weight, body surface area (BSA), and normal adult dose to reach the dosage that will most effectively achieve the desired therapeutic response in children.

Several formulas have been developed over the years to estimate pediatric dosages based on the adult dosage in combination with the child's weight (Clark's rule), the child's age in months (Fried's rule), and the child's age in years (Young's rule). Formulas based on a child's age assume, inaccurately, that all children have the same height, weight, and physiology at the same age. These assumptions make the formulas too imprecise for determining pediatric dosages, especially the minute dosages required for newborns and infants.

Another method is the calculation of dosages as a ratio of milligrams of medication per kilogram of body weight of the child. This is a simple means of dosage determi-

nation, and many medication manuals are published with dosages expressed in this way. However, this method is not ideal, because it does not consider maturational factors.

A more reliable dosage calculation method uses the BSA of the child, as BSA correlates more closely with the physiologic functions of the child than does age or weight. BSA is determined by plotting the child's height and weight on a nomogram, shown in Figure 7–1. A line is drawn between the two points. The point at which the line intersects the surface area is the child's BSA. The dosage formula is as follows:

$$\frac{BSA}{1.7} \times \text{adult dose} = \text{Pediatric dose}$$

It is evident that accurate and readily available documentation of height, weight, and BSA is important for precise calculation of pediatric dosages. Measurement of these factors should, therefore, be a high priority when admitting a neonate or pediatric patient and at regular intervals thereafter. It is wise to remember that most drugs are basically poisons and are safe only when administered in the correct dosage to reach the desired serum drug concentration.

Table 7–1. NURSING PROCESS FOR THE PEDIATRIC CLIENT

Assessment

Measure height, weight for calculation of body surface area/drug dosage.
Note developmental level.
Ascertain medication history, current drugs/dosage, length of treatment, drug form/route of administration, presence of side effects, allergies.
Evaluate family finances/ability to afford required therapy.

Nursing Diagnosis: Risk for Aspiration

RELATED TO: Inadequate swallowing and gag reflex.

Desired Outcomes/Evaluation Criteria

Swallows medication without choking.

Nursing Actions	Rationale
Choose form of oral drugs appropriate to developmental level.	Infant's tongue thrusts forward, pushing object out of the mouth, when it is touched. (Extrusion reflex, present from birth to age four months). Toddlers resist the unknown and may struggle and scream when approached with medication.
Place small amounts of liquid medications in the side of the mouth or pocket of the cheek. Do not introduce more medication until the infant has completely swallowed.	
Crush tablets, open capsules, dependent on pharmacotherapeutics of the drug.	Making medication easier to take facilitates administration.
Provide drug in firm, matter-of-fact approach.	Usually effective in gaining child's cooperation. Forcing drug ingestion by holding patient's nose increases danger of aspiration.

Nursing Diagnosis: Risk for Poisoning

RELATED TO: Type of drug, dosage.
AS EVIDENCED BY: Route of administration and storage method.

Desired Outcomes/Evaluation Criteria

Demonstrates beneficial effects of medication with no untoward side effects. Parents identity potential hazards and formulate plan to reduce risk factors.

Nursing Actions	Rationale
Calculate drug dosage correctly and double-check before administering.	Prevents errors with subsequent over/under medication.
Verify identity of patient via parent/ identification bracelet.	Assures that medication is administered to the right patient.
Thoroughly shake suspensions before measuring.	Provides for uniformity in dosage.
Administer liquids via calibrated medication spoon/dropper.	Allows for precise measurement of dosage.
Administer IM injections considering blood flow and muscle mass.	Affects rate of drug absorption.
Apply topical medications with care.	Stratum corneum is thinner in infants, allowing greater absorption of drug and increasing risk of undesirable systemic response.
Maintain hydration according to size and age of child.	Development of dehydration can increase risk of toxicity in infants as drug becomes more concentrated in extracellular fluid.
Evaluate therapeutic effectiveness of medication, monitor serum drug levels if available.	May need to alter drug dosage/choice to achieve desired effects.
Note development of side effects.	Side effects of medications are often difficult to evaluate but may require changes in timing (i.e., with/without food) or discontinuation dependent on type/severity of reaction.
Monitor body temperature.	Fluctuations alter metabolic rate, affecting drug half-life and duration of therapeutic effect.
Review safety precautions with parents/ care provider, e.g., proper storage and use of medications, availability of ipecac syrup, provision of emergency phone numbers.	Prevents accidental ingestion of drug. Provides for rapid action if accident occurs.

Nursing Diagnosis: Knowledge Deficit

RELATED TO: Lack of exposure/unfamiliarity of information resources.
AS EVIDENCED BY: Questions, verbalization of concerns.

Desired Outcomes/Evaluation Criteria

Verbalizes understanding of therapeutic regimen.

Nursing Actions	Rationale
Establish individual medication schedule based on drug absorption and feeding schedule.	Increases compliance in administering drug when schedule fits particular family's routine.

Continued on the following page

Table 7–1. NURSING PROCESS FOR THE PEDIATRIC CLIENT, *Continued*	
Nursing Actions	**Rationale**
Discuss timing of food, use of milk products, acidic liquids.	May prevent side effects, inactivation of drug.
Suggest combining crushed pills with jelly, applesauce, pudding, not liquids.	Powder often does not dissolve and a grainy residue remains in cup, reducing dosage delivered.
Recommend following drug with water, oral hygiene as indicated.	Clears drug and possible aftertaste, reduces potential for adverse dental effects.
Stress importance of continuing drug until completed or discontinued by physician.	Promotes optimal effect of medication.
Refer to social services as indicated.	May require financial assistance.

Other Suggested Nursing Diagnoses: Anxiety, Pain, and Risk for Fluid Volume Excess or Deficit.

USING THE NURSING PROCESS FOR THE PEDIATRIC PATIENT

ASSESSMENT

The nursing process begins with a comprehensive assessment of the patient that includes physical, developmental, and social factors, as shown in Table 7–1.

- **Obtain a physical assessment,** including measurement of height and weight because dosages will be calculated according to these parameters. Any physical handicaps that might affect the nurse's approach to medication administration and ongoing management should be noted. A comprehensive medication history is obtained from the care provider.
- **Obtain a developmental assessment,** which reveals the capabilities of the child. Growth and development have a predictable pattern that all children follow, cephalocaudal (head to toe) and proximodistal (near to far). Each child has his or her own individual schedule for reaching each developmental milestone. Knowledge of growth and development facilitates implementation of nursing actions and assists with predicting the child's response to those actions.
- **Obtain a social assessment,** including evaluation of the responses of the child and the family to their environment. It is important to remember that the child is never to be assessed in isolation but within the context of the family. The presence and effectiveness of family support systems and the nature of the child-parent relationship are integral components of the child's social well-being. Therefore, many of the data obtained from the assessment of the pediatric patient also include information concerning the parents and other family members.

    Children experience painful procedures and stress-provoking situations in the provision of well-child care as well as in management of acute or chronic illnesses. For this reason, children frequently develop a negative attitude toward health-care procedures. This may be exacerbated when parental anxiety, which is usually increased when a child is ill, is unknowingly transmitted. By reducing stressors such as pain and including a supportive parent in the treatment plan, the child's negative responses may be decreased.
- Assess the child's medication history. Ask the parent what drugs the child has received and why. Also ask about allergic reactions to medications.
- Assess the family's financial situation. Obtain help for them if needed.

NURSING DIAGNOSIS

Nursing diagnoses may be related to physical attributes of the child and/or psychosocial attributes that incorporate both the child and parents. Typical nursing diagnoses include Risk for Aspiration, Anxiety, Risk for Poisoning, and Knowledge Deficit (see Table 7–1).

PLANNING AND INTERVENTION

Data obtained during the nursing assessment are used in the development of nursing diagnoses and goals for the child (see Table 7–1). Because parents can have a significant impact on the emotional and psychological development of the child, involvement of the parents is an integral part of the nursing care plan.

General Guidelines

- Understand the action of the drug, correct dosage, and route of administration. If a unit dose is not available, determining the child's dose from the available form is a critical step in medication administration. It is at this point that medication errors frequently occur. Even the most conscientious nurse in a hectic pediatric unit can misplace a decimal point or calculate incorrectly. To ensure safety, calculations of drugs that bring about critical responses (e.g., aminophylline, digoxin, insulin, and morphine) are double-checked with another nurse prior to administration. Even a small error can be potentially lethal for the pediatric patient.
- Always properly identify the patient. In pediatrics, this often presents more of a challenge than in adult nursing. Infants are unable to identify themselves, young children may disavow their identity because they do not want the medication, and adolescents of-

ten find it fun to misidentify themselves to an adult authority figure. Therefore, the only acceptable means of identifying a pediatric patient is to check the identification bracelet and compare it to the medication record.

Administration Considerations

Oral Medications

The preferred route of administration of medication in the pediatric population is the oral route. This route is not always possible, however, because of malabsorption, vomiting, refusal, or severity of illness.

Children under the age of 5 years do not demonstrate the ability to swallow tablets and, for this reason, many pediatric drugs are available in liquid or chewable form. Medications that are supplied only in pill form may often be crushed and mixed with a palatable liquid for administration. It is important to determine if crushing the pill or tablet will interfere with the pharmacokinetics of the drug. If crushed, some enteric-coated pills are deactivated by the gastric acidity. Measurement of the dose is a potential problem with liquid preparations. Standardized medication spoons or oral syringes should be available for oral liquids. Parents are instructed not to use the household teaspoon because of variances of volume.

- Approach the child in a matter-of-fact manner. This usually results in his or her cooperation. If the child refuses to cooperate, the nurse must be firm and maintain control of the situation. Forcing a screaming child to swallow medication or pinching the nose is *never* an acceptable action and increases the risk of aspiration. Eliciting suggestions from the parents, who are familiar with what does and does not work with their child regarding medication administration, may be helpful.
- To administer liquid medication to an infant, small quantities of the liquid are directed toward the side of the mouth. Young infants may swallow the medication more readily if a nipple is placed in their mouth after medication administration. The use of the nipple to administer a drug is controversial because the infant may associate the nipple with medication and begin to refuse feeds.
- The Committee on Drugs of the American Academy of Pediatrics documents concern over undesirable effects such as neuronal dysfunction and hypoglycemia associated with ethanol-containing (i.e., alcohol-containing) liquid preparations. The committee, therefore, recommends that liquid preparations containing ethanol not be used in the pediatric population.

Eye, Ear, and Nose Medications

In administering eye, ear, or nose drops, restraint may be necessary for infants or children who do not cooperate.

- When administering eye drops, place the child in a supine position. Rest the heel of the hand on the child's forehead while holding the dropper with the forefinger and thumb. This is not only a safety precaution, but it also allows the nurse to move with the child and ensure that the medication goes into the child's eye and not onto the face. Gently separate the eyelids with the thumb and the index finger of the opposite hand, and place the medication along the conjunctiva of the lower lid. To prevent contamination of the remaining medication, the dropper or tip of the ointment tube should not touch any part of the eyelid.
- To administer ear drops, restrain the child with his or her head turned to the appropriate side. For children under three years of age, the pinna of the ear is pulled downward and back. Over three years of age, the pinna is pulled upward and back, as for adults. The child should remain in this position for a few minutes after instillation. Cotton placed in the ear must be loose enough to allow discharge of any drainage.
- Nose drops are instilled in the same manner as adults, with the head extending over the edge of the bed or examining table. The child should remain in this position for at least 1 minute following instillation.

Rectal Medications

- Lubricate the suppository with a water-soluble lubricant and insert beyond the rectal sphincter with a gloved index finger. The fifth finger is used for a child under age three. To prevent expulsion of the suppository, hold the buttocks together for several minutes.
- Absorption of rectal medication is not reliable in the child whose colon is packed with stool or in the child with active diarrhea.

Intramuscular Injections

- To determine proper injection sites for children, consult Table 7–2. In infants, their small muscle mass limits the choice of injection sites. The gluteus is not used in infants because it is small and the sciatic nerve is close to the muscle. The vastus lateralis is the first muscle of choice because it is well developed and does not have major nerves and blood vessels. The rectus femoris may be used as an alternative site or for rotating injection sites. It is a large muscle that promotes medication absorption. Both muscles are pinched firmly between the thumb and forefinger of one hand and the needle inserted at a 90° angle with the other hand. Using this method ensures that medication is instilled directly into the muscle without hitting the femur. When using the vastus lateralis in infants with small muscles, the needle may be inserted at a 45° angle toward the knee to keep the needle tip within the muscle. A maximum of 1.0 mL is given in this age group (a small muscle may tolerate only 0.5 mL). Even infants need to be restrained firmly by holding the knee down because they will react to the pain of the injection by trying to move their leg. After injection is completed, the child should be held and cuddled, preferably by the parents.
- The same muscles can be used for toddlers. The dorsogluteal muscle may be used once the child has been

Table 7–2. INTRAMUSCULAR INJECTION SITES

Age Group	Site	Needle Length	Needle Gauge	Max Sol
Infant	Vastus lateralis	⅝ in	25–27	1 mL
	Rectus femoris	⅝ in	25–27	1 mL
Toddler	Vastus lateralis	1 in	22–23	1 mL
	Rectus femoris	1 in	22–23	1 mL
	Dorsogluteal	1 in	22–23	1 mL
Preschool	Same as toddler; can also use	1 in	22–23	1.5 mL
	ventrogluteal, deltoid	1 in	22–23	1.5 mL
		1 in	22–23	1 mL
School-age and adolescent	Same as preschool-age child	1–1½ in	22–23	2 mL

walking for 1 year. Toddlers usually demonstrate resistance; therefore, the nurse will need assistance in restraining the child. As with infants, toddlers should be held and comforted after the injection.

• In preschoolers, the ventrogluteal muscle and the deltoid muscles can be used in addition to the muscles used in toddlers. The ventrogluteal muscle is relatively free of blood vessels and nerves.

▼ **CLINICAL ALERT**

Because of lack of development, the deltoid muscle is usually not used for injections prior to age 3 to 4 years. In addition, the radial and ulnar nerves and the brachial artery, which lie along the humerus bone in the upper arm, can be injured. To inject the deltoid muscle, the needle is angled toward the shoulder and no more than 1.0 mL is injected. The deltoid muscle is relatively small but has a rapid absorption rate.

Preschoolers may be very vocal and verbally lash out, in addition to physically kicking and hitting. Adequate restraint is required for preschoolers.

• The same muscles can be used in the school-aged child and the adolescent as are used in the adult.
• Assessment of the muscle size determines the needle size (1 to 1.5 inch), with no more than a 2.0 mL solution being administered in any one site. School-age children may show interest in the equipment, and they like to learn new words. Teaching them to use the word "syringe" rather than "needle" makes children feel important and may help to distract them during the injection. Many school-age children will need assistance by restraining, as they may forget their bravery once the needle is in the muscle. Adolescents generally react as adults.

Intravenous Medications

• When measuring intravenous (IV) doses, particularly for the neonate, the smallest hypodermic syringe available for the volume to be drawn up should be used to ensure that the dosage is accurate. Consid-

eration should be given to avoiding administration of drug located in the syringe dead space (hub and needle), especially in infants and young children. The potential for "dead space overdose" can be prevented by using the two-syringe method. This involves drawing the active drug up in one syringe and diluent into the second. The active drug is then transferred into the syringe of diluent and mixed, thus eliminating the potential of administering a higher dose than intended. A second method of preventing this potential problem is using syringes with permanently affixed hypodermic needles that have no dead space. Another potential source of measurement error exists when using drug preparations that result in a final dosage volume of less than 0.1 mL when the pediatric dose is measured. To ensure that measurement of such small volumes is precise, further dilution of the preparation is necessary to obtain a volume that is more easily measured and delivered.

• The common sites for IV infusions for infants and young children are shown in Figure 7–2. Scalp veins may be used in infants. These veins are covered with only a thin layer of subcutaneous tissue and are easily visualized. A small area of scalp is shaved to increase visualization and to allow tape to adhere to the scalp. It is preferable to insert the needle in the direction of venous flow, but it may be inserted in either direction, because scalp veins do not have valves.
• Veins in the feet, hands, and arms may also be used for IV infusions in infants and older children. If at all possible, avoid using the child's dominant hand or, in infants and young children, the thumb-sucking hand.
• Needle size is determined by the size of the vein and the solutions to be administered. Usually 21- to 27-gauge needles are used in neonates and children. Should blood products be administered at any time through the IV line, a 23-gauge needle or 24-gauge catheter is usually the smallest that can be used without damage to blood cells.
• Continuous IV infusions in pediatric patients should have in-line volume-control chambers (e.g., Volutrol or Soluset) and be controlled by infusion pumps. A volume-control chamber is a safety precaution to pre-

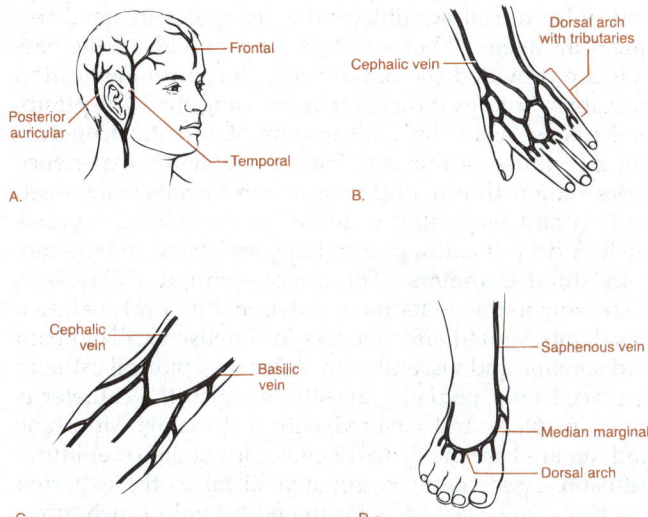

Figure 7–2. Vascular access sites in the neonate and pediatric patient. (A) Scalp. (B) Hand. (C) Antecubital fossa. (D) Foot.

vent accidental fluid overload. No more than 1 to 2 hours' worth of solution should be placed in the chamber at any one time. Medications may be added to the fluid chamber if they are compatible with the primary solution. If the medication is not compatible, it is mixed with a compatible solution and piggy-backed into the primary line. Following all drug infusions through the IV line, adequate amounts of fluid should be administered to flush the line, ensuring that all medication was administered.

The infusion pump ensures the accurate rate of infusion necessary to maintain the precise fluid balance needed in infants and children. Microinfusion and autosyringe pumps are available for delivery of small volumes of fluid and medications. These pumps are primarily used for the absolute control of delivery needed in neonates and infants. Autosyringe pumps are beneficial for controlled administration of particular drugs via heparin lock to avoid fluid overload due to unnecessary diluent or flush. Microinfusion pumps deliver fluid in micromilliliter increments and have safeguard mechanisms that prevent free flow of fluid and infusion of air.

- The four primary modes of intravenous medication administration for the pediatric patient are as follows: (1) intravenous push (IVP), (2) intravenous piggy-back (IVPB), (3) syringe pump, and (4) retrograde. The IVPB (or IV Soluset) method is generally safer than IVP for pediatric patients, because the drug is diluted and uses a slower infusion rate. However, it may require that more fluid be given than the fluid-restricted or neonatal patient can tolerate. In these cases, the syringe pump or careful IVP (with drugs that can be pushed) may be the method of choice. The retrograde method of drug administration refers to a system that incorporates a three-way stopcock within the intravenous line. Medication is administered in the line distal to the stopcock (away from the patient), and a syringe of equal amount of intravenous fluid is removed and discarded to maintain fluid balance.

The rate of flow should be calculated to infuse within a 30-minute period. The advantage to this method is maintenance of strict fluid intake, which is especially important in neonates.

- All medications must be properly diluted and should approximate an isotonic solution. An *isotonic solution* has the same osmotic pressure as plasma (280 to 290 mOsm/L), so no fluid will shift into or out of the cells. A *hypertonic solution*, which has an osmotic pressure greater than plasma, causes a fluid shift from the intracellular fluid space to the extracellular fluid space, in addition to being irritating to the vein. A *hypotonic solution*, which has an osmotic pressure less than plasma, causes a shift of fluid movement into the cells. A large amount of diluent presents the danger of fluid overload. It is especially important when caring for neonatal and pediatric patients to know the minimum recommended medication dilution amounts.

Alternative Routes of Drug Administration

Ommaya Reservoir The Ommaya reservoir, for the pediatric population, provides a drug-delivery mechanism for direct infusions into cerebral circulation of chemotherapy agents for oncology patients; withdrawal of cerebral spinal fluid for diagnostic purposes; for antibiotic therapy; and for analgesia for intractable pain. The Ommaya reservoir is a dome-shaped device connected to a catheter that is surgically implanted into the lateral ventricle.

- Advantages to this mechanism include a decrease of patient discomfort during chemotherapy, in contrast to lumbar punctures for intrathecal medication administration. Studies indicate a better clearing of cancer cells with the use of the intraventricular route.
- Complications associated with the Ommaya reservoir include infection, a malfunctioning reservoir, tissue damage, and a potential for neurologic complication such as seizures.

Intraosseous Infusions Intravenous access may be difficult to impossible in compromised infants or young children during an emergency situation. For emergency fluid and drug administration for children 6 years of age and younger, the intraosseous route is well established in pediatric emergency medicine. This large vascular bed contained within bony walls remains accessible when peripheral vasoconstriction thwarts attempts to attain venous access.

- Intraosseous access is accomplished by placing a 15- or 18-gauge Jamshidi needle into the bone marrow space of the femur or tibia. This technique uses specific landmarks that facilitate insertion with little risk. Any drugs and fluids given intravenously may be administered intraosseously.
- The positive patient outcomes in an emergency situation occurring as a result of using the intraosseous route greatly outweigh the risk of potential for infection. The intraosseous infusion is not a long-term strategy, however, and should be discontinued as soon as intravascular access is obtained.

Special Considerations

Analgesia

Pain management in infants and children is an especially challenging nursing goal. Because so many myths exist regarding pain in children, inadequate pain management is a common finding. There is no reason to believe that the experience of pain is any different in children than in adults. However, studies comparing analgesia administration in adults and children have revealed that adults are medicated for pain anywhere from 3 to 26 times more often than are children with similar diagnoses and medical situations.

The first step toward adequate pain management lies with assessment. Assessment of pain in children is challenging because the nurse must identify and interpret indicators that may be very subtle in a patient with few expressive skills. Fortunately, several pain assessment tools for children exist, which make use of colors and drawings. However, the developmental level of the child should be considered when selecting the instrument. For example, lack of verbal communication skills in the age group from birth to 2 years prevents the use of subjective assessment tools. In this age group, observation of such behavior cues as vital sign changes and irritability is valuable as these are ways in which infants and small children reveal pain.

In terms of planning and intervention, anticipation and recognition of pain-producing situations should guide nursing judgment in determining when analgesia is needed in patients who cannot or will not report their pain. A medication ordered prn may be administered—by nursing order—around the clock to maintain adequate analgesic blood levels. Around-the-clock dosing is especially important for the fresh postoperative or severely injured child. Scheduling the administration of analgesics at times of patient activities such as vital sign assessment, coughing and deep breathing, or ambulation ensures compliance during difficult procedures and provides comfort for the child.

▼ **CLINICAL ALERT**

Studies demonstrate that meperidine (Demerol), which is frequently used for pain control in the pediatric patient, may be ineffective for ongoing pain management. With regular dosing of meperidine, a metabolite called normeperidine is produced. Normeperidine occupies receptor sites for 18 to 30 hours. This occupation prevents the active drug from providing pain relief. The buildup of normeperidine causes central nervous system irritability, tremors, and (in some patients) seizures. Meperidine is also painful when injected. It is, therefore, recommended that meperidine be used for single-dose situations and not for postoperative or long-term pain.

Patient Controlled Analgesia Patient-controlled analgesia (PCA), a modality used extensively with adults, is also an effective method for controlling pain in the pediatric patient. The method permits patients 7 years of age and older to self-administer the analgesics in small frequent intravenous boluses. In younger children, the parents are provided the opportunity to control medication infusions. Studies indicate that by using the PCA pump, patients use a smaller total amount of narcotic drug during the course of therapy. Patients evidently experience less sedation, thus maintaining a more normal wake-sleep pattern and the ability to follow postoperative routines such as deep breathing, coughing, and early ambulation.

Epidural Catheters The use of epidural analgesia in increasing in the pediatric population. Epidural analgesia has demonstrated effectiveness for intense localized pain and somatic and visceral pain. After the epidural catheter is placed by a pediatric anesthesiologist, the catheter is taped in place and covered with a dressing. Morphine and fentanyl are the drugs of choice for pediatric epidural infusion. Assessment is initiated distal to the expected level of analgesia and is evaluated by light touch, pressure, or temperature. Potential complications related to medication infusion include respiratory depression, pruritus, urinary retention, and nausea and vomiting. Epidural catheter complications include epidural hematoma, arachnoiditis, neuritis, and spinal headache.

Emergency Situations

Management of infants and children in emergency situations is enhanced when the nurse is prepared in advance for the unique pharmacotherapeutic aspects of pediatric-neonatal resuscitation. Advance planning for an acute-care setting should include preparation of an emergency medication worksheet for those patients at higher risk for cardiopulmonary or respiratory arrest. This sheet might list, for each individual patient, the resuscitation drugs to be used and the appropriate dose to be given calculated from the patient's weight or BSA. Figure 7–3 is an example of such a worksheet. When such an emergency medication worksheet is posted on the patient's bed or in the chart, it permits rapid and accurate drug management by all members of the health-care team.

Some differences exist between the emergency pharmacologic management of the infant and child compared to that of the adult, and also between neonates and older children. The intraosseous route for drug administration is recommended for emergency vascular access in infants and children under the age of 6 years when venous access is unattainable within the first few minutes of resuscitation. Special implications relate to the use of sodium bicarbonate, calcium, and atropine in the resuscitation of infants and children. Sodium bicarbonate should be given only to correct documented metabolic acidosis, and when given to neonates, should be diluted to a 4.2% solution (0.5 mEq/mL) to prevent intraventricular hemorrhage. Atropine has not been found to be effective in treating bradycardia in the neonate; therefore, epinephrine is the drug of choice for asystole and bradycardia in the neonatal population. Calcium is indicated only for documented hypocalcemia.

Glucose is an important resuscitation drug for infants and children. Infants and small children have limited glycogen stores, which are rapidly depleted during stress. The resultant hypoglycemia inhibits the metabolic processes of vital organs and thus impedes resuscitation ef-

Name _____

Age _____ Diagnosis _____

Weight _____

Height _____ BSA _____

ET tube size _____ Date intubated _____

MEDICATION	USUAL DOSE	PATIENT'S DOSE (in mg)	PATIENT'S DOSE (in ml)
Adenosine (3 mg/ml)	50 μg/kg IV push over 1–2 sec; increase dose in 50 μg/kg increments q 2 min until return of sinus rhythm. Maximum dose 250 μg/kg. Flush with saline immediately. *Do Not Give ET.*		
Atropine (0.1 mg/ml)	0.01–0.03 mg/kg/dose IV over 1 min. Dose may be repeated q 10–15 min. Minimum dose 0.1 mg; maximum dose 0.04 mg/kg in children, 1 mg in adolescents. ET—Give increased dose.		
Ca Chloride 10% (100 mg/ml)	20 mg/kg/dose (0.2 ml/kg) q 10 min. *Do Not Give ET.*		
Dextrose 50% (0.5 g/ml)	0.5–1 g/kg. May repeat in 10–15 min.		
Dobutamine 12.5 mg/ml)	2–25 μg/kg/min. Prepare infusion in normal saline or D$_5$W.	Initial Rate = _____ Initial Dose = _____	Initial Rate = _____ Initial Dose = _____
Dopamine (40 mg/ml)	0.5–20 μg/kg/min. Prepare infusion in normal saline or D$_5$W.	Initial Rate = _____ Initial Dose =_____	Initial Rate = _____ Initial Dose =_____
Epinephrine for asystole and pulseless arrest	First dose—0.1 mg/kg (1:10,000 = 0.1 mg/ml) IV or IO (intraosseous); or 0.1 mg/kg (1:10,000 = 1 mg/ml) ET. Second dose and subsequent doses—0.1–0.03 mg/kg (1:1000 = 1 mg/ml) IV, IO, or ET. Doses up to 0.2 mg/kg of 1:1000 (1 mg/ml) may be effective. Repeat q 3–5 min.		
Epinephrine for bradycardia	0.01 mg/kg (1:10,000 = 0.1 mg/ml) IV or IO; or 0.1 mg/kg (1:1000) = 1 mg/ml) ET. Repeat q 5–10 min at same dose.		
Epinephrine infusion	Initial—0.1 μg/kg/min. Prepare infusion in normal saline or D$_5$W.	Initial Rate = _____ Initial Dose = _____	Initial Rate = _____ Initial Dose = _____
Isoproterenol (0.2 mg/ml)	0.05–0.5 μg/kg/min continuous IV infusion. Maximum dose 2 μg/kg/min.	Initial Rate = _____ Initial Dose = _____	Initial Rate = _____ Initial Dose = _____
Lidocaine 2% (20 mg/ml)	0.5–1 mg/kg/dose IV push over 5 min. May repeat in 10 min. Maximum bolus dose 5 mg/kg. Maintenance IV infusion—10–50 μg/kg/min. ET–Give increased dose.		
Naloxone (0.4 mg/ml)	Birth to 5 yr or weighing ≤20 kg—0.1–0.2 mg/kg IV, IM, or ET. > 5 years or weighing >20 kg—2 mg. May repeat in 3–5 min if no response.		
Sodium bicarbonate (1 mEq/ml)	1–2 mEq/kg/dose (1 ml/kg) IV push over 2 min or IO. *Do Not Give ET.*		
Succinylcholine (20 mg/ml)	1–2 mg/kg/dose. (*Give atropine first.*) Maintenance dose—0.3–0.6 mg/kg/dose q 5–10 min.		

Formula for infusions:

$$\frac{6 \times \text{pt. wt. (kg)} \times \text{desired dose (μg/kg/min)}}{\text{desired fluid rate (ml/min)}} = \text{mg of drug per 100 ml NS}$$

Figure 7–3. Emergency medication worksheet.

forts. Therefore, during resuscitation, the patient should be checked for hypoglycemia via a rapid bedside test (e.g., Chemstrip), and, if hypoglycemia is present, glucose should be administered. Because glucose is supplied as $D_{50}W$, it should be diluted with sterile water to at least a 25% solution ($D_{25}W$) before administering. Because $D_{25}W$ is hyperosmolar, care should be taken (1) to administer via a central line, if possible, to prevent peripheral venous irritation and (2) to monitor repeated administrations carefully to prevent a hyperosmolar state.

To speed delivery of all emergency drugs into the central circulation, intravascular and intraosseous lines should be flushed with 1 to 2 mL of normal saline in infants and 5 mL in older children.

Patient/Parent Teaching

- Identify to whom the teaching is to be directed. It is important to establish who the primary caregiver will be. Never assume that the parent who stays with the child in the hospital, or the parent who brings the child to the physician's office, is the person who is responsible for giving the medications in the home. Many children have medication regimens with drug administration times that occur while they are attending day-care centers or schools or while they are with baby-sitters or visiting a grandparent. When teaching the primary caregiver about the medication regimen, emphasize that all persons administering the drug must understand the importance of maintaining the medication schedule and must know the side effects to watch for.

- Obtain patient/parent compliance, which should be considered when teaching parents and families. Parents frequently stop a medication when the child's symptoms can no longer be seen. Emphasize the importance of continuing the drug until it is gone or until the physician determines it is not necessary to continue. By demonstrating concern for the child rather than just asking about family finances, the nurse can ascertain if cost of the medication will influence compliance. A parent may not be able to afford the medication, which would indicate the need for social service assistance. A parent may not be aware of the long-term physical consequences of a disease and may not realize that mild symptoms currently being exhibited may significantly affect long-term outcomes. By incorporating information from the initial assessment (such as meal times and school hours), compliance can be enhanced by establishing medication times that are convenient to home routines.

- Monitor the patient's progress and understanding of teaching. Even simple directions may require repeat sessions to ensure sufficient understanding. Active listening is a vital key to managing the positive progression of instruction about the drug regimen.

- Present information at the appropriate developmental level to decrease the child's anxiety level. Using various forms of puppet play, art, and graphic and audiovisual materials enhances the child's participation and helps to promote a more receptive atmosphere to learning. Children and adolescents frequently develop inaccurate concepts regarding their medications. Providing and reinforcing accurate information pertaining to purpose and side effects increases compliance and encourages children and adolescents to develop a sense of control over what is happening to their bodies.

Toddlers and preschoolers should not be told about medication administration procedures until just before they are performed. This prevents unnecessary anxiety and fantasizing. Adolescents and school-age children should be informed ahead of time to allow them the opportunity to prepare themselves. Explanations should be honest such as, "yes, an injection hurts for a short time." Reassuring children that "it is okay to cry, but it is very important to hold still" is helpful. Do not let children prolong the procedure by disruptive behavior. Medical interventions should not be used as a threat to correct behavior. Children who have been adequately prepared for a painful or difficult procedure tolerate the situation with decreased stress and anxiety. The instructional sessions should be directed to the immediate treatment and subsequently reinforced. Instruction must be provided to the parents as well as the children. When the parents have adequate and correct information, their actions will reinforce and support the teaching.

To help children view the parent as a source of comfort, parents should not be asked to help restrain their child for a painful procedure. If a child wishes the parents to be there, they should be allowed to stay, but only to give emotional support. Parents should be allowed to stand at the head of the bed where the child can see them and possibly hold their hands. Injection should never be given to a sleeping child without awakening him or her first, because the child may develop a fear of going to sleep. Allow children to view the procedure if they want to watch. Complete procedures as quickly as possible, as unnecessary delays only increase apprehension and anxiety. Give children an opportunity to express their feelings after the procedure and provide them with praise.

Medication Safety

Protection of the child from potentially fatal accidents is essential. The proper storage and use of medications is a simple safety precaution, but one that is not often practiced. Every year many children are treated for accidental ingestion of medications. Parents must be taught the following measures:

- Always replace childproof caps tightly on medicine bottles. These caps are not always an effective deterrent to a determined toddler, but may slow the child's progress in opening the bottle—this may give the parent time to intervene.

- In a home where there is a small child, store all medications in a locked container and hide the key. Placing drugs on a high shelf beyond the child's reach is not always a safe practice. Children watch their parents and remember where a good-tasting medication is stored. After children begin walking, they quickly learn to climb. They may open drawers to use as steps and maneuver chairs into a position that allows them to reach high shelves. Children may consume an entire bottle of pills before being found by a parent. Children also enjoy exploring a woman's purse that is within their reach. Many children are poisoned each year from the ingestion of birth control pills, diuretics, and antihypertensive drugs that were obtained from a purse.

- For emergency situations, keep the poison control telephone number (1-800-392-8548) available on all phones in the homes where children reside or frequently visit. Also, parents should also keep ipecac syrup, an emetic, in their home for accidental medication ingestion. The emetic is given if vomiting is not contraindicated. If given immediately, the emetic will prevent much of the medication from being absorbed by the child's body. The child should then be immediately taken to the emergency department to rule out systemic absorption.
- A medication in suspension must be shaken well before it is administered to ensure all the doses in the bottle are the same strength.
- Do not use household spoons to measure liquid medications. To ensure an accurate dose, always give liquid medications using a calibrated dropper or oral spoon.
- Do not crush or open capsules without discussing this with your child's physician.
- Administer the medication for the full time prescribed by the physician.

EVALUATION

During this phase, the nurse evaluates the effectiveness of the medications by assessing the patient's response. The data obtained during the initial assessment provide the baseline criteria for measuring therapeutic response.

- Evaluate effectiveness and toxicity in a number of ways. The effectiveness of drug therapy depends on the nurse's ability to assess and evaluate responses. For example, the degree of response to administration of furosemide (Lasix), a diuretic, is evaluated by accurate measurement of urinary output. For the asthmatic child, the response to the administration of theophylline, a bronchodilator, is evaluated by assessment of pulmonary status with an expected decrease in degree of wheezing.

  Frequently, the best method for evaluating therapeutic effectiveness is to obtain serum drug levels. However, because of individual and developmental limitations, many children do not demonstrate a positive response to a medication, even when their serum drug concentration is in the normal or above normal therapeutic range.
- Evaluate for the presence of side effects of medications. In the pediatric patient, this is often a difficult task. Infants not able to talk use crying and smiling as a means of communication. Young children often have difficulty expressing themselves due to their lack of vocabulary and lack of experience in knowing what is normal or abnormal. Assessment skills are extremely important for identifying the subtle changes that might occur with administration of potentially toxic drugs. For example, in the child receiving gentamicin (an ototoxic drug) the nurse may note the parents' concern that the child is not responding to them as the child did previously.
- Evaluate the child's pain. Infants and children do not pretend to have pain, so it is important to evaluate the child's complaints. Observe for signs such as a change in the sound of a cry or notice the child who is continuously crying. Vital signs also provide indicators of pain and therapeutic response in much the same way as they do for adults.

The bibliography for this chapter can be found in Appendix B, which begins on page 1054.

CHAPTER REVIEW QUESTIONS*

1. The physician orders morphine sulfate 0.8 mg IV push q 4 hr for abdominal pain for a one-year-old child. Administration should include all of the following *except:*
   a. Morphine sulfate is mixed in a compatible solution.
   b. IV line is flushed with adequate amount of fluid.
   c. Medication is drawn up in a 3-cc syringe.
   d. Two-syringe method is used to administer the medication.

2. The nurse recognizes the importance of adequate pain management for the pediatric patient. The most appropriate intervention for a young child includes:
   a. Using the pain assessment tool every 3 hours.
   b. Administering analgesics only at a parent's request.
   c. Administering analgesics infrequently because children counterfeit pain.
   d. Monitoring vital signs and behavior cues for discomfort.

3. Within 4 hours of admission, an emergency code was called for a young child whose IV had infiltrated. The child demonstrated symptoms of septic shock and respiratory depression. Which immediate intervention should the nurse anticipate?
   a. Assisting with intraosseous infusions of medications.
   b. Preparing the patient for immediate surgical intervention.
   c. Transferring the patient to the intensive care unit.
   d. Preparing to insert a nasogastric tube to decompress the stomach.

4. All of the following emergency pharmacologic interventions are appropriate for the pediatric patient *except:*
   a. Sodium bicarbonate should be administered to correct documented metabolic acidosis.
   b. Atropine is effective for treatment of bradycardia in the neonate.
   c. $D_{50}W$ should be diluted to $D_{25}W$ prior to administration.
   d. Calcium is indicated for documented hypocalcemia.

*See Appendix A, which begins on page 1051, for answers.

5. In the postoperative period, a one-year-old child is placed on intravenous gentamicin. The best criterion to use in evaluating the child's response to antibiotic therapy is:

   a. Therapeutic serum levels.
   b. Elevated urine output.
   c. Maintained normothermia.
   d. Elevated WBC count.

6. In teaching parents about medication safety and prevention of accidental ingestion of medications, the nurse might include all of the following information *except*:

   a. Use childproof caps, as they are effective in preventing ingestion errors.
   b. Store medications in a locked container and hide the key.
   c. Store medications in the mother's purse, because it is usually out of reach.
   d. Give liquid medications by a calibrated dropper or oral spoon.

CHAPTER 8

Drug Therapy and the Older Adult

Anne Marie Moraca-Sawicki, RN, MSN

KEY TERMS

Aged elderly	Lacrimation
Cardiotoxicity	Nephrotoxicity
Drug holiday	Polypharmacy
Extravasation	Tinnitus
Hangover	Vesicant
Homeostatic	

LEARNING OBJECTIVES

After reading this chapter, the student will be able to:

1. Discuss the normal physiologic changes of aging.
2. Describe how the physiologic changes of aging affect drug disposition in the body.
3. Explain how the age-related decreases in cardiac output and function affect other metabolic processes to alter drug disposition.
4. Discuss examples of how specific drugs may cause toxicity even when normal dosages are not exceeded.
5. Summarize necessary assessment data to obtain from older patients to formulate nursing diagnosis and to plan care with regard to a drug regimen.
6. List teaching strategies helpful in health-care teaching of older patients.
7. List types of assistive devices and aids and approaches available to help increase patient compliance with maintaining drug dosage schedules.

Older adults, those aged 65 and older, represent the fastest growing segment of the United States population. The average American will live to be 84 years old and suffer from three or more chronic diseases. Because cardiovascular disease is the number one cause of death, it is very likely that one disease this "average" American will have is a cardiovascular disorder. Other illnesses such as arthritis, cancer, respiratory disease, gastrointestinal disturbances, and sensory impairments are all associated with aging. Drug therapy is the primary mode of therapy in many illnesses. Those over age 65 constitute about 13% of the population; however, they consume about 30% of all prescription drugs. Eighty-six percent have a chronic health problem requiring medication and on average, elderly persons take four or more prescription drugs regularly, according to the U.S. Department of Health and Human Services. The elderly also consume the greatest number of over-the-counter drugs. Studies suggest up to 30% of older adults suffer adverse drug effects. Some studies have found 20% of hospitalizations of those over age 65 are due to the effects of prescription drugs. As a person ages, various anatomic and physiologic changes occur that are considered "normal." These changes can alter both therapeutic and adverse responses to drugs. Pathologic conditions can have an even greater effect on the patient's response to drugs.

DRUG THERAPY AND THE OLDER ADULT

Older adults are not a homogeneous group. Many older adults are healthy and are not major drug consumers. About 85% of older adults reside in their homes. The subgroups of elderly who are infirm, frail, the *aged elderly* (those 80 years and older), and the 15% who are residents of long-term care facilities are the primary consumers of medications. Several studies of medication-prescribing practices for residents of skilled-nursing-care facilities concluded that medications are overprescribed for the elderly. Often drug side effects are mistaken for signs of aging or illness. For example, lethargy may be caused by various tranquilizers; forgetfulness may be caused by barbiturates; confusion may be caused by several drugs including methyldopa, digoxin, or cimetidine; and weakness may be due to diuretic intake, which can deplete body potassium.

Drug therapy is one of the most important and often most risky components of patient care. Until recently, little has been done to identify the special needs of elderly patients relative to drug therapy. The surgeon general, along with the Public Health Service and Administration on Aging, has developed specific recommendations dealing with the elderly and health care, services, and medications. In the laws of the Omnibus Reconciliation Act of 1987 were new regulations on the use of psychotropic drugs, especially in nursing homes. Psychopathology is common in nursing home patients—studies show up to 94% have mental illness or developmental disability, and over 70% have dementias. Thus, use of psychotropic drugs (antipsychotics, antidepressants, anxiolytics, and hypnotics) in nursing home patients is common. However, recent studies show that these drugs are not always used appropriately or are overprescribed, contributing to patient falls and undesirable side effects and drug interactions.

These factors caused the Omnibus Budget Reconciliation Act (OBRA) to establish new regulations on the use of psychotropic drugs in nursing homes. The regulations went into effect in October 1990 to keep "each resident's drug regimen free from unnecessary drugs." They list drugs whose use is automatically considered inappropriate. Extended use of psychotropics or excessive dosages are monitored. Use of some drugs requires patient monitoring for tardive dyskinesia and periodic blood testing for drug level. Use of a psychotropic drug must be for the treatment of a diagnosis for which the drug is indicated and not merely for undesirable behaviors, such as pacing, fidgeting, or an uncooperative attitude. Also required by OBRA are dosage reductions, use of nondrug therapies like behavior modification, and *drug holidays* (skipping medication one day per week). Cardiac and anticonvulsant drugs are not included in drug holidays. Maximum dosages are listed in Table 8–1.

As an individual ages, there are gradual changes in the anatomy and physiology that may alter the therapeutic and toxic effects of drugs. Patients have the right to know about these and other significant aspects of drugs and their drug therapy so they can make informed choices regarding therapy. Patients do have the right to refuse a medication. To force a dose of medication upon an alert, cooperative patient constitutes battery. The nurse has a responsibility to act as patient advocate and provide ap-

Table 8–1. MAXIMUM DOSAGES OF SELECTED PSYCHOTROPIC DRUGS IN NURSING HOME PATIENTS ACCORDING TO OBRA		
Drug	**Usual Maximum Single Dose Age 12–65 Years**	**Usual Maximum Single Dose Age 65 and Older**
Antidepressants		
amitriptyline (Elavil)	300 mg	150 mg
desipramine (Norpramin)	300 mg	150 mg
imipramine (Tofranil)	300 mg	150 mg
nortnptyline (Aventyl)	150 mg	75 mg
trimipramine (Surmontil)	300 mg	150 mg
Anxiolytics		
chlordiazepoxide (Librium)	100 mg	40 mg
diazepam (Valium)	60 mg	20 mg
halazepam (Paxipam)	160 mg	80 mg
lorazepam (Ativan)	6 mg	3 mg
prazepam (Centrax)	60 mg	30 mg
Hypnotics*		
chloral hydrate (Noctec)	1,500 mg	750 mg
flurazepam HCL (Dalmane)	30 mg	15 mg
temazepam (Restoril)	30 mg	15 mg
triazolam (Halcion)	0.5 mg	0.25 mg

OBRA = Omnibus Budget Reconciliation Act of 1987.
*Use of hypnotic/sedative drugs beyond 7 days continuous use is considered unnecessary by OBRA unless special circumstances exist and are well documented (example: patient addicted and detoxification medically contraindicated).

Table 8–2. BILL OF RIGHTS FOR THE ELDERLY ON DRUG THERAPY

Right to take or not take medications.
Right to keep his or she faculties and not be chemically restrained.
Right to know what he or she is being medicated with and why.
Right to know the consequences of ingesting such chemicals into the body.
Right to express subjective response to drugs.
Right to have prescribed just enough of the drug needed for the ailment and not be made to buy more expensive drugs than necessary.
Right to use medicines he or she has purchased and not be coerced into buying a new supply of the same drug just because he or she is hospitalized or placed in a nursing home.
Right to take his or her own medications as long as he or she is capable and competent to do so.
Right to quality medicines at the least cost.
Right to nursing and medical caregivers getting at the root of his or her problems before medications are given.
Right to have medications prescribed, dispensed, administered, and evaluated by persons who have an up-to-date, broad yet specific, knowledge of geriatric pharmacology.

Source: Adapted from Alford DM: Bill of Rights for the elderly on drug therapy. Nurs Clin North Am 17:282, June 1982, with permission. Modified 1996.

propriate health teaching to all patients. Table 8–2, a bill of rights for the elderly on drug therapy, can serve as a model for nurse advocacy for older adults.

AGE-INDUCED BODY CHANGES AND THEIR EFFECT ON DRUG RESPONSE

Physiologic changes in the body that occur with aging include changes in body composition, cardiac function, GI function, hepatic function, renal function, and sensory and perceptual changes. These age-related body changes can alter a patient's response to medications.

CHANGES IN BODY COMPOSITION

As one ages, the relative proportions of fat, lean tissue, and water change. Total body mass and lean body mass tend to decrease with age while the proportion of body fat increases. There is a decrease in muscle mass and a loss of subcutaneous tissue. These changes in body composition vary from person to person; however, they definitely affect the relationship between a drug's concentration and solubility in the body. Because the normal aging process affects every body organ, every phase of drug pharmacokinetics in the body may be affected. Table 8–3 shows some examples of how aging can affect drug action.

Decreased lean body mass and water in the elderly contribute to undesired toxic drug effects. For example, a water-soluble drug such as gentamicin is distributed mostly to lean body tissue and aqueous parts of the body. Because the elderly have less lean tissue in which to distribute the drug, more drug remains in the bloodstream. This increased drug concentration can lead to gentamicin toxicity if dosage is not reduced. Measuring serum drug levels is important in determining dosages.

Just as changes in body composition may affect water-soluble drugs, they also may affect fat-soluble drugs. As the elderly body increases in fat composition, fat-soluble drugs are distributed to a greater volume of tissue. This initially results in lower drug concentration in the bloodstream. However, after body fat stores are saturated with a drug, it is slowly released back into the circulation. This results in increased duration of drug action. This phenomenon is a contributing factor in residual drowsiness caused by fat-soluble sleep medications the morning after drug ingestion, sometimes referred to as *hangover*. Other fat-soluble drugs such as chlorpromazine (Thorazine) and phenobarbital may have prolonged duration of action because of the increased fatty tissue available for drug distribution and storage.

The loss of subcutaneous tissue also affects the method and route of drug administration employed for the older patient. Loss of subcutaneous tissue occurs to a greater extent in the extremities than in the trunk of the body and especially on the dorsum of the hand. Special caution is needed to avoid excessive probing with the needle when using the blood vessels of the hand for intravenous injection. There is also a decline in the elastic fibers of the skin and vasculature which increases the risk of drug *extravasation* (leaking outside the vein). Thus, caution is observed when administering *vesicant* (damaging to tissues) drugs such as mechlorethamine (Mustargen), doxorubicin (Adriamycin), and vincristine (Oncovin).

CHANGES IN CARDIAC FUNCTION

As a person ages, myocardial contractile strength and efficiency decline. These age-associated changes are related to several factors: a decrease in cardiac muscle fiber, a reduction in mobilization of catecholamines, a decrease in amounts of adenosine triphosphate available in cardiac cells, and the inefficient utilization of oxygen. Between the third and eighth decade of life cardiac output can be reduced by up to 50%. Coronary artery blood flow also decreases and by age 60 is reduced by about 35%.

These normal cardiac changes may sound as if they would create significant functional impairments for older persons. However, most are not significantly affected by these age-related changes. Such normal alterations in cardiac function and output do create a potential for problems, which can readily occur when illness or stresses ap-

Table 8–3. PHYSIOLOGIC CHANGES OF AGING AND PHARMACOKINETICS

Physiologic Change	Pharmacokinetic Consequence	Examples Of Drugs Affected*
Changes in body weight and composition: reduced total body water and lean body mass per kg body weight and increased body fat.	Changes in drug distribution and action. With some drugs peak concentrations are greater and half-lives are prolonged, increasing drug effect. This may lead to toxicity.	Water-soluble drugs such as gentamicin; fat-soluble drugs such as pentobarbital: Check pharmacology reference for specific drug effects
Decreased cardiac output → increased circulation time.	Delayed onset of drug action. Prolonged drug effect.	All cardiac drugs
Altered circulation to liver, decline in hepatic blood flow. Decreased microsomal enzymatic activity and plasma protein synthesis.	Altered drug metabolism and detoxification by the liver. Biotransformation time is lengthened and both nonmetabolized drugs and active metabolites exert their effects for extended periods. Drug toxicity can occur more readily.	Acetaminophen, barbiturates, chlordiazepoxide, phenylbutazone, propranolol, oral anticoagulants, quinidine, tricyclic antidepressants, meperidine
Decrease in serum albumin.	Decreased availability of protein for binding. Increased serum concentration for free drug results in increased pharmacologic effects of some drugs. For some drugs, such as phenytoin, the increased free state causes faster drug clearance and lowers therapeutic effect.	Chlorthalidone, digitoxin, furosemide, hydralazine, prazosin, propranolol, quinidine, spironolactone, warfarin
Decreased renal function.	Impaired drug excretion, which can result in toxic buildup of drug levels in patient. Drug dose and patient response should be monitored closely. Some drug doses may need to be reduced in elderly patients.	Chlorthalidone, diazoxide, digoxin, ethambutol, furosemide, guanethidine, methyldopa, metolazone, methotrexate, phenobarbital, procainamide, tetracyclines (except doxycycline), the thiazides, and all aminoglycosides

*Aging can affect drug disposition in all phases; thus a drug may be listed in more than one category. Also, examples are of common drugs only and not meant to be all-inclusive. For more complete listings, consult a reference such as the American Hospital Formulary Service.

pear or in the presence of other variables, such as the ingestion of medications. Because the older person's *homeostatic* adaptabilities also slow with age, any illness or stress can more easily overwhelm the body's ability to cope.

The normal aging process also affects the blood vessels. The elastic fibers in the arteries lose about 30% of their stretch with age. There is also increased calcium deposition and collagen proliferation within the arterial walls, which further reduce the ability of the arteries to distend. These age-related changes result in an increased peripheral vascular resistance and pulse wave velocity, causing an increase in the systolic blood pressure. The normal cardiovascular changes associated with aging can also affect all other organs of the body. The reduced cardiac output causes a decreased blood flow to all organs, although the brain and cardiac muscle are the least affected by the decrease. Renal blood flow is especially affected: both glomerular filtration rate and renal plasma flow are significantly reduced. This can significantly alter drug distribution and excretion in the elderly.

The normal cardiovascular changes of aging with the pathologic changes of disease in the elderly can make drug therapy problematic. In many cases, early signs of drug toxicity are not as evident or are erroneously attributed to age-related changes when initially observed. Monitoring the elderly for drug-related side effects re-

quires careful consideration of these age-related changes. Drugs such as propranolol can induce congestive heart failure sooner and more suddenly in elderly patients than in younger patients.

Some drugs cause *cardiotoxicity* (toxic effects on the heart). Drugs such as the antineoplastic agents cyclophosphamide (Cytoxan), methotrexate (Mexate), daunorubicin (Cerubidine), and doxurubicin (Adriamycin) are all capable of causing serious cardiotoxic effects. The elderly patient experiencing age-related decreases in cardiac function and output is especially vulnerable to the toxic effects of such drugs.

CHANGES IN GASTROINTESTINAL FUNCTION

All body systems slow in function with normal aging. The elderly have decreased gastric acid secretion and decreased gastrointestinal motility. These changes cause slower emptying of the stomach and slower movement of intestinal contents through the gastrointestinal tract. A decrease in the body's ability to absorb medications can have a significant effect on drugs that have a narrow therapeutic range. Coadministration of certain drugs with food or other drugs can also affect the amount and speed of drug absorption.

CHANGES IN HEPATIC FUNCTION

The liver completely or partially biotransforms or metabolizes many drugs before they are excreted. The age-related decrease in cardiac output results in a decreased blood flow to the liver. Although decreased hepatic blood flow does not seem to cause significant reduction in hepatic function, there is an age-related decrease in the liver's ability to metabolize certain drugs.

There are other organic changes in liver function that occur in normal aging. Vitamins C, A, B$_{12}$, and folic acid are often deficient in older patients. These deficiencies may result from a decreased ability to absorb the vitamins, from dietary changes, or from a combination of these and other factors. Vitamin deficiencies and environmental pollutants can adversely affect liver function.

The metabolization and elimination of many drugs are highly dependent on adequate liver function. Decreased hepatic function can cause higher blood levels of drug, produce more intense drug effects, prolong drug effect due to prolonged blood concentrations of drug, and increase incidence of drug toxicity. Drugs affected by these age-related hepatic changes are oral anticoagulants, propranolol (Inderal), and chlordiazepoxide (Librium).

CHANGES IN RENAL FUNCTION

Decreased cardiac output in the elderly has a significant effect on the kidneys. Blood flow is especially adversely affected. Glomerular filtration rate and renal plasma flow are significantly reduced, and the number of intact nephrons is also reduced. Though renal function is generally sufficient to eliminate excess body fluids and wastes, the older patient's ability to eliminate some drugs may decrease by 50% or more.

The normal physiologic changes in the kidneys can have significant effects on drug distribution and excretion in the elderly. Some drugs, such as digoxin and procainamide (Procan, Pronestyl), are excreted primarily by the kidneys. Because the renal changes seen in normal aging can slow excretion and prolong high blood concentrations of drug, toxicity is common. Many elderly patients have cardiovascular problems and take drugs such as digoxin and procainamide. Thus, drug toxicity, especially of digoxin, is a particular problem. Careful monitoring is extremely important so drug dosages can be modified to compensate for decreases in renal function. Some drugs can cause *nephrotoxicity* (having a deleterious effect on the kidney). It is especially important to observe the elderly, who already have decreased renal function, for this adverse drug effect. The aminoglycoside antibiotics are excreted unchanged in the urine; hence, renal tissue is exposed to high concentrations of these drugs. Streptomycin is the least nephrotoxic, but is not very effective against gram-negative infections such as those caused by *Pseudomonas* species. Amikacin (Amikin), gentamicin (Garamycin), netilmicin (Netromycin), and tobramycin (Nebcin) are the most effective aminoglycosides against such organisms. Studies show that of these four drugs, tobramycin is the least nephrotoxic. Patients receiving any of these drugs must be observed for renal effects.

SENSORY AND PERCEPTUAL CHANGES

Sensory changes of normal aging present special problems in drug safety, effectiveness, and compliance with therapy. Generally, the sensory thresholds of response are higher in the elderly, and stimuli of greater intensity are needed, while the range and speed of responses become limited by the functional and structural decline in aging.

The normal aging process affects the sensory organs of the body in several ways. In the eye, the pupil becomes smaller and less responsive to light, color discrimination decreases, the lens becomes cloudy, the ability to focus on near objects is decreased, and *lacrimation* (tear formation and discharge) decreases. These visual changes can impair the patient's ability to distinguish between different drug tablets and his or her ability to clearly read the medicine label. Cataracts or other eye conditions common in older persons can have an even greater effect on the patient's ability to clearly see pills and read instructions.

Hearing acuity diminishes with age with decreased receptive and discriminative capacities. These changes may occur so gradually the person is either not fully aware of them or develops compensatory mechanisms to mask or hide the handicap so others are unaware of them. This can interfere with patient teaching and result in misinterpretation of instructions.

All hearing loss in older patients is not due to the changes of aging. Some drugs directly affect the ears to cause ototoxic effects—*tinnitus* (ringing in ears), vertigo, and hearing loss. All aminoglycoside antibiotics can cause ototoxicity. Most aminoglycosides are given intramuscularly or intravenously; hence, their use had been mostly confined to hospitals until the advent of intravenous home therapy. Other drugs can also have ototoxic effects. For example, when furosemide (Lasix) is given intravenously too rapidly, it can cause transient hearing loss. In addition, large doses of aspirin can cause tinnitus.

All senses are affected by the aging process. There are diminished taste and olfactory acuity, decreased sensitivity to touch (perception of pressure), and reduced manual dexterity (due to neuromuscular factors). These factors can uniquely limit the older person's ability to self-administer medications. At best they impose barriers that must be recognized and surmounted whenever a nurse is administering or teaching a patient to self-administer medications. At worst, they may preclude the patient from self-administering medications.

PHARMACOKINETICS AND THE AGING PROCESS

The pharmacokinetic process can be affected by normal, age-related changes that occur in major body systems and organs. Because normal age-related changes in physiology can influence the pharmacokinetic process, pathologic changes due to disease can have even more dramatic effects on drug therapeutics. It is therefore essential for appropriate nursing intervention in older patients that the nurse understand normal aging. The homeostatic mechanisms adapt less quickly in the elderly just at a time when many physiologic changes occur. Aging is often accompanied by environmental and social stresses as well (e.g., death of spouse or significant others, declining ability to care for self or home, illness, or infirmity.) As previously noted, the elderly suffer increased incidences of diseases and therefore consume about a third of all prescription drugs. When planning care of older patients on medications, it is important to consider the following factors:

1. Changes in the size and functional capabilities of major organs and transport systems impede drug disposition processes, making drug response less predictable.
2. Compensatory mechanisms become slower to respond, so side effects, toxicity, and interactions may occur that are disproportionate to actual drug dose.
3. Body tissue sensitivity and responsiveness decrease, making dosage and dose scheduling problematic.
4. The regulatory mechanisms that promote integrated activity of all body systems are less effective so that stimulation or depression of one organ may more readily affect many others.
5. The rate of readjustment to changes in the extracellular environment of the cells becomes substantially reduced so that even minor shifts in fluid-electrolyte balance can prove hazardous for the elderly.
6. Large variations in the rate of individual age-related changes make it extremely difficult to predict qualitative properties of drug response in elderly patients.

A discussion of the normal age-related changes in physiology relative to drug disposition follows. The reader is again reminded that normal changes are being discussed, and in the presence of pathology, even greater variations can occur. Every aspect of drug disposition (absorption, distribution, biotransformation/metabolism, and excretion) is affected by the changes that occur as a person ages.

DRUG ABSORPTION

Several factors may contribute to decreased drug absorption in older patients: a decrease in basal and maximal gastric acid output, which raises gastric pH and can affect the solubility of some drugs such as aspirin or barbiturates; a decrease in splanchnic blood flow, which could reduce or delay absorption; slower gastric emptying; and an increase in duodenal diverticula. Drugs with a narrow therapeutic range, such as digoxin, are most affected by any changes in drug absorption.

Esophageal motility decreases with age. Esophageal clearance time is lengthened because of weakened contractions of smooth muscle and failure of the lower esophageal sphincter to relax after swallowing. The nurse must take the physiologic effects of aging into account when giving pills and teaching medication administration to the patient or caregiver. Simple actions like having the patient sit fully upright during administration so gravity can aid the process and having the patient drink a full glass of water (half taken before the medicine) to ensure ease of drug passage can make administration much easier.

Gastric motility decreases with age, and gastric emptying time increases. These factors contribute to higher gastric pH, which can potentiate irritating effects of drugs such as aspirin (acidic) and phenytoin (strongly alkaline) due to the extended time they may be present in the stomach. Having the patient drink a full glass of water or eat a small, nonfat snack with the drug can decrease irritation to gastric tissue. The patient can also switch to enteric-coated aspirin to reduce gastric irritation.

Drug absorption following subcutaneous or intramuscular injection occurs by rapid diffusion from the injection site into the plasma. Both these injection routes ensure a more rapid onset of drug action than the oral route. The microcirculation in skeletal muscle promotes rapid drug absorption, although the age-related decrease in cardiac output can reduce blood flow to the muscles, thereby slowing drug absorption somewhat. Studies show that blood flow differs in muscle groups. It is important to select injection sites with care because older patients have some decrease in muscle mass, which may make a site unacceptable for injection of some drugs.

The age-related loss of subcutaneous tissues and increased fragility of the blood vessels can make administering intravenous drugs more problematic. Older patients also have increased risk of drug infiltration and extravasation due to decreased blood vessel wall elasticity and resiliency. While the infiltration of fluid-replacing IV solutions to a dehydrated patient generally produces no long-term effects, the infiltration or extravasation of antineoplastic drugs such as mechlorethamine (Mustargen), doxorubicin (Adriamycin), daunorubicin (Cerubidine), mitomycin (Mutamycin), vinblastine (Velban), and vincristine (Oncovin) can cause serious tissue damage (necrosis and sloughing).

Topical ointments and analgesic balms are often used by older patients because of their warming effect on sprains, strains, and inflamed arthritic joints; or for their numbing effect (hemorrhoid remedies). Though applied locally, systemic effects can occur from topical products if large enough amounts are applied and absorbed through the skin. For example, topical anesthetics can be absorbed systemically when applied to abraded skin or over large areas of the body. Hydrocortisone-containing creams can also be absorbed systemically, especially when applied over large areas of the body.

DRUG DISTRIBUTION

Physiologic changes that occur normally in aging can change drug distribution, causing higher blood levels of some drugs. There is also an increased potential for more intense drug effects, toxicity, and adverse drug reactions. Among the reasons for altered drug distribution are decreased cardiac output and changes in circulation, delayed onset of drug effect or prolongation of drug effect, changes in body weight and composition, changes in protein binding because of decreased albumin levels, and changes in red blood cell binding.

Probably the most important factor affecting drug distribution is the change in body composition that accompanies aging. Decreased lean body mass and increased fatty tissue can affect the action of many drugs, including chlorpromazine (Thorazine), diazepam (Valium), and phenobarbital. Increased distribution to fat cells can prolong drug action and increase drug sensitivity and/or toxic effects.

Elderly patients generally have higher plasma levels of drugs and more erratic distribution rates. Equal doses of digoxin given to a 70-year-old and a 40-year-old yield a higher blood level of drug in the older patient due to age-related changes in body size and drug distribution. Thus, loading doses of drugs equivalent to those given to young patients can be dangerous for older patients. Careful titration of drug doses can help reduce the number of undesirable drug reactions and toxicity in elderly patients.

DRUG BIOTRANSFORMATION/ METABOLISM

Drug metabolism as measured by prolonged drug elimination half-lives and reduced total drug clearance decreases with age. Other factors influence the rate of drug metabolism: exposure to alcohol; drugs; environmental pollutants; and nutritional deficits.

Aging decreases liver mass, reduces hepatic blood flow, and reduces protein synthesis and enzymatic activity. These changes prolong biotransformation, resulting in prolonged pharmacologic effects. Drugs quickly inactivated in the liver of a young person may have a prolonged effect in elderly patients. Examples of such drugs are meperidine (Demerol), barbiturates, propranolol (Inderal), and the tricyclic antidepressants.

Many drugs bind to protein in plasma and are therefore affected by decreases in serum protein levels. Hypoproteinemia increases the free, unbound fraction of circulating drug and results in a transient increase in intensity of pharmacologic action. Drugs highly bound to plasma protein readily affected by these alterations in metabolism include diazepam (Valium), meperidine (Demerol), phenytoin (Dilantin), furosemide (Lasix), tolbutamide (Orinase), and warfarin (Coumadin).

DRUG EXCRETION

The excretion rate of drugs is also affected by the aging process. Most drugs are excreted by the kidneys. Thus, excretion depends on renal blood flow, glomerular filtration rate, and urea clearance, all of which are decreased in aging. The excretion of water-soluble drugs depends on glomerular filtration rate. Fat-soluble drugs are reabsorbed by the tubular epithelium and excreted following their hepatic conversion to more water-soluble compounds.

Because elderly patients have reduced rates of renal excretion of drugs, the potential for adverse drug reactions and toxicity is increased. Disease and pathologic changes in the liver or kidneys can further increase these risks in the elderly. Examples of drugs that are renally excreted and are given in reduced doses to elderly patients include the aminoglycosides, digoxin, ethambutol (Myambutol), methotrexate (Mexate), phenobarbital, and the tetracyclines (except doxycycline).

NURSING PROCESS RELATED TO DRUG THERAPY IN THE OLDER ADULT

Major goals of drug therapy in the older adult are patient compliance, understanding how the aging process affects drug activity, enhancing the patient's ability to self-administer medication, and prevention of drug toxic effects.

Age-related physiologic changes can affect all phases of drug disposition—absorption, distribution, biotransformation/metabolization and excretion—increasing the risk of adverse effects or toxicity. When normal aging changes combine with multiple chronic illnesses and drug regimens, the potential for reduced drug effectiveness, increased side effects, and increased toxicity become greater. Understanding the processes that underlie the older patients' response to drugs results in better tailoring of nursing interventions to meet patient needs.

Major concerns related to drug therapy in the elderly are (1) preventing drug toxicity and complications due to normal age-related physiologic changes and (2) improving understanding of and compliance with therapy by health teaching appropriate to functional and sensory abilities. Table 8–4 provides a nursing process for an older adult on drug therapy.

ASSESSMENT

- Obtain a history before initiating the nursing assessment. Ask the patient about current prescriptions/medications, over-the-counter drugs taken (vitamins, supplements, aspirin, analgesics, laxatives), alcohol consumption, drug or alcohol abuse problems, and if he or she ever borrows drugs prescribed for others.
- Obtain an immunization history. Patients over age 65 should have annual pneumonococcal vaccine (Pneumovax). Hepatitis B immunization is recommeded for patients on dialysis or those who are immunocompromised. A tetanus booster, usually combined with diphtheria TD (tetanus/diphtheria), is needed every 10 years.
- Ask the patient about drug allergies and the exact reaction he or she had to the claimed allergy-causing drug. Patients often claim an allergy when only side effects such as stomach upset or diarrhea occur.
- Assess the patient's religious/ethnic background. Orthodox Jews and Muslims may reject pork-based insulins or vaccines. Mennonites and Christian Scientists may refuse vaccines. Ethnic, cultural, or folk remedies/herbal medicines can cause toxic effects when combined with other drugs.
- Assess the patient's psychosocial status, living conditions, structural barriers in the home, presence of caregivers, and self-esteem. Ask how often and from whom he or she seeks health care and where prescriptions are filled.
- Ask the patient about all doctors seen and prescriptions taken. Some people see several doctors to get multiple pain pill prescriptions or tranquilizers, a practice called *polypharmacy*. Such polypharmacy can lead to overdose or toxicity.

Table 8–4. NURSING FOR AN OLDER ADULT TAKING MEDICATIONS

Assessment

Assess drug use: current medicines being taken (drug name, dose, what the medicine is for, and side effects experienced); OTC, including vitamins, aspirin, analgesics, and laxatives; social, e.g., alcohol, nicotine and caffeine; street drugs.
Assess pattern of use: how often taken, what happens when taken, whether medication is borrowed from others.
Assess current status of immunizations.
Assess information about medical care: whom patient sees, how often, and where patient fills prescriptions.
Assess dietary restrictions/needs.
Assess sensory acuity, cognitive skills.
Assess availability of support system(s), need for assistance, living conditions.

Nursing Diagnosis: Noncompliance with Medication Regimen

RELATED TO: Financial concerns, health beliefs, inadequate knowledge.
AS EVIDENCED BY: Development of complications, failure to keep appointments, exacerbation of symptoms.

Desired Outcomes/Evaluation Criteria

Verbalizes accurate knowledge about disease and understanding of treatment regimen.

Nursing Actions	Rationale
Review drug regimen information, dietary intake, and financial considerations.	Identifies areas of concern and provides opportunity for giving new information/reinforcing previous knowledge.
Discuss reasons for taking medication as ordered and checking with physician before making changes.	Accurate information can enhance cooperation, preventing complications.
Encourage participation in problem-solving solutions to current situation.	Enhances feelings of self-worth and promotes sense of control over own life.
Demonstrate ways to open drug containers, obtain easy-open containers.	Administration of medication is easier when mobility/dexterity improves.

Nursing Diagnosis: Decreased Cardiac Output

RELATED TO: Drug-related alterations in rate/rhythm, electrical conduction.
AS EVIDENCED BY: Weight gain, dependent edema, and abnormal pulse.

Desired Outcomes/Evaluation Criteria

Maintains cardiac rate/rhythm within prescribed limits. Verbalizes understanding of desired effects and measures for control. Displays no toxic effects of medications.

Nursing Actions	Rationale
Teach how to take pulse daily before digoxin and caution against taking when pulse is below 60; have patient demonstrate skill.	Understanding of toxic effects and measures for controlling them reduces sequelae of these effects.
Report presence of dysrhythmias.	May indicate need for further evaluation and treatment.
Review diet and choices for supplemental K+.	Understanding which foods to choose will help to maintain proper K+ level.
Administer potassium replacement.	May be needed as additional K+ supplementation.

Nursing Diagnosis: Knowledge Deficit

RELATED TO: Lack of information or misinterpretation/unfamiliarity, cognitive limitation.
AS EVIDENCED BY: Questions, inaccurate follow-through of instructions, or development of preventable complications.

Desired Outcomes/Evaluation Criteria

Verbalizes understanding of medication regimen. Reports anxiety is decreased and is confident in own ability for self-care.

Nursing Actions	Rationale
Encourage verbalization of anxieties/fears.	Promotes recognition of concerns and steps that can be taken to manage own care.
Discuss normal aging process and symptoms needing physician.	Promotes understanding of differentiation between things that can be treated.
Emphasize importance of not taking OTC drugs or increasing prescribed dosage without contacting physician.	Beliefs about OTC drugs not being medicine and attitudes of "if one pill is good, two must be better" can lead to untoward complications.
Encourage patient to wear glasses during patient teaching sessions.	Reduces misunderstanding, speeds learning, and improves self-esteem.
Suggest ways to mark bottles to identify different drugs, e.g., a red paper heart on the digoxin bottle.	Developing a system helps patient identify correct medication and maintain independence and safety.
Identify possible side effects of ibuprofen. Instruct patient when to call physician.	Increasing aspirin or NSAID dosages may increase risk of GI complications such as ulcers and bleeding.
Give written materials for home review.	Information is remembered better when presented in more than one format.
Stress importance of follow-up care.	Monitoring physical status and medication regimen can prevent misunderstandings and complications.

Other Suggested Nursing Diagnoses: Risk for Injury (underdosing/overdosing of medications), Dysfunctional Grieving, Fear, and Sensory-Perceptual Alterations.

- Assess the patient for knowledge deficits in drug therapy/adverse side effects, impaired sensory acuity, noncompliant attitude, and dietary restrictions. These are potential problem areas to address in determining nursing diagnoses, goals, and interventions.

▼ **CLINICAL ALERT**

Patient misunderstanding of drug regimen and fear of adverse effects contribute to poor therapeutic response. Almost 60% of older adults fear adverse drug reactions or overmedication, leading to noncompliance in taking their medications. This fear discourages compliance more than the two other prime causes—advancing age and childproof containers.

- Assess the three basic areas of information gathering: (1) verbal and nonverbal data from the patient interview; (2) physical data from vital signs, inspection, palpitation, auscultation, and percussion; and (3) laboratory and x-ray reports, physician's history, and physical exam. Coordinating data from these areas helps with planning nursing intervention.

NURSING DIAGNOSIS

- Nursing diagnoses for the older adult on medications must be tailored to patient need. Examples of typical nursing diagnoses are as follows: Knowledge Deficit, Fear, Risk for Injury, Noncompliance with Medication Regimen, and Sensory-Perceptual Alterations (see Table 8–4).

PLANNING AND INTERVENTION

- Involve the patient in goal setting to foster patient compliance. Tailor the plan to individual need via creative problem solving. Remember, age-related physical changes may demand changes in the usual health teaching approach.
- Include a family member/significant other in the teaching phase to promote compliance and understanding.
- Encourage patient verbalization of fears and plan ways to overcome them.
- Allow the patient with sensory deficits to maintain as much independence as safely possible. For the patient with poor visual acuity, devise ways to help him or her tell similar-looking pills apart, or set up prepared drug trays or calendars, as shown in Figure 8–1.

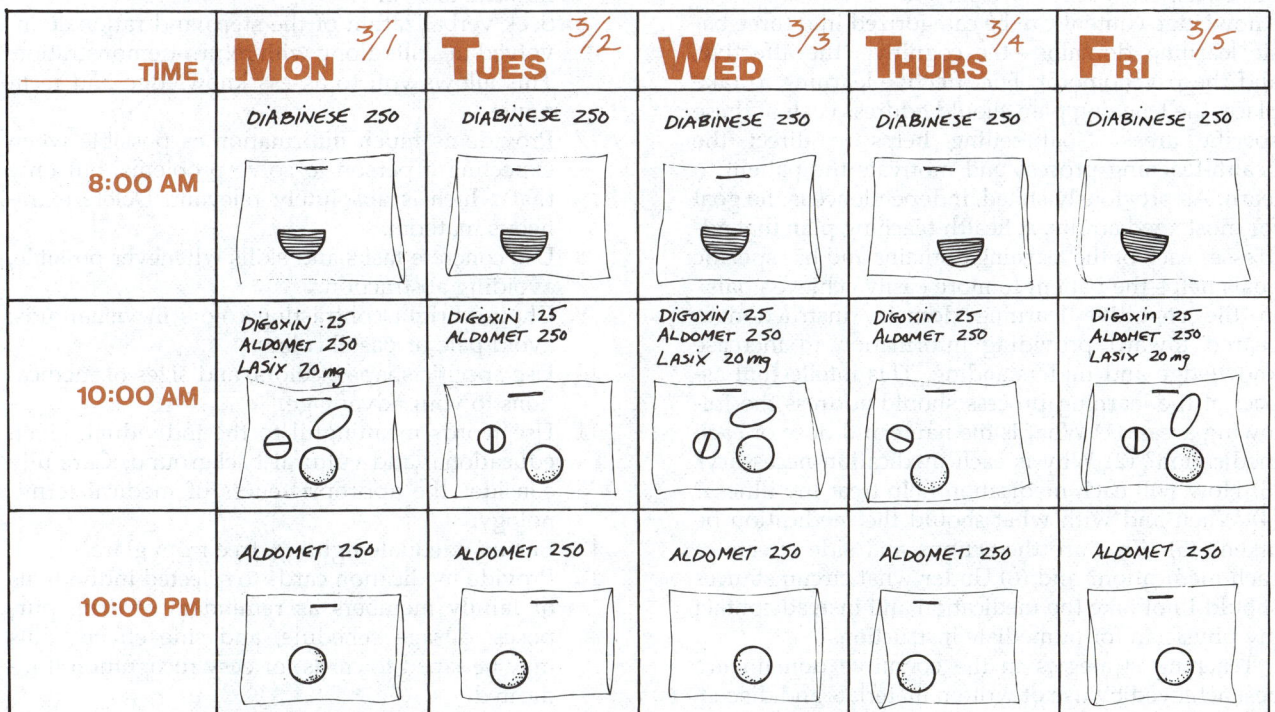

Figure 8–1. Sample drug regimen for patient using drug calendar with drugs attached. Medications are placed in plastic wrap or bags, which are stapled or taped to the correct time/date space.

- Stress that the patient must contact the physician before any change in drug dose to avoid overdosing. "If one pill is good, two is better" thinking can cause serious toxic effects.
- Discuss with the patient/caregiver what to do if a dose of medicine is missed. It is dangerous to "double up" on doses of some drugs such as cardiac glycosides or antineoplastics. Have a schedule/reminder system to help the patient remember medicines. Make a plan on how to adjust the drug schedule if a dose is missed.

Patient Teaching

Patient teaching is a primary concern for the nurse. The nurse must assess learning needs and then develop and implement a teaching plan. The following information deals with teaching strategies that are helpful in teaching the older adult.

- People can learn at any age. Memory may not be as sharp in old age as in youth, the attention span may be shortened, and vision and hearing less acute. These problems can be overcome via teaching strategies. The older patient may be a more motivated learner than the young patient because his or her health and independence—two of the most highly prized aspects of life—are at stake.
- Knowledge content can be categorized into three basic learning domains—the cognitive, the affective, and the psychomotor. For effective learning to take place, the teaching plan should address each of these specific areas. Goal setting helps to direct the health-teaching process and motivate the patient to learn. As previously stated, independence is the goal for most aged adults. A health-teaching plan that addresses each of the learning domains and has specific goals helps the patient to more easily achieve goals.
- In the cognitive learning domain, instruction is geared toward providing information to increase knowledge and understanding. This intellectual aspect of the learning process should address the following areas: (1) What is the name and dose of each medication? (2) Why is each medication necessary? (3) How will each medication help treat my illness? (4) When and with what should the medication be taken? (5) What are the actions and side effects of each medication? and (6) Under what circumstances should I not take the medication and instead contact my physician for immediate instructions?

Teaching strategies in the cognitive domain are best achieved by use of written materials and discussion with the patient. A one-to-one or small-group setting works best with elderly patients. Provide information as is necessary without too much technical or background information that can overwhelm, confuse, or obscure the teaching goal.

The affective domain encompasses patient attitudes toward illness, the treatment plan, and daily dependence on medications. The patient brings affective attitudes into all settings that can enhance or detract from willingness and ability to learn as well as compliance with the drug regimen. Patient attitudes must be recognized and problem areas overcome for information in the cognitive and psychomotor areas to be understood and used.

The psychomotor learning domain encompasses motor skills and performance ability. The learner must be able to translate knowledge gained in the cognitive domain into motor skills. Classic examples here are the ability to prepare and self-administer insulin or to take a pulse accurately. Psychomotor skills are best learned through demonstration and return-demonstration.

Dall and Gresham (1982) summarized the following effective teaching strategies for the older adult:

1. Begin teaching early.
2. Assess assets and liabilities in sensory perception, central processing and integration, and motor performance before initiating a teaching plan.
3. Encourage the use of effective adaptive devices (hearing aids, glasses) whenever possible.
4. Provide only general information in a group. Avoid group learning for individuals who find groups distracting. Provide specific drug information on an individual basis. Avoid mixing the very old with the "young" old in teaching groups.
5. Keep individual teaching sessions short, 15 to 20 minutes at a time.
6. Seek verbalization of the steps and rationale involved in skills along with return-demonstration. This allows you to assess knowledge and technique.
7. Provide as much information as possible when expecting a person to solve problems, but only that which is absolutely relevant. Delete extraneous material.
8. Use concrete tasks and skills whenever possible, avoiding abstraction.
9. Choose bright contrasting colors in visual aids; avoid pale or pastel colors.
10. Use specific shapes, colors, and sizes of medications to your advantage.
11. Use words meaningful to the individual, given educational and cultural background. Carefully consider the appropriateness of medical terminology.
12. Ensure adequate lighting, free from glare.
13. Provide medication cards to selected individuals or family members as reminders of drug purposes, dosage schedule, and side effects. Pills may be taped to cards for easy recognition if indicated.
14. Maintain a positive approach. Learning can and does occur in the older adult.

Medication Schedules and Assistive Devices

A persistent question for all those taking medication on a daily basis is, "Did I remember to take my pills today?" This is especially problematic for older people whose memory may not be as acute as in their youth. Assist the patient in developing a schedule plan and appropriate assistive aids. A simple device such as turning the medicine bottle upside down after a daily medicine has been taken and then righting the bottle at bedtime is a definite visual confirmation that the medicine has been taken. Patients on multiple drugs with more than a daily dosage require more elaborate aids.

When devising a dosage schedule with a patient, simplify the schedule as much as possible and schedule dosage times to coincide with routine daily activities to decrease chance of omission (e.g., upon arising, at mealtime, at bedtime). Some patients have wind-up alarm clocks to go off when the next dose is due.

- Alternate assistive aids/techniques include the following:
  1. A large calendar with room to write the drugs and dosing times each day, and on which the patient crosses off each dose as it is taken.
  2. A guide calendar with each day's drugs wrapped in cellophane and taped to the calendar. Such a device must be out of the way of access by visiting grandchildren.
  3. A cupcake tray with the drugs to be taken and the dosage schedule times clearly labeled on the tray.
  4. An egg container with the cups labeled and medications inserted in the appropriate cups. Be sure drugs will not lose potency if exposed to air or light. As with all open container systems, be sure tray is out of the reach of children.
  5. Obtain and organize a segmented commercial container. Braille and regular labels are available.
  6. The visually impaired diabetic patient can obtain a Monoject scale magnifier that magnifies the numbers printed on an insulin syringe or the Dos-Aid syringe filling device, which can be set to a precise insulin dosage on a U-100 syringe, which allows the visually impaired to draw the correct dosage.
  7. A well-informed family member or friend may assist the patient in maintaining the dosage schedule.
  8. If a hypnotic is required, it is best to take a single dose, then remove the bottle from the room to prevent patient from taking a repeat dose.

▼ CLINICAL ALERT

Special problems may be posed by residents of health-related facilities who are able to go outside the facility where they can purchase over-the-counter medicines. Use of a signed agreement between nurse and patient that spells out specific responsibilities in self-medication may help prevent such problems. The nurse's role is to interview the patient regularly to assess drug knowledge, evaluate compliance with the therapy regimen, and observe for clinical response to medications.

EVALUATION

- Review the patient's drug profile frequently. All members of the patient's health-care team should contribute toward devising a plan with which the patient can comply and which meets patient needs.
- Evaluate the patient for inappropriate drug usage and dosage. Most pharmaceutical experts agree that the best drug regimen is the fewest possible drugs at the minimum dosage. As previously discussed, with advancing age the margin of safety between therapeutic and toxic dose narrows. Therefore, the dose of a drug is often reduced. The development of geriatric dosage forms for drugs with age-dependent renal excretion is extremely helpful for patients. The dosage for drugs metabolized by the liver may also be reduced for elderly patients without altering blood levels of the drug.
- Evaluate the patient's ability to discriminate between the different drugs being taken. Many complain that "the pills all look alike." Consider the size, color, and shape of each drug when devising a drug regimen.
- Evaluate the patient's ability to self-administer the proper dose. If the medication is a liquid, evaluate whether the patient can correctly pour the proper dose. If tablets must be cut in half, scored tablets should be provided. If arthritic fingers find breaking tablets too difficult, it may be necessary for someone to break the tablets or for the patient to buy a commercial pill splitter. For patients who are extremely dysphagic, medication crushed and mixed with semisolid food such as applesauce is often safer to swallow than liquids. Care is taken not to crush enteric-coated or time-release tablets, however, because gastrointestinal side effects can result and drug effectiveness may be altered.
- Evaluate the patient/family's ability to recognize adverse drug effects. Increased risk of adverse reactions occurs with increasing age. The presence of multiple chronic illnesses, multiple drug therapy, and the effects of aging on drug pharmacokinetics all contribute to the problem. Thus, early recognition of adverse drug effects before they become toxic could prevent many problems and help reduce hospitalizations for drug toxicity treatment.

Certain drugs pose significant risk for older patients. Those causing the greatest potential hazard for these patients include the antidysrhythmics, the antimicrobials, digoxin, and the diuretics. These drugs are all commonly prescribed for older adults, and some have a high rate of adverse effects in this population. For example, about 20% to 30% of older patients taking digoxin experience adverse effects. Because these drugs are so essential for patients, the best way to reduce the risk of adverse effects is through patient teaching and frequent evaluation of continued patient understanding of what was taught.

- Monitoring of patient laboratory data can give important early warning signs of such impending problems as inadequate renal function or increasing serum drug levels. Serum drug levels allow for evaluation of whether or not the drug dose administered is within the therapeutic range for the patient. Physical assessment of the patient gives clues to drug effects. Close observation of the patient can also give important clues of beginning toxicity. Patients taking digoxin may experience anorexia, nausea, or vomiting. Thus, it is important not to dismiss physical signs (such as anorexia) as insignificant or attributable to moodiness. In the case of digoxin, such signs may indicate toxicity. It is likewise important to teach the patient or caregiver the signs that may indicate drug toxicity.

Drug side effects in the elderly are often mistaken for signs of aging. Among the drugs that can cause confusion are cimetidine (Tagamet), digoxin, and methyldopa (Aldomet). Depression may be an effect of digoxin or reserpine (Serpasil). Examples of drugs that can cause lethargy and drowsiness include analgesics (especially narcotics), sedative-hypnotics, and tranquilizers. Barbiturates can cause forgetfulness. Postural hypotension can result from antihypertensive therapy. Urinary urgency and incontinence may result from diuretic therapy. Furosemide (Lasix) is especially prone to cause urgency and incontinence in older patients. Examples of drugs that can cause ataxia include chlordiazepoxide (Librium), diazepam (Valium), and flurazepam (Dalmane). Gastrointestinal distress can be caused by drugs such as aspirin, ibuprofen (Motrin), indomethacin (Indocin), oral iron preparations, erythromycin, and piroxicam (Feldene).

As stated earlier, the elderly are frequent users of over-the-counter drugs. The availability of such drugs without a prescription lends a false sense of security about a drug's safety. All drugs can cause adverse effects and toxicity. Aspirin is frequently used for relief of arthritic symptoms. Aspirin must be taken in dosages of up to ten tablets per day to achieve adequate anti-inflammatory effects, and this can cause gastrointestinal distress, bleeding, and ulcers. Enteric-coated aspirin tablets decrease gastrointestinal distress.

- Careful evaluation of the older patient and questioning of patient/family can help to determine the cause of certain symptoms or behaviors. Because of the prolonged drug blood levels seen in elderly patients, the concept of a drug holiday has been advocated by some. Once a steady state of a drug is achieved, the patient skips a day of the drug (except cardiac and anticonvulsants). The drug holiday can reduce annual drug consumption with no loss of therapeutic effect or ill effects to patients and save money.

- Evaluate the patient's nutritional status. Some drugs, such as the antineoplastic cisplatin, can have a direct effect on the nutritional status of a patient and result in anorexia, nausea, and vomiting. Patients receiving antineoplastic chemotherapy may suffer from stomatitis and weight loss. Diarrhea, alterations in electrolytes, and interference in carbohydrate and fat metabolism can also result from other drug therapies. Patient weight loss may necessitate dose recalculation for drugs whose dose is given per kilogram of body weight. Malnutrition may prevent or impede drug absorption.

- Carefully evaluate the effectiveness of health teaching. Do not rely solely on the patient/family repeating instructions to you. Rote memory is generally a short-term memory pattern. When you are teaching a patient a medication regimen, it is the long-term memory (necessary for self-care at home) that is most essential. An excellent way to have the patient incorporate teaching into long-term memory is by having the patient demonstrate how medications are to be poured, taken, and remembered. You are not only evaluating the patient's technique but also the effectiveness of your health teaching.

Good health teaching is the key to ensuring patient compliance with a medication regimen. Also essential is patient trust and understanding of the value of the medication regimen so that compliance is motivated. Older patients are able to learn, but teaching strategies need to be modified according to the physical limitations that the aging process has imposed.

The bibliography for this chapter can be found in Appendix B, which begins on page 1054.

CHAPTER REVIEW QUESTIONS*

1. Which of the following statements is *not* correct with regard to aging and the drug response?
   a. Often signs of aging are mistaken for side effects of prescription drugs.
   b. In general, medications tend to be over-prescribed for the elderly.
   c. Drug therapy is often the most risky component of patient care in the elderly.
   d. Recommendations are in effect for medication use in the elderly.

2. Which of the following represents normal physiologic changes with aging?
   a. Lean body mass tends to decrease.
   b. Subcutaneous tissue tends to increase.
   c. Total body water in the elderly usually increases.
   d. Muscle mass proportionally increases.

3. In the older adult, fat-soluble drugs are:
   a. Distributed to a smaller portion of tissue than in young adults.
   b. Absorbed at a slow rate due to reduced fat stores.
   c. Released into circulation quickly after being absorbed.
   d. Associated with increased duration of drug action.

4. The effect of aging on hepatic function results in:
   a. Reduced blood levels of drugs.
   b. Prolonged drug effect.
   c. Reduced incidence of toxicity.
   d. Decreased intensity of drug effect.

5. Which teaching strategy is appropriate to gain medication compliance in the elderly?
   a. Mixing the older patients with those of younger age groups.
   b. Teaching at a rapid pace to cover all the material.
   c. Limiting teaching sessions to two-hour periods.
   d. Encouraging the use of adaptive devices when possible.

*See Appendix A, which begins on page 1051, for answers.

CHAPTER 9

Ethnic/Cultural Considerations for Drug Therapy

Carol Ann Maull, RN, PhD

CHAPTER OUTLINE

Ethnic/Cultural Assessment
Cultural Influences and Variations in Drug Response
   Among Four Major Ethnic Groups
Using the Nursing Process

KEY TERMS

Culture	Ethnic/cultural nursing care
Cultural assessment	Ethnicity
Culture distancing	Ethnocentrism

LEARNING OBJECTIVES

After reading this chapter, the student will be able to:

1. Explain the rationale for conducting an ethnic/cultural assessment on patients requiring drug therapy.
2. Use an assessment tool for collecting data regarding the patient's ethnic/cultural background.
3. Recognize differences in health beliefs, values, and practices among the four major subcultural groups in the United States and how these affect drug therapy.
4. Recognize the variations in drug response among the four major subcultural groups and understand how these affect drug therapy.
5. Describe the nursing implications for a patient from a specific subcultural group receiving drug therapy.

As the United States continues to become an increasingly diverse multicultural society, nurses are being challenged to learn more about how ethnic/cultural differences affect health and what potential impact those differences have on the health-care regimen. *Culture* is defined as a view of the world and a set of traditions used and transmitted from generation to generation. To deliver culturally diverse nursing care, nurses must become familiar with and better understand the *ethnicity* (a group's affiliation due to a shared linguistic or cultural background) of other people living in society, because health-care beliefs are generally culturally defined, learned, and practiced. To provide *ethnic/cultural nursing care*—the integration of the patient's ethnic/cultural background into a nursing-care plan to facilitate health care—nurses need to know how to perform a cultural assessment: how the cultural beliefs of the major ethnic/cultural subgroups in the United States—African-Amer-

icans, Hispanics, Asian-Americans, and Native Americans—can influence drug therapy; how ethnic and racial differences can affect drug response; and how to use the nursing process in monitoring drug therapy in patients from various subcultures.

ETHNIC/CULTURAL ASSESSMENT

A *cultural assessment* refers to a systematic appraisal or examination of individuals, groups, and communities as to their cultural beliefs, values, and practices to determine explicit nursing needs and intervention practices within the cultural context of the people being evaluated (Leininger, 1978). To assess the patient's cultural background during the initial assessment, a cultural assessment tool based on a broad cultural form of reference, such as Bloch's ethnic/cultural assessment guide, shown in Table 9–1, can be helpful. Bloch's assessment guide is presented as an example of a tool to systematically assess ethnic/cultural data based on four major categories of data collection—cultural, sociologic, psychologic, and biologic/physiologic—and may be used in combination with existing nursing collection instruments. Language, diet and food habits, ethics, rituals and taboos, and health/illness belief systems and practices are examples of important cultural manifestations that must be determined before involving the patient in drug therapy. The nurse may concentrate on a smaller segment of the tool, such as the health and illness belief section, if a complete cultural assessment is not required. The initial assessment should take into consideration the patient's ethnic/cultural background so that drug therapy interventions can be modified to make them compatible with the patient's value system. A strategy that takes into account a patient's belief in home remedies, herbal therapy, or traditional rituals is more likely to enhance the efficacy of the drug therapy, because it decreases the chances that the patient will avoid participating in the health-care regimen.

For example, the attitudes of the patient and family toward health, personal health habits, chronic illness, and the health-care team must be assessed before planning and interventions can proceed. Patients cannot be frightened, coerced, or threatened into adhering to a prescribed drug regimen. They can, however, be educated, advised, supported, and encouraged. By designing culture-specific care plans that take into consideration the patient's ethnic/cultural background, the nurse involves the patient as an active member of the health team, not as the passive recipient of a disease process. Members of the health team must acknowledge that merely telling a patient to follow a specific drug regimen does not guarantee compliance with the program.

GUIDING PRINCIPLES

Leininger has identified several guiding principles for the nurse to use while conducting a cultural assessment (Leininger, 1978). First, by maintaining a broad, objective, and open attitude regarding the patient's culture, the nurse is less apt to lean toward *ethnocentrism*, or to believe "that his or her own way is best" (Giger and Davidhizar, 1991). Ethnocentrism implies that other people's ideas and ways are inferior; it challenges the nurse to try to change the patient's belief system to match his or her own. Nurses must be made aware that their cultural behaviors are not always the best.

Second, the nurse should try to discern differences among individuals from the same cultural group rather than seeing them as alike. Classification of people into preconceived behavioral patterns greatly limits the identification of individual differences.

Third, to avoid the tendency for ethnocentrism, the nurse should assess a person from a culture other than his or her own, so that differences and similarities between the two cultures can be recognized and understood. *Cultural distancing* or "removing one's self from a given culture and studying it from a distance" helps the nurse be more objective and less ethnocentric.

Fourth, it is important for the nurse to reflect on all information obtained and behaviors observed during the cultural assessment to help accurately interpret cultural manifestations, particularly as they relate to the patient's health beliefs and care. As information is gathered, the nurse systematically documents what is heard and observed and then rechecks the findings with the patient to reaffirm that the interpretations are correct. Listening attentively to and observing the patient during the assessment phase helps the nurse to formulate and implement an effective plan of care.

ETHNIC AND RACIAL DIFFERENCES IN DRUG RESPONSE

A primary reason to conduct a cultural assessment when concerned with drug therapy is that significant differences among racial and ethnic groups may be responsible for observed variations in drug responses. DIFFERENCES in drug responses in various ethnic/cultural populations may be related to hereditary conditions (e.g., enzyme deficiencies such as lactase deficiency or glucose-6-phosphate deficiency) or altered biologic mechanisms that result in slower or faster rates of drug metabolism, defects in the structure of drug receptor sites within the body, or increased or decreased sensitivity to the side effects of some drugs. In addition, genetically susceptible groups can have altered drug responses caused by environmental factors.

Individuals who have a deficiency in the enzyme lactase, which is essential to the absorption of lactose, have lactase deficiency syndrome (hereditary or acquired). Patients with this syndrome are intolerant to lactose, a disaccharide found in milk and some dairy products that, when hydrolyzed in the body, yields glucose and galactose. Patients with lactose intolerance who ingest lactose-containing products display gastrointestinal symptoms, including abdominal cramps, bloating, and diarrhea. Ethnic/cultural groups with a high incidence of lactose intolerance include African-Americans, Asian-Americans, and Native Americans.

Glucose-6-phosphate dehydrogenase (G6PD) deficiency causes fragility of the red blood cells. Patients with this deficiency are prone to anemia when exposed to certain drugs, such as analgesics (aspirin), sulfonamides and sulfones, antimalarials (primaquine, quinacrine), antibacterials (nitrofurantoin, chloramphenicol, para-aminosalicylic acid), vitamin K, probenecid (Benemid) and quinidine (Giger and Davidhizar, 1991).

▼ **CLINICAL ALERT**

Chloroquine and antimalarial drugs impair red blood cell metabolism in patients with G6PD deficiency, and acute intravascular hemolysis may occur if these drugs are given (Kudzma, 1992). Ethnic/cultural groups with a high incidence of G6PD deficiency include African-Americans and Asian-Americans. To identify patients with this deficiency, the fluorescent spot test may be performed.

Table 9–1. BLOCH'S ETHNIC/CULTURAL ASSESSMENT GUIDE

Data Categories	Guideline Questions/Instructions	Data Collected
Ethnic origin	Does the patient identify with a particular ethnic group (e.g., Puerto Rican, African)?	
Race	What is the patient's racial background (e.g., African-American, Filipino, Native American)?	
Place of birth	Where was the patient born?	
Relocations	Where has the patient lived (country, city)? During what years did patient live there and for how long? Has he or she moved recently?	
Habits, customs, values, and beliefs	Describe habits, customs, values, and beliefs patient holds or practices that affect attitude toward birth, life, death, health and illness, time orientation, and health-care system and health-care providers. What is degree of belief and adherence by patient to his or her overall cultural system?	
Behaviors valued by culture	How does patient value privacy, courtesy, respect for elders, behaviors related to family roles and sex roles, and work ethics?	
Cultural sanctions and restrictions	*Sanctions*—What is accepted behavior by patient's cultural group regarding expression of emotions and feelings, religious expressions, and response to illness and death?	
	Restrictions—Does patient have any restrictions related to sexual matters, exposure of body parts, certain types of surgery (e.g., hysterectomy), discussion of dead relatives, and discussion of fears related to the unknown?	
Language and communication processes	What are some overall cultural characteristics of patient's language and communication process?	
Language(s) and/or dialect(s) spoken	Which language(s) and/or dialect(s) does patient speak most frequently? Where? At home or at work?	
Language barriers	Which language does patient predominantly use in thinking? Does patient need bilingual interpreter in nurse-patient interactions? Is patient non-English-speaking or limited-English-speaking? Is patient able to read and/or write in English?	
Communication process	What are rules (linguistics) and modes (style) of communication process (e.g., honorific concept of showing respect or deference to others using words only common to specific ethnic/cultural group)?	
	Is there need for variation in technique of communicating and interviewing to accommodate patient's cultural background (e.g., tempo of conversation, eye-body contact, topic restrictions, norms of confidentiality, and style of explanation)?	
	Are there any conflicts in verbal and nonverbal interactions between patient and nurse?	
	How does patient's nonverbal communication process compare with other ethnic/cultural groups, and how does it affect patient's response to nursing and medical care?	
	Are there any variations between patient's interethnic and interracial communication process or intracultural and intraracial communication process (e.g., ethnic minority patient and white middle-class nurse, ethnic minority patient and ethnic minority nurse: beliefs, attitudes, values, role variations, stereotyping [perception and prejudice])?	
Healing beliefs and practices		
Cultural healing system	What cultural healing system does the patient predominantly adhere to (e.g., Asian healing system, Hispanic curanderismo)? What religious healing system does the patient predominantly adhere to (e.g., Seventh Day Adventist, West African voodoo, fundamentalist sect, Pentecostal)?	
Cultural health beliefs	Is illness explained by the germ theory or cause-effect relationship, presence of evil spirits, imbalance between hot and cold (yin and yang in Chinese culture), or disequilibrium between nature and man?	
	Is good health related to success, ability to work or fulfill roles, reward from God, or balance with nature?	
Cultural health practices	What types of cultural healing practices does person from ethnic/cultural group adhere to? Does person use healing remedies to cure *natural* illnesses caused by the external environment (e.g., massage to cure *empacho* [a ball of food clinging to stomach wall], wearing of talismans or charms for protection against illness)?	
Cultural healers	Does patient rely on cultural healers (e.g., medicine men for Native American, curandero for Hispanic, Chinese herbalist, hougan [voodoo priest], spiritualist, or minister for African-American)?	
Nutritional variables or factors	What nutritional variables or factors are influenced by the patient's ethnic/cultural background?	
Characteristics of food preparation and consumption	What types of food preferences and restrictions, meaning of foods, style of food preparation and consumption, frequency of eating, time of eating, and eating utensils are culturally determined for patient? Are there any religious influences on food preparation and consumption?	

Continued on the following page

Table 9–1. BLOCH'S ETHNIC/CULTURAL ASSESSMENT GUIDE, *Continued*

Data Categories	Guideline Questions/Instructions	Data Collected
Influences from external environment	What modifications if any did the ethnic group patient identifies with have to make in its food practices in white-dominant American society? Are there any adaptations of food customs and beliefs from rural setting to urban setting?	
Patient education needs	What are some implications of diet planning and teaching to patient who adheres to cultural practices concerning foods?	
Economic status	Who is principal wage earner in patient's family? What is total annual income (approximately) of family? What impact does economic status have on lifestyle, place of residence, living conditions, and ability to obtain health services?	
Educational status	What is highest educational level obtained? Does patient's educational background influence ability to understand how to seek health services, literature on health care, patient teaching experiences, and any written material patient is exposed to in health-care setting (e.g., admission forms, patient-care forms, teaching literature, and lab test forms)?	
	Does patient's educational background cause him to feel inferior or superior to health-care personnel in health-care setting?	
Social network	What is patient's social network (kinship, peer, and cultural healing networks)? How do they influence health or illness status of patient?	
Family as supportive group	Does patient's family feel need for continuous presence in patient's clinical setting (is this an ethnic/cultural characteristic?) How is family valued during illness or death?	
	How does family participate in patient's nursing-care process (e.g., giving baths, feeding, using touch as support [cultural meaning], supportive presence)?	
	How does ethnic/cultural family structure influence patient response to health or illness (e.g., roles, beliefs, strengths, weaknesses, and social class)?	
	Are there any key family roles characteristic of a specific ethnic/cultural group (e.g., grandmother in African-American and other families) and can these key persons be a resource for health personnel?	
	What role does family play in health promotion or cause of illness (e.g., would family be intermediary group in patient interactions with health personnel and make decisions regarding care)?	
Supportive institutions in ethnic/cultural community	What influence do ethnic/cultural institutions have on patient receiving health services (i.e., institutions such as Organization of Migrant Workers, NAACP, Black Political Caucus, churches, schools, Urban League, community clinics)?	
Institutional racism	How does institutional racism in health facilities influence patient's response to receiving health care?	
Self-concept (identity)	Does patient show strong racial/cultural identity? How does this compare to that of other racial/cultural groups or to members of dominant society?	
	What factors in patient's development helped to shape his or her self-concept (e.g., family, peers, society labels, external environment, institutions, racism)?	
	How does patient deal with stereotypical behavior from health professionals?	
	What is impact of racism on patient from distinct ethnic/cultural group (e.g., social anxiety, noncompliance of health-care process in clinical settings, avoidance of using or participating in health-care institutions)?	
	Does ethnic/cultural background have impact on how patient relates to body image change resulting from illness or surgery (e.g., importance of appearance and roles in cultural group)?	
	Any adherence or identification with ethnic/cultural group identity (e.g., solidarity, "we" concept)?	
Mental and behavioral processes and characteristic of ethnic/cultural group	How does patient relate to external environment in clinical setting (e.g., fears, stress, and adaptive mechanisms characteristic of a specific ethnic/cultural group)? Any variations based on the life span?	
	What is patient's ability to relate to persons outside of his or her ethnic/cultural group (health personnel)? Is the patient withdrawn, verbally or nonverbally expressive, negative or positive, feeling mentally or physically inferior or superior?	
	How does patient deal with feelings of loss of dignity and respect in clinical setting?	
Religious influences on psychological effects of health/illness	Does patient's religion have a strong impact on how he relates to health/illness influence or outcomes (e.g., death/chronic illness, cause and effect of illness, or adherence to nursing/medical practices)?	
	Do religious beliefs, sacred practices, and talismans play a role in treatment of disease?	
	What is role of significant religious persons during health/illness (e.g., African-American ministers, Catholic priests, Buddhist monks, Islamic imams)?	

Continued on the following page

Table 9–1. BLOCH'S ETHNIC/CULTURAL ASSESSMENT GUIDE, *Continued*		
Data Categories	**Guideline Questions/Instructions**	**Data Collected**
Psychological/cultural response to stress and discomfort of illness (consideration of *norms* for different ethnic/cultural groups)	Based on ethnic/cultural background, does patient exhibit any variations in psychological response to pain or physical disability of disease processes?	
Racial-anatomical characteristics	Does patient have any distinct racial characteristics (e.g., skin color, hair texture and color, color of mucous membranes)? Does patient have any variations in anatomical characteristics (e.g., body structure [height and weight] more prevalent for ethnic/cultural group, skeletal formation [pelvic shape, especially for obstetrical evaluation], facial shape and structure [nose, eye shape, facial contour], upper and lower extremities)?	
	How do patient's racial and anatomical characteristics affect his or her self-concept and the way others relate to him or her?	
	Does variation in racial-anatomic characteristics affect physical evaluations and physical care, skin assessment based on color, and variations in hair care and hygienic practices?	
Growth and development patterns	Are there any distinct growth and development characteristics that vary with patient's ethnic/cultural background (e.g., bone density, fatfolds, motor ability)? What factors are important for nutritional assessment, neurologic and motor assessment, assessment of bone deterioration in disease process or injury, evaluation of newborns, evaluation of intellectual status, or capacity in relationship to motor/sensory development in children? How do these differ in ethnic/cultural groups?	
Variations in body systems	Are there any variations in body systems for patient from distinct ethnic/cultural group (e.g., gastrointestinal disturbance with lactose intolerance in African-Americans, nutritional intake of cultural foods causing adverse effects on gastrointestinal tract and fluid and electrolyte system, and variations in chemical and hematologic system [certain blood types prevalent in particular ethnic/cultural groups])?	
Skin and hair physiology, mucous membranes	How does skin color variation influence assessment of skin color changes (e.g., jaundice, cyanosis, ecchymosis, erythema, and its relationship to disease processes)?	
	What are methods of assessing skin color changes (comparing variations and similarities between different ethnic groups)?	
	Are there conditions of hypopigmentation and hyperpigmentation (e.g., vitiligo, Mongolian spots, albinism, discoloration caused by trauma)? Why would these be more striking in some ethnic groups?	
	Are there any skin conditions more prevalent in a distinct ethnic group (e.g., keloids in African-Americans)?	
	Is there any correlation between oral and skin pigmentation and their variations among distinct racial groups when doing assessment of oral cavity (e.g., leukoedema is normal occurrence in African-Americans)?	
	What are variations in hair texture and color among racially different groups? Ask patient about preferred hair-care methods or any racial/cultural restrictions (e.g., not washing hot-combed hair while in clinical setting, not cutting very long hair of Hispanic patients).	
	Are there any variations in skin-care methods (e.g., using Vaseline on African-American skin)?	
Diseases more prevalent among ethnic/cultural group	Are there any specific diseases or conditions that are more prevalent for a specific ethnic/cultural group (e.g., hypertension, sickle cell anemia, G6PD deficiency, lactose intolerance)?	
	Does patient have any socioenvironmental diseases common among ethnic/cultural groups (e.g., lead paint poisoning, poor nutrition, overcrowding [prone to tuberculosis], alcoholism resulting from psychologic despair and alienation from dominant society, rat bites, poor sanitation)?	
Diseases to which ethnic/cultural group has increased resistance	Are there any diseases that patient has increased resistance to because of racial/cultural background (e.g., skin cancer in African-Americans)?	

Source: Bloch, B: Bloch's assessment guide for ethnic/cultural variations. In Orque, M, et al (eds): Ethnic Nursing Care: A Multi-Cultural Approach, St Louis: CV Mosby Co. 1983, with permission.

Some individuals are fast or slow metabolizers. When drugs are metabolized too quickly, increased dosages may be required because the usual therapeutic effects may be below optimal or ineffectual. For example, African-Americans seem to require higher dosages of antihypertensive drugs—such as propranolol (In-deral)—to lower blood pressure. When drugs are metabolized too slowly, unbound or free drug may accumulate, leading to a greater drug effect. In this case, drug dosage may need to be decreased. Nine percent of African-Americans and Caucasians and 32% of Asian-Americans are considered to be slow metabolizers.

In some ethnic/cultural groups, drug tolerance may be related to defects in the structure of drug receptor sites within the body. These defects cause improper binding of the drug at the receptor site, and the drug will not be effective, despite the fact that serum drug levels will be adequate.

Habits such as smoking and drinking alcohol may increase the possibility of adverse drug reactions in genetically susceptible populations because of alterations in the absorption, distribution, and excretion of substances. For example, smoking has been known to alter the plasma concentration of chlorpromazine (Thorazine) and theophylline. A high alcohol level, which is known to speed drug metabolism, increases susceptibility to over-the-counter drugs and commonly prescribed medications.

CULTURAL INFLUENCES AND VARIATIONS IN DRUG RESPONSE AMONG FOUR MAJOR ETHNIC GROUPS

American society is primarily composed of four major ethnic groups: African-Americans, Hispanics, Asian-Americans, and Native Americans. Each of these groups shares culturally unique information that influences beliefs and effective interventions relative to health and illness. Table 9–2 identifies some traditional ethnic/cultural health interventions for each of these groups. Common treatment modalities may vary from culture to culture and include a combination of ritual and prayer, use of plant-based or vegetable drugs, use of Western medical practice (alone or in combination with folk practices), or adherence to dietary and environmental guidelines. The choice of treatment or cure is based in part on cultural beliefs regarding the etiology of the illness. Each of these groups may have unique responses to drug therapy, depending on the drug administered and the ethnic/cultural group involved.

The following section highlights some of the known beliefs and practices of these four ethnic populations to present an overview of how ethnic/cultural considerations may influence and/or affect drug therapy. By understanding how health and illness are influenced by ethnic/cultural orientations, the nurse is in an advantageous position to effectively assess, sensitively diagnose, and appropriately respond and intervene when dealing with patients who may have an ethnic/cultural value orientation that is different from that of the nurse.

This section also identifies physiologic differences common to each group that may cause variations in the usual or expected response to drugs. It also discusses types of reactions shared among members of each ethnic/cultural group to certain classes of drugs (or individual drugs).

None of the information presented is pertinent to all members of any one group, and cultural practices do differ among various subgroups in any one culture. The nurse is cautioned against overgeneralization. The *best* method of determining any one individual's health beliefs and practices is to carefully question that individual.

Table 9–2. TRADITIONAL ETHNIC/CULTURAL HEALTH INTERVENTIONS

Ethnic/Cultural Group	Health Intervention
African-American	Mixture of sugar and turpentine taken PO to treat worms or applied topically to cure a backache. Onion poultice used to heal infection; flaxseed poultice used to treat earache. Goldenseal root (herb) tea used to treat pain and to reduce fever; sassafras (herb) tea or mixture of hot lemon water and honey used to treat colds. Rubbing the chest with hot camphorated oil and wrapping the area with flannel used to treat cough and chest congestion; mixture of raw garlic, onion, parsley, and water used as an expectorant. Sour milk placed on stale bread and wrapped in cloth used to treat cuts and wounds.
Hispanic	Cinnamon used to treat cough. Chamomile tea used to relieve nausea or vomiting during pregnancy. Rosemary used to induce menstruation. Sweet basil used to ward off evil spirits or to treat infections and insomnia. Garlic used to treat earaches and toothaches.
Asian-American	Lime calcium used to treat excessive mucus. Quicksilver used to treat venereal disease. Turtle shells used to stimulate weak kidneys or to remove gallstones. Seahorses pulverized and used to treat gout. Snake flesh ingested to keep eyes healthy and vision clear.
Native American	Root of the globe mallow chewed to help mend broken bones. Leaves of the blue gillia boiled in water and ingested to treat digestive disorders. Blanketflower used as a diuretic to treat painful urination. Root of the bladderpod chewed to treat snakebite. Yucca plant stem used as a laxative.

Source: From Spector, RE: Cultural Diversity in Health and Illness, ed 3. Appleton & Lange, Norwalk, Conn., 1991, with permission.

AFRICAN-AMERICANS

Members of the African-American community have their origins in Africa, Haiti, or the Dominican Republic.

Cultural Influences

In some African-American subcultures, health is viewed as a state of harmony among body, mind, and spirit, and illness as a state of disharmony that results from natural causes or divine punishment. The focal point of health-related folk practices, therefore, is to restore harmony. This is carried out through the interaction and supportive efforts of the individual, family, and community. The art of healing practices stems from a fundamental belief that such power is a divine gift from God and certain persons within the community have been identified as having this power to cure. Further, some members of the African-American community are well versed in the use of home remedies, and frequently kitchen condiments are used in preparations to treat conditions such as respiratory illness, colds, fevers, open wounds, and boils. Prayer, alone or in combination with rituals, and the practice of laying on of hands are often used in conjunction with home remedies. Other forms of healing include spiritual healing, seeking advice from a voodoo practitioner, or wearing amulets and charms to protect against evil spirits and disease.

One type of folk practitioner is the "old lady" or the "granny," a person knowledgeable about different home remedies made from certain spices, herbs, and roots that can be used to treat common illnesses (see Table 9–2). When an illness or condition extends beyond her realm of practice, the granny makes appropriate referrals to another type of practitioner. The most prevalent and diverse type of folk healer is the spiritualist, who combines rituals, spiritual beliefs, and herbal medicines to effect a cure for specific illnesses.

Folk health and illness beliefs of some African-Americans are shown in Table 9–3. The African-American's use of folk medicine is respected, and every effort is made to assist the patient to combine folk treatment with traditional western medicine as long as the two are not antagonistic. People who have a strong belief in the healing power of folk medicines continue to use them at home with or without medical sanctions.

Table 9–3. FOLK HEALTH AND ILLNESS BELIEFS OF SOME AFRICAN-AMERICANS

Folk Illness	Etiology	Signs/Symptoms	Practitioner	Treatment
High blood (too much blood)	Diet very high in red meat and rich food. Belief that high blood causes stroke	Weakness Paralysis Vertigo or other signs/symptoms related to a stroke	Family member, friend, spiritualist, or self	Ingest lemon juice, vinegar, Epsom salts, or other astringent food to sweat out the excess blood. Treatment varies depending on what is appropriate according to the zodiac almanac.
Low blood (not enough blood—anemia is conceptualized)	Too many astringent foods, too harsh a treatment for high blood. Remaining on high blood pressure medications for too long.	Fatigue Weakness	Same as for high blood	Eat rich red meat, beets. Stop taking treatment for high blood. Consult the zodiac almanac.
Thin blood (predisposition to illness)	Occurs in women, children, and old people. Blood is thin until puberty and remains so until old age in women.	Susceptibility to illness	Self	Exercise caution in cold weather by wearing warm clothing or by staying indoors.
Rash appearing on a child after birth	Impurities within the body coming out. The body is being defiled and therefore produces skin rashes.	Rash anywhere on the body; may be accompanied by fever	Family member	Take catnip tea as a laxative or commercial laxative. The quantity and kind depend on the age of the individual.
Diseases of witchcraft, hex, or conjuring	Envy and sexual conflict are the most frequent reasons for hexing another person.	Unusual behavior Sudden death Symptoms related to poisoning (e.g., foul taste, weight loss, nausea, vomiting). A crawling sensation on the skin or in the stomach. Psychotic behavior	Voodoo priest(ess) Spiritualist	Treatment varies, depending on the spell cast. Conja is the help given the conjured person.

Source: Hautman MA: Folk health and illness beliefs. The Nurse Practitioner 4(4):27, 1979, with permission.

Variations in Drug Response

Seventy-five percent of African-Americans are affected with lactose intolerance, which causes gastrointestinal symptoms such as abdominal bloating, cramping, and diarrhea when products containing lactose are ingested. A hematologic problem present in about 35% of African-Americans is G6PD deficiency. African-Americans with G6PD deficiency should not be administered chloroquine and other antimalarial drugs because acute intravascular hemolysis may occur. If the African-American patient is receiving analgesics (aspirin), sulfonamides and sulfones, antimalarials (primaquine, quinacrine), antibacterials (nitrofurantoin, chloramphenicol, para-aminosalicylic acid), vitamin K, probenecid, or quinidine, monitor for signs of anemia.

Ethnic differences in responsiveness to certain antihypertensive agents have been demonstrated between African-Americans and Caucasians. Caucasians exhibit a greater average decrease in blood pressure with beta-adrenergic blocking drugs (e.g., propranolol [Inderal]) and angiotensin-converting enzyme (ACE) inhibitors (e.g., captopril [Capoten]) than do African-Americans (Kudzma, 1992). This suggests that higher doses of these drugs may be needed to lower blood pressure in African-Americans. An explanation for this difference may be that African-Americans have mostly low-renin hypertension, and beta-blockers and ace inhibitors reduce the activity of the renin-angiotensin system. On the other hand, African-Americans are more responsive to diuretics to control blood pressure, especially monotherapy with thiazide diuretics (Moser, 1989).

HISPANICS

Members of the Hispanic culture have origins in Spain, Cuba, South America, Mexico, Puerto Rico, and other Spanish-speaking countries.

Cultural Influences

Some Hispanics believe that a healthy state of being exists when the psychosocial, biologic, and spiritual nature are holistically balanced in relation to one's environment, wherein the focus of hot, cold, wet, and dry must be balanced. Within the body, humors or fluids are classified as either (1) blood (hot and wet), (2) yellow bile (hot and dry), (3) phlegm (cold and wet), or (4) black bile (cold and dry) (Spector, 1996). When the body is healthy, these four humors are in balance.

Disease occurs when there is a hot and cold imbalance among the body fluids. Treatment modalities are determined by whether the disease is classified as hot or cold. Foods and medicines or herbs also have hot or cold properties. (The hot or cold characteristics do not, however, necessarily denote actual physical temperature, color, or shape.) Treatments for hot or cold illnesses require selection of substances that counterbalance the hot or cold quality of that disease. For example, a hot illness such as an ulcer is treated with a cold medicine or herb, whereas a cold disease such as pneumonia is treated by the use of chili (considered a hot substance). Drugs may also be classified as either hot (e.g., penicillin) or cold (e.g., mannitol). With the hot-cold classification and treatment system, penicillin (a hot medicine) is not used to heal ailments also classified as hot, such as kidney problems, infections, or sore throat. The classification of a disease, food, or medicinal substance may vary from individual to individual because of a lack of consensus. Table 9–4 shows the hot-cold classification and treatment system. Table 9–5 provides examples of expected behaviors of patients subscribing to the hot-cold system.

The Hispanic may self-treat or consult a folk practioner. The belief that health is a matter of chance and controlled by sources in nature is known as "curanderismo." Curanderismo is a "medical system that combines spiritualistic, homeopathic, and scientific elements" (Spector,

---

Table 9–4. THE HOT-COLD CLASSIFICATION AND TREATMENT SYSTEM

Hot Conditions	Hot Foods	Hot Medicines and Herbs
Fever	Coffee	Penicillin
Infections	Chocolate	Aspirin
Ulcers	Garlic	Iron preparations
Sore throat	Cheese	Castor oil
Constipation	Eggs	Cod-liver oil
Diarrhea	Hard liquor	Vitamins
Rashes	Evaporated milk	Anise
Kidney problems	Kidney beans	Cinnamon
	Chili peppers	Gingerroot
	Cornmeal	

Cold Conditions	Cold Foods	Cold Medicines and Herbs
Cancer	Avocados	Bicarbonate of soda
Arthritis	Bananas	Milk of magnesia
Joint pain	Whole milk	Nightshade (yerba mora)
Headache	Honey	Linden flowers
Menstruation	Raisins	Orange flower water
Pneumonia	Sugar cane	Mannitol
Colds	Coconut	Sage

Source: Adapted from Wilson, H, and Kneisel, C: Psychiatric Nursing. Addison-Wesley, Reading, Mass., 1993.

Table 9–5. EXPECTED BEHAVIOR OF PATIENTS WHO ADHERE TO THE HOT-COLD SYSTEM

Patient's Condition	Expected Behavior
Common cold, arthritis, joint pains	Patient will not take cold-classified foods or medications but will accept those classified as hot.
Diarrhea, rash, ulcers	Patient will not take hot-classified medications and uses cool substances as therapy.
Requires a diuretic as part of a treatment regimen and has been told to supplement potassium intake by eating bananas, oranges, raisins, or dried fruit	Patient will not eat these cold-classified foods with a cold or other cold-classified condition (for female patients this includes the menses).
Requires penicillin or any other hot medication, particularly on an ongoing basis	Patient will stop taking hot medicine when suffering any hot-classified symptom (e.g., diarrhea, constipation, rash).
Infant requires formula, which contains hot-classified evaporated milk	Mother will put baby on cold-classified whole milk or will, after feeding formula, "refresh" the baby's stomach with various cool substances, some of which are diuretic.
Pregnant	Woman avoids hot medicine and hot foods and takes cool medicine frequently.
Postpartum and during menstruation	Woman avoids cool foods and medicines, particularly those that are acidic.

Source: Harwood, A: The hot-cold theory of disease: Implications for treatment of Puerto Rican patients. JAMA 216(7):1155, 1991, with permission.

1991). The curandero is a holistic folk healer who views illness from a religious and social perspective as opposed to the medical-scientific point of view. Imbalances between food, water, air, hot and cold, and God and man are thought to contribute to illness. To restore balance, treatments may include diet, herbs, suggestion, magic, prayers, and supernatural rituals. The curandero is often called upon to treat more serious physical and emotional illnesses and is frequently consulted before medical contact is made, or he may be consulted concurrently.

Other folk practitioners who may be consulted for healing purposes are the espiritualista, or spiritualist, and the yerbero, or herbalist (all folk healers). Herbal treatment, prayers, and the wearing of medals are common forms of interventions used by these folk healers to either prevent or cure the illness. See Table 9–2 for examples of traditional health interventions for Hispanics.

The nurse must assess whether the patient is using a curandero or other folk practitioner, what health interventions are being used, and whether the patient is self-medicating with other drugs. The nurse also must assess whether the Hispanic patient has received a BCG vaccine (a live attenuated vaccine prepared from *Mycobacterium bovis* that promotes active immunity to tuberculosis). BCG vaccine, which is not to be confused with bacillus Calmette-Guérin (BCG), is widely used in countries with a high incidence of tuberculosis, such as Mexico. When an individual is inoculated with BCG and then later given a purified protein derivative (PPD) skin test, an intense reaction to the combination of the BCG and the PPD generally occurs, resulting in possible skin necrosis and subsequent scarring of the infected area. If the nurse is unable to determine if the patient has had a BCG vaccination, a chest radiograph instead of a skin test is recommended (Giger and Davidhizar, 1991).

Variations in Drug Response

Because there are fewer studies of possible variations in drug response among Hispanics, less is known about whether members in this ethnic group share common altered physiologic responses to certain drug classes. However, it has been reported that Hispanic patients require lower doses of antidepressant medication than non-Hispanic patients. In addition, Hispanic patients taking tricyclic antidepressants are reported to experience side effects at half the dosages observed in Caucasians.

ASIAN-AMERICANS

Asian-Americans are a diverse group in the United States with origins in many Asian cultures, (i.e., Japanese, Chinese, Filipino, Korean, Vietnamese, and others). MOST ASIAN cultures have historically derived their traditional health-care beliefs and practices from China.

Cultural Influences

Many Asian-Americans believe that harmony with nature is essential for physical and spiritual well-being and that balance depends upon harmony between the elemental forces of fire, water, wood, earth, and metal. Regulation of these elements depends on the forces of yin and yang, the powers that regulate the universe. Yang represents the male, positive energy that produces light, warmth, and fullness; yin denotes the female, negative energy—the force of darkness, cold, and emptiness. Yin and yang exert power not only in the universe, but within humans as well. The imbalance of these forces causes physical disease.

Therapeutic options to restore the proper balance of yin and yang might include acupuncture, herbal medicines, massage, nutritional changes, and cupping. Acupuncture is used mainly in diseases in which there is an excess of yang and involves the practice of puncturing the body with needles to cure diseases such as stroke and asthma or to relieve pain. Moxibustion, the custom of applying heat to traditional acupuncture points, is used primarily in diseases in which there is an excess of yin and is often used during the labor and delivery period or to treat such illnesses as mumps or convulsions.

Herbals are often used to strengthen the body's natural healing forces. Herbal medicines are classified according to the properties of yin and yang and prescribed and used on the basis of the yin-yang nature of the particular illness. Many medicinal herbs are in use today for a variety of illnesses (see Table 9–2). Some herbs are used to treat more than one condition. Ginseng, for example, is recommended for use in more than two dozen illnesses, including anemia, colic, depression, indigestion, impotence, and rheumatism (Giger and Davidhizar, 1991).

Many Asian-Americans combine Western medical practices with traditional Asian folk medicine (primarily herbals). This may create problems of toxicity or interaction because the traditional drugs may have similar or antagonistic actions. For example, the medicinal herb ginseng is a tonic stimulant and an antihypertensive drug which, when taken concurrently with a Western-prescribed antihypertensive drug, may result in overmedication (Giger and Davidhizar,1991).

Variations in Drug Response

There are a variety of enzymatic and genetic variations among Asian-Americans, an example of which is glucose-6-phosphate dehydrogenase (G6PD) deficiency, a red blood cell defect that causes fragility of the red blood cells. To identify patients with this genetic deficiency, the fluorescent spot test may be performed. Asian-Americans with G6PD deficiency should not be administered chloroquine and other antimalarial drugs because acute intravascular hemolysis may occur. If the Asian-American patient is receiving analgesics (aspirin), sulfonamides and sulfones, antimalarials (primaquine, quinacrine), antibacterials (nitrofurantoin, chloramphenicol, para-aminosalicylic acid), vitamin K, probenecid, or quinidine, monitor for signs of anemia.

Caffeine, a component of many drugs as well as coffee, tea, and colas, appears to be excreted more slowly by Asian-Americans. The differences correlate with liver enzyme differences (Kudzma, 1992).

Alcohol, metabolized by the liver enzyme alcohol dehydrogenase in Caucasians, is metabolized by aldehyde dehydrogenase in Asian-Americans. Aldehyde dehydrogenase biotransforms alcohol more rapidly than alcohol dehydrogenase, often causing circulatory and unpleasant side effects such as flushing and palpitations (Kudzma, 1992).

Even after consideration of body surface area and weight, Asian-American men have been found to need half as much propranolol (Inderal) as Caucasian men, and they also require smaller doses of psychotropic medications. Awareness of the potential for unusually high plasma concentrations of psychotropic drugs such as lithium (Eskalith), haloperidol (Haldol), and alprazolam (Xanax) may alert the nurse to early detection and prevention of serious side effects, such as tardive dyskinesia in Asian-American patients (Kudzma, 1992). Asian-Americans are reported to better tolerate the sedating effects of diphenhydramine (Benadryl) and to be less sensitive to the cardiovascular and respiratory effects of analgesics such as morphine. Chinese-Americans are more sensitive to the sedative effects of benzodiazepines (e.g., diazepam [Valium]) and alprazolam (Xanax), and lower doses may be required.

NATIVE AMERICANS

The Native American population in the United States includes members of over 200 Indian tribes, and each Native American community is unique in its cultural beliefs. Therefore, the following discussion is intended only to present an overview of traditional beliefs and folk practices, although they may not be characteristic of all tribes.

Cultural Influences

The theme of total harmony with nature is a fundamental to Native American beliefs about health. The human body is considered one with the universe. Health depends on maintaining a state of equilibrium among the body, mind, and environment and is considered to be holistic in nature. Illness is believed to be a fact of life that occurs in relation to past or future events. One must deal, therefore, with the external event rather than the illness to effect improvement. Methods of intervention depend on this principle of cause and effect and traditionally are determined by the medicine man who diagnoses and recommends appropriate interventions. Treatment modalities include heat, herbs, sweat baths, prayers, massage, exercise, and diet modifications.

For many Native Americans, the medicine man is still the traditional healer, and he may perform special ceremonies to determine the cause and treatment of an illness or disease. The basis of treatment frequently lies in nature, hence, the use of herbal remedies to treat specific problems (see Table 9–2). Some Native Americans believe in the principle of "like cures like." Examples of this concept are the use of red plants to treat blood-related diseases or yellow plants to treat jaundice (Giger and Davidhizar, 1991). Experts in the medicinal use of native plants or animals are usually herbalists, although both the medicine man and the herbalist are believed to hold healing powers. Other Native American healers include sand painters, chanters, ceremonial specialists, and diagnosticians (Avery, 1994).

During the cultural assessment phase, the nurse should focus on tribe-specific beliefs and practices regarding health and illness rather than generalizing about all Native Americans (Antai-Otong, 1995).

Variation in Drug Response

About 85% to 90% of Native Americans have been found to have an intolerance to alcohol. Native Americans possess the high-activity variant of the ALDH enzyme, so consumed alcohol is rapidly converted to acetaldehyde. In 35% to 70% of Native Americans, the conversion of acetaldehyde to acetic acid (the next step in the metabolic process) is delayed. These enzyme differences cause most Native Americans to experience rapid onset of alcohol effects initially with a slow decrease in blood acetaldehyde levels thereafter.

Lactose intolerance occurs in 79% of Native Americans (Giger and Davidhizar, 1991). Patients with this disorder have an inherited or acquired deficiency in the enzyme (lactase) that converts lactose to glucose and galactose. When lactose (found in milk and some dairy products) is ingested, gastrointestinal symptoms—abdominal cramping, bloating, and diarrhea—occur.

Navajo Native Americans and Alaskan Eskimos are at greater risk for contracting invasive *Haemophilus influenzae* type b (Hib) infections. These groups may be targeted for inoculation with the Hib vaccine, which provides high immunogenity in all age groups.

USING THE NURSING PROCESS

ASSESSMENT

- Conduct a systematic assessment to integrate the patient's ethnic/cultural background into a nursing-process-based patient-care plan.
- Assess cultural, sociologic, psychologic, and biologic/physiologic aspects using an ethnic/cultural assessment tool such as Bloch's ethnic/cultural assessment guide. Combine this tool with existing assessment nursing collection instruments to identify key aspects of the patient's background that may influence his or her health care.
- Assess individual characteristics among patients from the same cultural group to design culturally specific care plans. Maintain an objective, open attitude regarding the patient's ethnic/cultural background to prevent ethnocentrism. Document all information heard and observed; confirm with the patient that the interpretations are correct.

NURSING DIAGNOSIS

- Establish nursing diagnoses that take into consideration the ethnic/cultural background of the patient. The patient is likely to disregard the medication regimen or combine it with traditional cultural health/illness practices if ethnic/cultural considerations are not accounted for. The blending of dissimilar types of therapy interventions may result in a variety of reactions, some of which may be detrimental to the patient's state of health or to the prescribed therapeutic drug program.
- Typical nursing diagnoses for a patient whose ethnic/cultural beliefs, values, and ideals are in conflict with the prescribed drug regimen include the following: Knowledge Deficit related to lack of exposure, information misinterpretation, and lack of interest in learning; Ineffective Management of Individual Therapeutic Regimen related to complexity of the therapeutic regimen and the health-care system, mistrust of the treatment and/or the health-care personnel; health belief conflicts and previous experiences with the health-care delivery system; and Noncompliance related to value system, health beliefs, cultural influences, and spiritual values.
- Involve the patient and family in the development of the nursing diagnoses. When the patient feels involved in the decision-making process and his or her ethnic/cultural heritage is considered in the prescribed drug therapy, the probability of patient satisfaction is enhanced because of shared patient interest.

PLANNING

- Design strategies for interventions that focus on the drug therapy as a central component of the plan or in conjunction with other therapies. During this phase all data regarding the patient's ethnic/cultural background are communicated and shared with the health-care team to ensure that cultural factors are an integral part of the plan. Record the information in the patient's chart or Kardex so that all personnel involved with the patient are appraised of the need for integration of ethnic/cultural influences into the plan of care.
- Obtain input from the patient and family. This is essential if a plan is to be effective and reflect the patient's cultural beliefs and values regarding health and illness. For example, if the patient uses folk medicine as part of his or her home treatment, the substance is included in the nursing care plan in conjunction with the proposed drug regimen whenever possible.

INTERVENTION

- Implement the nursing strategies listed in the nursing-care plan. Assess the patient for variant responses to drug therapy and make sure that modifications are made in the care plan based on these observations. For example:
  - Assess African-Americans for a lessened response to propanolol (Inderal) and angiotensin converting enzyme (ACE) inhibitors such as captopril (Capoten). This population also requires assessment for lactose intolerance and G6PD deficiency.
  - Hispanics may experience an increase in side effects when taking antidepressants and must be monitored for the appearance of these adverse drug responses.
  - Asian-Americans must be assessed for lactose and alcohol intolerance and G6PD deficiency. This cultural group may also require smaller doses of psychotropic medications and seem to be less sensitive to the cardiovascular and respiratory effects of mor-

phine. Chinese-Americans may be more sensitive to the sedative effects of diazepam (Valium) and alprazolam (Xanax) and require lower doses. Monitor Chinese-American male patients for adverse response to propranolol (Inderal), as they may require lower doses than Caucasian males.

○ Native Americans require monitoring for lactose and alcohol intolerance. All age groups of the Navajo Native Americans and Alaskan Eskimos are at a greater risk for contracting invasive *Haemophilus influenzae* type b (HIB) infections and need to be assessed regarding inoculations.

EVALUATION

- Evaluate the effectiveness of drug therapy. Drug regimens may have to be adjusted so they are not antagonistic with the patient's value system If the patient is discharged, schedule return visits at specified in-

tervals to the outpatient clinic where drug therapy interventions may be further evaluated. If the patient is unable to make follow-up visits or has never been hospitalized, a follow-up questionnaire may be a useful evaluation tool to obtain information and to appraise drug therapy effectiveness. In other cases, a home visit or phone call may be appropriate.

A drug therapy program that accommodates the patient's ethnic/cultural beliefs and practices regarding health and illness is likely to promote increased satisfaction with the traditional health-care delivery system in American subcultural groups. The nurse is in a pivotal position to ensure that these culture-dependent health assumptions are considered when designing a nursing care plan that involves drug therapy for the patient.

The bibliography for this chapter can be found in Appendix B, which begins on page 1054.

CHAPTER REVIEW QUESTIONS*

1. Mary Bell, RN, has been assigned to care for Mrs. Velasquez, a Hispanic admitted to the hospital for diabetic management. Perhaps the best method Mary may use to increase her knowledge of Mrs. Velasquez's cultural/ethnic background is to:
   a. Talk to other nurses who have had experience in caring for Hispanic Americans.
   b. Research information about Hispanics from reliable sources.
   c. Conduct an ethnic/cultural assessment and then reaffirm that interpretations of Mrs. Velasquez's needs are accurate.
   d. Read articles that deal with providing care for Hispanic patients.

2. Ted Jones, a 55-year-old African-American, has been admitted to your unit for management of hypertension. Which statement below indicates an *ethnocentric* response by the nurse caring for Mr. Jones?
   a. African-Americans exhibit a less than-average decrease in blood pressure when treated with beta-adrenergic blocking agents.
   b. Folk healing practices ought to be gently discouraged and replaced with modern medical treatments.
   c. African-Americans require higher doses of angiotension-converting enzyme inhibitors than Caucasians.
   d. Many African-Americans use home remedies and often seek the advice of "grannies."

3. Mr. Good, a Native American, has been admitted to your unit for treatment of alcoholism. Which statement below indicates a culturally sensitive nurse in discussing his alcohol problem?
   a. Join a support group to discuss your feelings about alcohol use and abuse.
   b. The 12-step Alcoholics Anonymous program is effective in treating people with alcohol problems.
   c. Seek out the traditional healer who will perform a special ceremony to cure your alcohol intolerance.
   d. Enzyme differences among Native Americans account for the rapid onset of alcohol effects.

4. As America continues to become a more multicultural society, nurses are being challenged to learn more about how ethnic/cultural differences affect health and health care. To develop a culture-specific care plan, the nurse:
   a. Uses culture distancing as a method of reinforcing ethnocentrism.
   b. Integrates the patient's ethnic/cultural background into a nursing-care plan.
   c. Considers his or her own cultural background, and then compares it with the patient's to promote ethnocentrism.
   d. Views people from the same ethnic/cultural group as alike, with few individual differentiations.

*See Appendix A, which begins on page 1051, for answers.

UNIT 4

DIAGNOSTIC AND NUTRITIONAL AGENTS

CHAPTER 10

Drugs Used in Diagnostic Testing

Merrily A. Kuhn, RNC, PhD

CHAPTER OUTLINE

KEY TERMS

Anergic
Angiography
Aortography
Arthrography
Candida
Cell-mediated immunity
Cholecystangiography
Extravasation
Fluoroscopy
Hysterosalpingography
Lymphography

Microcurie (μCi)
Millicurie (mCi)
Mycobacterium tuberculosis
Opaque
Radionuclide
Radiopaque compound
Radiopharmaceutical
Trichophyton
Urography
Venography
Vesiculation

LEARNING OBJECTIVES

After reading this chapter, the student will be able to:

1. Identify the major categories of diagnostic agents.
2. Differentiate among the common diagnostic agents the indication for use, mechanism of action, mode of administration, contraindications, precautions, adverse reactions, and interactions.
3. Identify the nursing implications for the common diagnostic agents.
4. Develop a nursing teaching plan for the patient undergoing diagnostic tests.

Diagnostic testing often involves the use of chemical substances to facilitate the diagnosis of illness or to aid in the visualization of various internal structures. Although the nurse usually does not administer these agents, knowledge of the agent's actions and potential adverse reactions is important in providing quality nursing care.

The diagnostic agents to be discussed are classified into the following general categories: radiopaque compounds used in diagnostic x-ray studies, agents used to stimulate glandular secretion (provocative agents), radioactive tracers used in nuclear imaging, nonradioactive dyes used in volumetric tests, and agents used in skin testing. The agents used most commonly are presented in Tables 10–1 to 10–3.

RADIOPAQUE COMPOUNDS

Conventional x-ray studies (plain film) visualize bone and other dense structures. *Radiopaque compounds* are substances that do not allow the passage of x-rays or other radiant energy. Because soft tissues (vascular structures and ductal systems, for example) have less absorption, they require the presence of a radiopaque compound as contrast for a definitive shape to be visualized on x-ray films. (Radiopaque areas appear white on exposed film.) The radiopaque contrast media used most commonly are barium sulfate and iodinated compounds.

Table 10–1. DIAGNOSTIC RADIOPAQUE COMPOUNDS

DRUG NAME/ROUTE AND DOSAGE	PHARMACOKINETICS/ DYNAMICS	NURSING IMPLICATIONS
barium sulfate **Adults and Children:** PO (tablets, suspension) or rectal (suspension) administration; dosage based on the region of GI tract being examined, degree of contrast needed, and technique used.	**Onset:** PO, immediate (esophagus and stomach), 15–90 min (small intestine); rectal, immediate (colon) **Peak:** not absorbed **Duration:** 24 hr after oral administration with normal GI function. In rectal administration barium expelled with enema, but some may persist for several weeks **½L:** NA **PB:** NA **B:** not biotransformed **E:** fecal	**ASSESSMENT:** Obtain patient history regarding GI dysfunction and previous reactions to barium. Assess potential for aspiration. Assess patient's ability to follow directions and tolerate procedure. Assess for pregnancy (a contraindication). Assess patient's understanding of pretest dietary and fluid restrictions. If performed on outpatient basis, assess patient's ability to self-administer suppositories or enemas. After test, assess bowel sounds to detect for possible bowel obstruction. Assess bowel movement to document barium evacuation and assess patient for signs of fluid volume deficit. Notify physician if abdominal pain, decreased bowel sounds, or constipation develop. **INTERVENTION: For barium swallow—**Patient is NPO for 8–12 hr before test. After test, cathartic is usually prescribed. Inform patient that stools will be chalky and light-colored for 24–72 hr. Record description for all stools passed. Barium should be expelled in 48–72 hrs. Mouth care to remove barium taste is also important. Encourage increased fluid intake to avoid dehydration. **For barium enema—**Tell patient to follow prescribed dietary restrictions. Give laxative, suppository, and/or enema as ordered. After test, patient is encouraged to defecate. Cathartic or cleansing enema is given. **EVALUATION:** Shows no adverse reaction to barium procedure. Bowel function returned to pretest condition.

IODINATED COMPOUNDS

diatrizoate sodium (Hypaque Sodium) **Adults:** 90–180 mL 25%–40% solution PO; 500–1000 mL 15%–25% solution rectally. For IV administration, dosage and concentration are individualized based on size of vascular region to be visualized and hemodilution in region. **Children:** 30–75 mL 20%–40% solution PO; 100–500 mL 10%–15% rectally. Dosage, mode of administration, and concentration based on body region to be examined, technique used, and contrast needed.	**Onset:** depends on mode and region to be visualized: PO, 30–40 min (stomach); Rectal, immediate (colon); IV, immediate **Peak:** as above **Duration:** NA **½L:** 30–60 min with normal renal function, 20–140 hr with severe renal impairment **PB:** <5% **B:** unchanged **E:** 95%–100% renal, 1–2% fecal; 20%–50% fecal with severe renal impairment.	**ASSESSMENT:** Obtain history regarding any reactions to diagnostic tests using radiopaque compounds and/or allergy to foods containing iodine (e.g., shellfish). Report positive history to physician immediately. Obtain menstrual history confirming nonpregnancy status. Assess vital signs and report any abnormalities. Assess for severe renal or liver impairment, hyperthyroidism, sickle cell anemia, multiple myeloma, congestive heart disease, and pheochromocytoma (all contraindications). **INTERVENTION:** Many techniques are used: IV, intra-arterial, or direct instillation. Patient preparation: Usually the patient is NPO at least 8 hr prior to the test to reduce aspiration risk. Clear fluids may be given, which may prevent dehydration. This is especially important in infants, young children, geriatric patients, or azotemic patients. A laxative at bedtime may also be ordered. Pretreatment with corticosteroids or antihistamines may be administered to patient with history of reactions to contrast media. Blood pressure and pulse are monitored during examination and for at least 30–60 min after test. **EVALUATION:** Patient shows no allergic or adverse reactions to test. Fluid status is normal. Patient understands test result and follow-up

iopanoic acid (Telepaque)		
oral cholecystographic agent **Adults:** 3 g (6 tablets) PO 10–14 hr prior to test, or 500 mg q 1 hr PO × 6 doses beginning 18 hr prior to test. Not to exceed 6 g/24 hr. **Children:** 50–150 mg/kg PO.	**Onset:** 5–6 hr **Peak:** 14–19 hr; children, 4–9 hr **Duration:** NA **½L:** 24 hr **PB:** 97% **B:** liver **E:** ⅓ renal, ⅔ fecal	**ASSESSMENT:** Check patient's history for iodine allergies or previous hypersensitivity reaction to contrast media. Assess for severe renal or hepatic impairment, malabsorption disorders, and pregnancy (all contraindications).

Continued on the following page

Table 10–1. DIAGNOSTIC RADIOPAQUE COMPOUNDS, *Continued*

DRUG NAME/ROUTE AND DOSAGE	PHARMACOKINETICS/ DYNAMICS	NURSING IMPLICATIONS
iopanoic acid (Telepaque), *continued*		
		INTERVENTION: Patient preparation—Normal diet with some fat for 1 or more days prior to test is usually prescribed to stimulate gallbladder. Evening meal before taking iopanoic acid tablets is low-fat or fat-free. Adult dose of 3 g (6 tablets) is administered with water after meal. Tablets are taken one at a time in 5-min intervals. Patient is NPO except for water until after test. Laxative may also be prescribed to be taken 4–6 hr before taking oral cholecystographic agent. Cleansing enema may be ordered morning of test to eliminate fecal contents or gas. Concomitant use of aspirin (600 mg) and repeated 2 hr later counteracts the uricosuric effects of iopanoic acid. Monitor blood pressure and pulse during and after test. Observe patient for allergic or adverse reactions. Epinephrine should be available to counteract severe reaction. **EVALUATION:** Patient understands pretest diet, is able to swallow and retain tablets, and shows no signs of adverse reactions. Patient understands diet modifications if gallstones are noted.

NA = not available.

Table 10–2. DIAGNOSTIC SECRETAGOGUES AND AGENTS FOR TESTING CARDIAC OR LIVER FUNCTION

SECRETAGOGUES

DRUG NAME/ROUTE AND DOSAGE	PHARMACOKINETICS/ DYNAMICS	NURSING IMPLICATIONS
histamine phosphate		
for gastric function Dosage expressed in terms of histamine. *Adults:* 0.01 mg/kg SC; 0.0145 mg/kg SC for augmented test. *Children:* No recommended dose stated.	**Onset:** immediate–15 min **Peak:** very transient **Duration:** up to 10 min **½L:** NA **PB:** NA **B:** NA **E:** renal	**ASSESSMENT:** Assess patient history, note particularly any history of dyspnea, wheezing, palpitations, syncope, or blood pressure problems. Assess patient's ability to follow dietary and activity restrictions. Assess for asthma or other severe allergies, pregnancy, cardiac abnormalities, hypotension or severe hypertension, and severe pulmonary or renal disease (all contraindications). **INTERVENTION: Patient preparation**—NPO including smoking 12 hr prior to test; bedrest. Hold medications that inhibit or stimulate gastric secretion, such as antacids, anticholinergics, adrenergic blockers, and H_2 antagonists. To inhibit adverse effects of histamine, simultaneous administration of antihistamine may be ordered. Monitor blood pressure and pulse during procedure and at least 30–60 min after test. A delayed response (60 min postinjection) may occur. **EVALUATION:** Shows no allergic or adverse reactions. Understands test results and follow-up.
secretin (Secretin-Kabi)		
for pacreatic function *Adults:* 1 CU/kg IV (pancreatic function); 2 CU/kg IV (gastrinoma).	**Onset:** NA **Peak:** 30 min **Duration:** 2 hr **½L:** 2–4 min **PB:** NA **B:** liver **E:** NA	Same as for histamine phosphate.

Continued on the following page

Table 10–2. DIAGNOSTIC SECRETAGOGUES AND AGENTS FOR TESTING CARDIAC OR LIVER FUNCTION, *Continued*		

SECRETAGOGUES, *Continued*

DRUG NAME/ROUTE AND DOSAGE	PHARMACOKINETICS/ DYNAMICS	NURSING IMPLICATIONS
sincalide (C8-CCK) (OP-CCK)		
for gallbladder function *Adults:* 02µg/kg IV. If contraction of the gallbladder does not occur in 15 min, second dose of 0.04 µg/kg may be given.	**Onset:** NA **Peak:** 5–15 min **Duration:** 1 hr **½L:** NA **PB:** NA **B:** NA **E:** NA	Same as for histamine phosphate plus: **INTERVENTION:** Administer slowly over 30–60 seconds.

AGENTS FOR CARDIAC OR LIVER FUNCTION: RADIOPHARMACEUTICALS

⁹⁹ᵐTc (technetium) sodium pertechnetate (⁹⁹ᵐTc-labeled RBC)		
for cardiac function *Adults:* 10–20 mCi IV (cardiac imaging). *Children:* Individualized.	**Onset:** immediately **Peak:** NA **Duration:** NA **½L:** 6.02 hr **PB:** high **B:** NA **E:** renal, about 39%/24 hr	**ASSESSMENT:** Assess history regarding past exposure to ionizing radiation and adverse reactions. Confirm nonpregnancy status; obtain menstrual history. **INTERVENTION:** Patient must follow directions regarding body position and motion during scanning. Post-test hydration to avoid accumulation of radioactivity in the bladder. Stress the necessity of proper hygiene after voiding to decrease contamination. **EVALUATION:** Patient shows no adverse reactions to procedure.
thallous chloride (Thallium 201)		
for cardiac function *Adults:* 1–2 mCi IV. *Children:* Individualized.	**Onset:** immediately–10 min **Peak:** NA **Duration:** NA **½L:** 1 hr **PB:** NA **B:** NA **E:** renal, 4–8%/24 hr	Same as for technetium.

AGENTS FOR CARDIAC OR LIVER FUNCTION: NONRADIOACTIVE DYES

indocyanine green (Cardio-Green)		
for cardiac function Given intracardiac via cardiac catheter. *Adults:* 5 mg. *Children:* 2.5 mg. *Infants:* 1.25 mg total dose not to exceed 2 mg/kg. **for liver function** *Adults:* 0.5 mg/kg IV.	**Onset:** 20 min **Peak:** NA **Duration:** NA **½L:** 1–4 min **PB:** 100% **B:** unchanged **E:** bile and fecal	**ASSESSMENT:** Assess patient history for allergy to iodine. Assess vital signs and note any cardiac irregularities prior to testing. **INTERVENTION: Cardiac studies**—Dye is injected rapidly through catheter into heart and timed blood measurements are made. Cardiac output is calculated using dilution of dye over time curve. After procedure, monitor blood pressure and pulse. Check incision for bleeding, leaking of dye, or hematoma formation. **Liver studies**—Patients should be in fasting, basal state. Venous blood sample taken before dye injected and blood samples taken at intervals following injection of dye. **EVALUATION:** Patient shows no signs of adverse reactions; understands test results and follow-up.

SC = subcutaneous; NA = not available; CU = clinical unit(s).

DIAGNOSTIC SECRETAGOGUES AND AGENTS FOR TESTING CARDIAC OR LIVER FUNCTION

Table 10–3. DIAGNOSTIC TUBERCULIN SKIN TEST AGENTS

DRUG NAME/ROUTE AND DOSAGE	PHARMACOKINETICS/DYNAMICS	NURSING IMPLICATIONS
purified protein derivative (PPD) *Adults:* Standard strength–5 TU/ 0.1 mL intradermally *First Strength*–1 TU/0.1 mL intradermally *Second Strength*–250 TU/0.1 mL intradermally	**Onset:** immediately–10 min **Peak:** NA **Duration:** NA **½L:** 1 hr **PB:** NA **B:** NA **E:** renal, 4%–8%/24 hr	**ASSESSMENT:** Assess history for positive skin test reaction, recent exposure to anyone with tuberculosis, or history of tuberculosis. Assess injection site for atopic dermatitis or other skin diseases. Assess for pregnancy (category C). **INTERVENTION:** Explain procedure to patient, reassure patient that test is relatively painless and injection is into only superficial layers of skin. Prepare injection site. Administer tuberculin by Mantoux method or by multiple-puncture devices method. Document location of injection on patient's chart. **Patient Teaching—**Patient to return within 48–72 hr to have skin reaction assessed. Inform patient that hard, red, raised area may appear at injection site, that it is temporary, and that it will resolve. Do not scratch area if pruritis develops. **EVALUATION:** Test site is examined 48–72 hr after administration. Skin induration and erythema are assessed. Induration is most significant clinical sign: <5 mm is negative; 5–9 mm is questionable; >10 mm is positive. Patients with positive skin test reactions should consult their physicians.

NA = not available.

BARIUM SULFATE

Barium sulfate is an inert, insoluble, nonabsorbable, *opaque* (impervious to light rays, x-rays, or other electromagnetic radiation) compound. It is used to visualize the gastrointestinal tract and is administered either orally (barium swallow test) or instilled rectally (barium enema). The barium swallow test is used for visualizing the upper gastrointestinal tract, the pharynx, esophagus, and the stomach. The barium enema is used to examine the lower gastrointestinal tract or the colon. Barium is eliminated unchanged in the feces and may require several days for complete evacuation. Therefore, if the patient is scheduled to have both a barium enema and barium swallow, the barium enema is performed before the barium swallow.

Contraindications and Precautions

Barium administration is contraindicated for use in patients with fistulas, perforations of the gastrointestinal tract, or known intestinal obstructions because resultant leakage of barium into the peritoneal cavity may cause peritonitis.

Adverse Effects and Interactions

The most common adverse reaction following barium administration is constipation. A cathartic or cleansing enema is given after the test. Abdominal distention, cramping, or diarrhea may also occur. The patient is assessed for signs of intestinal obstruction or perforation, which include abdominal pain, distention, rigidity, vomiting, and shock. Rectal administration of barium may stimulate a vagal response resulting in bradycardia (heart rate less than 50 beats per minute) and hypotension. This occurs more frequently in the older patient.

No known drug-drug interactions occur with barium sulfate.

Patient Preparation and Nursing Implications

In preparing the patient for gastrointestinal radiographic studies using barium, the nurse assesses the patient's history for past reactions to barium and present symptoms of gastrointestinal tract obstruction or perforation. The patient's ability to follow directions and tolerate the procedure is also assessed.

Barium Swallow For the barium swallow, the patient is allowed nothing by mouth (NPO) for 8 to 12 hours before the test. The patient is assessed for his or her ability to swallow and potential for aspiration. During the procedure, the patient is required to ingest 350 to 425 ml of barium, which has a milkshake consistency and a chalk-like taste. As the patient swallows the barium, a *fluoroscopy* (x-ray examination showing form and motion of the deep structures of the body) is performed, the image is observed, and films are obtained. After the barium swallow, a cathartic is usually prescribed. The patient is informed that barium will be expelled for the next 24 to 72 hours and stools will be chalky and light-colored. Retained barium may cause fecal impaction or obstruction; therefore, the nurse must note the passage of stool.

Barium Enema Patient preparation is rigorous, and acutely ill, debilitated, or geriatric patients may not tolerate the preparation. In addition, many patients fear this test and find it painful and embarrassing.

Preparation for the barium enema varies among hospitals. The nurse consults the policy and procedure manual for instructions. In general, the patient is put on a low-residue diet for 1 to 3 days or a clear liquid diet for 18 to 24 hours prior to the test. Laxatives are given the afternoon or evening before the test. The evening before the test or early in the morning on the day of the test, a suppository and/or enema is administered. After the test, the patient is encouraged to defecate and/or a cathartic or cleansing enema may be administered. The nurse records the passage of stool and/or the results of the enema. To avoid dehydration, the patient is encouraged to increase fluid intake.

IODINATED COMPOUNDS

The iodinated compounds are water-soluble, radiopaque agents that opacify structures and vessels upon contact. Visualization is maintained until significant hemodilution occurs. Iodinated compounds are used extensively as contrast media for a variety of diagnostic procedures involving x-ray-film visualization, including *angiography* (depicts vascular system), *venography* (depicts venous system), *lymphography* (depicts lymph vessels and lymph nodes), *aortography* (angiography of the aorta), *urography* (depicts urinary tract), *arthrography* (depicts joints), *cholecystangiography* (depicts gall bladder and bile ducts), and *hysterosalpingography* (depicts uterus and uterine tubes). Additionally, they are used in gastrointestinal radiography when barium is contraindicated. In computed tomography (CT) scans, iodinated contrast media are used to delineate soft tissue or vasculature. Depending on the area to be visualized and the method used, iodine preparations can be administered either orally or intravenously. Oral iodinated preparations are used to assess biliary and urinary function because after absorption they are concentrated by the biliary system and excreted via the kidneys. Commonly used iodinated compounds include **diatrizoate sodium *(Hypaque Sodium))*** and the oral cholecystographic agent **iopanoic acid *(Telepaque))*** (see Table 10–1).

Contraindications and Precautions

Diatrizoate sodium is contraindicated in patients with renal or hepatic impairment, as the kidney and liver are the organs of elimination/biotransformation, and in patients with hyperthyroidism, sickle cell anemia, multiple myeloma, heart disease, and pheochromocytoma because these conditions may worsen. Iopanoic acid is contraindicated in patients with severe renal or hepatic impairment, as the kidney and liver are the organs of elimination/biotransformation; in patients with malabsorption syndromes, as the dye needs to be absorbed; and in those who are pregnant, as fetal harm may occur.

Adverse Effects

The most common reactions following administration of intravenous iodinated compounds are pain and irritation at the injection site followed by a warm or burning sensation. Nausea, vomiting, diarrhea, sweating, and urticaria can also occur. Erythrocyte sludging and agglutination may occur, and normal coagulation may be inhibited. Children and elderly patients are most sensitive to this reaction.

▼ CLINICAL ALERT

Serious adverse reactions can occur in some individuals following the use of iodine contrast preparations. The most serious is anaphylaxis, which may result in cardiovascular collapse, central nervous system (CNS) depression, and, if untreated, death. Patients most at risk for anaphylaxis are those who are allergic to foods containing iodine, such as shellfish. During the history, make sure you ask the patient about previous allergic reactions to iodine-containing foods. (See Chapter 6 for discussion on drug-induced anaphylaxis and treatment.)

Interactions

There are many interactions to the iodinated preparations. Meperidine, morphine, and vasopressors may increase the hemodynamic and neurologic effects. Oral cholecystographic agents may cause renal toxicity when followed by intravenous (IV) diatrizoates. Concurrent use of IV diatrizoates with general anesthetics may increase the incidence of adverse reactions.

Possible drug-lab interactions include a decrease in leukocyte and red blood cell (RBC) counts, an increase in prothrombin time (PT) and partial thromboplastin time (PTT), an increase in serum protein-bound iodine (PBI), and a decrease in radioactive iodine uptake for a period of 1 week to 2 years. An increase in serum amylase may occur 6 to 18 hours after the administration of IV diatrizoates. Urine tests (e.g., protein, specific gravity, glucose) may be affected up to 2 days after the administration of IV diatrizoates.

Nursing Implications

Prior to any test using iodinated compounds, the patient's history is obtained and any previous exposure or reaction to iodinated compounds is assessed. Allergy to foods containing iodine (for example, shellfish) is also documented and reported to the physician. It is also important to determine if thyroid function tests are planned; iodine may interfere with thyroid tests.

AGENTS TO STIMULATE GLAND SECRETION

Agents used to stimulate glandular secretion are referred to as provocative agents because of a measurable physiologic response that is produced following their administration. There are two categories of these agents: tropic hormones, which stimulate endocrine glands to release their hormones; and secretagogues, which stimulate secretion of enzymes.

TROPIC HORMONES

Tropic hormones used in diagnostic testing include **adrenocorticotropic hormone** and **thyrotropin**. Adrenocorticotropic hormone stimulates the adrenal gland to release glucocorticoids and is used to diagnose adrenal insufficiency. The tropic hormone thyrotropin stimulates the thyroid gland to release thyroxine and thus aids in the differential diagnosis of primary thyroid disease versus pituitary dysfunction. Tropic hormones are discussed in Unit 11 (Drugs Affecting the Endocrine System).

SECRETAGOGUES

The secretagogous agents include **histamine phosphate**, which stimulates the production of gastric acid secretion; **secretin *(Secretin-Kabi)***, which stimulates pancreatic secretion; and **sincalide *(C8-CCK)***, which stimulates gallbladder contraction and bile release (see Table 10–2).

Adverse Effects and Interactions

The most common adverse effects include headache, hypertension, or hypotension. Patients may also experience dizziness, visual disturbances, syncope, tachycardia, palpitations, dyspnea, diarrhea, cramps, nausea, vomiting, and local erythema at the injection site. Allergic reactions, manifested by skin rash to anaphylaxis, may also occur.

There are no known interactions with the use of the secretagogues.

Patient Preparation and Nursing Implications

For each test a procedure protocol is used. Usually the patient is NPO for 12 to 24 hours prior to the test, an intravenous line is inserted, and with most gastrointestinal tests a nasogastric tube is also inserted. Following the administration of the provocative agent, the nurse is primarily responsible for obtaining gastric samples and/or blood samples at timed intervals.

Before the test is performed, the nurse obtains the patient's history, which includes information regarding the patient's underlying illness, previous history of exposure to the provocative agent, and associated adverse reactions. In collaboration with the physician, the test procedure and risks are reviewed with the patient and a written consent is obtained.

Most of these agents are administered systemically, after which they move to the specific target organ and induce a measurable response. The primary function of the nurse in caring for a patient who receives a provocative agent is to monitor for physiologic responses. The agent frequently exacerbates the patient's underlying illness. For example, the increased gastric acid secretion produced by the administration of histamine phosphate can cause perforation of a peptic ulcer; with administration of sincalide, acute cholecystitis may develop; and after the administration of secretin, acute pancreatitis may occur.

These are severe responses to the provocative secretogogue agents, and the nurse must know what signs and symptoms to anticipate. In addition, most secretagogues are protein substances that may stimulate an allergic reaction. Continual assessment of the patient during the testing procedure is essential.

RADIOACTIVE AGENTS

Radioactive compounds are referred to as *radiopharmaceuticals*, chemical compounds composed of two parts: a *radionuclide*, which is an unstable nucleus with orbiting radioactive electrons, and a chemical pharmaceutical with known physiologic properties. As the unstable nucleus rearranges to become more stable, energy is emitted. This energy is radiation and is either particulate or electromagnetic. Particulate radiation is the emission of alpha and beta rays. Electromagnetic radiation is the release of gamma rays or x-rays. In diagnostic radiology, the electromagnetic radiation is measured.

A radiopharmaceutical is chosen because of its selective affinity to localize in either normal or abnormal tissue. When a radiopharmaceutical is administered, the area is scanned with either a gamma camera or a rectilinear scanner, which detects specific localization of the drug. Pathologic findings are indicated as "cold" or "hot" spots. On the scan, an area with little uptake of the radioactive agent is called a cold spot, while an area with an increased uptake is a hot spot.

As a diagnostic agent, the dose of the radiopharmaceutical is lower than the therapeutic dose. Thus, there are no pharmacologic effects of the agent. The dosing unit for the radiopharmaceutical is usually the *millicurie (mCi)* or *microcurie (μCi)*, which is a measure of the radioactivity associated with a specific amount of the substance. Adverse reactions rarely occur, and the radiation risk to the patient is very low.

The radioactive agents commonly used include ^{99m}**Tc (technetium) sodium pertechnetate (*^{99m}TC-labeled RBC)** and **thallous chloride *(Thallium 201)*** (see Table 10–2). ^{99m}Tc sodium pertechnetate is used in cardiac blood pool imaging and as an adjunct in the diagnosis of pericardial effusion and ventricular aneurysm. Thallous chloride is used to assess coronary artery blood flow and myocardial perfusion and is often used in combination with a stress ECG to diagnose ischemic heart disease.

Contraindications and Precautions

Radioactive agents are contraindicated in pregnancy because they may be teratogenic. Therefore, prior to administration of these agents, it is important to ascertain whether the patient is pregnant.

Patient Preparation and Nursing Implications

Radioactive agents are prepared and administered by specially trained health care professionals such as physicians or nuclear medicine technicians under the direction of a physician. The nurse is primarily responsible for preparing the patient for the test and minimizing radiation contamination after the test. Patient preparation depends on the specific scan and the radioactive agent used (e.g., voiding just before a bone scan to decrease concentration of the radioactive agent in the bladder or fasting before a stress Thallium scan to decrease the risk of aspiration in case of cardiac arrest).

Many patients fear radiation. The purpose of the test is explained, and the procedure is described. Radionuclides are administered either orally or intravenously before scanning. The scan is done immediately or several hours later. More than one scan may be performed, so the patient is given written instructions regarding the specific time to return for the scan.

When a cardiac stress (exercise) test is combined with imaging, the patient is NPO for six hours before the test and the use of alcohol, tobacco, and nonprescription medication is restricted for 24 hours. The physician may also have the patient discontinue specific cardiac medication before the test.

After the test, the patient is instructed to increase fluid intake and void frequently to avoid accumulation of radioactivity in the bladder. Proper hygiene after voiding is important to decrease possible radioactive contamination.

For 24 hours after the procedure, pregnant nurses should avoid contact with the patient. For 1 to 2 days after injection of the radionuclide, rubber or plastic gloves are required when handling bedpans, urine specimens, or contaminated drainage bags.

NONRADIOACTIVE DYES

Nonradioactive dyes are used to measure organ function. Flow rates, diffusion, fluid volumes, and concentration parameters are obtained as the dye passes through the system. Because the dyes are relatively inert compounds, the distribution, metabolism, and excretion of the dye are the properties that make it useful as a diagnostic agent. The two dyes used most commonly are **bromosulfophthalein sodium (Bromsulphalein, BSP)**, which is used to assess liver function, and **indocyanine green (Cardio-Green)** used to measure cardiac output (see Table 10–2).

Adverse Effects

Nonradioactive dyes cause few and very mild effects, and allergic reactions are rare.

Interactions

Phenobarbital may decrease the half-life of indocyanine green. Hepatic excretion of bromosulfophthalein sodium is impaired with simultaneous administration of indocyanine green. Drug-lab interactions may cause a decrease in radioactive iodine uptake for at least 1 week following use of the dye, and there may be an increase in serum inorganic iodide concentrations.

Nursing Implications

Prior to the administration of the dye, the patient is assessed for dehydration or volume overload, which are both contraindications for use. Anaphylactic reactions are rare but may occur, especially following extravasation of bromosulfophthalein sodium. (*Extravasation* is the accidental escape of an intravenously administered drug into the surrounding tissues.) Thus, emergency equipment is always available.

DIAGNOSTIC SKIN TESTS

Skin testing for diagnostic purposes is performed to evaluate the cellular immune response of a patient upon injection of specific antigenic preparations. These tests are used to determine the presence of allergies, to diagnose infections, or to assess *cell-mediated immunity* (delayed immune response mediated primarily by T-cell lymphocytes rather than antibodies).

Three methods of skin testing are used: the patch test, wherein an adhesive patch impregnated with the antigenic substance is placed on the skin; the scratch test, wherein the skin is abraded and the testing substance is applied to the area; and the intradermal test, wherein the testing substance is injected intradermally.

The nurse is involved more frequently in administering skin tests for the diagnosis of infections such as tuberculosis (TB), coccidioidomycosis, and histoplasmosis. Skin tests with *Candida*—yeast-like fungi found in normal flora of the mouth, skin, intestinal tract, and vagina, which can cause a variety of infections—mumps virus, and *Trichophyton*—gaenus of fungi that causes infections of the skin, hair, and nails—are used to assess for the presence of cellular immunity. This chapter discusses tuberculin skin testing.

TUBERCULIN SKIN TESTING

The most common skin test is the tuberculin test used to detect exposure to the microorganism *Mycobacterium tuberculosis*, which causes tuberculosis. Skin testing involves injection of a known antigen into the superficial layers of the skin. In the tuberculin test, tuberculin purified protein derivative (PPD) or old tuberculin (OT) is the antigen (see Table 10–3). A hypersensitivity reaction evidenced by inflammation at the injection site indicates an immune response and recent or past exposure to the antigen.

Tuberculin skin testing is performed in a variety of settings: hospitals, clinics, schools, and places of employment. It is used most often as a screening test to detect carriers of tuberculosis. The nurse is the primary health professional involved in this testing; therefore, knowledge of the procedure and the interpretation of the results is important. Patients who are suspected of being immunosuppressed are often tested with three tests at once: PPD, mumps, and tetanus. If all three tests are negative, the patient is considered *anergic*, that is, he or she has an impaired or absent ability to react to common antigens.

Adverse Effects

The most common adverse effects include *vesiculation* (blister formation) and ulceration at the injection site. Patients may also experience pain and pruritis at the site. Anaphylactoid or acute hypersensitivity reactions are rare but can occur. Epinephrine should be readily available.

Interactions

Live or attenuated viral vaccines (e.g., measles, mumps, rubella, or influenza) given less than 6 weeks before the tuberculin test may suppress the skin test reaction. The tuberculin test may, however, be administered before or simultaneously with live viral vaccines. Patients taking systemic corticosteroids or aminocaproic acid may develop a false-negative reaction.

Patient Preparation and Procedure

A patient history is obtained to determine whether the patient has ever had a postive skin test reaction, has recently been exposed to anyone with tuberculosis, has had tuberculosis, or has had the bacillus Calmette-Guérin (BCG) vaccination. In all of these situations, the PPD results in a positive skin test. As a result, the TB test is contraindicated as it will not assist with a differential diagnosis. The injection site is assessed for atopic dermatitis or other skin disease prior to injection. The volar surface (inner aspect) of the upper one-third of the forearm is the recommended site; if this is unacceptable, the medial aspect of the thigh or the upper back is used.

The procedure is explained to the patient; the patient is reassured that the test is relatively painless and that the injection is into only the superficial layers of the skin. The injection site is cleaned with alcohol and allowed to dry before administration.

Mantoux Method For the intradermal injection of PPD by the Mantoux method, a tuberculin syringe with a ½-inch, 26 to 27-gauge needle is used to draw 0.1 mL solution of five tuberculin units (TU) of PPD. The solution is injected beneath the skin by holding the syringe nearly parallel to the skin with the bevel of the needle upward. When just the bevel becomes embedded, the solution is slowly injected and a wheal (raised area), 6 to 10 mm in diameter, is formed, as shown in Figure 10–1. If no wheal develops, the injection was given too deeply and must be

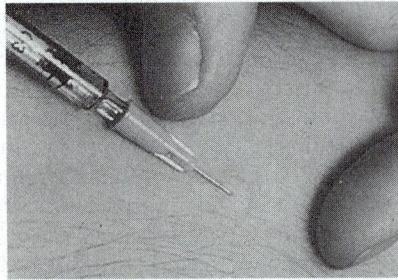

Figure 10–1. Intradermal injection on the volar surface of the forearm. Wheal forms with proper injection. (Courtesy of Parke-Davis, Division of Warner-Lambert Company, Morris Plains, NJ.)

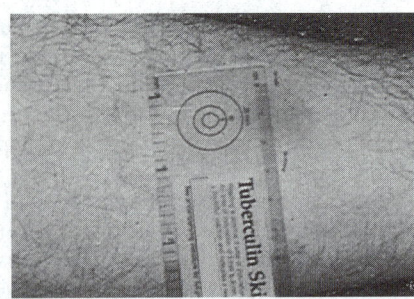

Figure 10–2. Measurement of induration. (Courtesy of Parke-Davis, Division of Warner-Lambert Company, Morris Plains, NJ.)

repeated at another site. The location of the injection is documented in the patient's chart.

Nursing Implications

The nurse is usually responsible for evaluating the results of the skin test and reporting these appropriately. Regardless of the procedure used, the test site is examined by the nurse 48 to 72 hours after the administration procedure. Skin induration and erythema are assessed. Induration is the most significant clinical sign. To evaluate the skin reaction, the site is inspected and palpated. The induration is measured transversely to the forearm and recorded in millimeters. A felt-tipped pen is used to draw a line on each side of the reaction along the transverse axis toward the induration. The edge of induration is indicated when the pen meets resistance. The distance between the lines is measured with a ruler, as shown in Figure 10–2.

With the Mantoux method, using 0.1 mL/5 TU, an induration that measures more than 10 mm in diameter is a positive reaction and a measurement of less than 5 mm is negative. An induration measuring 5 to 9 mm is often considered a questionable reaction, and the test may be repeated. In a patient who is immunosuppressed, such as with human immunodeficiency virus (HIV) infection, an induration as small as 5 mm may be considered positive. Even if a negative response is elicited in an immunosuppressed patient, all precautions are continued. A retest is often performed within 3 weeks.

In the Mantoux test, erythema is a secondary sign and as a single finding is not clinically significant. The degree of erythema is graded as follows: tr, trace discoloration; +, pink; ++, red; +++, purplish red; and ++++, vesiculation or necrosis.

Patients with positive skin test reactions require further diagnostic examinations to determine whether the reaction represents exposure to tuberculosis, dormant infection, or active infection.

USING THE NURSING PROCESS

Table 10–4 suggests assessment data to collect and summarizes the other steps of the nursing process for the patient undergoing diagnostic tests.

Table 10–4. NURSING PROCESS FOR PATIENT UNDERGOING DIAGNOSTIC TESTS

Assessment

Assess patient's ability to follow instructions.
Assess patient's reaction to previous diagnostic tests.
Assess allergies to iodine or iodine-containing foods, e.g., shellfish, and type of reaction.
Assess preexisting conditions, current drug therapy for possible interference with elimination of barium (e.g., ulcerative colitis, codeine, analgesics) or increased risk of dehydration (e.g., extremes of age; underweight patients or patients with preexisting conditions such as diarrhea, vomiting, bleeding; or diuretic therapy).
Assess menstrual history to confirm pregnancy status.

Nursing Diagnosis: Knowledge Deficit

RELATED TO: Lack of information regarding test procedures, preparation, and postprocedure care.
AS EVIDENCED BY: Questions and expressions of concern.

Desired Outcomes/Evaluation Criteria

Verbalizes understanding of test procedure and preparation.
Demonstrates ability to follow instructions.

Nursing Actions	Rationale
Assess patient's knowledge or previous experience with the diagnostic test.	Provides starting point for individual teaching program.
Provide materials regarding the test procedure and preparation.	Use of variety of materials, e.g., written, audio/visual aids, enhances learning and retention.
Clarify the information and provide follow-up to any questions.	Facilitates patient's understanding and includes patient as an active participant in the learning process.
Have the patient explain the test procedure and preparation.	Return-demonstration is used to document learning and patient understanding.

Nursing Diagnosis: Pain

RELATED TO: Test procedure and/or preparation.
AS EVIDENCED BY: Facial grimacing and complaints of discomfort.

Desired Outcomes/Evaluation Criteria

Verbalizes and demonstrates relief/control of pain or discomfort.
Acknowledges understanding that discomfort/pain is transient.

Nursing Actions	Rationale
Prepare patient for possible discomfort or pain (i.e., bowel preparation may include enemas that cause abdominal cramping).	Patients tolerate mild discomfort or pain if they have been prepared for it and know it will be transient.
Be available and provide support during uncomfortable procedures. Inform patient that any discomfort or pain felt will be transient, not long-lasting (e.g., pain, burning sensation at injection site of iodine compounds).	Support provides reassurance, facilitating the patient's coping with discomfort.
Tell patient to inform the medical/nursing staff of any discomfort or pain.	Presence of pain may indicate need for further intervention/medication to prevent complications.

Nursing Diagnosis: Risk for Fluid Volume Deficit

RELATED TO: Restricted intake, excessive fluid losses.
AS EVIDENCED BY: Denting of skin and dehydrated mucous membranes.

Desired Outcomes/Evaluation Criteria

Resumes normal fluid intake.
Demonstrates no signs or symptoms of dehydration/hypovolemia.

Nursing Actions	Rationale
Monitor development of thirst, presence of nausea/vomiting, changes in skin turgor and moisture of mucous membrane.	Signs suggesting changes in hydration status.
Maintain accurate intake/output.	Early recognition and prompt treatment of developing deficit may prevent serious complications.
Follow post-test procedure in resuming fluid intake.	Excessive fluid loss may occur secondary to enemas and suppositories used for bowel studies or reaction to injected iodinated compounds requiring adequate fluid replacement to prevent complications.
Provide oral hygiene after barium swallow.	Relieves aftertaste and may help alleviate feelings of nausea.

Other Suggested Nursing Diagnoses: Anxiety (specific level) and Constipation.

ASSESSMENT

- Assess the patient's emotional status before any diagnostic procedure. What does the patient know about the test to be performed? How does the patient relate this to the illness? Has the patient had the test previously and thus experienced its procedures and effects?
- Assess the patient's level of understanding before deciding what the preparation teaching is to include.
- Assess the patient's psychologic state to ascertain whether the individual fears the outcome of the test or the procedure itself, or whether the procedure is viewed as beneficial because the intent of the test is to reveal what is wrong. Assessment of the patient's feelings regarding the diagnostic procedure also helps the nurse to develop an appropriate teaching plan.
- Assess the physical status of the patient. How well will the patient tolerate the preparation for the procedure? The elderly patient with fluid and electrolyte problems may have difficulty tolerating the enemas and dehydration that some diagnostic tests require. Assessment of all systems just before testing is essential, as a patient's status can change suddenly. Unstable patients (medically or emotionally) may not be able to withstand the stress of the diagnostic procedure. The elderly patient or the patient experiencing pain will find some diagnostic procedures very difficult.
- Assess for allergies. The patient is questioned regarding a history of allergies or a reaction to a dye infusion test. If a positive response is obtained, the patient is asked to describe the reaction specifically. The development of nausea, vomiting, urticaria, pruritus, dyspnea, or tachycardia following the administration of a diagnostic agent is noted in the health history and reported to the physician. The physician determines whether the reaction is significant and another diagnostic agent needs to be selected. Iodine allergies are especially significant because most dye studies are performed with an iodine-based product. Many individuals allergic to fish or other seafood may actually have an iodine allergy.

NURSING DIAGNOSIS

Typical nursing diagnoses for a patient undergoing diagnostic tests include Knowledge Deficit, Pain, Risk for Fluid Volume Deficit, Constipation, and Anxiety. Many patients requiring diagnostic procedures are concerned about what the tests may reveal. The patient may fear that the tests will confirm the seriousness of the illness or the need for surgery. Also, waiting for the test results often produces anxiety for the patient. Support from the nursing staff at this time is very important.

PLANNING AND INTERVENTION

- Obtain data regarding the patient's response to the test to decrease patient anxiety and to prevent adverse effects. The nurse plays an integral role in preparing, supporting, and assessing the patient before, during, and after diagnostic tests.
- Explain the procedure and answer questions at the patient's level of understanding. Most patients undergoing a diagnostic procedure have questions and concerns. The patient must know the purpose of the test, how and where it is performed, the amount of discomfort associated with the procedure, and the specifics regarding scheduling and any special preparation needed.

Because many diagnostic procedures are performed on an outpatient basis, the time available for patient instruction prior to the procedure is limited. Preprinted instruction booklets for each procedure provide the patient with necessary information. The nurse reviews the instructions, clarifies any ambiguous information, and provides the telephone number of the outpatient clinic for further patient questions.

Scheduling Tests

The nurse may be responsible for scheduling diagnostic tests. For patient convenience, more than one test can be scheduled on a given day. The order in which procedures are scheduled is important to maintain accurate test results and avoid the need to redo tests because of compromised results. Thyroid studies are completed before using any iodine-based dye preparation because use of such dye can alter thyroid test results. Studies using barium are usually done last because retained barium can interfere with good visualization of other organs. Barium enemas are administered before an upper gastrointestinal series or a small bowel series. Special scheduling arrangements are often necessary for the diabetic patient undergoing diagnostic tests. Insulin is not given as long as the individual is NPO. Often, the diagnostic testing department takes diabetic patients first to prevent complications.

Special consideration is necessary for elderly patients undergoing diagnostic tests. For these patients, maintaining NPO status, waiting long periods in the diagnostic testing department, and assuming various positions during the test are uncomfortable and stressful. Thus, elderly patients are monitored closely. Dehydration can occur rapidly when elderly patients are NPO and undergoing numerous enemas. Following tests, it is very important to adequately replace fluids.

Physical preparation of the patient undergoing diagnostic tests is important. Effective bowel preparation permits better x-ray-film visualization. Hydration or dehydration orders for specific tests are followed precisely.

EVALUATION

- Evaluate the patient for any adverse effects following the administration of any diagnostic agent. The most significant reaction is anaphylaxis. Anaphylaxis may occur during diagnostic testing, especially when iodine-based dyes are used. If evidence of allergy is present, the physician and diagnostic department are notified. During the dye infusion, the patient is watched carefully for signs of respiratory distress, sudden diaphoresis, urticaria, or unstable vital signs. Diphenhydramine (Benadryl), epinephrine, oxygen, and resuscitation equipment are available, and all personnel are prepared in management of anaphylactic shock. Prior to testing, if a hypersensitivity reaction is anticipated, antihistamine preparations may be added to the dye preparations or a glucocorticoid may be administered to reduce the incidence of allergic response.

- Alter the patient's plan of care as needed after the diagnostic procedure. These alterations may include

increasing fluids to compensate for dehydration or to enhance removal of the dye, giving extra laxatives to prevent constipation, and providing extra attention to the patient waiting for test results. After the test results have been discussed with the patient, the nurse evaluates the patient's understanding of the results.

The bibliography for this chapter can be found in Appendix B, which begins on page 1054.

CHAPTER REVIEW QUESTIONS*

1. Iodine compounds may be:
   a. Administered only by the oral route.
   b. Administered to all patients without adverse reactions.
   c. Injected directly into the area to be visualized.
   d. Limited to use with patients allergic to barium.

2. Of the following statements regarding common diagnostic agents, which one is *not* correct?
   a. Radioactive isotopes localize only in abnormal tissue.
   b. The most common side effect following barium use is constipation.
   c. The most serious side effect of iodine testing is anaphylaxis.
   d. The diagnostic dosage of radiopharmaceuticals is lower than the therapeutic dosage.

3. In developing a nursing-care plan for the patient undergoing diagnostic testing, the nurse should *not*:
   a. Schedule barium studies last.
   b. Administer insulin to the NPO diabetic patient.

c. Assess the patient before, during, and after the procedure.
d. Explain the procedure at a level the patient can understand.

4. Diagnostic skin tests are performed for the diagnosis of all of the following *except*:
   a. Rheumatoid arthritis.
   b. Coccidiodomycosis.
   c. Histoplasmosis.
   d. Tuberculosis.

5. The diagnostic agent barium sulfate is:
   a. Administered via the intravenous route.
   b. Used to diagnose the presence of gastrointestinal fistulas.
   c. Absorbed through the gastrointestinal tract.
   d. Used to aid visualization of the gastrointestinal tract.

*See Appendix A, which begins on page 1051, for answers.

CHAPTER 11

Intravenous Therapy

Merrily A. Kuhn, RNC, PhD

CHAPTER OUTLINE

KEY TERMS

Anion	Iso-osmotic
Cation	Isotonic solution
Hyperosmotic	Osmolality
Hypertonic solution	Osmolarity
Hypo-osmotic	Pyrogens
Hypotonic solution	

LEARNING OBJECTIVES

After reading this chapter, the student will be able to:

1. Identify those fluids commonly administered intravenously, including dextrose and electrolyte solutions.
2. Differentiate among the IV solutions as to mechanism of action, adverse effects, contraindications and precautions, and interactions.
3. Identify specific areas to assess in the patient requiring IV solutions to formulate appropriate patient outcomes.
4. Plan the nursing interventions necessary to administer IV solutions.
5. Evaluate the patient at various stages of treatment to gauge nursing interventions.

Today, it is estimated that over half of the 50 million patients admitted to United States hospitals receive some form of intravenous (IV) therapy during their admission. Patients may require the administration of IV fluids because of (1) an inability to orally ingest adequate amounts of fluids, electrolytes, vitamins, or calories; (2) a fluid or electrolyte imbalance; or (3) a significant loss of blood volume.

IV therapy involves instilling many different types of fluids directly into the circulatory system. IV therapy has been used in humans for more than 300 years. IV therapy remained the responsibility of the physician until the mid-1960s, when state nurse practice acts began to issue policy statements pertaining to IV therapy. Today, state nurse practice acts serve as a general guide for the establishment of protocols and procedures. Each hospital or institution further clarifies these policies with specific guidelines or criteria essential for nursing personnel to insert and maintain the IV line, prepare and administer admixtures, and administer IV medications.

Further advances in the development of IV devices have enabled the delivery of IV therapy in the home. Commonly used for patients who require IV therapy but need no special monitoring, home IV therapy presents a unique nursing challenge (see Delivering Home Health Care box).

This chapter describes the administration of dextrose and electrolyte solutions. Electrolytes (as a group) are discussed in Chapter 12; vitamins and minerals, in Chapter 13; nutritional IV replacements, in Chapter 14; blood and blood components, in Chapter 34; and plasma expanders, in Chapter 68.

WATER BALANCE

The average adult human body is approximately 60% water. (Newborns contain 70% to 80% water.) Fat is mostly water free, so the lean individual has more water per ki-

---

DELIVERING HOME HEALTH CARE

IV Therapy

Home IV therapy differs little from hospital-based IV therapy, but does present a nursing challenge. Not all patients are candidates for home IV therapy. For example, the patient who needs meticulous or special monitoring or requires drugs that are used in emergencies, such as lidocaine or nitroprusside, would not be a good choice for home IV therapy. Not all patients are able to care for the IV site, maintain the equipment, or recognize potentially serious complications, such as drug hypersensitivity. Therefore, these patients require assistance at home from a home health nurse. Patients who are well suited to receive home IV therapy include those with long-term or chronic conditions and those who require prolonged chemotherapy, continuous pain control, or long-term parenteral nutrition.

DRUG PREPARATION AND ADMINISTRATION

Home health care patients are usually supervised by a home health care agency that typically is responsible for providing personnel who may administer drugs, check equipment, and provide necessary supplies. The preparation of drugs in the home for IV administration is the same as it is in the hospital. Plus, any of the various IV drug delivery systems and specialized infusion pumps—ambulatory or implantable infusion pumps, implantable access devices, or patient-controlled analgesia (PCA) pumps—can be adapted for home use. Most drugs administered intravenously in the hospital also can be given intravenously at home. These include fluids, antibiotics, nutritional agents, analgesics, and even some blood products, to name just a few.

PATIENT TEACHING

The success of home IV therapy depends on effective patient teaching, which begins in the hospital. Patient and significant-other teaching includes the following:

- Teach how to care for the IV site; how to recognize complications such as infection, irritation, or extravasation; and how to recognize when the physician or home health care nurse needs to be called (e.g., if redness, swelling, or pain develops at the insertion site; if the dressing becomes moist; or if blood is visible in the tubing).
- Review symptoms of drug toxicity and hypersensitivity. Do not forget that allergic reactions to a drug may be delayed for weeks after administration.
- Inform the patient with a peripheral IV line that the access site is changed at established intervals. Set up a changing schedule with the appropriate agency. Also establish a schedule for refilling the pump or medication cassette for patients with an ambulatory infusion device.
- Teach the patient how and when to flush a heparin or saline lock, as appropriate (e.g., the patient with an intermittent infusion device).
- Demonstrate to the patient with an implantable access how to access it for drug delivery, flushing, or heparinization; how to locate and stabilize the port by palpation; how to clean the site; how to attach a Huber needle to the syringe, extension, or IV tubing; how to insert the syringe into the port; how to apply a sterile dressing to the site; how to regulate, monitor, and discontinue the infusion; and how to flush the port. Stress the importance of aseptic technique

---

logram than the fat individual. The water is divided into intracellular water (approximately 45%) and extracellular water (approximately 15%), as shown in Figure 11–1. Intracellular fluid (ICF) is not a continuous fluid, but is divided into trillions of tiny cellular compartments, and its composition varies from cell to cell. Extracellular fluid (ECF) surrounds each cell in the body. ECF moves through the circulatory and lymphatic systems and contains, in solution or suspension, plasma, electrolytes, vitamins, minerals, protein, nutrients, and waste products. The water diffuses across cell membranes into the cells, where metabolic reactions occur that are essential to life; therefore, water balance is crucial to healthy living. Water balance is maintained through a dynamic balance of intake and output.

The kidney, the primary regulator of water balance, controls the amount of urine produced based on blood pressure and serum *osmolarity* (concentration of osmotically active particles in solution). Hormones released by the posterior pituitary—ADH (antidiuretic hormone or vasopressin)—and the adrenal cortex—aldosterone—assist in the regulation of fluid and electrolyte balance.

Water is an excellent solvent, allowing many substances to be dispersed within it. Water also permits electrolytes to ionize. Electrolytes are found in both ECF and ICF and include *cations* (positively charged ions) and *an-ions* (negatively charged ions). The major cation in ECF is sodium (Na^+), while the major cations in ICF are potassium (K^+) and magnesium (Mg^{++}). The anions in ECF are chloride (Cl^-) and bicarbonate (HCO_3^-) and proteins (see Fig. 11–1B). Small amounts of these ECF electrolytes are also found in the ICF and vice versa.

FLUID VOLUME IMBALANCES

Osmolality is a term used to describe the concentration of free particles, molecules, or ions (i.e., Na^+, K^+, glucose) in a solution. Osmolality is very important in classifying fluid imbalances. Dehydration and Overhydration are also useful, but incomplete because they do not specify the composition of the fluid lost or gained. The terms *iso-osmotic, hypo-osmotic,* and *hyperosmotic* are more exact in defining any loss or gain in ECF volume. An iso-osmotic solution contains a normal osmolality and neither draws nor loses water across a membrane. A hypo-osmotic solution contains abnormally low osmolality and loses water across a membrane until a similar osmolality is present on both sides of the membrane. A hyperosmotic solution contains abnormally high osmolality and draws water across a membrane until a similar osmolality is present on both sides of the membrane.

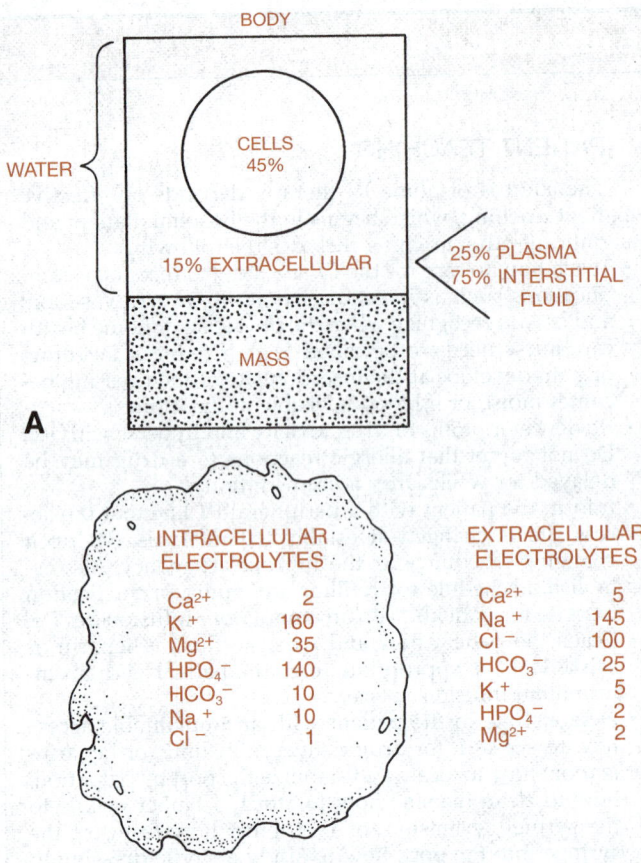

B

Figure 11–1. (a) Distribution of body water. The body is composed of 60% water; 45% is found in the cells (intracellular), while 15% is outside the cells (extracellular). (b) Body electrolytes. Primary intracellular electrolytes include K^+ (potassium), Mg^{2+} (magnesium), and HPO_4^- (phosphate); primary extracellular electrolytes include Na^+ (sodium), Cl^- (chloride), and HCO_3^- (bicarbonate). All values are listed in mEq/L.

Fluid Volume Contraction

Dehydration occurs when more fluid is lost from the body than is replaced. This occurs when the oral intake falls below normal, or when there is excessive loss of fluid from the body by evaporation from the skin or lungs or excretion of a very dilute urine. Fluid volume contraction, featured in Table 11–1, can be hyperosmolar or iso-osmotic.

A fluid volume deficit can be calculated from body weight. A liter of body fluid weighs 2.2 lb, and a kilogram also equals 2.2 lb; therefore, a loss of a liter of water equals a loss of 1 kg of weight. A mild loss is 2% of total body weight (5% in infants), a moderate loss is 2% to 5% of body weight (10% in infants), and a severe loss is more than 6% of total body weight (15% in infants).

To calculate these losses, it is useful to visualize a 154-lb (70-kg) man, as follows:

- A mild loss is about 2% of total body weight. Therefore, a 2% loss of body weight in a 70-kg man is 1.4 kg (or 1.4 kg times 2.2 lb = 3 lb) or 1.4 liters.
- A moderate loss is 2% to 5%. A 70 kg man losing 5% of total body weight loses 3.5 kg (7.7 lb) or 3.5 liters of fluid.

- A severe loss is more than 6% of total body weight. A 70-kg man losing 7% of his weight has a loss of 4.9 kg (10.78 lb) or 4.9 liters.

The very young and the very old are more threatened by small changes in water balance, so they must be monitored more closely and fluids replaced as needed. Patients who become dehydrated are generally treated with an isotonic solution (0.9% sodium chloride solution or 5% dextrose and water solution). IV solutions are discussed in more detail later in this chapter.

Fluid Volume Expansion

Edema, an increase in interstitial sodium with resultant increased reabsorption of fluid, may be local or generalized. Edema results from (1) increased hydrostatic pressure, (2) reduced oncotic pressure, (3) increased capillary permeability, (4) reduced lymphatic drainage, or (5) any combination of these circumstances. This state results when more sodium and fluid are retained by the body than excreted. This usually occurs in individuals with underlying heart, kidney, or liver disease who have an inability to excrete sodium and fluids. Expansion, featured in Table 11–1, can be hyperosmotic or hypo-osmotic.

Patients with a fluid volume excess are generally treated with fluid restriction and diuretics, which are discussed in Chapter 37. For a more detailed discussion of fluid imbalance, refer to a medical-surgical nursing text.

ELECTROLYTE AND ACID-BASE IMBALANCES

ELECTROLYTE IMBALANCES

Electrolytes are compounds that, when dissolved in water, separate into their component particles. Electrolyte imbalances may be more dangerous than water imbalances because electrolytes are able to change fluid distribution between body compartments and to cause other associated problems. The electrolytes are discussed in more depth in Chapter 12. Electrolytes can be lost excessively or retained by the body. Usually, one imbalance precipitates another if it is not treated promptly.

ACID-BASE IMBALANCE

Acid-base balance is an equilibrium between the total body bases and total body acids. Acid-base balance is a reflection of hydrogen-ion (H^+) concentration in the body. Hydrogen concentration is routinely described as pH, which reflects the relationship of acid to base. Normally, the body has one acidic ion for 20 base ions. Because pH is the negative logarithm of the concentration of hydrogen ions, the higher their concentration the lower the pH. Balance is accomplished by maintaining the arterial pH within a narrow range in the presence of acid or alkaline loads. Any change in acid or base concentration ultimately affects the pH. As the pH becomes less than 7.35, the patient becomes acidemic. As the pH becomes greater than 7.45, the patient becomes alkalemic. Note that increasing acidity is expressed as less than the neutral point of pH 7 (maximum acidity is pH 0) and that

Table 11–1. FLUID VOLUME CONTRACTION AND EXPANSION				
Disease Causes	Pharmacologic Causes	Laboratory Findings	Symptoms	Therapy
Fluid Volume Contraction:				
Sweating, adrenal insufficiency, burns, blood loss, diarrhea	Cathartics, diuretics	Lab little help, but with severe deficit Na$^+$ & Cl$^-$ are reduced in urine. Urine specific gravity increased. Hemoglobin increased, hematocrit increased, plasma protein increased. Serum Na$^+$ may be increased. BUN and creatinine may be increased.	Thirst, poor skin turgor, dry skin and mucous membranes; soft, sunken eyeballs; apprehension, restlessness; decreased urine	Replace ECF with isotonic or hypotonic solutions by any route.
Fluid Volume Expansion:				
Renal disease, liver disease, cardiac disease, Cushing's disease	Corticosteroids, excessive sodium intake, chlorpropamide	Hemodilution exists, hemoglobin decreased, hematocrit decreased, all electrolytes decreased, plasma protein decreased, urine specific gravity decreased.	Headache, nausea, vomiting, muscle pain, abdominal cramps, weakness, stupor, coma, respiratory congestion, absence of thirst	Withhold fluids temporarily, diuretics, low Na diet, dialysis.

increasing alkalinity is expressed as greater than pH 7 (maximum alkalinity is pH 14).

Acids donate hydrogen and bases receive hydrogen. Hydrogen ions are added to body fluids daily as metabolic by-products. To keep the pH within its normal range, the body must eliminate hydrogen ions at the same rate as they are produced. The hydrogen ion or acid produced daily in the body is either volatile or fixed. Volatile acid (carbon dioxide) is eliminated by the lungs. Fixed acids, such as hydrogen sulfate and hydrochloric acid, are excreted by the kidney. Both acids are chemically buffered to protect cells from dangerous concentrations of hydrogen ions.

The maintenance of this process is the result of a number of mechanisms: body buffers (extracellular and intracellular), respiratory regulation of carbonic acid, and renal regulation of bicarbonate.

Other Body Controls

Buffer systems in the body needed to maintain normal plasma pH include the phosphate system (in red blood cells and kidneys), the protein system (in tissue cells and plasma), and the hemoglobin system (in red blood cells). All of these systems work together.

THERAPEUTIC AGENTS FOR WATER AND ELECTROLYTE IMBALANCES

Many IV solutions are available, and a knowledge of the underlying fluid balance assists the nurse in understanding why a particular fluid is ordered. IV fluids are classified as hydrating, balanced, replacement, or carbohydrate solutions, and each has a place in treating water, fluid, and electrolyte imbalances.

All IV solutions contain solute particles that may be either electrolytes in their ionized form (Na$^+$, K$^+$, Cl$^-$, HCO$_3^-$) or particles of nonionizable urea, glucose, and others in solution or plasma.

Normally, in the healthy body, the number of cations equals the number of anions. When added together, they equal 310 mEq/liter in ECF. IV solutions may be equal to (isotonic), less than (hypotonic), or more than (hypertonic) 310 mEq/liter.

In *isotonic solutions*, the cations and anions approximate 310 mEq/liter (some sources use 280 mEq/liter), or the same osmotic pressure as body fluids. As an isotonic solution, 0.9% sodium chloride solution (normal saline) does not induce the osmotic movement of water into or out of cells. Although 0.9% sodium chloride solution is isotonic, it is not considered physiologic. This is because extracellular fluid normally contains 140 mEq/L of sodium and 103 mEq of chloride, while isotonic saline solutions contain equal proportions (154 mEq/L of sodium and chloride). Thus, isotonic saline imposes an appreciable load of chloride on the kidneys; if the kidneys cannot excrete chloride, hyperchloremic acidosis may follow.

Hypotonic solutions have an electrolyte content of cations and anions of less than 250 mEq/liter and therefore have a greater concentration of free water molecules than are found inside the cell. These solutions give up their water to a dehydrated cell so it can return to isotonic equilibrium.

▼ CLINICAL ALERT

Hypotonic solutions, such as 2.5% dextrose in 0.45% sodium chloride solution or 2.5% dextrose in 0.9% sodium chloride solution, are given slowly because a sudden shift of fluid into the cells can occur. Excessive use of hypotonic solutions can cause dilutional hyponatremia, especially in patients who tend to retain water.

Hypertonic solutions have an electrolyte content of greater than 375 mEq/liter and have a lower concentration of free water, but a higher osmotic weight, than do body fluids. These solutions, such as 10% or 50% dextrose

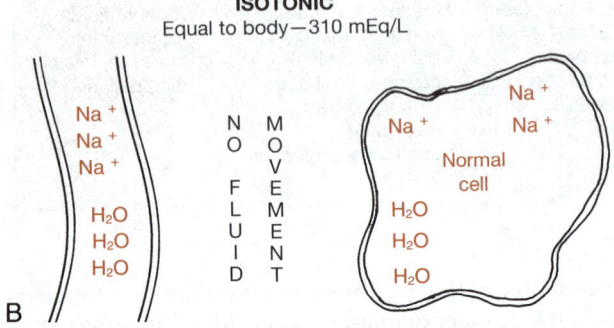

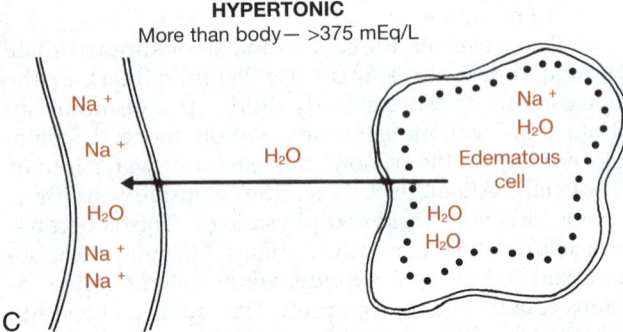

Figure 11–2. IV solutions. (a) *Hypotonic solutions* move from the vascular system into a dehydrated cell. (b) *Isotonic solutions* remain within the vascular system. (c) *Hypertonic solutions* pull free water from the edematous cell into the vascular system.

in water, 10% fructose in water, 3% saline solutions, or 5% dextrose in lactated Ringer's solution, are given slowly (usually not greater than 150 mL/hr) because they have the ability to pull water from the cell into the circulatory system, which can cause pulmonary edema and cardiac failure.

▼ **CLINICAL ALERT**

Hypertonic solutions should be used *only* in intensive care units because frequent monitoring of blood pressure, central venous pressure, lung sounds, and serum sodium must be done.

Figure 11–2 features isotonic, hypotonic, and hypertonic solutions and how they affect vascular volume.

HYDRATING SOLUTIONS

Hydrating solutions are composed of water, carbohydrate, and varying amounts of sodium chloride, as shown in Table 11–2. These solutions are used primarily for simple hydration and fluid replacement and to determine the adequacy of a patient's renal function. To determine if the kidneys are still functioning, a fluid challenge is administered. A fluid challenge is a large volume (250 to 1000 mL) of a hydrating solution given in a short period (10 to 45 minutes). During this time, urinary output and cardiac function are monitored closely. If the kidneys are still functional, urine appears before the fluid challenge is ended. If urine does not appear, the flow rate is slowed and continued for an additional hour. If at this point there is still no urine, it may indicate serious renal disease, and renal function studies (serum creatinine, blood urea nitrogen [BUN], and creatinine clearance) are indicated. Hydrating solutions are also used to increase renal function when a fluid deficit exists or is suspected. Hydrating solutions are potassium free. Potassium is essential to the body, but it can be toxic if the kidneys are not functioning effectively and are therefore unable to excrete the extra potassium.

BALANCED SOLUTIONS

Balanced solutions are composed of water, carbohydrate as an energy source, and both cations and anions in a balanced combination. Balanced solutions have fallen into disfavor, because they have too many unclear, unknown, and unrecognized ingredients and because their use may result in electrolyte disturbances. Examples of balanced solutions include 5% or 10% dextrose with electrolyte 48 or 75; and Isonosol B, MB, M, or P, all with 5% dextrose.

REPLACEMENT SOLUTIONS

Replacement solutions are a combination of water, carbohydrates, and electrolytes that are used to replace concurrent losses from the gastrointestinal (GI) system. Re-

Table 11–2. HYDRATING SOLUTIONS

Description	Cation Na (mEq/L)	Anion Cl (mEq/L)	Calories /L	mOsm/L
5% dextrose + 0.45% sodium chloride	77	77	170	405
5% dextrose + 0.33% sodium chloride	51–56	51–56	170	355–365
5% dextrose + 0.2% sodium chloride	34–38.5	34–38.5	170	320–330
2.5% dextrose + 0.45% sodium chloride	77	77	85	280

Solutions can be obtained in 250-, 500-, and 1000-mL sizes.

Table 11–3. REPLACEMENT SOLUTIONS

	Cations (mEq/L)				Anions (mEq/L)						
	Na⁺	K⁺	CA²⁺	Mg²⁺	Cl⁻	Lactate	Acetate	Gluconate (G) or Phosphate (P)	G/I Replacement	mOsm/L	Calories
10% Travert's (invert sugar) w/Electrolyte 2	56	25	—	6	56	25	—	12.5, P	G	726	384
Plasma-Lyte R + 5% dextrose	140	10	5	3	103	8	47	—	I	564	181
Ionosol MB w/10% dextrose	25	20	—	3	22	23	—	3, P	I	603	340
Normosol-R	140	5	—	3	98		27	23, G	I	294	15
Plasma-Lyte 148 5% dextrose	140	5	—	3	98		27	23, G	I	547	190
Lactated Ringer's (Hartmann's)	130	4	3	—	109	28	—	—	G/I	272	—

Most of these solutions are available in 500- and 1000-mL sizes.
G = gastric; I = intestinal.

placement solutions are listed in Table 11–3. These solutions are composed of various electrolytes that approximate losses from various GI areas through vomiting, diarrhea, fistulas, and suction. Table 11–4 describes body fluid production, composition, and probable imbalances. Replacement solutions are available in both 5% and 10% dextrose solutions. Lactated Ringer's solution (Hartmann's solution) is a good multipurpose solution and is considered to be almost physiologic. It is often used to correct isotonic fluid volume deficits (as in hypovolemia due to third-space fluid shift following major trauma or surgery). Its chief, but minor, disadvantage is its slight hypo-osmolarity; it furnishes 100 to 150 mL of free water/liter. In addition, it is low in potassium, and, therefore, supplemental potassium may need to be added to the infusion. Replacement solutions, other than lactated Ringer's, are declining in clinical use.

CARBOHYDRATE SOLUTIONS

Carbohydrate solutions contain a carbohydrate (e.g., dextrose [glucose] or fructose [levulose]) that assists with meeting the patient's energy requirements. Fructose offers no advantage over dextrose injection and has some disadvantages. It may increase serum levels of lactate and urate if given rapidly and it is considerably more expensive than dextrose. Travert contains both sugars. A liter of an IV solution of either water or normal saline with 5% dextrose has 170 calories per liter; 10% dextrose solution

has 340 calories; 20% dextrose has 680 calories; 50% dextrose has 1700 calories; 5% Travert (invert sugar, a combination of levulose and dextrose formed by inversion of sucrose by enzyme invertase) solution has 190 calories; 10% Travert solution has 380 calories; and 10% fructose solution has 380 calories. Five percent solutions are approximately isotonic compared to blood. As the percent of carbohydrate increases above 5%, they become hypertonic. Hypertonic dextrose solutions are infused in a high-flow vein to prevent irritation to the veins. The 5% and 10% solutions cannot meet the energy needs of a severely ill patient. A patient receiving 3000 mL of a 5% dextrose in water solution receives only about 600 calories. Protein catabolism and a state of metabolic acidosis soon develop if more calories are not added. This can be achieved through total parenteral nutrition (TPN), which is discussed in Chapter 14.

▼ CLINICAL ALERT

All dextrose solutions are acidic (pH 3.5 to 5.0) and may produce thrombophlebitis. Assess IV site at regular intervals for signs of thrombophlebitis.

The rate of utilization of dextrose varies considerably. The average maximal rate is 300 mg/kg per hr (5 ml/kg per min of dextrose injection 5%) over periods of less than 24 hours.

Table 11–4. BODY FLUID COMPOSITION AND LOSSES

	Volume (mL/24 hr)	pH	Composition (mEq/liter)				Probable Imbalance
			Na⁺	K⁺	Cl⁻	HCO₃⁻	
Gastric fluid	2500	1–3	10–115	1–35	90–150	0–15	Metabolic alkalosis, decreased K, decreased Na
Bile	500	7–8	130–160	3–12	90–120	40–50	Metabolic acidosis, decreased Na
Pancreatic fluid	700	8	115–150	3–8	55–95	60–120	Metabolic acidosis
Intestinal fluids	(3000 total)						
Jejunum	—	7.8–8	85–150	2–10	45–125	20–35ᵃ	Metabolic acidosis, decreased K, decreased Na
Ileostomy (old)	—	7.8–8	40–50	3–5	20–30	—	Imbalances are unlikely

Data are summarized from the literature for both average values and ranges and refer to an adult in a temperate climate engaging in mild physical activity.

▼ **CLINICAL ALERT**

If more dextrose is administered than the patient can utilize, hyperglycemia, glycosuria, and excessive diuresis can result. In addition, the dextrose is metabolized to carbon dioxide and water, leaving a solution physiologically equivalent to distilled water but without the hemolysis. The increase in carbon dioxide may lead to respiratory distress in some patients.

Carbohydrate in sodium chloride solution is best used when there has been an excessive loss of fluid through sweating, vomiting, or gastric suctioning. The sodium chloride solutions contain a combination of equal amounts of sodium and chloride. A 0.2% solution has 38.5 mEq of both Na and Cl, a 0.33% solution has 50 mEq of both Na and Cl, a 0.45% solution has 77 mEq of both Na and Cl, and a 0.9% solution has 154 mEq of both Na and Cl. Concentrations of 0.11% to 0.45% are hypotonic, 0.9% is isotonic, and concentrations of 3% to 5% are hy-

---

Table 11–5. NURSING PROCESS FOR PATIENT REQUIRING IV THERAPY

Assessment

Assess present illness including routes of fluid loss (e.g., vomiting, draining wound, diuretic use), characteristics of urine.
Assess ability to ingest and retain fluids.
Assess current vital signs, usual/current weight.

Nursing Diagnosis: Fluid Volume Deficit

RELATED TO: Excessive loss/inadequate intake.
AS EVIDENCED BY: Poor skin turgor, decreased urinary output, weight loss, decreased CVP, decreased blood pressure, confusion.

Desired Outcomes/Evaluation Criteria

Demonstrates improved fluid balance as evidenced by urine output of 35 cc/hour with normal specific gravity, stable vital signs, moist mucous membranes, good skin turgor, and capillary refill <3 sec.

Nursing Actions	Rationale
Begin/maintain intravenous fluid replacement therapy.	Replaces losses when oral route is not appropriate or rapid replacement is required.
Observe drip rate q hr.	Ensures accuracy of infusion preventing errors in intake.
Monitor vital signs and physical symptoms for deviation from assessed baseline. Record I/O and daily weight.	Adequate replacement of fluids should correct symptoms indicating deficit; however, continued losses and/or insufficient intake may worsen symptoms and increase imbalance between I/O and weight.
Note characteristics of urine and measure specific gravity.	Urine usually dark/concentrated with elevated specific gravity in presence of dehydration.
Review laboratory studies, e.g., Hgb/Hct, electrolytes, serum osmolality, and blood gases.	Useful in identifying type and amount of fluid needed for replacement.
Provide fluids for oral intake as appropriate.	Promotes patient comfort, and oral route is preferred for replacement as it reduces risks associated with invasive procedures.

Nursing Diagnosis: Knowledge Deficit

RELATED TO: Unfamiliarity with IV therapy.
AS EVIDENCED BY: Questions, statement of concern.

Desired Outcomes/Evaluation Criteria

Verbalizes understanding of condition and treatment.

Nursing Actions	Rationale
Provide information outlining current IV therapy to both patient and family. Allow time to ask questions and verbalize feelings/concerns.	Patient/family often have unspoken fears about what is happening, and accurate information and opportunity to discuss these fears promotes understanding and may enhance cooperation with therapy.

Nursing Diagnosis: Risk for Infection

RELATED TO: Invasive procedure
AS EVIDENCED BY: Elevated temperatures, warmth at IV site, pain at IV site.

Desired Outcomes/Evaluation Criteria

Demonstrates absence of edema, erythema, or purulent drainage at insertion site and is afebrile.

Nursing Actions	Rationale
Use aseptic technique for insertion of IV device. Cover with clear dressing and observe site hourly.	Eliminates skin contaminants, lowering risk of infection. Allows for early detection and prompt intervention to prevent serious complications.
Maintain integrity of IV system when changing bottles. Inspect bottle/bag and solution before adding to IV. Note expiration date.	Reduces risk of introduction of microbes into vascular system.
Change tubing and IV site at least every 72 hours or if signs of irritation/infection present.	Routine changing reduces potential for device-produced sepsis.

CVP = central venous pressure; Hgb = hemoglobin; hct = hematocrit; I/O = intake/output.

Table 11–6. FLUID AND ELECTROLYTE IMBALANCES: CAUSES, ASSESSABLE CLINICAL SIGNS AND SYMPTOMS, AND GOALS OF INTERVENTION

Imbalance	Clinical Causes	Assessable Clinical Signs and Symptoms	Goals of Intervention
Fluid volume deficit	Hypo-osmotic: adrenal insufficiency. (Addison's disease). Iso-osmotic: cholera, gastric suction, ulcerative colitis. Hyperosmotic: dehydration (i.e., fever), diabetic ketoacidosis, decreased protein intake	Dry skin and mucous membranes, longitudinal wrinkling of tongue, lack of sweating, poor skin turgor, decreased urinary output, decreased systolic blood pressure, lowered body temperature, weight loss, elevated pulse, decreased central venous pressure, depressed anterior fontanelle in infants	Restore volume to normal without altering electrolyte balance by administering balanced solutions.
Fluid volume excess	Hypo-osmotic: SIADH Iso-osmotic: edema Hyperosmotic: excessive administration of NaCl	Symptoms associated with congestive heart failure, edema, changes in vital signs	Restore volume to normal by correction of underlying cause, restricting fluids, diuretic therapy.
Respiratory acidosis	Oversedation, COPD, pulmonary infections	Respiratory embarrassment (shallow, slow breathing), weakness, coma, disorientation	Restore pH to normal by correction of underlying pathology.
Respiratory alkalosis	CNS disorders, sepsis, CNS stimulation, salicylate intoxication	Convulsions, unconsciousness, hyperventilation, possible tetany	Restore pH to normal by correcting underlying pathology.
Metabolic alkalosis	Vomiting, gastric suction, primary aldosteronism	Hyperactive reflexes, depressed breathing, muscle hypertonicity, possible tetany	Restore pH to normal by replacing nonbicarbonate ions. Fluid replacement with hydrating solutions, balanced solutions, GI replacement solutions, return Ca^{++} to normal.
Metabolic acidosis	Lactic acidosis, diabetic ketoacidosis, salicylate intoxication, renal failure, diarrhea	Disorientation, unconsciousness, stupor, coma, deep and rapid respirations	Restore pH to normal by correcting underlying pathology to provide bicarbonate ions and/or stop acid production. Replace fluids with hydrating solutions, balanced solutions, GI replacement solutions.

SIADH = syndrome of inappropriate antidiuretic hormone; COPD = chronic obstructive pulmonary disease; CNS = central nervous system.

pertonic. The 3% and 5% solutions are reserved for the treatment of severe symptomatic hyponatremia (serum Na level less than 120 mEq/mL).

USING THE NURSING PROCESS

ASSESSMENT

Assessment of the patient requiring IV therapy always begins with a thorough nursing history to develop the database needed for preparation of a nursing-care plan. Table 11–5 summarizes the nursing process.

- Obtain baseline laboratory data, particularly electrolytes, the patient weights, and assessment of water balance prior to beginning IV therapy.
- Assess for symptoms of fluid and electrolyte disturbances. Table 11–6 features the major volume and electrolyte imbalances with the most common symptoms and goals of nursing care. The nurse must further assess the patient for complications that can arise from IV therapy, which are discussed later in this chapter.
- Assess the patient's knowledge of IV therapy and

whether he or she (or a family member) is anxious or fearful about its use. IV therapy is a routine part of nursing. However, it may be a traumatic event for the patient and family, erroneously indicating serious illness or impending death. Share with the patient and family the reason for and the purpose of the IV and help them to recognize and allay their fears.

NURSING DIAGNOSIS

Typical nursing diagnoses for the patient receiving IV therapy include Fluid Volume Deficit, Risk for Infection, and Knowledge Deficit (see Table 11–5).

Table 11–7. PATIENT TEACHING INFORMATION—IV THERAPY

Dear Patient:
   IV therapy has been ordered for you to _____ (reason for therapy). Therapy is given to meet your average daily fluid, vitamin, and mineral needs. Medication can also be given IV. The most common site for the IV line is in your hand or arm. After the needle is put in, it is taped, and your hand or arm may be taped to a board to prevent movement. If you have any pain at the site of the IV line, please tell your nurse.

Table 11–8. IV THERAPY: A USER'S GUIDE

Type of Catheter*	Description/Uses	Flushing Catheter	Frequency of Flush	Dressing Change
Peripheral IV (Angicath, butterfly, microcath 20G or larger)	Peripheral venous access	Normal saline or 1.0 mL heparin (100 U/mL)	q 8 hr and after each use	Transparent dressing applied at time of catheter insertion per protocol
Hickman	Silicone central venous catheter, designed for long-term use for drugs and drawing blood, chemo, transfusions. May have 1, 2, or 3 lumens	2.5 mL heparin (100 U/mL)	q 24 hr and after each use	Hyperal protocol and PRN (3 times/wk)
Multi-lumen central catheter	*Lumen Size Color* Proximal 18G White *Use:* blood sampling, general access Middle 18G Blue *Use:* C-1800 or P-900 ONLY for general access Distal 16G Brown *Use:* CVP monitoring, blood products, general access	2.5 mL heparin (100 U/mL) Remove syringe as you inject last 0.5 mL ICU: May use above procedure or 2 U/mL heparin (5 mL of manifold flush)	q 12 hr and after each use q 6 hr	Hyperal protocol and PRN
Implantable vascular access device (Port-o-Cath, Mediport, etc.)	Implanted device that provides central venous access for drugs, fluids, and drawing blood	5 mL heparin (100 U/mL)	q 5 days and after each use, if not accessed at least once a month	q 5 days with needle change. Hyperal protocol and PRN. Support Huber needle with 2 × 2 and SteriStrips. Do not cover needle site with 2 × 2; should be visible through transparent dressing. No dressing when not accessed
Single-lumen central catheter	Central venous access	2.5 mL heparin (100 U/mL) ICU: May use above procedures or 2 U/mL heparin (5 mL of manifold flush)	q 12 hr q 6 h	Hyperal protocol and PRN (3 times/wk)
Pulmonary artery catheter	Thermodilution multilumen catheter, used to measure right, left heart and pulmonary artery pressure; IV access for IV fluids; measure mixed venous gases	PA distal port must be connected to continuous flushing and pressurized solution (heparin 1000 U/500 mL 0.9 NS) at all times		Hyperal protocol and PRN (3 times/wk)

Continued on the following page

...ving Blood	Special Notes	Change Caps	Removal of Lines	Troubleshooting Occlusions	Type of Catheter
...v blood with ...al insertion ...hing: If cathe- ...s in place, ...card 2 mL, in- ...1 mL heparin ...0 U/mL).		Change caps with device and PRN	Removal at RN's discretion. Change 72 hr unless order to leave in longer.	Replace catheter.	Peripheral IV (An-giocath, butterfly, microcath 20G or larger)
...ard 10 mL, ...w blood, in- ...5 mL NS ...n 2.5 mL hep- ...(100 U/mL).	Turn off IV fluids infusing into both lumens. Clamp before flushing and clamp port you are not drawing blood from. Do not attempt to flush against re-sistance or closed clamp. Do not leave clamped. Repair kits available in Central Supply for break or tear.	q week and PRN (for leaking or contamination)	Removal re-quires minor surgery.	Requires MD order. Instill 1 mL uro-klnase (5,000 U/mL), wait 30 min, withdraw, then flush. If no return, notify MD (Restricted to RNs certified in procedure.)	Hickman
...v blood ...ugh distal or ...ximal lumen, ...card 3 mL, ...w blood, in- ...3 mL NS ...n 2.5 mL hep- ...(100 U/mL). ...st turn off all ...sions and ...np prior to ...od draw.	If IV fluids that contain hyperal or electrolytes flow through promixal or mid-dle port, lab val-ues could be distorted. Need to stop fluids first.	q 5 days	Remove q 4 days; notify MD for order for re-placement.	Notify MD to re-place catheter.	Multi-lumen central catheter
...ard 10 mL, ...w blood, ...wly instill 20 ... NS over 5 ..., then 5 mL ...arin ...0 U/mL).	Flush *well* after drawing or infus-ing blood. Avoid excess pressure when giving meds or flush-ing.	Change caps on extension tubing PRN. Change extension tub-ing, dressing, and needle q 5 days	Removal re-quires minor surgery.	Requires MD order. Instill 1.5 mL uro-kinase (5000 U/mL), wait 30 min, aspirate uro-kinase; if no re-turn, notify MD.	Implantable vascu-lar access device (Port-a-Cath, Mediport, etc.)
...ntinuous IV ...in progress, ...card 5 mL, ...w blood, in- ...3 mL NS ...n 2.5 mL hep- ...(100 U/mL).		q week	RN removes q 4 days with MD order.	Notify MD.	Single-lumen cen-tral catheter
...CVP and VIP ...t, discard 5 ...and draw ...od. If continu- ...s IV not in ...gress, instill ...L NS then	Flush distal port with 1 mL hepa-rin (2 U/mL) af-ter drawing blood for mixed venous samples and PRN for	By hospital policy	MD or designate removes.	Flush gently with 1 mL heparin so-lution (2 U/mL) for damped wave-form PRN. Do NOT force flush! Notify MD.	Pulmonary artery catheter

Continued on the following page

Table 11–8. IV THERAPY: A USER'S GUIDE, *Continued*

Type of Catheter*	Description/Uses	Flushing Catheter	Frequency of Flush	Dressing Change
Pulmonary artery catheter (*continued*)		2.5 mL heparin (100 U/mL) or 2 U/mL heparin (5 mL of manifold flush)	q 12 hr (VIP, Paceport, Side-port, CVP port) q 6 hr (VIP, Paceport, Side-port, CVP port)	
"Vas-Cath" Quinfton double-lumen catheter	Large-bore, double-lumen catheter used for pheresis, hemodialysis; use red port access in emergency Red port: proximal lumen outflow port for blood Blue port: distal lumen return port for blood Place all IV infusions on infusion pumps	1. Wear mask 2. Remove cap/connect 3 mL syringe 3. Unclamp lumen 4. Aspirate 2 mL and discard 5. Clamp lumen 6. Instill 3 mL NS *quickly and forcefully* 7. Clamp lumen 8. Unclamp and instill *quickly and forcefully* 1500 U heparin (1000 U/mL) 9. Clamp lumen 10. Repeat steps 1–8 to flush other lumen. Replace clamps every flush	q 8 hr (instill both ports with each flush)	Hyperal protocol and PRN
Intrasil central venous catheter percutaneous (long line)	Central venous catheter inserted per brachial vein for long-term use for meds, chemo, transfusions, drawing blood, and fluids	2.5 mL heparin (100 U/mL)	q 12 hr days and after each use	Hyperal protocol and PRN
Groshong	Central venous catheter similar to Hickman, has special valves, to prevent backflow of blood from line or instillation of air	Saline only: 5 mL after meds. 20 mL after blood	q 7 days and after each use	Hyperal protocol and PRN
Hyperalimentation catheter	16G × 8 in catheter for hyperal infusion	Not done routinely	—	Hyperal portocol and PRN
Scribner shunt	Catheter inserted into artery and vein with catheter tubing exiting skin and joined together with T-tube connector or straight connector; the shunt is used for hemodialysis	Flushing required when T-tube in shunt 1. Wear mask 2. Vigorously scrub end of T-tube with providone-iodine swab 3. Aspirate 1 mL blood 4. Inject 3 mL NS 5. Inject 750 U heparin (1000 U/mL)	—	Sterile dressing change once a day. See P & P manual

Continued on the following page

rawing Blood	Special Notes	Change Caps	Removal of Lines	Troubleshooting Occlusions	Type of Catheter
2.5 mL heparin 100 U/mL) or nstill 5 mL manifold flush.	damped waveform. For supplemental ports (Paceport, VIP, Side-port, CVP port), instill 3 mL NS, then 2.5 mL heparin (100 U/mL) or instill 5 mL heparin flush solution (2 U/mL).				
scard 2 mL, raw blood, in-till 3 mL NS orcefully then 500 U heparin 000 U/mL), ap-ly sterile caps avoid taking amples for PT, TT from this ne.)	Use 10 mL slip tip syringes to obtain blood samples. Have patient cough to obtain blood sample. Catheter may be against wall of subclavian. Putting patient in Trendelenburg may help to obtain blood return.	q 8 hr flush	Remove q 2 weeks unless MD order.	Notify MD.	"Vas-Cath" Quinton double-lumen catheter
scard 5 mL, raw blood, in-till 5 mL NS en 2.5 mL hep-in (100 U/mL).	Do not attempt to repair.	q week and PRN	Remove in patient's room per MD or designate.	Notify MD.	Intrasil central venous catheter (long line)
card 10 mL, raw blood, in-ll 20 mL NS.	Repair kits available; contact Oncology CNS.	q week and PRN	Removal requires minor surgery.	As per Hickman.	Groshong
ver.	Placed initially only in the OR, Treatment Room, or ICU.	Not capped	If patient septic, change guidewire weekly, otherwise may stay in place indefinitely. Nurse may discontinue lines in patient's room with MD order.	Notify MD if unable to aspirate blood and line occluded.	Hyperalimentation catheter
sk preferred. gorously scrub d of tube with vidone-iodine ab. Discard 1 ., draw blood, still 2 mL NS en 750 U parin 000 U/mL).	Straight connector does not require flushing	—	MD removes.	—	Scribner shunt

Continued on the following page

Table 11–8. IV THERAPY: A USER'S GUIDE, *Continued*

Type of Catheter*	Description/Uses	Flushing Catheter	Frequency of Flush	Dressing Change
CAVH (continuous arteriovenous hemofiltration) femoral artery catheter, femoral vein catheter, Vygon catheter 8F	Large-bore catheters inserted into femoral artery and vein to provide a continuous method of dialysis for removal of water and toxins. Approx. 3 in long. These caths do *not* have a tapered end. High-blood catheters supplied by dialysis unit only	1. Wear mask 2. Clamp catheter tubing with tubing clamp supplied by dialysis unit or hemostat 3. Aspirate 2 mL blood; discard 4. Instill 2 mL NS 5. Instill 1.5 mL or 1,500 U heparin (1,000 U/mL), cap with red cap 6. Remove tubing clamp 7. Place bulldog clamp on tubing	—	Hyperal protocol and PRN

CHANGE q 24 HOURS **All IV Bags**		**CHANGE q 48–72 HOURS** **Cardiac output tubing**

- IV tubing (primary)
- IV tubing (secondary). NOTE: Use one secondary set for 48 hours for each individual drug ordered
- Buretrol
- All IV extensions (except hyperal)
- Med tubing
- PCA pump tubing. NOTE: If there is waste narcotic, tubing must be sent to Pharmacy
- Hyperal cassette

Source: American Journal of Nursing, Feb. 1990, with permission. Updated in 1996.

*Central venous catheters will have injection plugs placed on each port of catheter before patients are transferred out of ICUs (exception: hyperal catheters).

NS = normal saline

PLANNING AND INTERVENTION

To plan and intervene effectively,

- Understand the reason for use of IV therapy in the patient, the presenting symptoms of the condition, and the type of fluid used.
- Remember that the patient receiving IV fluids also has other nursing care problems. The IV therapy may have been instituted after surgery, after trauma, or after a medical emergency. This patient is usually acutely ill and needs additional emotional support as well as physical nursing care.

Nursing Responsibilities for IV Therapy

The professional nurse is most often responsible for starting an IV infusion. To accomplish this, the nurse must follow these steps:

1. **Explain the procedure to the patient.** Patient teaching information is provided in Table 11–7 on page 131.
2. **Elicit the patient's cooperation.** If this is not possible because the patient is confused or unconscious, the nurse may need assistance in the actual venipuncture.
3. **Verify the IV order.**

4. **Gather the equipment.** IV tray with alcohol or similar cleansing solution, tourniquets, adhesive bandages, tape, antiseptic ointment to apply over the site (if indicated by the hospital), a selection of needles, and an arm board. Appropriate IV tubing must also be selected as well as the correct solution.

IV tubing comes in three basic types: regular tubing with a drip factor of 10 to 15 drops per mL, minidrip tubing with a drip factor of 60 drops per mL, and Y tubing used for blood administration with a drip factor of 10 drops per mL.

Many types of IV lines are available. Table 11–8 compares the most commonly used products and includes such information as uses, flushing, dressing changes, ability to draw blood, removal of the line, and troubleshooting.

In-line filters, shown in Figure 11–3, may also be used. These devices help to eliminate particulate matter that may be introduced into the IV solution by opening and adding other fluids to the IV line such as from IV additives. Research has demonstrated that when IV medications are drawn from single-dose glass vials, macroparticles of glass can also be drawn into the syringe and administered to the patient. The use of any size filter traps these macroparticles. Filters come as part of the IV tubing or can be added to it. Filters are available in three

rawing Blood	Special Notes	Change Caps	Removal of Lines	Troubleshooting Occlusions	Type of Catheter
ot recommended hat blood sam- les be obtained rom these lines.	Bulldog clamps to be on catheters at all times.	q 12 h with flush-ing	MD removes.	Do NOT attempt to instill if blood will not aspirate from T-tube. If clot in T-tube, do not in-still NS or heparin. T-tube will require change (See pol-icy & procedure manual)	CAVH femoral ar-tery catheter, femoral vein catheter, Vygon catheter 8F

CHANGE q72 HOURS
Manifold system
including transducer,
monitoring kits and
pressure tubings

Wear gloves when handling blood samples. Do NOT recap needles.

CHANGE BLOOD COMPONENT RECIPIENT SETS AFTER q8 UNITS OF PLATELETS
Change per 1 unit of *single* donor platelets or per 8 small units of individual donor platelets. Change blood administration set after 2 units of blood or packed cells given consecutively.

---

sizes: 5 μm, 0.5 μm, or 0.22 μm. The 5-μm size fil-ters gross particulate material; the 0.5 μm size pre-vents passage of most bacteria, yeast, and particu-late matters; and the 0.22-μm filter (considered a sterilizing filter) removes nearly all bacteria, fungi, and particulate matter that find their way into IV fluids. The 0.5- and 0.22-μm filters require an in-fusion pump to administer fluids through them. Filters have been shown to reduce the incidence of infusion phlebitis to less than 10%. The incidence of phlebitis arising from IV infusions without filters ranges between 27% and 47%. Filters can also pre-vent the infusion of microorganisms and air emboli. Most solutions can be filtered, except suspensions such as fats and some cytotoxins. (Blood and blood products require their own special filters.) There is disagreement on the subject of in-line filters: The Centers for Disease Control does not recommend the use of filters as a routine infection control mea-sure, but the National Intravenous Therapy Asso-ciation believes that filters should be used for all IV therapy. It must be remembered, however, that IV filters do not remove endotoxins, nor do they re-duce the risk of contaminants entering the tubing below the filter. In addition, because some drugs bind to filters, using filters can reduce the drug's potency. In the final analysis, cost is a major factor

in deciding whether to use IV filters. Some hospi-tals compromise by using them only for IV prod-ucts that have a high concentration of particulate matter.

5. **Prepare the IV solution.** The solution may be a plain IV solution or an admixture. An admixture is the addition of one or more drugs and/or another solution to the main IV. Preparation of the admix-ture may fall under the scope of the pharmacy de-partment or may be within the realm of nursing. When the nurse is preparing an admixture, the IV must be labeled with the drug name and dose that was added, as well as the patient's name and room number, date and time, and the nurse's name.

Solutions come in various sizes: 100, 250, 500, and 1000 mL in either glass bottles or plastic bags. There are also 25-, 50-, and 100-mL bottles available for direct administration of IV medications.

As the nurse removes the solution from the shelf, it is inspected for clarity and lack of particulate matter. The nurse checks the expiration date and returns solution to the pharmacy if it is outdated. Next, the nurse checks for cracks in a glass bottle or leaks in a plastic bag. Any admixture must be prepared using sterile technique and labeled cor-rectly. The nurse connects the tubing to the IV con-tainer and runs fluid through the tubing to clear the

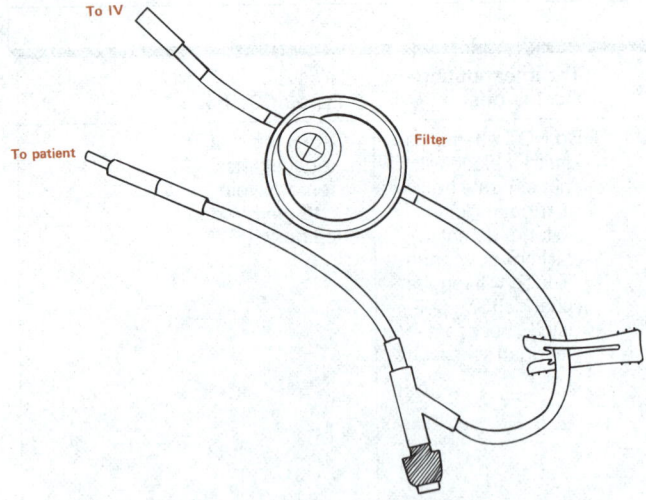

To IV

To patient

Filter

Figure 11–3. In-line IV filter.

air from the tubing. The solution and tubing are prepared in the medication room, where the nurse is free from distractions. (For review of medication preparation procedures, see a fundamental nursing text.)

6. **The nurse is now ready to enter the patient's room and perform the venipuncture.** (See a medical-surgical textbook for procedure.) After the venipuncture, the site is labeled with the time of insertion, the date, the needle size and type used, and the nurse's name.

7. **Regulate the IV.** The nurse calculates the IV flow rate and regulates the rate to the proper drops per minute. When infusion pumps are used, the nurse must understand the mechanics of operation. The drop rate is checked frequently and compared with the reading of the pump to ensure accuracy.

8. **Examine the IV site for complications.** At least once per hour, the nurse checks for complications at the site and on the extremity. Major complications include clotting, extravasation and infiltration, and thrombophlebitis. Extravasation and infiltration occur when fluid or blood enters the surrounding skin. The area becomes hard, swollen, and painful (toxic substances can even cause sloughing of the tissues). Thrombophlebitis is an inflammation at the insertion site, which may result from many possible causes including type, size, and site of the needle inserted; the fluid itself; and duration of time the IV remains in site. The site becomes red, swollen, and painful. (Refer to a medical-surgical nursing text for more detailed discussion of IV complications.)

9. **Inspect the patient for generalized complications and reactions.** These may include a pyrogenic reaction, which occurs when *pyrogens* (substances that produce fever) enter through the IV line and cause a systemic febrile reaction; infection, which results from the introduction of bacteria or fungi

through the IV line; an embolism, which may occur in any central location from part of a blood clot breaking off near the insertion site; and fluid overload, which results from too much fluid administered too quickly with the heart unable to manage the extra load. Symptoms of fluid overload are those of congestive heart failure.

10. **Inspect the patient for complications specific to the type of IV fluid.** For example, check for fluid shifts, dehydration, and overhydration.

11. **Administer additional IV medications as ordered.** Always ensure that the medications are compatible with the IV solution. (See Table 5–1 for IV drug compatibility.) The nurse may administer medications directly IV by push or bolus or through a device that allows a precise amount of medication to be given intermittently every 4 to 6 hours. The devices that can be used for this purpose include "piggybacks," partial fills, and volume control sets, shown in Figure 11–4. Antibiotics are often administered intermittently.

12. **Monitor intake and output and body weight on a daily basis.**

13. **Monitor laboratory reports for electrolyte balance.** Types of solutions may need to be changed daily.

Patients who will need IV therapy for more than 7 days, such as with long-term antibiotic therapy, chemotherapy, continuous narcotic infusions, long-term rehydration, or parenteral nutrition, benefit from central lines or peripherally inserted central (PIC) catheters. Central lines are reviewed in Chapter 14. PIC lines are often inserted by RNs who are certified to perform such insertion. The PIC lines are flexible, soft silicone catheters, inserted into either the basilic or cephalic vein via the antecubital space.

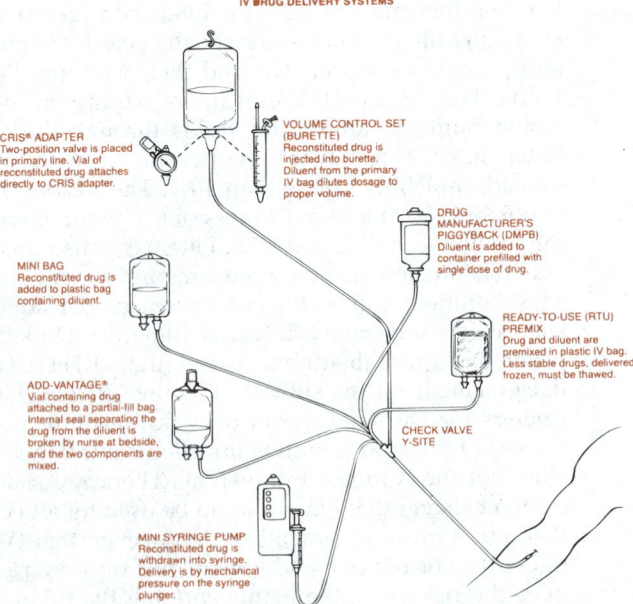

IV DRUG DELIVERY SYSTEMS

CRIS® ADAPTER
Two-position valve is placed in primary line. Vial of reconstituted drug attaches directly to CRIS adapter.

VOLUME CONTROL SET (BURETTE)
Reconstituted drug is injected into burette. Diluent from the primary IV bag dilutes dosage to proper volume.

MINI BAG
Reconstituted drug is added to plastic bag containing diluent.

DRUG MANUFACTURER'S PIGGYBACK (DMPB)
Diluent is added to container prefilled with single dose of drug.

READY-TO-USE (RTU) PREMIX
Drug and diluent are premixed in plastic IV bag. Less stable drugs, delivered frozen, must be thawed.

ADD-VANTAGE®
Vial containing drug attached to a partial-fill bag. Internal seal separating the drug from the diluent is broken by nurse at bedside, and the two components are mixed.

CHECK VALVE Y-SITE

MINI SYRINGE PUMP
Reconstituted drug is withdrawn into syringe. Delivery is by mechanical pressure on the syringe plunger.

Figure 11–4. IV delivery systems. (Adapted from In Vivo: The business and medicine report. 86(16):1–10, 1986, with permission.)

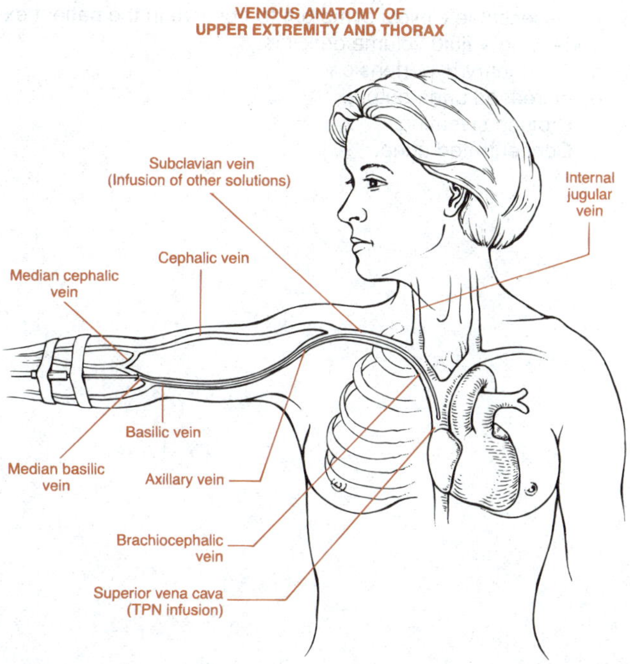

**VENOUS ANATOMY OF
UPPER EXTREMITY AND THORAX**

Subclavian vein
(Infusion of other solutions)

Internal
jugular
vein

Cephalic vein

Median cephalic
vein

Basilic vein

Median basilic
vein

Axillary vein

Brachiocephalic
vein

Superior vena cava
(TPN infusion)

Figure 11–5. Peripherally inserted central (PIC) catheter. The PIC catheter is inserted in the basilic or cephalic vein in the antecubital space and advanced until the catheter tip rests in the axillary, subclavian, or brachiocephalic vein.

The lines are then advanced until the catheter tip rests in the axillary, subclavian, or brachiocephalic vein, shown in Figure 11–5. PIC lines are less expensive than central lines, minimize the risk of phlebitis, and do not have to be immobilized, so patient comfort is greater. X-ray verification is required to assess the final location of the tip.

EVALUATION

- Evaluate the effectiveness of IV therapy. This evaluation is based on a predetermined list of outcome evaluation criteria that have been developed in relation to the goals determined by the nurse, patient, and family (see Table 11–5).
- Evaluate the patient for complications of IV therapy such as infiltration, extravasation, thrombosis, cellulitis, thrombophlebitis, pain at the administration site, fluid overload, pyrogenic reactions, and bacteremia, as well as for reactions to specific fluids. The IV site and drip rate are evaluated hourly or more often, if necessary. IV tubing and dressings must be changed according to the institutional policies. Research suggests that changing tubing and dressing every 72 hours is sufficient to prevent infection.

The longer the IV device remains in place, the greater the risk of infection. With appropriate infection control measures (such as aseptic initiation and maintenance of the IV system), few devices produce sepsis until they have been in place for at least 72 hours. Also, synthetic IV devices such as IV catheters have a greater risk of infection than smaller, steel "scalp vein" or "butterfly" needles—8% versus 0.1% to 0.2%.

There are three exceptions to the 72-hour interval for routine IV set changes: (1) during the administration of blood products and lipid emulsion, because both of these products enhance bacterial growth in parenteral solutions; (2) with arterial pressure monitoring, because of the high rate of arterial infusate contamination; and (3) in the presence of a suspected infusion-related septicemia epidemic. Because most U.S. hospitals try to replace IV cannulas every 3 days, researchers conclude that replacing the delivery sets along with the cannulas would be more time- and cost-effective.

- Evaluate the effectiveness of treatment by a return to normal homeostasis. This is evaluated through qualitative, quantitative, and laboratory findings.

The bibliography for this chapter can be found in Appendix B, which begins on page 1054.

CHAPTER REVIEW QUESTIONS*

1. An intravenous replacement solution is:
   a. A combination of water, carbohydrates, and electrolytes used to replace losses from the gastrointestinal tract.
   b. Available in both 10% and 20% dextrose solutions to correct losses due to hemorrhaging.
   c. High in potassium and sodium to approximate electrolyte loss through renal excretion.
   d. Used to promote renal function, when a fluid deficit exists, by using a balance among cations and anions.

2. Nursing responsibilities in caring for the patient receiving intravenous therapy include:
   a. Examining the intravenous sites at least once every four hours.
   b. Monitoring the patient's intake, output, and body weight daily.
   c. Preparing the solution and admixture using clean technique.
   d. Lowering the infusion rate if redness or swelling occurs at the intravenous site.

3. Lactated Ringer's solution (Hartmann's solution) is an example of the following type of solution:
   a. Hydrating.
   b. Carbohydrate.
   c. Balanced.
   d. Replacement.

4. A nursing goal for the patient with fluid volume deficit is to restore volume to normal by:
   a. Administering hypotonic solutions.
   b. Administering high glucose solutions.
   c. Monitoring hypertonic solutions.
   d. Restricting fluid intake.

*See Appendix A, which begins on page 1051, for answers.

5. A hydrating intravenous solution is:
   a. Composed of water, protein, and varying amounts of electrolytes.
   b. Isotonic, thus does not draw water from or pass into the cells.
   c. Composed of water, carbohydrate, and varying amounts of sodium chloride.
   d. High in potassium to replace electrolyte loss.

6. An assessable clinical symptom to observe in the patient experiencing a fluid volume deficit is:
   a. Pulmonary hypertension.
   b. Increased urine output.
   c. Profuse sweating.
   d. Concentrated urine.

CHAPTER 12

Major Body Electrolytes

Merrily A. Kuhn, RNC, PhD

CHAPTER OUTLINE

Sodium
Potassium
Calcium
Magnesium
Phosphorus
Using the Nursing Process

TABLES

Drug Tables
Nursing Process
Patient Teaching

KEY TERMS

Chvostek's sign
Electrolyte
Milk-alkali syndrome

Osteomalacia
Rhabdomyolysis
Trousseau's sign

LEARNING OBJECTIVES

After reading this chapter, the student will be able to:

1. Identify major body electrolytes commonly used as medications and select those specific to the patient requiring electrolyte medications.
2. Identify specific areas to assess in the patient requiring electrolytes to formulate appropriate patient outcomes.
3. Determine the nursing interventions necessary to administer electrolytes and choose appropriate teaching strategies to gain patient compliance.
4. Evaluate the patient at various stages of treatment to gauge nursing interventions.

*E*lectrolytes are substances capable of dissociating (or separating) in water into their component parts, carrying either a positive (cation) or a negative (anion) charge. The major electrolytes in the body are sodium (Na^+), potassium (K^+), calcium (Ca^{2+}), magnesium (Mg^{2+}), chloride (CL^-), phosphate (HPO_4^-), and bicarbonate (HCO_3^-). Electrolytes are found in varying concentrations inside and outside the cell, as shown in Figure 12–1. Other substances in the body that are not capable of dissociating are nonelectrolytes (glucose, proteins, urea, organic acids, and carbonic acid).

All electrolyte solutions are combination products; that is, they contain one cation for every anion. To prepare a solution, a stable solid composed of a combination salt such as KCl (potassium chloride), $MgSO_4$ (magnesium sulfate), or NaCl (sodium chloride) is diluted in a liquid vehicle. To make the solution stable, all of the cations must be neutralized by all of the anions.

SODIUM

Serum sodium is the major cation in the extracellular fluid (ECF). Normal serum sodium is 135 to 145 mEq/liter. Sodium maintains osmotic pressure and serum osmolarity (the concentration of osmotically active particles in solution) helps to maintain acid-base and water balance, contributes to nerve conduction and neuromuscular function, and plays a role in glandular secretions.

Sodium, when taken orally, is readily absorbed in the small intestine with small amounts excreted through the kidneys and the skin. Sodium is regulated in the kidney by several hormones: aldosterone, antidiuretic hormone (ADH), and the third factor—a kidney tubular enzyme. Sodium competes with both H^+ and K^+ ions in the renal tubule for excretion and reabsorption; 99% of the filtered sodium is reabsorbed in the kidney. Therefore, urinary sodium levels (when measured) are minimal.

Sodium replacement is necessary when there is rapid loss of fluid in the body—and thus a loss of sodium—as occurs with diarrhea, vomiting, trauma, adrenal insufficiency, inappropriate ADH secretion, or burns.

The most commonly used sodium preparation is **sodium chloride,** with several forms available for IV replacement. If oral intake is possible, table salt or **sodium bicarbonate** can be used for replacement. Sodium chloride is often used to correct an extracellular volume depletion.

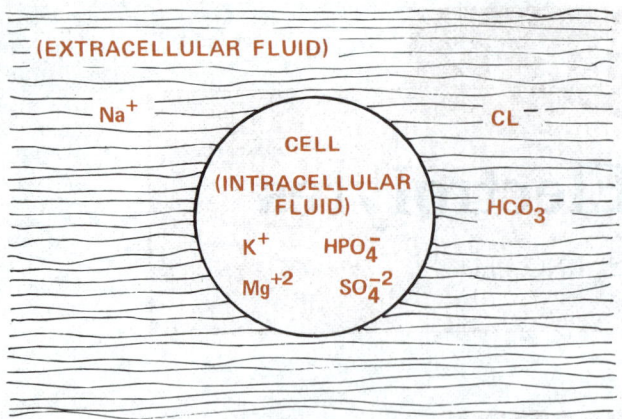

Figure 12–1. Electrolytes are found both inside and outside the cell in varying concentrations. The diagram shows where the major concentrations of each electrolyte are found.

○ **Sodium chloride** is available as a 0.45% hypotonic solution, a 0.9% isotonic solution, or a hypertonic solution of 3% (513 mEq sodium/liter) or 5% (855 mEq sodium/liter). Hypotonic solutions—with osmolarity less than plasma—are administered (often with dextrose) for maintenance therapy in patients unable to take anything by mouth for 3 days or less. Isotonic solutions—with the same osmolarity, as plasma—are infused when both sodium and water have been depleted in isotonic proportions; these solutions are used to maintain effective extravascular fluid volume and a stable circulation in many conditions. Hypertonic solutions—with osmolarity greater than plasma—are reserved for the treatment of severe symptomatic hyponatremia (serum sodium less than 120 mEq/liter) and only during the acute phase. In general, the hypertonic saline solutions are administered slowly to prevent fluid overload and the development of

Table 12–1. AGENTS USED TO MANAGE SODIUM AND POTASSIUM IMBALANCES

DRUG NAME/ROUTE AND DOSAGE	NURSING IMPLICATIONS
sodium bicarbonate	
metabolic acidosis ***Adults:*** 200–300 mEq as 7.5–8.4% solution by IV bolus; or, infuse 2–5 mEq/kg over 4–8 hr.	**ASSESSMENT:** Assess for alkalosis and hypocalcemia (contraindications). Assess for pregnancy (category C). **INTERVENTION:** Administer slowly IV. If extravasation occurs, inject area with lidocaine or hyaluronidase, elevate the affected area, and apply warm compresses to the site. **EVALUATION:** Evaluate for renal impairment, CHF, and edematous state.
potassium chloride usp (For list of oral products, see Table 12–2) Contains 2 mEq K⁺/mL	
hypokalemia ***Adults:*** Prevention–20 mEq/day PO. Treatment–40–100 mEq/day PO or 40–300 mEq/day IV (depending on serum potassium level). ***Children:*** Treatment–1–3 mEq/kg per day PO or IV.	**ASSESSMENT:** Assess baseline potassium level, urine output, and ECG and then periodically during therapy. Assess for pregnancy (category C). **INTERVENTION:** Administer PO with meals (may be irritating to GI tract). Dilute products well in ½–1 glass of water and sip over 5–10 min. Do not chew or crush tablets. Do not give until urine flow is reestablished in postoperative period. Give IV into large vein no faster than 10mEq/hr. *Never give IV push or IM.* Always dilute before IV administration. Add to new IV or turn IV off, turn upside down and mix before turning it on again. Do not add in a hanging position. **Patient Teaching**—Teach patient that the wax-matrix tablet of Slow-K may be found in the stool but that the medication has been absorbed.Teach patients about foods high in potassium. **EVALUATION:** Evalute for signs of hyperkalemia, increased fatigue, muscle weakness, cramps, nausea, vomiting, or black stools. Evaluate ECG and serum potassium periodically. Evaluate T and QRS wave changes on the ECG (see Fig. 13–2). These herald potassium toxicity and impending cardiac arrest.
sodium polystyrene sulfonate (Kayexalate) (Resonium A) (SPS)	
hyperkalemia ***Adults:*** 15–60 g/day PO (4 level tsp 1–4 times/day in 20–100 mL water or sorbitol); or 25–100 g in 100 mL sorbitol q 6 hr as a retention enema. ***Children:*** 1 g of resin PO or rectally for each mEq of potassium to be removed.	**ASSESSMENT:** Assess potassium and sodium serum levels frequently. Assess for pregnancy (category C). **INTERVENTION:** Use only fresh suspensions. Stir before use. Check for constipation. Do not expose to heat. **For retention enema**—Use warm fluid to prepare emulsion. Keep particles in suspension by continuous stirring. Flush suspension with 50–100 mL of fluid, then clamp tube and leave it in place. Urge patient to retain enema for 30–60 min or longer if possible. If leakage occurs, elevate hips on pillow or place patient temporarily in knee-chest position. May be given by rectum with Foley (30-cc balloon) catheter to prevent immediate expulsion of solution. After enema has been expelled, irrigate colon with 1–2 quarts of flushing solution. Allow drainage to return constantly through a Y tube connection. **EVALUATION:** Evaluate for the presence of hypokalemia or hypernatremia. Report to physician.

pulmonary edema. For additional information on IV solutions, see Chapter 11.

○ **Sodium bicarbonate** is used as a systemic alkalizer to correct metabolic acidosis, which may occur secondary to diabetic ketoacidosis, cardiac arrest, and vascular collapse. Sodium bicarbonate is rarely administered today unless the pH is less than 7.1 to 7.0 because it breaks down into hydrogen and water and makes the brain and tissues more acidic. Sodium bicarbonate is featured in Table 12–1.

CONTRAINDICATIONS AND PRECAUTIONS Sodium bicarbonate is contraindicated in patients with severe vomiting, metabolic or respiratory alkalosis, or hypocalemia and in patients receiving diuretics known to produce hypochloremic alkalosis. Use with caution in patients with impaired renal function, heart failure, or edematous states.

ADVERSE EFFECTS Excessive sodium bicarbonate may cause headache, dizziness, abdominal cramps, nausea, vomiting, and fluid retention. An alkalotic state may also ensue.

INTERACTIONS Do not mix with calcium, dopamine, or dobutamine as precipitation may occur. Sodium bicarbonate increases renal clearance of tetracyclines and doxycycline, which may reduce their effectiveness; it increases the half-life of quinidine, amphetamines, ephedrine, and pseudoephedrine, which may result in toxicity of these drugs.

POTASSIUM

Serum potassium is the most important intracellular cation. Ninety-eight percent of all potassium is found in intracellular fluid while only 2% is found in extracellular fluid. Normal plasma concentrations range from 3.5 to 5.0 mEq/liter. Potassium assists with the regulation of intracellular osmolality (the concentration of free particles, molecules, or ions in solution) and is necessary for cellular growth and metabolism. Potassium helps to maintain acid-base balance and enzyme action necessary to change carbohydrates into energy and to reassemble amino acids into protein. Potassium is also necessary for proper function of skeletal, cardiac, and smooth muscle.

Normally, 40 mEq of potassium is required daily; potassium cannot be stored in the body, so it must be consumed each day. Eighty to 90% of the ingested potassium is excreted in the urine under the influence of aldosterone while 10% to 20% is excreted in the stool. The kidney can conserve potassium to some degree when cellular potassium becomes depleted.

Potassium is moved into the cells during glucose metabolism and during beta-adrenergic stimulation. Potassium moves out of the cells during strenuous exercise, when cellular metabolism is impaired, and when cells die. When potassium is lost from cells, sodium and hydrogen ions shift into the cells to replace the lost potassium, making the cells more acid while the extracellular fluid becomes more alkaline.

HYPOKALEMIA

Hypokalemia (serum sodium less than 3.5 mEq/liter) occurs when there is inadequate intake of potassium through the diet such as in patients with nausea or anorexia or during extreme dieting, in acute alcoholism, and in patients maintained on intravenous therapy with no or low potassium levels. Potassium deficits can also occur when potassium utilization is increased during the healing phase of burns or secondary to excessive loss of potassium from vomiting, diarrhea, or fistulas, or secondary to therapies such as diuretics, antibiotics, corticosteroids, or nasogastric suction.

A host of symptoms threatens when the patient's potassium level deviates from the normal range, reflecting the importance of potassium. As the potassium decreases, symptoms—including weakness, speech changes, flaccid paralysis, shallow respirations, decreased intestinal motility, abdominal distention, anorexia, and paralytic ileus—occur because of decreased neuromuscular irritability. Dysrhythmias; a slow, weak, irregular pulse; hypotension; low, flat T waves and prominent U waves on the ECG, as shown in Figure 12–2, and cardiac arrest are all related to weakness of the cardiovascular smooth muscle and prolongation of myocardial repolarization. Polyuria and nocturia are related to the inability of the kidney to concentrate urine.

Potassium Products Used to Manage Hypokalemia

Potassium products—**potassium chloride *(Kaochlor)*, potassium bicarbonate *(K+ Care ET)*,** and **potassium gluconate *(Kaon)*—**vary in the amount of potassium they contain and are given orally, either for prevention of hypokalemia, as in a patient receiving diuretics, or for the actual treatment of hypokalemia (see Table 12–1). Potassium salts come in liquid form, as tablets—enteric-coated, wax matrix, and effervescent—or as powders that can be dissolved in water. Time-release products are also available, as listed in Table 12–2.

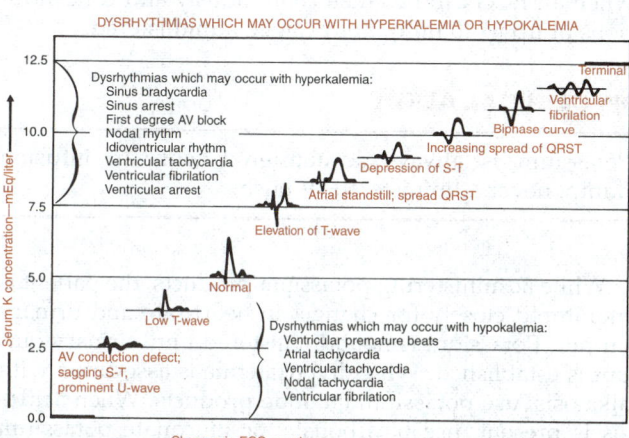

Figure 12–2. ECG changes at various levels of serum potassium concentration. (Used with permission from Krupp, MA and Chatton, MJ, eds. Current Medical Diagnosis and Treatment. Lange Medical Publications, Los Altos, CA, 1974.)

Table 12–2. SELECTED ORAL POTASSIUM AND CHLORIDE PREPARATIONS

Trade Name	Potassium (mEq)[a]	Chloride (mEq)[a]
Liquid Products		
Kaochlor 10% Liquid[b,c]	20	20
Kaochlor S-F 10% Liquid[b,c]	20	20
Kaon-Cl 20%[b]	40	40
Effervescent Products[d]		
Klorvess	20	20
K-Lyte/Cl	25	25
Time-Release Products[e]		
Kaon Cl[c]	6.7	6.7
Slow-K[f]	8	8

[a]Per 15 mL, packet, or tablet.
[b]Contains alcohol.
[c]Contains tartrazine, which may cause allergic reactions.
[d]Most effervescent formulas are sugar free. Completely dissolve and allow fizzing to stop, then sip slowly over a 5–10-minute period.
[e]Time-release products reduce the danger of bowel ulceration and potential complications.
[f]Slow-K uses a wax matrix as a carrier for the crystals. After absorption, the tablet carcass appears in the stool. There is no cause for alarm.

Potassium preparations for IV use come in vials of 10, 20, 30, 40, 60, 90, and 120 mEq per single-dose vial.

▼ **CLINICAL ALERT**

These vials are diluted in IV solution and given slowly into a large vein to prevent irritation. (A large vein, while not absolutely necessary, is recommended.)

The usual maintenance dose is 20 mEq per day, while the treatment dose can be 40 to 100 mEq per day. Generally, the maximum IV concentration is 40 mEq/liter at a rate of 10 mEq/hour, except in life-threatening hypokalemia when an ECG can be taken continuously and concentrations of up to 40 mEq/hour can be administered.

▼ **CLINICAL ALERT**

Potassium is always administered with an infusion pump, never administered IV push.

While administering potassium products, the patient is monitored closely for changes in heart rate and urinary output. Potassium is not administered until urinary output is established. When hypokalemia is associated with alkalosis, use potassium chloride products. When acidosis is present, use bicarbonate, or gluconate potassium salts.

Contraindications and Precautions Potassium products are contraindicated in severe renal impairment, such as with early postoperative oliguria, other oliguria and anuria; acute crushing injuries; Addison's disease; and acute dehydration, as all these conditions can lead to hyperkalemia. All potassium products are given cautiously to persons with cardiac disease, particularly patients taking digitalis glycosides, as there is increased risk of hyperkalemic adverse effects.

Adverse Effects Potassium products may cause adverse effects including nausea, vomiting, gastrointestinal disturbances, cardiac dysrhythmias, and muscle weakness. With oral administration, local gastrointestinal effects can be reduced by diluting oral products or by taking them with meals. With IV administration, local tissue necrosis can occur if extravasation occurs. Local infiltration of the affected area with 1% procaine hydrochloride with hyaluronidase often reduces venospasm and dilutes the potassium remaining locally in the tissues. Local application of heat may also be helpful.

Interactions Potassium products are not given concurrently with potassium-sparing diuretics such as spironolactone, triamterene, or amiloride as hyperkalemia can result. The angiotension converting enzyme inhibitors—captopril, enalapril, lisinopril, and others—may cause potassium retention resulting in hyperkalemia in 1 to 2 days due to lowering circulating aldosterone levels. Concurrent administration with anticholinergics, which slow gastrointestinal motility, can increase the likelihood of gastrointestinal erosion when solid potassium products are administered concurrently.

○ **Potassium chloride** (Kaochlor, Slow-K, and many others) is a combination of potassium and chloride. This combination is used because chloride depletion often occurs along with a potassium loss. Oral products are most often used concurrently when patients are taking potassium-depleting diuretics. Potassium chloride is generally used for intravenous replacement of potassium with 40 mEq/liter per bottle. Potassium chloride products are also available as liquids, soluble powders, and effervescent tablets (see Table 12–2).

○ **Potassium bicarbonate** (K + Care ET), with 20 mEq of potassium/15 mL, is available as an oral solution or as effervescent tablets. An oral dose of 25 to 50 mEq is dissolved in one-half to a whole glass of cold water and administered one or two times daily.

○ **Potassium gluconate** (Kaon), with 20 mEq of potassium/15 mL, is used to replace potassium levels. The usual dose is 5 to 20 mEq two to four times daily.

HYPERKALEMIA

Hyperkalemia is indicated when the serum potassium level is above 5.5 mEq/liter. Hyperkalemia has three major etiologies: (1) retention of potassium within the body, primarily due to poor renal function or adrenocortical insufficiency; (2) excessive release of potassium from the cells such as in patients with serious burns, traumatic injuries, infection, or acidosis; and (3) excessive intravenous infusion of potassium-containing fluids, even with normal renal function.

Assessment findings of hyperkalemia include intestinal colic, diarrhea, and muscle twitching proceeding to skeletal muscle weakness, flaccid paralysis, and cardiac arrhythmias. These are related to increased neuromuscular irritability in mild hyperkalemia and reduced neuromuscular irritability in more severe hyperkalemia. There is also altered cardiac muscle function.

Products Used to Manage Hyperkalemia

When the potassium level rises above 6.5 mEq/liter or there are significant ECG changes (see Fig. 12–2), treatment is instituted. Several treatment modalities are available. **Sodium polystyrene sulfonate *(Kayexalate)*,** an exchange resin, is administered either a 5% or 10% IV dextrose solution with 10 to 15 units of regular insulin is used, which will redistribute potassium from the plasma to the cells. The insulin causes potassium to enter the cells, while glucose prevents hypoglycemia caused by the insulin. The addition of sodium bicarbonate to the IV dextrose solution elevates blood pH, correcting acidosis that usually present in conjunction with hyperkalemia, which in turn promotes potassium movement into the cells in exchange for hydrogen ions. The additional amount of sodium also promotes potassium excretion.

○ **Sodium polystyrene sulfonate** (Kayexalate) is given orally or by rectum (see Table 12–1) to promote the excretion of potassium by acting as an exchange resin. Oral therapy takes several hours to work, but an enema effectively lowers the serum potassium level in about 1 hour. Sodium polystyrene can be administered with sorbitol to produce osmotic diarrhea and the passage of exchange resins through the GI tract.

CONTRAINDICATIONS AND PRECAUTIONS Sodium polystyrene sulfonate is contraindicated in patients with sodium restrictions as sodium serum levels increase. Because it can increase fluid levels, sodium polystyrene sulfonate is used cautiously in patients with heart failure, renal disease, or edema, and in elderly patients.

ADVERSE EFFECTS Most common adverse effects include changes in bowel habits (constipation, diarrhea), vomiting, gastric irritation, hypokalemia, hypocalcemia, and sodium retention.

INTERACTIONS Interactions of sodium polystyrene sulfonate include concurrent use of antacids containing calcium, which causes binding and may result in metabolic alkalosis.

CALCIUM

Serum calcium, the fifth most common element in the body, is primarily stored in the bones. The normal serum calcium level is rather narrow, 8.5 to 10.5 mg/dL. Calcium is necessary to support neuromuscular transmission, to promote muscle cell and cardiac contraction, to provide a component for coagulation, to promote normal neuromuscular irritability, to build bones and teeth, to assist with the secretion of many hormones, and to strengthen cell membranes.

The daily adult requirement for calcium is at least 0.8 g. Infants and children require 0.17 to 1.4 g/day, while pregnant and lactating women require 1.3 to 1.5 g/day. Calcium is supplied in the American diet primarily by milk and milk products, with a small amount being supplied by vegetables and fruit. Dietary calcium is absorbed in the gut in the presence of vitamin D and controlled by parathyroid hormone (PTH). When serum calcium levels are increased, PTH is decreased, causing increased excretion of calcium in the urine and decreased gastrointestinal absorption. When serum calcium levels decrease, PTH is increased, resulting in less calcium lost in the urine and an increase in bone resorption.

HYPOCALCEMIA

Hypocalcemia can occur when there is excessive loss or removal of calcium (serum level less than 8.5 mg/dL) from the body, which can result from acute pancreatitis, hypoparathyroidism, or renal disorders. Hypocalcemia can also occur secondary to damage or removal of the thyroid, resulting in parathyroid dysfunction. Hypocalcemia can also occur when there is inadequate intake of vitamin D, following the correction of acidosis, during alkalosis as more calcium is bound to protein, or in conjunction with hyperphosphatemia.

Assessment findings in hypocalcemia include tingling and numbness of the fingers and circumoral region; painful tonic muscle spasms; fatigue; a positive *Trousseau's sign* and *Chvostek's sign*, both shown in Figure 12–3; facial spasms; laryngospasm; and convulsions. All symptoms are related to increased neuromuscular irritability producing hyperaction of motor and sensory nerves to stimuli. Changes in the ECG and dysrhythmias occur due to altered cardiac muscle function.

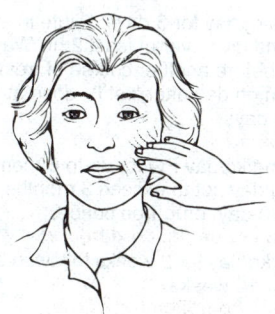

Chvostek's Sign

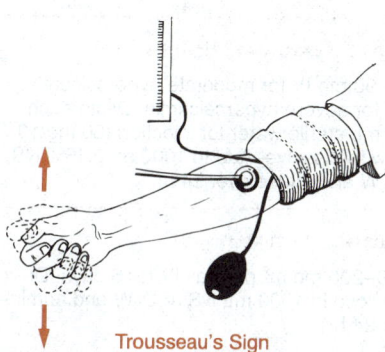

Trousseau's Sign

Figure 12–3. Signs of hypocalcemia. Chvostek's sign is positive when light stroking of the patient's cheek causes seventh cranial nerve stimulation and twitching of the cheek. Trousseau's sign is positive when a blood pressure cuff inflated on the arm for 10 seconds causes carpal spasm.

Table 12–3. CALCIUM PRODUCTS

DRUG NAME/ROUTE AND DOSAGE	NURSING IMPLICATIONS
PRODUCTS FOR HYPOCALCEMIA	
calcium gluconate Contains 10% Ca or 4.6 mEq/g (10 mL) *Adults:* 2.3–9.3 mEq (5–20 mL) IV. *Children:* 2.3 mEq/kg per day IV, in divided doses. **hypocalcemic emergency** *Adults:* 7–14 mEq IV. *Children:* 1–7 mEq IV. **hypocalcemic tetany** *Adults:* 4.5–16 mEq IV, repeated until tetany is controlled. *Children:* 0.5–0.7 mEq/kg IV 3–4 times daily until tetany is controlled. **prevention of hypocalcemia** *Adults:* 1–2 g/day PO. *Children:* 45–65 mg/kg per day PO.	**ASSESSMENT:** Assess baseline ECG (QT interval), muscle tone, and presence of Chvostek's and Trousseau's signs and monitor throughout therapy. **INTERVENTION:** Carefully monitor IV to avoid infiltration. If infiltration occurs, infiltrate area with 1% procaine and hyaluronidase and apply warm, moist compresses. Monitor digitalized patient carefully when giving calcium as calcium increases risk of digitalis toxicity. Do not put calcium in same IV bottle with bicarbonate or phosphate as a precipitate may form. Inject calcium gluconate IM into vastus lateralis in adults or lateral thigh in children in an emergency if IV administration is not feasible. After injecting calcium, keep patient recumbent for 15 min to prevent dizziness. Tablets are best administered after meals. **EVALUATION:** Evaluate ECG for prolonged QT interval and for signs of hypercalcemia.
calcium chloride Contains 27% Ca or 13.6 mEq/g (10 mL) *Adults:* 500 mg–1 g in 0.5% solution IV, given slowly (not to exceed 1 mL/min). *Children:* 25 mg/kg administered slowly. **calcium supplementation during tpn** *Adults:* 10–15 mEq IV daily. *Children:* 5–20 mEq IV daily.	Same as for calcium gluconate plus: **INTERVENTION:** Do not administer SC or IM. Avoid extravasation. Must not be injected into tissues because sloughing and severe necrosis may occur.
PRODUCTS FOR HYPERCALCEMIA	
etidronate disodium (EHDP) (Didronel) *Adults:* 7.5 mg/kg/day for 3 days. Dilute in at least 250 ml NS and give over at least 2 hr. Wait at least 7 days before another course of treatment. Start PO form on day after last IV dose at 20 mg/kg PO for 30 days. **paget's disease** *Adults:* 5–10 mg/kg/day PO for up to 6 months or 11–20 mg/kg/day not to exceed 3 months. Repeat only after a 90-day, drug-free period. **ossification due to spinal cord injury** *Adults:* 20 mg/kg/day for 2 weeks followed by 10 mg/kg/day for 10 weeks. **ossification as a complication of hip replacement** *Adults:* 20 mg/kg/day for 1 month before and 3 months after surgery.	**ASSESSMENT:** Assess GI function, dietary habits, and renal function before and during therapy. Assess for pregnancy (category C). **INTERVENTION:** Oral form—take on an empty stomach 2 hr before meals. May cause GI upset. Avoid food especially high in calcium and vitamins and minerals or antacids high in metals within 2 hr of dosing. Follow PO and IV administration under Drug Name/Route and Dosage column. Administer diluted IV solution slowly over at least 2 hr. **EVALUATION:** Evaluate for adverse reactions, including rash, pruritis, angioedema, and elevation of blood urea nitrogen (BUN) and creatinine levels.
pamidronate disodium (APD) (Aredia) *Adults:* 60–90 mg IV for moderate hypercalcemia; 90 mg IV for severe hypercalcemia. Dilute each vial in 10 mL sterile water for injection (30 mg/10 mL). Allow to dissolve. Add to 1000 ml 0.45% NS, NS, or D_5W and infuse over 24 hr.	Same as for etidronate disodium.
gallium nitrate (Ganite) *Adults:* 100–200 mg/m^2 per day IV for 5 days. Dilute daily dose in 1000 mL NS or D_5W and administer over 24 hr.	**ASSESSMENT:** Assess GI function, dietary habits, and renal function before and during therapy. Monitor BUN and serum creatinine before and frequently throughout therapy and serum calcium levels daily. Assess for pregnancy (category C). **INTERVENTION:** Dilute, mix and administer IV over a 24 hr period. **EVALUATION:** Evaluate patient for hypophosphatemia, renal toxicity, and hypocalcemia.

Calcium Products Used to Manage Hypocalcemia and Other Disorders

Calcium products, featured in Table 12–3, are available orally or intravenously to prevent or treat hypocalcemia and to relieve hypocalcemic tetany. Calcium products are also administered as nutritional supplements during pregnancy and lactation and for postmenopausal osteoporosis.

Oral calcium products include **calcium gluconate (Kalcinate), calcium lactate, calcium citrate (Citracal),** and **calcium carbonate (Os-cal, many others)**. The oral forms of calcium are usually administered three to four times daily during or after meals or with milk to avoid gastric upset. Many over-the-counter products are marketed today with various concentrations of calcium to prevent osteoporosis in women. Recent research indicates that calcium in any form alone does not prevent osteoporosis, but that coadministration of estrogen during and after menopause does help prevent osteoporosis.

The most potent calcium replacement preparations administered intravenously are **calcium chloride** (1 g provides 13.6 mEq calcium), **calcium gluceptate** (1 gm provides 4.1 mEq), and **calcium gluconate** (1 g provides 4.5 mEq). When administering intravenous calcium products, care must be taken that the needle does not slip out of the vein. If calcium salts infiltrate, they may cause serious tissue irritation. The IV preparations begin their action immediately and continue for 1 to 2 hours.

Pharmacokinetics

Oral calcium is readily absorbed from the duodenum and proximal jejunum in the presence of PTH and vitamin D. Absorption also depends on dietary factors. Calcium can bind to fiber, phytates, oxalates, and fatty acids to form insoluble nonabsorbable soaps. Calcium is excreted primarily in the feces (80%) and in the urine.

Contraindications and Precautions   Calcium products are given cautiously to patients with renal disease and to patients receiving cardiac glycosides as they potentiate the therapeutic and toxic effects of digitalis. Intravenous calcium is contraindicated in ventricular fibrillation occurring during cardiac resuscitation as it may increase ischemic tissue. Calcium products are also contraindicated in patients with hypercalcemia and renal calculi.

Adverse Effects   Adverse effects caused by calcium products include (1) constipation, decreased excitability of the nerves and muscles, and mental confusion as calcium acts as a sedative on the body, and (2) kidney stones as excess calcium is filtered and excreted by the kidney. Rapid IV administration can cause peripheral vasodilation and a local burning sensation.

Interactions   Calcium may antagonize the effects of calcium channel blockers. However, intravenous calcium chloride has been used as an antidote for verapamil-induced hypotension.

▼ CLINICAL ALERT

The combination of calcium and digitalis glycosides or administration of calcium to the digitalized patient may precipitate dysrhythmias. Also, coffee, tea and colas decrease the absorption of calcium. Intake should be separated by 2 hours.

○ **Calcium gluconate** (Kalcinate) is 9% calcium.
○ **Calcium lactate** contains 13% calcium. Calcium lactate tablets are best used as a supplement.
○ **Calcium citrate** (Citracal) is 21% calcium. Calcium citrate is better absorbed from the gastrointestinal tract than calcium carbonate. Tablets are administered 1 to 2 hours after meals three or four times daily.
○ **Calcium carbonate** (Calci-Chew, Os-Cal, BioCal, and many others) is 40% calcium. Calcium carbonate is the most efficient form of calcium available as both a regular and a chewable tablet. Five hundred mg is generally administered two to four times daily 1 to 2 hours after meals.
○ **Calcium gluceptate** contains 4.1 mEq of calcium per gram and is administered intravenously or intramuscularly.

HYPERCALCEMIA

Serum calcium acts as a sedative on the body. As serum calcium rises above 11 mg/dL, neuromuscular irritability is depressed. Hypercalcemia is most often associated with overactivity of the parathyroid gland, but may also occur secondary to immobilization and neoplastic disease in which there is increased movement of calcium out of the bones. Decreased renal excretion of calcium in renal disease can also account for hypercalcemia.

Hypercalcemia can also occur secondary to excessive ingestion of calcium or vitamin D or administration of thiazide diuretics, which decrease calcium excretion. Persons who have ulcers and who drink large amounts of milk and take various alkaline medications may also develop hypercalcemia as part of the *milk-alkali syndrome* (a syndrome of hypercalcemia, tissue calcification, renal insufficiency, and crystaluria occurring from the chronic administration of sodium bicarbonate with milk or calcium products).

Assessment findings in a patient with hypercalcemia include flank pain, kidney stones, and polyuria due to increased deposits of calcium in the renal pelvis and parenchyma, which results in the kidney's inability to concentrate urine. Lethargy, confusion, exhaustion, and loss of interest in surroundings occur because of neurologic hypofunction. Bone pain, osteoporosis, *osteomalacia* (adult rickets; a condition caused by vitamin D deficiency characterized by soft brittle bones, bone deformities, bone pain, and weakness), and pathologic fractures occur because of decalcification of the bones. Hypercalcemia also causes an increase in calcium ions in sympathetic ganglia, which impedes the transmission of stimuli, resulting in diarrhea, constipation, atony of the intestinal tract, peptic ulcer, anorexia, nausea, and vomiting.

Products Used to Manage Hypercalcemia

Hypercalcemia is treated with several different modalities. First, the cause is eliminated whenever possible, and renal excretion of calcium is increased. Intravenous saline solutions can be used to inhibit tubular reabsorption of calcium. Phosphate supplements are used to enhance calcium deposits in the bone and soft tissues and to reduce intestinal absorption of calcium. Glucocorticosteroids decrease calcium absorption from the intestinal tract and are often used to help control symptoms of lymphomas and multiple myloma. Mithramycin, a cytotoxic antibiotic discussed in detail in Chapter 55, is used when the hypercalcemia is due to malignancy. Other drugs used for hypercalcemia caused by malignancy include **etidronate disodium** *(EHDP)*, **pamidronate disodium** *(APD)*, and **gallium nitrate** *(Ganite)* (see Table 12–3). Calcitonin, a thyroid hormone discussed in detail in Chapter 46, is used when the hypercalcemia is related to excessive parathyroid activity.

○ **Etidronate disodium** *(EHDP)* **and pamidronate disodium** *(APD)* are biphosphates that act primarily in the bone. Etidronate disodium is also used to treat symptomatic Paget's disease of the bone.

CONTRAINDICATIONS AND PRECAUTIONS Etidronate disodium and pamidronate disodium are contraindicated in hypersensitivity. They are used cautiously in patients with impaired renal function or bowel disease. Safety in children and lactating women is unknown. Both drugs are pregnancy category B.

ADVERSE EFFECTS Etidronate disodium and pamidronate disodium may alter taste and cause rash, pruritis, urticaria, or angioedema. Pamidronate disodium is likely to cause fever, nausea, cough, fatigue, rhinitis, and somnolence. All adverse effects are dose dependent.

INTERACTIONS No interactions are known for etidronate disodium. Pamidronate disodium is not mixed in IV lactated Ringer's solution as a precipitate forms.

○ **Gallium nitrate** *(Ganite)* is also used to treat cancer-related hypercalcemia. The concurrent use of gallium nitrate and other nephrotoxic drugs (e.g., aminoglycoside, amphotericin B) increases the patient's risk of developing severe renal insufficiency. Serum creatinine levels are closely monitored.

CONTRAINDICATIONS AND PRECAUTIONS Gallium nitrate is contraindicated in patients with severe renal impairment as this is the organ of excretion. Use cautiously in patients with asymptomatic or mild hypocalcemia because of the large changes that can occur in calcium levels. Safety in children and lactating women is not established. Gallium nitrate is pregnancy category C.

ADVERSE EFFECTS Adverse effects include tachycardia, lower extremity edema, renal failure, transient hypophosphatemia, anemia, nausea, vomiting, diarrhea, and constipation.

INTERACTIONS Gallium nitrate combined with nephrotoxic drugs increases the likelihood of renal impairment.

MAGNESIUM

Serum magnesium, primarily found intracellularly, plays a critical role in the maintenance of normal muscle and nerve activity. It promotes regulation of blood phosphorus levels and activates many enzyme reactions important in carbohydrate metabolism. Normal serum levels are 1.5 to 2.5 mEq/liter. Symptoms of deficiency generally present below 1.0 mEq/liter; symptoms of excess, above 3.0 mEq/liter. Normal adults requirements are 200 to 300 mg/day. Magnesium is found abundantly in foods and is a vital constituent of chlorophyll.

Approximately 45% of ingested magnesium is absorbed. Parathyroid hormone increases the absorption of magnesium in the intestinal tract, while excessive fat, phosphates, calcium, and alkalosis inhibit magnesium absorption. Sixty-six percent is stored in the bone, 1% is found in the plasma and interstitial fluid, and the rest is found within the cells. Magnesium is excreted in both the urine and feces.

HYPOMAGNESEMIA

Major causes of hypomagnesemia (serum magnesium level less than 1.5 mEq/liter) are poor nutrition and either gastrointestinal or renal losses that were not replaced. Patients prone to magnesium deficiency are more likely to have one or more of the following: chronic and severe malnutrition, chronic renal disease, prolonged severe diarrhea, chronic alcoholism, intestinal malabsorption syndromes, prolonged diuretic therapy, acute renal failure in the diuretic phase, or prolonged intravenous therapy without magnesium replacement.

Assessment findings of hypomagnesemia include hyperactive reflexes, positive Chvostek's and Trousseau's signs, facial twitching, jerking, tetany, and convulsions. These symptoms are all due to increased neuromuscular irritability. Patients can also experience hallucinations, delusions, extreme confusion, and aggressive behavior due to increased stimulation of the central nervous system. Tachycardia and hypotension also occur due to decreased cardiac muscle function.

Magnesium Products Used to Manage Hypomagnesemia and Other Disorders

Magnesium is supplied as **magnesium sulfate,** which comes in both oral and intravenous forms. Magnesium products are featured in Table 12–4.

○ **Magnesium sulfate** (Epsom salt), when taken in its oral form, acts as an osmotic cathartic by retaining and drawing water into the bowel. The intravenous form depresses CNS activity and activity in smooth, skeletal, and cardiac muscles. In the CNS, it reduces acetylcholine at the neuromuscular junction, thereby producing neuromuscular blockade.

Magnesium sulfate can be mixed in total parenteral nutrition (TPN) solutions or be administered intravenously for magnesium deficiency. (For further dosing information, see Table 12–4.) Magnesium sulfate is also used to control seizures caused by hypomagnesemia, seizures secondary to hypomagnesemia in acute nephritis, and seizures in severe eclampsia or preeclampsia; to treat constipation and to evacuate the bowel before surgery or radiographic procedures (laxative); and to control paroxysmal atrial tachycardia that is unresponsive to other treatments.

Table 12–4. MAGNESIUM AND PHOSPHATE PRODUCTS	
DRUG NAME/ROUTE AND DOSAGE	**NURSING IMPLICATIONS**
MAGNESIUM PRODUCTS	
magnesium sulfate (MgSO$_4$) Contains 8 mEq Mg^{++}/g	
hypomagnesemia *Adults:* 3 g PO q 6 hr for 4 doses; 1 g IM as 25%–50% solution q 6 hr for 4 doses for a maximum of 2 mEq/kg IM; or 1–5 g IV as 10%–20% solution, not to exceed 0.2 mEq/kg per min. **preeclampsia** *Adults:* 4–5 g (up to 10 g) in each buttock undiluted solution IM, given deep gluteal with 1% procaine added to decrease pain; subsequent IM doses of 4–5 g q 4 hr, depending on patient response. Or, 4–5 g IV as 10%–20% solution at a rate not to exceed 150 mg/min followed by 1–2 g/hr IV.	**ASSESSMENT:** Frequently assess reflexes, serum levels, and vital signs (q 10–15 min) to monitor for hypermagnesemia. Assess for heart block (a contraindication) and pregnancy (category A). **INTERVENTION:** Oral form for laxative effect is best administered in the morning with a full glass of water or juice. Bitter, salty taste may be disguised by chilling medication or by adding ice chips. It may also be flavored with lemon or orange juice. Calcium neutralizes effects of parenteral magnesium sulfate. IM—inject deep IM in gluteal muscle. IV—painful and irritating so dilute at least 1:20 and do not exceed 0.2 mEq/kg per minute. **EVALUATION:** Monitor for signs of hypermagnesemia, profound thirst, feeling of warmth, sedation, and muscle weakness. When administering for preeclampsia: decrease in blood pressure and fluid retention. Absence of seizure activity.
PHOSPHATE PRODUCTS	
potassium phosphate Contains 3 mmol PO$_4$/mL; 4.4 mEq K/mL	
phosphorus supplementation in tpn *Adults:* 10–15 mmol phosphorus/liter of TPN solution IV. *Infants:* 1.5–2 mmol/kg per day phosphorus IV.	**ASSESSMENT:** Assess serum calcium and phosphorus levels and intake and output before and during therapy. Assess for severe renal impairment, hyperphosphatemia, and alkaline urine (all contraindications). Assess for pregnancy (category C). **INTERVENTION:** Do not give postoperatively until urine flow is reestablished. Give by IV infusion, never IV push or IM. **EVALUATION:** Evaluate for signs and symptoms of hyperphosphatemia. Report to physician.
sodium phosphate Contains 3 mmol PO$_4$/mL; 4.0 mEq Na/mL	
phosphorus supplementation in tpn *Adults:* 10–15 mmol phosphorus/liter of TPN solution IV. *Infants:* 1.5–2 mmol/kg per day phosphorus IV.	Same as for potassium phosphate plus: **ASSESSMENT:** Assess for hypernatremia (contraindication).
phosphorus (Uro-KP-Neutral)(Neutra-Phos-K) all contain 250 mg phosphorus and varying amounts of potassium or sodium	
Adults: 1–2 tablets or capsules PO with meals and at bedtime.	Same as for sodium phosphate except: **INTERVENTION:** Administer with meals and at bedtime. Mix with water for administration.

Magnesium sulfate can decrease overall mortality after acute myocardial infarction by a mechanism as yet undetermined and prevent episodes of variant angina. Much literature supports magnesium replacement therapy for patients on digoxin or long-term diuretics (especially of the loop and thiazide types). Magnesium sulfate is currently the standard of care for treating torsades de pointes and is useful in treating digitalis-related and ventricular dysrhythmias intractable to either potassium, lidocaine, or bretylium. Magnesium is used for treating reentrant supraventricular tachycardias (SVTs), especially in cardiac surgery patients. Magnesium has also been suggested as a secondary line of therapy for asthma and as prophylaxis against withdrawal seizures in alcoholics.

Several studies have examined the use of magnesium to decrease myocardial infarction size. Magnesium prevents damage by decreasing the influx of calcium into the cell and increasing the electrical excitation threshold. Magnesium also decreases systemic vascular resistance (SVR) and cardiac output without increasing myocardial oxygen consumption (MVO$_2$).

CONTRAINDICATIONS AND PRECAUTIONS Magnesium sulfate is contraindicated in patients with heart block as it may slow cardiac conduction. It is used cautiously in patients with decreased renal function because of possible toxicity as magnesium sulfate is renally excreted, and in patients with heart disease as peripheral vasodilatation may occur, resulting in hypotension. Use with caution in patients receiving cardiac glycosides and in persons with respiratory disease as their conditions may worsen. Magnesium sulfate is pregnancy category B or A, depending on the formulation.

ADVERSE EFFECTS   The most common adverse effects of magnesium sulfate include flushing, warmth, sweating, thirst, muscle weakness, dehydration, hyporeflexia, disorientation, somnolence, and decreased respiratory rate. Transient hypotension may also occur.

INTERACTIONS   Magnesium sulfate potentiates the neuromuscular blockade produced by tubocurarine, decamethonium, and succinylcholine. Because of the central nervous system effects of magnesium, there may be interactions between magnesium sulfate and barbiturates, narcotics, hypnotics, or systemic anesthetics. Calcium neutralizes effects of parenteral magnesium sulfate. With digitalis, glycoside cardiac conduction changes and heart block may occur.

HYPERMAGNESEMIA

Hypermagnesemia, a serum level greater than 2.5 mEq/liter, is generally associated with overdoses of magnesium, either orally or parenterally, or poor renal function. Typical assessment findings associated with hypermagnesemia include a warm sensation throughout the body, decreased deep-tendon reflexes, flaccid paralysis, hypotension, drowsiness, decreased respirations, and dysrhythmias. These symptoms are all related to a pronounced reduction in neuromuscular irritability.

Products Used to Manage Hypermagnesemia

The treatment of hypermagnesemia is aimed at correcting the underlying cause (such as renal failure). Patients are placed on dialysis, and foods and drugs containing magnesium are withheld. If magnesium toxicity occurs, the patient is given 10% calcium gluconate intravenously at a rate not to exceed 0.5 mL/min. The calcium gluconate slows the action of magnesium on the heart and reverses the symptoms of cardiotoxicity.

PHOSPHORUS

Phosphorus is a critical component of all body tissues and is essential for the proper functioning of muscle, red blood cells, and the nervous system, as well as for the metabolism of carbohydrates, fats, and protein. Eighty to 85% of all phosphorus is a component in the skeletal system. Phosphorus is a structural part of phospholipids in cell membranes that are responsible for nutrient transport. Phosphorus is part of the nucleic acids, both RNA and DNA. It is also part of the buffering system that helps to maintain acid-base balance. Normal serum phosphorus is between 2.5 and 4.5 mg/dL and may be as high as 6 mg/dL in children. The amount of phosphorus is higher in children because of the high rate of skeletal growth.

HYPOPHOSPHATEMIA

Hypophosphatemia occurs when the phosphorus level falls below 2.5 mg/dL. The most common cause for hypophosphatemia is severe protein-calorie malnutrition in which people are refed carbohydrates with inadequate phosphorus. Other causes of hypophosphatemia can include intense hyperventilation, alcohol withdrawal, poor dietary intake, diabetic ketoacidosis, and major thermal burns.

Most signs and symptoms that result from hypophosphatemia are caused by the deficiency of adenosine triphosphate (ATP) and 2,3-diphosphoglycerate (2,3-DPG). ATP is necessary for production of cellular energy. As ATP declines, muscle weakness, muscle pain, and at times *rhabdomyolysis* (rapid muscle breakdown) can occur. Weak respiratory muscles may impair respiratory function. Severe hypophosphatemia is dangerous and requires prompt attention. 2,3-DPG is necessary for oxygen to be unloaded from red blood cells at the tissue level. As 2,3-DPG decreases, tissue anoxia can result.

Phosphate Products

Phosphorus is obtained from phosphates, which come in combination with other electrolytes such as sodium—**sodium phosphate**—or potassium—**potassium phosphate**. Phosphates are available as tablets, capsules, or powders for oral solutions, or as intravenous solutions. Sodium phosphate and potassium phosphate are ordered and administered as millimoles (mmol) (see Table 12–4 for additional dosing information). The phosphates are used to restore a phosphate depletion syndrome to normal, to reduce hypercalcemia, to bind calcium orally in renal disease, or to act as effective saline cathartics.

Contraindications and Precautions   Phosphates are contraindicated in patients with high phosphorus or low calcium levels and in patients with Addison's disease. Potassium phosphate is contraindicated in patients with hyperkalemia and is used cautiously in patients with cardiac disease, particularly the digitalized patient. Sodium phosphate is contraindicated in patients with hypernatremia and used cautiously in patients with edema, sodium retention, cardiac failure, or cirrhosis. Both potassium phosphate and sodium phosphate are used cautiously in the renal patient.

Adverse Effects   Typical adverse effects of intravenous phosphate therapy include hypocalcemia and hyperphosphatemia. When oral phosphates are given, diarrhea and gastrointestinal upset may occur.

Interactions   When oral phosphates are administered, several interactions can occur. Antacids can combine with a phosphate preparation and prevent absorption. Calcium and vitamin D products may antagonize the effects of phosphates. Concurrent use of sodium phosphate products with antihypertensives or corticosteroids may result in hypernatremia.

HYPERPHOSPHATEMIA

Hyperphosphatemia, a serum level above 4.5 mg/dL, is most commonly associated with decreased renal excretion of phosphorus. Other causes include chemotherapy, high phosphorus intake, profound muscle necrosis, and increased phosphorus absorption.

As serum phosphorus levels rise, precipitation of calcium phosphate occurs in nonosseous sites. Also, because of the reciprocal relationship between phosphorus and calcium, a high serum phosphorus tends to lower serum calcium. Tingling sensations around the fingers and mouth and tetany can result.

Treatment of hyperphosphatemia is aimed at treating and eliminating the underlying cause. For patients with renal failure, several measures are indicated. These include the administration of phosphate-binding antacids to bind phosphorus in the gut, the restriction of dietary phosphorus, and dialysis.

USING THE NURSING PROCESS

Table 12–5 suggests assessment data to collect and summarizes the other steps of the nursing process for the patient with disturbances of major body electrolytes.

Table 12–5. NURSING PROCESS FOR PATIENT REQUIRING MAJOR BODY ELECTROLYTES

Assessment

Assess history of current illness, sources of fluid loss/shifts.
Assess complaints of muscle weakness/spasms, lethargy, fatigue.
Assess laboratory studies, e.g., serum electrolytes, osmolarity; urine pH, specific gravity.
Assess prescription and OTC drug use (especially diuretics, steroids).

Nursing Diagnosis: Risk for Fluid Volume Deficit

RELATED TO: Active loss and/or failure of regulatory mechanisms (specific to underlying disease process/trauma), inability to obtain/ingest fluids.
AS EVIDENCED BY: Poor skin turgor and hypotension.

Desired Outcomes/Evaluation Criteria

Displays moist skin/mucous membranes, stable vital signs, individually adequate urinary output; free of edema and excessive weight loss/inappropriate gain.

Nursing Actions	Rationale
Administer replacement via appropriate route (IV, PO) and dilute as indicated.	Corrects imbalance with minimal adverse reactions.
Routinely reevaluate for therapeutic response/adverse reactions.	Replacement may lead to excess and alter neurotransmission, reduced muscle strength, or impaired cardiac contractility.
Maintain accurate IO. Calculate fluid balance.	Indicators of fluid balance are important because either fluid excess or deficit can occur.
Weigh as indicated.	Sensitive indicator of fluid shifts. Loss/retention of 1 liter of fluid equals a weight change of 2.2 lb.
Monitor vital signs and CVP.	Changes may be indicators of imbalance.
Assess skin turgor and mucous membrane moisture.	Water deficit is manifested by signs of dehydration.
Give oral fluids with caution. If fluids are restricted, set up a 24-hr schedule for fluid intake.	Fluid restrictions and extracellular shifts can cause drying of mucous membranes, and patient may desire more fluids than are prudent.
Encourage coughing/deep breathing exercises.	Pulmonary fluid shifts potentiate respiratory complications.

Nursing Diagnosis: Knowledge Deficit

RELATED TO: Lack of exposure/recall, information misinterpretation, unfamiliarity with resources.
AS EVIDENCED BY: Questions, statement of concern, inaccurate follow-through of instruction/development of preventable complications.

Desired Outcomes/Evaluation Criteria

Verbalizes understanding of condition/disease process and treatment. Initiates necessary lifestyle changes and participates in treatment regimen.

Nursing Actions	Rationale
Discuss preventive measures to be taken, including adequate dietary intake or measures to replace losses associated with prescription drug use as indicated.	Understanding of these actions can avoid recurrence.
Review proper dosage, safe administration of oral electrolyte preparations.	Helps patient to maintain correct therapy regimen.
Stress necessity of strict adherence to therapeutic regimen.	Helps to achieve optimal results.
Identify signs/symptoms to be reported to physician, e.g., unusual thirst, edema, changes in mentation or muscle activity.	Prompt evaluation and intervention may prevent serious complications.

I/O = intake/output; CVP = central venous pressure.

ASSESSMENT

- Obtain a thorough nursing history to develop the database. Be sure to include the history of the current illness and sources of fluid losses or shifts.
- Assess laboratory tests to determine the degree of electrolyte imbalance. Laboratory tests might include examination of serum, for electrolytes and serum osmolarity; urine, for pH, specific gravity, electrolytes, and osmolality; and arterial acid-base measurement. When assessing serum calcium levels, it is also important to assess protein levels and pH. Serum calcium levels decrease in alkalosis, as more calcium is bound to protein. The additional bicarbonate ion in alkalosis attaches to free calcium and prevents it from fulfilling its normal metabolic function. In acidosis there is more ionized calcium (more free calcium), and serum calcium levels increase.
- Assess all patients for electrolyte imbalances. The nurse must also assess general parameters on each patient, including daily weight, intake and urine output, urinary pH, number and quality of stools, bowel sounds, and vital signs.

  The nurse also must be aware of which patients are more susceptible to electrolyte imbalances. These patients include the patient with decreased oral intake from age or debilitation; one with increased fluid losses from nasogastric suction, diarrhea, vomiting, or fistula drainage; one who has an altered metabolism from fever, diabetic ketoacidosis, or adrenal malfunction; the patient receiving diuretics, corticosteroids, IV solutions, or other drugs that may affect electrolyte balance; and finally, the patient with edema. The nurse must assess such patients frequently to prevent major complications of electrolyte imbalances, especially because one imbalance rarely occurs in isolation, but precipitates others.

NURSING DIAGNOSIS

- Typical nursing diagnoses for a patient with disturbances of major body electrolytes include Risk for Fluid Volume Deficit and Knowledge Deficit (see Table 12–5).

PLANNING AND INTERVENTION

- Teach patients how to prevent further episodes of imbalance, particularly those patients who take medications such as diuretics and steroids, which may precipitate electrolyte imbalances. (Chapter 37 provides additional important information on diuretics, and Chapter 44 provides more information on steroids.) If potassium-depleting diuretics are administered, the patient should increase daily intake of foods that are high in potassium unless contraindicated (1 banana provides 15 mEq; 2 to 3 apricots provide 7 mEq; 7 small dried figs provide 20 mEq; ½ cup dried peaches provide 28 mEq; ½ cup orange juice provides 6 mEq; and 1 tablespoon instant coffee provides 6 mEq.)

Nursing Responsibilities

- Administer electrolytes solutions at the recommended rate into a large vein and dilute the electrolyte in the recommended amount of diluent to prevent irritation of vessels. The patient is monitored closely for signs of toxicity. As an example, when electrolytes are given to a patient with hypocalcemia, the patient is observed closely for signs of hypercalcemia.

Potassium Products

- Teach patient about foods that are high in potassium. Hypokalemia, when mild, can usually be reversed by adding foods that are high in potassium to the diet. Salt substitutes contain a substantial amount of potassium and other electrolytes. Excessive use can be dangerous for the patient who is taking potassium products. Instruct the patient not to use any substitute unless it is specifically ordered by the physician. Co-Salt and Neocurtasal both deliver 50 to 60 mEq of potassium and 0.5 mg of sodium per teaspoon, while Morton's Lite Salt delivers 35 mEq of potassium and 1100 mg of sodium per teaspoon. Patients also must be aware that many over-the-counter products contain potassium, such as antacids (e.g., Alka-Seltzer) and multiple vitamin preparations.

  Patients with moderate hypokalemia, 3.5 mEq/ liter or lower, such as those on diuretic therapy, may have oral products ordered. Oral replacements generally prevent the rapid rise of potassium levels that can be associated with IV therapy. If rapid correction is necessary as in diabetic ketoacidosis, or if the patient is unable to take potassium orally, IV potassium is administered. Potassium chloride solutions are preferred to other salts because, if there is an associated metabolic alkalosis, this salt may correct both the hypokalemia and the metabolic alkalosis.
- Mix all IV preparations thoroughly before administering and put a maximum of 40 mEq in each liter. If more is ordered by the physician, mix and run half at a time or place on an IV pump. Administer slowly (10 mEq/hr) through a large vein to prevent irritation to the vein or the development of hyperkalemia. Never give potassium IV push. Intake and output are monitored closely to assess renal function. If urinary output drops below ½ ml/kg per hour for 1 hour, the nurse reports it immediately to the physician. The potassium is discontinued until urinary output returns to normal. The nurse monitors the electrocardiogram frequently to assess for the dangerous effects of hyperkalemia that can be detected more rapidly on the ECG (see Fig. 12–2) than by measuring serum potassium levels.
- If the patient is to go home taking potassium products, he or she needs teaching, featured in Table 12–6, prior to discharge.

Calcium Products

- Teach the patient at risk for calcium deficiency to eat plenty of dairy products, sardines, and other foods

Table 12–6. PATIENT TEACHING FOR POTASSIUM PRODUCTS

Dear Patient:

   This drug has been ordered for you. This is what you should know about your drug to get the most from your therapy.

☐ 1. Potassium products have been ordered for you to increase and/or maintain your blood potassium level within normal range.

☐ 2. Your potassium product is taken until your imbalance is corrected. (Potassium products may also be taken with certain medications such as digitalis products and diuretics. In this case, take your potassium products as long as you take your digitalis and diuretics.)

☐ 3. Oral liquids, effervescent (fizz) tablets, or powders are best diluted in 3–4 oz or more of cold water or juice. Larger doses may be mixed with 6 oz. Potassium salts taste bitter and are, therefore, best taken with meals or after meals. Allow the effervescent tablets to stop fizzing and then sip over 5–10 minutes. Some potassium products are contained in a wax pill. The drug is taken up by the body, but the wax pill is found in the stool. This is OK. Potassium tablets should not be taken dry, crushed, or chewed. Whole tablets should be swallowed with a full glass of water or juice.

☐ 4. Potassium products are not taken together with potassium-rich foods, which include bananas, orange juice, dried figs, peaches, and instant coffee. Also, the use of salt substitutes made from potassium salts (Diasal or CoSalt) should be limited, as a high potassium may result.

☐ 5. If you forget your potassium product through the next dose, do not take it. Do not try to catch up.

☐ 6. Do not suddenly stop your potassium product without checking with your doctor.

☐ 7. If the taste of a liquid product makes you want to stop taking the drug, check with your doctor. He or she can order a different potassium product, which may taste better.

☐ 8. If the following side effects occur, contact your doctor: nausea, vomiting, stomach upset, and muscle weakness.

☐ 9. Be alert for the following set of symptoms, which may indicate a high potassium level. If these occur, tell your doctor: cramps, diarrhea, irritability, nausea, weakness, and muscle cramps.

☐ 10. Store your medication in a tight, moisture-resistant container.

the skin. During IV administration, also monitor the ECG to detect QT interval lengthening that may proceed to more serious cardiac dysrhythmias like torsades de pointes and flattening of T-wave changes, which may indicate hypercalcemia.

• Assess the patient for both Chvostek's and Trousseau's signs, which indicate the development of hypocalcemia and tetany (see Fig. 12–3).

• Draw blood levels about 2 hours after finishing the infusion to assess serum calcium after calcium infusions. The body needs time to distribute the infused calcium.

• Administer calcium products carefully to the patient receiving digitalis glycosides as these may have an additive effect. In patients who are extremely cardiotoxic and have hyperkalemia, 5 to 10 mL of calcium gluconate 10% may be administered IV over a 3 to 5 minute period; this dose may be repeated once. During this therapy, the electrocardiogram is monitored constantly.

Magnesium Products

• Teach patients to increase their intake of meats, fish, dairy products, whole grains, green leafy vegetables, and other magnesium-rich foods to correct mild magnesium deficits. Dietary intake can be supplemented with magnesium-based antacids like Mylanta, Gelusil, or Maalox. Oral magnesium products are best ad-

Table 12–7. PATIENT TEACHING FOR CALCIUM PRODUCTS

Dear Patient:

   This drug has been ordered for you. This is what you should know about your drug to get the most from your therapy.

☐ 1. Calcium products have been ordered by your doctor to increase and/or maintain your blood calcium level within normal range.

☐ 2. You will take calcium products until your imbalance is corrected.

☐ 3. To increase gastrointestinal absorption, increase your intake of phosphate with either milk or dairy products and also limit the intake of foods such as spinach, rhubarb, bran, and whole cereals because of their ability to block calcium absorption.

☐ 4. Oral calcium (calcium gluconate and carbonate) is best taken with or following meals with water; calcium lactate is best taken with meals.

☐ 5. Calcium products are not taken together with tetracycline antibiotics. Additional interactions may occur. Please check with your doctor or pharmacist before taking other drugs.

☐ 6. If you forget your drug until the next dose, skip that dose. Do not try to catch up.

☐ 7. Do not stop taking your calcium products without checking with your doctor.

☐ 8. Side effects of calcium products include constipation, decreased appetite, muscle weakness, and some mental confusion. If these signs or symptoms are present, please contact your doctor.

☐ 9. If told by your doctor to increase your dietary intake of calcium, foods high in calcium include milk and dairy products, green leafy vegetables, and certain seafoods such as oysters, sardines, and clams.

☐ 10. Store your drug in a tight, moisture-resistant container.

rich in calcium and vitamin D to prevent hypocalcemia. Mild hypocalcemia can generally be relieved by dietary management. Tell the patient to restrict his or her intake of phosphorus—phosphorus competes with calcium for intestinal absorption. Additional teaching information for the patient requiring calcium products is provided in Table 12–7.

• Administer oral calcium products with or following meals with water. Oral calcium lactate is best administered with meals.

• The patient with moderate hypocalcemia receives calcium gluconate (9% calcium; 1 ampule raises the serum calcium level by 1 mEq) or calcium chloride (27% calcium; 1 ampule raises the serum calcium level by 10 mEq) IV at a rate not to exceed 1 mL/min of a 0.5% solution.

   Carefully monitor the IV to avoid its infiltration, which causes great irritation and possible necrosis of ministered in the morning in a full glass of ice water or juice to help disguise their bitter taste.

- Patients who have severe symptoms of hypomagnesemia are treated with IV magnesium sulfate given over 1 to 3 hours followed by continuous IV infusion. When administering magnesium sulfate intravenously, calcium gluconate is available to reverse the symptoms of potential magnesium toxicity. When the patient is receiving a maintenance dose (between 8 and 24 mEq/day), monitor serum levels daily. Also monitor blood pressure and respiratory rate, which may be depressed as a result of therapy.
- When magnesium levels are low, keep the patient supine to prevent hypotension; give soft foods to assist with chewing and swallowing as laryngeal and esophageal spasm may be present; and handle the extremities gently as muscle spasm may be present.
- Monitor for signs of hypermagnesemia (weakness, hypotension, flushed and hot skin), which occur when serum levels reach 3 to 5 mEq/liter; or abnormally weak deep-tendon reflexes, slurred speech, drowsiness, and dysrhythmias, which occur when serum levels reach 5 to 7 mEq/liter; or flaccid muscle paralysis, respiratory depression, and cardiac arrest, which occur when serum levels reach 10 mEq/L. The conditions that precipitate hypermagnesemia include chronic renal failure and, less commonly, adrenal insufficiency and overdosing on magnesium products.

EVALUATION

- Evaluate the effectiveness of the treatment. The evaluation of electrolyte disturbances is based on a list of outcome evaluation criteria that has been developed in relation to the goals determined through discussion among the nurse, patient, and family.
- Evaluate the patient for signs and symptoms of the imbalance and then observe for signs of improvement. Electrolyte imbalance can be mild or very severe. When the patient is acutely ill and in the hospital, the imbalance is corrected with IV therapy. If frequent monitoring is not done, the patient with an electrolyte deficit may show early signs of an electrolyte excess. Frequent laboratory studies do not prevent the condition; they calculate the degree of abnormality so the nurse can intervene to correct it.
- Teach the patient about the hazards of both overcompliance and noncompliance. Occasionally, patients develop an imbalance because they self-administer excessive amounts of sodium bicarbonate (baking soda) as an antacid. Sodium bicarbonate tends to produce a rebound acidity, which then prompts the patient to take another dose. This treatment eventually leads to sodium and bicarbonate excess and electrolyte imbalance. Noncompliance can also create a problem if the patient chooses not to follow the prescribed medication or diet regimen.
- When the patient is being prepared for discharge, review and update all previously taught material to ensure that the patient's knowledge base remains accurate. Also encourage the patient to keep all future physician visits.

The bibliography for this chapter can be found in Appendix B, which begins on page 1054.

CHAPTER REVIEW QUESTIONS*

1. Administration of potassium is contraindicated for patients taking the following medication:
   a. Aspirin.
   b. Spironolactone.
   c. Lithium.
   d. Tetracycline.

2. Which of the following is a correct nursing intervention associated with administration of sodium polystyrene sulfonate (Kayexalate)?
   a. Observe the patient for hyponatremia.
   b. Allow suspension to separate; do not stir.
   c. Urge patient to retain rectally for 30 to 60 minutes.
   d. Mix powder with an oil-base solution.

3. When administering intravenous or oral calcium products, the nurse monitors the patient for hypercalcemia, a sign of which is:
   a. Tetany.
   b. Trousseau's sign.

   c. Chvostek's sign.
   d. Lethargy.

4. Patients taking oral calcium should be taught to:
   a. Decrease intake of phosphate-containing foods.
   b. Take calcium chloride with meals.
   c. Avoid taking calcium with tetracycline antibiotics.
   d. Increase intake of spinach, rhubarb, and bran.

5. A patient with an electrolyte imbalance demonstrates a high peaked T wave on the ECG. Which electrolyte imbalance does this sign indicate?
   a. Hyperkalemia.
   b. Hyponatremia.
   c. Hypophosphatemia.
   d. Hypermagnesemia.

*See Appendix A, which begins on page 1051, for answers.

CHAPTER 13

Vitamins, Minerals, and Iron Products

Merrily A. Kuhn, RNC, PhD

CHAPTER OUTLINE

KEY TERMS

Chelating agent
Cones
Intrinsic factor
Kwashiorkor
Megaloblastic
Mineral

Provitamin
Refractory rickets
Rods
Tetany
Vitamin

LEARNING OBJECTIVES

After reading this chapter, the student will be able to:

1. Identify commonly used vitamins, minerals, and hematinics.
2. Differentiate among the various vitamins, minerals, and hematinics as to their function, source, deficiency state, toxic effects, route of administration, pharmacokinetics, contraindications and precautions, and interactions.
3. Identify specific areas to assess in the patient requiring vitamins, minerals, and hematinics to formulate appropriate patient outcomes.
4. Plan the nursing interventions necessary to administer vitamins, minerals, and hematinics and choose appropriate teaching strategies to gain patient compliance.
5. Evaluate the patient at various stages of treatment to gauge nursing interventions.

To maintain normal metabolic function, the human body needs a daily intake of both vitamins and minerals. It is estimated that 40% to 50% of adults in the United States take vitamin and mineral supplements. A *vitamin* is a biologically active, organic compound essential for human health and growth (its absence causing a deficiency disease or disorder). Vitamins are carried in small concentrations via the circulatory system and act on target organs or tissues. Thirteen vitamins have been identified as essential. A *mineral* is any naturally occurring nonorganic homogenous solid substance essential for human health and growth (its absence causing a deficiency disease or disorder), neither synthesized nor produced within the body, but available in the diet. Fifteen minerals are car-

ried in small amounts via the circulatory system and act on target organs or tissues.

VITAMINS

Vitamins are either fat soluble (vitamins A, D, E, and K) or water soluble (the B-complex vitamins—B_1, B_2, B_6, B_{12}, folic acid, pantothenic acid, niacin, and biotin—and vitamin C). Vitamins are essential for a healthy, normal life. Because some vitamins are not stored in the body in sufficient quantities and only a few vitamins are synthesized in the body, most vitamins must be consumed daily. Vitamin K and biotin are synthesized from bacteria in the small intestine, and vitamin D is produced by the skin in an inactive form on exposure to ultraviolet light.

In general, the body needs only small quantities of vitamins, which can easily be obtained from plant sources in a well-balanced diet. The sale of vitamins in the United States is a $4 billion business. Because of successful advertising, many individuals unnecessarily take supplemental vitamins, thinking that they improve normal health. However, vitamins are frequently misused and, if taken in large doses, may cause disease or vitamin toxicity. Toxic states can result from too much vitamin intake—generally vitamins A and D, and limited toxicity for E, K, niacin, C, and B$_6$. Education of the patient is important to prevent toxic vitaminosis.

It is important to understand the difference between the prophylactic use of vitamin supplements to prevent a deficiency and the therapeutic use of vitamins to treat a deficiency. Vitamin supplements are useful during periods of increased demand, as listed in Table 13–1. It is unusual for pronounced deficiencies such as pellegra, rickets, scurvy, and beriberi—found in underdeveloped or developing countries—to occur.

The United States Food and Drug Administration issues official United States Recommended Daily Allowances (U.S. RDAs), which represent the minimum daily dietary requirement needed to prevent the development of deficiency symptoms and to provide a standard for good nutrition. U.S. RDAs serve as a legal standard for labeling over-the-counter (OTC) vitamin supplements and foods. The U.S. RDAs are derived from the Recommended Dietary Allowances (RDAs) list, which is published and periodically revised by the Food and Nutrition Board of the National Academy of Sciences. The values in the RDA list indicate the quantity of nutrients needed to keep most people healthy. The reference male or female used in developing the RDAs is the average adult between 23 and 50 years old. These values should prevent deficiencies in 97% of the population. See a nutrition text for the RDA list of both vitamins and minerals.

Vitamin requirements and dosages are measured in several ways. Vitamins A, D, and E are measured in either USP units or international units (IU); biotin and vitamin B$_{12}$ are measured in micrograms (μg or mcg); and the remaining vitamins are measured in milligrams (mg). Allowances for Vitamins A, D, and E, and niacin may also be listed in other units of measurement. These are discussed in the individual sections for each vitamin.

FAT-SOLUBLE VITAMINS

The four fat-soluble vitamins—vitamins A, D, E, and K—require fat or bile salts for absorption. A patient with a biliary obstruction, which prevents bile from entering the duodenum, has difficulty absorbing these vitamins. Fat-soluble vitamins are stored in large quantities in both the liver and fatty tissues and are metabolized and excreted slowly. For this reason, a person develops deficiency states from lack of fat-soluble vitamins only after a long period of deprivation. Conversely, excessive intake of the fat-soluble vitamins, especially vitamins A and D, can lead to toxicity. Fat-soluble vitamins are featured in Table 13–2.

Interactions A patient taking mineral oil as a laxative on a regular basis or taking cholestyramine or colestipol, will have decreased absorption of all the fat soluble vitamins.

Vitamin A

Vitamin A (Aquasol A, Del-Vi-A, others), is referred to as retinol, A$_1$, A$_2$, or the anti-infective vitamin. Vitamin A is derived from animal sources, including butter, eggs, whole milk, and liver, which provide retinol; plant sources, including carrots, green leafy vegetables, squash, sweet potatoes, and pumpkins. Plant sources provide the provitamin A carotenoids—especially beta carotene—which are converted to retinol by cells of the intestinal mucosa. A *provitamin* is an inactive substance that is converted by the body to an active vitamin. Vitamin A is essential for growth in children and adolescents and is needed particularly for development and maintenance of epithelial tissues and bone. Vitamin A is needed to produce visual purple and to maintain function of both *rods* (cells in the retina responsible for vision in dim light) and *cones* (cells in the retina that receive color stimuli) in the eye. If vitamin A is lacking, night blindness ensues. Vitamin A is also needed to maintain the integrity of the skin and epithelial cells, helping to promote resistance to infection. In addition, vitamin A is necessary in the maintenance of the adrenal cortex and the synthesis of steroid hormones.

Uses Vitamin A is indicated only for treatment or prevention of vitamin A deficiency. It is also prescribed to treat or prevent hyperkeratotic dermatoses, including psoriasis, lichen planus, ichthyosis, and pityriasis rubra pilaris, even though vitamin A has not been proven effective for treatment of many of these conditions. Vitamin A cream, tretinoin or retinoic acid (Retin-A), and isotretinoin (Accutane), are available to treat acne vulgaris and wrinkling and are described in detail in Chapter 65.

Absorption and Storage When carotenoid pigments, especially beta carotene, are consumed by the human body, only about one-sixth to one-third are converted to vitamin A. Vitamin A is an unsaturated fat-soluble alcohol, which requires bile salts, pancreatic lipase, and dietary fat to be effectively absorbed. Current research also suggests that adequate amounts of zinc are necessary for mobilization of vitamin A. Orally ingested vitamin A is

---

Table 13–1. CONDITIONS FOR WHICH VITAMIN SUPPLEMENTS ARE APPROPRIATE

Adults	Children
Pregnancy	Acute/chronic illness
Lactation	Rapid growth phase
Acute/chronic illness	Malabsorption
Malabsorption	Regular, strenuous physical activity
Regular, strenuous physical activity	Neglect of diet
Neglect of diet	Breast-fed infants
Drug ingestion that increases vitamin requirements	Premature infants
	Vegetarian children
	Children receiving nonfortified skim milk

absorbed in the upper gastrointestinal tract, especially in the duodenum. This is also the primary site of conversion of carotene to vitamin A. Absorbed vitamin A is transported by the lymphatic system to the bloodstream where it is bound to retinal-binding protein (RBP) and transported to the liver for storage. A major portion of vitamin A is excreted in bile with a small amount excreted in the urine.

Toxic Effects   Vitamin A toxicity may occur in a few months in an infant or child, but may take years to manifest in an adult. The half-life of vitamin A is very long, weeks to months. Toxic side effects include increased in-

Table 13–2. FAT-SOLUBLE VITAMINS

VITAMIN/ROUTE AND DOSAGE	CAUSES AND SYMPTOMS OF DEFICIENCY	NURSING IMPLICATIONS
vitamin a (Aquasol, Del-Vi-A)		
severe deficiency with xerophthalmia ***Adults and Children over 8 yr:*** 500,000 IU/day PO for 3 days followed by 50,000 IU/day for 2 wk. Follow-up therapy: 10,000–20,000 IU/day for 2 mo. **severe deficiency** ***Adults:*** 100,000 IU IM for 3 days and 50,000 IU/day for 2 wk. ***Children 1–8 yr:*** 17,500–35,000 IU/day IM for 10 days. ***Infants:*** 7500–15,000 IU/day IM for 10 days.	**Causes:** interference with absorption or storage. Inadequate intake or conversion to vitamin A. Rapid loss of vitamin A **Symptoms:** night blindness (nyctalopia), hyperkeratosis (corneal softening), xerophthalmia (inflammation of the eye), dry skin, keratinized increased skin infection, diarrhea, kidney stones, slowed growth/development in children	**ASSESSMENT:** Assess for vitamin A deficiency. Assess for vitamin A intake in food and other multivitamins. Assess for pregnancy (category A). **INTERVENTION:** Vitamin A is never administered intravenous push because of possibility of anaphylaxis or anaphylactoid reactions. IV vitamin A is mixed in a large volume of fluid. Do not exceed RDA during pregnancy. **Patient Teaching**—Teach patient to avoid mineral oil, to protect vitamin A from light and heat, and to not megadose vitamin A. **EVALUATION:** Evaluate for signs of vitamin A toxicity and report to physician.
vitamin d₂ (ergocalciferol [Calciferol, Drisdol, Deltalin]) **vitamin d₃** (cholecalciferol [Delta-D]) **vitamin d metabolite** (calcifediol [Calderol]) **synthetic active form of vitamin d₃** (calcitriol [Rocaltrol, Calcijex]) **vitamin d analogue** (dihydrotachysterol [DHT, Hytakerol])		
ergocalciferol **vitamin d–resistant rickets** ***Adults:*** 50,000–500,000 IU/day PO. **hypoparathyroidism** ***Adults:*** 50,000–200,000 IU/day PO and 500 mg of elemental calcium administered 6 times/day PO. **vitamin d deficiency** ***Adults:*** 1000–2000 IU/day PO initially, then 400 IU/day maintenance. **familial hypophosphatemia** ***Adults:*** 10,000–80,000 IU/day PO plus 1–2 g/day elemental phosphorus. **cholecalciferol** **vitamin d deficiency** ***Adults:*** 400–1000 IU/day PO. **calcifediol** **chronic renal failure** ***Adults:*** 300–350 μg PO weekly administered on a daily or alternating day schedule. Dose may be increased at 4-wk intervals. **calcitriol** **chronic renal failure** ***Adults:*** 0.25–1 μg/day PO. **dihydrotachysterol tetany and hypoparathyroidism** ***Adults:*** 0.2–2.4 mg/day PO.	**Causes:** malabsorption, hypoparathyroidism **Symptoms:** rickets in children, osteomalacia in adults	**ASSESSMENT:** Assess for vitamin D deficiency. Assess for intake of vitamin D in foods and other multivitamins. Assess serum and urine calcium, albumin, serum phosphorous, magnesium, and BUN before and periodically during therapy. Assess urine for presence of casts and red blood cells in urine q 2 wk at least. Assess for pregnancy (category C). **INTERVENTION:** Margin of safety is very narrow, so very close monitoring is performed. Administer IV vitamin D in large volume of IV fluid only. **Patient Teaching**—teach patient to increase vitamin D foods in the diet, to take vitamin with food to avoid GI upset, and to swallow tablets or capsules whole (i.e., do not crush or chew). **EVALUATION:** Evaluate for toxic signs (dry mouth, nausea, vomiting, metallic taste in mouth, diarrhea, constipation) and report to physician.

Continued on the following page

Table 13–2. FAT-SOLUBLE VITAMINS, *Continued*

VITAMIN/ROUTE AND DOSAGE	CAUSES AND SYMPTOMS OF DEFICIENCY	NURSING IMPLICATIONS
vitamin e (Aquasol E, Alfacol E, others)		
Prevention of Deficiency *Adults:* 30 IU/day PO. *Premature or Low-Birth-Weight Neonates:* 5 IU/day PO. *Treatment of Deficiency Adults:* 60–75 IU/day PO. *Children:* 1 unit/kg per day PO.	**Causes:** malabsorption, abuse of oil-type laxatives. **Symptoms:** skin collagenosis, red cell hemolysis, xanthomatosis, cirrhosis, steatorrhea, creatinuria, possible inability to carry fetus to term	**ASSESSMENT:** Assess for signs of vitamin E deficiency. Assess for dietary intake of vitamin E. Assess for pregnancy (category A). **INTERVENTION:** Not for IV administration. The contents of capsules may be squeezed out and applied to the skin. **Patient Teaching**—Advise patient to swallow tablets or capsules whole (i.e., do not crush or chew); to store product in cool, dry place; and to not take megadoses of vitamin E. **EVALUATION:** Evaluate for signs of toxicity such as fatigue, weakness, nausea, or diarrhea, and report to physician.
vitamin K₁ (phytonadione [AquaMEPHYTON, Konakion, Mephyton]) **vitamin K₃** (menadiol sodium [Synkayvite])		
menadiol sodium **hypoprothrombinemia secondary to vitamin k malabsorption** *Adults:* 5–15 mg IM or SC once or twice daily or 5 mg/day PO. *Children:* 5–10 mg/day IM, SC, or PO. **phytonadione treatment of hypoprothrombinemia** *Adults:* 2.5–25 mg (up to 50 mg) PO, SC, IM, repeated if necessary 12–48 hr after oral dose or 6–8 hr after parenteral dose. **anticoagulant-induced prothrombinemia deficiency** *Adults:* 2.5–10 mg IM, SC or up to 25 mg (rarely, 50 mg). **hypoprothrombinemia from other causes (antibiotics, salicylates, or other drugs)** *Adults:* 2.5–25 mg (rarely 50 mg). **prevention of hypoprothrombinemia during tpn** *Adults:* 5–10 mg/wk IM. *Children:* 2.5 mg/wk IM. **prevention of hemorrhagic disease of the newborn** *Neonates:* 0.5–1 mg IM within 1 hr of birth, repeated in 6–8 hr, if needed (e.g., if mother received oral anticoagulants or long-term anticonvulsant therapy during pregnancy). **IV administration is not recommended,** but Aqua-MEPHYTON can be given IV in an emergency at a rate not to exceed 1 mg/min. Protect from light.	**Causes:** malabsorption, long-term use of parenteral nutrition without replacement, prolonged antibiotic therapy, chronic liver disease **Symptoms:** hypoprothrombinemia, increased bleeding and hemorrhage, increased clotting time. Hemorrhagic disease of the newborn	**ASSESSMENT:** Assess for signs of vitamin K deficiency. Assess for dietary intake of vitamin K. Assess PT before and during therapy. Improvement of PT takes 1–2 hr after IM, or 6–12 hr after PO administration. Cessation of bleeding occurs within 3–6 hr. Assess bilirubin in neonates receiving vitamin K. Assess for pregnancy (category C). **INTERVENTION:** Take PO vitamin K with food to reduce GI upset and promote absorption. Patients with biliary deficiencies may require oral bile salts to promote absorption of vitamin K. Assess for concurrent salicylates, oral antibiotics, quinidine, quinine, and sulfonamides as they may either inhibit or interfere with vitamin K activity. Follow mixing and administration instructions. **Patient Teaching**—Teach patient about increased dietary vitamin K. **EVALUATION:** Evaluate for continued signs of hypoprothrombinemia such as continued bleeding, oozing around IV catheters, petechiae, easy bruising. IV vitamin K can cause severe reactions including anaphylaxis, shock, and cardiac and respiratory arrest. Evaluate frequently.

BUN = blood urea nitrogen.

tracranial pressure, which can occur within 8 to 12 hours of overdose, diplopia, papilledema, skin changes (cutaneous desquamation follows within a few days), psychiatric symptoms, hepatic dysfunction (a cirrhotic-like syndrome), alopecia, and brittle nails. Fatigue, malaise, lethargy, anorexia, irritability, yellowing of the skin, and severe headaches also occur. Most symptoms disappear when the vitamin is discontinued, but permanent retardation of growth and premature epiphyseal closure may occur in children.

Patients are taught to report signs of overdose—nausea, vomiting, anorexia, drying/cracking skin/legs, loss of hair, and a bulging fontanelle in infants—to their physician.

Contraindications and Precautions Vitamin A is contraindicated in hypersensitivity. Oral administration of vitamin A is contraindicated in patients with malabsorption syndrome; if malabsorption is the result of inadequate bile secretion, the oral route may be used with concurrent administration of bile salts. Fetal abnormalities, growth retardation, and early epiphyseal closure have been reported in children whose mothers took excessive amounts (above 6000 IU) during pregnancy. Caution is recommended in nursing mothers, as vitamin A is excreted in breast milk; and in children, who are more sensitive to high doses of vitamin A. Use with caution in patients with impaired renal function, as vitamin A toxicity and elevated plasma calcium and alkaline phosphatase can occur.

Interactions Contraceptives may increase the plasma level of vitamin A.

Dosage Prescription forms of vitamin A, which are measured in USP units or IU, are available as capsules, tablets, oral solutions, and injections. OTC vitamin supplements are measured in IU or μg RE (retinol equivalents) where 1 RE equals 1 μg retinol or 6 μg beta carotene. Many vitamin A preparations are made from fish oils such as cod-liver oil, halibut-liver oil, or a combination of fish oils. Vitamin A is often combined with vitamin D, in both oral and topical forms.

Vitamin D

Vitamin D, a sterol compound, is a natural vitamin derived from fish liver oils or other provitamins. Other dietary sources include animal livers, egg yolks, butter, and oily fish. Two forms of vitamin D, calciferol or ergocalciferol (D_2) and cholecalciferol (D_3), are essential (along with parathyroid hormone) in regulating the absorption and excretion, in the gut and kidney, of calcium, phosphate, and magnesium. Vitamin D increases the intestinal absorption of calcium and, probably by directly influencing bone mineralization, also increases the rate of reabsorption of phosphate by the renal tubules. Because calcium and phosphate are inversely controlled by the body, vitamin D indirectly affects phosphate absorption and mobilization in the bone as well. Vitamin D may also reduce the risk of colon and breast cancer.

Absorption and Storage Vitamin D accumulates in the skin as the inactive form, 7-dehydrocholesterol. Upon exposure to sunlight, cholecalciferol (D_3) is produced and is transported to the liver to be hydroxylated to calcifediol (25 OHD$_3$). This product is converted into its active form (1,25-dihydroxycholecalciferol) in the kidney and is released into the bloodstream. It has a half-life of days to weeks in the normal adult. Because Vitamin D production depends on exposure to sunlight, people living in the northernmost latitudes, where daylight is shortest, are at a particular risk for Vitamin D deficiency.

Once vitamin D is consumed, absorption depends on the presence of bile and fats in the intestine and takes place in the jejunum and ileum in the presence of bile.

Uses Vitamin D is used to treat hypocalcemia, hypophosphatemia, and osteomalacia. It is also used to prevent and treat rickets, tetany, and vitamin D deficiency and to manage metabolic bone disease or hypocalcemia in patients on chronic renal dialysis.

Of the several forms of vitamin D that are available, **cholecalciferol (*D₃*, *Delta-D*)** is used as a daily vitamin D supplement or to treat vitamin D deficiency; **calcifediol (*Calderol*)** is used primarily to manage metabolic bone disease or hypocalcemia in patients with chronic renal disease; **ergocalciferol (*D₂*, *Drisdol*, *Calciferol*)** is used to treat familial hypophosphatemia or *refractory rickets* (rickets caused by a defect in renal tubular function); **calcitriol (*Rocaltrol*)** is used to manage hypocalcemia in patients with chronic renal failure; and **dihydrotachysterol (*DHT*, *Hytakerol*)** is used to treat *tetany* (syndrome characterized by intermittent painful tonic spasms of the extremities), in either acute or chronic forms, and hypoparathyroidism.

Toxic Effects As with other medications, when large doses of vitamin D (1000 to 3000 IU for a few weeks to months) are administered, toxic symptoms can occur. As toxicity develops, the patient may have symptoms resembling hyperparathyroidism (anorexia, nausea and vomiting, headache, drowsiness, diarrhea or constipation, polyuria, polydipsia, generalized weakness, stiffness, vague aches, and mild weight loss). Serum calcium and phosphate levels are increased, and correspondingly high concentrations of both are found in the urine, leading eventually to irreversible renal damage. Osteoporosis occurs with the simultaneous deposition of calcium in the heart, large blood vessels, lungs, renal tubules, and other soft tissues. Discontinuation of vitamin D is usually sufficient to control the symptoms.

Contraindications and Precautions Vitamin D is contraindicated in patients with hypersensitivity to the drug, hypercalcemia, or hyperphosphatemia. It is used cautiously in pregnant women, as it may suppress parathyroid function in the fetus, and in patients receiving digitalis glycosides, as hypercalcemia may precipitate dysrhythmias. Safety in children, above RDA requirements, has not been established.

Interactions Hydantoins and barbiturates may reduce the effectiveness of vitamin D. And, vitamin D may potentiate digitalis glycosides. Vitamin D may antagonize calcium channel blockers by increasing calcium levels.

Dosage Dosage is highly individualized and depends on the condition being treated. As soon as symptoms are relieved, vitamin D dosage is reduced to the RDA, as hypercalcemia and renal damage may result at higher levels. The FDA is attempting to place all vitamin D supplements containing over 400 IU/dosage unit on a prescription-only status. In some OTC products, vitamin D is measured in micrograms (μg) of cholecalciferol, where 10 μg cholicalciferol equals 400 IU vitamin D.

Vitamin E

Vitamin E actually refers to a group of naturally occurring fat-soluble substances known as tocopherols (alpha, beta, gamma, and delta). Alpha-tocopherol is the most physiologically active and abundant form of the group. Dietary sources include oils, margarine, mayonnaise, wheat germ, grains, seeds, nuts, fruits, vegetables, and eggs. Vitamin E, along with the mineral selenium, functions as a tissue antioxidant that protects polyunsaturated fatty acids from oxidative deterioration. It also appears to influence heme and porphyrin synthesis and, indirectly, the synthesis of several heme proteins and retards the hemolysis of red blood cells. Other functions of vitamin E include the enhancement of vitamin A utilization, stimulation of essential cofactors produced in steroid metabolism, maintenance of normal muscle metabolism, and inhibition of prostaglandin production. Vitamin E is believed to be needed for fertility and gestation.

Uses Vitamin E is indicated for prevention and treatment of vitamin E deficiency. It is also necessary in patients receiving total parenteral nutrition or who are undergoing rapid weight loss. Vitamin E has been found to be therapeutically useful in actual dietary deficiencies and in certain anemias (e.g., macrocytic and megaloblastic anemia often associated with the protein and calorie malnutrition of *kwashiorkor*). It can also be used topically to moisten dry and chapped skin and to relieve temporary skin irritation. Although many claims have been made, vitamin E has not been proven effective to treat inflammatory skin disorders, loss of hair, habitual abortion, heart disease, impotence, bursitis, liver spots, deterioration from aging, or to increase physical endurance or sexual ability.

Absorption and Storage Vitamin E is absorbed passively but relatively inefficiently from the gastrointestinal tract in the presence of bile, and incorporated into chylomicrons for lymphatic transfer. Vitamin E accumulates slowly in the muscle, liver, and fatty tissue, but can be stored for long periods of time, up to 4 years. If vitamin E is not stored, it has a half-life of about 2 weeks in the body and is primarily excreted in the bile and feces.

Toxic Effects Vitamin E appears to be relatively nontoxic at therapeutic doses. When excessive doses are administered for prolonged periods, the patient may develop skeletal muscle weakness, fatigue, disturbances in the reproductive system, and gastrointestinal upset. Symptoms generally subside within a few weeks after excessive doses are discontinued.

Interactions If administered concurrently, vitamin E may increase the hyperprothrombinemic effect of oral anticoagulants.

Dosage Several products are available, and dosage information is provided in Table 13–2. When vitamin E deficiencies are present, water-miscible oral products are preferred. The several forms of vitamin E (with varying potencies) are all standardized into international units (IU), as in the following examples:

> 1 mg dl-alpha tocopheryl acetate = 1 IU
> 1 mg dl-alpha tocopherol = 1.1 IU
> 1 mg d-alpha tocopheryl acetate = 1.36 IU
> 1 mg d-alpha tocopherol = 1.49 IU
> 1 mg d-alpha tocopheryl acid succinate = 1.21 IU
> 1 mg dl-alpha tocopheryl acid succinate = 0.89 IU

Some OTC products use alpha-tocopherol equivalents (α-TE) to measure vitamin E, where 1 α-TE equals 1 mg of d-α tocopherol (or 1.49 IU).

Free tocopherols are easily oxidized and destroyed when exposed to air and light. However, the ester acetate and succinate forms are more stable.

Vitamin K

Vitamin K was discovered accidentally in 1935 while researchers were studying newly hatched chicks with a fatal hemorrhagic condition and was identified as a compound needed for clotting factor synthesis. Vitamin K occurs naturally in two forms K_1 *(phytonadione)* and K_2, and synthetically as **vitamin K_3 (menadione)**. Dietary sources include most foods, green leafy vegetables, cauliflower, pork, spinach, organ meats, kidney, dairy products, seeds, and nuts. In most humans, intestinal bacteria can synthesize adequate amounts to meet daily requirements.

Orally ingested or bacteria-derived vitamin K is absorbed by the intestinal wall in the presence of bile and pancreatic juice. Because 50% of vitamin K is synthesized by bacterial flora of the intestine, when the patient is allowed nothing by mouth and is on antibiotics, vitamin K synthesis may cease. Vitamin K is needed by the body to synthesize prothrombin, and factors II, IX, X, and VII in the liver, although the exact mechanism of its action still remains unknown.

Uses Vitamin K is used to treat hypoprothrombinemia due to vitamin K deficiency. It can also be used when a deficiency has occurred secondary to the administration of one or more of the other fat-soluble vitamins in excessive doses. Newborn infants, especially those that are premature, have a low level of vitamin K–dependent clotting factors that decreases for a few days after birth. To prevent the occurrence, small doses of vitamin K are administered at birth.

Vitamin K is also effective in patients with bleeding disorders due to a low prothrombin level or bleeding disorders secondary to large doses or overdoses of salicylates, quinine, sulfonamides, arsenicals, or barbiturates. It is also the antidote for the oral anticoagulants, such as warfarin.

Absorption and Storage Vitamin K is unique because it is the only vitamin that is supplied almost totally by resident bacteria in the intestine. Like the other fat-soluble vitamins, vitamin K is passively absorbed (with carrier mediation—bile salts), incorporated into chylomicrons, and transferred to lymph and blood. It is stored in the liver for only a short time.

Toxic Effects Toxic effects include gastric upset, mild allergic reactions, and headache. When large doses are administered to a patient with liver disease, liver function may be depressed. When excessive amounts of vitamin K are administered to infants, particularly premature infants, hyperbilirubinemia, kernicterus, brain damage, and even death have occurred.

▼ CLINICAL ALERT

IV use of phytonadione may cause severe reactions, including death, during and immediately after IV injection. These reactions, which resemble anaphylaxis, include shock and cardiac and/or respiratory arrest.

Contraindications and Precautions   Vitamin K is contraindicated in patients hypersensitive to its components and in pregnant women, particularly during the last few weeks of pregnancy, or during labor, as hemorrhagic diseases of the newborn may occur. Although vitamin K crosses the placenta, teratogenic or other adverse effects on the fetus are unknown. Vitamin K is excreted in breast milk, so vitamin K is administered cautiously to nursing women. It is also administered cautiously to patients with impaired liver function. Generally, the hypoprothrombinemia caused by hepatocellular damage is not corrected with administration of vitamin K and, paradoxically, may even be worsened.

Interactions   Vitamin K antagonizes oral anticoagulants to the extent that the patient cannot become anticoagulated again for about a week.

Dosage   Several forms of vitamin K are available. Dosage information can be found in Table 13–2.

WATER-SOLUBLE VITAMINS

The water-soluble vitamins include the B-complex vitamins—vitamin B_1 (thiamine), vitamin B_2 (riboflavin), vitamin B_6 (pyridoxine), vitamin B_{12} (cyanocobalamin, hydroxocobalamin), folic acid (B_9), pantothenic acid (B_5, calcium pantothenate), niacin (B_3, nicotinic acid), and biotin—and vitamin C (ascorbic acid). Water-soluble vitamins are dissimilar in structure, but similar in action, to the fat-soluble vitamins. They all have a coenzyme action. This means that the vitamins function mainly as substances that activate the protein portion of enzymes. Vitamins assist in catalyzing the reactions of protein, fat, and carbohydrate metabolism. A very small quantity of vitamin as coenzyme is capable of catalyzing a great deal of biochemical activity. The water-soluble vitamins are not stored in the body in large quantities, so short periods of inadequate intake can result in deficiency states. Because these vitamins are not stored in the body, overdoses are not as much a problem as with the fat-soluble vitamins. Water-soluble vitamins are featured in Table 13–3.

Vitamin B_1

Vitamin B_1, or thiamine *(Thiamilate)*, functions as a coenzyme in pyruvate metabolism, which is necessary for carbohydrate metabolism, nerve conduction, energy production, and aerobic metabolism. Dietary sources include wheat germ, cereal, grains, nuts, yeast, meat, peas, and vegetables. Vitamin B_1 requirements are increased in untreated hyperthyroidism, heavy manual labor, malabsorptive syndromes, prolonged diarrhea, biliary disease, alcoholism, pregnancy, and when the carbohydrate content of the diet is high. A total absence of vitamin B_1 in the diet produces symptoms of deficiency in about 3 weeks.

Uses   Thiamine is indicated only in the treatment of a thiamine deficiency.

Absorption and Storage   Vitamin B_1 is absorbed in only small amounts from the jejunum by active transport and is stored in small amounts in the heart, liver, kidney, and brain.

Toxic Effects   In general, the incidence of toxic effects to thiamine is relatively low. Patients may complain of weakness or difficulty in breathing and may experience a slight fall in blood pressure. There are reports of anaphylactic reactions when vitamin B_1 is administered intravenously. Most likely, this is due to an allergic reaction to the preparation rather than to the vitamin B_1. Patients have also experienced a feeling of warmth, pruritis, urticaria, and nausea.

Dosage   In normal, healthy individuals consuming a normal diet, 5 mg per day is the most that is ever needed as a dietary supplement.

Vitamin B_2

Vitamin B_2, or riboflavin, has few tissue stores in the body and functions primarily as a coenzyme in various steps for energy to be produced in the mitochondrial energy system of the respiratory proteins. Vitamin B_2 also affects fetal growth and development and the maintenance of external tissues in the eyes and skin. Dietary sources include organ meats, yeast, green leafy vegetables, fruit, eggs, and dairy products. Human requirements are proportional to energy expenditures.

Uses   Vitamin B_2 is used primarily to treat and prevent riboflavin deficiencies.

Absorption and Storage   Vitamin B_2 is readily absorbed from both the GI tract (through facilitated diffusion) and parenteral sites. It is not stored in the body to any great extent and is excreted rapidly.

Toxic Effects   Vitamin B_2 is relatively nontoxic in normal and megadose quantities.

Interactions   Antidepressants, phenothiazines, or probenecid, when given concurrently, may increase requirements for riboflavin. Alcohol inhibits absorption of riboflavin. Riboflavin may cause false elevations of urinary catecholamines.

Dosage   Dosage information is included in Table 13–3.

Vitamin B_6

Vitamin B_6, or pyridoxine *(Nestrex, Beesix)*, functions as a coenzyme for a number of reactions associated with nitrogen metabolism. Vitamin B_6 also aids in the metabolism of tryptophan and enhances the transport of amino acids and potassium into cells. Dietary sources include liver, grains, yeast, vegetables, meat, and fish.

Table 13–3. WATER-SOLUBLE VITAMINS

VITAMIN	CAUSES AND SYMPTOMS OF DEFICIENCY	NURSING IMPLICATIONS
vitamin b₁ (thiamine hydrochloride [Apatate drops, Biamine]), thiamine chloride [Thiamilate])		
wet beriberi with chf *Adults:* 5–10 mg IV 3 times/day slowly. **wernicke's encephalopathy** *Adults:* 100 mg IV followed by 50–100 mg/day IV or IM until patient is consuming a regular balanced diet. **rda** *Adults:* 1–1.5 mg/day. *Children:* 0.3–1.5 mg/day. *Pregnant/Lactating Women:* 1.5–1.6 mg/day.	**Causes:** alcoholism, pregnancy, malabsorption syndromes, chronic diarrhea, liver disease, prolonged antacid therapy **Symptoms:** peripheral neuropathy (dry beriberi), fatigue, decreased attention spans, depression, loss of memory. CHF (wet beriberi), vomiting, diarrhea, polyneuritis, cardiac dysrhythmias, edema, Wernicke's encephalopathy, Korsakoff's psychosis	**ASSESSMENT:** Assess for thiamine deficiency. Assess for thiamine dietary intake. Due to possible anaphylaxis, interdermal testing is done prior to IV administration. Assess for pregnancy (category A). **INTERVENTION:** Administer IV slowly; do not mix in alkaline solutions or with sulfites in same IV. Have epinephrine on hand when giving larger parenteral doses. Take vitamin B₁ with food. Store in cool, dry place. Potency diminishes rapidly. Use in pregnant and lactating women only if clearly needed. Rotate IM sites and apply ice to reduce pain. **EVALUATION:** Evaluate for toxic effects such as weakness, labored breathing, pruritis, or nausea. Report to physician.
vitamin b₂ (riboflavin, vitamin G, lactoflavin [Riboderm])		
riboflavin deficiency states *Adults:* 5–30 mg/day PO given in divided doses. *Children:* 3–10 mg/day PO *RDA Adults:* 1.2–1.7 mg/day. *Children:* 0.4–1.8 mg/day. *Pregnant/Lactating Women:* 1.6–1.8 mg/day.	**Causes:** vegetarian diets, pregnancy, high-energy expenditures—fever and stress, liver disease, alcoholism **Symptoms:** photophobia, glossitis, stomatitis, dermatitis, corneal vascularization	**ASSESSMENT:** Assess for B₂ deficiency. Assess for B₂ intake in diet. Assess for increased need for vitamin B₂ with liver disease. Assess for pregnancy (category A). **INTERVENTION:** Take with food to enhance absorption. **Patient Teaching**—teach patient that vitamin B₂ colors urine bright yellow, and to store it in light-resistant container. Caution patient not to drink alcohol, as absorption is inhibited. **EVALUATION:** Evaluate for signs of overdose and notify physician.
vitamin b₆ (pyridoxine hydrochloride [Beesix, Hexa-Betalin, Nestrex, Rodex])		
dietary deficiency *Adults:* 2.5–10 mg/day PO, IM, or IV for 3 wk, then 2–5 mg/day for supplementation. Up to 600 mg/day in acute deficiencies. **isoniazid (inh) poisoning** *Adults:* 1–4 g IV followed by 1 g IM every 30 min until seizures stop. **deficiencies due to inh or penicillamine** *Adults:* Prophylaxis–10–50 mg/day PO. *Rx ment of established neuropathy–50–200 mg/day PO, IM, or IV.* **vitamin b₆ dependency syndrome** *Adults:* up to 600 mg/day PO, IM, or IV initially, then 30–50 mg/day PO for life. **rda** *Adults:* 1.6–2 mg/day. *Children:* 0.3–2 mg/day. *Pregnant/Lactating Women:* 2.1–2.2 mg/day.	**Causes:** inadequate intake, pregnancy, drug induced, inborn errors of metabolism. **Symptoms:** Convulsions, irritability, nervous disorders, neuritis, edema, seborrheic dermatitis, lesions on mucous membranes	**ASSESSMENT:** Assess for symptoms of deficiency. Assess for pregnancy (category A). **INTERVENTION:** Store in light-resistant container. Use with caution in lactating women; may depress lactation through inhibition of prolactin. Monitor for drug interactions: oral contraceptives, levodopa, INH, phenobarbital (see text). **EVALUATION:** Monitor for paresthesias (rare), somnolence, flushing, temporary burning at injection site. Report to physician.

Continued on the following page

Table 13–3. WATER-SOLUBLE VITAMINS, *Continued*

VITAMIN	CAUSES AND SYMPTOMS OF DEFICIENCY	NURSING IMPLICATIONS
vitamin b₁₂ (cyanocobalamin [Crystamine, Cyanoject, Cyomin, Rubesol-1000, and others], hydroxocobalamin [Droxomin, Hydrobexan, others])		
cyanocobalamin deficiency states *Adults:* 30 µg/day IM for 5–10 days, then 100–200 µg IM every mo. **pernicious anemia** *Adults:* 100 µg/day IM or deep SC for 6–7 days followed by 100 µg every other day for 7 more doses, then 100 µg q 3–4 days for 2–3 more wk initially, then 100–200 µg q month. *Children:* 30–50 µg/day deep IM for 2 wk or more (total dose 1–5 mg) initially, then 100 µg monthly. **hydroxocobalamin** *Adults:* 30–50 µg/day IM or SC for 5–10 days, then 100–200 µg monthly. Flushing dose for Schilling test is 1000 µg. *Children:* 30–50 µg/day IM or SC for 2 or more wk (total dose of 1–5 mg), then 100 µg monthly. **rda** *Adults:* 2 µg/day. *Children:* 0.3–2 µg/day. *Pregnant/Lactating Women:* 2.2–2.6 µg/day.	**Causes:** malabsorption syndromes **Symptoms:** retarded growth, megaloblastic or pernicious anemias, sprue, glossitis	**ASSESSMENT:** Assess for symptoms of deficiency. Assess for cobalt sensitivity. If patient is cobalt sensitive, do an intradermal test dose first. Assess blood folate levels before and during therapy with large doses (10 µg or more) as folate deficiency may occur. Assess serum potassium level during therapy if patient is taking concurrent cardiotonics. Assess for pregnancy (category C). **INTERVENTION:** Poor bioavailability from PO forms owing to inability of B₁₂ to absorb from GI tract. Parenteral medication is refrigerated and protected from light. Use cautiously in pregnant and lactating women. Monitor for drug interactions (aminoglycosides, anticonvulsants, colchicine, alcohol, cimetidine). **Patient Teaching—** Emphasize importance of monthly B₁₂ injection for patients with pernicious anemia, as neurologic damage can occur. **EVALUATION:** Evaluate for signs of toxicity such as hematologic, cardiovascular, and respiratory complications and report to physician.
folic acid (vitamin B₉, folate, Folvite) **leucovorin calcium** (Wellcovorin) (folinic acid)		
folic acid deficiency states *Adults and Children over 4 yr:* 0.25–1 mg/day. *Children up to 4 yr:* 0.3 mg/day PO. *Infants:* 0.1 mg/day PO. **leucovorin calcium folate-deficient megaloblastic anemia** *Adults:* up to 1 mg IM daily. (See Chapter 55 for other uses).	**Causes:** malnutrition, use of birth control pills, alcoholism, pregnancy **Symptoms:** macrolytic anemia, glossitis, diarrhea, malabsorption syndromes, sprue	**ASSESSMENT:** Assess for signs of folic acid deficiency. Assess dietary intake. Assess for pregnancy (category A). **INTERVENTION:** For IM use, do not mix with other medications. Protect from light. Monitor for drug interactions. Doses above 15–20 mg/day may increase metabolism of phenobarbital and phenytoin. Oral contraceptives may impair folate metabolism. Pyrimethamine, trimethoprim, triamterene may interfere with folate utilization. **Patient Teaching—**Inform the patient that folic acid needs are increased during pregnancy and that supplementation may be required. **EVALUATION:** Evaluate patient for allergic reactions and report to physician.
pantothenic acid (vitamin B₅, calcium panthothenate)		
deficiency *Adults and Children:* 5–10 mg.	**Causes:** aging, arthritis, stress, malabsorption **Symptoms:** neurologic disorders; irritability; fatigue; dry, scaly skin; adrenal hypofunction; muscle cramps	**ASSESSMENT:** Assess for symptoms of deficiency. Assess for pregnancy (category UK). **INTERVENTION:** Administer with food.

Continued on the following page

Table 13–3. WATER-SOLUBLE VITAMINS, *Continued*

VITAMIN	CAUSES AND SYMPTOMS OF DEFICIENCY	NURSING IMPLICATIONS
niacin (nicotinic acid, vitamin B₃ [Niac, Niacels, Nicobid, Nicolar, others]) **niacinamide** (nicotinamide)		
niacin **dietary supplementation** *Adults:* 10–20 mg/day PO. **treatment of pellegra** *Adults:* 300–500 mg/day PO in divided doses. *Children:* 100–300 mg/day PO in divided doses. **hyperlipidemia** *Adults:* 1.5–6 g/day in 2–4 divided doses. **niacinamide** **nicotinamide** **treatment of hartnup disease** *Adults:* 50–200 mg/day. **vasodilator** *Adults:* 100–150 mg 3–5 times/day or 300–400 mg as extended-release preparations q 12 hr.	**Causes:** malabsorption—alcoholism **Symptoms:** pellagra (red patchy skin eruptions, red swollen tongue, mental changes, dementia, diarrhea)	**ASSESSMENT:** Assess for symptoms of niacin deficiency. Assess liver function, blood glucose, and serum uric acid levels before and during therapy. Assess for aspirin or tartrazine sensitivity. Assess for pregnancy (category C). **INTERVENTION:** Start all oral doses in small doses and gradually increase. Administer with meals to minimize GI complaints. Suggest patient sit for 30–60 min after taking niacin to help eliminate dizziness and faintness due to the secondary vasodilating effect. With large doses (>1 g), administer 325 gr of ASA 30 minutes before niacin. Monitor for drug interactions (see text). Use cautiously in patients with anorexia, heartburn, impaired liver function. **EVALUATION:** Evaluate for signs of toxicity (flushing face, tingling, dryness of skin, headache, diarrhea, anorexia, heart burn, and liver disease) and report to physician.
biotin (vitamin H protective factor x) *Adults:* 100–200 μg/day PO or IV. *Children:* 65–120 μg/day PO.	**Causes:** malabsorption **Symptoms:** dermatitis, memory loss, mental depression	**ASSESSMENT:** Assess for signs of biotin deficiency. **INTERVENTION:** Monitor patient for dermatitis with IV administration. **Patient Teaching**—Caution patient to not take biotin and egg white together, as absorption of biotin is reduced.
vitamin c (ascorbic acid [Cecon, Dull-C, Flavorcee, many others])		
prevention of deficiency *Adults:* 55–60 mg/day PO. *Adolescents:* 55–60 mg/day PO. *Children:* 40 mg/day PO. *Infants:* 35 mg/day PO. *Pregnant/Lactating Women:* 60 mg/day and 80 mg/day PO, respectively. **prevention of scurvy** *Adults:* 70–150 mg/day PO. **treatment of scurvy** *Adults:* 300 mg to 1 g PO or 100–250 mg SC, IM, or IV once or twice daily up to 1–2 g. *Children and Infants:* 100–300 mg/day PO, SC, IM, or IV, in divided doses. **urine acidification** *Adults:* 4–12 g/day PO, in divided doses. **enhancement of wound healing** *Adults:* 300–500 mg/day SC, IM, or IV for 1 wk or 10 days to 1 g/day for 4–7 days. **burns** *Adults:* 200–500 mg/day up to 1–2 g/day are recommended PO, SC, IM, or IV.	**Causes:** poor dietary intake, decreased ability to metabolize amino acids, megalolastic anemia of infancy **Symptoms:** scurvy, slow healing of wounds	**ASSESSMENT:** Assess for signs of vitamin C deficiency. Assess for aspirin or tartrazine allergy. Give test dose of ascorbic acid to determine if allergic to this product. Assess for cigarette smoking and environmental stress; both increase vitamin C needs by 50% to 300%. Assess for pregnancy (category C). **INTERVENTION:** Ascorbic acid can interfere with urine testing for glucose or give false-positive results for occult blood in stool. After IV dose, mild soreness, dizziness, and faintness may occur. Avoid rapid IV infusion. **Patient Teaching**—Teach patient with diabetes or history of renal calculi that vitamin C intake should be limited. Tell patient to store in closed container away from heat and light. **EVALUATION:** Evaluate for signs of toxicity (hemolytic anemia in patients with G6PD deficiency, high acidification of urine, crystalluria) and report to physician.

Vitamin B_6 is needed in the formation of the heme part of erythrocytes. It also participates in the transfer of energy in the brain and in nervous tissue. Vitamin B_6 is a complex of three closely related compounds—pyridoxine, pyridoxal, and pyridoxamine. Pyridoxine is found in plants while pyridoxal and pyridoxamine are found in animals. All of these compounds are converted to physiologically active forms of vitamin B_6—pyridoxal phosphate (codecarboxylase) and pyridoxamine phosphate.

Uses Pyridoxine is indicated in pyridoxine deficiency associated with inborn errors of metabolism, inadequate diet, or drug-induced deficiencies (e.g., from isoniazid or oral contraceptives) causing peripheral neuritis.

Absorption and Storage Vitamin B_6 is readily absorbed after both oral and parenteral administration. Vitamin B_6 is absorbed throughout the intestine by simple diffusion and stored in skeletal muscle for 15 to 20 days.

Toxic Effects Toxic effects rarely occur in normal or even therapeutic doses. However, paresthesia, somnolence, flushing, and a feeling of warmth have been reported after large parenteral injections. Temporary burning or a stinging pain have also been reported after injections.

Contraindications and Precautions Vitamin B_6 is contraindicated in patients who are hypersensitive. It is also used with caution in lactating women as prolactin inhibition may decrease milk production.

Interactions Vitamin B_6, when taken in doses greater than 5 mg/day concurrently with levodopa (L-Dopa), enhances the peripheral metabolism of levodopa. This prevents it from having a therapeutic effect and may necessitate increasing the dose of levodopa. Special pyridoxine-free multivitamin preparations are available for those taking levodopa. Doses of vitamin B_6 greater than 80 mg/day enhance hepatic metabolism of phenobarbital or phenytoin by 40% to 50%. Isoniazid and penicillamine increase the urinary excretion of pyridoxine.

Dosage Dosage varies depending on the condition being treated. Dosage information is provided in Table 13–3.

Vitamin B_{12}

Vitamin B_{12} functions as a coenzyme in nucleic acid, protein, lipid, and red blood cell synthesis. It is necessary to maintain growth of epithelial cells and the nervous system, particularly the myelin sheath. Dietary sources include organ meats, egg yolk, and seafood.

Vitamin B_{12} is available as **cyanocobalamin (Crystamine)** or **hydroxocobalamin (Hydrobexan)**. Both cyanocobalamin and hydroxocobalamin are cobalt-containing substances produced from *Streptomyces griseus* or obtained from human liver.

Uses Vitamin B_{12} is used to correct and treat pernicious anemia, a megaloblastic anemia. *Megaloblastic* is the term used to describe most anemias characterized by large germ cells in the bone marrow as well as large immature red cells in the plasma (see Table 13–3). Pernicious anemia is due to the lack of *intrinsic factor*, which is a substance normally found in the gastric juice that makes the absorption of vitamin B_{12} possible. Without intrinsic factor, the absorption of vitamin B_{12} is reduced. Pernicious anemia occurs 3 months to 2 to 5 years after the onset of intrinsic factor deficiency. If not treated, pernicious anemia can result in neurologic degeneration such as degenerative spinal cord lesions.

Absorption and Storage Vitamin B_{12} is rapidly absorbed after an intramuscular injection. It is primarily stored in the liver (30% to 60%), lungs, kidneys, and spleen for up to 1 year.

Toxic Effects Vitamin B_{12} can precipitate an anaphylactic reaction with associated pulmonary edema and heart failure. Allergies to cobalt are determined before administration. Vitamin B_{12} can also cause optic nerve atrophy, so eye exams are necessary during administration. It can also precipitate mild transient diarrhea, itching, rash, and peripheral vascular thromboses.

Contraindications and Precautions Vitamin B_{12} is contraindicated in patients hypersensitive to cobalt or in those with hereditary optic atrophy, as the condition may worsen. It is used cautiously in pregnant and lactating women.

Interactions Neomycin, colchicine, para-aminosalicylic acid, potassium, and alcohol may cause malabsorption of vitamin B_{12}. Cimetidine impairs its absorption.

Dosage When a vitamin B_{12} deficiency exists, the treatment is parenteral administration of vitamin B_{12}. Of the two forms available, hydroxocobalamin is more highly protein bound than cyanocobalamin; however, it has no therapeutic advantage over cyanocobalamin. Oral vitamin B_{12} is poorly absorbed and has no valid therapeutic role. Additional dosage information can be found in Table 13–3.

Folic Acid

Folic acid, or **folate** or **vitamin B_9,** is an antianemic factor that is necessary for the synthesis of nucleic acid. It acts as a coenzyme in purine metabolism and is critical for red blood cell division. Dietary sources include liver, wheat, yeast, beans, green vegetables, nuts, and fruits.

Uses Folic Acid (Folvite) is used primarily to treat folic acid anemia, a megaloblastic anemia resulting from a deficiency in the vitamin folic acid. Folic acid is necessary to synthesize DNA within the red cell, and its lack inhibits normal hematopoiesis. Folate deficiencies are more common than vitamin B_{12} deficiencies, as folate stores are depleted rapidly in the presence of a dietary deficiency. Folic acid should not be used in patients with pernicious anemia who are not receiving vitamin B_{12}: the hematologic disorder will respond; however, the neurologic sequelae will continue to progress.

Folic acid is also used to treat megaloblastic or macrolytic anemias secondary to nutritional deficiency, hepatic disease, alcoholism, intestinal obstruction, or excessive hemolysis; to treat tropical sprue; and to prevent megaloblastic anemias in pregnancy.

Folic acid reduces the risk of neural-tube defects in the fetus, such as spinabifida and anencephaly. The benefits of folic acid occur primarily during the first trimester of pregnancy. Therefore, the U.S. Department of Health and

Human Services suggests that if women are planning pregnancy, they should take a supplement containing folic acid.

Absorption and Storage Folic acid is most commonly administered in its oral form. Approximately 65% of oral folic acid is quickly absorbed by the body from the proximal small intestine, converted to an absorbable complex by enzymes in the small intestine, and stored in the adrenal cortex and liver.

Toxic Effects Generally, folic acid is nontoxic, but mild allergic reactions are possible.

Contraindications and Precautions Folic acid is contraindicated in treatment of undiagnosed anemias, aplastic or normocytic anemias, or alone in the treatment of pernicious anemia, as it may mask neurologic damage.

Interactions Oral contraceptives may impair folate metabolism. Pyrimethamine, trimethoprim, and triamterene may interfere with folate utilization. Doses of folic acid greater than 15 to 20 mg daily may increase the metabolism of both phenobarbital and phenytoin, reducing their concentrations in serum.

Dosage Dosage information can be found in Table 13–3.

Pantothenic Acid

Pantothenic acid, or **calcium pantothenate** or **vitamin B$_5$,** occupies a key role in body metabolism. It is incorporated into coenzyme A, which is involved in many biochemical processes, including metabolism of fats, protein, and carbohydrates and the synthesis of steroids, porphyrins, acetylcholine, and other substrates. Dietary sources include liver, eggs, wheat germ, yeast, walnuts, and salmon.

Uses Pantothenic acid is indicated for the prevention and treatment of vitamin B deficiency. Special conditions that may require supplementation include stress, aging, arthritis, malabsorption, weakness, and depression.

Absorption and Storage Pantothenic acid is absorbed from the intestine and excreted fairly rapidly. About 25% of the daily intake is excreted within 24 hours after ingestion. Pantothenic acid is believed to be stored in the liver, heart, and kidneys. However, it is unknown in what quantities pantothenic acid is stored.

There are no known toxic effects, contraindications and precautions, or interactions for pantothenic acid.

Dosage Evidence indicates that dietary supplementation in a normal, healthy individual is not necessary. Dosage information can be found in Table 13–3.

Niacin

Niacin, or **nicotinic acid (Nicolar, Slo-Niacin, Nicobid, others),** is a water-soluble derivative of pyridine formerly called vitamin B$_3$. It occurs in two physiologically active forms that take part in many oxidation-reduction reactions: nicotinamide adenine dinucleotide (NAD) and nicotinamide adenine dinucleotide phosphate (NADP). These substances act as hydrogen acceptors, which ultimately help to convert protein, carbohydrate, and fat into energy through oxidation-reduction. At this time, there is no known biologic role for niacin other than this coenzyme function. Dietary sources include liver, peanuts, poultry, yeast, beans, nuts (particularly peanuts), fish, and meat.

Uses Nicotinic acid and nicotinamide are indicated for prevention or treatment of nicotinic acid deficiency and pellagra. Nicotinic acid is also used as adjunctive therapy in patients with significant hyperlipidemia who do not respond adequately to diet and weight loss to lower plasma cholesterol, triglycerides, and free fatty acids.

Absorption and Storage Niacin is readily absorbed, after both oral and parenteral administration, in the proximal jejunum through active transport. It is stored in the liver and the heart. It is metabolized by the liver, with small doses excreted as metabolites and large doses excreted unchanged in the urine. Approximately one third of the daily intake is excreted in 24 hours.

Toxic Effects Many adverse effects can be experienced, including flushing of the face and neck (as niacin stimulates histamine release), pruritus, dry skin, headache, dizziness, heartburn, anorexia, activation of peptic ulcer, vomiting, mild hypotension, impaired liver function, and allergic reactions. Flushing and itching reactions usually subside after about 3 days of therapy. Taking 325 grains of ASA (aspirin) 30 minutes before niacin also reduces flushing by reducing levels of prostaglandins.

Contraindications and Precautions Niacin is contraindicated in patients with hepatic dysfunction and in those with active peptic ulcer, as histamine release may activate bleeding. Caution is advised in patients with gout, as elevated uric acid levels occur, and in patients with gallbladder disease. Diabetics may have a decreased glucose tolerance and may need to have dietary or hypoglycemic therapy modification.

Interactions When niacin is given concurrently with adrenergic blocking drugs—particularly the ganglionic blockers—the vasodilating and hypotensive effects may be potentiated. Uricosuric effects of probenecid may be inhibited.

Dosage Dosage information can be found in Table 13–3.

Biotin

Biotin primarily functions as a coenzyme in the metabolism of proteins, fats, and carbohydrates. It is also important for the maintenance of skin, hair, nerves, and sex glands. Although biotin is still a little-known vitamin, it seems to have an important role in human growth. Dietary sources include yeast, liver, and egg yolks.

Uses Special conditions that may require dietary supplementation with biotin include certain cutaneous lesions, antibiotic and sulfonamide therapy, pregnancy, and excessive egg white ingestion. Egg whites contain avidin, a protein, which binds orally ingested and bacteria-produced biotin and prevents its absorption in the intestine.

Absorption and Storage Biotin is absorbed well. Its target tissues include the skin and the nervous tissue. It is stored in the liver and excreted slowly over 3 to 4 weeks. Much of the daily requirement of biotin is synthesized by intestinal flora and supplements oral intake.

There are no known toxic effects, contraindications and precautions, or interactions for biotin.

Dosage Dosage information can be found in Table 13–3.

Vitamin C

Vitamin C is a naturally occurring water-soluble vitamin that cannot be synthesized by the human body. It must be provided exogenously. It is available as **ascorbic acid, sodium ascorbate,** and **calcium ascorbate.** Dietary sources include fruits, fresh green vegetables, and rose hips. Vitamin C is probably the most controversial vitamin because of the claims by Linus Pauling that, when taken in megadoses, it relieves cold symptoms. Other researchers claim that vitamin C can treat cancer, heat rash, thrombophlebitis, and emotional illness and enhance wound healing. Primarily, vitamin C functions as an antioxidant that is essential to many enzymatic activities, particularly those of cellular respiration. It is also essential for the synthesis and maintenance of both collagen and intercellular substances, which ultimately are needed for wound healing. Vitamin C is also necessary for carbohydrate metabolism, the conversion of folic acid to folinic acid, the formation of serotonin, and the maintenance of vascular tone.

Uses Vitamin C is indicated for the prevention and treatment of scurvy. In large doses, vitamin C acts as a urinary acidifier; therefore, vitamin C is beneficial to bedridden patients with infectious diseases. Patients with severe infectious diseases such as tuberculosis, rheumatic fever, and pneumonia have an increased need for vitamin C. Failure to receive adequate vitamin C can result in delayed soft-tissue healing and disruption of the body's immune response.

Several studies have demonstrated that there is an association between high vitamin C concentrations and high plasma levels of high-density lipoprotein (HDL)—a blood protein that protects against coronary heart disease. Patients with atherosclerosis who have a diet rich in vitamin C and who monitor and eliminate risk factors such as smoking, hypertension, and excessive saturated fat intake may be able to slow the disease progress. Research is ongoing.

Absorption and Storage Vitamin C is readily absorbed after both oral and parenteral administration. Vitamin C is absorbed from the terminal ileum by active transport. It is stored in many tissues, particularly in the adrenal cortex, pituitary, ovaries, and connective tissue.

Toxic Effects With excessive oral doses, the patient may experience diarrhea (due to direct irritation of the intestinal mucosa) or strong acidification of the urine with possible precipitation of crystals of vitamin C or oxalate kidney stones. Hemolytic anemia may develop in patients who have a deficiency of glucose-6-phosphate dehydrogenase (G6PD).

Contraindications and Precautions Vitamin C is contraindicated in pregnancy. There are no studies that indicate whether or not fetal harm will occur. Vitamin C is used cautiously in patients with gout or crystalluria as the acidification of the urine from vitamin C may worsen these conditions. It is also used cautiously in lactating women as it is excreted in breast milk. The effects of vitamin C on the infant are unknown at this time.

Interactions Large doses of vitamin C, when taken concurrently with aminosalicylic acid and sulfonamides, may increase the possibility of producing urinary crystals of the other drugs because of urine acidification. Vitamin C increases serum levels of estrogen and oral contraceptives, which may result in adverse reactions. Vitamin C can interfere with the therapeutic effects of warfarin.

A patient taking large doses of vitamin C may have a false-negative or false-positive urinary glucose reading, depending on the type of glucose test used. The patient may also have false-positive tests for occult blood in the stool.

Dosage Dosage information can be found in Table 13–3.

ANTIOXIDANT VITAMINS

Several vitamins are antioxidants (agents that prevent or inhibit oxidation). These vitamins, particularly vitamins C, A (beta-carotene), and E, are being studied for their possible use in the prevention of cancer and heart disease. Researchers theorize that vitamins C and E may prevent cancer by protecting cells from the ravages of unstable molecules called free radicals, which are produced when cells are damaged or exposed to toxins such as cigarette smoke (Long, 1996). Vitamin E may prevent heart attack by blocking the oxidation and buildup on artery walls of low-density lipoproteins (LDLs)—the "bad" form of cholesterol. Adequate amounts of beta-carotene have been linked to a lower frequency of angina in men who have had a previous myocardial infarction (MI), and higher-than-normal serum levels of beta-carotene reduce the risk of MI. Because research studies are producing mixed results, additional studies are necessary before persons are encouraged to increase their daily intake of antioxidants.

MINERALS

Of the 15 minerals, five are considered macro (bulk essential) elements—calcium, magnesium, sodium, potassium, and phosphorus—and are needed daily by the body to maintain health. The remaining 10 minerals (iron, copper, manganese, zinc, iodine, selenium, molybdenum, chromium, cobalt, and fluorine) are termed micro (trace) elements. Iron is necessary for red blood cell production.

Minerals carry one or more charges in solution and are electropositive (cations) or electronegative (anions). They may be univalent (carrying one charge), bivalent (carrying two charges), or trivalent (carrying three charges). Ten minerals are cations: calcium (Ca^{++}), magnesium (Mg^{++}), sodium (Na^{+}), potassium (K^{+}), iron (Fe^{++}), copper (Cu^{++}), manganese (Mn^{++}), zinc (Zn^{++}), chromium (Cr^{+++}), and cobalt (Co^{++}); five minerals are anions: phosphorus (P^{-}), iodine (I^{-}), selenium (Se^{-}), molybdenum (Mo^{--}), and fluorine (F^{-}). Three of the anions are most commonly found as oxide complexes: phosphorus oxide (PO_4^{-}), selenium oxide (SeO_4^{--}), and molybdenum oxide (MoO_4^{++}).

The majority of mineral elements are soluble in the acid pH of the stomach. However, as the pH turns alkaline in the intestine, most of the divalent positive ions (Mg^{++},

Co^{++}, Fe^{++}, Cu^{++}, Mn^{++}, and Zn^{++}) become insoluble. This is especially true of the trace minerals, making it more difficult for metallic ions to be absorbed and necessitating special mechanisms for absorption, such as active transport, vitamin D, and bile salts.

The bulk minerals (also electrolytes) calcium, magnesium, sodium, potassium, and phosphorus are discussed in Chapter 12. Major trace elements—iron, copper, zinc, iodine, cobalt, chromium, and manganese—are discussed in the sections that follow.

IRON

Iron is present in every cell in the body and is a component of hemoglobin, myoglobin, and a number of enzymes necessary for oxygen transfer. About 30% of iron is stored as hemosiderin or ferritin, primarily in hepatic cells and reticuloendothelial cells of the spleen and bone marrow. The remaining two-thirds of iron circulates within the red cells as hemoglobin. Iron is made available for hemoglobin synthesis as needed through the aid of a beta-globulin transferrin. Transferrin carries iron released from old red blood cells (RBCs) to the bone marrow for storage and reuse. Transferrin also has specific binding capabilities that facilitate the transfer of iron across the membranes of immature RBCs. The total body content of iron is 50 mg/kg in men and 35 mg/kg in women. Iron is available in both oral and parenteral form. Both are discussed individually, and iron products are featured in Table 13–4.

Oral Iron Products

Oral iron products include **ferrous sulfate (Mol-Iron, others), ferrous gluconate (Fergon),** and **ferrous fumarate (Ircon, others)**. Iron is also available in combination with vitamin C for oral administration.

Uses Iron preparations correct erythropoietic abnormalities due to the deficiency of iron. Iron is of value only when the iron stores are depleted, as in hypochromic anemias. If iron supplements are given to a person with normal blood values, the hemoglobin content does not increase; there is, however, an increase in the reserve supply of iron. Iron deficiency anemia is the most common anemia today, affecting nearly 60% of all young women. As iron stores are reduced, cold intolerance and sleep disturbance may occur.

When iron is administered to a patient with hypochromic anemia, hematocrit and hemoglobin levels begin to increase in 3 days. The maximum response, however, does not occur until the second to fourth weeks. As the hemoglobin level increases, the patient notes less fatigue, improved appetite and nail condition, and improved sense of well-being.

Iron is also administered to patients receiving epoetin (Chapter 38), such as those with chronic renal failure.

Pharmacokinetics Iron preparations are absorbed best in the duodenum by active transport, and absorption continues until all of the transferrin is saturated, when iron absorption stops. As a rule, lower doses are better absorbed, so iron is best taken in divided doses. Iron is absorbed three times more readily in its ferrous form

(Fe^{++}), which is less ionized, than in its ferric form (Fe^{+++}). Sustained-release preparations are available; however, they have been shown to be poorly absorbed and produce poor clinical responses. Iron products may be combined with ascorbic acid (vitamin C), which helps to keep the iron in its ferrous form and enhances iron absorption. Oral preparations are best absorbed when taken between meals because food decreases absorption by 40% to 66%. However, many patients taking iron products complain of gastrointestinal irritation. If this occurs, the iron preparation is taken with a small snack.

Iron preparations have the same fate as dietary iron. Iron is removed through the loss of iron-containing cells from the bowel, skin, and genitourinary tract. Normal loss is 0.5 to 1 mg/day; in menstruating women the loss is 1 to 2 mg/day.

Contraindications and Precautions Oral iron is contraindicated in patients with primary hemochromatosis, hemolytic anemias, and hypersensitivity. Because it irritates the GI tract, oral iron is not given to patients with disorders such as peptic ulcer disease, regional enteritis, and ulcerative colitis. Iron is given cautiously to patients with renal and hepatic dysfunction as the kidney and liver are involved with elimination and storage of iron. Patients with sensitivity to tartrazine and sulfites (components of some preparations) should take forms that do not contain these ingredients.

Adverse Effects The local effects of orally administered iron include action as an irritant and astringent. Liquid iron preparations may stain the teeth, so they are given through a straw placed well back in the mouth. The oral inorganic iron acts with tissue proteins to form an insoluble iron compound that can irritate the gastrointestinal tract and contribute to nausea, vomiting, constipation or diarrhea, and abdominal distress. Rarely, this irritation can cause gastrointestinal (GI) bleeding and a positive test result for fecal occult blood. If symptoms of GI bleeding develop, the iron products are discontinued for several days until symptoms are relieved. Then, therapy with oral iron is resumed. More commonly, dark red or black stools can occur, resulting from the insoluble iron compound in the stool.

Interactions Iron is not given concurrently with antacids, because iron absorption is slowed due to its complexation with the antacid. Coffee and tea consumed with a meal or 1 hour after, eggs, and milk can also inhibit iron absorption. Administration is separated by at least 2 to 3 hours. Absorption can be enhanced slightly if iron is mixed with ascorbic acid (200 mg vitamin C/30 mg iron). Iron products can combine into an insoluble complex with tetracycline, decreasing its availability. They are administered 2 to 3 hours apart as well. Chloramphenicol delays iron clearance from plasma, delays iron incorporation into red blood cells, and interferes with erythropoiesis.

Dosage Dosages for several oral forms of iron can be found in Table 13–4.

○ **Ferrous sulfate** (Ferospace, Mol-Iron, others), the oldest iron product, is the standard iron preparation against which all other oral preparations are usually measured. The dosage is determined according to the severity of the anemia.

○ **Ferrous gluconate** (Fergon) causes less gastric irritation and is better tolerated than ferrous sulfate.

○ **Ferrous fumarate** (Femiron, Ircon) is comparable to the products previously described.

○ **Iron with Vitamin C** (Ferancee-HP, Mol-Iron with Vitamin C, others) Combining iron with vitamin C enhances the absorption of the iron. Several over-the-counter preparations are available in tablet, chewable tablet, or time-release products.

Parenteral Iron Products

The parenteral route is commonly used when the patient cannot tolerate or absorb oral iron. **Iron dextran injection (InFeD)** is the only parenteral iron product.

○ **Iron dextran injection** (InFeD) is a complex ferric hydroxide with dextran in a 0.9% sodium chloride solution for injection. Reticuloendothelial cells of the liver, spleen, and bone marrow separate the iron from the dex-

---

Table 13–4. IRON PREPARATIONS AND IRON ANTIDOTE

DRUG NAME/ROUTE AND DOSAGE	ADVERSE EFFECTS	INTERACTIONS	NURSING IMPLICATIONS
IRON PREPARATIONS			
ferrous sulfate (Ferospace, Mol-Iron, Fer-In-Sol) (20% iron)			
Adults: 300–1200 mg/day PO in divided doses. **Children 2–12 yr:** 10 mg/kg per day PO in divided doses.	**Common:** nausea, constipation/diarrhea, dark stools **Other:** anorexia, GI irritation, staining of teeth with liquid products, vomiting	**Drug-Drug:** Tetracyclines, antacids, coffee, tea, milk, or eggs inhibit iron absorption; separate administration times by 2–3 hr. Increased absorption of iron if administered with ascorbic acid. Chloramphenicol decreases iron clearance from serum. Iron may block the antihypertensive effect of methyl dopa. Iron decreases absorption of penicillamine and fluoroquinolones.	**ASSESSMENT:** Assess laboratory blood work, dietary intake, bowel function. Assess for tartrazine sensitivity. Assess for contraindications (primary hemochromatosis, hemosiderosis, and hemolytic anemias). **INTERVENTION:** Iron products should not be taken within 1 hr of bedtime because they are possibly corrosive to the stomach. For best absorption, all tablets or capsules are taken on an empty stomach between meals. If GI distress occurs, try enteric-coated tablets or give tablets after meals. Enteric-coated tablets are poorly absorbed and the entire tablet may be found in the stool of some patients (totally unabsorbed). Liquid preparations are well diluted and taken through a straw placed well back in the mouth to prevent damage to tooth enamel. Elixir cannot be mixed with milk or wine. Do not crush or chew sustained-release products. Stools may become dark green or black. **EVALUATION:** Iron therapy is continued 2–3 mo after hemoglobin returns to normal to assist in replenishing iron stores. Report severe constipation or diarrhea to physician.
polysaccharide-iron complex (Hytinic, Niferex Niferex-150, Nu-Iron 150) (Ferric, % depends on product)			
Adults: 150 mg PO 1–2 times/day. May be increased to 150 mg 4 times/day. **Children:** Therapeutic dosage not available.	Same as for ferrous sulfate	Same as for ferrous sulfate.	Same as for ferrous sulfate.
ferrous gluconate (Fergon) (11.6% iron)			
Adults: 300–640 mg PO 1–4 times/day. **Children 2 yr and over:** 8 mg/kg/day.	Same as for ferrous sulfate	Same as for ferrous sulfate.	Same as for ferrous sulfate.

Continued on the following page

Table 13–4. IRON PREPARATIONS AND IRON ANTIDOTE, *Continued*

DRUG NAME/ROUTE AND DOSAGE	ADVERSE EFFECTS	INTERACTIONS	NURSING IMPLICATIONS
ferrous fumarate (Ircon, Femiron) (33% iron)			
Adults: 200 mg PO 1–4 times/day **Children:** 3 mg/kg 3 times/day.	Same as for ferrous sulfate	Same as for ferrous sulfate.	Same as for ferrous sulfate.
iron dextran (InFeD) (1 mL = 50 mg elemental iron)			
Adults: IM or IV test dose of 25 mg (0.5 ml) is required before first dose. Dosage is based on weight. See manufacturer's instructions for formula. **IM (by Z-track):** If no reaction occurs after test dose, daily dosage should not exceed 50 mg (1 mL) for children weighing <9 kg; 100 mg (2 mL) for adults and children weighing 9–50 kg; and 25 mg (0.5 mL) for infants weighing >4 kg. **Direct IV:** after test dose, give undiluted at a rate of 1 mL/min. **IV infusion:** mix required dose in 250–1000 mL 0.9% sodium choride solution, give test dose first of 25 mg over 5 min, then infuse rest in 4–6 hr.	**Common:** chills, fever, flushing, hypotension, nausea, staining at IM site, tachycardia **Life-threatening:** anaphylactic reactions **Other:** abdominal pain, arthritis, bronchospasm, chest pain, convulsions, diarrhea, headache, hematuria, leukocytosis, lymphadenopathy, pain at IM site, phlebitis at IV site, shock, vomiting, weakness	None known.	**ASSESSMENT:** Assess for sensitivity. A skin test should be performed before first dose to detect for the presence of allergies. Administer 25 mg IM or IV 1 hr before first dose. If any reaction occurs, consult physician. Assess for renal and hepatic function and for significant allergies and asthma. Give cautiously in these conditions. **INTERVENTION:** No other medications are mixed in the syringe. Administer by Z-track technique in dorsal gluteal area of the buttock. Urine may turn dark brown or black on standing. Following IV administration, patient should remain on bed rest for 30 min. Do not administer with oral iron products. Give test dose at rate no faster than 50 mg/min. Administer to pregnant and lactating women only when clearly indicated. **EVALUATION:** Evaluate for anaphylactic reaction throughout therapy.
IRON ANTIDOTE			
deferoxamine (Desferal)			
acute iron intoxication **Adults and Children:** 1 g IM or IV followed by 500 mg every 4 hr for 2 doses, with subsequent 500 mg every 4–12 hr, not to exceed 6 g in 24 hr. IV rate not to exceed 15 mg/kg per hr. **chronic iron overload** **Adults:** 0.5–1 g IM and 2 g slow IV infusion in separate solution for each unit of blood; rate not to exceed 15 mg/kg per hr. Or, 20–40 mg/kg per day over 8–24 hr by continuous SC mini-infusion pump. **Children:** Safety and effectiveness under 3 years of age has not been established.	**With Short-Term Use:** blurred vision, cataracts, hearing loss, itching, pain and induration at injection site, itching, rash **With Long-Term Use:** dysuria, tachycardia **With Rapid IV Administration:** erythema, hypotension, shock, urticaria	None significant.	**ASSESSMENT:** Assess intake and output to ensure adequate renal function. Note urine color (often reddish). Assess stool for signs of occult bleeding. Assess eyes at baseline and periodically for cataracts. Assess for pregnancy (category C). **INTERVENTION:** Reconstituted solution should be stored for no longer than 1 wk. Protect from light. IV route is reserved for life-threatening poisoning. SC route is used to treat chronically elevated iron levels. **Patient Teaching**—Caution patient that urine may turn red.

tran complex and gradually release it; the iron then combines with transferrin for transport to the bone marrow. Iron dextran is used only after iron deficiency anemia has been confirmed and when oral therapy has failed or may further irritate gastrointestinal disease.

PHARMACOKINETICS Most iron dextran is well absorbed after IM injection within 72 hours, and the remaining drug is absorbed over the next 3 to 4 weeks. The half-life of iron dextran is 5 to 20 hours. Iron dextran is not easily eliminated, and accumulation, which may be toxic, may occur.

CONTRAINDICATIONS AND PRECAUTIONS Iron dextran is contraindicated in patients hypersensitive to it and in all anemias other than iron deficiency anemia. It is used cautiously with impaired liver and kidney function as these organs may be further damaged. Use during pregnancy and lactation only when clearly needed. Iron dextran is not recommended in infants less than 4 months of age.

▼ CLINICAL ALERT

Iron dextran has been associated with fatal anaphylactic reactions. Use caution when administering this drug to patients with significant allergies or asthma. Administer a test dose of 25 mg intramuscularly or intravenously to determine sensitivity and wait 1 hour before administering full dose. If any reaction occurs, consult the physician.

ADVERSE EFFECTS The adverse effects of parenteral administration of iron include pain at the injection site, temporary or permanent discoloration of the skin at the injection site, headache, nausea and vomiting, fever, and urticaria. Parenteral iron may be deposited in the liver or pancreas and may cause hemochromatosis.

DOSAGE The initial intramuscular dose in adults is 50 mg, with up to 250 mg administered every other day thereafter. The dosage is calculated to reconstitute the hemoglobin mass.

To avoid damage to the sensitive subcutaneous tissue, iron dextran is given by Z-track technique (see Chapter 3). Additional dosage information can be found in Table 13–4.

Iron Antidote

○ **Deferoxamine (*Desferal*),** a major *chelating agent* (a substance that binds with and removes certain metals, including iron, from the body system), has an affinity for ferric iron and low affinity for calcium. It binds ferric iron into a stable, water-soluble chelate readily excreted by the kidneys. Its main effect is to remove iron from ferritin, hemosiderin, and transferrin.

Deferoxamine is used to treat iron overload, which may result from overtreatment with iron products or with multiple blood transfusions, iron poisoning, or abnormally high levels injected over a long time. Iron poisoning is a common occurrence in children, as iron tablets may be readily accessible in the household. For example, many pregnant mothers take iron supplements during their pregnancy. Iron imparts a reddish color to the urine, indicating the presence of a high iron level and necessitating treatment with an antidote. For additional information see Table 13–4.

COPPER

Copper is necessary for hemostasis, for stabilization of hemoglobin in the red blood cell, and for the normal function of various enzymes involved in cellular respiration. It also helps to maintain the integrity of the myelin sheath on the spinal cord. Copper is an essential component of a number of proteins (e.g., erythrocuprein, hepatocuprein) and enzymes (e.g., lysyl hydroxylase, dopamine beta-hydroxylase). Copper is found in all tissues, but reaches its highest concentrations in the brain and liver.

Copper is richly present in foods (e.g., oysters, beef, liver, potatoes, sesame and sunflower seeds, cocoa), and virtually all soft water supplies contain large amounts of copper because of current use of copper piping. Therefore, copper deficiencies rarely occur, but may be found in infants and adults receiving copper-deficient parenteral nutrition. Copper deficiency is associated with hypochromic anemia, leukopenia, hypoproteinemia, and bone disease. Copper excess is possible in an American diet. An excess of copper antagonizes the effect of both iron and zinc, thereby resulting in deficiencies. Elevated copper levels may be produced by drugs such as estrogens, thyroid, and corticotropin. Acute toxicities are manifested by nausea and vomiting, epigastric pain, diarrhea, and malaise with hemolysis. Severe toxicity results in renal tubular disorders.

Copper is available in two forms for intravenous (IV) administration—**cupric chloride** and **cupric sulfate**. These IV forms are used to prevent copper deficiency in patients on long-term total parenteral nutrition (TPN). The dosage for adults is 0.5 to 1.5 mg/day; the dosage for children, 20 μg/kg per day. For supplementation, the RDA for adults is 1.5 to 3 mg.

ZINC

Zinc, needed for normal growth and development, is an essential cofactor for the proper functioning of over 100 enzymes required for metabolic processes. Zinc is involved in ribonucleic acid, protein, and carbohydrate metabolism. It acts as a stabilizer of cell membranes and interacts with insulin. Zinc is essential in maintaining health in the macula of the eye. Zinc is also essential for maintenance of arterial wall hemostasis, for brain development, and for stimulation of appetite, taste, and smell. It is also necessary for the maintenance of the sex glands, particularly the prostate. Zinc replacement is also important in wound healing.

Conditions that increase need for zinc include high stress, sepsis, and increased gastrointestinal fluid losses. Some current research indicates that a normal American diet may not contain sufficient zinc. Generally, such insufficiency can be corrected by increasing the intake of foods high in zinc, which include oysters, organ meats, sunflower seeds, cheese, wheat germ, and yeast.

Zinc is absorbed from the intestinal tract via active transport. Of the zinc consumed, only about 20% to 30%

is absorbed. This depends on a number of factors, including the source of zinc. Zinc from animal sources is generally better absorbed than zinc from plant sources. Absorption is also enhanced by pregnancy, corticosteroids, endotoxins, and leukocyte endogenous mediation (e.g., interleukin-2). Zinc is stored in the bones, spleen, and kidney.

Zinc deficiency causes growth failure, particularly in children; dermatitis; and sexual infantilism. With research indicating that zinc is responsible for stimulation of appetite, taste, and smell, deficiencies could be a cause of a child's poor eating habits and consequent poor growth. Signs of excessive zinc intake include lassitude, slow tendon reflexes, bloody enteritis, diarrhea, leukopenia, and central nervous system (CNS) depression.

The RDA for adults is 12 to 15 mg. Zinc is added to TPN solutions and to dialysate solutions to prevent deficiencies.

○ **Zinc sulfate** (*Zinc 15, Orazinc, and others*) is 23% zinc and is used primarily to treat zinc deficiency. It is available for both oral and intravenous administration. To supplement the diet, the average adult dose of zinc is 25 to 50 mg daily. When added to TPN solution, the usual dose is 2.5 to 6 mg IV daily.

○ **Zinc gluconate** is 14.3% zinc. This form of zinc is available only for oral administration. It is also administered in 25 to 50-mg doses for therapeutic use.

IODINE

Iodine, biologically inactive alone, is required by the body to produce the thyroid hormones T_3 (liothyronine) and T_4 (levothyroxine); thus, it is essential for the regulation of body metabolism. Iodine is distributed to all body cells, but it concentrates in the thyroid gland. Dietary sources of iodine include vegetables (especially those growing near the seacoast), seafood, kelp, cod-liver oil, mushrooms, and sunflower seeds. Adequate amounts of iodine can be obtained from iodized salt. In general, the average American diet does not need iodine supplementation.

If iodine deficiency exists, cretinism may occur. In this condition, thyroid gland secretions are reduced or lacking, resulting in the retardation of the physical, sexual, and mental development in children. Adults with iodine deficiency may develop an acquired form of cretinism, called myxedema, and hypothyroidism, with or without a simple endemic goiter. If iodine is excessive, the patient may develop signs of hyperthyroidism, including exophthalmic goiter or Graves' disease (thyrotoxicosis).

For adults the RDA for iodine is 150 μg. In the clinical setting, iodine is available for oral use as potassium iodide and for intravenous use as sodium iodide.

○ **Potassium iodide** (*Iostat, Pima, Thyro-Block, SSKI*) is supplied as a 130-mg tablet, a 300-mg enteric-coated tablet, an oral solution, a saturated oral solution (SSKI—saturated solution of potassium iodide), and a syrup. Doses are expressed in mg of potassium iodide. SSKI contains 1 g of iodine/mL. Potassium iodide is used to treat thyrotoxic crisis, to prepare patients for thyroidectomy, and to protect the thyroid gland from exposure to radiation.

○ **Iodine** (*Iodopen*) is an injectable form of iodine, which contains 100 μg of iodine/mL (as 118 μg of sodium iodide). It is used to prevent iodine deficiency in patients receiving long-term TPN. Iodopen is administered to metabolically stable adults in doses of 1 to 2 $\mu g/kg$ per day and to children and pregnant and lactating women in doses of 2 to 3 $\mu g/kg$ per day.

COBALT

Cobalt is essential for the production of vitamin B_{12} and thus for all of the functions of vitamin B_{12}. (See the vitamin B_{12} section in this chapter.) The daily requirements are easily obtained from a normal diet. Dietary sources of cobalt include seafood, liver, peanuts, butter, and grains. Cobalt is distributed to all tissues. It is stored in the kidney, liver, and bone marrow.

The deficiencies that develop (e.g., anemias) are those related to vitamin B_{12} deficiency. If supplemental cobalt must be administered, cobalt salts are avoided because they are absorbed readily and exert a competitive effect on the absorption of iron and manganese. Vitamin B_{12} is administered instead.

An excessive cobalt level causes the development of polycythemia (because excessive erythropoietin is excreted by the kidney), cardiomyopathies, and thyroid hyperplasia.

CHROMIUM

Normal glucose utilization in humans requires chromium, which affects the sensitivity of peripheral tissues to insulin. A diabetes-like syndrome has been observed in chromium deficiency. Chromium may also act to stabilize the tertiary structures of proteins and nucleic acids, and it apparently stimulates hepatic synthesis of fatty acids and cholesterol from acetate. Dietary sources of chromium include seafood, organ meats, peanuts, American cheese, wheat, and wheat germ. Chromium is stored in the skin, muscles, fat, testes, bone, liver, and spleen.

○ **Chromium** (*Chrometrace, chromic chloride*) is used to prevent deficiency in patients receiving TPN. The suggested daily intravenous intake of chromium is 10 to 20 μg. The oral dose is 50 to 200 μg daily. For supplementation, the RDA for adults is 0.29 mg/day.

MANGANESE

Manganese activates several enzymes, such as liver arginase and serum alkaline phosphatase. It is also involved in the synthesis of cholesterol, fatty acids, and mucopolysaccharides and in CNS function. Dietary sources of manganese include snails, peanuts, blueberries, olives, corn, corn germ, wheat, wheat germ, and tea. Manganese is stored in small amounts in the brain, kidneys, pancreas, and liver.

Symptoms of manganese deficiency include weight loss, transient dermatitis, occasional nausea and vomiting, slow growth, and changes in hair color. In animals, a diabetes-like glucose tolerance curve is seen in manganese deficiency. No RDA has been established for manganese, but an estimated safe and adequate daily intake of 2 to 5 mg has been recommended. This amount is usually provided by normal dietary intake.

○ **Chelated manganese** is administered as a dietary supplement only. The usual oral dose is 5 to 50 mg daily.

○ **Manganese sulfate** (*Mangatrace*) is administered parenterally to adults in doses of 0.15 to 0.8 mg/day and to children in doses of 2 to 10 μg/kg per day. It is also added to TPN solutions in doses of 0.15 to 0.8 mg per day.

USING THE NURSING PROCESS

ASSESSMENT

- Patients suspected of having vitamin or mineral excesses or deficiencies must have careful assessments. The information obtained is featured in Table 13–5.
- Obtain a diet history. It should include the intake of fortified foods, style of eating (e.g., one or several

meals daily), special diets (whether prescribed by physician or followed through religious or personal preference, such as kosher or vegetarian regimen), cultural background, economic status, the patient's personal views about nutrition, and the patient's smoking history.

- Obtain information on current use of self-administered or prescription vitamins and minerals including reasons for use, length of time used, dosage, frequency of administration, and who prescribed them. Also ask about the use of other medications or other dietary supplements. As an example, women taking oral contraceptives tend to have higher plasma levels of vitamin A, and if they were to take large supplemental doses of vitamin A, they might have a ten-

---

Table 13–5. NURSING PROCESS FOR PATIENT REQUIRING VITAMINS AND MINERALS

Assessment

Assess nutrition history, including style of eating, special diets (e.g., vegetarian), cultural eating patterns, personal food preferences. Assess socioeconomic status.
Assess current drug history and use of self-administered/prescribed vitamins/minerals and other medications used (including oral contraceptives.)
Assess presence of deficiency states.
Assess laboratory studies specific to the deficiency.

Nursing Diagnosis: Altered Nutrition, Less Than Body Requirements	**Desired Outcomes/Evaluation Criteria**
RELATED TO: Inability to ingest/digest food or to absorb nutrients because of biologic, psychologic, or economic factors. **AS EVIDENCED BY:** Reported inadequate food intake, altered taste sensation, poor muscle tone, sore/inflamed buccal cavity, capillary fragility.	Verbalizes understanding of causative factors and necessary interventions. Demonstrates change of nutritional habits to regain/maintain positive nutritional status and is free of signs of deficiency.

Nursing Actions	**Rationale**
Administer prescribed supplements as appropriate. Review usual daily dietary intake-patterns. Discuss dietary sources of specific deficient vitamins/minerals.	Provides for more rapid correction of identified deficiencies or may be used to prevent deficiency (e.g., prenatal). Useful for identifying strengths/deficiencies within diet. In most cases, once deficiency is corrected, ingestion of a balanced diet (possibly with an OTC daily product) will prevent recurrence and reduce likelihood of side-effects/adverse reactions related to drug therapy.

Nursing Diagnosis: Knowledge Deficit	**Desired Outcomes/Evaluation Criteria**
RELATED TO: Lack of exposure/recall, information misinterpretation, unfamiliarity with information resources. **AS EVIDENCED BY:** Questions, statement of concern, development of preventable complications.	Verbalizes understanding of condition/disease process and treatment. Takes vitamin/mineral supplements correctly and explains reasons for individual regimen.

Nursing Actions	**Rationale**
Provide information (verbal and written) concerning patient's individual deficiencies and treatment needs. Discuss specific factors for safe vitamin/mineral administration, e.g., some may be taken with food to enhance absorption or reduce gastric irritation; some may potentiate or interfere with other medications, laboratory tests; some may cause urinary stone formation. Discuss current beliefs of patient/significant other about vitamins/minerals and provide objective information.	Accurate information helps patient control own situation and prevents complications from inappropriate use. Helps to get the most from medication regimen and prevent untoward effects. Many individuals believe that most illness/conditions can be treated and cured with vitamin/mineral therapy, and correcting myths and misconceptions helps patient to deal with own situation more effectively.

dency to develop symptoms of vitamin A toxicity. Also, oral contraceptives can deplete vitamin C stores.

Many people know what they should eat even though they may not eat correctly. Take care during the diet history to assume a nonjudgmental attitude and to avoid leading questions so that the information will be as accurate as possible. Vegetarian diets using multiple food sources can provide essential nutrients if milk products or eggs are added to supply vitamin B_{12}. As vegetarian diets become more restrictive, the risk of nutritional inadequacies increases greatly, especially deficiencies of protein, vitamin B_{12}, calcium, vitamin D, and riboflavin. The Zen macrobiotic diets can endanger health. In particular, infants fed KoKoh, a Zen macrobiotic food mixture for infant feeding, grow poorly and become protein malnourished, which may lead to death. Most deficiency states develop from poor dietary habits; therefore, during the intervention phase, dietary management is stressed. Vitamin and mineral supplementation cannot make up for a poor diet.

- Assess the patient for vitamin deficiencies. The older, critically ill adult often is a candidate for vitamin deficiencies. Patients experiencing gum disease and loose teeth, bone pain, respiratory infections, spontaneous hemorrhages, and anemia may be exhibiting a vitamin C deficiency or other deficiency, which needs to be assessed and treated.

- Assess the patient who develops a deficiency of the fat-soluble vitamins A, D, E, or K for possible abuse of laxatives, particularly mineral oil. Oily laxatives prevent absorption of the fat-soluble vitamins in the intestine. Also, a patient who is allowed nothing by mouth and is taking antibiotics needs to be carefully assessed for vitamin K deficiencies.

- Assess the patient's need for supplemental vitamin or mineral therapy. Infants and children may need supplemental therapy, as well as pregnant and lactating women. In general, the physician prescribes vitamin or mineral supplements for these age groups. However, the physician may suggest a multivitamin and mineral preparation. The patient may ask the nurse's assistance in choosing an appropriate product. The pharmacist or registered dietitian may also be of help in selecting vitamin and mineral supplements. The nurse must be aware of the common OTC vitamin and mineral preparations and their primary ingredients to effectively suggest a preparation during the intervention phase.

The federal Food and Drug Administration divides vitamin and mineral products into three groups:

1. Supplemental—all ingredients are within established limits.
2. OTC proprietary—the vitamin/mineral content is above standard limits, but not excessive.
3. Prescription status—contents exceed OTC proprietary limits and are available by prescription only.

- Assess for hypersensitivity to aspirin, aspirin-like products, and products containing tartrazine before administering certain vitamins (e.g., C, D, or niacin) or minerals (e.g., potassium). Also, patients who will

Table 13–6. DRUGS THAT CAUSE HEMATOLOGIC TOXICITY

Drug	A	B	C	D	E
Antimalarials			x		
Antithyroid drugs	x				
Cephalosporins			x		
Chloramphenicol	x	x	x		x
Chlorpropamide		x			x
Diphenylhydantoin				x	
Folic acid antagonists				x	
Gold salts		x			x
Methyldopa			x		x
Phenothiazine tranquilizers	x				
Phenylbutazone	x	x			x
Sulfonamides	x	x	x		x
Thiazides	x				x

A = agranulocytosis; B = aplastic anemia; C = hemolytic anemia; D = megaloblastic anemia; E = thrombocytopenia.

be receiving iodine need to be assessed for an allergy to seafood.

- When anemia is diagnosed, assess both objective and subjective symptoms at the onset of treatment and periodically during treatment to determine the effectiveness of the therapy. Before therapy is undertaken, a definitive diagnosis of the anemia is essential, including its possible underlying cause. A thorough history to determine when symptoms began is important. Has the patient had a recent history of gastrointestinal tract disease, or bleeding in the lung, or epistaxis? Or, does he or she have a history of chronic disease, or drug therapy? Table 13–6 reviews drugs that are known to cause various types of hematologic toxicity. Also, it is important to determine how symptoms have changed over time.

- Assist with gathering laboratory data, such as red cell indices, blood smears, leukocyte count, differentials, reticulocyte count, and platelet count. Bone marrow aspiration may also be performed.

- Assess dietary intake to determine whether the cause of the anemia is diet related and whether dietary teaching is needed later during the intervention stage. Iron deficiency is the most common deficiency in the United States among children and young women. In men and postmenopausal women, the most common cause is abnormal bleeding, which may be obvious or occult—often a sign of bowel cancer. Folic acid deficiencies are less common than vitamin B_{12} deficiencies, and other hematopoietic deficiencies are rare.

NURSING DIAGNOSIS

- Possible nursing diagnoses for a patient with a vitamin and/or mineral imbalance include Altered Nutrition: Less than Body Requirements and Knowledge Deficit (see Table 13–5).

PLANNING AND INTERVENTION

- From the nursing diagnoses, develop the goals of the nursing intervention, which will, in turn, become the evaluation criteria (see Table 13–5). The more the patient and family are involved with the planning process, the more likely they are to comply with the treatment regimen.

Nursing Responsibilities in Administering Vitamins and Minerals

• It may be necessary to administer vitamins and minerals in a clinical setting to patients who cannot receive sufficient oral nourishment. Many vitamins and minerals can be administered both intramuscularly (IM) and IV.

Intravenous vitamins and minerals should not be mixed with other preparations in the same IV bottle unless doing so is known to be safe, as there may be drug interactions. For example, mixing vitamins B and C in the same IV bottle with antibiotics generally causes the antibiotic to be destroyed. Check with a pharmacist or other reliable reference before mixing any vitamin or mineral with another drug. Also check the expiration date to ensure that the vitamin or mineral preparation is effective.

All parenteral vitamins and minerals need to be well diluted to decrease vessel irritation. Solutions of vitamins and minerals are discarded after 24 hours if they are not used.

Vitamin mixtures, particularly those containing vitamins A, B_1, B_2, and B_6 , are light sensitive. Some authorities suggest that all IV bottles containing vitamin products should be covered with an ultraviolet filter (UVF) cover so the vitamins are not degraded by light.

• To administer vitamins and minerals to the patient safely, consider the following specific points:
  1. Mineral oil is avoided in all patients taking any of the fat-soluble vitamins.
  2. Mineral products, except for zinc, are best taken immediately after meals to prevent gastrointestinal upset.
  3. Zinc is not taken concurrently with dairy products or a high-fiber diet (fiber interferes with absorption of zinc).
  4. Liquid preparations are well diluted before administration to improve taste and decrease gastric irritation.
  5. Iron products (antianemic medications) may need to be administered parenterally. Remember that a skin test to detect allergies is performed before administering the first dose, as anaphylactic reactions can occur. Also, medications are administered deep IM to prevent irritation to the subcutaneous tissues. When the nurse administers iron dextran, a special Z-tract intramuscular injection technique is used (see Chapter 3).

Because the IM route is associated with several disadvantages, including pain and discoloration at the site, more physicians are ordering IV iron dextran (Imferon without preservative). The incidence of allergic reaction for both IM and IV administration is about the same. If the patient experiences vomiting, chills, fever, headache, joint pain, or urticaria, the infusion is stopped. Phlebitis is a common side effect of IV administration, but it can be minimized by mixing the iron dextran in normal saline solution and infusing the preparation at a rate of no faster than 50 mg/min (1 mL/min). Often, the entire iron deficit can be replaced in one infusion rather than in several IM injections.

For nursing interventions for specific vitamins, see Tables 13–2 and 13–3; for iron products, see Table 13–4.

Patient Teaching

• Many individuals have come to believe that just about any malady—from sexual difficulties to cancer—can be treated and cured with vitamin and mineral therapy. Most processed food, from breakfast cereals to frozen dinners, is enriched with vitamins and minerals. Some individuals may begin self-treatment with megadose vitamins and minerals to cure a problem that should have medical attention. Approximately 75% of the public believes that vitamins provide extra energy; however, no vitamin produces a rapid burst of energy. Vitamin supplements are also not effective in protecting against emotional stress. Interestingly, a recent survey of pharmacists indicated that they most often recommend vitamin and mineral supplements for complaints of fatigue and stress.As an educator, the nurse has a responsibility to be aware of the various claims for vitamin therapy, to evaluate the existing research, and then to disseminate objective information to patients.

• During the intervention phase the nurse emphasizes that diet is the treatment of choice—the five basic food groups using the food pyramid—for vitamin and mineral deficiencies. Teaching of proper dietary intake is of primary importance. Warn the patient that vitamins should not be used in place of a balanced diet. Before discharge, teach the patient that vitamins and minerals are best preserved by cooking foods in the smallest amount of water possible and that microwave cooking is an excellent way to preserve vitamins and minerals.

The bioavailability of a number of minerals may be altered by the special characteristics of a vegetarian diet. Plant-based diets may alter the levels of zinc, calcium, iron, manganese, selenium, and copper. Vegetarians can avoid potential problems in mineral status by limiting fiber, phytase, and oxalate to a reasonable degree; and eating a wide variety of nutrient-dense foods.

• It is important to discuss the use of vitamins for children with their parents. The American Academy of Pediatrics committee on nutrition states "there is no good evidence that suggests that supplements are necessary for the child who is steadily gaining height and weight." Because most vitamins are water soluble, once the body has enough to meet its needs and supply a small safety margin, the excess is flushed out as urine or perspiration. The fat-soluble vitamins—A, D, E, and K—if taken in excess, are stored in the liver and other organs and can cause toxic symptoms.

Children who take vitamins daily begin a "drug" habit in their early years. The chewable vitamins are thought of by children (or even suggested by parents) to be candy. Several surveys have found that 50% of 3-year-olds think it is okay to eat the entire bottle of chewables or other food-flavored medications.

- Vitamins and minerals are taken until the initial deficiency is treated. Daily multivitamin/mineral supplements may then need to be taken for life. If a dose is forgotten, tell the patient to skip it and to take the next dose at the regular time. Advise the patient not to stop his or her medication without checking with the physician.

- Vitamins and minerals can interfere with other medications, such as vitamin A with oral contraceptives; and 5 mg/day or more of vitamin B_6 (pyridoxine) may enhance the metabolism of levodopa (L-dopa), making it less effective in treating Parkinson's disease. Ensure that the patient knows of any such interactions.

- Vitamins and minerals can interfere with laboratory tests. For example, vitamin K can falsely elevate urinary steroids, and vitamin B_2 can cause false elevations of urinary catecholamines.

Table 13–7. PATIENT TEACHING— VITAMINS AND MINERALS

Dear Patient:

This drug has been ordered for you. This is what you should know about your drug to get the most from your therapy.

- ☐ 1. Vitamins and minerals are taken to return your own body levels to normal and to maintain that level.
- ☐ 2. Vitamins and minerals are taken until the initial deficiency is treated. Then, you may need to take multivitamin/mineral supplements daily for the rest of your life.
- ☐ 3. Vitamins and minerals can be taken with or between meals. Taking them with meals may prevent stomach upset. Mix liquids well to improve taste.
- ☐ 4. Vitamins and minerals can interfere with other medications or health problems. Check with your doctor or pharmacist before taking extra vitamins and minerals.
- ☐ 5. Vitamins and minerals can interfere with laboratory tests. Tell your doctor that you are taking vitamin and mineral products before blood or urine tests are done.
- ☐ 6. If you forget a dose, do not take it, but move on to the next dose.
- ☐ 7. Do not stop taking your vitamins and minerals without checking with your physician.
- ☐ 8. Vitamins lose stability and become less potent as they age. Vitamins may lose as much as one-third of their potency in 1 month and as much as 80% in 6 months. Look at expiration dates on vitamin bottles, and do not buy large quantities of vitamins that will not be taken until many months later.
- ☐ 9. Read vitamin labels and buy the least expensive one that meets your needs. The Food and Drug Administration requires that all vitamin labels have the amount of each ingredient and the amount of the recommended daily allowance (RDA) in each tablet.
- ☐ 10. Megadoses, those that far exceed the RDA, have as yet not been proven to be helpful and may even be harmful.
- ☐ 11. Store vitamins and minerals in tight, light-resistant, dry containers away from children. Adult vitamins, especially those with iron, can be toxic to small children.

Table 13–8. PATIENT TEACHING—ANTIANEMICS

Dear Patient:

This drug has been ordered for you. This is what you should know about your drug to get the most from your therapy.

- ☐ 1. Antianemic drugs, such as _____, are taken to improve your body's ability to make healthy blood.
- ☐ 2. You will take antianemics until your anemia is gone. (This may be 3 to 5 months or a lifetime depending on the anemia.)
- ☐ 3. Oral iron products are absorbed best when taken between meals; however, they may be irritating to the stomach, so you may find it better to take them with or immediately following meals.
- ☐ 4. Liquid products are diluted in a liquid and taken through a straw to avoid staining of your teeth. Rinse your mouth immediately after taking. (Feosol elixir can be mixed with water only—*not* with milk, fruit juice, or wine. Fer-in-Sol drops may be given in all liquids.)
- ☐ 5. Interactions between your drug and others may occur. Talk with your pharmacist or physician before taking other drugs.
- ☐ 6. If you forget a dose for more than 12 hours, skip it.
- ☐ 7. Do not stop taking your drugs without checking with your doctor.
- ☐ 8. Typical side effects of your drug are constipation, diarrhea, stomach pains, staining of the teeth, pain at the injection site, temporary or permanent skin color change at the injection site, headache, muscle ache, nausea and vomiting, fever, and mild itching.
- ☐ 9. Drugs may cause dark green or black stools.
- ☐ 10. Your diet is very important. It helps treat the present anemia and prevents further problems from occurring.
- ☐ 11. Reversal of symptoms usually begins to occur within 2 to 5 days after treatment is started. You may be asked to have frequent blood testing done to evaluate progress.
- ☐ 12. Store drugs in tight, light-resistant containers out of the reach of children.

- Vitamins lose stability and become less potent as they age. Vitamins may lose as much as one-third of their potency in 1 month and as much as 80% in 6 months. Advise the patient to check expiration dates on vitamin bottles and to discard old vitamins.

- Advise the patient to read vitamin labels. The Food and Drug Administration requires that all vitamin labels identify the amount of each ingredient and the proportion of the Recommended Dietary Allowance (RDA) or the United States Recommended Daily Allowance (U.S. RDA) in each tablet.

- Megadoses, doses that far exceed the RDA, have as yet not been proven to be helpful and may even be harmful. Vitamins that are the same as or only slightly higher than the RDA should be purchased. Caution any patient who is taking or planning to take vitamin C that megadoses may enhance crystal formation in the urine, which may cause dysfunctions for the patient, including hypervitaminosis and hypermineralosis.

- Warn the patient to keep all vitamins and minerals out of the reach of children. Tell the patient to store them in tight, light-resistant containers and to protect them from heat to prevent deterioration.

- Teach the patient the adverse effects of his or her medications. The patient should report symptoms to the physician or nurse.

Additional patient teaching information is provided in Tables 13–7 and 13–8.

EVALUATION

- Base the evaluation of the effectiveness of vitamin and mineral therapy on a predetermined list of evaluation criteria, which are developed on an individual basis through discussion among the nurse, patient, and family during the planning phase (see Table 13–5).
- Evaluate the patient to determine if he or she is taking the proper dosage of vitamins and minerals. Several vitamins are commonly abused.

- When anemia is the diagnosis, it is important to evaluate daily intake of all nutrients. Also evaluate the patient's dietary knowledge. The anemia may be the result of dietary deficiencies. Evaluate the patient for hematologic toxicity, which can occur secondarily to many drugs (see Table 13–7).
- Evaluate the patient's knowledge about the toxic or adverse effects of his or her medications.
- Before discharge, review and update all previously taught material, if necessary, to ensure that the patient's knowledge base remains accurate.

The bibliography for this chapter can be found in Appendix B, which begins on page 1054.

CHAPTER REVIEW QUESTIONS*

1. Which of the following is a fat-soluble vitamin?
   a. Biotin.
   b. Niacin.
   c. Vitamin K.
   d. Vitamin B$_{12}$.

2. Toxic side effects of vitamin A include:
   a. Insomnia
   b. Alopecia.
   c. Tetany.
   d. Hypomagnesemia.

3. Vitamin D is used in the treatment of:
   a. Hypercalcemia.
   b. Hypocalcemia.
   c. Hyperparathyroidism.
   d. Hypomagnesemia.

4. Which of the following reflects correct nursing practice when administering vitamins and minerals?
   a. Mineral oil should be avoided in patients taking the B vitamins.

   b. Intravenous solutions with multivitamins added should be protected from light.
   c. Vitamin D is best given on an empty stomach to enhance adsorption.
   d. The dosage of vitamin K is determined by PTT levels.

5. Vitamin C should be avoided in patients who are taking:
   a. Anticoagulants.
   b. Calcium agents.
   c. Penicillin antibiotics.
   d. Birth control pills.

6. A nursing responsibility associated with intravenous iron dextran administration is to:
   a. Administer a test dose before starting infusion.
   b. Give the drug at a rate of 100 mg/min.
   c. Reduce infusion rate if signs of allergy appear.
   d. Administer the drug undiluted to reduce phlebitis.

*See Appendix A, which begins on page 1051, for answers.

CHAPTER 14

Enteral and Parenteral Nutritional Agents

Merrily A. Kuhn, RNC, PhD

CHAPTER OUTLINE

Nutrition
Enteral Nutrition
Parenteral Nutrition
Using the Nursing Process

TABLES

Nursing Process
Nursing Process for Patient Requiring Enteral/Parenteral
    Nutrition, 193
Patient Teaching
Patient Teaching Information—Patients Requiring Feedings
    at Home, 199

BOXES

Delivering Home Health Care, 202
Building Your Critical Thinking Skills, 203

KEY TERMS

Anabolism
Anthropometric parameters
Aromatic amino acids
Branched-chain amino acids
Catabolism
Enteral
Gluconeogenesis
Glycolysis
Hydrolyzed
Hyperalimentation

Kilocalorie
Lipolysis
Malnutrition
Marasmus
Opsonic proteins
Protein-calorie malnutrition
Proteolysis
Somatic proteins
Visceral proteins

LEARNING OBJECTIVES

After reading this chapter, the student will be able to:

1. Compare and contrast states of nutrition and malnutrition.
2. Identify those agents commonly used as enteral and parenteral products.
3. Identify specific areas to assess in the patient requiring enteral and parenteral agents to formulate appropriate patient outcomes.
4. Plan the nursing interventions necessary to administer nutritional agents and choose appropriate teaching strategies to gain patient compliance.
5. Evaluate the patient at various stages of treatment to measure nursing interventions.

Nutrition is an important aspect of patient care. Many patients in hospitals and nursing homes suffer from *malnutrition*. Malnutrition is the loss of more than 10% lean body mass in 2 weeks. It is suggested that 69% of patients having an ICU admission leave the hospital in a malnourished state, and that 5% to 10% of these patients suffer from severe protein-calorie malnutrition. A well-nourished patient can usually tolerate 5 to 7 days of fasting, provided standard intravenous fluids are infused to maintain hydration. However, acutely ill patients have increased energy needs and may even need double their normal calorie requirements. For example, a 70-kg man who is undergoing surgery requires 2800 kcal/day, one

who has a trauma or sepsis requires 4200 kcal/day, and one who has extensive burns requires 5600 kcal/day.

Malnutrition is associated with increased length of hospital or nursing home stay resulting from poor wound healing, muscle atrophy, impaired immunocompetence related to depressed cell-mediated immunity and reduced lymphocyte count, septic syndrome, and sepsis. A reduction in plasma proteins leads to dry, flaky skin; peripheral edema; and even noncardiac pulmonary edema. Typical laboratory tests that indicate nutritional depletion are featured in Table 14–1.

If a patient enters the hospital in a malnourished state, he or she requires nutritional support immediately. A pa-

Table 14–1. LABORATORY TESTS AND VALUES INDICATING A MALNOURISHED STATE

Nutritional Status	Albumin (g/dL)	Transferrin (mg/dL)	TLC* (cells/mm³)	Prealbumin (mg/dL)
Normal	3.5+	200+	1800+	17–40
Mild malnutrition	3.0–3.5	150–200	1500–1800	14–16
Moderate malnutrition	2.1–3.0	100–150	900–1500	11–13
Severe malnutrition	<2.1	<100	<900	<10

*TLC = total lymphocyte count: $TLC = \dfrac{\%\ \text{lymphocytes} \times WBC}{100}$

tient may have nutritional needs met either by the *enteral* route, through the mouth or into the gastrointestinal tract, or by the *parenteral* route, through the vascular system.

The goals of nutrition support therapy are derived from the processes of the metabolic response to injury. The goals include the following: (1) to support current organ function and structure, (2) to prevent malnutrition from developing, (3) to treat malnutrition when present, and (4) to do no harm.

NUTRITION

Nutritional requirements vary according to a person's age, weight, and physical activity level and the rate and extent of metabolic activity within the body. The normal daily calorie requirement for a healthy adult between the ages of 20 and 50 is 1500 to 3000 calories. These calories are provided by the ingestion of foods, which contain nutrients—carbohydrate (45% to 60% or 380 to 504 g), protein (20% or 45 to 55 g), and fat (20% to 35% or 56 to 100 g)—that provide energy. These nutrients—along with the necessary vitamins and minerals—must be consumed daily to maintain normal body activities and constant body weight.

This chapter briefly reviews normal nutrition. For a more complete review, see a physiology nursing text. The main emphasis of discussion is affects of malnutrition and starvation on the body.

METABOLISM

There are two main phases of metabolism: catabolism and anabolism, featured in Table 14–2. *Catabolism* is the breaking down of complex substances into simpler constituents for use in energy production or excretion. *Anabolism* is the synthesis of cellular materials for growth, maintenance, and repair of body tissues, during which simple substances are combined to form more complex substances with a net result of new cellular material and the storage of energy. When anabolism exceeds catabolism, lean body mass (LBM) and fat are produced and growth occurs. When catabolism exceeds anabolism, tissue is lost and the body loses substance and weight. Hormones are activated by anbolism and catabolism. See Table 14–1 for a review of hormone stimulation.

When food is consumed and metabolized, the energy produced is measured in calories, or *kilocalorie* (kcal), the heat energy required to raise the temperature of 1 kg of water 1°C. The terms kcal and calorie are used interchangeably. Nutrients produce energy at various levels: 1 g of protein produces 4 calories, 1 g of fat produces 9 calories, and 1 g of carbohydrate produces 4 calories.

Carbohydrates

Carbohydrates, sugars composed of carbon, hydrogen, and oxygen, are oxidized through the process of *glycolysis*, the metabolic breakdown of complex carbohydrates into simpler sugars, that is, polysaccharides, disaccharides, and monosaccharides. The two important polysaccharides are starch and glycogen. The disaccharides are sucrose (equals glucose and fructose), lactose (equals glucose and galactose), and maltose. Monosaccharides, the

Table 14–2. ANABOLISM VERSUS CATABOLISM

Anabolism	Catabolism
Nitrogen Balance	
Positive	Negative
Simple > Complex	Complex > Simple
Hormones	
Insulin	Epinephrine
Growth hormone	Glucocorticoids
Anabolic steroids	Glucagon
Testosterone	
17-Ketosteroids	
Activated by	
Puberty	Fever
	Illness
	Stress
	Trauma
	Burns
Results in	
Weight gain	Weight loss
Growth and repair	Decreased wound healing
	Anemia
	Leukopenia
	Decreased immune function
	Muscle wasting
	Decreased mentation
	Increased temperature, pulse, and respiration
	Decreased level of consciousness
	Poor skin turgor
	Skin lesions
	Tissue edema, eczema

simplest sugars, include glucose, fructose, and galactose. Glucose is the preferred fuel for some tissues, such as the brain, and red blood cells.

Extra carbohydrate in the body is stored as glycogen in the liver and muscle. From these sites, glucose is immediately available for maintenance of blood sugar (liver) and anaerobic glycolysis for exercise (muscle). The amount of glycogen stored in the body is about 300 grams.

Lipids

Lipids, or fats, are composed of fatty acids and triglycerides (which transport and are the storage forms of fatty acids) containing carbon, hydrogen, and oxygen. Triglycerides are *hydrolyzed* (metabolically broken down by the chemical addition of water molecules) to form glycerol and fatty acids, which then are available for oxidation for energy. During starvation, fatty acid oxidation rates are high and the liver produces large quantities of ketones, which can be oxidized for energy in most tissues.

Fat, the principal form of energy storage in the body, is anhydrous and, therefore, can be stored without water. The amount of fat a person can store is unlimited. Fats are responsible for maintaining the lipid lining of cells and for the synthesis of immune response mediators such as prostaglandins and thromboxanes. Fats are also an appropriate fuel for hyperglycemic patients if peripheral tissues are insulin insensitive, reducing the usefulness of carbohydrate as an energy source.

Protein

Protein consists of amino acids that are unique in that they contain nitrogen along with carbon, hydrogen, and water. Body components, such as cells, enzymes, muscle fibers, collagen, and antibodies, are protein. All proteins in the body perform some structural or functional role. Protein is necessary to manufacture hemoglobin, maintain immunocompetence, and create and maintain gradient pressures. Unlike other nutrients, protein has no storage form and must be consumed on a daily basis. Protein consumed in excess of body requirements is converted to fat for storage.

Branched-chain amino acids (valine, leucine, and isoleucine) may be oxidized directly in skeletal muscle, which is a potential energy source for muscle. Patients with trauma, sepsis, or severe stress have greater branched-chain oxidation; therefore, requirements are increased.

Patients with liver disease ultimately have a change in the normal plasma amino acid profile with an increase in the aromatic amino acids, which may contribute to hepatic encephalopathy. *Aromatic amino acids* are amino acids that contain a benzene ring (e.g., phenylalanine, methionine, tryptophan).

RESPIRATORY QUOTIENT

The respiratory quotient (RQ) is the ratio of carbon dioxide production to oxygen utilization by the body. Carbon dioxide is a byproduct of metabolism that is eliminated by the lung. When carbohydrates are metabolized in the body, an average of 100 carbon dioxide molecules are formed for each 100 molecules of oxygen consumed; therefore, the RQ for carbohydrates is 1.0. The RQ for fat is 0.7, and the RQ for protein is 0.8. The RQs for fat and protein are lower because a large share of the oxygen metabolized with these foods is required to combine with the excess hydrogen ions present in them instead of forming carbon dioxide. The average RQ for a well-balanced diet is approximately 0.8.

NUTRITION IN ILLNESS

Persons may have difficulty digesting, absorbing, or metabolizing food, as with recent bowel surgery, a malabsorption syndrome such as sprue, or an enzyme deficiency or allergic reactions to food. For example, lactase (enzyme required for the digestion of milk) levels decrease with aging, causing intolerances to milk. In addition, persons may become undernourished with chronic illness like cancer, acute trauma, or severe burns. In each of these instances, catabolism is accelerated, and the individual loses weight and lacks energy for even normal metabolic functions. Signs and symptoms that can be observed in a patient in a catabolic state are featured in Table 14–2. At this point, the patient must receive additional nutrients either through tube feedings or by the parenteral route if the oral route is impossible or inadequate.

Starvation begins when nutrients are not supplied to the body in adequate amounts. A normal adult has about 200 g of glycogen (900 kcal) stored in the liver, 6000 g of protein (24,000 kcal) found in muscles and visceral proteins, and 15,000 g of fat (141,000 kcal) in storage, with fat content varying the most among individuals. When food no longer enters the body, these stores are utilized for energy production. Glycogen stores are used first, with primary glycogenolysis occurring in the liver to increase blood glucose. The glycogen stores are usually exhausted in 8 to 10 hours. Glucose requirements are then met by the initiation of *gluconeogenesis*, which is the formation of glucose from noncarbohydrate sources such as protein and fat. Although various substances are shuttled to the liver and kidneys for conversion to glycogen, amino acids derived from muscle and visceral proteins are the major substrate for this process. The protein must have the nitrogen (N) removed before it can be converted into glucose; the nitrogen is then excreted in the urine (1 g N equals 6.25 g of protein). Therefore, as urinary nitrogen increases, a negative nitrogen balance (catabolism) develops.

In the first few days of starvation, the body may break down up to 75 g of protein daily to meet energy requirements. At this rate of protein breakdown, a third of the body protein would be depleted in several weeks, leading to death. In addition, protein, although calorically important, is not accumulated or stored in humans purely as a nutritional reservoir. Each protein molecule serves a nonfuel function—as an enzyme or as a contractile, structural, or carrier protein. Because each molecule is already serving some nonfuel function, an adaptive process occurs to spare protein. Protein catabolism diminishes with prolonged starvation because of a change in fuel utilization. When food is consumed and glucose is available, the body, particularly the brain and nervous system, preferentially utilizes glucose for energy. In starvation, the body adapts to the lack of glucose and begins to break down fats (adipose tissue) to fatty acids and ketone bodies for energy to spare protein.

This adaptive process occurs through hormone-mediated changes. The amount of insulin secreted by a normal individual decreases during starvation. This decrease triggers the lipolytic release of fatty acids and glycerol from adipose tissue to be used either directly or indirectly as metabolic fuel. The oxidation of adipose tissue is also associated with a sharp rise in ketone bodies, as the body gradually enters a state described as "starvation ketosis." This ketosis is characterized by a decrease in endogenous protein catabolism as a fuel source and by a conversion of the central nervous system (CNS) to ketone body metabolism. Once this adaptive process occurs, protein breakdown decreases to 20 to 25 g daily, and urinary nitrogen excretion also decreases.

A feedback mechanism exists to prevent a pathologic ketosis from occurring, as is seen in diabetes. As ketone levels rise, insulin production is stimulated, and the lipolytic process is temporarily decreased.

With the adaptation to starvation ketosis, the fasting state can be prolonged, depending on the amount of body fat an individual has. Seventy percent of the brain's energy needs can be supplied by the oxidation of ketones, with glucose from amino acids supplying the rest. When fat stores are depleted, muscle and organ tissue are then sacrificed for energy. A normal healthy individual cannot tolerate a loss of more than 35% to 45% of his or her body weight.

A totally fasting healthy person adapts to an economical utilization of body fat and a conservation of body protein to the greatest possible extent. The person who is stressed (e.g., as a result of burns, surgery, trauma, infection, or shock) does not adapt as well to starvation. Starvation begins to occur as early as 24 hours after the initial stress when the patient has no oral intake and is being supported only with regular IV fluids such as dextrose and water, Ringer's lactate, or normal saline solutions.

When stress of disease or injury occurs, catabolism begins just after the onset because of the increased energy demands. Research has indicated that there is a 13% rise in metabolic rate for each 1°C (1.8°F) rise in temperature. Energy demands may be 60% above normal and higher. In addition to a negative nitrogen balance, deficiencies of potassium, magnesium, phosphate, sulfate, zinc, and other trace elements occur and can persist through convalescence. Stress, then, causes dramatic alterations in nutrient metabolism, as the normal adaptive processes that occur in starvation are prevented.

Glucose requirements increase as the body responds to the stress situation. A relative insulin resistance occurs, as the tissues are not as responsive to insulin in the uptake of glucose. This leads to greater production of insulin, which in turn decreases *lipolysis* (metabolic breakdown of fat). Because the body has only minimal glycogen stores and fat is not easily mobilized in this situation, protein catabolism increases to provide a substrate for gluconeogenesis as well as amino acids needed to synthesize blood cells, structural proteins, and enzymes. In addition to the

body's need for more nutrients during fever or infection, there are usually greater losses of body fluids and nutrients such as through vomiting or diarrhea, hemorrhage, transudation and exudation, wound drainage, and intestinal losses.

After several days, sufficient ketone bodies become available to decrease the demand on endogenous protein. However, the catabolism of protein continues with detrimental effects on the immune system, wound healing, the respiratory system, and lean body mass in general.

In a stress state, the bone marrow may be depleted of white blood cells (WBC), red blood cells (RBC), and platelets). It takes approximately 10 days to regenerate a supply of blood cells. If protein is not available, blood cells are not processed. The older adult is further compromised because aging results in one-third of the bone marrow going to fat. Therefore, instead of 3 liters of functional bone marrow, the older adult has only 2 liters.

Stress decreases bowel activity, secretions, and protective mechanisms and shuts down all alpha tone. Blood supply is rerouted to other more vital organs like the heart, brain, and kidney. Historically, the gut has been perceived as being dormant following stress because during the first 24 hours after surgery or trauma, the stomach does not empty normally. Nausea, vomiting, and acute gastric dilation may occur due to gastroparesis. Although gastric motility is abnormal for 1 to 2 days and colon peristalsis is impaired for 3 to 5 days following stress, small bowel motility and absorption are unaltered.

Paralytic ileus, which is usually confined to the stomach, is often cited as a contraindication for enteral feeding. However, because the small intestine still functions, feeding into the duodenum or jejunum is often successful, even in the absence of bowel sounds, because it bypasses the site of gastric ileus.

The villi, where nutrients are absorbed, are shed and rebuilt every 36 hours. To do this, the villi need a continuous supply of oxygen and glucose, which are both reduced or absent during stress. Many drugs and conditions also decrease the availability of oxygen and glucose to the gut. These include anesthetics, alpha-adrenergic agonists, digitalis glycosides, immunosuppressants, head and spinal cord injuries, hypotension, fluid and electrolyte imbalances, and anemia. The gut also needs glutamine, an amino acid, to assist with breakdown of ammonia. Immunosuppression with steroids decreases the bacteria in the gut by 30%, so colonization in the large bowel decreases. Antibiotics sterilize the gut, allowing the overgrowth and colonization of fungi and yeast, which usually are not affected by antibiotics.

In the critically ill, many factors upset normal flora. When the pH is 1, the stomach is sterile, and the high hydrochloric acid content helps to kill the bacteria in the food. Antacids and H_2 inhibitors raise the pH in the stomach to 4 to 8. As the pH rises, the normally sterile stomach becomes colonized. When a nasogastric (NG) tube or an intestinal tube is placed, it acts as a ladder and the bacteria crawl up, leading to sinusitis and pneumonias. Feeding the stomach, even if it is only 1 or 2 mL/hr, and administrating sucralfate (Carafate) begins the protection of the stomach and small intestine.

Infection or sepsis for which no clinical source can be

found is common in patients who experience surgery, burns, trauma, or shock. In these patients, bacteria or bacteria-derived toxins normally found in the gut may be responsible for sepsis and, in some cases, multiple organ failure. Sepsis may develop from translocation of bacteria or toxins across the gut wall ("leaky gut").

In addition to experiencing stress-associated reduction in gut-barrier function, critically ill patients who are not fed enterally may develop a decrease in gut mucosal integrity due to the lack of intraluminal nutrients. Starvation or parenteral nutrition may act in synergy with the stress response to decrease the integrity of the mucosal barrier, which, in turn, increases the risk of bacterial translocation from the gut. Furthermore, the supine position of the patient may augment ileus and facilitate overgrowth of pathogens in the colon and small intestine.

MALNUTRITION

Two major classifications of malnutrition can occur: protein-calorie malnutrition (marasmus) and protein malnutrition (kwashiorkor). Elements of both types may occur in a nutritionally compromised patient.

Protein-calorie malnutrition or *marasmus* is a manifestation of somatic protein deficiency. *Somatic protein* comprises muscle tissue. Patients who are at risk for this type of malnutrition have generally experienced a recent unplanned weight loss of 10% or more in less than 2 weeks. As this condition progresses, subcutaneous fat stores decrease, muscle mass atrophies, diarrhea occurs, and there is usually a diminished appetite or anorexia. A patient with marasmic type malnutrition does not usually experience edema.

Protein malnutrition or *kwashiorkor* has depressed visceral (endogenous) protein synthesis. Table 14–3 compares somatic and visceral proteins. *Visceral proteins*—proteins required for body functions—are divided into three groups: Group I proteins include the actual gut mass; group II includes proteins of homeostasis such as albumin, prealbumin, transferrin, and total protein; and group III includes the acute phase proteins such as fibronectin, C-reactive proteins, globulins, and *opsonic proteins* (proteins such as antibodies that are utilized to destroy microorganisms or make them more susceptible to phagocytosis). Visceral proteins are within normal range during health and are depressed during illness, especially infection. However, the acute phase proteins are low during health and rise during illness.

Albumin is responsible for maintaining plasma colloid osmotic pressure (COP). Fluid and metabolic flow from the interstitial fluid into the blood stream depends on COP. When kwashiorkor is present, edema and muscle wasting are usually present. The patient is generally apathetic and may claim to have an appetite, but often the foods that are eaten are high in carbohydrate and low in protein.

Patients with either type of malnutrition have a compromised muscle endurance and a decreased efficiency of the diaphragm, intercostal muscles, and accessory muscles of respiration. Loss of strength occurs in both inspiration and expiration. Chronically starved persons lack the periodic sighs that automatically provide for reinflation of atelectatic areas; therefore, respiratory failure may ensue.

Patients who are going to have surgery must be carefully assessed for the presence of either type of malnutrition. A surgeon who must perform surgery on a malnourished, protein-depleted patient, describes it as "suturing together a bowl of Jell-O." Jell-O does not hold sutures well. Surgical patients with malnutrition are at risk for poor wound healing, which in turn increases the threat of infection and dehiscence. Healing wounds and granulation tissue need amino acids and glucose as sources of energy. Ketones cannot be used. New granulation tissue also requires insulin to use glucose.

Malnutrition and the Immune System

Diet affects immune system function. Severe protein-calorie malnutrition increases the likelihood of a person developing pneumonia, bacteremia, or wound or urinary infections (see Table 14–1).

The body's first barrier to a foreign substance is provided by the intact skin and mucous membranes. Immunoglobulins, secreted in saliva and other external body fluids, as well as the total number of peripheral lymphocytes and T cells are lower in the malnourished. The thymus gland, an important regulator of cell-mediated immunity, may shrink with malnutrition.

A defect in fat (linoleic acid—found in soy, safflower, and corn oils) causes lymphoid tissues to atrophy and depresses antibody formation. Eicosapentaenoic acid (EPA), a lipid found in certain fish (tuna, salmon, and trout), appears to improve immune status. However, too much fat increases the risk of cancer of the colon, prostate, and breast.

Zinc also has an effect on the immune system. Too little zinc has an immunosuppressive effect, which increases susceptibility to skin lesions, poor wound healing, and

Table 14–3. COMPARISON OF SOMATIC AND VISCERAL PROTEINS	
Somatic Proteins	**Visceral Proteins**
Types of Protein	
Muscle proteins	Group I
	Gut mass protein
	Group II
	Homeostasis protein
	Albumin (½ liter 16–18 days)
	Transferrin (½ liter 6–8 days)
	Total protein
	Prealbumin (½ liter 20 hr)
	Group III
	Acute phase proteins
	Fibronectin
	C-Reactive proteins
	Globulins
	Opsonic proteins
Measurement	
Weight	Albumin
Fat-to-lean ratio	Transferrin
Urinary creatinine output	Total lymphocyte count
Anthropometric measurements	

immunodeficiency. Sepsis is associated with decreased serum zinc. However, too much zinc can interfere with the ability of lymphocytes to respond to an antigen and the ability of leukocytes to engulf bacteria.

Vitamin E can be administered in doses of 30 to 40 times RDA requirements as it boosts immune function and increases T-lymphocyte and neutrophil activity.

Glutamine, a nonessential amino acid, is an important fuel for rapidly dividing cells such as erythrocytes, lymphocytes, and macrophages. Glutamine plays a significant role in transfer of nitrogen between tissues. Glutamine is also important for renal ammoniagenesis and hepatic gluconeogenesis. Glutamine also prevents deterioration in gut permeability, prevents translocation of gut bacteria (discussed later), and preserves mucosal structure. Glutamine is also an important metabolic fuel for the colon. As illness increases, the need for glutamine also increases.

Arginine is an essential amino acid that may increase thymic weight, increase lymphocyte proliferation, and increase killer T-cell activity. It also enhances wound healing by increasing the synthesis of collagen.

Taurine, another essential amino acid, regulates the aggregation of platelets and aids in the function of neutrophils. Taurine is also involved in metabolic processes in the central nervous system and in the conjugation of bile.

Branched-chained amino acids (BCAAs) enhance the production of thymic and blood lymphocytes and increase the ability to fight infection.

Tryptophan and phenylalanine, also amino acids, enhance the immune response to antigens, enhance phagocytic activity, and enhance antibody production.

Beta-carotene has been shown to increase the percent of T-helper cells.

Carnitine, a conditional essential amino acid, is required to transfer long-chain fatty acids into the mitochrondria for energy production. Carnitine requirements increase after injury.

ENTERAL NUTRITION

Enteral nutrition is designed for patients who are unable to consume sufficient calories to maintain normal metabolic processes but who have a functional alimentary tract. Enteral nutrition is also used in a well-nourished patient who has eaten less than half his or her nutritional requirements for 7 to 10 days; in a patient with protein-calorie malnutrition; in a severely dysphasic patient; in a patient with full-thickness burns; in a patient with a massive small-bowel resection, as enteral nutrition speeds up regeneration of the remaining small intestine (the small intestine receives its nutrition from food, not blood); and in a patient with enterocutaneous fistulas that generate less than 500 mL of fluid/day, as feeding closes up the lesions. Indirectly, the use of enteral nutrition can prevent the development of hypermetabolism, translocation of GI flora in the GI tract with resulting immune incompetence, intestinal failure, and multiple organ failure in the critically ill patient. Enteral nutrition preserves production of humoral antibodies, the secretory immunoglobulin A

(sIgA); decreased sIgA production may allow antigens to imitate a systemic inflammatory response. Enteral nutrition allows the body to use nutrients efficiently and causes few metabolic problems. It also makes full use of the intact absorptive GI tract.

Enteral feedings are contraindicated in patients with total bowel obstruction, persistent vomiting, severe small-bowel ileus, malabsorption disease, or severe diarrhea.

Enteral nutrition begins when the patient is hemodynamically stable and after fluid resuscitation is complete. Either the stomach or the intestine may be appropriate sites. The decision for selecting the stomach versus the small intestine depends on several factors, including gastric function, presence of gastric outlet syndromes, presence of GI fistulas, and history of aspiration. The stomach may experience gastric arrest, but the small intestine has contractions until almost death. In patients with conditions mentioned previously, the small intestine is the best site.

Enteral formulas differ in many ways. Products contain minimally altered foods or processed or chemically isolated foods with various amounts of residue. Products also differ in their fat or protein content, viscosity, and osmolarity. Products may contain high or low levels of lactose (milk sugar) or be lactose free. Enteral products that contain intact proteins are more palatable than those made of crystalline amino acids or hydrolyzed protein.

TUBE FEEDINGS

A tube feeding is a method of administering adequate nutrition in a form that is easily digestible by the patient. Tube-feeding diets can be made from a mixture of foods served in an adequate normal diet, finely homogenized in a mechanical blender and strained to ensure passage through the tube. Commercial products contain varying amounts of electrolytes, vitamins, and trace elements and a known quantity of protein, carbohydrate, and fat. Many formulas are tailored to meet specific nutrient needs, for example, high-nitrogen formulas for stressed patients and low-fat formulas for patients with fat malabsorption. Commercial preparations have predominantly replaced blenderized diets.

Types of Tubes

When it is necessary to administer feedings via feeding tubes, the size of the tube is determined first. A smaller tube is more comfortable for transnasal feedings, but may require the use of a food pump to administer more viscous formulas.

Feeding tube, shown in Figure 14–1, may be inserted into the stomach through a nasogastric tube (NG), gastrostomy tube, or percutaneous endoscopic gastrostomy (PEG) tube; into the duodenum through a nasoduodenal tube; or into the jejunum through a nasojejunal tube or a jejunostomy tube. The nasoduodenal and nasojejunal tubes are usually placed under fluoroscopy. However, they may also be placed as an NG tube is, then allowed to pass by peristaltic action into the duodenum or jejunum. The PEG tube is placed under gastroscopic visualization. Both the gastrostomy and jejunostomy tubes are

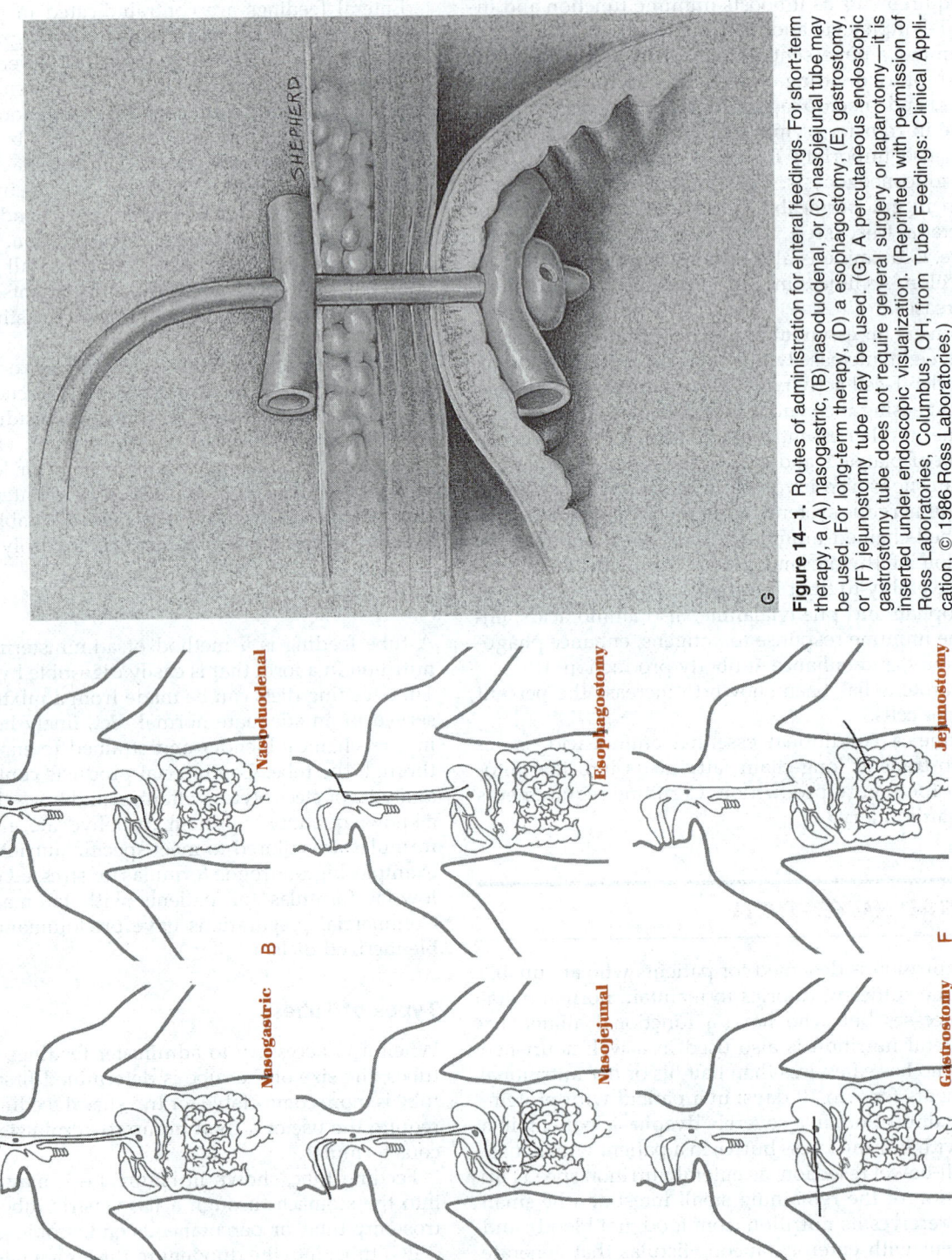

Figure 14–1. Routes of administration for enteral feedings. For short-term therapy, a (A) nasogastric, (B) nasoduodenal, or (C) nasojejunal tube may be used. For long-term therapy, (D) a esophagostomy, (E) gastrostomy, or (F) jejunostomy tube may be used. (G) A percutaneous endoscopic gastrostomy tube does not require general surgery or laparotomy—it is inserted under endoscopic visualization. (Reprinted with permission of Ross Laboratories, Columbus, OH, from Tube Feedings: Clinical Application, © 1986 Ross Laboratories.)

inserted through a surgical incision in the abdominal wall and sutured in place. Patients with either of these tubes may experience skin excoriation and infection. These complications are avoided with a cervical esophagostomy: a tube is passed through a surgically created, skin-line canal from the lower neck border extending to below the cervical esophagus. Nasogastric tubes have the highest risk for aspiration whereas the jejunostomy tube has the lowest risk.

Tubes used for these feedings are made from polyvinyl chloride (PVC) (e.g., Salem or Levin), polyurethane (e.g., Dobbhoff and Flexiflo), or silicone rubber (e.g., Keofeed). Feeding tubes come in various diameters ranging from a 5 to an 18, with a different number of holes at the end of the tube (one to four), with different size holes, different tip materials (tungsten or mercury), and different means of introduction into the patient (stiffer outer tube or a stylet). The weighted tip is intended to assist the movement of the tube through the pylorus into the duodenum within 24 hours. Polyvinyl chloride tubes are larger-bore nasogastric tubes, are more uncomfortable, and increase the risk of aspiration and other complications such as ulceration, fistulas, and tissue necrosis. Therefore, they should not be used for tube feedings.

The polyurethane and silicone rubber tubes have a mercury- or tungsten-weighted tip, and many have a guide wire included to aid in insertion. The silicone rubber and polyurethane tubes are better tolerated and produce fewer complications than the more rigid Levin tubes. These tubes do not harden in the presence of gastric juice nor do they need to be changed as frequently as PVC tubes. They are available as 5F or 18F tubes and vary in length from 36 to 45 inches.

The type of administered diet and its consistency may determine the tube size. For example, a home-prepared blenderized diet, because of its large particle size or consistency, can be inserted only through a 16 to 18 tube. Patients using an esophagostomy or gastrostomy tube can be given any consistency formula because these tubes are generally of a large diameter. The silicone rubber and polyurethane tubes can be used with any of the commercially prepared formulas. Feeding tubes may also be used to administer medications. Liquid forms of medication are used with these tubes whenever possible. However, avoid mixing medications with the formula, as this may lead to curdling of the formula or drug-nutrient interactions. Table 14–4 features a suggested procedure for administering medication through feeding tubes.

ENTERAL FORMULA CHARACTERISTICS

Osmolarity

Osmolarity is a measure of the osmotically active particles dispersed in solution. Tube feedings (400 to 1100 milliosmoles [mOsm]/liter H_2O) having osmolarity greater than body fluids (275 to 298 mOsm/liter H_2O), are hyperosmolar and have a tendency to draw water into the area where the solution is located. Hyperosmolar feedings (300 to 600 mOsm/liter H_2O) are started slowly at 25 mL/hr for the first 8 hours, increased to 50 mL/hr for the next

---

Table 14–4. SUGGESTED PROCEDURE FOR ADMINISTERING MEDICATIONS THROUGH FEEDING TUBES

1. Obtain drugs in liquid form if possible.
2. If the drug is not commercially available in liquid form, consult the pharmacy for extemporaneous formulations provided by American Society of Hospital Pharmacists in *Pediatric Extemporaneous Formulation List* or manufacturer's suggestions.
3. Calculate equivalent liquid dose carefully. Many liquid dosage forms are intended for pediatric use, and the dose of the drug must be appropriately adjusted for adults.
4. Administer crushed tablets only when no other alternatives are available.
5. If crushed tablets are administered, crush the tablet to a fine powder and mix in water. Do not crush any tablet on the list of oral drugs that should not be crushed or drugs with enteric coatings or sustained-release action. If in doubt, check with the pharmacy.
6. Stop the feeding, flush the tubing with 15–30 mL of water. Administer the medication and flush again.
7. Administer each drug separately. Do not mix all the medications for one dosing time in one container. Flush with at least 5 mL of water between medications.
8. If a drug is to be administered on an empty stomach, stop the feeding for 15–30 min. Then follow the above procedures.
9. Drugs that are hypertonic or irritating to the gastric mucosa such as potassium chloride should be diluted in at least 30 mL of water before administering to avoid gastric irritation and diarrhea.
10. Drugs that are usually administered with meals to avoid gastric irritation, such as indomethacin, should also be diluted with water prior to administering.
11. Slow- or sustained-release formulations of drugs that are used for once-daily dosing may need to have divided dosing schedules when administered in a liquid form. If you are uncertain about dosing schedule, contact the pharmacy.

Source: Wright, B, and Robinson, L: Enteral feeding tubes as drug delivery systems. Nutritional Support Services 6(2):37, 1986, with permission. Modified in 1996.

---

8 hours, and then increased to 75 mL/hr for the next 8 hours. Starting on day 2 they can be administered at full strength, 100 mL/hr, with the volume and rate adjusted to meet the specific nutritional goals of the patient. The more chemically simple the formula is, the higher the osmolarity. With hyperosmotic solutions (greater than 375 mOsm/liter) the patient is more likely to experience delayed gastric emptying, severe diarrhea, electrolyte depletion, and severe dehydration. Isotonic formulas (280 to 300 mOsm/liter) are available and may be better tolerated by some patients. Solutions with osmolarity less than body fluids are hypoosmotic and have a tendency to give up water.

Caloric Concentration

The commercially available tube-feeding products generally provide 0.5 to 2.0 calories per mL when mixed full strength according to the directions; therefore, to give 1000 calories of a 1 kcal/mL feeding, 1000 mL of fluid is administered. For patients with restricted fluid intake, high-calorie/low-volume formulas are available. Formulas such as Ensure Plus provide 1000 calories in only 676 mL; Magnacal and Two-Cal provide 2000 calories in 1000 mL. These high-calorie/low-volume formulas may also be helpful for the severely debilitated patient. Most patients require 25 to 30 kcal/kg of body weight.

ENTERAL NUTRITION FORMULA COMPONENTS

Enteral formulas may contain all or only one of the following components: protein, carbohydrates, fat, electrolytes, and vitamins and minerals. Enteral products are available as ready-to-use liquids or as powders for mixing.

Protein

The protein content ranges from 9% to 24% of the total calories and varies among products. Most patients require 0.8 to 1.5 g protein/kg of body weight. The protein content is derived from a variety of sources. Protein source may originate from milk, beef, egg albumin, skim milk powder, soy, hydrolyzed casein, or amino acids. The protein may be complete, partially hydrolyzed into peptides and amino acids, or administered as amino acids for easier digestion and absorption. Many formulas use a milk-based preparation, with casein as the primary protein source, because it is completely and easily digested. For persons with a milk intolerance there are lactose-free diets composed of soybean protein or other nonmilk products. Hydrolyzed protein and amino acids increase the osmolarity of the solution.

Crystalline amino acid formulas are usually composed of 30% to 50% branched-chain amino acids that require no digestion and are readily absorbed. There are also incomplete diets that have a high calorie-to-nitrogen ratio that are low in protein but high in carbohydrates and fats. These formulas are best for the patient with renal or hepatic disease.

Fat

The fat content in most commercial formulas is obtained from soy, corn, or safflower oil. Depending on the formula, it may be 1% to 47% of the total calories. Fats increase the calorie content of the formulas without increasing the osmolarity and give the patient a feeling of satiety. Several formulas contain medium-chain triglycerides (MCT), which are easier to digest and are used in patients with fat malabsorption syndromes. Digestion of fat usually requires bile, pancreatic enzymes, and normal intestinal flora. However, MCT are absorbed directly in the portal system. Fat-free formulas are also available. When fat-free formulas are used, small amounts of fat (10 g/liter) can be added to the feeding each day to increase fat intake gradually.

Carbohydrates

Assuming the patient has an intact endothelial brush border in the duodenum and sufficient absorptive capacity of the small bowel, carbohydrates (CHO) are easily digested and absorbed. Metabolism of CHO depends on the body having adequate amounts of insulin, glucagon, epinephrine, norepinephrine, the B vitamins, magnesium, chromium, zinc, and pyridoxine (vitamin B_6). When CHO is not absorbed or metabolized adequately, diarrhea, abdominal cramps, flatulence, fullness, and nausea develop.

Carbohydrates can be obtained from many sources including pureed fruits and vegetables, corn syrup, and sugars such as fructose, sucrose, and lactose. Fructose, a monosaccharide, is the sweetest sugar and is found in honey and fruit. Sucrose, ordinary table sugar, and lactose, the sugar found in milk, are disaccharides. Sucrose and lactose are hydrolyzed by digestive enzymes to the constituent monosaccharides before absorption into the body. Many individuals are lactose deficient, which leads to lactose intolerance and diarrhea. Thus, most enteral feeding formulas do not contain lactose. The carbohydrate source greatly affects the palatability of the formulas, with pureed fruits and vegetables being the best in taste. The amount and type of carbohydrates in the formulas also affect the osmolarity.

Electrolytes, Vitamins, and Minerals

Enteral feedings contain varying amounts of electrolytes: phosphorus, 0 to 1250 mg; sodium, 0 to 1915 mg; and potassium, 0 to 1670 mg.

Most commercially prepared formulas are fortified with vitamins and minerals. These usually meet the recommended daily allowances (RDA) when a specific volume is administered. The RDAs are designed for healthy individuals; therefore, requirements may be increased in an ill person, sometimes necessitating the administration of supplemental electrolytes, vitamins, and minerals.

Nitrogen to Nonprotein Calorie Ratio

The enteral nutrients include CHO, fat, and protein. The calories may be reported as either total kcal (that is, CHO plus fat plus protein), or nonprotein kcal (that is, CHO plus fat). In the absence of sufficient non-protein calories, protein is wasted as fuel.

Nitrogen can be used to evaluate nutritional status. This is discussed later. During a state of health (a positive nitrogen balance), a ratio of nitrogen (in grams) to nonprotein kcal is 1:350. During illness, protein requirements rise and the ratio of nitrogen to nonprotein kcal ranges from 1:100 to 1:200.

ENTERAL FORMULAS

A wide variety of commercially prepared enteral formulas are available. These formulas are categorized as polymeric, monomeric, specialized, or modular. All enteral diets can improve healing and promote tissue growth, and may be effective in restoring a positive nitrogen balance. Because there is little chance of sepsis with tube or oral formulas, they are safer for the individual than parenteral forms of nutrition. Patients have been maintained on these products for months, both in the hospital and at home, with no side effects.

Polymeric Formulas

Polymeric or nonelemental formulas contain protein, fat, and carbohydrate in high-molecular-weight form. They are low in osmolarity and are generally lactose free. These formulas can be used for most patients, but should not be used in patients with impaired processes of lipolysis or *proteolysis* (hydrolysis of protein). Polymeric formulas include blenderized diets and meal replacement formulas.

Blenderized Diets   Blenderized diets are generally high in residue and highly viscous with intact proteins. The blenderized diet is adequate for patients whose digestive and absorptive capacities are not impaired. For home patients, a blenderized diet can be achieved using a normal diet. For hospitalized patients, a commercial product is preferred.

Meal Replacement Formulas   Meal replacement formulas may either be milk based or lactose free. In milk-based formulas, the protein source is milk with or without soy protein. These formulas are nutritionally complete, generally meet the RDA for vitamins and minerals, and are palatable for oral ingestion. These products, which are high in lactose, should be avoided in patients known to be lactose intolerant.

Lactose-free formulas, listed in Table 14–5, contain casein, soy, or egg albumin as the protein source, plus complex carbohydrates. They vary in caloric content from the

Table 14–5. LACTOSE-FREE ENTERAL FORMULATIONS

Preparation	Comments
Attain Liquid	1 kcal/mL, isotonic
Criticare HN Liquid	1.06 kcal/mL
Ensure Liquid	1.06 kcal/mL, low residue
Ensure HN Liquid	1.06 kcal/mL, low residue
Ensure with Fiber Liquid	1.1 kcal/mL
Ensure Plus Liquid	1.5 kcal/mL, oral and tube feeding, low residue
Entrition 0.5 liquid	0.5 kcal/mL
Fiberlan Liquid	1.2 kcal/mL, gluten free
Isocal Liquid, Isocal HN Liquid	1.06 kcal/mL
Jevity Liquid, Jevity Osmolite Liquid	1.06 kcal/mL, isotonic, low residue
Osmolite HN Liquid	1.06 kcal/mL, oligomeric, fat free, low residue
Portagen Powder	1 kcal/mL
Pre-Attain Liquid	0.5 kcal/mL
Precision High Nitrogen Diet Powder	1.05 kcal/mL, protein from egg white solids
Profiber Liquid	1 kcal/mL, dietary fiber from soy, isotonic
Sustacal Basic Liquid, Sustacal Liquid	1 kcal/mL
Travasorb HN Powder	Oligomeric, low fat, low residue, gluten free
Travasorb MCT Powder, Travasorb STD Powder	1 kcal/mL, gluten free
Ultracal Liquid	1.06 kcal/mL
Vivonex T.E.N. Powder	1 kcal/mL, low fat, hypertonic

standard 1 kcal/mL to the high-density formulas with 1.5 to 2 kcal/mL. The high-density formulas are ideal for patients who are fluid restricted or catabolic and need additional calories and protein. The osmolality of these formulas ranges from 300 to 700 mOsm/kg. The lactose-free formulas also contain the RDA for vitamins and minerals in calorically adequate volumes. They are low in viscosity and may be administered through small-bore feeding tubes. Some of these formulas are flavored and can be administered orally.

Monomeric Formulas

Monomeric, elemental, or so-called chemically defined formulas provide nutrients in a form that requires little or no digestion and is usually incomplete. Monomeric diets are ideal for patients with digestive problems such as malabsorption syndromes, short-bowel syndrome, and antibiotic- or radiation-induced damage. Because monomeric formulas produce minimal stimulation of digestive secretions, they are also useful in treating chronic pancreatitis. Monomeric formulas are more expensive than polymeric formulas. They are considered clear liquid, low-residue, lactose-free diets. The protein source is crystalline amino acids and/or peptides. The main calorie source in most of these formulas is carbohydrate, which may be a problem in patients with respiratory insufficiency.

Monomeric formulas are generally low in fat. Some contain only minimal amounts of long-chain fatty acids and may require supplementation. Because they are low in fat, stomach emptying is not delayed. Many of these formulas are designed to be administered directly into the small intestine. Even though flavor packets are available to improve taste, they are generally unpalatable and best suited for tube feeding. When given in calorically adequate volumes, the RDAs for vitamins and minerals are met or exceeded. These formulas are higher in osmolality (450 to 900 mOsm/kg) than meal replacement formulas and, if started at full-strength concentration, generally produce diarrhea. Thus, they are gradually increased in strength and rate when initiating feeding.

Specialized Formulas

Specialized formulas are designed to fill specific needs in patients who have disease states such as renal failure, hepatic failure, pulmonary disease, or hypermetabolic states. These formulas, featured in Table 14–6, may be nutritionally incomplete and require vitamin and mineral supplementation.

The diets for renal failure, hepatic failure, and pulmonary disease contain crystalline amino acids (CAA) as the protein source, are hyperosmolar, and are available in various flavors. The renal-failure formulas contain only the eight essential amino acids plus histidine and have a high osmolality ranging from 590 to 1095 mOsm/kg. The hepatic-failure formulas are high in branched-chain amino acids and low in aromatic amino acids and have a high osmolality ranging from 560 to 690 mOsm/kg. Patients with pulmonary disease generally have normal ab-

Table 14–6. SPECIALIZED ENTERAL FORMULATIONS

Formula Types/Preparations	Comments
Renal Formulas	
Amin-Aid Instant Drink Powder	For acute or chronic renal failure, 2 kcal/mL, oral and tube feeding; protein content is 100% essential amino acids
Regain Medical Nutrition Bar	For renal impairment, 85-g bar, lactose free
Suplena Liquid	For renal conditions, 2 kcal/mL
Travasorb Renal Diet Powder	For acute renal failure, 1.35 kcal/mL, oral and tube feeding; protein content is 100% essential amino acids
Hepatic Formulas	
Hepatic-Aid II Instant Drink Powder	For chronic liver disease, 1.1 kcal/mL, oral and tube feeding; protein content is high in BCAA and low in aromatic amino acids
Travasorb Hepatic Powder	For hepatic failure, 1.1 kcal/mL, oral and tube feeding; protein content is high in BCAA and low in aromatic amino acids
GI Formulas	
Accupep HPF Powder	For GI conditions, protein source is hydrolyzed lactalbumin
Peptamen Liquid	For GI impairment, 1 kcal/mL
Immunosuppression Formulas	
Immun-Aid Powder	For immunocompromised patients, 500 kcal/mL
Stress Formulas	
Stresstein Powder	For moderately to severely stressed patients, 1.2 kcal/mL, tube feeding; protein content includes 44% BCAA
TraumaCal Liquid	For moderately to severely stressed patients, 1.5 kcal/mL, lactose free
Pulmonary Formulas	
Pulmocare Liquid	For pulmonary patients, 1.5 kcal/mL; oral and tube feeding; low carbohydrate, high fat
Respalor Liquid	For pulmonary patients, 1.5 kcal/mL, lactose free

sorptive and digestive capabilities, so pulmonary formulas are high in fat but low in carbohydrates. The metabolism of fat results in a lower respiratory quotient than the metabolism of carbohydrates, resulting in less carbon dioxide production and therefore less stress to the respiratory system. Pulmonary formulas are lactose free and have an osmolality of 490 mOsm/kg.

The formulas for hypermetabolic states (stresses like trauma, major surgery) contain CAA as the protein source. Although they are flavored, the taste of the amino acids is difficult to camouflage. These formulas generally have increased amounts of branched-chain amino acids, are also hyperosmolar (470 to 740 mOsm/kg), and vary in electrolyte and vitamin content. They are also lactose free.

Specialized formulas are also available for patients who

are immunosuppressed or stressed or who have vitamin B_6 nonresponsive hypermethioninemia, urea cycle disease, or abnormal glucose tolerance.

Modular Formulas

Modules or supplements are also available to supply a single nutrient and yield a higher calorie density. Modular formulas, featured in Table 14–7, are not designed to serve as a sole source of nutrition. Protein modules can be added to other products to help meet the extra nitrogen needs of a patient with burns or a severe trauma. Fat modules can be added to the formula of a ventilator-dependent patient to increase the ratio of fat to carbohydrate calories and thus decrease the respiratory quotient. Carbohydrate modules can be added to enteral formulas or foods to increase caloric intake.

PARENTERAL NUTRITION

For patients unable to eat or drink for longer than 7 days or for those with a dysfunction within the intestinal tract, some method of prolonged nutritional support must be maintained. Parenteral nutrition, also called total parenteral nutrition (TPN) or intravenous *hyperalimentation*, is a technique that can provide sufficient calories, amino acids, and other nutrients intravenously to achieve or maintain a positive nitrogen balance indefinitely. It may be administered peripherally or centrally, depending on the hypertonicity of the solution. Total parenteral nutrition promotes growth of tissue, improves wound healing, and

Table 14–7. MODULAR ENTERAL FORMULATIONS

Module/Product	Dosage/Content*
Protein	
Gevral Protein	26 g (⅓ cup) in 8 oz liquid (supplies 15.6 g protein)
Propac	Add 1 tablespoon (4 g) to liquid (supplies 3 g protein)
Carbohydrate (CHO)	
Polycose Liquid	Add to foods or beverages or mix in water (supplies 50 g CHO/100 mL)
Sumacal Powder	Add to foods or beverages or mix in water (supplies 95 g CHO/100 g powder)
Fat	
Lipomul	45 mL 2–4 times daily after or between meals (supplies 10 g corn oil/15 mL)
Microlipid	Give by tablespoon or add to patient's tube-feeding formula (contains 500 g fat/liter)

These products are not balanced and must not be used as a sole source of nutrition.

*Only the specific nutrient is listed, but products contain other nutrients.

often results in a weight gain of as much as a pound per day.

Total parenteral nutrition is also indicated for individuals who have lost 10% or more of their normal body weight and are unable to obtain adequate nutrition orally, or by tube enteral nutrition, or by peripheral intravenous fluids; and for those who have a caloric need of greater than 50% greater than normal. A patient receiving TPN may receive 3000 or more calories per day. Individuals who are unable to eat, digest, and absorb ingested nutrients usually become debilitated or malnourished. Conditions such as Crohn's disease, ulcerative colitis, burns, diverticulitis, hypermetabolic states, or cancer; severe gastrointestinal side effects from surgery, chemotherapy, or radiation; acute hepatic or renal failure; or prematurity may cause a need for nutritional support, often for months. Sepsis is also a unique use for TPN. In sepsis, there is increased breakdown of muscle tissue that is used for energy and a decrease in glucose utilization due to an increase in insulin resistance. Septic patients should be placed on TPN solution early to prevent nitrogen imbalance, to supply an available energy source, and to improve their recovery time. Total parenteral nutrition should not be used in patients with untreatable end-stage disease or in those who decline aggressive interventions.

Researchers are investigating the disadvantages of TPN, which may outweigh the benefits in certain patients. Sepsis, catheter displacement, metabolic complications, and mechanical problems occur in up to 10% of patients. Total parenteral nutrition also encourages the passage of gut bacteria and endotoxins into portal circulation, which increases the risk of sepsis and shock. Many large-scale trials have found few clinical benefits for TPN in surgical patients and recommend using enteral rather than parenteral products. Cost is also a consideration: Parenteral nutrition can cost up to 74% more than enteral nutrition.

The three major parenteral systems for nutritional support are as follows:

1. protein-sparing nutrition (PSN)
2. peripheral-vein total parenteral nutrition (PTPN)
3. central venous hyperalimentation (central TPN)

PROTEIN-SPARING NUTRITION

In protein-sparing nutrition (PSN), an isotonic solution of 3% to 5% essential and nonessential amino acids, carbohydrate-free fluids, vitamins, minerals, and electrolytes is administered through a peripheral vein. Protein-sparing nutrition prevents protein catabolism for short periods of time in patients with adequate body fat and with no clinically significant protein malnutrition. Solutions provide approximately 400 to 600 kcal/day. Energy requirements are met by the use of free fatty acids and ketone bodies derived from endogenous adipose tissue, thus preserving the body's protein compartment. Depending on the amount of calorie supplementation, the protein solutions provide a substrate for protein synthesis or anabolism; or enhance conservation of existing body protein, which is a protein-sparing effect. Numerous amino acid solutions are available today (see Table 14–8).

Table 14–8. AMINO ACID SOLUTIONS

Solution*	AAC[†] (%)	Uses[‡] PTPN	CTPN	PPSN
Aminosyn	3.5	X	—	X
Aminosyn II	3.5	X	—	X
Aminosyn II	5	X	X	X
Aminosyn	5	X	X	X
Aminosyn II	7	X	X	X
Aminosyn	7	X	X	X
Aminosyn II	8.5	X	X	X
Aminosyn	8.5	X	X	X
Aminosyn	10	X	X	X
Aminosyn II	10	X	X	X
FreAmine III[§]	10	X[§]	X	X
ProcalAmine	3	X	—	X
Travasol	5.5	X	X	X
Travasol	8.5	X[¶]	X	X
Travasol	10	X[¶]	X	X
Novamine	11.4	X[¶]	X	X
Novamine	15	X	X	—

*Other products available; this is not a complete list.
[†]AAC = amino acid concentration.
[‡]PTPN = Peripheral total parenteral nutrition; CTPN = central total parenteral nutrition; PPSN = peripheral protein sparing nutrition.
[§]Contains electrolytes.
[¶]Before peripheral administration, these products must be diluted.

PERIPHERAL-VEIN TOTAL PARENTERAL NUTRITION

Peripheral-vein total parenteral nutrition (PTPN) is indicated in patients when central access cannot be obtained or is not appropriate; supplemental feedings are required; the GI tract cannot be used; GI absorption is impaired; bowel rest is needed; or metabolic requirements for protein are substantially increased.

The major development in PTPN is the use of lipid as a nonprotein calorie source. Lipids (discussed later) are used to increase the caloric density of the formula, to supply a source of energy, to decrease the osmolarity, and to buffer the vein. Because calorie-dense 20% lipid solutions are available, it is possible to provide nearly 2000 kcal/day by a peripheral vein in a volume tolerated by most patients. A crystalline amino acid solution is mixed with dextrose to supply protein and energy requirements. However, the final dextrose concentration must be limited to 10% because the peripheral vein will sclerose at higher concentrations. Vitamins, electrolytes, and trace elements are added to this solution. This admixture is continuously infused with the lipid emulsion continuously through a Y-connector. Some centers mix all the hyperalimentation components into one bag, which allows the infusion of the mixture without the need for a Y-connector. The concentration of potassium and calcium must be limited to prevent sclerosis and irritation to the vein. A PTPN solution usually contains about 200 nonprotein calories, 35 to 50 grams of protein per liter, and may contain lipids.

When possible, it is advantageous to administer PTPN

because there is less risk of catheter placement, care of the infusion site is simpler, and the complications associated with a hyperosmolar solution are avoided. The limitations associated with PTPN include the need for several peripheral veins, as the catheter is rotated on a regular basis. The veins must also be of adequate size to accommodate the catheter. In addition, in a stressed or hypermetabolic patient, calorie requirements may exceed those that can be delivered by PTPN. Another limitation is the patient's inability to utilize lipids as an energy source. If the patient has a disorder of lipid metabolism, hypertonic dextrose through a central line may be necessary.

CENTRAL VENOUS HYPERALIMENTATION

In central venous hyperalimentation (central TPN), a hypertonic, concentrated solution of both crystalline amino acids and nonprotein calories (given as dextrose and lipid emulsion) is administered through a central vein. Vitamins and minerals are added to the preparation to meet all daily nutritional requirements. In general, the nitrogen-to-calorie ratio is 1:150 to 1:200, which is ideal for maximum utilization, anabolism, and protein synthesis. Highly stressed patients require a 1:80 to 1:100 nitrogen-to-calorie ratio.

The caloric source for central TPN is 12.5% to 50% dextrose in water, usually in a volume of 500 to 1000 mL. This solution is a concentrated calorie source of relatively small volume. Hypertonic concentrations greater than 10% necessitate that the TPN infusion be given through a central line at a regular rate.

PARENTERAL NUTRITION SOLUTION COMPONENTS

The following components are available for parenteral solutions: carbohydrates, protein, electrolytes, and vitamins and minerals. Fat is supplied by parenteral fat emulsions (discussed later in the chapter). Special formulations are available for patients with renal failure, hepatic failure, or hypermetabolic states.

Carbohydrates

The most common carbohydrate source is dextrose derived from cornstarch. Dextrose is an inexpensive and readily available source that provides 3.4 kcal/g. A TPN solution that begins with 25% to 50% dextrose is diluted with the amino acid mixture to yield a final concentration of 12.5% to 25%. If patients are allergic to dextrose, which is rare, invert sugars, derived from beet or cane sugar, are available. TPN solutions are given cautiously to diabetics, in patients with fluid overload, during pregnancy (category C), during lactation, or to infants of diabetic mothers. Maximum infusion rate without causing glycosuria is 0.5 g/kg per hour.

Protein

In the majority of TPN solutions used today, the protein source is crystalline amino acids (CAA). Crystalline amino acid solutions have a defined amount of essential and nonessential amino acids, but the CAA content is different among brands and among concentrations within a brand. However, the nitrogen content is completely utilizable and does not vary from one manufacturing lot to the next. Most products contain both the eight essential amino acids and the nonessential amino acids. If the solution is for children, it also contains two semiessential amino acids that cannot be synthesized in adequate amounts during growth periods. (Ten amino acids are considered essential in children.)

As with enteral formulas, parenteral formulas contain various types of protein. Critically ill patients require about twice the normal nitrogen intake, as long as no hepatic or renal failure coexists. In general, the goal is to provide a protein intake of approximately 15% to 20% of the kilocalorie intake in a calorie-to-nitrogen ratio of 150:1. The calories can be supplied by carbohydrates, but these increase the ratio, and respiratory insufficiency or failure may be precipitated. To solve this problem, half of the nonprotein calories can be supplied by lipid emulsion.

Most patients require 2 to 3 liters of TPN per day to meet their protein requirements, which are 0.5 to 1.5 grams per kilogram of body weight. Severely stressed patients may require 2 to 3.5 g/kg. Infants require at least 2.5 to 3 grams per kilogram of body weight.

Electrolytes

The crystalline amino acid solutions contain small amounts of sodium, potassium, phosphate, chloride, and acetate. Additional electrolytes are added according to patient need to prevent deficiencies. Potassium, phosphate, and magnesium are particularly important, as requirements of each increase as the patient enters the anabolic state. Potassium (important in protein synthesis) and phosphate also move intracellularly due to the effect of the hypertonic glucose. Phosphate is an essential component in the production of adenosine triphosphate diphosphoglycerate (2,3-DPG), phospholipids, and nucleic acids. Magnesium is needed for a number of enzyme reactions. Calcium is added to balance the phosphate infusion, as well as to meet body needs for calcium. Sodium, chloride, sulfate, and acetate are also needed to help maintain normal serum levels and to maintain acid-base balance.

Vitamins and Minerals

For those patients whose only nutritional intake is the TPN solution, adequate vitamin supplementation is also important. Vitamins such as A, C, D, E, K, B complex, and folic acid may be added to the TPN solution, or administered intravenously or through another IV line. The addition of vitamins can be made by daily alternating the administration of 5 mL of a multiple vitamin infusion (MVI) with 2 mL of a product containing B and C vitamins. This regimen provides vitamin A 10,000 IU, vitamin D 1,000 IU, vitamin E 5 IU, thiamine 50 mg, riboflavin 10 mg, pyridoxine 15 mg, niacin 100 mg, pantothenic acid 25 mg, and vitamin C 100 mg. With this method, folic acid, vitamin B_{12}, and vitamin K are not included. Folic acid (1 mg/day) and vitamin K (5 to 10 mg/week) can be added daily to the TPN solution or given weekly intramuscularly. Vitamin B_{12} (1000 μg) should be given intramuscularly monthly.

The preferred method for providing adequate vitamins is to use an MVI-12 product daily. Fat- and water-soluble vitamins are provided in smaller amounts on a daily basis. MVI-12 contains vitamin A 3300 IU, vitamin D 200 IU, vitamin E 10 IU, thiamine 3.0 mg, riboflavin 3.6 mg, pyridoxine 4.0 mg, vitamin B_{12} 5 μg, niacin 40 mg, pantothenic acid 15 mg, biotin 60 μg, folic acid 400 μg, and vitamin C 100 mg. Vitamin K must be administered separately. Iron dextran can be used to prevent iron deficiency.

When TPN is given for prolonged periods, trace elements such as copper, zinc, manganese, iodine, chromium, and others also must be administered to prevent deficiency syndromes.

SPECIALIZED PARENTERAL FORMULATIONS

Specialized formulations for parenteral use are available for patients with renal failure, hepatic failure, or hypermetabolic states. These formulations are similar to their enteral counterparts.

Renal-failure formulas (Aminess, Aminosyn-RF, NephrAmine, RenAmin) are generally mixed with 70% dextrose and 250 to 300 ml of amino acid solution to provide a high-calorie, low-protein feeding. Vitamins, trace elements, and electrolytes are added as needed. Generally, this type of formula is infused at a low rate, according to the patient's fluid tolerance.

The hepatic-failure formula (HepatAmine) contains all the amino acids but has increased amounts of branched-chain amino acids and decreased amounts of aromatic amino acids. The amino acid solution (500 mL) is mixed with dextrose 50% (500 mL), depending on the patient's needs. Electrolytes, vitamins, and minerals are added as needed. Depending on protein and fluid tolerance, 1 to 3 liters/day may be infused.

Hypermetabolic formulas (Aminosyn-HBC, 4% BranchAmin, and FreAmine HBC) are similar to the hepatic-failure formulas but do not have decreased amounts of aromatic amino acids. These amino acid solutions are mixed with concentrated dextrose (up to 70%) to form a high-protein, low-carbohydrate formula. Again, electrolytes, vitamins, and minerals are added as needed. Administration depends on fluid tolerance.

PARENTERAL FAT EMULSIONS

Parenteral fat emulsions (PFEs) are prepared from soybean oil (Interlipid, Nutrilipid, Soyacid, Liposyn III) or soybean and safflower oil (Liposyn II) and provide a mixture of neutral triglycerides, mostly unsaturated fatty acids. Parenteral fat emulsions also contain 1.2% egg yolk phospholipids as an emulsifier and glycerol to adjust tonicity. They are isotonic and may be given intravenously either centrally or peripherally. Parenteral fat emulsions

are needed in patients who require parenteral nutrition for longer than 5 days.

Of the total daily calories, 4% to 8% must be endogenous fatty acids (EFAs) to prevent EFA deficiency. Parenteral fat emulsions are used in conjunction with TPN as a source of essential fatty acids or as a calorie source. Most studies indicate that 20% to 40% of the total daily calories should be fat. Minimal fat requirements can be met with two or three 500-mL bottles of 10% fat per week. Infants have substantially less essential fatty acid stores than adults and often require supplemental fat administration at the onset of parenteral therapy. Parenteral fat emulsions are also used as a calorie source in patients who do not tolerate the amount of dextrose used in central TPN solutions. This intolerance is seen as hyperglycemia, as the development of fatty liver from increased glycogen deposits, or as an increased production of carbon dioxide.

Pharmacokinetics

It is thought that PFEs are metabolized by the body in the same manner as ingested fats. As the PFE enters the bloodstream, the protein in blood acts as an emulsifier. The fat particles are coated with a hydrophilic layer, forming lipid-protein complexes. These complexes are carried to the liver, adipose tissue, muscle, and other cells, where they are hydrolyzed to fatty acids and glycerol, transported into cells, resynthesized as triglycerides, and stored. When needed for energy, the triglycerides are mobilized and oxidized. The PFEs have a protein-sparing effect like that of dextrose and may be administered concurrently with amino acid–dextrose solutions to ensure that the amino acids are utilized properly.

Contraindications and Precautions

Parenteral fat emulsions are contraindicated in patients with disturbances in normal fat metabolism, such as acute pancreatitis associated with hyperlipemia, because they tend to augment the dysfunction. They are administered with caution when there is a risk of fat embolism, as in a patient with long bone fractures, and when the patient has severe hepatic damage, anemia, or blood coagulation disorders. Because egg yolk phospholipids are used to stabilize the PFE, a history of severe egg allergy precludes their use. Safe use in pregnancy (category C) has not been established.

▼ CLINICAL ALERT

Assess benefit versus risk before administering PFE to premature and low birth weight infants. Deaths in premature infants have occurred after infusion of PFE because of intravascular fat accumulation in the lungs. Do *not* exceed recommended total daily dosage. Infuse slowly and do not exceed 1 g/kg in 4 hours. Monitor triglyceride or plasma free fatty acid levels to ensure that the infant can eliminate the infused fat from the circulation.

Adverse Effects

Acute adverse effects, which can develop from the administration of any of the PFEs, are associated with an allergy to the egg protein in the fat emulsion and include chills, fever, flushing, diaphoresis, dyspnea, cyanosis, allergic reactions, chest and back pain, headache, a feeling of pressure over the eyes, dizziness, and sleepiness. Signs of thrombophlebitis at the injection site can also occur. Most acute reactions necessitate discontinuation of the PFE solution. Adverse effects seen with chronic administration include deposition of IV fat pigment in Kupffer's cells of the liver and a decrease in hemoglobin concentration. These effects are reversible after discontinuation of the PFE.

Dosage

The usual dose of PFE in adults is 500 mL/day of a 10% formula 2 or 3 times weekly for the prevention or treatment of EFA deficiency. As a calorie source, these emulsions may be used daily in infants and adults, providing up to 60% of the total daily caloric needs. The remaining calories are supplied by carbohydrates. It is recommended that the daily dose of PFE not exceed 2 g/kg of body weight in an adult. These emulsions are relatively expensive compared with the cost of dextrose and therefore may not be routinely used in adults on short-term (less than 3 weeks) parenteral therapy.

Fat emulsions are available as either 10% or 20% emulsions. Usually, only 500 mL is infused the first day. The first day, patients should receive only 250 mL (Liposyn II) or 500 mL (Intralipid). Fat emulsions can be administered alone. Heparin (1 or 2 units/mL) is added to the emulsions, as it clears the triglycerides. The nurse follows specific guidelines (described later) to administer fat emulsions safely. Fat emulsions can also be mixed with TPN and administered slowly over 24 hours. This technique is discussed later.

USING THE NURSING PROCESS

ASSESSMENT

- Obtain a thorough nursing assessment of the patient history to develop a database. Patients requiring these feedings may be in the hospital or may be maintained on these therapies at home. Information to be obtained from the patient and/or family is featured in Table 14–9.
- Assess for the presence of underlying diseases of the heart, kidney, or liver, which may limit the type or the amount of the feedings or the amount of weight the patient can safely gain. Often the current symptoms of malnutrition are produced by medications or other forms of therapy, such as radiation therapy for cancer treatment. If the malnourished state is due to current therapy, there may be no additional need for supplemental feeding after therapy is discontinued. If, however, the reason for the malnutrition is found

to be a lack of understanding about proper nutrition or poor nutritional habits, this problem must be resolved during the intervention phase. Additional causes of a poor nutritional state may be the result of psychologic status, sensory deficits, chronic conditions such as cancer, drug or alcohol dependence, abuse of cathartics, or increases in metabolism. All underlying conditions must be carefully assessed and treated to prevent further recurrences.

- Assess for food allergies. Enteral products are derived from real food; thus, if the patient has food allergies, care must be taken to ensure that those foods are not part of the feeding.
- Assess for a history of lactose intolerance. African-Americans, Asian-Americans, Native Americans, and Jews are particularly prone to lactase deficiencies. Lactase is found in the intestinal brush border and is necessary for lactose (milk sugar) absorption. If a lactose intolerance is present, the patient experiences varying degrees of diarrhea, abdominal cramps, bloating, and flatulence after consuming milk or milk products. Most enteral formulas are lactose free.
- Assess for objective symptoms of a catabolic state (see Table 14–2).
- Assess daily weight at the same time every morning. Weight may provide a means of assessing whether calorie and fluid needs are being met or exceeded (tissue gain versus edema).
- Discuss calorie needs with other members of the health team, such as the registered dietitian. The registered dietitian uses formulas that take into account age, weight, diagnosis, and stressors to help determine caloric needs. If the patient continues to lose weight after several days of nutritional support, the formula must be adjusted, possibly by increasing the protein and calories.
- Assess other parameters indicating fluid balance, including jugular vein distention, dependent edema, lung sounds, mucous membrane moisture, presence of thirst, and skin turgor. The medical team often must distinguish between edema of hypoproteinemia and edema of heart failure (HF). The following are several discriminating findings: central venous pressure is up in HF and low in hypoproteinemia; chest x-ray films in hypoproteinemia have a ground glass appearance in the bottom half of the lung and are clear at the top; the heart size is enlarged in HF and normal-sized or small in size in hypoproteinemia. Hypoproteinemia is treated with albumin for several days until the patient begins diuresis.
- Assess respiration function. A direct correlation exists between nutritional status and proper lung function. If nutritional status is compromised, the muscles involved in respiration are without adequate food supply. Clinically, malnourished patients have fewer deep breaths per hour and smaller tidal volumes than those who are properly nourished. Poor ventilation can result from poor nutrition. A decrease in respiratory function can be particularly devastating to a patient with chronic obstructive pulmonary disease and/or a patient who is critically ill.

Table 14–9. NURSING PROCESS FOR PATIENT REQUIRING ENTERAL/PARENTERAL NUTRITION

Assessment

Review nutritional history, assess cultural, economic and religious variables; housing and cooking facilities; where meals are taken; likes and dislikes of food; allergies.

Assess history of illness/treatment (e.g., cancer/chemotherapy, renal or liver failure), extent of weight loss.

Assess psychologic status.

Nursing Diagnosis: Altered Nutrition Less Than Body Requirements

RELATED TO: Conditions that interfere with nutrient intake or increase nutrient need/metabolic demand (massive burns, cancer and associated treatments, surgical procedures, dysphagia/difficulty swallowing, depressed mental status/level of consciousness).

AS EVIDENCED BY: Body weight 10% or more under ideal, decreased subcutaneous fat/muscle mass, changes in gastric motility and stool characteristics.

Desired Outcomes/Evaluation Criteria

Demonstrates stable weight or progressive weight gain toward goal with normalization of laboratory values and free of signs of malnutrition.

Nursing Actions	Rationale
Consult with dietitian/nutritional support team.	Useful in calculating individual needs and appropriate formula/product.
Document oral intake by use of 24-hr recall, food history, calorie counts as appropriate.	Identifies imbalance between estimated nutritional requirements and actual intake.
Administer nutritional solutions at prescribed rate via infusion control device. Adjust rate to prescribed hourly rate but never "catch up."	Nutrition support prescriptions are based on estimated caloric and protein requirements. A consistent rate of nutrient administration ensures proper utilization with fewer side effects.
Be familiar with electrolyte content of nutritional solutions.	Metabolic complications of nutritional support often result from a lack of appreciation of changes that can occur as a result of refeeding.
Schedule activities with adequate rest periods. Promote relaxation techniques.	Conserves energy/reduces calorie needs.
Monitor nutritional status routinely.	Provides the opportunity to observe deviations from normals/patient baseline and influences choices of interventions.
Weigh daily and compare with admission weight.	Establishes baseline, aids in monitoring effectiveness of therapeutic regimen and alerts nurse to inappropriate trends in weight loss/gain.
Monitor for development of diarrhea with enteral feedings.	Changes in intestinal flora, hyperosmolar solutions, or lactose intolerance may necessitate changes in drug therapy or type of formula/rate of administration to improve patient tolerance.

Nursing Diagnosis: Risk for Fluid Volume Deficit

RELATED TO: Active loss and/or failure of regulatory mechanisms, complications of nutrition therapy, e.g. high-glucose solutions, hyperglycemia, inability to obtain/ingest fluids.

Desired Outcomes/Evaluation Criteria

Displays moist skin/mucous membranes, stable vital signs, individually adequate urinary output, and is free of edema and excessive weight loss/inappropriate gain.

Nursing Actions	Rationale
Incorporate knowledge of caloric density of enteral formulas into assessment of fluid balance.	Enteric solutions are usually concentrated and do not meet free water needs.
Provide additional water/flush tubing as indicated.	With higher calorie formula, additional water is needed to prevent dehydration/HHNK.
Record intake and output, calculate fluid balance. Measure urine specific gravity.	Excessive urinary losses may reflect developing hyperglycemia. Specific gravity is an indicator of hydration and renal function.
Monitor laboratory studies, e.g., serum potassium/phosphorus.	Hypokalemia/phosphatemia can occur because of intracellular shifts during initial refeeding and may compromise cardiac function if not corrected.
Monitor hematocrit (Hct).	Reflects hydration/circulating volume.
Monitor serum albumin.	Hypoalbuminemia/decreased colloidal osmotic pressure leads to decreased circulating volume as fluid shifts into the tissues.
Monitor peripheral blood sugars with TPN.	Hyperglycemia can occur because of increased stress on the pancreas.

Other Suggested Nursing Diagnoses: Knowledge Deficit and Risk for Injury.

- Assess for the presence of subjective symptoms such as thirst, fatigue, and anorexia. Thirst may be one of the first signs of impending dehydration from the administration of hyperosmolar enteral preparations. The nurse may also assist with determining how the patient is to receive the additional nourishment, such as with supplemental oral feedings between meals, tube feedings, or TPN.
- Assess for essential fatty acid deficiency. The signs to observe for include thrombocytopenia; increased hemolysis; impaired wound healing; light, flaky, and reddened skin lesions, often appearing on the scalp, arms, and legs; and growth retardation in infants and children. The dermatologic signs are usually noted first.
- Assess various laboratory and x-ray tests ordered by the physician: endocrine, renal, and hepatic function are often assessed. Laboratory tests examine various hormones, total proteins, albumin, blood urea nitrogen (BUN), electrolytes, minerals, and vitamins (see Table 14–1). All individuals have frequent assessments of their blood glucose level, as hyperglycemia can precipitate osmotic diuresis and hyperosmolar dehydration. Patients in need of nutritional support need to have their serum protein levels assessed often. When malnutrition is present, the liver's ability to synthesize albumin is reduced. Nitrogen balance studies—the balance between nitrogen intake and output—may also be obtained. This is done by assessing a 24-hour urine for urea, the major form of nitrogen loss. All urine for the 24-hour period is saved for this analysis. Nitrogen balance can be calculated using the following formula:

$$\text{N balance} = \frac{\text{Protein intake (g)}}{6.25}$$
$$- \text{ (urinary urea nitrogen} + 4)$$

A value below 0 indicates negative nitrogen balance.
- Assess before and during enteral or parenteral nutrition the following laboratory tests, which may be ordered daily until a constant volume of nutrition is being delivered and then reduced to once a week or even monthly with chronic use: hematocrit, sodium, potassium, chloride, carbon dioxide, calcium, phosphate, albumin, total protein, creatinine, blood sugar, and BUN. Additional laboratory tests are generally ordered weekly, including magnesium level, complete blood count, prothrombin time, and liver function tests.
- Obtain a complete nutritional assessment, including *anthropometric parameters* (a measure of nutritional status that evaluates a patient's height, weight, and body proportions in relation to the patient's age and/or population averages); biochemical data; physical findings; medical or surgical interventions; and diet, drug, and socioeconomic histories.
- Estimate the patient's ideal weight. This can be done from weight charts or by estimation, as follows:
  Men: 106 lb (48 kg) for first 5 ft (150 cm) + 6 lb (2.7 kg) for each in (2.5 cm) over 5 ft (±10%)

Table 14–10. ACTIVITY AND INJURY FACTORS AND VALUES FOR ESTIMATING CALORIC REQUIREMENTS

Factor	Value
Activity:	
Confined to bed	1.2
Ambulatory	1.3
Injury:*	
Surgery:	
Minor	1.1
Major	1.2
Trauma:	
Skeletal	1.35
Head injury with steroid therapy	1.6
Blunt	1.35
Infection:	
Mild	1.2
Moderate	1.4
Severe	1.8
Burns:	
40% BSA†	1.5
100% BSA	1.95

Source: Tube Feedings: Clinical Application. Ross Laboratories, Columbus, Ohio, 1986, with permission.
*The magnitude of the injury factor decreases as metabolic responses return to normal, nonstressed levels during recovery.
†BSA = body surface area.

  Women: 100 lb (45 kg) for first 5 ft + 5 lb (2.2 kg) for each in over 5 ft (±10%)
- Estimate energy requirements. The Harris-Benedict equation is available for calculation of precise energy requirements. The Harris-Benedict equation is as follows:
  Men: (66.47 + 13.75 weight in kgs + 5.0 height in cms − 6.76 age in yr) × activity factor × injury factor
  Women: (65.10 + 9.56 weight in kilograms + 1.85 height in centimeters − 4.68 age in years) × activity factor × injury factor

Activity factor and injury factor and their values for calculating caloric requirements are featured in Table 14–10.

Another method to determine caloric requirements is the use of a simple rule-of-thumb relation. Generally, patients experiencing mild stress require 25 to 35 kcal/kg per day; those with moderate stress, 30 to 40 kcal/kg per day; and those with severe stress, 40 to 45 kcal/kg per day. The degree of stress can be estimated from the clinical setting or from collection of a 24-hour urine with determination of nitrogen excretion. Patients excreting less than 10 grams of nitrogen per day can be classified as having mild stress; those with 10 to 15 g/day, moderate stress; and those with greater than 15 g/day, severe stress.

NURSING DIAGNOSIS

- Typical nursing diagnoses for a patient requiring enteral and parenteral feedings are Altered Nutrition, Risk for Injury, Fluid Volume Deficit, and Knowledge Deficit (see Table 14–9).

PLANNING AND INTERVENTION— ENTERAL NUTRITION

- Three modalities of intervention that the nurse frequently uses in malnutrition states are education, nutritional modifications, and medications. These responsibilities are shared with the dietitian and physician.

   Patients may require nutritional support both in the hospital and at home. Some patients may require only supplemental support through the administration of between-meal high-protein or high-calorie preparations. Other patients may need to be totally maintained with tube feedings. When long-term tube feedings are required, the patient is discharged with tubes in place.

Supplemental Feedings

- Record the exact amount of formula taken for supplemental feedings between meals. Supplemental feedings must be administered between meals so they do not interfere with normal food intake. Patients often need encouragement to take this formula, as they may not feel well or do not have big appetites. Enteral feedings are available in various flavors—strawberry, vanilla, chocolate, and others—and only those appealing to the patient, assuming an absence of allergy, are ordered. In general, formulas taste like milkshakes and are best served very cold. To calculate the amount of supplement feeding the patient needs, the following calculation is used:
  1. Determine patient's total caloric need.
  2. Determine amount of calories the patient is actually eating.
  3. Provide enough calories to make up the difference between need and intake.

Tube Feedings

The nurse may be responsible for inserting the feeding tube or for teaching the patient how to insert his or her own tube. See a nursing fundamentals text for the procedure.

- Care for the tube and the affected part of the body daily. The nose is washed and dried, and fresh tape is applied. The nose is carefully observed for skin breakdown; if the nose begins to show signs of inflammation, the tube is taped to the forehead or the cheek. Surgically placed tubes, such as gastrostomy tubes, also need daily attention. The skin is inspected daily to determine if there is breakdown from contact with gastrointestinal secretions. Initially, the skin is cleansed with half-strength hydrogen peroxide daily. Once healing has occurred, soap and water is sufficient. A dressing is avoided if possible. If a dressing is used, it must be changed immediately if it becomes wet. If there is gastric leakage around the tube, the skin must be protected with a skin barrier (ointment

or commercial disk). An enterostomal therapist can help to determine the cause of the leakage and to provide suggestions for skin care.

- Administer tube feedings by the appropriate method: slow intermittent feeding, continuous feeding, or continuous interrupt or cyclic feeding.

   The slow intermittent feeding delivers approximately 200 to 400 mL of formula over a period of 20 minutes to 1 or 2 hours, depending on patient tolerance. It is usually administered every 3 to 4 hours, depending on patient need. It may be administered either by gravity drip or pump delivery. Pump delivery is more likely if the patient must receive a prescribed amount over 1 or 2 hours.

   The continuous feeding method is administered over 24 hours. Usually 50 to 125 mL/hour is administered, depending on patient tolerance and needs. Pumps are usually necessary.

   The continuous interrupt or cyclic feeding is administered continuously over 12 to 16 hours. This allows the patient a period of rest from the feeding. Some feel this method holds metabolic advantages. It is also helpful with transitional feeding. For example, feeding the patient by tube 12 hours overnight and allowing the patient to eat during the day helps to wean the patient from tube feeding.

   Regardless of the method used, start gradually and increase the rate and strength of formula, if applicable, as tolerated by the patient.

   It is also important to determine the patient's total fluid needs (e.g., 30 mL/kg of body weight) and to determine how much water is in the formula. (E.g., 1 kcal/mL formula has approximately 840 mL water/liter, while 1.6 kcal/mL has approximately 770 mL water/liter.) Calculate how much additional water is needed and administer it throughout the day.

- Elevate the head of the patient to at least 45° from the horizontal for the feeding. The patient must remain elevated for at least 1 hour after the feeding. This helps prevent aspiration of the formula into the lungs. Before administering a tube feeding, tube placement is checked. Stomach contents are aspirated before the intermittent feeding, or approximately every 4 hours during continuous feedings, to ensure or assess presence of minimal residue from the previous feeding. Once the full feeding rate is achieved for 24 to 48 hours and residues are minimal, aspirations are abandoned in the stable patient. Excessive residue (over 400 mL) may indicate an obstruction or digestive problem that should be resolved before the feeding is continued. A general rule of thumb is that the volume aspirated should not exceed the infusion rate. The gastric aspirate should be returned to the stomach, not discarded. After each feeding, the tube is carefully rinsed with about 30 mL of water to prevent contamination and plugging of the tube. Protein in the feedings has a tendency to coagulate when it comes in contact with hydrochloric acid in the stomach. Flushing the tubing with 20 to 30 mL of water every 4 hours or each time the feeding is interrupted helps keep the tube patent. The delivery set is changed every 24 to 48 hours (depending on institution policy) to control bacterial growth.

- Closely monitor the respiratory rate and status of the patient. Respiratory distress may indicate the feeding was given too quickly, pushing the stomach up into the chest cavity and compromising chest expansion, or that the patient has aspirated.
- Dilute hypertonic formulas with water to half-strength at the onset of the tube feeding. After several hours, if there are no complications (diarrhea, nausea, vomiting, or glucosuria), the rate and strength (full) are increased (100 to 125 ml/hr). This half-strength administration helps the patient develop a gradual tolerance to the hyperosmolarity of the formula. Hyperosmolar solutions draw water into the intestinal tract, and patients are likely to complain of cramping or diarrhea or both. Debilitated patients, patients with gastrointestinal disorders, patients who have not had food for a long time, and patients who are being fed via gastrostomy and jejunostomy tubes are more likely to be intolerant of hyperosmolar formulas. When patients are fed half-strength or reduced-strength formulas because of problems with cramping or diarrhea, they are not receiving the full supply of nutrients, vitamins, and minerals. Supplemental intravenous preparations may need to be administered to ensure proper nutrition. Isotonic solutions can be started and run at full strength.
- Encourage patients who are alert and being tube-fed by the nurse to help with the feeding. If the patient is receiving several administrations of tube feedings daily, feedings should arrive at normal meal times in an attractive container on a clean, neat tray. When caring for a patient with enteral feedings, there are many items to check and monitor. Table 14–11 briefly reviews the monitoring summary and check list.
- Administer oral medications as ordered (see Table 14–4). Medication should not be added directly to the feeding formula as drug-nutrient interactions can occur. Also be aware of feeding-medication interactions. Much of the diarrhea previously thought to be a complication of enteral feeding may really be associated with the concurrent administration of oral medication. Never administer medications while a feeding is infusing. Stop the feeding, flush the tube with 15 to 30 ml of water, administer the medication, and flush again. If the drug should be administered on an empty stomach, stop the feeding for 15 to 30 minutes, then follow the previous procedure. If administering antacids, wait 30 to 60 minutes before administering other drugs that interact with antacids (e.g., tetracycline, cimetidine, iron supplements, and digoxin; see additional list in Chapter 50). Sorbitol, which increases osmolarity and may result in diarrhea, is a common component of elixirs (e.g., acetaminophen, theophylline, and cimetidine) and manufacturers do not have to reveal the amount. Seek an alternative dose form or similar product, as needed, for medications that cannot be crushed or opened; these medications are listed in Table 14–12. When administering phenytoin (Dilantin), administer the whole dose once daily. Stop the feeding for 2 hours,

Table 14–11. MONITORING SUMMARY AND CHECKLIST

Monitoring Summary	Checklist
When initiating a new or intermittent feeding	Check tube placement. Check amount of residual. If greater than 100 mL, delay feeding for approximately 0.5–1 hr. Consider possible reasons for delayed gastric emptying. Possibly pass tube into intestine.
Every half hour and PRN—intermittent feeding	Check gravity drip rates and patient response.
Every hour and PRN—continuous pump feeding	Check pump functioning and patient response.
Every 2–4 hr of continuous feeding for first 24–48 hr	Check residuals. When stable, residuals assessment may be abandoned.
Every 4 hr	Check vital signs, including blood pressure, temperature, pulse, and respiration.
Every 6 hr	Check blood sugar. (In nondiabetic patient, checks can be discontinued after 48 hr if consistently negative.)
Every 8 hr	Check fluid intake and output. Check specific gravity of urine. Hang new formula for continuous feeding.
Every day	Change feeding container and pump or gravity tubing. Check patient's weight. Check electrolytes, BUN, and blood glucose until stabilized.
PRN	Repeat nutrition assessment. Observe patient for any negative response to tube feeding (e.g., nausea, vomiting, diarrhea). Check tube placement (nasogastric). Calculate nitrogen balance. Conduct delayed hypersensitivity skin testing. Check laboratory data as ordered by physician. Change feeding tube. Clean pump.

Source: Tube Feeding: Clinical Application. Ross Laboratories, Columbus, Ohio 1986, with permission. Modified in 1996.

flush with 30 to 60 mL of water, administer suspension of 1:2 with water, flush with 30 to 60 mL of water, and withhold feeding for 2 more hours.

Another problem associated with oral drug administration is the osmolality of the drug. Table 14–13 provides the osmolality of various medications. Bolus administration of some medications via a feeding tube

Table 14–12. MEDICATIONS THAT CANNOT BE CRUSHED OR OPENED

aspirin, enteric-coated (Ecotrin)
benzonatate (Tessalon)
bisacodyl (Dulcolax)
diclofenac (Voltaren)
diltiazem, sustained-release (Cardizem SR)
diltiazem, controlled-delivery (Cardizem CD)
docusate (Colace)
erythromycin base (Ery-Tab, others)
erythromycin ethylsuccinate (E.E.S. 400, others)
estrogen, conjugated (Premarin)
ferrous sulfate (Feosol, Mol-Iron, others)
indomethacin (Indocin, others)
isotretinoin (Accutane)
morphine sulfate, sustained-release (MS Contin, Roxanol SR)
nifedipine, sustained-release (Procardia XL)
omeprazole (Prilosec)
orphenadrine (Norflex)
pancreatic enzyme (Pancrease, Viokase)
pentoxifylline (Trental)
phenytoin (Dilantin)
piroxicam (Feldene)
potassium chloride, sustained-release (Slow-K, K-Tab, others)
procainamide, sustained-release (Procan SR, others)
propranolol, sustained-release (Inderal LA, others)
quinidine gluconate (Quinaglute, others)
theophylline, sustained-release (Theo-Dur, Slo-Bid, others)
valproic acid (Depakene)
verapamil, sustained-release (Calan SR, Isoptin SR)

presents a high osmotic load to the GI tract and may precipitate diarrhea. These medications are diluted before administration to reduce their osmolality.

Use of Enteral Pumps

Today, numerous enteral pumps are available. The pump should have enough force to push the solution through the tubing even in the presence of small twists in the tubing and there should be alarms for an empty bag, obstruc-

Table 14–13. OSMOLALITY OF VARIOUS MEDICATIONS

Medication	Osmolality (mOsm/kg)
cefaclor suspension (Eli Lilly)	2430
cephalexin suspension (Distal)	2445
cimetidine (Tagamet liquid) (Smith Kline Beecham)	4035
digoxin elixir* (Burroughs Wellcome)	3865
furosemide solution (Hoechst-Roussel)	3375
Neutra-Phos oral solution (Willen)	2500
phenytoin injection (Parke-Davis)	9120
phenytoin suspension (Parke-Davis)	1725
potassium chloride injection (2 mEq/mL)	3600
potassium phosphate injection (3 mEq/mL)	5450
sodium bicarbonate injection (1 mEq/mL)	1730
sodium chloride injection (4 mEq/mL)	7090
theophylline elixir* (Rhone-Poulenc Rorer) 300 mg/liter of enteral feeding	6760
trimethoprim/sulfamethoxazole suspension (Roche)	4560

*Elixirs often contain sorbitol, which can cause diarrhea.

tion, and low battery. The pump should be light so it can easily be carried over a shoulder. Flow accuracy should be within 10%. Rate should be controllable in increments of at least 5.0 mL to optimize flow and adjust for changes in rate-prescription. The pump should be sturdy, resist bumps, and be easily cleaned. A rechargeable battery should last several hours. And, finally, the pump should be simple to operate.

Complications of Enteral Feedings

One of the most common complications of enteral feedings is diarrhea. Diarrhea may be associated with too rapid an infusion rate, lactose intolerance, osmolarity intolerance, low serum albumin levels, vitamin B deficiencies, change in intestinal bacterial, concurrent antibiotic administration, lack of fiber, fat intolerance, too much fluid, or medications. Table 14–14 reviews these problems, their possible causes, and their management and/or prevention.

Measurement of Gastric Intramucosal pH

It is important to determine if the gut is functioning properly or if there is hypoperfusion and hypoxia of the vascular bed in the GI tract. Gastrointestinal tonometry (measurement of the partial pressure of gas) uses a noninvasive device to measure the partial pressure of PCO_2 of the GI mucosa. Intermucosal pH of the gut decreases with hypoxia. Changes in pH may provide an early warning sign of impending shock and the inability of the GI tract to utilize enteral nutrition.

Patient Teaching

Patients going home on tube feedings must have the information presented in Table 14–15 included in their teaching plan. Patients being fed via a tube are deprived of the personal gratification of the act of eating. Studies indicate the most distressing experience of patients who are tube-fed is related to thirst and having an unsatisfied taste for food. Thirst can be eliminated by providing additional water, rinsing the mouth with water, or by chewing gum or sucking on hard candy. Lubricating the lips with petroleum jelly also enhances comfort. Patients and families must have the opportunity to discuss their feelings. Patients are encouraged to join their family at meal times for the social interactions. If the patient prefers not to be present when others are eating, then other provisions for social activities are important.

- Stress the importance of cleaning the teeth, gums, and tongue at least twice a day and as needed to decrease the amount of bacteria in the mouth. Rinsing with a warm water and mouthwash solution both cleans and refreshes. Anesthetic spray and lozenges may also help alleviate any discomfort. Chewing sugarless gum or sucking on hard candy may help keep the mouth moist and satisfy the urge to eat.
- Teach the patient and family the rationale for the feeding, the proposed length of time that this method is necessary, and what is to be expected from these feedings.

Table 14–14. ENTERAL NUTRITION COMPLICATIONS

Complication	Possible Cause	Management
Tube obstruction	Pill fragments, formula residue, physical incompatibilities, slow formula flow	• When possible, use polyurethane feeding tube. • Flush q 4 hr with 30 mL of water during continuous feedings after medications or after intermittent feedings. • Use controller pump. • Use liquid forms of medications. • Irrigate tube with only water if obstruction occurs. Avoid meat tenderizer and pancreatic enzyme, as they can cause lung damage if aspirated.
Pulmonary complications	Improper tube placement Aspiration	• Assess tube position on x-ray film. • Use small-bore feeding tube. • Add food coloring to formula, which allows aspirate to be seen. • Monitor residuals. • Monitor bowel sounds.
Skin/mucous membranes		• Tape tube to minimize pressure on nares. • Keep nares lubricated with water-soluble lubricant. • Oral care at least two times per day and as needed.
Diarrhea	Concomitant drug therapy	• Restore normal flora with *Lactobacillus acidophilus.* • Dilute hypertonic solutions or elixirs. • Alternate magnesium-containing antacid with calcium- or aluminum-containing antacid.
	Formula-related causes	• Avoid lactose formulas. • Temporary use of elemental formulas are helpful (e.g., Ensure, Protain XL, Jevity). • Use low-fat content if possible. • Use formulas high in fiber (e.g., Ensure, Protain XL, Jevity).
	Bacterial contamination	• Use prefilled, ready-to-use containers. • Use good hand-washing technique. • Avoid touching inside of delivery set. • Rinse delivery set with water before adding new formula. • Hang only for 8–12 hr.
	B_6 deficiency Change in bacterial flora Malabsorption	• Administer supplemental B_6. • Restore normal flora. • Discontinue causative agent if possible. • Maintain serum albumin levels. • Monitor brush border of intestine (walls should be like bristles of a brush, not a waxed floor) • Temporary use of elemental formulas is helpful.
Cramps and diarrhea	Cold feeding	• Administer at room temperature. • Never heat a formula.
Nausea	Odor of feeding Too rapid administration	• Use flavored feedings. • Slow feeding.
Constipation	Lack of fluid/fiber	• Administer adequate fluid and fiber in feeding. (Low residue formulas reduce bowel movements—do not confuse with constipation.)
Hyperglycemia	High caloric density formulas	• Monitor blood and/or urine glucose q 4–6 hr. • Monitor for signs and symptoms of hyperglycemia. • Administer insulin as ordered. • Use controller pump.
Hypercapnia	High CHO feedings	• Use low CHO feedings when possible. • Monitor respiration quotient.

• Teach the patient and family how to prepare and administer the feedings and how to care for the tubing. Both patients and their families have to learn what to do if the patient aspirates, what to do if the tube comes out, and what to do in case of any other complications. Patients need to know whom to call and what is and is not an emergency. Both verbal and written instructions are given to the patient and family.

The patient may a have permanent feeding tube that is changed only by the nurse or physician. Or, the patient may be educated to insert his or her own tube. Several manufacturers make small (6F to 8F) diameter, flexible tubes that are ideal for this purpose. Having the patient learn to insert his or her own feeding tube allows the patient to look "normal" when going to work or shopping. The feeding tube is inserted each evening when the feeding is done.

Most enteral formulas are thick and if spilled act as a very strong glue and are difficult to clean up. Pa-

Table 14–15. PATIENT TEACHING INFORMATION—PATIENTS REQUIRING FEEDINGS AT HOME

Dear Patient:

SUPPLEMENTAL FEEDINGS

☐ 1. You will have to use supplemental feedings for _____.
☐ 2. Mix the feeding exactly as instructed in the hospital.
☐ 3. Take the extra feeding between meals.
☐ 4. Keep any leftover feeding solution in the refrigerator.

TUBE FEEDINGS

☐ 1. You will have to use tube feedings for _____.
☐ 2. Mix the feeding exactly as instructed in the hospital.
☐ 3. Administer the tube feeding as taught in the hospital.
☐ 4. Sit up when receiving the tube feeding.
☐ 5. If you have a change in bowel habits (diarrhea or constipation), notify your physician.
☐ 6. Keep any leftover feeding solution in the refrigerator.

PARENTERAL FEEDINGS

☐ 1. You will have to use parenteral feedings for _____.
☐ 2. Make the feeding exactly as instructed in the hospital, or use a ready-made solution.
☐ 3. Administer the parenteral feeding as taught in the hospital.
☐ 4. Care for the IV line as you were shown by the nurse.
☐ 5. If you see any redness or swelling at the site, or if you get a fever, notify your physician.
☐ 6. Keep your parenteral solution in the refrigerator after mixing, and use it within 24 hours.

tients who receive tube feeding during the night should tape all the connections and place papers or plastic under the bottles. To allow the patient to turn at night, suggest that he or she tape the feeding tube to the forehead and place the feeding and the pump at the head of the bed.

Poles are difficult to push around in most homes, particularly up and down stairs, so all apparatus should be wearable.

PLANNING AND INTERVENTION—PARENTERAL NUTRITION

Patients may need parenteral nutritional support both in the hospital and at home. In general, most patients are hospitalized during the initial stage of parenteral nutrition. Later, they may be discharged to home with the feedings. Patients and their families need a great deal of education and support to continue parenteral nutrition at home.

The intervention phase can be divided into four stages: (1) product preparation, (2) preparation of the patient and insertion of the catheter (for TPN) or peripheral IV line (for PTPN), (3) the administration of the solution, and (4) the care of the catheter line.

Preparing the Solution

• Mix TPN solutions in sterile conditions under a laminar flow hood and according to written hospital protocols. Ideally, the solution is prepared in the pharmacy and then sent to the nursing unit. The ambient air found on a busy nursing unit does not provide a

satisfactory environment for preparing sterile TPN solutions. Contamination rates of 10% to 18% have been reported when TPN is mixed without a laminar flow environment. No additives are added to the solution once it is on the nursing unit.

Most pharmacies use commercially prepared TPN solutions. These contain a dextrose bottle and bottle of amino acid solution, which are mixed together. The exact mixing of TPN solutions is done according to individual institutional policies. Any additives are generally added to the dextrose bottle. Insulin may be added to control hyperglycemia, and it can be added at any time. Many authorities today recommend that insulin not be placed in the bottle. Instead, blood is assessed for sugar, and insulin administered every six hours as needed. Some medications are incompatible with TPN solution and are never administered through the same central line.

Administer the TPN solution immediately after mixing or store it in a refrigerator at 4° to 8°C. The solution must generally be used within 7 days of its preparation, although home IV suppliers give a 30-day expiration date.

When parenteral fat emulsions (PFEs) are used, maintain the stability of the lipid emulsion before and during the infusion. Parenteral fat emulsions have an unconventional, milklike appearance. Never agitate the bottle, because the fat globules may aggregate. Inspect the bottle carefully before infusion for cracks and any signs of altered stability. Do not use the PFE if the oil has separated out or if there is an inconsistent texture or color. Discard unused portions within 30 minutes. Nothing except heparin, 1 or 2 units/mL, is ever added to a lipid emulsion. Lipid emulsions may be stored at room temperature.

Inserting the Lines

• Explain the entire procedure to the patient before the catheter is inserted. The patient understands what is going to be done, where the catheter is to be inserted (the subclavian vein is most common), why this particular form of therapy was selected, and the approximate duration of the therapy. Before the procedure begins, the patient, if alert, is also taught how to do the Valsalva maneuver (unless it is contraindicated) and allowed to practice. A properly timed Valsalva maneuver prevents air from entering the catheter and vascular system during the threading maneuver. (See a procedure manual for proper insertion technique.) Whenever possible, the catheter insertions are performed in the operating room to maintain sterility.

Implantable ports or Hickman, Broviac, Portacath, or Groshong catheters are central lines for long-term use that can be used for infusion of drugs, parenteral feedings, or other therapies. These catheters are designed so that the ends may be capped between infusions. Several catheters have a Dacron cuff that is placed under the skin in a tunnel, as shown in Figure 14–2, which decreases the risk of infection and prevents the catheter from becoming dislodged. If this catheter is severed or cut, repair kits are available. The Broviac catheter has a small diameter and

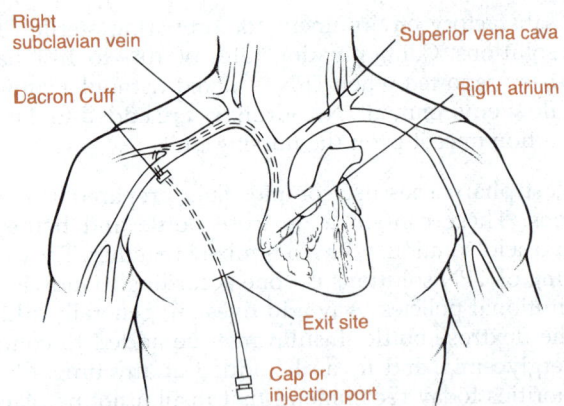

Figure 14–2. Double-lumen catheter. The catheter has a Dacron cuff, that is placed in a tunnel under the skin. This cuff prevents the catheter from becoming dislodged or infected.

it is particularly suitable for children. The Groshong catheter has 1, 2, or 3 lumens and also has a Dacron cuff that is tunneled under the skin. An advantage of the Groshong catheter is that a heparin flush is required only once weekly. When the patient is to receive PFE, a peripheral line may be used with any needle size greater than 20 gauge. For short-term use, a double- or triple-lumen central catheter is preferred.

Administering the Solution

- Administer solutions *steadily*, always with an infusion pump. Patients receiving TPN solutions must be checked at least hourly to observe the infusion rate and to prevent changes in the drip rate, which may be caused by changes in body position or by kinked tubing. Because TPN solutions contain great quantities of glucose, the balance between insulin release and glucose infusion is best achieved by a constant infusion rate. If a TPN solution containing over 20% dextrose must be suddenly interrupted, it is recommended that a 5% dextrose solution with appropriate electrolytes be substituted either through the central catheter or via a peripheral vein to run at the same rate as the previous TPN solution.
- Initiate TPN solution slowly at a rate of 40 to 50 mL/hr and increase the rate over a 24-hour period until the desired rate is reached. The solution is started slowly to allow for the stimulation of the microsomal proteins within the body to utilize the TPN products. In addition, the pancreas is stimulated slowly to increase its release of insulin. To avoid the possibility of contamination and degradation of vitamins, TPN solutions are changed at least every 24 hours. Tubing is changed every 1 to 3 days depending on policy. In-line filters may be used to prevent infection, although their effectiveness has not been conclusively substantiated by research. The filter, if used, is changed daily. If a TPN administration is interrupted for more than 1 hour, the remaining solution is discarded. Usually the TPN solution is tapered slowly.

Before starting the first lipid emulsion, take baseline vital signs and perform a test administration as previously discussed. Monitor vital signs every 10 minutes during this period and observe the patient for the presence of chills, fever, flushing, diaphoresis, chest or back pain, nausea, vomiting, or any other signs of an allergic reaction. If problems arise, the infusion is stopped and the physician is notified.

It is recommended that the lipid emulsion be inserted into a Y-connector or sterile stopcock of the primary tubing closest to the catheter insertion site. This reduces the time the PFE is in contact with a foreign substance, which may affect its stability. Because the lipid particles are very large, an in-line filter is *never* used with PFE. Heparin may be given during the PFE to help speed clearance of the lipids from the patient's plasma.

When the PFE is completed, the bottle is removed, a bottle of 5% dextrose solution is added, and the tubing is flushed. This part of the Y line can then be turned off, but it is left intact until the next lipid infusion, tube, or dressing change. Blood, IV fluids, and some medications are administered through a separate site to avoid contamination of the TPN catheter. Routine blood work is not done until 2 to 6 hours after a PFE so the extra fat in the bloodstream will not distort results. During an infusion of a PFE, a patient is not moved anywhere, as this causes agitation of the bottle.

Care of the Catheter or Line

- Always take special care of the TPN line to ensure its sterility. Infection at the insertion site can progress to colonization of the catheter tip and cause sepsis. Care consists of either daily or alternate-day site care, which may be performed by either the nurse or a physician, depending on institutional policy. A TPN line is generally left in place until it is no longer needed. If a patient has some distant infection in the body, the line may be changed routinely every 1 to 2 weeks to prevent spread of the local infection; however, unless the line is clearly the source of infection, it is better to leave the line in place than to expose the patient to risks of reinsertion.

A line used for PFE is cared for in the same way as any other peripheral line.

Total Nutritional Admixtures

Currently, three-in-one or all-in-one total nutritional admixtures are being used. This mixture is a 24-hour supply of dextrose, crystalline amino acids, and lipids in one container. By mixing these products, all are absorbed evenly over the 24-hour period. Because the lipid is in the combination, piggyback attachments and additional peripheral lines are not necessary. Less frequent manipulation of the lines may reduce the possibility of infection. Only one container is hung every 24 hours, so mixing time is saved. And, fewer administration sets are used. The admixture is opaque, which prevents the nurse from visually checking for suspended particles, fine precipitates, or

Table 14–16. PARENTERAL NUTRITION COMPLICATIONS		
Complication	**Related To**	**Management**
Hepatic dysfunction Fluid and electrolyte imbalances	Substrate intolerance Faulty absorption	• Administer hepatic formulas temporarily. • Monitor F & E balance often. • Monitor patient's weight and urinary output. • Prevent loss of body fluid from high osmolar products.
Infection	Contaminated solution or lines	• Maintain sterile technique when mixing solution. • Change dressing. • Remove lines and reinsert after afebrile for 48 hr.
Aspiration pneumonia	High gastric pH when antacids or H_2 antagonists are administered	• Prevent ulcers with sucralfate (Carafate) while patient is NPO, as sterile pH is maintained in stomach.
Hyperglycemia	High glucose content in formula, diabetes	• Administer less than 25% dextrose solution whenever possible. • Monitor blood glucose levels q 6 hr until stable. • Administer insulin by drip to maintain blood sugar at 100–200 mg/dL
Refeeding Syndrome	TPN forces electrolytes Mg^{++}, PO_4^{++}, Ca^{++} to shift into the cell, thus resulting in hypostates leading to acute heart failure, pulmonary edema, or myocardial infarction.	• Starting TPN 1000 kcal in 24 hr and increasing gradually. • Monitor electrolytes. • Administer electrolytes as needed to correct imbalance.

microbial growth. Also, because of the fat, an in-line filter cannot be used.

Infusion Interrupts

As the patient becomes stabilized on the parenteral feeding, better utilization of nutrients occurs if the infusion is interrupted or cycled for a period each day. The infusion interrupt is started for 2 hours. The IV that is hung during the interrupt can be 5% dextrose/water with half of all the additives in the TPN bottle. The interrupt time is gradually increased to 8 hours. Interruption of the TPN allows for better utilization of nutrients and allows any fat that has accumulated in the liver to be utilized.

Complications of Parenteral Nutrition

As with enteral nutrition, patients receiving parenteral nutrition can experience complications. These complications are described in Table 14–16.

Drug incompatibilities can also occur with TPN solutions. The field of compatibilities is complex and confusing. As administration systems and solutions change, so do the medications that can be safely mixed with them. In the early 1980s, TPN solutions were mixed with only vitamins and minerals. Now admixtures of dextrose, amino acids, fats, and vitamins are becoming more common. Also, TPN solutions are known to be compatible with some medications (e.g., aminophylline, cimetidine, albumin, heparin, hydrocortisone, and insulin, to name a few), but frequent updating on drug compatibilities is necessary.

EVALUATION

• Evaluate the effectiveness of the enteral and parenteral feedings. This evaluation is based on a list of evaluation criteria that has been developed in relation to the goals determined by the nurse, patient, and family. The database obtained in the original assessment and used to formulate the nursing diagnoses provides useful criteria for measuring treatment effectiveness. The typical goals of enteral and parenteral feedings are included in Table 14–9.

• Evaluate all objective symptoms of the patient to ensure that they are returning to normal. Skin turgor, the presence of abnormal thirst, the presence of edema, growth (in infants), changes in weight, urine characteristics (such as amount and specific gravity), and the conditions of the mucous membranes (dry, moist, pink, and so on) indicate changes in hydration level. The older, unconscious, semicomatose, confused, sedated, or intubated patient requires closer evaluation because he or she is unable to convey the presence of thirst.

• Evaluate patients with cardiac disease closely when nutritional support is administered. Approximately 20% of all cardiac output (CO) goes to the GI tract for normal function. When enteral nutrition is administered, CO to the GI tract may increase to 30%, putting an excess burden on the already compromised heart.

• Evaluate liver function studies. Patients with liver disease may have problems related to increased protein intake. A compromised liver cannot make aromatic amino acids and depends on branched-chained amino acids (BCAA) derived from skeletal muscle.

• Evaluate the septic patient for glucose use. Septic patients cannot utilize glucose well. They may need more BCAA for use as energy. Actually, 12 hours prior to developing sepsis, patients usually start to spill glucose in the urine and their WBCs become elevated.

• Evaluate the patient's psychologic response to therapy. Does the patient accept the therapy? How does the patient plan on coping with not eating regular foods (if therapy is long term)? Will the patient comply with the therapy?

- Evaluate blood glucose levels on a routine basis, usually every 6 hours until blood sugar stablizes (about 100 to 200 mg/dL during TPN). The patient may be receiving insulin in the TPN solution or be covered with insulin injections (never bolus insulin, always use a drip). Stress to the patient that he or she will not be permanently diabetic. After TPN is stopped, blood and urinary glucose levels usually fall to normal levels within several days.
- Evaluate laboratory tests for electrolytes and to detect the presence of infection. If infection at the insertion site or due to the catheter, is suspected, all lines are removed and their tips cultured. New lines are inserted in different locations.
- Evaluate subjective symptoms such as anorexia, pain, discomfort, and any emotional complications. Patients receiving parenteral nutrition for long periods may need much skilled emotional support. "Food" is normally associated with eating, and not eating can have major psychologic effects on some people, even to the point of hallucinating about food. Patients must be reassured that their appetites and normal bowel activity will return to normal after parenteral feedings have been stopped. Patients have very few, small

stools, possibly only once a week while TPN is being used.
- Evaluate for side effects of TPN and teach the patient and family what to look for if the patient is being discharged on TPN. The most common side effects of TPN include sensitivity of the patient to the solution manifested by fever or allergic reactions such as itching and hives; metabolic abnormalities noted by glucose intolerance with a blood sugar greater than 200 mg/100 mL or urine glucose of 3 to 4 or more, or hyperosmolar hyperglycemic nonketotic coma (HHNK); electrolyte disorders, or elevated blood urea nitrogen (BUN) or ammonia; mineral deficiencies, including hypocalcemia, hypophosphatemia, and hypomagnesemia, trace mineral deficiencies; and sepsis, for which no other source of contamination can be identified, which necessitates removal of the catheter. The most common side effects of PFE include fever, chills, shivering, vomiting, a sensation of warmth, and pain in the chest and back.

The bibliography for this chapter can be found in Appendix B, which begins on page 1054.

DELIVERING HOME HEALTH CARE

Parenteral Nutrition

Patients requiring total parenteral nutrition (TPN) and parenteral fat emulsions (PFE) are generally in the hospital at the initiation of the therapy. However, because of the prolonged duration of the therapy, patients without other problems may be sent home with a TPN line in place. Policies differ among institutions concerning the discharge care of the individual. Three distinct policies may occur: (1) Some hospitals may send a nurse to the home daily with the premixed TPN solution, and the nurse continues to care for the line and observe the patient for complications; (2) a public health nurse assumes responsibility for visiting the patient, mixing the solution and changing the dressings; or (3) the patient and family are taught how to mix the solutions, how to administer them, how to care for the line(s), what side effects to observe for, and how to handle complications. If the third option is chosen, the nurse has the responsibility of ensuring that the patient's level of knowledge is adequate for self-care at home. Patients on home TPN may infuse their feedings only at

night. This technique enhances patient mobility during the day.

Before infusing TPN solutions:

- Assess patient weight, nutritional status, skin turgor (for hydration), and any complaints the patient may have.

To administer the TPN solution:

- Set up the feeding and start the infusion, maintaining sterile technique.

During the infusion:

- Monitor the patient during the beginning of PFE administration (as described in the text). Teach the patient and family how to perform the procedure.

After the infusion:

- Evaluate for complications (see Table 14–16).

CHAPTER REVIEW QUESTIONS*

1. Which of the following statements is *correct* regarding the process of metabolism?
   a. Anabolism is the breaking down of complex cellular materials.
   b. Catabolism is the synthesis of cellular materials for growth.
   c. If food intake exceeds metabolic demands, anabolism occurs.
   d. If food intake is less than metabolic demands, weight is gained.

2. A general principle concerning the administration of commercial feeding formulas is that:
   a. Hypo-osmolar formulas have a tendency to cause diarrhea.
   b. Protein content is 50% of the total calories.
   c. Fats increase calories without increasing osmolarity.
   d. Most formulas provide 20 calories per mL when fixed full strength.

3. When assessing the patient receiving enteral or parenteral feedings, the nurse is aware that:

a. Thirst may be a sign of dehydration from hyperosmolar enteral feedings.
b. Light, flaky, reddened skin may indicate impending hyperosmolar shock.
c. Patients with food allergies can tolerate enteral feedings without reactions.
d. Hyperosmolar-induced edema occurs as a result of fluid overload.

4. A possible reason for respiratory distress during administration of continuous tube feeding is that:
a. The feeding tube may be in the duodenum.
b. The patient is allergic to the tube feeding formula.
c. A distended stomach interferes with diaphragmatic excursion.
d. A small-bore feeding tube may impede ventilations.

5. Which of the following is a sign or symptom of a catabolic state?
a. Decreased temperature.
b. Tissue edema.
c. Decreased respirations.
d. Elastic skin turgor.

6. An important guideline to teach families of patients who will receive tube feedings at home is to:
a. Store tube feeding at room temperature.
b. Give 100 cc of feeding over a 15-minute period.
c. Stop tube feeding if greater than three stools per day.
d. Place patient in a sitting position for feeding.

*See Appendix A, which begins on page 1051, for answers.

BUILDING YOUR CRITICAL THINKING SKILLS

NUTRITION

Patient 1

Hilda, a 25-year-old woman severely debilitated because of chemotherapy and radiation treatments for ovarian cancer, has recently lost 20% of her body weight. Ensure Plus is started via feeding tube at a rate of 2000 mL/24 hr.

Focus of Inquiry: Within 36 hours of beginning the tube feeding, Hilda has severe, liquid diarrhea.

Analysis and Synthesis: Recall the diarrhea is a complication of tube feeding for several reasons: too much free water in the feeding, high osmolarity of the feeding, poor quality of villi from malnutrition, reduction of bacterial flora of the gut, high osmolarity drugs, and lack of fiber.

New Supposition: Tests for albumin and prealbumin levels are performed, and both indicate severe malnutrition.

Resolution: The tube feedings are slowed to 500 mL/day and parenteral protein solutions are administered IV to restore the function of the villi.

Patient 2

Emily is a 50-year-old woman recently admitted to the intensive care unit (ICU) after an auto accident. She has multiple fractures of both legs, head injury, a cervical neck injury, and a ruptured spleen that was removed on admission. Enteral feeding was started on day 2 of hospitalization.

Focus of Inquiry: On day 7, severe diarrhea has developed.

Analysis and Synthesis: Recall the diarrhea is a complication of tube feeding for several reasons: too much free water in the feeding, high osmolarity of the feeding, poor quality of villi from malnutrition, reduction of bacterial flora of the gut, high osmolarity drugs, and lack of fiber. Examine the patient's oral drugs. Emily is receiving cimetidine q 12 hr and phenytoin 3 times per day.

New Supposition: The diarrhea is most likely due to the administration of both drugs, as they have very high osmolarity (cimetidine 4035 mOsm/kg and phenytoin 9120 mOsm/kg).

Resolution: The nursing order is written to administer the cimetidine mixed with 30 mL of water and the tube flushed with 30 mL after the drug. The physician is consulted, and the phenytoin dosage is changed to 1 time per day mixed with 60 mL of water, followed by a 60 mL flush and the tube clamped for 2 hours. After 3 days, the diarrhea resolves.

UNIT 5

DRUGS AFFECTING THE NERVOUS SYSTEM

CHAPTER 15

Overview of the Anatomy and Physiology of the Nervous System

Merrily A. Kuhn, RNC, PhD
Jeremiah T. Herlihy, PhD
Barbara L. Herlihy, RN, PhD

CHAPTER OUTLINE

Central Nervous System
Peripheral Nervous System

KEY TERMS

Axon
Blood-brain barrier
Effector organ
Ganglia

Interneurons
Neuron
Neurotransmitter

LEARNING OBJECTIVES

After reading this chapter, the student will be able to:

1. Describe the purpose and function of neurotransmitters.
2. Describe the blood-brain barrier.
3. Differentiate between the somatic and autonomic nervous systems.
4. Differentiate between the parasympathetic and sympathetic nervous systems.
5. Differentiate between adrenergic and cholinergic fibers.
6. Describe the adrenergic receptor subtypes (alpha and beta) and the cholinergic receptor subtypes (muscarinic and nicotinic).

This chapter provides a brief and selective review of the nervous system, focusing primarily on those structures and functions affected by neuropharmacologic agents. In general, the nervous system controls and coordinates bodily functions. It receives vast amounts of information and very quickly sorts and integrates this information to determine appropriate responses. In addition to sensation and movement, this highly complex interconnected network of nervous tissue functions in consciousness, thought, memory, learning, emotions, and behavior.

DIVISIONS OF THE NERVOUS SYSTEM

The nervous system is divided into the central nervous system (CNS) and the peripheral nervous system (PNS).

The CNS is composed of the brain and spinal cord, as shown in Figure 15–1. The peripheral nervous system is composed of afferent and efferent systems, which contain the somatic nervous system (SNS) and the autonomic nervous system (ANS). There are two divisions of the ANS: the sympathetic division and the parasympathetic division.

CENTRAL NERVOUS SYSTEM

BRAIN

The main divisions of the brain are the cerebrum, diencephalon (thalamus, hypothalamus), brain stem (mid-

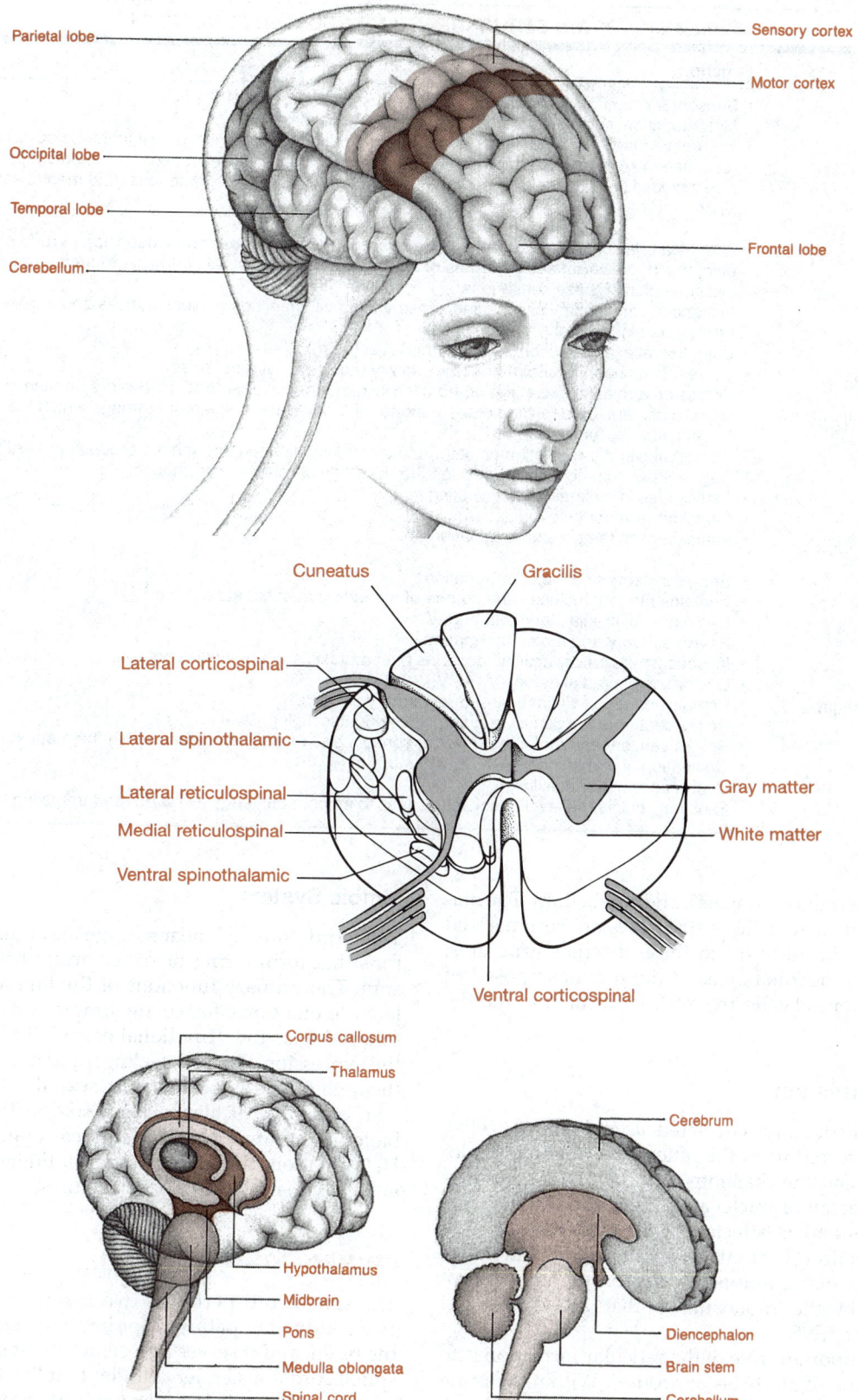

Figure 15–1. Structures of the central nervous system. The cross-section of the spinal cord indicates some of the major ascending (sensory) and descending (motor) tracts.

Table 15–1. BRAIN STRUCTURES AND RELATED FUNCTIONS

Structure	Function
Cerebrum	• Sensory function: awareness and analysis of sensory input. • Motor function: initiation and control of voluntary movement. • Integrative functions: a nebulous term referring to all events that occur within the cerebral cortex in response to sensory input. In addition to the appropriate motor responses (to sensory input), this term also includes consciousness, memory, learning, use of language, emotions, and mental activities of all kinds.
Diencephalon Thalamus	• Acts as a relay center for sensory information. Produces a conscious recognition of rude sensations of pain, touch, pressure, and extremes of temperature. The cerebral cortex is required for finer discrimination of these sensations. • Influences emotions by associating sensory input with feelings of pleasantness and unpleasantness. • Plays a role in the arousal mechanism. • Complex reflexes are coordinated at this level (pain).
Hypothalamus	• Serves as a coordinator of autonomic activity (i.e., visceral responses). • Serves as a relay between the cerebral cortex and the lower autonomic centers and the spinal cord somatic centers. This "linking of the mind to the body" provides a route through which the mind can influence bodily function. • Participates in the regulation of water and electrolyte balance through the production of ADH. • Regulates endocrine function through the secretion of releasing hormones. • Participates in maintaining the waking state. • Participates in appetite regulation. • Participates in temperature regulation.
Brain stem Midbrain	• Relays sensory and motor information. • Contains the red nucleus—the source of the extrapyramidal tracts. • Origination of cranial nerves III and IV.
Pons	• Relays sensory and motor information. • Influences respiratory activity (contains pneumotaxic and apneustic centers). • Origination of cranial nerves V, VI, VII, and VIII.
Medulla oblongata	• Contains cardiac, vasomotor, and respiratory centers. • Reflex center for vomiting, coughing, sneezing, hiccuping, swallowing. • Relays sensory and motor information; sensory and motor tracts cross within the medulla. • Origination of cranial nerves IX, X, XI, and XII.
Cerebellum	• Coordinates motor activity. • Functions below the level of consciousness to smooth out jerky, awkward, and trembling movements.

brain, pons, medulla oblongata), and cerebellum. The major functions of each of these structures are summarized in Table 15–1. In addition to these discrete structures, there are two functional areas of the brain composed of diffuse collections of cells: the reticular formation and the limbic system.

Reticular Formation

Groups of functionally associated *neurons* (nerve cells), collectively referred to as the reticular formation, are located throughout the thalamus and brain stem. Because of its diffuse array of nuclei and fibers, the reticular formation affects and is affected by all CNS activity. The reticular formation (1) modulates both sensory and motor activity, (2) regulates autonomic responses, and (3) produces most of the monoamines that are distributed throughout the CNS.

The most important role of the reticular formation is to maintain a state of alertness or arousal. Within the brain stem reticular formation is the reticular activating system (RAS). The RAS receives impulses from the spinal cord and relays them to the thalamus and from there to all areas of the cerebral cortex. Thus, the reticular formation is the arousal or alerting system for the cerebral cortex; its functioning is crucial for maintaining consciousness. The reticular formation is sensitive to the action of many pharmacologic agents.

Limbic System

The word "limbic" means fringe and refers to those neurons that form a ring or fringe around the corpus callosum. The primary functions of the limbic system are related to emotions; hence, the limbic system is sometimes referred to as the "emotional brain." It is concerned with the expression of mood, feelings, and emotions, especially those emotions associated with sexual behavior, pleasure, fear, and rage. It also plays a role in the regulation of biologic rhythms, appetite, and learning. Like the reticular formation, the limbic system influences and is influenced by many other CNS structures.

SPINAL CORD

The spinal cord performs two major functions: it serves as a conducting pathway for impulses going to and from the brain, and it serves as a center for spinal reflexes. The spinal cord is a slender cylinder that lies within the spinal cavity and extends from the medulla to approximately the second lumbar vertebra. As shown in cross section in Figure 15–1, it consists of an H-shaped inner gray area composed primarily of cell bodies of motor neurons and *interneurons* (neurons that carry impulses from one part of the CNS to another) that is surrounded by an outer area of white matter. The white matter is composed primarily of interneurons, with the majority of their *axons* (processes of a neuron that conduct impulses away from the cell body) covered by a white myelin sheath, hence the designation white matter.

The white matter is arranged in pathways or tracts. Each tract is composed of individual fibers that possess similar anatomic and functional characteristics. For example, the fibers that comprise the spinothalamic tract have the same origin and destination and are concerned with the same general function—the sensations of crude touch, pain, and temperature. Tracts are classified as either ascending (sensory) or descending (motor). Ascending tracts conduct impulses up the spinal cord toward the brain. Descending tracts conduct impulses down the spinal cord from the brain and toward the periphery.

BLOOD-BRAIN BARRIER

The brain is perfused by two fluids: blood and cerebrospinal fluid (CSF). A rich arterial blood supply is provided by the circle of Willis, an interconnecting arrangement of vessels under the cerebrum.

The major sites of nutrient and end-product exchange are the cerebral capillaries. However, the exchange of substances between the blood and nervous tissue differs from the diffusion of nonprotein substances in other capillary beds. The *blood-brain barrier* is the barrier separating the parenchyma of the CNS from blood. It controls both the type and rate of diffusion. This barrier to exchange is both anatomic (i.e., created by brain capillaries and astrocytes) and physiologic (i.e., has physiologic transport systems that handle substances in different ways). The blood-brain barrier presents a formidable barrier to the diffusion of various toxins and pharmacologic agents. The ability of a drug to cross the blood-brain barrier is an important therapeutic consideration. For instance, high plasma levels of an antibiotic may prove ineffective for the treatment of an infection within the CNS if the antibiotic is unable to cross the barrier. Generally, the blood-brain barrier is permeable to water, oxygen, carbon dioxide, and most lipid-soluble substances, including alcohol and anesthetics.

The cells of the CNS are perfused by a second fluid, the CSF. Cerebrospinal fluid is formed by the choroid plexuses and flows through the ventricles and central canal of the spinal cord and throughout the subarachnoid space. The CSF protects the brain and spinal cord from mechanical damage. A barrier also exists within the choroid plexus; secretion is therefore selective and accounts for the difference in electrolyte concentrations of the CSF and plasma. The CSF eventually drains into the dural venous sinuses and finally into the internal jugular veins.

NEUROTRANSMITTERS

Information is transferred centrally and peripherally in the form of electrical impulses. The process involves both electrical conduction of the signal down the axon and chemical transmission of the signal from one neuron to another or from a neuron to an *effector organ* (a structure such as a muscle or gland that produces an effect when stimulated) across the neural synapse or across the effector cell junction, respectively. The chemical transmission of the signal is accomplished by chemicals called neurotransmitters. A *neurotransmitter* is a chemical substance released by a neuron that acts on another neuron, a muscle fiber, or gland to initiate or modulate an action potential.

Common neurotransmitters include norepinephrine, serotonin, dopamine, and acetylcholine, featured with other neurotransmitters in Table 15–2. Disturbances in the levels of various neurotransmitters have been implicated in certain disease states. For instance, a deficiency of do-

Table 15–2. NEUROTRANSMITTERS AND NEUROHORMONES

Transmitter	Type	Characteristics
Acetylcholine	Excitatory (primarily)	Found in autonomic nervous system. Facilitates transmission over the myoneural junction. Inactivated by cholinesterase.
Norepinephrine	Excitatory	Distributed throughout brain; lower in putamen and caudate, also in the postganglionic synapse of the sympathetic division of autonomic nervous system. Inactivated by MAO.
Dopamine	Excitatory	Highest concentration in caudate and putamen. Implicated in regulation of emotional responses and complex movements. Inactivated by MAO.
Serotonin	Inhibitory	Concentrated in pons, upper brain stem, and hypothalamus. Acts as a vasoconstrictor and vasopressor and may play a role in temperature regulation, sensory perception, and the onset of sleep.
Gamma-aminobutyric acid (GABA)	Inhibitory	Present largely in gray matter of brain and cord. Influences brain activity. Hyperpolarizes postsynaptic membranes.
Glutamic acid	Excitatory	Amino acid present throughout nervous system, unequally distributed in the spinal cord, and released by primary afferent nerve endings.
Neuropeptides (enkephalins and endorphins)	Inhibitory	Found in some sensory neurons at their synapses with spinal cord neurons. In the brain, may be involved with perception and integration of pain and emotional responses.

pamine within the basal ganglia has been associated with Parkinson's disease, while dopamine excess within the limbic system has been implicated in schizophrenia. Alterations in neurotransmitter levels have obvious pathophysiologic and pharmacologic implications.

PERIPHERAL NERVOUS SYSTEM

AFFERENT DIVISION

The afferent division of the PNS is composed of nerves that convey sensory information (pain, sound, and so on) from the sensory receptors to the CNS. The cell bodies of the afferent nerves lie outside, but near, the CNS. Action potentials are initiated by the receptors and are conducted via these afferent neurons to the CNS.

EFFERENT DIVISION

The efferent division of the PNS, more diverse than the afferent division, includes the SNS and the ANS, the latter being further subdivided into the sympathetic and parasympathetic divisions.

Anatomy

Somatic efferent nerves innervate only skeletal (voluntary) muscle. The cell bodies of these neurons are grouped within the brain and spinal cord and synapse directly with skeletal muscle cells. Action potentials initiated by local reflexes or by the activity of descending central pathways are rapidly conducted via the large-diameter, myelinated axons of these motor neurons to their respective skeletal muscles.

Autonomic efferent nerves innervate cardiac and smooth muscle as well as glands. Unlike the somatic efferent neurons that synapse directly with their respective effector organ (skeletal muscle), preganglionic autonomic nerve fibers, originating in the spinal cord or brain, synapse with cell bodies of postganglionic neurons arranged in clusters (*ganglia*) located outside the CNS. At the synapse a neurotransmitter is released and moves (diffuses) across the synapse. An action potential is initiated in the postganglionic fiber and is conducted to the effector organ (heart, intestine, and so on).

Several anatomic features distinguish the parasympathetic from the sympathetic divisions of the ANS. First, these divisions differ in the location of their respective ganglia. The parasympathetic ganglia are situated mainly within the effector organ, while most of the sympathetic ganglia lie close to the spinal cord (paravertebral ganglia), as shown in Figure 15–2. Thus, the parasympathetic nervous system possesses long preganglionic and short postganglionic nerve fibers, while the sympathetic nervous system consists of short preganglionic and long postganglionic nerve fibers.

The sympathetic and parasympathetic divisions also differ in the location from which the preganglionic fibers exit the CNS. Sympathetic fibers emerge from either the thoracic or lumbar sections (thus the thoracolumbar system) of the spinal cord. In contrast, the parasympathetic

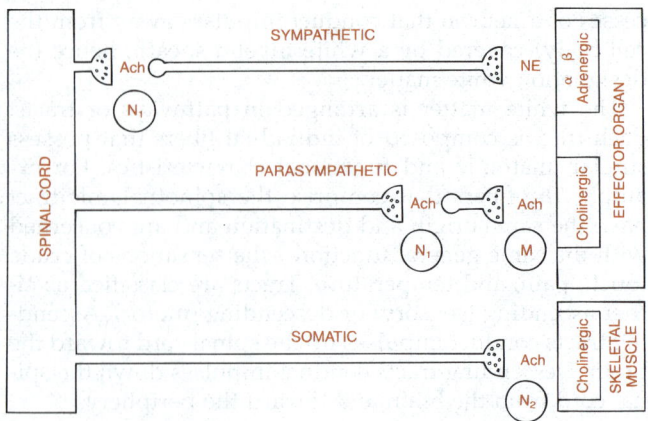

Figure 15–2. Schematic of the autonomic and somatic nervous systems. Ach = acetylcholine. NE = norepinephrine. N_1 = nicotinic type 1 receptors. N_2 = nicotinic type 2 receptors. M = muscarinic receptors. α, β = alpha- and beta-adrenergic receptors, respectively. (From Herlihy & Herlihy, Critical Care Nurse 6(17), 1986, with permission.)

preganglionic fibers (the craniosacral system) originate in either the subcortical axis (brain) or the sacral portion of the spinal cord.

Finally, the ratio of preganglionic to postganglionic fibers differs between the two systems. In general, in the sympathetic nervous system, one preganglionic fiber activates many postganglionic fibers. In the parasympathetic system, one preganglionic fiber may activate one postganglionic fiber. The result of this difference is that sympathetic outflow tends to cause widespread effects whereas parasympathetic activity causes more localized effects.

Physiology

The function of the somatic motor system is simply to initiate contraction of skeletal muscle. Without somatic motor impulses, voluntary muscle cannot contract. Because an individual neuron may innervate several skeletal muscle fibers, the functional motor unit consists of the somatic motor nerve fiber and its respective skeletal muscle fibers. Somatic motor nerves are only excitatory; that is, their activation inevitably leads to contraction of the skeletal muscle. No inhibitory somatic motor nerves have been described.

The function of the ANS differs in several ways from the SNS. First, activation of the ANS generally does not initiate activity in the effector organs. Instead, it modulates the spontaneous activity arising from the organ itself. Second, activation of the ANS is not confined exclusively to excitation: it can enhance or inhibit the intrinsic activity of the effector organs. Whether activity is enhanced or inhibited depends on the organ itself and which of the autonomic nerves (sympathetic or parasympathetic) is exerting the major influence on that organ.

Much of the functional complexity of the ANS resides in the great diversity of effector organ responses to sympathetic and parasympathetic nerve stimulation. Table 15–3 lists the predominant effects of sympathetic and parasympathetic nerve stimulation on the function of many major organs and tissues. Note that these two sys-

Table 15–3. SYMPATHETIC AND PARASYMPATHETIC RESPONSES OF SELECTED EFFECTOR ORGANS TO AUTONOMIC NERVE STIMULATION

Organ System	Receptor Subtype	Sympathetic Response	Parasympathetic Response
Cardiovascular system			
Heart rate	Beta$_1$	Increase	Decrease
Atrioventricular conduction	Beta$_1$	Increase	Decrease
Contractility	Beta$_1$	Increase	Decrease
Blood vessels*	Alpha	Contract	Relax
	Beta$_2$	Relax	—
Pulmonary system			
Bronchial muscle	Beta$_2$	Relax	Contract
Bronchial glands	—	—	Stimulate
Gastrointestinal system			
Motility	Alpha and beta$_2$	Decrease	Increase
Sphincters	Alpha	Contract	Relax
Secretion	—	—	Stimulate
Urinary bladder			
Detrusor	Beta$_2$	Relax	Contract
Trigone and sphincter	Alpha	Contract	Relax
Miscellaneous			
Male sex organs	Alpha	Ejaculation	Erection
Uterus (pregnant)	Alpha	Contract	Variable
Uterus (nonpregnant)	Beta	Relax	Variable
Sweat glands	Alpha	Secretion	Secretion
Liver	Alpha	Glycogenolysis	Glycogen synthesis
	Beta	Gluconeogenesis	—
Fat cells	Alpha and beta	Lipolysis	—
Salivary gland secretions	Alpha	K$^+$ and H$_2$O	K$^-$ and H$_2$O
	Beta	Amylase	

*The sympathetic system in skeletal muscle is cholinergic and elicits vasodilation.

tems often exert opposite effects on a given organ. In general, the sympathetic system activates those organs necessary for physical activity, including the "fight-or-flight" reaction. Increase in heart rate and contractility, shunting of blood from skin and viscera to working skeletal and cardiac muscle, and mobilization of glucose to supply an acute demand for energy—all of these arise from enhanced sympathetic outflow. The parasympathetic system, on the other hand, regulates normal activity in a nonstressful situation. Under its influence, heart rate declines, blood is shunted away from the resting muscle to the viscera and kidney, and food absorption is enhanced by activation of the gastrointestinal system.

Peripheral Neurotransmitters

The efferent division of the peripheral nervous system utilizes many neurotransmitters, but only acetylcholine (Ach) and norepinephrine (NE) are discussed here. Neurons that release Ach and receptors that bind Ach are referred to as cholinergic nerve fibers and cholinergic receptors, respectively. Neurons that release NE and receptors that bind NE are referred to as adrenergic nerve fibers and adrenergic receptors, respectively.

The SNS is completely cholinergic; that is, it utilizes only acetylcholine as the neurotransmitter across the myoneural junction, as shown in Figure 15–3. Acetylcho-

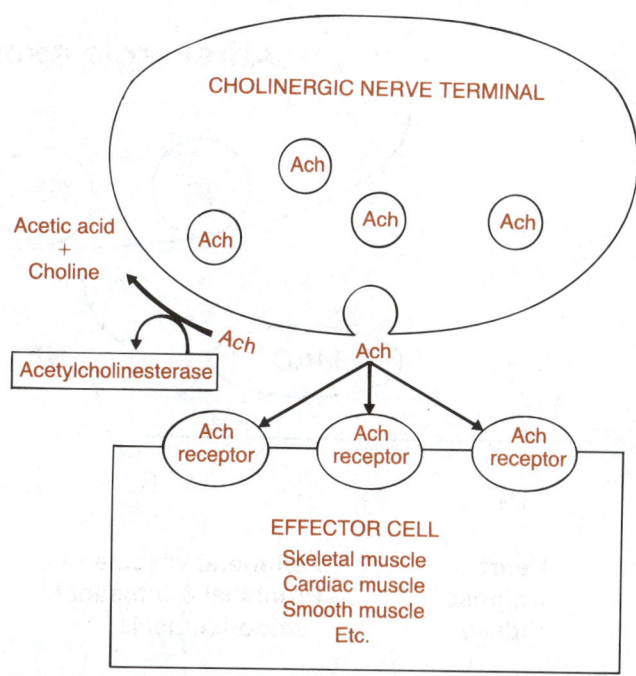

Figure 15–3. Schematic of the cholinergic axon terminal and effector cell. Ach = acetylcholine. Acetylcholinesterase, located on the postsynaptic membrane, catalyzes the degradation of Ach to acetic acid and choline.

line is synthesized in the somatic axon terminal and stored in synaptic vesicles. An action potential arriving at the nerve terminal causes the vesicular and plasma membranes to fuse and break down. Acetylcholine is released from the axon terminal, diffuses across the synapse, binds to the postsynaptic receptor, and initiates a new action potential in the skeletal muscle fiber. Contraction then ensues. The removal of Ach from the myoneural junction and postjunctional membrane terminates its action. This removal occurs through (1) degradation by acetylcholinesterase and (2) diffusion into the plasma compartment for processing by other organs of the body.

The effective Ach concentration can, therefore, be altered in several ways. Any agent that decreases Ach synthesis or release, or increases its degradation, compromises the action of somatic nerves on skeletal muscle. Conversely, agents that increase Ach synthesis or release, or decrease its degradation, enhance the action of the SNS on skeletal muscle (see Chapter 22).

The ANS consists of both cholinergic and adrenergic nerve fibers and receptors and utilizes both acetylcholine and norepinephrine as neurotransmitters, as shown in Figure 15–4. It is imperative to note that all preganglionic nerve fibers (whether sympathetic or parasympathetic) are cholinergic; that is, Ach is the neurotransmitter released from preganglionic axon terminals. Thus, agents that interfere with the synthesis, release, or inactivation of Ach affect both the sympathetic and parasympathetic systems. The situation differs quite markedly with regard

to the postganglionic cells. The parasympathetic postganglionic neurons are cholinergic and release Ach, as do the preganglionic autonomic axon terminals and the somatic axon terminals. However, most sympathetic postganglionic nerve fibers are adrenergic and release NE as the neurotransmitter.

The synthesis, storage, release, and degradation of Ach in the ANS are identical to those described above for the SNS. In the sympathetic system, NE is synthesized in the postganglionic cell body and packaged in storage vesicles that flow to the axon terminals. An action potential releases NE from the sympathetic neuron in a manner analogous to that described above for Ach. NE diffuses across the synaptic cleft, binds to the postsynaptic receptor, and modulates the activity of the effector organ. The action of NE can be terminated by (1) diffusion into the plasma compartment for processing by other organs of the body, (2) reuptake into the presynaptic terminal for repackaging or further metabolism by monoamine oxidase (MAO) or catechol O-methyltransferase (COMT), or (3) uptake by the effector cell and degradation by COMT and MAO.

As with cholinergic transmission, adrenergic transmission can be inhibited by agents that decrease synthesis or release or enhance degradation. Conversely, adrenergic transmission can be enhanced by agents that increase synthesis or release or decrease degradation. The adrenal medulla, which can be considered a specialized ganglion of the sympathetic nervous system, is innervated by cholinergic preganglionic fibers and releases mainly epineph-

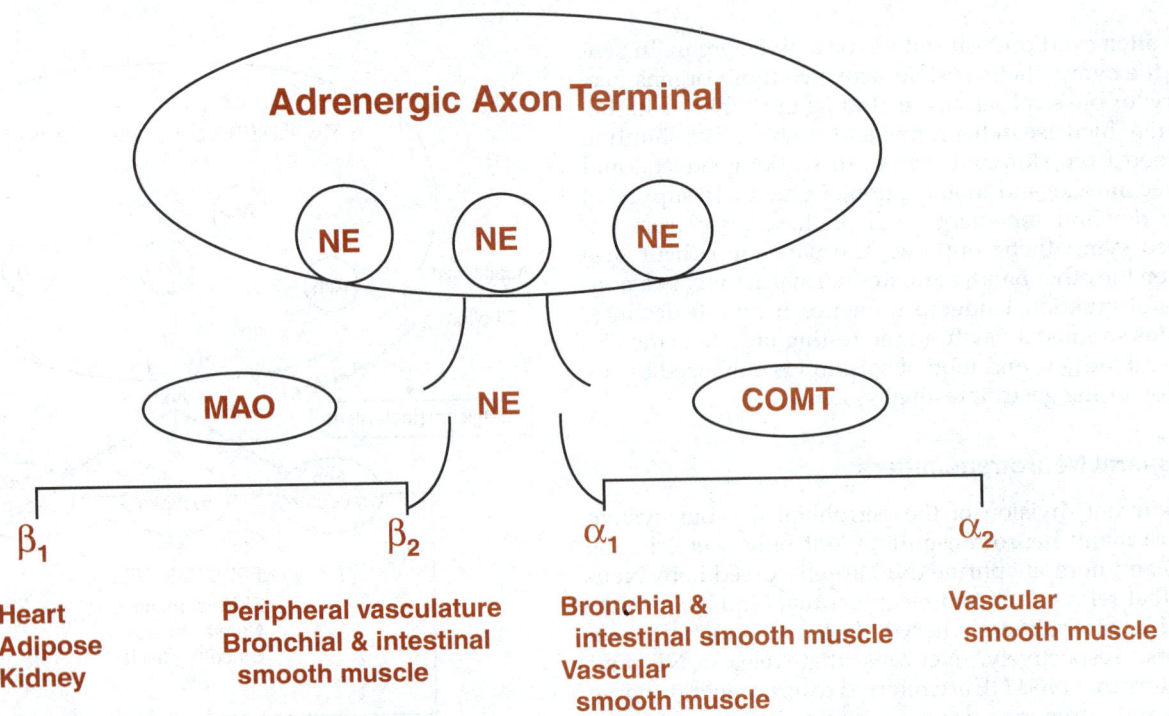

Figure 15–4. Schematic of the adrenergic axon terminal and effector cell. NE = norepinephrine. α_1 = alpha$_1$ receptor. α_2 = alpha$_2$ receptor. β_1 = beta$_1$ receptor. β_2 = beta$_2$ receptor. COMT (catechol-O-methyl transferase) and MAO (monamine oxidase) are enzymes responsible for the degradation of NE.

rine (and some NE) directly into the blood, which in turn stimulates adrenergic receptors.

Receptors

Although the efferent peripheral system contains many other types of receptors (serotoninergic, dopaminergic, purinergic, etc.), only the cholinergic and adrenergic receptors are discussed here. Cholinergic receptors specifically bind Ach, whereas adrenergic receptors specifically bind NE (and epinephrine). Agents that bind to cholinergic receptors and elicit effects similar to Ach are termed cholinomimetic agents. Agents that bind to adrenergic receptors and elicit effects similar to NE are called sympathomimetic agents. These major receptor types are divided into subtypes. A given agonist or antagonist may bind to only one receptor subtype, or it may bind more broadly to more than one receptor subtype. Many of the adverse and side effects of drugs arise from the tendency of a drug to interact with more than one receptor subtype.

The cholinergic receptors are subdivided into muscarinic and nicotinic subtypes. This division is based on the observation that certain cholinergic receptors are activated by muscarine, whereas other cholinergic receptors are activated by nicotine. Muscarinic receptors are located only on the effector cell membranes innervated by parasympathetic postganglionic fibers (see Fig. 15–2). In contrast, nicotinic receptors are found in the somatic nervous system as well as in the ganglia of the autonomic (both sympathetic and parasympathetic) nervous system. The distinction between muscarinic and nicotinic receptors has important ramifications for drug therapy. Muscarinic antagonists (e.g., atropine) exert limited effects, which remain confined to the parasympathetic postganglionic nerve transmission. On the other hand, ganglionic antagonists (e.g., mecamylamine), which block nicotinic receptors, exert effects beyond ganglionic transmission. When ganglionic transmission is blocked, both cholinergic (muscarinic) and adrenergic postganglionic fibers remain quiescent, affecting the whole ANS.

Nicotinic receptors are further subdivided into nicotinic type 1 (N_1) and nicotinic type 2 (N_2). Neuromuscular blocking agents such as pancuronium, which are relatively specific for cholinergic N_2 receptors, exert very little effect on autonomic ganglionic transmission (cholinergic N_1). Other neuromuscular blocking agents such as tubocurarine block both N_1 and N_2 receptors and therefore exert a broader inhibition of the ANS.

The adrenergic receptors are subdivided into alpha and beta subtypes (see Figs. 15–2 and 15–4). An organ's response to adrenergic stimulation is highly dependent on whether alpha or beta receptors are primarily activated. For example, although NE can affect the activity of both alpha and beta receptors, its release produces different effects in the different organs, depending on the concentration of receptors. Cardiac muscle possesses mainly beta receptors with few (if any) alpha receptors, which results in increased contactibility and heart rate. Therefore, the effect of NE released from the cardiac sympathetic nerves is mediated primarily by stimulation of beta receptors. However, in the peripheral vasculature, because the alpha receptor is the major receptor subtype, the release of NE from peripheral sympathetic nerves causes vascular smooth muscle contraction. Norepinephrine (as well as epinephrine) is often referred to as a catecholamine because of its chemical structure. Synthetic catecholamines can activate predominantly either alpha receptors or beta receptors. For example, phenylephrine activates predominantly alpha receptors, whereas isoproterenol activates beta receptors.

Both alpha- and beta-adrenergic receptors are further subdivided into subtypes 1 and 2 (see Fig. 15–4). $Beta_1$ receptors are located in heart, adipose tissue, and kidney. Activation of these receptors causes an increase in heart rate and contractility, adipocyte lipolysis, and release of renin from the kidney. $Beta_2$ receptors are located primarily in the peripheral vasculature and in bronchial and intestinal smooth muscle. Activation of $beta_2$ receptors causes vasodilation, bronchodilation, and inhibition of intestinal motility. Naturally occurring compounds like epinephrine, or synthetic beta-agonists like isoproterenol, have both $beta_1$ and $beta_2$ activity. Some synthetic compounds, like albuterol, have only $beta_2$ activity. Synthetic antagonists possess similar specificities. For example, propranolol blocks both $beta_1$ and $beta_2$ receptors, while atenolol is relatively specific for $beta_1$ receptors.

The alpha-adrenergic receptors are subdivided into $alpha_1$ and $alpha_2$ receptor subtypes (see Fig. 15–4). The $alpha_1$ receptor is located on effector cell membranes innervated by sympathetic nerves. In vascular smooth muscle, $alpha_1$ adrenergic stimulation leads to vasoconstriction; in bronchial and intestinal smooth muscle it causes relaxation. The $alpha_2$ receptor subtype is located on both the presynaptic sympathetic nerve terminal and the postsynaptic membrane. When activated, the presynaptic $alpha_2$ receptor inhibits the further release of NE from the nerve terminal (see Fig. 15–4). Postsynaptic $alpha_2$ stimulation causes constriction of vascular smooth muscle. Recent evidence suggests that activation of postsynaptic $alpha_2$ receptors plays a major role in control of blood flow.

The bibliography for this chapter can be found in Appendix B, which begins on page 1054.

CHAPTER REVIEW QUESTIONS*

1. Alpha$_1$ adrenergic stimulation causes:
   a. Bronchial constriction.
   b. Vascular vasodilation.
   c. Constriction of intestinal smooth muscle.
   d. Bronchial dilation.

2. Beta$_1$ receptors are located in all of the following sites *except*:
   a. Bronchial smooth muscle.
   b. Heart.
   c. Adipose tissue.
   d. Kidney.

3. Nerve receptors that bind with norepinephrine are:
   a. Cholinergic.
   b. Adrenergic.
   c. Dopaminergic.
   d. Purinergic.

4. Which of the following statements is *correct* concerning peripheral neurotransmitters?
   a. The somatic nervous system utilizes only acetylcholine as the neurotransmitter.
   b. All autonomic preganglionic nerve fibers release norepinephrine as the neurotransmitter.
   c. The parasympathetic postganglionic nerve fibers release norepinephrine.
   d. The sympathetic postganglionic nerve fibers release only acetylcholine.

*See Appendix A, which begins on page 1051, for answers.

CHAPTER 16

Drugs Affecting the Parasympathetic Nervous System

Merrily A. Kuhn, RNC, PhD

CHAPTER OUTLINE

Cholinomimetic Agents
Anticholinergic Agents
Nursing Implications for Administering Drugs Affecting the
   Parasympathetic Nervous System

KEY TERMS

Anticholinesterases

Cholinomimetic agents

LEARNING OBJECTIVES

After reading this chapter, the student will be able to:

1. Discuss the similarities and differences between the cholinergic drugs—the direct-acting cholinomimetics, the indirect-acting cholinomimetics (anticholinesterases), and anticholinergic agents.
2. Describe general drug action, therapeutic uses, pharmacokinetics, contraindications and precautions, and adverse effects of each of the classifications.
3. Understand general nursing implications for cholinergic medications.

The parasympathetic nervous system works with the sympathetic nervous system to maintain homeostasis. (See Chapter 15 for a review of the parasympathetic nervous system.) Because autonomic drugs affect multiple systems and organs of the body, the parasympathetic drugs are discussed in detail in chapters corresponding to the affected body systems. For example, the medications used for myasthenia gravis, glaucoma, and hypertension are discussed in separate chapters. This chapter presents only an overview of each class of the parasympathetic agents. It does not contain a nursing process section because these drugs are used for such varied conditions; however, a short section on nursing care is included. Table 16–1 references chapters in which the nursing process sections for specific parasympathetic agents can be found.

The parasympathetic agents are classified into four types: (1) cholinomimetic agents (direct-acting), (2) anticholinesterases (indirect-acting cholinomimetic agents,

cholinesterase inhibitors), (3) anticholinergic agents (muscarinic blockers, antimuscarinics), and (4) neuromuscular blockers. Neuromuscular blockers are discussed in Chapter 22.

CHOLINOMIMETIC AGENTS

Cholinomimetic agents are substances that elicit a similar response and mimic the action of acetylcholine. The cholinergic receptor categories are nicotinic, muscarinic, and neuromuscular (see Chapter 15). The cholinergic receptor can be stimulated by (1) direct activation with a cholinergic agonist; (2) the release of acetylcholine; and (3) inhibition of the breakdown of acetylcholine, allowing for the buildup of endogenous acetylcholine (indirect-acting).

In a patient with myasthenia gravis, drugs that stimulate the nicotinic neuromuscular receptors are of therapeutic value. In patients with urinary retention, intestinal atony, or glaucoma, drugs that stimulate muscarinic

The publisher gratefully acknowledges the contribution of Barbara K. Clark, RN, MN, CCRN, to the third edition.

Table 16–1. NURSING PROCESS REFERENCES FOR PARASYMPATHETIC DRUGS

Drug	Classification	Indications	Nursing Process Chapter Reference
Carbachol	Cholinomimetic	Simple glaucoma	63
		Stimulates bladder and intestine	50
Bethanechol	Cholinomimetic	Open-angle glaucoma	63
		Prevention and treatment of postoperative bowel distention, gastric atony, and congenital megacolon	50
Pilocarpine	Cholinomimetic	Decreases intraocular pressure in simple glaucoma and in treatment of detached retina	63
Neostigmine (Prostigmin)	Cholinesterase inhibitor	Myasthenia gravis	23
		Esophageal dilation and initiation of peristalsis postoperatively	50
		Potentiation of narcotics, including morphine	18
Physostigmine (Eserine)	Cholinesterase inhibitor	Miotic to treat glaucoma	63
Atropine sulfate	Anticholinergic	Preoperative medication to diminish secretions and block cardiac vagal reflexes	21
		Dilate pupil in eye surgery	63
Propantheline bromide (Pro-Banthine)	Anticholinergic	Reduces gastric acid secretion	50
		Decreases spasm of the gastrointestinal tract	50
		Decreases rigidity of Parkinson's disease	23

receptors are beneficial because muscarinic agonists decrease gastrointestinal (GI) secretions, decrease gut motility, and induce pupillary constriction. Other cholinomimetics are nonselective, limiting the effects of acetylcholine at the cholinergic receptors.

DIRECT-ACTING CHOLINOMIMETICS

The direct-acting cholinomimetics directly bind to and activate muscarinic or nicotinic receptors. The cholinomimetics are divided into two groups: the choline esters similar to acetylcholine—including **acetylcholine, carbachol (Miostat, Isopto Carbachol)**, and **bethanechol (Urecholine, Duvoid)**—and the alkaloids, derived from plant sources—including **muscarine, pilocarpine (Ocusert, Pilo-20, Pilo-40)**, and **nicotine**.

Action

The parasympathetic nervous system can modify organ function in two ways. First, acetylcholine can activate muscarinic receptors on the effector organ, thus altering organ function. Second, acetylcholine can interact with muscarinic receptors on sympathetic nerve terminals, thereby blocking the release of norepinephrine.

Activation of nicotinic receptors results in depolarization of the nerve cell. Activation of this receptor causes structural changes that allow sodium and potassium ions to diffuse down the concentration gradients. Table 16–2 shows the effects of cholinomimetic drugs on different systems in the body.

Uses

The major uses of muscarinic agonists are for diseases of the eye (glaucoma, accommodative esotropia), the gastro-

intestinal and urinary system (postoperative atony, neurogenic bladder), and the heart (atrial dysrhythmias).

Pharmacokinetics

The choline esters are lipid insoluble, so they are poorly absorbed and distributed in the central nervous system. The cholinomimetic alkaloids are absorbed from most sites of administration, including the gastrointestinal tract. Because these alkaloids are not esters, they escape the enzymatic destruction by cholinesterases, therefore increasing the duration of action. Excretion of these agents is through the kidneys.

Contraindications and Precautions

Contraindications to the use of cholinomimetics include diabetes mellitus, coronary artery disease, myocardial infarction, heart block, and gangrene, as these conditions are aggravated by the effects of the drugs. Caution is used if these drugs are given to patients with respiratory disorders or asthma because the cholinomimetic effect can exaggerate bronchial constriction and increase secretions. The gastrointestinal tract has increased contractile activity and increased gastric secretions; therefore, the cholinominetics are contraindicated in patients with mechanical obstruction of the intestine, ulcerative colitis, or upper gastrointestinal disease such as peptic ulcer. Cholinomimetics are also contraindicated in patients with preexisting muscle-weakening disorders such as myotonia congenita and myotonia atrophica. Safe use in pregnancy (category C), lactation, and children has not been established.

Adverse Effects

The adverse effects of these drugs include the development of increased bronchial secretions and respiratory

Table 16–2. EFFECTS OF CHOLINOMIMETIC, ANTICHOLINESTERASE, AND ANTICHOLINERGIC AGENTS ON BODY SYSTEMS

Tissue or System	Effects of Direct-Acting Cholinomimetics	Effects of Indirect-Acting Cholinomimetics (Anticholinesterases)	Effects of Anticholinergics
Skin	Increased sweating, dilation of blood vessels	Sweating	Inhibition of sweating (hyperpyrexia may result); flushing
Eye	Contraction of iris and ciliary muscle	Lacrimation, miosis, blurred vision, accommodative spasm	Cycloplegia (relaxation of ciliary muscle); mydriasis (relaxation of sphincter pupillae muscle); increase in aqueous outflow resistance (increases introcular pressure in many cases of glaucoma)
Digestive	Increased motility; relaxes sphincters; stimulates secretions	Salivation; increased gastric, pancreatic, and intestinal secretions; increased tone and motility in gut (abdominal cramps, vomiting, diarrhea, and defecation)	Decreased salivation; reduced tone and motility in the gastrointestinal tract; decrease in vagus-stimulated gastric, pancreatic, intestinal, and bilary secretions
Urinary	Urinary frequency (contraction of detrusor muscle), relaxation of sphincter	Urinary frequency and incontinence	Urinary retention (relaxation of the detrusor muscle); relaxation of ureter and urinary sphincter
Respiratory	Bronchoconstriction; stimulates bronchial glands	Increased bronchial secretions, bronchoconstriction, weakness or paralysis of respiratory muscles	Bronchial dilation and decreased secretions
Skeletal muscle	No effect	Fasciculations, weakness, paralysis (depolarizing block)	No effect
Cardiovascular	Decrease in rate (negative chronotropy); decrease in atrial contractile strength (negative inotropy); decrease in refractory period; decrease in conduction velocity (negative dromotropy); small decrease in contractile strength of ventricles	Bradycardia (due to muscarinic predominance), decreased cardiac output, hypotension; effects due to ganglionic actions and activation of adrenal medulla also possible	Bradycardia at low doses (may be a CNS effect) and tachycardia at higher doses (peripheral effect); increased cardiac output if patient is recumbent
Central nervous system	Tremor, anxiety, restlessness, disrupted concentration and memory, confusion, sleep disturbances, desynchronization of electroencephalogram, convulsions, coma, circulatory and respiratory depression	Tremor, anxiety, restlessness, disrupted concentration and memory, confusion, sleep disturbances, desynchronization of electroencephalogram, convulsions, coma, circulatory and respiratory depression	Decreased concentration and memory, drowsiness, sedation, excitation, ataxia, asynergia; decrease in alpha electroencephalogram and increase in low-voltage slow waves (as in drowsy state); hallucinations, coma

embarrassment. In addition, the cholinomimetics may cause diarrhea and increased GI secretion.

INDIRECTING-ACTING CHOLINOMIMETICS

Indirect-acting cholinomimetics, or *anticholinesterases* (cholinesterase inhibitors), are agents that inhibit the action of acetylcholinesterase, an enzyme that degrades acetylcholine. Anticholinesterases interact with cholinesterase enzymes and block their catalytic activity. Acetylcholinesterase (AChE) normally destroys acetylcholine at various cholinergic nerve endings. Because of the blocking ability of anticholinesterase agents, acetylcholine accumulates at the cholinergic receptor sites and contributes to stimulation of the cholinergic receptors in the central and peripheral nervous systems. These drugs not only serve as therapeutic agents but also are used in agricultural insecticides and in chemical warfare. Because anti-

cholinesterases prolong the action of acetylcholine, they are also called indirect-acting cholinoceptor stimulants. Table 16–2 lists the effects of anticholinesterase agents on various body systems.

The cholinesterase inhibitors fall into three chemical groups: simple alcohols having a quaternary ammonium group—including **ambenonium chloride (Mytelase)**, **edrophonium (Tensilon)**, and **pyridostigmine bromide (Mestinon)**; carbamic acid esters of alcohols having quaternary or tertiary ammonium groups—including **neostigmine (Prostigmin)** and **physostigmine (Isopto-Eserine)**; and organic derivatives of phosphoric acid—including **isoflurophate (Floropryl)**.

Uses

Anticholinesterase agents have a variety of clinical uses. Neostigmine, pyridostigmine, and edrophonium are used in anesthesia to reverse the neuromuscular blockade caused by nondepolarizing muscle relaxants. Anticholinesterases are used to improve muscle strength in myasthenia gravis, a disease in which neurotransmission at skeletal muscles is impaired. Anticholinesterase agents can also be used to treat glaucoma, strabismus, smooth muscle atony, and antimuscarinic toxicity. If these agents fail to lower intraocular pressure, then a long-acting anticholinesterase agent such as isoflurophate is used. Marked ciliary spasm can occur with this agent. Strong miotics can also produce iris cysts, which disappear if the agents are discontinued.

Pharmacokinetics

The quaternary compounds, because they are lipid insoluble, are poorly absorbed from the conjunctiva, GI tract, skin, and lungs. With the exception of physostigmine, the quaternary compounds require larger doses when given by the oral route. Physostigmine, a tertiary amine, is absorbed well from the gastrointestinal tract.

Most of the organophosphate cholinesterase inhibitors are absorbed well from the skin, gut, lungs, and conjunctiva. These agents are excellent insecticides, but are very dangerous to humans. The thiophosphate insecticides (parathion, malathion) are lipid soluble and are absorbed well from all sites. Some of these agents are used by the general public as insecticides. Metabolites of these agents are eliminated in the urine.

Contraindications and Precautions

Although anticholinesterases are used in the treatment of atony of the bladder, they are contraindicated in patients with mechanical obstructions of the intestine or urinary tract. Diabetes, gangrene, coronary artery disease, heart block, ulcerative colitis, upper gastrointestinal disease, hypothyroidism, myotonia congenita, and myotonia atrophica are contraindications to anticholinesterase therapy as they are all worsened. Caution must be used if these drugs are given to patients with asthma or respiratory disorders that would further constrict the smooth muscles of the bronchioles and increase secretions.

Adverse Effects

General adverse effects of anticholinesterases involve their actions on muscarinic receptors and on the autonomic and central nervous systems. Table 16–3 lists specific toxic effects.

Interactions

Anticholinesterases potentiate the neuromuscular blocking effects of succinylcholine (an adjunct to general anesthesia) by inhibiting its breakdown. If anticholinesterases are used with ganglionic blocking agents, severe hypotension may result.

Table 16–3. TOXIC EFFECTS OF ANTICHOLINESTERASE DRUGS (CHOLINERGIC CRISIS)

Autonomic Effects
- Miosis
- Hypotension
- Vasodilation
- Bradycardia
- Salivation
- Intestinal spasm
- Nausea/vomiting
- Bronchial secretions and spasm
- Muscle fasciculations
- Blockage of neuromuscular junctions, causing paralysis of all muscles including diaphragm

CNS Effects
- Respiratory arrest

ANTICHOLINERGIC AGENTS

The anticholinergic agents, sometimes called muscarinic antagonists, compete with acetylcholine for binding sites on the muscarinic receptors. These drugs have little effect on the actions of acetylcholine at nicotinic receptor sites. Table 16–2 lists the effects of anticholinergic drugs on different systems in the body.

The anticholinergic agents reviewed in this section include **atropine, scopolamine _(Hyoscine, Transderm-Scop)_, glycopyrrolate _(Robinul)_,** and **propantheline bromide _(Pro-Banthine)_.**

USES

There are various therapeutic applications for anticholinergic agents. Atropine increases heart rate and cardiac output by blocking the vagus nerve. Atropine, scopolamine, and glycopyrrolate dry up secretions of the respiratory tract and are used in anesthesiology to prevent anesthesia-induced bradycardia. These anticholinergic agents also inhibit gastric secretions and gastrointestinal motility and are used therapeutically for peptic ulcer disease and irritable bowel syndrome. Anticholinergic drugs such as atropine, scopolamine, homatropine, cyclopentolate, and tropicamide are used to determine the refractory state of the eye. When there is inflammation of the eye, anticholinergics may be used to relax the iris and ciliary body. Anticholinergic agents are also used in the treatment of parkinsonism (see Chapter 23) and as antidotes for certain types of poisoning. Atropine is used as an antidote for cholinesterase inhibitor poisoning.

PHARMACOKINETICS

The tertiary amines (atropine and scopolamine) are absorbed well from the gut and conjunctiva, and they cross the blood-brain barrier. The excretion of the tertiary amines occurs in the urine. The quaternary amines, in belladonna alkaloid derivatives, and the synthetic quaternary amines (glycopyrrolate) are poorly absorbed from the gut and do not cross the blood-brain barrier. Large amounts of these compounds are found in the feces.

CONTRAINDICATIONS AND PRECAUTIONS

Use of anticholinergic agents is contraindicated in patients with glaucoma because they may precipitate an attack by dilating the pupil and narrowing the iridocorneal angle. Anticholinergics are also contraindicated in patients who have demonstrated previous hypersensitivity to the preparations and in patients who have accelerated heart rates. Caution is used in patients with chronic lung disease, hepatic and renal disease, myasthenia gravis, cardiac disease, prostatic hypertrophy, paralytic ileus, pyloric stenosis, and severe ulcerative colitis. Anticholinergic agents are administered cautiously to elderly and debilitated patients and to children under 6 years of age.

ADVERSE EFFECTS

Anticholinergic agents affect several body systems at the same time. Many of the adverse effects depend on the drug selected and dosage used. Some of the general adverse effects include dry mouth, blurred vision, constipation, difficult urination, and tachycardia, which are collectively identified as "anticholinergic side effects." This group of side effects is also common to many other drug categories. Other side effects include contact dermatitis of the eyelids and conjunctiva and central nervous system effects. The cause of the contact dermatitis of the eyelids and conjunctiva is unknown.

These agents produce an inhibitory effect on the digestive system, which is under the influence of the vagus nerve, a parasympathetic nerve. This results in a decrease in saliva production, gastric secretion, and gastrointestinal motility. Anticholinergic agents can cause an increase or decrease in heart rate. At low doses, these agents block the parasympathetic input to the sinoatrial node, causing tachycardia and palpitations. Anticholinergic agents produce vasodilation, resulting in flushing, headache, and a decrease in sweating. Allergic reactions may also occur. Anticholinergic agents block the excitatory effects of acetylcholine on the detrusor muscle of the bladder, resulting in urinary retention. In toxic doses rash, restlessness, excitement, disorientation, delirium, hallucinations, hyperthermia, respiratory depression, and death can occur. Atropine has a mild stimulant effect on the central nervous system, causing restlessness and agitation.

INTERACTIONS

Additive adverse reactions from cholinergic blockade can occur when anticholinergics are administered with the phenothiazines, amantadine, antiparkinson drugs, glutethimide, meperidine, tricyclic antidepressants, quinidine, disopyramide, and some antihistamines. Concurrent use of propantheline and slow-dissolving tablets of digoxin may result in increased digoxin absorption, placing the patient at risk for digoxin toxicity. Antacids decrease the extent of absorption of oral anticholinergics. It is important to give the anticholinergic 1 hour prior to use of antacids. Concurrent administration of glycopyrrolate and sustained-release potassium has been shown to increase the severity of potassium chloride–induced gastrointestinal mucosal lesions.

NURSING IMPLICATIONS FOR ADMINISTERING DRUGS AFFECTING THE PARASYMPTHETIC NERVOUS SYSTEM

When administering drugs that affect the parasympathetic nervous system, it is essential for the nurse to follow the nursing process (assessment, intervention, evaluation). Careful assessment is needed prior to administration of parasympathetic agents. The direct-acting cholinomimetics can activate or aggravate peptic ulcers, so monitoring of complaints of a gnawing, aching, burning, or epigastric pain is important.

Visual changes occur with the administration of direct-acting cholinomimetics and anticholinergics (antimuscarinics). Miosis, impaired accommodation, blurred vision, and impaired night vision occur with direct-acting cholinomimetics. Mydriasis is common with antimuscarinic agents. When using direct-acting cholinomimetics, anticholinesterases, and anticholinergics, assessment of bowel function (abdominal distention, bowel sounds, constipation, diarrhea) and bladder function (urinary output, urinary retention, urinary frequency) is essential. Monitoring of vital signs is important during administration of neuromuscular blockers.

When administering the cholinergic agents, it is important to know which drugs can reverse their effects. When administering anticholinesterases, atropine is administered to lessen the muscarinic effects. When administering the direct-acting cholinomimetics and anticholinergic agents, it is important to watch for cholinergic toxicity.

The nurse is also responsible for patient teaching. Patients are taught to recognize the side effects of cholinergic agents and to know when to report them. Because many of these agents affect vision, patient safety is an important consideration. The nurse should warn patients to use caution when driving.

The evaluation of cholinergic agents is based on the therapeutic response. When administering the anticholinesterases, evaluate for an improvement in muscular function and a decrease in fatigue. When administering anticholinergic agents, evaluate for a decrease in spasms of the gastrointestinal tract. It is also important to evaluate patients for allergic reactions to these drugs and for the degree of side effects. Dry mouth is a common side effect, and the patient is taught to take fluids frequently, to chew gum, to suck on hard candy, or to perform frequent oral hygiene.

The bibliography for this chapter can be found in Appendix B, which begins on page 1054.

CHAPTER REVIEW QUESTIONS*

1. Which of the following statements is *not* correct regarding the classification of cholinergic medications?
   a. Cholinergic agents mimic the effects of the parasympathetic system.
   b. Indirect-acting cholinomimetic agents are cholinesterase inhibitors.
   c. Anticholinergic drugs neutralize the effects of the parasympathetic system.
   d. Depolarizing neuromuscular blockers are reversed by anticholinesterase.

2. Scopolamine, an anticholinergic agent used in the treatment of motion sickness, is contraindicated in patients with:
   a. Bradycardia.
   b. Angle-closure glaucoma.
   c. Hypersensitivity to cholinergics.
   d. Excessive salivation.

3. All of the following conditions are contraindications to the use of cholinomimetics *except*:
   a. Neurogenic bladder.
   b. Myocardial infarction.
   c. Asthma.
   d. Peptic ulcer disease.

4. Jane, who has myasthenia gravis, is experiencing a cholinergic crisis. A cholinergic crisis produces all of the following effects *except*:
   a. Intestinal spasm.
   b. Hypotension.
   c. Mydriasis.
   d. Muscle fasciculations.

5. Mr. Perry had an endoscopic examination that revealed peptic ulcer disease. Which of the following drug therapies are contraindicated for Mr. Perry?
   a. Anticholinergics.
   b. Cholinesterase inhibitors.
   c. Parasympatholytics.
   d. Muscarinic blockers.

*See Appendix A, which begins on page 1051, for answers.

CHAPTER 17

Drugs Affecting the Sympathetic Nervous System

Merrily A. Kuhn, RNC, PhD

CHAPTER OUTLINE

Adrenergic Agonist Agents
Adrenergic-Blocking Agents
Ganglionic Blockers

TABLES

Drug Tables
Beta-Adrenergic Blockers, 225
Patient Teaching
Patient Teaching—Beta-Blockers, 233

BOXES

Building Your Critical Thinking Skills, 235

KEY TERMS

Dopaminergic receptors   Dromotropic effect

LEARNING OBJECTIVES

After reading this chapter, the student will be able to:

1. Compare and contrast the sympathetic medications—the adrenergic agonist agents and the adrenergic blocking agents.
2. Describe general drug action, therapeutic uses, pharmacokinetics, contraindications and precautions, adverse effects, and interactions of the beta-adrenergic blockers.
3. Understand general nursing implications for sympathetic medications.

The sympathetic nervous system works with the parasympathetic nervous system to maintain homeostasis. A large number of adrenergic fibers synthesize and release norepinephrine. This chapter reviews drugs that mimic the sympathetic nervous system (adrenergic agonists or sympathomimetic agents) and drugs that block it (adrenergic blocking or sympatholytic agents). It also reviews the ganglionic blockers, which affect both the sympathetic and parasympathetic nervous systems. A brief overview of each of these drug groups is presented; however, the primary discussion of these drugs occurs later in the text. A complete discussion of beta-adrenergic blockers is found in this chapter.

Because of the multiple body systems and organs affected by medications, the nursing process approach to the use of these drugs has been developed in detail in the chapter corresponding to the particular body system. Chapter references are listed in Table 17–1.

Adrenergic agonist agents mimic the effects of the sympathetic nervous system by acting on alpha-adrenergic, beta-adrenergic, and *dopaminergic receptors* (receptors of the autonomic nervous system that are specifically stimulated by dopamine). Adrenergic blocking agents inhibit the effects of the sympathetic nervous system by blocking alpha- and beta-adrenergic receptors.

The alpha-adrenergic receptors are found primarily in blood vessels, most abundantly in the resistance vessels of the skin, mucosa, intestine, and kidney. Drugs with a positive effect on the alpha-adrenergic receptors, such as norepinephrine, cause greater vasoconstriction, whereas alpha-adrenergic blockers, including drugs used for hypertensive crisis such as phentolamine, have a relaxant effect and produce vasodilation.

Two subtypes of beta-adrenergic receptors have been identified: beta$_1$ receptors, found primarily in the heart, and beta$_2$ receptors, found primarily in the lung and peripheral blood vessels, particularly in skeletal muscle. In general, drugs that act positively on the beta$_1$ receptor sites (e.g., epinephrine and isoproterenol) increase cardiac contractility and heart rate and accelerate atrioventricular conduction in the heart, while drugs that act positively on the beta$_2$ receptor sites may cause some vasodilatation in the arterioles of skeletal muscle and mesenteric vascular beds and bronchiolar dilation. The beta-adrenergic blockers have a negative effect, causing profound slowing of the heart as well as inhibiting the force of contraction,

Table 17–1. MEDICATIONS AFFECTING THE SYMPATHETIC NERVOUS SYSTEM

Classification	Drug	Indication	Chapter Reference
Adrenergic stimulant (sympathomimetic)	Epinephrine (Adrenalin)	Allergic states	41
	Isoproterenol hydrochloride (Isuprel)	Asthma, heart failure	40
	Norepinephrine (Levophed)	Hypotension, as vasoconstrictor, cardiac arrest	68
	Ephedrine	Bronchodilator, nasal decongestant, allergic states	40
	Phenylephrine hydrochloride (Neo-Synephrine)	Bronchodilator, nasal decongestant, vasoconstrictor, allergic states	40
Alpha-adrenergic blockers	Phenoxybenzamine (Dibenzyline)	Peripheral vascular disorders, Raynaud's disease, frostbite	32
	Dihydrogenated ergot alkaloids (Hydergine)	Confused elderly persons	19
	Prazocin (Minipress) Terazocin (Hytrin) Doxazocin (Cardura)	Mild to moderate hypertension and congestive heart failure	30
Beta-adrenergic blockers	Propranolol hydrochloride (Inderal)	Hypertension, migraine headache control, dysrhythmia control	30, 31
	Metoprolol (Lopressor)	Hypertension, acute myocardial infarction	30, 31
	Nadolol (Corgard)	Hypertension	30
	Timolol maleate (Blocadren)	Myocardial infarction: acute and prophylaxis	30, 31
	Timolol maleate ophthalmic (Timoptic)	Glaucoma	63
	Atenolol (Tenormin)	Myocardial prophylaxis, hypertension, angina, dysrhythmia control	30, 31
	Pindolol (Visken)	Hypertension	30
	Labetalol (Trandate, Normodyne)	Hypertension, angina	30
	Acebutolol (Sectral)	Hypertension, angina, dysrhythmia control	30
	Sotaloll (Betapace) Esmolol (Brevibloc)	Dysrhythmia control	31
	Bisoprolol (Zebeta)		30
Ganglionic blockers (block both sympathetic and parasympathetic ganglia)	Mecamylamine hydrochloride (Inversine)	Hypertension	30

and include agents to control angina or lower blood pressure such as propranolol (Inderal) or metoprolol (Lopressor).

Two subtypes of dopaminergic receptors have been identified: DA-1 and DA-2. The DA-1 receptors are found primarily in the renal and mesenteric vascular beds, with a few in the coronary and cerebral circulation. Smaller arteries are more sensitive to the vasodilating actions of dopamine than are larger vessels, suggesting that greater numbers of receptors are located in smaller vessels. The DA-2 receptors are located on postganglionic sympathetic nerve terminals. When these receptors are activated, norepinephrine release is inhibited. Dopamine (Intropin) is a dopaminergic-stimulating drug that affects both DA-1 and DA-2 receptors.

ADRENERGIC AGONIST AGENTS

The adrenergic drugs (sympathomimetic agents), which mimic the sympathetic nervous system, act in three different ways. They act directly on the adrenergic alpha or beta receptors; they act indirectly, by first releasing a catecholamine from their storage sites, which in turn activates the alpha and beta sites; or they act by a mixed direct and indirect effect.

DIRECT-ACTING ADRENERGIC AGENTS

Action

The direct-acting adrenergic medications, described in more detail in Chapter 68, include the catecholamines— **dopamine *(Intropin)*, norepinephrine *(Levophed)*, dobutamine *(Dobutrex)*, isoproterenol *(Isuprel)*,** and **epinephrine**. These agents produce many physiologic responses, including a marked inotropic effect (by increasing cardiac contraction); a marked chronotropic effect (by increasing cardiac rate); a positive *dromotropic effect* (an effect related to conductivity of a nerve, which, with drugs in this class, results in an increase in cardiac conduction); and a stimulatory effect on the Purkinje fibers, possibly resulting in ventricular dysrhythmias. Some direct-acting adrenergic agents may elevate blood pressure because of increased peripheral resistance. The catecholamines increase contractility, thus reducing preload as in cardiac failure.

Sympathomimetics can increase anxiety, increase alertness, and cause respiratory stimulation. The catecholamines also exert an effect on all nonvascular smooth muscle, in most cases leading to relaxation and less peristalsis in the gastrointestinal tract. The urinary bladder relaxes, delaying the need to void. The pupils dilate, giving the patient a wide-staring appearance.

Some catecholamines, particularly isoproterenol and epinephrine, have a pronounced effect on the bronchial smooth muscle through beta$_2$-agonist stimulation, which results in bronchodilation. Epinephrine also constricts the bronchial vessels and inhibits bronchial secretions, which makes it effective in the management of bronchial asthma.

The catecholamines inhibit or stimulate metabolic activity (e.g., insulin secretion), depending on the sympathetic nervous system receptors stimulated. However, in a stress situation, they make more energy available to the body by stimulating glycogen release from the liver and skeletal muscles and fatty acid release as a result of lipolysis in the adipose tissue.

INDIRECT- AND MIXED-ACTING ADRENERGIC AGENTS

The indirect- and mixed-acting adrenergic drugs—**ephedrine** and **phenylephrine hydrochloride (Neo-Synephrine)**—indirectly affect adrenergic receptor, or act either directly or indirectly on the receptors. More information on these agents is found in Chapter 40.

○ **Ephedrine,** an indirect adrenergic stimulant affecting both alpha and beta receptors, is similar to epinephrine but is less potent, with slower onset and more prolonged action. It acts indirectly by releasing tissue stores of norepinephrine. Bronchodilation is less pronounced but more sustained than with epinephrine. Ephedrine is used parenterally to correct acute hypotension (e.g., from spinal anesthesia or overdosage with antihypertensive agents), to support ventricular rate in Adams-Stokes syndrome, and to manage acute attacks of asthma. Topically and orally, it is used for bronchodilation or nasal decongestion.

○ **Phenylephrine hydrochloride** (Neo-Synephrine) is a potent, synthetic, noncatecholamine adrenergic agonist stimulator that is chemically related to epinephrine. Phenylephrine hydrochloride acts primarily on the alpha receptors, with little or no effect on beta receptors. Because of its alpha effect, it is a potent vasoconstrictor that elevates both the systolic and diastolic blood pressures during anesthesia. It has no effect on the central nervous system and little effect on the heart. It does, however, cause a reflexive bradycardia as a result of stimulation of the cardioreceptors, baroreceptors, and increased vagal activity. For this reason, it has been useful in converting paroxysmal atrial tachycardia to a normal rate. Topically and orally, it is used for allergic rhinitis and sinusitis. Ophthalmically, it is used as a mydriatric in open-angle glaucoma and in eye examinations.

ADRENERGIC-BLOCKING AGENTS

The adrenergic-blocking agents (sympatholytics) are a group of medications that interfere with the transmission of nerve impulses to adrenergic neuroeffectors. The adrenergic-blockers occupy the adrenergic receptor sites (alpha or beta) without evoking any response from the effector muscle or gland. As long as the adrenergic-blocking drugs occupy these receptors sites, all normal neural or hormonal activity is blocked. The adrenergic-blocking agents include both alpha- and beta-blocking agents.

ALPHA-ADRENERGIC BLOCKING AGENTS

The alpha-adrenergic blocking agents inhibit the effects of alpha receptors primarily in vascular smooth muscle. These agents are more effective against the action of circulating catecholamines than against catecholamines released from storage sites, and they have relatively limited usefulness. The alpha-adrenergic blockers are obtained from natural sources such as ergot and its derivatives, or they are synthetically prepared. Additional information on these agents can be found in Chapter 19.

BETA-ADRENERGIC BLOCKING AGENTS

The beta-adrenergic blockers were first introduced in the 1960s. Until 1978, the only beta-blocker approved by the Food and Drug Administration in the United States was **propranolol (Inderal)**. Since 1978, many new beta-blockers have been released, including **propranolol long-acting (Inderal LA)**, **metoprolol (Lopressor)**, **metoprolol long-acting (Lopressor SR, Toprol XL)**, **nadolol (Corgard)**, **timolol maleate (Blocadren)**, **atenolol (Tenormin)**, **pindolol (Visken)**, **acebutolol (Sectral)**, **labetalol (Trandate, Normodyne)**, **betaxolol hydrochloride (Kerlone)**, **penbutolol (Levatol)**, **esmolol hydrochloride (Brevibloc)**, **carteolol (Cartrol)**, **bisoprolol fumarate (Zebeta)**, **carvedilol (Coreq)**, and **sotalol hydrochloride (Betapace)**. Beta-blockers are classified by receptor affinity, which refers to their selectively acting on the beta$_1$ or on beta$_2$ receptors. General receptor selectivity is identified for approved generic drugs and investigational agents in Table 17–2. Specific receptor selectivity appears in Table 17–3, along with dosages, pharmacokinetics, and nursing implications for selected beta-blockers.

Action

The beta-adrenergic blockers compete with norepinephrine for available beta-receptor sites. These medications inhibit the response to adrenergic stimuli in either the beta$_1$ or beta$_2$ receptors or both. Blocking the beta$_1$ adrenergic receptor sites in the heart results in a decrease in heart rate during both rest and exercise and a decrease in myocardial contractility and ultimately in cardiac output. It is through these mechanisms that angina is most likely controlled. Conduction velocity through the atrioventricular node and the firing rate in the sinoatrial node also

Table 17–2. CLASSIFICATION OF BETA-ADRENERGIC RECEPTOR BLOCKING AGENTS

Action	Approved Generic Drugs	Unapproved Generic Drugs
Nonselective beta-blockade	Carteolol Nadolol Penbutolol Pindolol Propranolol Sotalol Timolol	
Selective beta$_1$-blockade	Acebutolol Atenolol Bisoprolol Betaxolol Esmolol Metoprolol	
Membrane-stabilizing activity	Acebutolol—low Betaxolol—low Pindolol—low Propranolol—moderate	
Intrinsic sympathometic activity	Acebutolol—low Carteolol—moderate Penbutolol—low Pindolol—high	
Beta-blockade and vasodilation secondary to beta$_2$ receptor stimulation	Pindolol	Dilevalol Celiprolol
Beta-blockade and vasodilation secondary to alpha$_1$ receptor blockade	Labetalol Carvedilol	
Beta-blockade and direct vasodilation effects (nonreceptor mediated)		Bucindolol
Beta-blockade and intrinsic sympathomimetic activity (both beta-blocking and beta-activating properties)		Xamaterol

decrease. These effects assist in preventing exercise-induced increases in the heart rate and in effectively treating various dysrhythmias. Beta$_2$ receptor blockade causes bronchoconstriction in the lung, which can aggravate any type of chronic lung disease. Beta-blockers do not abolish the response to catecholamines, but simply require that a higher concentration of catecholamine be present to be effective. This activity is known as competitive inhibition. Beta-blockers may have intrinsic sympathetic activity and/or membrane-stabilizing activity. In Table 17–2, these activities are identified for each drug.

Intrinsic Sympathetic Activity Several beta-blockers—pindolol, carteolol, penbutolol, and acebutolol—have intrinsic sympathetic activity (ISA) or partial beta-agonist activity. Because of the beta-agonist activity, the negative chronotropic and inotropic activity of the beta-blockers is reduced. Thus, beta-blockers with ISA may have little effect on resting heart rate or may reduce it by an average of 4 to 8 beats per minute. Drugs with ISA may also reduce exercise-stimulated cardiac output. A drug's ISA can be either low, moderate, or high. Because of their low level of cardiac stimulation, beta-blockers with high ISA are useful in patients with bradycardia or borderline heart failure.

Membrane-Stabilizing Activity Membrane-stabilizing activity (MSA) is a quinidine-like effect that is exhibited by propranolol and to a lesser extent by acebutolol, betaxolol, and pindolol. MSA suppresses excitation of the cardiac cell. MSA was once thought to be responsible for the antidysrhythmic effectiveness of these agents; however, MSA appears to occur only with doses that far exceed those used in the treatment of dysrhythmias. A drug's MSA can be either low or moderate.

Uses

Over the last 30 years, beta-blockers have been used to treat cardiovascular, endocrine, neurologic, psychiatric, and gastrointestinal diseases, as listed in Table 17–4. Several beta-blockers are equally effective in reducing the frequency and severity of anginal episodes, as shown in Figure 17–1, the consumption of nitroglycerin, and the electrocardiographic evidence of ischemia; and they are effective in increasing exercise performance in patients with chronic stable angina pectoris. Most beta-blockers are effective antihypertensive agents for managing mild, moderate, and severe hypertension but not for hypertensive emergencies. They lower systolic and diastolic su-

Table 17–3. BETA-ADRENERGIC BLOCKERS

DRUG NAME/ROUTE AND DOSAGE	PHARMACOKINETICS/ DYNAMICS	BLOCKING ACTIVITY	NURSING IMPLICATIONS
all beta-adrenergic blockers			**ASSESSMENT:** Assess cardiac rhythm including rate (particularly bradycardia), regularity, quality of the pulse, ECG, neurologic symptoms, urinary output, and level of anxiety. Assess electrolytes, particularly potassium and calcium. May be discontinued prior to cardiac diagnostic tests or surgery. Assess presence of diabetes. Assess for pregnancy (category B or C). **INTERVENTION:** May produce drowsiness, dizziness, lightheadedness, and blurred vision; may decrease libido. **Patient Teaching**—Advise patient to observe caution in driving or performing tasks requiring alertness. Teach patient to monitor own blood pressure and pulse. Caution patient not to smoke (regular cigarettes and marijuana), because this may raise the blood pressure. Teach patient *to not discontinue beta-blockers abruptly*. Instruct patient to take at appropriate times in relation to food (see propranolol and metoprolol). Teach patient to check with physician or pharmacist before taking OTC drugs. **EVALUATION:** Evaluate for effectiveness, sensitivity, and adverse effects. Evaluate weight (report weight gain of 2 lb/week) and check frequently for signs of edema and shortness of breath. Monitor blood sugar in diabetic patients carefully. Notify physician if HF occurs or if a slowed pulse rate, confusion, skin rash, fever, sore throat, or unusual bleeding or bruising occur.
propranolol hydrochloride (Inderal, Inderal LA)			
hypertension ***Adults:*** Initially 40 mg/day PO bid or 80 mg ER form once daily; increase to 120–240 mg bid or tid. **angina** ***Adults:*** 80–320 mg PO in divided doses; or 120–160 mg ER daily. **dysrhythmias** ***Adults:*** 10–30 mg PO tid or qid, up to 160–480 mg/day; or 1–3 mg IV bolus not to exceed 1 mg/min. **migraine prophylaxis** ***Adults:*** 160–240 mg/day PO in divided doses; or 80 mg (extended release) daily, up to 240 mg/day.	**Onset:** PO, 30 min; IV, immediate **Peak:** PO, 1–1.5 hr; IV, 1 min **Duration:** PO, 6–12 hr; ER, 24 hr; IV, 4–6 hr ½**L:** 3–6 hr **PB:** 90% **B:** liver **E:** urine	β_1 and β_2 MSA ++ ISA 0	Same as for all beta-adrenergic blockers plus: **INTERVENTION:** Regular PO form can be crushed. Do not open extended-release capsules. **Patient Teaching**—Instruct patient to take at the same time each day in relation to food. Food enhances bioavailability.

Continued on the following page

Table 17–3. BETA-ADRENERGIC BLOCKERS, *Continued*

DRUG NAME/ROUTE AND DOSAGE	PHARMACOKINETICS/ DYNAMICS	BLOCKING ACTIVITY	NURSING IMPLICATIONS
timolol maleate (Blocadren)			
hypertension *Adults:* 10–60 mg PO daily in divided doses. **myocardial prophylactic** *Adults:* 10 mg PO bid. **migraine prophylaxis** *Adults:* 10–30 mg PO daily in single or divided doses.	**Onset:** 30 min **Peak:** 1–2 hr **Duration:** 12–24 hr **½L:** 3–4 hr **PB:** 10% **B:** liver **E:** liver	β_1 and β_2 MSA 0 ISA 0	Same as for all beta-adrenergic blockers
metoprolol (Lopressor, Toprol XL)			
hypertension *Adults: Initial dose*–100 mg/day PO in single or divided doses. *Maintenance dose*–100–450 mg/day. ER tablets (Toprol XL) given once daily. **myocardial infarction** *Adults:* As soon as patient is hemodynamically stable three 5-mg IV boluses at 2-min intervals; then after 15 min start 50 mg PO q 6 hr for 48 hr; then 100 mg PO bid for 1–3 yr. ER tablets (Toprol XL) given once daily. **angina** *Adults:* 100 mg PO daily in 2 divided doses. Range is 100–400 mg/day. *Heart failure* 6.25 mg once or twice daily, Dose doubled each week till maximum of 50 mg daily.	Maximum effect about 1 wk after 1st dose **Onset:** PO, 15 min; IV, 5 min **Peak:** PO, 1 hr; XL, 6–12 hr; IV, 20 min **Duration:** PO, 6–12 hr; XL, 24 hr; IV, 5–8 hr **½L:** 3–7 hr **PB:** 12% **B:** liver **E:** urine	β_1 (low doses only) MSA 0 ISA 0	Same as for all beta-adrenergic blockers plus: **INTERVENTION:** Should be taken at same time in relation to food. Food enhances bioavailability.
atenolol (Tenormin)			
hypertension *Adults:* 50–100 mg PO once daily **myocardial infarction** *Adults:* As soon as patient is hemodynamically stable 5 mg IV over 5 min, wait 5–10 min, 5 mg IV again, then start 50 mg PO bid for 2 yr. **angina** *Adults:* 50–100 mg PO once daily.	**Onset:** PO, 1 hr; IV, 5 min **Peak:** PO, 2–4 hr; IV, 5 min **Duration:** PO, 24 hr; IV, <12 hr **½L:** 6–7 hr **PB:** 6%–16% **E:** 50% unchanged in feces	β_1 (low doses) MSA 0 ISA 0	Same as for all beta-adrenergic blockers plus: **INTERVENTION:** Does not potentiate insulin-induced hypoglycemia or delay return of blood glucose to normal. Often administered with a diuretic. Administer 50-mg dose after renal dialysis.

Table 17–3. BETA-ADRENERGIC BLOCKERS, *Continued*

DRUG NAME/ROUTE AND DOSAGE	PHARMACOKINETICS/ DYNAMICS	BLOCKING ACTIVITY	NURSING IMPLICATIONS
labetalol hydrochloride (Normodyne, Trandate)			
hypertension *Adults:* Initial dose–100 mg PO bid; increase in increments of 100 mg bid every 2–3 days. *Maintenance dose–*200– 400 mg bid up to 2400 mg/day. **severe hypertension** *Adults:* 20 mg IV bolus slowly over 2 min; additional injections of 40–80 mg every 10 min up to total of 300 mg; or 2 mg/min (total dose not to exceed 300 mg).	**Onset:** PO, 20 min–2 hr; IV, 2–5 min **Peak:** PO, 1–4 hr; IV, 5–15 min **Duration:** PO, 8–12 hr; IV, 2–4 hr (up to 24 hr) **½L:** 6–8 hr **PB:** 50% **E:** unchanged in urine (55–60%)	β_1 and β_2, alpha blocker MSA 0 ISA 0	Same as for all beta-adrenergic blockers plus: **INTERVENTION:** Administer on an empty stomach. During IV administration, always keep patient supine. Measure blood pressure immediately before and 5–10 min after injection. Do not administer with sodium bicarbonate.
acebutolol (sectral)			
hypertension *Adults:* 200–1200 mg PO single or divided doses. **ventricular dysrhythmias** *Adults:* Initial dose–200 mg PO bid. *Maintenance dose–*600– 1200 mg PO single or divided doses. **angina** *Adults:* 200 mg PO bid, up to 800 mg daily.	**Onset:** 1–1.5 hr **Peak:** 2–8 hr **Duration:** 12–24 hr **½L:** 3–4 hr **PB:** 26% **B:** liver **E:** urine 30%–40%, bile 50%–60%	β_1 (low doses) MSA + ISA +	Same as for all beta-adrenergic blockers plus: **INTERVENTION:** May be taken without regard to meals.
esmolol hydrochloride (Brevibloc)			
Adults: Loading dose–500 μg/kg/min for 1 min, then 50 μg/kg for 4 min continued until effect reached. *Maintenance dose–*25–50 μg/kg per min ideally used for 48 hr or less.	**Onset:** 1 min **Peak:** 5 min **Duration:** 20 min **½L:** 9–15 min **PB:** 55% **B:** in red blood cell **E:** urine	β_1 MSA 0 ISA 0	Same as for all beta-adrenergic blockers plus: **INTERVENTION:** Have emergency equipment present. Dilute prior to administration (2.5 g esmolol in 250 ml dilutant or 5 g in 500 mL to achieve a dilution of 10 mg/mL). Not compatible with bicarbonate. Use of central line preferable. Wean when discontinuing. Avoid concurrent vasoactive drugs (dopamine, epinephrine, and norepinephrine). Monitor for hypotension. **EVALUATION:** Evaluate ECG for AV block and bradycardia. Consider discontinuing drug if they occur.

ER = extended release; MSA = membrane stabilizing activity: 0 = none, + = low, ++ = moderate; ISA = intrinsic sympathomimetic activity: 0 = none, + = low, ++ = moderate; ECG = electrocardiogram; AV = atrioventricular.

pine and standing blood pressures at rest and during exercise. Possible mechanisms of action include a reduction in cardiac output, a reduction in plasma renin activity, and a CNS sympatholytic action. Persons more likely to respond favorably to beta-blockers are those who are young, white, nonsmoking men who have a higher-than-normal plasma renin level, increased sympathetic activity with higher cardiac output, normal left ventricular function, and labile hypertension. Patients over age 60 may have a response rate as low as 20%.

Table 17–4. USES OF BETA-ADRENERGIC BLOCKING AGENTS

Drug Name	Use
Acebutolol	Hypertension Premature ventricular contractions
Atenolol	Hypertension Angina pectoris Supraventricular dysrhythmias/tachycardias* Ventricular dysrhythmias/tachycardias* Myocardial infarction Migraine prophylaxis* Alcohol withdrawal syndrome* Anxiety (including situational)*
Betaxolol	Hypertension
Bisoprolol	Hypertension Angina pectoris* Supraventricular dysrhythmias/tachycardias* Premature ventricular contractions*
Carteolol	Hypertension Angina pectoris*
Esmolol	Angina pectoris* Supraventricular dysrhythmias/tachycardias Sinus tachycardia
Labetalol	Hypertension Pheochromocytoma*
Metoprolol	Hypertension Angina pectoris Ventricular dysrhythmias/tachycardias* Atrial ectopy* Myocardial infarction Migraine prophylaxis* Tremors (essential)* Aggressive behavior* Enhanced cognitive performance*
Nadolol	Hypertension Angina pectoris Ventricular dysrhythmias/tachycardias* Migraine prophylaxis* Tremors (essential, lithium-induced, Parkinsonism)* Aggressive behavior* Antipsychotic-induced akathisia* Esophageal varices rebleeding* Anxiety (including situational)* Intraocular pressure reduction*
Penbutolol	Hypertension
Pindolol	Hypertension Ventricular dysrhythmias/tachycardias* Antipsychotic-induced akathisia* Anxiety (including situational)*
Propranolol	Hypertension Angina pectoris Supraventricular dysrhythmias/tachycardias Ventricular dysrhythmias/tachycardias Premature ventricular contractions Digitalis-induced tachydysrhythmias Myocardial infarction Pheochromocytoma Migraine prophylaxis

Table 17–4. USES OF BETA-ADRENERGIC BLOCKING AGENTS, *Continued*

Drug Name	Use
Propranolol (continued)	Hypertrophic subaortic stenosis Tremors (essential) Tremors (parkinsonism)* Alcohol withdrawal syndrome* Aggressive behavior* Antipsychotic-induced akathisia* Esophageal varices rebleeding* Anxiety (including situational)* Schizophrenia/Acute panic* Gastric bleeding in portal hypertension* Vaginal contraceptive* Thyrotoxicosis symptoms*
Sotalol	Ventricular dysrhythmias/tachycardias
Timolol	Hypertension Ventricular dysrhythmias/tachycardias* Myocardial infarction Migraine prophylaxis Tremor (essential)* Anxiety (including situational)* Intraocular pressure reduction*

*Unlabeled use

▼ CLINICAL ALERT

African-American patients do not always respond well to beta-blocker monotherapy. However, when a diuretic is added, the combination is usually effective. The reason for this racial difference in drug response is not well understood. A pragmatic rule is that if a standard dose of a beta-blocker does not work within a week, it is useless to try another.

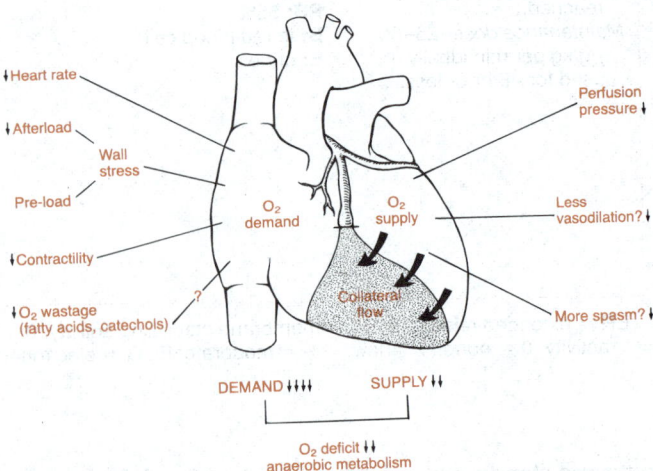

Figure 17–1. Effects of beta blockade on ischemic heart. Beta blockade has a beneficial effect on the ischemic myocardium, unless (1) the preload rises substantially as in left heart failure or (2) there is vasospastic angina when spasm may be promoted in some patients. (From Opie, LH: Drugs for the Heart. Grune and Stratton, FL, 1991, p 2, with permission.)

Beta-blockers (propranolol, atenolol, bisoprolol, esmolol, metoprolol, nadolol, pindolol, timolol, sotalol, and acebutolol) are used to treat various dysrhythmias, including fast supraventricular rhythms, atrial fibrillation and flutter, and atrial and ventricular ectopic beats. Beta-blockers are particularly effective in dysrhythmias caused by increased circulating catecholamines or by increased cardiac sensitivity to catecholamines.

Beta-blockers (atenolol, metoprolol, propranolol, timolol) are also used for cardiac protection during a myocardial infarction by decreasing infarct size, the incidence of ventricular dysrhythmias, and creatinine phosphokinase levels. Findings indicate that beta-blockers are best administered within 12 hours to a patient with myocardial infarction with no failure and whose heart rate is above 75 beats per minute. Ideally, beta-blockers are administered IV in the emergency room at the time of admission to the hospital. Beta-blockers are then continued for 6 months to 2 years. Research indicates that these drugs decrease myocardial oxygen consumption, decrease sympathetic nervous system effects on the heart, decrease overall mortality by 8% to 10%, and decrease the incidence of sudden death by 45%.

Beta-blockers (propranolol) are also used in both hypertrophic and congestive cardiomyopathies. They decrease contractility and heart rate, which results in an improvement of left ventricular filling pressure. Thus, cardiac output is improved.

Beta-blockers (atenolol and metoprolol) are used to improve cardiac function in patients with severe heart failure. Progressive heart failure (HF) is associated with a reduction in the number of beta adrenoceptors. The degree of impairment of adrenoceptor activity is related to the severity of the HF. Paradoxically, blockade of cardiac beta adrenoceptors by specific beta-blockers in severe HF is associated with an increase in the number of $beta_1$ receptors and may be accompanied by an improvement in cardiac function (Fitzgerald and Singh, 1994). Therapy with beta-blockers should be initiated only after standard therapy, including angiotensin converting enzyme (ACE) inhibitors, is maximized.

Beta-blockers (propranolol) are also used to control chest pain and dysrhythmias in patients with ballooned mitral valve syndrome (prolapsed mitral valve). And, beta-blockers palliatively relieve the hypoxia and cyanosis seen with tetralogy of Fallot by reducing sympathetic effects in the right ventricle.

Beta-blockers (propranolol, timolol, nadolol, metoprolol, and atenolol) are effective in the prevention but not in the treatment of migraines. The exact mechanism of action is unknown, but it may result from the effect of beta-blockers on peripheral resistance.

Beta-blockers (propranolol) are effective in treating the symptoms of hyperthyroidism. They may inhibit the conversion of T_4 to T_3 as well as acting as a nonspecific antiadrenergic to inhibit sympathetic activity.

The beta-blockers nadolol, timolol, and others (as eyedrops) are used to manage glaucoma. They decrease the production of aqueous humor, thus reducing pressure in the eye.

Because of their constrictor effect in the arterial circulation, nonselective beta-blockers (propranolol, nadolol, and atenolol) are used to control bleeding from portal hypertension and esophageal varices.

Lastly, beta-blockers (propranolol, timolol, metroprolol, nadolol, atenolol, and pindolol) are used in a variety of neurologic and psychiatric disorders including tremor, anxiety, alcohol withdrawal syndrome, and neuroses. The mechanism of action is probably through their depressive effect on the CNS.

Pharmacokinetics

The beta-blockers are either lipid or water soluble in the body. The solubility affects the pharmacokinetics and possibly the adverse effects of the drug. Figure 17–2 identifies the lipid- and water-soluble beta-blockers.

Absorption   The lipid-soluble products are more readily and more completely absorbed from the gastrointestinal system than are the water-soluble products. Ingestion with food enhances the bioavailability of propranolol and metoprolol and reduces the absorption of sotalol; however, this effect is not noted with nadolol, carteolol, pindolol, bisoprolol, or betaxolol.

Distribution   The lipid-soluble products are approximately 90% plasma bound and are widely distributed to tissues. They readily cross the blood-brain barrier. All products reach maximal plasma concentrations within 1 to 3 hours. Propranolol (Inderal) and metroprolol (Lopressor) are found in the CNS in concentrations many times higher than in the serum. This fact accounts for the adverse effects on the CNS, although some recent research suggests that there is no difference in CNS effects between lipid- and water-soluble beta-blockers.

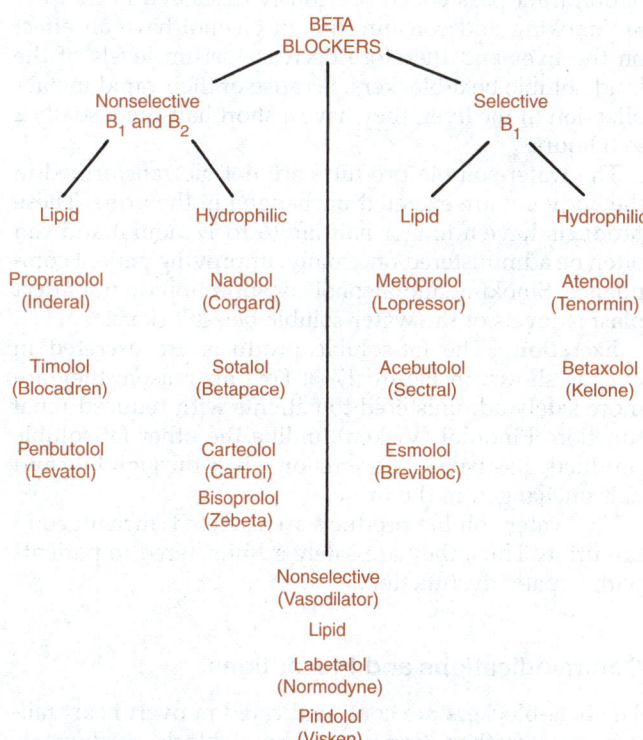

Figure 17–2. Beta-blockers are divided into selective B_1, nonselective B_1 and B_2, or nonselective (vasodilator) products.

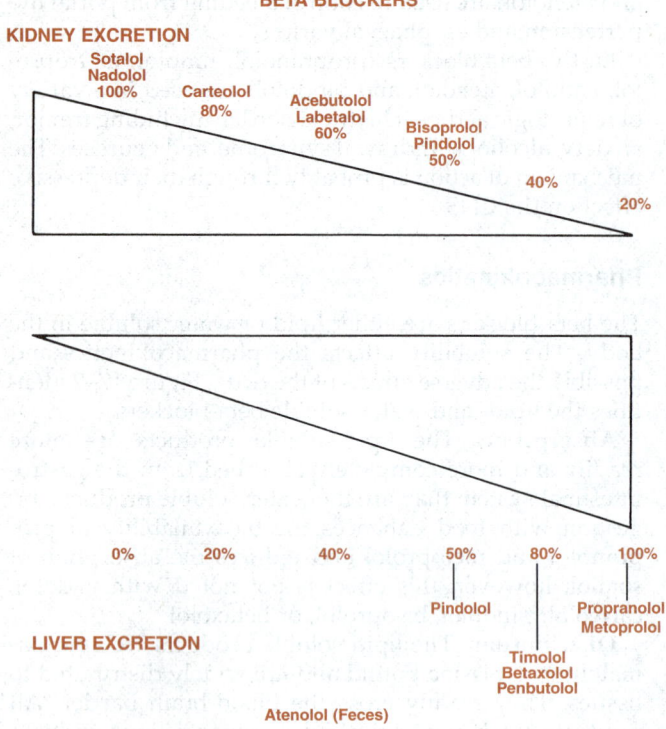

Figure 17–3. Routes of elimination of beta-blockers. The hydrophilic beta-blockers are excreted unchanged by the kidneys. The lipophilic beta-blockers are largely metabolized by the liver. Esmolol is metabolized by esterases within the red blood cell.

The water-soluble products are only 3% plasma bound and do not cross the blood-brain barrier and therefore have few CNS effects.

Biotransformation The lipid-soluble products are metabolized in the liver, often through presystemic elimination (first-pass effect, previously discussed in Chapter 6). Smoking and consumption of alcohol have an effect on the liver and therefore decrease serum levels of the lipid-soluble beta-blockers. Because of their rapid metabolization in the liver, they have a short half-life, usually 2 to 6 hours.

The water-soluble products are not biotransformed in the body but are excreted unchanged in the urine. These products have a longer half-life (6 to 17 hours) and can often be administered once daily, improving patient compliance. Smoking and alcohol consumption do not affect plasma levels of the water-soluble beta-blockers.

Excretion The fat-soluble products are excreted in bile, as shown in Figure 17–3. For this reason, they are more safely administered to patients with reduced renal function. Pindolol (Visken), unlike the other fat-soluble products, has balanced excretion—half through bile and half unchanged in the urine.

The water-soluble products are excreted unchanged in the urine. Thus, they are safely administered to patients with hepatic dysfunction.

Contraindications and Precautions

The beta-blockers are contraindicated in overt heart failure, greater than first-degree heart block, cardiogenic shock, sinus bradycardia, and hypersensitivity. In addition, many of the beta-blockers (propranolol, nadolol, timolol, penbutolol, carteolol, and pindolol) are contraindicated in patients with bronchial asthma because of their beta₂-blocking effects.

▼ **CLINICAL ALERT**

Beta-blockers, especially the nonspecific drugs, are given cautiously to patients with peripheral vascular insufficiency because they decrease blood flow to the extremities through peripheral vasoconstriction; to patients with renal or hepatic impairment, because of their serum accumulation in these diseases; and to patients with hypoglycemia, because they block the normal sympathetic response to the development of hypoglycemic symptoms. Because of their effect on blood glucose, beta-blockers are also given cautiously to patients with diabetes who are taking insulin or oral hypoglycemic drugs. The medications should not be stopped abruptly, particularly in a patient with ischemic heart disease. They are titrated down slowly, usually over a week or two, to avoid the increased sensitivity to catecholamine, which could result in an acute myocardial infarction. Abrupt discontinuation of beta-blockers has been associated with a fourfold risk of having an anginal attack or a mild myocardial infarction within 30 days when drugs are taken to treat angina.

Renal and hepatic disease are also cautions for beta-blocker use. The water-soluble products are administered cautiously in patients with renal disease, because they are excreted primarily in the kidneys. The lipid-soluble products are administered cautiously in patients with liver disease, because they are excreted primarily in the liver.

Safety in pregnancy (category B or C, depending on the specific drug) has not been established, so use only when clearly indicated. Beta-blockers should not be administered to nursing mothers, and the efficacy in children has not been established. Beta-blockers are given cautiously to patients with diabetes who are taking insulin or oral hypoglycemic drugs.

Adverse Effects

For most patients receiving beta-blockers, the incidence of adverse effects is relatively low. Major mechanisms of adverse effects include (1) smooth muscle spasm, (2) CNS penetration, and (3) exaggeration of cardiac therapeutic effects. The blockade of the beta$_2$ receptors, primarily those located in the lung, results in bronchospasm, particularly in patients with any form of chronic obstructive pulmonary disease, including asthma. Propranolol hydrochloride, nadolol, and timolol maleate are beta$_1$- and beta$_2$-blockers. Metoprolol and acebutolol, administered in low doses, are highly selective beta$_1$-blockers. In larger doses, however, they also block beta$_2$ receptors and thus must be used cautiously in patients with lung disease. Fatigue, a common complaint, may result from the hemodynamic effects of these agents or from peripheral metabolic effects, such as inhibition of lactic acid release from skeletal muscle. Patients with peripheral vascular impairment experience a decreased blood flow in muscles by 30%, which may worsen existing conditions. Exercise performance may decrease. This effect is dose dependent. Chronic therapy does not impair submaximal exercise performance, but does reduce maximal exercise performance (atenolol causes less of a reduction than propranolol). Central nervous system complaints of vivid dreams, insomnia, depression, hallucinations, and dizziness may be more common with the lipid-soluble beta-blockers. Additional adverse effects include bradycardia, drug fever, nausea, vomiting, diarrhea, transient thrombocytopenia, agranulocytosis, and sleep disorders.

Beta-blockers may affect glucose levels. Although the blood glucose level is usually normal at rest, it may drop during exercise. This is because the glycogenolytic and lipolytic actions of endogenous catecholamines, normally released in response to the increased energy requirements during exercise and in response to hypoglycemia, are inhibited by beta-blockade. However, this does not appear to occur in practice. Therefore, beta-blockers are given cautiously to patients with diabetes who are taking insulin or oral hypoglycemic drugs. (Atenolol does not potentiate insulin-induced hypoglycemia). Beta-blockers may also mask the clinical signs of hypoglycemia: tachycardia, diaphoresis, and a slightly decreased diastolic pressure. In fact, the opposite clinical signs may appear, including increased diastolic pressure and bradycardia. Beta-blockers may also precipitate hyperglycemia because they block the release of insulin.

▼ CLINICAL ALERT

Beta-blockers (except pindolol, carteolol, bisoprolol, and acebutolol) tend to elevate plasma levels of triglycerides and very low density lipoproteins, which may contribute to the development of atherosclerotic heart disease and lower plasma levels of high-density lipoproteins (HDLs),

which have a protective effect. Pindolol is associated with an increase in HDL levels. Atenolol is associated with a decrease in HDL levels, but after a year of therapy HDLs return to pretreatment levels. The clinical importance of these findings is still under investigation.

Interactions

Interactions include an increased potential for bradycardia, hypotension, and cardiac depression when cardiac glycosides, calcium channel blockers, birth control pills, flecainide, disopyramide, haloperidol, hydralozine, monoamine oxidase (MAO) inhibitors, or quinidine are given concurrently. There is also an increased hypotensive effect with diuretics. Concurrent phenothiazine administration may result in increased effects of both drugs. Beta-blockers may decrease the clearance of acetaminophen and lidocaine, possibly leading to toxicity. Bioavailability may be decreased with concurrent administration of aluminum and calcium salts, barbiturates, cholestyramine, colestipol, penicillin, rifampin, the salicylates, and sulfinpyrazone, thus decreasing the pharmacologic effect of the beta-blocker. The presence of food greatly decreases the bioavailability of both propanolol and metoprolol. Food decreases the absorption of sotalol by 20%. The absorption of carteolol and penbutolol are slowed by food but not reduced. Beta-blockers may produce hypoglycemia and interfere with glucose and insulin tolerance tests. The beta-blockers may falsely increase creatinine and alkaline phosphatase.

○ **Propranolol hydrochloride** (Inderal, Inderal LA) is the oldest and most widely used of all the beta-blockers. Propranolol is often considered the standard beta-blocker to which each new beta-blocker is compared. Along with all the uses and actions of beta-blockers already discussed, propranolol produces significant enhancement of functional capacity during exercise training in the patient with coronary artery disease.

Patients receiving propranolol are cautioned to limit smoking because of reports that smoking can elevate blood pressure in these patients. Patients are also taught to take their drug at the same time each day and to always take with or without food (their choice) as food enhances bioavailability.

○ **Metoprolol** (Lopressor, Toprol XL) is administered to hypertensive patients and to patients who have had a myocardial infarction and for myocardial infarction prophylaxis. Like propranolol, metoprolol inhibits response to adrenergic stimuli by competitively blocking beta$_1$-adrenergic receptors within the myocardium. Unlike propranolol, however, metoprolol blocks beta$_2$-adrenergic receptors within bronchial and vascular smooth muscle only in high doses.

○ **Timolol maleate** (Blocadren) has pharmacologic actions similar to those of other beta-adrenergic blocking agents. Unlike atenolol and metoprolol, timolol is not a beta$_1$-selective adrenergic blocking agent; it is a nonselective beta-adrenergic blocking agent, inhibiting both beta$_1$- and beta$_2$-adrenergic receptors.

Timolol maleate is similar to propranolol hydrochloride. It has a 50% first-pass effect in the liver. Timolol maleate is used for the secondary prophylaxis of myocardial infarction and is started within 1 to 4 weeks following acute myocardial infarction. It is also used as eyedrops to treat glaucoma.

○ **Atenolol** (Tenormin), in low doses, inhibits beta$_1$ receptors while having little effect on beta$_2$ receptors. At high doses (over 100 mg/day orally or 10 mg/daIV), this selectively diminishes and the drug competitively blocks both beta$_1$- and beta$_2$-adrenergic receptors.

Atenolol is also administered as soon as possible after an myocardial infarction. Dosage adjustment is required for persons with renal impairment, because atenolol is excreted via the kidneys.

○ **Labetalol** (Trandate, Normodyne) is a nonselective lipid-soluble agent with both beta- and alpha$_1$-adrenergic (postsynaptic) blocking features. The principal physiologic action of labetalol is to competitively block beta$_1$ and beta$_2$ receptors and alpha$_1$ receptors within vascular smooth muscle. In addition to inhibiting access of endogenous or exogenous catecholamines to beta-adrenergic receptors, labetalol exhibits some intrinsic beta$_2$-agonist activity in animals; however, the drug exerts little, if any, intrinsic beta$_1$-agonist activity.

Labetalol produces marked vasodilation and decreased afterload with acute initiation of therapy and maintains the cardiac output despite the usual negative inotropic effects. Severe bradycardia, peripheral vascular symptoms, and heart failure occur less frequently with labetalol.

○ **Acebutolol** (Sectral), an oral drug for both hypertension and ventricular dysrhythmia, is a beta$_1$-selective adrenergic blocking agent. It has pharmacologic activity similar to that of other beta-adrenergic blocking agents. At low dosages, acebutolol selectively inhibits response to adrenergic stimuli by competitively blocking beta$_1$-adrenergic receptors while having little effect on the beta$_2$-adrenergic receptors of bronchial and vascular smooth muscle. At high dosages (greater than 800 mg daily), the selectivity of acebutolol for receptors usually diminishes, and the drug competitively blocks both beta$_1$- and beta$_2$-adrenergic receptors. In addition to inhibiting access of physiologic or synthetic catecholamines to the beta-adrenergic receptors, acebutolol exhibits mild ISA.

○ **Esmolol hydrochloride** (Brevibloc) is a rapid-onset, ultra-short-acting agent that has pharmacologic actions similar to those of other beta-adrenergic blocking agents. Esmolol selectively inhibits response to adrenergic stimuli by competitively blocking cardiac beta$_1$-adrenergic receptors while having little effect on the beta$_2$-adrenergic receptors of bronchial and vascular smooth muscle. At high doses (greater than 300 μg/kg per minute), this selectivity usually diminishes, and the drug competitively inhibits beta$_1$- and beta$_2$-adrenergic receptors.

At usual clinical doses, esmolol does not exhibit appreciable ISA or MSA, nor does the drug exhibit alpha-adrenergic blocking activity. It is used effectively to decrease blood pressure, ventricular heart rate in patients with acute atrial fibrillation and flutter, and the rate in noncompensatory sinus tachycardia. Esmolol has an elimination half-life of only 9 to 15 minutes, which allows for a rapid, controlled titration to a desired effect and prompt reversal of beta-blockade if necessary.

To discontinue esmolol, the infusion rate is decreased by 50% 30 minutes after transitioning to another agent such as digitalis, propranolol, quinidine, verapamil, or metoprolol. One hour after the second dose of the alternative agent, esmolol is discontinued if adequate response is achieved.

Esmolol is rapidly and extensively metabolized via esterases that are principally found in erythrocytes and in highly perfused tissues that contain esterases, such as the liver and kidneys. Methanol is formed as a by-product of metabolism, but the amount of methanol does not appear to be clinically significant. Ideally, esmolol is used for 24 hours or less.

Other Beta-Adrenergic Blocking Agents

○ **Nadolol** (Corgard) is similar to propranolol in its action. It is used as an antihypertensive and antianginal medication. Nadolol is also used for migraine prophylaxis, to control tremors, to control and treat aggressive-violent behavior, and to decrease intraocular pressure. It may also reduce extrapyramidal symptoms. It is administered orally in doses of 40 to 320 mg once daily. It has a half-life of 20 to 24 hours. It has beta$_1$ and beta$_2$ blocking activity, no MSA, and low ISA. It may be taken without regard to meals.

○ **Pindolol** (Visken) is a nonselective beta-adrenergic blocking agent, inhibiting both beta$_1$- and beta$_2$-adrenergic receptors. In addition to inhibiting access of physiologic or synthetic catecholamines to the beta-adrenergic receptors, pindolol causes slight activation of the beta receptors, making the drug a partial beta-agonist. Pindolol has the highest ISA of all beta-blockers. It has pharmacologic actions similar to those of other beta-adrenergic blocking agents with ISA. However, other beta-adrenergic blocking agents can block pindolol's ISA. Pindolol has low MSA.

The blunting of stress- and exercise-stimulated tachycardia by pindolol, however, is similar to that of the other beta-blockers. Pindolol also slows conduction in the atrioventricular node but usually to a lesser extent than do the other beta-adrenergic blocking agents. Pindolol reduces exercise-stimulated cardiac output, but has a slightly lesser effect on cardiac output than do other beta-adrenergic blockers. Pindolol is probably not effective in patients who develop angina at rest or at low exercise levels.

Pindolol is administered 15 to 60 mg/day in divided doses (two to three per day) for the control of hypertension. Pindolol is less effective for angina, but is a better choice of drug when the patient also has peripheral vascular disease because there is less vasoconstriction. It has a half-life of 3 to 4 hours and is only 40% protein bound. It may be taken without regard to meals.

○ **Carteolol** (Cartrol) is similar to propranolol and has little therapeutic gain over other beta-blockers to treat mild to moderate hypertension. It has beta$_1$- and beta$_2$-receptor blocking activity, low MSA, and moderate ISA. Carteolol is administered orally in doses of 2.5 to 5.0 mg/day. It has a long half-life of 6 hours and is only 25% to 30% protein bound. It is not biotransformed and is excreted unchanged in the urine (50% to 70%).

○ **Penbutolol** (Levatol) is almost identical to carteolol. It is used for mild to moderate hypertension. It has no MSA and moderate ISA. It is administered orally, 20 mg once daily. The hypertensive effect is not seen until after 2 weeks of therapy. It is 80% to 90% protein bound and has a half-life of 5 hours.

○ **Betaxolol hydrochloride** (Kerlone), a beta₁-specific blocker with low lipid solubility, no ISA, and low MSA, is primarily used to treat hypertension (in doses of 10 mg/day). Because of its long half-life (14 to 22 hours), betaxolol hydrochloride can be administered once daily. The full effect may not be seen for 7 to 14 days. It is 50% protein bound, metabolized in the liver, and excreted in the urine (80%). When discontinuing betaxolol hydrochloride, reduce dose gradually over a 2-week period.

○ **Bisoprolol fumarate** (Zebeta) is used alone or in combination to treat hypertension. The initial dose oral is 2.5 to 5.0 mg once daily with a maintenance dose of 5 to 20 mg once daily. It has a half-life of 9 to 12 hours and is excreted unchanged in urine (50%). It is a beta₁-selective drug with no MSA or ISA.

○ **Carvedilol** (Coreg), a nonselective beta-adrenoreceptor and alpha-adrenergic blocker with no ISA, is used primarily as an antihypertensive (6.25 to 25 mg twice a day). It is also being studied to treat heart failure (12.5 to 50 mg twice a day), angina pectoris (25 to 50 mg twice a day), and idiopathic cardiomyopathy (6.25 to 25 mg twice a day). Caution is used in the elderly as plasma levels may average about 50% higher and in patients with hepatic impairment because the liver is the organ of biotransformation and elimination.

○ **Sotalol hydrochloride** (Betapace), a competitive nonselective beta-blocker, is primarily used to treat life-threatening ventricular dysrhythmias. It has a proarrhythmic effect (1.5% to 2% rate of torsades de pointes) and is therefore not recommended in patients unless other drugs have been unsuccessful in controlling the dysrhythmia. Sotalol is not metabolized but is excreted unchanged in the urine. Sotalol has no MSA or ISA. It is administered orally starting at 80 mg twice a day and increased every 2 to 3 days to a maximum of 240 to 320 mg/day. If renal dysfunction is present, the dose is reduced. Before starting sotalol, withdraw other antidysrhythmics for a minimum of two to three half-lives, if condition permits. Monitor the QT interval before and after 8 hours; if it lengthens beyond 50% of the beginning QT, stop the drug. Have emergency equipment nearby. It is important to report any increased dysrhythmia to the physician.

○ **D-Sotalol,** chemically similar to sotalol, has less beta-blocking activity and therefore exhibits little or no negative inotropic action and less beta-blocker side effects. And, d-sotalol is less likely to induce torsades de pointes. D-sotalol is not yet approved in the United States.

Nursing Considerations for Beta-Adrenergic Blockers

As the nurse administers any of the beta-blockers, vital signs including cardiac rate and rhythm are assessed. Baseline weight is obtained. Because beta-blockers are taken at home possibly for the rest of the patient's life,

---

Table 17–5. PATIENT TEACHING— BETA-BLOCKERS

Dear Patient:
This drug has been ordered for you. This is what you should know about your drug to get the most from it.

☐ 1. Beta-blockers work by controlling certain nerve impulses. Beta-blockers are used to treat many conditions; the most common are high blood pressure, anginal pain, after a heart attack to help prevent another, irregular heartbeats, migraine headaches, and many others.

☐ 2. Beta-blockers generally will be taken for a long time and perhaps for the rest of your life.

☐ 3. Try to take your drug at the same time each day. You may be asked to take your heart rate or your blood pressure before you take your drug.

☐ 4. Do not take your beta-blocker with antacids. There are many drugs that interact with beta-blockers, so always check with your physician before taking any other drug.

☐ 5. If you forget to take your drug, take the next dose. *Do not* double dose.

☐ 6. *Do not* stop the drug on your own. If your physician does stop it, the dose is decreased gradually over several weeks.

☐ 7. Do not change the dose on your own.

☐ 8. Several beta-blockers are best taken between meals. _____ is best taken (between meals) or (whenever it is convenient, food does not matter). Do not drink beer, whiskey, or wine while taking your beta-blockers because these may lead to low blood pressure and dizziness. Limit your caffeinated beverages to 2/day.

☐ 9. Several side effects may occur. If any unusual symptoms occur, call your doctor. The most common side effects include dizziness and light-headedness, unusually slow pulse, tiredness, breathing difficulties, and reduced alertness. Be careful when operating heavy equipment or driving a car.

☐ 10. Store the drug in a dry, tight, moisture-resistant container and place out of the reach of children.

☐ 11. Do not take hot baths or showers or sit in a hot tub. Limit your exposure to the sun to short periods. Weigh yourself weekly.

---

much teaching is needed. Table 17–5 describes general patient teaching for beta-blockers. Patients are taught the best time to administer their beta-blocker. Propranolol and metoprolol have enhanced bioavailabilities when taken with food, so they are taken at the same time each day. Sotalol is taken on an empty stomach. Nadolol, pindolol, acebutolol, atenolol, carteolol, bisoprolol, and penbutolol are taken without regard to meals. It is extremely important that patients are taught not to discontinue their medications abruptly, as sudden cessation may precipitate angina, hypertensive crisis, or even an acute myocardial infarction. The patients are also taught information pertaining to drug interactions, typical side effects, and the importance of always remembering to take their medication.

Treatment of Overdose Clinical presentation and management of beta-blocker overdose, although rare, vary from person to person. Treatment priorities in the emergency department are directed toward reversal of life-threatening complications, including cardiovascular depression, respiratory compromise, and CNS disturbances. The major difficulty in treating these patients has been their refractoriness to treatment with catecholamines and parasympatholytic agents. Glucagon, a polypeptide hormone historically used to manage hypoglycemia, has demonstrated an ability to enhance myocardial contractility in the presence of massive beta-blockade. The recommended dosage of glucagon is 5 to 10 mg IV bolus over 30 seconds, followed by continuous infusion at 5 mg/hour, titrated to the desired patient response. Effects occur in 1 to 3 minutes, with peak action being reached in 5 to 7 minutes and lasting 15 to 20 minutes. The most commonly reported adverse effects are nausea and vomiting.

Selection of a Beta Blocker The major difference between the beta-blockers is their site of action. Beta-blockade is a very effective treatment, alone or in combination with other drugs, in 70% to 80% of patients with classic angina and in 50% to 70% of those with mild to moderate hypertension. Propranolol is likely to remain the gold standard because it is still so widely used and approved for so many different indications. However, propranolol is not beta$_1$-selective and being lipid soluble, it has a high brain penetration and undergoes an extensive hepatic first-pass effect. Propranolol has a short half-life and requires dosing two to four times daily; however, a sustained-release form, administered twice a day, is available. Today, other beta-blockers are being used because of their specific attractive properties: cardioselectivity (atenolol, metoprolol, acebutolol); lipid insolubility and no hepatic metabolism (atenolol, nadolol); long acting (nadolol, atenolol); ISA to help avoid myocardial depression (pindolol, carteolol, acebutolol, and penbutolol); and added alpha-blockade to achieve more arterial dilation (labetalol). When side effects are encountered, they may be avoided by switching to another beta-blocker. If one product is not working, another beta-blocker probably will not either. Two beta-blockers should never be administered together in hopes of improving therapeutic response. In general practice, the differences between beta-blockers are slight.

Combination Therapy Combining beta-blockers with diuretics, hydralazine, methyldopa, calcium antagonists, angiotensin converting enzyme inhibitors, and alpha-adrenergic blockers have all been successful in the therapy of hypertension. In general, when combining a beta-blocker and a thiazide diuretic, the dose of the thiazide need be no more than 12.5 to 25 mg daily. A combination of a beta-blocker and nifedipine is also hemodynamically sound; the afterload reduction of nifedipine offsets the bradycardia and negative inotropic effects of beta-blockade. A combination of quinidine with propranolol may improve the likelihood of converting atrial fibrillation to sinus rhythm.

GANGLIONIC BLOCKERS

The ganglionic blockers prevent transmission of both sympathetic and parasympathetic nerve impulses through the ganglia. They appear to compete with acetylcholine to occupy the cholinergic synapse of the autonomic ganglia. This competition makes it impossible for the vasoconstrictive impulses to then be transmitted across the neuromuscular junction; therefore, blood vessels dilate and arterial pressure is decreased.

Ganglionic blockers are most useful in the treatment of advanced stages of hypertension (including hypertensive crisis) when other medications are not effective. However, other more potent and more selectively acting drugs with fewer side effects have been developed, and the ganglionic blockers are seldom used today. Only one ganglionic blocker is still available in the United States—mecamylamine hydrochloride (Inversine).

The bibliography for this chapter can be found in Appendix B, which begins on page 1054.

CHAPTER REVIEW QUESTIONS*

1. Drugs acting positively on the beta-adrenergic receptor sites:
   a. Decrease cardiac contractility.
   b. Constrict bronchial smooth muscle.
   c. Increase cardiac rate.
   d. Constrict arterioles of skeletal muscle.

2. Which statement is *correct* regarding drugs acting as adrenergic stimulants?
   a. Norepinephrine (Levophed) increases blood flow to the kidney and skeletal muscles.
   b. Isoproterenol hydrochloride (Isuprel) produces bronchial constriction and peripheral vasodilation.
   c. Dobutamine hydrochloride (Dobutrex) causes the release of endogenous norepinephrine from adrenergic fibers.
   d. Epinephrine (Adrenalin) causes vasodilation in the blood vessels of muscle fibers with mostly beta$_2$ receptors.

3. Atenolol and metoprolol are used to improve cardiac function in patients with heart failure because they:
   a. Decrease further the number of beta$_1$ receptors.

   b. Block sympathetic activity.
   c. Increase the likelihood of ventricular dysrhythmias.
   d. Protect the myocardium.

4. In the event of beta-blocker overdose, the following drug has been shown to be useful in reversal of life-threatening complications:
   a. Protamine sulfate.
   b. Phenotolamine.
   c. Atropine.
   d. Glucagon.

5. The beta-adrenergic blocker propranolol (Inderal) has all of the following effects *except*:
   a. Slow the heart rate.
   b. Increase the SA node cycle.
   c. Control supraventricular dysrhythmias.
   d. Lower the blood pressure.

*See Appendix A, which begins of page 1051, for answers.

BUILDING YOUR CRITICAL THINKING SKILLS

β-ADRENERGIC BLOCKING AGENTS

A 52-year-old patient with a 4-year history of angina pectoris has been well controlled on propranolol hydrochloride (Inderal), 40 mg qid. He comes to the emergency room early one morning stating that he has had several severe anginal attacks during the night. The patient states he has been worried lately because he has been without a job for 4 weeks.

1. How might the patient's psychosocial data relate to his symptoms?
2. What additional assessments should the nurse make?
3. What discharge teaching and planning should be done for this patient?

Drugs That Provide Pain Relief

Merrily A. Kuhn, RNC, PhD

CHAPTER OUTLINE

KEY TERMS

Acute pain
Addiction
Chronic pain
Cephalad
Dependence
Endogenous peptides
Endorphins
Enkephalins
Epidural analgesia
Intrathecal analgesia

Migraine
Miosis
Nociceptors
Opiate
Opiate agonist
Opiate agonist-antagonist
Opiate antagonist
Opiate receptors
Photophobia

LEARNING OBJECTIVES

After reading this chapter, the student will be able to:

1. Identify medications commonly used as pain relievers.
2. Differentiate among the pain relievers' mechanisms of action, routes of administration, pharmacokinetics, adverse effects, contraindications and precautions, and interactions.
3. Identify specific areas of assessment in the patient requiring pain relievers to formulate appropriate patient outcomes.
4. Plan the nursing interventions necessary to administer pain relievers, and choose appropriate teaching strategies to gain patient compliance.
5. Evaluate the patient at various stages of treatment to measure the effectiveness of nursing interventions.

Pain has been described as an ambiguous puzzle, humanity's unremitting companion and inescapable end. Pain is beneficial because it alerts us to impending harm from the environment. It protects us from extreme temperatures, mechanical pressure, and penetrating wounds (e.g., stepping on a piece of glass). Beyond this warning purpose, pain becomes meaningless and causes suffering. The total pain experience involves both the perception of pain and the associated sensations, emotional reactions, effects, and psychophysiologic responses that result. Pain is one of the most frequently encountered patient problems. It is often difficult to assess and is frequently unyielding to treatment. The nurse must view the patient with pain holistically and believe that the patient has pain.

Pain can be either *acute* or *chronic*. Both of these types of pain alter the comfort level of the patient but cause different pain reaction behaviors, which affect the nature of the nursing assessment. Table 18–1 compares acute and chronic pain.

 The publisher greatly acknowledges the contribution of Barbara K. Clark, RN, MN, CCRN, to the third edition.

Table 18–1. DIFFERENTIATING BETWEEN ACUTE AND CHRONIC PAIN

	Acute Pain Characteristics	Chronic Pain Characteristics
Time, course	Transient, lasts less than 6 mo; pain subsides as healing occurs; has an ending.	Prolonged; lasts longer than 6 mo; may be intractable; ending is not always in sight.
Location	Localized.	Diffuse, difficult to localize.
Purpose	Warns one of impending or actual tissue damage.	Serves no purpose; depletes one of energy; pain becomes the pathology.
Characteristics	Sharp, various intensity (mild to severe), can radiate; comes and goes in accordance with pathology.	Aching, burning, dull, cramping, nagging, persistent; lasts after recovery from injury/disease.
Emotional response to pain	Positive; pain is experienced on a short-term basis.	Negative; pain serves no purpose; patient is emotionally distressed and may experience alterations in lifestyle.
Signs/symptoms	Sympathetic activation (increased blood pressure, tachycardia, increased respirations, diaphoresis, pallor, dilated pupils, increased muscle tone, increased concentration, anxiety, weakness), facial expression.	Compensatory responses (in sympathetic response), sleep disturbances, anorexia, listlessness, apathy, personality changes (anger, withdrawal, helplessness, hostility, hopelessness, irritability, depression).

PAIN PATHWAYS

Pain is detected by free nerve endings called *nociceptors* found in the skin, tissues, and organs. The nociceptors respond to mechanical, thermal, and chemical stimuli and convey these stimuli electrically via sensory (afferent) neurons to the central nervous system (CNS). The axons of these neurons are either myelinated (A-delta) fibers or unmyelinated (C) fibers. A-delta fibers transmit rapid pain sensations described as pricking or searing, such as

occurs when a person touches a hot flame. The C fibers carry impulses associated with slow, dull, aching, diffuse pain, such as occurs when a person suffers sunburn or headache. When pain fibers are stimulated by noxious stimuli, the information is sent to the dorsal horn of the spinal cord or brain stem, where it is then conveyed to higher centers in the brain. Pain impulses are carried along three major pain pathways: the spinothalamic (shown in Figure 18–1), spinoreticular, and spinomesen-

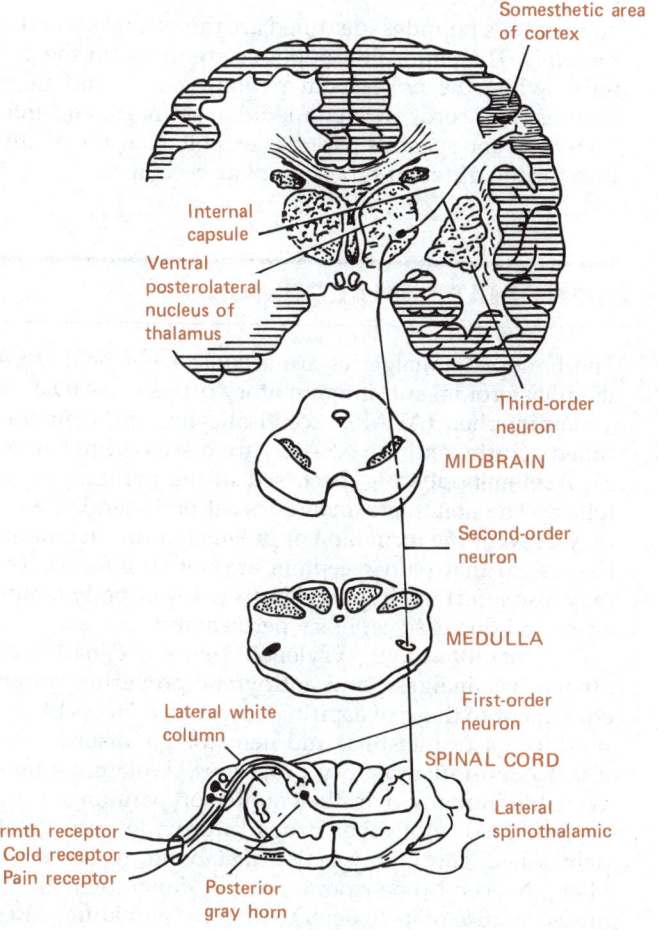

Figure 18–1. Sensory pathway for pain and temperature—the lateral spinothalmic pathway.

cephalic. Specific nuclei of the brain, such as the reticular formation, also are components of pain pathways.

DRUG INFLUENCES OVER PAIN

Major groups of drugs administered to control pain include the nonopiate (non-narcotic) analgesics and the opiate (narcotic) analgesics. The ergot alkaloids and sumatriptan, a selective serotonin receptor agonist, are used to control pain from *migraine* (paroxysmal attacks of headache thought to be the result of vasodilation of extracerebral cranial arteries). These drugs influence the pain experience in several ways. The first alteration to the pain experience is an interruption of the peripheral pain receptors at the free nerve endings. Nonopiate analgesics (salicylates, aniline derivatives, indene derivatives, and alkylanoic acid compounds) play a critical role in interrupting pain impulses in the periphery. The second mechanism by which analgesics alter the pain experience is by modifying pain perception at the level of the CNS. Opiate analgesics and some non-narcotic analgesics interfere with the perception of pain. Finally, drugs interfere with the pain experience by changing one or more of the three major types of pain reactions: (1) autonomic response—changes in palmar sweat index or blood pressure; (2) skeletal muscle response—increased muscle tension, tense facial expressions; and (3) psychologic response—suffering of pain. The suffering of pain is greatly modified by opiate analgesics, whereas the other two types of pain reactions can be influenced by either opiate or nonopiate analgesics, depending on the intensity of the pain experience. Ergot alkaloids affect pain relief through their action as alpha-adrenergic blockers. They are effective in reducing extracranial blood flow, thereby decreasing the pain associated with vascular headaches. Sumatriptan acts as a selective agonist at specific vascular serotonin receptor sites, causing vasoconstriction in large arterial arteries. This results in pain relief of acute migraine attacks.

Opiate Receptors In The Central Nervous System

Opiates (substances derived from opium), or opiate analgesics, alter the perception of pain through their interaction with opiate receptors. *Opiate receptors* are receptors that interact in a highly selective, stereospecific manner with morphine and other opiate drugs and with endogenous peptides. The density of opiate receptors varies in different regions of the brain and spinal cord. This variation in opiate receptors is important to the mechanism of action of opiate drugs. Binding studies have identified the following receptor types: (1) mu receptor, (2) kappa receptor, (3) sigma receptor, (4) delta receptor, and (5) epsilon receptor. Table 18–2 summarizes the relationship between the receptors and various drugs that interact with a particular group of receptors.

Endogenous Peptides

The opiate receptors interact not only with opiate drugs but also with *endogenous peptides,* morphine-like peptides that modulate pain and serve as neurotransmitters. The

Table 18–2. OPIATE RECEPTORS

Receptor Type	Physiologic Effect	Opiate/Endogenous Peptide—Type of Activity
Mu	Bradycardia, bradypnea, analgesia	Morphine (agonist) Meperidine (agonist) Methadone (agonist) Codeine (agonist) Fentanyl (antagonist) Levorphanol (agonist) Buprenorphine (agonist) Naloxone (antagonist) Dezocine Enkephalin Endorphin
Kappa	Spinal analgesia, miosis, sedation	Morphine (agonist) Pentazocine (agonist) Naloxone (antagonist) Dynorphin
Sigma	Dysphoria, hallucinations, respiratory and vasomotor stimulation	Pentazocine (agonist)
Delta	Unknown	Enkephalin Endorphin
Epsilon	Unknown	Endorphin

endogenous peptides identified are the *endorphins* and *enkephalins.* The endorphin peptides are found in the pituitary, while the enkephalin peptides are found in the brain, spinal cord, adrenal medulla, stomach, and intestines. The endogenous peptides exhibit a variety of affinities for the different types of opiate receptors.

NONOPIATE ANALGESICS

The nonopiate analgesics are acetylsalicylic acid (ASA), the nonsteroidal anti-inflammatory drugs (NSAIDs), and acetaminophen (APAP). Acetylsalicylic acid, commonly called aspirin, and the NSAIDs are discussed in Chapter 57. **Acetaminophen** is discussed in the paragraphs that follow. The nonopiate analgesics act peripherally, where they prevent the formation of prostaglandins in inflamed tissues, so that pain receptors are not stimulated. They may also affect the hypothalamus to lower body temperature and decrease capillary permeability.

○ **Acetaminophen** (Tylenol, Tempra, Panadol, and others) has analgesic and antipyretic properties roughly equivalent to those of aspirin. However, it is less likely to produce gastrointestinal and hematologic disorders and it lacks anti-inflammatory properties. Acetaminophen is available in many over-the-counter preparations. It may be combined with other drugs to provide even greater pain relief. The highly active metabolite of acetaminophen, N-acetyl-p-benzoquinone, is dangerous in high doses because of its toxicity to the liver and kidney. Refer

Table 18–3. NONOPIATE ANALGESICS

DRUG NAME/ROUTE AND DOSAGE	PHARMACOKINETICS/ DYNAMICS	NURSING IMPLICATIONS
acetaminophen (Anacin-3) (Panadol) (Tempra) (Tylenol) and many others		

oral administration	**Onset:** PO and rectal, 0.5–1 hr **Peak:** PO and rectal, 1–3 hr **Duration:** PO and rectal, 3–4 hr **½L:** 1–4 hr **PB:** 25% **B:** liver **E:** urine	**ASSESSMENT:** Assess hepatic, hematologic, and renal function periodically during the course of prolonged, high-dose therapy. Assess patient's overall health status and alcohol usage before administering this medication. Patients who are malnourished or who are chronic alcohol abusers are at a higher risk of developing hepatotoxicity with chronic use of usual dose of this drug. Assess for pregnancy (category B).
Adults and Children over 12 yr: 325–1000 mg PO (tablet, capsule, syrup) q 4–6 hr not to exceed 4 g/day, or 2.6 g/day chronically.		
Children 11–12 yr: 480 mg PO q 4–6 hr as needed.		**INTERVENTION:** Many OTC products contain acetaminophen; be aware of this when calculating daily dosage.
Children 9–10 yr: 400 mg PO q 4–6 hr as needed.		**Patient Teaching**—Teach patient to avoid alcohol when taking drug and to not use for more than 10 days (5 days in children) without medical supervision.
Children 6–8 yr: 320 mg PO q 4–6 hr as needed.		**EVALUATION:** Evaluate for adverse effects such as rash, urticaria, or hepatic or renal dysfunction. Notify physician if these occur.
Children 4–5 yr: 240 mg PO q 4–6 hr as needed.		
Children 2–3 yr: 160 mg PO q 4–6 hr as needed.		
Children 1–2 yr: 120 mg PO q 4–6 hr as needed.		
Children 4–11 mo: 80 mg PO q 4–6 hr as needed.		
Children under 3 mo: 40 mg PO q 4–6 hr as needed.		
rectal administration		
Adults and Children over 12 yr: 325–650 mg rectally q 4–6 hr as needed, not to exceed 6 doses in 24 hr.		
Children 6–12 yr: 355 mg rectally q 4–6 hr as needed, not to exceed 2.6 g/24 hr.		
Children 3–6 yr: 120 mg rectally q 4–6 hr as needed, not to exceed 720 mg/24 hr.		
Children under 3 yr: Consult physician.		

to Table 18–3 for specific drug dosages, pharmacokinetics, and nursing implications.

CONTRAINDICATIONS AND PRECAUTIONS Because the liver and kidney contain the enzymes that convert the cytotoxic metabolite in acetaminophen to a nontoxic metabolite, acetaminophen is not given to patients with renal or liver disease. When large doses of acetaminophen are administered to children under the age of 12, a rare complication—methemoglobinemia—can occur. Children tend to form methemoglobin more readily than adults, which results in cyanosis of the skin, mucosa, and fingernails and is a sign of acute *p*-aminophenol derivative toxicity. This is a rare complication, however, and acetaminophen is the drug of choice for children.

ADVERSE EFFECTS Adverse effects occur with hypersensitivity reactions and overdose. Rare hypersensitivity reactions may produce laryngeal edema, skin rash, fever, angioedema, and mucosal lesions. Signs of overdose include nausea, vomiting, pain, and chills, as well as blood dyscrasias, methemoglobinemia, psychologic changes, renal and hepatic damage, hypoglycemic coma, and myocardial dysfunction. Acute poisoning may be manifested

by dizziness, nausea, vomiting, palpitations, and sweating. A single dose of 25 g or more can be fatal, causing fulminating hepatic failure. Acute renal failure is also possible. Both the liver and the kidney contain the enzyme systems for converting acetaminophen to the cytotoxic metabolite that causes cellular necrosis.

INTERACTIONS Antipyretics may cause severe hypothermia when used with phenothiazine antipsychotics. Hepatotoxicity may be additive with other hepatotoxic substances, including alcohol. Phenobarbital may increase liver toxicity if overdosage occurs. Cholestyramine and colestipol decrease acetaminophen's absorption and may decrease its effectiveness. False-positive results of plasma amylase and lipase levels have occurred. Acetaminophen may produce a slight increase in responsiveness to oral anticoagulants. It may also cause a false increase in urinary 5-HIAA (5-hydroxyindoleacetic acid) test results. Persons taking acetaminophen should refrain from drinking alcohol. There have been reports in the literature that even as few as one or two drinks a day, combined with acetaminophen, may precipitate hepatic or renal disease.

ACETAMINOPHEN OVERDOSE   If overdose of acetaminophen is suspected, syrup of ipecac is administered to the patient or gastric lavage is performed. The antidote for an overdose of acetaminophen is acetylcysteine (Mucomyst). The loading oral adult dose is 140 mg/kg of body weight. The maintenance oral adult dosage is 70 mg/kg every 4 hours for 17 doses. Acetylcysteine is most effective when it is started within 10 hours after the overdose. Acetylcysteine substitutes for a lack of glutathione and forms an inactive compound with the reactive metabolite.

○ **Tramadol**   (Ultram), a centrally acting analgesic, is used to treat moderately severe pain. Despite some opioid activity, tramadol is not a controlled substance. Tramadol binds with the mu-opioid receptors and inhibits the reuptake of norepinephrine and serotonin. The analgesic effects are only partly antagonized by naloxone. Many side effects can occur including seizures and anaphylaxis, nausea, vomiting and constipation. Dependence can occur, so careful administration is necessary. Fifty to 100 mg (PO, IM, IV, SC, rectal, or epidural) every 4 to 6 hours up to a maximum of 400 mg/day (300 mg for older patients) is the recommended dose. Dosing intervals are increased for patients with hepatic or renal dysfunction.

OPIATE ANALGESICS

Opiate or narcotic analgesics are drugs that are the natural, semisynthetic, or synthetic alkaloid derivatives of opium that mimic the actions of morphine. Opiate analgesics are classified as either opiate agonists, partial agonists, or opiate agonist-antagonists, based on their activity at the opiate receptor. An *opiate agonist* is a drug or endogenous substance that stimulates opiate receptors. A partial agonist stimulate some receptors but do not have any antagonistic qualities. An *opiate agonist-antagonist* is a drug or substance that stimulates certain opiate receptors but antagonizes other opiate receptors. Opiate analgesics, featured in Tables 18–4 to 18–6 are well known for their clinical use for pain relief. Other clinical uses include providing sedation and controlling diarrhea and cough. The opiate analgesics are Schedule II controlled substances. Combination products that contain opiate analgesics may be Schedule III, IV, or V, depending on the amount of the narcotic.

ACTION

Sites throughout the body that have a high affinity for opiate analgesics also have high concentrations of endogenous peptides (endorphins). These drugs suppress the opioid receptors within the limbic system of the brain, thus inhibiting the unpleasant emotional responses to pain. Certain receptors in the midbrain are also activated, which in turn relay inhibitory impulses down the dorsolateral tracts to the dorsal horn neurons. Thus, the ascent of the pain stimuli to the brain is stopped when the dorsal horn neurons receive pain stimuli from the periphery.

Opiate analgesics inhibit neuronal firing in specific areas of the brain, thus decreasing the release of certain neurotransmitters. The release of transmitter substances is associated with calcium entry into the neuron. This action alters activation of postsynaptic sites. The person is aware of pain but states that its intensity is no longer bothersome.

Organ-System Effects of Opiate Analgesics

The systemic effects described below include the opiate agonists. The effects of the opiate agonist-antagonists are described later in the chapter.

Central Nervous System Effects   The opiate analgesics have an affinity for the mu receptors. The major effects are analgesia, euphoria, sedation, respiratory depression, cough suppression, miosis, truncal rigidity, and emesis. The euphoria is characterized by a floating sensation and a feeling of freedom from anxiety and distress. This effect contributes significantly to the addictive use of these agents. The sedative effect is a result of drowsiness and clouding of mentation. Patients may experience some impairment of reasoning ability. Patients, especially the elderly, may feel the need to sleep as a result of these drugs. Table 18–7 reviews a sedation scale. Patients with a rating of four are difficult to arouse and require immediate attention. The respiratory depression caused by the administration of opiate analgesics is a result of a depression in the respiratory centers in the pons and medulla, caused by a depressed response to a carbon dioxide challenge. This is one reason why patients with increased intracranial pressure, asthma, chronic obstructive pulmonary disease (COPD), or cor pulmonale cannot tolerate opiate analgesics. Respiratory depression is a decrease in rate or depth of respirations, not necessarily a specific number of respirations per minute. This means that patients breathing less than 10 times per minute may not have respiratory depression if they are breathing deeply. It takes more opiate to produce respiratory depression than sedation, so patients with respiratory depression are very sleepy and hard to arouse. Patients who are recovering from anesthesia, are heavy smokers, or have COPD or renal dysfunction are more at risk for respiratory depression than other patients. Cough suppression occurs because of the depressive effects of opioid analgesics on the brain stem. *Miosis* (constriction of the pupil) is a hallmark of opiate use. Miosis is blocked by atropine and opiate antagonists. Truncal rigidity is believed to be the result of opiate action at the level of the spinal cord. The large trunk muscles have increased tone while the drug is in the system. Emesis is a result of activation of the chemoreceptor trigger zone in the medulla. Prolonged use of the opiate analgesics leads to tolerance to these effects.

Peripheral Effects   Generally opiate analgesics do not have a direct effect on cardiac rate, rhythm, or blood pressure. Some opioids stimulate histamine release, which can result in orthostatic hypotension, especially if the cardiovascular system is stressed by disease. The histamine release may also be responsible for the pruritis that is so common with opiates, particularly morphine, and the

Table 18–4. OPIATE AGONIST ANALGESICS

DRUG NAME/ROUTE AND DOSAGE	PHARMACOKINETICS/ DYNAMICS	NURSING IMPLICATIONS
NATURAL ALKALOIDS		
morphine (Duramorph) (MS Contin) (RMS) (Oramorph) (Roxanol)		
Adults: 10–30 mg PO or rectally q 4 hr or 30–60 mg PO (ER tablets) 8–12 hr; 5–20 mg IM or SC q 4 hr; or 2.5–15 mg IV q 4 hr, or IV infusion initated at 1–10 mg/hr increased as needed (large doses of 10–60 mg/hr have been used). *Children:* 0.1–0.2 mg/kg SC or IM q 4 hr or 0.05–0.1 mg/kg IV. **epidural analgesia** *Adults:* 2–10 mg/day initially or 2–4 mg/day as a continuous infusion. **intrathecal analgesia** *Adults:* 0.2–1 mg for up to 24 hr.	**Onset:** PO, within 1 hr; IM, 10–30 min; SC, 20 min; IV, rapid; epidural, 6–30 min; intrathecal, rapid **Peak:** PO, 60 min; IM, 30–60 min; SC, 50–90 min; rectal, 20–60 min; IV, 20 min **Duration:** PO, IM, SC, rectal, and IV, 4–5 hr; ER, 8–12 hr; epidural and intrathecal, up to 24 hr **½L:** 2–3 hr **PB:** 33% **B:** liver **E:** urine, feces	**ASSESSMENT:** Prolonged use may lead to dependence and tolerance. This should not prevent patient from receiving adequate analgesia. Assess for head trauma; increased intracranial pressure; severe renal, hepatic, or pulmonary disease; hypothyroidism; adrenal insufficiency; alcoholism; undiagnosed abdominal pain; or prostatic hypertropy. Assess bowel function routinely. Increased intake of fluids and bulk, stool softeners, and laxatives may minimize constipating effects. Assess blood pressure, pulse, and respiratory rate before and periodically during administration. Assess for pregnancy (category C; D for prolonged use or high doses given near term). **INTERVENTION:** Explain therapeutic value of medication prior to administration to enhance the analgesic effect. Regularly administered doses may be more effective than PRN administration. Medication may cause drowsiness. Oral doses may be administered with food or milk to minimize GI irritation. ER preparations should not be crushed or chewed. Dilute for IV administration with at least 5 mL sterile water or 0.9% NaCl. Administer slowly, 15 mg of morphine or equivalent or fraction thereof, over 3–5 min. Rapid administration may lead to increased respiratory depression, hypotension, and circulatory collapse. May be added to IV solutions for continuous infusion. This method requires close titration and an infusion pump to control the rate. Dose is titrated to ensure adequate pain relief without excessive sedation, respiratory depression, or hypotension. Medication is discontinued gradually after long-term use to prevent withdrawal symptoms. **Patient Teaching**—Advise patient to call for assistance when ambulating or smoking. Advise patient to make position changes slowly to minimize orthostatic hypotension. **EVALUATION:** Pain is relieved without major side effects. Report severe sedation to physician.
codeine		
analgesia *Adults:* 15–60 mg PO, SC, IM, or IV q 4–6 hr as needed, not to exceed 360 mg/24 hr. *Children 1 yr and over:* 0.5 mg/kg PO, SC, or IM q 4–6 hr as needed. IV use is not recommended in children. **antitussive** *Adults:* 10–20 mg PO q 4–6 hr as needed (not to exceed 120 mg/day). *Children 6–12 yr:* 5–10 mg PO q 4–6 hr as needed (not to exceed 60 mg/day). *Children 2–6 yr:* 2.5–5 mg PO q 4–6 hr (not to exceed 30 mg/day).	**Onset:** PO, 30–45 min; IM and SC, 10–30 min **Peak:** PO, 60–120 min; IM, 30–60 min **Duration:** PO, IM, and SC, 4 hr **½L:** 2.5–4 hr **PB:** 50% **B:** liver **E:** urine (5%–15% unchanged)	**ASSESSMENT:** Prolonged use may lead to dependence and tolerance. This should not prevent patient from receiving adequate analgesia. Potential for dependence is less than with morphine. Progressively higher doses may be required to relieve pain with long-term therapy. Assess bowel function routinely. Increased intake of fluids and bulk, stool softeners, and laxatives may minimize constipating effects. Assess cough and lung sounds during antitussive use. Assess for pregnancy (category C; D for prolonged use or high doses given near term). **INTERVENTION:** Food or milk may minimize GI irritation with oral doses. Medication is discontinued gradually after long-term use to prevent withdrawal symptoms. **Patient Teaching**—Caution patient to avoid driving and activities that require alertness until effects of drug are known. **EVALUATION:** Suppression of cough or relief of pain determines effectiveness.

Continued on the following page

Table 18–4. OPIATE AGONIST ANALGESICS, *Continued*

DRUG NAME/ROUTE AND DOSAGE	PHARMACOKINETICS/DYNAMICS	NURSING IMPLICATIONS
SEMISYNTHETIC ANALOGS		
hydromorphone (Dilaudid) (Dilaudid-HP)		
analgesia **Adults:** 2–4 mg PO, IM, or SC q 4–6 hr as needed; 1–2 mg slow IV q 4–6 hr; or 3 mg rectally q 6–8 hr as needed.	**Onset:** PO, IM, and SC, 15–30 min; IV, 10–15 min; rectal, 15–30 min **Peak:** PO, IM, and SC, 30–90 min; IV, 15–30 min; rectal, 30–90 min **Duration:** PO, SC, and IM, 4–5 hr; IV, 2–3 hr; rectal, 4–5 hr **½L:** 2–4 hr **PB:** UA **B:** liver **E:** urine	**ASSESSMENT:** Assess for hypersensitivity. Use cautiously in severe renal, hepatic, or pulmonary disease. Assess organ function often. Assess for pregnancy (category B; D for prolonged use or high doses given near term). **INTERVENTION:** Food or milk may minimize GI irritation with oral doses. Dilute for IV administration with at least 5 mL sterile water or 0.9% NaCl. Administer slowly at a rate not to exceed 2 mg over 3–5 min. Rapid administration may lead to increased respiratory depression, hypotension, and circulatory collapse. Do not use IV administration without having antidote available. **EVALUATION:** Relief of pain demonstrates effectiveness. Report side effects to physician.
SYNTHETIC COMPOUNDS		
meperidine (Demerol)		
analgesia **Adults:** 50–150 mg PO, IM, or SC q 3–4 hr. **Children:** 1.1–1.8 mg/kg PO, IM, or SC q 3–4 hr. **preoperative sedation** **Adults:** 50–100 IM or SC 30–90 min before anesthesia. **Children:** 1–2 mg/kg IM or SC 30–90 min before anesthesia (not to exceed adult dose).	**Onset:** IV, immediate; PO, 15 min; IM and SC, 10–15 min **Peak:** IV, 5–7 min; PO, 60 min; IM, 35–50 min; SC, 40–60 min **Duration:** IV, PO, IM, and SC, 2–4 hr **½L:** 4–8 hr (prolonged in hepatic or renal dysfunction) **PB:** 60–80% **B:** liver **E:** urine (5% unchanged)	**ASSESSMENT:** Same as for morphine. **INTERVENTION:** Oral doses may be administered with food or milk to minimize GI irritation. Syrup is diluted in a half glass of water. Oral dose is less than 50% as effective as parenteral. When changing to oral administration, dosage may need to be increased. IM is the preferred parenteral route for repeated doses. SC administration may cause local irritation. If IV administration is required, dilute with at least 5 mL sterile water or 0.9% NaCl. Administer slowly, at a rate not to exceed 25 mg over 1 min. Rapid administration may lead to increased respiratory depression, hypotension, and circulatory collapse. Do not use IV administration without having antidote available.
methadone hydrochloride (Dolophine)		
analgesia **Adults:** 2.5–10 mg PO, IM, or SC q 3–4 hr, up to 5–20 mg q 6–8 hr. **Pediatric:** Not recommended for use in children. **detoxification** **Adults:** 15–40 mg/day PO. Should not exceed 21 days. *Maintenance dose*—20–120 mg/day PO.	**Onset:** PO, 30–60 min; IM and SC, 10–20 min **Peak:** PO, 90–120 min; IM and SC, 60–120 min **Duration:** PO, 4–12 hr; IM and SC, 4–6 hr **½L:** 25 hr **PB:** 90% **B:** liver **E:** urine, bile	**ASSESSMENT:** Same as morphine plus assess for pregnancy (category B). **INTERVENTION:** Food or milk may minimize GI irritation with oral doses. IM is the preferred route for repeated doses. SC administration may cause local irritation. Administered only in an approved drug rehab program. **Patient Teaching**—Advise patient to avoid concurrent use of alcohol or CNS depressants.

ER = extended release; NA = not available.

bronchospasm. Thus, opiates are administered cautiously to patients with known allergies or respiratory disease. Morphine sulfate is used as a preload and afterload reducer in myocardial infarction. This reduction in vascular tone is secondary to a decrease in central sympathetic outflow or splanchnic pooling.

PHARMACOKINETICS

The opiate analgesics are absorbed well from mucosal surfaces of the nose and gastrointestinal tract as well as from subcutaneous and intramuscular sites. The absorption from the gastrointestinal tract may be rapid, but the potency of some compounds may be lower because of the

Table 18–5. OPIATE ANTAGONIST ANALGESICS: PHENYLPIPERIDINES		
DRUG NAME/ROUTE AND DOSAGE	**PHARMACOKINETICS/ DYNAMICS**	**NURSING IMPLICATIONS**
fentanyl transdermal (Duragesic)		
Adults: Apply one patch, releasing 25, 50, 75, or 100 μg/hr. Change q 3 days.	**Onset:** 7–8 hr **Peak:** 12–24 hr **Duration:** 72 hr (while patch is worn) **½L:** 13–22 hr after patch is removed **PB:** 79%–87% **B:** liver **E:** urine	**ASSESSMENT:** Prolonged use may lead to dependence and tolerance. This should not prevent patient from receiving adequate analgesia. Assess for head trauma; increased intracranial pressure; severe renal, hepatic, or pulmonary disease; hypothyroidism; adrenal insufficiency; alcoholism; undiagnosed abdominal pain; or prostatic hypertrophy (all cautions). Assess bowel function routinely. Increased intake of fluids and bulk, stool softeners, and laxatives may minimize constipating effects. Assess blood pressure, pulse, and respiratory rate before and periodically during administration. Assess for pregnancy (category C). **INTERVENTION:** Explain therapeutic value of medication prior to administration to enhance the analgesic effect. Regularly administered doses may be more effective than PRN administration. High addiction potential. Protect from light. **Transdermal patch—**Apply to nonirradiated, nonshaved skin as absorption may be altered. Change dose no more often than q 3 days; patients may require supplementation with other narcotics during the dose titration phase. Best applied to hairless area of upper torso; hair may be clipped but not shaved if necessary. Apply new patches to sites different from old patch. To discard, remove patch, fold in half, and flush down toilet. **EVALUATION:** Evaluate for sedation, confusion, hypotension, constipation—report to physician. Evaluate respiratory rate. Administer antidote naloxone if needed.
fentanyl, parenteral (Sublimaze)		
Adults: 0.05–0.1 mg IM 30–60 min prior to surgery. **Adults:** 0.025–0.1 mg IM or slow IV (over 1–2 min) as adjunct to surgery. **Children 2–12 yr:** 2–3 μg/kg IV for induction and maintenance.	**Onset:** IV, 1–2 min; IM, 7–15 min **Peak:** IV, 3–5 min; IM, 20–30 min **Duration:** IV, 0.5–1 hr; IM, 1–2 hr **½L:** 3–6 hr **B:** liver **E:** kidney	Same as for fentanyl transdermal plus: **INTERVENTION:** Often used for open heart surgery and other major surgical procedures to protect the myocardium from excessive oxygen demand. Only staff trained in administering anesthetics and managing their potential adverse effects should administer parenteral fentanyl. Administer only in monitored anesthesia care settings.

first-pass metabolism in the liver after absorption. The oral dosage of these compounds is higher than that required when parenteral administration is used. Table 18–8 details the potency of these agents.

The opiate analgesics are distributed to a variety of tissues, such as the lungs, liver, kidneys, and spleen. The skeletal muscle and fatty tissue are storage sites for these compounds, and concentrations in the brain are low compared with concentrations in other organs. The opiates are converted to metabolites and are excreted by the kidneys.

CONTRAINDICATIONS AND PRECAUTIONS

Opiate analgesics are contraindicated in those with known hypersensitivity. The drugs have a high abuse potential. They are used cautiously in patients with head injury and increased intracranial pressure. If they are used in these circumstances, the patient's intracranial pressure should be monitored because these agents depress consciousness, decrease respirations, increase carbon dioxide partial pressure, increase intracranial pressure, and alter pupil reaction to light. Opiate analgesics are also used with caution in the elderly and in patients who have severe renal, hepatic, or pulmonary disease, hypothyroidism, adrenal insufficiency, alcoholism, undiagnosed abdominal pain, or prostatic hypertrophy. Safe use in pregnancy (category C) has not been established. A 4-hour interval is recommended between drug administration and infant nursing.

ADVERSE EFFECTS

The most common adverse effects of opiate analgesics are constipation, urinary retention, nausea, and vomiting. In the ambulatory patient, restlessness, dizziness, and light-

Table 18–6. OPIATE AGONIST-ANTAGONIST ANALGESICS AND OPIATE ANTAGONISTS		
DRUG NAME/ROUTE AND DOSAGE	**PHARMACOKINETICS/ DYNAMICS**	**NURSING IMPLICATIONS**
OPIATE AGONIST-ANTAGONISTS		
pentazocine hydrochloride and lactate (Talwin) (Talwin-Nx [pentazocine, 50 mg, with naloxone, 5 mg])		
Adults: 50 mg PO q 3–4 hr; maximum dose of 600 mg/24 hr; or 30 mg IM, SC, or IV q 3–4 hr (excluding patients in labor); not to exceed 60 mg IM or SC or 30 mg IV each dose. **patient in labor** *Adults:* 20–30 mg IM; 20 mg may be repeated 1–2 times at 2–3 hr intervals if needed.	**Onset:** PO, IM, or SC, 15–30 min; IV, 2–3 min **Peak:** PO, 1–3 hr; IM, 60 min; IV, 15 min **Duration:** PO, 4–5 hr; IM, 2–3 hr: IV, 1 hr **½L:** 2–3 hr **PB:** 60% **B:** liver **E:** kidney	**ASSESSMENT:** Assess for head injury, increased intracranial pressure, or history of drug abuse, and emotionally unstable patients (all contraindications). Safe use during pregnancy or in children under 12 years of age has not been established. Assess for impaired renal or hepatic function, respiratory depression, biliary surgery, and in those with myocardial infarction who have nausea and vomiting (all cautions). Assess for pregnancy (category C). **INTERVENTION:** Pentazocine may cause acute withdrawal symptoms in patients regularly receiving opioids. Observe for chills, abdominal and muscle cramps, yawning, rhinorrhea, lacrimation, itching, restlessness, anxiety, and drug-seeking behavior. Monitor injection sites for signs of irritation or inflammation. Do not mix pentazocine in the same syringe with barbiturates because this causes precipitation. Pentazocine can cause withdrawal symptoms. **EVALUATION:** Report severe nausea, vomiting, and respiratory depression to physician.
nalbuphine hydrochloride (Nubain)		
Adults: 10–20 mg IM, SC, or IV q 3–6 hr (maximum 160 mg).	**Onset:** IM and SC, 15 min; IV, 2–3 min **Peak:** IM, 60 min; IV, 30 min **Duration:** IM, SC, and IV, 3–6 hr **½L:** 5 hr **PB:** <30% **B:** liver **E:** urine, kidney	**ASSESSMENT:** Assess blood pressure, pulse, and respiration before and periodically during administration. Nalbuphine produces respiratory depression, but this does not markedly increase with increased doses. This drug has a low potential for dependence, but prolonged use may lead to physical and psychologic dependence and tolerance. **INTERVENTION:** Explain therapeutic value of medication prior to administration to enhance effectiveness. Regularly administered doses may be more effective than PRN administration. Caution ambulatory patients against operating a car or hazardous machinery after taking the drug. Administer IM injections. May give IV undiluted. Administer slowly, each 10 mg over 3–5 min. Antagonistic properties may induce withdrawal symptoms in narcotic-dependent patients. **EVALUATION:** Report severe nausea, vomiting, and respiratory depression to physician.
butorphanol (Stadol) (Stadol NS)		
Adults: 1–4 mg IM q 3–4 hr as needed (not to exceed 4 mg in a single dose); 0.5–2.0 mg IV q 3–4 hr as needed; or 1 spray into one or both nostrils q 3–4 hr PRN. *Pediatric:* Not recommended in children under 18 yr.	**Onset:** IM, 1–30 min; IV, 1 min; intranasal, 15 min **Peak:** IM, 30–60 min; IV, 4–5 min; intranasal, 1–2 hr **Duration:** IM and IV, 3–4 hr; intranasal, 4–5 hr **½L:** 3–4 hr **PB:** 96% **B:** liver **E:** urine, feces	**ASSESSMENT:** Same as for nalbuphine except pregnancy category unknown. **INTERVENTION:** Butorphanol, 2 mg, has approximately the same respiratory depression as 10 mg of morphine, but respiratory depression does not increase in amount, only in duration with increased dosage. Prolonged use may lead to physical and psychologic dependence and tolerance. Abrupt withdrawal following chronic administration may produce vomiting, restlessness, abdominal cramps, and increased blood pressure and temperature. Administer IM injections deep into well-developed muscle. Rotate sites of injections. May give IV undiluted. Administer over 3–5 min. Encourage patient to turn, cough, and breathe deeply every 2 hr to prevent atelectasis. Antagonistic properties may induce withdrawal symptoms in opiate-dependent patients. **EVALUATION:** Report severe nausea, vomiting, and respiratory depression to physician.

Chapter 18 • DRUGS THAT PROVIDE PAIN RELIEF

OPIATE AGONIST-ANTAGONIST ANALGESICS AND OPIATE ANTAGONISTS

Table 18–6. OPIATE AGONIST-ANTAGONIST ANALGESICS AND OPIATE ANTAGONISTS, *Continued*

DRUG NAME/ROUTE AND DOSAGE	PHARMACOKINETICS/ DYNAMICS	NURSING IMPLICATIONS
dezocine (Dalgan) ***Adults:*** 2.5–10 mg IV q 2–4 hr; or 5–20 mg IM q 3–6 hr, up to maximum 120 mg in 24 hr.	**Onset:** IV, 15 min; IM, 30 min **Peak:** IM, 30–150 min **Duration:** IV and IM, 2–4 hr (dose dependent) **½L:** 2–4 hr **PB:** NA **B:** liver **E:** kidney (<1% unchanged)	Same as for pentazocine plus: **ASSESSMENT:** Assess for metabisulfite allergy. Do not administer if present. Assess for previous dependency on narcotics. Antagonistic properties of drug may induce withdrawal symptoms in opiod-dependent patients. **INTERVENTION:** Do not administer with alcohol or other CNS depressants. Do not administer SC because it is extremely irritating. Administer IM or IV and adjust dose according to weight, pain, physical status, and other medication. **EVALUATION:** Evaluate respiratory rate and depth periodically.
buprenorphine (Buprenex) ***Adults and Children over 13 yr:*** 0.3 mg IM, IV (bolus, PCA), epidurally, or intrathecally q 6 hr; maximum dosage is 0.6 mg q 6 hr.	**Onset:** IM, 15 min; IV rapid **Peak:** IM, 60 min; IV, rapid **Duration:** 6 hr **½L:** 2–3 hr **PB:** 96% **B:** liver **E:** urine	Same as for pentazocine.

OPIATE ANTAGONISTS

naloxone hydrochloride (Narcan)		
narcotic-induced respiratory depression ***Adults:*** 0.4–2 mg IV, IM, or SC. May repeat q 2–3 min to a total dose of 10 mg. IV Infusion—0.4 mg IV loading dose, then 0.4 mg/hr. May also be given IM or SC if IV is not available. ***Children:*** 0.01 mg/kg IV; if no response, increase dose to 0.1 mg/kg; may also give IM or SC if IV is not available. ***Neonates:*** 0.01 mg/kg IV into umbilical vein; may repeat q 2–3 min; additional doses may be needed at 1–2 hr intervals. May also give IM or SC if IV is not available. **postoperative respiratory depression** ***Adults:*** 0.1–0.2 mg IV q 2–3 min as needed, or continuous infusion of 0.5 mg/hr. ***Children:*** 0.005–0.01 mg IV; may repeat q 2–3 min. Additional doses may be needed at 2–3 hr intervals (up to 0.1 mg/kg may be required).	**Onset:** IV, 1–2 min; IM and SC, 2–5 min **Peak:** NA **Duration:** IV, IM, and SC, 1–4 hr **½L:** 60–90 min **PB:** 50% **B:** liver **E:** urine	**ASSESSMENT:** Assess respiratory rate, rhythm, and depth; pulse, blood pressure, and level of consciousness frequently until effects of narcotic wear off. The effects of some narcotics may outlast the effects of antagonist and repeat doses may be necessary. Assess patient for signs and symptoms of narcotic withdrawal. Symptoms may occur within a few min to 2 hr. Severity varies. Lack of significant improvement indicates that symptoms are due to other non-narcotic CNS depressants that are not affected by antagonist or due to disease process. Use cautiously in patient with cardiovascular disease. May antagonize postoperative analgesia. Use cautiously in narcotic-dependent patients—may precipitate severe withdrawal. Safety in pregnancy (category B) and lactation has not been established. **INTERVENTION:** May be given as direct IV, undiluted, at a rate of 0.4 mg over 15 sec. Titrate to patient response. For IV infusion, dilute 5% dextrose in water or 0.9% NaCl. The standard dilution varies according to individual hospitals. Mixture is stable for 24 hours; discard unused solution. Incompatible with preparations containing bisulfite and sulfite and solutions with an alkaline pH. **Patient Teaching**—As medication becomes effective, explain purpose and effects of naloxone to patient. **EVALUATION:** Clinical response is demonstrated by adequate ventilation and alertness without significant pain.

NA = not available.

Table 18–7. SEDATION SCALE

S Sleep, easily aroused
1 Awake and alert
2 Occasionally drowsy, easy to arouse
3 Frequently drowsy, arousable, drifts off to sleep during conversation
4 Somnolent, minimal or no response to stimuli

Source: Pasero, C and McCaffery, M: Avoiding opioid-induced respiratory depression. Am J Nurs 94(4):29, 1994, with permission.

headedness may occur because of central brain stimulation. The typical pupillary constriction is caused by stimulation of the oculomotor center. The patient may experience reddened eyes as a result of cerebral vessel dilatation. This dilatation occurs secondary to respiratory depression (increased carbon dioxide and decreased oxygen), which causes cerebral vessels to dilate. As cerebral vessels dilate, intracranial pressure increases and may result in mood changes, confusion, and flushing. Opiate analgesics may interfere with a patient's ability to drive, operate machinery, and use accurate judgment. Subcortical and spinal centers are also depressed, which leads to the suppression of the cough reflex. Opiate analgesics produce some degree of depression of the respiratory center in the medulla. Breathing becomes slowed and shallow, and may even become irregular, as the respiratory center fails to respond adequately to blood carbon dioxide levels.

The opiate analgesics affect the gastrointestinal system in various ways. First, there is decreased peristaltic motility and decreased glandular secretion, which can lead to constipation. Second, there is increased spasticity of sphincters, which can lead to biliary colic.

Table 18–8. COMPARISON OF OPIATE ANALGESICS WITH RESPECT TO DOSAGE, POTENCY, AND DURATION OF ACTION

Analgesic	Usual Adult Therapeutic Dose (mg)	Equizanalgesic Dose (IM)* (mg)	Duration of Action (hr)
morphine	5 (sublingual) 5–15 (IM, SC) 2.5–15 (IV) 10–30 (oral)	10	4–5
codeine	15–60 (oral)	120–130	4–6
oxymorphone (Numorphan)	10 (oral) 1–1.5 (IM)	1–1.5	3–6
hydromorphone (Dilaudid)	1–2 (IV) 2 (IM) 2–3 (oral)	1.3–2	3–4
meperidine (Demerol)	50–150 (IM) 50–150 (oral)	75–100	2–4
methadone (Dolophine)	10–15 (oral) 2.5–10 (IM)	8–10	4–12
levorphanol (Levo-Dromoran)	2–3 (SC, oral)	2–2.3	6–8
fentanyl (Sublimaze)	0.05–0.1 (IM, IV)	0.2	0.5–1
pentazocine (Talwin)	30–50 (IM) 50 (oral)	30	3–5
propoxyphene (Darvon)	30–60 (oral)	32–65	2–4
oxycodone (Percodan) (Percocet)	30 (oral)	10	4–5
nalbuphine (Nubain)	10 (IM, SC, IV)	10	3–6
butorphanol (Stadol)	0.5–2 (IV) 1–4 (IM)	10	3–4
buprenorphine (Buprenex)	0.3 (IV, IM)	0.3	4–5
dezocine (Dalgan)	2.5–10 (IV) 5–20 (IM)	10	3–6

*Compared with morphine.

The effect of the opiate analgesics on the cardiovascular center in the medulla is minimal, although cardiac dysrhythmias can occur. In the periphery, there is vasodilatation, which may lead to postural hypotension, dizziness, weakness, and fainting in ambulatory patients.

An increase in urethral sphincter tone occurs, which contributes to urinary retention in the postoperative patient. The use of narcotic-opiate analgesics in the obstetric patient can prolong labor.

Common signs of narcotic analgesic toxicity include pinpoint pupils, shallow respiration, and coma. Other conditions that mandate caution in administering narcotic analgesics include cardiac dysrhythmias, Addison's disease, and hypothyroidism, because further depression of body systems may occur; increased intracranial pressure, increased cerebrospinal fluid (CSF) pressure, seizures, and head injury, because pressure may be increased, further worsening symptoms; acute abdominal disease, because symptoms may be masked; severe hepatitis and alcoholism, because these drugs are detoxified in the liver; and prostatic hypertrophy and urethral stricture, because urinary function may be further impaired.

Opiate analgesics may lead to drug tolerance, *dependence* (craving for a drug that may or may not be accompanied by a physiologic component), and *addiction* (compulsive need to use a drug, evidence of tolerance, and/or withdrawal). Studies have found few people become addicted. Studies have shown that newborns of mothers regularly taking opiates will become drug dependent. The first sign of tolerance is the patient's report that the analgesic effect is not lasting as long as it had previously. One possible solution is to switch the patient to an alternate opiate. It is also important to use nonpharmacologic approaches to pain relief, such as imagery, relaxation therapy, transcutaneous electrical nerve stimulation (TENS), biofeedback, and distraction.

INTERACTIONS

The opiate analgesics interact with alcohol, antianxiety drugs, phenothiazines, sedative-hypnotics, barbiturates, anesthetics, and monoamine oxidase (MAO) inhibitors to exaggerate or prolong the CNS effects of analgesia. Concurrent use of skeletal muscle relaxants can enhance their neuromuscular blocking action. Smoking may decrease the analgesic effect.

DOSAGE

Dosages of opiate analgesics are not interchangeable from one type of drug to another, nor are dosages of oral and parenteral forms of the same drug. Table 18–8 lists the equianalgesic effects of selected opiate analgesics as compared with the standard, morphine. Note, for instance, that 10 mg of morphine given intramuscularly is equianalgesic to 100 mg of meperidine. Also note that 10 mg of morphine given intramuscularly is comparable in effect to 30 mg of morphine taken orally. Response to narcotics is highly individualized. Not every patient responds favorably to 75 mg of meperidine given intramuscularly every 4 hours as needed for pain. Some adjustment in dosage and timing may be necessary to gain optimum pain relief for each patient.

OPIATE AGONISTS

The opiate agonists include natural opium alkaloids—**morphine** and **methylmorphine (codeine)**; semisynthetic analogs—**hydromorphone (Dilaudid)**, **oxycodone hydrochloride (Percocet, Percodan)**, and **oxymorphone hydrochloride (Numorphan)**; and synthetic compounds—**meperidine (Demerol)**, **methadone hydrochloride (Dolophine)**, **levorphanol tartrate (Levo-Dromoran)**, **propoxyphene (Darvon, Darvocet)**, and the phenylpiperidine compounds, which include **fentanyl (Duragesic)**, **sufentanil (Sufenta)**, and **alfentanil (Alfenta)**. The opiate agonists have their activity at the mu and kappa receptors, the same receptors as endogenous opioid peptides (enkephalins or endorphins). Refer to Table 18–4 for specific drug dosages, pharmacokinetics, and nursing implications.

Opiate Agonists—Natural Alkaloids

○ **Morphine sulfate** (Duramorph, MS Contin, RMS, Oramorph SR, Roxanol, and others) is one of the most widely used and potent of the narcotic analgesics. The routes of administration are intramuscular (IM), subcutaneous (SC), intravenous (IV), oral (PO), rectal, and epidural. Morphine is also being used in a gelatin sponge (Gelform, 10-mm thickness, soaked with 2 to 4 mg preservative-free morphine) that is left in place at the site of a laminectomy. Patients ambulate more quickly, have little or no pain and go home more quickly (Gibbons et al., 1994). Preservative free morphine is used for epidural administration.

○ **Methylmorphine (Codeine)** provides analgesia through intramuscular, subcutaneous, intravenous, and oral routes of administration. There is a ceiling effect to pain relief with codeine. When combined with aspirin or tylenol, codeine exerts an additive effect for pain relief.

Opiate Agonists—Semisynthetic Analogs

○ **Hydromorphone** (Dilaudid) is a semisynthetic derivative of morphine and may cause tolerance, dependence, and addiction. It is 7–10 times more potent than morphine.

○ **Oxycodone hydrochloride** (Percocet, Percodan) is available as a single agent or combined with aspirin and caffeine (Percodan) or acetaminophen (Tylox and Percocet-5) in tablet form. A Percodan-Demi tablet is available for pediatric use. Oxycodone is classified as pregnancy category B.

○ **Oxymorphone hydrochloride** (Numorphan) is similar to morphine in structure and potency. It is 10 times as potent as codeine. Oxymorphone is classified as pregnancy category B.

Opiate Agonists—Synthetic Compounds

❍ **Meperidine** (Demerol) is a synthetic narcotic that is used to relieve pain, as a preoperative and intraoperative medication, and during labor to ease the pain of uterine contractions.

Meperidine is commonly underdosed. The common postoperative order of 75 mg IM every 4 hours as needed is inadequate. Meperidine produces clinical analgesia for only 2.5 to 3.5 hours, and a dose of 75 mg every 4 hours is equivalent to only 5 to 7.5 mg morphine. To produce pain control with morphine requires 10 mg morphine every 4 hours. Therefore, the equivalent analgesic dose is 100 to 150 mg meperidine every 3 hours.

Meperidine is biotransformed in the liver. If respiratory depression occurs within 3 to 4 hours of administration, naloxone hydrochloride (Narcan) is administered. The active, toxic metabolite of meperidine is normeperidine, which circulates for 15 to 20 hours. Normeperidine is a cerebral irritant and may cause agitation, jerky movements, and seizures. Patients with renal insufficiency and the elderly are at the greatest risk, as normeperidine is excreted by the kidney. Naloxone hydrochloride will not reverse these symptoms and may in fact worsen them. The best way to prevent the accumulation of normeperidine is to use meperidine for only 48 hours.

INTERACTIONS Solutions of meperidine and barbiturates are chemically incompatible and should not be mixed in the same syringe. Meperidine should not be used together with, or within 14 days after therapy with, MAO inhibitors because the combination may be lethal. Other interactions are similar to those of all opiate analgesics.

❍ **Methadone hydrochloride** (Dolophine) is a synthetic opiate that resembles morphine and is used to relieve pain in the terminally ill, and to maintain the person attempting to overcome addiction. Because methadone has a different method of metabolism in the body than morphine, it is often administered to patients with chronic, severe cancer pain who no longer respond to morphine. Methadone is very effective after an oral administration and has a long duration of action. It is classified as pregnancy category B.

❍ **Levorphanol tartrate** (Levo-Dromoran) is a derivative of morphine.

❍ **Propoxyphene hydrochloride** (Darvon) and **propoxyphene napsylate** (Darvon-N) are synthetic narcotics used alone or in combination with other drugs to relieve pain. These agents are Schedule IV narcotics used for chronic pain. Propoxyphene is usually not effective for single or acute dosing, but may be effective with chronic dosing. These drugs are classified as pregnancy category C.

CONTRAINDICATIONS AND PRECAUTIONS Propoxyphene is contraindicated in those with hypersensitivity and in children. Combination products containing aspirin (Darvon Compound-65) are contraindicated in patients with hypersensitivity to aspirin or caffeine. Propoxyphene may produce drug dependence when taken in higher than recommended dosages.

▼ **CLINICAL ALERT**

Propoxyphene products, alone or in combination with other CNS depressants (e.g., alcohol), are a major cause of drug-related deaths.

Propoxyphene is not prescribed for the suicidal or addiction-prone patient. It is given with caution to those taking tranquilizers or antidepressants and for alcohol abusers. The drug may impair the patient's ability to drive or operate machinery.

ADVERSE EFFECTS Less than 1% of patients experience side effects. Adverse effects that do occur are similar to those of other opiate analgesics. Propoxyphene napsylate has a lower incidence of gastrointestinal side effects than propoxyphene hydrochloride.

Phenylpiperidine Compounds

These synthetic opiates include rapid-onset, short-acting, and highly potent agents such as fentanyl (Duragesic), sufentanil (Sufenta), and alfentanil (Alfenta) (meperidine is also a phenylpiperdine compound). Fentanyl is approximately 80 times more potent than morphine. Sufentanil is related to fentanyl and is seven times more potent than fentanyl. Alfentanil, an analog of fentanyl, has one-fourth the potency of fentanyl. These products are lipophilic, that is, they readily dissolve in fatty tissue. Lipophilic drugs penetrate fatty membranes better than hydrophilic products such as morphine and cross the blood-brain barrier more readily. Less than 1% of morphine enters the CNS. These phenylpiperidine compounds have a much shorter time to onset and peak and a shorter duration of action than morphine.

The phenylpiperidine compounds are used in the induction and maintenance of regional, and spinal anesthesia. Recently, these agents have been used to treat a variety of postoperative pain with systemic devices (i.e., patient-controlled analgesia). These drugs can be administered alone or in combination with other agents (e.g., droperidol, benzodiazepine). They are classified as pregnancy category B. Refer to Table 18–5 for additional drug information.

When fentanyl is administered alone, it has a short plasma half-life (20 minutes), and an intravenous dose can be titrated to counter the patient's perception of pain. This is an advantage over morphine or meperidine.

Adverse Reactions Adverse reactions are similar to those for morphine. Fentanyl is known to cause muscle rigidity and apnea and more nausea and vomiting than morphine (particularly with the transdermal patch).

Interactions The interactions are similar to those of morphine. See Chapter 21 on general anesthesia for an in-depth discussion of these agents.

❍ **Fentanyl transdermal** (Duragesic) is primarily used in patients with chronic, severe pain requiring extended management. The patch is *not* to be used in acute or postoperative pain control, in mild or intermediate chronic pain control, in starting doses higher than 25 μg/hr, or in children. The skin acts as both a barrier and a reservoir, causing the drug to be slowly absorbed and released. This produces a relatively constant blood concentration over a long period, so the pharmacokinetics differ among patch, IV, epidural, or intrathecal routes.

Available patches release 25, 50, 75, or 100 μg/hr. Serum concentration takes 12 to 24 hours to build up, with maximal concentration reached in 24 to 78 hours. Patches are worn on a flat body surface for up to 72 hours. The site is washed with water only; if there is excessive hair, it is clipped, not shaved. If the skin is abraded, the drug is absorbed more rapidly. Heating pads are never used near or over the patch. When the patch is removed, the elimination half-life depends on the length of time the patch was worn: 8 hours for a patch worn 24 hours and up to 22 hours for a patch worn 72 hours or longer. After removal, patches are folded in half and flushed down the toilet. Any residual drug is a hazard to pets and children.

○ **Fentanyl, parenteral** (Sublimaze) is an excellent choice for continuous IV or patient-controlled analgesia administration because it lacks the associated histamine release. Single bolus doses can be used for procedures such as insertion or removal of chest tubes or changing burn dressings.

○ **Fentanyl-Bupivacaine** is a combination of fentanyl with the anesthetic agent bupivacaine for epidural or intrathecal administration. The pharmacy mixes a solution of fentanyl and bupivacaine, with the dose dependent on the patient and the type of pain. Adding bupivacaine lessens the amount of fentanyl needed for effective analgesia. When the rate of this combination is increased, it must be titrated carefully as increasing the amount of fentanyl also increases the bupivacaine, which increases the chance of sympathetic blockade.

To assess for motor blockade, ask if the patient can feel you touching his or her toes, feet, legs. Motor blockade is evident if the patient says the legs feel heavy or he or she has difficulty lifting them. Call the physician if motor blockade occurs.

OPIATE AGONIST-ANTAGONISTS

Opiate agonist-antagonists (partial agonists) are valuable in a wide variety of situations because of their combined agonist and antagonist action. Drugs in this class include **pentazocine *(Talwin)*, nalbuphine hydrochloride *(Nubain)*, butorphanol *(Stadol)*, dezocine *(Dalgan)*,** and **buprenorphine *(Buprenex)*.** Refer to Table 18–6 for specific drug dosages, pharmacokinetics, and nursing implications for all these drugs.

Action

The agonist-antagonists are believed to combine opiate receptors in the brain, producing generalized CNS depression and altering the perception of and response to pain. These drugs have an affinity for mu and possibly kappa opiate receptors. The significance of these agents is their antagonistic property, which reduces their abuse potential. If the agonist-antagonists are used by a person addicted to potent narcotic analgesics, the antagonistic property causes a withdrawal effect. Opiate agonist-antagonists are useful for relief of moderate to severe pain.

Contraindications and Precautions

Opiate agonist-antagonists are used cautiously in patients with known hypersensitivity or in those with cardiovascular and pulmonary conditions because these drugs can increase pulmonary artery pressure and systemic vascular resistance. These agents can also worsen intracranial pressure associated with head injury. The drugs are used cautiously in patients who have impaired hepatic or renal function and in patients with a history of depression or other emotional instability. Safety in pregnancy (category B or C), lactation, and children has not been established.

Adverse Effects

Adverse effects of the opiate agonist-antagonists are similar to those of morphine sulfate and other opiate agonists.

○ **Pentazocine** (Talwin, Talwin-Nx) is a synthetic narcotic agonist-antagonist that is available in oral form (Talwin-Nx) and for parenteral use (Talwin). It has relatively weak antagonistic activity. Talwin-Nx combines pentazocine hydrochloride with naloxone (an opiate antagonist) to prevent its abuse. Pentazocine does cause a high rate of psychominetic side effects.

▼ CLINICAL ALERT

Talwin-Nx is intended for oral use only. When ingested orally, the naloxone is rapidly metabolized by the liver. However, if the tablet is used to prepare an injection, the naloxone produces potentially life-threatening withdrawal effects in persons dependent on opiates.

Pentazocine is also available in combination with aspirin (Talwin Compound) or acetaminophen (Talacen) when an antipyretic as well as anti-inflammatory effect is desired.

CONTRAINDICATIONS AND PRECAUTIONS Pentazocine has the same contraindications as the other opiate agonist-antagonists. Pentazocine is administered cautiously to patients with recent myocardial infarction and heart failure because it elevates systemic vascular resistance, pulmonary artery pressure, and left ventricular end-diastolic pressure, increasing the workload of the heart.

INTERACTIONS The effects of pentazocine are additive with those of other CNS depressants (including alcohol), general anesthetics, phenothiazines, and sedative-hypnotics.

○ **Nalbuphine hydrochloride** (Nubain) is a synthetic opiate agonist-antagonist analgesic. It is a very potent drug that has an analgesic effect equivalent to that of morphine. Nalbuphine does not have a significant effect on cardiac workload.

○ **Butorphanol** (Stadol) is a potent synthetic opiate agonist-antagonist analgesic that is 3.5 to 7 times more potent than morphine sulfate. Its potential for addiction is similar to other opiate agonist-antagonists. Butorphanol does increase the workload of the heart.

○ **Dezocine** (Dalgan) is a potent opiate agonist-antagonist that relieves pain as effectively as morphine. It may be better tolerated than other opiate agonist-antagonists. It is not classified as a controlled substance.

○ **Buprenorphine** (Buprenex) is a semisynthetic opiate partial agonist that is 30 times as potent as morphine sulfate. Buprenorphine has a low potential for abuse and is classified as a Schedule V controlled substance.

OPIATE ANTAGONISTS

The *opiate antagonists* are used to reverse narcotic-induced CNS and respiratory depression. These drugs precipitate withdrawal in persons physically dependent on opiates. They are largely metabolized in the liver and are excreted in the urine. Drugs in this class include **naloxone hydrochloride (Narcan)** and **nalmefene hydrochloride (Revex)**.

Correct administration of opiate antagonists reverses the sedative and respiratory effects of opiate analgesics, but not the analgesia. Observe the patient closely while administering these drugs. The reversal of sedation should occur within 1 to 2 minutes and the patient should be able to open his or her eyes and to talk. When the patient is awake, the dose is stopped. However, because of the short duration of action, a repeat dose may be necessary in 30 to 60 minutes.

○ **Naloxone hydrochloride** (Narcan) is used in adults, children, and neonates. It may be used to counteract adverse effects of epidural morphine sulfate administration. Refer to Table 18–6 for drug dosages, pharmacokinetics, and nursing implications.

CONTRAINDICATIONS AND PRECAUTIONS Naloxone hydrochloride is contraindicated in patients with known hypersensitivity. It is used with caution in patients with cardiac irritability because tachycardia and circulatory depression may occur and in patients with pulmonary edemas because respiratory depression may occur. Naloxone hydrochloride is ineffective in cases of non-narcotic respiratory depression.

ADVERSE EFFECTS Naloxone hydrochloride has few adverse effects, unless the patient is receiving narcotics. In those who are receiving narcotics, naloxone hydrochloride can precipitate withdrawal symptoms and cause reversal of analgesia. Withdrawal symptoms may occur in newborns of addicted mothers as well as in addicts themselves. No drug interactions are known at this time.

○ **Nalmefene hydrochloride** (Revex) is an analog of naltrexone with a longer duration of action at fully reversing doses. It has no pharmacologic activity when administered in the absence of opiate agonists. As with other opioid antagonists, nalmefene can produce acute withdrawal symptoms in opioid-dependent persons. Nalmefene is administered primarily as an IV bolus, but can be given intramuscularly or subcutaneously if venous access cannot be established. Safety in pregnancy (category B), lactation, and children has not been established. Contraindications, precautions, and adverse reactions are similar to those of naloxone. Nalmefene may not completely reverse buprenorphine-induced respiratory depression.

INTERACTIONS With coadministration of flumazenil and nalmefene, there is a potential risk of seizures.

ANTIMIGRAINE AGENTS

Agents prescribed to abort or prevent vascular headaches such as migraine or migraine variant and cluster headache (histaminic cephalalgia) include the ergot alkaloids and the serotonin receptor agonist sumatriptan.

ERGOT ALKALOIDS

The ergot alkaloids—**ergotamine tartrate (Ergomar)**, **ergotamine with caffeine (Cafergot)**, **dihydroergotamine mesylate (D.H.E. 45)**, and **methysergide maleate (Sansert)**—are derived from a fungus grown on rye. Besides being alpha-adrenergic blockers that reduce extracranial blood flow, the ergot derivatives constrict the vascular smooth muscle of the uterus. The gravid uterus is more sensitive to these effects. Specific drug dosages, pharmacokinetics, and nursing implications are provided in Table 18–9.

Contraindications and Precautions

The ergot alkaloids are contraindicated in known hypersensitivity, sepsis, vascular disease, hepatic or renal disease, marked atherosclerosis, hypertension, and anemia because all of these conditions may be worsened. These agents are contraindicated in pregnancy (category X) because it is a powerful uterine stimulant and may cause fetal harm. These drugs are administered cautiously to lactating women, elderly patients, and children.

Adverse Effects

The most common side effect is *ergotism*. Early signs of ergotism include nausea, vomiting, and complaints of abdominal cramps. Sometimes the patient may have a headache and show signs of confusion. More serious signs are circulatory stasis, including itching, tingling, numbness, and coldness in the fingers and toes. This can lead to gangrene of the nose, digits, and ears. Patients may also experience seizures; rapid, weak, or irregular pulse; and confusion. Patients are encouraged to report these symptoms, and the medication is discontinued.

Interactions

An interaction occurs between ergotamine tartrate and nitroglycerin, increasing the availability of ergot products and decreasing the effectiveness of nitrates. When beta blockers and macrolide antibiotics are used concurrently, the likelihood of peripheral ischema increases. Concurrent use of vasodilators increases the pressor effect and may cause dangerous hypertension.

○ **Ergotamine tartrate** (Ergostat) is a natural amino acid alkaloid of ergot that has alpha-adrenergic blocking properties. It is used primarily in the acute treatment of vascular headaches, including migraines and cluster headaches with a clear-cut prodrome (a symptom indic-

Table 18–9. ANTIMIGRAINE AGENTS

DRUG NAME/ROUTE AND DOSAGE	PHARMACOKINETICS/ DYNAMICS	NURSING IMPLICATIONS
ERGOT ALKALOIDS		
ergotamine tartrate (Ergostat) (Medihaler Ergotamine)		
Adults: 2 mg sublingual at onset, repeated q 30 min, for a total of no more than 3 tablets/day or 5 tablets/wk; or 2 mg PO, then 1–2 mg q 30 min until attack subsides or a total of 6 mg has been given; or 1 inhalation (0.36 mg/dose) from Medihaler, repeated in 5 min, for a total of 6 inhalations in 24 hr or 15 inhalations/wk	**Onset:** PO, 1–2 hr **Peak:** PO, 1–5 hr **Duration:** NA $\frac{1}{2}$**L:** α 2.7 hr, β 21 hr **PB:** NA **B:** liver **E:** urine (trace)	**ASSESSMENT:** Assess for known hypersensitivity, vascular disease, hepatic or renal impairment, and pregnancy (all contraindications). **INTERVENTION:** Drug therapy is begun as soon as possible after onset of headache. Patient should lie down in dark, quiet room for 2–3 hr after taking drug. Do not increase dose without consulting physician. Do not administer more than specifically ordered. Monitor for ergotism: mild—nausea, vomiting, abdominal cramps, headache, signs of confusion; severe—tingling, numbness, cold extremities, rapid, irregular pulse, confusion. Report to physician at once. **EVALUATION:** Notify physician of irregular heartbeat, tingling and numbness in fingers and toes, or pain and weakness of extremities.
ergotamine with caffeine (Cafergot)		
Adults: 1–2 PO tablets at onset, repeated at 30 min, for a total of 6 tablets/24 hr not to exceed 10 tablets/wk. Suppository—2 mg rectally at onset of headache	Same as for ergotamine tartrate	Same as for ergotamine tartrate.
methysergide maleate (Sansert)		
Adults: 4–8 mg PO daily in divided doses	**Onset:** 1–2 days **Peak:** NA **Duration:** 1–2 days $\frac{1}{2}$**L:** 10 hr **PB:** NA **B:** liver **E:** urine	**ASSESSMENT:** Assess for heart and blood vessel disease, impaired liver and kidney function, and serious infection (all contraindications). Assess frequently for edema. Assess for pregnancy (category X) **INTERVENTION:** Position changes should be made slowly. Drug is withdrawn slowly to prevent headache rebound. There must be a drug-free interval for 3–4 wk every 6 mo. **Patient Teaching**—Instruct patient to take medication with meals and to use caution when operating heavy equipment. Teach patient about likelihood of insomnia, drowsiness, dizziness, ataxia. **EVALUATION:** Evaluate for peripheral circulation, paresthesia, and edema. If these occur, report to physician.
SELECTIVE SEROTONIN AGONIST		
sumatriptan succinate (Imitrex)		
Adults: 6 mg SC with one additional dose after a minimum of 1 hr (maximum dose in 24 hr is 2 injections); or 25–100 mg PO taken with fluids, repeated q 2 hr to a maximum of 300 mg/24 hr	**Onset:** SC, 30 min; PO, 60–90 min **Peak:** SC, 1–2 hr; PO, 2–4 hr **Duration:** up to 24 hr $\frac{1}{2}$**L:** 15 min (distribution); 115 min (terminal) **PB:** 14%–21% **B:** liver **E:** urine, feces	**ASSESSMENT:** Assess for underlying ischemic heart disease and Prinzmetal's angina (both contraindications). Do not administer to patients with basilar or hemiplegic migraine. Assess for hepatic and renal impairment (cautions). Assess for pregnancy (category C). **INTERVENTION:** Teach patient how to give injections. An autoinjection device is available to facilitate self-injection. If the first dose is ineffective, the efficacy of a second dose is questionable. Administer as soon as symptoms of headache appear. Do not take drug if pregnant or nursing. Redness at injection site usually disappears within 1 hr. Administer oral sumatriptan only to patients who have a diagnosis of migraine. **EVALUATION:** Monitor for side effects such as chest tightness, tachycardia/bradycardia, hypertension/hypotension. Report skin rash, hives, heart throbbing, or swelling face and eyelids to physician immediately.

NA = not available.

ative of an approaching disease). It is available in oral or sublingual tablets and as an aerosol inhaler.

○ **Ergotamine with caffeine** (Cafergot) contains 1 mg of ergotamine tartrate and 100 mg of caffeine in each tablet. The caffeine, as a cerebral vasoconstrictor, probably increases the effectiveness of the ergotamine.

○ **Dihydroergotamine mesylate** (D.H.E. 45) is a hydrogenated ergotamine derivative that has a direct constricting effect on smooth muscle of peripheral and cranial blood vessels. Administered intramuscularly or intravenously, it is used to prevent or relieve vascular headaches.

○ **Methysergide maleate** (Sansert) is an semisynthetic ergot derivative, but unlike ergotamine it has weak vasoconstrictor and oxytocic actions. It inhibits or blocks the effects of serotonin (a potent vasoconstrictor), which may be implicated in the mechanism of vascular headaches. Methysergide is not useful in treating acute migraine attacks, only in prophylaxis.

▼ **CLINICAL ALERT**

Methysergide is reserved for patients whose vascular headaches are severe or frequent and/or uncontrollable because pulmonary fibrosis and fibrotic thickening of cardiac valves may occur in patients receiving long-term therapy.

ADVERSE EFFECTS Methysergide has many severe adverse effects, including fibrosis of the retroperitoneal area (causing fatigue, flank pain, dysuria, increased blood urea nitrogen), chest pain, and tachycardia. To prevent these complications, the drug is usually stopped for 4 weeks every 6 months. When the medication is stopped, the dosage is titrated down slowly to prevent a rebound of migraine or cluster headaches. Other adverse effects include coldness and numbness in the fingers and toes, gastrointestinal complaints, flushing, and insomnia.

SELECTIVE SEROTONIN AGONIST

○ **Sumatriptan succinate** *(Imitrex)* is a selective agonist for a vascular serotonin receptor subtype—5-hydroxytryptamine$_1$, probably 5-HT$_1$ D. The 5-HT$_1$ D receptor subtype is present on the basilar artery and in the vasculture of the dura mater. Sumatriptan activates the receptors in these tissues, causing vasoconstriction, which correlates with the relief of migraines in some patients.

Sumatriptan succinate is available as a subcutaneous (SC) injection or an oral tablet. The SC injection may be administered in two doses at least 1 hour apart to treat migraine with or without an aura. If the patient is not helped by the first dose, the added efficacy of a second dose is only 5%. Sumatriptan has also been used to treat cluster headaches, although safety and efficacy for this indication have not been established. Sumatriptan may also relieve the *photophobia* (abnormal intolerance to light), phonophobia (sound sensitivity), and nausea and vomiting that are associated with migraine attacks. Onset of relief from migraine pain with SC sumatriptan occurs within 10 minutes of a single 6-mg dose in most patients;

and with oral sumatriptan, within 60 to 90 minutes of a single 25-, 50-, or 100-mg dose.

CONTRAINDICATIONS AND PRECAUTIONS Sumatriptan succinate is contraindicated in patients with ischemic heart disease, Prinzmetal's angina, or uncontrolled hypertension because of its ability to cause a small increase in heart rate and transient increases in both systolic and diastolic pressure. It is also contraindicated in patients with hypersensitivity or hemiplegic or basilar migraine and in those taking ergot-containing agents or MAO inhibitors. Sumatriptan should not be administered intravenously because of its potential to cause coronary vasospasm.

Sumatriptan succinate is given cautiously to patients with kidney or liver impairment, as these are the organs of elimination/biotransformation. In addition, in patients with liver disease, the bioavailability of oral sumatriptan in markedly increased, leading to possible toxicity. Use in pregnancy (category C) and lactation only if clearly indicated. Safety and efficacy in children have not been established.

ADVERSE EFFECTS Patients may experience cardiovascular adverse effects such as hypertension, hypotension, bradycardia, tachycardia, palpitations, and transient ECG changes (nonspecific ST- or T-wave changes, prolonged PR or QT intervals, ectopic beats). Patients may experience chest discomfort that is similar to angina, even if ischemic heart disease is not present. In addition, patients often experience pain and redness at the injection site and flushing and discomfort of the mouth and tongue. Other adverse effects include mental confusion, euphoria, agitation, facial pain, sleep disturbance, simultaneous hot and cold sensations, dysarthria, and dystonia. Adverse effects from oral sumatriptan are generally milder than those from SC sumatriptan.

INTERACTIONS Concurrent ergotamine or other ergot derivatives may result in prolonged vasospastic effects from sumatriptan. It is recommended that 24 hours separate the administration of ergot-containing drugs and sumatriptan. MAO inhibitors can affect the elimination of sumatriptan, increasing its half-life. Do not use sumatriptan within 14 days of MAO inhibitor therapy.

ANALGESIC THERAPY

SELECTION OF AN ANALGESIC

Because each patient perceives and responds to pain differently and the analgesic effects of pain medications vary for each patient as well, it is often difficult to pharmacologically manage pain effectively. The controversies surrounding the administration of opioids include the following: choice of opiate analgesic, method of drug administration, route of drug administration, development of tolerance, and risk of substance abuse and addiction. Selection of an appropriate analgesic depends on several factors, including the nature of the pain (i.e., acute or chronic), the patient's age and general health, and the disease process causing the pain.

Severe pain of short duration (e.g., from surgery or trauma) is generally managed initially with nonsteroidal anti-inflammatory drugs (NSAIDs) and parenteral opiate analgesics, followed by oral opiate analgesics, and finally acetaminophen or aspirin compounds as pain lessens with recovery.

▼ CLINICAL ALERT

Use of a nonsteroidal anti-inflammatory drug with an opiate analgesic may lessen pain to such an extent that the dosage of the opiate can be reduced.

Pain associated with biliary spasm or pancreatic disease responds best to an opiate agonist-antagonist because these agents do not produce additional spasm, as is frequently experienced with morphine and codeine and, to a lesser extent, meperidine.

Chronic pain (e.g., from arthritis or low back pain) responds well to nonsteroidal anti-inflammatory drugs, aspirin, or acetaminophen. Less commonly, opiate analgesics are used with this type of pain.

The progressive pain of cancer is best managed with a step approach. Initially, a nonsteroidal analgesic and aspirin or acetaminophen may be used to act at peripheral nerve endings. As pain becomes more severe, the addition of a mild opiate analgesic such as codeine may be added. As the disease process increases the intensity of the pain, potent opiates such as morphine are needed. The use of heroin to relieve the most severe, unrelenting forms of cancer pain is receiving very favorable response from many researchers.

METHODS OF DRUG ADMINISTRATION

One major issue related to method of administration is the use of a fixed or an as needed (PRN) schedule. When a fixed schedule is used, the patient experiences continuous pain relief and the pain is kept from resurfacing.

This approach can be dangerous in the patient who has had no previous narcotic exposure. Repeated doses of long-acting opiate analgesics can lead to drug accumulation and side effects. In the PRN approach, the drug is administered when there is recurrence of pain. This seems to work well for patients with chronic pain, although not for those with chronic acute pain (e.g., pain occurring during exacerbation of a chronic illness such as pancreatitis). One disadvantage is that the patient may experience a delay in receiving the medication. The most appropriate means of administration is individualization of timing. If patients are not receiving relief from their pain, then the nursing assessment becomes a critical intervention.

Patient-Controlled Analgesia

In patient-controlled analgesia (PCA) therapy, illustrated in Figure 18–2, the patient self-administers analgesic medications as needed. This system consists of an infusion pump that is electronically controlled and connected to a timing device. When a patient experiences pain, he or she (or family member for a child) presses a thumb button located on the end of a cord extending from the pump. The pump releases the preset amount of analgesia through the patient's indwelling intravenous catheter. The timer is programmed to lock out supplemental doses until the first dose has had time to reach its peak pharmacologic effect. The loading dose, lockout interval, dose volume, and maximum volume allowed are prescribed by the physician. A wide variety of analgesic drugs— morphine, meperidine, fentanyl, hydromorphone, methadone, oxymorphone, sufentanil, buprenorphine, nalbuphine, and pentazocine—are used in PCA therapy. See Table 18–10 for common bolus doses. Patients have an opportunity to actively participate in their care and as a result exhibit decreased anxiety. Patients control their own care by being able to minimize the time interval between the perception of pain and the administration of the analgesic.

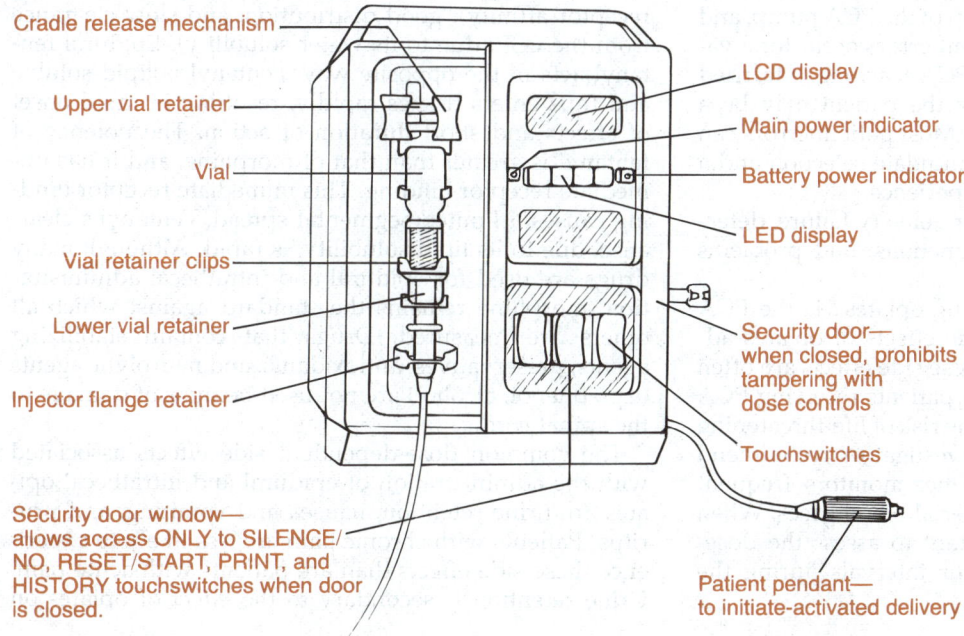

Cradle release mechanism

Upper vial retainer

Vial

Vial retainer clips

Lower vial retainer

Injector flange retainer

Security door window— allows access ONLY to SILENCE/ NO, RESET/START, PRINT, and HISTORY touchswitches when door is closed.

LCD display

Main power indicator

Battery power indicator

LED display

Security door— when closed, prohibits tampering with dose controls

Touchswitches

Patient pendant— to initiate-activated delivery

Figure 18–2. Patient-controlled analgesia pump. (From Brunner and Suddarth's Textbook of Medical Surgical Nursing, ed 7. JB Lippincott, Philadelphia, 1992, with permission.)

Table 18–10. COMMON BOLUS DOSES FOR PCA THERAPY

Drug	Bolus Dose (mg)	Lockout Interval (min)
Buprenorphine hydrochloride (A-A)	0.03–0.2	10–20
Fentanyl citrate (A-A)	0.02–0.1	3–10
Hydromorphone hydrochloride (A)	0.1–0.5	5–15
Meperidine hydrochloride (A)	5–30	5–15
Methadone hydrochloride (A)	0.5–3	10–20
Morphine sulfate (A)	0.5–3	5–20
Nalbuphine hydrochloride (A-A)	1–5	5–15
Oxymorphone hydrochloride (A)	0.2–0.8	5–15
Pentazocine hydrochloride (A-A)	5–30	5–15
Sufentanil citrate (A)	0.003–0.015	3–10

A-A = agonist-antagonist; A = agonist.

Research indicates that patients using PCA therapy require less narcotic; experience less sedation, fewer pulmonary complications, and less postoperative fever; and increase their postoperative physical activity. When patients experience less pain and sedation, they are able to move around in bed and ambulate more easily.

Problems encountered with PCA fall into three areas: operator errors, patient errors, and mechanical errors. Operator errors, very common in clinical practice, consist of misprogramming the PCA device, improper loading of syringe/cartridge, failure to clamp/unclamp tubing, inability to respond to safety alarms, and misplacement of the PCA pump key. It is critical for the nursing staff to understand the concept of PCA therapy and how the system works.

Patient errors include failure to understand PCA therapy, confusion about the operation of the PCA pump, and intentional analgesia abuse. Patient errors occur for a variety of reasons, such as lack of PCA teaching, a hurried teaching/learning experience, or the patient may be a poor candidate for PCA therapy. Most patient errors can be overcome with appropriate candidate selection and a nonhurried teaching/learning experience.

Mechanical errors include drug delivery failure, defective one-way valves, lock malfunctions, and problems with the alarms.

The side effects of administering opiates via the PCA pump are similar to the systemic effects of opiates administered by other methods. These side effects are often dose-related and reported less in patients receiving PCA therapy. However, to minimize the risk of life-threatening respiratory depression, many investigators recommend the use of precautions such as apnea monitors, frequent respiratory assessment, serial arterial blood gases. When using PCA therapy, it is important to assess the dose-effect relationship at 1- to 3-hour intervals during the early postoperative period.

Continuous Intravenous Infusion

Opiate analgesics may also be administered by continuous intravenous infusion. The same opiate analgesics used in PCA therapy are also used with this method. An advantage of continuous intravenous infusion of opiate analgesics is better control of the pain because of a continuous infusion of the opiate. However, with this type of delivery system, more nursing care is required for monitoring the patient. Continuous intravenous infusion of opioid drugs such as morphine and fentanyl is being used increasingly for postoperative and chronic cancer pain.

Epidural and Intrathecal Analgesia

Epidural and intrathecal analgesia, shown in Figure 18–3, are being used increasingly in the management of acute and chronic pain. *Epidural analgesia* is the administration of an analgesic drug directly onto, but not into, the outer membrane of the spinal cord. *Intrathecal analgesia* is the injection of an analgesic drug directly into the cerebrospinal fluid (CSF) in the subarachnoid space. Properly managed, both of these types of analgesic administration offer dependable, long-acting, site-specific pain relief with lower doses of analgesics.

When the epidural or intrathecal routes are used, the pharmacologic aspects of the opiates must be considered. Important pharmacologic characteristics include lipid solubility, molecular weight and volume, specific receptor affinities (which influence opiate spread), and rate of opiate clearance from the central nervous system. Knowledge of these characteristics enables the nurse to monitor the clinical effects of the opiates. It is important to predict the onset, duration of action, analgesic potency, CSF distribution, and clearance of the opiate because all of these factors determine clinical outcomes. The following examples illustrate how differences in physical properties of the drug change clinical effects. Epidural morphine is more water soluble, demonstrating a slow onset of action (takes time to diffuse through the lipid neural membranes), a long duration of action, a high potency (strong receptor affinity), good distribution, and slow clearance from the CSF (due to its water solubility). Epidural fentanyl acts in the opposite way. Fentanyl is lipid soluble and thus enters tissues rapidly, resulting in rapid onset of effects and short duration of action. The potency of fentanyl is greater than that of morphine, and it has immediate receptor binding. This immediate receptor binding causes a limited segmental spread. Fentanyl's clearance, due to its lipid solubility, is rapid. Although many drugs are used for epidural and intrathecal administration, morphine remains the standard against which all others are measured. Drugs that contain stabilizing agents, preservatives, antioxidants, and neurolytic agents (e.g., phenol, alcohol) are not used because of damage to the spinal cord.

The common dose-dependent side effects associated with the administration of epidural and intrathecal opiates are urine retention, nausea and vomiting, and pruritus. Patients with chronic pain are less likely to experience these side effects than are patients with acute pain. Urine retention is secondary to the effect of opiates on

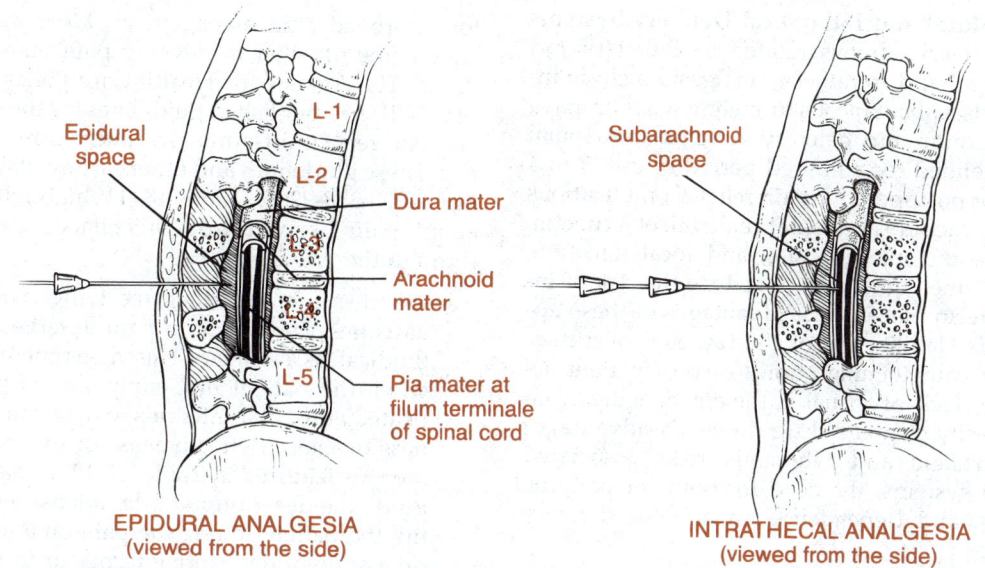

Figure 18–3. How epidural and intrathecal analgesia are administered. Epidural analgesia (also called epidural block) is administered by inserting a spinal needle between the thoracic or lumbar verebrae (the position is dependent on the location of the pain). The client is positioned in the flexed lateral position with the back arched and the chin tucked to the chest.

For epidural analgesia, the needle is inserted to the surface of the dura mater, and a pain-blocking agent is injected—sometimes through an indwelling catheter—into the epidural space. For intrathecal analgesia, a large spinal needle is inserted to the surface of the dura mater, and a second, smaller needle is passed through the first to penetrate the dura mater and arachnoid mater. A pain-blocking agent is injected—sometimes through an indwelling catheter—directly into the cerebrospinal fluid in the subarachnoid space. (From Ignatavicius and Bayne, Medical-Surgical Nursing: A Nursing Process Approach. WB Saunders, Philadelphia, 1991, with permission.)

spinal nerves innervating the bladder and the influence of opiate-mediated ADH release, causing oliguria. Nausea and vomiting are the result of the stimulation of the vomiting center in the medulla and the spinal suppression of visceral inhibitory fibers that act to suppress the vomiting center. Pruritus may be related to histamine release, cephalad spread of opiates, and/or disturbances in cutaneous sensation due to opiate receptor binding. Respiratory depression is an unusual but potentially lethal complication and may be identified by frequent respiratory assessment. This problem occurs early or late following administration of the opiate and may be dose-related. The early development of respiratory depression is related to plasma uptake, drug shunting via epidural circulation, or changes in CSF bulk flow. A late onset of respiratory depression (up to 12 hours after administration) is due to opiate penetration and distribution in the CSF and movement of the opiate via the CSF to the receptors in the medulla. These side effects can be reduced by the use of antiemetics, antipruritics, and small doses of naloxone or naloxone infusions, without reversing analgesia. As with PCA therapy, precautions (e.g., apnea monitors and serial arterial blood gas analysis) minimize the risk of respiratory depression.

The other complications associated with epidural and intrathecal therapy are technique-related. These include catheter malposition, catheter malfunction, and infection. Catheters can migrate from the epidural space into the subarachnoid space or from the epidural space into the vascular system. Or, the catheter may come into contact with neural tissues (e.g., nerve roots) or compress the spinal cord. As part of assessment, it is important for the nurse to recognize the signs and symptoms of dural puncture (e.g., aspiration of CSF; wet catheter dressing; patient complaining of a continuous, throbbing, occipital headache) and intravascular placement (e.g., aspiration of blood from the catheter; the patient experiences sudden nausea and vomiting, hypotension, and respiratory depression after administration of epidural opiates). The nurse is also alert to signs and symptoms of paresthesia, motor weakness, paralysis, and bowel/bladder dysfunction, which indicate compression of nerve tissue from the catheter. If these problems arise, the physician is notified.

Catheter malfunction occurs as a result of catheter kinking, knotting, compression, slippage, or shearing. Indications of catheter malfunction include patient difficulty in administering the opiate and reports of poor pain relief. Medication is never forced through the epidural/intrathecal catheter. If difficulty occurs, the patient is repositioned with the spine slightly flexed. This flexion of the spine increases the intervertebral spaces and frees the catheter if it is compressed. If problems with administration remain after the patient has been repositioned, the physician is notified. When the epidural catheter is removed, the nurse checks it to make sure that it is intact and that the holes are not occluded. In many hospitals, removing an epidural catheter is a nursing function, but removing an intrathecal catheter is not. If part of the catheter is missing, the physician is notified. Surgery may be required to retrieve the missing part of the catheter.

Types of Epidural and Intrathecal Delivery Systems
Examples of delivery options related to catheters and pumps in epidural and intrathecal analgesia include intraspinal conduits, subcutaneous tunneling (i.e., Ommaya reservoir), and continuous delivery systems. Intraspinal conduits are intended for a limited period of use (3 to 4 days), such as for postoperative pain relief. Complications with this system include accidental removal, obstruction, kinking, pain at the injection site, and local infection. Subcutaneous tunneling is used to reduce the risk of infection of long-term placement. Advantages of these approaches include stabilization of the catheter (decreases the potential of catheter migration), ease of patient access to the site, lack of visual catheters hanging from the skin, and easily changed drug doses. Disadvantages include hemorrhagic and infectious risks associated with implanted systems, the need for bolus or periodic reservoir refills, and dependence on a bolus delivery mode.

A continuous implantable infusion pump, similar to the insulin delivery device, is approved for morphine delivery. The pump is placed in a subcutaneous pocket and anchored. The pump's catheter is then connected to a tunneled intrathecal or epidural catheter.

USING THE NURSING PROCESS

ASSESSMENT

- Every nurse has an obligation and is qualified to actively assess pain, document pain, and evaluate the effectiveness of treatment. Pain can be experienced by many patients, especially after surgery, trauma, or delivery or with cancer. Research indicates that as many as 42% of patients receive no analgesia the day of surgery and that oral analgesics are given infrequently (Maxam-Moore et al., 1994). Pain is a major complaint for about 50% of cancer patients who are in active stages of the disease and are still receiving chemotherapy, radiation, or other therapies. Unrelieved pain takes its toll in physical and physiologic consequences: reluctance to cough, to breathe deeply, and to move and ambulate. Immobility can lead to complications such as pneumonia, thrombophlebitis, or ileus.

The elderly patient may be more likely to have cognitive impairment from unrelieved pain rather than as a side effect of medication to control pain (Duggleby and Lander, 1994). Pain control in the older adult has been found to be inferior to that in younger adults.

The common practice of ordering pain medications intramuscularly as needed (PRN) leaves about half of adults and children in pain after surgery. IM injections cause pain, are often absorbed poorly, and can predispose some patients to infection. Alternate methods, such as PCA pumps or epidural analgesia, are much better. If IM injections must be administered, apply ice first or use the Z-track method to minimize discomfort (Beard, 1994).

The American Pain Society has been a leader in the fight for improved pain management. Medicine and nursing have come together to develop pain management standards. The Agency for Health Care Policy and Research (AHCPR) has published guidelines for the control of pain after surgery and trauma, in cancer care, and in pediatrics. These guidelines and others are available free by calling 1-800-358-9295. Table 18–11 highlights some facts about pain derived from a collaborative drug study through the AHCPR.

- Whether the patient is receiving narcotics or nonnarcotics, the patient in pain deserves a careful, methodical assessment. This assessment is performed when the patient first complains of pain and is repeated at regular intervals to determine the effectiveness or lack of effectiveness of the medication regimen, as featured in Table 18–12. It may be helpful to guide the description of the intensity of pain by asking the patient to rate the pain on a numerical scale, on a scale of descriptive terms, or in relation to past experience. In determining the quality of the pain or

Table 18–11. FACTS ABOUT PAIN CONTROL

☐ A patient's report of pain is the determinant of pain control and should be requested not only when the patient is at rest, but during routine activity, such as turning in bed. Ideally, both pain intensity and pain distress are assessed.

☐ Assess and reassess pain frequently during the immediate postoperative period; for example, after major surgery, every 2 hours.

☐ Patients given epidural anesthesia before elective limb amputation for vascular insufficiency are less likely to feel phantom limb pain afterwards.

☐ Preoperative ibuprofen appears to delay the onset of postoperative dental pain and lessen its severity.

☐ Pain is assessed differently in children than it is in adults, and different tools are used. Moreover, children in pain may regress, requiring a different scale of assessment. Parents' assessment of their child's pain may underestimate moderate to severe pain and overestimate lesser pain. Children as young as 7 years of age can use patient-controlled analgesia.

☐ Elderly patients are at risk for undertreatment and overtreatment of pain; treatment may be influenced by institutionalized elders' tendency to be stoic. Elderly patients are also at greater risk for gastric and renal toxicity from nonsteroidal anti-inflammatory drugs (NSAIDs). If gastric ulceration is a concern, coadministered misoprostol (Cytotec) or "platelet-sparing" NSAIDs should be considered. Elderly patients also are more sensitive to analgesia from opiates, experiencing both higher peak and longer duration of pain relief.

☐ The risk of opioid-naive patients abusing the drugs is low.

☐ Phenytoin enhances the biotransformation of meperidine, causing faster elimination and necessitating higher doses of the analgesic.

☐ The sedative effects of opioids and psychotropic drugs may be additive if the drugs are combined. For example, amitriptyline can raise morphine levels. Meperidine, in particular, can lead to effects that mimic malignant hyperthermia, causing death in patients on monoamine oxidase inhibitors.

☐ Contrary to the myth that "third-degree burns don't hurt," evidence shows that after a brief period of endogenous analgesia evoked by the stress of injury, pain can be excruciating for months as tissue regenerates.

Source: Jacox, A, et al: Facts about pain control. Am J Nurs, May 1992:53, with permission.

Table 18–12. NURSING PROCESS FOR PATIENT REQUIRING PAIN MEDICATION

Assessment

Assess OTC analgesic use; other drugs (including alcohol, street drugs).

Assess allergic reactions/hypersensitivity, previous response to drugs.

Assess pain characteristics–dull, throbbing, sharp, constant, or intermittent—and review previous experiences with pain, attitudes toward pain.

Assess preexisting medical conditions, e.g., GI bleeding/ulcer, impaired renal or hepatic function, respiratory disease, cardiac dysrhythmias.

Assess current physical status/condition, including pregnancy.

Nursing Diagnosis: Knowledge Deficit

RELATED TO: Unfamiliarity with prescribed medication(s) and therapeutic needs.

AS EVIDENCED BY: Questions, statement of concerns.

Desired Outcomes/Evaluation Criteria

Verbalizes understanding of drug regimen.

Nursing Actions	Rationale
Provide verbal and written information about pain medication, including action, use, dose, common side effects (e.g., nausea/vomiting, sedation).	Understanding promotes safe/effective drug use and reduces risk of untoward actions/effects.
Discuss possible/frequent drug interactions and encourage reading of ingredient labels for OTC medications. Discuss time frame of absorption of prescribed medication.	Knowledge of potential interactions can help patient optimize drug effect/prevent adverse reactions. Allows patient to gain maximum benefit from drug and lessen undesired side effects.
Stress importance of notifying physician if side effects persist/impair activities or desired lifestyle, or adequate pain control is not achieved.	Provides for change in prescribed regimen when necessary.

Nursing Diagnosis: Pain (acute/chronic)

RELATED TO: Injuring agents (specify).

AS EVIDENCED BY: Verbal complaints, alteration in muscle tone, guarding behavior, autonomic responses.

Desired Outcomes/Evaluation Criteria

Reports pain is relieved/controlled. Follows prescribed pharmacologic regimen. Discusses/demonstrates ways in which pain can be minimized by own actions.

Nursing Actions	Rationale
Provide comfort measures, e.g., backrub, change of position.	Promotes relaxation and may reduce perception of severity of pain.
Encourage use of relaxation exercises, distraction techniques, visualization.	Helps to refocus attention and enhances sense of self-control.
Administer pain medication through appropriate routes, e.g., oral, IM, IV/PCA (patient-controlled analgesia).	Properly administered medication enhances drug effectiveness and provides for optimal pain management.
Explore the way in which the patient copes with pain. Discuss alternate strategies. Explore ways patient does have control over situational factors, e.g., splinting of incision during cough, use of firm mattress/proper supporting shoes for low back pain.	Identifies possibilities of ways in which patient may minimize own suffering and pain behavior. Promotes control over self, reducing sense of powerlessness.
Assist patient to evaluate drug regimen; encourage decreasing dosage, alternate route, increased time span as pain lessens.	Promotes active patient participation/control in therapeutic regimen and may reduce risk of drug tolerance/dependence.

Nursing Diagnosis: Constipation

RELATED TO: Changes in usual pattern of activity, reduced dietary/fluid intake, side effects of opiate analgesics.

AS EVIDENCED BY: Hard stools.

Desired Outcomes/Evaluation Criteria

Maintains adequate fluid/fiber intake. Establishes/returns to normal patterns of bowel functioning.

Nursing Actions	Rationale
Provide information about adequate fluid intake. Identify foods high in fiber.	Adequate fluid intake and fiber in the diet normalize consistency/amount of stool to decrease side effects of constipation.
Encourage increased activity/exercise within the limits of individual ability.	Stimulates bowel motility, enhancing transit time through the bowel and reducing opportunity for excessive reabsorption of fluid from stool.
Discuss use of stool softeners and bulk laxatives.	Provides for normalization of stool consistency and amount to promote elimination and may decrease discomfort associated with gas, decreasing the experience of pain.

Other Suggested Nursing Diagnoses: Sleep Pattern Disturbance; Altered Nutrition, Risk for More Than Body Requirements; and Risk for Trauma.

what the pain is like, it may be helpful to read off terms that describe pain (e.g., intermittent, continuous, sharp, dull, stabbing, annoying, and unbearable), and allow the patient to pick those most applicable to the situation. Other examples of such terms can be found in the McGill-Melzack Pain Questionnaire, shown in Table 18–13.

The nurse's attitude in assessing the patient with pain can make a great difference between an accurate and inaccurate database. Psychogenic pain is as real to the patient as any physiologic trauma. Pain tolerance is highly individualized, and comparisons among patients in differing situations with varying conditions are not accurate. A patient's lack of expression of pain does not necessarily mean lack of pain but is, instead, a reflection of cultural, personal, and physiologic adaptation. Health-care team members are not the experts on the specific pain of an individual patient and tend, in fact, to assess the patient as experiencing less pain than the patient actually has.

Table 18–13. THE MCGILL-MELZACK PAIN QUESTIONNAIRE

McGill-Melzack PAIN QUESTIONNAIRE

Patient's name _____ Age _____
File No. _____ Date _____
Clinical category (eg. cardiac, neurological, etc.):
_____

Diagnosis: _____
_____

Analgesic (if already administered):
1. Type _____
2. Dosage _____
3. Time given in relation to this test _____
Patient's intelligence: circle number that represents best estimate
1 (low)   2   3   4   5 (high)
* * * * * * * * * * * * * * * *

This questionnaire has been designed to tell us more about your pain. Four major questions to ask are:
1. Where is your pain?
2. What does it feel like?
3. How does it change with time?
4. How strong is it?
It is important that you tell us how your pain feels now. Please follow the instructions at the beginning of each part.

© R. Metzack, Oct. 1970

Part I.   Where is your Pain?

Please mark, on the drawings below, the areas where you feel pain. Put E if external, or I if internal, near the areas which you mark. Put EI if both external and internal.

Part 2.   What Does Your Pain Feel Like?

Some of the words below describe your present pain. Circle ONLY those words that best describe it. Leave out any category that is not suitable. Use only a single word in each appropriate category—the one that applies best.

1	2	3	4
Flickering	Jumping	Pricking	Sharp
Quivering	Flashing	Boring	Cutting
Pulsing	Shooting	Drilling	Lacerating
Throbbing		Stabbing	
Beating		Lancinating	
Pounding			

5	6	7	8
Pinching	Tugging	Hot	Tingling
Pressing	Pulling	Burning	Itchy
Gnawing	Wrenching	Scalding	Smarting
Cramping		Searing	Stinging
Crushing			

9	10	11	12
Dull	Tender	Tiring	Sickening
Sore	Taut	Exhausting	Suffocating
Hurting	Rasping		
Aching	Splitting		
Heavy			

13	14	15	16
Fearful	Punishing	Wretched	Annoying
Frightful	Gruelling	Blinding	Troublesome
Terrifying	Cruel		Miserable
	Vicious		Intense
	Killing		Unbearable

17	18	19	20
Spreading	Tight	Cool	Nagging
Radiating	Numb	Cold	Nauseating
Penetrating	Drawing	Freezing	Agonizing
Piercing	Squeezing		Dreadful
	Tearing		Torturing

Part 3.   How Does Your Pain Change With Time?

1. Which word or words would you use to describe the pattern of your pain?

1	2	3
Continuous	Rhythmic	Brief
Steady	Periodic	Momentary
Constant	Intermittent	Transient

2. What kind of things relieve your pain?

3. What kind of things increase your pain?

Part 4.   How Strong Is Your Pain?

People agree that the following 5 words represent pain of increasing intensity. They are:

1	2	3	4	5
Mild	Discomforting	Distressing	Horrible	Excruciating

To answer each question below, write the number of the most appropriate word in the space beside the question.

1. Which word describes your pain right now?   _____
2. Which word describes it at its worst?   _____
3. Which word describes it when it is least?   _____
4. Which word describes the worst toothache you ever had?   _____
5. Which word describes the worst headache you ever had?   _____
6. Which word describes the worst stomach-ache you ever had?   _____

The American Pain Society's guideline is very clear: "Do not use placebos to assess the nature of pain. The deceptive use of placebos and the misinterpretation of the placebo response to discredit the patient's pain report are unethical and should be avoided" (American Pain Society, 1992).

▼ **CLINICAL ALERT**

Researchers now feel that placebos actually enhance the endogenous curative mechanisms of the body.

Placebos provide relief in patients of all types; there is no "placebo personality." In addition, about 30% to 75% of patients may respond to placebos. The nurse should not judge a patient's pain as imaginary just because the patient responds to a placebo. Placebos are given to produce a therapeutic response, lessening the patient's pain and improving the patient's quality of life.

NURSING DIAGNOSIS

- Establish the nursing diagnoses based on the nursing assessment to begin the planning of interventions. Typical nursing diagnoses for a patient with pain include Pain, Chronic Pain, Anxiety, Fear, and Impaired Physical Mobility (see Table 18–12).

PLANNING AND INTERVENTION

- Medicate the patient in anticipation of pain. If the patient is allowed to experience severe pain, the length of time needed for the analgesic to become effective increases and the overall analgesic effectiveness decreases.
- Provide information to the patient and to the family regarding the nature of pain, analgesics, and common adverse effects. It is not necessary for the patient to "hang in there" or "keep a stiff upper lip" or to suffer. It is necessary for the patient to achieve pain control, maintain alertness, and participate in daily activities as much as possible.

Nursing Responsibilities

- Take advantage of the placebo effect of all drugs. The placebo effect can be heightened if the therapeutic value of the medication and the drug action are explained and the positive aspects of the medication are stressed.
- Determine which, if any, nonpharmacologic interventions for pain relief are suitable for the patient. Nonpharmacologic methods to lessen pain include the following: relaxation, imagery, music distraction, biofeedback, therapeutic touch, application of heat or cold, massage, exercise, immobility, and TENS. These methods increase the effectiveness of pain-relieving medications, providing the patient with optimum pain control.
- Administer nonsteroidal anti-inflammatory drugs

(NSAIDs) such as indomethacin or ketorolac IM as ordered. NSAIDs reduce the dosage requirements of both opiate and nonopiate analgesics. Pain that does not respond to routine measures prompts a search for infection, osteitis, peripheral nerve injury, or the emergence of psychologic and behavior changes consistent with the development of chronic pain syndrome.

- Carefully monitor pain medication administration in the elderly patient. Older adults often have an increased fat-to-lean mass ratio and reduced renal function. Opiate analgesics often cause confusion, as the toxic metabolites increase in the brain. The high prevalence of visual, hearing, and motor impairments in the elderly may impede the use of universal pain scales, making pain monitoring more difficult. Cognitive impairment, delirium, and dementia also represent serious barriers to pain control.
- When the patient requires intramuscular (IM) injections, rotate sites and observe proper technique. Two weeks is the maximum period that IM injections are given on an every-4-hour basis. When using parenteral forms of narcotics, consult the pharmacist before mixing the narcotic with another drug (such as an anticholinergic, a tranquilizer, or a barbiturate) because the drugs often are not compatible when combined.
- Understand and monitor all equipment used to administer pain medications. It is important to monitor the patient's respiratory status as well as other side effects of opiate administration.
- Always administer preservative-free preparation when administering a bolus or continuous drip of opiate via the epidural or intrathecal route. The tubing, infusion bag, and pump are labeled with tape reading "epidural" or "intrathecal." This alerts all caregivers to the type of infusion line to minimize confusion with similar-looking lines. Injection ports are taped over or capped to prevent accidental injection into the epidural or intrathecal lines. Prior to administering drugs, aspirate the catheter to determine whether there is a clear fluid or bloody return. If the catheter is in the epidural space, no fluid is aspirated. The presence of CSF or blood signifies a migrated catheter; the physician is notified, and the drug not given. When working with the epidural or intrathecal system, strict aseptic technique is observed. The tubing and filter of a continuous infusion are changed in accordance with hospital policy. Monitor the patient for infection (fever, excessive pain or tenderness at the catheter site, redness at the catheter site, headache, stiff neck, photophobia, mental changes).
- Understand the equianalgesic doses and individualize the dosage to the patient's need. If the patient is receiving intravenous or intramuscular medication and is switched to oral medication prior to discharge, allow sufficient time to test the oral route for successful home therapy.

To provide adequate analgesia for patients in severe pain, much larger dosages of drugs than are normally considered therapeutic are required. For such patients, medication given on a scheduled round-the-clock basis rather than every 3 to 4 hours as needed is the more effective dosage schedule.

Patient Teaching

- Provide the required health teaching about analgesic medications, including over-the-counter (OTC) analgesics (Table 18–14). Because many OTC analgesics contain ingredients other than aspirin, the patient with medical problems (such as liver or kidney disease) and the patient who is receiving several medications should consult with a health-care team member before selecting such an analgesic. Attractive packaging and flavorings of aspirin and acetaminophen may lead to ingestion by children, resulting in accidental overdosage. Special precautions are maintained in the storage of these preparations.

- Teach patients about their unique type of therapy. Patients must understand the concept of PCA therapy and know how to work the pump. For many patients, this is a new approach to pain management, and they are not aware of their role in this type of therapy. Patients must understand that they control the frequency at which the analgesic is received. Emphasize the degree of control the patient has over the pain and what to expect in relation to the activities of daily living.

Patients receiving long-term epidural or intrathecal analgesia receive instruction prior to discharge. This teaching protocol includes self-medication regimen, signs and symptoms of infection, procedures to follow if an infection occurs, and catheter care. Many of the subcutaneous tunneling and implanted systems are easily accessible to the patient. If patients are unable to self-administer their medication and to perform catheter care, a family member or other caregiver is taught to do so.

Explain to patients and families that pain will not be totally absent with any of these treatment modalities. However, as partners in pain control, nurses and patients can work together to maximize pain relief—a more realistic and achievable goal.

EVALUATION

- Determine the effectiveness of the analgesic medications during the evaluation phase of the nursing process. Outcome goals for the patient requiring analgesics are included in Table 18–12.
- Evaluate the development of adverse effects. The most common adverse effects of the non-narcotic analgesics include gastrointestinal irritation and subsequent bleeding, prolonged bleeding time, and development of analgesic nephropathy, which may result in renal failure. Signs of gastrointestinal irritation include nausea, vomiting, tarry stools, anemia, and positive results of a test for occult blood in the stool. Irritation may be prevented or reduced by administering buffered products or by administering the analgesics at mealtime, with food, or shortly after eat-

---

Table 18–14. PATIENT TEACHING INFORMATION—PAIN MEDICATIONS

Non-narcotic Analgesics and Nonsteroidal Anti-inflammatories

Dear Patient:

This drug has been ordered for you. This is what you should know about your drug to get the most from your therapy.

Non-narcotic analgesics and nonsteroidal anti-inflammatories are used to alleviate mild pain. Examples are aspirin, acetaminophen, ibuprofen, and indomethacin.

- ☐ 1. Take by mouth every 4 to 6 hours.
- ☐ 2. Try not to forget a dose. Do not play catch up with missed doses.
- ☐ 3. If the drug is relieving the pain at the ordered dose and time, continue the pain medication. If not, call your physician before stopping the drug.
- ☐ 4. Always check with your physician before changing the dose of the drug or taking over-the-counter medications with your ordered drug.
- ☐ 5. Side effects include stomach upset and possible stomach bleeding, prolonged bleeding time, blood problems, allergic reaction, sodium and water retention, and kidney and liver problems with long-term use.
- ☐ 6. Chronic or excessive use of acetaminophen and alcohol (beer, wine, hard liquor) can cause liver problems. Oral anticoagulants and aspirin and/or acetaminophen can increase the bleeding effect. Birth control pills and acetaminophen cause a decrease in pain effect. Take your medication with food to reduce stomach upset.
- ☐ 7. Keep medication tightly covered in a light-resistant container, at room temperature. Keep out of the reach of children.

Opiate Analgesics

Dear Patient:

This drug has been ordered for you. This is what you should know about your drug to get the most from your therapy.

Opiate analgesics are used to reduce moderate or severe pain. Examples of medication that relieve moderate pain are codeine, codeine and aspirin, codeine and acetaminophen, propoxyphene, oxycodone, and hydrocodone. Medications that relieve severe pain include morphine, hydromorphone, methadone, and levorphanol.

- ☐ 1. Take by mouth every 4 to 6 hours or every 6 to 8 hours as prescribed.
- ☐ 2. Try not to forget a dose. Do not play catch up with missed doses.
- ☐ 3. If the drug is relieving the pain at the ordered dose and time, continue the pain medication. If not, call your physician before stopping the drug.
- ☐ 4. Always check with your physician before changing the dose of the drug or taking over-the-counter medications with your ordered drug
- ☐ 5. Alcohol (beer, wine, hard liquor) increases sedation, dizziness, lightheadedness, and inability to concentrate.
- ☐ 6. Side effects include constipation, nausea and vomiting (first 2 weeks of therapy), and drowsiness.
- ☐ 7. Interactions vary with each opiate analgesic.
- ☐ 8. Keep drug tightly covered at room temperature and out of the reach of children.

---

ing. Prolonged bleeding time is manifested by easy bruising or profuse bleeding of minor cuts and may indicate a need for a change in analgesic. Analgesic nephropathy develops after chronic long-term use or abuse of analgesics. Research suggests that the risk of analgesic nephropathy can be minimized through use

DELIVERING HOME HEALTH CARE

Administration of Pain Medications

Caring for patients with chronic pain is becoming more prevalent in the home. Home care, particularly Hospice, for dying patients is cost effective and more comfortable for both the patient and family.

Before administering pain medications, do the following:
- Assess the patient's and family's knowledge of pain control.
- Assess the patient's allergy history.
- Assess baseline vital signs.
- Assess when pain is present (e.g., all the time, in relation to activities, at night).
- Assist with determining the best route of drug administration (PO, IV, intrathecal, intraspinal, and so on).
- Assist the patient/family in obtaining doctor's order and medication.
- Determine who will be responsible for drug administration.

To administer medications, perform the following:
- Select an appropriate site and insert the IV line if needed.
- Teach the patient/family how to care for the injection site.
- Teach the patient and family the side effects and monitoring implications of the specific drug(s).
- Prepare handouts to be left with the patient and family.

During administration, perform the following:
- Ensure that the line is in the proper position and is working normally.
- Monitor the patient closely for adverse reactions and side effects.
- Monitor respiratory rate and vital signs.

After drug administration:
- Continue to monitor the patient's respiratory rate closely.
- Determine when pain relief occurs and for how long.
- Determine if the patient is able to participate in his or her normal activities of daily living.
- Evaluate the patient's ability to problem solve. For example, what happens if IV line becomes dislodged? What does patient do if there is blood in the IV line? What does patient do if skin around the IV line becomes red and swollen? Can medication be increased or decreased to control pain?
- Chart the drug administration correctly according to agency policy.

---

of one analgesic rather than combination forms and by increasing fluid intake.

Patients receiving epidural or intrathecal opiate analgesia are monitored for nausea and vomiting, urinary retention, pruritus, and respiratory depression. Anticipating *cephalad* (toward the head) spread of opiates (i.e., morphine) as evidenced by increasing segmental analgesia, miosis, and changes in mentation is also important. The incidence of respiratory depression with this type of therapy is low, but constant nursing surveillance is required. Evaluate respiratory function (respiratory rate, volume, quality of effort, auscultation of lungs, apnea, skin color changes, arterial blood gas analysis). Apnea monitors are used but not relied on solely. See Table 18–15 for nine ways to prevent opioid respiratory depression.

Common adverse effects of opiate analgesic therapy include constipation, urinary retention, nausea and vomiting, orthostatic hypotension, sedation, and addiction. Constipation may be relieved by a prophylactic bowel-management plan. This plan provides the patient with information about fluid, food, and exercise as well as stool softeners and cathartics. Neostigmine or pyridostigmine may also be used because they enhance peristalsis, which decreases the likelihood of constipation. Urinary retention generally subsides during the first 24 to 48 hours of narcotic treatment. Warm baths and neostigmine may be useful in preventing and treating the spasm that causes urinary retention. Nausea and vomiting are common adverse effects in patients receiving narcotics, particularly

ambulatory patients, but may also be a sign of poorly controlled pain. Restricting ambulation may be helpful to some patients or an antiemetic (an antihistamine or a phenothiazine) may be given. The antihistamine antiemetics act on vestibular sensitivity, whereas phenothiazines act on medullary trigger areas for nausea and vomiting. If initial doses of one type of antiemetic are unsuccessful, adding the other type of antiemetic to the regimen may be more helpful than increasing the dosage of the original drug. Narcotics may be routinely accompanied by antiemetics to prevent nausea and vomiting. Orthostatic hypotension is also common in ambulatory patients. Patients are reminded to rise slowly from the supine position. Drugs such as the phenothiazines, which might potentiate this adverse effect, are used cautiously. Sedation also occurs initially, but usually subsides within 2 or 3 days if narcotics are given on a regular schedule. Sedation may necessitate a slight reduction in analgesic dosage. Sedation is never automatically linked with overdosage because it may be the result of many factors, including the analgesic and the pain itself. Addiction, physical dependence, tolerance, and withdrawal syndrome are possible sequelae of treatment with narcotics and are reviewed in Chapter 67.

- Evaluate for potential drug interactions. The depressant effects of other drugs in the medication regimen (e.g., hypnotics, sedatives, anxiolytics) that may be used concurrently with opiates must be recognized. Reports of respiratory depression have discouraged concurrent use of parenteral opiates and sedatives.

Table 18–15. NINE WAYS TO PREVENT OPIOID-INDUCED RESPIRATORY DEPRESSION

Clinically significant respiratory depression is preventable. In fact, its prevention is easier than its management. Here are nine suggestions to prevent respiratory depression from reaching clinical significance:

1. Assess risk.	Determine on admission if your patient is at high or low risk for opioid-induced respiratory depression. During the admission interview, ask your patient to describe past experiences with surgery, anesthesia and analgesics, and current opioid use. Ask specific questions about the effects of the analgesics they have taken, including the level of pain relief and the adverse effects. Make sure that an opioid antagonist is ordered along with the analgesic in case it is needed.
2. Communicate.	The information you obtain in the admission interview is very important for everyone involved in managing your patient's pain. If your patient has a history of sensitivity, inform the pain service nurse, the anesthesiologist, and the physician of this opioid sensitivity so that less-sedative drugs can be used before, during, and after surgery, and so the postoperative opioid dose can be reduced.
3. Anticipate pain.	Whenever possible, address your patient's postoperative analgesic needs during preoperative preparation. Nonsteroidal anti-inflammatory drugs (NSAIDs), for example, are capable of producing analgesia without sedation and respiratory depression. When NSAIDs are administered in combination with opioids, the opioid dose often can be reduced. Patients then will experience pain relief but with less risk of sedation and respiratory depression. If your patient is at high risk for opioid-induced respiratory depression, request an order from the physician to administer an NSAID preoperatively and to continue the administration of the NSAID around-the-clock postoperatively, using an opioid to provide additional analgesia if needed.
4. Watch for additive effects.	Be aware of other drugs that your patient is receiving. For all patients receiving opioid analgesia, carefully assess the need for antiemetics and sedatives. Avoid routinely adding phenothiazines (e.g., promethazine [Phenergan]) and benzodiazepines (e.g., midazolam [Versed] or diazepam [Valium]). These drugs provide little, if any, pain relief but they can increase respiratory depression, sedation, and hypotension—effectively limiting the dose of opioid you can safely give.
5. Adjust initial doses.	If your patient is at risk for respiratory depression and a range of dosage has been prescribed, administer the lowest amount and titrate upward to effectiveness. If your patient is not at high risk, start in the middle of the range for your patient and titrate upward to effectiveness. Remember, the first dose will reveal your patient's ability to tolerate opioids. It is up to you to evaluate these effects and make arrangements to adjust the dose or interval if needed. Continue to assess the appropriateness of dose and interval for as long as your patient is receiving opioid analgesia.
6. Act on response, not amount.	Increase or decrease the dose of opioid based on your assessment of the patient's response. Patients' responses and therefore their requirements vary widely, even when they have identical diagnoses or surgical procedures, so it is less important to focus on the amount given. To determine what dose your patient needs after the initial dose, always look at the effect the opioid has had on your patient's pain rating, sedation level, and respiratory status.
7. Adjust maintenance doses.	The safest way to increase the dose of opioid is gradually, by percentage of the previous dose or the current opioid infusion dose, and after the peak effect. If your patient is not at high risk for respiratory depression, reports pain, and has no intolerable adverse effects, the dose can be increased by 10% to 50%. If your patient is at high risk for opioid-induced respiratory depression, reports pain, and has no intolerable adverse effects, increase the dose by only 25%.
8. Be aware of pharmacokinetic differences.	Learn the peak times for the various opioids and other sedative drugs you administer and monitor your patient closely when those peak times are reached. It is also wise initially to stagger the times you give other sedative drugs so that all the effects do not peak at the same time.
9. Plan ahead.	Known high-risk patients need more frequent monitoring. The busiest times on surgical units are when most of the patients are in their first 24 postoperative hours. These busy times are often predictable because most major surgeries are done on a known, regular schedule. Whenever possible, work with your nursing administrators to ensure adequate staff on those days that are the busiest and require the closest patient monitoring. Communicate staffing needs as soon as you are aware of them. Accountability for providing patients with effective, safe pain relief begins at the administrative level in the hospital, but they need information from the front line to provide support. Also, be willing to be part of the team to manage the demands on nurses caring for high-risk patients. Through teamwork, nurses can protect their patients from developing clinically significant respiratory depression.

Source: Pasero, C, and McCaffery, M: Avoiding opioid-induced respiratory depression. Am J Nurs 94(4):28–31, 1994, with permission.

The elderly patient is susceptible to this effect. Infusions of opiate antagonists (e.g., naloxone) can reverse respiratory depression.

- Maintain a current working knowledge of analgesia information helps the nurse perfect the process of nursing the patient with pain. This includes familiarity with recent advances in the body of knowledge regarding pain, such as the development of theories of pain, the discovery of endogenous agents that mediate pain, and development of assessment tools to determine levels of pain.

The bibliography for this chapter can be found in Appendix B, which begins on page 1054.

CHAPTER REVIEW QUESTIONS*

1. All of the following are opiate agonist-antagonists *except*:
   a. Nalbuphine hydrochloride (Nubain).
   b. Butorphanol tartrate (Stadol).
   c. Naloxone hydrochloride (Narcan).
   d. Pentazocine (Talwin).

2. Which of the following statements regarding methylmorphine (codeine) is *not* correct?
   a. Codeine is contraindicated in patients with high intracranial pressure.
   b. The average adult dosage is 15 to 60 mg four times daily PRN.
   c. The drug is classified as a Schedule II controlled substance.
   d. Common side effects include constipation, drowsiness, and nausea.

3. A 55-year-old male, 36 hours post abdominal perineal resection, is alert and complaining of severe pain. The patient has an epidural catheter in place. Vital signs are blood pressure—135/75; pulse—86, regular; and respirations—7, regular, good breath sounds. Fentanyl is ordered for pain. What is your nursing action?
   a. Administer the prescribed dose of fentanyl.
   b. Withhold the fentanyl because of the respiration rate.
   c. Administer naxolone, which is ordered to reverse the respiratory depression.
   d. Call the physician.

4. The antidote for an overdose of acetaminophen (Tylenol) is:
   a. Propanolol (Inderol).
   b. Sodium bicarbonate.
   c. Naloxone hydrochloride.
   d. Acetylcysteine.

5. Which statement is *correct* regarding narcotic agents?
   a. Common signs of narcotic toxicity include dilated pupils and agitation.
   b. Dosages of oral and parenteral forms of the same drug are interchangeable.
   c. Intramuscular injection of narcotics is recommended for cancer patients.
   d. Narcotics interfere with the perception of pain at higher brain centers.

*See Appendix A, which begins on page 1051, for answers.

BUILDING YOUR CRITICAL THINKING SKILLS

EPIDURAL ANALGESIA

A 52-year-old patient returns from surgery after a hysterectomy. She has epidural morphine infusing at 2 mg/hr for pain control. Currently she is stable, awake, oriented, and pain-free. Two hours after admission the patient states her pain has increased, and an order is obtained to increase the epidural morphine dose to 4 mg/hr. The nurse increases the flow rate and repositions the patient. One hour later, the patient is obtunded and has a respiratory rate of 6/min.

1. What is the nurse's priority concern for this patient?
2. What factors are contributing to the patient's change in condition?
3. What would the nurse expect the physician to order for this patient?
4. What additional assessments should be made once the patient is stable?

CHAPTER 19

Central Nervous System Stimulants

Merrily A. Kuhn, RNC, PhD

CHAPTER OUTLINE

KEY TERMS

Asthenia
Cataplexy
Depolarizing postsynaptic
potential
Drug holiday
Hyperactivity
Hyperpolarizing potential
Opisthotonos

LEARNING OBJECTIVES

After reading this chapter, the student will be able to:

1. Identify those medications commonly used as central nervous system stimulants.
2. Differentiate among the central nervous system stimulants as to mechanism of action, route of administration, pharmacokinetics, adverse effects, contraindications and precautions, and interactions.
3. Identify specific areas to assess in the patient requiring central nervous system stimulants to formulate appropriate patient outcomes.
4. Plan the nursing interventions necessary to administer central nervous system stimulants and choose appropriate teaching strategies to gain patient compliance.
5. Evaluate the patient at various stages of treatment to measure the effectiveness of nursing interventions.

The central nervous system (CNS) stimulants are a diverse group of pharmacologic drugs whose first action is stimulation of the central nervous system. CNS stimulation is demonstrated through a change in the patient's usual behavior: mild elevations of alertness, increased restlessness, irritability, euphoria, nervousness, and anxiety. The patient can also experience increased muscle tone and seizures. The degree of the CNS stimulation caused by a certain drug depends on both the area in the brain or spinal cord that is affected by the drug and the cellular mechanism fundamental to the increased excitability.

There is a fine balance between excitation and inhibition in the CNS. Information is transmitted along neurons by action potentials. A *depolarizing postsynaptic potential* (an action potential produced in a nerve of such magnitude that it depolarizes the next neuron and allows for conduction) is an excitatory postsynaptic potential (EPSP), which produces an all-or-nothing response in the second (postsynaptic) neuron. The *hyperpolarizing potential* (an action potential produced in a nerve of such magnitude that it excessively depolarizes the next neuron and prevents conduction), on the other hand, is inhibitory and prevents the action potential of the second neuron. The purpose of the inhibitory postsynaptic potential (IPSP) is to decrease the number of nerve impulses generated per unit of time. If this did not occur, the CNS would be in a constant state of stimulation.

The publisher greatly acknowledges the contribution of Barbara K. Clark, RN, MN, CCRN, to the third edition.

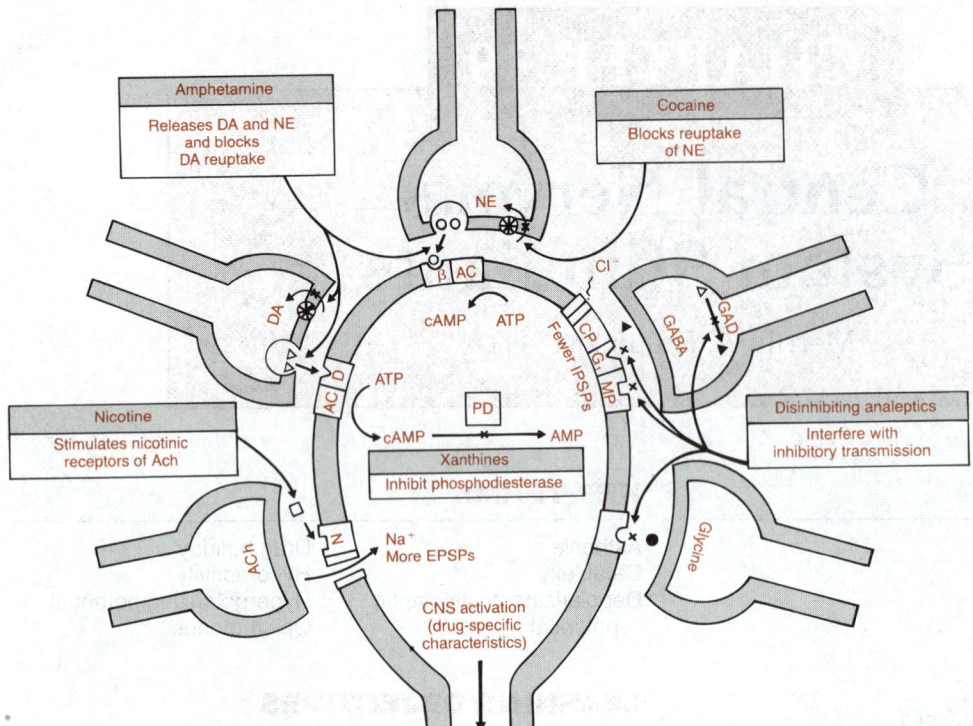

Figure 19–1. Neurochemical mechanisms of stimulants. AC = adenyl cyclase; ACh = acetylcholine; AMP = adenosine monophosphate; ATP = adenosine triphosphate; cAMP = cyclic adenosine monophosphate; β = Beta-adrenergic receptor: D = dopamine receptor; DA = dopamine; EPSP = excitatory postsynaptic potential; GABA = gamma-aminobutyric acid: G_1 = GABA receptor, type 1; GAD = glutamic acid decarboxylase; IPSP = inhibitory postsynaptic potential; MP = modulatory protein; NE = norepinephrine; PD = phosphodiesterase. (From Swonger, AK and Matejski, MP: Nursing Pharmacology: An Integrated Approach to Drug Therapy and Nursing Practice. Scott, Foresman and Company, 1988, p 202, with permission.)

ACTION

Altering the fine balance between excitatory and inhibitory influence at the level of the neuron explains how CNS stimulants produce their pharmacologic action. This action is produced by one or more of the following mechanisms: (1) increasing the effect of excitatory neurotransmission (e.g., doxapram); (2) decreasing or opposing inhibitory neurotransmission (e.g., strychnine); (3) blocking the uptake of catecholamines at adrenergic synapses (e.g., cocaine); or (4) modifying neurotransmitter response by altering cyclic 3,5 adenosine monophosphate (cAMP) (e.g., methylxanthines). A review of the neurochemical mechanisms of CNS stimulants is shown in Figure 19–1.

In general, when given in small doses, CNS stimulants increase mental alertness and capacity for work, improve motor performance, impart a feeling of well-being, and stimulate the respiratory and cardiac systems and general metabolism. In large doses, these agents cause tremor, restlessness, and insomnia and result in deterioration of motor performance. Prolonged use can lead to hypertension and exhaustion. With continued use, abuse, or overdose, toxicities develop, which result in hallucinations, seizures, and cardiac dysrhythmias.

There are two main groups of CNS stimulants: analeptic stimulants and psychomotor stimulants. This division of groups is based on mechanism of action or chemical composition. Descriptions of each group of stimulants and some specific agents are reviewed. Table 19–1 features selected analeptic and psychomotor stimulants.

ANALEPTIC STIMULANTS

The agents in this group—**caffeine**, **doxapram** *(Dopram)*, and the **methylxanthines**—are very different in chemical composition, which makes it difficult to classify each one in reference to absorption, distribution, and metabolism. Most of these agents are absorbed orally and have short duration of action. These products have a generalized effect on the brain stem, spinal cord, and higher centers in the brain, which makes dosing especially difficult. Today, analeptics have limited usefulness.

ADVERSE REACTIONS

This group of agents produces adverse reactions that are exaggerations of their therapeutic effect. They produce life-threatening clonic-tonic seizures that can lead to death. Prior to these seizures, there may be an increase in respiration, tachycardia, and severe hypertension. Patients also experience extreme *opisthotonos* (a severe muscular spasm characterized by the head and heels being bent backward and the body bent forward so that only the head and heel remain in contact with the ground) and increased sensitivity to sensory-stimuli-induced seizures.

○ **Caffeine** is absorbed from the gut and distributed in tissues. Low to moderate amounts of caffeine intake produce stimulation of the cerebral cortex, increasing alertness and decreasing fatigue. However, 250 mg or more of caffeine (two to three cups of coffee) increases the chances of developing signs of excessive CNS stimulation—nervousness, restlessness, insomnia, and tremors. Table 19–2 lists caffeine levels in various drugs and beverages.

Caffeine exerts a positive inotropic effect on the myocardium and a positive chronotropic effect at the sinoatrial node, resulting in transient increases in heart rate, force of contraction, and cardiac output. In larger amounts (more than 250 mg), the centrally mediated vagal effects of caffeine can be masked with increased sinus rates, extrasystole, or ventricular dysrhythmias.

Table 19–1. CENTRAL NERVOUS SYSTEM STIMULANTS

DRUG NAME/ROUTE AND DOSAGE	PHARMACOKINETICS/ DYNAMICS	NURSING IMPLICATIONS
all central nervous system stimulants		
		ASSESSMENT: Neurologic assessment establishes a baseline for mental, behavioral, and motor functioning prior to initial therapy. It is important to obtain a drug history prior to amphetamine therapy. **INTERVENTION:** Monitor the patient for therapeutic response and possible adverse effects. Monitor blood pressure, pulse, and respiratory status while patient is receiving amphetamine therapy. Monitor the weight and height of children. **EVALUATION:** Patients experience minimal side effects.
ANALEPTIC STIMULANTS		
caffeine (various combination products)		
mild cns stimulation *Adults:* 65–325 mg PO tid **cns stimulation** *Children:* 8 mg/kg PO or SC every 4 hr PRN. **neonatal apnea** *Children <6 months:* loading dose of 5–10 mg/kg, PO followed by 2.5–5 mg/kg daily.	**Onset:** 30–45 min **Peak:** 50–75 min **Duration:** NA **½L:** 3–4 hr for adults; 80 hr for neonates **PB:** 17% **B:** liver **E:** kidneys	**ASSESSMENT:** Monitor vital signs closely. CNS effects of caffeine are more severe in children. Obtain history of caffeine intake. Assess for pregnancy (category C). **INTERVENTION:** IM injections are painful. Explain this to the patient prior to administration. Administer IV caffeine slowly. Overdosage can be treated with a short-acting barbiturate. **EVALUATION:** Patients experience minimal side effects. If given as an analgesic, ask patient whether relief is obtained.
PSYCHOMOTOR STIMULANTS		
methamphetamine hydrochloride (Desoxyn) (Methampex)		
attention deficit disorder *Adults:* 5 mg PO daily or bid; increase 5 mg/wk to 20–25 mg daily (usual effective dose). **obesity** *Adults:* 10–15 mg extended-release tablet before breakfast daily; this treatment is used for only about 2 wk.	**Onset:** 1–2 hr **Peak:** NA **Duration:** 2–10 hr **½L:** 4–5 hr; 6.8 hr in children **PB:** NA **B:** liver **E:** kidneys	Same as for all plus: **ASSESSMENT:** Assess for pregnancy (category C). **EVALUATION:** Therapeutic effectiveness is the desired effect from the agent with minimal or no side effects.
methylphenidate (Ritalin)		
attention deficit disorder *Children 6 yr and over:* 5 mg PO bid before breakfast and lunch; increase by 5–10 mg at weekly intervals (maximum 60 mg/day). **narcolepsy** *Adults:* 10 mg PO bid or tid (60 mg/day maximum). Administer 30–45 min before meals.	**Onset:** 1 hr **Peak:** 1–3 hr **Duration:** 4–6 hr; ER, 8 hr **½L:** 1–3 hr **PB:** NA **B:** liver **E:** kidneys	**ASSESSMENT:** Assess patient's behavior prior to and periodically throughout therapy. Therapy may be interrupted at intervals to determine if symptoms are sufficient to continue therapy. Monitor CBC and differential and platelet count periodically throughout therapy. Assess blood pressure and pulse periodically throughout therapy. **INTERVENTION:** Growth, including height and weight, is monitored in children on long-term therapy. The drug may be administered with meals if GI irritation becomes a problem. ER tablets are swallowed whole; the patient should not crush, break, or chew. Take last dose 6 hr before bedtime. **EVALUATION:** In children with hyperkinetic syndrome, effectiveness is demonstrated by calming effect with decreased hyperactivity and prolonged attention span. In narcolepsy, effectiveness of therapy is demonstrated by increased motor activity, increased mental alertness, diminished sense of fatigue, and brighter outlook.

Continued on the following page

Table 19–1. CENTRAL NERVOUS SYSTEM STIMULANTS, *Continued*

DRUG NAME/ROUTE AND DOSAGE	PHARMACOKINETICS/ DYNAMICS	NURSING IMPLICATIONS
pemoline (Cylert)		
attention deficit disorder ***Children 6 yr and over:*** *Initial dose*–37.5 mg PO administered in the morning. The daily dose is increased by 18.75 mg weekly. *Usual effective range*–56.25—75 mg daily. Dosage for children should not exceed 112.5 mg daily.	**Onset:** 30–45 min (blood levels); effects in 2–**4** weeks **Peak:** 2–4 hr **Duration:** 8 hr **½L:** 9–14 hr in adults: nonlinear kinetics in children increase the half-life. **PB:** 50% **B:** liver **E:** kidneys	**ASSESSMENT:** Monitor liver function tests in long-term therapy. Assess for pregnancy (category B). **INTERVENTION:** Administer pemoline in the morning to provide maximal effectiveness during waking hours and to avoid insomnia. Insomnia and anorexia are dose-dependent. If these side effects occur, the dose may need to be reduced. Drug holidays prescribed by the physician can determine the effectiveness of therapy and the need for continuation. Monitor height and weight in children. **EVALUATION:** Child's attention span is longer, concentration on tasks is greater, and hyperactivity is decreased, indicating that the therapy is effective. Side effects from pemoline are minimal.

NA = not available; ER = extended release; CBC = complete blood count.

Caffeine possesses the properties of a weak diuretic. It increases renal blood flow and glomerular filtration rate and decreases proximal tubular reabsorption of sodium and water. Caffeine has been shown to increase the basal metabolic rate. The intake of 3 to 9 mg/kg of body weight (225 to 675 mg caffeine, or two to six cups of coffee) can raise the basal metabolic rate about 10%.

CONTRAINDICATIONS AND PRECAUTIONS Caffeine is contraindicated in persons with a hypersensitivity to caffeine. Safe use during pregnancy (category C) has not been established. Caffeine crosses the placenta and achieves fetal serum levels similar to maternal concentrations. Caution is used when administering caffeine to patients with peptic ulcer or coronary heart disease.

○ **Doxapram** (Dopram) produces respiratory stimulation via the peripheral carotid chemoreceptors. As the dosage level increases, the respiratory centers in the medulla are stimulated along with other parts of the CNS. This agent is used for postanesthesia respiratory depression, drug-induced CNS depression, and chronic pulmonary disease with hypercapnia (temporary measure only). The value of analeptics in the therapy of pulmonary disease is very limited today.

Administration of doxapram is not a substitute for a patent airway. It is important to administer the minimum effective dosage to avoid side effects. To avoid overdosage, it is necessary to observe blood pressure and deep tendon reflexes. Intravenous short-acting barbiturates, oxygen, and resuscitative equipment should be available to manage overdose. Rapid infusion of doxapram can result in hemolysis. If sudden hypotension or dyspnea develops, doxapram should be discontinued.

○ **Methylxanthines** (caffeine, theophylline, aminophylline) are xanthine derivatives that are used primarily in respiratory disease. Theophylline relieves paroxysmal dyspnea associated with left heart failure and is used alone with aminophylline as a bronchodilator to treat asthma, bronchospasm, and paroxysmal dyspnea. All of the methylxanthines are capable of producing some degree of diuresis. The methylxanthines are discussed in detail in Chapter 40.

PSYCHOMOTOR STIMULANTS

Many of the psychomotor agents—**dextroamphetamine sulfate** *(Dexedrine)*, **methamphetamine hydrochloride** *(Desoxyn)*, **methylphenidate hydrochloride** *(Ritalin)*, **pemoline** *(Cylert)*, and **cocaine**—have pharmacologic activity similar to amphetamine (see Table 19–1). Methylphenidate and pemoline have different chemical structures in comparison with the amphetamines.

USES

The therapeutic uses of the psychomotor stimulants are very limited. They are used in the management of attention deficit disorder with hyperactivity and narcolepsy.

▼ **CLINICAL ALERT**

Amphetamines have a high potential for abuse. When administered for prolonged periods, dependency may occur. They are used in weight reduction programs only when alternative therapy has been ineffective.

Attention Deficit Disorder A common pediatric behavior disorder is attention deficit disorder with hyperactivity (ADDH), which has a prevalence rate range from 1.2% to 20%. This disorder has a male predominance of 6:1. The etiology is obscure, but there is some evidence that supports genetic transmission. There is a higher incidence of *hyperactivity* (a level of activity that is excessive for the circumstances) in parents of children with ADDH than in parents of children without this disorder. The di-

Table 19–2. CAFFEINE LEVELS IN DRUGS AND BEVERAGES

Drug/Beverage	Prescription (P) or Over-the-Counter (OTC)	Amount of Caffeine (mg)
Analgesics		
Anacin Maximum Strength	OTC	32
Cafergot	P	100
Darvon	P	32.4
Excedrin	OTC	65
Fiorinal	P	40
Stimulants		
Cafedrine	OTC	200
No-Doz	OTC	100
Menstrual Drugs		
Aqua-ban	OTC	100
Aqua-ban Plus	OTC	200
Midol	OTC	32.4
Cold Tablets		
Dristan Decongestant Tablet and Dristan-AF Tablet	OTC	16.2
Duradyne Forte	OTC	30
Chocolate and Cocoa		**Average**
Cocoa (150 mL/5 oz)		4
Chocolate milk (240 mL/8 oz)		5
Chocolate syrup (30 mL/1 oz)		4
Milk chocolate		6
Chocolate cake and frosting (1/12 of cake)		15.8
Dark, semi-sweet chocolate (30 mL/1 oz)		20
Baker's chocolate (30 mL/1 oz)		26
Coffee*		
Brewed, drip method		115
Brewed, percolator		80
Instant		65
Decaffeinated, brewed		3
Decaffeinated, instant		2
Tea		
U.S. brands, brewed		40
Imported brands, brewed		60
Instant		30
Iced (360 mL/12 oz)		70
Soft Drinks†		
Coca-Cola		45
Dr. Pepper		40
Mountain Dew		53
Pepsi		41
Diet Pepsi		38

*150 mL/5 oz.
†360 mL/12 oz.

fore age 6. A large percentage of children with ADDH respond well to psychomotor stimulants. The stimulants used most frequently are methylphenidate, dextroamphetamine, and pemoline. The stimulant is given in the morning and at lunch. Usually, the drug is given only on school days, and *drug holidays* (prescribed omission of one or more doses of medication) are used to evaluate behavioral response to the use of psychomotor stimulants. Reduced growth may occur if stimulants are used over long periods.

Narcolepsy Approximately 250,000 Americans suffer from narcolepsy. This sleep disorder results from abnormal timing of rapid eye movement (REM) sleep. The symptoms associated with narcolepsy are sleep attacks, cataplexy, sleep paralysis, and hallucinations. The sleep attack is identified by the sudden overwhelming desire to sleep, which lasts from 5 to 20 minutes. The narcoleptic patient can be doing anything at the time the sleep attack occurs with no warning. The second symptom associated with narcolepsy is *cataplexy,* a sudden loss of muscle tone that is often associated with emotions. Many times the narcoleptic patient slumps in a chair or falls to the ground during the episode of cataplexy. Sleep paralysis, another symptom of narcolepsy, is muscle paralysis that occurs during the interval between sleep and wakening. The sleep paralysis lasts for approximately 1 minute. The attack of immobility can be terminated by touch. Hallucinations are auditory or visual and, like the sleep paralysis, occur in the interval between sleep and wakening. The narcoleptic is aware of his or her environment at the time of the hallucinations. The psychomotor stimulants used to treat this disorder include methylphenidate, amphetamine, and dextroamphetamine.

ACTION

Amphetamines act by releasing catecholamines (norepinephrine) from adrenergic nerve terminals, which directly stimulates the alpha and beta receptor sites in the cerebral cortex and the reticular-activating system. By inhibiting the action of amine oxidase, mood elevation occurs. The overall effects of amphetamine are CNS and respiratory stimulation, mydriasis, bronchodilation, hypertensive response, anorexigenic effect, and contraction of the urinary bladder sphincter.

CONTRAINDICATIONS AND PRECAUTIONS

Amphetamines are contraindicated in patients with hyperthyroidism, advanced arteriosclerosis, agitated states, moderate to severe hypertension, cardiovascular disease, drug abuse, glaucoma, concurrent use or use within 14 days of administration of MAO inhibitors, and hypersensitivity to amphetamines. Most of these contraindications are based on the mechanisms of action of amphetamines, such as the release of catecholamines, the pressor effect, and the direct action on alpha and beta receptor sites in the body. Amphetamines have an abuse potential and are frequently abused with alcohol or barbiturates.

Amphetamines are used with caution in situations that require the person to be mentally alert or coordinated.

agnosis of ADDH relies on a history of inattention, impulsivity, and hyperactivity. Neurologic "soft" signs may be present, such as problems with motor coordination or perceptual difficulties. Onset of ADDH usually occurs be-

Performing hazardous activities (e.g., operating machinery, driving a car) is postponed until the peak effect of the drug has occurred or the person is adjusted to a particular dose. Amphetamines are administered cautiously to persons with hyperexcitability states or who are concurrently receiving medications that produce hyperexcitability. Amphetamines are administered with caution in elderly or debilitated patients or in those with *asthenia* (weakness). These groups of patients may require more individualized dosages of amphetamines based on their particular situations. Caution is also used when administering amphetamines to persons with psychopathic personalities or a history of suicidal or homicidal tendencies. The psychic stimulation produced by amphetamines is followed by depression and fatigue. The psychic effects of amphetamines depend on dose, mental state, and personality of the individual. When administering amphetamines to children, there may be a temporary suppression of normal weight gain and growth. Amphetamines may also aggravate motor and vocal tics.

ADVERSE REACTIONS

The number or combination of side effects the patient may experience varies considerably among patients. The following adverse effects and side effects are reported with the use of amphetamines: nervousness, irritability, talkativeness, insomnia, dizziness, headaches, increased motor activity, mydriasis, hyperexcitability, depression, hypertension, tachycardia, palpitation, cardiac dysrhythmias, nausea, anorexia, vomiting, abdominal cramping, diarrhea, constipation, dry mouth, metallic taste, and increased libido, which is related to the release of catecholamines and direct action on alpha and beta receptors. Late evening doses are avoided as nighttime insomnia may occur.

INTERACTIONS

Various drug interactions occur with amphetamines. Concurrent use of an amphetamine with guanethidine, tricyclic antidepressants, MAO inhibitors, furazoladone, phenothiazines, lithium carbonate, and sodium bicarbonate are avoided. Guanethidine is displaced from its site of action, resulting in hypotension. Sodium bicarbonate cause alkalinization of the urine, decreasing the renal excretion of amphetamines and resulting in an increase in the amphetamine effect. Tricyclic antidepressants release norepinephrine, decreasing the effects of amphetamines. An increased dose of amphetamine may be necessary. Concurrent MAO inhibitors may increase the pressor response to the amphetamines, possibly resulting in hypertensive crisis and intracranial hemorrhage. An antimicrobial with MAO inhibitor activity, furazolidone, may also cause this interaction, so combining this drug with amphetamines should be avoided. The phenothiazines and lithium carbonate cause a decreased amphetamine response. Oral dextroamphetamine–nicotine induces a dose-related increase in cigarette smoking in ''normal'' smokers. Evidence supports this premise because dextro-

amphetamine is a behavioral stimulant—it increases the rate of a variety of learned and stereotypic behaviors.

Drug-laboratory interactions also occur. These include elevated serum and urinary cortisol levels. Foods that acidify the urine (e.g., cranberry juice) can enhance the effect of amphetamines.

Refer to Table 19–1 for dosages of individual amphetamines.

○ **Amphetamine sulfate** is given before breakfast and lunch for the treatment of narcolepsy. It is administered in the morning to children with attention deficit disorders.

○ **Methamphetamine hydrochloride** (Desoxyn) is given for the treatment of attention deficit disorder and obesity.

○ **Dextroamphetamine sulfate** (Dexedrine, Oxydess II, Spancap No. 1) is used for attention deficit disorder in children and narcolepsy in both children and adults.

○ **Methylphenidate** (Ritalin) is different from the amphetamines in chemical structure, but its action is similar. It also shares the same therapeutic uses, contraindications and precautions, adverse reactions and side effects, and interactions. Methylphenidate is the drug of choice for attention deficit disorders in children and narcolepsy in adults.

○ **Pemoline** (Cylert) is similar to that of amphetamines. However, it differs from amphetamines in pharmacokinetics, pharmacodynamics, dosage, contraindications and precautions, and interactions. It is used primarily in children with ADDH, but it is not as effective as other drugs.

CONTRAINDICATIONS AND PRECAUTIONS Many of the contraindications and precautions are the same as those for amphetamines, but some differences do exist. Pemoline is not used in the following situations: hypersensitivity or idiosyncrasy to the drug; impaired hepatic function because the liver metabolizes this agent; and children under 6 years of age. Pemoline is used cautiously in children and in patients with renal dysfunction. The drug is excreted by the kidneys, leading to the accumulation of pemoline and toxicity.

INTERACTIONS Pemoline may alter the requirements of antidiabetic agents, insulin, and hypoglycemics. After several months of treatment, it may also elevate aspartate aminotransferase (AST), alanine aminotransferase (ALT), and alkaline phosphatase levels. Patients should have periodic liver function tests. If these tests are abnormal, the drug is discontinued.

NONAMPHETAMINE ANOREXIANTS

Nonamphetamine anorexiants, used to suppress the appetite, are pharmacologically similar to amphetamines. These agents—**diethylpropion (Tenuate, Tepanil), fenfluramine (Pondimin), phenmetrazine (Preludin), mazindol (Mazanor, Sanorex), phentermine (Fastin, Phentrol), benzphetamine (Didrex), dexflenfluramine (Redux),** and **phendimetrazine tartrate (Bacarate, Metra, Trimstat)**—stimulate the CNS and can elevate blood pressure. These, featured in Table 19–3, agents are also sympathomimetics. Some tolerance develops with all of these agents after

Table 19–3. NONAMPHETAMINE ANOREXIANTS

DRUG NAME/ROUTE AND DOSAGE	CSA SCHEDULE	NURSING IMPLICATIONS
phentermine hydrochloride (Fastin) (Phentrol) and many others **Adults:** 8 mg PO tid 30 min before meals or 24–30 mg 2 hr after breakfast.	Schedule IV	**ASSESSMENT:** Assess weight before administration. Assess for presence of heart disease, hypertension, glaucoma, hyperthyroidism (all contraindications). **INTERVENTION:** May produce blurred vision, insomnia. Time prescribed is usually 6–12 wk. SR tablet should not be crushed or chewed. **Patient Teaching**—Teach patient about dietary restrictions. Instruct patient to not take drug more frequently than prescribed and to not take within several hours of sleep because it causes insomnia. Tell patient to observe caution when driving. **EVALUATION:** Notify physician of palpitations, nervousness, or dizziness.
benzphetamine hydrochloride (Didrex) **Adults:** 25–50 mg PO 1–3 times daily. Give single dose mid-morning.	Schedule III	Same as for phentermine plus: **ASSESSMENT:** Assess for pregnancy (category X).
phenmetrazine hydrochloride (Preludin) **Adults:** 75 mg PO once daily.	Schedule II	Same as for phentermine.
phendimetrazine tartrate (Melfiat) (Trimstat) and many others **Adults:** 35 mg PO 2–3 times daily 1 hr before meals or 105-mg SR tablet once daily 30–60 min before breakfast. Do not exceed 70 mg tid.	Schedule III	Same as for phentermine.
diethylpropion hydrochloride (Tenuate) **Adults:** 25 mg PO tid 1 hr before meals or 75-mg SR tablet once daily midmorning.	Schedule IV	Same as for phentermine plus: **ASSESSMENT:** Assess for pregnancy (category B).
mazindol (Sanorex) **Adults:** 1 mg PO tid 1 hr before meals or 2 mg once daily.	Schedule IV	Same as for phentermine.
fenfluramine hydrochloride (Pondimin) **Adults:** 20 mg PO tid before meals. May increase dose 20 mg/day until 120 mg/day is reached.	Schedule IV	Same as for phentermine plus: **ASSESSMENT:** Assess for pregnancy (category C). **INTERVENTION:** Monitor for pulmonary hypertension, a rare adverse effect. **Patient Teaching**—Advise patients to immediately report any deterioration in exercise tolerance.
dexflenfluramine (Redux) **Adults:** 15 mg BID with meals.		Same as for phentermine plus: **INTERVENTION:** Monitor for hypertension and pulmonary hypertension. **Patient Teaching**—false positive urine tests for amphetomine can occur.

CSA = Controlled Substances Act; SR = sustained release.

a period of 6 to 12 weeks. They are not administered in pregnancy (category X), and safety in lactation and children has not been established.

STIMULANT ABUSE

Like many drugs, stimulants can be abused. Three categories of drugs are examined in this discussion of stimulant abuse: caffeine, amphetamines, and cocaine. Drug abuse is discussed in detail in Chapter 67.

The use of caffeine is so customary in most cultures that it is easy not to think of it as a drug. Caffeine appears in over-the-counter medications for pain and for allergy and cold relief, and it is contained in our favorite beverages (coffee, tea, cocoa, soft drinks) and food (chocolate) (see Table 19–2). There is probably no question that the use of caffeine is habituating and that certain symptoms result when intake of caffeine is reduced (headache, feeling of fatigue). There is a lack of evidence to support the development of tolerance to the CNS effects of caffeine. Like other drugs used to excess, caffeine can be lethal.

Amphetamines have been produced since the 1920s. Abuse of this type of drug began in the 1940s when amphetamines were present in inhalers and nasal decongestants. One appealing effect of stimulants was anorexia. Before amphetamines were removed from over-the-counter diet pills, they were a popular method of weight control. By the 1960s, the common route of administration became intravenous injection. Amphetamines are among the drugs most frequently abused by health-care professionals. When amphetamines were outlawed except for legitimate medical practice, more dangerous drug abuse was introduced.

Cocaine is one of the more commonly abused drugs today. Research suggests that approximately one million people are addicted to cocaine and that at least 15 to 21 million Americans have tried cocaine once. Cocaine was once the preferred drug for the well-to-do, sophisticated social circles. Now this recreational drug is encountered in all circles of society. The half-life of cocaine is short, and single-dose effects persist for about 2 hours. Cocaine can be used many times during the day or night. The repetitive use of cocaine has been shown to have destructive effects on the individual, family, friends, and society. Addiction to cocaine involves physical and psychologic dependence. Overdoses of cocaine can be lethal.

USING THE NURSING PROCESS

ASSESSMENT

- Obtain a complete assessment. Information to be obtained is found in Table 19–4. With patients receiving amphetamines, obtain an accurate psychologic and sociologic history and, in particular, a history of previous drug abuse. Because the amphetamines have a high abuse potential, patients who might become abusers must be identified early and monitored carefully. See Chapter 67 for further details on assessment. In female patients, determine current pregnancy and future plans for childbearing because the safety of these drugs in pregnancy has not been established. Prior to initiating amphetamine therapy in children, gather growth and development data for comparison after therapy has begun.

Narcolepsy

If amphetamines are being used to treat the patient with narcolepsy, an additional specific assessment must be made.

- When taking the patient history, make special note of seizure disorders, sleep irregularities, obesity, nervous disorders, depression, or endocrine disorders in both the patient and family.
- Obtain additional information leading up to the present illness by questioning the patient about previous head trauma, infections, and occlusive vascular disorders that may be related to the narcolepsy. The exact nature of the narcolepsy—including frequency and duration as well as regular sleep and arousal patterns—is noted.
- Obtain a history of past medications, including stimulants and inhibitory agents.
- Perform a baseline neurologic check, noting movement of the eyes, pupillary reaction and symmetry; assess motor and sensory function. Any deviations from normal are recorded.

Obesity

If amphetamines are being used to treat the patient with obesity, an additional specific assessment must be made.

- Obtain information regarding height, weight, and bone structure to determine the degree of obesity.
- Assess the diet history and ask the patient to keep a diet diary for several weeks to record information about usual patterns of intake, exercise, and activity.
- Assess the patient for physical problems including high blood pressure, cardiac irregularities, or diabetes, which may restrict the diet/drug/exercise options. A social and psychologic profile may reveal the rationale for present habits of overeating and may provide clues as to how to adjust that pattern. The patient may offer insight about why he or she overeats and what he or she feels may be the best method of weight reduction to fit his or her lifestyle.

Attention Deficit Disorder with Hyperactivity

When the patient receiving amphetamines is a child with attention deficit disorder with hyperactivity (ADDH), an additional specific assessment must be made.

- Obtain the health history, physical examination, family dynamics, and previous assessments of the child's

Table 19–4. NURSING PROCESS FOR PATIENT REQUIRING CNS STIMULANTS

Assessment

Assess mental/cognitive status, affect, and general behavior.
Note support systems, family interactions, and use of coping mechanisms.
Ascertain self-image.
Assess effects of illness/condition on lifestyle, activity/sleep.
Assess current and past drug history, including drug abuse.
Assess blood pressure, pulse, respiratory rate.

Nursing Diagnosis: Altered Thought Processes

RELATED TO: Pharmacologic effects of stimulants.
AS EVIDENCED BY: Short attention span, inability to concentrate, and restlessness.

Desired Outcomes/Evaluation Criteria

Displays usual mentation, cognitive ability, and affect with absence of adverse behaviors, e.g., restlessness, agitation, tremor, hyperactivity, insomnia, or dizziness.

Nursing Actions	Rationale
Maintain a calm, supportive environment. Reduce external stimuli (TV, radio, others talking).	Stimulation of the central nervous system is the action of these drugs. Prevention of overstimulation allows patient to focus on desired activity and may enhance intake of information.
Keep instructions, conversations, and commands simple, short, and concrete.	Sensory overload alters patient's ability to process information and respond appropriately.
Repeat information or redirect patient as necessary. Allow the patient sufficient time to answer questions or follow directions.	May experience a short attention span or have difficulty concentrating.
Observe for therapeutic or adverse response to medication.	Drug choice/dosage depends on effect of the drug.

Nursing Diagnosis: Impaired Adjustment

RELATED TO: Disability requiring change in lifestyle and impaired cognition.
AS EVIDENCED BY: Emotional outbursts, poor behavioral reports from school and parents, falling asleep during the day.

Desired Outcomes/Evaluation Criteria

Verbalizes positive attitude toward situation. Demonstrates increased interest in self-care activities.

Nursing Actions	Rationale
Encourage discussion of concerns related to disability. Active-listen to feelings.	Promotes clarification of problems and possible solutions.
Discuss expected actions of the prescribed drug.	Understanding reasons drug is being taken enhances cooperation, e.g., to prevent sleepiness in narcolepsy, to decrease appetite and complement weight-loss program, and to lengthen a hyperactive child's attention span.
Plan other activities for patient, e.g., diet and exercise, training in effective parenting skills, use of adjunct services.	Promotes nonpharmacologic solutions to problems, which can maximize the effectiveness of the drugs.

Nursing Diagnosis: Sleep Pattern Disturbance

RELATED TO: Illness, side effects of medications, intake of caffeine/other stimulant drugs.
AS EVIDENCED BY: Verbal complaints of difficulty falling asleep, falling asleep during activities, irritability, not feeling well rested.

Desired Outcomes/Evaluation Criteria

Verbalizes understanding of sleep disorder. Reports decrease in narcoleptic attacks and increased sense of well-being and feelings.

Nursing Actions	Rationale
Provide quiet environment. Administer last dose of medication before evening.	Conditions such as narcolepsy, ADDH, and high intake of caffeine or other stimulant drugs can interfere with ability to sleep. The patient with narcolepsy can drop off to sleep, but the sleep pattern is different from continual sleep at night. Also these patients may experience vivid dreams, nightmares, and hallucinations that alter the sleep pattern. The child with ADDH is constantly in motion and has great difficulty taking naps or sleeping at night. These drugs may overstimulate the CNS and may result in insomnia.
Discuss which foods/beverages contain caffeine.	A high intake of caffeine, especially when consumed during the evening/night, may interfere with ability to sleep.

Other Suggested Nursing Diagnoses: Knowledge Deficit

behavior, activity level, and school performance when the patient is to receive amphetamines for ADDH. History taking includes prenatal, perinatal, and postnatal information.

- Question the parents about maternal infection, uterine bleeding, maternal use of drugs with teratogenic effects, and difficulties during labor and delivery with this child. Answers to these questions may offer reasons for the development of ADDH. A history of the achievement of developmental tasks may indicate the sequence of development of the symptoms of ADDH. Family history may reveal a familial pattern of the syndrome.
- During the physical examination, observe for external characteristics such as enlarged thyroid and exophthalmos, which may suggest hyperthyroidism.
- Assess the child for clumsiness, motor incoordination, difficulties with right/left discrimination, and involuntary movements or tremors. Nursing observations of difficulties in reading, writing, and speaking may be validated by school performance reports from teachers and by discussion with the family. Objective and subjective data regarding behavior patterns and activity level are recorded. Family interaction patterns are assessed to give as complete a picture as possible.

Analeptic Stimulants

- Obtain a baseline assessment of the following parameters: blood pressure, heart rate, deep tendon reflexes, and oxygen and carbon dioxide levels of arterial blood when using the analeptic agents. In addition, before using the analeptics, adequacy of airway and oxygenation must be ensured.

NURSING DIAGNOSIS

- Establish the nursing diagnoses to begin planning interventions. Some typical nursing diagnoses for patients receiving CNS stimulants include Altered Thought Processes, Impaired Adjustment, Sleep Pattern Disturbance, and Knowledge Deficit.

PLANNING AND INTERVENTION

- Monitor the patient frequently for habituation, tolerance, and/or dependence. Because of the excitatory and euphoric effects of the amphetamines, they have a high abuse potential. In administering these medications, the lowest possible dose is used initially and then increased gradually. Chapter 67 describes interventions and precautions in detail. Because amphetamines may cause insomnia, the last amphetamine dose is scheduled no later than 6 hours before bedtime. The nurse instructs the patient and family to follow a similar pattern at home. If the amphetamine is not being used specifically for an anorexiant effect, anorexia and weight loss may be undesirable side effects.
- Monitor the patient's weight weekly and review intake records to make certain that adequate nutrients are being ingested.
- Teach the patient and family the importance of good nutrition; the elements of a basic, healthy diet; and the need to weigh the patient weekly, reporting weight loss to the health-care team.

Narcolepsy

- Observe the patient to identify the times of the patient's peak sleepiness when these drugs are used to

---

Table 19–5. PATIENT TEACHING INFORMATION (CHILDREN)—STIMULANT THERAPY FOR NARCOLEPSY OR ATTENTION DEFICIT DISORDER WITH HYPERACTIVITY

Dear Patient:
This drug has been prescribed for you. This is what you should know about your drug to get the most from your therapy.

☐ 1. This stimulant is taken to improve your attention span, decrease your excessive activity, *or* decrease your sleep attacks (narcolepsy).
☐ 2. This stimulant may be ordered by your doctor for you to take for several years. There will be days you will not take the drug. The drug may be ordered to take on school days. Over the weekend or during vacation you may not take the drug. It is very important to read the directions on the label to know when to take the medication (attention deficit disorder). If you have narcolepsy, you will be taking the drug daily.
☐ 3. Take this drug as ordered by the doctor. Take this drug 30 to 45 minutes prior to meals. Try not to take this drug after 4:00 PM because it might interfere with your sleep at night.
☐ 4. Avoid taking other drugs unless you tell your doctor.
☐ 5. Always check with your doctor or pharmacist before taking over-the-counter drugs for colds, pain, allergy, upset stomach, or obesity.
☐ 6. Do not stop your drug unless directed by your doctor.
☐ 7. If you forget a dose of your drug, eliminate that dose. Do not try to catch up by taking two doses at once.
☐ 8. If you experience any side effects from your drug, notify your doctor. Side effects can include the following: altered mood, dizziness, irritability, restlessness, the shakes (tremor), inability to sleep, headache, seizures, fast heart rate, high blood pressure, palpitations, loss of appetite, stomach pains, dry mouth, unpleasant taste, and itching skin. Keep a written record of the side effects that you have and time of day.
☐ 9. Loss of appetite and weight loss may be common the first 3 weeks of starting this drug.
☐ 10. Obtain a weekly height and weight and keep a record of this to show your doctor.
☐ 11. Limit the intake of coffee, tea, cocoa, chocolate, and caffeinated soft drinks. They can increase the side effects.
☐ 12. Good mouth care and rinsing of the mouth can decrease the dry mouth and/or bad taste in your mouth.
☐ 13. If you are a diabetic, stimulants can change your requirements for insulin or oral hypoglycemic drug.
☐ 14. Store in a tight, light-resistant container out of the reach of other children.

Table 19–6. PATIENT TEACHING INFORMATION (ADULTS)—STIMULANT THERAPY FOR NARCOLEPSY

Dear Patient:
This drug has been prescribed for you. This is what you should know about your drug to get the most from your therapy.

☐ 1. This stimulant is taken to diminish your sleep attacks.
☐ 2. This stimulant may be ordered by your doctor for you to take for several years. Please read the directions on the label for the frequency of taking the drug.
☐ 3. Take this drug as ordered, usually 30–45 minutes before meals. Try taking your last dose prior to the evening hours. Stimulants can interfere with sleeping at night.
☐ 4. Avoid taking other drugs unless you tell your doctor.
☐ 5. Always check with your doctor or pharmacist before taking over-the-counter medications for colds, pain, allergy, upset stomach, or obesity.
☐ 6. Do not stop your drug unless so directed by your doctor.
☐ 7. If you forget a dose of your drug, eliminate that dose. Do not try to catch up by taking two doses at one time.
☐ 8. If you have any side effects from your drug, call your doctor. Side effects include the following: altered mood, dizziness, irritability, restlessness, the shakes (tremor), inability to sleep, headache, seizures, fast heart rate, high blood pressure, palpitations, loss of appetite, stomach pain, dry mouth, unpleasant taste, and itching skin. Keep a written record of your side effects.
☐ 9. Loss of appetite and weight loss may be common the first 3 weeks of starting this drug.
☐ 10. Limit the intake of coffee, tea, cocoa, chocolate, and caffeinated soft drinks. They can increase the side effects.
☐ 11. This drug does not replace the body's requirement of rest and sleep.
☐ 12. Good mouth care and rinsing your mouth can decrease a dry mouth or bad taste in your mouth.
☐ 13. If you are a diabetic, stimulants can change your requirements for insulin or oral hypoglycemic drugs.
☐ 14. Store this drug in a tight, light-resistant container out of the reach of children.

treat narcolepsy. Doses of the amphetamine are scheduled to coincide with these times to achieve maximum therapeutic effect.

- Provide a varied and interesting daily routine, using available diversions such as recreational therapy and volunteer visitors to decrease the possibility of narcoleptic attacks.
- Teach the patient to avoid monotony and boring routines at home and at work that are likely to precipitate narcoleptic attacks.
- Teach the patient to avoid shift work and frequent air travel because both can precipitate more frequent attacks. There is some indication that obesity contributes to narcolepsy. If the narcoleptic patient is obese, a sensible program of diet and exercise is initiated by the nurse and patient and is continued at home on a regular basis. Because narcolepsy may present serious social problems, compromising the patient's ability to interact as a family member or to perform at work, the nurse may refer the patient for personal counseling. Additional patient teaching for narcolepsy can be found in Tables 19–5 and 19–6.

Obesity

- Teach the patient that amphetamines used as anorexiants are one-third of the plan, which also includes diet and exercise. This information is shared with the patient, who needs to understand that the medication alone does not produce long-lasting results.
- Help the patient to establish a realistic weight-loss goal. Reinforcement of the weight-loss plan is important for compliance.
- Monitor the patient's daily diet and exercise habits and observe for drug response.
- Weigh the patient weekly and provide verbal support and encouragement during the weight-loss program. Take into account the patient's normal dietary pat-

terns and schedule drug administration accordingly. Because amphetamines suppress appetite for a limited time (they peak in 1 hour), doses are scheduled 30 to 90 minutes before meals. If the patient skips a meal, it is senseless to take the amphetamine prior to that meal. If needed, refer the patient for behavior modification and personal counseling to enhance the weight-loss plan.

Attention Deficit Disorder with Hyperactivity

- Inform the family that the CNS stimulants are therapeutic in every case, but that a clinical trial of several weeks with dosages adjusted by the physician should clearly indicate whether the drug benefits the child with ADDH. Teaching of the family assumes major importance (see Table 19–5). Use of the drug may enhance peer relationships, the child's self-image, and the child's ability to find satisfaction in learning.
- Instruct the parents that the drug is not a panacea but improves the child's ability to pay attention and to be more physically coordinated. The nurse, family, and other health-team members may identify a need for adjunct services to deal with related problems. These adjunct services include family and personal counseling, psychologic testing and evaluation, and special education classes. The nurse and physician, along with the family, may plan for drug-free holidays. These holidays should fall on weekends or school vacations and should allow time to evaluate the effectiveness of and continued need for the drug. Scientific literature indicates that habituation and dependence do not occur in children when amphetamines are used for treatment of ADDH. Reasons cited for this exception include the finding that children under the age of 11 or 12 do not view medications as desirable and that therapy usually ceases before adolescence,

when a child might tend to experiment with excessive dosages and abuse the drug.

Caffeine

- Educate the patient about the implications of caffeine intake, because caffeine is a substance that is ingested in large quantities through foodstuffs and over-the-counter (OTC) medications in the United States. In providing care for the patient with gastritis or ulcers, teach the patient to substitute other beverages in the meal plans.
- Caution the patient to decrease caffeine intake slowly, because abrupt cessation may result in withdrawal symptoms. Because caffeine may adversely affect the cardiovascular system of some patients with heart disease and hypertension, explore ways of modifying caffeine intake with these patients as well. Many OTC products containing caffeine are ingested to provide pep and to perk up a sleepy or tired person. If the patient's history indicates a pattern of caffeine use for this reason, teach the patient the importance of adequate rest and sleep.
- Stress the fact that caffeine is never used as a substitute for sleep. Excess ingestion of caffeine-containing products such as chocolate, colas and other soft drinks, and cocoa has been implicated in hyperactivity and behavioral problems in children. Until this research is refined, counsel parents to limit the intake of such snacks, replacing them with fruit juices and "natural" snacks and using carob as a replacement for chocolate flavor.

EVALUATION

- Determine the effectiveness of CNS stimulants.
- Evaluate the adverse effects of the CNS stimulants.

Patient compliance with amphetamine therapy can be increased by stressing the need for continued health-care follow-up and by periodic review of health teaching and treatment goals.

- Evaluate overcompliance or abuse of amphetamines, as well as signs of developing tolerance, habituation, or dependence. Patients receiving long-term amphetamine therapy may develop psychiatric syndromes, which can be evidenced by increasing irritability, paranoia, or frank psychosis.
- Evaluate the patient for signs of noncompliance or withdrawal. When high-dose amphetamines are prescribed, withdrawal symptoms include headache, difficulty breathing, sensations of hot and cold, muscle cramps, and gastrointestinal cramps. The patient may also experience a paradoxic situation in which incredible hunger is coupled with an inability to eat, which is caused by muscular weakness. The patient may also act out aggressive impulses; may be irritable and demanding; and may experience fatigue, anxiety, nightmares, and suicidal ideation.
- Continually stress the need for regular follow-up and periodically review all previously taught material to ensure that the patient's knowledge base remains accurate.

The bibliography for this chapter can be found in Appendix B, which begins on page 1054.

CHAPTER REVIEW QUESTIONS*

1. Central nervous system stimulants produce their pharmacologic action by:
   a. Decreasing the effect of excitatory neurotransmission.
   b. Increasing or stimulating inhibitory neurotransmission.
   c. Enhancing the uptake of catecholamines at adrenergic synapses.
   d. Modifying neurotransmitter response by altering cAMP.

2. When administering amphetamines, which statement is correct?
   a. The use of amphetamines for weight loss is safe for 3–4 months.
   b. When treating narcolepsy, amphetamines are administered before breakfast and lunch.
   c. With attention deficit disorder, administered at bedtime.
   d. With obesity, administered in morning.

3. Jane is going home on anorexiants for weight reduction. What information is included in her teaching?
   a. Take these products 6 hours before bedtime.
   b. Anorexiants are helpful taken when a meal will be skipped.

   c. Anorexiants can safely be administered to patients with cardiovascular disease and hypertension.
   d. Sustained-release products can be taken at dinnertime.

4. Which of the following statements is *correct* with regard to drug interactions with amphetamines?
   a. Sodium bicarbonate increases the amphetamine effect by altering renal excretion of amphetamine.
   b. The use of amphetamines with guanethidine results in severe hypertension.
   c. The use of phenothiazines causes an exaggerated amphetamine response.
   d. Tricyclic antidepressants increase the effects of amphetamines.

5. Caffeine produces all of the following actions *except*:
   a. Exerting a positive chronotropic effect.
   b. Stimulating pepsin secretion.
   c. Depressing the cerebral cortex.
   d. Decreasing reabsorption of sodium.

*See Appendix A, which begins on page 1051, for answers.

Agents Used to Treat Seizure Disorders

Merrily A. Kuhn, RNC, PhD

CHAPTER OUTLINE

KEY TERMS

Absence seizure	Morbilliform
Aphasia	Postictal period
Aura	Scarlatiniform
Convulsion	Seizure
Ictal period	Stevens-Johnson syndrome

LEARNING OBJECTIVES

After reading this chapter, the student will be able to:

1. Identify those medications commonly used to control and treat seizures.
2. Differentiate among the antiseizure drugs as to mechanism of action, route of administration, pharmacokinetics, adverse effects, contraindications and precautions, and interactions.
3. Identify specific areas to assess in the patient requiring antiseizure medication to formulate appropriate patient outcomes.
4. Plan the nursing interventions necessary to administer anticonvulsants and choose appropriate teaching strategies to gain patient compliance.
5. Evaluate the patient at various stages of treatment to measure the effect of nursing interventions on antiseizure therapy.

Epilepsy is a group of neurologic disorders that has as its hallmark recurring seizures. A *seizure* is a sudden, uncontrolled burst of neuronal firing is a symptom of central nervous system (CNS) dysfunction. The seizure process starts with synchronous, high-frequency discharge from a group of neurons, called a focus. If the electrical activity from the discharge is not inhibited, it spreads to other areas in the brain by recruiting other neurons to also discharge. The abnormal spread of electrical activity causes a variety of signs and symptoms, including *convulsions* (paroxysms of involuntary muscular contractions and relaxations). No two seizures are alike.

The publisher gratefully acknowledges the contribution of Barbara K. Clark, RN, MN, CCRN, to the third edition.

Approximately 1% of the population in the United States has epilepsy. It is the second most common neurologic disorder after cerebrovascular accident. Epilepsy can affect any age population and occur at any time. Epilepsy may be a result of birth trauma or an inherent imbalance in CNS activities. However, late onset in adults may indicate the development of a cerebral tumor or other organic brain disease. Approximately 80% of persons with epilepsy are controlled with antiseizure medications, but there are 500,000 people in the United States with uncontrolled epilepsy.

CLASSIFICATION OF SEIZURES

Seizures can be classified by cause or by seizure type. Seizures that do not have an identifiable cause are called

Table 20–1. EPILEPTIC SEIZURE CLASSIFICATIONS

Seizure Classification	Age	Clinical Characteristics

Generalized Seizures (Convulsive or Nonconvulsive)
A. Absence seizures (petit mal seizures)
   1. Atypical absence seizure
   Duration: 10–30 sec
	Onset usually occurs between 4 and 8 yrs; rarely occurs before age 3 or after age 15	An absence attack is an abrupt, brief loss of consciousness, amnesia, or unawareness characterized by staring and a 3-sec spike-and-wave pattern in the EEG, which may be associated with mild clonic movements (eye-blinking, jerking movements), automatisms, or changes in postural tone. No postictal or confused state follows attack. May occur as frequently as 50–100 times a day.

B. Myoclonic seizures Duration: 1–5 sec	Late childhood, adolescence	Single or multiple sudden, brief, shocklike contractions may be generalized or confined to the face and trunk or to one or more extremities. Many cases of myoclonic jerks and action myoclonus are not classified as epileptic seizures.
C. Clonic seizures Duration: few seconds	Early childhood	Clonic seizures are characterized by repetitive clonic jerks that lack a tonic component. Clonic jerks may be symmetrical, asymmetrical, rhythmic, or dysrrhythmic; these seizures are relatively rare.
D. Tonic seizures Duration: 10 sec	Any age	Tonic contraction of certain muscle groups is accompanied by altered consciousness, but there is no progression to clonic phase. Ocular phenomena are common and include fixation of the eyes, eyelid retraction, superior ocular deviation, nystagmus, and mydriasis. Autonomic signs include tachycardia, hypertension, respiratory distress, and capillary restriction with cyanosis. Seizures are usually activated by sleep.
E. Tonic-clonic seizures Duration: 2–5 min	Any age	These types of seizures are the most commonly encountered primary and secondary generalized seizures and can occur at any age. While some patients experience a vague aura, the majority lose consciousness without premonitory signs. Seizures begin with a sudden tonic contraction of muscles (if the respiratory muscle is affected, there is stridor); the patient falls to the ground and remains rigid (10–30 sec). The tonic phase gives way to the clonic phase (30–50 sec), and muscle relaxation interrupts tonic contraction. Muscle tone returns in rhythmic flexor spasms, which become less frequent as the seizure subsides. Following this, the patient remains unconscious for variable periods. Urinary and fecal incontinence may occur in the clonic phase.
F. Atonic seizures Duration: 10–30 sec	Infants and children	Sudden reduction of muscle tone may selectively affect muscle groups leading to head drop with slackening of the jaw, the dropping of a limb, or loss of all muscle tone, leading to a slumping to the ground. When attacks are brief, they are called drop attacks. Other conditions, such as narcolepsy-cataplexy syndrome and brain stem ischemia, also cause drop attacks.

Partial Seizures (Focal Seizures)
A. Simple partial seizures
   1. With motor symptoms
   2. With somatosensory or special sensory symptoms
   3. With autonomic symptoms
   4. With psychic symptoms
   Duration: 1–2 min
	Most commonly occurs in older children and adults	Consciousness usually is not impaired. Paroxysmal attacks are limited to functional disturbances of sensory, motor, and/or autonomic nerves and to anatomic regions of the brain, depending on the particular cortical area of involvement. Seizures with motor (Jacksonian seizure) and special sensory symptoms (odor, taste) are most common.

B. Complex partial seizures
   1. Simple partial onset followed by impairment of consciousness
   2. With impairment of consciousness at onset
   Duration: minutes
	Any age	Daily episodes of impaired consciousness (e.g., amnesia, unresponsiveness), usually characterized by brief (1–2 min) loss of contact with environment. Clinical manifestations are varied; they most commonly consist of automatisms (e.g., staring, chewing movements or smacking of lips, bizarre purposeless motor or psychic performances, mumbled speech or unintelligible sounds). Confusion may persist for 1–2 min after attack subsides. The EEG is helpful for diagnosis because unusual variants of this disorder may be extremely difficult to distinguish from purely functional psychiatric disorders.

Table 20–1. EPILEPTIC SEIZURE CLASSIFICATIONS, *Continued*

Seizure Classification	Age	Clinical Characteristics

C. Partial seizures evolving to secondarily generalized seizures
  1. Simple partial seizures evolving to generalized seizures
  2. Complex partial seizures evolving to generalized seizures
  3. Simple partial seizures evolving to complex partial seizures evolving to generalized seizures
  Duration: minutes
	Any age	On occasion, partial seizures may spread and become generalized tonic-clonic seizures.

Unclassified Epileptic Seizures Duration: 10–30 sec	Neonate	Inadequate data for classification. This category includes some neonatal seizures (e.g., rhythmic eye movements, chewing, and swimming movements).

idiopathic or primary seizures. Idiopathic seizures often start in childhood or adolescence. With symptomatic or secondary seizures, the cause can be determined: congenital defects, hypoxia at birth, head injury, brain tumors, CNS infections or abscesses, vascular insufficiency, substance abuse, metabolic causes (e.g., electrolyte and glucose imbalances, hypoxia, vitamin deficiencies), and drug interactions. The Commission of Classification and Terminology of the International League against Epilepsy classifies epilepsy into two broad groups: partial seizures and generalized seizures, featured in Table 20–1. Partial (focal) seizures are localized to one area of the brain, whereas generalized seizures involve both cerebral hemispheres of the brain. Each seizure is a single event.

OVERVIEW OF ANTISEIZURE DRUGS

Antiseizure drugs (or anticonvulsants) possess the ability to depress abnormal neural discharges in the CNS. The antiseizure drugs discussed in this chapter include the hydantoins (phenytoin, mephenytoin, and ethotoin), the barbiturates (phenobarbital), the succinimides (ethosuximide, methsuximide, and phensuximide), the benzodiazepines (clorazepate and diazepam), the oxazolidinediones (paramethadione and trimethadione), and the miscellaneous agents (carbamazepine, primidone, valproic acid, gabapentin, lamotrigine, and felbamate). Magnesium sulfate, used to prevent or control preeclamptic and eclamptic seizures, is reviewed in Chapter 48.

ACTION

Antiseizure drugs influence seizure activity in two ways: (1) by suppressing the focus of neuronal discharge so excessive discharge is reduced or abolished and (2) by preventing the spread of neural excitation. This is often referred to as the "neuronal membrane stabilizing effect."

These actions modify sodium, calcium, and potassium ion transport, which stabilizes the cell membrane.

The exact mechanisms of drug action are unknown, but gamma-aminobutyric acid (GABA) is involved. Some of the therapeutic agents used to treat epilepsy enhance the GABA-mediated inhibitory system (clonazepam, diazepam, felbamate, phenobarbital, valproic acid) by influencing chloride ion influx through chloride channels, leading to greater inhibition of the postsynaptic neuron. Lamotrigine, phenytoin, and carbamazepine block voltage-dependent sodium channels, resulting in decreased release of stimulating neurotransmitters such as glutamate. A new agent being evaluated—progabide, gamma-vinyl GABA (Vigabatrin)—boosts GABA-mediated inhibition. Others, such as eterobarb (an agent similar to phenobarbital in action) and stirpentol (an ethylene alcohol), are showing promise in clinical trials.

Other neurotransmitter defects may exist in epilepsy. Enkephalin, a pain-relieving neuropeptide found in the pituitary gland, brain, and gastrointestinal tract, may be involved in absence seizures (a type of generalized seizure; see Table 20–1). In an *absence seizure*, the person experiences an abrupt, brief loss of consciousness, amnesia, or unawareness.

DRUG SELECTION

When selecting an antiseizure agent, many factors are considered: seizure type; the patient's medical history, age, sex, occupation, fatigue and stress levels; cost of medications; ingestion of large quantities of caffeine and/or alcohol; and patient acceptance of the treatment plan. Successful treatment includes consideration of the quality of the patient's life. The goal of pharmacotherapy is to reduce or eliminate seizures with minimal side effects.

Generally, therapy is started with an appropriate dose for the patient's age and weight. Loading doses of the medications are usually necessary only with acute seizures or frequent attacks. To evaluate the effectiveness of

Table 20–2. DRUGS FOR TREATMENT OF SEIZURE DISORDERS

Seizure Type	Drug of Choice	Alternative
Absence (petit mal)	Ethosuximide Valproic acid	Clonazepam Lamotrigine
Atypical absence Myoclonic Atonic	Valproic acid	Clonazepam Felbamate (as adjunct)
Primary generalized tonic-clonic	Valproic acid Carbamazepine Phenytoin	Lamotrigine Primidone Phenobarbital
Partial, including secondary generalized	Carbamazepine Phenytoin Valproic acid	Primidone Phenobarbital Lamotrigine (as adjunct) Gabapentin (as adjunct)

therapy, a serum drug level is obtained when the steady state for that particular medication is reached.

The trend for the selection of antiseizure agents is in the direction of monotherapy. A growing number of neurologists are selecting carbamazepine for women and for children over 5 years of age because it does not cause coarsening of facial features, hirsutism, or gingival hyperplasia. Phenobarbital is used initially in children under 5 years of age. The long-term use of phenobarbital in young children is being reexamined because of the evidence that phenobarbital affects cognitive ability in children and adults.

Drugs that are effective in absence seizures include ethosuximide, valproic acid, and clonazepam. If seizures remain uncontrolled, a second agent is added to the therapy. Combination therapy is more difficult to manage because of drug interactions. Table 20–2 lists the recommended drugs of choice and alternative drugs for generalized and partial seizures.

Nonepileptic Seizures

Nonepileptic seizures include febrile seizures, seizures caused by drug withdrawal, and seizures induced by trauma. Phenobarbital is the agent of choice for febrile seizures. It is given in doses that produce a serum level of 15 μg/mL. Children between the ages of 3 months and 3 years are at risk for a febrile seizure. There is a fever but no evidence of neurologic origin. These children are at a higher risk of having another febrile seizure (30% to 40%) and a slightly increased risk of epilepsy. Seizure prophylaxis is not routinely instituted unless a neurologic origin is determined: febrile seizures lasting longer than 15 minutes with transient or persistent neurologic deficit; genetic origin of febrile seizures in a sibling or parent; and seizures in very young children, who have the highest risk of recurrence.

Phenobarbital or benzodiazepines are used to relieve the signs and symptoms of drug withdrawal syndrome in persons who are physically dependent on barbiturates, alcohol, benzodiazepines, and nonbarbiturate-nonbenzodiazepine antianxiety and hypnotic drugs. The selection of the antiseizure agent depends on the cause.

Data are inconclusive on the effectiveness of antiseizure drug therapy in the treatment of post-traumatic seizures. Patients who may benefit from therapy fall into four groups: (1) those with penetrating head injuries, (2) those with closed head injuries with neurologic deficit and abnormal electroencephalogram (EEG), (3) those with closed head injury with coma lasting longer than 3 hours, and (4) those with a family history of seizures or a history of abnormal delivery or febrile seizures in childhood.

Status Epilepticus

Status epilepticus occurs when seizures are repeated so frequently that the person does not regain his or her pre-seizure state. There are a variety of reasons why a person experiences status epilepticus: noncompliance, abrupt withdrawal of antiseizure medication, withdrawal of alcohol or other drugs, fever, metabolic-induced deficiencies (hypoglycemia, hypocalcemia, hyponatremia), and deficits of neurologic origin (stroke, meningitis, head injury).

The treatment for status epilepticus is immediate drug therapy and supportive care. The supportive care is directed at maintaining a patent airway, providing ventilatory support if needed, establishing an intravenous route for administering drugs, and ensuring patient safety. After obtaining a serum sample for glucose, a 50-mL bolus of 50% dextrose is given. Drug selection varies, but intravenous diazepam is usually the drug of choice. Lorazepam (Ativan) is being used more frequently because of its longer duration of action. A loading dose of phenytoin is usually given intravenously as well. If seizures continue despite drug therapy, general anesthesia is used. See Table 20–3 for information about parenteral therapy for status epilepticus.

MONITORING DRUG CONCENTRATIONS

Measuring the drug concentration in plasma can help in the overall management of the patient. There is a relationship between the serum concentration of an antiseizure drug and its therapeutic effect. This measurement is especially helpful with initial dosage adjustment, use of multiple agents, providing an index of patient compliance, and monitoring toxicity. Because serum values vary from different institutions and laboratories, as well as among patients, the therapeutic range should serve only as a guideline. It is important to treat the patient and not just the drug level. The most important issue is to maintain a steady plasma level. The enteric-coated capsules and controlled-release products assist with steady plasma levels.

Two pharmacokinetic factors are important when examining drug levels and drug interactions. One factor is the administration of carbamazepine. After about two weeks of administration, carbamazepine induces hepatic enzymes that are then responsible for the carbamazepine's own biotransformation and enhanced excretion. Usually an increase in the dosage of the drug is required.

Table 20–3. PARENTERAL THERAPY FOR STATUS EPILEPTICUS	
Drug	**Dosage/Route**
Diazepam (Valium)	**Intravenous:** *Adults,* 5–10 mg given at a rate of 1 mL (5 mg)/min, repeated at 5–10 minute intervals (maximum, 30 mg). This dose may be repeated in 2 to 4 hours if necessary. For intravenous drip, diazepam 100 mg is diluted in 500 mL of 5% dextrose in water and given at a rate of 40 mL/hr to maintain a serum concentration of 0.2–0.8 μg/mL. *Children 5 years or older,* 1 mg every 2–5 min (maximum, 10 mg), repeated in 2–4 hours if necessary. *Infants over 30 days and children under 5 years,* 0.2–0.5 mg every 2–5 min (maximum, 5 mg).
Lorazepam (Ativan)	**Intravenous:** *Adults,* although no dosage or rate of administration has been firmly established, 4 mg given at a rate of 1 mL (2 mg)/min has been effective. This dose can be repeated at 10-min intervals if needed. *Children,* experience is limited.
Phenytoin (Dilantin)	**Intravenous:** *Adults and children,* a loading dose of 15–18 mg/kg undiluted is administered at a rate not to exceed 50 mg/min. (Pediatric loading dose also may be calculated on the basis of 250 mg/m² given at a rate of 1–2 mg/kg per min.) An additional 5 mg/kg is given after 12 hr. With either regimen, therapeutic serum concentrations are between 10 and 25 μg/mL at 24 hr in most patients. Phenytoin should be administered in an intensive care unit so that heart rate, blood pressure, and ECG activity can be monitored.
Phenobarbital	**Intravenous, Intramuscular:** *Adults,* the loading dose is 5–10 mg/kg. One fifth of the total dose given intravenously undiluted at a rate of less than 50 mg/min every 5–10 min helps to prevent respiratory depression. If the patient has previously been given phenytoin without success or an unknown serum level of phenobarbital is present, 2 mg/kg of phenobarbital should be administered intravenously every 15 min until adequate response is obtained, hypotension and/or respiratory depression develops, or a cumulative dose of 1 g/24 hr has been given. IV administration is preferred, but IM administration may be used if necessary, the initial dose is 3–5 mg/kg. *Children,* 10–15 mg/kg. One fifth of total dose given intravenously undiluted at a rate of less than 50 mg/min every 5–10 min helps to prevent respiratory depression. Dosage is adjusted to maintain serum concentration of 15–40 μg/mL. If patient had previously been given phenytoin without success or an unknown serum level of phenobarbital is present, a dose of 2 mg/kg of phenobarbital should be administered intravenously every 15 min until an adequate response is obtained or hypotension and/or respiratory depression develops. IV administration is preferred, but IM administration may be used if necessary; the initial dose is 3–5 mg/kg. *Neonates,* the loading dose is 15–20 mg/kg.

The degree of autoinduction is variable. Autoinduction contributes to drug interactions. The second factor to consider is related to the biotransformation of phenytoin, which involves dose-dependent kinetics. As the metabolism of phenytoin approaches saturation, even small dosage increases may cause unexpected toxicity as a result of disproportionately large increases in the serum concentration and half-life of the drug. Also, the biotransformation of phenytoin can be inhibited by a number of drugs, causing phenytoin toxicity. Table 20–4 shows therapeutic serum concentration ranges and signs and symptoms associated with elevated serum concentrations for commonly used antiseizure drugs.

ADVERSE EFFECTS

Drowsiness is a common adverse reaction caused by all antiseizure medications. It may be transient or long term, depending on the drug. If single daily doses of the antiseizure agent are used, drowsiness may be managed by giving the dose at bedtime. If multiple daily doses are being used, drowsiness may be managed by giving the largest dose at bedtime.

Behavioral and cognitive disturbances associated with antiseizure medications may be seen in children. These disturbances include hyperactivity, disrupted sleep, irritability, and emotional liability. The development of behavioral disturbances may be more readily apparent and easily attributed to the antiseizure medications. These problems are most commonly associated with phenobarbital use and tend to be idiosyncratic but not dose-related. Other anticonvulsants may cause either idiosyncratic or dose-related behavioral disturbances. Carbamazepine and valproic acid seem to be relatively free of many of these adverse neuropsychologic effects and thus are the preferred anticonvulsants in children.

Teratogenic effects are associated with both epilepsy itself and the perinatal use of most of the antiseizure medications. See the Use in Pregnancy section for additional information.

The estrogen and progesterone components of oral contraceptives may be metabolized more rapidly in a patient whose hepatic enzymes have been induced by an antiseizure drug. Some women have become pregnant because of this interaction; breakthrough bleeding may be a sign that the oral contraceptive is not providing adequate coverage. Alternative methods of contraception may be necessary in these patients (Steiner, 1994).

Use In Pregnancy

Women of childbearing age who are receiving antiseizure drugs should be informed that there is a risk of congenital malformation in their children. The chance of bearing a normal child is greater than 90%, but the risk for producing a child with birth defects is approximately 7%, com-

Table 20–4. COMMONLY USED ANTISEIZURE DRUGS—SERUM CONCENTRATIONS AND SIGNS AND SYMPTOMS OF TOXICITY

Drug	Signs and Symptoms Usually Associated with Elevated Serum Concentrations or Toxicity	Usual Therapeutic Serum Concentration Range (μg/mL)
Carbamazepine (Tegretol)	Vertigo, lethargy, nystagmus, blurred vision, diplopia, confusion, ataxia, stupor	4–12
Clonazepam (Klonopin)	Sedation, confusion, slurred speech, somnolence, respiratory depression, coma, hypotension	0.02–0.08
Ethosuximide (Zarontin)	Nausea, vomiting, gastric distress, drowsiness, ataxia	40–100
Felbamate (Felbatol)	Fatigue, headache, somnolence, nausea, vomiting	No value established
Gabapentin (Neurontin)	Slurred speech, drowsiness, lethargy	No value established
Lamotrigine (Lamictal)	Rash, dizziness, headache	No value established
Phenobarbital	Sedation, drowsiness, slurred speech, nystagmus, confusion, somnolence, ataxia, respiratory depression, coma, hypotension	15–40
Primidone (Mysoline)	Same as phenobarbital	5–12
Phenytoin (Dilantin)	Vertigo, ataxia, slurred speech, nystagmus, diplopia, somnolence, coma (dysrhythmias with rapid intravenous administration)	5–20
Valproic acid (Depakene, Depakote)	Sedation, gastric disturbance, diarrhea, ataxia, somnolence, coma	50–150

pared with the 2% to 3% for the general population. It is difficult to determine the exact cause(s), but the birth defects could be due to the effects of repeated seizures, to the teratogenic effects of antiseizure agents, or to genetic factors. The common malformations are cleft lip and/or palate and congenital heart disease. Trimethadione is a very potent teratogen; birth defects or spontaneous abortions have occurred in 90% of fetuses exposed to this agent in utero. Spina bifida has been reported with the use of valproic acid. Most of the congenital malformations have occurred with the use of phenytoin or phenobarbital, either used alone or concurrently. This may be due to the fact that these two agents are used most frequently. The pattern of some of the abnormalities has been referred to as the "fetal hydantoin syndrome" or the "fetal barbiturate syndrome." These syndromes are discussed later in the chapter.

It is recommended that antiseizure agents not be discontinued during pregnancy. With abrupt discontinuation, the risk of status epilepticus is greater, and dangerous outcomes for both mother and fetus may occur. Serum concentrations of antiseizure drugs tend to decrease during pregnancy. Drug levels must be monitored frequently and the dosage adjusted when necessary. Monitoring is continued for about 6 weeks in the postpartum period.

Antiseizure agents can cause a vitamin K deficiency, leading to the depression of clotting factors and the potential for hemorrhage. This is the greatest risk for mothers who receive phenobarbital, primidone, or phenytoin during pregnancy. Fetal monitoring is used during labor, and bleeding can be prevented by the administration of vitamin K (phytonadione).

INTERACTIONS

Antiseizure agents have a high potential for drug interactions for three main reasons. The first reason is that many of the antiseizure agents are enzyme inducers and/or inhibitors of hepatic microsomal enzymes involved in biotransformation. If they are enzyme inducers, they stimulate the synthesis of new drug-metabolizing enzymes in the liver, and the new drug is metabolized at a faster rate. Enzyme inhibitors act the opposite way and cause drugs to compete with each other. Some drugs may be toxic to enzymes and inhibit their activity. Alternatively, the drug may bind to enzymes, inhibiting their actions. The second reason is that antiseizure medications alter the protein binding of other anticonvulsants used in combination for mixed epilepsies. The last reason for a high potential for drug interaction is the fact that antiseizure agents are administered over long periods. The end result is that the drug interactions can cause toxicity or reduce the therapeutic effectiveness of the drug. It is critical that the patient be monitored for signs and symptoms of toxicity and that the serum concentration of the drug also be monitored (see Table 20–4). Table 20–5 identifies some antiseizure drug-drug interactions.

Table 20–5. SOME ANTISEIZURE DRUG INTERACTIONS*

Interacting Drugs	Adverse Effects (Probable Mechanism)	Comments and Recommendations
Carbamazepine with: Phenytoin	Decreased carbamazepine effect (increased metabolism) Altered phenytoin effect (mechanism not established)	Monitor carbamazepine and phenytoin concentrations both increased and decreased phenytoin concentrations have been reported.
Primidone	Decreased primidone effect and increased phenobarbital effect (increased conversion of primidone to phenobarbital)	Monitor primidone and phenobarbital concentrations.
Valproic acid	Decreased valproic acid effect (increased metabolism)	Monitor valproic acid concentration.
Clonazepam with: Phenobarbital	Decreased clonazepam effect (increased metabolism)	Monitor clonazepam concentration.
Phenytoin	Decreased clonazepam effect (increased metabolism) Variable effect on phenytoin concentration (mechanism not established)	Monitor clonazepam and phenytoin concentrations.
Valproic acid	Clonazepam may precipitate absence status (mechanism not established)	Avoid concurrent use.
Diazepam with: Valproic acid	Increased IV diazepam effect (displacement from binding and decreased metabolism)	Use IV diazepam with caution.
Ethosuximide with: Valproic acid	Possible increased ethosuximide effect (decreased metabolism)	Highly variable, clinical significance not established; monitor ethosuximide concentration.
Phenobarbital with: Clonazepam	Decreased clonazepam effect (increased metabolism)	Monitor clonazepam concentration.
Valproic acid	Increased phenobarbital effect (decreased metabolism)	Monitor phenobarbital concentration.
Phenytoin with: Clonazepam	Decreased clonazepam effect (increased metabolism) Variable effect on phenytoin concentration (mechanism not established)	Monitor clonazepam and phenytoin concentrations.
Primidone	Decreased primidone effect and increased phenobarbital effect (increased conversion of primidone to phenobarbital)	Monitor primidone and phenobarbital concentrations.
Valproic acid	Increased phenytoin toxicity (displacement from binding)	Conflicting reports; monitor phenytoin concentration and clinical status.
Primidone with: Carbamazepine	Decreased primidone effect and increased phenobarbital effect (increased conversion of primidone to phenobarbital).	Monitor primidone and phenobarbital concentrations.
Phenytoin	Decreased primidone effect and increased phenobarbital effect (increased conversion of primidone to phenobarbital).	Monitor primidone and phenobarbital concentrations.
Valproic acid with: Carbamazepine	Decreased valproic acid effect (increased metabolism).	Monitor valproic acid concentration.

Continued on the following page

Table 20–5. SOME ANTISEIZURE DRUG INTERACTIONS*, *Continued*

Interacting Drugs	Adverse Effects (Probable Mechanism)	Comments and Recommendations
Clonazepam	Clonazepam may precipitate absence status (mechanism not established).	Avoid concurrent use.
Diazepam	Increased IV diazepam effect (displacement from binding and decreased metabolism).	Give IV diazepam with caution.
Ethosuximide	Possible increased ethosuximide effect (decreased metabolism).	Highly variable; clinical significance not established; monitor ethosuximide concentration.
Phenobarbital	Increased phenobarbital effect (decreased metabolism).	Monitor phenobarbital concentration.
Phenytoin	Increased phenytoin toxicity (displacement from binding).	Conflicting reports; monitor phenytoin concentration and clinical status.
Gabapentin with: Antacids	Decreased bioavailability of gabapentin by 20%.	Separate administration by at least 2 hr.
Cimetidine	Alters renal excretion of gabapentin.	Separate administration by 2 hr.
Lamotrigine with: Phenobarbital, primidone, phenytoin	Lamotrigine is decreased by 40%–45%.	Separate administration by 2 hr.
Valproic acid	Lamotrigine is increased twofold, while valproic acid is decreased by 25%.	Avoid concurrent administration.
Carbamazepine	Lamotrigine is decreased by 70%.	Avoid concurrent administration.

Source: Abramowicz, M (ed): The Medical Letter on Drugs and Therapeutics 28: 723, 1986, with permission modified in 1996.
*For interactions of anticonvulsants with other drugs, see the most recent edition of *The Medical Letter Handbook of Adverse Drug Interactions.*

WITHDRAWAL OF MEDICATION

Many of the seizures that start in childhood have the potential for a spontaneous remission. Other types of seizures that have an underlying pathology (head injury, brain tumor, arteriovenous malformations, and so on) may not have a remission. Guidelines for discontinuation of therapy, especially in children, are very controversial. However, it is agreed that antiseizure agents are tapered off and never abruptly discontinued because of the risk of status epilepticus. It is also agreed that epilepsy of long duration (e.g., 6 years) prior to control and the presence of partial seizures, mixed seizures, and atypical febrile seizures warrant continuation of therapy.

HYDANTOINS

Hydantoins are antiseizure agents that stabilize neurons in the CNS to reduce the spread of abnormal electrical discharges from a seizure focus. Through an effect on sodium, there is a reduction of activity in the synapse that prevents the seizure foci from spreading to adjacent cortical areas. The most commonly used drugs in this group are **phenytoin** *(Dilantin)*. Mephenytoin (Mesantoin) and ethotoin (Peganone) are also available but are not as widely used.

○ **Phenytoin** (Dilantin) is the primary drug used in the treatment of all types of seizures except absence seizures. Phenytoin is also used in the treatment of trigeminal and related neuralgias, digitalis-induced cardiac dysrhythmias, and for the treatment of compulsive thought disorder. Drug dosages, pharmacokinetics, and nursing implications for phenytoin are given in Table 20–6.

CONTRAINDICATIONS AND PRECAUTIONS This agent is contraindicated in patients with hypersensitivity and in those with sinus bradycardia and heart block because of its effect on ventricular automaticity. Phenytoin is used cautiously in patients with liver disease, as it is metabolized in the liver. Phenytoin-induced hepatitis is one of the more commonly reported hypersensitivity syndromes. This drug is usually discontinued if a rash appears (hypersensitivity). When given intravenously, the drug is administered slowly (50 mg/min) because it can cause hypotension and dysrhythmias. Phenytoin is excreted in breast milk and may cause serious adverse effects in nursing infants. Either the drug or lactation should be discontinued.

ADVERSE EFFECTS At normal therapeutic doses, phenytoin is relatively safe with few reported side effects. The CNS, skin, GI system, endocrine system, and hematologic system are usually involved in adverse phenytoin reactions.

Phenytoin has an excitatory effect on the cerebellar-vestibular system. The result of this action is nystagmus,

Table 20–6. ANTISEIZURE DRUGS: HYDANTOINS AND BARBITURATES

DRUG NAME/ROUTE AND DOSAGE	PHARMACOKINETICS/ DYNAMICS	NURSING IMPLICATIONS
HYDANTOINS		
phenytoin (Dilantin)		
anticonvulsant **Adults:** *Loading dose*–10–15 mg/kg PO *Maintenance dose*–300–400 mg/day PO (once daily as ER capsules or in 3–4 divided doses); usual maximum dose is 600 mg/day. **Children:** initially 5 mg/kg PO *Maintenance dose*–4–8 mg/kg per day PO in divided doses q 8–12 hr. Maximum dose 300 mg/day. **status epilepticus** **Adults:** 150–250 mg IV; may repeat 100–150 mg IV after 30 min or up to 15–18 mg/kg (rate not to exceed 25–50 mg/min) **Children:** 15–20 mg/kg per day in divided doses.	**Onset:** PO, 2–24 hr; IV, 1–2 hr; IM, erratic **Peak:** PO, 1.5–3 hr; ER, 12 hr; IV, rapid **Duration:** PO: 6–12 hr; ER, 12–36 hr; IV, 12–24 hr; IM, 12–24 hr (based on loading dose) **½L:** dose dependent **PB:** 90% **B:** liver **E:** kidneys	**ASSESSMENT:** Assess location, duration, and characteristics of seizure activity. CBC and platelet count, serum calcium, urinalysis, and hepatic and thyroid function tests are monitored prior to therapy and monthly for the first several months, then periodically throughout the course of therapy. Patient should have routine physical examinations, especially monitoring of skin and lymph nodes and EEG testing. Dental examinations, including teeth cleaning and reinforcement of plaque control for inhibition of gingival hyperplasia, should be performed at 3-mo intervals. Assess for pregnancy (category C). **INTERVENTION:** Administer with or immediately after meals to minimize GI irritation. Shake liquid preparations well before pouring. Chewable tablets must be crushed or chewed well before swallowing. Immediate-release capsules may be opened and mixed with food or fluids for patients who have difficulty swallowing. ER capsules are not opened, but swallowed whole. To prevent direct contact of alkaline drug with mucosa, have patient swallow a fluid first, follow with mixture of medication, then follow with a full glass of water or milk, or food. The 100-mg tablets and capsules contain 95 mg of phenytoin and are not interchangeable with two 50-mg tablets or capsules. Capsules labeled "extended" may be used for once-a-day dosage; those labeled "prompt" may result in toxic serum levels if used for once-a-day dosage. Administer direct IV at a rate not to exceed 50 mg over 1 min (25 mg/min in elderly patients). Rapid administration may result in severe hypotension or CNS depression. Administer as intermittent infusion by mixing with 0.9% NaCl in a concentration of less than 6.7 mg/mL. Administer immediately following admixture. Use tubing with a 0.22-μm in-line filter. Complete infusion within 4 hr at a rate not to exceed 50 mg/min. Monitor cardiac function and blood pressure throughout infusion. To minimize local venous irritation, follow infusion with 0.9% NaCl. Avoid extravasation; phenytoin is caustic to tissues. Do not admix with other solutions or medications, especially dextrose, because precipitation will occur. Slight yellow color will not alter solution potency. If refrigerated, may form precipitate, which dissolves after warming to room temperature. Discard solutions that are not clear. Implement seizure precautions. **EVALUATION:** Effectiveness of therapy can be demonstrated by decrease or cessation of seizures without excessive sedation.
BARBITURATES		
phenobarbital (Luminal)		
anticonvulsant **Adults:** 100–300 mg/day PO in 2–3 divided doses; or 100–300 mg IV repeated as necessary to a total of 600 mg IV/24 hr period.	**Onset:** PO, 30–60 min; IM and SC, 10–30 min; IV, 5 min **Peak:** IM, SC, and IV, 4–6 hr; PO, 8–12 hr (several weeks unless loading dose used)	**ASSESSMENT:** Assess sleep patterns prior to and periodically throughout the course of therapy. Patient may experience an increase in dreaming on discontinuation of medication. Monitor respiratory status, pulse, and blood pressure frequently in patients receiving pheno-

Continued on the following page

Table 20–6. ANTISEIZURE DRUGS: HYDANTOINS AND BARBITURATES, *Continued*

DRUG NAME/ROUTE AND DOSAGE	PHARMACOKINETICS/ DYNAMICS	NURSING IMPLICATIONS
BARBITURATES		
phenobarbital (Luminal)		
anticonvulsant *Children:* 3–5 mg/kg per day PO in divided doses; or 20 mg/kg IV as a single loading dose, followed by maintenance dose of 1–6 mg/kg per day IV. **status epilepticus** *Children:* 20 mg/kg IV then 6 mg/kg IV q 20 min as needed to a maximum of 40 mg/kg in 24 hr.	**Duration:** PO, 6–24 hr; IM, SC, and IV: 4–6 hr **½L:** 2–6 days **PB:** 40%–60% **B:** liver **E:** urine (25%)	barbital IV. Equipment for resuscitation and ventilatory support should be available. Prolonged therapy may lead to psychologic or physical dependence. Restrict amount of drug available to patient if patient is depressed, suicidal, or has a history of addiction. Patients on prolonged therapy should have hepatic and renal function and CBC evaluated periodically. Assess for pregnancy (category D). **INTERVENTION:** Tablets may be crushed and mixed with food or fluids (do not administer dry) for patients who have difficulty swallowing. Oral solution may be taken straight or mixed with water, milk, or fruit juice. Sterile phenobarbital sodium powder may be administered SC after reconstitution, but prediluted phenobarbital sodium injection is not recommended for SC use. IM injections should be given deep into the gluteal muscle to minimize tissue irritation. Reconstitute sterile powder for IV dose with a minimum of 10 mL of sterile water for injection. Dilute further with 10 mL of sterile water. Administer each 60 mg over at least 1 min. Titrate slowly for desired response. Rapid administration may result in respiratory depression. Solution is highly alkaline; extravasation may cause tissue damage and necrosis. Do not use solutions that are discolored or contain particulate matter. Do not mix with other medications. Discard powder or solutions that have been exposed to air for longer than 30 min. Supervise ambulation and transfer of patients following administration. Remove cigarettes. **Patient Teaching**—Teach patient to carry or wear ID indicating medication usage and epilepsy. **EVALUATION:** Several weeks may be required to achieve maximum anticonvulsant effects. Effectiveness may also be demonstrated by sedation when used for this purpose.

ER = extended release.

ataxia, diplopia, and vertigo. Other CNS effects include blurred vision, mydriasis, hyperactive tendon reflex, hyperactivity, silliness, confusion, inattention, drowsiness, dullness, headache, and coma (large doses). These side effects may disappear with a reduced dose.

▼ **CLINICAL ALERT**

Gingival hyperplasia occurs frequently with chronic therapy and is a common manifestation of toxicity in children and adolescents. This occurs only in portions of the gum that have teeth. This side effect is due to the overgrowth of tissue caused by altered collagen metabolism. This side effect can be minimized by good oral hygiene.

Hirsutism and coarsening of facial features are induced by phenytoin. These effects are probably due to altered androgen levels that result secondarily from use of the drug.

Gastrointestinal problems include nausea, vomiting, anorexia, weight loss, and epigastric pain. Many of these reactions are caused by taking phenytoin on an empty stomach. To reduce these reactions, administer the drug with food or in more frequent divided doses.

Endocrine effects such as hyperglycemia, glycosuria, and osteomalacia have been reported. The hyperglycemia and glycosuria occur secondarily to the inhibition of insulin secretion. The osteomalacia, with hypocalcemia and increased alkaline phosphatase activity, has been reported to be due to altered metabolism of vitamin D and the inhibition of intestinal absorption of calcium. Hypersensitivity reactions include the *morbilliform* (resembling measles) rash, *Stevens-Johnson syndrome* (erythema multiforme), systemic lupus erythematosus, and hepatic necrosis. Phenytoin is usually discontinued if a skin rash appears so more serious skin problems do not develop. These reactions are idiosyncratic in origin.

Hematologic reactions include fever, neutropenia, leukopenia, red cell anemia, aplastic anemia, hypoprothrombinemia, and hemorrhage in newborns of mothers who received phenytoin. A marked phagocytosis of myeloid precursors by bone marrow histiocytes occurs in agranulocytosis. In vitro studies suggest that phenytoin-induced red cell aplasia is immunologic in nature, mediated through an immunoglobulin inhibitor, requiring the presence of phenytoin to suppress erythroid colony formation. The megaloblastic anemia has been associated with altered folate absorption and metabolism. The lymphadenopathy is a secondary result of the reduction in immunoglobulin A production. The hypoprothrombinemia and hemorrhage are secondary to the vitamin K deficiency.

DRUG CONCENTRATIONS Therapeutic effectiveness is obtained with concentrations over 10 μg/mL (total concentration of phenytoin), whereas toxic effects such as nystagmus develop at about 20 μg/mL; ataxia is present at 30 μg/mL; and lethargy at 40 μg/mL. The serum level assumes a normal albumin, renal function and protein binding. If these are abnormal, free phenytoin levels are a better test. The clinical signs of toxicity are correlated with the concentration of the unbound drug. This varies considerably among patients, so drug concentrations should serve only as a general guideline (see Table 20–4). Switching between phenytoin products could have an effect on drug serum concentration levels. Nurses should assess the patient for signs of toxicity. Monitoring drug concentration is important for the patient on anticonvulsants because it can help in individualizing therapy to provide minimal benefit and to decrease dose-related side effects.

INTERACTIONS Many of the drug interactions connected with phenytoin are secondary to effects on its metabolism. Some agents decrease the effects of phenytoin by increasing its metabolism by inducing hepatic microsomal enzymes, decreasing its absorption, or through some unknown mechanism. For example, the chronic use of alcohol stimulates phenytoin-metabolizing enzymes, causing a decrease in antiseizure effect. Other drugs increase phenytoin's effects by competitively inhibiting its microsomal metabolism, displacing phenytoin from its protein-binding sites, or through some unknown mechanism. The phenytoin-phenobarbital interaction is complex. Phenobarbital can be either an enzyme inducer (by increasing the biotransformation of phenytoin) or an enzyme inhibitor (by decreasing phenytoin activity). Phenytoin can also decrease the effects of other drugs by increasing their metabolism or through some unknown mechanism. These drug-drug interactions are detailed in Table 20–7.

There are also phenytoin–enteral nutrition interactions. Phenytoin elixir is very high in osmolarity and therefore may cause diarrhea. (See Chapter 14 for guidelines for administering phenytoin with enteral formulas.)

○ **Fosphenytoin,** a prodrug of phenytoin, is being investigated for intravenous (IV) or intramuscular (IM) use in patients who are unable to receive oral phenytoin therapy. It can also be used in situations where injectable phenytoin may be necessary. Fosphenytoin is designed to overcome some of the disadvantages associated with the current phenytoin formulations (e.g., poor solubility in aqueous solution, slow IV administration, poor bioavailability).

Fosphenytoin is completely absorbed (98% to 99%) following IM administration and is rapidly and completely converted to phenytoin by phosphatases following both IV and IM administration.

Phenytoin-related adverse drug reactions have occurred, including paresthesia, drowsiness, dizziness, light-headedness, headache, nausea, and dysrhythmias. However, when administered IV, fosphenytoin is associated with less pain and less phlebitis than phenytoin. In addition, it is safer than phenytoin when given IV or IM.

The equimolar dose of fosphenytoin is 1.5 mg for every 1 mg of phenytoin sodium (375 mg dose of fosphenytoin should be equivalent to 250 mg of phenytoin sodium).

BARBITURATES

○ **Phenobarbital** *(Luminal)* inhibits the spread of seizure activity from a focus by increasing the threshold for neuronal firing. It might also enhance GABA-ergic inhibition. It is also thought that phenobarbital reduces the excitatory effects of glutamate. Between 40% and 60% of phenobarbital is bound to plasma proteins. Phenobarbital is metabolized by microsomal enzyme systems. Phenobarbital is described in detail in Chapter 26, so only information that pertains to its antiseizure activity is presented here. Additional pharmacokinetic and drug dosage information is given in Table 20–6.

USES Phenobarbital is effective in the treatment of generalized and partial seizures. It is an alternative in the treatment of status epilepticus, and it is used in the treatment of febrile seizures in infants and children.

CONTRAINDICATIONS AND PRECAUTIONS Phenobarbital is contraindicated in patients with hypersensitivity. It should not be used in comatose patients, those with preexisting CNS depression, or in patients with acute porphyria. Phenobarbital is used cautiously in patients who have hepatic dysfunction or severe renal impairment. Because phenobarbital is biotransfomed in the liver and excreted by the kidneys, any impairment in these organ functions could lead to poor seizure control or toxicity. These agents are used cautiously in pregnant patients. The possibility of congenital malformations or coagulation defect and hemorrhage in the newborn exists.

Research indicates that exposure to phenobarbital in the womb causes lower (by an average seven points) intelligence scores. If children were socially and economically deprived or born as a result of unwanted pregnancy, the intelligence score dropped by 20 points. Phenobarbital can have important benefits during pregnancy, but the risks and benefits need to be balanced. (Reinisch et al., 1995). Nursing infants must be monitored for excessive sedation because phenobarbital concentrations in milk may exceed those in maternal plasma. Dosage may need to be reduced in the elderly and children due to their high susceptibility to CNS adverse effects.

Table 20–7. DRUGS THAT INTERACT WITH PHENYTOIN AND OTHER HYDANTOINS

Interacting Drugs	Effects	Mechanisms	Comments
Antacids, charcoal, sucralfate	Decreased hydantoin effects	Decreased absorption	
Barbiturates, carbamazepine, diazoxide, ethanol (chronic ingestion), rifampin, theophylline	Decreased hydantoin effects	Increased metabolism	*Barbiturates'* effect on phenytoin is variable and unpredictable. Addition of phenytoin generally increases phenobarbital serum concentrations. Individual monitoring is needed, especially when starting or stopping either drug. *Carbamazepine's* effect on phenytoin is variable. Carbamazepine serum levels may also be decreased.
Antineoplastics, folic acid, influenza virus vaccine, loxapine, nitrofurantoin, pyridoxine	Decreased hydantoin effects	Unknown	*Influenza virus vaccine* may increase, decrease, or have no effect on total serum phenytoin concentrations.
Allopurinol, amiodarone, benzodiazepines, chloramphenicol, cimetidine, disulfiram, ethanol (acute ingestion), fluconazole, isoniazid, metronidazole, miconazole, omeprazole, phenacemide, phenylbutazone, succinimides, sulfonamides, trimethoprim, valproic acid	Increased hydantoin effects	Inhibited metabolism	*Valproic acid* affects phenytoin disposition in different ways. Displacement of phenytoin from plasma proteins increases free friction and decreases total phenytoin levels; concentration of unbound phenytoin is not significantly altered. Increased levels may result from inhibition of phenytoin metabolism. Conversely, phenytoin increases metabolism of valproic acid.
Salicylates, tricyclic antidepressants, valproic acid	Increased hydantoin effects	Displaced anticonvulsant	*Salicylates* displace phenytoin from its plasma protein binding sites in a dose-dependent manner; no significant change occurs in free phenytoin concentration. *Valproic acid* affects phenytoin disposition in different ways. Displacement of phenytoin from plasma proteins increases free friction and decreases total phenytoin levels; concentration of unbound phenytoin is not significantly altered. Increased levels may result from inhibition of phenytoin metabolism. Conversely, phenytoin increases metabolism of valproic acid.
Chlorpheniramine, ibuprofen, phenothiazines	Increased hydantoin effects	Unknown	
Acetaminophen, amiodarone, carbamazepine, cardiac glycosides, corticosteroids, dicumarol, disopyramide, doxycycline, estrogens, haloperidol, methadone, metyrapone, mexiletine, oral contraceptives, quinidine, theophylline, valproic acid	Decreased effects of other drugs	Increased metabolism by phenytoin	*Acetaminophen:* Although therapeutic effects of acetaminophen may be reduced by concomitant phenytoin use, potential hepatotoxicity of acetaminophen may be increased, especially with chronic phenytoin administration.
Cyclosporine, dopamine, furosemide, levodopa, levonorgestrel, mebendazole, nondepolarizing muscle relaxants, phenothiazines, sulfonylureas	Decreased effects of other drugs	Various	

ADVERSE EFFECTS The major adverse effect of the barbiturates is neurotoxicity. This is due to the depressive effect on the brain. The side effects include cognitive and behavioral manifestations, with children and the elderly being most susceptible. Signs and symptoms include drowsiness, depression, inattention, impaired memory, confusion, excitation, delirium, ataxia, and nystagmus. Because barbiturates depress the brain stem, respiratory depression can be seen, especially with high doses. Tolerance can develop after long-term therapy.

Another group of adverse reactions are skin rashes, thought to be an allergic reaction. These rashes are *scarlatiniform* (resembling scarlet fever) or morbilliform in nature. If rashes occur, discontinuation of the drug is considered.

Hematologic adverse reactions include megaloblastic anemia, osteomalacia, and hypoprothrombinemia with hemorrhage in the newborn.

DRUG CONCENTRATIONS A precise relationship between therapeutic results and concentration of phenobarbital in plasma does not exist, but it is recommended that serum levels be monitored and serve as a guideline for treatment. For the control of seizures, plasma levels of 10 to 25 μg/mL are recommended. For the prophylaxis of febrile seizures, 15 μg/mL is the minimum level. Levels higher than 60 μg/mL may be associated with marked toxicity (see Table 20–4).

INTERACTIONS Drug interactions occur between phenobarbital and many other drugs. See Chapter 26 for a complete discussion.

SUCCINIMIDES

The succinimide derivatives are **ethosuximide (Zarontin)** (Table 20–8), **methsuximide (Celontin)**, and **phensuximide (Milontin)**. The mechanism of action of succinimides is unknown, but it is related to enhancement of central inhibitory pathways.

○ **Ethosuximide** (Zarontin), **methsuximide** (Celontin), **and phensuximide** (Milontin) are used primarily in the treatment of absence seizures. Ethosuximide is the drug of choice because methsuximide is more toxic and phensuximide is less effective.

CONTRAINDICATIONS AND PRECAUTIONS The succinimides are contraindicated in patients with a history of hypersensitivity to succinimide drugs. Ethosuximide is metabolized in the liver and excreted from the kidneys; therefore, caution is used when administering this drug to patients with hepatic or renal disorders. Ethosuximide has not been proven safe for use during pregnancy (category C) and lactation. Methsuximide is classified as pregnancy category C and phensuximide as category D.

ADVERSE EFFECTS The most common side effects of these succinimides are gastrointestinal disturbances and CNS effects. The gastrointestinal reactions include anorexia, gastric upset (epigastric pain), nausea, vomiting, cramping, weight loss, diarrhea, and hiccups. The CNS effects include drowsiness, headaches, euphoria, irritability, hyperactivity, dizziness, blurred vision, inability to

concentrate, aggressiveness, anxiety, and restlessness. The exact cause of complaints is unknown. With ethosuximide, the presence of behavioral alterations may necessitate discontinuing the drug. If discontinued, ethosuximide is withdrawn slowly.

Some hematologic reactions—aplastic anemia, agranulocytosis, leukopenia, and eosinophilia—have also been reported. These may be idiosyncratic reactions.

DRUG CONCENTRATIONS The plateau state is reached in about 4 to 6 days in children and in a longer period for adults. For control of absence seizures, a serum level of 40 to 100 μg/mL for methsuximide, and 4 to 8 μg/mL for phensuximide is recommended (see Table 20–4).

INTERACTIONS When the succinimides are administered with other anticonvulsants (hydantoin, primidone, and valproic acid), monitor serum levels carefully, as all drugs may be affected (see Table 20–5).

BENZODIAZEPINES

The benzodiazepines used most frequently in treating seizure disorders include **diazepam (Valium)**, **clonazepam (Klonopin)** (see Table 20–8), and **clorazepate dipotassium (Tranxene)**. Some benzodiazepines are not useful as sole therapy, but are used in combination with other antiseizure agents.

○ **Diazepam** (Valium), **clonazepam** (Klonopin), and **clorazepate dipotassium** (Tranxene) potentiate GABA-ergic neurotransmission at various levels of the brain and spinal cord. These receptor areas include the spinal cord, hypothalamus, hippocampus, substantia nigra, cerebellar cortex, and cerebral cortex. The efficiency of GABA-ergic synaptic inhibition (which leads to decreased firing rate of neurons) is enhanced with use of the benzodiazepines. These agents have broad antiseizure properties.

USES Clonazepam and clorazepate have been approved for the treatment of absence and myoclonic seizures. Clorazepate is used concurrently with other antiseizure agents for treatment of partial seizures. Diazepam is currently used for the treatment of status epilepticus. The other uses of the benzodiazepines are relief of anxiety, hypnosis, preoperative sedation, balanced anesthesia, control of withdrawal states, muscle relaxation, and diagnostic aids or treatment in psychiatry. These drugs are discussed in detail in Chapter 25.

OXAZOLIDINEDIONES

The oxazolidinediones—**trimethadione (Tridione)** and **paramethadione (Paradione)**—increase the presynaptic and postsynaptic inhibition in synapses that utilize GABA as a neurotransmitter. Both of these drugs are used to treat refractory absence seizures. Trimethadione was previously the agent of choice for absence seizures, but it has been replaced by newer agents such as ethosuximide and valproic acid.

Table 20–8. ANTISEIZURE DRUGS: SUCCINIMIDES AND BENZODIAZEPINES

DRUG NAME/ROUTE AND DOSAGE	PHARMACOKINETICS/ DYNAMICS	NURSING IMPLICATIONS
SUCCINIMIDES		
ethosuximide (Zarontin)		
Adults and Children over 6 yr: 250 mg PO bid initially; may be increased by 250 mg/day q 4–7 days up to 1.5 g/day given in 2 divided doses. **Children 3–6 yr:** 250 mg/day PO as a single dose or 20 mg/kg per day given in 2 divided doses.	**Onset:** hours–days **Peak:** days **Duration:** days **½L:** 40–60 hr (adults); 30 hr (children 7–9 yr) **PB:** not protein bound **B:** liver **E:** 10% by kidneys	**ASSESSMENT:** Assess location, duration, and characteristics of seizure activity. CBC and platelet count, serum calcium, urinalysis, and hepatic and thyroid function tests are monitored prior to therapy and monthly for first several months, then periodically throughout course of therapy. Patient should have routine physical examinations, especially monitoring of skin and lymph nodes and EEG testing. Assess patient's mood, behavior patterns, and facial expressions. Patients with history of psychiatric disorders have increased risk of developing behavioral changes. These symptoms may necessitate withdrawal of the medication. Assess for pregnancy (category C). **INTERVENTION:** Administer with food or fluids to minimize GI irritation. Available in capsules and liquid preparations. Implement seizure precautions. **Patient Teaching**—Advise patient to carry or wear ID indicating medication and diagnosis of epilepsy. **EVALUATION:** Effectiveness of therapy can be demonstrated by decrease or cessation of seizures without excessive sedation.
BENZODIAZEPINES		
clonazepam (Klonopin)		
Adults: Initial daily dose not to exceed 1.5 mg PO given in 3 divided doses. May increase by 0.5–1 mg q 3 days until therapeutic response is achieved. Total daily maintenance dose not to exceed 20 mg. **Children under 10 yr or 30 kg:** Initial daily dose 0.01–0.03 mg/kg PO (not to exceed 0.05 mg/kg) given in 2–3 divided doses. Increase by no more than 0.5 mg q 3 days until therapeutic levels are reached. Daily dose not to exceed 0.2 mg/kg.	**Onset:** 20–60 min **Peak:** 1–2 hr **Duration:** 6–12 hr **½L:** 18–60 hr **PB:** 50%–85% **B:** liver **E:** urine, feces	**ASSESSMENT:** Assess patient for drowsiness, unsteadiness, and clumsiness. These symptoms are dose related and are most severe during initial therapy; may decrease in severity or disappear with continued or long-term therapy. Prolonged high-dose therapy may lead to psychologic or physical dependence. Restrict amount of drug available to patient. Pregnancy category unknown. **INTERVENTION:** Administer with food to minimize gastric irritation. Tablets may be crushed if patient has difficulty swallowing. Institute seizure precautions for patients on initial therapy or undergoing dosage manipulations. **EVALUATION:** Dosage adjustments may be required after several months of therapy.

▼ **CLINICAL ALERT**

Because of their potential to cause fetal malformations and serious side effects, the oxazolidinediones are used only when other less toxic drugs have been ineffective.

MISCELLANEOUS ANTISEIZURE DRUGS

Many antiseizure drugs are classified as miscellaneous agents. These include **primidone** *(Mysoline)*, **carbamazepine** *(Tegretol)*, **valproic acid** *(Depakene)*, **lamotrigine**

(Lamictal), **felbamate** *(Felbatol)*, and **gabapentin** *(Neurontin)*. Each of these drugs is discussed individually and drug dosages, pharmacokinetics, and nursing implications are featured in Table 20–9.

○ **Primidone** (Mysoline) is metabolized by the liver to phenobarbital and can be substituted for phenobarbital in the treatment of seizure activity. The exact mechanism of action is unknown but may be similar to that of phenobarbital. Primidone may produce more undesirable effects than either phenytoin or phenobarbital.

USES   Primidone is used for the treatment of all seizures except absence seizures. Some reports indicate that primidone is especially useful in the management of partial seizures. Primidone may be used concurrently with phenytoin or carbamazepine.

Chapter 20 • AGENTS USED TO TREAT SEIZURE DISORDERS **291**

MISCELLANEOUS ANTISEIZURE DRUGS

Table 20–9. MISCELLANEOUS ANTISEIZURE DRUGS

DRUG NAME/ROUTE AND DOSAGE	PHARMACOKINETICS/ DYNAMICS	NURSING IMPLICATIONS
all miscellaneous anticonvulsants		**ASSESSMENT:** Assess location, duration, and characteristics of seizure activity. CBC and platelet count, serum calcium, urinalysis, and hepatic and thyroid function tests are monitored prior to therapy and monthly for first several months, then periodically throughout course of therapy. Patient should have routine physical examinations, especially monitoring of skin and lymph nodes and EEG testing.
primidone (Mysoline) *Adults and Children over 8 yr:* *Initial dose*—100–125 mg PO at bedtime for 3 days, then 100–125 mg bid for 3 days. *Maintenance dose*—250 mg tid (not to exceed 2 g/day). **Children under 8 yrs:** *Initial dose*—50 mg PO at bedtime for 3 days, then 50 mg bid for 3 days, then 100 mg bid for 3 days. *Maintenance dose*—125–250 mg tid (10–25 mg/kg per day). Dosage adjustment required in severe liver disease.	**Onset:** 4–7 days **Peak:** 3 hr **Duration:** 8–12 hr **½L:** 5–15 hr; PEMA (metabolite), 10–18 hr; PB (metabolite), 53–140 hr **PB:** 20%–25% **B:** liver (to PEMA and PB) **E:** urine (40%)	Same as for all plus: **ASSESSMENT:** Assess patient for allergy to phenobarbital. Assess patient for signs of folic acid deficiency (mental dysfunction, unusual tiredness or weakness, psychiatric disorders, neuropathy, megaloblastic anemia). May be treated with folic acid. **INTERVENTION:** May be administered with food to minimize GI irritation. Tablets may be crushed and mixed with food or fluids for patients who have difficulty swallowing. Shake liquid preparations well before pouring. Implement seizure precautions. **Patient Teaching—** Advise patient to carry or wear ID indicating medication and epilepsy. **EVALUATION:** Effectiveness of therapy can be demonstrated by decrease or cessation of seizures without excessive sedation. May require week or more of therapy before therapeutic response is seen.
carbamazepine (Tegretol) *Adults:* Start with 200 mg PO bid, increase by 200 mg/day until therapeutic levels are achieved. Usual dose is 800–1200 mg/day in divided doses given q 6–8 hr. In 12–15-year-olds, do not exceed 100 mg/day. **Children 6–12 yr:** 20–30 mg/kg per day PO in 3–4 divided doses. Usual therapeutic dose is 400–800 mg/day.	**Onset:** 2–4 days **Peak:** 2–8 hr **Duration:** 6–12 hr **½L:** 10–54 hr initially, then 10–20 hr **PB:** 75% **B:** liver **E:** urine (72%), feces (28%)	Same as for all plus: **ASSESSMENT:** Monitor CBC, including platelet count, reticulocyte count, and serum iron during the first 3 mo and monthly thereafter for evidence of potentially fatal blood dyscrasias. Liver function tests, eye examinations, urinalysis, and BUN should be routinely performed. Assess for pregnancy (category C). **INTERVENTION:** Administer medication with food to minimize gastric irritation. Tablets may be crushed if patient has difficulty swallowing. Also available in chewable tablets and suspension. Do not discontinue this medication abruptly because this may precipitate seizures. **EVALUATION:** Clinical response is indicated by an absence or reduction of seizure activity. Report increasing tiredness, abnormal bruising or bleeding, and increased infection to doctor.
sodium valproate **valproic acid** (Depakene) **divalproex sodium** (Depakote) *Adults and Children:* Initial dose is 15 mg/kg per day PO, increased by 5–10 mg/kg per day at weekly intervals until therapeutic levels are reached (not to exceed 60 mg/kg per day). When dosage exceeds 250 mg, give in divided doses.	**Onset:** Liquid, capsule, and enteric-coated tablet, 2–4 days for therapeutic effect, then 1–2 hr **Peak:** Liquid, 15–20 min; capsule, 1–4 hr; enteric-coated tablet, 2–5 hr (blood levels) **Duration:** 24 hr **½L:** 5–20 hr **PB:** 80%–94% **B:** liver **E:** urine	Same as for all plus: **ASSESSMENT:** Therapeutic blood levels should be monitored periodically. Assess for pregnancy (category D). **INTERVENTION:** Administer with or immediately after meals to minimize GI irritation. Single daily doses are usually administered at bedtime because of sedation. Capsules and enteric-coated tablets should be swallowed whole; patient should not break or chew, as this will cause irritation of mouth and throat. Administering tablets with milk causes premature dissolution of tablets. Implement seizure precautions. **EVALUATION:** Report yellow skin, pregnancy, tremor, difficulty with vision, abnormal bleeding to physician.

Continued on the following page

Table 20–9. MISCELLANEOUS ANTISEIZURE DRUGS, *Continued*

DRUG NAME/ROUTE AND DOSAGE	PHARMACOKINETICS/ DYNAMICS	NURSING IMPLICATIONS
gabapentin (Neurontin)		
Adult: 900–1800 mg/day PO in 3 divided doses. Start at 300 mg on day 1 and increase 300 mg/day. Maximum time between doses should not be more than 12 hr.	**Onset:** rapid **Peak:** several hours **Duration:** 10–15 hr **½L:** 5–7 hr **PB:** 3% **B:** not biotransformed **E:** renal	Same as for all plus: **ASSESSMENT:** Assess for pregnancy (category C). **INTERVENTION:** May cause drowsiness. **Patient Teaching**—Caution patient about driving or operating heavy equipment. Warn patient not to suddenly stop drug. Tell patient not to take gabapentin within 2 hours of antacids. **EVALUATION:** Report somnolence and dizziness to the physician if they become severe.
lamotrigine (Lamictal)		
With valproic acid and enzyme-inducing antiepileptic drug(s): *Adults:* Initial dose—25 mg PO every other day for 2 wk, then 25 mg/day for 2 wk. Maintenance dose—100–150 mg/day in 2 divided doses. With enzyme-inducing antiepileptic drug(s) but no valproic acid: *Adults:* Initial dose—50 mg/day PO for 2 wk, then 50 mg bid for 2 wk. Maintenance dose—300–500 mg/day in 2 divided doses.	**Onset:** 1–2 hr **Peak:** 1.5–5 hr **Duration:** 24–36 hr **½L:** 24 hr **PB:** 55% **B:** liver **E:** urine	Same as for all plus: **ASSESSMENT:** Assess for skin rash or previous skin condition. Assess for pregnancy (category C). **INTERVENTION:** Lamotrigine may cause drowsiness and somnolence. Caution patient about driving or operating heavy equipment. **Patient Teaching**—Teach not to suddenly stop drug, as severe seizures may occur. Warn patient about photosensitivity. Protect skin from sun. Notify physician if pregnancy occurs. **EVALUATION:** Report skin rash to physician at once.

PB = phenobarbital; BUN = blood urea nitrogen.

CONTRAINDICATIONS AND PRECAUTIONS Primidone is contraindicated in patients with hypersensitivity or porphyria. This agent, like the barbiturates, exerts depressive effects on the brain. This drug should be used with caution in patients who have liver disease as the liver is the site of metabolism. The use of this agent during pregnancy (category D) can result in hemorrhage in the newborn. Excessive drowsiness and somnolence can occur in newborns during lactation, so nursing is discontinued.

ADVERSE EFFECTS The most common adverse effects are caused by the depressive effects of primidone and its two metabolites (phenobarbital and phenylethylmalonamide [PEMA]) on the brain. Signs and symptoms of these effects include sedation, vertigo, dizziness, ataxia, diplopia, nystagmus, and an acute feeling of intoxication.

Gastrointestinal manifestations—nausea and vomiting—disappear as therapy continues or if the agent is taken with food. A maculopapular and morbilliform rash can occur. Rash is viewed as a drug allergy, and the drug is discontinued if it occurs.

Hematologic adverse reactions include leukopenia, thrombocytopenia, systemic lupus erythematosus, lymphadenopathy, hemorrhagic disease in the newborn, megaloblastic anemia, and osteomalacia. These occur by mechanisms similar to those of phenytoin.

DRUG CONCENTRATIONS Plasma concentrations greater than 12 μg/mL are associated with significant toxic side effects (see Table 20–4). Phenobarbital, at steady state, varies from 15 to 30 μg/mL. Doses of 10 to 20 mg/kg per day are necessary to maintain these levels. It is important to remember that the parent drug reaches its steady state in 40 hours, whereas the steady state of the active metabolites is reached in 4 to 20 days.

INTERACTIONS Drug interactions are the same as those for phenobarbital (see Table 20–5).

○ **Carbamazepine** (Tegretol) acts by reducing polysynaptic responses and blocking the posttetanic potentiation. This agent has the capacity to increase discharge of nonadrenergic neurons, which may contribute to its antiseizure actions.

USES Carbamazepine is used for the treatment of partial, mixed, and generalized seizures. It is not used for absence seizures. This drug is recommended for patients whose seizures are difficult to control or those experiencing marked side effects from other agents. Carbamazepine is also used for the management of pain associated with trigeminal and glossopharyngeal neuralgia.

CONTRAINDICATIONS AND PRECAUTIONS Carbamazepine is contraindicated in patients with hypersensitivity to this agent or to tricyclic antidepressants as it is structurally related to tricyclic compounds. It is not used in patients with a history of bone marrow depression. Serious and sometimes fatal abnormalities of blood cells have occurred with use of carbamazepine. Concurrent use of MAO inhibitors is not recommended. Carbamazepine inhibits the uptake and release of norepinephrine from brain synapses. Patients with liver or kidney dysfunction are monitored closely for toxic effects as these are the organs of biotransformation/elimination.

Carbamazepine has some anticholinergic properties, so patients with glaucoma are monitored closely. Carbamazepine is used with caution in patients with mixed seizures because an increased frequency of generalized seizures have been reported. Children and the elderly are potentially at risk for developing cognitive and behavioral reactions to this drug (latent psychosis in elderly patients on other tricyclic agents), and dosage may need to be reduced. Carbamazepine is used with caution in patients with cardiac disease. There may be retention of water along with decreased osmolarity and concentration of sodium in plasma related to the inappropriate secretion of antidiuretic hormone (ADH). This agent is also used with caution by patients who need to be mentally or physically active because drowsiness, dizziness, and unsteadiness can occur. Patients are cautioned about the hazards of operating machinery or performing other dangerous tasks.

ADVERSE EFFECTS Early adverse reactions are related to the depressive and anticholinergic effects of carbamazepine on the CNS. These reactions include drowsiness, fatigue, vertigo, unsteadiness, ataxia, diplopia, hyperirritability, and psychosis. Starting this agent at a low dosage can minimize these reactions.

Gastrointestinal reactions can also occur early in treatment with carbamazepine. These include nausea, vomiting, dry mouth, and hepatitis. Dry mouth is due to the anticholinergic properties of the drug, while the other reactions are idiosyncrasies of the drug.

The most severe reactions to this drug affect the skin and cardiovascular and hematologic systems. Frequent skin reactions include rashes, uriticaria, photosensitivity, and alteration in skin pigmentation. More rarely, severe reactions that have been reported with the use of carbamazepine include epidermal necrosis and Stevens-Johnson syndrome. These reactions signal hypersensitivity and are difficult to predict.

The reactions of the cardiovascular system include congestive heart failure, syncope, hypertension, and hypotension. Some of these reactions are made worse by the hyponatremia and water retention that result from the inappropriate secretion of ADH.

The mechanisms responsible for adverse effects in the hematologic system are unknown and may be idiosyncratic. These reactions include aplastic anemia, agranulocytosis, thrombocytopenia, leukopenia, leukocytosis, and eosinophilia. Monitoring the complete blood count (CBC), platelet and reticulocyte counts, and serum iron level is essential. The patient is instructed to report the early toxic signs and symptoms of hematologic dysfunction: fever, sore throat, ulcers in the mouth, easy bruising, petechial or purpuric hemorrhage.

DRUG CONCENTRATIONS Monitoring of the drug level of carbamazepine is important for management, particularly when multiple drugs are being used concurrently. The usual therapeutic level of carbamazepine ranges from 4 to 12 μg/mL for adults. It must be remembered that these levels are variable and should serve as a guideline. CNS side effects are seen with levels above 9 μg/mL (see Table 20–4).

INTERACTIONS See Table 20–5 for interacts among anticonvulsants. In addition, carbamazepine decreases the serum levels of warfarin, doxycycline, theophylline, and haloperidol. Because carbamazepine is an enzyme inducer, it speeds up the metabolism of these agents. Carbamazepine's metabolism is inhibited by erythromycin, desipramine, isoniazid, cimetidine, propoxyphene, and calcium channel blockers. These agents raise serum carbamazepine levels, resulting in toxicity. Dangerous interactions have occurred between tricyclic antidepressants and MAO inhibitors. Because carbamazepine is related to tricyclic agents, the potential for these interactions exists.

○ **Valproic acid** (Depakene and others) is an analogue of the inhibitory neurotransmitter GABA. Although the exact mechanism of action is unknown, valproic acid is an enzyme inhibitor, resulting in an increase in the concentration of GABA in the synapses. Derivatives of valproic acid include sodium valproate (sodium salt) and divalproex sodium (Depakote), which contains both valproic acid and sodium valproate.

USES Valproic acid is very effective for treatment of a variety of seizures and is the drug of choice for absence seizures. It is also effective in treating myoclonic seizures, generalized tonic-clonic seizures, and atonic attacks (see Table 20–1). Valproic acid is less effective with partial seizures. Valproic is also used for migraine prophylaxis.

CONTRAINDICATIONS AND PRECAUTIONS Valproic acid is contraindicated in hypersensitivity. It should be used cautiously in patients with hepatic disease or significant impairment because valproic acid is hepatotoxic. Children under age 2 are at increased risk of developing fatal hepatotoxicity. Valproic acid is also contraindicated in patients with bleeding disorders; it prolongs bleeding time by inhibiting platelets aggregation.

ADVERSE EFFECTS Gastrointestinal disturbances—nausea, vomiting, indigestion, hepatotoxicity, pancreatitis, hypersalivation, anorexia, increased appetite, diarrhea, abdominal cramps, and constipation—are the most common side effects of the valproates (valproic acid and its derivatives). These effects can be minimized by administering the drug with food and by beginning therapy with a low dose. The increase in appetite is thought to be secondary to the GABA-enhancing effects. The hepatotoxicity may be an idiosyncratic reaction rather than a dose-related event. Hepatic biopsy in fatal cases reveals centrilobular necrosis and severe fatty changes in the liver.

CNS depressive effects are less severe for the valproates than for other antiseizure agents. Side effects include drowsiness, sedation, headache, dizziness, ataxia, incoordination, confusion, and visual disturbances.

Hematologic reactions include thrombocytopenia and hemorrhage. These reactions are secondary to the inhibition of the secondary phase of platelet aggregation. Thrombocytopenia may also be due to an autoimmune mechanism.

DRUG CONCENTRATIONS Therapeutic values of valproic acid range from 50 to 100 μg/mL. Some patients may require and tolerate levels in excess of 100 μg/mL. Again, this therapeutic range should be used only as a guideline. The clearance of valproic acid is dose dependent, because of the changes in clearance and protein binding. At a low dose, valproic acid inhibits its own metabolism, decreasing the intrinsic clearance. At higher doses, there is more free valproic acid, resulting in lower serum levels. It is useful to measure the total and free drug levels (see Table 20–4).

INTERACTIONS Valproic acid has many drug interactions, see Table 20–5.

The use of valproic acid can alter several laboratory tests. These include increased alkaline phosphatase levels, false-positive urine glucose test, false-positive urine ketone test, prolonged bleeding time, elevated liver function tests, and altered thyroid function tests.

○ **Lamotrigine** (Lamictal), a phenyltrazine derivative, is approved for adjunctive therapy (usually administered with either carbamazepine or phenytoin) in the treatment of partial seizures in adults with epilepsy. Because this diagnostic category includes the largest number of patients with intractable epilepsy, new drugs with antiseizure activity are usually tried first for this indication. Lamotrigine has a broad spectrum of antiseizure activity. Its precise mechanism of action is unknown, but the drug apparently blocks voltage-dependent sodium channels, resulting in decreased release of stimulatory neurotransmitters such as glutamate and aspartate. Phenytoin and carbamazepine have similar activity.

CONTRAINDICATIONS AND PRECAUTIONS Lamotrigine is contraindicated in hypersensitivity. Lamotrigine is administered cautiously to persons with underlying skin rash or skin condition. Approximately 10% of all patients receiving lamotrigine develop a rash. Maculopapular or erythematous eruptions are common, but more serious rashes with systemic involvement can occur. If rash is severe, therapy may need to be discontinued. Care is taken in patients with underlying renal and hepatic disease as the liver and kidneys are the organs of biotransformation/elimination. Safety in lactation and children has not been established.

ADVERSE EFFECTS Typical adverse effects seen with lamotrigine include dizziness, diplopia, ataxia, blurred vision, nausea, vomiting, and headache. All these effects are due to its activity in the brain. Rash can also occur. Evidence indicates that the inclusion of valproate in a multidrug regimen increases the risk of serious, life-threatening rash. Photoallergy or phototoxicity may also occur.

INTERACTIONS Lamotrigine apparently does not induce or inhibit cytochrome P450 isoenzymes. See Table 20–5 for other anticonvuls and interactions.

○ **Gabapentin** (Neurontin) is structurally related to the neurotransmitter GABA. The exact mechanism of activity is unknown. It is used as an adjunct in the treatment of partial seizures with and without secondary generalization in adults with epilepsy. Pharmacokinetics and drug dosages are given in Table 20–9.

CONTRAINDICATIONS AND PRECAUTIONS Gabapentin is contraindicated in patients with hypersensitivity. It should not be discontinued suddenly due to the possibility of status epilepticus. Safety in children has not been established.

ADVERSE EFFECTS The most common adverse effects include somnolence, dizziness, ataxia, fatigue, and nystagmus.

INTERACTIONS Because gabapentin is not metabolized, it does not interfere with metabolism of coadministered antiseizure drugs. Antacids reduce the bioavailability of gabapentin by about 20%. Thus, antacids are not administered within 2 hours of gabapentin.

○ **Felbamate** (Felbatol), a phenyl dicarbamate structurally similar to meprobamate (Equanil and others), is indicated for use alone or with other drugs in adults with partial seizures with or without secondary generalization. It is also approved for use in addition to other drugs in children with the multiple types of seizures associated with the Lennox-Gastaut syndrome, a severe epileptic encephalopathy. Felbamate's mechanism of action is unknown, but in neuronal cultures it blocks sustained repetitive neuronal firing, possibly through an effect on sodium channels.

▼ **CLINICAL ALERT**

Since the release of felbamate there have been reports of numerous cases (including several deaths) of aplastic anemia and several cases of acute liver failure (including several deaths). An FDA advisory committee recommends felbamate only for second-line therapy. Felbamate is used only if the well-being of the patient is judged so dependent on continuous therapy that withdrawal is deemed to pose a greater threat.

USING THE NURSING PROCESS

Nurses play a vital role in the care of the patient with seizures. The nurse has continuous interactions with the patient and is in a unique position to recognize abnormal behavior patterns, to witness the seizure, and to assess and monitor the postseizure behavior. In the hospital, the nurse has the opportunity to plan care for the patient and to establish a teaching plan that can assist the patient and family in planning for a normal life. When treatment is initiated with an antiseizure agent, the goal is to control the seizures without causing intolerable adverse reactions.

ASSESSMENT

- Obtain a nursing history. Because alteration in consciousness often accompanies a seizure, information about patient activities prior to, during, and after the seizure may be obtained from family or friends. If the patient can remember events prior to, during, or after a seizure, obtain the data from him or her. Table 20–10 summarizes the nursing process for the patient requiring antiseizure medications.
- Establish a trend of the patient's behavior prior to a seizure as well as during and after the seizure. Nurs-

Table 20–10. NURSING PROCESS FOR PATIENT REQUIRING ANTISEIZURE MEDICATIONS

Assessment

Assess mentation (response to environment, orientation), noting drowsiness, confusion, restlessness; dizziness.
Assess muscle strength and coordination; balance, gait and movement.
Assess respiratory rate, rhythm, and depth during seizure activity.

Nursing Diagnosis: Risk for Trauma

RELATED TO: muscle weakness, balancing difficulties, loss of large or small muscle coordination, cognitive changes, altered consciousness.

Desired Outcomes/Evaluation Criteria

Verbalizes understanding of safety measures. Remains free from injury.

Nursing Actions	Rationale
Encourage patient to keep a log of activities that occur prior to a seizure.	Provides information about factors that can lead to injury.
Discourage smoking in bed.	Drowsiness and lack of coordination may lead to dangerous situation.
Discuss seizure precautions, e.g., reduce the amount of sensory stimuli; leave the patient in one location; remove harmful objects from the environment or pad objects/areas as possible; take axillary temperature in patient with uncontrolled seizures.	Helping the patient/family identify ways to reduce risks promotes control of situation and prevents injury. Depending on the site of the foci, the motor system can be directly involved and during the postictal period, a motor deficit may occur.
Assist patient to a safe place if aura develops. Encourage the patient to rest following the seizure activity.	Prevents fall with possibility of injury. May experience extreme fatigue and exhaustion impairing function/reflexes.

Nursing Diagnosis: Self-Esteem Disturbance

RELATED TO: Stigma of epilepsy, perception of loss of control, long-term need for medications.
AS EVIDENCED BY: verbalization about changed lifestyle, fear of rejection, negative feelings about body/self, withdrawal, lack of follow-through/nonparticipation in therapy.

Desired Outcomes/Evaluation Criteria

Identifies feelings and methods for coping with negative perceptions of self. Verbalizes increased sense of self-esteem in relation to current situation.

Nursing Actions	Rationale
Encourage expression of feelings. Determine patient's perception of the effect of a seizure disorder on daily life/future expectations.	Acceptance of self is important to maintenance of self-esteem and to motivation and the success of therapy.
Provide information related to developmental issues, e.g., overprotection by family, cognitive abilities, issues of dependence/independence.	Enhances ability to manage situation more effectively and may improve cooperation with treatment regimen.
Give age-appropriate information.	Patient will understand information more readily when it is given on his or her age/developmental level.
Explore with patient current/past successes and strengths.	Focusing on positive aspects can help to alleviate feelings of guilt/self-consciousness and help patient begin to accept managability of condition.

Nursing Diagnosis: Risk for Poisoning

RELATED TO: narrow therapeutic range of medications, emotional difficulties.

Desired Outcomes/Evaluation Criteria

Demonstrates decrease or cessation of seizures without excessive sedation, hypotension, or dysrhythmias.

Nursing Actions	Rationale
Discuss reasons for administering drug as prescribed.	Having information helps patient to recognize importance of following medication regimen.
Discuss side effects, differentiating between common and life-threatening effects.	Early identification of undesired side effects allows for prompt intervention, change in drug dosage/choice.
Stress importance of avoiding CNS depressants such as alcohol.	Can potentiate effects of the drugs.

Other Suggested Nursing Diagnoses: Ineffective Airway Clearance and Knowledge Deficit.

ing observation plays a critical role in seizure management. These observations may aid the physician in diagnosing the type of seizures the patient experiences. Nursing assessment and documentation during the *ictal period*—the time encompassing an epileptic seizure—and *postictal period*—the time beginning at the conclusion of an epileptic seizure and ending with establishment of full recovery—include the following pertinent information: data related to the precipitating event, presence of an *aura* (a sensation that precedes a seizure, migraine headache, or other recurrent condition), body area where seizure activity starts, progression of the seizure (i.e., leg jerking, lip smacking, grimacing, talking, and so on), duration of the seizure, alterations in consciousness and their duration, eye movement during ictal and postictal periods, presence of tongue biting, incontinence, periods of apnea or cyanosis, head deviations, falls, behavior changes, motor weakness or paralysis, ataxia, and headache.

- Assess the impact of a seizure on the patient's psyche. The process of diagnosis of uncontrolled seizure activity are a very difficult time for the patient and family.
- Establish an effective nurse-patient relationship so that the patient feels free to discuss his or her feelings about the seizures or about his or her treatment plan. The patient's approval of and cooperation in the treatment plan are essential to successful management of the seizures.

NURSING DIAGNOSIS

Establish the nursing diagnoses. Once a nursing diagnosis has been made, the nurse plans appropriate nursing interventions for the patient. Typical nursing diagnoses for the patient with seizure activities include Knowledge Deficit; Risk for Trauma; Self-Esteem Disturbance; Ineffective Airway Clearance; and Risk for Poisoning (see Table 20–10).

INTERVENTION

- The patient with seizures is managed medically with specific agents that are designed to control the seizures. Monitoring is an ongoing part of the management of the seizure patient. Other nursing measures center on the medication regimen, seizure precautions, and the psychosocial needs of the patient. Antiseizure agents can be administered with food to minimize gastric distress. If the patient has difficulty swallowing pills, other options are available. Many antiseizure agents are available in liquid, chewable tablet, capsule, and intravenous forms. Capsules can be opened and mixed with food. Liquids are shaken well to ensure proper mixing prior to administration. When administering an antiseizure agent intravenously, check the rate to be administered over 1 minute to avoid unpleasant or dangerous side effects.
- Allow time for the drug to reach steady state prior to

evaluating its effectiveness. It is recommended that at least five drug half-lives pass before the steady-state serum concentrations are drawn (unless loading has occurred). Peak levels are usually measured after the drug distribution is complete to determine whether the drug level is within therapeutic range. Trough levels are measured to ensure that the serum level is above the minimum effective concentration and that the drug is being eliminated at the correct rate. Sometimes frequent recurring seizures may require that steady state be achieved more quickly. This is accomplished by giving a loading dose. When an agent is inadequate and the patient is still having seizures with the maximal tolerated dose, another agent is substituted or a second drug is added to the regimen. Unless serious side effects occur, the ineffective drug is reduced gradually to minimize the risk of precipitating status epilepticus.

- Know the therapeutic range for particular antiseizure agents, potential drug interactions, and side effects of these agents.
- Inform patients about side effects and monitor for side effects or signs and symptoms of toxicity.
- Implement seizure precautions as needed depending on the type of seizure the patient experiences.
- Approach seizure patients in a holistic manner.
- Address patient concerns about having a seizure disorder, the medication regimen, and other social matters. Seizures can have a significant effect on the patient's self-esteem, socialization, employment, school, and other activities. If seizures are predictable and controlled, the patient can have a flexible lifestyle. Seizures that are partially controlled or uncontrolled can alter one's lifestyle considerably.

Patient Teaching

- Involve the patient in the treatment plan.
- Teach the patient and family as much as possible about the treatment plan. Teaching the patient and family about the action of the medication, its interactions with other drugs, and side effects is essential. It is important for the patient to understand the methods for taking his or her medications and to avoid the concurrent use of over-the-counter medications.
- Teach patients to keep a seizure diary. This diary includes a calendar in which the patient records the type of seizure, number of times it occurred, the time it happened, and how long it lasted. The diary must provide space to record factors that might have precipitated the seizure.
- Teach women taking oral contraceptives the specific risks of becoming pregnant.
- Teach patients the importance of routine examinations to monitor progress. They also need to know to report certain signs and symptoms to the physician. These include skin rash, severe nausea or vomiting, drowsiness, slurred speech or *aphasia* (complete or partial loss of the ability to comprehend or express

Table 20–11. PATIENT TEACHING INFORMATION—ANTISEIZURE MEDICATION

Dear Patient:

This drug has been ordered for you. This is what you should know about your drug to get the most from your therapy.

1. Anticonvulsants are taken to decrease the number of or to stop your seizures.
2. Anticonvulsants are taken for about 2 years and then you are examined by your physician. You may stay on the drug, or the drug may be slowly stopped.
3. Phenytoin (Dilantin), phenobarbital (Luminal), primidone (Mysoline), carbamazepine (Tegretol), valproic acid (Depakene, Depakote), ethosuximide (Zarontin), and clonazepam (Clonopin) can be taken with meals. Do not take with milk, calcium, antacids, or milk of magnesia because these products decrease absorption of the drug.
4. Do not take your anticonvulsants with alcohol, antidepressants, phenothiazines, barbiturates, antihistamines, narcotics, sedative-hypnotics, monoamine oxidase inhibitors, and over-the-counter medications unless prescribed by your physician.
5. Always check with your physician or pharmacist before taking other drugs as interactions may occur. Medications known to cause interactions include over-the-counter products for nasal congestion, allergy, pain, or obesity. Drugs of abuse such as marijuana may interact with your drug by increasing the side effects or lowering the seizure threshold, causing you to be at risk for seizures.
6. If you forget to take your anticonvulsant, take your forgotten dose (unless it is almost time for the next dose) to maintain your blood level. Do not try to catch up by taking two doses at the same time.
7. Do not stop your drug because this causes an increase in seizures and/or status epilepticus.
8. Do not alter the drug dosage yourself. Changes may need to be made under conditions of increasing physical stress, such as infection, or emotional stress, such as a loss of a loved one. However, the drug dosage is never changed without talking with your physician because either underdosage or overdosage can be hazardous.
9. Alcohol or alcohol withdrawal may precipitate seizures.
10. Drowsiness and unsteadiness are frequent side effects for all patients; be cautious when operating vehicles or machinery or when engaging in possibly hazardous activities. Often, drowsiness is an initial problem when you first begin anticonvulsant therapy; however, as therapy continues, the drowsiness lessens in severity.
11. If you have any adverse effects from your drug, talk with your physician. Side effects to antiseizure medications include drowsiness, slurred speech, dizziness, swollen glands, bleeding or tender gums, skin rash, severe nausea or vomiting, yellow skin or eyes, joint pain, fever, sore throat, unusual bleeding or bruising, and headache.
12. It is important for you to maintain good oral care and to see the dentist frequently for teeth cleaning to prevent tenderness, bleeding, and gum overgrowth.
13. Some antiseizure medications decrease the effectiveness of oral contraceptives. If you are taking oral contraceptives, consult your physician.
14. Some antiseizure medications cause sensitivity to the sun. Use sunscreen and protective clothing when outdoors.
15. Patients receiving antiseizure therapy should carry identification with this information at all times.
16. It is important for you to continue your follow-up visits to your physician to monitor the effectiveness of your drug.
17. Store these products in a tight, light-resistant container to prevent deterioration.

language), ataxia, swollen glands, tender gums, easy bruising, mouth ulcers, nosebleeds, sore throat, chills, and fever. Because many of the antiseizure agents cause drowsiness, patients must be cautioned to avoid activities that require alertness (driving, using power tools, and so on). It is also important for patients to be advised not to use alcohol or CNS depressants concurrently with these agents.

• Obtain the patient's approval of and commitment to the treatment plan, which is essential for obtaining and maintaining seizure control. The patient must live with this treatment plan and his or her cooperation is essential. A major reason for treatment failure is lack of patient compliance. As many as 40% to 60% of adults and 25% to 75% of pediatric patients have been reported to be noncompliant (Steiner, 1994). Monotherapy and once-daily dosing, when possible, may aid in compliance. Education is an important factor to enhance compliance. Support groups may help also. See Table 20–11 for specific patient teaching for antiseizure drugs.

EVALUATION

• Evaluate patient outcomes. As a member of the health team, the nurse's observations provide needed information that enables the physician to adjust drugs and dosages.

Some causes of failure of antiseizure medication are as follows: improper diagnosis of the type of seizure, incorrect choice of drug, inadequate or excessive dosage, too frequent changes in medication without regard to the time required for transition between plateau states, failure to fully use the advantages of a multiple-drug regimen, inattention to ancillary aspects of therapy, and poor compliance by the patient.

• Evaluate the patient continually for adverse effects and signs and symptoms of toxicity.
• The bibliography for this chapter can be found in Appendix B, which begins on page 1054.

CHAPTER REVIEW QUESTIONS*

1. Which agents of the following blocks enkephalinergic-induced seizures?
   a. Phenytoin.
   b. Phenobarbital.
   c. Diazepam.
   d. Valproic acid.

2. Shelly has had tonic-clonic seizures for 7 years. She has been well controlled on phenobarbital. She is now pregnant and near term. Close monitoring during labor of women is important because of the potential for:
   a. Toxicity.
   b. Hemorrhage.

*See Appendix A , which begins on page 1051, for answers.

   c. Withdrawal symptoms.
   d. Febrile seizures.

3. Which of the following is true of phenobarbital?
   a. Phenobarbital is useful in the control of absence seizures.
   b. Phenobarbital should not be given to comatose patients.
   c. A decrease in drug level occurs with propoxyphene.
   d. The dosage should be increased in the elderly patient.

4. Lamotrigine (Lamictal) is being considered for Jane to control her partial seizures. With which of the following may lamotrigine be administered?
   a. Liver and kidney disease.
   b. Lactation.
   c. History of skin rashes.
   d. Heart disease.

BUILDING YOUR CRITICAL THINKING SKILLS

STATUS EPILEPTICUS

A 32-year-old patient is admitted to the emergency department in status epilepticus. A friend states the seizures have lasted for 30 minutes. The patient has a 5-year history of insulin-dependent diabetes and a 9-year history of idiopathic seizure disorder for which he takes phenytoin (Dilantin). The patient is given 15 mg of diazepam (Valium) IV, and the convulsions terminate. When the patient is alert, he relates a 3-day history of flulike symptoms including nausea and vomiting. As a result, he missed three or four doses of his Dilantin.

1. What are the possible causes of seizure disorder in this patient?
2. What laboratory tests should be performed?
3. What precautions should the nurse observe when administering IV Dilantin?
4. What patient teaching needs to be done?

CHAPTER 21

Drugs in Anesthesia

Anne Moraca-Sawicki, RN, MSN

CHAPTER OUTLINE

KEY TERMS

Anesthesia
Balanced anesthesia
Certified registered nurse
   anesthetist (CRNA)
Depolarizing neuromuscular
   blockade
Dissociative anesthesia
General anesthesia
Induction

Inhalation anesthetic
Local anesthesia
Neuroleptic analgesia
Nondepolarizing
   neuromuscular blocking
   agents
Regional anesthesia
Volatile anesthetics

LEARNING OBJECTIVES

After reading this chapter, the student will be able to:

1. Identify those medications commonly used as
   anesthetics.
2. Differentiate among the intravenous general anesthetics
   as to mechanism of action, route of administration, pharmacokinetics, adverse effects, contraindications, interactions, advantages, and disadvantages.
3. Identify specific areas to assess in the patient requiring
   anesthetics to formulate appropriate nursing outcomes
   relative to type of anesthesia administered.
4. Plan the nursing interventions necessary to facilitate administration of anesthetics and choose appropriate
   teaching strategies to facilitate patient compliance.
5. Evaluate the patient at various stages of treatment to
   gauge nursing interventions.

This chapter deals with anesthetic agents. Basic information on the types of anesthesia, stages of general anesthesia, anesthetic drugs, and anesthetic adjuncts is included. Discussion of these agents is limited to their use
in facilitating, enhancing, or maintaining anesthesia.
Nurses do not administer anesthetics unless they are specially trained and certified to do so as *certified registered
nurse anesthetists* (CRNA). However, nurses play an integral role in administering perioperative care. Thus, it is
essential that nurses understand the types and stages of
anesthesia as well as the effects of anesthetics to ensure
the delivery of optimum patient care. The word *anesthesia*
literally means "without sensation" and is derived from
the Greek words for "negative sensation." Oliver Wen-
dell Holmes is credited with coining the term "anesthe-

sia" and, in so doing, naming the specialty responsible
for painless surgery. The history of modern anesthesia
began in 1840 with the use of nitrous oxide for dental
extractions by Drs. Morton and Wells. The first successful
general anesthetic was ether. Dr. William Morton first
demonstrated the use of ether on October 16, 1846, at
Massachusetts General Hospital. Since then the science of
anesthesia has developed into a medical specialty, and
more recently a nursing specialty, of considerable complexity.

There are three basic categories of anesthesia: general,
local, and regional. Different modes of administration exist within each category. General anesthesia may be
achieved through inhalation or intravenous drug administration. *Local anesthesia* may be achieved by topical drug

application or injection, producing anesthesia of small body areas such as a finger. *Regional anesthesia* is used to negate sensation in large areas of the body such as in spinal anesthesia.

GENERAL ANESTHESIA AND ANESTHETICS

General anesthesia is the progressive, reversible stage of central nervous system depression that occurs following the administration of drugs used for this purpose. General anesthetics may be given by the intravenous or inhalation route. Many different drugs may be used to achieve patient anesthesia, each with individual characteristics, side effects, and contraindications. The ideal agent should be nonflammable, nonexplosive if given by inhalation, and relatively nontoxic. It should achieve its desired effect without causing tissue hypoxia, laryngospasm, excessive tracheobronchial secretions, or respiratory depression. Many useful anesthetics do not meet all these criteria. Thus, it has become common practice to combine small amounts of several intravenous drugs to achieve the most beneficial drug characteristics with a minimum of toxicity. This practice is known as *balanced anesthesia* and allows the anesthetist to select drug combinations tailored to individual patient needs relative to the surgery to be performed. Balanced anesthesia can also be achieved by using narcotics with inhalation gas. Balanced anesthesia is typically achieved with a combination of inhalation, narcotic, and neuromuscular blocking agents (muscle relaxants).

The anesthesia process is divided into three phases: *induction*, maintenance, and recovery. The induction phase is analogous to climbing up a mountain. It requires a comparatively large amount of anesthetic to reach the height of anesthesia, just as it requires a large energy expenditure to reach the mountaintop. The maintenance dose required to remain on top, or at the desired level, is much less. In the recovery phase, anesthetic administration is stopped, or an antidote given and anesthesia is reversed as the drugs wear off.

STAGES AND CLASSIFICATION OF GENERAL ANESTHESIA

When a general anesthetic is administered, anesthesia is not achieved immediately. Induction occurs in a definite order, as the patient passes from one level of central nervous system depression to the next until adequate surgical anesthesia occurs. Although passage from one level (stage) of anesthesia to the next occurs rapidly because of rapid onset of action of barbiturates used, progressive signs of central nervous system depression do occur at each stage. The combination of two or more drugs is often needed to achieve and maintain the triad of anesthesia: amnesia, analgesia, and muscle relaxation.

The exact mechanism of action of general anesthetic drugs is unknown. There are several theories of anesthetic action. One theory is that anesthetics change the cell's permeability, surface tension, electrical stability, and/or cy-

Table 21–1. STAGES AND PLANES OF ANESTHESIA

Stage and Plane	Characteristics	Special Considerations
Stage I: Analgesia Plane 1 Plane 2 Plane 3	Conscious. Partial analgesia; total amnesia, conscious, breathing slows. Complete analgesia and amnesia, conscious.	Patient may be quiet or euphoric. Because cortex is depressed in this state, it is sometimes called the cortical stage. This stage ends when consciousness is lost.
Stage II: Delirium (dream)	Conscious is lost; excitement and muscle activity may be marked or minimal; breathing is irregular. Incontinence or vomiting may occur.	Because of hyperexcitability that may occur in this transition stage, it is generally kept to minimum. Depression of midbrain occurs in this stage. This stage ends when automatic breathing occurs.
Stage III: Surgical Plane 1 Plane 2 Plane 3 Plane 4	Rhythmic breathing occurs. Hypoactivity to painful stimuli. Assisted respiration necessary from this point on. Somatic response to pain lost. Progressive intercostal paralysis occurs; visceral response to pain is lost. Intercostal paralysis complete; diaphragmatic breathing occurs.	Moderate depression of subcortex occurs. Light anesthesia. Predominant control is by midbrain. Moderate level of anesthesia. Moderate depression of midbrain occurs. Moderate level of anesthesia. Continued depression of midbrain; deep level of anesthesia. Approaching toxic level of anesthesia. State ends with apnea.
Stage IV: Medullary paralysis Plane 1 Plane 2	Respiratory paralysis (arrest) occurs; blood pressure falls; pupils dilate. Cardiovascular collapse (arrest) occurs; pupils fully dilated; muscles flaccid.	Moderate depression of pons occurs; toxicity is reversible at this level; this level ends when circulatory collapse occurs. Irreversible level of anesthesia. Death results.

toplasm. These agents act on the central nervous system: brain, medulla, and spinal cord. The cerebral cortex and midbrain control consciousness are affected first. The spinal cord, involved in both sensory and motor functions, is the next site of drug action. The third site of action is the blocking of the medulla, which controls respiratory and cardiovascular functions.

Guedel devised a classification (Gilman et al., 1990) of the stages and planes of anesthesia in 1920, using ether as his model. Table 21–1 features the stages and planes of anesthesia.

Today, most patients receive barbiturate induction to general anesthesia. Because these drugs have a rapid onset of action, it is not possible to observe each individual sign of the stages outlined by Guedel. However, his classification system is of value in understanding how anesthesia occurs.

An *inhalation anesthetic* is sometimes used in children to induce anesthesia. Because inhalation induction is slower than that achieved with intravenous agents, it is sometimes possible to observe the signs Guedel outlined. Inhalation anesthesia is also used when an intravenous route is not readily available, such as in patients with sclerosed veins due to intravenous chemotherapy for cancer or in intravenous drug abusers.

INHALATION ANESTHETICS

Commonly used inhalation agents include **halothane (Fluothane)**, **methoxyflurane (Penthrane)**, **enflurane (Ethrane)**, **isoflurane (Forane)**, **desflurane (Suprane)** and **sevoflurane (Ultane)**. Inhalation anesthetics are not given in pure form but are mixed with oxygen or nitrous oxide. Liquid inhalation agents are vaporized by an anesthesia machine for administration via mask or endotracheal tube. Once vaporized and mixed with oxygen or nitrous oxide, anesthesia is given and transported to the patient's lungs. These drugs may be given by open system, closed systems, or nonrebreathing systems. The nonrebreathing valve-type delivery is used most commonly in the United States. The other methods are seldom used today.

Inhalation agents are also referred to as *volatile anesthetics*, that is, liquid or solution forms that are evaporated into a vapor for administration. Absorption, distribution, and excretion of these drugs depend on the pressure concentration gradients, moving from the area of higher concentration to the area of lower concentration. This gradient is responsible for moving oxygen from the alveoli to the arterioles and carbon dioxide from the venules back to the alveoli. Once gas exchange occurs in the lungs, the heart circulates the anesthetic to the brain and other organs. Once biotransformation occurs, most of the inhaled anesthetic is excreted in the form of exhaled gases. Most of the inhalational agent is excreted by the time the patient returns to the unit, unless surgery lasts more than a few hours. All are nonexplosive and nonflammable. Malignant hyperthermia may be triggered by any of these agents.

○ **Nitrous oxide** was the first modern anesthetic agent used. It is commonly referred to as "laughing gas" because inhaling small amounts mixed with air has an intoxicating effect: The patient feels happy, giddy, and laughs. Nitrous oxide was first used to produce analgesia

and amnesia during dental procedures, and it remains popular for this purpose today. Because it has only relatively mild anesthetic properties, it is rarely used alone, except for dental and minor surgical procedures and during the second stage of labor. Nitrous oxide is often used in combination with other anesthetics for its analgesic/amnesic effects and to provide rapid induction. The major advantages of this agent is that it has no clinically significant effect on the cardiovascular system as long as the patient is adequately ventilated. Nitrous oxide is relatively free from major toxicities and side effects, but chronic use may cause leukopenia. The major disadvantages are that it is too weak to produce anesthesia beyond stage II (delirium); it rapidly diffuses out of the lungs once it is discontinued, so a diffusion hypoxia oxygen deficiency may occur; and it tends to diffuse into open cavities, making it unacceptable for surgeries involving gastrointestinal obstruction, pneumothorax, or ear procedures.

○ **Halothane** (Fluothane) is a halogenated hydrocarbon anesthetic five times more potent than the obsolete anesthetic ether. It is one of the most commonly used inhalation anesthetics. The major advantages of halothane are its pleasant, rapid induction and rapid recovery. Major disadvantages are its narrow safety range and strong circulatory, myocardial, and respiratory depressant effects. It is the only inhalation agent that can cause bradycardia. It produces poor skeletal muscle relaxation and profound uterine relaxation. Halothane sensitizes the heart to epinephrine, causing dysrhythmias, and can cause hepatotoxicity and halothane hepatitis. It is not recommended for routine obstetric use, in cases where epinephrine may be used, or in patients with hepatic disease. Despite its narrow safety range, halothane remains a widely used anesthetic, especially for children, because they seem less susceptible to halothane hepatitis. It is the most commonly used pediatric induction agent because it is the least noxious smelling and smoothest induction agent. Specially calibrated vaporizers are available for use with halothane to ensure drug delivery within the safe limit range.

○ **Methoxyflurane** (Penthrane) is the most potent inhalation anesthetic. However, it has several important disadvantages that severely limit its use, including numerous side effects, slow induction and recovery times, narrow margin of safety, and low vapor pressure. Methoxyflurane, like halothane, sensitizes the heart to the effects of epinephrine, depresses the respiratory system (more so than halothane), and produces cardiovascular effects (less severe than halothane). It can also cause high-output renal failure. Methoxyflurane has a high lipid and blood solubility, which slows induction and recovery time. It is not readily vaporized, which further delays induction. Thus, when used, methoxyflurane is used mainly to maintain anesthesia induced by other agents such as nitrous oxide and is supplemented with muscle relaxants. The long recovery period of methoxyflurane decreases the need for narcotic analgesics in the first few hours postoperatively. The long recovery following use of this drug makes it a poor agent for patients having same-day surgery who are discharged shortly after surgery.

○ **Enflurane** (Ethrane) is a fluorinated ether inhalation anesthetic. This drug and its effects are very similar to halothane. It does not cause renal or hepatic toxicity or cardiovascular depression as do other fluorinated ethers, but it does sensitize the heart to the effects of epinephrine and may cause dysrhythmias. This cardiac effect occurs much less often with enflurane than with halothane. Enflurane gives good muscle relaxation, although its analgesic effects are not as great as some other anesthetics.

○ **Isoflurane** (Forane) is a halogenated ether inhalation anesthetic. It is thought by many anesthetists to be an ideal agent because it has no apparent side effects. Isoflurane is less potent than halothane. There is good patient acceptance of this anesthetic, despite its slightly pungent odor. Induction is smooth when the patient is premedicated and nitrous oxide and oxygen are given concomitantly. Isoflurane markedly potentiates effects of neuromuscular blocking agents; for example, tubocurarine dosage must be decreased by one-third when isoflurane is given.

Isoflurane does not produce the renal, hepatic, or cardiotoxic effects seen with other gases. There is little or no cardiovascular depression with this agent and less tendency to develop dysrhythmias than with enflurane or halothane. Assisted ventilation is recommended with isoflurane because it may depress respiratory rate. No central nervous system stimulation is evident, even with deep isoflurane anesthesia. The drug has no adverse effect on intracranial or intraocular pressure as long as adequate ventilation is maintained. However, isoflurane can cause marked tachycardia at higher doses.

Postanesthesia nausea, vomiting, and excitation are rare after use of this anesthetic. Mental alertness is generally depressed 2 to 3 hours after use of isoflurane; thus it reduces patient perception of pain in the immediate postoperative period.

○ **Desflurane** (Suprane) and sevoflurane (Ultane) are slightly pungent volatile liquid almost structurally identical to isoflurane (Forane). They are highly stable, has low solubility, rapid induction time, and short postanesthesia recovery time, making it an excellent choice for ambulatory surgery patients. They resist metabolism/biodegradation. Deep anesthesia is readily achieved, and reawakening time is almost twice as fast with desflurane as compared to isoflurane. Organ specific toxicity is minimal or absent. Both are mild airway irritants and can cause dose-dependent respiratory depression. Like isoflurane, they decrease systemic vascular resistance and mean arterial blood pressure; do not sensitize the myocardium to catecholamines, and cardiac rhythm stability is unchanged during anesthesia. Both significantly depress neuromuscular function, but cause no renal or hepatic effects.

INTRAVENOUS ANESTHETICS

The intravenous route is commonly used to induce or maintain anesthesia. Drugs commonly used are the ultra-short-acting barbiturates and the neuroleptics. The ultra-short-acting barbiturates include **thiopental sodium (Pentothal)**, **methohexital sodium (Brevital Sodium)**, and **thiamylal sodium (Surital)**. The neuroleptic agents used in anesthesia or, in some cases, as adjuncts to anesthesia are **ketamine hydrochloride (Ketalar)**, **droperidol/fentanyl (Innovar)**, **alfentanil hydrochloride (Alfenta)**, and **sufen-**

tanil citrate **(Sufenta)**. In addition, a short-acting benzodiazepine midazolam HCL (Versed), a sedative hypnotic propofol (Diprivan), and a butyrophenone derivative droperidol (Inapsine) are frequently used for short procedures such as intubation, or for conscious sedation. Remember that these products provide for conscious sedation, but have no affect on pain. Therefore, if a painful procedure is to be performed, the patient will also need pain medication. These agents, especially the ultra-short-acting barbiturates, are excellent for inducing anesthesia because they give pleasant, rapid induction; are easily administered; have no explosive properties; cause no respiratory tract irritation; and have rapid recovery periods. In addition to the intravenous route, barbiturates can also be given orally (common, but not for anesthesia) and rectally (less common). The barbiturates have a rapid onset of action (within a few seconds) and a duration of 1 hour or less when administered intravenously. These drugs are metabolized mainly in the liver and excreted in the urine.

▼ **CLINICAL ALERT**

Disadvantages of barbiturates are their poor analgesic and skeletal muscle relaxation properties. These drugs are generally used in combination with potent analgesics and muscle relaxants; they give good anesthesia for short surgical and diagnostic procedures. As with all barbiturates, the "hangover" side effect may occur.

○ **Thiopental sodium** (Pentothal) is an ultra-short-acting barbiturate with a rapid onset and a short duration of action (15 minutes or less). It is one of the most widely used barbiturate anesthetics. Its major use is for induction of anesthesia, but it may be used as a sole agent for short procedures. It is sometimes used to control drug-induced convulsions resulting from allergy to local anesthetics. Adverse effects include respiratory depression, bronchospasm, cardiac depression, and hypotension. Use of thiopental sodium is contraindicated in patients with asthma or porphyria. Most of the complications seen with this drug are iatrogenic, the result of poor drug administration technique. Skin sloughing, edema, chemical arteritis, or gangrene can result if this drug is not properly given and is delivered into subcutaneous tissues or into an artery.

○ **Methohexital sodium** (Brevital Sodium) is an ultra-short-acting barbiturate that has five times the strength of thiopental sodium. It is also shorter acting than thiopental sodium. And, as it is less likely to cause bronchospasm, methohexital sodium may be administered cautiously to patients with asthma. Its disadvantages are similar to those of thiopental sodium and include respiratory depression. It also is not a good skeletal muscle relaxant or analgesic. Methohexital sodium is especially useful in examination under anesthesia procedures, oral surgery, and the setting of fractures. Intra-arterial administration of this agent can cause gangrene. Because of a shorter duration of action than thiopental, this drug is especially useful for outpatients. It is also used for patients undergoing electroconvulsive therapy.

○ **Thiamylal sodium** (Surital) is the last of the ultra-short-acting barbiturates commonly used to induce anesthesia. Thiamylal sodium is also similar to thiopental in its rapid onset, short duration of effect, and recovery time. It is used as a short-duration anesthetic for diagnostic procedures. It shares the same limitations and disadvantages as other ultra-short-acting barbiturates.

○ **Ketamine hydrochloride** (Ketalar) is a synthetic nonbarbiturate agent that can be administered either intravenously or intramuscularly. It is metabolized by the liver and excreted primarily in the urine, with small amounts eliminated in the stool. Ketamine produces a state known as *dissociative anesthesia* because the patient feels dissociated or detached from the environment during induction. The exact mechanism of dissociative anesthetic action is not fully understood. Ketamine selectively interrupts the higher brain centers of the cerebral cortex, causing a generalized sensory blockade that produces anesthesia. This drug has a rapid induction and produces good analgesia and amnesia but poor muscle relaxation. Ketamine does not depress the respiratory system. This drug actually increases the tone of skeletal, cardiac, and respiratory muscles and can thus raise blood pressure and heart and respiratory rates. Ketamine produces good anesthesia for 5 to 25 minutes with stable cardiovascular activity and good airway status. Intubation is not necessary when this drug is administered, because of its negligible effect on the pharyngeal and laryngeal reflexes. This agent is often used in combination with other low-potency drugs like nitrous oxide to produce balanced anesthesia. It is a good drug of choice for short surgical or diagnostic procedures (except those involving the pharyngeal-laryngeal areas). Ketamine is often used in burn units where patients require frequent, repetitive anesthesia for procedures and dressing changes.

▼ **CLINICAL ALERT**

The major disadvantage of ketamine is its prolonged (up to several hours) recovery period and the occurrence of emergence reactions. About 12% of those receiving ketamine have disturbing dreams and/or hallucinations as the drug wears off. This may occur more often in adults than children.

Diazepam (Valium) administration is recommended in conjunction with ketamine to help reduce emergence reactions. Ketamine is contraindicated in patients with hypertension or alcoholism, in those who will undergo intracranial surgery, and in those who have bad dreams, like psychiatric patients. Safe use of ketamine in pregnancy and delivery has not yet been established.

○ **Droperidol/Fentanyl** (Innovar) is the combination of a potent opioid analgesic (fentanyl) with the anesthetic/antipsychotic agent droperidol available under the trade name Innovar in a 50:1 fixed ratio. Innovar produces *neuroleptic analgesia*: The patient is psychologically indifferent to the environment, pain free, but not necessarily asleep (depending on the dose administered). Thus, it can be useful for patients undergoing endoscopic procedures where some degree of patient cooperation may be needed. It is also an excellent adjunct to more potent general anesthetics for both induction and maintenance.

Droperidol/fentanyl may be given intramuscularly (45 to 60 minutes preoperatively) or intravenously. Droperidol/fentanyl can be used alone for short surgical or diagnostic procedures or in combination. In addition to anesthetic effects, it produces excellent antiemetic effects, beta-adrenergic blocking effects, and antidysrhythmic effects. Its major disadvantages are the slow onset of anesthesia and degree of postoperative respiratory depression produced. Analgesic effects may linger several hours following surgery, so it is essential to reduce doses of all central nervous system depressant drugs, like narcotic analgesics, by one-third to one-half for 8 hours after anesthesia.

▼ **CLINICAL ALERT**

Droperidol/fentanyl can cause bradycardia, bronchospasm, apnea, and muscle rigidity, which is usually due to the fentanyl component in the drug. Thus, it is essential to have available atropine (for bradycardia) and cardiopulmonary resuscitation and airway intubation equipment, neuromuscular blockers, and narcotic antagonists (for respiratory complications); and to check vital signs frequently.

○ **Alfentanil hydrochloride** (Alfenta) is an opioid analgesic with a rapid onset of action. It is an excellent induction agent and can also be a component of balanced opioid anesthesia. Alfenta is useful for (1) incremental injection as an analgesic adjunct for short surgical procedures (less than 1 hour); (2) continuous infusion as a maintenance analgesic with nitrous oxide/oxygen for general surgical procedures; and (3) for general anesthesia (by intravenous injection) for procedures at least 45 minutes long. Because opioid analgesics tend to produce some muscle rigidity, use of a neuromuscular blocking agent is necessary with Alfenta.

The dose of Alfenta is individualized according to ideal body weight, physical status, underlying pathologic status, and the type and duration of surgical procedure and anesthesia. Dosage should be reduced in elderly or debilitated patients and not used in children under age 12. Alfenta should be used with caution in patients with pulmonary disease, decreased respiratory reserve, potentially compromised respiration, or impaired renal or liver function. When Alfenta is given in combination with other CNS depressants, the magnitude and duration of central nervous system and cardiovascular effects may be enhanced, necessitating a reduction in dose of one or both agents.

○ **Sufentanil citrate** (Sufenta) is an opioid analgesic with an immediate onset of action. It is used as an adjunct in maintenance of balanced general anesthesia or as a primary anesthetic for induction and maintenance of anesthesia with 100% oxygen in patients undergoing major surgery. Sufenta is useful in cardiovascular or neurosurgical procedures and provides favorable myocardial and cerebral oxygen balance. It is also useful when extended postoperative ventilation is anticipated. A neuromuscular blocking agent is needed with Sufenta because of the muscle rigidity this opioid produces.

Sufenta dosages are based on lean body weight and are

reduced in elderly or debilitated patients and used with caution in those with pulmonary disease, compromised pulmonary status, or liver or renal impairment. When used in combination with other CNS depressants, the magnitude and duration of central nervous system and cardiovascular effects may be enhanced; thus the dosage of one or both agents should be reduced.

○ **Midazolam HCL (Versed)** is a short-acting benzodiazepine CNS depressant, three times more potent than Valium. It is used for short procedures where memory impairment of the procedure is desired. Midazolam is administered in a 1 mg dose over 2 minutes, then wait at least 2 minutes before another dose is administered to evaluate the effect. Respiratory depression can occur if drug is administered too much, too quickly. Reduce the dose by 1/3 if a narcotic premedication was administered.

○ **Profofol (Diprivan)** is a sedative hypnotic used for induction and maintenance of anesthesia, as well as for conscious sedation. The dose range is from 0.5 to 8 mcg/ml. Small doses are administered with a 3 to 5 minuite waiting period between doses to evaluate effects. Profofol is used only if the patient is mechanically ventilated.

○ **Droperidol (Inapsine),** a butyrophenone derivative, which produces tranquilization, sedation, and an antiemetic effect. The onset of action is 3 to 10 minutes with the full effect occuring in about 30 minutes.

ADJUNCTS TO ANESTHESIA

In addition to the various anesthetic agents already discussed, several other drugs may be given in the perioperative period to facilitate and/or augment the anesthetic process. These drugs will be considered only in relation to their status as anesthetic adjuncts. Preoperative adjuncts to anesthesia include **atropine, promethazine hydrochloride (Phenergan)**, and **glycopyrrolate (Robinul)**. Neuromuscular blocking agents are administered intraoperatively. Drugs administered in the postoperative period include reversal agents—**naloxone (Narcan)** and **neostigmine (Prostigmin)**.

Preoperative Agents

○ **Atropine,** a parasympatholytic or cholinergic blocking agent, is frequently administered as a preanesthetic medication. The main reasons for its preanesthesia use are its ability to decrease respiratory tract secretions and prevent anesthesia-induced bradycardia. Atropine produces many effects, including mydriasis, reduced secretion of certain glands, relaxation of smooth muscles, and vagolytic activity. The usual adult dose given is 0.4 to 0.6 mg intramuscularly 30 to 60 minutes preoperatively. Because many anesthetics currently used are relatively nonirritating to the respiratory tract, use of atropine may not be as common as in the past. For further information on atropine, see Chapter 17.

○ **Promethazine hydrochloride** (Phenergan) is a phenothiazine-derivative antihistamine with anticholinergic, antiemetic, antipruritic, and sedative properties. Promethazine is a phenothiazine, so precautions and warnings applicable to phenothiazines apply to this drug as well. (For further information, see phenothiazines in Chapter 27.) Promethazine is thought to potentiate analgesia, although scientific data does not support this notion. It is used preoperatively for its sedative effect. The usual adult preoperative dose is 50 mg, combined with an atropine-like drug. Postoperatively, promethazine is given to combat nausea and as an adjunct to analgesics, especially narcotics, given for postoperative pain. The usual adult dose is 12.5 to 50 mg intramuscularly.

○ **Glycopyrrolate** (Robinul) is a synthetic anticholinergic used for preoperative medication and to help counteract adverse effects of anticholinergics given to reverse neuromuscular blockade. It decreases the volume and acidity of respiratory tract secretions. Glycopyrrolate is not believed to cross the blood-brain barrier. Robinul is used because of its low level of toxicity and better ability to reduce respiratory secretions. Usual adult preoperative dose is 0.002 mg per pound of body weight intramuscularly 30 to 60 minutes preoperatively. To help reverse adverse effect of neuromuscular blockade, the adult dose is 0.2 mg intravenously for each 1 mg neostigmine or equivalent dose of pyridostigmine. There are no significant interactions, but use of this drug is contraindicated in narrow-angle glaucoma, unstable cardiovascular status, myasthenia gravis, and obstructive urologic or gastrointestinal diseases, as glycopyrrolate worsens these conditions.

Intraoperative Agents

Neuromuscular Blocking Agents Neuromuscular blocking agents are commonly used as adjuncts to other anesthesia-producing drugs to facilitate endotracheal intubation and to help maintain sufficient anesthesia for procedures requiring deep muscle relaxation, like abdominal surgery. Although commonly referred to as muscle relaxants, this term is a misnomer. Neuromuscular blocking agents paralyze skeletal muscle by peripherally blocking nerve impulses to skeletal muscle at the neuromuscular junction, which results in muscle relaxation. Many general anesthetics have minimal muscle-relaxing properties. During surgery, it is usually desirable for the patient to be paralyzed. Neuromuscular blockers are powerful drugs that produce apnea and paralysis. To produce sufficient muscle relaxation for surgery, a deep level of anesthesia must be achieved. Specific neuromuscular blocking drugs able to produce enough muscle paralysis for surgery while maintaining a lighter level of anesthesia are often combined with anesthetics.

Two types of neuromuscular blockers used are the depolarizing and nondepolarizing agents. Both types paralyze the neuromuscular junction, but accomplish this by different mechanisms. A detailed description of how these drugs work appears in Chapter 22.

NONDEPOLARIZING AGENTS *Nondepolarizing* (also called competitive) *neuromuscular blocking agents* work by competitive inhibition on the postsynaptic membrane. Nondepolarizing neuromuscular blockers include tubocurarine chloride (Tubarine), rocuronium bromide (Zemuron), mivacurium chloride (Mivacron), vecuronium bromide (Norcuron), pancuronium bromide (Pavulon), and atracurium besylate (Tracrium).

Table 21–2. POSSIBLE REACTIONS TO GENERAL ANESTHESIA DUE TO PREOPERATIVE MEDICATION/DRUG USE

Drug	Use/Action	Potential Effect(s)
Hydralazine (Apresoline)	Antihypertensive—produces peripheral blood vessel and some smooth muscle relaxation.	Hypertensive crises. Rebound hypotensive crisis may occur 48 hr following anesthesia.
Methyldopa (Aldomet)	Antihypertensive—"false transmitter" for norepinephrine at CNS nerve ending.	Hypertensive crisis.
Reserpine (Serpasil)	Antihypertensive—depletes the stores of catecholamines.	Hypertensive crisis.
Guanethidine (Ismelin)	Antihypertensive—depresses postganglionic sympathetic nerve fiber function.	Hypertensive crisis.
Propranolol (Inderal)	Antidysrhythmic; antihypertensive β-blocking drug whose effects persist for 24 hr after discontinuing therapy.	Hypotension.
Glucocorticoids	Anti-inflammatory, multiple uses.	Hypotension.
Oral contraceptives	Birth control—impairs biotransformation of meperidine (Demerol).	Decreased effectiveness of meperidine (Demerol).
Tricyclics	Antidepressants—produce sympathetic effects.	Hypotension/hypertension, junctional rhythms.
Digoxin (Lanoxin)	Cardiotonic—positive inotropic effect.	Increased sympathetic effect of this drug on the heart.
Cocaine	Drug abuse.	Cardiac arrest in patients given lidocaine with epinephrine for local anesthesia. Risk not associated with plain lidocaine.
Marijuana/THC/Nabilone	Drug abuse; control of nausea/vomiting associated with cancer chemotherapy.	Potentiates the effects of barbiturates.
Cimetidine (Tagamet)	Duodenal and gastric ulcers. Inhibits histamine action to decrease gastric acid secretions.	Prolongs duration of action of succinylcholine.

Patients taking specific medication to control conditions such as hypertension may be more susceptible to certain reactions following general anesthesia. Drug abuse may also precipitate certain postanesthesia side effects.

DEPOLARIZING AGENTS *Depolarizing* (or noncompetitive) *neuromuscular blockade* is achieved with succinylcholine (Anectine, Quelicin, Sucrostrin), the only drug of this type currently used. Succinylcholine is a potent skeletal muscle relaxant that achieves its effect rapidly through depolarization of the motor end-plate. It is especially useful in facilitating endotracheal intubation. After administration of this drug, muscle fasciculations occur and potassium is forced out of the muscle cells into the circulation. Cimetidine (Tagamet) apparently intensifies the action of succinylcholine. Combining these drugs may lead to prolonged respiratory depression and extended periods of apnea. Table 21–2 lists potential effects of preoperative drugs.

Postoperative Reversal Agents

○ **Naloxone** (Narcan) is a narcotic antagonist frequently used to reverse the effects of opioids. Naloxone has no respiratory depressant or agonist activity of its own and is the most frequently used narcotic antagonist. The usual adult dose is 0.1 to 0.2 mg intravenously every 2 to 3 minutes as needed to reverse the effects of perioperatively administered narcotics. There are no significant interactions with Narcan. Once the effects of narcotics are reversed, the patient can experience intense pain.

○ **Neostigmine** (Prostigmin) is an anticholinesterase agent used to reverse the effects of nondepolarizing neuromuscular blocking agents after surgery. It enhances cholinergic action by facilitating the transmission of impulses across neuromuscular junctions. Neostigmine is contraindicated in patients with known hypersensitivity to this drug and those with peritonitis or mechanical obstruction of the intestinal or urinary tract. Adverse effects are usually due to an exaggeration of pharmocologic effects like salivation and muscle fasciculation. Cardiac dysrhythmias, dizziness, allergic reactions and anaphylaxis, diaphoresis, and urinary frequency can also occur. Overdosage can cause cholinergic crisis. When neostigmine is used to reverse nondepolarizing neuromuscular blockade, it is recommended that atropine also be administered (use separate syringes). Neostigmine causes a build-up of acetylcholine to reverse the block, and atropine minimizes the side effects of acetylcholine buildup. These side effects include bradycardia, bronchospasm, and excessive salivation at the muscarinic sites.

Other Adjuncts to Anesthesia

There are numerous other drugs that may be used for facilitating anesthesia and for their effects during and after anesthetic administration. Antianxiety agents such as diazepam (Valium), hypnotic sedatives such as pentobarbital sodium (Nembutal), and narcotics such as meperidine (Demerol) and midazolam (Versed) are all commonly used perioperative agents. They may be used before surgery to facilitate anesthesia; during surgery to augment anesthesia/analgesia; and after surgery to relieve nausea, promote sedation, and/or provide analgesia. (For further information on any of these drugs, turn to their respective chapters.)

LOCAL/REGIONAL ANESTHESIA AND ANESTHETICS

Like general anesthetics, local anesthetics are not administered by nurses (except for specially trained certified registered nurse anesthetists). However, nurses administer care to patients who have received local anesthesia and are responsible for monitoring for adverse effects and promoting safe recovery. Local anesthetics stabilize nerve cell membranes to sodium and potassium exchange to block the conduction of impulses in nerve fibers without depolarizing the cell membrane. As anesthetic concentration increases, the threshold for excitation increases. These drugs can act on any part of the central nervous system and on any type of nerve cell. Onset of effect is first on small nonmyelinated autonomic fibers; next, ability to sense cold, warmth, pain, and touch is affected; and finally, motor function is affected. Sensation returns in reverse order.

There are several different techniques of local (sometimes called conduction) anesthesia. The types of local anesthesia and their sites of actions are as follows:

1. Topical (surface) anesthesia is application of a readily absorbed drug to the skin or mucous membranes. Cocaine and tetracaine are topical anesthetics.
2. Infiltration anesthesia is produced by injecting the agent throughout the area to be desensitized. This is commonly done by injecting a drug along the line of an incision or the edges of a laceration to be sutured. The drug is injected into the tissue in the area and not into any specific nerves.
3. Field block anesthesia is accomplished by infiltrating the tissue around the area to be made insensitive without infiltrating the area itself. This technique is commonly used in the excision of sebaceous cysts.
4. Nerve block is the injection of the drug close to a mixed nerve so that the area innervated by that nerve will become insensitive.
5. Spinal anesthesia is achieved by injecting a local anesthetic into the subarachnoid space. Epidural anesthesia is the technique of injecting the drug between the vertebral spines and beneath the ligament into the extradural space. There are fewer complications, such as headache, following epidural anesthesia. Spinal and epidural anesthesia, whose sites are shown in Figure 21–1, are sometimes called regional anesthesia techniques.
6. Caudal anesthesia is produced by injecting local anesthetic lower in the spinal canal or sacral canal. Caudal anesthesia is a variation of epidural anesthesia commonly used in obstetric patients.
7. Intravenous regional anesthesia is anesthesia of the entire distal part of an extremity. This is achieved by elevating the extremity, producing exsanguination with tourniquets, and injecting the drug in the distal part of the limb. This technique is commonly used in hand surgery (the Bier block) and foot surgery. Maximum length of anesthesia is 1.5 hours due to use of tourniquets.

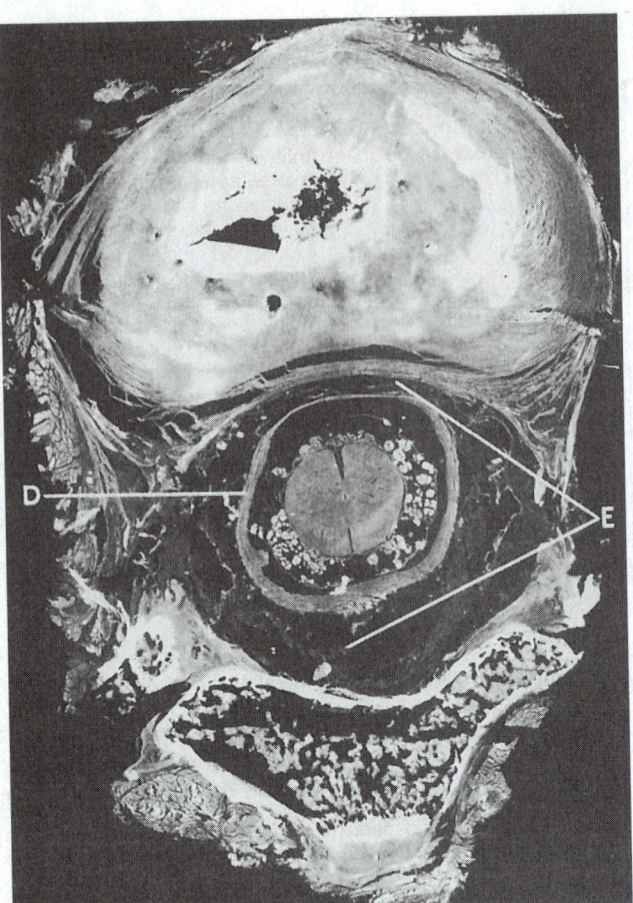

Figure 21–1. Sites of anesthetic administration in the spinal canal. Traverse section of spine between first and second lumbar vertebrae. **E** is the epidural space where local anesthetic agent is placed for epidural anesthesia. **D** is the dural and arachnoid layers separating it from the subarachnoid space. The subarachnoid space is where anesthetic is injected to achieve spinal anesthesia. (From Norris, W, and Campbell, D: A Nurses' Guide to Anesthetics, Resuscitation and Intensive Care, ed 5. Williams & Wilkins, Baltimore, 1972, p 11, with permission.)

Desirable characteristics of a good local anesthetic include complete reversibility, low systemic toxicity, action confined principally to nerve tissue, short onset time, sufficiently long duration, solubility in saline solution and water, sterilizability and storability without deterioration, compatibility with vasoconstrictor drugs, and lack of tissue irritation.

There are two types of local anesthetics, the amides and the esters. Determination of anesthetic type depends on the kind of chemical bond in the drug's molecular structure. Epinephrine, because of its vasoconstrictor effects, is often combined with local anesthetic drugs to slow absorption and prolong anesthetic effect. Speed of drug absorption depends on drug dose, site of injection, technique of anesthesia used, and local conditions at the site of administration. Table 21–3 summarizes local anesthesia drugs.

Amide-type local anesthetics include **bupivacaine (Marcaine, Sensorcaine)**, **dibucaine (Nupercainal)**, **etidocaine (Duranest)**, **lidocaine (Xylocaine, others)**, **mepivacaine (Carbocaine)**, and **prilocaine (Citanest)**. These agents are

Table 21–3. LOCAL ANESTHETICS

DRUG NAME/ROUTE AND DOSAGE	PHARMOKINETICS/DYNAMICS	NURSING IMPLICATIONS
all local anesthetics		
		INTERVENTION: Protect anesthesized area from trauma while numb. Monitor for return of sensation and motor function. **EVALUATION:** Monitor for adverse effects, anaphylaxis, allergy, respiratory distress.
AMIDE TYPE		
bupivacaine hydrochloride (Marcaine) (Sensorcaine)		
Available with or without epinephrine. All doses given for drug without epinephrine. Contraindicated in children under 12 yr. ***Epidural:*** 0.50% sol, 75–100 mg. ***Caudal:*** 0.50% sol, 75–100 mg. ***Peripheral Nerve Block:*** 0.50% sol, 24–400 (max).	**Onset:** 4–17 min **Peak:** NA **Duration:** 3–6 hr **PB:** 52%–96% **½L:** 1.5–5.5 hr **B:** liver **E:** urine	Same as for all plus: **INTERVENTION:** Observe patient for signs of adverse effects, anaphylaxis. After spinal anesthesia, use spinal headache precautions: patient lies flat 8–12 hr postoperatively. **Patient Teaching**—Inform patient duration of action is 3–6 hr but can be up to 16 hr. **EVALUATION:** Patient has pain-free procedure with sensory return afterwards. Health teaching is effective and patient complies. In spinal anesthesia, headache is avoided. No preventable adverse effects occur.
etidocaine hydrochloride (Duranest)		
Infiltration: 0.5% sol, 4–400 mg. ***Peripheral Nerve Block:*** 0.5% sol, 25–400 mg. ***Caudal:*** 0.5% sol, 50–150 mg. ***Vaginal:*** 0.5% sol, 50–150 mg.	**Onset:** 2–8 min **Peak:** NA **Duration:** 3–6 hr **PB:** 94%–96% **½L:** 1–2 hr **B:** liver **E:** urine	Same as for all plus: **ASSESSMENT:** Ask women if any chance of pregnancy because safe use in pregnancy not established. **INTERVENTION: Patient Teaching**—Tell patient drug action can be up to 13 hr (usually 3–6 hr) so ambulatory patients know drug lasts longer than lidocaine or typical dental anesthesia.
lidocaine hyprochloride (Xylocaine) (Nervocaine) (Ultracaine)		
Available with and without epinephrine; safe dose 7 mg/kg; maximum 200 mg without epinephrine, 500 mg with epinephrine. ***Caudal (obstetric use) or Epidural (thoracic):*** 1% sol, 200–300 mg. ***Caudal (surgery):*** 1.5% sol, 225–300 mg. ***Spinal Surgical Anesthesia:*** 5% sol, with 7.5% dextrose, 75–100 mg.	**Onset:** 5–10 min **Peak:** NA **Duration:** 1 hr without epinephrine; 2–3 hr with epinephrine **PB:** 60%–80% **½L:** 100 min **B:** liver **E:** urine	Same as for all plus: **ASSESSMENT:** Ask whether patient is taking MAO inhibitors or tricyclic antidepressants; severe hypertension can occur if drug containing epinephrine is given to patients on these drugs. **INTERVENTION:** Drug has moderate potency for surface anesthesia and is available in 4% topical form, but duration is short in this form. **Patient Teaching**—Tell patient duration of drug action is 1–3 hr when used as local anesthetic. Instruct patient to use spinal headache precautions. Caution ambulatory patients with local anesthetic to protect area of anesthesia from trauma while numb. Most patients are familiar with the effects of lidocaine, so this enhances patient teaching.
mepivacaine (Carbocaine)		
Doses listed are for drug without levonordefrin (a vasoconstrictor). ***Nerve Block:*** 1% sol, 5–200 mg. ***Transvaginal Block:*** 1% sol, 400 mg max. ***Caudal or Epidural:*** 1% sol, 150–300 mg. ***Therapeutic Block:*** 1% sol, 10–50 mg.	**Onset:** 15 min **Peak:** NA **Duration:** 3 hr **PB:** 60%–80% **½L:** 100 min **B:** liver **E:** urine	Same as for all plus: **ASSESSMENT:** Observe pregnant patients closely—drug can cross placenta and cause fetal bradycardia, neonatal depression. Monitor fetal heart rate when used in delivery. Ask patients about drugs they are taking, because severe hypertension can occur if drug with levonordefrin is given to those on MAO inhibitors or tricyclic antidepressants. **INTERVENTION: Patient Teaching**—Tell patient onset of drug action rapid (within 15 min) and duration about 3 hr.

Continued on the following page

Table 21–3. LOCAL ANESTHETICS, *Continued*

DRUG NAME/ROUTE AND DOSAGE	PHARMOKINETICS/DYNAMICS	NURSING IMPLICATIONS
AMIDE TYPE		
prilocaine (Citanest)		
Used with caution in children under 10 yr. **Infiltration:** 1%–2% sol, 200–600 mg. **Peripheral Nerve Block (intercostal or paracervical):** 1%–2% sol, 30–100 mg. **Peripheral Nerve Block (surgery):** 2% sol, 400–600 mg. **Caudal Nerve Block (obstetrics):** 1% sol, 200–300 mg. **Epidural:** 1% sol, 200–300 mg.	**Onset:** 10–15 min **Peak:** NA **Duration:** 1–3 hr **PB:** 60%–85% **½L:** NA **B:** liver **E:** urine, lungs (5%)	Same as for all plus: **INTERVENTION:** Drug is about 40% less toxic than lidocaine and is not used topically. **Patient Teaching—**Tell patient onset of drug action is slower than lidocaine, but duration may be longer.
ESTER TYPE		
chloroprocaine hydrochloride (Nesacaine) (Nesacaine-CE)		
Drug available without epinephrine. **Infiltration Nerve Blocks:** 1% sol, 30–200 mg; 2% sol, 20–400 mg. **Caudal and Epidural:** 2%–3% sol, 300–750 mg.	**Onset:** within minutes **Peak:** NA **Duration:** 30–60 min **PB:** NA **½L:** NA **B:** plasma **E:** urine	Same as for all plus: **INTERVENTION:** Discard any partially used vials of drug without preservatives; do not reuse. **Patient Teaching—**Tell patient that duration of action is 30–60 min.
tetracaine hydrochloride (Pontocaine)		
Low Spinal (for vaginal delivery): 2–5 mg, 15 mg max. **Spinal up to Costal Margin:** 15–20 mg; spinal doses generally do not exceed 15 mg. **Topical Anesthesia of the Eye:** 0.5% sol or ointment.	**Onset:** within 15 min **Peak:** NA **Duration:** 2–3 hr **PB:** NA **½L:** NA **B:** liver **E:** urine	Same as for all plus: **INTERVENTION:** This is the most frequently used drug for spinal anesthesia. **Patient Teaching—**For topical eye anesthesia, patient should not touch or rub eye and should stay indoors away from wind, drafts until numbness is gone. Instruct patient to use spinal headache precautions.
piperocaine hydrochloride (Methycaine)		
Caudal: 1.5 % sol, 450 mg: can give additional 300 mg q 30–40 min for maintenance: 0.5% sol, 1000 mg max; 1% sol, 800 mg min 1%–2% sol. Also used in dental and IV infiltration.	**Onset:** within minutes **Peak:** 20–30 min **Duration:** decreases after peak **PB:** NA **½L:** NA **B:** NA **E:** NA	Same as for all plus: **INTERVENTION: Patient Teaching—**Tell patient anesthetic effect peaks at 20–30 min then begins to wear off.
procaine hydrochloride (Novocain)		
Spinal: Dose depends on nerves to be blocked. Drug supplied in 2 mL vials of 200 mg and is diluted for use with sterile H_2O, normal saline, dextrose, or spinal fluid. **Caudal:** 0.5% sol, up to 50 mg. **Epidural:** 1% sol, up to 100 mg. **Spinal up to Costal Margin:** 2% sol, up to 400 mg.	**Onset:** 2–5 min **Peak:** NA **Duration:** about 60 min; longer if solution with epinephrine is used for local nerve blocks of infiltration **PB:** NA **½L:** NA **B:** plasma **E:** urine	Same as for all plus: Procaine is the prototype local anesthetic and one of the most commonly used. Drug not irritating to soft tissues or nerves, and not effective as surface anesthetic. **INTERVENTION: Patient Teaching—**Instruct patient to use spinal headache precautions.

NA = not available.

metabolized almost totally by the liver and excreted in the urine.

Ester-type local anesthetics are **chloroprocaine (Nesa-caine)**, **tetracaine (Pontocaine)**, **piperocaine (Methy-caine)**, and **procaine (Novocaine)**. Ester-type anesthetics are rapidly and almost completely metabolized by blood pseudocholinesterase. The rest of the drug is metabolized in the liver, and drug metabolites are excreted in the urine.

PHARMACOKINETICS

The onset of action for both amide and ester types of local anesthetics is within 15 minutes of administration. The duration of action varies according to the agent used, dose, technique of administration, and local tissue conditions. For example, the presence of local infection changes the tissue pH, causing less anesthetic to enter the cells, and results in less effective anesthesia.

ADVERSE EFFECTS

Adverse reactions to all local anesthetic drugs may occur. They can result from toxic effects produced by an excess of drug entering the systemic circulation. Toxicity can also occur in elderly, debilitated, or acutely ill patients in whom drug metabolism is impaired. If a toxic reaction to a local anesthetic is going to occur, it usually happens within 10 minutes of administration but can occur as long as 45 minutes later.

▼ CLINICAL ALERT

Local anesthetics of the amide and ester types can interfere with the function of any organ or system that is dependent on the conduction or transmission of impulses, for example, the central nervous, respiratory, and cardiovascular systems. These drugs can produce dysrhythmias, bradycardia, hypotension, cardiac arrest, or respiratory failure.

Local anesthetics work directly on the myocardium, decreasing electrical excitability, conduction rate, and the force of contractions. This is the rationale for the clinical use of lidocaine to control an irritable heart. However, a toxic dose of lidocaine can produce cardiac arrest in a normal heart.

Hypersensitivity reactions to local anesthetics may occur, but are relatively uncommon. Most reactions of this type occur with the ester rather than the amide group. Anaphylactic reactions are theoretically possible but extremely rare. Early signs and symptoms of allergic reaction to local anesthesia include rash, erythema, hives, itching, and edema. Treatment includes airway maintenance and administration of oxygen and diphenhydramine (Benadryl) 50 mg intravenously.

USING THE NURSING PROCESS IN PATIENTS RECEIVING ANESTHETICS

The nursing process that follows focuses on care of the patient relative to the anesthetic drugs being administered. For other perioperative patient-care details, consult a comprehensive surgical nursing text. The nursing process is summarized in Table 21–4.

PREOPERATIVE ASSESSMENT

Preoperative care begins with the initial nursing assessment. For the hospitalized patient, this means the admission nursing assessment. In the ambulatory (outpatient) surgical patient, this assessment may be done just before the procedure or during the patient's preoperative visit for tests. In ambulatory or outpatient surgery, the patient arrives shortly before surgery and leaves after sufficiently recovering from the anesthetic.

Ambulatory care units are popular for several reasons: the rising cost of all phases of health care and the relative safety of certain routine procedures. Newer general anesthetics with rapid onset of action and rapid recovery make it possible to discharge patients the day of surgery. Many insurance companies no longer pay for hospitalization after procedures deemed outpatient or same-day surgical procedures that do not require skilled nursing care in the immediate postoperative period. Exceptions are patients at high risk for complications. Because of the shortened preoperative contact and interaction in this surgery, the nursing assessment is more important than ever. Postoperative patient contact is likewise abbreviated at a time when patient/family teaching is essential to patient observation and care.

- Initial patient assessment includes health history and psychosocial assessment, personal health habits, eating and sleeping patterns, and drinking and smoking habits.
- Information such as when the patient last ate or took fluids (especially walk-in patients), and concurrent conditions or diseases are noted prominently on the chart because they can influence the choice of anesthetics. For example, succinylcholine is contraindicated in patients with glaucoma. Conditions like hypertension or alcoholism (chronic or acute) contraindicate use of ketamine. The following are also important:
  - Ask about allergies. For example, if a patient had a hypersensitivity reaction to procaine, the physician may avoid other ester-type local anesthetics as a precaution. Ask about previous reactions to anesthetic agents.
  - Ask if any drugs or medications (prescriptions, over the counter, or recreational) have been taken within the 72 hours preceding surgery, because this may influence anesthesia choice or preclude use of other drugs. For example, marijuana potentiates barbiturates (see Table 21–2).

Table 21-4. NURSING PROCESS FOR PATIENT RECEIVING ANESTHETIC MEDICATION

Assessment (Preoperative)

Assess what patient knows/has been told about surgery and type of anesthesia planned.
Assess ability to understand.
Assess medication history, drugs patient currently taking (include alcohol or recreational drug use), noting date/time and amount of last ingestion/use.
Assess history for renal, hepatic impairment; pulmonary disease; glaucoma; other factors that affect choice of anesthetic agents.

Nursing Diagnosis: Knowledge Deficit

RELATED TO: Unfamiliarity with drug therapy and possible interactions.
AS EVIDENCED BY: Questions and statement of concern.

Desired Outcomes/Evaluation Criteria

Verbalizes understanding of preoperative restrictions for general anesthesia or restrictions and effects of any local anesthesia used. Complications minimized or prevented.

Nursing Actions	Rationale
Explain necessity/time of fluid restrictions and which routine drugs should be held or continued.	Patient will be more likely to comply with restrictions if he or she understands the reasons for them.
Stress that patient should not make any major decisions or drink alcoholic beverages for 48 hr and should avoid driving for 24 hr after procedure.	Complications and undesired drug interactions can occur if drug/alcohol use is inappropriate. Post-general-anesthesia drowsiness can contribute to auto accidents.
Local anesthesia: Tell patient/family to protect area of local anesthetic.	Numbness can last for several hours, increasing risk of injury.

Assessment (Postoperative)

Assess level of consciousness, ability to follow instructions (e.g., turn, cough, after general anesthesia).
Assess patient's breathing pattern, rate and depth of respirations.
Assess skin/mucous membrane color.
Assess characteristics of pain, noting nonverbal cues as well.

Nursing Diagnosis: Ineffective Breathing Pattern

RELATED TO: Effects of general complications of anesthesia or other perioperative drug(s).

Desired Outcomes/Evaluation Criteria

Displays usual/effective respiratory pattern free of hypoxia, cyanosis, or signs/symptoms of such as atelectasis and pneumonia.

Nursing Actions	Rationale
Monitor respiratory rate and depth. Assess for signs of air hunger, hypoxia, cyanosis.	Evaluates effectiveness of respiratory effort and identifies need for intervention.
Encourage patient to cough and deep breathe.	Helps to expel anesthetic gases and prevent pooling of secretions.
Evaluate effectiveness of cough and expelling of secretions. Suction as needed, as anesthesia may impair cough for several hours.	Ineffective coughing and deep breathing predispose to retained secretions and complications such as atelectasis, pneumonia.
Demonstrate use of spirometry device if ordered.	Promotes maximal inspiratory effort to open collapsed airways and mobilize secretions.
Administer supplemental oxygen as needed.	Maximizes oxygen available for circulatory uptake, especially when respiratory effort is depressed.

Nursing Diagnosis: Acute Pain

RELATED TO: Postoperative pain.
AS EVIDENCED BY: Complaints, muscle tension, restlessness, nonverbal cues.

Desired Outcomes/Evaluation Criteria

Reports pain is relieved/controlled. Displays relaxed manner and is able to mobilize, sleep/rest, appropriately.

Nursing Actions	Rationale
Give ordered pain medications.	Some patients are reluctant to ask for medication even when needed. Patients having severe pain move less and may develop complications of immobility.
Provide routine comfort measures, e.g., position change, back rub.	Helps relieve muscle tension and facilitate rest.
Encourage appropriate diversionary activities (radio/TV).	Promotes relaxation, comfort by distracting attention from pain and may help reduce need for medication.
Elevate affected extremity if local anesthesia or if regional limb anesthesia such as Bier block was given. Apply ice packs to surgical site as indicated/ordered.	Can reduce swelling and associated pain and protect anesthetized limb from trauma.
Keep patient supine for 8–12 hr after spinal anesthesia.	Helps prevent spinal headache.

Other Suggested Nursing Diagnoses: Preoperative—Anxiety, Body Image Disturbance, Anticipatory Grieving, and Spiritual Distress. Postoperative—Sensory-Perceptual Alterations, Urinary Retention, Constipation, and Altered Tissue Perfusion.

- Patients on cardiac medications should take them as usual, even when they are allowed nothing by mouth (NPO) before surgery; take such necessary drugs with as little fluid as possible.
- Patients to be discharged after the procedure must be accompanied by a responsible adult, even if only local anesthesia is planned.
- Assess the patient's psychologic and physiologic status to determine patient understanding of surgery and anxiety level. Physiologic baseline data include vital signs, routine laboratory test reports, radiographs, and electrocardiograms. Abnormalities are reported promptly to the physician, anesthetist, or both, because they may cause changes in the surgical plan.

NURSING DIAGNOSIS

- Nursing diagnoses based on assessment data may relate to physical or psychologic findings. A nursing diagnosis of High Level of Anxiety may be appropriate for the excessively apprehensive patient. Other potential nursing diagnoses include Knowledge Deficit, Sensory-Perceptual Alterations, and Ineffective Breathing Pattern (see Table 21–4).

PREOPERATIVE NURSING INTERVENTIONS

- Give an explanation of preoperative procedures, anesthesia recovery, equipment likely to be in use, and the postoperative routine. An ideal time for this is when the patient comes to the hospital for preoperative tests several days before surgery. Adequate explanations in this first contact help allay patient/family fears. Table 21–5 lists general patient teaching information. The surgeon should have prepared the patient by giving specifics about the planned surgery.
- Give printed instructions to the patient to help ensure that instructions are understood. Figure 21–2 is an example of preoperative patient instructions for use after podiatric surgery.
- When the patient is admitted, check laboratory data and tests and perform other presurgical tasks. Report any abnormalities or problems at once.
- Take vital signs, administer the preanesthetic injection, and document the patient's chart appropriately.
- Administer ordered barbiturates, analgesics, and/or cholinergic blockers to dry secretions, sedate the patient, and facilitate anesthetic induction. Because it is common for more than one drug to be ordered, always check the compatibility of the drugs to be administered before mixing them.

▼ **CLINICAL ALERT**

Some drugs, such as diazepam (Valium), are highly incompatible and should not be mixed with other drugs.

When in doubt about the compatibility of drugs, check with the pharmacist. Do not administer any drugs that appear cloudy or have precipitate matter present.

Once the medication is given, have the patient lie quietly with side rails up until transport to the operating room to promote safety and facilitate drug effectiveness.
- Give psychologic and emotional reassurance, as appropriate, to the patient. Studies show that patients having repeat procedures do not necessarily experience less anxiety. Patients having surgery generally experience two major fears—fear of death and fear of cancer. It is common for patients having general anesthesia to fear "not waking up," even though anesthesia deaths are quite rare.

Table 21–5. PATIENT TEACHING INFORMATION—ANESTHETIC DRUGS

Dear Patient:
   Anesthetic drugs will be administered prior to your surgery. This is what you should know about your planned anesthesia to avoid possible complications from your anesthesia.

FOR PATIENTS RECEIVING GENERAL ANESTHESIA

☐ 1. Food and fluid will be restricted preoperatively; usually no food or fluids are allowed from midnight before your operation.
☐ 2. Preanesthetic medication will be administered 30–60 minutes preoperatively. For safety reasons, do not get out of bed after this medication is given.
☐ 3. Following surgery, there may be additional food or fluid restrictions depending upon the procedure performed.
☐ 4. Following surgery, there may be activity restrictions until full recovery from the anesthetics has occurred.
☐ 5. Following surgery, some nausea may be experienced because of medications given. This can be controlled by medication that the physician will order.
☐ 6. Pain will be controlled by the administration of ordered analgesics.

FOR PATIENTS HAVING OUTPATIENT SURGERY OR AMBULATORY SURGERY

☐ 1. There may be food or liquid restrictions prior to the procedure. Follow physician's orders.
☐ 2. Do not come alone; have a family member or friend accompany you, even if a local anesthetic is planned.
☐ 3. Bring in bottles of all medications you are currently taking so that the physician and/or anesthetist is aware of them.
☐ 4. If taking regular medications, check with physician to determine if alteration in dose or schedule will be necessary because of surgery. (For example, patients with diabetes may have to alter their insulin regimen.)
☐ 5. If a local anesthetic is used, protect the area from trauma because it will be numb for several hours, and injury may occur without being felt.
☐ 6. Have prescriptions for postoperative medications filled and follow postoperative instructions regarding rest, food/fluid restrictions, wound care, elevations of extremity (if appropriate), and return visits for postoperative physician care.

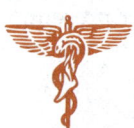

DR. RICHARD L. SAWICKI
8657 Buffalo Ave.
Niagara Falls, NY 14304
Tel. (716) 283-3338

PODIATRY POST-OP INSTRUCTIONS

1. Call Dr's. office for follow-up appointment when you get home. Make appt. for

   _____

2. Keep operative foot clean at all times. Wear protective cover-slippers, socks, etc.
3. Keep dressing or cast dry unless Dr. instructs otherwise.
4. If given a post-op wooden bottom shoe, be sure to *wear it at all times when walking*.
5. Keep operative foot elevated when sitting to decrease swelling and pain.
6. Apply an ice pack to the foot while awake. Place ice pack on for 30 minutes, then leave off for 30 minutes. Do this for the first 3 days post-op.
7. Watch for & notify Dr.'s office right away if there is increasing redness with swelling and/or pain. Call the regular office phone #283-3338.
8. Take any medications Dr. Sawicki ordered for you exactly as written.
9. If you plan convalescing at a place other than your home, please notify the Dr's. office of a phone number you can be reached at.
10. A local anesthesia has been used to numb the foot and its effect will last several hours. Protect the area from trauma (bumps, etc.) since you will not be able to feel any injury while the area is numb.
11. TAKE IT EASY. REST. This is very important to your recovery. Adequate rest and proper diet promote healing. *DO NOT* do any yardwork or extensive housework.

_____   _____
         NAME   DATE

Figure 21–2. Same-day surgery postoperative instructions. This is a copy of instructions given to patients who have undergone podiatric surgery. The Surgical Coordinating Nurse explains the preoperative testing and other requirements and makes the necessary appointment for the patient during a preoperative visit to the physician's office about 10 days before surgery. The podiatrist reviews the surgery with the patient (and family) and answers questions. The postoperative routine is also explained. If necessary, arrangements are made at this time for crutch-walk training or for the procurement of assistive devices such as crutches or a walker if needed. The surgeon obtains informed patient consent at this time. (Courtesy of Dr. Richard L. Sawicki, Niagara Falls, NY.)

PREOPERATIVE NURSING EVALUATIONS

Preoperative nursing evaluations include the following:

- Checking vital signs to be sure they are stable.
- Checking preoperative medication effectiveness.
- Making a final physical check to determine if the patient is properly prepared for surgery.
- Documenting patient status on a preoperative checklist and in the regular nurse's notes.

Patient care during surgery and anesthesia recovery in the postanesthesia recovery room is generally done by specially trained nurses and technicians. Nursing care in the anesthesia recovery period focuses on facilitating respirations and frequent monitoring of vital signs.

PLANNING AND INTERVENTION

Following surgery, the patient is transferred to the postanesthesia room where frequent monitoring by specially trained nurses occurs. Respiratory status and vital signs are checked frequently. Return of the gag reflex and coughing signals that extubation is necessary. Once the anesthetist extubates the patient, respiratory status is monitored to be sure it remains adequate. For the staff nurse, the postoperative nursing assessment begins when the patient arrives from the recovery room. The nurse takes vital signs, assesses level of consciousness, and inspects the operative area. If the patient received local anesthesia, take care to protect the area from injury and be sure limbs are in correct alignment. Observe for color, temperature changes, and signs of returning sensation.

▼ CLINICAL ALERT

Once patient transfer to the patient-care unit occurs, complete neuromuscular function and satisfactory respiratory status should be present. The patient should be able to lift his or her head and hold it up for 10 seconds, should be able to grasp with a fairly firm grip, and gag/cough reflex should be present. Notify the anesthetist if these signs are absent.

- Caution patients who had long-acting local anesthetics to rest and protect the operative area from trauma for up to 8 to 10 hours after leaving the surgical unit for home.
- After spinal anesthesia, headaches can occur that can be severe and persist up to 36 hours.
- Patients may have nausea, vomiting, or both after general anesthesia. This usually subsides within 24 hours. Most physicians include an antiemetic in routine postoperative orders and this can be given if needed.
- Pain occurs with recovery from anesthesia. This is especially true after recovery from inhalation anesthetics, because these drugs leave the patient's system more rapidly and have less lingering effects than agents administered by other modes. As recovery from anesthesia progresses, the patient is aware of pain and requires analgesic administration as ordered. During the initial postoperative period, the hospitalized patient may need parenterally administered narcotic analgesics or other analgesics. Ambulatory/outpatient surgery patients will have oral analgesics prescribed.
- Frequency of assessment of vital signs and other status parameters depends on type of surgery performed, patient status, and anesthetic used. Progressive changes (like gradually declining blood pressure) or abrupt, dramatic changes are reported to the physician.

- Because anesthetics and other perioperative drugs depress the central nervous system, observe the patient for respiratory depression and hypoventilation, which predispose to pooling of secretions. Encourage the patient to cough and breathe deeply to help expel anesthetic gases and to prevent pooling of secretions. Because hypotension can also occur, mobilize the patient carefully to prevent syncopal episodes.
- The deep muscle relaxation in general anesthesia can cause bladder atony or decreased intestinal motility. Anesthetics can depress renal function temporarily and may prevent voiding for several hours after surgery. If a patient has not voided within 8 hours after surgery, catheterization is done.
- Tell patients who are discharged the same day as general anesthesia administration to notify the surgeon if they void only in small amounts (urinary retention with overflow) or are unable to void. Patients are generally not discharged until after they void; however, a patient can still experience urinary retention, especially those with a history of urinary or prostrate problems.
- Abdominal distention can result from the decreased intestinal motility caused by anesthetic and muscle-relaxant drugs. Patients may have discomfort from flatus distension. Mobilizing the patient as soon as permissible after surgery helps relieve this discomfort. If the discomfort persists, notify the surgeon to obtain further orders.
- Early patient mobilization also helps prevent other immobility-related problems. Immobility predisposes to hazards including urinary, circulatory, and pulmonary stasis that contribute to complications like thrombi, emboli, and pneumonia. Providing adequate pain relief before mobilization/ambulation activities can greatly enhance patient compliance and comfort. (For information on analgesic drugs, see Chapter 18).

Patient Teaching

Next-day discharge after many surgical procedures and outpatient surgery have combined to shift the nurses' care focus from giving care to teaching the patient/family how to give immediate postoperative care. For example, after outpatient surgery on an extremity (arm, hand, foot), the patient is usually advised to elevate the part to reduce pain and swelling and to protect the part from bump-ing/trauma if a local anesthetic was given. If a long-acting anesthetic like bupivacaine (Marcaine) was given, be sure the patient knows sensation will be absent longer than if lidocaine (Xylocaine) had been given, because most people know the duration of Xylocaine. Ice packs may be applied intermittently to reduce pain and swelling. Patients who are discharged the day after surgery may have to continue certain treatments at home. For example, iced compresses are often ordered for 3 to 5 days after cosmetic facial surgery to reduce pain and swelling. Ideally, adequate preoperative teaching is done so patient/family are prepared for needed aftercare. Routine care measures are outlined relative to patient surgery and signs and symptoms that should be reported to the surgeon right away. All instructions should be verbally explained and provided in a printed list. The caregiver should repeat instructions so the nurse can tell if a clear understanding exists. See Table 21–5 for sample patient teaching information provided for patients following foot surgery.

POSTOPERATIVE EVALUATION

Postoperative evaluation of nursing interventions to prevent or minimize side effects of anesthetic/analgesic drugs is an ongoing process. Patient responses (objective and subjective) are evaluated for effectiveness of interventions. Once this output information is evaluated, the pertinent information becomes new input for the problem-solving nursing process.

- Many postoperative interventions are preventive care measures that aim to prevent complications like respiratory or urinary tract problems and are judged effective in the absence of these problems.
- Some nursing interventions are planned as problem-solving rather than preventive measures. For example, when a patient has pain or nausea postoperatively and an ordered medication is given, evaluation is based on symptom relief.
- For ambulatory/outpatient surgery patients, a surgical coordinating nurse will call the patient at home within 24 hours of surgery to evaluate patient status. The trend of short hospital stays and the increase in outpatient surgery challenge the nurse to assess and plan care to meet patient needs efficiently and effectively.

The bibliography for this chapter can be found in Appendix B, which begins on page 1054.

CHAPTER REVIEW QUESTIONS*

1. Bob Wills, a 40-year-old, received halothane (Fluothane) as an induction agent. All of the following can occur with halothane administration *except*:
   a. Hepatotoxicity.
   b. Skeletal muscle relaxation.
   c. Respiratory depression.
   d. Bradycardia and dysrhythmias.

2. Amy Pallet is recovering from abdominal surgery in which isoflurane (Forane) was used as the anesthetic agent. All of the following can occur after Forane administration *except*:
   a. Nausea and vomiting.
   b. Postoperative excitation.
   c. Dysrhythmias.
   d. Depressed mental alertness.

*See Appendix A, which begins on page 1051, for answers.

3. Mrs. Reeves received ketamine hydrochloride (Ketalar) for debridement of a burn. Potential effects of the drug include:
   a. Frequent urination.
   b. Constipation.
   c. Disturbing dreams.
   d. Decreased muscle control.

4. Mr. Steiner received naloxone (Narcan) 0.1 mg IV to reverse the effects of narcotics during surgery. Which of the following should be assessed after Narcan administration?
   a. Respiratory difficulty.
   b. Dry mouth.
   c. Intense pain.
   d. Urine output.

5. For an endoscopic procedure, a patient received droperidol/fentanyl (Innovar). Which of the following drugs may be given if the patient develops Innovar-induced bradycardia?
   a. Atropine.
   b. Demerol.
   c. Lidocaine.
   d. Compazine.

6. The anesthesiologist administered succinylcholine to Mr. Judd to facilitate endotracheal intubation. The electrolyte that is affected by this drug is:
   a. Sodium.
   b. Calcium.
   c. Magnesium.
   d. Potassium.

7. Mrs. Hayes is scheduled for removal of ganglionic cyst, using lidocaine hydrochloride (Xylocaine) with epinephrine for a field block. Patient teaching instructions with Mrs. Hayes will include all of the following *except*:
   a. Estimated length of time area will be numb.
   b. An okay for her to drive herself home because only local anesthesia was given.
   c. Instructions to protect area from trauma while numb.
   d. The use of ice packs to decrease pain as anesthetic wears off.

8. Mr. Dominick is scheduled for surgery using alfentanil hydrochloride (Alfenta) as an analgesic adjunct. Which of the following is *not* true in reference to Alfenta use?
   a. This drug is especially useful for pediatric patients and infants.
   b. Dose is reduced to elderly or debilitated patients.
   c. Drug is not a good choice for patients with renal failure.
   d. Alfenta is an opiate analgesic.

CHAPTER 22

Skeletal Muscle Relaxants and Neuromuscular Blocking Agents

Merrily A. Kuhn, RNC, PhD

CHAPTER OUTLINE

Skeletal Muscle Relaxants
Neuromuscular Blocking Agents
Nursing Process Related to Movement Disorders

TABLES

Drug Tables

Nursing Process

Patient Teaching

KEY TERMS

Depolarizing neuromuscular blocking agents
Muscle fasciculation
Neuromuscular junction
Nondepolarizing neuromuscular blocking agents
Pseudocholinesterase
Spasticity
Spasm

LEARNING OBJECTIVES

After reading this chapter, the student will be able to:

1. Describe specific disorders that could require the use of skeletal muscle relaxants.
2. Differentiate among the skeletal muscle relaxants as to mechanisms of action, routes of administration, metabolism, adverse effects, contraindications and precautions, and interactions.
3. Prepare a specific plan to assess the patient requiring the use of skeletal muscle relaxants to formulate an appropriate patient outcome.
4. Plan the nursing intervention necessary to counsel the family of a patient who requires a skeletal muscle relaxant.
5. Evaluate the patient at various stages of treatment to gauge nursing intervention.

Muscle relaxants affect skeletal muscles, which are striated (striped) muscles attached to the skeleton. Skeletal muscles are able to contract, causing and allowing movement of the skeleton. In many cases, skeletal muscle relaxation is a desired therapeutic effect, achieved phar-

macologically with skeletal muscle relaxants or neuromuscular blocking agents. Skeletal muscle relaxants and neuromuscular blocking agents produce their pharmacologic effects through very different mechanisms of action. Thus, their clinical uses also vary considerably. Skeletal muscle relaxants are used to control skeletal muscle hyperactivity. Neuromuscular blocking agents are used to induce muscle relaxation during surgery, intubation, and mechanical ventilation.

The publisher gratefully acknowledges the contribution of Barbara K. Clark, RN, MN, CCRN, to the third edition.

SKELETAL MUSCLE RELAXANTS

Skeletal muscle relaxants produce their therapeutic effect by acting on the central nervous system (CNS) or by acting directly on skeletal muscle.

SKELETAL MUSCLE HYPERACTIVITY

Skeletal muscle hyperactivity is characterized by skeletal muscle *spasticity* or *spasm*. Spasticity is a form of increased muscle tone, or hypertonicity, that results in increased resistance to passive movement of an extremity. As increased force is applied to a joint or extremity, it is matched by resistance to movement. Muscle spasticity may interfere with rehabilitation and may result in contractures, pain, and psychosocial problems.

Muscle spasticity originates within the central nervous system. It is associated with a number of clinical conditions, such as upper motor neuron disorders, multiple sclerosis, cerebral palsy, cerebrovascular accidents, amyotrophic lateral sclerosis (Lou Gehrig disease), and spinal cord injuries. The damage (or lesion) from any of these conditions causes an interruption of normal excitatory or inhibitory responses with abnormal nerve transmission resulting in sustained muscle contraction, relaxation, or both.

Muscle spasm, an involuntary contraction of a muscle or muscle group, is elicited by acute muscle injury, severe cold, or lack of blood flow to the muscle. Spasm occurs when the impulses from the muscle are transmitted to the spinal cord and back to the muscle, causing a reflex contraction. The central-acting skeletal muscle relaxants are believed to break the cycle by acting as CNS depressants.

CENTRAL-ACTING MUSCLE RELAXANTS

The central-acting skeletal muscle relaxants include **carisoprodol (Soma)**, **baclofen (Lioresal)**, **cyclobenzaprine hydrochloride (Flexeril)**, **methocarbamol (Robaxin)**, and **chlorzoxazone (Paraflex)**. See Table 22–1 for dosage, pharmacokinetics, and nursing implications.

Action

The mechanism of action of most of the central skeletal muscle relaxants has not been clearly identified. As a group they do not directly relax tense muscles, but their action may be through their sedative properties. Chlorzoxazone (Paraflex) acts at the spinal cord level, inhibiting the multisynaptic reflex arcs that produce and maintain skeletal muscle spasm. Cyclobenzaprine (Flexeril) acts within the CNS at the brain stem.

Uses

Central skeletal muscle relaxants are used in combination with rest, physical therapy, and other measures for the relief of discomfort associated with acute, painful musculoskeletal conditions caused by inflammation or trauma. These agents are only slightly effective in treating spasticity related to cerebrospinal trauma, cerebral palsy, or demyelinating disorders such as multiple sclerosis. Diazepam, a benzodiazepine, is used in the treatment of muscle spasm of local origin and muscle spasticity caused by upper motor neuron disorders. (For more information on diazepam, see Chapter 25).

Contraindications and Precautions

Safe use in pregnancy, lactation, and children has not been established. Cyclobenzaprine is classified as pregnancy category B; the other skeletal muscle relaxants are classified as category C.

Because these drugs act centrally, drowsiness and dizziness frequently occur. Therefore, patients receiving skeletal muscle relaxants should use caution when performing activities that require mental alertness.

Although psychic and physical dependence is rare, it may develop after long-term use of large doses. Discontinuation should be gradual to prevent withdrawal symptoms, which may include seizures.

Because central skeletal muscle relaxants are biotransformed in the liver and excreted in urine, use cautiously in patients with hepatic or renal dysfunction.

Adverse Effects

Central skeletal muscle relaxants cause drowsiness, dizziness, and light-headedness. Elderly or debilitated patients may exhibit increased sensitization to the usual adult dosage and, therefore, are started on lower doses and are assessed more closely during initial therapy. Occasional gastrointestinal complaints such as nausea, vomiting, abdominal distress, constipation, and diarrhea also occur. Taking the drug with food may minimize gastrointestinal complaints.

Interactions

Caution is used when these drugs are administered with CNS depressants such as alcohol, anxiolytics, or antipsychotic drugs because the effects are additive.

○ **Carisoprodol** (Soma, Rela) has a chemical structure similar to that of meprobamate, a CNS depressant.

CONTRAINDICATIONS AND PRECAUTIONS Carisoprodol is contraindicated in patients with suspected or acute intermittent porphyria because it may increase porphyrin synthesis, thereby exacerbating symptoms.

▼ CLINICAL ALERT

Observe the patient receiving carisoprodol for idiosyncratic reactions after first to fourth dose (extreme weakness, quadriplegia, dizziness, ataxia, dysarthria, visual disturbances, agitation, euphoria, confusion and disorientation) or severe reactions, including bronchospasm, hypotension, and anaphylactic shock. Withhold dose and notify the physician immediately of any unusual reactions.

○ **Baclofen** (Lioresol), a chemical analog of the inhibitory neurotransmitter, gamma-aminobutyric acid (GABA), inhibits the release of excitatory transmitters at the spinal level. Baclofen is used to relieve spasticity, and it is more effective than dantrolene and diazepam in treating patients with multiple sclerosis. Baclofen is most effective in treating patients with reversible spasm. It may be of some value in treating patients with spinal cord injury or disease. Baclofen is the only skeletal muscle relaxant that can be administered intrathecally (within the spinal canal).

CONTRAINDICATIONS AND PRECAUTIONS Patients with seizure disorders may have a lowered seizure threshold, possibly requiring an increase in their anticonvulsant medication. Patients in whom spasticity is used to maintain posture and balance may experience a loss of muscle tone or function while on baclofen therapy.

▼ **CLINICAL ALERT**

Abrupt withdrawal of baclofen may precipitate an acute withdrawal reaction (hallucinations, increased spasticity, seizures, mental changes, restlessness).

○ **Cyclobenzaprine hydrochloride** (Flexeril), both structurally and pharmacologically related to the tricyclic antidepressants (TCAs), acts within the brain stem to decrease tonic somatic motor activity. It relieves skeletal muscle spasm of local origin without interfering with muscle function.

CONTRAINDICATIONS AND PRECAUTIONS Cyclobenzaprine hydrochloride is contraindicated in patients who have received monoamine oxidase (MAO) inhibitors within 14 days; during acute recovery phase of myocardial infarction; or in patients with dysrhythmias, heart block or conduction disturbances, or heart failure as all these conditions can worsen. Cyclobenzaprine is contraindicated in patients hypersensitive to TCAs as it is structually and pharmacologically related to the tricyclics. Because of this drug's anticholinergic effect, use cautiously in patients with a history of urinary retention, angle-closure glaucoma, and increased intraocular pressure. Cyclobenzaprine hydrochloride should be used only for short-term (2 to 3 weeks) therapy.

ADVERSE EFFECTS Adverse effects are the same as for all skeletal muscle relaxants, especially drowsiness, plus the following: ataxia, disorientation, dysarthria, paresthesia, vertigo, dysrhythmias, tachycardia, dry mouth (common), gastritis, and sweating.

○ **Methocarbamol** (Delaxin, Marbaxin, Robaxin, Robomol) reduces transmission of impulses from the spinal cord to skeletal muscle. Methocarbamol is also used as an adjunct in treating tetanus.

CONTRAINDICATIONS AND PRECAUTIONS Contraindications also include hypersensitivity to polyethylene glycol, the vehicle for the parenteral form. Because polyethylene glycol is nephrotoxic, the parenteral form is contraindicated in patients with renal impairment. The parenteral form should also be used cautiously in patients with seizure disorders.

ADVERSE EFFECTS Adverse effects from intravenous and intramuscular injection include anaphylaxis and seizures. Intravenous injection may also cause hypotension and bradycardia. Monitor the patient closely during administration. Urine may turn brown, black, or green, so warn the patient about this possibility. Other adverse effects include blurred vision, nasal congestion, urticaria, and rash. Notify the physician if any of these occurs.

○ **Chlorzoxazone** (Paraflex, Parafon Forte DSC, Remular-S) is chemically distinct from other muscle relaxants but shares all other properties. Monitor patients with known allergies for hypersensitivity reactions such as urticaria, redness or itching, and possibly angioedema. Chlorzoxazone may also cause malaise and urine discoloration.

Central-acting skeletal muscle relaxants not discussed in this chapter include chlorphenesin carbamate (Maolate), metaxalone (Skelaxin), and orphenadrine citrate (Banflex, Flexon, Myolin, Norflex).

DIRECT-ACTING SKELETAL MUSCLE RELAXANTS

The only available direct-acting skeletal muscle relaxant. See Table 22–1 for dosage, pharmacokinetics, and nursing implications.

○ **Dantrolene sodium** (Dantrium) acts at the muscle and interferes with the intramuscular release of calcium ions from the sarcoplasmic reticulum, thus weakening the force of contraction. It does not interfere with nerve impulse transmission as the central-acting muscle relaxants do. Dantrolene is effective in treating the spasticity of spinal cord and cerebral injuries, multiple sclerosis, cerebral palsy, and possibly stroke. It is particularly useful in treating spasm that causes pain.

Dantrolene is also administered to patients with a diagnosis of malignant hyperthermia. Malignant hyperthermia is an autosomal dominant trait characterized by possibly fatal hyperthermia with rigidity of the muscles occurring in affected people exposed to certain anesthetic agents, particularly halothane, succinylcholine, and methoxyflurane. Dantrolene prevents a severe catabolic process associated with this condition.

CONTRAINDICATIONS AND PRECAUTIONS Dantrolene is contraindicated in active hepatic disease such as hepatitis and cirrhosis, in patients in whom spasticity is used to maintain posture and balance, and in the treatment of skeletal muscle spasm resulting from rheumatic disorders. Because dantrolene produces muscle weakness, it is used cautiously in patients with borderline strength. It should also be used cautiously in patients with pulmonary dysfunction.

ADVERSE EFFECTS Besides adverse effects common to all skeletal muscle relaxants, CNS side effects—depression, confusion, visual and speech disturbances, and headache—may occur. Other reactions are GI bleeding, urinary frequency, impotence, photosensitivity, and rash. Advise the patient to wear protective clothing when in the sun. Notify the physician of persistent rash or bloody or tarry stool. Dantrolene also has a potential for hepatotoxicity. Notify the physician of yellow discoloration of skin or eyes.

Table 22–1. SKELETAL MUSCLE RELAXANTS

DRUG NAME/ROUTE AND DOSAGE	PHARMACOKINETICS/ DYNAMICS	NURSING IMPLICATIONS
CENTRAL-ACTING SKELETAL MUSCLE RELAXANTS		
carisoprodol (Soma) (Rela) ***Adults:*** 350 mg PO 3–4 times daily. ***Pediatric:*** Not recommended in children under 12 years.	**Onset:** 30 min **Peak:** 4 hr **Duration:** 4–6 hr **½L:** 8 hr **PB:** NA **B:** liver **E:** urine	**ASSESSMENT:** Assess neuromuscular status before and during therapy. Assess bowel and bladder function and hepatic and renal function. **INTERVENTION:** Drug dependence may occur; monitor patient closely. Do not abruptly discontinue drug. **Patient Teaching**—Advise patient to take drug with food to prevent GI upset and to avoid alcohol and activities requiring alertness. **EVALUATION:** Report rash, pruritus, and other evidence of hypersensitivity to physician. If symptoms are not relieved in 30–40 days, notify physician.
baclofen (Lioresal) ***Adults:*** 5 mg PO tid; may increase q 3 days by 5 mg/dose to maximum of 80 mg/day; or 300–800 μg/day intrathecally (IT).	**Onset:** PO, varies from hours to weeks; IT, 0.5–1.0 hr **Peak:** PO, 2–3 hr; IT, 4 hr **Duration:** PO, 8 hr; IT, 4–8 hr **½L:** 2.5–4 hr **PB:** 30% **B:** liver **E:** urine	Same as for carisoprodol plus: **ASSESSMENT:** Assess for pregnancy (category C). **EVALUATION:** Notify physician if patient complains of frequent urge to urinate or painful urination.
cyclobenzaprine hydrochloride (Flexeril) ***Adults:*** 20–40 mg PO in 2–4 divided doses, not to exceed 60 mg/day.	**Onset:** 1 hr **Peak:** 4–6 hr **Duration:** 12–24 hr **½L:** 1–3 days **PB:** 93% **B:** liver **E:** urine, feces	Same as for carisoprodol plus: **ASSESSMENT:** Assess for pregnancy (category B). **INTERVENTION:** Use for short-term (2–3 wk) therapy only. **EVALUATION:** Evaluate for urinary output and urinary retention.
methocarbamol (Delaxin) (Marbaxin) (Robaxin) (Robomol) ***Adults:*** *Initial dose*—1.5 g PO qid for 2–3 days; or 1 g IM or IV, up to 1 g every 8 hr for 3 days. *Maintenance dose*—4–4.5 g PO daily in 3–6 divided doses.	**Onset:** PO, 30 min; IV, immediate **Peak:** PO, 2 hr **Duration:** NA **½L:** 1–2 hr **PB:** NA **B:** liver **E:** urine	Same as for carisoprodol plus: **INTERVENTION:** During IV administration, patient should be recumbent. Urine may turn dark brown, black, or green when standing. **EVALUATION:** Notify physician if skin rash, fever, or nasal congestion occurs.
DIRECT-ACTING SKELETAL MUSCLE RELAXANTS		
dantrolene sodium (Dantrium) **spasticity** ***Adults:*** 25 mg PO once daily up to 100 mg 2–4 times daily; or 2.5 mg/kg IV over 1 hr. **malignant hyperthermia** ***Adults:*** 2.5 mg/kg IV over 1 hr. ***Children over 5:*** 0.5 mg/kg 3–4 times daily. Do not exceed 100 mg qid.	**Onset:** PO, 1 hr (blood levels); 1 wk (therapeutic effect) **Peak:** PO, 4–6 hr **Duration:** PO, 6–12 hr **½L:** 9 hr **PB:** highly **B:** liver **E:** urine	**ASSESSMENT:** Assess baseline liver function, ALT, AST, and total bilirubin. **INTERVENTION:** Monitor liver function closely. If no benefit has been obtained within 45 days, discontinue drug. Difficulty in swallowing may occur. Reconstitute with 60 mL sterile water, not bacteriostatic water, or 0.9% NaCl or D₅W when administering drug IV. **Patient Teaching**—Warn patient to wear protective clothing when in sun. **EVALUATION:** Notify physician of persistent rash, bloody or tarry stool, or yellow discoloration of skin or eyes.

NA = not available; ALT = alanine aminotransferase (serum); AST = aspartate aminotransferase (serum).

The incidence of symptomatic hepatitis (fatal and nonfatal) is much higher in patients taking 800 mg or more of dantrolene sodium per day, even for short courses of therapy. Risk of hepatic injury is greater in women, in patients more than 35 years of age, and in patients taking other medicines concurrently. Hepatitis most frequently occurs between the 3d and 12th months of therapy and is generally preceded by anorexia, nausea, vomiting, and abdominal discomfort. Patients should notify the physician immediately if any of these symptoms occur.

INTERACTIONS   Avoid concurrent use of alcohol or other CNS depressants with dantrolene sodium because of additive CNS depression. Monitor the patient on verapamil therapy. An increased risk of dysrhythmias occurs. Concurrent use with other hepatotoxic agents or estrogen may increase the possibility of hepatotoxicity. Warfarin and clofibrate decrease plasma protein binding; tolbutamide increases it.

NEUROMUSCULAR BLOCKING AGENTS

Although neuromuscular blocking agents are commonly referred to as muscle relaxants, the term is a misnomer. Neuromuscular blocking agents work peripherally by blocking the transmission of impulses at the *neuromuscular junction* (the area where a motor neuron terminates on the muscle fiber). True muscle relaxants (such as those discussed earlier in this chapter) work centrally to reduce the transmission of impulses from the spinal cord to skeletal muscle and thereby provide relief from muscle strain. There are two types of neuromuscular blocking agents: nondepolarizing and depolarizing. Both effectively induce paralysis, but produce this effect through different mechanisms of action.

ACTION

Neuromuscular blocking agents work by interrupting or preventing the electrochemical transfer of information at the point at which the axon of a neuron meets a muscle fiber, that is, at the neuromuscular (myoneural) junction. At this junction, the axon of the motor neuron divides to form branching terminals that are enfolded in muscle fibers. These axon terminals are separated from the fibers by the synaptic cleft or synapse. Impulses do not "jump across" these synapses. Instead, the electrical conduction of a signal down the axon occurs as an action potential (a series of polarizations and depolarizations). As the action potential invades the nerve ending, a chemical presynaptic neurotransmitting substance—in this case acetylcholine—is released into the synapse. The acetylcholine diffuses (moves) across the synapse to act on the postsynaptic membrane to produce a new action potential or modulate a preexisting action. Neuromuscular blocking agents act at the neuromuscular junction by competing with acetylcholine for the receptor sites or by blocking depolarization. Figure 22–1 shows where neuromuscular blockers act in neurons.

Because neuromuscular blocking agents cannot readily cross membranes, they must always be administered parenterally. And, because of their inability to cross the blood-brain barrier, they have no effect on the central nervous system. Thus, neuromuscular blockers do not diminish consciousness or the perception of pain.

These drugs must be accompanied by adequate anesthesia during surgery to prevent patient distress. Neuromuscular blocking agents are administered after unconsciousness is induced. For painful procedures, opioid narcotics or sedatives are administered concurrently.

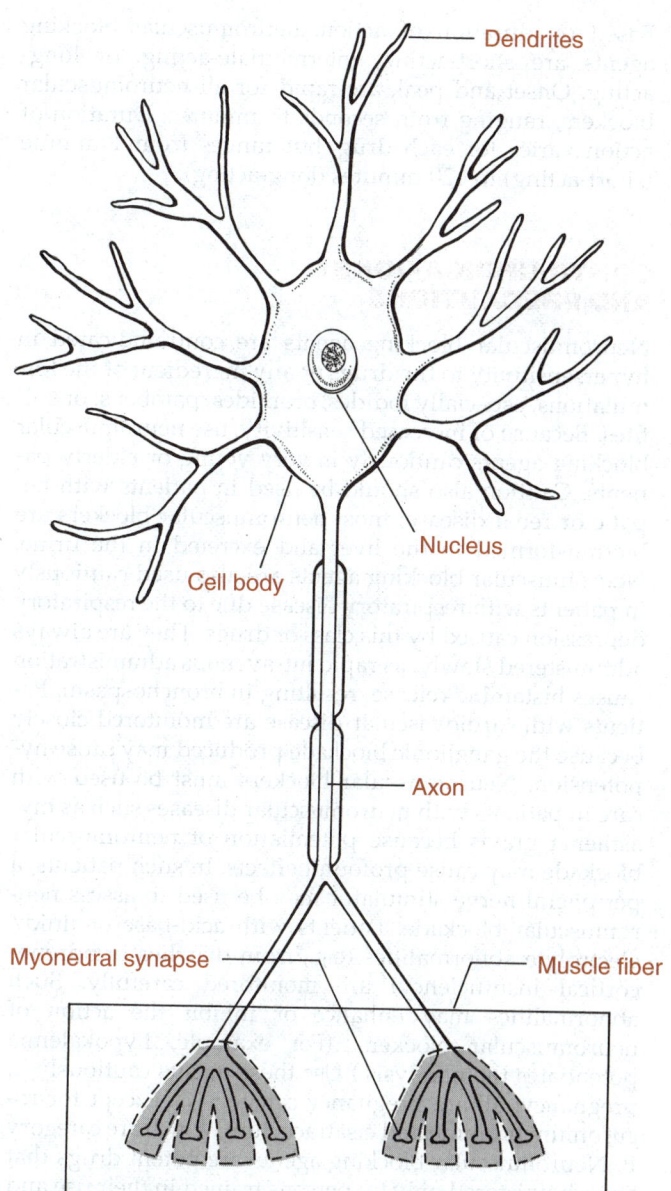

Figure 22–1. Location of neuromuscular blocking drug action in neurons.

USES

Neuromuscular blocking agents are used to induce sufficient muscle relaxation to assist with various surgical procedures. As an adjunct to anesthesia, neuromuscular blockers can decrease the dosage of the general anesthetic, providing a greater margin of safety for the patient. There is less risk of respiratory depression, and recovery from anesthesia occurs more quickly. Neuromuscular blockers also help maintain anesthesia sufficient for the performance of surgery requiring deep muscle relaxation, such as abdominal procedures. Other drugs used in anesthesia are discussed in Chapter 21. Neuromuscular blocking agents can also be used to manage the muscle spasms of tetanus and to prevent convulsive muscular activity during electroshock therapy.

PHARMACOKINETICS

Based on duration of action, neuromuscular blocking agents are short-acting, intermediate-acting, or long-acting. Onset and peak are rapid for all neuromuscular blockers, ranging from seconds to minutes. Duration of action varies for each drug, but ranges from 1 minute (short-acting) to 120 minutes (long-acting).

CONTRAINDICATIONS AND PRECAUTIONS

Neuromuscular blocking agents are contraindicated in hypersensitivity to the drugs or any ingredient of the formulations, especially iodides, bromides, parabens, or sulfites. Because of increased sensitivity, use neuromuscular blocking agents cautiously in very young or elderly patients. Caution also should be used in patients with hepatic or renal disease; most neuromuscular blockers are biotransformed in the liver and excreted in the urine. Neuromuscular blocking agents are also used cautiously in patients with respiratory disease due to the respiratory depression caused by this class of drugs. They are always administered slowly, as rapid intravenous administration causes histamine release, resulting in bronchospasm. Patients with cardiovascular disease are monitored closely because the ganglionic blockade produced may cause hypotension. Neuromuscular blockers must be used with care in patients with neuromuscular diseases such as myasthenia gravis because potentiation of neuromuscular blockade may cause profound effects. In such patients, a peripheral nerve stimulator may be used to assess neuromuscular blockade. Patients with acid-base or fluid/electrolyte abnormalities (e.g., from diarrhea or adrenocortical insufficiency) are monitored carefully. Such abnormalities may enhance or inhibit the action of neuromuscular blockers. (For example, hypokalemia potentiates the paralysis.) Use these agents cautiously in pregnancy: all are pregnancy category C, except for rocuronium bromide and cisatracurium, which are category B. Neuromuscular blocking agents are potent drugs that are administered only by persons trained in their use and under conditions in which the patient can receive constant close monitoring. Adequate equipment for endotra-cheal intubation, ventilation, oxygen therapy, and reversal agents must be available.

ADVERSE EFFECTS

All of the neuromuscular blocking agents interfere with respiratory function, progressing to respiratory paralysis. Most of these agents produce residual muscle weakness. Muscle testing (5-second head lifts, hand grips, inspiring with force against a closed glottis) is performed at frequent intervals to assess recovery of neuromuscular function (see Nursing Process section). The use of a twitch monitor also gives information about the recovery of neuromuscular function. One adverse effect common to most neuromuscular blockers is hypersensitivity reactions. Some neuromuscular blocking agents cause hypotension, bronchospasm, and cardiac disturbances. The hypotension is due to ganglionic blockade, which decreases sympathetic tone to arterioles and veins, and histamine release, which promotes vasodilation. The bronchospasm is secondary to histamine release. The cardiovascular effects are due to histamine release, blocking acetylcholine at sites other than the neuromuscular junctions, and stimulation of the sympathetic nervous system. Histamine release also may cause rash, urticaria, and pruritus. The newer products—rocuronium, vecuronium, and cisatracurium—do not cause histamine release, so side effects from these drugs are minimal.

INTERACTIONS

Prolonged intensity and duration of paralysis may occur when neuromuscular blocking agents are used with aminoglycosides, polymyxin B, lincosamides, inhalation anesthetics, magnesium, and thiazide diuretics. A reversal of neuromuscular blockade may occur with concurrent use of theophylline. Neuromuscular blockers are not to be mixed with alkaline solutions such as barbiturates in the same syringe or administered simultaneously during IV infusion through the same needle.

NONDEPOLARIZING AGENTS

Nondepolarizing (also called competitive) *neuromuscular blocking agents* include **tubocurarine chloride *(Tubarine)*, atracurium *(Tracrium)*, cisatracurium besylate *(Nimbex)*, vecuronium bromide *(Norcuron)*, rocuronium bromide *(Zemuron)*, doxacurium chloride *(Nuromax)*, metocurine iodide *(Metubine Iodide)*, pipecuronium bromide *(Arduran)*, gallamine triethiodide *(Flaxedil)*, pancuronium bromide *(Pavulon)*, and mivacurium chloride *(Mivacron)*.** See Table 22–2 for dosages, pharmacokinetics, and nursing implications.

Action

All nondepolarizing neuromuscular blocking agents work by competitive inhibition of the postsynaptic membrane at the neuromuscular junction. Nondepolarizing neuromuscular blockers do not change muscle membrane

Table 22–2. NEUROMUSCULAR BLOCKING AGENTS

DRUG NAME/ROUTE AND DOSAGE	PHARMACOKINETICS/ DYNAMICS	NURSING IMPLICATIONS
NONDEPOLARIZING NEUROMUSCULAR BLOCKING AGENTS		
tubocurarine (Tubarine)		
adjunct to general anesthesia *Adults:* 6–9 mg IV followed by 3–4.5 mg in 3–5 min if necessary. Additional doses of 3 mg may be necessary for longer procedures. **adjunct for electroconvulsive therapy** *Adults:* 0.165 mg/kg slowly IV. **diagnoses of myasthenia gravis** *Adults:* 0.004–0.033 mg/kg IV.	**Onset:** 15 sec–2 min IV **Peak:** 2–5 min IV **Duration:** 20–90 min **½L:** 2 hr **PB:** 40%–45% **M:** liver **E:** urine (33%–75%) excreted unchanged and 11% excreted in bile	**ASSESSMENT:** Assess respiratory status during and following use. Monitor neuromuscular response intraoperatively with peripheral nerve stimulator. Monitor cardiac activity with ECG; monitor blood pressure. Assess for residual muscle weakness. Assess bladder and bowel function. Assess for pregnancy (category C). **INTERVENTION:** Maintain hemodynamic monitoring postoperatively until patient is stable. For continuous infusion, monitor fluid and nutritional status, maintain intake and output, turn patient every 1–2 hr, provide active and passive range of motion (ROM), orient frequently to person, place, and time. Monitor electrolyte status. Provide for methods of communication. Provide support to patient and family. Drug should be used only by persons trained in endotracheal intubation, and equipment should be readily available. **EVALUATION:** Report evidence of hypersensitivity. Evaluate return of neuromuscular function.
atracurium (Tracrium)		
Adults: 0.08–0.1 mg/kg IV intermittently; or 9–10 μg/kg per min continuous IV infusion, followed by maintenance rate of 5–9 μg/kg per min. **intubation** *Adults:* 0.4–0.5 mg/kg IV. *Children 2 yr and over:* Doses are the same as for adults.	**Onset:** 2–2.5 min **Peak:** 5 min **Duration:** 20–35 min **½L:** 20 min **PB:** 82% **M:** spontaneous degradation **E:** urine, feces	Same as for tubocurarine plus: **ASSESSMENT:** Assess for pregnancy (category C). **INTERVENTION:** Best administered through central line, as the low pH (3.5) can cause phlebitis. Administer small doses over 60 sec. If patient is acidatic or hypothermic, drug action is delayed.
pancuronium bromide (Pavulon)		
Adults: 0.04–0.1 mg/kg IV push.	**Onset:** 30–45 sec. **Peak:** 3–15 min **Duration:** 35–45 min **½L:** 2 hr **PB:** 87% **B:** liver (small amounts) **E:** urine and bile (small amounts)	**ASSESSMENT:** Assess for pregnancy (category C). **INTERVENTION:** Drug interaction: prior administration of succinylcholine has been reported to increase the intensity and duration of neuromuscular blockade produced by pancuronium.
rocuronium bromide (Zemuron)		
intubation *Adults:* Initial dose–0.6–1.2 mg/kg IV. *Maintenance dose*–0.1–0.2 mg/kg. *Continuous infusion*–0.01–0.012 mg/kg per min.	**Onset:** 1 min **Peak:** 1–2 min **Duration:** 22–30 min **½L:** biphasic, 1–2 min; 14–18 min **PB:** 30% **M:** liver **E:** urine	Same as for tubocurarine plus: **ASSESSMENT:** Assess for pregnancy (category B).
vecuronium bromide (Norcuron)		
Adults: Initial dose–0.08–0.1 mg/kg IV bolus. *Maintenance dose*–1 μg/kg per min by continuous infusion for long surgical procedures.	**Onset:** 1–3 min **Peak:** 3–5 min **Duration:** 15–25 min **½L:** 65–75 min **PB:** 60%–90% **M:** liver **E:** feces, urine	Same as for tubocurarine plus: **ASSESSMENT:** Assess for pregnancy (category C).

Continued on the following page

Table 22–2. NEUROMUSCULAR BLOCKING AGENTS, *Continued*

DRUG NAME/ROUTE AND DOSAGE	PHARMACOKINETICS/ DYNAMICS	NURSING IMPLICATIONS
DEPOLARIZING NEUROMUSCULAR BLOCKING AGENTS		
succinylcholine (Anectine) (Quelicin) (Sucrostin)		Same as for tubocurarine.
Adults: 0.3–1.1 mg/kg IV push over 10–30 sec for short surgical procedures; 2.5–4.3 mg/min IV for long surgical procedures.	**Onset:** 0.5. sec–1 min **Peak:** 1 sec–2 min **Duration:** 8–10 min **½L:** NA **PB:** NA **M:** pseudocholinesterase in plasma (90%) **E:** urine (10%)	

NA = not available; ECG = electrocardiogram.

potential, and they affect only skeletal muscles. These agents block the action of the neurotransmitter acetylcholine by binding to the receptors on the muscle end-plate that are usually occupied by acetylcholine. If more than 60% of the acetylcholine receptors are occupied by nondepolarizing agents, the action potential of the muscle cells cannot reach threshold level and muscle contraction cannot occur. As the concentration of drug at the muscle membrane receptors decreases and sufficient receptors become available to acetylcholine, muscle contraction is possible again. When the nondepolarizing block is no longer needed, it can be reversed by administering anticholinesterase agents such as neostigmine, edrophonium, or pyridostigmine. Anticholinesterase agents antagonize the effects of nondepolarizing neuromuscular blocking agents, allowing a buildup of acetylcholine. Atropine is usually administered prior to or concurrently with anticholinesterase agents to minimize the side effects (bradycardia, bronchospasm, and excessive salivation) of acetylcholine buildup.

Intermediate-Acting Products

○ **Tubocurarine chloride** (Tubarine) reduces the intensity of muscle contractions during electroshock therapy. Tubocurarine is also used as a diagnostic agent for myasthenia gravis when test results are inconclusive. Both ganglionic blockade and histamine release occur with this drug.

CONTRAINDICATIONS AND PRECAUTIONS In addition to the general contraindications and precautions, tubocuranine is also contraindicated in patients sensitive to histamine release (e.g., asthmatics). In addition, tubocurarine is used cautiously in patients with hypothermia, endocrine disorders, lung cancer, bronchogenic carcinoma, fractures, or muscle spasms.

ADVERSE EFFECTS Tubocurarine's effects on respiration include apnea and bronchospasm. Adverse cardiovascular effects include dyshythmias, hypotension, and bradycardia. Other reactions include excessive salivation and hypersensitivity.

○ **Atracurium** (Tracrium) is eliminated rapidly, there is no progressive or cumulative effect when given in repeated doses. Ganglionic blockade, antimuscarinic effects, and sympathetic stimulation are absent with atracurium.

ADVERSE EFFECTS In addition to adverse effects for all neuromuscular blockers, atracurium can cause bradycardia and tachycardia as well as changes in blood pressure.

○ **Cisatracurium besylate** (Nimbex) has a potency three times that of atracurium. It is used to provide skeletal muscle relaxation during surgery, endotracheal tube insertion, or mechanical ventilation in the intensive care unit and as an adjunct to general anesthesia.

○ **Vecuronium bromide** (Norcuron) does not cause histamine release and has minimal cardiovascular effects.

CONTRAINDICATIONS AND PRECAUTIONS Airway or ventilatory problems may occur in patients with severe obesity, requiring special care before, during, and after the use of vecuronium.

ADVERSE EFFECTS The major CNS side effects are skeletal muscle weakness or paralysis. Vecuronium can cause prolonged apnea.

Short-Acting Products

○ **Rocuronium bromide** (Zemuron) has no effect on the cardiovascular system. Rocuronium also causes no histamine release and, therefore, no histamine-related hypersensitivity reactions.

CONTRAINDICATIONS AND PRECAUTIONS Rocuronium is contraindicated in patients hypersensitive to bromides.

ADVERSE EFFECTS Rarely, tachycardia, abnormal ECG, nausea, vomiting, asthma, rash, edema, and pruritus may occur.

Other Nondepolarizing Agents

These agents share the same mechanism of action as the other nondepolarizing neuromuscular blockers. They differ in time course of action and cardiovascular effects.

Long-Acting Agents

○ **Doxacurium chloride** (Nuromax) has no adverse cardiovascular effects. Dosage is usually 0.025 mg/kg every 30 minutes in maintenance therapy.

○ **Metocurine iodide** (Metubine Iodide) is one of the neuromuscular blockers used to induce muscle relaxation during electroshock therapy. With rapid administration of large doses, the patient may exhibit signs of histamine release. Metocurine has fewer cardiovascular effects than equally potent doses of tubocurarine or gallamine.

○ **Pipecuronium bromide** (Arduran) is recommended only for procedures lasting 90 minutes or longer. The drug does not release histamine. Adverse cardiovascular effects are rare but include hypotension, bradycardia, and hypertension. Maintenance dose is 10–15 μg/kg.

Intermediate-Acting Agents

○ **Gallamine triethiodide** (Flaxedil) does not cause histamine release or ganglionic blockade, so hypotension does not occur. It can cause tachycardia. The IV dose is 1–1.5 mg/kg.

○ **Pancuronium bromide** (Pavulon) does not cause ganglionic blockade. Therefore, it does not induce hypotension. Its action decreases with hypothermia. Pancuronium has a long lag time between administration and onset and thus cannot be used for acute emergency procedures such as intubation. It has a potential for accumulation, so it should not be administered by continuous infusion. Pancuronium has the same adverse effects as all neuromuscular blockers. In addition, it can cause tachycardia, hypertension, and increased cardiac output.

Short-Acting Agents

○ **Mivacurium chloride** (Mivacron) release of histamine is related to dose and speed of injection. The most common adverse effect is cutaneous facial flushing. Other cardiovascular effects are minimal but can include bradycardia, tachycardia, and hypotension. Mivacurium is metabolized by *pseudocholinesterase*, in plasma (an enzyme that speeds up the breakdown of noncholine esters as well as acetylcholine). In patients with low pseudocholinesterase levels, metabolism is delayed, prolonging neuromuscular blockade. Before administering the drug, ask the patient about any history of genetic low plasma pseudocholinesterase disorders.

DEPOLARIZING AGENTS

The only *depolarizing* (or noncompetitive) *neuromuscular blocking agent*—**succinylcholine (Anectine)**—differs from nondepolarizing neuromuscular blocking agents in its mechanism of action and in its interactions with anticholinesterase agents.

○ **Succinylcholine** (Anectine, Quelicin, Sucrostin) is a short-acting drug that rapidly produces skeletal muscle relaxation through depolarization of the muscle endplate. Succinylcholine stimulates the muscle in a fashion similar to the action of the natural substance acetylcholine, producing transient *muscle fasciculation* (the involuntary contraction or twitching of muscle fibers). The drug prolongs depolarization because it does not disso-

ciate rapidly from the receptor, which prevents the endplate from repolarizing and, therefore, prevents further muscle contraction. Paralysis persists until the drug dissociates from its receptors, which occurs when plasma levels of the drug decline.

There is no specific antidote to succinylcholine. Anticholinesterase drugs such as neostigmine or edrophonium are not used as reversal agents. Anticholinesterase agents decrease the activity of pseudocholinesterase, the enzyme that breaks down succinylcholine. This results in a delay in the biotransformation of succinylcholine, which prolongs the drug's pharmacologic effect. However, the prolonged apnea caused by administration of a large dose may be reversed by neostigmine.

Because of its brief duration of action, succinylcholine is used primarily for muscle relaxation during endotracheal intubation, electroconvulsive therapy, endoscopy, and other short procedures.

CONTRAINDICATIONS AND PRECAUTIONS Succinylcholine is contraindicated in patients with low plasma pseudocholinesterase levels because they experience prolonged (3 to 24 hours) paralysis after a single intubation dose of succinylcholine. These patients may require prolonged ventilatory support and close monitoring until the effects of the drug have worn off. Before administration, ask the patient about history of genetic disorders of low plasma pseudocholinesterase.

Succinylcholine raises intraocular pressure and is contraindicated in patients with acute narrow-angle glaucoma or penetrating eye injuries; it is used cautiously in patients with recent eye surgery.

Succinylcholine is also contraindicated in patients with personal or familial malignant hyperthermia, a rare and potentially fatal condition (associated with dangerous temperature elevation), which can be triggered by this drug (and inhalation anesthetics).

▼ CLINICAL ALERT

Because succinylcholine can trigger malignant hyperthermia, make sure the patient is assessed for history of this condition prior to administration. Monitor the patient for the following signs throughout therapy: tachycardia, tachypnea, hypercarbia, jaw muscle spasm, lack of laryngeal relaxation, and hyperthermia. If these signs occur, succinylcholine and the accompanying anesthetic are discontinued, the patient is cooled with ice or an infusion of iced saline, and dantrolene sodium is administered.

Succinylcholine may cause hyperkalemia, especially in patients with severe burns, trauma, or neurologic disorders such as myasthenia gravis. Neuromuscular blockade is prolonged in hypokalemic or hypocalcemic patients, so use cautiously in those with electrolyte imbalances.

In patients with fractures or muscle spasms, muscle fasciculation caused by the antagonistic pharmacologic effect of succinylcholine may result in additional trauma. Muscle fasciculation may also force potassium out of muscle cells and into the circulation, resulting in digitalis toxicity in patients taking cardiac glycosides. Safe use of succinylcholine in pregnancy has not been established; this drug is pregnancy category C.

ADVERSE EFFECTS Muscle fasciculation may be responsible for the postoperative muscle pain that is experienced by most patients. A small dose of a nondepolarizing agent may be used prior to succinylcholine to decrease the severity of muscle fasciculation. The patient on succinylcholine may exhibit signs of profound respiratory depression and apnea. Adverse cardiovascular effects include bradycardia, tachycardia, hypertension, hypotension, and dysrhythmias. Therefore, patients with underlying cardiac or neurologic disease are monitored closely. Hypersensitivity reactions are rare. Other adverse effects include myoglobinemia and excessive salivation. To prevent excessive salivation, patients may be premedicated with atropine or scopolamine.

SELECTION OF A NEUROMUSCULAR BLOCKING AGENT

The choice of drug depends on several considerations. First, the indication of the patient, for short-, immediate-, or long-term therapy; the speed of onset; the potential for adverse effects; the organs of biotransformation and excretion; ease of antagonism or reversal; and rate of recovery after discontinuation. Most drugs today are administered by continuous IV drip, which assists with achieving a steady-state level.

NURSING PROCESS RELATED TO MOVEMENT DISORDERS

A major goal of therapy for the patient with a skeletal muscle disorder is to maintain or improve the patient's independent functioning.

The patient with skeletal muscle problems may require hospitalization if there is a need for dosage adjustments, nonmedical therapy such as traction or physical therapy, or surgical intervention. Hospitalization may also be needed if the patient experiences a worsening of the ability to carry out activities of daily living (i.e., walking, in-

---

Table 22–3. NURSING PROCESS FOR PATIENT REQUIRING SKELETAL MUSCLE RELAXANTS

Assessment

Assess muscle strength, gait, level of comfort.
Assess tremor, rigidity, spasticity, fasciculation, dystonia, fatigue.
Assess voice characteristics for speech pattern alterations.
Assess history for other disease or illness.
Assess emotional stress, level of anxiety, and/or behavior reflective of ineffective coping skills.

Nursing Diagnosis: Impaired Physical Mobility

RELATED TO: Spasm and resistance to movement.
AS EVIDENCED BY: Immobility, decreased daily activity, and decreased ability to provide own care.

Desired Outcomes/Evaluation Criteria

Achieves maximum amount of mobility possible. Displays no complications associated with muscle spasticity.

Nursing Actions	Rationale
Administer medication prior to initiating morning self-care activities.	Promotes independence within the individual situation.
Allow time for medication to take effect before beginning activities.	Helps to relieve symptoms so activities can be undertaken, maximizing ability to participate in activity.
Assist with activities of daily living.	Provides assistance while maintaining independence.
Monitor level of fatigue or pain with activity.	Ability to perform desired activities is a good way to monitor effectiveness of the medication.
Promote rest periods between activities.	Prevents undue fatigue and strain on affected muscles.
Provide exercise as indicated to affected area.	Helps maintain joint and muscle mobility.

Nursing Diagnosis: Pain

RELATED TO: Inflammation associated with muscle spasm.
AS EVIDENCED BY: Facial grimacing and inability to participate in daily activities.

Desired Outcomes/Evaluation Criteria

Reports less pain (rated on scale from 1–10) from muscle spasm.

Nursing Actions	Rationale
Administer medication throughout a 24-hr period.	Maintains consistent level of muscle relaxation.
Position patient to support area affected by muscle spasticity.	Helps promote comfort by decreasing strain of affected muscle groups; maintains good body alignment.
Apply hot and cold packs; massage affected muscles.	Helps promote comfort by decreasing tenseness of affected muscles.

Other Suggested Nursing Diagnoses: Ineffective Coping, Self-Care Deficit, Sleep Pattern Disturbance, and Risk for Trauma.

itiating volitional movements, dressing, and so on).

The major concerns related to motor dysfunction are alterations in daily living, self-concept, and client safety. Table 22–3 suggests how the nursing process can be applied to the patient with a movement disorder who requires skeletal muscle relaxants.

ASSESSMENT

- Obtain a history including specific routines or needs the patient has, such as sleep patterns, eating habits, and bowel and bladder routines. Obtain data related to the patient's ability to tolerate activity. Knowledge of the patient's fatigue level is important for planning activities effectively. A psychosocial assessment and drinking and smoking habits are included.
- Perform and record a basic neurologic assessment, including a basic screening for sight, eating, swallowing, facial expression, general movements, initiation of volitional movements, gait, and walking. If deficits appear during the screening, perform a more detailed neurologic assessment.
- Assess the patient 1 hour after the administration of medication to observe for effects.
- With neuromuscular blocking agents, the nurse assesses the procedure to determine if there will be pain. Because neuromuscular blocking agents do not have an effect on consciousness, pain threshold, or cerebration, opioids or anesthetics are administered concurrently.

NURSING DIAGNOSIS

Nursing diagnoses may relate to physical or psychosocial findings. Suggested nursing diagnoses include Impaired Mobility, Pain, Risk for Trauma, Self-Care Deficit, Sleep Pattern Disturbance, and Ineffective Coping (see Table 22–3).

PLANNING AND INTERVENTION

- Plan interventions to minimize the patient's discomfort and altered mobility. Nurses are critical thinkers solving patient problems. For example, the nurse can help the patient obtain self-help devices, which may help to maintain or improve his or her activity level.
- Assess deficits related to walking on the basis of observations. Include posture, muscle tone, arm swing, rhythm, gait, coordination, and the ability to move freely in the environment. When a motor dysfunction related to walking occurs, consider the effects this deficit has on the patient's ability to perform self-care activities. This has relevance in the planning of care and in giving discharge instructions.
- Consider the influence of the deficit on the patient's self-concept. How does the patient view himself or herself? Does the deficit influence how the patient interacts with other people? Does the alteration in mobility affect the patient's ability to work?

- Consider concerns related to the patient's safety such as in ambulation environment? If not, how much assistance will be needed?
- Administer IV products carefully. Extravasation may cause thrombophlebitis and sloughing.
- Monitor train-of-four (TOF) testing to assess for the desired amount of neuromuscular blocking action when drugs are administered continuously in the ICU setting. A peripheral nerve stimulator delivers a mild electrical current to a motor nerve (usually the ulnar is used, but facial or superficial peroneal nerve in feet can be used). The response to four consecutive stimuli (train of four) predicts the depth or extent of neuromuscular blockade. TOF response is as follows:
  one twitch = 90% blocked
  two to three twitches = 75% to 90% blocked
  4 twitches indicate no block
  The TOF can be visually observed or palpated. Increasing the current does not increase the response. TOF is assessed every 15 minutes during drug initiation and every 4 hours thereafter. The desired level of blockade is usually 85% to 90%, reflecting one or two twitches on the TOF. Too much medication can result in prolonged paralysis (hours to days) when the neuromuscular blockers are discontinued. If patients do not respond to the TOF, the dose of the neuromuscular blocker is reduced until a response is elic-

Table 22–4. PATIENT TEACHING—SKELETAL MUSCLE RELAXANTS

Dear Patient:

This drug has been prescribed for you for _____. To get the most from your drug therapy, you should know the following:

☐ 1. Skeletal muscle relaxants are used to relieve muscle pain due to injury.

☐ 2. Skeletal muscle relaxants may be taken for a short time for acute injuries or indefinitely for chronic problems.

☐ 3. Your drug is best taken at the same time each day and with food.

☐ 4. If you forget to take your drug for a dose, skip it; do *not* try to catch up.

☐ 5. Do not omit or stop taking your drug without telling your physician.

☐ 6. These drugs help to make an injury feel better. Do not push your recovery. Lifting weight of any kind or exercising too early may cause further tissue injury. Follow your physician's instructions carefully.

☐ 7. Notify your physician if side effects—dry mouth, headache, difficulty in urination, or constipation—are severe. Also notify your physician if skin rash occurs.

☐ 8. Change body position slowly to prevent sudden dizziness. Be careful when climbing stairs because of possible muscle weakness.

☐ 9. Do not drink beer, wine, or alcohol because these may make you very dizzy.

☐ 10. Be careful when driving a car or operating heavy machinery.

☐ 11. Do not adjust your drug dose yourself. Take your drug exactly as prescribed.

☐ 12. Your urine may turn orange, purple, red, brown, black, or green while you are taking these drugs.

ited. It is important to keep a few receptors unblocked so the neuromuscular blocker can be reversed. Reversal drugs must have a free receptor site to work on.

- Monitor cerebral function with monitors when available. Computer-processed electroencephalograms (EEG)s are derived from external monitoring of the frontal cerebral area. If a patient is receiving adequate neuromuscular blockers, seizure activity cannot be assessed. If status epilepticus occurs, the brain may be destroyed.
- When neuromuscular blockers are administered, they cause only paralysis. Conscious sedation is achieved by administering other drugs such as morphine, fentanyl (Sublimaze), or the benzodiazepines. Monitor the patient's response to these drugs carefully.
- Monitor for adequate reversal of neuromuscular blockers. If the patient can lift his or her head off the bed and sustain the lift for 5 seconds, the reversal is considered adequate.
- Place a card indicating the reversing agent over the patient's bed for emergency use.
- Refer to Table 22–4 for the teaching plan for patients requiring skeletal muscle relaxants.

EVALUATION

The effectiveness of therapy is determined by the success of nursing interventions to maintain or improve the patient's independent functioning.

- Evaluate mobility, pain, activities of daily living, and psychosocial status.
- Evaluate for unusual or idiosyncratic reactions, which usually appear within the 1st hour (extreme weakness, dizziness, ataxia, dysarthria, visual disturbances, confusion).
- Evaluate other therapies (physical therapy, heat, cold, transcutaneous electrical nerve stimulation, and so on) for effectiveness.
- Evaluate for increased range of motion or a return to normal movement.
- Evaluate for relief of symptoms to determine if dosage can be reduced.

With the use of neuromuscular blockers, the therapeutic goal is to restore normal muscle functioning. (Refer to Chapter 21, Anesthetics, for information on applying the nursing process to patients receiving neuromuscular blockers.)

The bibliography for this chapter can be found in Appendix B, which begins on page 1054.

CHAPTER REVIEW QUESTIONS*

1. Central-acting skeletal muscle relaxants are *most* effective in relieving muscle spasm caused by:
   a. Multiple sclerosis.
   b. Cerebral palsy.
   c. Pain receptor stimulation.
   d. Inflammation or trauma.

2. Which of the following is an example of a direct-acting skeletal muscle relaxant?
   a. Diazepam (Valium).
   b. Methocarbamol (Robaxin).
   c. Dantrolene sodium (Dantrium).
   d. Carisoprodol (Soma).

3. When monitoring train-of-four response in a patient receiving neuromuscular blockers, the most appropriate response is:
   a. one to two twitches.
   b. two to three twitches.
   c. three to four twitches.
   d. No twitches.

* See Appendix A, which begins on page 1051, for answers.

4. Which is an important nursing consideration when caring for a patient on neuromuscular blockers?
   a. Monitor urinary output closely.
   b. Maintain conscious sedation at an appropriate level.
   c. Monitor respiratory function.
   d. Maintain adequate level of deep tendon reflexes.

5. John, who is receiving carisoprodol (Soma), is assessed for what idiosyncratic reaction?
   a. Hypotension, bronchospasm.
   b. Weakness, ataxia, visual disturbances.
   c. Psychic dependence.
   d. Constipation.

Drugs for Parkinson's Disease, Myasthenia Gravis, Alzheimer's Disease, and Multiple Sclerosis

Merrily A. Kuhn, RNC, PhD

CHAPTER OUTLINE

Drugs for Parkinson's Disease
Drugs for Myasthenia Gravis
Drugs for Alzheimer's Disease
Drugs for Multiple Sclerosis
Nursing Process Related to Movement Disorders

TABLES

Drug Tables

Nursing Process

Patient Teaching

KEY TERMS

Akinesia
Bradykinesia
Bulbar
Decarboxylase
Dyskinesia
Erythromelalgia
Extrapyramidal system
Fasciculation
Ptosis
Thymectomy
Tremor

LEARNING OBJECTIVES

After reading this chapter, the student will be able to:

1. Describe the specific nervous system disorders discussed in this chapter and the various medications that are commonly used to treat them.
2. Differentiate among the medications for specific nervous system disorders as to mechanisms of action, routes of administration, metabolism, contraindications and precautions, adverse effects, and interactions.
3. Identify specific areas to assess in the patient with a specific nervous system disorder to formulate appropriate patient outcomes.
4. Plan the nursing interventions necessary to safely administer drugs for specific nervous system disorders and choose appropriate teaching strategies to gain patient compliance.
5. Plan the nursing intervention necessary to counsel the families of patients who have disorders of the nervous system.
6. Evaluate the patient at various stages of treatment to measure the effects of nursing interventions.

The publisher greatly acknowledges the contribution of Barbara K. Clark, RN, MN, CCRN, to the third edition.

This chapter discusses the common pharmacologic agents used to treat several specific disorders of the nervous system—Parkinson's disease, myasthenia gravis, Alzheimer's disease, and multiple sclerosis. The pharmacologic products discussed include dopaminergic and anticholinergic agents for treating Parkinson's disease, cholinesterase inhibitors and immunosuppressive agents for myasthenia gravis, tacrine hydrochloride for Alzheimer's disease, and interferon beta-1b for multiple sclerosis.

DRUGS FOR PARKINSON'S DISEASE

Parkinson's disease is a chronic, progressive neurologic disorder of the extrapyramidal system. The *extrapyramidal system* is a complex network of neurons located in the basal ganglia, thalamic and subthalamic nuclei, red nucleus, substantia nigra, and parts of the reticular formation, cerebellum, and cerebrum that helps regulate movement. When this system is disrupted, the result is *dyskinesias* (disorders characterized by abnormal involuntary movement). The dyskinesias that characterize Parkinson's disease include *bradykinesia* (a condition characterized by slow voluntary movements), *akinesia* (a condition characterized by the inability to make voluntary movements), *tremor* (an involuntary trembling or shaking movement), rigidity, and postural instability. Associated symptoms include delayed reaction time, lack of autonomic movements, depression, and dementia.

The cause of this movement disorder is neuronal degeneration of the nigrostriatal pathway. There is a loss of dopaminergic neurons in the substantia nigra and a reduction in the concentration of dopamine in the striatum and the substantia nigra. There is also a loss of the dopaminergic receptors in the striatum, which further limits the dopaminergic action. This loss of dopaminergic action causes an imbalance between dopamine (an inhibitory transmitter) and acetylcholine (an excitatory transmitter). This imbalance results in the enhancement of the cholinergic activity and the signs and symptoms of Parkinson's disease. The course of Parkinson's disease is variable. In general, parkinsonism leads to motor, posture, and tone dysfunction.

Drug therapy is directed at balancing striatal activity by enhancing dopaminergic function with dopaminergic agents or by reducing cholinergic activity with anticholinergics. Sometimes, a combination of anticholinergic and dopaminergic agents is used. The choice of drug therapy depends on the severity of the disease, its progression, and the patient's ability to tolerate adverse reactions.

As drug therapy for Parkinson's disease does not provide a cure, the goal of therapy is to provide relief of symptoms and to maintain maximum independence of movement for as long as possible. In addition to drug therapy, nonpharmacologic measures such as exercise, speech therapy, physical therapy, psychotherapy, and family support are critical in the management of patients with this disorder.

DOPAMINERGIC AGENTS

The dopaminergic agents, which enhance dopaminergic function by a variety of mechanisms, include **levodopa (Dopar)**, **carbidopa (Lodosyn)**, **amantadine (Symmetrel)**, **bromocriptine (Parlodel)**, **pergolide (Permax)**, and **selegiline hydrochloride (Eldepryl)**. The major symptomatic relief is associated with bradykinesia, rigidity, and to a lesser extent, tremor. They also reported to improve the problems connected with balance, posture, gait, and handwriting. These drugs are featured in Table 23–1.

○ **Levodopa** (Dopar, Larodopa) is a precursor to dopamine. Dopamine does not cross the blood-brain barrier, but levodopa does. Once levodopa is converted to dopamine in the central nervous system (CNS), it serves as a neurotransmitter that facilitates movement and postural reflexes.

Levodopa does not stop the progression of the pathology associated with parkinsonism, but it does improve symptoms and the quality of life for most patients.

Levodopa is rarely used today alone but used in combination with carbidopa. Although carbidopa is available separately, a combination product with the trade name Sinemet, which contains both carbidopa and levodopa, is generally used.

USES Sinemet is the drug of choice for the treatment of Parkinson's disease. It is also used to manage postencephalitic parkinsonism; and symptomatic parkinsonism after carbon monoxide or manganese intoxication or in association with cerebral atherosclerosis. Sinemet is not useful in controlling drug-induced extrapyramidal reactions.

PHARMACOKINETICS Sinemet is well absorbed from the small bowel. The rate of absorption is influenced by the rate of gastric emptying, acidity of gastric juice, and competition for amino acids. Administration with food or dietary protein slows the absorption of sinemet and therefore lowers peak absorption.

CONTRAINDICATIONS AND PRECAUTIONS Sinemet is contraindicated in patients with narrow-angle glaucoma because it produces mydriasis, which would aggravate the glaucoma. It is the precursor of skin melanin which induces or stimulates the growth of cutaneous melanomas. Thus, it is contraindicated in patients with undiagnosed skin lesions or a history of melanoma. Sinemet is not used during lactation. Safety and effectiveness during pregnancy (category C) and in children under 12 have not been established.

○ **Carbidopa** (Lodosyn) is a decarboxylase inhibitor that, when combined with levodopa, diminishes the decaboxylation of levodopa in peripheral tissues. This allows more levodopa to reach receptor sites in the nigrostriatum. Carbidopa does not cross the blood-brain barrier and thus does not interfere with the decarboxyation of levodopa in the brain. By using carbidopa with levodopa (1) the effective dose of levodopa is reduced by 75%; (2) the stimulation of the receptors in the medullary emetic center is decreased, thereby decreasing nausea and vomiting; (3) the antagonsim of the therapeutic efficacy of levodopa by pyridoxine is avoided; (4) the frequency

Table 23–1. ANTIPARKINSON DRUGS: DOPAMINERGIC AGENTS

DRUG NAME/ROUTE AND DOSAGE	PHARMACOKINETICS/ DYNAMICS	NURSING IMPLICATIONS
all antiparkinson agents		
		ASSESSMENT: Assess parkinsonian symptoms prior to and throughout course of therapy. Assess blood pressure during period of dose adjustment. **EVALUATION:** Effectiveness of therapy can be demonstrated by a resolution of parkinsonian signs and symptoms.
levidopa (Dopar) (L-Dopa) (Larodopa) **carbidopa/levodopa** (Sinemet) (Sinemet CR)		
levodopa *Adults:* *Initially*–500–1000 mg PO given in divided doses every 6–12 hours; increase by 100–750 mg/day every 3–7 days until response occurs or dose of 8000 mg/day is reached. Usual maintenance dose is 2000–8000 mg/day. **carbidopa/levodopa** (Tablets contain 10/100, 25/100, or 25/250 mg of carbidopa and levodopa, respectively.) *Adults:* 75/300–150/1500 mg/day PO in 3–4 divided doses; can be increased up to 200/2000 mg/day. **sinemet cr** (Contains 25/100 or 50/200 mg of carbidopa and levodopa, respectively.) *Adults:* 100/400–400/1600 mg/day PO in divided doses q 4–8 hr.	**Onset:** 10–15 min **Peak:** 0.5–2 hr **Duration:** 5–24 hr (up to 3–5 days with prolonged therapy) **½L:** 1–3 hr **PB:** NA **B:** GI tract and liver **E:** kidney **Onset:** rapid **Peak:** 2 hr **Duration:** 5–24 hr (up to 3–5 days with prolonged therapy) **½L:** 1–2 hr, carbidopa; 2 hr, levodopa **PB:** 36%, carbidopa; NA, levodopa **B:** GI tract and liver **E:** kidney	Same as for all plus: **ASSESSMENT:** In patients receiving long-term therapy, CBC and serum glucose should be monitored periodically. **INTERVENTION:** Administer food shortly after medication to minimize GI irritation; taking food before or concurrently may retard levodopa's effect. If patient has difficulty swallowing, confer with pharmacist. In the carbidopa/levodopa combination, the number following the drug name represents the mg of each respective drug. Wait 8 hours after last levodopa dose before switching patient to carbidopa/levodopa. Administering carbidopa shortly after full dose of levodopa may result in toxicity. In preoperative patients who are NPO, confer with physician about continuing medication administration. **Patient Teaching**—Caution patient to avoid vitamin B_6 in diet and to monitor protein intake (divide among 6 small meals). Tell patient that drug may darken sweat or urine. Advise patient to use caution when driving or doing activities requiring alertness and to avoid sudden changes in posture. **EVALUATION:** Therapeutic effects usually become evident after 2–3 weeks of therapy, but may require up to 6 months. Patients who receive this medication for several years may experience a decrease in its effectiveness. An increased response to the drug may occur after a drug holiday. Evaluate for signs of toxicity (involuntary muscle twitching, facial grimacing, spasmodic winking, exaggerated protrusion of tongue, or behavioral changes). Consult physician promptly if these symptoms occur.
DOPAMINE RECEPTOR AGONISTS		
amantadine (Symmetrel)		
parkinson's disease *Adults:* 100 mg PO twice daily increased to 200 mg bid if no response after 1 wk.	**Onset:** 48 hr **Peak:** 2–4 hr **Duration:** 12–24 hr **½L:** 11–15 hr **PB:** NA **B:** liver **E:** kidneys	Same as for all plus: **ASSESSMENT:** Monitor blood pressure periodically. Assess patient for drug-induced postural hypotension. Advise patient to make position changes slowly. Assess patient for confusion, hallucinations, and mood changes. Notify physician if these occur. Assess patient for the appearance of a diffuse purple mottling of the skin. This common side effect disappears with continued therapy, but may not completely resolve until several weeks after therapy has been completed. Assess renal function; reduce dose with renal dysfunction. Assess for pregnancy (category C).

Continued on the following page

Table 23–1. ANTIPARKINSON DRUGS: DOPAMINERGIC AGENTS, *Continued*

DRUG NAME/ROUTE AND DOSAGE	PHARMACOKINETICS/ DYNAMICS	NURSING IMPLICATIONS
amantadine (Symmetrel)		
		INTERVENTION: Do not administer last dose of medication near bedtime, because this drug may produce insomnia in some patients. Administering drug in divided doses tends to decrease CNS side effects. The contents of capsules may be mixed with food or fluids if patient has difficulty swallowing pills. Drug is also available as syrup. **EVALUATION:** Therapeutic effects are usually apparent by end of first week of therapy.
bromocriptine (Parlodel)		
parkinsonism *Adults:* 1.25 mg PO twice daily; increased by 2.5 mg/day in 2 to 4 wk intervals (usual dosage range is 30–90 mg/day in 3 divided doses).	**Onset:** 30–90 min **Peak:** 1–2 hr **Duration:** 8–12 hr **½L:** biphasic: first phase, 4–4.5 hr; terminal phase, 45–50 hr **PB:** 90% to 96% **B:** liver **E:** feces 84%, urine 2.5%–5%	Same as for all plus: **ASSESSMENT:** Assess patient for allergy to ergot derivatives. **INTERVENTION:** Administer with food or milk to minimize gastric distress. Tablets may be crushed if necessary. Supervise ambulation and transfer during initial dosing to prevent injury from hypotension. Monitor blood pressure prior to and frequently during drug therapy. Instruct patient to remain supine during and for several hours after first dose, because severe hypotension may develop. Monitor patient's mental status frequently. Psychotic symptoms have been reported with this drug.
pergolide (Permax) *Adults:* 0.05 mg PO once/day for 2 days, then increased by 0.1–0.15 mg/day every 3rd day for 12 days, then increased by 0.25 mg every 3rd day until optimal response obtained; usual maintenance dose, 3 mg/day in 3 divided doses.	**Onset:** NA **Peak:** NA **Duration:** NA **½L:** NA **PB:** 90% **B:** liver **E:** kidney (55%)	Same as for all plus: **ASSESSMENT:** Assess patient for allergy to ergot derivatives. Monitor blood pressure and ECG frequently during drug therapy. Monitor patient's mental status frequently. Assess for pregnancy (category B) **INTERVENTION: Patient Teaching—**Instruct patient to take medication as prescribed. Tell patient to report side effects to physician. Teach patient to change position slowly to minimize hypotensive effects. Caution patient that medication may cause drowsiness.
MONOAMINE OXIDASE TYPE B INHIBITOR		
selegiline hydrochloride (Eldepryl) *Adults:* 5 mg PO at breakfast and lunch.	**Onset:** 1 hr **Peak:** 0.5–2 hr **Duration:** 1–3 days **½L:** 0.15 hr; up to 20 hr for active metabolites **PB:** NA **B:** liver to N-desmethyldeprenyl, amphetamine, and methamphetamine **E:** urine	Same as for all plus: **ASSESSMENT:** Assess symptoms carefully after therapy starts. Assess for pregnancy (category C). **INTERVENTION:** Concurrent use of meperidine and selegiline should be avoided. **Patient Teaching—**Inform patient that doses of levodopa may need to be reduced. Teach patient signs and symptoms of tyramine reactions and foods to avoid. **EVALUATION:** Evaluate for increased blood pressure. If present, report to physician.

NA = not available; CBC = complete blood count; ECG = electrocardiogram.

and intensity of daily variation in control of symptoms by levodopa are reduced; and (5) the degree of clinical improvement is greater than with levodopa alone.

Carbidopa is used only with levodopa. The combination product Sinemet is used in most patients. Carbidopa is available separately for the patient who requires separate titration of both carbidopa and levodopa.

Because the effects of carbidopa are related to the potentiation of levodopa's effects, the contraindications and precautions, adverse effects, and interactions are the same as those of levodopa. However, abnormal involuntary movements and psychiatric disturbances may be more intense and may occur sooner than when levodopa is given alone.

○ **Carbidopa/levodopa** (Sinemet) is the combination product that contains both drugs. The optimal daily dose (Table 23–1) is carefully titrated for each patient.

▼ CLINICAL ALERT

Levodopa is discontinued at least 8 hours before therapy with carbidopa/levodopa is started. In addition, the total daily dose of levodopa in the carbidopa/levodopa combination must be reduced by 20% to 25% to prevent toxicity.

Sinemet is used with caution in patients with cardiac, psychiatric, or peptic ulcer disease. The cardiac irregularities are due to the beta-adrenergic action of dopamine on the heart and the direct beta-adrenergic receptor stimulation by other catecholamine metabolites of this agent. Persons with psychiatric disturbances, especially psychosis, should be monitored closely because levodopa can enhance hallucinations, paranoia, mania, insomnia, anxiety, nightmares, and depression, especially in the elderly.

There have been some reports of GI bleeding in patients. Patients with peptic ulcer disease are monitored closely. Dark-colored sweat and red-tinged urine have been reported, but are not indications for discontinuation of the drug.

ADVERSE EFFECTS The adverse reactions to the dopaminergic agents fall into two categories: reactions that occur early in therapy and to which a tolerance may develop, such as gastrointestinal effects and cardiovascular effects; and reactions that occur after long-term therapy—the dyskinesias and behavior disturbances.

▼ CLINICAL ALERT

To reduce the high incidence of adverse reactions, therapy is individualized and dosage is gradually increased to the desired therapeutic level.

The GI reactions—anorexia, nausea, and vomiting—are caused by overstimulation of the chemoreceptors in the medulla by the newly formed dopamine. This reaction is easily prevented by increasing the dosage slowly. The common cardiovascular effects are orthostatic hypotension and dysrhythmias. Some of the dysrhythmias reported include sinus tachycardia, atrial and ventricular extrasystoles, atrial flutter or fibrillation, and ventricular tachycardia. These dysrhythmias are caused by the beta-adrenergic action of dopamine on the heart and beta-adrenergic receptor stimulation by other catecholamine metabolites of the drug.

The adverse reactions that occur after long-term therapy include abnormal involuntary movements (dyskinesias), akinetic spells, and behavioral disturbances. The

dyskinesias appear several months after starting sinemet. These abnormal movements usually occur at either the time of peak drug action or at the end of the period of drug action. This particular side effect is referred to as the "end-of-dose failure" because it reflects the tapering of effectiveness. These abnormal involuntary movements vary in type but might include faciolingual tic, grimacing, head bobbing, and rocking movements of the arms, legs, or trunk. Tolerance does not develop to this side effect, and it can become worse if the amount of medication is not reduced. Approximately 15% to 40% of patients develop this phenomenon after 2 to 3 years of treatment, and frequency increases after 5 years. The abnormal involuntary movements are thought to be caused by hypersensative dopamine receptors. Another group of side effects seen as a complication of long-term therapy are akinetic spells during which the patient is immobilized. This is part of the "on/off" phenomenon in which there are periods in which the patient experiences functional ability (often with abnormal involuntary movements) alternately with periods of akinetic attacks. These attacks may be accompanied by tremor and rigidity. Tolerance does not develop to this side effect. However, effects may be decreased by adding amantadine or bromocriptine to the therapy and adjusting the diet and times of meals. Amantadine augments the release of dopamine. Bromocriptine affects a different group of dopamine receptors. The cause of the on/off phenomenon is not fully understood but data suggest an imbalance in physiologic regulatory mechanisms; the phenomenon usually occurs when the blood levels of levodopa are in the low therapeutic range. Behavioral disturbances also occur as side effects of long-term therapy with levodopa. The drug-induced psychosis in parkinsonism patients usually occurs after 2 to 5 years of dopaminergic therapy. These patients can experience vivid dreams or nightmares, hallucinations, confusion, delusions, insomnia, and depression. The only treatment is to reduce the amount of the dopaminergic agent, use a drug holiday, or withdraw the agent. The exact cause of the mental side effects is unknown.

INTERACTIONS Certain drugs can interfere with the effectiveness of sinemet. Pyridoxine (vitamin B_6), a cofactor in the decarboxylation of levodopa to dopamine, can reverse the effectiveness of levodopa by promoting a rapid conversion of levodopa to dopamine in the periphery. This causes a decrease in the amount of levodopa transported to the brain. Patients are instructed to avoid multivitamin preparations and nutritional supplements that contain more than 5 mg of pyridoxine. When levodopa is administered with carbidopa, this antagonistic effect of pyridoxine is lost.

Nonspecific MAO inhibitors interfere with the inactivation of dopamine, norepinephrine, and other catecholamines. They amplify the central effects of sinemet and its catecholamine metabolites, leading to hypertensive crisis and hyperpyrexia. MAO inhibitors are withdrawn at least 14 days prior to the administration of a dopaminergic agent.

The effectiveness of sinemet is decreased when it is combined with benzodiazepines, hydantoins, reserpine, methionine, papaverine, and metoclopramide. Many of these agents deplete stores of central dopamine (reserpine), whereas other agents block dopaminergic receptors. Tricyclic antidepressants (TCAs) can delay absorption and decrease bioavailability of it, reducing its effectiveness. Concurrent therapy with TCAs has also caused hypertensive episodes. Concurrent antacids increase levodopa's bioavailability and possibly increase its efficacy.

Anticholinergic agents such as trihexyphenidyl, benztropine, and procyclidine act synergistically with dopa-

---

Table 23–2. GUIDELINES FOR PATIENTS ON DRUG HOLIDAY

1. Tapering medications:
   - Carbidopa/levodopa: Total dose decreased by one-half every 3 days (may begin as an outpatient) to 5/50 at 7 AM; 5/50 at 11 AM before total withdrawal
   - Bromocriptine: taper and discontinue
   - Anticholinergics: taper and discontinue
   - Amantadine: discontinue
2. Duration goal of drug holiday = 14 days off carbidopa/levodopa
3. Daily assessment to include:
   - Functional abilities (out of bed, chair, roll over, and so on)
   - Ambulation
   - Tremor
   - Rigidity (cogwheeling vs. plastic; unilateral or bilateral; which extremities, trunk, and so on)
   - Mental status
   - Speech
   - Swallowing
   - Expression
   - Respiratory function
   - Circulation
   - Sleep pattern
   - Any dyskinesia/dystonia
   - Emotional response to immobility
4. If on day 7 of drug holiday, there are no major problems with swallowing, respiratory, or circulatory systems, then continue off carbidopa/levodopa until day 10. If still no problems at day 10, continue until day 14.
5. During drug holiday, to avoid problems of decreased mobility:
   - Change of diet to soft, mechanical soft, etc.
   - Subcutaneous heparin, 5000 units, every 12 hours
   - Water mattress
   - Elastic stockings
   - Turning assistance every 2 hours
   - Physical therapy
   - Occupational therapy
   - Recreational therapy
6. Restarting carbidopa/levodopa after a drug holiday: (Regardless of preholiday dose, *note:* doses are given 30 to 40 minutes *before* meals)
   Day 1 = 5/50 at 7 AM; 5/50 at 11 AM
   Day 3 = 5/50 at 7 AM; 5/50 at 11 AM; 5/50 at 4 PM
   Day 6 = 10/100 at 7 AM; 5/50 at 11 AM; 5/50 at 4 PM
   Day 9 = 10/100 at 7 AM; 10/100 at 11 AM; 5/50 at 4 PM
   If still in need of additional medication, the last increase is to 10/100 three times daily before discharge. (Increments can be given after discharge according to functional requirement.) During increases, assessment should be made each day of items listed in (3).
7. Maintenance dose is established after discharge according to targets of therapy and to avoid symptoms of excess dopaminergic stimulation.

Source: Lannon, MC, et al: Comprehensive care of the patient with Parkinson's disease. J Neurosci Nurs 18(3):121–131, 1986, with permission. Updated in 1996.

---

mineric agents to improve certain symptoms associated with parkinsonism. Large doses of the anticholinergic agents can slow gastric emptying, causing a delay in the absorption and possibly a decrease in effectiveness.

Sinemet can transiently elevate serum asparate aminotransferase (AST), serum alanine aminotransferase (ALT), lactate dehydrogenase, bilirubin, blood urea nitrogen (BUN), and protein-bound iodine. White blood count (WBC), hemoglobin, and hematocrit show transient reductions.

DRUG HOLIDAYS When there is a loss of the therapeutic efficacy of dopaminergics and the patient is experiencing the long-term side effects previously mentioned, the carbidopa/levodopa dosage is tapered and the drug withdrawn for up to a 14-day period. The loss of efficacy is caused by the desensitization of receptors for dopamine. The goals of drug holidays are to eliminate or reduce the adverse drug effects and to restore receptor sensitivity to dopamine. After "resensitization," lower doses of dopamine seem sufficient to alleviate symptoms of parkinsonism. During the period of the drug holidays, the patient must be monitored closely. Table 23–2 lists guidelines for patients on drug holidays.

Dopamine Receptor Agonists

The gradual loss of responsiveness to dopaminergics that occurs with long-term therapy has led to the investigation of specific agonists that act directly on striatal dopamine receptor sites. The three major agents available for the treatment of parkinsonism are amantadine (Symmetrel), bromocriptine (Parlodel), and pergolide (Permax).

○ **Amantadine** (Symmetrel) is an antiviral agent that has been found to relieve symptoms associated with parkinsonism. Amantadine is thought to increase dopaminergic activity in the peripheral and central nervous systems by increasing the synthesis, facilitating the release, and inhibiting the cellular reuptake of dopamine. This agent may also have anticholinergic effects.

USES In the early stages of Parkinson's disease when tremor is not the major symptom, amantadine is the drug of choice. In the advanced stages of parkinsonism, it is used concurrently. This agent is not as effective as dopaminergics, but it produces a more rapid response and fewer side effects. See the antibiotic chapter for more information.

○ **Bromocriptine** (Parlodel) is a direct-acting dopamine receptor agonist that is used clinically for the treatment of parkinsonism and also for hyperprolactinemia of various causes. Bromocriptine is an ergot derivative with a preference for dopamine receptors different from those of levodopa. This agent acts on the postsynaptic dopamine receptors. The pharmacologic action of bromocriptine results from stimulation of dopamine receptors in the CNS, cardiovascular system, pituitary-hypothalamic axis, and GI tract.

USES Bromocriptine is more effective than the anticholinergic drugs and amantadine in treating parkinsonism. It is an adjunct to levodopa/carbidopa in patients experiencing significant fluctuations in therapeutic response and end-of-dose akinesia. The decrease in fluctuations may be caused by bromocriptine's longer duration of action, or it may result because the dopamine receptor sites affected by bromocriptine are different from those affected by levodopa.

CONTRAINDICATIONS AND PRECAUTIONS Bromocriptine is contraindicated in patients hypersensitive to bromocriptine or ergot alkaloids. This agent is used cautiously in patients with a history of cardiac disease or psychic disturbances. This is due to the dopaminergic effect. The dose of bromocriptine is reduced in patients with liver impairment because the metabolism of the drug is affected. Safety in pregnancy or children under the age of 15 years has not been established.

ADVERSE EFFECTS The response and tolerance to bromocriptine vary among patients. The drug is carefully titrated to determine the maximum benefit-to-risk ratio. The adverse reactions are generally related to its activity as a dopaminergic agonist. The adverse reactions are classified into two groups: effects with initial therapy and long-term effects. Initial effects include nausea, vomiting, and postural hypotension. The gastrointestinal effects can be decreased by administering bromocriptine with food or by reducing the dose. Long-term effects include constipation, *erythromelalgia* (a condition characterized by recurrent episodes of peripheral vasodilation accompanied by burning pain, redness, and increased skin temperature; erythromelalgia is usually most pronounced in the feet), mental disturbances (confusion, vivid dreams, delusions, hallucinations), dyskinesia, alcohol intolerance, and digital vasospasm. All of these adverse reactions can be reversed by decreasing the dose or discontinuing the drug.

INTERACTIONS Concurrent use of bromocriptine and antihypertensive agents results in additive hypotension. The use of bromocriptine with CNS depressants (antihistamines, alcohol, sedative-hypnotics) increases sedation. Concurrent administration of phenothiazines, haloperidol, methyldopa, reserpine, and TCAs reduces bromocriptine's ability to decrease prolactin levels, so they are not administered concurrently.

○ **Pergolide** (Permax) is a dopamine agonist that stimulates postsynaptic dopaminergic receptors. When used in conjunction with levodopa/carbidopa, pergolide provides continued relief from the symptoms of Parkinson's disease at lower dosages of levodopa/carbidopa.

CONTRAINDICATIONS AND PRECAUTIONS Pergolide is contraindicated in patients hypersensitive to the drug or ergot derivatives. The drug is used cautiously in patients who have a history of dysrhythmias because of the dopaminergic effect on the heart. Safety during lactation and in children has not been established. Pergolide is classified as a pregnancy category B agent.

ADVERSE EFFECTS Adverse effects of pergolide are related to its dopaminergic agonist activity. The most frequent side effects include nausea, constipation, orthostatic hypotension, hallucinations, dyskinesia, somnolence, and rhinitis. Other adverse effects include dysrhythmias, diarrhea and abdominal pain, confusion, and dyspnea.

INTERACTIONS The effectiveness of pergolide is reduced by the phenothiazines, metoclopramide, and thioxanthines, because these agents antagonize the effects of dopamine.

Monoamine Oxidase Type B Inhibitor

○ **Selegiline hydrochloride** (Eldepryl) is an adjuvant agent to levodopa or levodopa/carbidopa used in the management of Parkinson's disease (see Table 23–1). Selegilene is a monamine oxidase type B inhibitor that was initially approved for use with patients showing a decreased response to levodopa/carbidopa therapy. More recent evaluations indicate that selegiline demonstrates an ability to delay the onset of disability in the early onset of Parkinson's disease.

ACTION Selegiline inhibits the action of the enzyme monoamine oxidase (MAO) in the brain, thereby resulting in a reduction of dopamine catabolism and an increase in the concentration of dopamine in the brain synapses.

CONTRAINDICATIONS AND PRECAUTIONS Selegiline is contraindicated in patients hypersensitive to the drug or its metabolites.

ADVERSE EFFECTS Adverse reactions of selegiline are similar to those of levodopa, occur for the same reasons, and include gastrointestinal reactions such as nausea and anorexia and the cardiovascular effects of orthostatic hypotension, angina, and dysrhythmias. Neurologic reactions include increased tremor, restlessness, chorea, dyskinesias, loss of balance, hallucinations, confusion, anxiety, mood changes, and headache. Selegiline may exacerbate the adverse effects of levodopa/carbidopa, requiring a reduction in dose by 10% to 30%.

INTERACTIONS Selegiline increases the effect of levodopa, meperidine, and fluoxetine. If doses of selegiline exceed 10 mg per day, a hypertensive crisis may occur if the drug is used in combination with a nonselective MAO inhibitor or tyramine-containing foods.

ANTICHOLINERGIC AGENTS

The anticholinergic agents atropine and scopolamine were the first to be used in the treatment of parkinsonism. These agents have been replaced by synthetic drugs—**trihexyphenidyl (Artane)**, **benztropine (Cogentin)**, **biperiden (Akineton)**, **procyclidine (Kemadrin)**, and **ethopropazine hydrochloride (Parsidol)**—that are equally as effective but have fewer adverse reactions. After dopaminergic agents were discovered, anticholinergics played a supportive role in the treatment of parkinsonism. However, these agents are still very useful for patients who have minimal symptoms and for those unable to tolerate levodopa or levodopa/carbidopa because of the adverse reactions or contraindications. Trihexyphenidyl and benztropine are featured in Table 23–3.

Action

The anticholinergic agents inhibit the actions of endogenous acetylcholine and muscarinic agonists at the muscarinic receptors of peripheral effector tissues and in the CNS. Muscarinic receptors are distributed at sites of cholinergic transmission. The decreased amounts of dopamine in the striatum of parkinsonian patients create an intensified excitatory effect of the cholinergic system within the striatum. Anticholinergic agents block the excitatory effect of the cholinergic system.

Table 23–3. ANTIPARKINSON DRUGS: ANTICHOLINERGIC AGENTS

DRUG NAME/ROUTE AND DOSAGE	PHARMACOKINETICS/ DYNAMICS	NURSING IMPLICATIONS
all antiparkinson agents		**ASSESSMENT:** Assess parkinsonian symptoms prior to and throughout course of therapy. Assess blood pressure during period of dose adjustment. **EVALUATION:** Effectiveness of therapy can be demonstrated by a resolution of parkinsonian signs and symptoms.
trihexyphenidyl (Artane) (Artane Sequels) *Adults:* Initially 1 mg/day PO; increase by 2 mg every 3–5 days. Usual maintenance dosage is 5–15 mg/day in 3–4 divided doses. Extended-release (ER) preparations (Artane Sequels) may be given every 12–24 hr once the daily dose has been determined using conventional tablets or liquids.	**Onset:** PO, 1 hr **Peak:** PO, 1–1.5 hr **Duration:** PO, 6–12 hr; ER, 12–24 hr **½L:** 5.6–10.2 **PB:** NA **B:** NA **E:** urine	Same as for all plus: **ASSESSMENT:** Assess blood pressure and pulse frequently during period of dose adjustment. Assess for pregnancy (category C). **INTERVENTION:** Usually administered after meals. May be administered before meals if patient suffers from dry mouth, or with meals if gastric distress is a problem. ER capsules should be swallowed whole; do not crush, break, or chew.
benztropine (Cogentin) **parkinsonism** *Adults:* 0.5–6 mg/day PO in 1–2 divided doses. Start with 0.5–1.0 mg, increase by 0.5 mg every 5–6 days until response is obtained. If given as single daily dose, administer at bedtime. **acute dystonic reactions** *Adults:* 1–2 mg IM or IV.	**Onset:** PO, 1–2 hr; IM and IV, few min **Peak:** 2–3 days (clinical effects) **Duration:** PO, 24 hr; IM and IV, 24 hrs **½L:** NA **PB:** NA **B:** NA **E:** NA	Same as for all plus: **ASSESSMENT:** Assess bowel function daily. Monitor for constipation, abdominal pain, distention, or the absence of bowel sounds. Report abnormal findings promptly. Monitor intake/output ratios and evaluate patient for urinary retention (dysuria, distended abdomen, infrequent voiding of small amounts, overflow incontinence). Patients with mental illness are at risk for developing exaggerated symptoms of their disorder during early therapy with this medication. Withhold drug and notify physician if significant behavioral changes occur. Assess for pregnancy (category C). **INTERVENTION:** Administer with food or immediately after meals to minimize gastric irritation. May be crushed and administered with food if patient has difficulty swallowing. Parenteral doses of the drug are used only in acute situations. **EVALUATION:** Effectiveness of therapy can be demonstrated by decrease in drooling and rigidity and improvement in gait and balance. Therapeutic effects are usually seen 2–3 days after initiation of therapy.

NA = not available

Uses

The anticholinergic agents are used in the early stages of Parkinson's disease. Many times these agents are used to treat younger patients who require long-term therapy and for patients who are experiencing tremor. Tremor and rigidity respond well to the anticholinergic agents. There is less of a response in patients with bradykinesia and loss of the postural reflexes. Anticholinergic agents are also beneficial in the treatment of drug-induced parkinsonism. As parkinsonism progresses, the patient becomes refractory to the effects of anticholinergic agents. Responsiveness to these agents can occur by increasing the dose or by substituting another class of anticholinergic agent. These agents are well absorbed from the gastrointestinal tract and can cross the blood-brain barrier.

Contraindications and Precautions

Anticholinergic agents are contraindicated in patients with hypersensitivity to these drugs, narrow-angle glaucoma, and tachycardia. Anticholinergic agents can block the parasympathetic input to the sinoatrial node, producing tachycardia. The mydriatic effect of anticholinergic agents can precipitate an attack of acute glaucoma. These agents also increase aqueous outflow resistance, increasing intraocular pressure.

Anticholinergic agents are used with caution in patients with abdominal obstruction, prostatic hypertrophy, and in the elderly or very young because of susceptibility to adverse reactions. These agents block the excitatory effect of acetylcholine on the detrusor muscle of the bladder, causing urinary retention. Patients with prostatic hypertrophy are observed for urinary retention. Anticholinergic agents impair gastric secretion and gastrointestinal motility, so patients with abdominal obstruction are observed for signs of constipation and intestinal obstruction. Safe use in pregnancy (category C) and lactation has not been established.

Adverse Effects

The most common reactions—dry mouth, mydriasis, cycloplegia, tachycardia, constipation, urinary retention, and psychic disturbances—are all due to the anticholinergic effects. Anticholinergic agents inhibit salivation (which is helpful in the parkinsonism patient, because excessive salivation may be a problem). Some of the frequent CNS reactions include mental confusion, hallucinations, delirium, sedation, nervousness, dizziness, and headache. These reactions are especially troublesome to the elderly patient.

Interactions

Concurrent use of anticholinergic agents with amantadine, TCAs, antihistamines and phenothiazines have an additive anticholinergic effect. Digoxin levels may be increased. And, when haloperidol is administered concurrently, a worsening of schizophrenic symptoms may occur. The use of anticholinergic agents can alter the absorption of other drugs (levodopa, carbidopa) by slowing motility of the GI tract. All of these agents counteract the cholinergic effects of drugs such as bethanechol.

DRUGS FOR MYASTHENIA GRAVIS

Myasthenia gravis is an autoimmune neuromuscular disease that presents clinically as fluctuating weakness of one or more skeletal muscle groups. Weakness becomes more severe with activity and improves with rest. The myasthenic patient can present with an acute or subacute onset precipitated by infection or emotional stress. One of the confusing aspects of myasthenia gravis is the course of the disease. It may advance irregularly, remain static for years, or spontaneously remit. Signs and symptoms are variable, fluctuating from hour to hour. They can range from mild *ptosis* (drooping of the upper eyelid) to respiratory and *bulbar* (relating to the medulla oblongata) failure.

The pathophysiology of myasthenia gravis involves the postjunctional receptors. There is a reduced availability of receptor sites for acetylcholine (ACh) on the postjunctional membrane caused by their blocking by antibody and the C9 component of complement to the ACh receptors. Antigenic modulation also leads to a reduction in postjunctional ACh receptors. With this process, postsynaptic receptors are cross-linked, degraded, and cleared at a faster rate than normal. As a result of these pathophysiologic processes, the number of interactions between the ACh release by nerve impulses and the receptors is reduced, which results in decreased muscle strength or progressive failure of contraction from repeated nerve stimulation.

Drug therapy is the focus of this discussion, but other measures include *thymectomy* (surgical removal of the thymus gland) and plasmapheresis. The management of myasthenia gravis depends on the severity of the disease, the age and lifestyle of the patient, and the type of myasthenia. The types of myasthenia gravis include ocular myasthenia, generalized myasthenia with ocular signs, generalized myasthenia with bulbar and ocular signs, and generalized myasthenia with bulbar and respiratory complications.

The goals of pharmacotherapy in myasthenia gravis are twofold: Cholinesterase inhibitors are used to enhance cholinergic nerve transmission, and immunosuppressive agents are used to repair or reverse the immunologic flaw. The two groups of immunosuppressive agents are corticosteroids (prednisone) and cytotoxic agents (azathioprine, cyclophosphamide, and cyclosporine).

CHOLINESTERASE INHIBITORS

Action

Acetylcholine (ACh) is the neurotransmitter that is released at the skeletal neuromuscular junction (see Chapter 16). Cholinesterase inhibitors, also called anticholinesterase agents, inhibit the breakdown of acetylcholine, allowing it to accumulate at the cholinergic receptor sites. The increased level of ACh results in the stimulation of cholinergic receptors throughout the central and peripheral nervous systems, producing an increase in muscle strength. For a review of the cholinergic synapse, see Figure 23–1.

The three classes of cholinesterase inhibitors are the quaternary ammonium compounds, carbamates, and organophosphates. This discussion addresses the ammonium compounds and carbamates. Blockage at the anionic or esteratic site of the acetylcholinesterase (AChE) molecule prevents the hydrolysis of ACh. These two sites on the AChE molecule are chemically different. The quaternary ammonium amines, **edrophonium (Tensilon)** and **ambenonium chloride (Mytelase Caplets)**, compete with ACh for binding at the anionic site of the active center on the AChE molecule. The carbamates, **neostigmine (Prostigmin)** and **pyridostigmine bromide (Mestinon)** form a covalent bond with the esteratic site of the AChE molecule. Pyridostigmine bromide is the drug of choice unless the patient is sensitive to bromide. The end result is inhibition of the enzyme AChE. These two classes of AChE inhibitors are reversible inhibitors. The sites of action include the neuromuscular junction, adrenal medulla, autonomic ganglia, cholinergic synapses at effector tissues of the autonomic nervous system, and cholinoceptive cells of the CNS. For a review of the effects of anticholinesterase agents on various body systems, see Table 23–4. These drugs are featured in Table 23–5.

Uses

The cholinesterase inhibitors have therapeutic uses in a variety of clinical situations. They are used in the diagnosis and treatment of myasthenia gravis. They are also used in the reversal of neuromuscular blockade and smooth muscle atony.

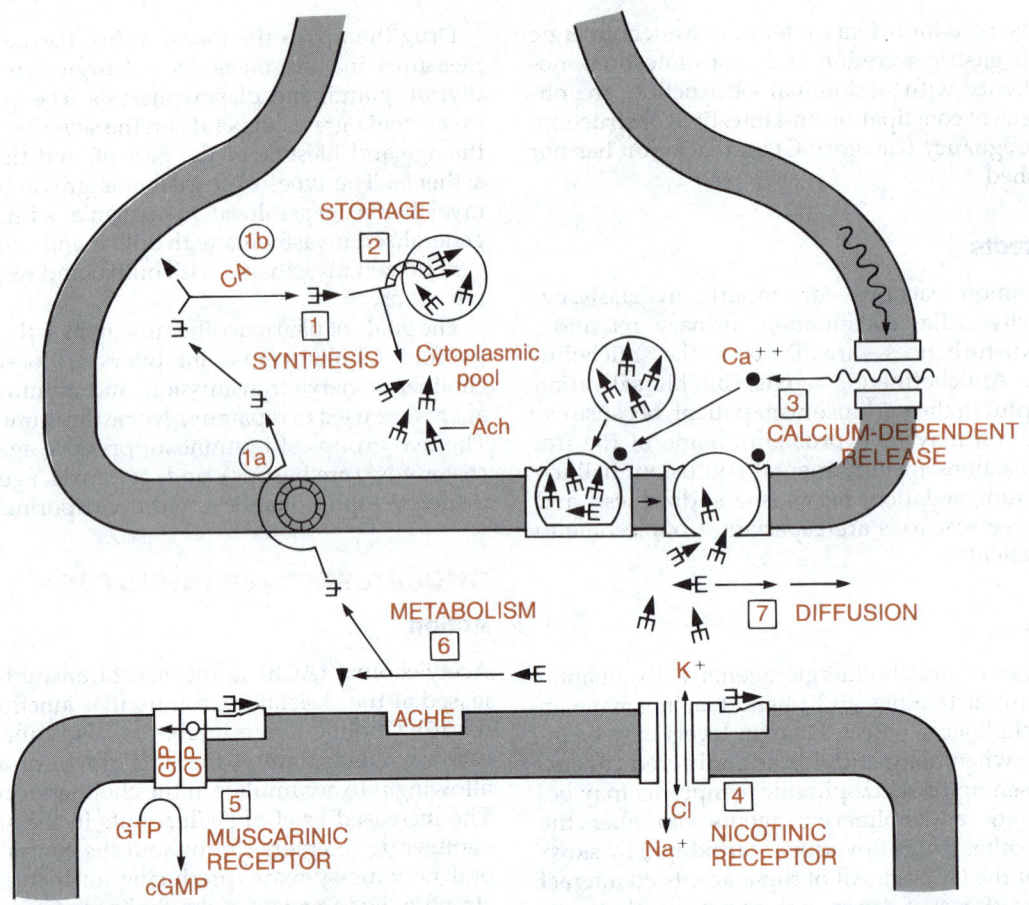

Figure 23–1. Cholinergic synapase. (1) Synthesis of acetylcholine (ACH), including (1a) choline uptake and (1b) acetylation of choline by choline acetylase (CA); (2) storage in vesicles; (3) calcium-dependent release; (4) interaction with a nicotinic receptor; (5) interaction with a muscarinic receptor linked by a coupling protein (CP) with guanadyl cyclase (GC), which catalyzes formation of cyclic-guanadly monophosphate (cGMP) from guanadyl triphosphate (GTP); and (6) hydrolysis of ACH by acetylcholinesterase (ACHE). (From Swonger, AK and Matejski, MP: Nursing Pharmacology. Scott, Foresman & Co, Boston, 1988, with permission.)

Table 23–4. EFFECTS OF ANTICHOLINESTERASE AGENTS

Tissue or System	Effects
Skin	Sweating
Visual	Lacrimation, miosis, blurred vision, accommodative spasm
Digestive	Salivation; increased gastric, pancreatic, and intestinal secretions; increased tone and motility in gut (abdominal cramps, vomiting, diarrhea, and defecation)
Urinary	Urinary frequency and incontinence
Respiratory	Increased bronchial secretions, bronchoconstriction, weakness or paralysis of respiratory muscles
Skeletal muscle	Fasciculations, weakness, paralysis (depolarizing block)
Cardiovascular	Bradycardia (due to muscarinic predominance), decreased cardiac output, hypotension; effects due to ganglionic actions and activation of adrenal medulla also possible
Central nervous system	Tremor, anxiety, restlessness, disrupted concentration and memory, confusion, sleep disturbances, desynchronization of electroencephalogram, convulsions, coma, circulatory and respiratory depression

Source: Craig, CR, and Stitzel, RE: Modern Pharmacology. Little, Brown, Boston, 1986, with permission.

Table 23–5. DRUGS FOR MYASTHENIA GRAVIS: CHOLINESTERASE INHIBITORS

DRUG NAME/ROUTE AND DOSAGE	PHARMACOKINETICS/ DYNAMICS	NURSING IMPLICATIONS
all cholinesterase inhibitors		**ASSESSMENT:** Assess neuromuscular status (ptosis, diplopia, vital capacity, ability to swallow, extremity strength) prior to and immediately after administration of medications. **EVALUATION:** Effectiveness of therapy can be demonstrated by relief of ptosis and diplopia and improvement in chewing, swallowing, extremity strength, and breathing without the appearance of cholinergic symptoms.
edrophonium (Tensilon)		
diagnosis of myasthenia gravis Anticholinesterase agents should be discontinued for 8 hours prior to administration. **Adults:** IV–2 mg IV; if no response, administer 8 mg more. May repeat test in 30 min. If cholinergic response occurs, administer atropine, 0.4–0.5 mg IV. IM–10 mg IM; if cholinergic response occurs, repeat 2-mg dose in 30 min to rule out false-negative reaction. **Children Under 34 kg:** IV–1 mg IV; if no response, administer 1 mg every 30–45 sec to total dose of 5 mg. If cholinergic response occurs, administer atropine IV. IM–2 mg IM. **Children Over 34 kg:** IV–2 mg IV; if no response, administer 1 mg every 30–45 sec to total of 10 mg. If cholinergic response occurs, administer atropine IV. IM–5 mg IM. **assessment of anticholinesterase therapy** **Adults:** 1–2 mg IV 1 hr after oral anticholinesterase dose. **differentiation of cholinergic from myasthenic crisis** **Adults:** 1 mg IV; may give additional 1 mg 1 min later.	**Onset:** IM, 2–10 min; IV, 30–60 sec **Peak:** NA **Duration:** IM, 5–30 min, IV, 5–10 min **½L:** NA **PB:** NA **B:** NA **E:** NA	Same as for all plus: **ASSESSMENT:** To differentiate myasthenic from cholinergic crisis, assess for increased weakness, diaphoresis, increased saliva and bronchial secretions, dyspnea, nausea, vomiting, diarrhea, and bradycardia. If these symptoms occur, patient is in cholinergic crisis. Monitor pulse, blood pressure, and ECG (for supraventricular tachycardia) before and throughout administration of this drug. Assess for pregnancy (category C). **INTERVENTION:** Usually administered by a physician for myasthenia gravis patients. IV doses are administered undiluted with a tuberculin syringe. A dose of 2 mg is given over 15 sec; wait 45 sec while assessing neuromuscular status, and if cholinergic symptoms have not appeared, remaining dose is administered slowly. As a curare antagonist, administer 10 mg IV slowly over 30–45 sec. **EVALUATION:** Notify physician of excessive weakness, bradycardia, excessive secretions, vomiting, diarrhea, or sweating.
pyridostigmine bromide (Mestinon) (Mestinon Timespan) (Regonol)		
myasthenia gravis **Adults:** 60–180 mg PO 2–4 times daily (up to 1500 mg/day); or 2 mg or 1/30 of oral dose IM or IV, repeated every 2–3 hr as needed. 180–540 mg PO qid or bid sustained-release (SR) form. **Children:** 7 mg/kg per day PO in 5–6 divided doses.	**Onset:** PO, 20–30 min; SR, 30–60 min; IM, 15 min; IV, 2–5 min **Peak:** NA **Duration:** PO, 3–6 hr; SR, 6–12 hr; IM, 2–4 hr, IV, 2–4 hr **½L:** PO, 3.7 hr; IV, 1.9 hr **PB:** NA **B:** plasma cholinesterase and liver **E:** urine	Same as for all plus: **ASSESSMENT:** Patients with myasthenia gravis may be advised to keep a daily record of their condition and the effects of this medication. Assess patient for overdose, which may induce cholinergic crisis, and underdose or resistance. Both have similar symptoms (muscle weakness, dyspnea, dysphagia). Symptoms of overdose usually occur within 1 hr after administration. Cholinergic symptoms may also include increased respiratory secretions and saliva, nausea, vomiting, cramping, diarrhea, and diaphoresis. Assess for pregnancy (category C).

Continued on the following page

Table 23–5. DRUGS FOR MYASTHENIA GRAVIS: CHOLINESTERASE INHIBITORS, *Continued*

DRUG NAME/ROUTE AND DOSAGE	PHARMACOKINETICS/ DYNAMICS	NURSING IMPLICATIONS
pyridostigmine bromide (Mestinon) (Mestinon Timespan) (Regonol)		
		INTERVENTION: Administer drug with food or milk to minimize side effects. SR tablets do not affect potency. To facilitate chewing, pyridostigmine may be administered 30 min before meals. Administer IV doses undiluted. Do not add to IV solutions. For myasthenia gravis, administer each 0.5 mg over 1 min. For use as muscle-relaxant antagonist, administer each 0.5 mg over 1 min. Oral dose is not interchangeable with IV dose. Parenteral form is 30 times more potent.
neostigmine (Prostigmin) (Prostigmin Bromide)		
myasthenia gravis *Adults:* 15–30 mg PO tid increased at daily intervals until response is achieved (up to 375 mg may be needed); or 0.5–2.5 mg IV, IM, or SC every 1–3 hr. *Children:* 7.5–15 mg PO 3–4 times a day, up to 45 mg every 2 hr.	**Onset:** PO, 45–75 min; IM, 20–30 min; IV, 4–8 min **Peak:** PO, 1–4 hr (highly variable); IM, 20–30 min; IV, 20–30 min **Duration:** PO, IM, or IV, 2–4 hr **½L:** PO and IV, 40–60 min; IM, 50–90 min **PB:** 15%–20% **B:** plasma cholinesterase and liver **E:** urine	Same as for pyridostigmine.
ambenonium chloride (Mytelase) *Adults:* Initially, 5 mg PO 3–4 times daily with daily dosage gradually increased at 48-hr intervals; usual adult dosage ranges from 15–100 mg/day. With doses over 200 mg/day, watch for cholinergic reactions. *Children:* Initially, 0.3 mg/kg per day PO or 10 mg/m² per day, 3–4 times a day. The maintenance dosage is 1.5 mg/kg per day or 50 mg/m² daily in divided doses 3–4 times a day.	**Onset:** 20–30 min **Peak:** NA **Duration:** 3–8 hr **½L:** NA **PB:** NA **B:** NA **E:** NA	Same as for pyridostigmine except: **ASSESSMENT:** Pregnancy category unknown.

NA = not available; ECG = electrocardiogram.

Contraindications and Precautions

Cholinesterase inhibitors are not used in patients who are hypersensitive. These agents are contraindicated in patients with mechanical obstruction of the gastrointestinal or genitourinary tracts. These agents enhance gastric contractions and increase the secretion of gastric acid. They also increase motor activity in the small and large bowel. This effect is a combination of actions at the ganglion cells of Auerbach's plexus and at the muscle fibers, as a result of the preservation of ACh.

Caution is used in patients with a history of asthma, ulcer disease, cardiovascular disease, seizure disorders, and hyperthyroidism. The cholinesterase inhibitors cause smooth muscle constriction of the bronchioles and increase respiratory secretions. The effects of accumulated ACh on the heart and blood vessels are complex because of the involvement of both ganglionic and postganglionic fibers. The major effects are bradycardia and decreased cardiac output. The effect of ACh on the GI tract is an increase in gastric acid secretion and contraction. The overall effect of ACh on the CNS is excitation, which can potentiate seizures. In general, the accumulation of ACh causes an increase in secretory glands that are innervated by postganglionic cholinergic fibers, as in the case of the thyroid gland. In hyperthyroidism there is already increased secretion without more ACh. Safe use in pregnancy (category C), lactation, and children has not been established.

There is a fine line between the therapeutic dose and undermedication or overdose of cholinesterase inhibitors. Myasthenic weakness can occur suddenly because of the disease or undermedication or overmedication. Some of the exacerbations are due to a decrease in the responsiveness to cholinesterase inhibitors that cannot be overcome by a higher dose. Myasthenic crisis is characterized by increased weakness. The muscles affected are those associated with respiration, chewing, swallowing, and the muscles of the head and neck. The goal at this point in treatment is respiratory support, which may require patency of airway and ventilatory support.

When too many cholinesterase inhibitors are in the system, cholinergic crisis occurs. The cholinesterase inhibitors occupy the same receptors as ACh, and their excess reduces neuromuscular transmission. The signs and symptoms of overdose are similar to those for myasthenia crisis. The goal is the same: patency of the airway and respiratory support.

Adverse Effects

The majority of adverse reactions are caused by excessive cholinergic stimulation of the muscarinic and nicotinic receptors. The muscarinic side effects include abdominal cramps, nausea, vomiting, diarrhea, increased salivation, increased bronchial secretion, lacrimation, miosis, and diaphoresis. These side effects are uncomfortable, but usually a tolerance develops. If tolerance does not occur, the agent can be taken with food, the dose adjusted, or atropine added to the drug regimen. Atropine can alleviate these reactions, but it may also mask warning signs associated with overdosage. Masking these side effects can inadvertently lead to cholinergic crisis. The nicotinic adverse reactions are muscle cramps, *fasciculation* (small, local, involuntary muscle contraction), and muscle weakness.

Interactions

There are many drugs that enhance or induce neuromuscular blockade (trimethaphan, neomycin sulfate, quinidine). Most of these drugs present a threat to the myasthenic because of the problems at the neuromuscular junction. Other drugs (curare, succinylcholine) induce muscle weakness in normal persons. Myasthenics are very sensitive to the normal doses of these agents. Cholinergic effects are antagonized by other drugs such as antihistamines, antidepressants, atropine, haloperidol, phenothiazines, quinidine, and disopyramide, which have anticholinergic properties.

Some drug interactions occur in the myasthenic because use of cholinesterase inhibitors with drugs such as corticosteroids, analgesics, and over-the-counter drugs that contain ephedrine can exacerbate the signs and symptoms of myasthenia gravis. Some agents, such as corticosteroids, can cause a refractoriness to cholinesterase inhibitors; other agents, such as aminoglycoside antibodies, beta-blockers, and phenytoin, cause the presynaptic action of depressing ACh formation and/or release. Another problem encountered with aminoglycoside antibodies is that they reduce the sensitivity of the postjunctional membrane to ACh, accentuating blockade. Some agents are competitive neuromuscular blockers, such as curare, succinylcholine, lidocaine, trimethaphan, quinidine (large doses), and chlorpromazine. Other agents potentiate hypokalemia. The diuretics are noted for this problem. As hypokalemia develops, there is mus-

Table 23–6. DRUGS USED WITH CAUTION OR CONTRAINDICATED IN MYASTHENIA GRAVIS

Alcohol
Analgesics (narcotics)
Anesthetics
Antibiotics
    Aminoglycosides (neomycin, streptomycin, amikacin, tobramycin, netilmicin, gentamicin, kanamycin)
    Clindamycin
    Polymyxin B
    Sulfonamides
Anticonvulsants (Dilantin, phenobarbital, and others)
Antimalarials
Quinine in tonic water
Antirheumatics (D-penicillamine, colchicine, chloroquine)
Cardiovascular
    Quinidine, lidocaine, procainamide
    Beta blockers (Inderal and others)
    Lidocaine
Diuretics
Laxatives
Magnesium preparations
Over-the-counter cold preparations (antihistamines)
Psychotropics (lithium carbonate, haloperidol, benzodiazepines, and others)
Sedative-hypnotics
Thyroid preparations

Source: Adapted from Adams, SL, et al: Drugs that may exacerbate myasthenia gravis. Ann Emerg Med 13(7):532, 1984, with permission. Modified in 1996.

cle weakness. This clouds the picture for the myasthenic because it is difficult to determine the cause of the muscle weakness (the disease or the hypokalemia). Laxatives are problematic because they can render the patient weak after straining or diarrhea. See Table 23–6 for a summary of agents that are contraindicated or to be used with caution.

Dosage

Dosage does not lend itself to the "cookbook" approach. Myasthenia gravis can be aggravated by factors such as upper respiratory infection, general fatigue, excitement, loss of sleep, menstruation, high-carbohydrate meals, hyperthyroidism, and alcohol intake. Requirements change based on the patient's signs and symptoms. Usually, cholinesterase inhibitors are started in a low dose, with no attempt made to reach maximal muscle strength in the initial regimen. The daily doses are divided into three or four equal dosing intervals. Patients are encouraged to keep a diary of dosing times, periods of peak effect, periods of worsening, and side effects. This helps the physician to know how effective the particular cholinesterase inhibitor is for the patient. Some myasthenics become progressively refractory to these agents, and drug holidays can restore their effectiveness. Dosage is titrated against the response of the most important muscle group. It is not uncommon for the patient's response to the cholinesterase inhibitors to be an increase in muscle strength in one group of muscles and a decrease in muscle strength in other muscle groups. Oral and parenteral doses are not equal. Changing from the oral to parenteral route of administration requires reducing the dose of the agent.

CORTICOSTEROIDS

The use of corticosteroids has been beneficial in the treatment of myasthenia gravis. There are several indications for using corticosteroids: (1) inadequate control with a cholinesterase inhibitor; (2) older adults with moderate to severe disease; (3) short-term use following thymectomy, because there is a delayed response associated with the procedure; (4) patients who refuse a thymectomy or do not respond to a thymectomy; (5) maintenance therapy following a thymectomy (long-term use of corticosteroids); (6) maintenance following crisis; or (7) preoperative use to prepare patients for thymectomy.

It is thought that corticosteroids act by suppressing the immune system. A proposed mechanism of action is interference with the cell cycle of activated lymphoid cells, especially lymphocytes. There are also possible lysis of the suppressor or helper T cells, decreased antibody response, and lowered concentration of specific antibody populations. Corticosteroids also provide anti-inflammatory action.

Approaches to dosage are based on low-dose or high-dose therapy. A short-acting corticosteroid (prednisone) is the drug of choice. With low-dose therapy, the agent is administered on a daily or an alternate-day basis. The dose is increased every third dose to the maximal dosage (25 mg daily or every other day, increased 12.5 mg every third dose to 100 mg). The advantage of this approach is that it minimizes the severity of early-worsening episodes. Early worsening is a worsening of the signs and symptoms of myasthenia gravis 3 to 14 days after the initiation of corticosteroids. This response may be due to enhancing the mollification of sensitized lymphocytes. The disadvantage of this approach is that it takes weeks or months to achieve maximal dose and maximal clinical benefit. The high-dose approach also involves administration of the agent on a daily or an alternate-day basis. The dose of the agent is introduced at its high dose, which is usually 80 to 100 mg. The advantage is that initially there is rapid improvement in the patient's clinical presentation. The disadvantage is that early worsening is more common and can be more severe. The patient can also experience a period in which the myasthenia gravis is refractory to cholinesterase inhibitors.

Other specific information on related corticosteroids is provided in Chapter 44.

CYTOTOXIC AGENTS

When a myasthenic patient remains unresponsive to the conventional measures described previously, cytotoxic agents may be used. The most frequently used cytotoxic agents are azathioprine (Imuran), cyclophosphamide (Cytoxan), and cyclosporine (Sandimmune). As with corticosteroids, the benefits from this mode of therapy occur after months (4 to 15) of therapy. The major disadvantage of these agents are the serious side effects.

The proposed mechanisms of action for cytotoxic agents include interference with nucleic acid metabolism, DNA replication and RNA transcription, destruction of proliferating lymphoid cells, and alteration of antibody formation. These agents are discussed in further detail in Chapters 54, 55, and 56.

DRUGS FOR ALZHEIMER'S DISEASE

Alzheimer's disease, a commonly occurring neurologic disorder, causes severe cognitive dysfunction, generally in the older adult. The most common dementia, Alzheimer's disease is a chronic condition characterized by declining intellectual capacity, memory loss, and loss of other cognitive functions, such as language or spatial orientation. Eventually, the patient loses motor function as well. The exact cause is unknown, but several possible theories are under investigation. Drug therapy for the patient with Alzheimer's disease may include **tacrine hydrochloride (Cognex)** to help treat memory deficits; cerebral vasodilators such as ergot derivatives, isoxsuprine, and cyclandelate to enhance cerebral circulation; psychostimulators such as methylphenidate to improve mood; and antidepressants to manage depression (if it seems to exacerbate the patient's dementia).

○ **Tacrine hydrochloride** (Cognex) is a centrally acting reversible cholinesterase inhibitor. Deficiency of cortical acetylcholine is believed to account for some of the clinical manifestations of mild-to-moderate dementia. Tacrine hydrochloride is thought to improve cognitive function by elevating ACh concentrations in the cerebral cortex and by slowing the degradation of ACh release by still intact cholinergic neurons. As the disease progresses, there are fewer cholinergic neurons remaining intact, and the effects of tacrine hydrochloride may lessen.

Pharmacokinetics and dosages are listed in Table 23–7.

CONTRAINDICATIONS AND PRECAUTIONS Tacrine hydrochloride is contraindicated in patients who are hypersensitive to the drug and those with liver diseases. Caution is advised in patients with underlying cardiac disease due to tacrine hydrochloride's cholinomimetic action on the heart rate (bradycardia). Patients with previous ulcer disease or those taking nonsteroidal anti-inflammatory drugs are monitored closely because tacrine hydrochloride causes an increase in gastric acid secretion.

▼ **CLINICAL ALERT**

Patients with normal liver function may experience an elevation of ALT and AST levels. If the drug is withdrawn promptly, no liver injury will occur.

Based on current experience, 50% of patients experience an ALT elevation at least double that of normal, and 25% develop a three-times-normal level. The usual rise begins about week 6, and 95% of the elevations occurs within the first 18 weeks of therapy. If the ALT level returns to normal after a stoppage of tacrine hydrochloride, the patient may be rechallenged with the drug.

Table 23–7. DRUG FOR ALZHEIMER'S DISEASE

DRUG NAME/ROUTE AND DOSAGE	PHARMACOKINETICS/ DYNAMICS	NURSING IMPLICATIONS
tacrine hydrochloride (Cognex) **Adults:** Initially, 10 mg PO qid for at least 6 wk. If no increase in ALT, increase to 20 mg qid. Dose may be increased q 6 wk. Maximum dose 160 mg/day.	**Onset:** rapid (2 wk for clinical effect) **Peak:** 1–2 hr **Duration:** NA **½L:** 2–4 hr **PB:** 55% **B:** liver **E:** urine	**ASSESSMENT:** Assess baseline symptoms, including cognitive ability. Assess for pregnancy (category C) as needed. **INTERVENTION:** Administer between meals. If GI upset occurs, take with meals. Administer as directed on a regular schedule. Food may reduce plasma levels by 30%–40%. Titrate dose upwards at 6-week intervals only. Do not abruptly discontinue doses of more than 50 mg/day, as a decline in cognitive function and behavioral disturbances may occur. Monitor ALT weekly for 18 wks, then every 3 mo. If dose increases, resume weekly testing for at least 6 wk. **Patient Teaching—** Teach caregivers to monitor patient for side effects. Warn patient to not abruptly discontinue drug, because a rapid decline in cognitive function may occur. **EVALUATION:** If rash, change in color of stools, or jaundice occur, notify physician. Evaluate for changes in cognitive function. Evaluate urinary output—drug may lead to outflow obstruction.

NA = not available.

Tacrine hydrochloride is also used with caution in patients with respiratory disease because of its cholinomimetic action. Safety in pregnancy (category C), lactation, and children has not been established.

ADVERSE EFFECTS The most common adverse effects to tacrine hydrochloride are ALT elevations, nausea, vomiting, diarrhea, dyspepsia, and anorexia. These effects are primarily dose dependent; if the dose can be lowered, they may disappear. Patients may also experience myalgia and ataxia.

INTERACTIONS Tacrine hydrochloride is primarily eliminated by hepatic metabolism via the cytochrome P-450 liver enzyme system. Thus, drug interactions may occur with drugs such as phenytoin and theophylline, which undergo extensive metabolism by the same system. For example, with concurrent theophylline, blood levels of theophylline are increased, causing possible toxicity.

Tacrine hydrochloride interferes with the activity of all anticholinergic agents, possibly decreasing their effects. A synergistic effect occurs that increases activity of all cholinergics (e.g., bethanachol) and cholinesterase inhibitors. And, cimetidine increases the serum level of tacrine hydrochloride. Therefore, it is recommended that these agents not be taken concurrently with tacrine hydrochloride.

DRUGS FOR MULTIPLE SCLEROSIS

Multiple sclerosis (MS) is a chronic, autoimmune disease that results from progressive demyelination of the white matter of the brain and spinal cord. MS is characterized by widespread neurologic dysfunction marked by periods of exacerbation and remission. Symptoms range from mild tiredness to severe immobility. **Interferon beta-1b (Betaseron)** reduces the incidence of relapse in patients with relapsing-remitting MS. Corticosteroids may relieve symptoms of exacerbation and hasten remission, but do not prevent future exacerbations. Other drugs that may be used include chlordiazepoxide to mitigate mood swings, baclofen or dantrolene to relieve spasticity, bethanechol or oxybutynin to relieve urinary retention and minimize urinary frequency and urgency, and immunosuppressants such as cyclophosphamide and azathioprine.

○ **Interferon beta-1b** (Betaseron) is an analog of human interferon beta produced in *Escherichia coli*. It is being used to treat relapsing-remitting multiple sclerosis (MS), the most common form of the disease. The mechanism of action of interferon beta-1b in MS is unknown. Interferons generally have antiviral, antiproliferative, and immune-modulating effects. Interferon beta-1b decreases T-cell proliferation, blocks synthesis of interferon gamma (thought to be involved in attacks of MS), inhibits release of other cytokines that damage oligodendrocytes, and increases suppressor T-cell activity. The interferons are discussed in detail in Chapter 56. In patients with mild to moderate relapsing-remitting MS, interferon beta-1b given by injection every other day can decrease both the number and severity of attacks of neurologic dysfunction. It appears to be well tolerated. Its effect on the progression of disability, however, remains to be established.

○ **Glatiramen acetate** (Copaxone), is the first non-steroid, non interferon, approved to treat chronic relapsing-remitting MS. The most common side effects include flushing, chest pain, palpitations, anxiety, dyspnea, urticaria and constriction of the throat. These side effects are transient and self-limiting and do not require specific treatment.

Table 23–8. NURSING PROCESS FOR PATIENT WITH MOVEMENT DISORDERS

Assessment

Assess muscle strength, ability to initiate volitional movement, gait.
Assess tremor, rigidity, bradykinesia, akinesia, dystonia, fatigue.
Assess strength of voice, ability to swallow, presence of coughing/choking following fluids/foods.
Assess for a history for chronic diseases, use of immunosuppressive agents.
Note psychologic, emotional distress and/or behavior reflective of ineffective coping skills.

Nursing Diagnosis: Impaired Physical Mobility

RELATED TO: Decreased strength/endurance, neuromuscular impairment.
AS EVIDENCED BY: Tremor, rigidity, and difficulty in movement/inability to perform desired activities.

Desired Outcomes/Evaluation Criteria

Achieves the maximum amount of mobility possible. Reports improved level of comfort. Displays no complications associated with immobilization.

Nursing Actions

Administer medication prior to initiating morning self-care activities or feeding. Allow time for the medication to take effect before beginning activities. Assist with activities of daily living as necessary.
Monitor level of fatigue or tolerance to activity and care.

Promote rest periods between activities.
Provide range of motion on all extremities. Obtain physical/occupational therapy consult if indicated.
Assist with/encourage frequent change of position (at least q 2 hr).

Rationale

Promotes independence within the individual situation. Helps to relieve symptoms so activities can be undertaken, maximizing ability to participate in activity. Provides assistance while maintaining independence.

Ability to perform desired activities is a good way to monitor the effectiveness of the medication. There is a fine line between therapeutic response to the medications and toxicity.
Prevents undue fatigue.
Maintains/improves joint flexibility and ability to participate in activities.

Helps prevent muscle fatigue and complications of immobility.

Nursing Diagnosis: Impaired Verbal/Written Communication

RELATED TO: Decreased muscle strength/voice volume, hand tremors.
AS EVIDENCED BY: Impaired articulation, inability to modulate speech, illegible handwriting, frustration.

Desired Outcomes/Evaluation Criteria

Establishes method of communication by which needs can be expressed.

Nursing Actions

Identify appropriate form of alternate means of communication.
Massage neck and facial muscles.

Encourage a deep breath prior to speaking. Verify meaning of patient's words/sounds. Obtain speech therapy consultation.

Rationale

Frustration can be reduced by establishing a means of letting others know needs and thoughts.
Relieves tension and assists patient to express words more easily. May help to relax muscles and aid in vocal expression.
Promotes understanding and sense of worth. May need additional assistance to help patient be more expressive.

Nursing Diagnosis: Impaired Adjustment

RELATED TO: Presence of permanent disability requiring change in lifestyle.

Desired Outcomes/Evaluation Criteria

Assumes responsibility for personal needs. Initiates lifestyle changes that permit adaptation to present life situations. Acknowledges own limitations and identifies ways to cope with them.

Nursing Actions

Provide information for patient/family regarding disease and management.
Provide time for expression of feelings.
Discuss ways to change lifestyle in least disruptive manner.
Provide opportunity for discussion of the impact of immobility on self-concept. Actively listen to patient.
Discuss fluctuation of the course of the disease and effectiveness of medications.

Rationale

Helps to develop effective coping mechanisms to deal with chronic illness.

Promotes identification of concerns and ways of dealing with them.
Helps to develop a way of living with problems without altering normal routine significantly.
Inability to do own self-care can result in feelings of dependency and powerlessness. Communicates caring and unconditional acceptance of the patient.

Understanding the nature of chronic disease helps with dealing with therapeutic regimen, which affects all areas of life.

Other Suggested Nursing Diagnoses: Risk for Trauma, Sleep Pattern Disturbance, and Knowledge Deficit.

NURSING PROCESS RELATED TO MOVEMENT DISORDERS

A major goal of therapy in the patient with movement disorders is to maintain or improve his or her independent functioning. Motor system dysfunction is problematic. With many of the diseases described in this chapter, chronicity, variability, and progression of the disease are common. There is rarely a classic case, and a cookbook approach to these patients is not recommended.

ASSESSMENT

- Obtain a nursing history. It is important to address specific routines or needs the patient has. Such activities as sleep pattern, eating, and bowel/bladder routines are specifically addressed, as featured in Table 23–8.
- Perform and record a basic neurologic assessment. Basic screening for seeing, eating, swallowing, expressing (facially), general movements, initiating volitional movements, gait, and walking is performed. If deficits appear during this screening session, a more detailed neurologic assessment is performed. In addition to these baseline data, it is important to assess the patient 1 hour after the administration of medications.
- Assess patient's ability to tolerate activity. The patient's fatigue level is important to know when planning activities.
- Obtain other assessments, such as cognitive ability, as needed. For example, baseline levels of cognitive ability are important to obtain before administering tacrine hydrochloride to the patient with Alzheimer's disease.
- Assess results of baseline laboratory tests when needed. For example, liver function studies, particularly ALT levels, are important before starting tacrine hydrochloride.
- Assist the patient with other diagnostic tests, such as the Tensilon test for mysthenia gravis.

NURSING DIAGNOSIS

- Develop the nursing diagnosis and the patient outcomes. Nursing diagnoses typical for the patient with disorders of the nervous system may include Impaired Physical Mobility, Risk for Trauma, Impaired Communication, Sleep Pattern Disturbance, Impaired Adjustment, and Dysreflexia (see Table 23–8).

PLANNING AND INTERVENTION

- Monitor the patient's deficits as to their progression. It is important to plan specific nursing interventions based on the patient's problem. For example, if deficits related to walking are determined, many factors must be considered when planning interventions. Initially, walking is assessed on the basis of observations made by the nurse. These observations include posture, muscle tone, arm swing, rhythm, gait, coordination, and the ability to move freely in the environment. When a motor dysfunction occurs related to walking, the nurse must consider the effects this deficit has on the patient's ability to perform self-care activities. This has relevance in planning care as well as in the patient's going home. The next concern is the influence of the deficit on the patient's self-concept. How will the patient view himself or herself? Will this deficit influence how he or she interacts with other people? Other concerns relate to the patient's safety. Will the patient be able to navigate safely in the environment? If not, how much assistance is needed for this patient?

Patient Teaching

- Determine the patient's (and caregiver's) level of knowledge about the disease, treatment plan, and drug regimen.
- Develop teaching plans about drug therapy as needed. Tables 23–9, 23–10, and 23–11 feature patient teaching information for drugs used in parkinsonism, myasthenia gravis, and Alzheimer's disease.

Table 23–9. PATIENT TEACHING—ANTIPARKINSON DRUGS

Dear Patient:
  This drug has been ordered for you. This is what you should know about your drug to get the most from your therapy.

- ☐ 1. You will take antiparkinson drugs for the remainder of your life. Antiparkinson drugs are administered to _____.
- ☐ 2. It is best to take antiparkinson drugs during or shortly after meals to decrease upset stomach and lack of appetite. This also aids in preventing dryness of the mouth.
- ☐ 3. Many interactions occur. Please consult your doctor or pharmacist before taking any other medication.
- ☐ 4. If you forget a dose, take it, and then delay the next dose for several hours. Always take all of your drugs.
- ☐ 5. Do not stop taking your drug.
- ☐ 6. Typical side effects that may occur from your drug include: _____.
- ☐ 7. Protein prevents the absorption; therefore, decrease your intake of high-protein foods (milk, meat, eggs, fish, poultry, nuts). Also, spread the protein intake over four or more small meals rather than two or three large meals. Pyridoxine (vitamin B_6) limits the amount of levodopa available to the brain. Multiple vitamins containing pyridoxine (vitamin B_6) as well as foods high in pyridoxine (yeast, whole-grain cereals, potatoes, bananas, pork, glandular meats such as liver, and oatmeal) are avoided. (Patients taking a combination drug such as Sinemet do not need to limit pyridoxine.) Alcohol (wine, beer, hard liquor) in large amounts antagonizes dopamine, and alcohol intake should be limited to one or two drinks a day.
- ☐ 8. It is important to maintain a normal weight. Levodopa carbidopa is absorbed by fat deposits, and obese people do not receive the full effect of the dose.
- ☐ 9. Store in a tightly closed, dry container away from heat.

Table 23–10. PATIENT TEACHING—DRUGS FOR MYASTHENIA GRAVIS

Dear Patient:
This drug has been ordered for you. This is what you should know about your drug to get the most from your therapy.

☐ 1. The patient is an individual. Avoid evaluating your drug regimen in relation to other myasthenic patients.
☐ 2. Take your drugs on time. Avoid skipping doses. If you miss a dose of your drug, avoid doubling up on the next dose.
☐ 3. Know the action and the side effects of your drugs. If you have side effects, call your doctor. Keep a diary of the drug, time taken, your activity level, and the side effect(s).
☐ 4. Taking the drug with meals can decrease stomach discomfort.
☐ 5. Check with your doctor and/or pharmacist before taking any over-the-counter drug for colds, allergy, sleep, laxatives, or pain.
☐ 6. Take steroids during early morning hours to correspond to the natural release of cortisol.
☐ 7. If you are on alternate-day steroids and you miss the morning dose and remember it that afternoon, wait until the next morning and take it at that time. Rearrange the steroid schedule accordingly.
☐ 8. Avoid taking alcohol while on the drugs.
☐ 9. Avoid abruptly stopping your drugs without doctor's order.
☐ 10. Call the M. G. Foundation and obtain a list of drug banks in your area.
☐ 11. Tell your dentist that you have myasthenia gravis and whether or not you are taking steroids.
☐ 12. Always check the labels of your drugs to make sure you are taking the right drug at the right time.
☐ 13. Use a calendar to schedule all your drugs especially if you are on an alternate-day or alternate-dose schedule.
☐ 14. Keep drugs out of the reach of children.
☐ 15. Destroy leftover drugs by flushing them down the toilet.
☐ 16. If you have weakness, ask the pharmacist for a regular container instead of a childproof container.
☐ 17. Refill your drugs on time so that you will not run out.
☐ 18. When traveling, carry a supply of your drugs in your purse or carry-on luggage.
☐ 19. If you are traveling, carry a copy of your medical records and additional prescriptions.
☐ 20. Keep your drugs in a cool place. They should be stored in a dry, light-sensitive container.
☐ 21. Watch for signs of infection (fever, chills, sore throat, frequency of urination, low back pain).
☐ 22. Lab work should be checked periodically if on steroids or other immunosuppressive agents.
☐ 23. Know other prescribed drugs you are taking.
☐ 24. Obtain a medical alert bracelet.

Source: Myasthenia Gravis Foundation, 53 W. Jackson Blvd., Suite 909, Chicago, IL 60604.

• Teach the patient taking dopaminergics about dietary modification. As Parkinson's disease progresses and natural levels of dopamine continue to diminish, the patient must increasingly rely on levodopa carbidopa to boost dopamine levels. As a result, the parkinsonian patient often suffers periods of erratic, uncontrollable tremors, rigidity, and/or loss of movement—"off" phases when dopamine levels drop—alternating with "on" phases when the patient feels in control of his or her muscles because the levodopa carbidopa apparently is working.

Researchers are now finding that it may be possible to prolong levodopa's carbidopa positive effects, and the solution they are looking at involves diet—the timing of meals and the foods chosen. It is recommended that patients who begin to suffer the on-off syndrome start taking their levodopa carbidopa 45 minutes to an hour before eating, because food can interfere with the drug's ability to make it to the brain. Another, more controversial, dietary recommendation is to keep protein consumption to a minimum. Protein poses a particular problem for the parkinsonian patient because during digestion, protein components, amino acids, enter the bloodstream and are taken from the blood to the brain via the same carrier that transports levodopa. That is, the more amino acids present at the time the patient takes levodopa carbidopa, the harder it is for the drug to get a "seat" on the carrier that goes to the brain. And if the drug cannot get to the brain, the patient is likely to slip into an off phase.

To get around the problem, many experts are now recommending the careful distribution of protein throughout the day—enough for a levodopa carbidopa taker to meet nutritional needs but not enough to interfere with the body's ability to carry the drug to the brain. Some recent research suggests that meals with seven parts carbohydrate to one part protein help prevent off phases. A breakfast meeting the seven-to-one ratio might include two pancakes with margarine, syrup, a piece of fruit, a small glass of milk, and a cup of coffee or tea. By follow-

Table 23–11. PATIENT TEACHING—DRUGS FOR ALZHEIMER'S DISEASE

Dear Patient:
This drug has been prescribed for you. This is what you should know about your drug to get the most from your therapy:

☐ 1. Tacrine is designed to improve your ability to think and function.
☐ 2. Tacrine is generally taken for several months to years, depending on your response.
☐ 3. Take as directed. Tacrine is best taken on an empty stomach between meals. However, if GI upset occurs, take it with meals.
☐ 4. When the drug is working, cognitive ability, memory, and concentration abilities should improve.
☐ 5. Most common side effect include headache, increased agitation and nervousness, nausea, vomiting, and possibly abdominal pain. If your skin turns yellow or you have difficulty urinating, please notify your physician.
☐ 6. If you forget a dose, do not double your next dose. Just take your next pill.
☐ 7. It is important for you to continue taking your medication. Do not stop taking this drug without first consulting your physician.
☐ 8. Store your medication where others, particularly small children, cannot reach it.

ing such a regimen, many people report they feel better within a few days.

Patients with Parkinson's disease who decide to try the seven-to-one diet may have to experiment, with the help of a physician and a dietitian. A different ratio of carbohydrate to protein, possibly five to one or eight to one, may be more effective than the seven-to-one ratio. In addition, such a regimen requires careful planning to prevent nutrient deficiencies and weight loss. Caloric intake is important in patients with Parkinson's disease, because these patients not only have poor appetites in many instances but also tend to have slightly faster metabolisms than other people. Therefore, they need more calories to keep up their weight (Tufts University Diet and Nutrition Letter, 1994).

EVALUATION

- Evaluate the patient outcomes on a regular basis. The primary goal is to maintain or enhance the patient's level of independent functioning. The major concerns related to motor dysfunction are alterations in daily living, self-concept, and client safety. Nurses have a major impact in all of these areas.
- Evaluate the patient for effectiveness or ineffectiveness of the drug regimen. Effectiveness results in a controlling or a reduction in symptoms with minimal side effects. If drug therapy is ineffective, work with the patient, family, and physician to modify the drug regimen.
- Evaluate the patient for side effects of the drug therapy. When these become apparent, make sure the patient has a consultation with his or her physician.
- Evaluate the overall progress of the patient. All of the conditions discussed in this chapter are chronic and often relapsing. Encouraging a positive outlook is very important.

The bibliography for this chapter can be found in Appendix B, which begins on page 1054.

CHAPTER REVIEW QUESTIONS*

1. Cholinesterase inhibitors used to treat myasthenia gravis:
   a. Are well absorbed from the gastrointestinal tract.
   b. Lead to cholinergic crisis if given in excess.
   c. Stimulate the breakdown of acetylcholine.
   d. Produce tolerance and an end-of-dose failure.

2. Amantadine (Symmetrel):
   a. Is an antiviral agent.
   b. Is used alone in the advanced stages of Parkinson's disease.
   c. Is excreted in an alkaline urine.
   d. Is a direct dopamine agonist.

3. James, newly diagnosed with Alzheimer's disease, is placed on tacrine hydrochloride. It is important to teach the patient that:
   a. The drug is taken with meals for best results.
   b. Nausea, vomiting, diarrhea are common problems and will never be relieved.

   c. When the drug is to be stopped, it will be stopped abruptly.
   d. Blood tests will be done for at least 18 weeks to monitor liver function.

4. A patient taking tacrine hydrochloride should be cautioned not to take concurrent:
   a. Antibiotics.
   b. Digoxin.
   c. Propranolol.
   d. Cimetidine and theophylline.

5. Kim is being changed from levodopa (L-Dopa) to carbidopa/levodopa (Sinemet). What nursing consideration is important?
   a. Discontinue the L-Dopa at least 8 hours before the first dose of Sinemet.
   b. Continue both drugs together for 48 hours.
   c. Administer both drugs with a high-protein diet.
   d. Discontinue the L-dopa for 24 hours before starting Sinemet.

See Appendix A , which begins on page 1051, for answers.

PSYCHOBIOLOGY AND PSYCHOTHERAPEUTIC DRUGS

Pharmacotherapeutics and Principles of Psychobiology

Mary C. Townsend, RN, MN, CS
Meredith A. Davison, PhD

CHAPTER OUTLINE

Review of the Nervous System
Neuroendocrinology
Genetics
Psychoimmunology

KEY TERMS

Circadian rhythm   Psychoimmunology
Neuroendocrinology   Synapses
Neurotransmitters

LEARNING OBJECTIVES

After reading this chapter, the student will be able to:

1. Discuss the physiology of neurotransmission within the central nervous system and identify the role of neurotransmitters in human behavior.
2. Discuss the association of endocrine functioning and genetics to the action of psychotherapeutic drugs.
3. Discuss the correlation of alteration in brain functioning to various psychiatric disorders.
4. Discuss the influence of psychologic factors on the immune system.
5. Discuss the implications of psychobiologic concepts to the mechanisms of actions of psychotherapeutic drugs.

The role of neurobiologic mechanisms in explaining the biologic basis of behavior is undisputed. Peschel and Peschel (1991) state, "The revolution occurring in neurobiology and molecular biology has documented that serious mental illnesses are, in fact, physical illnesses characterized by, or resulting from, malfunctions and/or malformations of the brain."

This is not to imply that psychosocial and sociocultural influences are totally discounted. A multifaceted, transactional model of stress/adaptation is the cornerstone of understanding mental illness. But a study of the organic basis for psychiatric illness is necessary to understand the mechanisms of action of psychoactive drugs.

To understand how psychoactive drugs produce their effects, it is necessary for the nurse to know about the structure and functioning of the brain, including the pro-cess of neurotransmission and the function of various neurotransmitters. The nurse must also understand the role of the endocrine system in human behavior, the role of genetics in psychiatric illness, and the impact of psychologic factors on the immune system.

REVIEW OF THE NERVOUS SYSTEM

THE BRAIN

The brain has three major divisions: the forebrain, midbrain or mesencephalon, and hindbrain. Each of these structures is discussed briefly.

Forebrain The forebrain consists of the cerebrum and diencephalon.

CEREBRUM The cerebrum is comprised of two hemispheres separated by a deep groove that houses a band of 200 million neurons called the corpus callosum. The outer shell is called the cerebral cortex. It is extensively folded and consists of billions of neurons. The left hemisphere appears to be dominant in most people. It controls speech, comprehension, rationality, and logic. The right hemisphere is nondominant in most people. It may be called the "creative" brain and is associated with affect, behavior, and spatial perceptual functions. Masses of gray matter called basal ganglia are found deep within the cerebral hemispheres. They are responsible for certain subconscious aspects of voluntary movement, such as swinging the arms when walking, gesturing while speaking, and the regulation of muscle tone.

Each hemisphere of the cerebrum is divided into four lobes: the frontal, parietal, temporal, and occipital (Fig. 24–1). Voluntary body movement is controlled by the impulses through the frontal lobes. The frontal lobe may also play a role in the expression of feelings, as evidenced by changes in mood and character after damage to this area, and may be involved in thinking and perceptual interpretation of information.

Somatosensory input, including touch, pain, pressure, taste, temperature, perception of joint and body position, and visceral sensations, occurs in the parietal lobe area of the brain. The parietal lobes also contain association fibers linked to the primary sensory areas through which interpretation of sensory-perceptual information is made. Language interpretation is associated with the left hemisphere of the parietal lobe.

Auditory processing, short-term memory, and language interpretation are functions of the temporal lobes. The temporal lobes also play a role in the expression of emotions and the sense of smell.

The occipital lobes are the primary area of visual reception and interpretation. Language interpretation is also influenced by the occipital lobes through an association with the visual experience.

DIENCEPHALON The diencephalon connects the cerebrum with lower structures of the brain. The major components of the diencephalon include the thalamus, the hypothalamus, and the limbic system.

The thalamus integrates all sensory input (except smell) on its way to the cortex. This helps the cerebral cortex interpret the whole picture very rapidly, rather than experiencing each sensation individually. The thalamus is also involved in temporarily blocking minor sensations.

The hypothalamus is located just below the thalamus and just above the pituitary gland. It has diverse functions, including regulation of the pituitary gland, neuronal control over the autonomic nervous system, regulation of appetite, and regulation of temperature.

The limbic system consists of portions of the cerebrum and the diencephalon. The major components include the medially placed cortical and subcortical structures and the fiber tracts connecting them with one another and with the hypothalamus. The limbic system has been called "the emotional brain" and is associated with feelings of fear and anxiety; anger, rage, and aggression; love, joy, and hope; and with sexuality and social behavior.

Midbrain The mesencephalon, or midbrain, extends from the pons to the hypothalamus and is responsible for integration of various reflexes, including visual reflexes (e.g., automatically turning away from a dangerous object when it comes into view), auditory reflexes (e.g., automatically turning toward a sound that is heard), and righting reflexes (e.g., automatically keeping the head upright and maintaining balance).

Hindbrain The hindbrain consists of the pons, medulla, and cerebellum.

PONS The pons is a bulbous structure between the midbrain and medulla that is composed of large bundles of fibers, which form a major connection between the cerebellum and the brain stem. It also contains the central connections of cranial nerves V through VIII and centers for respiration and skeletal muscle tone.

MEDULLA The medulla is the connecting structure between the spinal cord and the pons, and all of the ascending and descending fiber tracts pass through it. It contains vital centers that regulate heart rate, blood pressure, and respiration. The medulla also contains reflex centers for swallowing, sneezing, coughing, and vomiting, as well as nuclei for cranial nerves IX through XII. The medulla, pons, and midbrain form the structure known as the brain stem.

CEREBELLUM The cerebellum has connections to the brain stem through bundles of fiber tracts. The functions of the cerebellum are concerned with involuntary movement, such as muscular tone and coordination and the maintenance of posture and equilibrium.

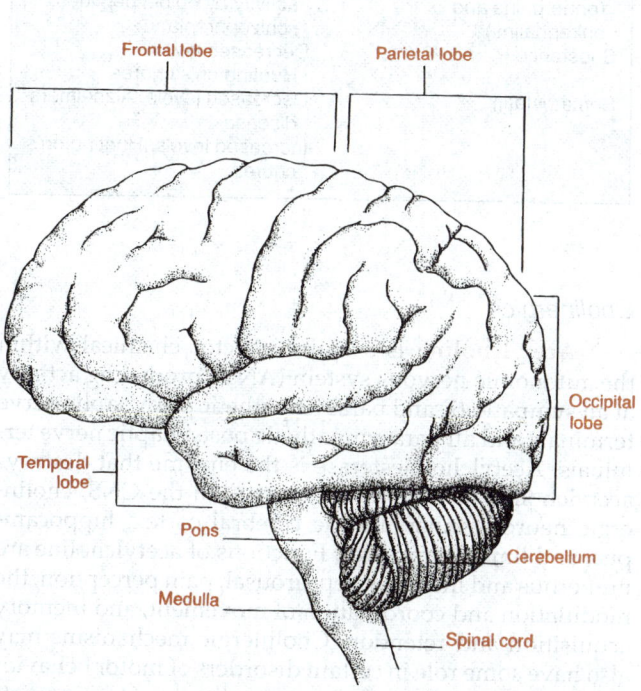

Figure 24–1. The brain: cerebral lobes, cerebellum, and brain stem. (From Scanlon, VC and Sanders, T: Essentials of Anatomy and Physiology, ed 2. FA Davis, Philadelphia, 1995, with permission.)

NEUROTRANSMISSION AND NEUROTRANSMITTERS

The tissue of the central nervous system consists of nerve cells called neurons that generate and transmit electrochemical impulses. The three classes of neurons include afferent (sensory), efferent (motor), and interneurons. The afferent neurons carry impulses from receptors in the internal and external periphery to the central nervous system (CNS), where they are then interpreted into various sensations. The efferent neurons carry impulses from the CNS to effectors in the periphery, such as muscles (that respond by contracting) and glands (that respond by secreting). Interneurons exist entirely within the CNS, and 99% of all nerve cells belong to this group. They may carry only sensory or motor impulses, or they may serve as integrators in the pathways between afferent and efferent neurons. They account in large part for thinking, feelings, learning, language, and memory.

Synapses

When information is transmitted through the body from one neuron to another, the neurons do not actually touch each other. The junction between two neurons is called a *synapse*. Neurons conducting impulses toward the synapse are called presynaptic neurons and those conducting impulses away are called postsynaptic neurons.

When a *neurotransmitter* stored in the axon terminals of the presynaptic neuron is released, it diffuses (moves) across the synaptic cleft and combines with receptor sites that are situated on the cell membrane of the postsynaptic neuron. The result of the combination of neurotransmitter-receptor site is the determination of whether or not another electrical impulse is generated. If one is generated, the result is called an excitatory response, and the electrical impulse moves on to the next synapse. If another electrical impulse is not generated by the neurotransmitter-receptor site combination, the result is called an inhibitory response, and synaptic transmission is terminated. After the neurotransmitter has performed its function in the synapse, it either returns to the vesicles to be stored and used again or it is inactivated and destroyed by enzymes in the postsynaptic neuron. The process of being stored for reuse is called reuptake, a function that holds significance for understanding the mechanism of action of certain psychotropic drugs.

Neurotransmitters

Neurotransmitters play an important role in human emotion and behavior and are the target for mechanisms of action of many of the psychotropic medications. Major categories of neurotransmitters that have implications for psychiatry include cholinergics (acetylcholine), monoamines (norepinephrine, dopamine, serotonin, histamine), amino acids (inhibitory—gamma-aminobutyric acid, glycine; excitatory—glutamate, aspartate), and neuropeptides (opioid peptides, substance P, somatostatin). Each of these is discussed separately and summarized in Table 24–1. The locations of acetylcholine, dopamine, norepinephrine, and serotonin neurons in the brain are illustrated in Figure 24–2.

Table 24–1. NEUROTRANSMITTERS IN THE CENTRAL NERVOUS SYSTEM

Neurotransmitter	Possible Implications for Mental Illness
Cholinergics Acetylcholine	Decreased levels: Alzheimer's disease, Huntington's chorea, Parkinson's disease Increased levels: Depression
Monoamines Norepinephrine	Decreased levels: Depression Increased levels: Mania, anxiety states, schizophrenia
Dopamine	Decreased levels: Parkinson's disease and depression Increased levels: Mania and schizophrenia
Serotonin	Decreased levels: Depression Increased levels: Anxiety states
Histamine	Decreased levels: Depression
Amino Acids Gamma-aminobutyric acid (GABA)	Decreased levels: Huntington's chorea, anxiety disorders, schizophrenia, and various forms of epilepsy
Glycine	Decreased levels: Spastic motor movements Toxic levels: Glycine encephalopathy
Glutamate and Aspartate	Increased levels: Huntington's chorea, temporal lobe epilepsy, spinal cerebellar degeneration
Neuropeptides Opioid peptides (endorphins and enkephalins)	Modulation of dopamine activity by opioid peptides: schizophrenia
Substance P	Decreased levels: Huntington's chorea
Somatostatin	Decreased levels: Alzheimers disease Increased levels: Huntington's chorea

Cholinergics

○ **Acetylcholine** is a major effector chemical within the autonomic nervous system (ANS), producing activity at all sympathetic and parasympathetic presynaptic nerve terminals and all parasympathetic postsynaptic nerve terminals. Acetylcholinesterase is the enzyme that destroys acetylcholine or inhibits its activity. In the CNS, cholinergic neurons innervate the cerebral cortex, hippocampus, and limbic structures. Functions of acetylcholine are numerous and include sleep, arousal, pain perception, the modulation and coordination of movement, and memory acquisition and retention. Cholinergic mechanisms may also have some role in certain disorders of motor behavior and memory, such as Parkinson's disease, Huntington's chorea, and Alzheimer's disease. For example, in Alzheimer's disease, regions in the brain experience a decline in

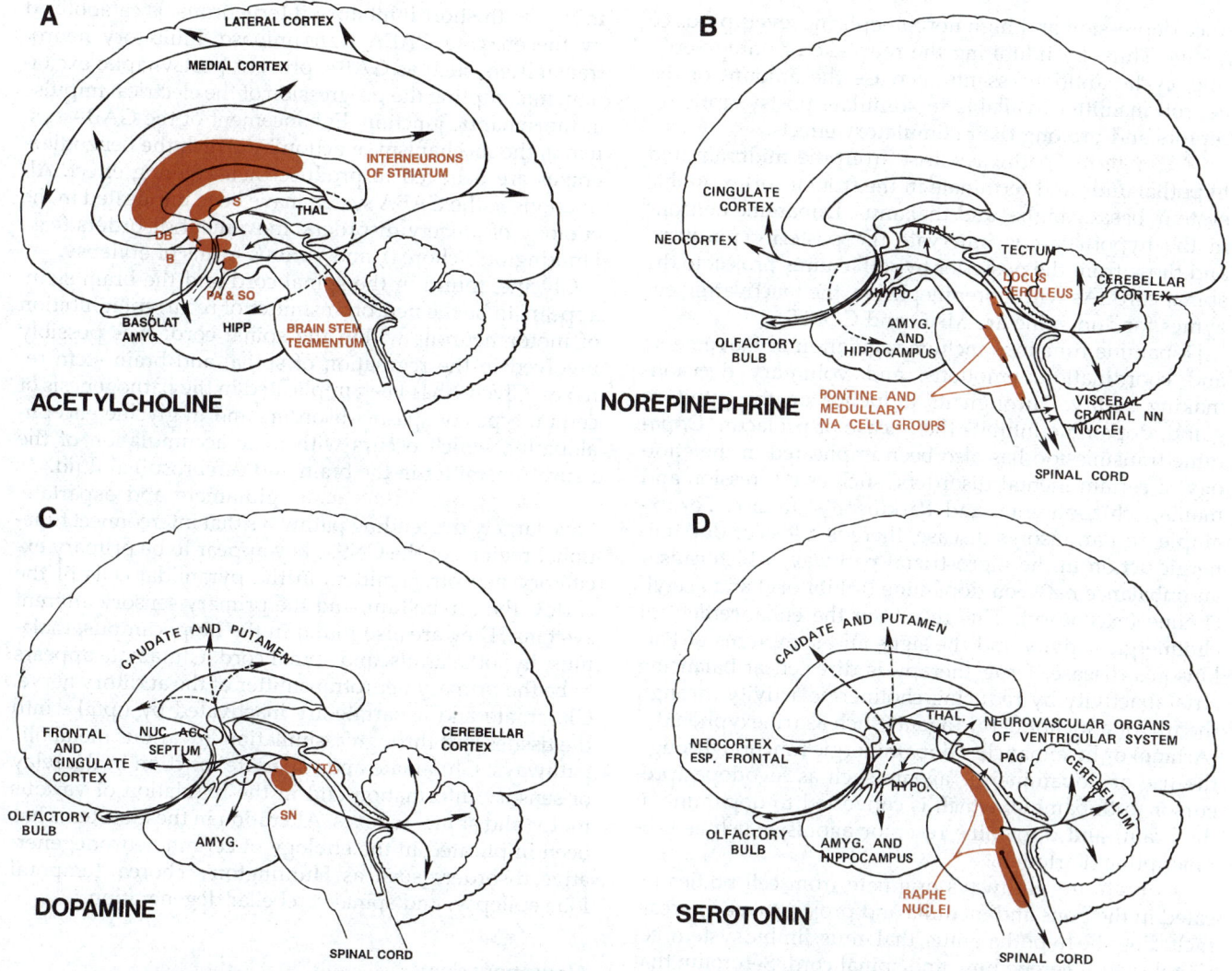

Figure 24–2. The locations and projections of neurotransmitters—acetylcholine, norepinephrine, dopamine, and serotonin—in the brain and/or brain stem. Areas containing cell bodies are shown (and labeled) in gold, and the projections pathways are indicated with gold arrows. (A) Acetylcholine. The areas that receive the cholinergic input are labeled in black. DB = diagonal band of Broca; HYPO = hypothalamus; IPN = interpeduncular nucleus; THAL = thalamus. (B) Norepinephrine. AMYG = amygdala; HYPO = hypothalamus; NA = norepinephrine; THAL = thalamus. (C) Dopamine: two major systems. AMYG = amygdala; NUC ACC = nucleus accumbens; VTA = ventral tegmental area. (D) Serotonin: fibers arising from the raphe nuclei. AMYG = amygdala; HYPO = hypothalamus; SUB NIGRA = substantia nigra; THAL = thalamus. (From Gilman, S and Newman, SW: Manter and Gatz's Essentials of Clinical Neuroanatomy and Neurophysiology, ed 8. FA Davis, Philadelphia, 1992, with permission.)

the neurotransmitters acetylcholine and norepinephrine. Thus, tacrine hydrochloride (Cognex), a potent centrally acting anticholinesterase agent, is used to help improve memory deficits. Tacrine hydrochloride produces its therapeutic effect by inhibiting the action of the enzyme acetylcholinesterase, which results in an increased concentration of acetylcholine.

Monoamines

○ **Norepinephrine** is the neurotransmitter that produces activity at the sympathetic postsynaptic nerve terminals in the ANS, resulting in the "fight or flight" responses in the effector organs. In the CNS, norepineph-

rine pathways originate in the pons and medulla and innervate the thalamus, dorsal hypothalamus, limbic system, hippocampus, cerebellum, and cerebral cortex. When norepinephrine is not returned for storage in the vesicles of the axon terminals, it is metabolized and inactivated by the enzymes monoamine oxidase (MAO) and catechol-O-methyl-transferase (COMT).

The functions of norepinephrine include the regulation of mood, cognition, perception, locomotion, cardiovascular functioning, and sleep and arousal. The mechanisms of norepinephrine transmission have also been implicated in certain disorders of mood, such as depression and mania, in anxiety states, and in schizophrenia. For example, it has been suggested that low norepinephrine levels produce depression and high norepinephrine levels produce mania. Thus, by inhibiting the reuptake of norepinephrine, cyclic antidepressants increase the amount of the neurotransmitter available to stimulate postsynaptic receptors and prolong their stimulatory effects.

○ **Dopamine** pathways arise from the midbrain and hypothalamus and terminate in the frontal cortex, limbic system, basal ganglia, and thalamus. Dopamine neurons in the hypothalamus innervate the posterior pituitary, and those from the posterior hypothalamus project to the spinal cord. As with norepinephrine, the inactivating enzymes for dopamine are MAO and COMT.

Dopamine functions include regulation of movements and coordination, emotions, and voluntary decision-making ability. Through its influence on the pituitary gland, dopamine inhibits the release of prolactin. Dopamine transmission has also been implicated in the etiology of certain mental disorders, such as depression and mania, schizophrenia, and Parkinson's disease. For example, in Parkinson's disease, there is a loss of dopaminergic action in the nigrostriatal pathway, which causes an imbalance between dopamine (inhibitory) and acetylcholine (excitatory). This results in the enhancement of cholinergic activity and the signs and symptoms of Parkinson's disease. Drug therapy is directed at balancing striatal activity by reducing cholinergic activity through the use of anticholinergic agents such as trihexyphenidyl (Artane) or by enhancing dopaminergic function through the use of dopaminergic agents such as levodopa (precursor to dopamine, which is converted to dopamine in the brain) and dopamine receptor agonists such as bromocriptine (Parlodel).

○ **Serotonin** pathways originate from cell bodies located in the pons and medulla and project to many areas, including the hypothalamus, thalamus, limbic system, cerebral cortex, cerebellum, and spinal cord. Serotonin that is taken back into the presynaptic terminal is catabolized by MAO. Serotonin may play a role in sleep and arousal, libido, appetite, mood, aggression, pain perception, coordination, and the ability to pursue goal-directed behavior. The serotonergic system has been implicated in the etiology of certain psychopathologic conditions including anxiety states and mood disorders.

○ **Histamine** has a well-documented role in mediating allergic and inflammatory reactions, but its role in the CNS as a neurotransmitter has only recently been confirmed. The highest concentrations of histamine are found within various regions of the hypothalamus. Histamine is catabolized by MAO. Although the exact processes mediated by histamine in the CNS are uncertain, data suggest that histamine may play a role in depressive illness.

Amino Acids

○ **Inhibitory amino acids** implicated as neurotransmitters include gamma-aminobutyric acid (GABA) and glycine. GABA has a widespread distribution in the CNS with high concentrations in the hypothalamus, hippocampus, cortex, cerebellum, and basal ganglia of the brain, in the gray matter of the dorsal horn of the spinal cord, and in the retina. GABA, which is associated primarily with short inhibitory interneurons, is catabolized by the enzyme GABA transaminase. Inhibitory neurotransmitters such as GABA prevent postsynaptic excitation, interrupting the progression of the electrical impulse at the synaptic junction. Enhancement of the GABA system is the mechanism of action by which the benzodiazepines are believed to produce their calming effect. Alterations in the GABA system have been implicated in the etiology of anxiety disorders, movement disorders (e.g., Huntington's chorea), and various forms of epilepsy.

Glycine, found in the spinal cord and the brain stem, appears to be the neurotransmitter of recurrent inhibition of motor neurons within the spinal cord. It is possibly involved in the regulation of spinal and brain stem reflexes. Glycine has been implicated in the pathogenesis of certain types of spastic disorders and in glycine encephalopathy, which occurs with toxic accumulation of the neurotransmitter in the brain and cerebrospinal fluid.

○ **Excitatory amino acids,** glutamate and aspartate, have largely descending pathways that interconnect functional regions of the CNS. They appear to be primary excitatory neurotransmitters in the pyramidal cells of the cortex, the cerebellum, and the primary sensory afferent systems. They are also found in the hippocampus, thalamus, hypothalamus, and spinal cord. Glutamate appears to be the primary neurotransmitter of the auditory nerve. Glutamate and aspartate are inactivated by uptake into the tissues and through assimilation in various metabolic pathways. Glutamate and aspartate function in the relay of sensory information and in the regulation of various motor and spinal reflexes. Alteration in these systems has been implicated in the etiology of certain neurodegenerative disorders such as Huntington's chorea, temporal lobe epilepsy, and spinal cerebellar degeneration.

Neuropeptides

It is known that neuropeptides often coexist with the classical neurotransmitters within a neuron, but their role has not been clearly established.

○ **Opioid peptides,** which include the endorphins and enkephalins, are found in various concentrations in the hypothalamus, thalamus, limbic structures, midbrain, and the brain stem. Opioid peptides are released in response to painful stimuli and are thought to have a role in pain modulation, with their morphinelike properties. Opioid peptides alter the release of dopamine and affect the spontaneous activity of the dopaminergic neurons. These findings may have some implication for opioid peptide–dopamine interaction in the etiology of schizophrenia.

○ **Substance P** is present in high concentrations in the hypothalamus, limbic structures, midbrain, brain stem, thalamus, basal ganglia, and spinal cord. Substance P is found in high concentrations in sensory fibers and is thought to play a role in sensory transmission and the regulation of pain. Decreased concentrations have been found in the substantia nigra of the basal ganglia of patients with Huntington's chorea.

○ **Somatostatin,** also called growth hormone release inhibitory hormone, is found in the cerebral cortex, hippocampus, thalamus, basal ganglia, brain stem, and spinal cord. It exerts inhibitory effects on the release of norepinephrine and excitatory effects of serotonin. It also stimulates the turnover and release of dopamine in the basal ganglia and acetylcholine in the brainstem and hippocampus. High concentrations of somatostatin have been reported in brain specimens from patients with Huntington's chorea and low concentrations in patients with Alzheimer's disease.

AUTONOMIC NERVOUS SYSTEM

The autonomic nervous system (ANS) has two divisions: the sympathetic and the parasympathetic. The ANS is actually part of the peripheral nervous system, but its regulation is integrated by the hypothalamus. Therefore, the emotions exert a great deal of influence over its functioning, and the ANS has been implicated in the etiology of a number of anxiety disorders. The sympathetic division is dominant in stressful situations and prepares the body for the fight or flight response. This results in an increase in heart rate and respirations and a decrease in digestive secretions and peristalsis. Blood is shunted to the vital organs and to skeletal muscles to ensure adequate oxygenation. The parasympathetic division dominates when an individual is in a relaxed, nonstressful condition. The heart and respirations are maintained at a normal rate and secretions and peristalsis increase for normal digestion. Elimination functions are promoted.

ACTIONS OF DRUGS ON THE CNS

CNS drugs have actions that can be generally considered as either specific or nonspecific. A drug effect is specific if its action is attributable to a distinct molecular mechanism of action. There are receptor mechanisms that are specific to a drug's action on target cells. For example, the effects of opioid analgesics are thought to be produced by interaction with specific opioid receptors in the CNS and peripheral tissues. Conversely, drugs with nonspecific actions generally produce their effects on numerous target cells and act by diverse mechanisms. Many sedative-hypnotic drugs, such as the barbiturates and alcohol, are believed to cause a generalized depression of CNS neurons. However, the distinction between drugs that appear to have either specific or nonspecific actions may be one of degree rather than an absolute difference. For instance, nonspecific-acting drugs may not have equivalent effects on all parts of the CNS, but may preferentially affect the brain stem or the cerebrum.

Frequently CNS drugs that are termed nonspecific in their action are classified as either CNS depressants or CNS stimulants. While this may be a useful classification, it also oversimplifies a frequently complex mode of action. Because CNS stimulation can be caused by either stimulation of excitatory neurons or depression of inhibitory neurons, a CNS depressant may cause stimulation in certain doses. The "stimulant" effects of alcohol are an example of this type of CNS depression.

NEUROENDOCRINOLOGY

Neuroendocrinology is the study of the endocrine influence on the nervous system or the influence of the nervous system on endocrine function. Endocrine functioning has a strong foundation in the CNS under the direction of the hypothalamus. The hypothalamus has direct control over the pituitary gland, which is sometimes called the "master gland." Hormones and their circadian rhythm of regulation significantly influence a number of physiologic and psychologic life-cycle phenomena, such as moods, sleep and arousal, stress response, appetite, libido, and fertility. *Circadian rhythm* refers to regular, cyclical, daily fluctuations in activity. See Table 24–2 for a discussion of hormones under hypothalamus-pituitary regulation that may have implications for behavioral function.

GENETICS

Behavior genetics has been described as a science that combines aspects of psychology, psychiatry, physiology, and genetics with the goal of clarifying the role that genetic factors play in the determination of behavior. It is likely that most psychiatric disorders are the result of a combination of genetics and environmental influences.

Investigators who study the etiologic implications for psychiatric illness may explore several risk factors. Familial studies estimate the prevalence of psychopathology among relatives and make predictions about the predisposition to an illness based on familial risk factors. Schizophrenia, bipolar disorder, major depression, anorexia nervosa, panic disorder, somatization disorder, antisocial personality disorder, and alcoholism are examples of psychiatric illnesses in which familial tendencies have been implicated.

Studies that are purely genetic in nature search for a specific gene that is responsible for an individual having a particular illness. A number of disorders exist in which the mutation of a specific gene or change in the number or structure of a chromosome has been associated with the etiology. Examples include Huntington's chorea, cystic fibrosis, phenylketonuria, Duchenne's muscular dystrophy, and Down syndrome. The search for genetic links to certain psychiatric disorders continues.

In addition to familial and purely genetic investigations, other studies have been conducted to estimate the existence and degree of genetic and environmental contributions to the etiology of certain psychiatric disorders. Twin studies and adoption studies have been successfully used for this purpose. Disorders in which twin studies have suggested a possible genetic link include alcoholism, schizophrenia, major depression, bipolar disorder, anorexia nervosa, panic disorder, and obsessive compulsive disorder. Adoption studies have found a possible genetic link for alcoholism, schizophrenia, major depression, bipolar disorder, somatization disorder, and antisocial personality disorder.

Table 24–2. HORMONES OF THE NEUROENDOCRINE SYSTEM

Hormone	Location and Stimulation of Release	Target Organ	Function	Possible Behavioral Correlation to Altered Secretion
Antidiuretic Hormone (ADH)	Posterior pituitary Release stimulated by dehydration, pain, stress	Kidney (causes increased reabsorption)	Conserves body water and maintain blood pressure	Polydipsia, altered pain response, modified sleep pattern
Oxytocin	Posterior pituitary Release stimulated by end of pregnancy, stress, during sexual arousal	Uterus, breasts	Contraction of uterus for labor, release of breast milk	May play role in stress response by stimulation of ACTH
Growth Hormone (GH)	Anterior pituitary Release stimulated by growth hormone releasing hormone from hypothalamus	Bones, tissues	Growth in children, protein synthesis in adults	Anorexia nervosa
Thyroid Stimulating Hormone (TSH)	Anterior pituitary Release stimulated by thyrotropin releasing hormone from hypothalamus	Thyroid gland	Stimulates secretion of thyroid hormones needed for metabolism of food and regulation of temperature	Increased levels: insomnia, anxiety, emotional lability Decreased levels: fatigue, depression
Adrenocorticotropic Hormone (ACTH)	Anterior pituitary Release stimulated by corticotropin releasing hormone from hypothalamus	Adrenal cortex	Stimulates secretion of cortisol, which plays a role in response to stress	Increased levels: mood disorders, psychosis Decreased levels: depression, apathy, fatigue
Prolactin	Anterior pituitary Release stimulated by prolactin releasing hormone from hypothalamus	Breasts	Stimulates milk production	Increased levels: depression, anxiety, decreased libido, irritability
Gonadotropic Hormones	Anterior pituitary Release stimulated by gonadotropin releasing hormone from hypothalamus	Ovaries and testes	Stimulates secretion of estrogen, progesterone and testosterone; role in ovulation and sperm production	Decreased levels: depression and anorexia nervosa Increased testosterone: increased sexual behavior and aggressiveness
Melanocyte-Stimulating Hormone (MSH)	Anterior pituitary Release stimulated by onset of darkness	Pineal gland	Stimulation secretion of melatonin	Increased levels: depression

Recent studies have also indicated a familial factor in responsiveness to various antidepressant medications. A summary of various psychiatric disorders and the possible biologic influences discussed in this chapter is presented in Table 24–3.

PSYCHOIMMUNOLOGY

Psychoimmunology is the study of the influence of stress on the immune system and its role in the susceptibility to illness. In studies of the biologic response to stress, it has been hypothesized that individuals become more susceptible to physical illness following exposure to a stressful stimulus or life event. This response is thought to be due to the effect of increased glucocorticoid release from the adrenal cortex following stimulation from the hypothalamic-pituitary-adrenal axis during stressful situations. The result is a suppression in lymphocyte proliferation and function.

Growth hormone, which may be released in response to certain stressors, may enhance immune functioning, while testosterone is thought to inhibit immune functioning. Increased production of epinephrine and norepinephrine occurs in response to stress and may decrease immunity. Serotonin has demonstrated both enhancing and inhibitory effects on immunity.

Studies have correlated a decrease in lymphocyte functioning with periods of grief, bereavement, and depression, associating the degree of altered immunity with severity of the depression. A number of research studies have attempted to correlate the onset of schizophrenia to abnormalities of the immune system. These studies have considered autoimmune responses, viral infections, immunogenetics, and food allergies. The role of these factors in the onset and course of schizophrenia remains unclear. Immunologic abnormalities have also been investigated in a number of other psychiatric illnesses, including alcoholism, Alzheimer's disease, autism, cerebral atrophy, criminal behavior, dementia, mental retardation, and Parkinson's disease.

Table 24–3. BIOLOGIC IMPLICATIONS OF PSYCHIATRIC DISORDERS

Anatomic Brain Structures Involved	Neurotransmitter Hypothesis	Possible Endocrine Correlation	Implications of Circadian Rhythms	Possible Genetic Link
Schizophrenia Frontal cortex, temporal lobes, limbic system	Dopamine hyperactivity	Decreased prolactin levels	May correlate antipsychotic medication administration to times of lowest level	Twin, familial, and adoption studies suggest genetic link
Depressive Disorders Frontal lobes, limbic system, temporal lobes	Decreased levels of norepinephrine, dopamine, and serotonin	Increased cortisol levels, thyroid hormone hyposecretion, increased melatonin	DST used to predict effectiveness of antidepressants; melatonin linked to depression during periods of darkness	Twin, familial, and adoption studies suggest genetic link
Bipolar Disorder Frontal lobes, limbic system, temporal lobes	Increased levels of norepinephrine, dopamine, and serotonin in acute mania	Some indication of elevated thyroid hormones in acute mania		Twin, familial, and adoption studies suggest genetic link
Panic Disorder Limbic system, midbrain	Increased levels of norepinephrine, decreased GABA activity	Elevated levels of thyroid hormones	May have some application for times of medication administration	Twin and familial studies suggest genetic link
Anorexia Nervosa Limbic system, particularly the hypothalamus	Decreased levels of norepinephrine, serotonin, and dopamine	Decreased levels of gonadotropins and growth hormone, increased cortisol levels	DST often shows same results as in depression	Twin and familial studies suggest genetic link
Obsessive Compulsive Disorder Limbic system, basal ganglia (specifically caudate nucleus)	Decreased levels of serotonin	Increased cortisol levels	DST often shows same results as in depression	Twin studies suggest possible genetic link
Alzheimer's Disease Temporal, parietal, and occipital regions of cerebral cortex; hippocampus	Decreased levels of acetylcholine, norepinephrine, serotonin, and somatostatin	Decreased corticotropin releasing hormone	Decreased levels of acetylcholine and serotonin may inhibit hypothalmic-pituitary axis and interfere with hormonal releasing factors	Familial studies suggest genetic predisposition; early onset disorder linked to marker on chromosome 21

DST = dexamethasone suppression test. Dexamethasone is a synthetic glucocorticoid that suppresses cortisol secretion via the feedback mechanism. In this test, 1 mg of dexamethasone is administered at 11:30 PM and blood samples are drawn at 8:00 AM, 4:00 PM, and 11:00 PM on the following day. A plasma value greater than $5\mu g/dL$ suggests that the individual is not suppressing cortisol in response to the dose of dexamethasone. This is a positive result for depression and may have implications for other disorders as well.

Evidence also exists to support a correlation between psychosocial stress and the onset of illness. However, research is still required to determine the specific processes involved in stress-induced modulation of the immune system.

The evidence for the interaction between physical and mental factors in the development and management of psychiatric illness is obvious. The increasing role of psychotropic medication in the treatment of psychiatric illness demands that nurses understand the biology of the central nervous system so that they may predict outcomes and safely manage the administration of psychotropic medications. Further research into the role of neurobiologic mechanisms in explaining the biologic basis of behavior offers great promise for alleviating the suffering associated with psychiatric disorders.

The bibliography for this chapter can be found in Appendix B, which begins on page 1054.

CHAPTER REVIEW QUESTIONS*

1. Which of the following systems of the brain has been referred to as the emotional brain and is associated with feelings of fear, anxiety, anger, rage, love, and sexuality?
   a. Basal ganglia.
   b. Cerebral cortex.
   c. Limbic system.
   d. Autonomic nervous system.

2. Which neuropeptide is released in response to painful stimuli and alters the release of dopamine?
   a. Substance P.
   b. Opioid peptide.
   c. Somatostatin.
   d. Norepinephrine.

3. Which of the following neurotransmitters is implicated in certain disorders of moods, such as depression and mania?
   a. Gamma-aminobutyric acid (GABA).
   b. Norepinephrine.

   c. Glutamine.
   d. Opioid peptide.

4. An example of a class of drugs that has a *nonspecific* action on the CNS is:
   a. Opioids.
   b. Barbiturates.
   c. Phenothiazines.
   d. MAO Inhibitors.

5. Adoption studies have found a possible genetic link for the following psychiatric disorder(s):
   a. Bipolar disorder.
   b. Schizophrenia.
   c. Major depression.
   d. All of the above.

*See Appendix A, which begins on page 1051, for answers.

CHAPTER 25

Sedative, Hypnotic, and Anxiolytic Drugs

Meredith A. Davison, PhD

CHAPTER OUTLINE

KEY TERMS

Abuse
Anterograde amnesia
Anxiolytic
Cross-tolerance
Dependence
Hypnotic
Paradoxic reactions

Porphyria
Rebound
Reinforcement
Sedative
Somnambulism
Tolerance
Withdrawal syndrome

LEARNING OBJECTIVES

After reading this chapter, the student will be able to:

1. Identify medications commonly used as sedative, hypnotic, and anxiolytic agents.
2. Differentiate among the sedative, hypnotic, and anxiolytic medications as to use, mechanism of action, route of administration, pharmacokinetics, adverse effects, contraindications and precautions, and interactions.
3. Identify specific nursing assessments for the patient requiring sedative, hypnotic, and anxiolytic medications and formulate appropriate patient outcomes.
4. Plan the nursing interventions necessary to administer sedative, hypnotic, and anxiolytic medications; choose appropriate teaching strategies; and help develop the patient's goals.
5. Evaluate the patient at various stages of treatment to gauge the effectiveness of nursing interventions.

The sedative, hypnotic, and anxiolytic drugs belong to a group of agents that depress the central nervous system (CNS) in a more or less nonselective, dose-dependent fashion. A *sedative* calms the recipient and reduces activity. A *hypnotic* produces drowsiness and induces sleep. An *anxiolytic* reduces anxiety, an apprehensive uneasiness of mind usually regarding an impending or anticipated misfortune. Sedative and anxiolytic drugs usually produce hypnosis as the dosage is increased. Disagreement exists as to whether antianxiety effects are the same as or different from sedative effects.

All of these drugs alleviate only specific symptoms such as anxiety or sleep problems but do not alter the factors that cause them. Therefore, these medications are used for symptomatic, noncurative treatment and as aids to minimize feelings of distress so that the patient may cope with the underlying causes.

When taken chronically, almost all of the sedative, hypnotic, and anxiolytic agents can produce physiologic *dependence,* a compulsive need to repeatedly use the drug.

The publisher gratefully acknowledges the efforts of Frances C. Schneider in the preparation of this chapter.

Table 25–1. SEDATIVE, HYPNOTIC, AND ANXIOLYTIC DRUGS: BENZODIAZEPINES

DRUG NAME/ROUTE AND DOSAGE	PHARMACOKINETICS/ DYNAMICS	NURSING IMPLICATIONS
all benzodiazepines		**ASSESSMENT:** Assess for pregnancy (category D).
diazepam (Valium) (Valrelease) (Vazepam) (Zetran)		
sedation **Adults:** 2–10 mg PO 2–4 times daily or 15–30 mg of extended-release capsule once daily. **Chidren age 6 and over:** 1–2.5 mg PO 3–4 times/day. **alcohol withdrawal** **Adults:** 20 mg PO 3–4 times/day on day 1, then decrease to 5 mg 3–4 times/day; or 10–20 mg IM or IV initially, then 5–10 mg in 3–4 hr PRN. **convulsions** **Adults:** 2–10 mg PO 2–4 times daily. **status epilepticus** **Adults:** 5–10 mg IV, repeated at 10–15 min intervals to maximum of 30 mg in 2–4 hr. Repeat regimen if necessary. **Children > 5 yr:** 1mg IM or IV q 2–5 min to a maximum of 10 mg. Repeat q 2–4 hr PRN. **Children 1 mo–5 yr:** 0.2–0.5 mg IM or IV q 2–5 min to a maximum of 5 mg. **skeletal muscle relaxation** **Adults:** 2–10 mg PO 3–4 times daily or 15–30 mg of extended-release capsule once daily; or 5–10 mg IM or IV, repeated in 2–4 hr PRN. **Geriatric:** 2–2.5 mg PO 1–2 times daily, increased as tolerated. **psychoneurotic reactions** **Adults:** 2–5 mg IM or IV repeated in 3–4 hr PRN. **cardioversion** **Adults:** 5–15 mg IV 5–10 min before procedure. **endoscopic procedures** **Adults:** Up to 20 mg IV just before procedure; or 5–10 mg IM 30 min before procedure if IV route cannot be used.	**Onset:** PO and IM, 15–45 min; IV, 1–3 min **Peak:** PO and IM, 0.5–2 hr; IV, 20 min **Duration:** variable **½L:** 20–80 hr (30–200 hr desmethyldiazepam) **PB:** very high **B:** hepatic (active metabolites) **E:** renal	**ASSESSMENT:** Assess whether PRN dose is necessary. Assess possibility of using nonpharmacologic therapies. **INTERVENTION:** Drug dependence may occur; monitor patient closely. Do not abruptly discontinue drug. **Patient Teaching—**Advise patient that drowsiness, light-headedness, or dizziness may occur. Remind patient to avoid alcoholic beverages. Note policies and legal restrictions applying to benzodiazepines. **EVALUATION:** Look for characteristics of tolerance to same dose (higher doses needed), physical dependence, paradoxic reactions (excitement), withdrawal reactions (REM rebound).
flurazepam (Dalmane) **Adults:** 15–30 mg PO hs. **Geriatric:** 15 mg PO hs.	**Onset:** 15–45 min **Peak:** 0.5–1 hr **Duration:** 7–8 hr (hangover effect for up to 2 days) **½L:** 47–100 hr. **PB:** 97% **B:** hepatic (active metabolites) **E:** renal	Same as for diazepam.

Table 25–1. SEDATIVE, HYPNOTIC, AND ANXIOLYTIC DRUGS: BENZODIAZEPINES, *Continued*

DRUG NAME/ROUTE AND DOSAGE	PHARMACOKINETICS/ DYNAMICS	NURSING IMPLICATIONS
triazolam (Halcion) ***Adults:*** 0.125–0.5 mg PO hs. ***Geriatric:*** 0.125–0.25 mg PO hs.	**Onset:** 15–30 min **Peak:** 0.5–2 hr **Duration:** NA **½L:** 1.5–5.5 hr **PB:** 78%–89% **B:** hepatic, no active metabolites **E:** renal	Same as for diazepam plus: **INTERVENTION:** Monitor patient closely for possible memory problems or CNS side effects for first 2 weeks.
alprazolam (Xanax) ***Adults:*** 0.25–0.5 mg PO 3 times/ day up to 4 mg/day. ***Geriatric:*** 0.25 mg 2–3 times/day (increased as tolerated). **panic disorder** ***Adults:*** up to 10 mg/day.	**Onset:** 15–60 min **Peak:** 1–2 hr **Duration:** NA **½L:** 12–15 hr **PB:** high **B:** hepatic **E:** rapid renal clearance after discontinuance	Same as for diazepam plus: **INTERVENTION: Patient Teaching**—Caution patient that abruptly stopping drug can precipitate CNS excitation and seizures.
lorazepam (Ativan) **sedation** ***Adults:*** 1–3 mg PO 2–3 times daily. ***Geriatric:*** 0.5–2 mg PO 2–3 times daily. **anxiety** ***Adults:*** 2–3 mg/day given in 2–3 divided doses. **preoperative sedation** ***Adults:*** 0.05 mg/kg IM 2 hr before surgery, not to exceed 4 mg total; or 0.044 mg/kg IV 15–20 min before surgery, not to exceed 2 mg. **for operative amnesia** ***Adults:*** up to 0.05 mg/kg IV, not to exceed 4 mg.	**Onset:** PO, 15–60 min; IM, 15–30 min; IV, 5–15 min **Peak:** PO, 1–6 hr; IM, 1–1.5 hr; IV, immediate **Duration:** 6–10 hr **½L:** 10–20 hr **PB:** 91% **B:** hepatic, no active metabolites **E:** renal	Same as for diazepam plus: **INTERVENTION:** Inject undiluted deep into muscle mass for IM administration. IV must be diluted with equal volume of sterile water for injection, normal saline solution, or D₅W. Do not exceed 2 mg/min.

NA = not available.

Some individuals resort to these medications to help them cope with the stresses of everyday life. The relief provided by these drugs may lead to reinforcement of their use without any resolution of the cause of the stress. *Reinforcement* is the provision of positive rewards (relief) that strengthens, augments, or increases the probability that the behavior will occur again. If one drug becomes unavailable, a similar CNS depressant can be substituted because of *cross-tolerance*, a situation in which the development of tolerance to one drug creates a tolerance to other drugs with similar pharmacologic effect. This practice has contributed to the problems with *abuse* (misuse or excessive use) sometimes associated with these drugs, particularly if they are combined with alcohol. The patterns of drug abuse range from chronic use for anxiety and insomnia to episodes of intoxication to compulsive daily use of large quantities of CNS depressants.

BENZODIAZEPINES

Benzodiazepines are a large group of drugs used primarily to treat anxiety and insomnia. The group includes **diazepam** *(Valium)*, **triazolam** *(Halcion)*, **chlordiazepoxide hydrochloride** *(Librium)*, **alprazolam** *(Xanax)*, **clorazepate dipotassium** *(Tranxene)*, **flurazepam** *(Dalmane)*, **lorazepam** *(Ativan)*, **estazolam** *(ProSom)*, **halazepam** *(Paxipam)*, **oxazepam** *(Serax)*, **prazepam** *(Centrax)*, **quazepam** *(Doral)*, and **temazepam** *(Restoril)*. Another benzodiazepine, **clonazepam** *(Klonopin)* is used for the treatment of seizure disorders and panic disorders. **Midazolam** *(Versed)* is a benzodiazepine used as a preoperative medication. Benzodiazepines are classified as Schedule IV controlled substances because of their abuse potential. Specific information about selected benzodiazepines can be found in Table 25–1.

Table 25–2. FDA-APPROVED USES OF BENZODIAZEPINES

	Anxiety*	Anxiety†	Epilepsy	Insomnia	Muscle Spasm	Panic Disorder	Preop. Med.
Alprazolam		X				X	
Clorazepate	X	X	X				
Chlordiazepoxide	X	X					X
Clonazepam			X			X	
Diazepam	X	X	X		X	X	X
Estazolam				X			
Flurazepam				X			
Halazepam	X						
Lorazepam	X	X					X
Midazolam							X
Oxazepam	X	X					
Prazepam		X					
Quazepam				X			
Tamazepam				X			
Triazolam				X			

*Not associated with depression.
†Associated with depression.
Preop. Med. = preoperative medication.

ACTION

Benzodiazepines are believed to act on the benzodiazepine receptor, which is closely linked with the gamma-aminobutyric acid (GABA) receptor. Stimulation of the benzodiazepine receptor leads to GABA receptors producing stronger inhibition of the postsynaptic neuron. This hypothesis is supported by numerous behavioral and electrophysiologic studies. However, the participation of other neuronal mechanisms of action has not been excluded.

USES

The uses of benzodiazepines include sleep induction, anxiety reduction, muscle relaxation, seizure control, acute alcohol withdrawal, phobias, and premedication for surgery and diagnostic procedures. Benzodiazepines are not effective for severe psychotic disorders or psychiatric depression but may be useful adjuncts to antidepressant therapy for severe anxiety accompanying depression. Some benzodiazepines are, however, approved by the Food and Drug Administration (FDA) for prevention of panic attacks. The uses of benzodiazepines approved by the FDA are listed in Table 25–2.

PHARMACOKINETICS

The benzodiazepines, which can be administered either orally or parenterally, are characterized by high lipid solubility. Rates of absorption following oral adminstration are variable. The time for peak plasma concentration occurs ½ hour after diazepam administration to 6 hours after prazepam. Following intramuscular administration, absorption is slower and more erratic, depending on the site of injection. Intravenous administration of benzodiazepines is used to treat status epilepticus and to induce anesthesia.

Benzodiazepines and their metabolites are widely distributed into body tissues. They cross the blood-brain barrier and the placenta and are distributed into breast milk. They are highly bound to plasma proteins. Steady-state plasma levels may be obtained after 5 days to 2 weeks.

As illustrated in Figure 25–1, the benzodiazepines share similar metabolic pathways. Diazepam, chlordiazepoxide, prazepam, clorazepate, and halazepam are all converted to desmethyldiazepam, which must be further metabolized by the liver. During chronic administration, the accumulation of desmethyldiazepam, which has a long half-life, may lead to excessive sedation and ataxia. This is especially problematic for elderly patients with liver dysfunction. Alprazolam, flurazepam, and triazolam

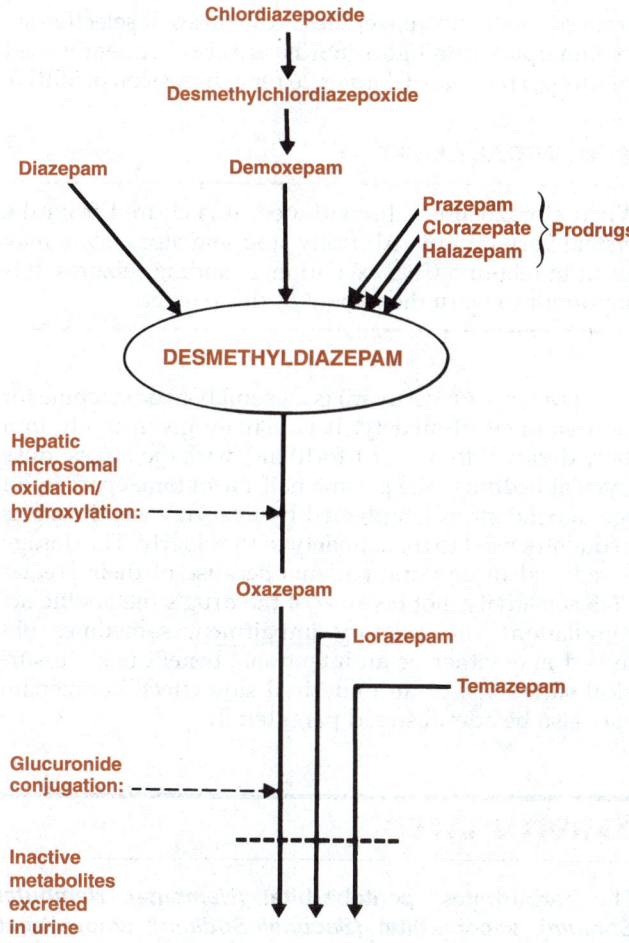

Figure 25–1. Common metabolic path of many benzodiazepine drugs.

are all metabolized to active metabolites that have relatively short half-lives (1 to 6 hours). Oxazepam, temazepam, and lorazepam have shorter half-lives; they produce no active metabolites and therefore do not produce problems resulting from metabolite buildup.

CONTRAINDICATIONS AND PRECAUTIONS

Benzodiazepines potentiate the effects of other CNS depressants (including alcohol, narcotics, antihistamines, and barbiturates) and should not be used in combination with these agents. Although benzodiazepines are relatively safe drugs, the problems of tolerance and dependence, both psychologic and physical, are possible. *Tolerance* occurs when the patient requires larger doses of the drug to obtain the same effect. A *withdrawal syndrome*, which often mimics the symptoms of anxiety syndrome, occurs with abrupt cessation of the drug and is most prominent with the use of short-acting drugs such as triazolam. The dosage of benzodiazepines should be tapered slowly over 6 to 8 weeks to minimize *rebound* or withdrawal symptoms.

▼ **CLINICAL ALERT**

Benzodiazepines are believed to cause fetal deformities, but definitive studies are not available. Unless there are strong maternal indications, their use is not recommended during pregnancy. Chronic use of benzodiazepines during late pregnancy may cause physical dependence in the neonate, resulting in withdrawal symptoms.

ADVERSE REACTIONS

Sedation and ataxia are the most common side effects of benzodiazepines. The elderly are especially sensitive to these effects, which increase the risk of falls. Gastrointestinal disturbances, anticholinergic side effects, headache, incontinence, jaundice, and rashes can also occur. Rarely, *paradoxic reactions* (responses to a medication that are opposite those which would be predicted by the drug's pharmacology) have been observed. The most commonly observed paradoxic reaction occurring with the use of benzodiazepines is increased excitation. An infrequent but potentially disturbing effect of benzodiazepines is *anterograde amnesia*, an inability to remember events that occur for a period after drug administration. Anterograde amnesia may be of benefit when the drug is given before an unpleasant experience (e.g., surgery or chemotherapy).

Isolated benzodiazepine abuse is relatively uncommon. When an individual abuses a benzodiazepine, it is seldom the drug of choice. The most likely groups of people found to abuse benzodiazepines include past or current abusers of other psychoactive substances, including alcohol.

Overdose of benzodiazepines is rarely lethal unless other CNS depressant drugs (i.e., alcohol, opioids, barbiturates, and so on) are taken concomitantly. A benzodiazepine receptor antagonist, flumazenil (Mazicon), is available to reverse the effects of benzodiazepine overdose. It appears to be effective but can also precipitate convulsions in some patients.

INTERACTIONS

The benzodiazepines produce fewer problematic interactions with other drugs than do older sedatives and hypnotics. The primary interaction occurs when these drugs are combined with another CNS depressant, such as alcohol. Such combinations tend to produce oversedation and motor impairment and may, in rare instances, lead to impaired respiratory function and death. Fluvoxamine and sertraline (selective serotonin reuptake inhibitors) may decrease the metabolism of benzodiazepines.

▼ **CLINICAL ALERT**

Benzodiazepines metabolized by oxidation or hydroxylation (including alprazolam, chlordiazepoxide, diazepam, and others with the desmethyldiazepam metabolite) have an increased elimination half-life when administered with cimetidine (but not with ranitidine). This enzyme-inhibition problem does not affect oxazepam and lorazepam. Because cimetidine is now available without prescription, it is imperative to question the patient about possible use of this drug.

The benzodiazepines can also decrease the elimination of digoxin, increasing risk of toxicity. This class of drugs alters the results of some laboratory tests, such as elevating the results of serum bilirubin, aspartate aminotransferase (AST), and alkaline phosphatase tests.

○ **Diazepam** (Valium), the prototype of the benzodiazepine drugs, is used for sedation, sleep induction, anxiety, status epilepticus, skeletal muscle relaxation, acute alcohol withdrawal, and preoperative sedation. It is taken orally in daily doses of 4 to 40 mg. Its intramuscular or intravenous dose is usually 5 to 10 mg every 3 to 4 hours. If diazepam must be given intramuscularly, the preferred site is the deltoid muscle, as absorption from this site is less erratic. When administered intravenously, the rate of infusion should not exceed 5 mg/min. Diazepam should not be mixed with other injectable solutions or drugs. Its plasma half-life increases based on the age of the recipient, ranging from approximately 20 hours for young adults to several days for elderly patients.

○ **Flurazepam** (Dalmane) is an effective hypnotic, and its usual oral bedtime dose is 15 to 30 mg. The elderly patient should be given the lower dose. It promotes drowsiness within 15 to 45 minutes of ingestion. This effect lasts for 7 to 8 hours with minimal sleep disruption. Flurazepam is converted in the liver primarily to the active metabolite desalkylflurazepam, which has a plasma half-life of 47 to 100 hours. This metabolite tends to accumulate with repeated doses. Because of this effect, flurazepam is not maximally effective for the first few nights, but dosage should not be increased during the initial treatment period. Flurazepam has been shown to be effective treatment for insomnia for up to 28 days. A disadvantage of flurazepam (and other benzodiazepines with long half-lives) is the frequent occurrence of prolonged sedation or "hangover." This is especially prevalent in elderly patients.

○ **Triazolam** (Halcion), a short-acting benzodiazepine hypnotic, is one of the most widely prescribed sedative-hypnotic agents in the United States. Because triazolam is rapidly absorbed, has no active metabolites, and does not accumulate, residual daytime sedation is less of a problem than with longer-acting benzodiazepines. The usual dosage of triazolam is 0.125 to 0.25 mg, given orally. Triazolam is different from other benzodiazepines in that it does not suppress stage IV (deep) sleep; therefore, it is not used to treat *somnambulism* (sleep walking).

After its introduction there was much controversy regarding the use of triazolam in regard to anterograde amnesia and psychiatric side effects. Following a review in 1992, the FDA declared triazolam to be a safe and effective medication, although it recommended that caution regarding possible memory problems be exercised.

○ **Alprazolam** (Xanax) is the only benzodiazepine with FDA indications for both anxiety and panic disorders. It appears to have some actions resembling the tricyclic antidepressants while maintaining the anxiolytic properties of benzodiazepines. Low doses of selective serotonin uptake inhibitors (SSRIs) are also frequently used for this purpose (see Chapter 26 for a discussion of SSRIs).

▼ **CLINICAL ALERT**

When alprazolam is discontinued, it is cleared from the system very rapidly. Abruptly stopping alprazolam may result in rebound CNS excitation, including seizures. It is important to warn the patient of this danger.

○ **Lorazepam** (Ativan) is a useful benzodiazepine for the treatment of anxiety. It is usually given orally in a daily divided dosage of 1 to 10 mg, with the largest dose given at bedtime. The plasma half-life of lorazepam is not age dependent or lengthened by liver disease; thus, it is frequently used to treat anxiety in the elderly. The dosage is reduced in geriatric patients because of their greater CNS sensitivity, not because of the drug's metabolite accumulation. The memory impairment sometimes observed may either be an intentional benefit (e.g., in surgical situations) or an undesired side effect. Lorazepam may also be administered parenterally.

BARBITURATES

The barbiturates—**pentobarbital (Nembutal, Nembutal Sodium), secobarbital (Seconal Sodium), amobarbital (Amytal, Amytal Sodium), aprobarbital (Alurate), butabarbital (Butisol Sodium), mephobarbital (Mebaral),** and **phenobarbital (Barbita, Solfoton)**—are a large class of drugs derived from barbituric acid that produce a nonspecific CNS depression. Although still used for treatment of insomnia, anxiety, and daytime sedation, barbiturates have generally been replaced by the much safer benzodiazepines. Table 25–3 features nursing implications for the barbiturates and provides dosage and pharmacokinetic information for secobarbital.

ACTION

All barbiturates are derived from the same substance, barbituric acid, and have similar mechanisms of action and side effects. Barbiturates are capable of producing all levels of CNS depression, from mild sedation to hypnosis to death by respiratory depression. Their precise effect on neurotransmitters is unclear, but they apparently decrease the excitability of both presynaptic and postsynaptic membranes in the cerebral cortex and reticular formation. Relatively low doses of barbiturates depress the sensory cortex, decrease motor activity, and produce sedation and drowsiness. In some individuals, however, drowsiness is preceded by transient elation, confusion, or excitement, which increases the abuse potential of these drugs.

Barbiturates also reduce random eye movement (REM) sleep and decrease sleep stages III and IV. Sleep disruption due to REM rebound is common following discontinuation of barbiturates.

Table 25–3. SEDATIVE, HYPNOTIC, AND ANXIOLYTIC DRUGS: BARBITURATES

DRUG NAME/ROUTE AND DOSAGE	PHARMACOKINETICS/ DYNAMICS	NURSING IMPLICATIONS
secobarbital (Seconal Sodium)		
sedation **Adults:** 30–50 mg PO 3–4 times daily. **hypnotic** **Adults:** 100 mg PO hs; 100–200 mg IM; or 50–250 mg IV. **Children:** 3–5 mg/kg IM, not to exceed 100 mg; or 4–5 mg/kg rectally. **Geriatric:** lower dose may be needed. **preoperative sedation** **Adults:** 200–300 mg PO 1–2 hr before surgery; or 1.1–1.6 mg/kg IM 10–15 min before surgery (light sedation). **Children:** 2–6 mg/kg PO 1–2 hr before surgery, not to exceed 100 mg/dose; or 4–5 mg/kg rectally.	**Onset:** PO, 10–15 min **Peak:** PO, 2–4 hr; IM, 7–10 min; IV, 1–3 min **Duration:** 3–4 hr **½L:** about 30 hr **PB:** 30%–45% **B:** hepatic **E:** renal	**ASSESSMENT:** Assess the patient's suicide potential. Assess respiratory status, pulse, and blood pressure frequently in patients receiving barbiturates IV. Assess for pregnancy (category D). **INTERVENTION:** Most barbiturates are absorbed rapidly and quickly promote calmness and sleep. Drug dependence may occur; monitor patient closely. Do not abruptly discontinue drug. Watch depressed, suicidal, or drug-dependent patient for signs of barbiturate toxicity: coma, pupillary constriction, cyanosis, clammy skin, and hypotension. **Patient Teaching**—Advise patient that drowsiness, light-headedness, or dizziness may occur. Caution patient to avoid activities requiring mental alertness such as driving or operating machinery until CNS effects are known. Warn patient to avoid alcoholic beverages and other CNS depressants. Note policies and legal restrictions applying to barbiturates. **EVALUATION:** Look for characteristics of tolerance to same dose, which can occur within 7–14 days. Evaluate patient routinely for signs of dependency; and elderly patient for paradoxic reactions (excitation). Report skin eruptions to physician, as these may proceed potentially fatal reactions.

USES

Besides their occasional use for insomnia and anxiety, some barbiturates are indicated as anticonvulsants; they are also used as preoperative medications. A discussion of these uses can be found in Chapters 20 and 21, respectively.

PHARMACOKINETICS

All of the barbiturates are absorbed both orally and rectally. The rate of absorption after oral ingestion is rapid, but slows with the presence of food in the stomach. Rapid absorption leads to a rapid onset of action, which causes initial feelings of dizziness and excitement.

Major differences among barbiturates occur in the onset of action and duration of effect, as shown in Table 25–4.

Table 25–4. TIME COURSE OF ACTION FOR BARBITURATES

Barbiturate	Onset (min)*	Duration (hr)*
Short Acting		
Pentobarbital	10–15	3–4
Secobarbital	10–15	3–4
Intermediate Acting		
Amobarbital	45–60	6–8
Aprobarbital	45–60	6–8
Butabarbital	45–60	6–8
Long Acting		
Mephobarbital	60+	10–12
Phenobarbital	60+	10–12

*For oral dosage forms.

The barbiturates are distributed throughout the tissues and fluids of the body. Lipid solubility is the dominant reason that high concentrations are found in the brain. Barbiturates that are most lipid soluble (e.g., thiopental) are suitable for use as anesthetics because they penetrate the blood-brain barrier rapidly (see Chapter 21 for a discussion of preanesthetic medications). Less lipophilic barbiturates such as phenobarbital penetrate and leave the brain more slowly and therefore have a slower onset and longer duration of action. Barbiturates cross the placental barrier and pass into the milk of nursing women.

The barbiturates are metabolized in the liver and excreted as inactive metabolites in the urine. These drugs stimulate microsomal enzymes in the liver; continued use may increase the rate of metabolism of certain other drugs. A tolerance to the effects of barbiturates develops, usually within 7 to 14 days, and use of barbiturates for a period of only 1 month may lead to dependence. Barbiturates with long half-lives tend to have a cumulative effect, creating the feeling of a hangover upon awakening.

CONTRAINDICATIONS AND PRECAUTIONS

Patients with pulmonary disorders and debilitated patients suffering from pulmonary insufficiency are not given barbiturates because they are extremely sensitive to the respiratory depressant action of these drugs. Barbiturates must be used with extreme caution in patients with decreased hepatic or renal function because of alterations in the rate of metabolism and excretion of the drug, which increases the possibility of overdose.

▼ **CLINICAL ALERT**

Geriatric and debilitated patients are more likely to react to usual doses of barbiturates with excitement (paradoxic reaction), confusion, or mental depression. Therefore, lower doses are always advised if and when barbiturates are prescribed for geriatric patients. Unless analgesics are also given, barbiturates are contraindicated in patients with pain, because they may increase the reaction to painful stimuli.

Barbiturates (pregnancy category D) have been shown to cause an increased incidence of fetal abnormalities; risk-to-benefit ratio must be carefully considered in life-threatening situations or serious conditions for which other medications cannot be used or are ineffective. Use of barbiturates in the third trimester of pregnancy may cause physical dependence in the newborn. Withdrawal symptoms such as seizures and hyperirritability may have a delayed onset of up to 14 days after birth.

Barbiturate use is also contraindicated in patients with intermittent *porphyria* (a disorder of porphyrin metabolism). Administration of a barbiturate to a patient with this condition causes an increase in the level of porphyrins, leading to paralysis and death.

ADVERSE REACTIONS

The most frequent adverse effects are the neurologic extensions of CNS depression. Infrequent side effects include nausea, diarrhea, headache, joint or muscle pain, vomiting, dyspnea, hives, sore throat, fever, angioedema, bradycardia, wheezing, and jaundice. Paradoxic reactions of excitement, confusion, and hostility may be seen, mainly in elderly patients and in patients with severe pain.

INTERACTIONS

The barbiturates interact problematically with many other drugs. They should not be given concurrently with any other CNS depressant, because this combination creates further depressant effects, especially respiratory depression. Barbiturates may also decrease the effectiveness of estrogens, estrogen-containing contraceptives, anticoagulants (coumarin or indanedione derivatives), steroids, digitoxin, and quinidine. Barbiturates, especially phenobarbital, stimulate the microsomal enzymes responsible for metabolizing these drugs. When these drugs are metabolized faster, lower blood levels result and their pharmacologic effects are shortened.

○ **Secobarbital** (Seconal Sodium) is a short-acting barbiturate used for sedation, insomnia, preoperative sedation, status epilepticus, and acute tetanus convulsions. Secobarbital can be administered orally, parentally, or rectally. It promote sleepiness within 10 to 15 minutes following an oral dose of 200 to 300 mg. A single oral dose has a duration of 4 to 6 hours, but residual sedative effects may last as long as 48 hours. It is a Schedule II controlled substance.

OTHER BARBITURATES

Pentobarbital (Nembutol, Nembutal Sodium), amobarbital (Amytal, Amytal Sodium), butabarbital (Butisol), and aprobarbital (Alurate) have all been used as hypnotics. These barbiturates produce sleep within 45 to 60 minutes. A single dose usually has a duration of 6 to 8 hours, but the residual sedative effects may last up to 2 days. Amobarbital is also used for daytime sedation in lower, divided doses. Pentobarbital and amobarbital are both Schedule II controlled substances; aprobarbital and butabarbital are Schedule III. Phenobarbital (Barbita, Solfoton) is a slow-onset, long-acting barbiturate frequently used for its anticonvulsant action (see Chapter 20). Even when administered intravenously, it may take 15 or more minutes to reach peak concentration in the brain.

MISCELLANEOUS SEDATIVE, HYPNOTIC, AND ANXIOLYTIC DRUGS

Besides the benzodiazepines and the barbiturates, numerous drugs from a variety of chemical classes have been used as CNS depressants. These include **busprione (BuSpar), zolpidem tartrate (Ambien), diphenhydramine (Benadryl), doxylamine (Doxysom, Sleep Easy, Unisom), hydroxyzine (Atarax, Vistaril), chloral hydrate (Noctec, Somnos), ethchlorvynol (Placidyl), glutethimede (Doriden), meprobamate (Equanil, Miltown), paraldehyde,** and **propranolol (Inderal)**.

In addition, antidepressants (discussed in Chapter 27) are sometimes used for anxiety, including panic attacks, as are monoamine oxidase inhibitors. Neuroleptics have not been found effective in the treatment of anxiety unless the anxiety is associated with dementia, delirium, or psychosis.

○ **Buspirone** (BuSpar), a nonbenzodiazepine antianxiety drug, is the first drug of the azapirone class to become available for clinical use. It does not cause sedation and has no known potential for abuse.

ACTION Buspirone does not bind to the GABA–benzodiazepine receptor complex and appears to act via partial stimulation of the serotonin ($5-HT_{1A}$) receptors. Cross-tolerance to benzodiazepines, alcohol, and other CNS agents does not occur. No withdrawal or rebound effects are associated with buspirone discontinuation.

USES Buspirone is approved for the treatment of generalized anxiety and anxiety with coexisting depressive symptoms. It is primarily used to treat chronic anxiety, and its efficacy is comparable to that of the benzodiazepines, although the onset of clinical effects is more gradual. Buspirone may offer several advantages over both the barbiturates and the benzodiazepines. It appears to cause less sedation and less impairment of motor skills, does not potentiate the effects of alcohol, and has no apparent abuse potential. Withdrawal symptoms are not reported after discontinuation of therapy. Because it takes 1 to 4 weeks to work, it is not indicated for acute anxiety or panic attacks.

ADVERSE EFFECTS Adverse reactions to buspirone are infrequent and have a distinctly different profile than those of other CNS depressants. Dizziness, lightheadedness, nausea, headache, and paradoxic excitement are the most commonly observed side effects. The absence of noticable side effects, combined with the nonsedating, nonrewarding, and nonreinforcing profile of buspirone have tended to raise concerns about efficacy and decreased patient satisfaction. The gradual onset of effects and the absence of sedation may lead patients to believe that the drug is ineffective.

The safety of buspirone in pregnancy (category B) and lactation has not been established. It is also unknown whether it crosses the placenta or is excreted in breast milk. Pharmacokinetics, dosages, and nursing implications for buspirone are listed in Table 25–5.

○ **Zolpidem tartrate** (Ambien), a nonbenzodiazepine of the imidazopyridine class, is indicated for the short-term management (7 to 10 days) of insomnia.

ACTION Zolpidem interacts with and modulates the action of the GABA–benzodiazepine receptor complex (thought to be responsible for sedative, anticonvulsant, and anxiolytic drug properties) by binding to and activating omega receptor subtypes. Although chemically unrelated to benzodiazepines, barbiturates, and other known hypnotics, it shares some of the pharmacologic properties of the benzodiazepines. Zolpidem generally preserves all stages of sleep, including deep sleep. This effect is thought to be related to zolpidem's preferential binding to omega$_1$ receptors.

CONTRAINDICATIONS AND PRECAUTIONS Use zolpidem cautiously in patients with compromised respiratory status because hypnotics may depress respiratory drive. Also use cautiously in patients with a history of alcohol or drug abuse or in those with depression. Use during pregnancy only if clearly needed. Zolpidem is excreted in breast milk, so its use in lactation is not recommended. Safety in children has not been established.

ADVERSE EFFECTS Most adverse effects are dose related; use the smallest effective dose, especially in elderly

Table 25–5. MISCELLANEOUS SEDATIVE, HYPNOTIC, AND ANXIOLYTIC DRUGS

DRUG NAME/ROUTE AND DOSAGE	PHARMACOKINETICS/ DYNAMICS	NURSING IMPLICATIONS
buspirone (BuSpar)		
Adults: 5 mg PO tid up to 60 mg/day.	**Onset:** 1–2 wk (therapeutic effect); 3–4 wk (optimal effect) **Peak:** 0.6–1.5 hr (blood level) **Duration:** 4–8 hr **½L:** 2–3 hr **PB:** 95% **B:** hepatic (active metabolites) **E:** renal	**ASSESSMENT:** Assess degree and manifestations of anxiety before and periodically throughout therapy. Assess for pregnancy (category B). **INTERVENTION:** Patients switching from another sedative need to taper it, because buspirone does not prevent withdrawal symptoms. **Patient Teaching**—Advise patient that drug has no sedative actions and that it may take a few weeks before effects are noticed. Caution patient to avoid activities requiring alertness until CNS effects (dizziness, restlessness) of drug are known. Tell patient to notify physician if pregnancy is suspected. **EVALUATION:** Notify physician if dystonia, motor restlessness, or involuntary movements of facial or cervical muscles occur.
zolpidem tartrate (Ambien)		
Adults: Dosage is individualized. Usual dose is 10 mg PO just before bedtime. *Geriatric:* Initially, 5 mg just before bedtime.	**Onset:** NA **Peak:** 1.6 hr (blood level) **Duration:** NA **½L:** 2.5 hr **PB:** 92.5% **B:** hepatic **E:** renal	**ASSESSMENT:** Assess respiratory, renal, and hepatic function (dosage reduction recommended in hepatic dysfunction). Assess history of drug abuse (including alcohol) and suicide potential. Assess for pregnancy (category B). **INTERVENTION:** Zolpidem is used only for short-term management of insomnia, usually 7–10 days. Patient should be reevaluated if drug is taken for more than 2–3 weeks. Monitor patients at risk of habituation and dependence closely. Monitor elderly or debilitated patients as they may be more sensitive to the effects of zolpidem. Do not abruptly discontinue drug. **Patient Teaching**—Advise patient that drowsiness or dizziness may occur. Caution patient to avoid activities requiring mental alertness such as driving or operating machinery until CNS effects are known. Warn patient to avoid alcoholic beverages and other CNS depressants because effects are additive. For faster sleep onset, instruct patient to not take drug with or immediately after a meal. **EVALUATION:** Evaluate for effectiveness of therapy and adverse effects. Report amnesia or excessive drowsiness or dizziness to physician.

NA = not available.

or debilitated patients, because they may be more sensitive to the effects of zolpidem. The most common adverse effects observed with short-term zolpidem therapy are drowsiness, dizziness, and diarrhea. Other adverse effects include amnesia, headache, hangover effect, and vomiting. Abrupt discontinuation of zolpidem rarely may produce withdrawal signs and symptoms: fatigue, nausea, flushing, light-headedness, uncontrolled crying, emesis, stomach discomfort and cramps, panic attack, and nervousness.

Refer to Table 25–5 for pharmacokinetics, dosages, and nursing implications.

○ **Diphenhydramine** (Benadryl), **doxylamine** (Unisom Nighttime Sleep Aid), and **hydroxyzine** (Vistaril, Atarax) are antihistamines that may be useful for treating insomnia because of their sedative actions, but they are not very effective in reducing anxiety. Diphenhydramine and doxylamine are mild sedatives available over the counter as sleeping aids for the treatment of insomnia. Use of these drugs in the treatment of individuals with anxiety associated with pruritic dermatosis may produce desired results. Hydroxyzine is also used as an adjunct to anesthesia because of its antiemetic effects and additive effects with CNS depressants and anticholinergics.

○ **Chloral hydrate** (Noctec, Somnos) is one of the oldest hypnotics and is well tolerated by elderly patients. It is absorbed rapidly when given orally and is converted to the active metabolite, trichloroethanol, in the liver. This metabolite produces the hypnotic effect. This drug can produce side effects of nausea, vomiting, and flatulence. Its taste is unpleasant; therefore, it is given with food or in capsule form with plenty of water. Chloral hydrate may also produce tolerance and drug dependency.

○ **Ethchlorvynol** (Placidyl), **glutethimide** (Doriden), and **meprobamate** (Equanil, Miltown) are nonbarbiturate CNS depressants that were previously used as hypnotics. These drugs cause both physical and psychologic dependence and have been the cause of overdose and suicide. Their use as sedative-hypnotics is not recommended.

○ **Paraldehyde** is an older drug that is an effective CNS depressant for use as an anxiolytic and for alcohol withdrawal syndrome. One unique property is that it is not dependent on the kidneys for elimination; thus, it is suitable for administration to patients with poor renal function.

○ **Propranolol** (Inderal, Inderal LA, Detensol) is a beta-adrenergic blocking agent that is sometimes used for treating specific symptoms of anxiety. However, the FDA has not approved propranolol for this indication. With beta-blockers, patients often feel a rapid resolution of their physical anxiety symptoms. The suggested anxiolytic daily dose is 10 to 120 mg given orally.

USING THE NURSING PROCESS

Use of sedative, hypnotic, or anxiolytic medications is a difficult process because each individual has a unique pattern of response to increased levels of anxiety. Patients who receive the maximum therapeutic benefit from these

Table 25–6. ASSESSMENT OF LEVELS OF ANXIETY	
Level	Characteristics
Mild (+)	Perceptual field is broadened: perceptual abilities are intensified. Learning and problem-solving abilities are enhanced. Able to connect feelings, thoughts, and actions. Motivated to focus on the here-and-now problems. Able to make cause-and-effect relationships. Appears calm.
Moderate (++)	Perceptual field is narrowed. Experiences selective inattention—fails to notice what goes on in situations peripheral to the immediate focus, but can attend to the stimuli if they are pointed out. Alertness is increased, reaching its highest, most efficient level. Able to connect feelings, thoughts, and actions. Experiences feelings of tension and challenge. Uses ego defense mechanisms. May appear tense and restless.
Severe (+++)	Perceptual field is greatly decreased. Selective inattention continues, but forces the person to focus on one small part of the problem or environment. Dissociation may occur. Learning and problem-solving abilities are decreased. Unable to connect feelings, thoughts, and actions. Behaviors are aimed at obtaining immediate relief from the anxiety. Appears tense and manifests cues of physiologic response to anxiety, such as increased respirations, pulse, and blood pressure.
Panic (++++)	Person experiences intense feelings of panic, awe, dread, terror, gloom and doom. Dissociation continues. Perception of reality becomes difficult: details within the environment may appear enlarged or scattered and spinning. Learning and problem-solving abilities are nonexistent. Behavior is focused on gaining or maintaining control. Symptoms of helplessness, hopelessness, rage may be observed. Symptoms of physiologic response to anxiety such as hypertension and hyperventilation syndrome may occur.

medications are those who demonstrate both psychologic and physiologic symptoms of anxiety. An increase in a person's level of anxiety creates physiologic, cognitive, behavioral, and emotional changes. Table 25–6 reviews the response categorization to anxiety levels and highlights the physiologic, cognitive, behavioral, and emotional characteristics of each of the four levels of anxiety.

ASSESSMENT

• Following an estimate of the patient's level of anxiety, determine associated factors, everyday stress, and how the increased level of anxiety is affecting the patient's ability to manage activities of daily living. Assessment information is provided in Table 25–7.

Table 25–7. NURSING PROCESS FOR PATIENTS REQUIRING SEDATIVES, HYPNOTICS, AND ANXIOLYTICS

Assessment

Assess sleeping patterns during both day and night, including presleep activities/rituals, and effects of pattern on patient's life.
Assess history of past and current health problems.
Assess mental status and level of anxiety, noting presence of phobias, obsessions, compulsions.
Assess current/past coping behaviors.

Nursing Diagnosis: Sleep Pattern Disturbance

RELATED TO: Anxiety/depression, inactivity, illness/pain.
AS EVIDENCED BY: Difficulty falling asleep, awakening earlier or later than desired, interrupted sleep, complaints of feeling tired.

Desired Outcomes/Evaluation Criteria

Reports improvement in sleep/rest pattern with increased sense of well-being/feeling rested upon awakening.
Appears relaxed. Vital signs are within normal limits.

Nursing Actions	Rationale
Recommend avoidance of caffeine-containing substances at least 2 hr before bedtime.	Stimulation may interfere with REM sleep.
Decrease environmental stimuli. Encourage use of relaxation techniques prior to bedtime.	Reduces muscle tension, aids in refocusing attention, promoting rest/sleep.
Acknowledge difficulty and frustration of insomnia.	Communicates empathy and aids in reduction of associated anxiety.
Administer medication as indicated.	Short-term use of antianxiolytics, sedatives, hypnotics may help until other problems are resolved.
Evaluate whether desired therapeutic effect is achieved.	Promotes optimal medication response with minimal side effects.

Nursing Diagnosis: Anxiety, moderate level

RELATED TO: Stressful event.
AS EVIDENCED BY: Increased tension, feelings of helplessness, inability to sleep and eat, weight loss/gain.

Desired Outcomes/Evaluation Criteria

Reports anxiety is reduced to manageable level.
Identifies stress situations and specific actions to deal with them.

Nursing Actions	Rationale
Encourage patient to acknowledge and express feelings.	Helps to identify and deal with underlying feelings.
Use problem-solving techniques to help patient to make appropriate choices for individual situation. Actively listen to patient.	Promotes adaptive coping behaviors that may have been impaired by high anxiety level.
Provide accurate information about situation.	Promotes dealing with realities.

Other Suggested Nursing Diagnoses: Severe to Panic-Level Anxiety and Knowledge Deficit.

- Ask the patient about sleep habits and whether or not a specific event or problem is causing the sleep disturbance. Observe the patient during sleep if possible.
- Listen to the patient's cues regarding the ability to sleep and his or her preferences for medication.
- The practice of giving hypnotics on an as-needed (PRN) basis to promote sleep when patients are admitted is not recommended.
- Determine whether the patient is experiencing the desired effect from the same dosage or has developed a tolerance to the drug.
- Be alert to cues of physical dependency. Many of these drugs are addictive. Complete withdrawal from certain benzodiazepines may not occur for 7 to 10 days after the last dose because of the relatively long half-lives of some of these drugs.
- Recognize the potential for these drugs to cause paradoxic reactions, such as hallucinations, hostility, insomnia, and confusion.

- Assess the patient's suicide potential because death may result from sedative-hypnotic overdose. Pay special attention to alcohol use and the availability of other sleeping or anxiolytic medications, including over-the-counter medications.

NURSING DIAGNOSIS

- Nursing diagnoses focus on each patient's and family's responses to anxiety disorders and/or sleep problems. Possible nursing diagnoses include Sleep Pattern Disturbance, Moderate-Level Anxiety, Severe to Panic-Level Anxiety, and Knowledge Deficit (see Table 25–7).

PLANNING AND INTERVENTION

- Recommend interventions to promote good sleep habits: Avoid caffeine-containing substances, decrease environmental stimuli, maintain regular bedtime, avoid daytime naps, develop a bedtime ritual, and avoid alcohol. Help the patient maximize the effects of hypnotic drugs by suggesting sleep habits that minimize insomnia.

- Encourage the patient to acknowledge and express feelings underlying anxiety. Problem-solving techniques can be used to assist the patient to make appropriate choices. Assist in providing accurate information about the situation and be an active listener.
- Administer medications as prescribed. Encourage the use of relaxation exercises 30 minutes after drug administration. Stay with the severely anxious patient for a short while after administering the medication if possible; a calm, supportive manner promotes the maximal effect of the medication.
- Monitor the patient's level of anxiety and insomnia because both tend to fluctuate according to changes in circumstances and the environment. The frequency of checks is correlated with the severity of the patient's symptoms. Recognize the early cues that indicate a patient's level of anxiety is rising.
- Teach the patient the information covered in the teaching plan, as shown in Table 25–8.

EVALUATION

The effectiveness of therapy is based on an appraisal of the reduction of target symptom(s) and the patient's understanding of the treatment regimen.

- Evaluate the patient's level of anxiety. Has it decreased? Is he or she able to focus on the current situation and to connect current feelings and thoughts with actions?
- Evaluate the patient's physical symptoms of anxiety such as pulse rate and blood pressure. Evidence of decreased anxiety is usually observed within 1 hour of an oral dose of most of these drugs.
- When the patient is being treated for insomnia, evaluate the individual's sleep patterns by observation in the hospital and by patient assessment in outpatient settings. Determine any positive changes in sleep habits. Determine whether the person wakes up feeling rested or "hung over." Listen for remarks by the patient about dreaming during the night.
- Evaluate the patient's knowledge about the medication.
- Watch for signs of increased suicide potential. Many of these medicines, when combined with other CNS depressants, may be used as a means of suicide.

Patients Receiving Benzodiazepines

- Evaluate the patient both for signs of a favorable response to the anxiolytic drug and for side effects. Drowsiness and ataxia are most common. Recognize how frustrating these side effects can be to the patient and reassure him or her that the effects tend to decrease as the body becomes adjusted to the drug.
- Encourage the patient to take the drug during or immediately following meals to alleviate the intensity of gastrointestinal discomfort, nausea, or vomiting that may develop.
- Evaluate whether the patient is experiencing any of the infrequently reported side effects, such as blurred vision, hypotension, depression, urinary retention, or incontinence. If these symptoms occur, consult the physician.
- Evaluate the patient for symptoms of paradoxic reactions: excitement, hostility, rage, confusion, hallucinations, and acute hyperpyrexia. If these symptoms appear, withhold the medication and contact the physician immediately.

Patients Receiving Barbiturates

- Observe the patient to determine whether he or she is experiencing side effects such as nausea, drowsiness, and slurred speech.

Table 25–8. PATIENT TEACHING INFORMATION—SEDATIVES, HYPNOTICS, AND ANXIOLYTICS

Dear Patient:
This drug has been prescribed for you. This is what you should know about your drug to get the most from your therapy:

☐ 1. This drug will help you to relax. Or, this drug will help you to sleep.

☐ 2. This drug is usually not to be taken for more than a few months. Check with your physician to make sure you need to continue taking it.

☐ 3. Take this medication only as directed by your physician. Do not take more of it or take it more frequently or for a longer period than your physician ordered. It may become habit forming (causing psychologic or physical dependence) if too much is taken.

☐ 4. This drug will add to the effects of alcohol and other drugs that slow down the nervous system, such as antihistamines, pain medications, seizure medication, tranquilizers, and other sedatives. Check with your physician before taking this with any of these medications.

☐ 5. If you forget to take a dose (while taking it regularly) and if you remember the missed dose within an hour of missing it, take it immediately. However, if you do not remember until later, skip the dose and go back to your regular schedule. Do not double the dose.

☐ 6. Do not stop taking this medicine without first discussing this with your physician. Your physician will want you to gradually reduce the amount you are taking. Stopping this medicine suddenly may cause serious side effects.

☐ 7. When you begin taking this medicine, it may take a few days before you receive the full effects of the medicine. This is especially true for patients taking buspirone (BuSpar).

☐ 8. Do not drink beer, wine, or alcohol while you are taking this medicine. The effects of the alcohol will be intensified.

☐ 9. This drug may cause you to feel drowsy, dizzy, or lightheaded. Be sure you know how the drug affects you before you drive or participate in other activities that require you to be alert, such as operating machinery.

☐ 10. Keep this medicine out of reach of children because overdose may be especially dangerous to children.

- Evaluate the patient for less frequent side effects such as mental confusion, depression, sore throat, fever, angioedema, wheezing, and paradoxic reactions of excitement or hostility. If these symptoms are observed, consult the physician.
- Monitor the patient carefully for overdose and suicide potential because barbiturates can be extremely dangerous.

- Determine whether the patient has experienced any symptoms of physical or psychologic dependence, such as reports of decreased effect of the same dose or a desire to increase dosage.

The bibliography for this chapter can be found in Appendix B, which begins on page 1054.

CHAPTER REVIEW QUESTIONS*

1. The effects of benzodiazepines are believed to result from:
   a. Stimulation of a neuronal receptor, which is closely linked with the neurotransmitter, gamma-aminobutyric acid (GABA).
   b. Cumulative effects on the neurotransmitter norepinephrine.
   c. Blockage of the neurotransmitter dopamine, which results in lower levels of dopamine at the synapse.
   d. An overall increase in neuronal inhibition in the central nervous system, especially the cortical areas.

2. Benzodiazepines are useful for all the following indications *except*:
   a. Short-term treatment of insomnia.
   b. Anxiety.
   c. Psychiatric depression.
   d. Severe anxiety with depression.

3. In comparing the use of benzodiazepines with that of barbiturates, the following is *correct*:
   a. Benzodiazepines are used less frequently than barbiturates.

b. Benzodiazepines are more likely to be fatal in overdose.
   c. Benzodiazepines are contraindicated in patients with pulmonary disorders, but barbiturates are considered safe.
   d. Benzodiazepines are believed to act via a specific receptor.

4. The benzodiazepine that has been most frequently associated with memory impairment is:
   a. Chlorazepate dipotassium (Tranxene).
   b. Chloral hydrate (Noctec).
   c. Oxazepam (Serax).
   d. Triazolam (Halcion).

5. Alprazolam (Xanax) is the only benzodiazepine with FDA indications for
   a. Anxiety associated with depression.
   b. Both anxiety and panic disorders.
   c. Sleep disturbances.
   d. Anxiety, muscle spasm, and epilepsy.

*See Appendix A, which begins on page 1051, for answers.

CHAPTER 26

Drugs Used to Treat Mood Disorders

Meredith A. Davison, PhD

KEY TERMS

Bipolar disorder
Cyclic antidepressant
Depression
Enterohepatic recycling
Extrapyramidal syndrome
Hepatic first-pass effect
Mania
Monoamine oxidase (MAO) inhibitor
Selective serotonin reuptake inhibitors
Tricyclic antidepressant

LEARNING OBJECTIVES

After reading this chapter, the student will be able to:

1. Identify medications commonly used to treat mood disorders.
2. Differentiate among the drugs used to treat mood disorders as to mechanism of action, route of administration, pharmacokinetics, adverse effects, contraindications and precautions, and interactions.
3. Identify nursing assessments for the patient who requires drugs to treat mood disorders to formulate appropriate patient outcomes.
4. Plan the nursing interventions necessary to administer drugs used to treat mood disorders, and choose appropriate teaching strategies for the patient and family.
5. Evaluate the patient routinely during treatment to assess response to medication and nursing interventions.

Mood is defined as a conscious state of mind or predominant emotion. This term is used to refer to an individual's prevailing emotional attitude on which life events impinge. Mood fluctuates continually as part of our response to the world on a continuum from normal and functional to what is termed dysfunctional. Mood disorders are disturbances in mood that generally have to do with affective dysfunction.

Mood disorders are classified as depressive or bipolar. The essential feature of depressive disorder is major depression. *Depression* is an emotional state characterized by extreme dejection; gloomy ruminations; and feelings of worthlessness, hopelessness, and often apprehension. *Bipolar disorder* is characterized by mood swings from profound depression to extreme mania, with intervening periods of normalcy. In *mania*, the predominant mood is elevated, expansive, or irritable. The *Diagnostic and Statis-*

The publisher gratefully acknowledges the efforts of Mark D. Watanabe in preparation of this chapter.

Table 26–1. DEPRESSION
Definition Emotional state characterized by extreme dejection, gloomy ruminations, feelings of worthlessness, hopelessness, and often apprehension.
Types Grief reactions Pathologic grief reactions Adjustment reaction Major depression with melancholia Bipolar disorder, depressed Severe depression
Etiology The specific etiology of depression is unknown. There are numerous current theories relating to psychoanalytic, cognitive, psychodynamic, biologic, and sociocultural concepts. Currently, many researchers believe depression may result from a combination of many interrelated variables.
Symptoms The major symptoms include: a. A change in feelings toward sadness, loneliness, and apathy b. Vegetative physical changes (anorexia, constipation, fatigue, and changes in sleeping patterns) c. Changes in the level of activity ranging from psychomotor retardation to agitation d. Lowered self-esteem e. Suicidal thoughts
Treatment The goal of treatment is to have the person experience relief from the symptoms of depression. The type of treatment used depends on the differential diagnosis of the patient's depression. The major forms of treatments include: 1. Psychotherapy 2. Tricyclic antidepressants 3. Tetracyclic and other new types of antidepressants 4. Monoamine oxidase inhibitors 5. Amphetamines 6. Electroconvulsive therapy

tical Manual—IV (American Psychiatric Association, 1994) identifies a number of clinical conditions characterized by depression and/or mania that are not secondary to any other physical or mental disorder. Summaries of clinical depression and bipolar disorder are presented in Tables 26–1 and 26–2, respectively.

The drugs used to alleviate the symptoms of depression are called antidepressants. Lithium carbonate is the drug of choice for acute manic episodes in bipolar disorder and for the prevention or diminishment of subsequent manic episodes.

ANTIDEPRESSANTS

The current theory for the cause of depression is that supersensitivity of catecholamine receptors in the presence of low serotonin level permits the expression of the affective state governed by norepinephrine—low norepinephrine produces depression; high norepinephrine produces

mania. Antidepressants alter this biochemical imbalance of norepinephrine, serotonin, or both to alleviate depression. Figure 26–1 is a schematic diagram of the normal neurotransmitter system affected by these drugs.

Antidepressants fall into one of four major groups: cyclic antidepressants, selective serotonin reuptake inhibitors, monoamine oxidase inhibitors, or miscellaneous or atypical antidepressants.

CYCLIC ANTIDEPRESSANTS

Cyclic antidepressants, which include the tricyclic and tetracyclic antidepressants, are named as such because of their chemical structure—they are composed of one or more rings. For example, the *tricyclic antidepressants* have a three-ringed nucleus. The tricyclic antidepressants include **impramine *(Tofranil)*, doxepin *(Adapin, Sinequan)*, amitriptyline *(Elavil, Endep)*, desipramine *(Norpramin)*, nortriptyline *(Pamelor)*, protriptyline *(Vivactil)*, amoxapine *(Asendin)*, trimipramine *(Surmontil)*,** and **clomipramine *(Anafranil)*. Maprotiline *(Ludiomil)*** is a tetracyclic antidepressant. The cyclic antidepressants all share similar pharmacologic and toxicologic properties.

Action

Cyclic antidepressants are believed to potentiate the effects of norepinephrine and serotonin by blocking the reuptake of these neurotransmitters at nerve terminals. Through this blockade, more neurotransmitter is available to stimulate postsynaptic receptors, prolonging the stimulatory effects. Figure 26–2 illustrates how cyclic antidepressants may affect the functioning of the normal neurotransmitter system.

Table 26–2. BIPOLAR DISORDER
Definition Group of psychotic illnesses characterized by periods of elation and overactivity and/or by periods of depression and decreased activity levels or by alternation of the two.
Types Manic Depressed Mixed
Symptoms *Manic Type:* increased elation and optimism; talkative, boisterous; decreased ability to concentrate; distractibility; may develop delusions of grandeur *Depressed Type:* symptoms similar to ones listed in Table 26–1. *Mixed Type:* symptoms demonstrated depend on whether the person is in a period of the manic type or the depressed type
Treatment Lithium carbonate or lithium citrate is the treatment of choice. It is given to decrease symptomatology during an acute episode and prophylactically to prevent recurrence of symptoms. Usually the patient and family should have supportive psychotherapy to help them to develop insights into the illness and to cope adaptively with its long-term effects.

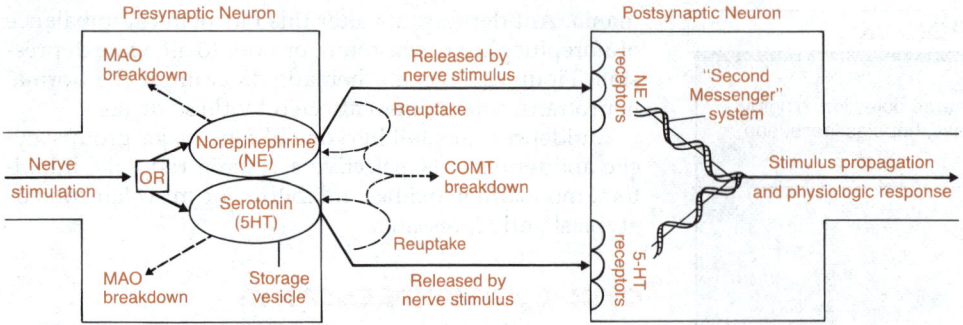

Figure 26–1. Schematic diagram showing normal release and metabolism of catecholamines at synaptic junctions.

Uses

Cyclic antidepressants are effective in relieving symptoms of depression in most patients. However, because of their numerous adverse side effects and the potential for overdose, these drugs are no longer considered the initial drug of choice for depression. But for patients who do not respond to other antidepressant medications, they are an excellent second choice.

Pharmacokinetics

Absorption The cyclic antidepressants are generally absorbed completely from the gastrointestinal system after oral administration. The rate of absorption varies: amoxapine (Asendin) reaches its peak plasma level within 90 minutes, whereas maprotiline (Ludiomil) does not do so for 8 to 24 hours. Absorption rates of other cyclic antidepressants are between these two extremes. Extent of absorption is reduced by significant hepatic first-pass effect, which reduces the average bioavailability of many of these agents. In *hepatic first-pass effect*, a drug that has been absorbed into the gastrointestinal system is extensively metabolized by the liver prior to reaching the systemic circulation. Concurrent ingestion of food appears to have minimal effects on bioavailability and peak concentration of these drugs.

Distribution Once absorbed, cyclic antidepressants (which are lipophilic compounds highly bound to plasma proteins and body tissues) are extensively distributed throughout the body. Very little accumulation occurs in adipose tissue; therefore, in obese patients the cyclic antidepressants will probably not have longer half-lives as the result of a larger volume of distribution. Measurement of concentrations of cyclic antidepressants in blood may be useful in determining optimal treatment levels or in predicting toxicity.

Metabolism All cyclic antidepressants undergo extensive hepatic metabolism, first being oxidized by microsomal enzymes, then being conjugated with glucuronic acid. Concurrent administration of phenobarbital or cigarette smoking may induce microsomal enzyme activity, resulting in an increase in metabolites. Many of the antidepressants are metabolized to clinically active substances. For example, imipramine is transformed to desipramine, which is available in addition to the parent compound. The extent of the contribution of the active metabolites to the overall clinical effect is not fully known.

Excretion Elimination of cyclic antidepressants occurs over a period of several days. The elimination rate slows once the plasma concentration has been stabilized. The cyclic antidepressants are primarily eliminated by a combination of hepatic metabolism and renal excretion of the conjugate. Some of the parent drug and its metabolites may be excreted in the feces via the bile. There is also some evidence of enterohepatic recycling. In *enterohepatic recycling*, a drug is secreted in the bile into the intestine, where it is reabsorbed into the systemic circulation. Because of the slow elimination, the drug sometimes may be detected in the urine for months after its discontinuation.

Contraindications and Precautions

Absolute contraindications to cyclic antidepressants include acute myocardial infarction and hypersensitivity. Caution must be taken in prescribing these drugs to patients with severe coronary artery disease. Most of the cyclic antidepressants lower the seizure threshold, so care must be taken when prescribing these agents to patients with a preexisting seizure disorder. The anticholinergic side effects of these drugs require caution in treating patients with angle-closure glaucoma, benign prostatic hy-

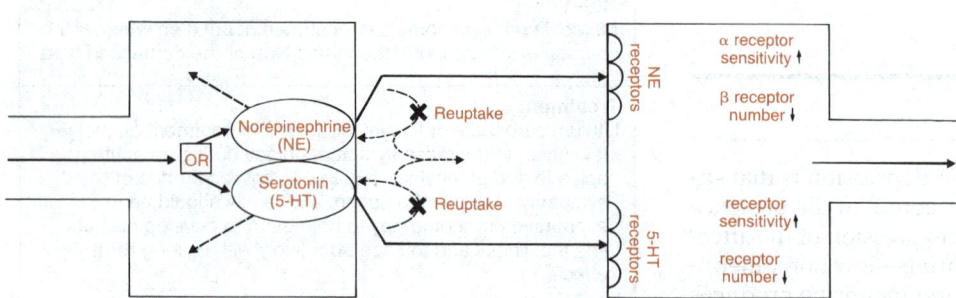

Figure 26–2. Proposed mechanism of action for antidepressants: blockade of catecholamine reuptake and regulation of postsynaptic receptor activity. (Compare with Fig. 26–1.)

pertrophy, and urinary retention. Experience with the use of these agents in pregnant women is limited, and the relative safety of these drugs is undefined. Cyclic antidepressants should be used only when the therapeutic benefits clearly outweigh the potential risks to the fetus.

Adverse Effects

Adverse reactions from cyclic antidepressants are common and range from mildly annoying to incapacitating and life threatening. If severe, the drug may need to be discontinued.

Disturbances of neurotransmission at noradrenergic, serotonergic, dopaminergic, histaminergic, and cholinergic nerve terminals are the biologic basis of the adverse reactions. The most troubling constellation of adverse reactions is due to cholinergic blockade: dry mucous membranes (especially dry mouth), blurred vision, urinary hesitancy, and constipation. Fortunately, tolerance to these effects usually develops, and starting therapy at lower doses minimizes anticholinergic reactions.

Most cyclic antidepressants cause orthostatic hypertension, a problem most significant in elderly and underweight patients. Sedation is also commonly reported, particularly with imipramine, amitriptyline, doxepin, and trimipramine. In patients with insomnia, this side effect may be beneficially exploited by giving the medication at bedtime.

Headaches, including migraines, can be caused by all antidepressants. Miscellaneous side effects include what has been described as the "switch process," a transition in certain patients from depression to mania or hypomania. In addition, confusion and/or delirium may be observed, most commonly in patients over age 50. These symptoms are secondary to central anticholinergic activity. A fine tremor is not unusual in patients receiving antidepressants. Other individuals may experience photosensitivity reactions.

Toxicity

Acute poisoning by cyclic antidepressants is not uncommon. The drugs given to treat severe depression are potentially lethal, especially as they are given to individuals with a high risk of suicide. Cardiovascular symptoms are predominant in cyclic antidepressant overdose and include depression of myocardial contractility, heart rate, and coronary blood flow; cardiac irregularities are frequent. Excessive anticholinergic activity of the central nervous system (CNS) may manifest as confusion or delirium, agitation, hallucinations, hyperpyrexia, and bowel or bladder paralysis. Other CNS effects may include seizures, ataxia, coma, and respiratory depression. Even when the phase of delirious intoxication has passed, the risk of life-threatening cardiac dysrhythmias continues. Cardiac symptoms are often difficult to manage and must be treated aggressively in cyclic antidepressant overdose.

Interactions

Cyclic antidepressants may interact with a wide variety of other medications. Concurrent use with monoamine oxidase (MAO) inhibitors causes hypotension and tachycardia. Cyclic antidepressants should not be used within two weeks of MAO inhibitor therapy. Cyclic antidepressants may prevent therapeutic responses to most antihypertensives. When used with clonidine, severe hypertension can occur, so concurrent use is avoided. Additive CNS depression can occur when cyclic antidepressants are taken with other CNS depressants, including alcohol, antihistamines, opiate analgesics, and sedative-hypnotics. Serum levels of cyclic antidepressants can be increased by concurrent use with cimetidine, fluoxetine, the phenothiazines, or oral contraceptives. This could lead to toxicity. Concurrent disulfiram may produce organic brain syndrome.

Cyclic antidepressants can also interfere with the results of laboratory tests. These agents can elevate serum bilirubin, alkaline phosphatase, and blood glucose; decrease urinary 5-hydroxyindoleacetic acid (5-HIAA) and vanillylmandelic acid (VMA) excretion; and falsely increase excretion of urinary catecholamines.

○ **Imipramine** (Tofranil), the oldest tricyclic antidepressant, is the prototype to which other antidepressants are compared. Since 1958, when imipramine was first reported to be effective in the treatment of depression, no other antidepressant has been consistently shown to be more effective. However, side effects from imipramine are often quite bothersome, particularly the anticholinergic effects and sedation, which are predominant when the medication is initiated. Refer to Table 26–3 for drug dosages, pharmacokinetics, and nursing implications for imipramine.

○ **Doxepin** (Adapin, Sinequan) is another tricyclic antidepressant that has a similar profile to that of imipramine. Sedation is quite prominent; thus, this drug may be preferred for a patient with agitated depression.

○ **Maprotiline** (Ludiomil) is a tetracyclic antidepressant that has significant anticholinergic properties. Refer to Table 26–3 for drug dosages, pharmacokinetics, and nursing implications for maprotiline.

SELECTIVE SEROTONIN REUPTAKE INHIBITORS

The role of serotonin in the pathophysiology of depression has been increasingly recognized in the last decade. This has lead to the development of antidepressants that produce selective blockade of serotonin reuptake. These antidepressants, called *selective serotonin reuptake inhibitors* (SSRIs), include **fluoxetine (Prozac), paroxetine (Paxil), sertraline hydrochloride (Zoloft)**, and **fluvoxamine (Luvox)**.

Action

The SSRIs are potent and selective inhibitors of serotonin reuptake in neurons in the CNS. They also have weak effect on norepinephrine and dopamine reuptake. However, there is no evidence of a direct relationship between the plasma concentration of the SSRIs, the changes in platelet serotonin transport, and clinical response to treatment. Long-term administration of these drugs to depressed patients actually increases the serotonin uptake.

Table 26–3. DRUGS USED TO TREAT DEPRESSION

DRUG NAME/ROUTE AND DOSAGE	PHARMACOKINETICS/DYNAMICS	NURSING IMPLICATIONS
TRICYCLIC ANTIDEPRESSANTS		
imipramine(Tofranil) **Adults:** 25–50 mg PO 3–4 times daily. Do not exceed 500 mg (100 mg in elderly). **childhood enuresis** **Children 6–12 yr:** 10–30 mg PO daily in 2 divided doses. **Adolescents:** 25–50 mg/day in divided doses (not to exceed 100 mg/day). **enuresis** **Children over 6 yr:** 25 mg once daily 1 hr before bedtime; increase if necessary by 25 mg at weekly intervals to 50 mg in children under 12 years, up to 75 mg in children over 12 years.	**Onset:** 2–4 weeks or longer (therapeutic effect) **Peak:** PO and IM, 2–4 hr **Duration:** PO and IM, 6–20 hr **½L:** 11–25 hr **PB:** 90% **B:** liver **E:** urine	**ASSESSMENT:** Assess patient's suicide potential routinely. Patient's risk may increase as he or she feels better. Monitor serum bilirubin, alkaline phosphatase, blood glucose, urinary catecholamines, urinary 5-HIAA and VMA excretion levels. Assess patient's responsiveness to the drug beginning at 2–3 weeks. Assess compliance with treatment regimen, nutritional intake, sleep patterns, and ability to function in activities of daily living. Assess supine and standing blood pressure daily. Assess for pregnancy (category B). **INTERVENTION:** Administer with or immediately following a meal to minimize gastric irritation. Monitor vital signs, ECGs, and mental status. **Patient Teaching**—Tell patient that desired response may not occur for 2–3 weeks. Teach patient to make position changes slowly to minimize orthostatic hypotension. **EVALUATION:** Evaluate for effectiveness and side effects of therapy.
TETRACYCLIC ANTIDEPRESSANTS		
maprotiline (Ludiomil) **Adults:** 75–225 mg/day PO.	**Onset:** 2–4 weeks or longer (therapeutic effect) **Peak:** 8–24 hr **Duration:** 51 hr **½L:** 51 hr **PB:** 90% **B:** liver (active metabolite) **E:** urine	Same as for imipramine.
SELECTIVE SEROTONIN REUPTAKE INHIBITOR		
fluoxetine (Prozac) **Adults:** 10–80 mg/day PO.	**Onset:** 2–4 weeks or longer (therapeutic effect) **Peak:** 6–8 days **Duration:** 10–21 hr **½L:** 2–3 days (fluoxetine); 7–9 days (norfluoxetine) **PB:** 90% **B:** liver (to active metabolite) **E:** urine, feces	Same as for imipramine plus: **ASSESSMENT:** Assess patient for alcohol intake and whether pregnant or breast feeding. **INTERVENTION:** Motor skills, judgment, and thinking may be impaired. **Patient Teaching**—Caution patient about performing tasks requiring coordination or judgment until effects of drug are known. Advise patient to limit alcohol intake. **EVALUATION:** Periodically evaluate the long-term (>1 yr) efficacy of this drug. Monitor patient for side effects.
MONOAMINE OXIDASE INHIBITOR		
tranylcypromine (Parnate) **Adults:** 30 mg/day PO in 2 divided doses (morning and afternoon). After 2 wk, dose can be increased by 10 mg/day, at 1 to 3-wk intervals (up to 60 mg/day). **Geriatric:** 2.5–5 mg/day PO, increased q 3–4 days up to 45 mg/day.	**Onset:** 2–4 weeks or longer (therapeutic effect) **Peak:** 1–3.5 hr (plasma level) **Duration:** 10–21 days (recovery of MAO activity after therapy discontinued) **½L:** NA **PB:** NA **B:** NA **E:** urine, feces	**ASSESSMENT:** Assess patient's suicide potential daily. Assess blood pressure and heart rate on a routine basis as well as patient's knowledge of dietary restrictions. Also monitor patient's laboratory values for hepatic function. **INTERVENTION:** Do not give at bedtime. Maintain patient on low-tyramine diet. Observe for signs of hypertension/hypotension. Protect patient from self-harm. **Patient Teaching**—Instruct patient to not take other medications because severe adverse effects can occur

Table 26–3. DRUGS USED TO TREAT DEPRESSION, *Continued*		
DRUG NAME/ROUTE AND DOSAGE	**PHARMACOKINETICS/ DYNAMICS**	**NURSING IMPLICATIONS**
		if MAO inhibitors are taken with CNS stimulants or vasoconstrictors; or OTC cold, hay fever, or diet preparations. Warn patients with angina to moderate activities to avoid overexertion (MAO inhibitors may alleviate chest pain). **EVALUATION:** Evaluate patient for signs of drug-drug and drug-food interactions, adverse drug reactions, and overdose.

ECG = electrocardiogram; NA = not available.

Uses

An SSRI is now generally the drug of first choice for treatment of mild to moderate depression. In addition to their proven clinical efficacy, the SSRIs are better tolerated by the patient because of their more acceptable side-effect profile. The SSRIs used for depression include fluoxetine, paroxetine, and sertraline. Fluoxetine and fluvoxamine are indicated for the treatment of obsessive-compulsive disorder.

Pharmacokinetics

The SSRIs have a slow rate of absorption, typically between 4 and 8 hours. Nausea can occur within 1 hour, suggesting a direct gastric effect. Substantial differences exist among the SSRIs in regard to their half-life, ranging from 13.5 hours for fluvoxamine to 4 to 15 days for fluoxetine (including its active metabolite norfluoxetine). Time to achieve a steady state in young, physically healthy adults is long: 7 days for fluvoxamine and sertraline, 10 days for paroxetine, and 28 to 35 days for fluoxetine.

Norfluoxetine, fluoxetine's active metabolite, is equipotent to the parent drug. Fluoxetine and paroxetine produce clinically meaningful inhibition of the hepatic isoenzyme IID6, leading to increased plasma levels of drugs metabolized via this enzyme, such as phenothiazines and group Ic antidysrhythmics. Age has a negligible effect on plasma sertraline levels, but a greater effect on paroxetine and fluoxetine levels.

Contraindications and Precautions

SSRIs are contraindicated in patients known to be hypersensitive to these agents. Also, SSRIs should not be used in combination with an MAO inhibitor or within 14 days of discontinuing therapy with an MAO inhibitor because of serious, sometimes fatal, reactions. Because SSRIs have very long elimination half-lives, it is *recommended* that at least 5 weeks be allowed after stopping an SSRI before prescribing an MAO inhibitor.

SSRIs are used with caution in patients with anxiety because this is a common side effect. Caution is also used in patients with altered appetite and weight because SSRIs can cause significant weight loss. SSRIs are administered cautiously to patients with a history of mania, as SSRIs can activate mania/hypomania. Because SSRIs may cause seizures, caution is used when these agents are given to patients with seizure disorders. Close supervision of patients at risk for suicide should accompany initial drug therapy, because the possibility of suicide is inherent in depression.

Adverse Effects

All of the SSRIs are well tolerated with a low incidence of life-threatening side effects. Nausea occurs quite frequently as a result of increased serotonergic activity in the gastrointestinal tract and possibly via central serotonin receptors; vomiting may also occur. Nausea usually dissipates after the first weeks of treatment.

Although anticholinergic effects are less common with the SSRIs than with the cyclic antidepressants, they may also accompany the use of these drugs, especially paroxetine. Cardiovascular side effects are not common with the SSRIs.

The CNS is affected by the SSRIs. Although both sedation and activation have been reported, SSRIs commonly cause activation overstimulation, or jitteriness, especially during the initial stage of treatment. This side effect may be more likely to occur in patients who have panic disorder. Antidepressant insomnia appears to be common with SSRIs. Antidepressant-associated sexual dysfunction, which may begin later rather than earlier during the course of therapy, is associated with SSRIs, particularly sertraline. In contrast to the cyclic antidepressants, SSRIs cause decreased appetite and/or weight loss. SSRIs are associated with a higher incidence of headache than other antidepressants. Two other rarely encountered adverse reactions to SSRIs include mild cognitive impairment and parathesias.

The safety and prolonged efficacy of the SSRIs render them particularly beneficial for the long-term treatment of depressed patients. In clinical trial experiences, the rate of early treatment discontinuations from adverse effects with a tricyclic antidepressant was seven times higher than that seen with the SSRIs.

Interactions

SSRIs must not be combined with MAO inhibitors, and at least 14 days should separate use of these drugs because of the risk of potentially fatal reactions. These reactions include hyperthermia, rigidity, myoclonus, rapid fluctuations of vital signs, confusion, delerium, and coma.

○ **Fluoxetine** (Prozac) was the first SSRI introduced. It has assumed enormous popularity, both with clinicians and the lay public, as the premier antidepressant. The favorable side-effect profile, coupled with efficacy on par with the older antidepressants, has led to this position. Fluoxetine and the other SSRIs have a large safety advantage over the traditional antidepressants, a distinct plus when treating potentially suicidal patients. Refer to Table 26–3 for drug dosages, pharmacokinetics, and nursing implications for fluoxetine.

MONOAMINE OXIDASE INHIBITORS

The *monoamine oxidase inhibitors* are a chemically diverse group of drugs that share the ability to interfere with the effects of monoamine oxidase (MAO) and alleviate clinical depression. The MAO inhibitor antidepressants include **phenelzine** *(Nardil)* and **tranylcypromine** *(Parnate)*.

Action

MAO inhibitors block the action of monoamine oxidase in the presynaptic nerve terminals and thus increase the concentration of these amines in CNS neurons. "Monoamine oxidase" refers to a number of enzymes present in cells within the brain, blood platelets, liver, spleen, and kidneys. The major function of these enzymes is to metabolize biogenic amines, such as the neurotransmitters epinephrine, norepinephrine, and serotonin. The action of the MAO inhibitors lends credence to the hypothesis that depression results from low levels of norepinephrine and/or dopamine. Figure 26–3 is a schematic diagram of this proposed mechanism of action.

Uses

The use of MAO inhibitors is usually limited to patients not responding to cyclic antidepressants, selective serotonin reuptake inhibitors, or electroconvulsive shock therapy. The MAO inhibitors are probably as effective as the cyclic antidepressants in the treatment of major depression, but because of their potentially severe and frequently unpredictable side effects, their medical use is limited.

Pharmacokinetics

The MAO inhibitors are well absorbed through the gastrointestinal tract when given orally. The maximum enzyme inhibition is observed within 5 to 10 days, but therapeutic effects may not be observed until 1 to 4 weeks following the start of therapy. The reason for this delay in response is unknown. Its similarity to the response observed with other antidepressants suggests that it may be due to reestablishing a new set-point for CNS emotional functioning.

The MAO inhibitors are rapidly metabolized by means of hepatic oxidation and acetylation. The metabolites are excreted quickly through the gastrointestinal tract. Because of the irreversible nature of MAO inactivation by phenelzine, up to 2 weeks may be required to restore amine metabolism after therapy with this drug is discontinued. Restoration following withdrawal of tranylcypromine is only slightly more rapid. Behavioral effects of tranylcypromine are also produced more rapidly, probably because of its amphetamine-like stimulant properties.

Contraindications and Precautions

Most of the contraindications to MAO inhibitors are related to the ability of these agents to increase circulating sympathomimetic amines. Caution should be exercised when using MAO inhibitors in patients with cardiovascular disease, hypertension, liver dysfunction, severe renal impairment, pheochromocytoma, and/or an inability to adhere to the required dietary and drug restrictions.

The effects of these agents on the developing fetus or on breast milk have not been determined, so their use in either pregnant or lactating women is avoided.

Adverse Effects

Orthostatic hypotension, weight gain, sexual dysfunction, and edema are the most common adverse reactions. These tend to diminish as the patient adjusts to the medication. Anticholinergic effects may occur, but not as frequently as with the cyclic antidepressants.

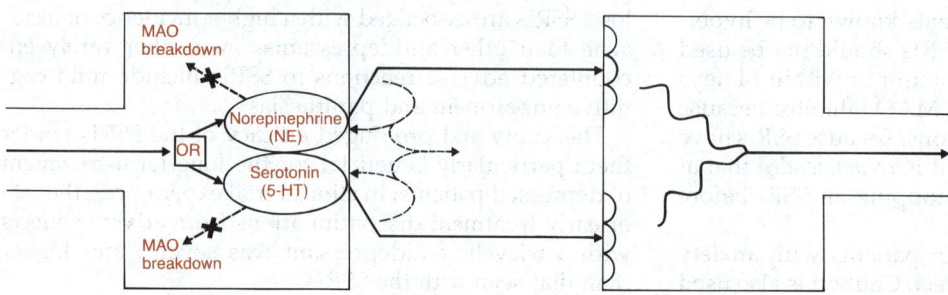

Figure 26–3. Proposed mechanism of monoamine oxidase inhibitors: decreased presynaptic metabolism of catecholamines results in increased availability in synapse. (Compare with Fig. 26–1.)

Toxicity

Toxic reactions from overdose may occur within hours despite the delay in therapeutic response. The most dangerous toxic effects are those involving the liver, the brain, and the cardiovascular system. The incidence of hepatotoxicity is low, but when it occurs, the damage can be quite severe.

Excessive CNS stimulation may result in insomnia, agitation, confusion, and convulsions. Sweating, miosis, acidosis, and hyperthermia are also sometimes seen. Treatment for overdose is primarily supportive, but may include hemodialysis and peritoneal dialysis.

Interactions

Significant interactions involving MAO inhibitors result in either a potentiation of pharmacologic effects or a hypertensive response brought about by the release of catecholamine stores from presynaptic nerve endings. The lack of obvious signs of MAO inhibition in the patient taking these agents is deceptive, as a variety of changes have occurred.

▼ **CLINCAL ALERT**

Hypertensive crisis following the ingestion of certain foods containing tyramine is the most serious toxic effect of MAO inhibitors. Foods with high tyramine content (e.g., cheeses, smoked meats, red wines) must be avoided, and intake of caffeine must be limited as both may precipitate a hypertensive crisis. A hypertensive crisis is serious and may be fatal. Table 26–4 provides a list of dietary restrictions.

Concomitant use of sympathomimetics (e.g., amphetamines, phenylpropanolamine, ephedrine, pseudoephedrine, phenylephrine) and certain antihypertensive drugs may also be contraindicated because of the risk of a hypertensive crisis.

Coadministration of MAO inhibitors and meperidine (Demerol) is contraindicated because it may result in hypertension or hypotension, coma, convulsions, and death. This adverse effect is possible weeks after MAO inhibitor therapy is discontinued. At least 14 to 21 days should separate administration of these drugs. Other opiate analgesics may cause this reaction, so they are administered cautiously.

Dosage

Measurement of platelet MAO activity is usually recommended before MAO inhibitor therapy is initiated. A low monoamine diet for 1 to 2 weeks before the initiation of drug therapy and for 1 week after its termination is suggested. The dose of MAO inhibitor should be adjusted to result in 85% to 90% of MAO inhibition. Care should be taken not to exceed 95% platelet enzyme inhibition, at which level the risk of serious food and drug interactions increases.

As with the cyclic antidepressants, at least 2 to 4 weeks should pass before a clinical response is anticipated. If no clinical improvement is seen by 4 weeks, continuation of therapy is unlikely to help, and an alternative antidepressant therapy may be tried.

MISCELLANEOUS ANTIDEPRESSANTS

Miscellaneous antidepressants include **bupropion (Wellbutrin), nefazodone (Serzone), trazodone (Desyrel)**, and **venlafaxine hydrochloride (Effexor)**. Because SSRIs are generally the first choice for mild or moderate depression, and cyclic antidepressants (and to a lesser extent, MAO inhibitors) are reserved for more severe depression, these miscellaneous antidepressants are alternatives for patients who do not respond adequately or are unable to tolerate side effects of other agents.

○ **Bupropion** (Wellbutrin), a member of the aminoketone class, inhibits reuptake of dopamine and may

Table 26–4. DIET RESTRICTIONS FOR PATIENTS RECEIVING MONOAMINE OXIDASE INHIBITORS	
Foods	**Restrictions**
Do not eat cheese except as noted. Avoid sour cream and yogurt.	Processed cheese, cream cheese, and cottage cheese are allowed. One slice of pizza with mozzarella is believed to be safe.
Avoid stews or drinks made with meat extracts.	Meats and natural gravies are safe.
Avoid foods made with yeast extracts such as marmite.	Baked goods made with yeast are allowed.
Avoid foods that have been aged without refrigeration, especially meats, poultry, or fish.	Freshly prepared frozen or tinned meats, poultry, or fish are safe.
Avoid sausages, such as bologna, salami, and pepperoni.	
Avoid pickled herring.	
Avoid chicken livers, goose livers, and pâté de foie gras.	
Avoid broad bean pods, including Java beans.	These are frequently served in Chinese dishes.
Avoid avocados, raisins, figs.	Controversy exists as to whether bananas should be limited.
Avoid soy sauce.	
Restrict intake of alcohol.	Limit intake of beer to 1–2 glasses per day. Limit intake of whiskey, gin, rum, and so on to 3 oz/day.
Avoid red wines (e.g., Chianti) and sherry.	Limit intake of white wine to 4–8 oz per day.
Limit intake of foods containing caffeine.	Chocolate, coffee, cola, and tea in small amounts are considered safe.
Avoid any foods or drinks that have caused problems, including allergies, in the past.	

work in patients refractory to other classes. The short half-life of bupropion (1 to 3 hours) is associated with the onset of several effects, such as nausea and CNS stimulation. Bupropion-induced seizures are also most likely to occur in this interval. Bupropion has three biologically active metabolites—hydroxybupropion, threohydrobupropion, and erythrohydrobupropion—which all have half-lives considerably longer than that of the parent compound. However, there are no data at this time to suggest that the metabolites contribute to the antidepressant efficacy of the drug. Bupropion undergoes extensive biotransformation in the liver prior to elimination. Bupropion's side effects include CNS activation, agitation, insomnia, decreased appetite, and weight loss. It is also associated with a higher incidence of headache.

○ **Nefazodone** (Serzone) inhibits neuronal reuptake of serotonin and norepinephrine and also acts as an antagonist at alpha$_1$-adrenergic and serotonin receptors. Nefazodone is rapidly and completely absorbed after oral administration, reaching peak plasma concentrations in 1 to 3 hours. Food delays absorption of the drug and decreases its bioavailability. Nefazodone undergoes metabolism in the liver, resulting in three active metabolites, one of which is also a major metabolite of trazodone. The half-life of nefazodone is 2 to 4 hours, but active metabolites persist longer. Clearance of nefazodone may decrease in elderly patients and in those with hepatic dysfunction. Side effects of nefazodone include headache, somnolence, dry mouth, nausea, dizziness, postural hypotension, and blurred vision. Sexual dysfunction has also been reported, but is less common than with SSRIs.

○ **Trazodone** (Desyrel), an antidepressant of the triazolopyridine or phenylpiperazine class, acts to block serotonin receptors. Trazodone is rapidly absorbed following oral administration and has a relatively short half-life (5 to 9 hours). However, lower and delayed peak concentrations of trazodone may occur when the drug is taken with food. Trazodone has an active metabolite, m-chlorophenylpiperazine (mCPP), which may be responsible for the drug's anxiogenic effects. Adverse effects that occur commonly include drowsiness, hypotension, and dry mouth. Less common adverse effects are priapism, irregular heartbeat, fainting, confusion, dizziness, headache, constipation, diarrhea, muscle aches, skin rash, and tremors.

○ **Venlafaxine hydrochloride** (Effexor), a phenethylamine antidepressant, strongly inhibits both norepinephrine and serotonin uptake. Venlafaxine hydrochloride has a rapid onset of action that makes it unique among the antidepressants. Side effects include nausea, somnolence, dizziness, dry mouth, and sweating. Headaches and nausea are also commonly experienced. A dose-dependent increase in blood pressure may also occur.

SELECTION OF AN ANTIDEPRESSANT

The selection of a particular antidepressant is empiric. If one agent does not work after full dosage, another agent with a different neurotransmitter blocking effect and an acceptable side-effect profile should be tried. Because the choice of an antidepressant cannot be based on superior efficacy, it is usually based on the agent's side-effect profile. When a patient has responded positively to a particular antidepressant in the past, that drug is generally chosen for subsequent therapy.

▼ **CLINICAL ALERT**

Lack of therapeutic response to antidepressant medication usually results from inadequate dosing or too brief a therapeutic trial. Maximal clinical improvement usually does not occur until 4 to 8 weeks following initiation. Administration ordinarily begins at the lower end of the dosage range, and as tolerance to side effects develops, the dosage is increased to obtain maximum effectiveness.

Decreased drug metabolism in older patients may require lower doses, and subsequently, slower increases. Lower dosages may also be warranted in patients with hepatic impairment and reduced renal function. Because of the high rate of relapse, treatment is usually continued for several months following recovery from an acute depressive episode. After the initial dosing period, these agents can be given in a single dose at bedtime to minimize sedation and CNS side effects.

USING THE NURSING PROCESS WITH ANTIDEPRESSANTS

ASSESSMENT

- Begin the assessment of the depressed patient with a thorough history to determine suicide risk. The potential for suicide is always present in a patient experiencing depression. Evaluation of suicide risk must continue during the period after onset of medication when the patient begins to feel better physically and emotionally.
- Assess the symptoms of depression that the patient is experiencing. Table 26–5 lists these symptoms and can act as a guide for the nurse as the patient is assessed. Table 26–6 identifies information needed in the nursing database.
- Obtain a drug history regarding treatment with medications for depression and the patient's response to the therapeutic agent. A therapeutic response to antidepressants is often realized slowly and requires concurrent individual and/or family counseling.

NURSING DIAGNOSIS

Nursing diagnoses focus on the individual and family responses to the depression and the treatment regimen. Examples of nursing diagnoses related to using antidepressants include Risk for Violence Directed at Self, Individual Ineffective Coping, and Knowledge Deficit (see Table 26–6).

Table 26–5. ASSESSMENT OF SYMPTOMS OF MOOD DISORDERS

Mode	Depression	Bipolar Reaction, Manic State
Physiologic:		
Rest and exercise	Extreme fatigue	Hyperactivity
	Insomnia	Restlessness
	Early morning awakening	Irritability
	Diurnal rhythm of symptoms	No time to sleep
	Decreased motivation of any activity	Constant initiation of activities, but no completion
	Psychomotor retardation	Frequent clothes changes
Oxygenation and circulation	Decreased pulse	Increased pulse
	Deep sighing	Increased blood pressure
Fluid and electrolytes	Decreased fluid intake	Frequent dehydration
Nutrition	Anorexia	No time to eat
	Bloated feeling	Weight loss
	Weight loss	
Elimination	Constipation	Constipation and impaction
	Decreased urine output	Bladder distention
Skin	Decreased interest in hygiene	No time for personal hygiene
		Frequent use of excessive makeup
		Frequent accidental injuries
Regulation and senses	Decreased taste (food tastes "like straw")	Hypersensitivity to environmental stimuli
	Colors all appear gray tinged	Irritability
	Decreased awareness	
	Decreased attention span	
Endocrine	Amenorrhea	Increased sexual activities
	Impotence	
	Frigidity	
Neurologic	Decreased responses to pain	Ignoring of cues to pains
	Complaints of many vague pains	Decreased attention span
	Thought retardation	
Self-concept:		
Body image	Self-depreciation	Loves self
	Feeling of loss of control	Delusions of grandeur
	Disgust with body	
	Self-mutilation	
Moral/ethical self	Extreme guilt feelings	Decreased moral and ethical standards
	Delusions of sin and guilt	Impulsive behaviors
Self-consistency	Loss of interest in all previous concerns and motivations	Unpredictability
		Fight of ideas
	Self-centered preoccupations	
	Delusions of poverty	Pressured speech
Self-ideal and expectancy	Hopelessness	Hopefulness
	Helplessness	Powerfulness
	Powerlessness	
	Suicidal ideation	
Self-esteem	Denial of past accomplishments	Increased delusions of grandeur
	Very low self-esteem	
	Feeling of worthlessness	
	Self-consciousness	
	High sensitivity to criticism	
Role function	Role failure	No time to fulfill responsibilities
	Decreased motivation to fulfill responsibilities	Role failure
Interdependence	Withdrawal	Independence
	Dependency	Manipulative behavior
	Clinging	Seductive behavior
	Feels unloved	Refusal of offers of help
	Views self as a burden to others	

PLANNING AND INTERVENTION

- Help the patient and family understand that antidepressants are only a part of the overall treatment plan. One goal of therapy is to strengthen coping mechanisms so that the patient handles future crises more adaptively.
- Work closely with the patient's family members to help them understand the depressed patient and their reaction to feelings of guilt.

Patient Teaching

- Teach the patient and family to expect a delay in therapeutic response and assist the patient in maintaining the motivation needed to continue treatment. Table 26–7 features other necessary information for patients receiving cyclic antidepressants.
- Teach patients taking MAO inhibitors about the low-tyramine diet outlined in Table 26–4. Consultation with a registered dietitian is arranged to assist

Table 26–6. NURSING PROCESS FOR PATIENT REQUIRING ANTIDEPRESSANT MEDICATIONS

Assessment

Assess mood, coping abilities, personality styles, i.e., temperament, aggression, impulsive behavior, level of self-esteem.
Assess feelings of hopelessness, sense of being overwhelmed.
Assess plan of suicide, e.g., telling people goodbye, giving away possessions, expressions of despair.
Assess degree of risk/suicidal potential and reevaluate periodically.

Nursing Diagnosis: Risk for Violence, directed at self

RELATED TO: Depressed mood, self-destructive behavior with indicators of expression of intent to harm self, increased anxiety, sudden mood elevation.

Desired Outcomes/Evaluation Criteria

Verbalizes understanding of behavior and precipitating factors.
Demonstrates evidence of planning for the future.

Nursing Actions

Observe patient frequently, especially as mood lifts and physical/emotional state improves.
Encourage verbalization of feelings. Apply active listening to patient concerns. Administer drug trial of tricyclic antidepressants (TCA) or monoamine oxidase (MAO) inhibitors.

Rationale

Provides for external control until patient regains internal control. As lifts, patient is more likely to have the ability to carry out suicide plan.

Promotes understanding and clarification of reasons for depression. TCAs are generally considered safer and easier to manage and are given first. If a positive response is not noted in 4 to 6 wk, an MAO inhibitor may be the drug of choice.

Nursing Diagnosis: Coping, ineffective, individual

RELATED TO: Personal vulnerability, multiple life changes, unmet expectations, actual/perceived loss.
AS EVIDENCED BY: Perception of events and stressors in a manner that precipitates depressive episode, areas of life are seen as losses or as unfulfilled, weeping/labile affect.

Desired Outcomes/Evaluation Criteria

Verbalizes understanding of relationship between feelings and antecedent events. Identifies coping patterns previously used and alternative strategies to cope with this/other situations

Nursing Actions

Encourage verbalization of and assist in identification of feelings and relationship between feelings and event/stressor, when known.
Use crisis or social skills model to teach and appropriately reinforce more effective problem-solving/coping strategies.
Involve in activities, e.g., OT/RT, brisk walks, punching bag.

Rationale

Talking about and labeling the feelings helps patient begin to deal with them more effectively.

These models can be used effectively to increase patient's repertoire of coping techniques.

Provides safe, effective methods for releasing endorphins and discharging pent-up tensions, learning to trust self, and enhancing self-esteem.

Other Suggested Nursing Diagnoses: Knowledge Deficit.

the patient with meal planning. Until the patient experiences relief of depression, the nurse or family member must carefully monitor dietary intake. All health-care providers must be informed that the patient is taking MAO inhibitors. The precaution about diet and medication must be adhered to for 2 weeks before the drug's initiation and for 2 weeks following its discontinuation. Table 26–8 presents other information for health teaching about the MAO inhibitors.

- Explain the importance of not taking any other prescription medications or over-the-counter (OTC) preparations without first checking with the physician.

EVALUATION

The effectiveness of therapy is determined by the success of nursing interventions to alleviate the symptoms of depression.

- Ascertain that the patient realizes that even after the depressive episode has improved, he or she may still feel sad, depressed, or blue on occasion, as these feelings are within the normal range of emotions.
- After the patient has been on cyclic antidepressants for 7 to 10 days, assess how he or she is responding. Although the patient may not report a response, the family members may observe that the patient appears to be improving. If the patient exhibits no progress after a trial of 3 to 4 weeks at optimum dosage, consider another antidepressant agent.
- Evaluate patients receiving antidepressants for the presence of side effects. Anticholinergic reactions are common, especially to cyclic antidepressants, but patients generally experience tolerance over time. Also evaluate the patient taking cyclic antidepressants for cardiovascular side effects, especially tachycardia and orthostatic hypotension. Also ask the patient about any changes in sexual function, such as impotence, decrease in libido, or priapism.
- Evaluate patients receiving MAO inhibitors frequently because these drugs have potentially serious food and drug interactions. Because hypertensive cri-

Table 26–7. PATIENT TEACHING INFORMATION— CYCLIC ANTIDEPRESSANTS

Dear Patient:

This drug has been prescribed by your doctor. The following information will assist you to receive the most help from your total program of therapy. If you have any additional questions about the drug, please consult your doctor, nurse, or pharmacist.

☐ 1. This drug will help decrease your symptoms of depression.

☐ 2. This medicine may cause you to have feelings of dizziness and light-headedness when you stand up. Changing positions slowly and gradually will help prevent these feelings.

☐ 3. This drug may cause you to feel drowsy. Be sure you know how the drug affects you before you drive or do other activities that require you to be alert.

☐ 4. This medicine may need to be taken for 2–3 weeks or longer before you begin to have its positive effects.

☐ 5. Do not drink alcohol (beer, wine, hard liquor) while you are taking this drug.

☐ 6. Do not change the dose or number of times when the medicine is taken. A missed dose may be taken if you remember within 1 hour of the scheduled time. Otherwise check with your physician as soon as possible before continuing your regular schedule.

☐ 7. Do not stop taking this medicine without first talking with your physician. It is important to continue taking the medicine even when you begin to feel better.

☐ 8. Before having any kind of surgery (including dental surgery) or emergency treatment, inform the physician or dentist that you are taking this medication.

---

sis is one of the most dangerous side effects, the patient's blood pressure is monitored regularly. The patient's level of knowledge of a low-tyramine diet and compliance with the dietary restrictions are also evaluated.

TREATMENT OF BIPOLAR DISORDER

The lithium salts—**lithium carbonate *(Eskalith, Lithane, Lithonate, and others)*** and **lithium citrate *(Cibalith-S)***—are particularly effective in bipolar affective disorders. Other drugs that may also be used to treat bipolar disorder include the neuroleptics and anticonvulsants.

LITHIUM SALTS

Action

Lithium, a group IA alkali metal, was discovered to have a calming effect in guinea pigs by an Australian psychiatrist in 1949. The effectiveness of lithium in the long-term management of manic-depressive disorder was established in the 1950s. In 1970, the U.S. Food and Drug Administration approved the use of lithium carbonate for the treatment of mania.

The mechanisms by which lithium produces its therapeutic effects are largely unknown. Lithium is believed to antagonize actions at synapses mediated by catecholamines in the brain. This effect includes inhibition of re-

lease of both norepinephrine and dopamine, as well as an increase in reuptake and turnover of catecholamine transmitters. Lithium may also decrease the synthesis and release of acetylcholine and affect the metabolism of glutamate and gamma-aminobutyric acid (GABA), which are suspected neurotransmitters. The molecular basis for lithium's effects may be related to its inhibition of receptor-mediated synthesis of cyclic adenosine monophosphate (cAMP) by antagonism of the enzyme adenyl cyclase. This action may also provide a basis for some of lithium's side effects. Figure 26–4 is a schematic diagram of lithium's proposed mechanism of action.

Uses

Lithium is the treatment of choice for bipolar illness in the manic or depressed stages. Subsequent manic episodes are prevented or diminished in frequency and intensity

Table 26–8. PATIENT TEACHING INFORMATION— MONOAMINE OXIDASE INHIBITORS

Dear Patient:

This drug has been prescribed by your doctor. The following information will assist you to receive the most help from your total treatment program. If you have any additional questions about the drug, please consult your doctor, nurse, or pharmacist.

☐ 1. This drug will help reduce your symptoms of depression.

☐ 2. Some foods contain tyramine and may cause a rapid rise in your blood pressure: cheese, yogurt, sour cream, stews or drinks made from meat extracts, foods made with yeast extracts, foods aged without refrigeration (especially meats, poultry, and fish), sausages (bologna, salami, and pepperoni), pickled herring, chicken and goose livers, pâté de foie gras, Java beans (often found in Chinese food), avocados, raisins, figs, soy sauce, red wines, sherry, and foods containing caffeine. You *must* avoid eating the foods listed or foods not allowed by a registered dietitian.

☐ 3. Do not take any other medicine, including over-the-counter agents, without first talking to your doctor.

☐ 4. This drug may cause you to feel dizzy and light-headed when you stand up. Changing positions slowly and gradually will help.

☐ 5. This drug needs to be taken for 1–2 weeks or longer before you begin to have its positive effects.

☐ 6. These precautions about your diet and other drugs need to be followed for 2 weeks before beginning this drug and for 2 weeks after you stop taking this drug.

☐ 7. Be certain you tell all other doctors and dentists who may treat you that you are taking this drug or have taken it in the last 2 weeks.

☐ 8. Do not change the dose or number of times the medicine is taken. If a dose is missed and you remember it within 2 hours of the scheduled time, take the dose and continue the regular schedule. If you remember after 2 hours, skip the dose and continue the regular schedule. Do not stop taking this drug without first checking with your doctor, even when you begin to feel better.

☐ 9. This drug may cause some people to become drowsy or less alert than usual. Be certain you know how you react to this medicine before you drive, use machinery, or engage in other activities that require you to be alert.

☐ 10. Check with your doctor or hospital emergency room immediately if severe headache, stiff neck, chest pains, rapid heartbeat, or nausea and vomiting occur while you are taking this medicine. These may be symptoms of a serious reaction that requires medical help.

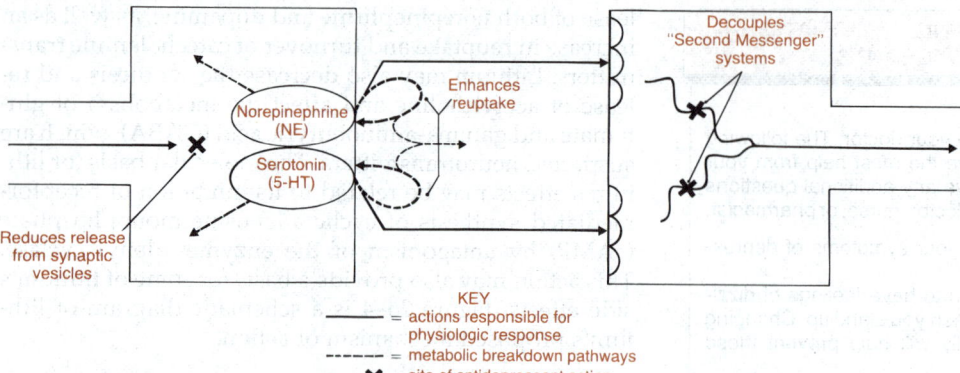

KEY
——— = actions responsible for physiologic response
----- = metabolic breakdown pathways
✗ = site of antidepressant action

Figure 26–4. Hypothesized mechanism of action sites for lithium salts. (Compare with Fig. 26–1.)

by prophylactic maintenance therapy. Acute mania and the prevention of recurrences of bipolar manic-depressive illness are the only indications for lithium currently approved in the United States. Significant clinical improvement is seen in 70% to 80% of patients after 1 to 2 weeks.

Pharmacokinetics

Lithium is well absorbed from the gastrointestinal tract without regard to food intake. Peak concentrations usually occur in 1 to 3 hours after the oral dose, with complete absorption in 8 hours. Slow-release preparations peak at 4 to 12 hours.

Initially, lithium is distributed to extracellular fluid and then gradually accumulated in various tissues. Distribution into the brain is slow, but cerebrospinal fluid concentrations approach 40% of that found in plasma. Lithium does not bind to plasma proteins.

Lithium is not metabolized, but excreted unchanged in the urine. Renal excretion of lithium is biphasic, with two-thirds of an acute dose excreted in 6 to 12 hours, followed by the slow excretion of the remaining one-third over the next 10 to 14 days. The half-life is 18 to 20 hours in healthy young adults, but it increases in elderly patients or those with decreased renal function.

Contraindications and Precautions

Lithium is contraindicated in patients with a history of leukemia, because this condition may be reactivated upon initiation of therapy. Extreme caution must be taken in patients with significant renal or cardiovascular disease, with severe dehydration or sodium depletion, or on diuretic therapy. These patients are at highest risk of developing lithium toxicity. Also, the decreased renal function of geriatric patients predisposes them to a higher incidence of lithium toxicity. Lower doses and frequent monitoring are necessary. The patient should also maintain a normal diet with adequate fluid and salt intake.

Long-term lithium therapy can also result in hyperthyroidism. Many patients develop a transient decrease in serum bound iodine and free thyroxine, but only about 5% of patients develop clinical hyperthyroidism. Lithane

tablets may contain tartrazine dye, which may cause allergic reactions in some individuals.

The use of lithium in pregnant women must be carefully considered. Lithium crosses the placenta, and fetal lithium levels approximate those of the mother. Serious cardiac abnormalities, especially Ebstein's anomaly, have resulted from lithium administration in the first trimester. In general, lithium should not be used in pregnant women unless the clinical benefits clearly outweigh the potential risks. Because lithium is excreted in human breast milk, breast feeding should not be undertaken during lithium therapy.

Adverse Effects and Toxicity

Most patients experience side effects when lithium is administered at therapeutic levels. Central nervous system reactions, including dysphoria, slowed reaction time, and intellectual sluggishness, are common early in treatment but tend to diminish over time. Most adverse reactions appear to be dose related. Toxicity is a function of both the level and the duration of therapy. Because toxic lithium levels are close to accepted therapeutic values, careful monitoring of plasma concentrations is considered standard clinical practice.

At concentrations of less than 1.5 mEq/L, mild toxicity may cause gastrointestinal upset, fine tremor, and urinary frequency. Some of these symptoms may occur initially, but usually abate over time. Taking lithium with food or milk often relieves gastrointestinal symptoms.

As serum levels rise above 1.5 mEq/L, lithium toxicity may cause coarse tremor with twitching, a recurrence of gastrointestinal distress, slurred speech, vertigo, sedation, lethargy, and confusion. Severe toxic responses generally occur at lithium blood concentrations that exceed 2.5 mEq/L. These toxic concentrations can lead to coma, cardiovascular collapse, and death. Lithium toxicity can resemble the confusion and agitation of an acute manic state. Lithium levels should always be checked before administering lithium to a patient with increasing mania. Table 26–9 summarizes the side effects associated with serum lithium levels.

Some reactions that have been reported that are unrelated to dosage include hypothyroidism, leukocytosis,

Table 26–9. SIDE EFFECTS AND TOXICITY OF LITHIUM

Mild (<1.5 mEq/L)	Moderate (1.5–2.5 mEq/L)	Toxicity (2.5–7.0 mEq/L)
Metallic taste in the mouth	Severe diarrhea	Nystagmus
Fine hand tremor (resting)	Nausea and vomiting	Coarse tremor
Nausea	Mild to moderate ataxia	Dysarthria
Polyuria	Incoordination	Fasciculations
Polydipsia	Dizziness, sluggishness, giddiness, vertigo	Visual or tactile hallucinations
Diarrhea or loose stools	Slurred speech	Oliguria, anuria
Muscular weakness or fatigue	Tinnitus	Confusion
	Blurred vision	Impaired consciousness
	Increasing tremor	Dyskinesia—chorea, athetoid movements
	Muscle irritability or twitching	Tonic-clonic convulsions
	Asymmetric deep tendon reflexes	Coma
	Increased muscle tone	Death

Source: Adapted from Harris, E: Antipsychotic Medications. Am J Nurs 81(7):1320–1323, 1981, with permission.

headache, weight gain, edema, metallic taste, and a symptomatic nephrogenic diabetes insipidus. The diabetes insipidus normally resolves within 3 weeks after discontinuing the drug.

Mild adverse reactions are usually managed by either reducing the dose or discontinuing administration of lithium. Treatment can be reinstated in 24 to 48 hours.

Patients with toxicity from lithium overdose may deteriorate rapidly and should be observed closely. Gastric lavage to facilitate removal of lithium combined with good supportive care is indicated. In patients with severe intoxication (serum concentrations greater than 3.5 mEq/liter), hemodialysis is considered an effective intervention.

Interactions

A variety of drugs affect lithium concentration by altering renal clearance. Agents that reduce lithium levels by increasing renal excretion include methylxanthines, urinary alkalinizers, osmotic diuretics, and sodium chloride. Conversely, agents that increase lithium concentrations by decreasing its renal excretion include thiazide diuretics, spironolactone, methyldopa, and several nonsteroidal anti-inflammatory drugs.

Severe neurotoxicity, manifested as either a severe extrapyramidal syndrome or an organic brain syndrome, has been reported when lithium has been taken concomitantly with antipsychotic medications or some anticonvulsants (phenytoin or carbamazepine). In addition, lithium potentiates the effects of neuromuscular blocking agents.

Dosage

Lithium dosage is determined by the patient's clinical presentation. For a patient with normal renal function, 900 to 1800 mg/day in divided doses generally produces serum lithium levels within a range of 1.0 to 1.5 mEq/L. Initial doses are lower for hypomanic patients or in patients taking concomitant antipsychotics. Current data suggest that a plasma level of 0.8 to 1.2 mEq/L is appropriate for prophylaxis. Monitoring of lithium levels should be done as often as the clinical situation dictates.

○ **Lithium carbonate** (Eskalith, Lithane, Lithonate, and others) and **lithium citrate** (Eskalith-S) are the solid and liquid dosage forms of lithium, respectively. Lithium carbonate is more commonly used, having a longer shelf-life and more lithium on a percentage weight basis than the citrate salt.

OTHER AGENTS USED IN TREATMENT OF BIPOLAR DISORDER

Lithium clearly remains the primary therapy for bipolar disorder because it both acts against acute manic episodes and provides prophylaxis against recurrence of both phases of bipolar illness. Many patients, however, respond inadequately to lithium and require adjunctive or alternative medication.

Neuroleptics (e.g., chlorpromazine, haloperidol) are widely used either concurrently with lithium therapy or singularly in treating manic episodes. Neuroleptic medication has a significant antimanic benefit, but appears to worsen depressive episodes. Despite the usefulness of neuroleptics in the treatment of bipolar disorder, there are significant disadvantages associated with their use. The presence of affective disorder increases the risk of neuroleptic-induced tardive dyskinesia and acute extrapyramidal syndromes.

Neuroleptic medication is rationalized clinically because the potentially adverse consequences have to be weighed against the high cost of uncontrolled bipolar disorder. A more complete discussion of neuroleptics can be found in Chapter 27.

Several anticonvulsant drugs show promise as potential adjuncts or alternatives to lithium therapy in treatment of bipolar disorders. Most research on anticonvulsants has centered on carbamazepine (Tegretol) for the treatment of acute mania. Data from controlled studies suggest that carbamazepine may be comparable to lithium in the treatment of mania, at least in relatively treatment-refractory patients. Other structurally dissimilar anticonvulsants such as valproic acid and clonazepam are

Table 26–10. CRITICAL PATHWAY OF CARE FOR THE MANIC PATIENT

Estimated Length of Stay: 14 days—Variations from designated pathway should be documented in progress notes

Nursing Diagnoses and Categories of Care	Time Dimension	Goals and/or Actions	Time Dimension	Goals and/or Actions	Time Dimension	Discharge Outcome
Risk for injury/ violence	Day 1	Environment is made safe for patient and others.	Ongoing	Patient does not harm self or others.	Day 14	Patient has not harmed self or others.
Referrals	Day 1	Psychiatrist. Clinical nurse specialist. Internist (may need to determine if symptoms are caused by other illness or medication side effects). Neurologist (may want to check for brain lesion). Alert hostility management team.			Day 14	Discharge with follow-up appointments as required.
Diagnostic studies	Day 1	Drug screen. Electrolytes. Lithium level.	Day 5 Day 10	Lithium level Lithium level	Day 14	Lithium level and discharge with instructions to return monthly to have level drawn.
Additional assessments	Day 1 Ongoing Ongoing	Vital signs q 4 hr. Restraints PRN. Assess for signs of impending violent behavior: Increase in psychomotor activity, angry affect, verbalized persecutory delusions, or frightening hallucinations.	Day 2–14	Ongoing assessments		
Medications	Day 1	Antipsychotic medications, scheduled and PRN. Lithium carbonate 600 mg tid or qid.	Day 2–14	Administer medications as ordered and observe for effectiveness and side effects.	Day 14	Patient is discharged on maintenance dose lithium carbonate.
Patient education			Day 9	Teach about lithium: Continue to take medication even when feeling okay. Teach signs and symptoms of toxicity. Emphasize importance of monthly blood levels.	Day 14	Patient is discharged with written instructions and verbalizes understanding of material presented.
			Day 12	Reinforce teaching.		
Altered nutrition: Less than body requirements					Day 14	Nutritional condition and weight have stabilized.
Referrals	Day 1	Consult dietitian.	Day 1–14	Fulfill nutritional needs.		

Table 26–10. CRITICAL PATHWAY OF CARE FOR THE MANIC PATIENT, *Continued*

Estimated Length of Stay: 14 days—Variations from designated pathway should be documented in progress notes

Nursing Diagnoses and Categories of Care	Time Dimension	Goals and/or Actions	Time Dimension	Goals and/or Actions	Time Dimension	Discharge Outcome
Diet	Day 1	High-protein, high-calorie, nutritious finger foods. Juice and snacks as tolerated.	As mania subsides	Regular diet with foods of patient's choice.		
Diagnostic studies	Day 1	Chemistry profile. Urinalysis.	Day 2–13	Repeat of selected diagnostic studies as required.		

Source: Townsend, M.: Psychiatric Mental Health Nursing: Concepts of Care. FA Davis, Philadelphia, pp 374, 375, 1996.

also reported to have antimanic effects. See Chapter 20 for a further discussion of antiseizure drugs.

USING THE NURSING PROCESS WITH LITHIUM

The signs and symptoms of patients experiencing acute manic episodes include elevated and/or irritable mood, an increase in activity, and excessive verbalizations. The patient also exhibits increased feelings of self-esteem with grandiose ideation, frequently causing the person to exercise a lack of judgment. A Critical Pathway of Care for the Patient with Manic Disorder is presented in Table 26–10.

ASSESSMENT

- Assess the symptoms of mania according to the criteria outlined in DSM-IV.
- Determine whether any other family members have demonstrated similar patterns of mood swings. Also determine if these relatives were ever treated with lithium and the effectiveness of the treatment.
- Establish baseline data on lithium levels prior to the start of therapy by determining that the laboratory work is completed as ordered.
- Discuss both the patient's and the family members' feelings about the disorder and their expectations of treatment.
- Be certain that legal safeguards of patients' rights are observed.

NURSING DIAGNOSIS

Examples of typical nursing diagnoses for a patient being treated for bipolar disorder with lithium include the following: Risk for Injury/Violence; Risk for Trauma; Risk for Poisoning; and Altered Nutrition, Less than Body Re-

Table 26–11. PATIENT TEACHING INFORMATION—LITHIUM

Dear Patient:
  This drug has been ordered by your doctor. The following information will assist you to get the most help from your total treatment program. If you have any additional questions about the drug, please consult your doctor, nurse, or pharmacist.

☐   1. This drug will help you stop your mood swings.
☐   2. You will need to take this drug for an indefinite period, even after your mood swings have stabilized.
☐   3. This drug should be taken with food or milk to prevent stomach upset.
☐   4. Drink 2–3 quarts of water per day. Avoid large amounts of food and drinks that have caffeine.
☐   5. Do not alter salt intake without talking to your doctor.
☐   6. You need to take this drug on a regular schedule. The dose should never be doubled. If you miss a dose, it should be taken as soon as possible unless you remember 2 hours or less before the next scheduled dose.
☐   7. During your first weeks on this drug, you may have nausea, malaise, and very frequent urination. These problems will decrease in a few weeks.
☐   8. Call your doctor if you have any of the following symptoms: vomiting, diarrhea, fine hand tremors, muscle weakness, or ringing in the ears.
☐   9. You should carry with you at all times an ID card that says you are taking lithium.
☐ 10. You will need to have your lithium blood levels checked on a routine basis. *Do not fail* to get this done when ordered by your doctor.
☐ 11. This drug may make you feel drowsy, so you should check your reaction to this medicine before participating in activities that require you to be alert, for example, driving a car or operating machinery.

quirements. The nursing goals and/or actions for the nursing diagnoses Risk for Injury/Violence and Altered Nutrition, Less than Body Requirements, are shown in the critical pathway of care (see Table 26–10).

PLANNING AND INTERVENTION

- Assist the patient and family members in understanding the illness. The nursing goals for caring for a patient with bipolar disorder include (1) reducing current symptoms, (2) preventing relapses, and (3) educating the patient and family members about the illness. Table 26–11 presents information for patient teaching about lithium therapy.

- Monitor plasma levels of lithium during the initial stage of treatment. Blood tests are ordinarily scheduled for early in the morning, before the initial dose of lithium and 8 to 12 hours after the patient's last dose of lithium, to help ensure that the lithium levels will be relatively stable.
- Assess the patient for symptoms of lithium toxicity (see Table 26–9), regardless of plasma levels.
- Anticipate that the patient may decide to discontinue therapy against medical advice. This is a major problem in prophylactic lithium treatment, occurring in up to 50% of patients. Multiple reasons have been cited for noncompliance, including discomfort with the drug's side effects, intellectual and physical sluggishness, and curbing of the high level of creativity and energy previously experienced. Actively encourage the patient's and family's understanding of the role of medication in preventing the complications associated with relapses.

EVALUATION

The effectiveness of lithium therapy is determined by whether the symptoms of the acute bipolar episode have been reduced.

- Evaluate the patient to determine if anxiety, excessive talking, insomnia, and agitation have decreased.
- Evaluate the effectiveness of patient and family education on an ongoing basis.
- Evaluate the development of side effects and signs of lithium toxicity (see Table 26–9). Most patients initially experience side effects of nausea, polyuria, thirst, mild diarrhea, and a fine resting tremor of the hands. These symptoms usually subside after the first few weeks of treatment, when the dosage may be decreased.

The bibliography for this chapter can be found in Appendix B, which begins on page 1054.

CHAPTER REVIEW QUESTIONS*

1. The action of antidepressants is thought to be most closely related to which neurotransmitters?
   a. Acetylcholine and norepinephrine.
   b. Gamma-aminobutyric acid and acetylcholine.
   c. Norepinephrine and serotonin.
   d. Serotonin and acetylcholine.

2. In which of these patients might a monoamine oxidase (MAO) inhibitor antidepressant be appropriate?
   a. A 24-year-old female college student newly diagnosed with moderate depression.
   b. A suicidal man who has not responded to a selective serotonin reuptake inhibitor, a tricyclic antidepressant, or electroconvulsive shock therapy.
   c. A 54-year-old man who is experiencing a manic episode.
   d. An individual taking lithium chronically for bipolar disorder who is experiencing a mild depression.

3. The most common side effect associated with selective serotonin reuptake inhibitors involve which body system?
   a. Cardiovascular.
   b. Renal.
   c. Musculoskeletal.
   d. Central nervous.

4. Which of the following statements is *correct* with regard to drug interactions when tricyclic antidepressants are given?
   a. A decreased effectiveness of antidepressants is seen when given with phenothiazines.
   b. Ammonium chloride increases the effect of tricyclic antidepressants.
   c. CNS depression is increased when alcohol is taken with tricyclic antidepressants.
   d. A decreased effectiveness of antidepressants is seen when given with acetazolamide.

5. Which of the following is a symptom of severe lithium toxicity:
   a. Coarse tremor.
   b. Vertigo.
   c. Polydipsia.
   d. Muscle weakness.

6. Fluoxetine and other selective serotonin reuptake inhibitors have large safety advantages over the traditional antidepressants, a distinct plus when treating:
   a. Elderly patients.
   b. Potentially suicidal patients.
   c. Bipolar patients.
   d. Manic patients.

*See Appendix A, which begins on page 1051, for answers.

DEPRESSION

Case Study 1: Tricyclic Antidepressants

A 27-year-old patient is admitted to the emergency department with cardiac irregularities, delirium, agitation, hallucinations, and respiratory depression. His wife reports that he has been depressed for several months and has been taking medication for this condition, but she cannot remember the type, nor did she bring the bottle with her. She also states that her husband did not seem to be responding to this medication.

1. What additional information should the nurse gather regarding this patient?
2. What should the nurse suspect as the result of this patient's history and present condition?

Case Study 2: Lithium

A 45-year-old woman with a history of bipolar disorder was brought to the mental health clinic by the police after being arrested for disturbing the peace in a local shopping center. The patient is wearing an identification bracelet indicating that she takes lithium. She is angry, agitated, and denies that anything is wrong. She loudly asserts that she is not a manic-depressive. The patient's family is contacted who state that her mood has been "going up" for the last week and that she became irrational last night and left the house.

1. What additional data does the nurse need to complete this patient's clinical picture?
2. What is the expected treatment for this patient?

CHAPTER 27

Antipsychotic Medications

Meredith A. Davison, PhD

CHAPTER OUTLINE

KEY TERMS

Akathisia
Antipsychotic
Delusion
Dysphagia
Dystonia
Extrapyramidal reaction
Galactorrhea
Gynecomastia
Hallucination

Neuroleptic
Neuroleptic malignant
   syndrome
Parkinsonism
Perioral tremor
Poikilothermia
Schizophrenia
Tardive dyskinesia

LEARNING OBJECTIVES

After reading this chapter, the student will be able to:

1. Identify commonly used antipsychotic medications.
2. Differentiate among the antipsychotic medications as to mechanism of action, route of administration, disposition in the body, adverse effects, contraindications and precautions, and interactions.
3. Identify areas of nursing assessment in the patient requiring antipsychotic medications to formulate appropriate patient outcomes.
4. Plan the nursing interventions for patients requiring antipsychotic medications.
5. Evaluate the patient at various stages of treatment to gauge the effectiveness of the nursing interventions.

Antipsychotic medications, also called *neuroleptics*, have assumed a prominent role in the treatment of major mental illnesses in the last half of the 20th century. The term *antipsychotic* is derived from the drug's ability to effectively relieve certain symptoms of acute and chronic psychoses including thought disorders, *hallucinations* (visual, auditory, or olfactory perceptions having no relation to reality), *delusions* (false beliefs that are inconsistent with the patient's own knowledge and experience), and agitation. Antipsychotic medications are very effective in treating the symptoms of *schizophrenia*, featured in Table 27–1.

The antipsychotic drugs are not curative, but they have proven effective in the control of symptoms to a degree that allows many patients a much improved quality of life. Since chlorpromazine (Thorazine) was introduced in 1954, many patients who would previously have spent long years as patients in institutional settings have been able to successfully live outside of hospitals. However, a "perfect" antipsychotic drug has not yet been discovered. Adverse effects continue to affect many individuals, and a significant minority fail to achieve benefit from the use of antipsychotic drugs.

Antipsychotic drugs fall into two main groups: the phenothiazines and the nonphenothiazines. Table 27–2 features selected drugs from each group. Drugs in both groups block dopamine receptors in the central nervous system (CNS), and they can all cause serious extrapyra-

   The publisher gratefully acknowledges the efforts of Loretta L. Smith in the preparation of this chapter.

Table 27–1. SCHIZOPHRENIA

Definition
A disturbance that lasts for at least 6 months and includes at least 1 month of active-phase symptoms (i.e., two or more of the following: delusions, hallucinations, disorganized speech, grossly disorganized or catatonic behavior, negative symptoms). Schizophrenic subtypes: paranoid, disorganized, catatonic, undifferentiated, and residual.

Etiology
Unknown: Many theories about physical, psychologic, and social causations abound. Evidence also suggests that genetic factors are important.

Characteristic Symptoms (Criteria A)
Two (or more) of the following, each present for a significant portion of time during a 1-month period (or less if successfully treated):
1. Delusions
2. Hallucinations
3. Disorganized speech (e.g., frequent derailment or incoherence)
4. Negative symptoms, i.e., affective flattening, alogia, or avolition

Note: Only one criteria A symptom is required if delusions are bizarre, hallucinations consist of a voice keeping up a running commentary on the person's behavior or thoughts, or two or more voices are conversing with each other.

Duration
Continuous signs of the disturbance persist for at least 6 months. This 6-month period must include at least 1 month of symptoms (or less if successfully treated) that meet criteria A and may include periods of prodromal or residual symptoms. During these prodromal or residual periods, the signs of the disturbance may be manifested by only negative symptoms or two or more symptoms listed in criteria A in an attenuated form (e.g., odd beliefs, unusual perceptual experiences).

Source: Adapted from American Psychiatric Association: Diagnostic and Statistical Manual of Mental Disorders: IV. The Association, Washington, DC, 1994.

midal reactions. *Extrapyramidal reactions* are movement disorders (e.g., parkinsonism) resulting from the effect of antipsychotic drugs on the extrapyramidal tracts in the CNS.

PHENOTHIAZINES

The major antipsychotic drugs of the phenothiazine class include **chlorpromazine (Thorazine, Ormazine), fluphenazine hydrochloride (Prolixin, Permitil), mesoridazine (Serentil), perphenazine (Trilafon), prochlorperazine (Compazine), promazine (Sparine), trifluoperazine (Stelazine),** and **thioridazine (Mellaril)**. The phenothiazine class contains the vast majority of the currently used drugs as well as the original antipsychotic drug, chlorpromazine, the standard to which all antipsychotic drugs are compared.

The phenothiazines are divided into three distinct chemical categories: aliphatic, piperidine, and piperizine.

The aliphatic phenothiazines—chlorpromazine and promazine—often produce strong sedative effects and moderate-to-strong extrapyramidal side effects. They are particularly effective in controlling the psychotic symptoms of hallucinations and delusions.

The piperidine phenothiazines—thioridazine and mesoridazine—have moderate-to-strong anticholinergic effects, strong sedative effects, and minimal extrapyramidal side effects. The drugs in this group are sometimes used for short-term treatment of major depression, sleep disturbances, severe behavioral problems in children, and organic brain disorders in the elderly.

The piperazine group of phenothiazines—trifluoperazine, fluphenazine hydrochloride, perphenazine, and prochlorperazine—contains the largest number of drugs in current use. These drugs cause less sedation and appear to be effective, particularly for withdrawn, apathetic patients.

ACTION

The mechanism of action of the various antipsychotics is not definitively understood. The link between the positive effect of the antipsychotic drugs and the production of unwanted extrapyramidal movement disorders suggests a mechanism of dopamine blockade in the midbrain and basal ganglia. The basal ganglia play a crucial role in the control of posture and the involuntary (extrapyramidal) aspects of movement. Dopamine, a biogenic amine that acts as a neurotransmitter, has been demonstrated to vary in level as a function of antipsychotic drug potency. Selective blockade of subtypes of dopamine receptors in different areas of the brain has been strongly implicated in the explanation for the differences. Clozapine (Clozaril), however, an atypical nonphenothiazine antipsychotic drug, appears to have minimal extrapyramidal side effects. It is thought that its unique pattern of dopamine blockade may be responsible.

Antipsychotic medications also have numerous other effects on the central nervous system. These drugs inhibit the chemoreceptor trigger zones in the medulla through dopamine-receptor blockade and are thus useful for their antiemetic properties, especially prochlorperazine (Compazine). Sedative effects of the antipsychotics are believed to result from indirect reduction of stimuli to the brain stem reticular system and central alpha-adrenergic blocking effects. Muscarinic receptor blockade of the cholinergic autonomic receptors is responsible for many of the unpleasant side effects experienced by patients taking antipsychotic medications, such as dry mouth, constipation, and so forth.

USES

Phenothiazine antipsychotic drugs remain the mainstay of treatment for schizophrenia. They are also useful in the treatment of acute mania and psychotic depressions or as replacement for maintenance lithium in unresponsive bipolar disorder. Neuroleptics continue to be widely used in the treatment of psychoses and behavioral dysregulation that occur in association with a variety of organic

Table 27–2. ANTIPSYCHOTIC MEDICATIONS

DRUG NAME/ROUTE AND DOSAGE	PHARMACOKINETICS/ DYNAMICS	NURSING IMPLICATIONS
PHENOTHIAZINES: ALIPHATIC		
chlorpromazine (Ormazine) (Thorazine) (Thor-Prom)		
Adults: Initial dose–10–25 mg PO 2–4 times daily, increasing dosage by 25–50 mg twice weekly (extended-release [ER] capsules given 1–3 times daily); or 25–50 mg IM q 1–4 hr PRN. Maintenance dose–200–1000 mg/day PO (up to 2 g may be needed). **Children 6 Months and Over:** 0.5 mg/kg PO; 1 mg/kg rectally q 6–8 hr; or 0.5 mg/kg IM q 6–8 hr. IM dose not to exceed 40 mg/day in children 6 mo–5 yr or 75 mg/day in children 5–12 yr.	**Onset:** PO, 30–60 min; ER, 30–60 min; rectal, 1–2 hr **Peak:** PO, 2–4 hr **Duration:** PO, 4–6 hr; ER, 10–12 hr; IM, 4–8 hr; rectal, 3–4 hr **½L:** 10–20 hr (metabolites in urine 6 mo after last dose) **PB:** 92%–97% **B:** liver, kidney **E:** urine (<1% within 72 hr)	**ASSESSMENT:** Assess behavioral and physiologic status. Liver function tests, ophthalmoscopic exam, complete blood count, and ECG should be completed and reviewed periodically. Assess prior responses to prescribed medications. **INTERVENTION:** Administer oral concentrate with at least 4 oz of tomato or fruit juice, carbonated beverages, coffee, tea, or water. Avoid irritating subcutaneous tissues during intramuscular injection. **Patient Teaching**—Emphasize the need for taking the drug to help the patient avoid the merry-go-round syndrome. Inform the patient and family that the full therapeutic response may not occur for 3 wk after therapy begins. Explain to patient that these drugs are not potentially addicting and how they differ from the antianxiety agents. Teach patient precautions to follow to avoid problems resulting from orthostatic hypotension. Teach patient about extrapyramidal reactions and other adverse effects and to call health-care provider if such effects are experienced. Instruct patient to take medication as ordered, to not take antacids with the medication, and to not take unprescribed medications without first consulting the physician. Caution patient about photosensitivity reactions and to avoid exposure to sunlight. Warn patient to avoid activities such as driving until response to drug is known. **EVALUATION:** Observe for decreased primary symptoms. Be aware of and observe for the possibility of secondary anxiety reactions. Evaluate for early symptoms of extrapyramidal reactions and collaborate early with physician to begin treatment as soon as possible.
PHENOTHIAZINES: PIPERAZINE		
fluphenazine hydrochloride (Permitil) (Prolixin)		
fluphenazine hydrochloride **Adults:** Initial dose–0.5–10 mg PO 3–4 times daily; or 1.5–2.5 mg IM q 6–8 hr. Maintenance dose–1–5 mg/day PO. **Geriatric:** Initial dose–1–2.5 mg/day PO or IM. **fluphenazine enanthate or decanoate** **Adults:** Initially, 12.5–25 mg IM or SC every 3–4 wk; adjust subsequent injections and dosage interval according to patient response. Do not exceed 100 mg.	**Onset:** PO and IM, 60 min; IM (enanthate and decanoate), 24–72 hr **Peak:** IM, 1.5– 2 hr; IM (enanthate), 48–72 hr; IM (decanoate), 24–48 hr **Duration:** PO and IM, 6–8 hr; IM (enanthate), 3 wk; IM (decanoate), >4 wk **½L:** HCl, 4.7–15.3 hr; enanthate, 3.5–4 days; decanoate, 6.8–9.6 days **PB:** 92%–97% **B:** liver **E:** feces, urine	Same as for chlorpromazine except: **INTERVENTION:** Administer oral concentrate with at least 4 oz of apricot, grapefruit, orange, prune, pineapple, tomato, or V8 juice; 7UP; carbonate orange beverage; milk; or water. Do *not* mix with beverages containing caffeine (e.g., coffee, cola, tea) or pectinates (e.g., apple juice).
trifluoperazine (Stelazine)		
Adults: 2–5 mg PO bid (up to 40 mg/day); or 1–2 mg IM q 4–6 hr (up to 10 mg/day). **Children 6–12 yr:** 1 mg once or twice daily PO or IM.	**Onset:** 20–30 min **Peak:** 2–3 hr **Duration:** PO, 12–24 hr; IM, 4–6 hr **½L:** NA **PB:** 92%–97% **B:** liver **E:** urine (<1% within 72 hr)	Same as for chlorpromazine.

Table 27–2. ANTIPSYCHOTIC MEDICATIONS, *Continued*

DRUG NAME/ROUTE AND DOSAGE	PHARMACOKINETICS/ DYNAMICS	NURSING IMPLICATIONS
PHENOTHIAZINES: PIPERIDINE		
thioridazine (Mellaril) **Adults and Children over 12 yr:** *Initial dose*—50–100 mg PO tid. *Maintenance dose*—10–200 mg PO qid (up to 800 mg/day). **Children 2–12 yr:** 0.5–3 mg/kg daily.	**Onset:** 1 hr **Peak:** 4 hr **Duration:** 8–12 hr **½L:** 26–36 hr **PB:** NA **B:** liver, GI mucosa **E:** urine	Same as for chlorpromazine.
NONPHENOTHIAZINES		
thiothixene (Navane) **Adults:** 2 mg PO tid or 5 mg PO bid (not to exceed 60 mg/day); or 4 mg IM 2–4 times daily (not to exceed 30 mg/day).	**Onset:** PO, days–weeks (effects); IM, 1–6 hr **Peak:** PO, 1–3 hr; IM, 1–6 hr **Duration:** NA **½L:** 30 hr **PB:** NA **B:** liver **E:** feces	Same as for chlorpromazine.
haloperidol (Haldol) (Haldol Decanoate) (Halperon)		
haloperidol **Adults:** 0.5–5 mg PO 2–3 times daily or 2–5 mg IM q 1–8 hr (up to 100 mg/day PO or IM). **Children 3–12 yr:** 0.05–0.075 mg/kg/day in 2–3 divided doses. **haloperidol decanoate** **Adults:** 50–100 mg IM q 4 wk (not to exceed 300 mg).	**Onset:** PO, 2 hr; IM, 20–30 min; IM (decanoate), 3–9 days **Peak:** PO, 3–5 hr; IM, 20 min; IM (decanoate), 4–11 days **Duration:** PO, 8–12 hr; IM, 4–8 hr (effect may persist for several days); IM (decanoate), 4 wk **½L:** 12–38 hr PO (avg 24), 13–36 hr IM; decanoate 3 wk **PB:** 92% **B:** liver **E:** urine, bile	Same as for chlorpromazine.

NA = not available.

mental disorders. Phenothiazines are also used to treat behavioral disturbances in children.

Beside their use in psychiatry, phenothiazines are employed in the treatment of nausea and vomiting, intractable hiccups, and preoperatively for relaxation.

Available data suggest that all antipsychotic drugs (with the possible exception of clozapine) are equally efficacious. However, the finding that 70% to 80% of a sample of patients respond well to various neuroleptics does not necessarily mean that a given individual will respond equally well to each drug. Neuroleptic drugs do appear to differ in their profiles of adverse effects, and such differences may be the reason for prescribing a particular medication for a patient with a known vulnerability to a particular adverse effect. The patient's previous therapeutic response to specific antipsychotic drugs or the response of a first-degree relative with the same illness is

also a major consideration. A comparison of the effects of the antipsychotic drugs is presented in Table 27–3.

PHARMACOKINETICS

Antipsychotic medications tend to have erratic and unpredictable patterns of absorption, especially after oral administration. Intramuscular administration provides four to ten times more active drug than oral administration. As a group, these drugs are lipophilic, are strongly membrane or protein bound, and accumulate in tissues with a high blood supply (e.g., brain, lung). The considerable variability among individuals in peak plasma concentrations results from genetic differences in metabolism and biodegradation of the drugs. Therapeutic ranges for drug concentrations have not been clearly established.

Table 27–3. COMPARISON OF EFFECTS OF ANTIPSYCHOTIC AGENTS

Classification and Generic Names	Trade Name	Effects							Dosage Ranges*	
		EPS	Sedation	Anti-cholinergic	Hypo-tension	Anti-emetic	Traditional Equivalence		Acute Dose (mg/day)	Maintenance Dose (mg/day, PO)
Phenothiazines										
Aliphatics:										
Chlorpromazine	Thorazine	++	+++	+++	+++	Strong	100		400–1500†	200–1000
Promazine	Sparine	++	+++	+++	+++	Moderate	100		50–800	200–800
Piperidines:										
Thioridazine	Mellaril	+	+++	+++	+++	Weak	100		400–800	25–800
Mesoridazine	Serentil	+	+++	++	++	Weak	NA		20–600	10–400
Piperazines:										
Perphenazine	Trilafon	+++	+	++	+	Weak	10		12–24	reduce
Trifluoperazine	Stelazine	+++	+	+	+	Weak	5		20–100	10–40
Fluphenazine HCl	Prolixin	++++	+	+	+	Weak	2		20–80	1–40
Prochlorperazine	Compazine	+++	++	+	+	Strong	NA		50–150	20–100
Nonphenothiazines										
Thiothixine	Navane	+++	+	+	+	0	4		6–30†	5–40
Haloperidol	Haldol	++++	+	+	+	0	2		6–15	reduce
Loxapine	Loxitane	+++	++	+	++	0	10		50–250†	25–100
Molindone	Moban	+++	+	+	+	0	50		50–400	25–100
Clozapine‡	Clozaril	+	+++	+++	+++	0	50		25–50	300–450; max 900

++++ = very frequent/strong; +++ = high incidence; ++ = moderate incidence; + = low incidence.
*Children, adolescents, and the elderly require smaller doses. Dosages for these age groups are not established.
† = Dosage can be exceeded with caution.
‡Clozapine has a distinct profile of drug actions. See text for more detailed explanation.

The phenothiazines are extensively metabolized in the liver, and many active metabolites are produced.

Most metabolites of antipsychotic medications are excreted in urine and feces; however, some remain in the body for months after discontinuation of the drug. The pharmacokinetics of antipsychotics usually follow a multiphasic pattern with the half-life typically between 20 and 40 hours. Because the drugs are highly lipophilic, the phenothiazines are stored in the fatty tissues until a point of saturation is reached. When the drug is discontinued, the stored drug is then slowly released, metabolized, and excreted. Repository preparations of neuroleptic drugs are much more slowly absorbed and eliminated than are oral preparations. For example, whereas half of an oral dose of fluphenazine hydrochloride (Prolixin HCL) is eliminated in about 20 hours, the elimination half-time for a depot of the decanoate ester of fluphenazine is 7 to 10 days. This characteristic of fluphenazine allows the drug to be administered by injection every 4 weeks, allowing many patients to remain outside the hospital.

CONTRAINDICATIONS AND PRECAUTIONS

Phenothiazines are contraindicated in cases of known hypersensitivity. Cross-sensitivity among phenothiazines may occur.

Phenothiazines are classified as pregnancy category C compounds, indicating that risk to the fetus from these drugs cannot be ruled out. In pregnant women, the phenothiazines cross the placental barrier and reach significant plasma levels in the fetus. Although the drugs do not appear to cause congenital malformations, infants born to mothers taking the drug in their last trimester may exhibit jaundice and extrapyramidal and/or anticholinergic side effects at birth. Phenothiazines are also excreted in human breast milk. Table 27–4 features a list of medical conditions in which phenothiazines should be used cautiously.

Table 27–4. ANTIPSYCHOTICS SHOULD BE USED WITH CAUTION WHEN THE FOLLOWING MEDICAL CONDITIONS EXIST

- Bone marrow depression (could mask or exacerbate drug-induced agranulocytosis)
- Cardiovascular disease (complicated by cardiovascular effects of antipsychotics)
- Myocardial infarction
- Alcoholism
- Hepatic function impairment (could mask or exacerbate hepatic hypersensitivity to drug)
- Hypoparathyroidism (may mask endocrine effects of drugs)
- Parkinson's disease (symptoms worsened by neuroleptics)
- Glaucoma (because anticholinergic drug effects are likely to exacerbate the symptoms of this disorder)
- Gastrointestinal disturbances (as drug's antiemetic effect may mask symptoms)
- Peptic ulcer (same as glaucoma)
- Prostatic hypertrophy (same as glaucoma)
- Urinary retention (same as glaucoma)
- Respiratory problems (especially in children; some of these products contain the dye tartrazine, which may cause allergic reactions in sensitive patients)
- Reye's syndrome (because antiemetic and extrapyramidal effects may obscure the diagnosis of Reye's syndrome)

ADVERSE EFFECTS

Phenothiazines are remarkably safe drugs, have a relatively flat dose-response curve and can be prescribed over a wide range of doses. Most side effects are extensions of the drugs' pharmacologic actions. In general, there are six extrapyramidal reactions that are of most concern. Four of these reactions—*acute dystonia, parkinsonism, akathisia,* and the rare *neuroleptic malignant syndrome*—usually occur early in therapy. Two other reactions, *perioral tremor* and *tardive dyskinesia,* usually appear after prolonged treatment. Table 27–5 describes the primary characteristics of each syndrome and provides times of onset and points for nursing assessment.

Approximately one-third of all patients who receive phenothiazines experience these neurologic syndromes, which are the result of the effects of the phenothiazines on the dopaminergic extrapyramidal tracts of the CNS. Extrapyramidal symptoms can be mistaken for clinical psychiatric symptoms: parkinsonian rigidity resembles catatonia, and akathisia may be confused with psychotic agitation or anxiety. The best preventive practice is to use the minimum effective dose of an antipsychotic drug in combination with short-term use of anticholinergic antiparkinsonian agents (see Chapter 23 for a discussion of these drugs).

The pathophysiology of tardive dyskinesia remains somewhat obscure, but abundant data now support the concept of disuse supersensitivity of dopaminergic systems in the brain. The longer a patient takes antipsychotic medications, the greater the possibility this syndrome will occur. It is also more frequent among older patients and is correlated with higher doses of medication. Extrapyramidal side effects and tardive dyskinesia have been ob-

Table 27–5. EXTRAPYRAMIDAL REACTIONS TO NEUROLEPTIC DRUGS

Type	Symptoms	Time of Onset	Points for Nursing Assessment
Acute dystonia	Uncoordinated jerking or spastic movements of the neck, face, eyes, tongue, and limbs; oculogyric crisis; torticollis; respiratory distress; dysphagia; opisthotonos; carpal spasms	1–5 days	1. Patient complains of having problems chewing and/or swallowing food. 2. Patient complains of "eyes rolling in head." 3. Patient has a look of terror and fear as symptoms develop.
Akathisia	Restlessness, agitation, compulsion to walk, facial tics, insomnia, fine hand tremor	5–60 days	1. Assess for feelings of fear, anger, and/or terror when patient experiences these symptoms. 2. Person views these symptoms as being ego-alien (unlike his or her usual behavior and outside of his or her control). 3. Symptoms increase after a dose of a neuroleptic.
Parkinsonism	Akinesis, muscle rigidity, stooped posture, shuffling gait, tremors, masklike facies, decreased or absent swing, hypersalivation, drooling, pill-rolling tremor, listlessness, unusual numbness or tingling sensations	5–30 days	1. Cues of feeling weak, like a zombie, apathetic, being slowed down. 2. Test to see if strength in both hands and arms has decreased. 3. Passive range of motion exercises produce lead-pipe or cogwheel rigidity. 4. Person uses methods other than facial gestures to express emotion. 5. Walks with forearms perpendicular to trunk of body. 6. Increasing dose of neuroleptic produces catatonic-like symptoms.
Neuroleptic malignant syndrome	Catatonia, stupor, fever, unstable blood pressure, myoglobinemia	Weeks after initiation of therapy	1. Patient exhibits muscle rigidity, fever, alterations in consciousness. 2. Evaluate blood pressure, heart rate. 3. Dysphagia, dyspnea, diaphoresis, and incontinence may be present. 4. Leukocytosis ranging from 15,000 to 30,000 have been reported and CPK elevations as high as 15,000 units.
Perioral tremor (rabbit syndrome)	Perioral tremor similar to parkinsonism	After months or years of treatment	1. Often categorized with tardive dyskinesia, but unlike tardive dyskinesia, this syndrome responds to antiparkinson drugs and removal of the offending agent. 2. Assess for a tremor with a frequency of 5 to 6 Hz.
Tardive dyskinesia	Bucco-linguo-masticatory syndrome, choreiform movements of the extremities, grimacing, tongue protrusion, rocking movements	After months or years of treatment	1. Assess for earliest cues: blinking, vermiform movements of the tongue. 2. Patient may view the symptoms as being embarrassing. 3. Symptoms worsen with withdrawal of medication.

served with all antipsychotic medications except clozapine (discussed under Nonphenothiazines).

Phenothiazines, especially aliphatic phenothiazines with low potency (such as chlorpromazine), lower the seizure threshold and induce discharge patterns in the electroencephalogram (EEG) that are associated with epileptic seizure disorders. Patients with seizure disorders may require higher doses of prophylactic antiseizure medication concurrent with phenothiazine administration. Sedation is also a common side effect, especially with chlorpromazine and thioridazine.

Autonomic side effects are frequent, especially early in therapy. Anticholinergic effects resulting from muscarinic receptor blockade include blurred vision, dry mouth, constipation, and urinary retention. Cardiovascular effects, such as orthostatic hypotension and tachycardia, are believed to be due to alpha-receptor blockade. Mild changes in the electrocardiogram (ECG) are also observed.

Endocrine system side effects, primarily an increase in prolactin secretion, may also develop. Phenothiazines induce secretion of prolactin from the anterior pituitary by inhibiting dopamine receptors in the pituitary and hypothalamus. Elevated prolactin levels may stimulate the development of *galactorrhea* (lactation not associated with childbirth or nursing) or breast engorgement in both men and women. Women may also experience amenorrhea with long-term antipsychotic therapy.

Phenothiazines can also cause thermoregulatory problems *(poikilothermia)*, particularly in the elderly. Hypothermia or hyperthermia may be induced by environmental temperature deviations from normal room temperature. Men may also experience ejaculation difficulties and *gynecomastia*, the abnormal enlargement of one or both breasts. These two side effects are most prominent with thioridazine. Both males and females may experience a decreased libido as a result of phenothiazine use.

A skin/eye syndrome may also occur rarely. The colored areas of the skin exposed to sunlight may change to brown, gray, metallic blue, and/or purple. The color change is caused by the drug's reacting within the body to create melanin-like granules that are deposited within the skin tissues, and also in the conjunctiva, sclera, lens, and cornea of the eye. A more serious visual side effect that may cause blindness (pigmentary retinopathy) occurs with the use of thioridazine in daily doses of 800 mg or more. Other side effects involving the skin include increased photosensitivity. The patient may develop a severe sunburn after only brief exposure to the sun.

Some reactions may occur that stimulate specific allergic or toxic effects. Systemic dermatosis, usually a maculopapular rash on the face, neck, chest, arms, and legs, tends to develop 2 to 8 weeks after the initial dose. Two rare but extremely serious allergic syndromes associated with the use of phenothiazines are agranulocytosis and cholestatic jaundice.

Side effects that mimic psychiatric states may also occur, including an atropine-like psychosis. Rarely, patients using neuroleptics demonstrate symptoms of depression. The phenomenon of secondary anxiety reaction may also appear, manifested by a rise instead of a decrease in the patient's level of anxiety shortly after a dose of a neuroleptic. The neuroleptic agents are not addicting, but patients may experience gastrointestinal symptoms such as nausea, vomiting, and/or diarrhea when the drug is withdrawn.

▼ **CLINICAL ALERT**

Patients over 60 years of age appear to experience a greater incidence of side effects. Part of the explanation for this increase is that the half-life of phenothiazines is prolonged in the elderly when compared with younger patients. In addition, the elderly may be inherently more sensitive to the anticholinergic effects of these drugs. Elderly patients, and those with organic brain syndromes, are highly susceptible to pseudo-psychotic symptoms from central effects of excessive anticholinergic drug action.

INTERACTIONS

Phenothiazines can strongly potentiate CNS depressant drugs such as sedatives, opiate analgesics, alcohol, and antihistamines. Interactive effects on the cardiovascular system can occur because of alpha-adrenergic blocking actions and the quinidine-like action, which can cause myocardial depression. The antimuscarinic action of phenothiazines also results in numerous potential interactions. Potential drug interactions are presented in Table 27–6.

O **Chlorpromazine** (Thorazine, Ormazine, ThorProm) is the prototype for the phenothiazine class of antipsychotics. It is an aliphatic phenothiazine that is frequently used to calm extremely agitated patients because of its potent sedative effect. Chlorpromazine is available in various forms that permit optimal dosage modalities for particular patients. Liquid concentrate forms may be prescribed for patients who experience difficulty in swallowing *(dysphagia)* or who have been noncompliant in swallowing pills. The intramuscular route of administration results in the most rapid calming effect and is frequently chosen when chlorpromazine is administered in an emergency situation. The injectable form tends to irritate the subcutaneous tissues locally. Rectal chlorpromazine is frequently used to treat severe nausea and vomiting when patients are unable to tolerate oral agents. Chlorpromazine is approved for use in children over 6 years of age.

O **Fluphenazine** (Permitil, Prolixin) is a member of the piperazine class of phenothiazines that is available in three chemical formulations, as the hydrochloride, the decanoate, and the enanthate. Fluphenazine hydrochloride is available for oral use, while the decanoate and enanthate salts are used for intramuscular and subcutaneous injection. Because intramuscular injections of fluphenazine are formulated with an oil-based preparation, the active drug is slowly absorbed over a 2-week (fluphenazine enanthate) to 4-week (fluphenazine decanoate) period. This characteristic allows patients to be easily maintained on antipsychotic medication in an outpatient treatment situation. However, a disadvantage of using IM injections of long-acting fluphenazine is that the drug causes a high level of extrapyramidal effects that

Table 27–6. DRUGS THAT INTERACT WITH ANTIPSYCHOTICS

Medication	Type of Interaction
Alcohol	Potentiates and prolongs the effects of the neuroleptics and vice versa.
Amphetamines	Neuroleptics decrease the effects of the amphetamines.
Antacids or antidiarrheal suspensions	Concurrent administration blocks the absorption of the neuroleptics.
Anticonvulsants	Neuroleptics decrease the seizure threshold; therefore, the dosage of anticonvulsants may have to be increased.
Antimuscarinics, especially atropine	Effects of these drugs are potentiated with concurrent use; these drugs may reduce the plasma levels of neuroleptics.
Antiparkinson drugs	Anticholinergic effects of these drugs may be potentiated.
Levodopa	Antiparkinsonian effects are inhibited with concurrent use.
Epinephrine	Neuroleptics may block the α-adrenergic effects of this drug, producing severe hypotension.
Guanethidine and related drugs	Neuroleptics block the antihypertensive effects of these drugs.
Central nervous system depressants	Potentiate and prolong the effects of these drugs; concurrent use with some drugs (e.g., meperidine) may produce severe respiratory depression.
Monoamine oxidase inhibitors and tricyclics	Concurrent use prolongs and potentiates the sedative effects of these drugs; potentiation of the anticholinergic effect also occurs.
Diuretics	Volume depletion produces orthostasis.
α-Blocking antihypertensives (Prazosin) and α- and β-blockers (Lubetolol)	α Blockade produces orthostasis.

cannot be rapidly alleviated by discontinuation of the medication.

○ **Trifluoperazine** (Stelazine, Suprazine), a piperazine phenothiazine, causes significantly less sedation than chlorpromazine, but is more prone to precipitate extrapyramidal side effects. Both oral and injectable forms of the drug are available. Trifluoperazine has been approved for use in children over the age of 6 years.

○ **Thioridazine** (Mellaril) is a frequently used phenothiazine that belongs to the piperadine classification. It produces a low incidence of extrapyramidal side effects, but does cause significant sedation. The sedative effect usually dissipates within a few days or weeks. Thioridazine differs from other phenothiazines by lacking antiemetic effects. It also has little, if any, effect on seizure threshold. Thioridazine has been approved for use in children over the age of 2 years.

NONPHENOTHIAZINES

○ **Thiothixene** (*Navane*) belongs to a separate class of antipsychotic drugs called thioxanthines. Drugs in this class have weak anticholinergic, hypotensive, and sedative properties. They are usually prescribed to treat chronic schizophrenic patients who have not responded to other drugs.

○ **Haloperidol** (*Haldol*), a member of the butyrophenome class, has very strong extrapyramidal side effects and weak anticholinergic effects. Because of haloperidol's high incidence of extrapyramidal reactions, it is contraindicated in patient's with Parkinson's disease or in those displaying symptoms of parkinsonism. Haloperidol is available in a variety of dosage forms, including haloperidol decanoate, a long-acting depot form for intramuscular use that requires dosing only once a month. Haloperidol is also approved for use in children ages 3 to 12 years.

○ **Clozapine** (*Clozaril*), a member of the dibenzodiazepine group, is indicated for patients with schizophrenia who have not responded to traditional antipsychotic drugs. It has strong anticholinergic effects and is believed to exert greater serotonergic, adrenergic, and histaminergic effects relative to its dopamine-blocking effects. Before the introduction of clozapine, all antipsychotic drugs had neuroleptic properties, meaning that all were associated with acute extrapyramidal side effects and the long-term development of tardive dyskinesia. Clozapine has relatively few extrapyramidal side effects, and a substantially reduced risk of tardive dyskinesia is expected. Current clinical experience suggests that clozapine has superior antipsychotic efficacy in treatment-refractory schizophrenia. However, clozapine's major adverse effect—agranulocytosis—may limit its clinical usefulness.

▼ CLINICAL ALERT

To ensure the earliest possible detection of agranulocytosis, clozapine is dispensed only if a patient undergoes appropriate weekly blood tests. Treatment must be interrupted at the first sign of significant bone marrow suppression (total white blood cell count [WBC] less than 3000/mm³ or a granulocyte count of less than 1500/mm³). Early detection of agranulocytosis can prevent fatalities.

The most common adverse effects of clozapine therapy include drowsiness/sedation, seizures, dizziness/syn-

Table 27–7. NURSING PROCESS FOR PATIENT REQUIRING ANTIPSYCHOTIC MEDICATIONS

Assessment

Assess baseline data, e.g., TPR, BP (sitting and standing); liver function tests, ophthalmoscopic exams, CBC and ECG.
Assess prior responses to prescribed medications.
Assess presence of delusions, hallucinations, sleep disturbances, paranoia.
Assess affect, mood swings, unpredictable behaviors (withdrawal, aggression, agitation, and restlessness) and note how these affect patient's life.
Assess presence of preexisting physical conditions, e.g., pregnancy/lactation, hepatic and cardiovascular disorders.

Nursing Diagnosis: Knowing Deficit

RELATED TO: Lack of information/misinterpretation, cognitive limitation.
AS EVIDENCED BY: Inaccurate statements, questions, refusal of medication.

Desired Outcomes/Evaluation Criteria

Displays decrease in primary symptoms. Correctly explains reasons for medication/treatment regimen. Takes medications as prescribed.

Nursing Actions	Rationale
Discuss reasons for taking prescribed medication, e.g., reduction of target symptoms, decreased level of anxiety/agitation, maintaining control of behavior.	Understanding why medication is needed helps patient to participate with treatment.
Review expectations of drug administration, e.g., therapeutic response may not occur for 3 wk, drugs are not addicting.	Knowing what to expect helps the patient to feel in control and may enhance participation in medication regimen.
Caution against sudden changes in position, unprotected exposure to sunlight.	Orthostatic hypotension may occur with these drugs. Sensitivity to the sun may result in severe sunburn.
Identify adverse symptoms that need to be reported to health-care giver. Distinguish between significant toxic effects (e.g., onset of extrapyramidal side effects) and uncomfortable but benign side effects (e.g., dry mouth, oral lesions).	Provides for timely evaluation and intervention to adjust drug regimen/prevent serious complications.
Emphasize that unprescribed medications/OTC drugs, especially antacids, should not be taken with antipsychotic drugs.	Untoward interactions may interfere with absorption and desired effect of drug.
Active-listen to patient feelings and concerns.	Clarifies patient/family expectations and promotes sense of control of own treatment.
Encourage continuation of antipsychotic medication as prescribed.	May be needed to control symptoms on long-term basis.

Nursing Diagnosis: Risk for Injury

RELATED TO: Side effects of prescribed pharmaceutical agents (e.g., antipsychotic drugs).
AS EVIDENCED BY: Clinical indications of adverse reactions.

Desired Outcomes/Evaluation Criteria

Reports reduction of psychotic symptoms/absence of serious side effects.

Nursing Actions	Rationale
Monitor medication regimen, observing for therapeutic effect.	Enables identification of the minimal effective dose with least adverse effects.
Identify/review adverse effects of medications, hemorrhagic gingivitis, sedation, hormonal effects, reduction of seizure threshold, agranulocytosis, and extrapyramidal symptoms (tremors, akinesia/akathisia, dystonia, oculogyric crisis, and tardive dyskinesia).	Anticholinergic effects of psychotropics (and antiparkinson drugs that may be given concomitantly) alter autonomic nervous system functioning. Most side effects occur within the first few weeks of treatment and subside with time. Signs indicative of agranulocytosis (sore throat, malaise), extrapyramidal symptoms, and tardive dyskinesia need immediate attention.
Emphasize importance of immediate medical attention for onset of high fever/severe muscle stiffness and to discontinue the medication until seen by the doctor.	Severe muscle stiffness and high fever are the hallmarks of neuroleptic malignant syndrome, which can usually be effectively treated before it becomes life-threatening if it is detected early.
Administer antiparkinson drugs as indicated.	Used for relief of drug-induced extrapyramidal reactions.

Other Suggested Nursing Diagnoses: Risk for Violence, directed at self or others; Impaired Adjustment; Personal Identity Disturbance; and Altered Thought Processes.

cope, hypersalivation, tachycardia, hypotension, constipation, nausea, vomiting, leukopenia, and fever.

○ **Molindone** *(Moban)* is one of the two marketed members of the dihydroindolone drug class. It may cause less weight gain during long-term use, a disturbing side effect of most other neuroleptics. Molindone is available in tablets for oral administration.

○ **Loxapine** *(Loxitane, Loxitane-C)* is a dibenzoxazepine antipsychotic with effects comparable to those of haloperidol. Its metabolite, amoxapine, is marketed separately as an antidepressant. Thus, loxapine may be useful for patients who have both psychosis and features of depressive illness.

USING THE NURSING PROCESS

The goals of nursing intervention for the patient being treated with an antipsychotic medication include reducing the target symptoms, decreasing the level of anxiety and agitation, maintaining patient control of personal behavior, and educating the patient about the diagnoses, the treatment regimen, and potential adverse effects. When the patient is able to participate, his or her personal care goals should be made central to the planning process.

ASSESSMENT

- Before initiating the nursing assessment, obtain a history to establish the database. The person may be experiencing some or all of the following symptoms: delusion, hallucination, blunted or flat affect, mood swings, sleep disturbances. Feelings of paranoia, withdrawal from activities, and difficulties in relationships are also often present.
- Assess the length of time the patient has been experiencing these feelings and symptoms and how the symptoms affect his or her daily life. Question whether the patient has previously experienced similar episodes, and if so, how long they lasted.
- Assess whether the patient or other family members have ever been treated with antipsychotic medications, and if so, which ones. Determine the response to these medications and side effects experienced.
- Prior to the administration of the initial dose, thoroughly assess the patient's overall physical health and emotional state. Data to collect during the assessment appear in Table 27–7.

NURSING DIAGNOSIS

- Nursing diagnoses may relate to physical or psychosocial findings. Suggested nursing diagnoses include Knowledge Deficit, Risk for Violence Directed at Self or Others, and Risk for Injury (see Table 27–7).

PLANNING AND INTERVENTION

- Anticipate the potential for a wide range of side effects that accompany antipsychotic drug therapy. Pa-

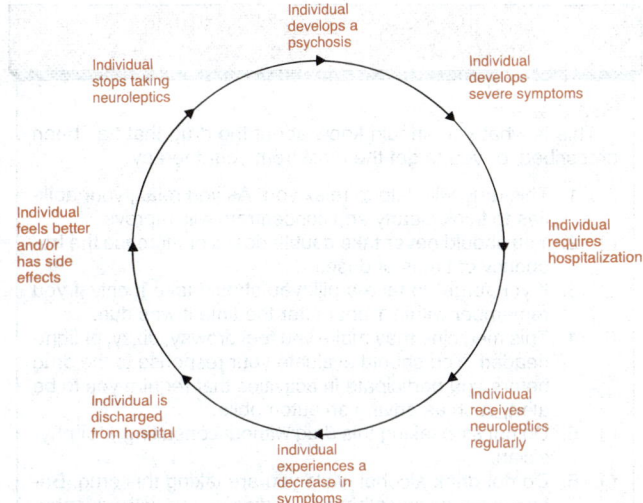

Figure 27–1. Merry-go-round syndrome associated with the use of neuroleptics to treat long-term psychosis.

tients may become upset with the sedation and extrapyramidal symptoms that are often experienced, and many stop taking the medicine as prescribed. Discuss with the patient the expectations of drug administration and identify adverse symptoms that need to be reported to the health-care provider.

- When a patient leaves the inpatient treatment facility and begins to feel well, he or she may decide to discontinue medication or counseling. Because virtually all patients not treated with antipsychotic medication will relapse within about 3 years, the "merry-go-round syndrome" occurs, as shown in Figure 27–1. Focus patient teaching on the positive effects of treatment and distinguishing significant toxic effects from annoying but benign side effects. Important information the nurse should teach the patient who is receiving antipsychotic medication is featured in Table 27–8.

EVALUATION

- Evaluate whether the patient has demonstrated a positive response to the antipsychotic medication. If the response is not positive, consider whether the patient may have stopped taking the medication. Use of a different form of the medication (e.g., injectable) may be indicated for the patient who is compromised in decision making. If the patient has taken the medication appropriately and still not had a positive response after two weeks, evaluate whether an increase in dosage or another antipsychotic drug should be tried.
- Evaluate the patient for potential side effects. Symptoms considered indicators of problems include fever, sore throat, nausea, upper right quadrant abdominal pain, pruritus, dark-colored urine, light-colored stools, sunburn, orthostatic hypotension, pulse rate greater than 120 bpm, brownish skin coloration, a brownish cast to vision, or extrapyramidal reactions.

Table 27–8. PATIENT TEACHING INFORMATION—ANTIPSYCHOTICS

Dear Patient:

This is what you should know about the drug that has been prescribed for you to get the most from your therapy.

☐ 1. This drug will help to relax you. As you relax, your abilities to think clearly and concentrate will improve.

☐ 2. You should never take double doses or increase the frequency of times of doses.

☐ 3. If you forget to take a pill, you should take it only if you remember within 1 hour after the time it was due.

☐ 4. This medicine may make you feel drowsy, dizzy, or lightheaded. You should evaluate your response to the drug before you participate in activities that require you to be alert, such as driving an automobile.

☐ 5. Do not stop taking this drug without consulting your physician.

☐ 6. Do not drink alcohol while you are taking this drug. Before you take any other drugs, discuss this with your physician.

☐ 7. This drug may increase your sensitivity to the sun. You should use a sunscreen graded R-15 or greater and wear protective clothing when in the sun.

☐ 8. If you feel restless or excited soon after taking the medicine, or develop a sore throat with no other cold symptoms or muscle stiffness, contact your physician.

☐ 9. You should not take any antacids within 1 hour of ingesting this drug.

☐ 10. This drug may be taken with food or 8 ounces of water or milk.

☐ 11. If you are using the liquid concentrate, avoid getting it on your skin or clothing.

☐ 12. This medicine may cause your urine to become pinkish red, red, or reddish brown. This effect is harmless.

• Evaluate the patient for extrapyramidal reactions, which can frequently be difficult to differentiate from the symptoms of psychoses. Recognize the reactions early as the proper intervention can usually control these side effects. Extrapyramidal reactions are generally treated by one or more of the following: lowering the dose of the antipsychotic agent, using an antiparkinson medication, or replacing the drug with one that produces a lower level of extrapyramidal effects. (Refer to Chapter 23 for information about use of the antiparkinson medications for the treatment of extrapyramidal reactions induced by antipsychotic medications.)

• Provide the patient with supportive, honest education about the extrapyramidal side effects of the drug. If patients continue to experience extrapyramidal side effects despite dosage changes, antiparkinson medications, and a trial of various antipsychotic drugs, consider use of the atypical neuroleptic, clozapine.

• Evaluate the patient for sedation during the first weeks of treatment when this side effect is frequently severe. Control sedation by administering a single dose of the medication shortly before bedtime.

• Evaluate the patient for the potentially serious effect of agranulocytosis, which tends to occur within the first 6 months of treatment. The WBC declines ordinarily over a period of weeks, but cases may also develop precipitously within 1 week. The decline in WBC may or may not be associated with symptoms of infections, although the first indication of agranulocytosis is often a complaint of sore throat or fever. Medical treatment is vigorous and includes discontinuing the neuroleptic agent while using antibiotics and plasmapheresis. Patients who survive this reaction should never receive the same neuroleptic agent again.

• Evaluate patients receiving antipsychotic medication for early symptoms of cholestatic jaundice and cardiovascular side effects. Orthostatic hypotension is a common side effect, especially in the elderly, and tachycardia may also occur.

• Evaluate the patient's skin and eyes frequently because of the possibility of the skin/eye syndrome. Side effects of hypothermia and, rarely, hyperthermia also may occur. This reaction appears more frequently in elderly patients.

• Evaluate the patient for weight gain as this side effect is found in most patients receiving antipsychotic medication. A well-balanced, nutritional diet that minimizes sweets may reduce this tendency.

• Evaluate the patient for endocrinologic side effects such as amenorrhea, galactorrhea, gynecomastia, and ejaculation difficulties. Lowering the dosage of the medication may alleviate these effects.

After recognizing all the problems inherent in the use of antipsychotic agents, the nurse may question the rationale for their use. However, the risks and disability caused by the psychotic state far outweighs the risks of using the drugs. Many individuals who would previously have been confined to mental hospitals are now able to successfully lead a relatively normal life because of the use of antipsychotic medication.

The bibliography for this chapter can be found in Appendix B, which begins on page 1054.

CHAPTER REVIEW QUESTIONS*

1. The antipsychotic drugs have proven to be effective in the treatment of schizophrenia by:
   a. Controlling symptoms.
   b. Reducing side effects.
   c. Producing a sense of euphoria.
   d. Preventing psychosis.

2. Tardive dyskinesia, a syndrome associated with antipsychotic drugs, is most likely related to:
   a. Cholinergic receptor blockade.
   b. Dopaminergic receptor blockade.
   c. Short-term drug use.
   d. Subtherapeutic drug levels.

*See Appendix A, which begins on page 1051, for answers.

3. Which of the following descriptions is *correct* concerning the extrapyramidal side effects of antipsychotic medications:
   a. Akathisia is characterized by a shuffling gait.
   b. Acute dystonic reactions are characterized by abnormal facial grimacing and/or eye movements.
   c. Parkinsonism is characterized by torticollis.
   d. Tardive dyskinesia is characterized by difficulty sitting still.

4. Haloperidol is contraindicated in patients with:
   a. Parkinson's disease.
   b. Severe anxiety reaction.
   c. Senile dementia.
   d. Alzheimer's disease.

5. Current clinical experience suggests that clozapine has superior antipsychotic efficacy in:
   a. Patients over the age of 60.
   b. Adolescent schizophrenia.

   c. Patients who have features of depressive illness and psychosis.
   d. Treatment-refractory schizophrenia.

6. Repository preparations of neuroleptic drugs are much more slowly absorbed and eliminated than are oral preparations. For example, the elimination half-time for a depot of fluphenazine is:
   a. 24 hours.
   b. 25 to 30 days.
   c. 7 to 10 days.
   d. 6 months.

BUILDING YOUR CRITICAL THINKING SKILLS

EXTRAPYRIMIDAL SIDE EFFECTS

Case Study 1: Chlorpromazine (Thorazine)

A 34-year-old man began taking chlorpromazine (Thorazine) last month when he was diagnosed with schizophrenia. He was hospitalized for 2 weeks, then discharged home. Currently he comes to the emergency room complaining of restlessness, agitation, compulsive walking, and insomnia. The patient is anxious that his schizophrenia is returning, and his family wants him admitted.

1. What could be the possible cause of the patient's symptoms?
2. What course of action should the health-care team take for this patient?
3. What teaching should the nurse do for this patient?
4. Is it necessary for the patient to be admitted? Why or why not?

Case Study 2: Haloperidol (Haldol)

A 56-year-old homeless woman enters the free clinic and indicates she has "strange movements of her arms and legs." The nurse notes rhythmic rocking movements, tongue protrusion, and grimacing during the interview. The patient has been in and out of mental health institutions since the age of 28. She is currently receiving "some type of shot" once a month at the local mental health clinic. She says she has been taking this medication for years. The nurse calls the clinic and is told the patient is taking haloperidol (Haldol).

1. Describe the basis of the patient's symptoms.
2. What interventions should the nurse initiate for this patient?

UNIT 7

DRUGS AFFECTING THE CARDIOVASCULAR SYSTEM

UNIT OUTLINE

CHAPTER 28

Overview of the Anatomy and Physiology of the Cardiovascular System

Merrily A. Kuhn, RNC, PhD

CHAPTER OUTLINE

Structure and Function of the Heart
Electrophysiology of the Heart
Systemic Circulation and Blood Pressure
The Conduction System and the Electrocardiogram
Dysrhythmias

KEY TERMS

Absolute refractory period	Dysrhythmias
Action potential	Ectopic beat
Afterload	Mean arterial pressure
Automaticity	Peripheral resistance
Capillary blood pressure	Preload
Colloid osmotic pressure	Relative refractory period
Conductivity	Resting membrane potential
Contractility	Stroke volume
Diastole	Systole
Diastolic pressure	Systolic pressure

LEARNING OBJECTIVES

After reading this chapter, the student will be able to:

1. Diagram the heart, identify all four chambers, and recognize the normal pressures within the heart.
2. Understand the characteristics of the action potential curve and the normal conduction through the heart muscle.
3. Explain the concepts of preload, contractility, and afterload.
4. Identify characteristics of dysrhythmias including the following: sinus bradycardia and tachycardia, atrial flutter and fibrillation, sick sinus syndrome, supraventricular tachycardias, premature atrial and ventricular beats, ventricular tachycardia and fibrillation, and the conduction defects—first-, second-, and third-degree AV block.

The heart does an enormous amount of work for its size. With an average of 72 beats per minute, the heart will beat 4320 beats per hour, 103,680 beats per day, 37,843,200 beats per year, and 2,649,024,000 beats per lifetime of 70 years. This does not take into account the daily increases of heart rate caused by exercise and stress. The heart is responsible for supplying oxygenated blood to all cells of the body through about 60,000 miles of blood vessels and for returning oxygen-poor blood to the lungs to be reoxygenated. This chapter discusses the anatomy and phys-

iology that is pertinent to drug administration. For additional information on anatomy and physiology, see other textbooks.

STRUCTURE AND FUNCTION OF THE HEART

The heart, a four-chambered muscular organ weighing about 300 g, is located behind the sternum and is con-

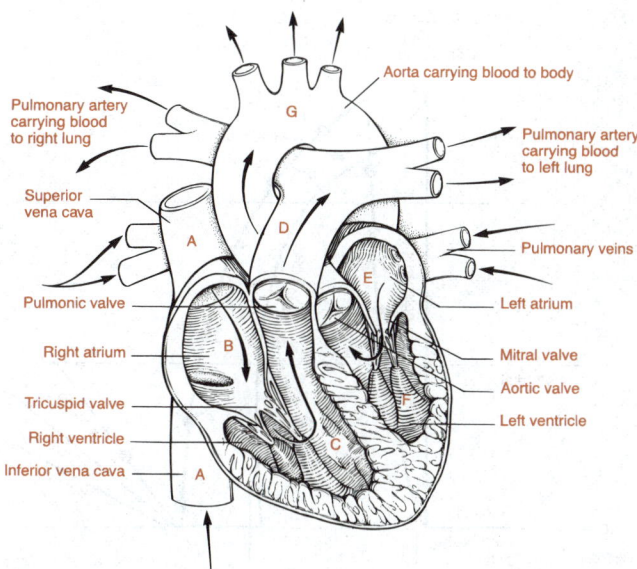

Figure 28–1. Frontal section of the heart demonstrating directional flow of blood and pressures. (A) Superior/inferior vena cava 5 to 15 cm H$_2$O. (B) Right atrial pressure 5/0 mm Hg. (C) Right ventricle 25/5 mm Hg. (D) Pulmonary artery 25/10 mm Hg. (E) Left atrium 10/0 mm Hg. (F) Left ventricle 120/5 mm Hg. (G) Aortic pressure carrying blood to body.

tained in the pericardial sac. Figure 28–1 shows a cross section of the heart. The heart generates pressure, which pushes blood throughout the vascular system. For normal pressures found in each chamber, refer to Figure 28–1.

CORONARY CIRCULATION

Located just above the aortic valve are the two orifices of the coronary arteries, as shown in Figure 28–2. The right coronary artery and the left coronary artery branch into

two vessels that supply blood to the entire heart. Of all coronary perfusion to the left heart, 70% to 80% occurs during cardiac *diastole* (the part of the cardiac cycle during which the entire heart is at rest), whereas the right heart is perfused during both diastole and *systole* (the part of the cardiac cycle during which a chamber is in contraction).

CARDIAC CELLS

The heart muscle is made of individual cardiac muscle cells called myocytes. Contained within each myocyte are two types of contractile proteins—the actin (thin) filaments and the myosin (thick) filaments. During contraction, large amounts of energy are released from the splitting of adenosine triphosphate (ATP), allowing the actin and myosin to slide past each other and form crossbridges. In order for the actin and myosin to slide, calcium must be present in the fiber. Calcium enters the myocardial fiber through the calcium channels in the sarcolemma. Calcium combines with a protein—troponin—found bound to actin. Normally, troponin prevents the sliding; however, when bound with calcium, sliding or contraction occurs.

CARDIAC OUTPUT

Cardiac output (CO) is the total volume of blood ejected by a ventricle per unit of time.

Cardiac output can be calculated by using the following formula:

Cardiac output = Stroke volume × heart rate

If stroke volume is 75 mL per beat and heart rate is 70 beats per minute, then

CO = 75 mL per beat × 70 beats per minute

= 5250 mL

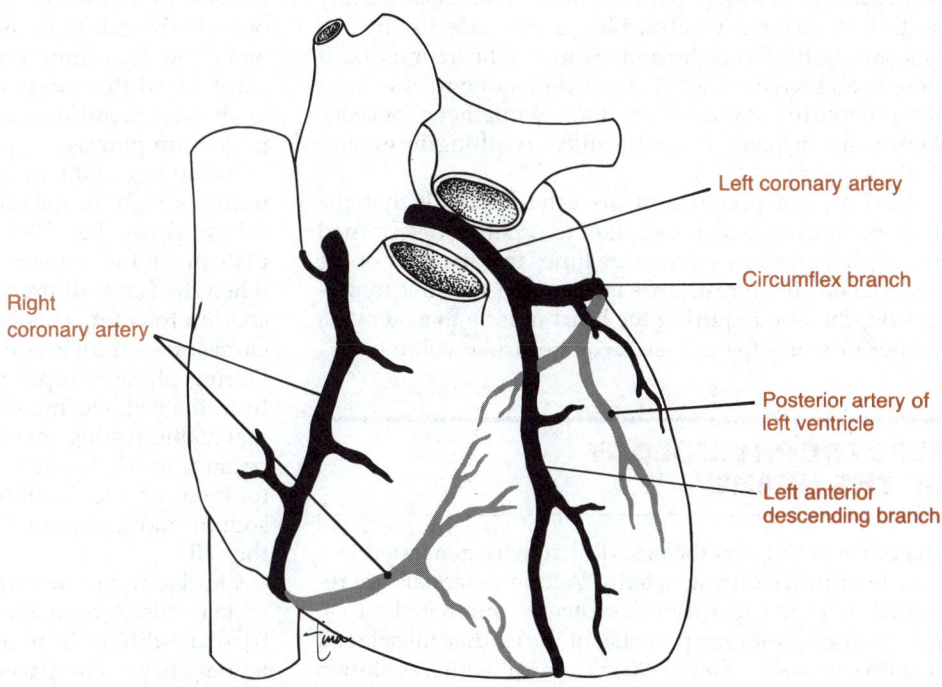

Figure 28–2. Coronary arteries.

or about 5 to 6 L/min. Cardiac output varies with the size of the individual, approximately in proportion to the body surface area. Cardiac output can increase by four to five times with strenuous exercise or other forms of physical or emotional stress. Cardiac output is often expressed in terms of cardiac output per square meter of body surface area, or cardiac index (cardiac output in liters per minute divided by the body surface area). The normal adult cardiac index averages 2.5 to 4.0 L/m^2 per minute. A cardiac index below 2.5 is abnormal.

The ejection fraction is the amount of blood ejected per beat, usually 70%. Each heartbeat ejects approximately 60 to 80 mL of blood, called the *stroke volume*, which depends on three factors: preload, contractility, and afterload.

Preload is stretch (Frank-Starling curve) of the myocardial fibers at the onset of contraction and is measured by blood volume in the ventricle at the end of diastole. When the heart is functioning properly, the length of heart muscle fibers is proportional to (or a function of) the amount of blood in the ventricle at the end of diastole (end-diastolic volume). Therefore, stroke volume is directly related to the end-diastolic volume. If stretch or preload decreases, the amount of blood in the ventricle at the end of diastole decreases (decreased end-diastolic volume), and therefore stroke volume decreases. The end-diastolic volume is also determined by three additional factors:

1. the amount of venous return to the atria
2. the strength of atrial contraction that is responsible for pushing blood into the ventricle (atrial contraction adds 20% to 25% to cardiac output)
3. the amount of blood that was ejected from the ventricle during the last contraction.

If any of these three factors is reduced, then stroke volume in turn is reduced.

Contractility is the ability of the ventricle to generate a force to eject the blood at particular fiber length. If a heart chamber is dilated or enlarged over its maximum because of disease, it contracts with less force and consequently ejects less volume. Contractility is also affected by the concentration of catecholamines in the heart muscle. If there is an increased level of catecholamine release (e.g., norepinephrine released by the sympathetic nerves), there is an increase in contractility, resulting in greater stroke volume.

Afterload, the pressure in the arterial circuit that the heart must overcome for ejection to occur, is determined by *peripheral resistance* (pressure times the diameter of the vessel). Peripheral resistance increases in systemic hypertension, thereby requiring the heart muscle to generate a greater pressure to eject an adequate stroke volume.

ELECTROPHYSIOLOGY OF THE HEART

The *action potential* is the electrical activity generated in a muscle or nerve during activity. Action potentials are recorded in a cardiac cell in four phases, numbered 1 to 4. The resting membrane potential of the cardiac muscle cell is approximately −80 to −90 mV, or millivolts, as shown in Figure 28–3. *Resting membrane potential*, the potential

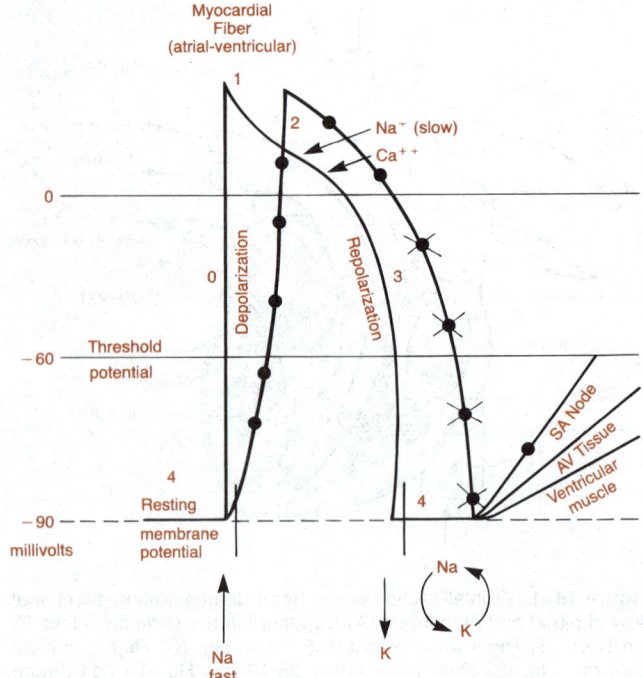

Figure 28–3. The solid line represents the action potential of cardiac cells. Phase 0—Sodium rapidly influxes through the fast sodium channels and cell depolarization begins. Phase 1—The fast sodium channels close. Phase 2—The plateau phase occurs as sodium enters slowly along with Ca^{++} through the slow Ca^{++} channels. Phase 3—K$^+$ effluxes from the cell and late repolarization occurs. Phase 4—The cell returns to its original resting membrane potential. There is activation of the Na$^+$-K$^+$ pump's mechanism, which actively pumps K$^+$ into the cell and Na$^+$ out of the cell. The action potential curve of a pacemaker cell is represented by the x-x-x portion of the curve.

difference across the membrane of a normal cell at rest, is a result of the distribution of ions inside and outside the cell. Inside the cell there is a high concentration of potassium and a low concentration of sodium, whereas outside the cell there is a high concentration of sodium and a low concentration of potassium (a reverse relationship). The difference in ion concentration on the two sides of the cell membrane is maintained by the sodium and potassium pumps.

At the beginning of rapid depolarization there is a fast influx of sodium ions through the fast sodium channels (phase 1) (see Fig. 28–3). Phase 2, often described as the plateau of the transmembrane action potential, occurs when the fast sodium channels close and no longer allow sodium to enter. This is followed by a slow influx of calcium and sodium ions through the slow calcium channels. During phase 3, rapid repolarization potassium effluxes from the cell. During phase 4, the cell returns to its original stable resting membrane potential, that is, with potassium inside the cell and sodium outside the cell. Restoration of the sodium-potassium gradient occurs as sodium moves out of the cell and potassium moves into the cell.

Cardiac tissue contains both pacemaker and nonpacemaker cells. A nonpacemaker cardiac cell—atrial or ventricular—differs from a pacemaker cell in its action potential curve. The pacemaker cell (automatic cell) has a spontaneously depolarizing phase 4 (see Fig. 28–3). This excitation allows the pacemaker cell to reach threshold and depolarize spontaneously. The sinoatrial (SA) nodal tissue has the steepest phase 4, and the automatic cells in ventricular muscle have the shallowest phase 4. The excitation allows the SA nodal tissue to reach threshold potential before other cells as sodium is entering the cell; therefore, the SA node is the pacemaker of the heart. Pacemaker, or automatic, cells are found only in the conduction pathway of the heart. All of the conduction pathway except the cells in the center of the atrioventricular (AV) node is made of automatic cells.

SYSTEMIC CIRCULATION AND BLOOD PRESSURE

Blood pressure, the pressure the blood exerts on the blood vessel walls, is generated by the left ventricle during contraction (systole). As the vessels age and lose their elasticity, more pressure is required to pump blood through them. Blood pressure is lowest at birth and increases with age and during stress or exercise.

Arterial pressure is composed of the systolic and diastolic pressures, which are measured in millimeters of mercury (mm Hg), or torr. The *systolic pressure* is the maximum pressure generated by the left ventricle during its contraction and ranges from 100 to 125 mm Hg (torr). The *diastolic pressure* is the pressure exerted on the artery walls during ventricular diastole and is usually 80 mm Hg. *Mean arterial pressure* (MAP) (usual range is 70 to 90 mm Hg) is a relationship between arterial and diastolic pressure, as follows:

$$\text{MAP} = \text{Cardiac output (CO)} \times \text{total peripheral resistances}$$

or

$$\text{MAP} = \text{Systolic pressure} + \frac{2\ (\text{diastolic pressure})}{3}$$

The pulse pressure is the difference between the systolic and diastolic pressures and is generally about 40 mm Hg.

Capillary blood pressure (the force generated by the blood flowing through the capillaries, which causes fluid to shift from the capillary to the interstitium) ranges from 30 mm Hg at the arterial end to 10 mm Hg at the venous end, with an overall average of 25 mm Hg. Capillary blood pressure is opposed by *colloid osmotic pressure* (oncotic or protein pressure maintained primarily by albumin). The higher blood pressure at the arterial end is the driving force for the movement of nutrients through the capillary membrane into interstitial space, as shown in Figure 28–4A. When the capillary blood pressure is normal or elevated or colloid osmotic pressure is low, capillary filtration increases and more fluid shifts from the vascular system to the interstitial tissues, a condition called edema (Fig. 28–4B). Conversely, if colloid osmotic pressure is high and capillary blood pressure is low, capillary filtration decreases, causing fluid to shift from the interstitial space to the circulatory system, increasing the blood volume and producing cellular dehydration (Fig. 28–4C). The maintainence of systemic blood pressure depends

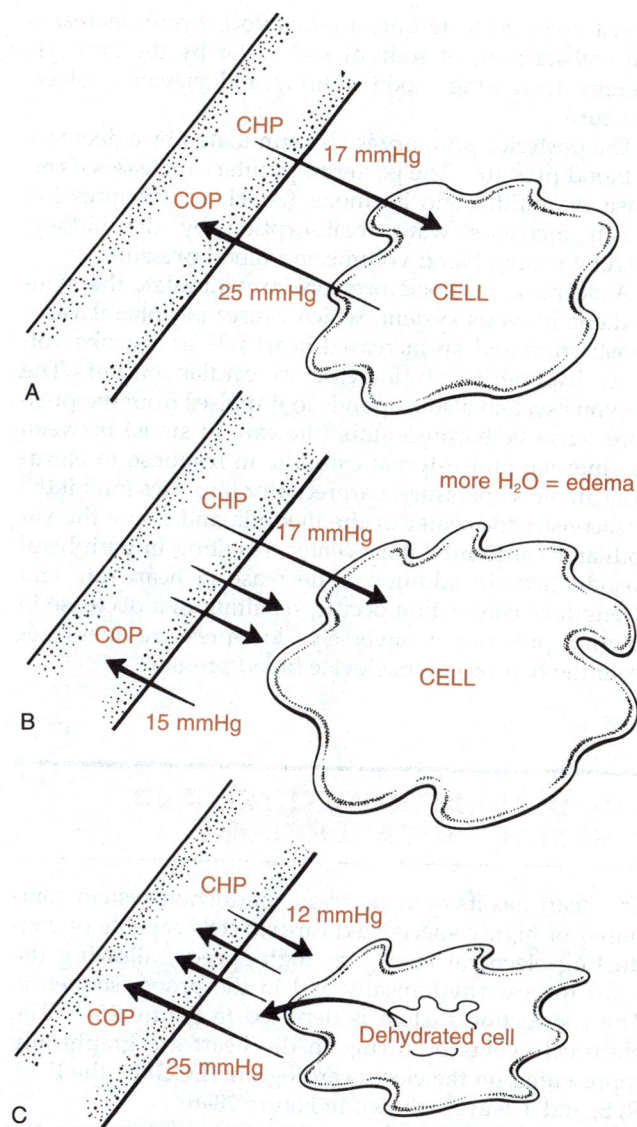

Figure 28–4. Fluid movement. (A) Normal venous capillary. Capillary blood pressure generated in the venous system is approximately 17 mm Hg. This pressure forces plasma and nutrients into the cell. Colloid osmotic pressure (COP) is pressure generated by protein that pulls plasma and waste products back into the vessel. When total protein is normal (about 7.2 mg/dl), a COP of 25 mm Hg is generated in the venous system. Therefore, the net pull is always back into the vessel. (B) When capillary blood pressure is normal or rises and colloid oncotic pressure (COP) is low, capillary filtration increases and more fluid shifts from the vascular system to the interstitial tissues. Thus, edema ensues. (C) When CHP is lower than normal, capillary filtration decreases, causing fluid to shift from the interstitial space into the circulation, increasing blood volume and producing interstitial and ultimately cellular dehydration.

on renal, endocrine, neurologic, and cardiovascular factors. The kidneys produce renin, which is released into the bloodstream in response to a decrease in blood pressure and renal ischemia. In the circulatory system, renin reacts with angiotensinogen, a plasma protein synthesized by the liver, to form angiotensin I. Angiotensin I is converted to angiotensin II by a converting enzyme found, in highest quantities, in the lung. Angiotensin II causes vasoconstriction, which raises blood pressure. Angiotensin II also stimulates the adrenal cortex to release aldosterone. Aldosterone, a mineralocorticoid, increases the reabsorption of sodium and water by the kidneys, thereby increasing blood volume and elevating blood pressure.

The posterior pituitary is also stimulated by a decrease in blood pressure. The posterior pituitary increases its release of antidiuretic hormone (ADH, or vasopressin), which increases water reabsorption by the kidney, thereby raising blood volume and blood pressure.

A decrease in blood pressure can stimulate the sympathetic nervous system, which causes peripheral vasoconstriction and an increased heart rate and stroke volume, leading to an increase in cardiac output. The nervous system also responds to impulses from the pressure-sensitive baroreceptors (the carotid sinus) between the internal and external carotids. In response to elevations in blood pressure, baroreceptor impulses inhibit the vasoconstrictor center of the medulla and excite the vasodilator cardioinhibitory center, resulting in peripheral vasodilation. In addition, a decrease in heart rate and strength of contraction occurs, resulting in a decrease in arterial pressure. Conversely, low-pressure messages from the baroreceptors elevate blood pressure.

THE CONDUCTION SYSTEM AND THE ELECTROCARDIOGRAM

The heart has its own electrical conduction system composed of highly specialized cardiac cells capable of conducting electrical energy at high speeds, allowing the heart to beat rhythmically and in the proper sequence. The conduction system is depicted in Figure 28–5. The electrical events occurring in the heart are graphically represented on the electrocardiogram (ECG) by the P, Q, R, S, and T waves, shown in Figure 28–6.

Although there are three potential backup systems, the SA node located high in the right atrium near the entrance of the superior vena cava is usually the pacemaker of the heart. It initiates each heartbeat and is under the direct influence of both the sympathetic and parasympathetic nervous systems. The SA action potential exits the node and travels through the atria, causing the atria to contract (usually 60 to 100 beats per minute). Depolarization of the atria is represented on the ECG by the P wave.

The impulse moves into the AV node, where it is slowed so the atria and ventricles do not contract simultaneously. The AV node has no pacemaking cells of its own. The junctional area generates impulses when the SA node fails to function. The junctional area has an inherent rate of 40 to 60 beats per minute. Atrial depolarization and the movement of the impulse through the AV node are represented by the PR interval on the electrocardiogram. The normal PR interval is 0.12 to 0.20 seconds in duration.

The impulse proceeds through the bundle of His to the right and left bundle branches and then to the ventricles. The impulse is transmitted rapidly throughout the ventricular muscle by way of the Purkinje fibers. The ventricles then depolarize and contract. The ventricular depo-

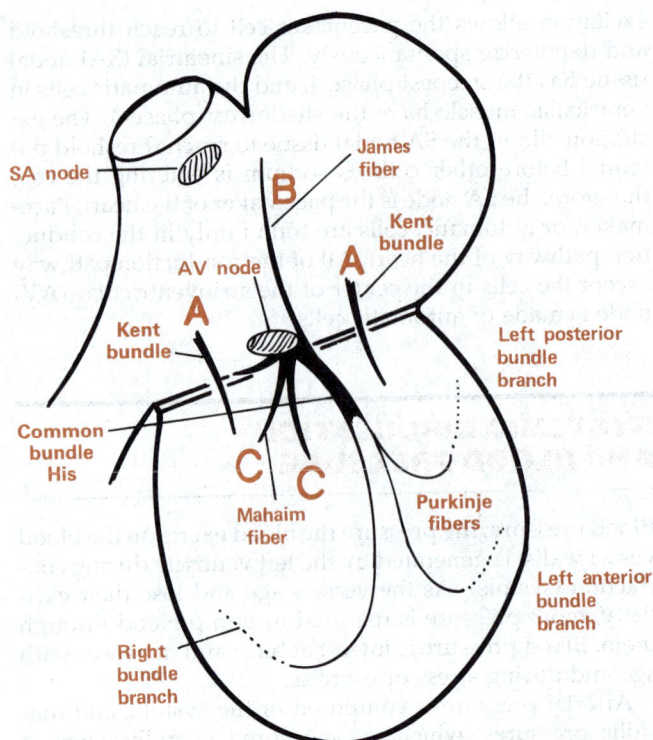

Figure 28–5. Conduction system. The normal impulse originates in the SA nodes, moves through the atrial tissue to the AV node, down the common bundle of His into the bundle branches (right bundle branch, left anterior bundle branch, left posterior bundle branch), and to the Purkinje fibers. Several abnormal accessory bundles can exist: A, the Kent bundle, when activated results in Wolf-Parkinson-White syndrome; B, the James fiber, when activated results in the Lawn-Ganong-Levine syndrome; and C, the Mahaim fiber.

larization is represented by the QRS wave on the ECG. The Purkinje fibers in the ventricular muscle are also capable of generating an electrical impulse if the higher pacemakers (SA node and junction) fail to generate an impulse. Their inherent rate is 20 to 40 beats per minute.

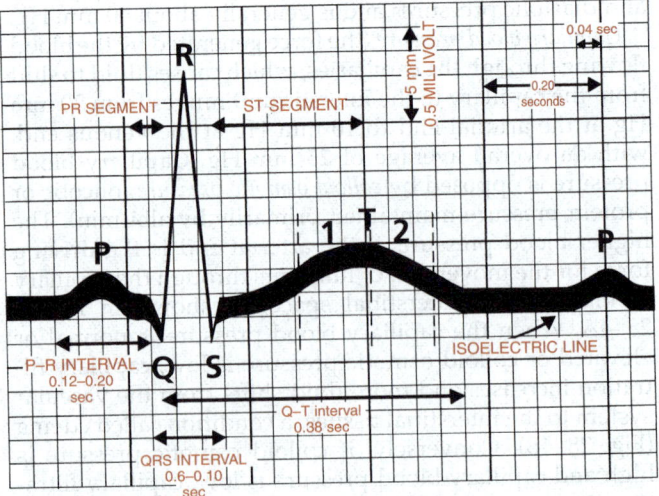

Figure 28–6. Normal electrocardiogram wave deflection and intervals. Phase 1 of the T wave represents the absolute refractory period; phase 2 of the T wave, the relative refractory period.

The ventricular muscle now enters its repolarization phase. This is represented by the T wave on the ECG. The T wave is composed of two phases: the absolute refractory period and the relative refractory period, as shown in Figure 28–6. The *absolute refractory period* is the interval during which no impulse can reexcite an already excited area of cardiac muscle. The *relative refractory period* is the interval during which the heart can respond to an electrical stimulation if the stimulation is greater than normal. If any electrical impulse stimulates the heart during the relative refractory period, an abnormal rhythm may occur.

Between the end of the T wave and the beginning of the next QRS, the ventricles, in diastole, are filling with blood. Most of the flow into the coronary arteries occurs at this time also. Therefore, in tachycardias, there is less time for coronary perfusion, leading to myocardial ischemia in patients with coronary obstruction. In a normal, healthy person, the decrease in coronary perfusion occurs at a pulse rate above 210 beats per minute. In an individual with heart disease, the decrease in coronary perfusion may become significant at a pulse rate over 120 beats per minute.

DYSRHYTHMIAS

Dysrhythmias are disorders of the heart rate and rhythm. Any change of rate is considered a change of rhythm. Generally, two factors account for cardiac dysrhythmias:

Table 28–1. DYSRHYTHMIAS AND DISORDERS OF IMPULSE FORMATION/CONDUCTION

Type of Dysrhythmia/Description	Etiology	Hemodynamic Consequences	Management
DYSRHYTHMIAS			
Sinus bradycardia: Rhythm is regular, but heart rate is slower; SA node discharge <60 beats/min.	Digoxin toxicity Late hypoxia Vagal hyperactivity Hyperkalemia slows depolarization	Decreased mean arterial pressure Increased preload	If hypotensive, treat cause and support Follow with sympathomimetics, cardiotonics, and pacer Vagolytics
Sinus tachycardia: Rhythm is regular, but heart rate is faster; SA node discharge 100–150 beats/min.	Lung disease Hypoxic cell metabolism Catecholamines Fever Hypercalcemia Digoxin toxicity	Increased myocardial demand Decreased filling times Decreased mean arterial pressure	Oxygen, bed rest Calcium channel blockers Pacer override Vagus stimulation Control ventricular rate
Atrial tachycardia (AT): rapid, regular atrial rhythm arising from atrial tissue; rate of 200 +/−50 beats/min.			
Premature atrial contractions (PACs): Atrial beat arising in atria before normal impulse.	Electrolyte disturbances Hypoxia and elevated preload Hypercalcemia	Occasional decreased filling time and mean arterial pressure	Treat underlying cause Digoxin
Atrial flutter: Atria beat at rate of 300 +/−50 beats/min; some degree of AV block exists.	Same as atrial tachycardia, plus aging	Decreased filling time Decreased mean arterial pressure	Same as atrial tachycardia Synchronous cardioversion Digoxin
Atrial fibrillation: Atria no longer contract but quiver at rate of 400 +/−beats/min.	Dysrhythmia	Dysrhythmia	Dysrhythmia
Premature ventricular contractions (PVCs): Contraction of ventricle before normal time; caused by electrical impulse, which originates in cell outside normal conduction system and spreads through muscle tissue.	Same as PACs, plus aging Induction of anesthesia Hypertrophy	Occasional decreased filling time and mean arterial pressure	Pharmacology to change thresholds and refractory periods, to reduce myocardial demand, and to increase O$_2$ supply Removal of cause
Agonal rhythm/electromechanical dissociation or pulseless electrical activity (PEA): Depolarization and contraction not coupled.	Usually caused by profound hypoxia	Absent or barely present cardiac output and pulse Not compatible with life	Vigorous pharmacology aimed at restoring rate and force Usually ineffective May attempt to pace
Ventricular fibrillation (Asystole): No cardiac activity.	Profound ischemia Hyperkalemia Acidosis	No cardiac output No coronary perfusion Not compatible with life	Same as agonal rhythm, plus electrical defibrillation
DISORDERS OF IMPULSE FORMATION/CONDUCTION			
AV (atrioventricular) blocks—first, second, or third (complete): Delay or blockage in transmission of impulses from atria to ventricles.	Local hypoxia Scarring of intra-atrial conduction pathways Electrolyte imbalances Increased atrial preload Hyperkalemia (>7 mEq/L) Hypokalemia (>3.5 mEq/L) Formation of myocardial abscesses in endocarditis	Occasional decrease in cardiac output Increase in preload for the following beat	Pharmacologic treatment includes vagolytics, sympathomimetics, pacing Discovery and correction of cause

(1) an increase in automaticity and (2) a disturbance in conduction from the SA node, or through the AV node or accessory bundles. As *automaticity* (the ability of the cells to develop an action potential spontaneously) is increased, tachydysrhythmias or *ectopic* (at or from an abnormal location) *beats* are produced, such as atrial or ventricular tachycardia and atrial or ventricular premature beats. When automaticity is decreased, bradydysrhythmias, such as sinus bradycardia, develop. Altered *conductivity* (the ability of the heart to conduct impulses in an orderly fashion throughout the heart muscle) is associated with either a change in conduction in normal pathways or conduction through an abnormal accessory bundle. Accessory bundles are outside the normal conduction system and are known as the Kent, James, and Mahaim fibers. When these accessory bundles are present, the patient may experience tachydysrhythmias such as the Wolff-Parkinson-White syndrome, due to activation of the Kent bundles (Fig. 28–5A), or the Lown-Ganong-Levine syndrome, due to activation of the James fibers (Fig. 28–5,B).

Dysrhythmias are classed as to disorders of impulse formation, such as bradycardias, tachycardias, premature beats, flutters, or fibrillation; or disorders of impulse conduction such as first-, second-, or third-degree AV blocks, or incomplete or complete bundle branch blocks. The dysrhythmias are reviewed in Table 28–1. For a more complete review, see a pathophysiology text.

CHAPTER REVIEW QUESTIONS*

1. Which of the following statements is *correct* regarding the action potential curve of the cardiac cell?
   a. During phase 1, a fast influx of potassium ion moves into the cell.
   b. During phase 4, only a strong stimulus will precipitate an action potential.
   c. During phase 2, a slow influx of calcium ions moves into the cell.
   d. During phase 3, a fast influx of sodium ions moves into the cells.

2. The following description applies to the conduction system of the heart and the ECG pattern:
   a. The P wave reflects ventricular depolarization.
   b. The PR interval represents atrial contraction.
   c. The QRS complex represents ventricular depolarization.
   d. The T wave represents ventricular depolarization.

3. Cardiac output is calculated by multiplying stroke volume by:
   a. Preload.
   b. Heart rate.
   c. Conductivity.
   d. Elasticity.

4. The sequence of normal electrical conduction through the heart is:
   a. SA node, bundle branches, AV node, bundle of His, Purkinje fibers.
   b. SA node, AV node, bundle of His, bundle branches, Purkinje fibers.
   c. SA node, AV node, bundle branches, Purkinje fibers, bundle of His.
   d. SA node, bundle of His, AV node, bundle branches, Purkinje fibers.

5. Which of the following is *correct* with regard to second-degree AV block:
   a. These are absent or barely present P waves.
   b. May be associated to hyper- or hypokalemia.
   c. Cardiac output increases in response to greater cardiac demand.
   d. Has a decreased filling time.

*See Appendix A, which begins on page 1051, for answers.

CHAPTER 29

Cardiac Glycosides and Other Positive Inotropic Agents

Merrily A. Kuhn, RNC, PhD

CHAPTER OUTLINE

KEY TERMS

Chromatopsia   Positive inotropic agents
Chronotropic   U wave

LEARNING OBJECTIVES

After reading this chapter, the student will be able to:

1. Identify those medications commonly used as cardiac glycosides.
2. Differentiate among the cardiac glycosides as to mechanism of action, route of administration, pharmacokinetics, adverse and toxic effects, contraindications and precautions, and interactions.
3. Identify specific areas to assess in the patient requiring cardiac glycosides to formulate appropriate patient outcomes.
4. Plan the nursing interventions necessary to administer cardiac glycosides and choose appropriate teaching strategies to gain patient compliance.
5. Evaluate the patient at various stages of treatment to measure the effectiveness of nursing interventions.

---

*P*ositive inotropic agents are medications that increase the contractile force of the heart, causing the ventricles to empty more completely and thus improving cardiac output. Positive inotropic agents include the cardiac glycosides and bipyridine derivatives. The cardiac glycosides are the oldest positive inotropics and have been in recorded use since 1775. They were first used by William Withering of England as a "cure" for dependent edema in the lower extremities caused by heart failure, referred to as dropsy in older literature. Cardiac glycosides are all produced from a natural source, either *Digitalis purpurea*, the purple foxglove, or *Digitalis lanata*, the white foxglove, both beautiful flowering plants native to the northern United States. Thus, cardiac glycosides are also known as digitalis glycosides.

Approximately 10% of all hospitalized patients receive cardiac glycosides. Many patients receiving cardiac glycosides are rehospitalized for medical problems, many of which are due to lack of patient compliance with their medical and nursing regimens or to the very narrow therapeutic index of the digitalis glycosides. Some hospitalizations could be eliminated with proper patient and family education.

CARDIAC GLYCOSIDES

Both of the cardiac glycosides—**digoxin (Lanoxin)** and **digitoxin (Crystodigin)**—are potent in very low doses, and their therapeutic effects on the heart are qualitatively similar. Cardiac glycosides are composed of three parts:

a sugar, a steroid, and a lactone. The sugar affects kinetics and potency and thus increases the water solubility and absorption and modifies toxicity. The steroid is similar to the sex hormones and corticosteroids. The lactone is responsible for the cardiac effects.

Digoxin is used to represent the cardiac glycosides, as it is the prototypical drug in this class. The cardiac glycosides are featured in Table 29–1.

ACTION

The cardiac glycosides have both a direct effect on cardiac muscle and the conduction system and an indirect action on the cardiovascular system mediated through the autonomic nervous system. These effects are dose related. Digitalis glycosides have both positive inotropic and negative *chronotropic* (reduction of heart rate) effects on the muscle cells of the myocardium. These effects are present on both the failing and nonfailing heart, although a greater magnitude of effect is usually seen on the failing heart.

The positive inotropic effect causes a more complete emptying of the ventricles during systole, which is more pronounced in patients with failing hearts. The improved emptying increases the cardiac output (CO) and helps to decrease systemic venous pressure (preload reduction). This, in turn, reduces the symptoms of heart failure such as dyspnea, ascites, and dependent edema. A review of management of heart failure is featured in Table 29–2.

The digitalis glycosides exert an inotropic effect on the heart through the inhibition of the adenosine triphosphatase (ATPase) enzyme, depicted in Figure 29–1, required for the movement or active transport of sodium and calcium across the cell membrane into the cardiac cell and for the movement of potassium out of the cell (often referred to as the sodium-potassium pump mechanism). By inhibiting ATPase, digitalis causes an accumulation of sodium within the cell. The intracellular sodium is exchanged for extracellular calcium through the T tubules. This calcium current moves along the T tubule, causing the cell to contract more rapidly and forcefully, thus increasing the inotropic action of the heart. The inhibition of ATPase is the reason that digitalis, at toxic levels, causes dysrhythmias. When ATPase is inhibited, more calcium is allowed to enter the cell, rendering it more irritable and thus causing it to contract more frequently. ATPase is further inhibited if the serum potassium level is low. Digitalis dysrhythmias can be prevented by adequate monitoring and replacement of potassium. ATPase activity is also maintained by magnesium. When magnesium levels are lower (as in acute pancreatitis, chronic alcoholism, chronic diarrhea, or chronic diuretic therapy), ATPase is inhibited further, possibly leading to dysrhythmias. The administration of magnesium sulfate may alleviate these dysrhythmias.

Secondary to the increase in contractility is a decrease in preload and end-diastolic volume. Also, a secondary concomitant reduction in the sympathetic tone with an increased sensitization of the myocardium to acetylcholine (the neurotransmitter from the vagus nerve) decreases the heart rate, thereby exerting a negative chronotropic effect.

The primary site of chronotropic action of the digitalis glycosides is the atrioventricular (AV) node. Conduction through the AV node and bundle of His is slowed due to an increase in the refractory period of the AV node and also because vagal tone is increased. The sinoatrial (SA) and AV nodes have enhanced sensitivity to acetylcholine and reduced sensitivity to norepinephrine. As repolarization is lengthened, fewer impulses are allowed to pass through the AV node at any given time.

The digitalis glycosides also decrease the heart size in patients with cardiomegaly and heart failure that occurs secondary to an increase in workload. Digitalis glycosides increase the stroke volume and improve ventricular emptying, decreasing workload, and leaving less blood in the ventricle to dilate the heart during diastole.

The digitalis glycosides also have a mild, indirect diuretic effect. This diuretic effect results from improved cardiac output, which increases blood flow to the kidney, thus improving filtration and ultimately increasing urinary output. In addition, the production of renin and thus angiotensin decreases, and afterload is reduced.

The digitalis glycosides have an effect on the electrocardiogram (ECG). The most prominent and consistent effects produced by the cardiac glycosides at therapeutic levels are changes in the (1) T wave, (2) PR interval, (3) ST segment, and (4) U wave, all shown in Figure 29–2. Clinically, T wave and ST segment changes are taken as evidence that the heart has been affected by the cardiac glycosides. The T wave shows a decrease in its amplitude, the ST segment sags below the baseline, and relatively high *U waves* (an electrocardiographic wave, occurring after the T wave, which is secondary to the effects of digitalis) may begin to appear. These changes do not correlate with either the optimum or the toxic effects of the cardiac glycosides. The PR interval is slightly prolonged because of the delayed conduction in the AV node. The digitalis glycosides have a direct effect on the action potential curve. They shorten phase 3, as shown in Figure 29–3, which has a shortening effect on the QT interval as the ventricular cells are stimulated by digitalis.

As serum levels of the cardiac glycosides begin to increase, conduction velocity through the AV node is further delayed. As a toxic serum level is approached, the patient may develop heart block (see Chapter 28).

Digitalis glycosides cause a slight increase in blood pressure by several mechanisms: increasing cardiac output; exerting a direct vasoconstrictor effect on arteriolar smooth muscle; and sensitizing the baroreceptors in the carotid sinus and aortic arch. The baroreceptors are stimulated even though blood pressure is not high. This is especially true following rapid IV bolus administration.

USES

The digitalis glycosides are currently used to treat or control systolic heart failure and dysrhythmias, including atrial fibrillation, atrial flutter, and supraventricular tachycardias. (See Chapter 28 for review of dysrhythmias.) If heart rates are not slowed with digitalis glycosides, magnesium levels are assessed and corrected.

By increasing the force of contraction, which improves cardiac output, these drugs relieve the symptoms of sys-

Table 29–1. CARDIAC GLYCOSIDES AND DIGOXIN ANTAGONIST

DRUG NAME/ROUTE AND DOSAGE	PHARMACOKINETICS/ DYNAMICS	NURSING IMPLICATIONS
CARDIAC GLYCOSIDES		

digoxin (Lanoxin) (Lanoxicaps)
therapeutic serum level: 0.5–2 ng/mL.   **Toxicity:** >2.5 ng/mL.

Adults: Loading dose–0.5–1 mg PO in divided doses over 24 hr. *Maintenance dose*–0.125–0.5 mg PO or IV slowly over 5–30 min (depending on renal function; see text). *Children over 5–10 yr: Loading dose*–15–30 μg/kg IV or 20–35 μg/kg PO. *Maintenance dose*–6–10 μg/kg PO. *Children 2–5 yr: Loading dose*–25–35 μg/kg IV or 30–40 μg/kg PO in divided doses. *Maintenance dose*–8–12 μg/kg PO per day. *Children 1 mo–2 yr: Loading dose*–35–60 μg/kg PO or IV in divided doses. *Maintenance dose*–20%–30% of loading dose. *Full-term Newborns (under 1 mo): Loading dose*–25–35 μg/kg in divided doses over 24 hr or 20–30 mg/kg IV. *Maintenance dose*–25%–35% of loading dose. *Premature Infants: Loading dose*–20–30 mg/kg PO or 15–25 mg/kg IV. *Maintenance dose*–20%–30% of loading dose.	**Onset:** PO, 1 hr; IV, 5–30 min **Peak:** PO, 2–6 hr; IV, 1–5 hr **Duration:** 2–6 days **½L:** 30–40 hr **PB:** 25% **B:** minimally in liver **E:** kidney	**ASSESSMENT:** Assess cardiac rate and rhythm and determine the presence of dysrhythmias. Obtain baseline serum and periodic levels of potassium, serum creatinine, BUN, and liver studies. Assess digitalis serum levels. Assess for pregnancy (category C). **INTERVENTION:** Take apical pulse for 1 full min before administering (range should be 60–110/min). Administer at the same time each day (noon or 6 PM is best). Administering with food delays but does not reduce absorption. Determine pulse deficit as ordered. Administer PO or IV (IM and SC irritating to tissues). Full loading dose is not given if other digitalis product is given within 1 wk or digitoxin given within 2 wk. Administer IV bolus over at least 10–30 min to avoid increases in blood pressure. IV solutions stable for 6 hr at room temperature. **Patient Teaching**—Tell patient to store drug in tightly closed containers and to protect from excessive heat and light. Caution patient to not discontinue medication without checking with physician. Teach patient how to take pulse and inform about his or her pulse limits. **EVALUATION:** Weigh patient weekly to evaluate fluid retention. Notify physician if loss of appetite, lower abdominal pain, nausea, vomiting, diarrhea, unusual tiredness or weakness, drowsiness, headache, blurred or yellow vision, skin rash or hives, or mental depression occur.

digitoxin (Crystodigin)
therapeutic serum level: 14–26 ng/mL.   **Toxicity:** >35 ng/mL.

Adults: Loading dose–1.2–1.6 mg PO in divided doses in 24 hr. *Maintenance dose*–0.05–0.3 mg PO daily. *Children over 2 yr: Loading dose*–0.03 mg/kg PO. *Maintenance dose*–10% of loading dose. *Children 1–2 yr: Loading dose*–0.04 mg/kg PO. *Maintenance dose*–10% of loading dose. *Children under 1 yr: Loading dose*–0.045 mg/kg PO. *Maintenance dose*–10% of loading dose.	**Onset:** 1–4 hr **Peak:** 8–12 hr **Duration:** 1–3 wk **½L:** 5–7 days **PB:** 97% **B:** liver **E:** urine	Same as for digoxin.

DIGOXIN ANTAGONIST		

digoxin immune Fab (Digibind)

Adults: 40 mg IV binds 0.6 mg/of digoxin. Dose varies according to amount of digoxin to be neutralized. See package insert for dosing.	**Onset:** 1 min **Peak:** 15–30 min **Duration:** NA **½L:** 15–20 hr **B:** not biotransformed **E:** kidney	**ASSESSMENT:** Draw digitalis level and K$^+$ before administration. Obtain baseline temperature, blood pressure, and ECG. Assess for pregnancy (category C). **INTERVENTION:** Dissolve 1 vial in 4 mL sterile water; use immediately or refrigerate up to 4 hr. Use 0.22-μm membrane filter. Infuse over 30 min. **EVALUATION:** Evaluate ECG and K$^+$ level. Administer K$^+$ as needed.

BUN = blood urea nitrogen.

Table 29–2. HEART FAILURE

Definition
Clinical syndrome that occurs when the heart cannot pump enough blood to meet the body's needs, resulting in intravascular/interstitial volume overload and inadequate tissue perfusion.

Types
Systolic ejection heart failure (chronic/acute)
Diastolic filling heart failure
Mixed systolic and diastolic failure

	Systolic Failure	Diastolic Failure	Mixed Systolic and Diastolic Failure
Etiology	• Coronary heart disease • Acute ischemia with injury	• LV hypertrophy • Chronic hypertension • Aortic stenosis • Hypertrophic cardiomyopathy • Aging	• Dilated cardiomyopathy • Aortic/mitral insufficiency • Long-term diabetes • Viral myocarditis • Postpartum myocarditis • Hypothyroid state • Secondary drugs (doxorubicin)
Pathophysiology	LV loses ability to eject blood effectively; problem of contractility	Problem of relaxation and filling	Poor systolic function is further compromised by dilated LV walls, which are unable to reflex owing to chronic volume overload
Diagnostic Findings	• ↓ LV ejection fraction • ↑ LVEDP • ↑ PCWP • Pulmonary edema • ↓ CO	• Normal systolic function • Pulmonary congestion • Low LV pressure • High atrial pressure • Pulmonary edema • PCWP	• Pulmonary congestion • ↑ PCWP • ↓ CO • Pulmonary edema
Sexual Predisposition	Male	Female	—

Symptoms	Systolic Failure	Diastolic Failure	Mixed Systolic and Diastolic Failure
Pulmonary congestion	X	X	X
Shortness of breath	X	X	X
Weakness/Fatigue	X	X	X
Peripheral edema	—	X	—
Dyspnea/Crackles/Hypoxia	X	X	X

Management: Acute	Systolic Failure	Diastolic Failure	Mixed Systolic and Diastolic Failure
Balanced vasodilators like sodium nitroprusside (Nipride) (may increase ST so monitor closely)	X	—	X
Nitroglycerin IV (reduces preload and SVR)	X	X	X
Dobutamine (Dobutrex)	X	—	—
Loop diuretics	X	X (Careful use)	X
Dopamine (Intropin) in low doses	X	X	X
Maintain PCWP/PAOP above 14	X	X	X

Management: Chronic	Systolic Failure	Diastolic Failure	Mixed Systolic and Diastolic Failure
ACE inhibitors	X	—	—
Na+-restricted diet to 3 g/day	X	X	X
Home exercise regimen	X	X	X
Diuretics	X	X	X
Long-acting nitrates	X	—	—
Cardiac glycosides	X	—	X
Amrinone/Milrinone	X	—	—
O$_2$	X	X	X
Morphine	X	X	
Calcium channel blockers	—	X	X (Careful use)
Beta-blockers	—	X	X (Careful use)

X = symptoms applicable to condition. LV = left ventricle; LVEDP = left ventricular end-diastolic pulse; PCWP = pulmonary capillary wedge pressure; SVR = systemic vascular resistance.

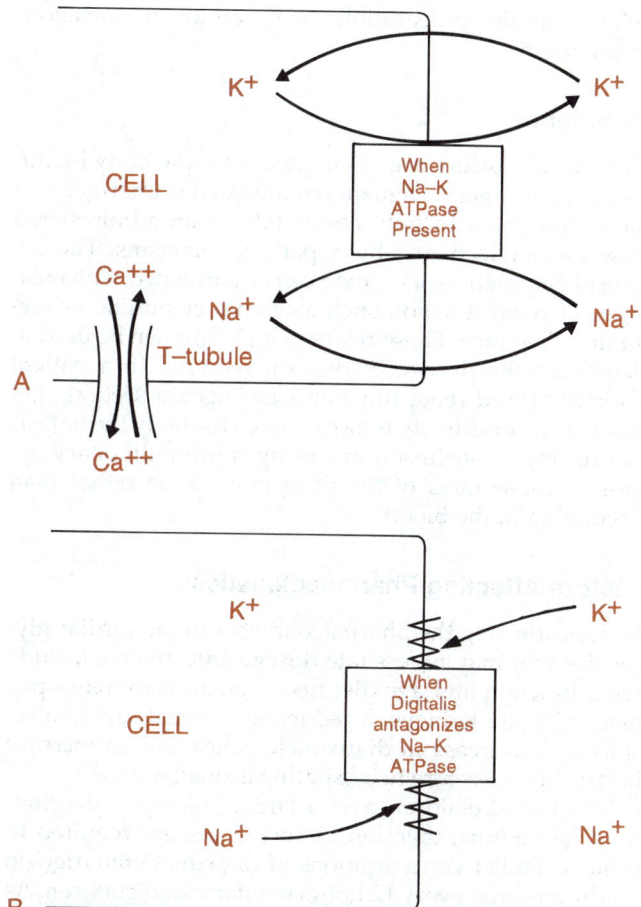

Figure 29–1. (A) Adenosine triphosphates (ATPase), the enzyme that surrounds each cardiac cell and is maintained by magnesium, is responsible for active transport of sodium and calcium across the cell membrane. (B) When digitalis is administered, the Na–K ATPase is depressed, and Na^+ remains in the cell and K^+ remains outside, as the Na–K pump mechanism does not work effectively.

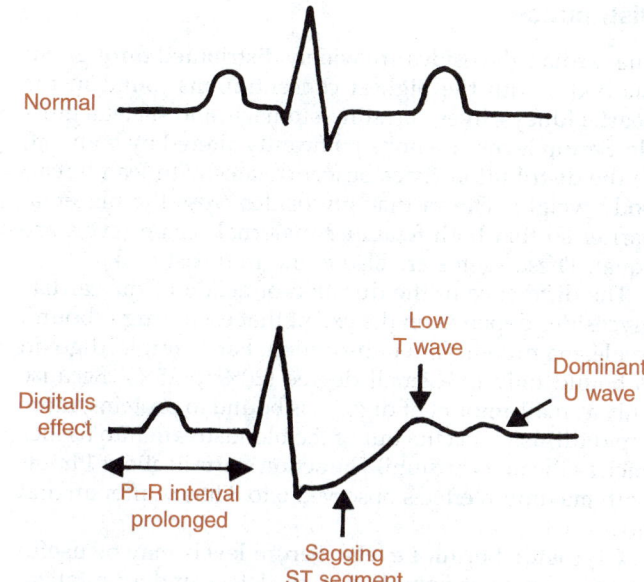

Figure 29–2. Normal ECG and effect of digitalis on the ECG.

atrial fibrillation. If the atrial fibrillation is due to heart failure, digitalis may be appropriate as a single drug. But if failure is not present, other drugs such as verapamil may be added to the drug regimen to obtain better control.

PHARMACOKINETICS

Absorption

The metabolic handling, excretion, and duration of action of the cardiac glycosides depend on the glycoside being administered. Most digitalis preparations can be absorbed from the gastrointestinal system, primarily from the jejunum. The extent of absorption (bioavailability) for the various preparations ranges from 20% to 100% (see Table 29–1 for specific information) and varies from patient to patient, from manufacturer to manufacturer, and even from dose to dose in the same patient. When oral digoxin is taken with meals, the rate of absorption is slowed; however, the total amount absorbed is unchanged. The variability of absorption, particularly of digoxin, can lead to problems for patients who have been stabilized on one tablet brand and then switch to another.

tolic heart failure. Through their effect on cardiac output, the cardiac glycosides improve both oxygen delivery to the tissues and blood flow to the kidney, which increases renal filtration and increases urinary output. Total circulating blood volume is thereby reduced. Coronary perfusion is improved by decreasing the heart rate and increasing the diastolic filling time, the period during which the coronary arteries are perfused.

The cardiac glycosides are most effective in systolic heart failure associated with the inability of the heart to pump enough blood volume. They are less effective in diastole failure caused by hypertrophy, hypertension, or ischemia, which are associated with the heart's ability to relax. The cardiac glycosides are commonly used concomitantly with diuretics and/or vasodilators to treat the patient in heart failure.

The cardiac glycosides are also used to slow the heart rate by causing decreased conduction through the AV node of certain dysrhythmias such as atrial flutter, fibrillation, or atrial tachycardias such as paroxysmal atrial tachycardia (PAT). However, newer research indicates that digitalis may not always be the best drug for treating

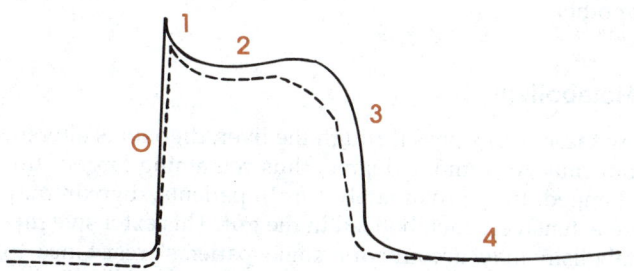

Figure 29–3. Action potential curve. A normal curve *(solid line)* with changes due to cardiac glycosides *(dashed line)*.

Distribution

The cardiac glycosides are widely distributed throughout the body, with the highest concentrations found in the heart, kidneys, liver, intestine, stomach, and skeletal muscle. Serum levels are not significantly altered by body fat, so the distribution space best correlates with lean (ideal) body weight. The cardiac glycosides cross the placental barrier so that both fetal and maternal serum levels are equal. These agents are also found in breast milk.

The difference in the duration of action of the cardiac glycosides depends on the extent that each drug is bound to plasma proteins after absorption. For example, digoxin is bound only to a small degree (20% to 25%). Because only a small amount of digoxin is bound to proteins, more rapid diffusion occurs out of the bloodstream into tissues such as the myocardium. The action starts in about 1 hour, with maximum effects observed 6 to 8 hours after an oral dose.

Glycoside Serum Levels Serum levels may be useful to assess patient compliance, to detect underdigitalization, to monitor patients who may be at risk for becoming toxic, and to detect problems in bioavailability caused by gastrointestinal disorders, concurrent use of other drugs, or poor tablet dissolution (see Table 29–1).

The time that the blood sample is obtained is taken into consideration, because serum levels are high during the absorptive and distributive phases. A delay of 3 to 4 hours after an intravenous dose of digoxin and up to 11 hours after an oral dose is recommended. Obtaining samples earlier results in values that do not reflect physiologic effects and is the most common cause of misinterpretation of serum concentrations. Most of the inotropic effects of digoxin are achieved at a serum level of 1 to 1.5 ng/mL. Levels up to 2 ng/mL are better for treating atrial fibrillation.

Rather than just administering digoxin alone to control atrial fibrillation, calcium channel blockers (e.g., verapamil [Calan], diltiazem [Cardizem]) or beta-adrenergic blockers (e.g., atenolol [Tenormin], pindolol [Visken]) are added. These drugs act directly to increase the refractoriness of the AV node, whereas digoxin largely has an indirect effect that can be suppressed by sympathetic activity during stress or fever.

Serum levels often do not correlate well with actual clinical events. Serum levels are evaluated in conjunction with current symptoms, laboratory test results, and ECG findings. Even if serum levels are in the toxic range, digitalis should not be discontinued in the absence of other signs of toxicity. A serum level that is effective and safe for one patient may be excessive or inadequate for another.

Metabolism

As these drugs pass through the liver, digoxin is altered, but only to a minor degree, thus remaining largely unchanged. In approximately 1 in 10 patients, digoxin may be extensively metabolized in the gut. This extensive metabolism may account for some patients' resistance to therapy and unusually high dose requirements. Encapsulated liquid preparations may minimize metabolic inactivation.

Elimination

Digitalis glycosides are eliminated from the body by different mechanisms. Digoxin is eliminated primarily by renal excretion, with only about 14% of an administered dose metabolized first by hepatic mechanisms. The degree of elimination of digoxin can be correlated with measures of renal function such as serum creatinine or creatinine clearance. These relationships can then be used to determine the dosage of digoxin required in a patient with decreased renal function (see Digoxin section). Digoxin is not effectively removed from the body by dialysis or exchange transfusion or during cardiopulmonary bypass, because most of the drug is in tissue rather than circulating in the blood.

Factors Affecting Pharmacokinetics

Factors affecting the pharmacokinetics of the cardiac glycosides that may necessitate dosage adjustments include renal function and age. Because digoxin is excreted primarily by the kidneys, a reduction in renal function results in a decrease in digoxin clearance and an increase in half-life, therefore necessitating a smaller dose.

Infants and children have a larger volume of distribution than adults; therefore, larger doses are required to achieve similar concentrations of digoxin. Often digoxin is administered every 12 hours to infants and children. As a person ages, there is decrease in volume of distribution, primarily because of a decrease in muscle mass. A decrease in renal clearance also occurs. Therefore, in the elderly patient the maintenance dose is reduced.

Digoxin levels are quite low in fatty tissue, so obesity does not affect dosing. The dosage of digoxin is calculated on lean body mass rather than total body weight.

CONTRAINDICATIONS AND PRECAUTIONS

The contraindications for all cardiac glycosides include idiopathic hypertrophic subaortic stenosis (IHSS), diffuse cardiomyopathies, and constrictive pericarditis, as the drugs increase the workload of the heart and worsen these conditions. Cardiac glycosides are contraindicated in patients with Wolff-Parkinson-White (WPW) syndrome, because administration may aggravate tachydysrhythmias by depressing AV nodal function and allowing accessory bundle activation. They are also contraindicated in patients with heart block because of the possibility of further slowing of AV conduction. Ventricular tachycardia and fibrillation are also contraindications to cardiac glycosides.

Precautions include hypothyroidism because such patients may suffer severe bradycardia and are more sensitive to digitalis effects; impaired renal function because of delayed excretion and possible toxic effects; and hypokalemia, hypomagnesemia, and hypercalcemia because these all favor the development of digitalis toxicity.

Pregnant women or nursing mothers are also given the drug cautiously because of its passage across the placenta and into breast milk. The cardiac glycosides are pregnancy category C. Cardiac glycosides are given cautiously to patients with acute or toxic myocarditis as there may be an increased incidence of digitalis-induced tachydysrhythmias. The elderly are also given these products cautiously because of the increased possibility of digitalis intoxication from decreases in either liver or kidney function. Also, because the increased force of contraction raises myocardial oxygen consumption, which may increase infarct size, the cardiac glycosides are given cautiously in patients with an acute myocardial infarction.

ADVERSE EFFECTS

Digitalis side-effects are the same for all preparations and can be categorized according to noncardiac and cardiac effects. Digitalis toxicity can be life threatening, but its incidence is declining. The factors most likely responsible for this decline are a decrease in the use of digoxin and the careful selection of patients who will respond best to therapy. To identify potential toxicity in patients, it is important to understand predisposing factors and the signs and symptoms of digitalis toxicity, which are listed in (Table 29–3).

Noncardiac Effects

Gastrointestinal (GI) effects such as anorexia, nausea, vomiting, and diarrhea are activated by the irritation of the chemoreceptor trigger zone in the medulla. These GI effects are frequently self-limiting and disappear after continued therapy. However, these symptoms reappear in digitalis toxicity. Visual disturbances can manifest as blurred vision, white dots, halos, yellow or green tint to vision (*chromatopsia*—a condition in which colors are incorrectly perceived), double vision, and flickering. These GI and central nervous system (CNS) side effects, although bothersome, are not life threatening. They may occur at lower serum concentrations and usually precede the more serious cardiac side effects.

Gynecomastia, the enlargement of breast tissue, although rare, can be seen in both men and women. It is related to the steroid component of digitalis glycosides and is more common with digoxin use. Other less common side effects include mental depression, respiratory depression, and pruritus.

Cardiac Effects

Digitalis glycosides produce the expected ECG changes. The effect of slowing conduction through the AV node, although beneficial and desired in the treatment of some rhythm disturbances (see Uses), can produce varying degrees of heart block, ranging from prolongation of the PR interval to Mobitz type I heart block (the PR interval gets progressively longer until a beat is missed) to complete heart block. By slowing conduction through the AV node, accessory bundles can be activated, causing supraventricular tachycardias.

Table 29–3. DIGITALIS TOXICITY

Predisposing Factors
Electrolyte disturbances:
   Hypokalemia
   Hypomagnesemia
   Hypercalcemia
Acid-base imbalances
Hypothyroidism
Renal impairment
Hepatic impairment
Elderly patients
Too-rapid IV administration
Dehydration

Signs and Symptoms
Gastrointestinal:
   Anorexia*
   Nausea*
   Vomiting*
   Diarrhea*
   Abdominal pain
Neurologic:

Drowsiness	Lassitude
Fatigue	Confusion
Dizziness	Disorientation
Headache	Insomnia
Restlessness	Psychosis
Irritability	Convulsions
Depression	Coma
Personality change	

Cardiac:
   New bradycardia
   New tachycardia
   Paroxysmal atrial/junctional rhythms[†]
   Atrial ectopic rhythms[†]
   Onset of regularity and/or irregularity
   Atrial tachycardia with varying AV block[†]
   Ventricular bigeminy or trigeminy*
   Ventricular tachycardia
   Second-degree AV block (Wenckebach)[†]
   AV dissociation
   Complete AV block[†]
Visual:
   Blurred or yellow vision
   Flickering lights
   White borders on dark objects
   Colored dots
   Halos
   Double vision

Management
Mild overdose:
   Withhold digitalis products for several days or up to 3 wk
   Correct magnesium/potassium deficit
   Reinstitute a lower maintenance dose
Severe toxicity:
   Hospitalize at once
   Support ventilation/give oxygen as necessary
   Continuously monitor ECG
   Administer potassium as needed
   Administer phenytoin or lidocaine (Dilantin) for degenerating ventricular dysrhythmias
   Support blood pressure
   Insert a temporary demand pacemaker
   Administer digoxin antibody

*Most common early symptom in adults.
[†]Most common early symptom in children.

Dysrhythmias such as premature ventricular contractions (PVCs), premature atrial contractions (PACs), ventricular tachycardia, and supraventricular dysrhythmias can be caused by disturbances in automaticity. A combination of these disturbances with delayed AV conduction can be seen. Children receiving digitalis glycosides are more likely to experience ectopic, junctional, or atrial beats. Because almost any dysrhythmias can present as digitalis intoxication, a good rule to use is to assume that any new rhythm disturbance observed in a patient receiving a digitalis preparation is caused by digitalis until proven otherwise.

Digitalis Toxicity

Predisposing Factors Various factors may predispose the patient to digitalis toxicity (see Table 29–3). These include electrolyte disturbances such as hypokalemia, hypomagnesemia, and hypercalcemia; acid-base imbalances; and hypothyroidism. Renal dysfunction and aging also may predispose some patients to toxicity.

Potassium loss may be caused by a number of conditions—vomiting; diarrhea; administration of certain diuretics, steroids, laxatives, or certain antibiotics (carbenicillin, ticarcillin, piperacillin, mezlocillin, amphotericin B) that increase renal potassium excretion; poor dietary intake of potassium; and continuous use of potassium-free intravenous solutions. If any of these conditions exists and the patient is receiving a digitalis glycoside, he or she may be more prone to developing digitalis toxicity. A low serum potassium level enhances digitalis toxicity by making the Na-K ATPase enzyme system more susceptible to inhibition by digitalis.

Hypomagnesemia, as is commonly seen in alcoholics and those taking diuretics, tends to increase sensitivity to digitalis. It can be easily corrected by administering soluble, absorbable magnesium salts.

Hypercalcemia may be seen in the immobile patient, in persons with hyperparathyroidism, and in patients with certain malignant tumors that cause calcium to leave the bone. Hypercalcemia tends to cause increased automaticity, leading to tachydysrhythmias and ectopic beats. Rapid intravenous administration of calcium may also cause digitalis toxicity.

▼ **CLINICAL ALERT**

In patients with one or more predisposing factors, careful monitoring of serum concentrations and appropriate dosage adjustments can prevent toxicity. Rapid intravenous administration, another cause of toxicity, should be avoided.

Signs and Symptoms When a patient experiences high serum concentrations of digitalis (e.g., >2.5 ng/mL for digoxin), the chemoreceptor trigger zone in the medulla is stimulated, resulting in nausea and possible emesis. In addition, anorexia, increased salivation, abdominal pain, and diarrhea can be seen.

In high doses, cardiac glycosides increase sympathetic outflow from the CNS to both cardiac and peripheral sympathetic nerves. This increase in sympathetic activity is an important factor in digitalis toxicity, because most of the extracardiac manifestations are mediated by the CNS. Typical symptoms that may be associated with increased sympathetic tone include drowsiness, fatigue, dizziness, changes in vision, and, in elderly patients, confusion, delirium, and hallucinations.

Digitalis toxicity also enhances cardiac automaticity, so many dysrhythmias may occur. No single dysrhythmia is unique to digitalis toxicity, but the possibility of toxicity should be considered in the presence of sudden cardiac rhythm change from the baseline rhythm. ECG changes, such as ST and T wave changes, are not diagnostic of toxicity in most patients.

In children, vomiting, diarrhea, and neurologic and visual disturbances are rarely seen initially. The most common and reliable signs of toxicity are atrial dysrhythmias such as atrial ectopic rhythms, paroxysmal atrial tachycardia (PAT), and AV block. Ventricular dysrhythmias are rarely seen.

Treatment When digitalis toxicity is diagnosed, the digitalis preparation is discontinued; or if the toxicity is severe, digoxin immune Fab (Digibind) may be administered (to be discussed later). Electrolytes (potassium, calcium, magnesium) and acid-base states are checked and returned to normal. It is critical that the serum level of potassium be monitored closely and if low, administration of potassium can suppress many of the dysrhythmias. On the other hand, if the potassium level is high, administration of potassium may potentiate or intensify AV block, with the potential for the occurrence of complete AV block and cardiac arrest. Severe digitalis toxicity can cause an elevated serum potassium.

If ventricular dysrhythmias (premature ventricular contractions, ventricular tachycardia) or atrial dysrhythmias (PAT with block, atrial tachycardia) are present, they can usually be effectively suppressed by using lidocaine or phenytoin. The antidysrhythmics quinidine, procainamide, lidocaine, and propranolol may also be effective; however, they may also cause dysrhythmias. Because cardioversion in the presence of digitalis causes dysrhythmias, it is not usually used to treat digitalis-induced dysrhythmias.

Bradydysrhythmias, sinoatrial arrest, and AV block can be treated with atropine. Temporary pacing may be required to maintain an adequate heart rate until digoxin levels are within the therapeutic range.

Digitalis toxicity, in addition to being a significant cause of morbidity, also adds substantially to health-care costs. Patients with cardiac toxicity frequently require hospitalization and intensive monitoring until therapeutic levels have been attained and an appropriate dosage regimen achieved. Because all digitalis glycosides have long serum half-lives, this stabilization can take several days. For example, if a patient is admitted with digoxin toxicity with a serum digoxin level of 5.0 ng/mL and the drug has a half-life of 3 days, the serum concentration will be 2.5 ng/mL 3 days after admission and 1.25 ng/mL 6 days after admission. This, together with the seriousness of the cardiac side effects, has led researchers to investigate methods that can enhance the removal of digitalis glycosides from the body.

Traditional methods of drug removal such as hemodialysis, charcoal hemoperfusion, and peritoneal dialysis are generally ineffective because of the wide tissue distribution of the cardiac glycosides. Administration of digoxin- or digitoxin-specific antibodies, known as Fab fragments, is helpful when digoxin levels are very high. Fab fragments bind very tightly to digoxin, resulting in an inactive digoxin-antibody complex that is excreted renally. This produces high serum concentrations of the complex, but very low concentrations of active digoxin. Fab fragments are discussed later in this chapter.

INTERACTIONS

Cardiac glycosides adsorb to aluminum-containing antacids (e.g., Amphojel, Mylanta-II, Gelusil-II, and Maalox), kaolin-pectin preparations (e.g., Kaopectate), and bran, forming an insoluble complex in the gut that is not absorbed. Binding resins such as cholestyramine and colestipol can reduce the absorption of cardiac glycosides by a similar mechanism. The administration of digitalis glycosides should be separated by 2 hours when used concurrently with any of these products. Oral aminoglycosides (e.g., neomycin, kanamycin, paromomycin, and sulfasalazine) also inhibit the absorption of cardiac glycosides. Also, combination chemotherapy regimens (several drugs together), such as bleomycin, cyclophosphamide, and procarbazine, can decrease digoxin absorption 20% to 50%.

Metoclopramide (Reglan) or propantheline (Pro-Banthine) may alter the bioavailability of cardiac glycosides. Administering digoxin as an elixir or as gel caps may reduce this interaction.

Administration of quinidine with digoxin increases serum digoxin concentration, producing a twofold increase on the average and an increase in the risk of toxicity . This results from quinidine's tendency to cause tissue displacement of digoxin with reequilibration into serum, a reduction in the ability of the kidney to remove digoxin from serum, a decreased volume of drug distribution; and possible increased absorption. The digoxin dose may need to be reduced by as much as 50% when quinidine is added. A similar interaction occurs with administration of the calcium antagonists verapamil (Isoptin) and others. The magnitude of increase in digoxin level, however, is not as great as that observed with quinidine.

Amiodarone (Cordarone), indomethacin (Indocin), propafenone (Rhythmol), and quinine interfere with the elimination of digoxin, necessitating the reduction of digoxin dose by one-fourth to one-half.

Drugs that decrease impulse formation from the sinus node, such as the beta-adrenergic blockers or calcium channel blockers, or increase vagal activity, such as edrophonium or succinylcholine, may increase the possibility of bradycardia. The concurrent administration of drugs that increase heart rate and contractility, such as isoproterenol and other sympathomimetics (dopamine, dobutamine, epinephrine, ephedrine), and thyroid preparations may enhance the potential for developing tachydysrhythmias and ectopic dysrhythmias. Intravenous

administration of calcium salts, as previously discussed, can potentiate toxicity. Drugs that can cause hypokalemia, like diuretics, increase the likelihood of digoxin toxicity.

Patients receiving cardiac glycosides also may have altered laboratory test results. Serum iodine[131] uptake may be reduced. Serum creatine kinase increases after IM administration. Digitalis may increase levels of estrone and estrogen and decrease levels of luteinzing hormone and testosterone. Digitalis may alter urinary levels of 17-hydroxycorticosteroids, 17-ketosteroids, and glucose.

○ **Digoxin** (Lanoxicaps, Lanoxin) is the most commonly used form of digitalis because of its rapid onset of action and short duration. It is available as tablets, capsules, or elixir and for IV administration.

Digoxin can be administered as a loading dose (digitalization) if a rapid onset of action is desired. The loading dose saturates the nonspecific myocardial receptor sites. Either the oral or intravenous route can be used. The digitalizing dose in adults is approximately 0.010 to 0.020 mg/kg ideal body weight (total of 0.5 to 1.0 mg) administered as three to four equally divided doses over 24 hours. Intramuscular injection is not recommended because it is painful and causes muscle fasciculations and necrosis.

If the effects of digitalis are not needed quickly, a daily maintenance dose may be administered. It will take an average of 11 days to reach steady state with this method of administration. Additional dosing information can be found in Table 29–1.

Because of varying bioavailability, oral and intravenous doses are not equal. Lanoxicaps (gelatin capsules) have greater bioavailability than standard tablets. The 0.2-mg capsule is equivalent to the 0.25-mg tablet; the 0.1-mg capsule, to the 0.125-mg tablet; and the 0.05-mg capsule, to the 0.0625-mg tablet. The maintenance dose is based on the patient's renal function, as this is the primary route of digoxin elimination.

○ **Digitoxin** (Crystodigin), available in crystalline form, is readily absorbed from the intestinal tract. Digitoxin is given orally, intramuscularly, or intravenously. It has the longest duration of action of the digitalis glycosides, ranging from 1 to 3 weeks.

DIGOXIN ANTAGONIST

Digoxin immune Fab (Digibind) is an orphan drug used in the treatment of life-threatening digoxin and digitoxin intoxications.

○ **Digoxin immune Fab** (Digibind) contains antigen binding fragments (fab) derived from specific antidigoxin antibodies (IgG) produced in sheep. Digoxin immune Fab is administered intravenously, distributes widely to tissues, and binds avidly with digoxin and digitoxin; it is excreted by the kidneys in 15 to 20 hours. As a result, serum levels of digoxin and digitoxin are eventually reduced. (See Table 29–1 for dosing information.)

Life-threatening episodes of digoxin or digitoxin intoxication are indicated by shock, impending shock, cardiac arrest, serious ventricular dysrhythmias, bradycardia, blocks unresponsive to atropine, and potassium levels above 6 mEq/L.

CONTRAINDICATIONS AND PRECAUTIONS No contraindications are known at this time. Caution must be used, as cardiac function may decrease rapidly and even cardiac arrest may occur. Use caution when administering digoxin immune Fab during pregnancy (category C) or lactation and in children.

ADVERSE EFFECTS The adverse effects of digoxin immune Fab include a mild increase in congestive heart failure and an increase in the ventricular rate with atrial fibrillation. There are rapid shifts of potassium in digoxin toxicity. At first, with a high digoxin level, potassium shifts from the cell to the extracellular fluid, causing hyperkalemia. The potassium is then lost through normal renal excretion, leading to hypokalemia. Digoxin immune Fab allows potassium to move back into the cell, so serum potassium levels become even lower. Potassium levels must be monitored and potassium given cautiously.

BIPYRIDINE DERIVATIVES

The bipyridine derivatives—**amrinone (Inocor)** and **milrinone (Primacor)**—are positive inotropic agents with vasodilator activity. These two drugs are featured in Table 29–4.

ACTION

The bipyridine derivatives relax vascular smooth muscle and increase cardiac output and stroke volume, thus reducing afterload and preload. These agents increase myocardial contractility by inhibiting cyclic adenosine monophosphate phosphodiesterase, which increases the intracellular mediator cyclic adenosine monophosphate (cAMP). The bipyridine derivatives also enhance calcium ion movement into or storage within the myocardial cell. Heart rate and systemic blood pressure remain unchanged, as the increase in cardiac output compensates for the lowered vascular resistance. Pulmonary artery occlusive pressure (PAOP) or pulmonary artery wedge pressure (PAWP) and total peripheral resistance show dose-related decreases.

USES

The bipyridine derivatives are indicated for short-term management of patients with congestive heart failure who can be closely monitored and who have not responded adequately to digitalis glycosides, diuretics, dobutamine, or other vasodilators. It is important to return fluid volume and electrolytes to normal before therapy is begun if the patient has been treated vigorously with diuretics; the patient may have insufficient cardiac filling pressures to respond adequately.

CONTRAINDICATIONS AND PRECAUTIONS

The bipyridine derivatives are contraindicated in patients experiencing hypersensitivity reactions to these products or bisulfites (a preservative used in amrinone solution). The bipyridine derivatives are given cautiously to pa-

---

Table 29–4. OTHER POSITIVE INOTROPIC AGENTS: BIPYRIDINE DERIVATIVES

DRUG NAME/ROUTE AND DOSAGE	PHARMACOKINETICS/ DYNAMICS	NURSING IMPLICATIONS
amrinone (Inocor) ***Adults:*** 0.75 mg/kg IV bolus slowly over 2–3 min, repeated in 30 min; 5–10 μg/kg per min IV drip, not to exceed 10 mg/kg 24 hr. ***Children:*** Dosage has not been established.	**Onset:** immediate **Peak:** 10 min **Duration:** 0.5–2 hr **½L:** 3.6–5.8 hr **PB:** 10%–49% **B:** conjugative pathways in liver **E:** kidney(63%), feces(18%)	**ASSESSMENT:** Assess fluid balance and electrolytes and maintain near normal so as not to precipitate reduced filling pressure and hypotension. Assess platelets weekly, particularly with amrinone. Assess for pregnancy (category C). **INTERVENTION:** Take blood pressure often. Do not mix in glucose solutions for IV drip, because chemical reaction occurs slowly over 24-hr period. Bolus administration in glucose is permissible. Protect ampules from light. Furosemide and amrinone are incompatible. **EVALUATION:** Evaluate cardiac rhythm for supraventricular tachycardia and ventricular dysrhythmias. Treat them appropriately.
milrinone (Primacor) ***Adults:*** *Loading Dose*—50 μg/kg IV infused over 10 min. *Maintenance dose*—0.375–0.75 μg/kg/min IV infusion.	**Onset:** immediate **Peak:** 10 min **Duration:** 8 hr **½L:** 2–3 hr **PB:** 70% **B:** liver (minimally) **E:** kidney	Same as for amrinone.

tients with outflow obstruction such as occurs in aortic valvular disease, severe pulmonic valvular disease, and hypertrophic aortic stenosis, because these drugs may aggravate such problems. With amrinone, platelet counts are reduced because of decreased platelet survival. These agents are not currently recommended for use in patients with an acute myocardial infarction. Safety in pregnancy (category C), lactation, and children has not been established.

○ **Amrinone** (Inocor) is primarily prescribed for patients who have not responded to therapy with digitalis glycosides, diuretics, and vasodilators.

ADVERSE EFFECTS   The most common adverse effects from amrinone include supraventricular and ventricular dysrhythmias related to the increased inotropic cardiac effect; thrombocytopenia, which is often dose dependent and probably related to decreased platelet survival time; and hypotension related to vasodilation effects. Other minor side effects include nausea, vomiting, abdominal pain, anorexia, hepatotoxicity, chest pain, and fever. Reduce dosage or discontinue the drug if severe or debilitating GI side effects occur. Delayed hypersensitivity reactions (2 weeks after therapy) have been reported.

INTERACTIONS   When amrinone is given concurrently with disopyramide (Norpace), excessive hypotension may occur. Inotropic effects may be additive with cardiac glycosides.

DOSAGE   Amrinone is best diluted in a normal saline solution. A chemical reaction occurs slowly over a 24-hour period when amrinone is mixed in solutions containing glucose. However, amrinone can be injected into a running glucose solution through a Y-connector or directly into the tubing.

○ **Milrinone** (Primacor), structurally similar to amrinone, is available as an intravenous solution for short-term use or as oral doses (in Europe) for chronic therapy.

ADVERSE EFFECTS   Cardiovascular adverse reactions include supraventricular dysrhythmias and ventricular dysrhythmias (ventricular ectopic activity, nonsustained and sustained ventricular tachycardia, and ventricular fibrillation), hypotension, angina pectoris, and chest pain. With chronic therapy, milrinone may cause headache and aggrevate angina.

OTHER DRUGS USED TO TREAT HEART FAILURE

Digitalis has been a primary treatment for heart failure for over 200 years. But, other drugs such as angiotensin converting enzyme (ACE) inhibitors (captopril [Capoten], enalapril [Vasotec], lisinopril [Prinivil], and qiunapril [Accupril]) are currently being used as first-line therapy for heart failure. ACE inhibitors shift blood flow to the kidneys, heart, and brain; increase sodium excretion; dilate the renal bed; block sympathetic vasoconstrictor activity; prevent ventricular remodeling; and may reduce the rate of sudden death. ACE inhibitors are discussed in more detail in Chapter 30.

Dobutamine, a beta$_1$-adrenergic agonist, promotes vasodilation in the peripheral vessels and reduces the heightened sympathetic drive seen in heart failure. Dobutamine also improves renal blood flow and promotes an increase in urinary output. It is used to control symptoms of heart failure both acutely and chronically. More information on dobutamine can be found in Chapter 68.

Additional medications are also used in selected patients with heart failure. These include calcium channel blockers, nitrates, sodium nitroprusside, and hydralazine (all discussed in detail in other chapters).

USING THE NURSING PROCESS

ASSESSMENT

- Obtain a thorough nursing history to develop the database from which to individualize drug therapy and to monitor therapeutic response, adverse reactions, and signs of toxicity. Table 29–5 summarizes the nursing process for patients requiring cardiac glycosides. If the patient has been or is currently taking cardiac glycosides, it is important to learn how and when the glycosides are taken and if there are any adverse effects.
- Obtain a current drug history to determine if there are any possible drug interactions with digitalis glycosides.
- Assess objective and subjective symptoms associated with the patient's medical condition.
- Assess ECG tracings and laboratory tests, including serum electrolytes (potassium, calcium, magnesium); serum creatinine levels to evaluate kidney function; liver function studies; and serum digitalis levels if toxicity is suspected. The serum digitalis level is generally checked about 6 to 8 (up to 11) hours after an oral dose of a digitalis glycoside, as that is when the drug equilibrates with the heart and other tissues. See Table 29–1 for levels.

NURSING DIAGNOSIS

Establish the nursing diagnoses based on the information obtained during the assessment (see Table 29–5). Typical nursing diagnoses for the patient taking cardiac glycosides include: Decreased Cardiac Output; Fluid Volume Excess; Impaired Adjustment; and Knowledge Deficit.

INTERVENTION

- Develop both short- and long-term goals (see Table 29–5).

Nursing Responsibilities when Administering Cardiac Glycosides

The nurse in the hospital situation has several nursing responsibilities when administering cardiac glycosides.

Table 29–5. NURSING PROCESS FOR PATIENT REQUIRING CARDIAC GLYCOSIDES

Assessment

Ascertain current/past medication history, response to drug(s), and any side effects including use of OTC drugs.
Assess concurrent health problems, e.g., impaired renal/hepatic function, electrolyte imbalances, history of hypothyroidism, pregnancy, or prior myocardial infarction/heart block.
Assess blood pressure, skin color/temperature, peripheral pulses, mental status.
Assess signs of congestion (liver/lung) and urinary output.
Assess nutritional history (particularly use of foods high in sodium and cholesterol).
Assess current lifestyle/activities and effect of current health status on desired lifestyle.
Assess emotional and psychologic significance of illness.

Nursing Diagnosis: Decreased Cardiac Output

RELATED TO: Mechanical factors (e.g., inotropic changes in heart)/electrical changes in rate, rhythm, conduction).
AS EVIDENCED BY: Fatigue, variations in hemodynamic readings, dysrhythmias, edema, dyspnea.

Desired Outcomes/Evaluation Criteria

Reports decreased episodes of dyspnea, angina, and/or dysrhythmias. Displays a reduction in frequency/duration or severity of dysrhythmias. Demonstrates an increase in activity tolerance.

Nursing Actions	Rationale
Administer cardiac glycoside, e.g., Lanoxin.	Increases the force of myocardial contraction; reduces preload; prolongs refractory period of AV junction, decreases conduction through SA node and AV junction, reducing heart rate; improves cardiac output.
Monitor vital signs, cardiac rhythm, fluid balance, and daily weight. Restrict fluid intake as indicated. Plan fluid schedule with patient.	Indicators of need for/effectiveness of therapy. Tachycardia and lower blood pressure may indicate worsening congestive heart failure. Fluid restriction (if needed) minimizes risk of fluid overload. Body weight reduction reduces myocardial workload.
Promote adequate rest periods, assist with self-care activities as necessary.	Prevents undue fatigue/reduces cardiac workload.

Nursing Diagnosis: Knowledge Deficit

RELATED TO: Lack of recall, information misinterpretation, unfamiliarity with resources, possible cognitive limitations.
AS EVIDENCED BY: Questions, statement of concern, development of preventable complications.

Desired Outcomes/Evaluation Criteria

Verbalizes understanding of disease process and measures needed to maintain/improve current health state.

Nursing Actions	Rationale
Provide information (verbal and written formats) about cardiac glycosides including action, use, dosage, side and toxic effects (e.g., nausea/vomiting, anorexia, weakness, headache, blurred vision or yellow halos, change in cardiac rate or rhythm) and potential interactions, especially with OTC drugs.	Understanding can facilitate adherence to prescribed regimen and prevent drug interactions/complications.
Discuss normal heart function. Include information regarding patient's variance from normal.	Helps patient to understand significance of own situation and need for continued therapy.
Stress importance of not discontinuing/altering drug dosage without first consulting with physician.	Prevents untoward responses that could be life threatening.
Recommend storage of drug in tightly closed container, protected from excessive heat/light.	Maintains potency of the drug.
Review administration routine/proper timing of drug, e.g., same time every day (noon often best), set pattern (with or without food).	Provides for consistent release and absorption of drug.
Identify foods low in sodium and cholesterol (within economic means) that can be used while maintaining a well-balanced diet.	Increased sodium expands fluid volume and further aggravates congestive heart failure. Decreased cholesterol levels may prevent further arteriosclerotic heart disease development.

Other Suggested Nursing Diagnoses: Impaired Adjustment and Fluid Volume Excess.

(These are featured in the Nursing Implications column in Table 29–1.)

- Assess the heart rate apically for one full minute and chart along with the rhythm. The specific pulse limitations must be known for each patient. The physician is consulted, and the limitations are written in the patient's Kardex. If the pulse rate falls below the pulse limitation set by the physician, contact the physician to determine the recommended action. A fall in pulse rate is associated with increased digitalis levels. The physician may order an ECG or blood work to assess for signs of toxicity. If the cardiac glycoside digoxin is stopped for longer than 3 days (duration of action averages about 3 days [half-life 1.5 to 3 days]), the body would have excreted most of the digitalis and there would no longer be a therapeutic blood level. The patient may then experience an exacerbation of previous symptoms, that is, heart failure. If the pulse rate goes above the limitation, the physician is also consulted. A rapid pulse may indicate the patient needs more of his or her digitalis glycoside. Weight is usually measured daily to check for fluid retention. In general, if the pulse rate is less than 60 but the patient has a sinus rhythm, it is safe to administer digoxin. If the pulse rate is less than 50 with atrial fibrillation or flutter, withhold the digoxin and contact the physician. Digitalis increases the refractoriness of the AV node and may set the patient up for ventricular rhythms.

  Determine pulse deficits (apical pulse minus radial pulse) as ordered for the patient with atrial flutter or fibrillation. A pulse deficit occurs when a weak cardiac contraction cannot be felt in the periphery, indicating a poor cardiac output. A goal of digitalis therapy is to lower the pulse deficit to zero.
- Administer digitalis glycosides at approximately the same time each day. Noon is best, since it allows the patient time to be up and active before the pulse is taken. This is of particular importance in the older adult whose resting heart rate may be low.
- Administer oral medications with or between meals, but follow the same routine each day. The absorption rate is slowed with food, but the total amount absorbed is not affected. However, when oral medications are taken with meals high in bran fiber, the amount may be reduced.
- Use the IM or IV route only when oral administration is not possible. The cardiac glycosides are irritating to both the subcutaneous and muscular tissues, and digoxin in particular may cause muscle fasciculations and necrosis. These drugs are administered only into the gluteus maximus or ventrogluteal sites and never into the deltoid. In a patient experiencing the current signs of heart failure, the absorption rate of an intramuscular injection is uncertain because of decreased perfusion to the periphery; therefore, the IV route is more certain. The IV route is best in an emergency.
- Administer intravenous cardiac glycosides over 10 to 30 minutes. Slow administration helps to prevent arteriolar vasoconstriction or an increase in afterload and thus hypertension. It allows the positive inotropic effect to keep pace with the peripheral effects.

Digitalization

Digitalization is the administration of enough digitalis to reach therapeutic blood level and to eliminate the signs and symptoms of heart failure or to control dysrhythmias with as few side effects as possible. During the period of digitalization, the serum digitalis levels may be checked to help evaluate the patient's response to therapy. Serum potassium and calcium are also checked.

Elderly patients are more sensitive to the effects of the cardiac glycosides and need lower doses and closer monitoring. Infants, however, usually need larger amounts of digoxin than expected, that is, greater than normal adult doses. This results from the increased elimination of water-soluble drugs in infants.

Patient Teaching

General information about all cardiac glycosides that is included by the nurse-educator in the teaching plan for each patient is presented in Table 29–6.

- Teach the patient about signs and symptoms related to heart failure that occur (pulmonary congestion, weight gain, and so on) or symptoms that indicate aggravation of his or her dysrhythmia.
- Establish a medication schedule that will not be forgotten by an older adult (see Chapter 8 for more information on the older adult). Also, ensure that the patient does not confuse the cardiac glycoside, "little white pills," with other "little white pills," which may be diuretics or antidysrhythmics. Also check to see if the patient can open the childproof caps. If not, the patient needs a regular cap on the medications.
- Teach the patient to store medications in a safe place out of the reach of small children. Older adults may leave their medication on a counter when their grandchildren come to visit. However, digitalis products can be toxic, especially to small children.

EVALUATION

- Evaluate the effectiveness of cardiac glycosides on a predetermined list of evaluation criteria. Generally, these criteria include (1) a well-informed patient and family who understand the disease and the medical and nursing regimens; (2) a reduction in the symptoms; (3) medication compliance; (4) dietary compliance; (5) understanding of and compliance with the exercise regimen; (6) minimal side effects related to medications; and (7) the maintenance of a therapeutic blood level of digitalis.
- Enhance patient compliance. Compliance is often a problem with patients on cardiac glycosides, usually because the patient does not have enough knowledge about the condition or the medication regimen. It is the nurse's responsibility to educate the patient to

Table 29–6. PATIENT TEACHING INFORMATION— CARDIAC (DIGITALIS) GLYCOSIDES

Dear Patient:

This drug has been ordered for you. This is what you should know about your drug to get the most from your therapy.

☐ 1. Digitalis products improve the strength and efficiency of your heart and control abnormal heart rhythms.

☐ 2. Cardiac glycosides will generally be taken for the rest of your life.

☐ 3. Take your pulse, noting both rate and rhythm, before taking your drug (pulse should be between 50 and 110 beats per minute). If the pulse is above or below this limit, or is different in rhythm, call your doctor before taking your medication.

☐ 4. Digitalis glycosides can be taken with or between meals. Try to take this medication at the same time each day. Do not alter the dose.

☐ 5. Do not take your cardiac glycosides together with antacids, antidiarrheals, or laxatives. If you must take these medications, take them at least 2 to 3 hours before or after your digitalis glycoside.

☐ 6. Always check with your physician or pharmacist before taking other drugs, as an interaction may occur. Drugs known to interfere with the effectiveness of digitalis glycosides include quinidine and verapamil.

☐ 7. If you forget to take your digitalis glycosides for a whole day, skip the dose. *Do not* try to catch up by taking two doses in the same day.

☐ 8. Do not stop taking your cardiac glycosides without checking with your physician.

☐ 9. If you have any side effects from your digitalis glycosides or if you develop symptoms you think may be caused by these drugs, consult your physician. Common side effects include loss of appetite, nausea, vomiting, weakness, diarrhea, abdominal pain, fatigue, visual changes, and irregular pulse.

☐ 10. Weigh yourself weekly. A gain of 1 to 2 pounds a week may indicate fluid retention. Also check your feet and ankles for swelling. Notify your physician if swelling or weight gain occurs.

☐ 11. If persistent cough and shortness of breath occur, notify your physician.

☐ 12. Store these drugs in a tight, light-resistant, moisture-resistant container to prevent deterioration. Store out of the reach of children.

prevent future need for rehospitalization to control untoward effects. (See Chapter 2 for more information on patient compliance.)

- Evaluate for hypersensitivity reactions when the digitalis glycosides are being administered for the first time. Hypersensitivity may not be observed for 5 to 7 days after therapy is initiated. Observe for toxic reactions, which may result from the patient's taking too many tablets, from diminishing renal functioning, from drug interaction, or from hypokalemia. The elderly patient may experience CNS symptoms early, along with anorexia. The neonate may show a slowing of the sinus rate and a prolongation of the PR interval.

- Evaluate the patient for adverse effects. The effects of the cardiac glycosides are cumulative, and most effects can usually be eliminated by suspension of the dose for several days. Older adults are much more likely to develop toxic side effects. It is imperative that they be evaluated more closely for signs and symptoms of toxicity. If digitalis toxicity is suspected, a serum digitalis level is measured. A blood serum creatinine level may be ordered to evaluate kidney function. If the patient is found to have toxicity, the cardiac glycosides are withheld until the drug serum level returns to normal limits. The serum electrolytes, particularly serum potassium and calcium, are also evaluated at this time. If the potassium level is low, the patient often experiences dysrhythmias such as premature ventricular contractions (either singly or in ventricular bigeminy) and ventricular tachycardia. When these dysrhythmias develop from digitalis toxicity, they are treated, preferably with specific antidysrhythmic medications. Ventricular tachycardia from digitalis toxicity may be treated with IV phenytoin. (See Chapter 31 for more information on antidysrhythmic drugs.) In conjunction with administration of antidysrhythmics, potassium chloride (KCl) is given slowly IV to increase the serum potassium level.

Digitalis rarely produces sinus bradycardia. It is much more likely to produce AV block as a manifestation of cardiotoxicity. In the presence of atrial fibrillation (AF), a junctional escape rhythm may develop because, in AF, digitalis may produce complete AV block. (Digitalis rarely converts AF to sinus rhythms.) If the junctional rate is over 60, then automaticity may have been increased. In patients being treated with digitalis who have a sinus rhythm, a slight first-degree AV block may occur. Again, withholding the medication for several days usually resolves these problems. The patient is usually then placed on a lower maintenance dosage.

There is also an increased risk for digitalis toxicity when patients are also receiving quinidine or verapamil (see Chapters 30 and 31). Quinidine and verapamil increase the serum digoxin level, possibly by displacing digoxin from tissue binding sites. This interaction leads to greater potential for GI disturbances and ventricular dysrhythmias. When starting quinidine or verapamil in patients already receiving a digitalis glycoside, the clinical course, ECG, and serum digitalis levels are followed closely. Consequently, when the quinidine or verapamil is discontinued, close observation of digitalis levels is also necessary to prevent a decrease in the therapeutic blood level of digitalis.

- Review and update all previously taught material with the patient and family, if necessary, to ensure that their knowledge base is still accurate.

- Encourage the patient to keep scheduled visits to the physician. The patient requiring cardiac glycosides may have some physical limitations. With help from the nurse, physician, and family, it is hoped that the patient is able to live fully within these restrictions.

The bibliography for this chapter can be found in Appendix B, which begins on page 1054.

CHAPTER REVIEW QUESTIONS*

1. As a class of drugs, the cardiac glycosides:
   a. Are produced from synthetic sources.
   b. Increase the rate of ventricular ejection.
   c. Are effective within a wide therapeutic range.
   d. Increase the force of cardiac contraction.

2. Which of the following statements is *correct* regarding the effect of cardiac glycosides?
   a. These agents have an indirect effect on the cardiac conduction system.
   b. Digitalis glycosides have a negative chronotropic effect on the cardiac muscle cells.
   c. The glycosides exert direct action on the heart through the autonomic nervous system.
   d. A greater magnitude of therapeutic effect is seen on the nonfailing heart than on the failing heart.

3. Which of the following is *not* an outcome associated with digoxin therapy?
   a. Increased heart size.
   b. Increased urine output.
   c. Reduced afterload.
   d. Increased stroke volume.

*See Appendix A, which begins on page 1051, for answers.

4. Which of the following dysrhythmias can be corrected with digitalis glycosides?
   a. Ventricular tachycardia.
   b. Sinus bradycardia.
   c. First-degree AV block.
   d. Paroxysmal atrial tachycardia.

5. When adding quinidine therapy to patients who are on digoxin, the following may occur:
   a. Ventricular dysrhythmias.
   b. Reduced digoxin levels.
   c. Mental status changes.
   d. Elevated potassium levels.

6. Which of the following statements is *correct* regarding digoxin immune Fab (Digibind)?
   a. This agent is derived from foxglove as an antidote for digoxin toxicity.
   b. Digibind is a cost-effective agent that has a wide variety of side effects.
   c. A potentially dangerous side effect of this antidigoxin drug is hyperkalemia.
   d. Derived from antidigoxin antibodies, this agent is used to treat emergency digoxin toxicities.

CHAPTER 30

Antihypertensive Agents

Merrily A. Kuhn, RNC, PhD

KEY TERMS

Coarctation
Funduscopic exam
Hypertension
Orthostatic

Prodrug
Pheochromocytoma
Raynaud's phenomenon

LEARNING OBJECTIVES

After reading this chapter, the student will be able to:

1. Identify medications commonly used as antihypertensives.
2. Compare and contrast the differences and similarities among antihypertensive medications.
3. Identify mechanisms of action, routes of administration, pharmacokinetics, adverse effects, and interactions common to the antihypertensive medications.
4. Formulate a plan to assess the patient requiring antihypertensive medications to develop appropriate patient outcomes.
5. Plan the nursing interventions necessary to administer antihypertensive medications safely and choose appropriate teaching strategies to gain patient compliance.
6. Evaluate the patient at various stages to assess nursing interventions.

*H*ypertension, a disease of the circulatory system affecting about 60 million adults in North America, is characterized by persistently elevated systolic or diastolic pressure or both. In 95% of patients, the specific cause of the elevated blood pressure cannot be determined. This is termed essential, or primary, hypertension. In secondary hypertension, the causes can be identified and include renal artery stenosis, renal disease, primary hyperaldosteronism, *pheochromocytoma* (a tumor of the adrenal medulla characterized by hypersecretion of epinephrine and norepinephrine, causing persistent or intermittent hyperten-

sion), and *coarctation* (stricture or contracture) of the aorta. Figure 30–1 and Chapter 28 review blood pressure control.

Hypertensive persons often have an early increase in cardiac output followed by adaptive changes in the media of resistance vessels. These changes eventually cause an increase in systemic vascular resistance. In the United States, it is estimated that more than 1 million deaths occur each year as a consequence of hypertension and hypertension-related events, including myocardial infarction, cerebrovascular accident, and renal failure. Despite

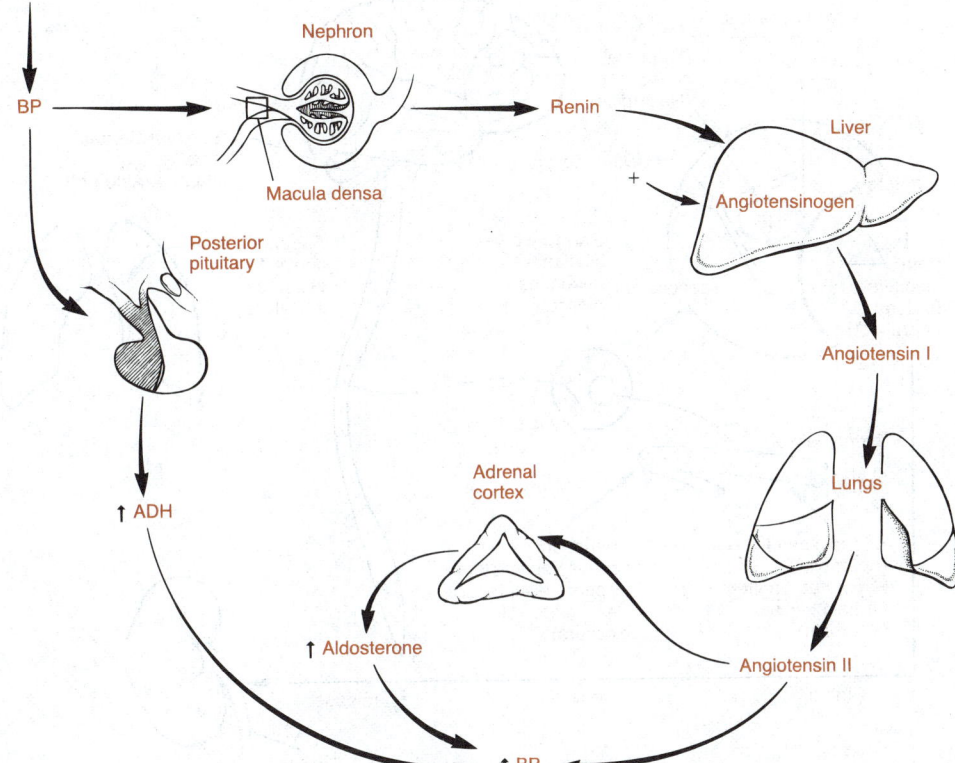

Figure 30–1. Blood pressure control. Several systems regulate blood pressure in the body. The renal system conserves volume and releases renin from the macular densa cells. Renin is eventually converted to angiotensin II, a powerful vasoconstrictor. The endocrine system releases antidiuretic hormone (ADH) from the posterior pituitary, which conserves volume, and aldosterone from the adrenal cortex, which conserves sodium. The nervous system, through the vasomotor center in the medulla, controls the size of the blood vessels.

these complications many hypertensive patients continue to lack awareness of their disease and/or do not comply with therapy.

Medications on the market today have a variety of actions that can be used in the treatment of hypertension. The antihypertensive medications do not cure hypertension; they merely lower the blood pressure, which helps to control complications. Therefore, the diagnosis of hypertension having been made, patients are likely to be under treatment for the remainder of their lives.

The actions of antihypertensives can be divided into four types: (1) centrally or peripherally acting sympathetic nervous system inhibitors, such as ganglionic blockers, neuroeffector-transmission blockers, and beta-blocking agents; (2) peripheral vasodilators, such as arterial dilators or mixed arterial and venous dilators; (3) inhibitors of the renin-angiotensin system; and (4) diuretics, which are discussed fully in Chapter 37. Regardless of the method of action, the majority of antihypertensives eventually contribute to the development of peripheral vasodilation, resulting in decreased blood pressure.

The antihypertensives are used to lower blood pressure to a normal level or to the lowest level tolerated. A diastolic pressure of less than 90 mm Hg usually can be achieved without producing intolerable adverse effects.

To facilitate successful management of the disease and its consequences, treatment protocols for hypertension should consider the pathophysiologic change. Hemodynamic derangements seen in hypertension have traditionally been viewed in terms of abnormalities in cardiac function (cardiac output) or as derangements of systemic resistance. Hypertension of cardiac origin is dominated by beta-subtype adrenoreceptors and responds best with beta-adrenergic receptor antagonists. The beta-adrenoreceptors are primarily found in the autonomic nervous system (beta$_1$ receptors in the heart, beta$_2$ receptors in the blood vessels and lungs) where inhibitory responses occur when adrenergic agents such as norepinephrine and epinephrine are released. Hypertension of vascular origin is modulated by alpha-subtype adrenoreceptors and responds best to direct alpha-adrenergic receptor antagonists. The alpha-adrenoreceptors, found in the autonomic nervous system primarily in blood vessels, release norepinephrine and epinephrine when excited.

Because each type of antihypertensive agent is so different, each group of drugs is discussed individually as to its action, specific use, contraindications, precautions, adverse effects, and interactions. Tables 30–1 through 30–4 feature dosages, pharmacokinetics, and nursing implications for selected antihypertensive medications. Nursing implications are also discussed in the nursing process section of this chapter. Figure 30–2 reviews the general sites of action of each of these groups of medications. Table 30–7 summarizes the general drug classification, use, and action for most antihypertensive agents.

ANTIADRENERGICS

Antiadrenergics inhibit the sympathetic nervous system through central or peripheral action.

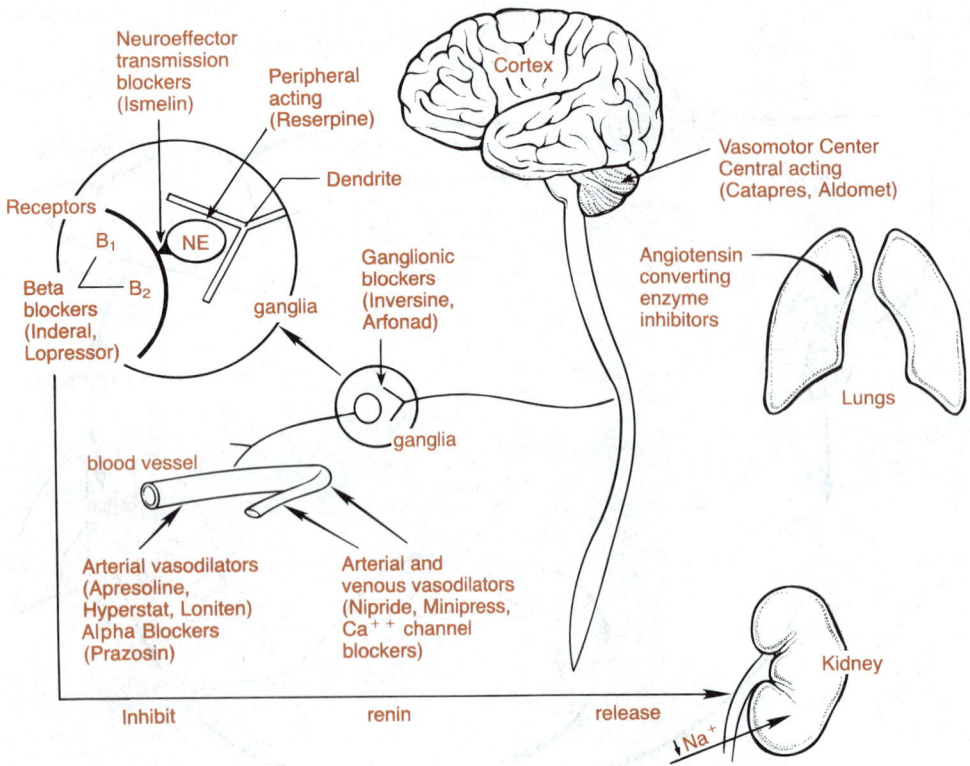

Figure 30–2. Sites of action of anti-hypertensives.

CENTRALLY ACTING SYMPATHETIC NERVOUS SYSTEM INHIBITORS

Sympathetic nervous system inhibitors, in addition to their use as antihypertensives, are used for a variety of other conditions. This chapter primarily reviews their actions only in relation to their ability to control hypertension. (See Chapter 17 for additional information on other uses of these drugs.) Commonly prescribed centrally acting sympathetic nervous system inhibitors are **clonidine hydrochloride (Catapres)** and **methyldopa (Aldomet)**. Pharmacokinetics and dosages are presented in Table 30–1. Other centrally acting inhibitors include **guanabenz (Wytensin)** and **guanfacine (Tenex)**.

Action

The centrally acting alpha$_2$-adrenergic agonists stimulate receptors located primarily in the medulla oblongata. This central activity results in inhibition of peripheral sympathetic activities and vasodilatation in the peripheral blood vessels due to a reduction in sympathetic tone. These drugs have little effect on cardiac output. All drugs in the group are lipid neutral and have no effect on total cholesterol, high-density lipoprotein, low-density lipoprotein, or triglycerides.

Uses

The centrally acting alpha$_2$-adrenergic agonists are used in the treatment of mild to moderate hypertension. They lower both the supine and standing blood pressures and, therefore, may produce orthostatic hypotension. They are more often used in combination with diuretics or other antihypertensive medications to achieve a greater reduction in blood pressure. These drugs are often third-step drugs. (Step-care therapy is discussed later.)

Adverse Effects

The most disturbing side effects of the alpha-adrenergics are related to the central nervous system (CNS). These include drowsiness, decreased intellectual drive, sedation, inability to concentrate, depression, forgetfulness, and vivid dreams. However, these tend to diminish as therapy continues. Because these drugs decrease salivary flow, dry mouth is a frequent adverse effect. Impotence and decreased libido occur frequently. Other less common adverse effects are anorexia, vomiting, rash, heart failure, *orthostatic* (relating to standing upright; in orthostatic hypotension, the blood pressure is normal while the patient is reclining but low while he or she is standing) symptoms, change in heart rate, and *Raynaud's phenomenon* (a syndrome characterized by recurring attacks of diminished blood supply to the fingers and toes). Symptoms of Raynaud's phenomenon, which are often precipitated by exposure to cold or emotional stress, include pain, numbness, tingling, pallor, and cyanosis. As with other antihypertensives, sodium and fluid accumulation often occurs, necessitating the administration of a diuretic.

Table 30–1. ANTIHYPERTENSIVE DRUGS: ANTIADRENERGIC AGENTS

DRUG NAME/ROUTE AND DOSAGE	PHARMACOKINETICS/ DYNAMICS	NURSING IMPLICATIONS

CENTRALLY ACTING ANTIADRENERGIC AGENTS

clonidine hydrochloride (Catapres, Catapres-TTS)

Adults: *Initial dose*—0.1 mg PO bid with increments of 0.1–0.2 mg/day. *Maintenance dose*—0.2–0.8 mg PO in 2 doses. Or, apply transdermal patch q 7 days; patch delivers 0.1, 0.2, or 0.3 mg/24 hr. **Children:** 5–25 mg/kg per day PO divided q 6 hr. Increase at 5–7 day intervals.	**Onset:** PO, 30–60 min; patch, 30–60 min **Peak:** PO, 2–4 hr (may be 8 hr); patch, 2–3 days (changed every 7 days) **Duration:** PO, 12–24 hr; patch, 7 days and 8 hr after removal **½L:** 12–16 hr; in renal disease may increase to 25–40 hr **PB:** NA **B:** liver (50%) **E:** urine (40%–60% unchanged)	For all antihypertensives: **ASSESSMENT:** Thorough nursing history including history of hypertension; complete drug history including OTC, diet pills, and decongestants. Assess current smoking habits, including use of marijuana. Obtain baseline blood pressure, pulse, weight, and renal function studies. Assess for pregnancy (category C). **INTERVENTION:** Check blood pressure in both the supine and standing positions. Patients on tricyclic antidepressants with history of mental depression require close supervision, as their depression may increase. Tolerance may develop in some patients. Withdrawal of drug should occur over 2–4 days. Do not discontinue abruptly; abrupt withdrawal may lead to increased blood pressure. **Patient Teaching**—Instruct patient to take medication every day near the same time, to take as directed, and, if a dose is forgotten, to skip that dose. Warn patient not to take 2 doses next time. Early AM and bedtime administration helps prevent drowsiness that may occur. Advise patient to be cautious for at least 2 hr after taking medication while driving or working around heavy equipment until effects of drug are known. Tell patient to avoid hot baths or showers. Warn patient to sit first when moving from supine to standing position. Tell patient to avoid excessive tea, coffee, and cola (more than 4 cups per day); and to avoid excessive sweating and dehydration, which may lead to excessive fall in blood pressure. Warn patient to not stop medication without physician's approval and to consult pharmacist before taking OTC products. Inform patient that good oral hygiene may help to prevent dry mouth. Tell patient to store drug in tight container. **EVALUATION:** Notify physician of any change in mood or sleep habits. Evaluate weight at least twice a week to closely monitor fluid retention.

methyldopa (Aldomet)

Adults: 250–500 mg PO 1–4 times daily, not to exceed 750 mg/day for first 2 days or 3 g/24 hr maintenance (tablets can be crushed); or 250–500 mg IV q 6 hr diluted in 100 ml of D₅W administered over 30–60 min. Cannot be used to treat hypertensive crises. **Children:** 10 mg/kg PO 2–4 times daily; or 20–40 mg/kg per day IV q 6 hr. Maximum dosage 65 mg/kg per day or 3 g/day.	**Onset:** PO, 1–2 hr (2 days when starting therapy); IV, 2–3 min **Peak:** PO, 4–6 hr **Duration:** PO, 12–24 hr **½L:** 2 hr **PB:** weakly **B:** liver **E:** feces (10%–20%); urine (60%–70%); removed by dialysis	Same as for clonidine hydrochloride plus: **ASSESSMENT:** Assess for pregnancy (category B). **INTERVENTION:** During early drug therapy to 15 weeks, patient should have periodic blood counts and liver function tests to assess for adverse effects. Drug may cause urine to darken on standing. Approximately 2 days of therapy is required to establish maximal antihypertensive effects. Drug is removed by dialysis.

Continued on the following page

Table 30–1. ANTIHYPERTENSIVE DRUGS: ANTIADRENERGIC AGENTS, *Continued*

DRUG NAME/ROUTE AND DOSAGE	PHARMACOKINETICS/ DYNAMICS	NURSING IMPLICATIONS
PERIPHERALLY ACTING ANTIADRENERGIC AGENTS		
reserpine (Serpasil) (Serpalan) *Adults:* Initial dose–0.1 mg PO daily. *Maintenance dose*–0.1–0.25 mg PO daily.	**Onset:** days **Peak:** 6–12 hr **Duration:** 6–24 hr **½L:** 33 hr (stored in adipose tissue) **PB:** 96% **B:** liver **E:** feces (50%), urine (small amounts)	Same as for all antihypertensives: **ASSESSMENT:** Assess for pregnancy (category C). **INTERVENTION:** May cause GI upset, so give with food or milk. Crosses blood-brain and placental barriers. Effects are cumulative; full antihypertensive effects may not be seen for 3 wk. **EVALUATION:** Notify physician if mental depression or early morning insomnia occurs.
ALPHA₁-ADRENERGIC BLOCKING DRUGS		
prazosin (Minipress) *Adults:* Initial dose–1 mg PO at hs. *Maintenance*–6–15 mg PO daily in divided doses.	**Onset:** 120–130 min **Peak:** 1–3 hr **Duration:** 6–12 hr **½L:** 2–3 hr **PB:** 92%–97% **B:** liver **E:** bile/feces 90%, urine 10%	Same as for all antihypertensives plus: **ASSESSMENT:** Assess for pregnancy (category C). **INTERVENTION:** Food does not affect absorption.
terazosin (Hytrin) *Adults:* Initial dose–1 mg PO hs. *Maintenance dose*–1–5 mg PO up to 20 mg/day.	**Onset:** 15 min **Peak:** 1–2 hr **Duration:** 12–24 hr **½L:** 9–12 hr **PB:** 90%–94% **B:** minimally **E:** bile/feces (60%), urine (40%)	Same as for prazosin.
doxazosin (Cardura) *Adults:* Initial dose–1 mg PO hs. *Maintenance dose*–1–8 mg PO once/day.	**Onset:** 2 hr **Peak:** 4–8 hr **Duration:** 24 hr **½L:** 22 hr **PB:** 98%–99% **B:** liver **E:** urine (9%), feces (63%)	Same as for prazosin except: **ASSESSMENT:** Assess for pregnancy (category B).

NA = not available.

Contraindications and Precautions

The centrally acting alpha₂-adrenergic agonists cause sedation or drowsiness because of their effect on the CNS. During initial therapy, the patient is cautioned against driving or operating heavy equipment to prevent injury or accident. All centrally acting drugs are given cautiously to patients with severe coronary insufficiency and recent myocardial infarction, as the vasodilatation in the peripheral circulation may necessitate an increased heart rate and cardiac output and thus may aggravate these conditions. Patients with cerebral/vascular disease may also have their symptoms worsened by the vasodilatation. Caution is also used in patients with renal or hepatic disease, as these drugs are metabolized and excreted by these routes. Safety in pregnancy (category B or C), lactation, and children has not been established.

Abrupt cessation of alpha₂-adrenergic agonists can result in increased plasma and urinary catecholamine levels, increases in blood pressure (often to levels significantly higher than before treatment was instituted), and increased nervousness and anxiety. Dosage of these products should be slowly tapered rather than abruptly stopped.

○ **Clonidine hydrochloride** (Catapres), along with its hypertensive use, is currently being investigated for the prophylaxis of migraine headache and episodes of menopausal flushing, the treatment of dysmenorrhea, the reduction of intraocular pressure in open-angle and secondary glaucoma (topical application), and the prevention of asthma attacks by relaxing bronchial smooth muscle when the drug is nebulized and inhaled. Clonidine is also used to assist with postoperative pain relief. Intravenous clonidine (not available in the United States) is added to morphine, and the combination relieves pain better than morphine alone. It is also currently being used for treatment of opiate withdrawal and to detoxify patients from chronic methadone administration. Sublingual clonidine may prove useful in treating hypertension in patients unable to take oral medications.

▼ **CLINICAL ALERT**

If clonidine therapy is to be discontinued, as for elective surgery or substitution of other antihypertensives, the dose is to be tapered off over several days to a week.

Patients who have taken clonidine for blood pressure control and who stop the medication abruptly are at risk for clonidine withdrawal symptoms, including rebound hypertension, agitation, restlessness, and tachycardia. Patients are warned about the severity of this reaction and counseled to adhere strictly to their prescribed regimen.

INTERACTIONS Tricyclic antidepressants (imipramine, desipramine, amitriptyline, nortriptyline, doxepin, and protriptyline) are alpha-adrenergic antagonists. At least two of these, imipramine and desipramine, negate the hypotensive effects of clonidine. In addition, depressed patients with hypertension should receive a different antihypertensive, as their depression may worsen. CNS depression may be potentiated by other CNS-depressant drugs such as barbiturates, alcohol, and tranquilizers. Alcohol may increase clonidine's hypotensive effects secondary to its vasodilatory effects. Also, when clonidine is combined with cardiac glycosides and other antihypertensives, there may be an increased bradycardic effect.

○ **Methyldopa** (Aldomet) is structurally related to the other alpha-adrenergics. The exact mechanism of action is unknown. Methyldopa does, however, reduce the tissue concentration of serotonin, dopamine, and epinephrine. Withdrawal symptoms are significantly less with methyldopa than with clonidine.

ADVERSE EFFECTS Along with the group's adverse effects, the urine may also darken. In 20% of patients, a positive direct Coombs' test occurs. This is an incidental finding. However, in 1% to 5% of patients with a positive Coombs' test, hemolytic anemia will develop. Hepatic dysfunction, which can resemble either acute hepatitis or chronic active hepatitis, is sometimes seen. Although this reaction is usually reversible on discontinuation of the drug, overt hepatic failure leading to death has been reported. Liver function tests and complete blood counts

(CBCs) are to be monitored on a routine basis. Lactation, associated with high prolactin concentrations, can occur in either sex.

INTERACTIONS When methyldopa is administered concurrently with amphetamines and tricyclic antidepressants, the antihypertensive effect of methyldopa is decreased. Concurrent administration of methyldopa with propranolol or phenothiazines may result in a paradoxic hypertensive effect. Fenfluramine and verapamil may potentiate the effects of methyldopa. Tolbutamide metabolism may be impaired by methyldopa, resulting in enhanced hypoglycemic effect. Several laboratory tests—uric acid, serum glutamic oxaloacetic transaminase (SGOT), and serum creatinine—are also altered.

○ **Guanfacine** (Tenex) is a centrally acting alpha₂-adrenergic receptor agonist similar to clonidine and methyldopa that is used to treat hypertension in patients already receiving a thiazide-type diuretic. It is not a single-control agent.

○ **Guanabenz acetate** (Wytensin), decreases both supine and standing blood pressures. However, normal postural mechanisms remain unchanged, so there is little postural hypotension, and a slight reduction in heart rate occurs. Monitor renal function, as the kidney is the organ of this drug's excretion.

An advantage of guanabenz is that it needs to be taken only two times daily. Also, it may cause less reactive fluid retention than others in the group. The major disadvantage is the common side effect of sedation and dry mouth.

PERIPHERALLY ACTING SYMPATHETIC NERVOUS SYSTEM AGENTS

The peripherally acting drugs exert their effects in the peripheral resistance arterioles and capacitance (vein) vessels. Both supine and standing blood pressures are lowered, with a more pronounced effect on the diastolic pressure. The peripherally acting agents include the rauwolfia compound—**reserpine (Serpasil)**; the antiadrenergic sulfate drugs—**guanethidine monosulfate (Ismelin)** and **guanadrel sulfate (Hylorel)**; and the alpha-adrenergic blocking drugs—**prazosin (Minipress), terazosin (Hytrin)**, and **doxazosin (Cardura)**. These drugs have a mixed effect on heart rate and cardiac output. Prazosin, terazosin, and doxazosin lower total cholesterol and raise high-density lipoprotein. They have a duration of action between 6 and 24 hours; therefore, once or twice a day dosing is possible.

Rauwolfia Compounds

The rauwolfia compounds are the most commonly available peripheral sympathetic vasoconstriction inhibitors. Used for many years as a tranquilizer in India, rauwolfia compounds were finally introduced in the United States in the 1950s. In 1953, researchers clearly demonstrated that rauwolfia had antihypertensive qualities as well as sedative effects, and they developed reserpine, a single pure alkaloid of *Rauwolfia serpentina*.

○ **Reserpine** (Serpasil, Sandril), considered the most potent of the rauwolfia compounds, presumably exerts its antihypertensive effects by depleting the stores of catecholamines in the sympathetic nerve ending. It may inhibit the active transport of norepinephrine to the storage site, thus further impairing its storage mechanism. The net effect is a reduction in sympathetic output, which reduces total peripheral resistance and decreases cardiac output. Both the cardiovascular and the CNS effects may persist following withdrawal of these drugs.

USES Reserpine is used in the treatment of mild to moderate hypertension. It is often combined with diuretics or other antihypertensive agents to lower blood pressure more effectively. It is used in step 3 of step-care therapy (discussed in Nursing Process section).

All pharmacokinetic and dosage information is presented in Table 30–1.

CONTRAINDICATIONS AND PRECAUTIONS Reserpine is contraindicated in acute peptic ulcer and acute ulcerative colitis because it causes gastric and intestinal irritation. It is given cautiously to persons with renal and hepatic insufficiency as it is biotransformed and excreted in these organs and to patients with cardiac damage and dysrhythmias as there is a decrease in peripheral vascular resistance and the decreased cardiac output may worsen these conditions. A parkinsonian state may occur in debilitated or elderly patients.

▼ **CLINICAL ALERT**

Reserpine is not used in patients with depression because it reduces norepinephrine levels in the brain, increasing depression. Reserpine is also discontinued 7 days prior to electroshock therapy to allow brain norepinephrine levels to return to normal.

ADVERSE EFFECTS The most common adverse effects include drowsiness and sleep changes due to norepinephrine blockade, weight gain, and nasal stuffiness. Increased gastrointestinal (GI) motility, abdominal cramps, and diarrhea are also seen. Reserpine can increase gastric acid secretion and exacerbate peptic ulcer disease. In high doses, reserpine can cause GI bleeding and can produce nightmares and depression severe enough to cause a suicide attempt. As many as 40% of patients taking reserpine complain of depression and sexual problems. Less common effects include angina symptoms, bradycardia, and blurred vision. Despite these adverse effects, reserpine is still used because of its low cost.

INTERACTIONS Interactions include increasing the sedative effects of barbiturates and alcohol and decreasing the effectiveness of amphetamines and ephedrine. There may be an additive hypotensive effect when reserpine is given with diuretics, along with an increased risk of cardiac dysrhythmia when it is given concurrently with digitalis or quinidine. Concurrent theophylline can result in tachycardia.

Patients on reserpine have decreased urinary excretion of catecholamines, 17-ketosteroids, and vanillylmandelic acid because reserpine depletes the tissue stores of these substances.

Peripherally Acting Sulfate Antiadrenergics

Peripherally acting sulfate antiadrenergics include guanethidine monosulfate and guanadrel sulfate.

○ **Guanethidine monosulfate** (Ismelin) acts as a neuroeffector-transmission blocker, producing a selective blockade of efferent, peripheral sympathetic pathways. Administration of this medication slowly reduces the catecholamine stores from the adrenergic nerve endings, producing a prolonged decrease in blood pressure. Guanethidine sulfate lowers upright blood pressure more than supine; therefore, it can cause postural hypotension. Frequently, it also causes sexual dysfunction.

Guanethidine is used in the treatment of severe hypertension that does not respond to other drug regimens. It is generally used when other drugs have been ineffective in controlling blood pressure. As do certain other antihypertensives, it causes renal retention of sodium and water. It is not commonly used today because the dosage is difficult to regulate without causing orthostatic hypotension.

○ **Guanadrel sulfate** (Hylorel) is structurally and pharmacologically similar to guanethidine, but has a more rapid onset and shorter duration of action after withdrawal. Guanadrel does not readily cross the blood-brain barrier; therefore, there is less sedation and there are fewer CNS effects than with guanethidine.

USES Guanadrel is usually reserved for patients with severe hypertension and is used in step 3 of step-care therapy. It is considered as effective as guanethidine and more effective than methyldopa. An advantage of guanadrel is that it has no CNS effects. A disadvantage is the frequent orthostatic hypotension and occasional diarrhea that is experienced (pregnancy category B).

Peripherally Acting Alpha-Adrenergic Blocking Drugs

The alpha$_1$-adrenergic blockers—**prazosin *(Minipress)*, terazosin *(Hytrin)*,** and **doxazosin *(Cardura)***—are structurally unrelated to other antihypertensives, but act as other peripherally acting alpha-adrenergic drugs. Heart rate, renal blood flow, and glomerular filtration are not significantly changed, but fluid retention does occur. Thus, alpha-adrenergic blockers are often given concurrently with a diuretic.

The advantage of the alpha$_1$-adrenergic blockers is that they lack sedation dry-mouth, and sexual side effects, they decrease peripheral resistance with a decrease in cardiac output, and they may benefit plasma lipid levels. The disadvantage is the hypotension, general lassitude, and tolerance that occurs with the administration of the first dose, which may require titration.

Uses

The alpha$_1$-adrenergic blockers are useful in treating mild to moderate hypertension. They can increase cardiac output by reducing preload and afterload and, therefore, can be used in the treatment of heart failure with coexisting hypertension. Prazosin and terazosin are generally used in step 2 or step 3 of step-care therapy. Drug resistance frequently develops after weeks or months when these products are administered alone. Prazosin is also used to treat Raynaud's phenomenon, and prazosin and doxazosin are used as adjuncts in treating heart failure with concurrent digoxin and diuretics. Prazosin and doxazosin improve cardiac output and thus relieve pulmonary congestion.

Doxazosin also quickly relieves urination problems caused by benign prostatic hypertrophy. Doxazosin allows the bladder to empty completely so frequent nighttime urination is eliminated. It improves urinary flow in about 1–2 weeks.

Pharmacokinetics

All drugs are well absorbed from the GI tract and are all highly bound to plasma protein. All are biotransformed in the liver and excreted in the urine. For specific pharmacokinetic information, see Table 30–1.

Contraindications and Precautions

Safety in pregnancy (category C for prazosin and terazosin, category B for doxazosin) and in children has not been established.

Adverse Effects

The most significant adverse effects of the alpha$_1$-adrenergic blockers, orthostatic hypotension and syncope, occur early in therapy and are common. These effects are particularly common in patients who are dehydrated and volume depleted. The orthostatic hypotension and syncope, which may be caused by an inadequate venous return to the right side of the heart, are generally not seen in patients with an increased venous return, as in those with heart failure. These effects are minimized by administering the first dose, of no larger than 1 mg, at bedtime. Other adverse effects include dizziness, drowsiness, headache, palpitations, and nausea. Adverse effects usually disappear with continued therapy.

Interactions

Concurrent beta-adrenergic blockers and calcium channel blockers may enhance postural hypotension. Because alpha$_1$-adrenergic blockers are highly protein bound, they theoretically may interact with other highly protein-bound drugs.

BETA-ADRENERGIC BLOCKING DRUGS

Beta-adrenergic blockers—**propranolol hydrochloride (Inderal)**, **acebutolol (Sectral)**, **metoprolol (Lopressor)**, **nadolol (Corgard)**, **atenolol (Tenormin)**, **pindolol (Visken)**, **betaxolol (Kerlone)**, **carteolol (Cartrol)**, **penbutolol (Levatol)**, and **timolol (Blocadren)**—compete with epinephrine for available beta-receptor sites, thereby inhibiting the response to beta-adrenergic stimuli. Beta receptors are typically classified as beta$_1$ receptors, found primarily in the heart, and as beta$_2$ receptors, located primarily in the lung. By blocking the beta-adrenergic receptor sites in the heart, these drugs decrease heart rate, myocardial contractility, and ultimately cardiac output. Conduction ve-

locity through the atrioventricular (AV) node and firing rate in the sinoatrial (SA) node also decrease. These effects prevent exercise-induced increases in the heart rate. The mechanisms through which they lower blood pressure are by reducing cardiac output, reducing plasma renin activity, by sympatholytic action in the CNS, by stimulating synthesis of vascular prostacyclin (a major vasodilating prostaglandin) and/or inhibiting the synthesis of thromboxane A$_2$ (a powerful vasoconstrictor), and by resetting the arterial baroreceptors. Beta-adrenergic blockers are often administered in combination with diuretics or other antihypertensive drugs and are used in step 1 and step 2 of the antihypertensive regime. Some beta-adrenergic blockers, because of their rapid antihypertensive effect, are useful in emergency management of hypertension. The beta-adrenergic blockers are discussed in depth in Chapter 17.

Using beta-adrenergic blockers to treat hypertension has many advantages. Beta-adrenergic blockers allow once-a-day dosing for many patients, provide relief from anxiety-related symptoms, cause little volume retention, have antianginal and antidysrhythmic properties, and have postinfarction protection and reverse left-ventricular hypertrophy.

However, there are also disadvantages to using beta-adrenergic blockers. These include serious side effects such as bronchospasm, masked hypoglycemia in the diabetic patient, heart failure, impotence, cold extremities, and associated increases in triglycerides with a decrease in high-density lipoprotein.

In patients with mild to moderate hypertension, 50% to 70% respond to average doses of beta-adrenergic blockers. Optimal doses are sometimes hard to predict. A general rule is that if a standard beta-adrenergic blocker dose does not work within a week, it is useless to try another beta-adrenergic blocker. When using a beta-adrenergic blocker to treat an African-American patient, labetalol may be the best choice, as it also has vasodilatory effects. (African-Americans often have a higher vascular pressure.)

ALPHA- AND BETA-ADRENERGIC BLOCKING DRUG

○ **Labetalol** (Normodyne, Trandate) is an alpha- and beta-adrenergic blocking agent that combines both selective postsynaptic alpha$_1$-adrenergic blocking plus nonselective beta-blocking actions. Because of these actions, it is used primarily to reduce hypertension. Labetalol mildly decreases cardiac output, decreases total peripheral resistance, and reduces levels of renin (enzyme produced by the kidney that acts on angiotensin to form angiotensin I). Standing blood pressure is lowered more than supine; therefore, patients may experience postural hypotension. Labetalol is available in intravenous and oral forms. Intravenous labetalol has a rapid onset of action (5 to 7 minutes) and is titratable for predictable results. Initially, labetalol 20 mg is injected slowly (over 2 minutes). Maximum effect usually occurs within 5 minutes. Blood pressure is measured every 5 to 10 minutes. Additional injections of 40 to 80 mg may be given at 10-minute intervals until desired blood pressure is achieved or a total of 300 mg has been administered. Slow continuous infusion can also be used. Orally, labetalol is started at 100 mg twice a day with a maintenance dose of 400 to 800 mg daily. Severe hypertension may require up to 1.2 grams daily in two or three divided doses. Concomitant diuretic therapy enhances the therapeutic response. For more information see Chapter 17.

DIRECT-ACTING VASODILATORS

The direct-acting vasodilators act directly on the peripheral blood vessels, either on the arteries alone (arterial vasodilator) or on the arteries and veins together (mixed arterial and venous vasodilator). Both groups of drugs lower blood pressure by decreasing peripheral vascular resistance. This reduction in blood pressure can consequently stimulate the baroreceptors and, in turn, increase the heart rate, cardiac output, and force of contraction. This effect may prove dangerous for a patient with underlying ischemic cardiac disease. The peripheral vasodilators are generally given in combination with beta-adrenergic blockers to reduce the adverse effects related to baroreceptor stimulation.

ARTERIAL VASODILATORS

The arterial vasodilators reduce blood pressure by directly relaxing the arteriolar smooth muscle. The increased caliber of the blood vessel reduces total periph-

eral resistance, which lowers blood pressure, decreasing afterload. Cardiac output is increased as afterload is reduced and renal and cerebral blood flow is maintained or increased. Arterial vasodilators include **hydralazine hydrochloride (Apresoline)** and **minoxidil (Loniten)**, featured in Table 30–2. **Diazoxide (Hyperstat)**, also an arteriolar dilator, is used primarily for emergency reduction of blood pressure in short-term, malignant hypertension. Diazoxide is featured in Table 30–3.

○ **Hydralazine hydrochloride** (Apresoline) is used in the chronic management of moderate to severe hypertension. It can be used intravenously to decrease blood pressure rapidly in hypertensive emergencies. It is also used alone or in combination with nitrates to increase cardiac output (by reducing afterload) in patients with heart failure. The reflex catecholamine response can result in tachycardia and increases in heart rate. It is also used to treat hypertension in both preeclampsia and eclampsia of pregnancy. Hydralazine hydrochloride is usually a step-3 or -4 drug in step-care therapy. Hydralazine with a diuretic is often an effective, well-tolerated treatment for hypertensive elderly patients because they are less likely to develop a reflex tachycardia.

CONTRAINDICATIONS AND PRECAUTIONS Hydralazine is contraindicated in coronary artery disease because it can produce anginal attacks and in patients with mitral valvular disease because the hyperdynamic state (increased heart rate and cardiac output) may accentuate or aggravate the valvular disease. Hydralazine is used with caution in patients with cerebral vascular accidents because of the possibility of increased cerebral ischemia,

Table 30–2. ANTIHYPERTENSIVE DRUGS: DIRECT-ACTING ARTERIAL VASODILATORS

DRUG NAME/ROUTE AND DOSAGE	PHARMACOKINETICS/ DYNAMICS	NURSING IMPLICATIONS
hydralazine hydrochloride (Apresoline)		
Adults: Initial dose—10 mg PO qid (can be crushed). Maintenance dose—50–300 mg PO daily in divided doses; 5–40 mg IV or IM, repeat as necessary. **Children:** 0.75 mg/kg PO per 24 hr q 60 hr. Maximum dose 7.5 mg/kg PO per 24 hr or 200 mg/day; 0.1–0.2 mg/kg IV q 4–6 hr.	**Onset:** PO, 20–30 min; IV, 5–20 min, IM, 10–30 min **Peak:** PO, 1–2 hr; IV, 10–80 min; IM, 1 hr **Duration:** PO, 6–12 hr; IV, 4–6 hr **½L:** 3–7 hr **PB:** 87% **B:** liver **E:** urine (13%)	Same as for other antihypertensives plus: **ASSESSMENT:** LE prep and antinuclear antibody titer are done prior to and periodically during treatment. Assess for pregnancy (category C). **INTERVENTION:** Observe mental status carefully. Monitor intake and output. Pyridoxine (vitamin B_6) may be ordered for patient experiencing peripheral neuritis due to hydralazine. Take with meals. Use hydralazine injection immediately after withdrawing from vial. Drug changes color when in contact with metal filter. **EVALUATION:** Report any prolonged tiredness, fever, muscle or joint aching, or chest pain.
minoxidil (Loniten)		
Adults: Initial dose—5 mg PO per day. Maintenance dose—2.5–20 mg PO once daily or bid, dose adjustments at least 3-day intervals. Maximum dose 100 mg/day. **Children under 12 yr:** Initial dose—0.2 mg/kg PO. Maintenance dose—0.25–1 mg/kg PO per day in 1–2 divided doses.	**Onset:** 30 min **Peak:** 2–3 hr **Duration:** 24–72 hr **½L:** 4.2 hr **PB:** not bound—concentrates in arteriolar smooth muscle **B:** 90% by conjugation **E:** urine	**ASSESSMENT:** Same as for other antihypertensives. **INTERVENTION:** Weigh patient daily. Suggest cosmetics to mask hypertrichosis. Auscultate lungs frequently. **EVALUATION:** Notify physician of unusual swelling of extremities, severe indigestion, dizziness, lightheadedness, or fainting.

Table 30–3. VASODILATORS USED IN EMERGENCY TREATMENT OF MALIGNANT HYPERTENSION

DRUG NAME/ROUTE AND DOSAGE	PHARMACOKINETICS/ DYNAMICS	NURSING IMPLICATIONS
ARTERIAL VASODILATORS		
diazoxide (Hyperstat) **Adults:** 1–3 mg/kg IV bolus over 30 sec or less, may repeat in 5–15 min; do not use longer than 10 days.	**Onset:** 1–2 min **Peak:** 5 min **Duration:** 3–12 hr **½L:** 28 +/−8 hr **PB:** 90% **B:** not biotransformed **E:** urine, excreted unchanged	Same as for all antihypertensives plus: **ASSESSMENT:** Assess for pregnancy (category C). **INTERVENTION:** Monitor IV site closely for extravasation. Monitor blood glucose level. Have patient remain recumbent for at least 1 hr after injection. Administer IV bolus over 1 min to decrease excessive hypotension. Start oral therapy as soon as blood pressure is controlled.
MIXED ARTERIAL AND VENOUS VASODILATORS		
sodium nitroprusside (Nipride) **Adults:** 0.5–10 μg/kg per min by IV infusion. Mix only in D₅W. Do not exceed 10 μg/kg per min infusion rate. See package insert for dosing table.	**Onset:** 0.5–1 min **Peak:** 30–60 sec **Duration:** 3–5 min after infusion is stopped **½L:** 2 min **PB:** NA **B:** liver to cyanide **E:** urine	Same as for antihypertensives: **ASSESSMENT:** Assess for pregnancy (category C). **INTERVENTION:** Solutions are freshly prepared every 24 hr and mixed with only dextrose and water. They are light sensitive and are covered with foil wrapper that comes in box. Carefully monitor the patient every 5–10 min when beginning or stopping the medication and every 15 min during maintenance. The blood pressure range for the patient and how fast the blood pressure is to be lowered must be known. Administered IV through infusion pumps and microdrip regulators. No other drug is added to the IV bottle or to the IV line. Oral medications are started as soon as possible so that IV medication can be discontinued. **EVALUATION:** Evaluate for thiocyanate and cyanide toxicities after 1–2 days.

NA = not available.

which may be precipitated. Safe use in lactation and in children also has not been established.

ADVERSE EFFECTS Common adverse effects include headache caused by cerebral vasodilatation, palpitation caused by reflex increase in heart rate, anorexia and nausea caused by GI congestion, and sweating caused by increased caliber of peripheral vessels. These cardiac effects can be controlled with concurrent administration of beta-adrenergic blockers. Less common effects are nasal congestion, flushing, lacrimation, conjunctivitis, paresthesias, edema, tremors, and muscle cramps. Tolerance to these effects can occur with continued therapy. Adverse effects that require discontinuation of therapy include rash, drug fever, polyneuritis, GI hemorrhage, anemia, and pancytopenia (a reduction of all cellular components of blood).

▼ **CLINICAL ALERT**

A drug-induced systemic lupus erythematosus (SLE) syndrome can develop with hydralazine therapy. This syndrome usually presents with myalgias, arthralgias, and/or pleuritis. The antinuclear antigen (ANA) test is positive. Renal and CNS involvement is rare with drug-induced SLE. This syndrome is seen more commonly in

slow acetylators (hydralazine is subject to polymorphic acetylation) and in patients receiving dosages greater than 400 mg/day. The syndrome disappears upon discontinuation of the drug, but residual effects have been detected years later.

INTERACTIONS Interactions include an increased hypotensive effect when other antihypertensive agents, diuretics, quinidine, and monoamine oxidase inhibitors are given concurrently.

○ **Minoxidil** (Loniten) is a very potent oral vasodilator with an action similar to that of hydralazine. Renal vascular resistance is reduced, and glomerular filtration rate is not decreased.

The advantage of minoxidil is its once-a-day dosing, greater potency, and effectiveness in renal failure. The disadvantage is that fluid retention may occur, as well as reflex sympathetic stimulation. In addition, hirsutism occurs in 80% of patients. A topical formulation of minoxidil (Rogaine) is available over the counter (OTC) for treatment of baldness.

USES Because of serious adverse effects, the use of minoxidil is limited to patients with severe hypertension and is generally considered a step-4 or -5 drug in step-care therapy. Minoxidil is useful for long-term therapy in patients refractory to maximum doses of standard drugs. Both a diuretic and a beta-adrenergic blocker or other sympathetic depressant drug are given concurrently to control fluid retention, prevent tachycardia, and enhance minoxidil's therapeutic effectiveness. This drug appears to be effective in the treatment of hypertensive patients with severe renal failure.

CONTRAINDICATIONS AND PRECAUTIONS Minoxidil is contraindicated in pheochromocytoma because it may stimulate catecholamine release from the tumor, elevating blood pressure. Minoxidil is also contraindicated in myocardial infarction and dissecting aortic aneurysm because reflex cardiac stimulation may occur, aggravating these conditions.

Minoxidil is administered cautiously to patients after a myocardial infarction because the reduction in arterial pressure may further limit blood flow to the myocardium. In patients with renal disease, smaller doses may be necessary and close medical supervision is required. Safety in pregnancy (category C), lactation, and children has not been established.

ADVERSE EFFECTS The most common adverse effects are related to reflex activation of the sympathetic nervous system, resulting in palpitations, tachycardia, exacerbations of angina pectoris and increased myocardial workload. These are unwanted effects in patients with ischemic heart disease that can be effectively controlled with beta-blockade. Changes in direction and magnitude (flattening or inversion) of T waves also occur. Fluid accumulation caused by the reduction in arterial pressure can be effectively managed with diuretics.

▼ CLINICAL ALERT

A common adverse effect of minoxidil is hair growth (80%), most prominent on the face, arms, and back. Hair growth may take up to 6 months to disappear after the drug is stopped.

Minoxidil does not cause impotence and may occasionally alleviate it.

▼ CLINICAL ALERT

It has been recommended that patients be monitored by echocardiography for the development of pericardial effusion, a serious adverse effect that may be produced by minoxidil.

Pulmonary hypertension has also occured with the use of this drug and may be secondary to increased cardiac output.

INTERACTIONS Concurrent administration with guanethidine can result in orthostatic hypotension.

○ **Diazoxide** (Hyperstat), a thiazide derivative, has no diuretic activity but does have a direct vasodilating effect on the arteries. Increased heart rate and cardiac output occur as blood pressure is reduced.

USES Diazoxide is used effectively to treat patients with severe, malignant hypertension and hypertensive crisis. The advantages of diazoxide over other antihypertensives include its rapid action time, its ability to not cause sedation or extreme hypotension, and its ability to not need a continuous infusion. Diazoxide is also used to treat hypoglycemia.

CONTRAINDICATIONS AND PRECAUTIONS Excessive hypotension and reflex sympathetic stimulation can produce myocardial ischemia in susceptible patients. It is also contraindicated in aortic coarctation or arteriovenous shunt and dissecting aortic aneurysm because the cardiac stimulation may aggravate these conditions. It should also be used with caution in patients with renal disease as prolonged hypotension may precipitate renal failure. Safe use in pregnancy (category C) and lactation has not been established.

ADVERSE EFFECTS The most common adverse effect from diazoxide is hypotension followed by nausea and vomiting, dizziness, and weakness. Diazoxide also causes sodium and water retention. It is fairly common practice to administer a 20 to 40-mg IV dose of furosemide (Lasix) concurrently with diazoxide to overcome this adverse effect. Diazoxide can also decrease glomerular filtration rate by reducing blood pressure and renal plasma flow. Hyperglycemia can occur if diazoxide is used for several days. Under these circumstances, blood glucose levels are monitored. If used chronically, hypertrichosis and hyperuricemia can develop.

INTERACTIONS Diazoxide may increase hepatic metabolism of hydantoins. Concurrent thiazides or other diuretics may potentiate hyperglycemia and hyperuricemia. Diazoxide appears to inhibit insulin release from pancreatic islet cells and may antagonize sulfonylureas.

MIXED ARTERIAL AND VENOUS VASODILATORS

Sodium nitroprusside (Nipride) is a balanced arterial and venous vasodilator (see Table 30–3).

○ **Sodium nitroprusside** (Nipride) acts directly on both arteries and veins. By reducing afterload and preload, sodium nitroprusside improves cardiac performance and may increase cardiac output, particularly in the patient with left ventricular failure. Nitroprusside increases renal blood flow, but it also increases cerebral blood flow, a potential problem in the patient with intracranial hypertension.

USES Nitroprusside is indicated for rapid reduction of blood pressure in patients in hypertensive crisis and to maintain blood pressure at a given level by simple titration of the dose. Nitroprusside has also been shown to be effective in treating refractory heart failure. Patients with increased pulmonary artery obstructive pressure (pulmonary capillary wedge pressure) greater than 15 mm Hg and a decreased cardiac output are the most suitable candidates. Unlike the other vasodilators, nitroprusside causes minimal reflex tachycardia because of its balanced effects on preload and afterload. This results in an increase in cardiac output.

Sodium nitroprusside is a very potent agent and must be used carefully to avoid causing inadvertent hypotension. Both reflex catecholamine activity and renin-angiotensin release interfere with the drug's action and may lead to rebound hypertension.

PHARMACOKINETICS Nitroprusside is used only by the IV route. It has an immediate onset of action with blood pressure reductions occurring in 30 to 60 seconds. Maximal effects occur within 1 to 2 minutes. The infusion flow rate is titrated until the desired results are achieved. Nitroprusside has a very short plasma half-life (about 2 minutes).

▼ **CLINICAL ALERT**

Nitroprusside is metabolized to cyanide, which is metabolically converted in the liver to thiocyanate. The thiocyanate metabolite is excreted renally with a half-life of 4 days and can accumulate and cause significant adverse effects in patients receiving prolonged infusions or those with renal failure.

CONTRAINDICATIONS AND PRECAUTIONS Nitroprusside is contraindicated in arteriovenous shunt or coarctation of the aorta, as the reduction in flow may worsen these conditions. Nitroprusside is also contraindicated in patients with pulmonary embolism, as it interferes with the normal intrapulmonary shunting that occurs in the lung. Nitroprusside is given with caution to patients with hepatic or renal disease. Because thiocyanate can interfere with the transport of iodine into the thyroid gland, resulting in hypothyroidism, nitroprusside should be given with care to patients with hypothyroidism. Administer to pregnant (category C) and lactating women with extreme caution and only if clearly needed.

ADVERSE EFFECTS Common adverse effects include nausea, abdominal pain, headache, diaphoresis, restlessness, agitation, chest pain, and palpitations, all related to vasodilatation and its effects within the body. These effects usually go away when the drug is discontinued. Thiocyanate toxicity, although rare, may occur if the infusion is prolonged or when renal failure is present. Symptoms include confusion, slurred speech, weakness, muscle twitching, and tinnitus. Thiocyanate levels are monitored in patients receiving nitroprusside for more than 1 to 2 days. The thiocyanate level is maintained under 10 mg/dL. Cyanide toxicity with subsequent methemoglobinemia can occur if infusion rates exceed 10 μg/kg per minute for 10 minutes. Cyanide toxicity, if serious enough, can be treated by removing the compound by hemodialysis. Symptoms include myocardial ischemia and even infarction, ataxia, seizures, and stroke. Cyanide toxicity may be prevented by adding sodium thiosulfate to nitroprusside (10:1 ratio).

An important concern is the risk of myocardial ischemia caused by diastolic hypotension and increased cardiac output. Arterial oxygen tension can decrease in patients on nitroprusside related to the increased intrapulmonary shunting. This is usually about 10 mm Hg of oxygen and may be of significance in patients with compromised respiratory function or localized lung lesions.

INTERACTIONS Concurrent ganglionic blockers, volatile liquid anesthetics, circulatory depressants, and other antihypertensives all augment the hypotensive effects of nitroprusside.

DOSAGE Nitroprusside is mixed with D_5W and given by IV infusion in doses of 0.5 to 10 μg/kg per minute. Do not infuse above 10 μg/kg per min. If blood pressure is not adequately reduced within 10 minutes, administration should be stopped.

The infusion rate is usually titrated by the individual patient's response. An infusion pump is required to ensure appropriate dosage of this medication. The IV bottle is protected from light by the tinfoil wrapper included in each package. When deterioration by light occurs, the solution turns blue, green, or dark red. The solution is changed every 24 hours. The patient's blood pressure and the flow rate of the infusion must be monitored continually. When no longer needed, nitroprusside must be tapered and not abruptly reduced. The use of nifedipine for acute afterload reduction, and nitrates and furosemide for preload reduction, have tended to decrease the indications for nitroprusside, as it must be more carefully monitored than the other agents because of its very rapid onset and cessation of activity. Nonetheless, nitroprusside is still the vasodilator of choice in many acute emergency situations.

Nitroprusside may be combined with inotropic agents such as dopamine and dobutamine and with digitalis to optimize the hemodynamic benefit. It is important to maintain an adequate ventricular filling pressure to maximize effectiveness.

CALCIUM CHANNEL BLOCKERS

The calcium channel blockers, or calcium antagonists, are a group of medications used for the treatment of hypertension, dysrhythmias, and angina pectoris. They include **nicardipine (Cardene)**; **verapamil (Calan, Isoptin)**, **sustained-release verapamil (Calan SR, Isoptin SR, Verelan)**, and **controlled-release verapamil (Covera HS)**; **diltiazem (Cardizem)** and **sustained-release diltiazem (Cardizem SR, Cardizem CD, Dilacor-XR, Tiazac)**; **isradipine (Dynacirc)**, **felodipine (Plendil)**; **nisoldipine (Sular)**; and **amlodipine (Norvasc)**. The calcium channel blockers are discussed in more detail in Chapters 31 and 32 (see Table 32–3, which describes dosages, pharmacokinetics, and nursing implications for calcium channel blockers).

ACTION

The calcium channel blockers have several modes of action in hypertension. In general, these agents block the slow calcium channel in the cell membrane and prevent calcium entry into the cell. This blocking action reduces the mechanical activity of vascular smooth muscle and leads to a decrease in peripheral vascular resistance, usually without reflex tachycardia. The calcium channel blockers also block norepinephrine-mediated vasoconstriction. This may occur because alpha-sympathetic vasoconstriction is produced by enhanced calcium influx into the cell. If calcium influx is decreased, then norepinephrine vasoconstriction is reduced. Another system regulated by intracellular calcium is the release of renin by the juxtaglomerular cells of the kidney. Because calcium channel blockers inhibit renin release, the renin-angiotensin system is also suppressed. The natriuretic (sodium-excreting properties) properties of calcium blockers, enables them to be effective in the absence of diuretic therapy. They also have a potential to prevent the formation of atheromatous lesions in peripheral vascular tissue, which are often accelerated in some hypertensive patients. These products can all cause the regression of left ventricular hypertrophy and improvement of left ventricular diastolic function. And, unlike other antihypertensives (e.g., beta-adrenergic blockers, diuretics), the calcium channel blockers are lipid neutral.

USES

Calcium channel blockers are used to control mild to moderate hypertension, alone or in combination with diuretics. Calcium channel blockers are most efficacious in persons with low renin production, and are also useful in hypertensive patients who also have chronic stable angina or spastic angina. The vasodilating properties of the calcium channel blockers lead to a reduction in afterload, and their regional smooth muscle relaxant properties are useful in relieving coronary spasm. Calcium channel blockers are also useful in treating patients who cannot take beta-adrenergic blocking agents. The degree of blood pressure reduction is related to the pretreatment blood pressure.

Short acting nifedpidine has never been approved for treatment of hypertensive emergencies. If hypertension in a symptomatic patient without target organ disease is lowered fast, a real emergency could occur. In 1985, the FDA committee concluded to abandon the practice of their oral capsule (Grossman, E, et al., 1996).

The advantage of the calcium channel blockers is that they also act as antianginal agents and are lipid neutral. They combine well with beta-adrenergic blockers and diuretics and are effective in all populations (e.g., Caucasians, African-Americans, the young, the elderly). Their major disadvantage is the headache, negative inotropic effect, and AV block that can occur.

ANGIOTENSIN CONVERTING ENZYME INHIBITORS

The angiotensin converting enzyme (ACE) inhibitors block conversion of angiotensin I to angiotensin II by inhibiting angiotensin converting enzyme (see Fig. 30–1). Examples of ACE inhibitors include **captopril** *(Capoten)*, **enalapril** *(Vasotec)*, **enalaprilat** *(Vasotec IV)*, **lisinopril** *(Prinivil)*, **ramipril** *(Altace)*, **benazepril** *(Lotensin)*, **quinapril** *(Accupril)*, **fosinopril** *(Monopril)*, **moexipril hydrochloride** *(Univasc)*, **spirapril** *(Renormax)* **trandolapril** *(Mavik)*, and **moexipril** *(Univasc)*. Selected ACE inhibitors

are in Table 30–4 along with their pharmacokinetics and dosages. Because angiotensin II is a powerful vasoconstrictor, interfering with its production can reduce total peripheral resistance and hence blood pressure. In addition, angiotensin II also acts on the adrenal cortex to stimulate the release of aldosterone, which increases sodium and water reabsorption. Angiotension II may also stimulate growth factors in the heart muscle, which can lead to hypertrophy. The ACE inhibitors also prevent degradation of the vasodilator bradykinin and increase the urinary excretion of prostaglandins. In contrast to direct vasodilators, such as hydralazine and minoxidil, ACE inhibitors do not cause reflex tachycardia nor do they induce sodium and water retention to any substantial extent. ACE inhibitors are most effective in patients who tend to respond favorably to beta-adrenergic blockers. The hemodynamic effects of ACE inhibitors differ from those of other antihypertensive agents and are beneficial in patients with hypertensive and diabetic damage to the kidneys and heart.

Studies of male Caucasian hypertensive patients suggest that the use of the ACE inhibitor captopril (Capoten) is associated with a better quality of life than treatment with the beta-blocker propranolol or the antiadrenergic methyldopa. Patients taking captopril displayed the greatest improvement in standardized measures of general well-being and satisfaction with life. They also reported the most freedom from physical symptoms and the least decline in sexual function.

In patients with heart failure, captopril, enalapril, lisinopril, and ramipril significantly decrease systemic vascular resistance (SVR), blood pressure (afterload), pulmonary capillary obstructive pressure (PAOP or PCWP) (preload), pulmonary vascular resistance (PVR), and heart size; and increase cardiac output, stroke index, and exercise tolerance time. These effects start with the first dose and continue during therapy.

ACE inhibitors also block the sympathetic nervous system and therefore prevent ventricular remodeling. (Remodeling is thought to be responsible for the development of end-stage heart disease after a myocardial infarction, or MI). The remodeled myocyte (cardiac cell) develops a different shape and size, becomes stretched and elongated, and eventually fails (Foy, S, et al., 1994; and Moyle, LA, et al., 1994).

The advantage of the ACE inhibitors is that there is no sedation and they are lipid neutral. Patients also experience a good quality of life. The major disadvantage is the cough, rash, and loss of taste that can occur.

Diuretics given prior to and during ACE inhibitor therapy enhance the responsiveness to these drugs. In addition, ACE inhibitors blunt the hypokalemic effect of diuretics. The combination of a thiazide-type diuretic with an ACE inhibitor is generally well-tolerated and highly effective in the treatment of the younger hypertensive patient who has no symptoms of coronary artery disease.

USES

The ACE inhibitors are part of initial therapy in mild to moderate hypertension. They are also effective as a vasodilator for the treatment of moderate to severe heart failure and are used to prevent ventricular remodeling

Table 30–4. ANTIHYPERTENSIVE DRUGS: ANGIOTENSIN CONVERTING ENZYME INHIBITORS

DRUG NAME/ROUTE AND DOSAGE	PHARMACOKINETICS/ DYNAMICS	NURSING IMPLICATIONS
captopril (Capoten)		
hypertension *Adults:* 25 mg PO bid or tid; increase to 50 mg after 1–2 wk, to maximum 100–150 mg tid to daily maximum of 450 mg. **malignant or accelerated hypertension** *Adults:* 25 mg PO tid with increases q 24 hr until blood pressure is controlled. **congestive heart failure** *Adults: Initial dose*–6.25–12.5 mg PO tid. *Maintenance dose*–50–100 mg PO tid. Reduce dose with renal dysfunction. **remodeling** *Adults:* 6.25 test dose, followed by 12.5 mg 3 times daily, increased up to 50 mg PO tid; started 48 hr after MI and continued for 44–48 months as above.	**Onset:** 0.25 hr **Peak:** 0.5–1.5 hr **Duration:** 6–12 hr **½L:** 1.7 hr **PB:** 25%–30% **B:** not biotransformed **E:** urine (40%–50% unchanged)	**ASSESSMENT:** Assess CBC frequently—every 2 wk for 3 mo, then monthly. Assess patient carefully for signs of infection such as sore throat and fever. Assess for pregnancy (category C). **INTERVENTION:** Monitor serum potassium levels. May reduce dosage with renal disease and in patients on dialysis. Administration of diuretics can increase efficacy. **Patient Teaching**—Teach patient to avoid all NSAIDs, K^+ supplements, and cough and cold medications. Caution patient against excessive sweating and dehydration, which may lead to excessive fall in blood pressure, and advise him or her to change body position slowly. Advise patient not to stop medication without physician's approval. Tell patient not to take drug with antacids. **EVALUATION:** Notify physician if mouth sores, fever, chest pain, swelling of hands and feet, or skin rash occur. A persistent, dry cough may occur and does not usually subside unless the medication is discontinued.
enalapril (Vasotec) *Adults: Initial dose*–2.5–5 mg PO per day increase dose at 1- to 2-wk intervals. *Maintenance dose*–10–40 mg PO per day. Reduce dose in renal impairment and in dialysis patients.	**Onset:** 1 hr **Peak:** ½–1½ hr **Duration:** 24 hr **½L:** 1.3 hr **PB:** NA **B:** not biotransformed **E:** urine (54% unchanged)	Same as for captopril except: **ASSESSMENT:** Assess for pregnancy (category D).
enalaprilat (Vasotec IV) *Adults:* 0.625–1.25 mg IV over 5 min q 6 hr; if also receiving diuretic, dose is 0.625 mg.	**Onset:** 5–15 min **Peak:** 3–4 hr **Duration:** 6 hr **½L:** 11 hr **PB:** greatly **B:** liver **E:** urine (90%)	Same as for captopril except: **ASSESSMENT:** Assess for pregnancy (category D).
lisinopril (Prinivil) (Zestril) *Adults: Initial dose*–10 mg PO once daily. *Maintenance dose*–20–40 mg PO once daily. Reduce dose with renal impairment.	**Onset:** 1 hr **Peak:** 7 hr **Duration:** 24 hr **½L:** 12 hr **PB:** UA **B:** not biotransformed **E:** unchanged in urine (100%)	Same as for captopril except: **ASSESSMENT:** Assess for pregnancy (category D).
ramipril (Altace) *Adults: Initial dose*–2.5 mg PO daily. *Maintenance dose*–2.5–20 mg PO daily.	**Onset:** 1–2 hr **Peak:** 1 hr **Duration:** 24 hr **½L:** ramipril, 1–2 hr; ramiprilat, 23.5 hr **PB:** ramipril (73%); ramiprilat (56%) **B:** liver **E:** urine (22%), feces	Same as for captopril except: **ASSESSMENT:** Assess for pregnancy (category D). **INTERVENTION:** Food slows the rate, but not the extent of absorption.

NA = not available.

after an MI. ACE inhibitors are effective alone but, in general, patients (because of their previous difficulty in controlling blood pressure) are generally placed on diuretics as well.

PHARMACOKINETICS

All ACE inhibitors are absorbed in varying amounts from the GI tract. Captopril is best administered 1 hour before meals, as the presence of food reduces absorption. The other ACE inhibitors are not affected by food. With the exception of captopril and lisinopril, all others are prodrugs. *Prodrugs* are administered in an inactive form and made active after absorption into active compounds. Captopril and lisinopril, therefore, do not require biotransformation. All ACE inhibitors are bound to plasma protein in varying amounts (25% to 95%). Onset of activity begins in approximately 1 hour and lasts 12 to 24 hours. All are excreted in the urine, and their half-life is prolonged in renal disease.

CONTRAINDICATIONS AND PRECAUTIONS

ACE inhibitors are contraindicated in persons hypersensitive to these products or who have experienced angioedema related to previous ACE inhibitor therapy. ACE inhibitors may cause a first dose effect—a profound fall in blood pressure. This is more likely to occur in patients severely salt or volume depleted, such as those pretreated with diuretics. Blood pressure needs to be monitored closely. Safety in lactating women and in children has not been established.

▼ CLINICAL ALERT

The use of ACE inhibitors during the second and third trimesters of pregnancy is associated with fetal injury and death. And, although there is no evidence that this adverse effect occurs during the first trimester, ACE inhibitors should be discontinued as soon as possible after pregnancy is diagnosed.

ACE inhibitors are given cautiously to patients with impaired renal function, because elevated blood urea nitrogen (BUN) and serum creatinine levels have been induced after a reduction in blood pressure. Total urinary protein above 1 g is frequently seen with captopril patients. Nephrotic syndrome occurs in 20% of these patients. In most cases, the proteinuria clears within 6 months regardless of whether captopril was continued. Proteinuria generally occurs about the eighth month of therapy.

▼ CLINICAL ALERT

Patients started on ACE inhibitors outside the hospital must return to the office within 3 to 4 days to have renal function reassessed.

Patients may also experience hyperkalemia, particularly if they have renal insufficiency or diabetes. Serum potassium levels must be monitored.

ADVERSE EFFECTS

ACE inhibitors have been found to cause serious adverse effects. Patients taking ACE inhibitors are monitored closely. Several patients have developed proteinuria, neutropenia, and agranulocytosis with captopril and decreased hemoglobin and hematocrit with enalapril or lisinopril. Rash, often with pruritus and fever (rash is usually mild and disappears within a few days with dose reduction and short-term therapy with an antihistamine), tachycardia, and chest pain may occur. Gastrointestinal symptoms such as abdominal pain, vomiting, nausea, and diarrhea may also occur.

▼ CLINICAL ALERT

A dry, hacking cough appears in 15% to 20% (possibly up to 39%) of patients and is associated with the inhibition of the degradation of endogenous bradykinins. The cough has a higher incidence in women. The use of nebulized cromolyn (Intal) may be effective in managing the cough in selected patients. In some cases, the cough may necessitate discontinuing the drug.

Patients receiving ACE inhibitors may also experience elevations of liver enzymes, transient elevations of BUN and serum creatinine, and increases in serum potassium concentration.

Patients placed on ACE inhibitors after an MI to prevent remodeling may have a lowering of the blood pressure below 80 mm Hg. If the patient remains warm and dry and can "read the newspaper," he or she is fine regardless of what his or her blood pressure is. However, if the patient becomes restless, cool, ashen, and clammy, he or she is *not* fine. These findings are reported to the physician and the ACE inhibitor may be temporarily stopped or the dose reduced.

INTERACTIONS

Concurrent ACE inhibitors enhance the hypotensive effects of diuretics and other antihypertensive medications. Potassium-sparing diuretics and potassium supplements should be given only for documented hypokalemia, as they may interact to cause a significant increase in serum potassium. Nonsteroidal anti-inflammatory drugs block prostaglandin production and can, therefore, blunt the effects of ACE inhibitors.

○ **Captopril** (Capoten) is used to treat patients with hypertension and heart failure and to prevent remodeling following MI. It can also be used, in reduced dosages, in patients with renal impairment. A loop diuretic is generally administered with captopril in patients with renal impairment. In addition, captopril is also used to slow the progression of and to manage diabetic nephropathy, rheumatoid arthritis, or idiopathic edema and for the symptomatic relief of Raynaud's syndrome.

○ **Enalapril** (Vasotec) is a long-acting ACE inhibitor with pharmacologic actions similar to the other ACE inhibitors. Enalapril is useful in treating mild to severe essential hypertension and renovascular hypertension. Enalapril also can decrease mortality in patients with both acute and chronic heart failure, as it decreases the heart size and reduces the need for other drugs for heart failure. Enalapril is more effective in Caucasians and younger patients than in African-Americans and older patients.

○ **Enalaprilat** (Vasotec IV) is used to reduce blood pressure in an emergency.

○ **Lisinopril** (Prinivil, Zestril) is used to manage essential hypertension and heart failure. If blood pressure is not controlled with lisinopril alone, a low dose of a thiazide diuretic may be added.

○ **Ramipril** (Altace) is also similar to enalapril and indicated for the treatment of hypertension. It is administered once daily.

○ **Benazepril** (Lotensin), a highly protein-bound prodrug, is used to treat hypertension alone or in combination with thiazide diuretics.

○ **Fosinopril** (Monopril), like benazepril, is a prodrug that is highly protein bound. It is used to treat hypertension, with or without a thiazide diuretic. Fosinopril is metabolized in the liver.

○ **Quinapril** (Accupril) is as effective as captopril and enalapril for treating hypertension and heart failure.

○ **Moexipril hydrochloride** (Univasc) may be administered alone or in combination with a low-dose thiazide diuretic for better hypertension control. Daily or twice-daily dosing is appropriate.

○ **Spirapril** (Renormax) may be administered alone or in combination with a low-dose thiazide diuretic for better hypertension control. Daily or twice-daily dosing is appropriate.

○ **Trandolapril** (Mavik) is approved for hypertension. The minimum dose for caucasians is 1 mg/day and for blacks is 2 mg/day.

○ **Moexipril** (Univasc) is administered for hypertension. It is administered before meals with the initial dose of 7.5 mg and the maintenance dose of 7.5–30 mg/day.

ANGIOTENSIN II ANTAGONISTS

The angiotensin II antagonist—**losartan potassium (Cozaar)**—blocks the vasoconstriction and aldosterone-secreting effects of angiotensin, selectively blocking the binding of angiotensin II to angiotensin receptors. Contraindications and precautions, use during pregnancy, and use in children are the same as those for the ACE inhibitors.

○ **Losartan potassium** (Cozaar) is primarily used as an antihypertensive. It is well absorbed, reaches a peak in 1 to 4 hours and has a half-life of 2 hours (6 to 9 hours for the metabolite). It has a substantial first-pass metabolism in the liver and is excreted in the urine. It is more effective in Caucasians than in African-Americans.

ADVERSE EFFECTS The most common adverse effects of losartan are angioedema, diarrhea, dyspepsia, dizziness, and cough. Cough, however, occurs less often than with ACE inhibitors.

INTERACTIONS Concurrent losartan and phenobarbital leads to reduction of losartan levels, probably due to the enzyme induction effects of phenobarbital in the liver.

DOSAGE Inital starting dose is 50 mg daily with maximal maintenance dosage from 50 to 100 mg/day.

GANGLIONIC BLOCKERS

Only one ganglionic blocker—**mecamylamine hydrochloride (Inversine)**—is available today. It blocks transmission of both sympathetic and parasympathetic nerve impulses through the ganglia. It appears to compete with acetylcholine to occupy the cholinergic receptors of the autonomic ganglia. When this drug interacts with cholinergic receptors instead of acetylcholine, sympathetic impulses transmitted from the ganglia to the vascular bed are blocked, causing blood vessels to dilate and arterial pressure to fall. Since 1961, more potent and selectively acting drugs with fewer adverse effects have been developed.

SEROTONIN RECEPTOR BLOCKING AGENTS

The serotonin receptor blocking agents, still investigational in the United States, block the effect of serotonin at the peripheral receptor sites and thus prevent serotonin-induced vasoconstriction. Total peripheral resistance, and thus blood pressure, are reduced.

The prototype of these agents is ketanserin, which also has antiplatelet activity. Ketanserin is more effective in older patients, and the full effect may not be seen until after 12 weeks of treatment. Ketanserin has also been shown to lower pulmonary vascular resistance in patients with acute respiratory failure while decreasing the pulmonary shunt fraction. In addition, ketanserin decreases portal hypertension in patients with alcoholic cirrhosis.

DOPAMINE RECEPTOR STIMULATORS

Several of these agents, of which fenoldopam is the prototype, are available in oral form outside the United States. The dopamine receptor stimulators have a prominent renal vasodilation effect, which enables them to reduce blood pressure in severe hypertension with an additional sodium duiresis. In contrast, sodium nitroprusside is a superior drug to reduce severe hypertension, but it is associated with sodium retention.

HYPERTENSIVE EMERGENCIES

True hypertensive emergency (blood pressure 200/130 mm Hg) occurs in many conditions, including hypertensive encephalopathy, acute heart failure, intracranial hemorrhage with hypertension, aortic dissection, acute myocardial infarction or unstable angina, acute pulmonary edema with hypertension, acute renal failure, malignant hypertension, severe hypertension after surgery, and toxemia of pregnancy. Patients with continued severe hypertension are prone to develop cerebrovascular occlusion, intracerebral bleeding, or subarachnoid hemorrhage. These patients often complain of headache, dizziness, occasional blurred vision, paralysis, convulsions, vomiting, and stupor. The optic fundi have hemorrhages, exudates, and papilledema. Immediate reduction in blood pressure is necessary, but an excessive decrease may be dangerous. Usually a decrease of 20% to 30% in the mean arterial pressure is safe, with a minimum diastolic pressure of 100 mm Hg. Table 30–5 features drugs commonly used in hypertensive emergencies and their advantages and disadvantages. Table 30–6 features two drugs used to control the persistent or intermittent hypertension caused by a pheochromocytoma: **phenoxybenzamine (Dibenzyline)** and **phentolamine mesylate (Regitine)**.

SELECTION OF AN ANTIHYPERTENSIVE

After analyzing the patient's history, physical, and laboratory findings, the choice of a pharmacologic agent is based on patient demographics, sequelae, concomitant diseases, and other risk factors such as cholesterol levels. Only diuretics and beta-adrenergic blockers have been shown in large-scale clinical trials to decrease mortality in patients with hypertension. ACE inhibitors, calcium channel blockers, and alpha-adrenergic blockers, how-

Table 30–5. DRUGS FOR HYPERTENSIVE EMERGENCIES

Drug	Class	Uses*	Advantages	Disadvantages
Parenteral Nitroprusside (Nipride, others)	Arteriolar and venous vasodilator infusion	1, 2, 3, 4, 5, 6, 8	Rapid onset and resolution of action; no tachyphylaxis; no sedation; decreases preload and afterload	Requires continual arterial pressure monitoring. Prolonged use can lead to thiocyanate toxicity.
Diazoxide (Hyperstat)	Arteriolar vasodilator	1, 2, 7, 8	No sedation	Hypotension with previously recommended dosage (300-mg bolus); hyperglycemia; increases heart rate with exacerbation of MI and aortic dissection. Avoid in MI, aortic aneurysm, pulmonary edema.
Labetalol (Trandate; Normodyne)	α- and β-adrenergic blocker	1, 2, 3, 5, 7	No tachycardia	Contraindicated in patients with asthma, > 2nd or 3rd degree heart block, severe sinus bradycardia, congestive heart failure, and pheochromocytoma.
Propranolol (Inderal, others)	β-adrenergic blocker	5, 6, 8	Useful as adjunct to prevent or treat excessive tachycardia	Will not lower blood pressure acutely.
Oral Diltiazem (Cardizein)	Calcium channel blocker	2, 4, 5, 8	Rapid onset (10 min), easily administered	Somewhat variable response.
Captopril (Capoten)	Angiotensin converting enzyme (ACE) inhibitor	4	Easily administered	Variable, sometimes excessive response.
Enalapril (Vasotec)	Angiotensin converting enzyme (ACE) inhibitor	2, 4, 5	Little sedation; rapid onset of action	Doses must be reduced in renal disease. Additive hypotension with other drugs. May require volume expansion.

Source: Adapted from Drugs for Hypertensive Emergencies. Med Lett 29(733), 1987, modified in 1996.
*1-hypertensive encephalopathy, 2-malignant hypertension, 3-subarachnoid hemorrhage, 4-acute heart failure, 5-acute myocardial infarction or unstable angina, 6-aortic dissection, 7-acute renal failure. 8-post-operative hypertension.

Table 30–6. DRUGS TO MANAGE HYPERTENSION IN PHEOCHROMOCYTOMA		
DRUG NAME/ROUTE AND DOSAGE	**PHARMACOKINETICS/ DYNAMICS**	**NURSING IMPLICATIONS**
phenoxybenzamine (Dibenzyline)		
Adults: Initial dose—10 mg PO bid; increase every other day as needed. *Maintenance dose*—20–40 mg PO bid/tid. *Children:* 1–2 mg/kg PO per day divided q 6–8 hr.	**Onset:** 2 hr **Peak:** 2–3 hr **Duration:** 30–36 hr **½L:** unknown **PB:** urine, feces, bile **B:** NA **E:** NA	**ASSESSMENT:** Assess for postural hypotension. Closely observe blood pressure when administering. Assess for pregnancy (category C). **INTERVENTION: Patient Teaching**—Advise patient to avoid cough and cold medication and alcohol. Tell patient to administer with milk or food to lessen GI upset. Warn patient to change position slowly to prevent orthostatic hypotension. Inform patient to protect drug from light. **EVALUATION:** Evaluate for side effects, which usually subside with use.
phentolamine mesylate (Regitine)		
Adults: 5 mg IV or IM. *Children:* 1 mg IV or IM. **diagnosis of pheocromocytoma** *Adults:* 5 mg IV. *Children:* 1 mg IV.	**Onset:** immediately **Peak:** NA **Duration:** NA **½L:** NA **PB:** NA **B:** NA **E:** urine	Same as for phenoxybenzamine plus: **ASSESSMENT:** Assess patient's condition carefully during administration.

NA = not available.

ever, have a more favorable effect on some cardiovascular risk factors. Table 30–7 reviews all antihypertensive medications and their actions and uses. The typical young, Caucasian male or female with normal renal function is started on ACE inhibitors or calcium channel blockers. Beta-adrenergic blockers—because of their ability to reduce exercise tolerance and their tendency to raise serum triglycerides and lower high-density lipoprotein (HDL) levels—are often not advocated for initial therapy. African-Americans are not as effectively treated with beta-adrenergic blockers as Caucasians, but do well with sustained-release verapamil, calcium channel blockers, the alpha- and beta-adrenergic blocker labetalol, and/or diuretics. Smoking, while generally an adverse factor in patients with hypertension, seems specifically to interfere with the effects of propanolol in African-Americans. If cost is a factor, reserpine and a diuretic are as effective as a beta-adrenergic blocker plus a diuretic.

Older patients are less responsive to beta-adrenergic blockers and more responsive to calcium channel blockers and diuretics. Combination therapy with the potassium-sparing drug Dyazide (hydrochlorothiazide/triamterene) and the drug methyldopa is successful therapy in many elderly patients. When treating the elderly patient, it is important not to lower diastolic pressure too much so that tissue perfusion is at risk.

Patients with underlying angina pectoris are best treated with beta-adrenergic blockers, calcium channel blockers, ACE inhibitors, or alpha-adrenergic blockers, as they all have a favorable effect on myocardial oxygen consumption. Beta-adrenergic blockers, however, do have an adverse effect by raising triglycerides and lowering HDL levels. Because abnormal lipid profile can worsen coro-

nary artery disease, beta-adrenergic blockers are not advocated for initial therapy. Whatever drug is ordered, evaluation of blood lipid levels is essential in all patients with hypertension, and the effects of the agents chosen on the lipid profile need to be considered. Patients with hyperlipidemia are best placed on an ACE inhibitor, alpha-adrenergic blocker, or calcium channel blocker because of their negative effect on lipids.

▼ CLINICAL ALERT

A patient with a large MI should be started on an ACE inhibitor or a beta-adrenergic blocker (to decrease the incidence of another MI), even if his or her ejection fraction is not markedly abnormal. ACE inhibitors prevent ventricular remodeling.

When hypertension is complicated with heart failure, ACE inhibitors are indicated. Beta-adrenergic blockers and calcium channel blockers are contraindicated, as they have negative inotropic properties and worsen the heart failure.

Hypertension is twice as common among diabetic patients as in the general population. Research shows that a combination of propanolol and hydrochlorothiazide increases the blood sugar by 56%. ACE inhibitors appear to be the drugs of choice in the diabetic patient because they may have a beneficial effect on insulin sensitivity and on renal function in diabetic nephropathy. Captopril is better than nifedipine in reducing exercise-induced microalbuminuria.

Table 30–7. SUMMARY OF ANTIHYPERTENSIVE DRUGS

Drug Classification	Drug	Antihypertensive Action and Use
Centrally Acting Drugs	Clonidine Methyldopa Guanabenz Guanfacine	Drugs inhibit sympathetic outflow from brain by stimulating alpha receptors in vasomotor center of medulla. Result is decrease in peripheral resistance. Slowed mental functioning limits their usefulness.
Centrally and Peripherally Acting Drug	Reserpine	Drug depletes norepinephrine stores peripherally and centrally, resulting in decreased peripheral resistance.
Neuroeffector-Transmission Blockers (Peripherally Acting Antiadrenergics)	Guanethidine Debrisoquinet† Guanadrel	Loss of peripheral sympathetic tone decreases peripheral resistance by reducing cardiac output and peripheral resistance. Used for severe hypertension.
Alpha-Adrenergic Receptor Antagonists (Alpha-Adrenergic Blockers)	Prazosin Terazosin Doxazosin	Drugs block vasoconstrictive action of norepinephrine, thereby decreasing peripheral resistance. Used for moderate to severe hypertension.
Beta-Adrenergic Receptor Antagonists (Beta-Adrenergic Blockers)	Acebutolol Atenolol Betaxolol Carteolol Metoprolol Nadolol Oxprenolol Penbutolol Pindolol Propranolol Sotalol Timolol	Drugs reduce cardiac output by reducing renin release from kidney. May have central antihypertensive action. Preferred drugs for individuals with high renin levels, typically young whites. These agents decrease incidence of sudden death in patients with recent heart attacks. Cardioselective (beta$_1$-adrenergic receptors) drugs are acebutolol, atenolol, and metoprolol. Not recommended for diabetic patients with elevated cholesterol level.
Alpha- and Beta-Adrenergic Receptor Antagonist	Labetalol	Both alpha- and beta-receptor antagonistic actions apply. Alpha-receptor antagonist actions predominate. Excellent for severe hypertension.
Arterial Vasodilators	Hydralazine Minoxidil Diazoxide	Drugs relax arterial smooth muscle to lower peripheral resistance. When used alone, these agents cause rebound tachycardia (increased heart rate) and edema. Used for moderate to severe hypertension.
Mixed Arterial and Venous Vasodilator	Nitroprusside	Drug dilates blood vessels. It is useful in hypertensive emergencies.
Calcium Channel Blockers	Diltiazem Felodipine Isradipine Nicardipine	Drugs reduce tone of blood vessels by reducing intracellular calcium, thereby causing arteriolar dilation and decreased total peripheral resistance. Often used in first-line therapy.
Angiotensin Converting Enzyme (ACE) Inhibitors	Benazepril Captopril Enalapril Fosinopril Lisinopril Quinapril Ramipril Trandolapril	Drugs reduce peripheral resistance in individuals with high plasma renin levels. Excellent for patients who also have diabetes or associated MI.
Ganglionic Blocking Drugs	Mecamylamine	Drug blocks nicotinic receptors of autonomic ganglia to inhibit sympathetic and parasympathetic functions. Peripheral resistance is decreased. Used in severe hypertension.

Listing includes most drug classes.
†Available in Canada only.

When hypertension occurs concurrently with chronic pulmonary disease, ACE inhibitors, calcium channel blockers, peripherally acting alpha-adrenergic blockers, and centrally acting agonists are the best choices.

In the patient with chronic renal failure and hypertension, ACE inhibitors are associated with prevention of renal deterioration and reduction of proteinuria. Diuretics may be added to this regimen.

Hypertension in obese individuals is associated with an increase in cardiac output that is thought to result from plasma volume expansion; thus, diuretics are recommended as first-line therapy if weight loss and sodium restriction are unsuccessful. Diuretics can aggravate insulin resistance and hyperinsulinemia and stimulate the sympathetic nervous system. When diuretics are inappropriate, ACE inhibitors and calcium channel blockers, as well as sympatholytics, can be used. Beta-adrenergic blockers are relatively undesirable because they may aggravate metabolic factors.

The primary aim of antihypertensive therapy is to prevent or cause the regression of left ventricular hypertrophy (LVH). By controlling LVH, complications of dyspnea, and overt congestive heart failure can be avoided. Recent studies demonstrate that propanolol and labetalol reduce left ventricular wall thickness, which ultimately decreases the likelihood of heart failure.

It is important that the patient maintains his or her intellectual function. Beta-adrenergic blockers have subtle detrimental effects on intellect and cause increased drowsiness. Calcium channel blockers and ACE inhibitors seem to have the least effect on intellectual activity and memory.

Physical activity must be maintained. Beta-adrenergic blockers are known to induce fatigue and limit physical exercise capacity. Calcium channel blockers, ACE inhibitors, and diuretics allow the patient to maintain physical activity.

It is also important to maintain sexual function. Almost all antihypertensives have been reported to reduce sexual function. However, calcium channel blockers and ACE inhibitors seem to cause the fewest sexual side effects.

Many combination products are available: Lexxel (enalapril and felodipine), tarka (tranclolapril/verapamil) and thiazide and potassium-sparing diuretics as fixed-dose combinations with antihypertensive drugs (e.g., Ziac, a combination of the beta-blocker bisoprolol and the thiazide diuretic hydrochlorothiazide). Generally, it is best to adjust the dosage of each drug separately. However, when the optimum maintenance doses correspond to the ratio in a combination product, then taking one tablet is better for patient compliance than taking two.

USING THE NURSING PROCESS

ASSESSMENT

- Develop a thorough nursing history to create a database. The information to obtain is featured in Table 30–8. The diagnosis of mild to moderate hypertension is made only after three consecutive tests, taken on three different days, show blood pressure to be elevated. Both standing and supine blood pressures are assessed, as well as pulse pressures. Both diastolic and systolic numbers are considered. Pulse rate is also recorded because the hypertensive patient who is tachycardic needs different drugs from the hypertensive patient who is bradycardic.
- Assess current and past medication that have been taken to control blood pressure. Ask the patient what drugs he or she is taking, for how long, and whether there are any adverse effects. Also obtain a thorough OTC medication history. Patients can experience hypertension from combining OTC diet pills and decongestants. If such a combination is found, the medication is discontinued to determine if the blood pressure will return to normal.
- Assess the current exercise level of the patient. What are the usual type, frequency, and duration of sporting activities? How does the patient get to work? Is there job-related physical activity? How many flights of stairs does the patient climb per day? The answer to these questions will help to identify patients with infrequent exercise in their lifestyle.
- Assess current smoking habits, including the use of cigarettes, cigars, and marijuana. All types of smoking are eliminated because of the untoward side effects that can be experienced. During the intervention phase, help the patient devise a method to reduce or eliminate smoking.
- Assess the dietary profile. Dietary habits may have a profound effect on blood pressure and may affect the action of antihypertensive drugs. Dietary manipulations alone can often provide effective therapy for hypertension and may be prescribed alone or in addition to medications. The most important dietary factors are calorie, alcohol (ethanol), and sodium intake. Because obesity is strongly associated with hypertension, weight loss can decrease or even cure hypertension. The average hypertensive person can expect to decrease systolic blood pressure by 1 mm Hg and diastolic blood pressure by ¾ mm Hg for every pound lost. The consumption of three or more alcoholic drinks per day is associated with an increase in mean blood pressure. Approximately 5% of the cases of hypertension in the United States may be associated with increased alcohol ingestion.
- Assess family profile. Because hypertension frequently is familial, the whole family, not just the patient, is assessed to determine possible contributing factors to the development of hypertension.
- Assist with the collection of laboratory data. Typical lab tests that may be ordered include serum potassium; cholesterol and triglycerides to rule out risk factors for coronary artery disease; thyroid studies, if indicated, to rule out hyperthyroidism; chest radiography and electrocardiogram (ECG) to determine heart size; and urine studies such as urine steroids and vanillylmandelic acid to rule out secondary causes of hypertension.
- Assess blood pressure standing and supine and in the arms and legs using the correct size blood pressure cuff. Height and weight are important, and any recent changes are noted. Lungs are auscultated, and a *funduscopic exam* (examination of the posterior portions of the eye utilizing a special instrument called a funduscope) of the eyes is performed to determine the presence of papilledema or retinal changes such as hemorrhages or exudates that occur as hypertension progresses.

Patients with "borderline" hypertension (diastolic blood pressure 90 to 94 mm Hg) are generally considered at low risk. It is recommended that they be assessed periodically for 4 months before any form of therapy is initiated. If pharmacologic therapy is postponed, it is important to reexamine untreated patients about every 6 months, as their hypertension may progress or their risk profile may worsen.

NURSING DIAGNOSIS

- Develop the nursing diagnoses with the help of the patient and family. Possible nursing diagnoses for the patient with hypertension include the following: Knowledge Deficit; Altered Nutrition, More than Body Requirements; Impaired Adjustment; De-

Table 30–8. NURSING PROCESS FOR PATIENT REQUIRING ANTIHYPERTENSIVE MEDICATIONS

Assessment

Assess blood pressure (standing and supine) and heart rate.
Assess smoking habits, including cigarettes, cigars, and marijuana.
Assess current weight and height.
Assess usual dietary pattern, including intake of sodium and use of alcohol.
Assess medication history (including OTC, prescription, and any other antihypertensive medication).

Nursing Diagnosis: Knowledge Deficit

RELATED TO: Unfamiliarity with resources, misunderstanding.
AS EVIDENCED BY: Questions, statement of concern, poor control of condition, development of preventable complications.

Desired Outcomes/Evaluation Criteria

Verbalizes understanding of condition and therapy needs. Demonstrates behavior (e.g., monitoring of blood pressure, diet modifications designed to maintain blood pressure at an optimal level).

Nursing Actions	Rationale
Define and state the limits of normal blood pressure. Explain hypertension and its effects on the heart, blood vessels, kidneys, and brain.	Provides basis for understanding elevations of blood pressure and that it can be elevated without symptoms.
Avoid saying "normal" blood pressure, and use the term "well-controlled" when describing blood pressure within desired limits. Define and state the limits of normal blood pressure. Explain hypertension and its effects on the heart, blood vessels, kidneys, and brain.	Because treatment is lifelong, conveying the idea of control helps the patient to understand the need for continued treatment/medication. Provides basis for understanding elevations of blood pressure and that it can be elevated without symptoms.
Provide information (verbal and written) about antihypertensives including action, use, dose, adverse effects, and interactions.	Enhances knowledge base so patient is capable of making educated decisions about therapy.
Discuss possible drug interactions and how and when to take antihypertensive medications.	Enhances success of drug therapy. Drugs that could possibly increase blood pressure or counteract antihypertensives are eliminated.
Assist the patient in identifying modifiable cardiovascular risk factors, e.g., obesity, diet high in saturated fats and cholesterol, sedentary lifestyle, smoking, alcohol intake, stressful lifestyle.	These risk factors have been shown to contribute to hypertension and cardiovascular/renal disease.
Discuss importance of eliminating smoking and assist patient in formulating a plan to quit.	Nicotine increases catecholamine discharge, resulting in increased heart rate, blood pressure, and vasoconstriction, reducing tissue oxygenation, and increasing the myocardial workload.
Establish an individual exercise program incorporating aerobic exercise within patient capabilities. Stress the importance of avoiding isometric activity.	Besides helping to lower blood pressure, aerobic activity aids in toning the cardiovascular system. Isometric exercise can increase serum catecholamine levels, further elevating blood pressure.
Instruct and demonstrate technique of self-monitoring of blood pressure.	Teaching the patient/significant other to monitor blood pressure is reassuring to the patient, provides visual/positive reinforcement for patient efforts, and helps in guiding therapy.

Nursing Diagnosis: Altered Nutrition More than Body Requirements

RELATED TO: Excessive intake in relation to metabolic need.
AS EVIDENCED BY: Reported dysfunctional eating patterns, percentage of body fat greater than 18%–20% for trim women; 10%–12% for trim men.

Desired Outcomes/Evaluation Criteria

Identifies inappropriate behaviors associated with weight gain or overeating. Maintains optimal individual diet and exercise program.

Nursing Actions	Rationale
Review individual nutritional needs and appropriate food selection within economic means. Discuss need for reduction of sodium intake, alcohol consumption, caloric intake; and importance of exercise program.	Faulty eating habits contribute to weight gain, sodium retention, and atherosclerosis. Exercise can assist with weight reduction, improved mental outlook, and reduction in blood pressure.
Encourage weekly monitoring of weight.	Useful in evaluating therapy needs and effectiveness.

Other Suggested Nursing Diagnoses: Impaired Adjustment; Decreased Cardiac Output; and Noncompliance with Medication, Exercise, and Diet Regimen.

creased Cardiac Output; and Noncompliance (see Table 30–8).

PLANNING AND INTERVENTION

- Short-term goals include patient education and blood pressure control; long-term goals include changes in lifestyle to help reduce blood pressure.
- Know the target blood pressure that the physician and the patient have agreed on.
- Teach the patient and family about the physiology of this disease; the dietary regimen (usually sodium restriction and limited alcohol) and ideal weight maintenance; the medication regimen, including adverse effects that may be experienced; and how stress and anxiety relate to the condition and how they can be controlled. Exercise counseling may be necessary based on the information obtained in the assessment phase. Suggest various relaxation techniques to the patient, including biofeedback, transcendental meditation, mind control, and yoga, as necessary. All these methods have been proven effective in lowering blood pressure to some extent in selected patients. Stress that these methods can be used in conjunction with medications but should not be a substitute for medical therapy.

Step-Care Therapy

The patient who is newly diagnosed with mild hypertension usually progresses through a stepped-care method of treatment for hypertension. The stepped-care method has been developed by the Joint National Committee on the Detection, Evaluation, and Treatment of High Blood Pressure. (Patients with moderate to severe hypertension are started directly on antihypertensive medications.) The stepped-care method, shown in Figure 30–3, is supported by many clinical trials in which it has been found both effective and well tolerated over the long term in most patients.

The stepped-care method begins with nonpharmacologic approaches such as weight loss, if indicated, and dietary restriction of sodium (step 1). If this treatment is not totally successful, drug therapy, or step 2, is started with a single drug. (See Chapter 37 for more information on diuretics.) The physician may choose a diuretic, a beta-adrenergic blocker, an ACE inhibitor, an alpha-adrenergic blocker, or a calcium channel blocker. If the patient is under 50 years of age or has ischemic heart disease, the physician may prescribe a beta-adrenergic blocker initially. Beta-adrenergic blockers usually reduce blood pressure to the level achieved with diuretics.

If the first drug has some efficacy and is well tolerated but target blood pressure has not been reached, the drug dose may be increased, another single agent may be substituted for the initial first drug, or a second drug with a different pharmacologic effect is added (step 3). Smaller doses of two drugs with different mechanisms of action may prove more effective than larger doses of a single drug. Drugs may be substituted or added as necessary until the blood pressure is controlled. The use of antihypertensive drugs without diuretics is generally followed by reflex sodium and water retention and loss of antihypertensive effect (this is not true, however, with ACE inhibitors and calcium channel blockers). Loop diuretics are usually required in the presence of renal insufficiency or poor left ventricular function. Because of the differences in responsiveness, the regimen must be individualized. It may be necessary to try various drugs or combinations of drugs until the optimal effect is obtained. This process is often very depressing for the patient, and he or she may begin to lose confidence in the medical and nursing personnel. It is imperative that the patient have good explanations of why the drug regimen is being altered.

If the patient has not responded favorably to drug therapy in steps 2 and 3, step 4 begins. If the patient began therapy with a beta-adrenergic blocker but did not respond, a diuretic is added. If this regimen does not effectively control blood pressure, a direct vasodilator, calcium channel blocker, ACE inhibitor, alpha₁-adrenergic

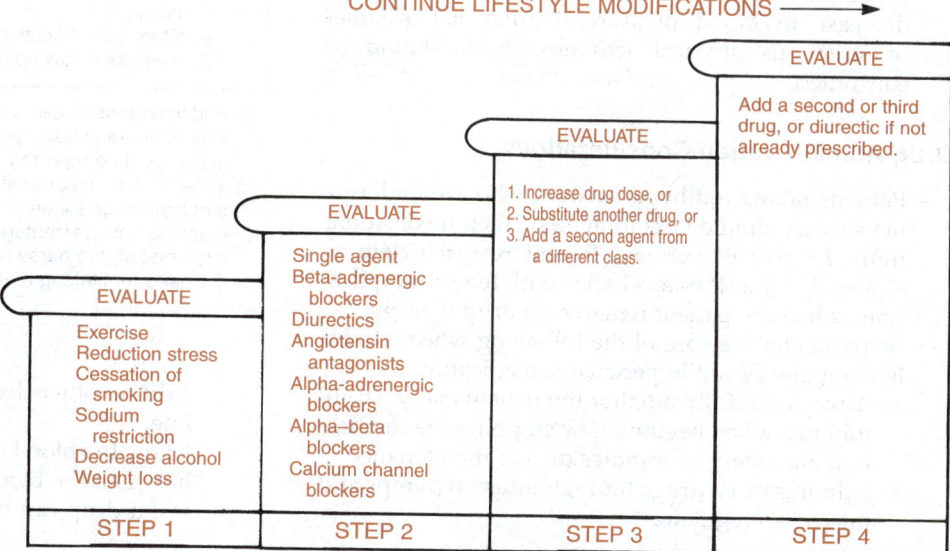

Figure 30–3. Stepped-care protocol for treating hypertension. (Revised by the Joint National Committee on Detection, Evaluation, and Treatment of High Blood Pressure, in 1993.)

blocker, or rauwolfia product is added. This approach frequently minimizes adverse reactions without significantly reducing effectiveness. If blood pressure is not reduced to a satisfactory level, a third drug such as hydralazine or guanethidine is added in step 4. These drugs are added to or substituted for one of the drugs already being administered from steps 2 and 3. Guanethidine is held in reserve for patients who fail to respond to anything else.

The interval between drug or dosage modification is determined by the severity of the hypertension: in mild hypertension, adjustments are made at 2 to 3 month intervals; in moderate hypertension, adjustments are made every 2 to 6 weeks; and in severe hypertension, adjustments may be made within hours to days depending on the blood pressure range. When the blood pressure goal is achieved, medication may be titrated down to avoid unnecessary overmedication of the patients.

The effective doses may vary considerably from patient to patient. Therapy usually is initiated with a single drug and, if additional agents are needed, they are added to the regimen one at a time. If the patient requires more than one drug, the use of a fixed-dose combination drug may improve compliance. Drugs with similar mechanisms of action (e.g., clonidine, methyldopa) are not used together.

Patients who suffer from both angina and hypertension often benefit from treatment with beta-adrenergic blockers and calcium channel blockers, as they are also antianginal agents. African-American and elderly patients may have blunted antihypertensive effect from beta-adrenergic blockers alone. Elderly patients also are particularly sensitive to the blood pressure–lowering effects of the calcium channel blockers.

Patient Teaching

- Ensure that the patient has adequate knowledge to administer the medications safely. The information to be taught to all patients requiring antihypertensives is presented in Table 30–9.
- Teach patients to maintain their fluid balance and prevent dehydration, which may lead to an excessive decrease in blood pressure. During hot weather or strenuous physical activities, fluids should be consumed.

Drug Administration Considerations

- Patients taking antihypertensives who are undergoing surgery should be continued on their medications until the day of surgery. Recent research demonstrates that anesthesia is easier with fewer complications when the patient remains on drug therapy.
- Be particularly aware of the following when administering any IV antihypertensive medication:
  1. Always carefully monitor the patient every 5 to 10 minutes when beginning or stopping the medication and every 15 minutes during maintenance.
  2. Administer IV drugs through infusion pumps and microdrip regulators.

Table 30–9. PATIENT TEACHING—ANTIHYPERTENSIVES

Dear Patient:
This drug has been prescribed for you. This is what you should know about your drug to get the most from your therapy.

- ☐ 1. _____ is taken to lower your blood pressure. Specifically _____ works by _____.
- ☐ 2. Medications are taken every day, most likely for the rest of your life.
- ☐ 3. Most antihypertensives can be taken with or between meals. (To nurse: If different instructions are needed, fill in.)
- ☐ 4. Alcohol (beer, wine, whiskey) intake is limited because of its vasodilator effect.
- ☐ 5. All other over-the-counter and prescription drugs should be checked by your doctor or pharmacist before they are taken.
- ☐ 6. If you forget a dose, do not take it later. Never take 2 doses the next time.
- ☐ 7. Medication should *not* be stopped abruptly as blood pressure tends to rise higher because of increased sensitivity to substances within the body. Do not delay in refilling your prescriptions.
- ☐ 8. If dizziness or faintness is experienced, you should lie down or sit with your head down for a few minutes. The dizziness usually goes away.
- ☐ 9. If you experience any side effects from your medications, call your doctor. (A new drug or a change in dosage will most often stop side effects.)
- ☐ 10. Use caution for at least 2 hours after taking the medication, especially while driving or working around heavy equipment. Medications may make you drowsy, but this is usually transient and stops within a month.
- ☐ 11. Do not take hot baths or showers, as this may cause further vasodilation and fainting.
- ☐ 12. Careful exposure to sun is important, as heat increases peripheral blood flow, and some antihypertensives decrease sweating; therefore, hypotension and heat stroke may occur.
- ☐ 13. Change body position slowly to prevent fainting. When moving from a lying position to standing, sit first.
- ☐ 14. Check your weight at least twice a week, and closely watch for fluid retention.
- ☐ 15. Avoid too much tea, coffee, and cola (more than 4 cups per day), because caffeine has been shown to raise blood pressure.
- ☐ 16. Blood pressures may be taken at home. Records that are kept should be reviewed periodically by the doctor or nurse.
- ☐ 17. Carry an ID card identifying the drug, dose, and the time taken.
- ☐ 18. Store all medications in a tight, light-resistant container.
- ☐ 19. Keep all follow-up appointments.

In addition to these items, the specific drug's actions and side effects are discussed with the patient as well as symptoms that should be reported. Recent studies show that 40%–70% of hypertensive patients stop taking their medication for a variety of reasons. With good health teaching, this percentage can be reduced. Through the intervention, the nurse must continually stress and reinforce the need for lifelong therapy.

3. Add no other drug(s) to the IV bottle or to the IV line.
4. Know the blood pressure range for the patient and how fast the blood pressure is to be lowered. Too fast a drop can be just as dangerous as sustained

hypertension. Patients can experience angina pectoris and possibly even a myocardial infarction.

5. Start oral medication as soon as possible so that IV medication can be discontinued.

- Hospitalized patients in hypertensive crisis may need to have immediate reduction in their blood pressure. Hypertensive crises occur in various pathologic conditions, including accelerated essential hypertension, secondary hypertension, and malignant hypertension, as well as in hypertension associated with renal disease and pregnancy. (See Table 30–3, which features vasodilators used in the emergency treatment of malignant hypertension.) Hypertensive emergencies are situations in which the blood pressure must be lowered within 1 hour. (See Table 30–5, which features drugs for hypertensive emergencies.) The nurse is primarily responsible for lowering the blood pressure to the predetermined levels. During this period of crisis, check for and be alert for changes in other body systems including the brain, kidney, and lung. To prevent cerebral hypoperfusion from occurring because of too rapid a blood pressure reduction, it is suggested that mean blood pressure be lowered no more than 20% to 30% in the first 24 hours.

- Secondary hypertension, often associated with pheochromocytoma, is best treated with phentolamine (Regitine), an alpha-adrenergic blocking agent, phenoxybenzamine (Dibenzyline), an irreversible alpha-adrenergic receptor blocking agent, or metyrosine (Demser), which decreases endogenous levels of catecholamines (see Table 30–6). Phentolamine is described in Chapter 20 and is only an antihypertensive agent when there are large amounts of circulating catecholamines, as produced by a pheochromocytoma or in a patient who suddenly discontinues centrally acting antihypertensives (e.g., clonidine).

EVALUATION

- Evaluate the effectiveness of antihypertensive therapy based on a predetermined list of evaluation criteria, which are developed on an individual basis through discussion among the nurse, patient, and family (see Table 30–8).
- Work with the patient and family to ensure their complete assistance and support. A frequent problem with hypertensive patients is lack of compliance. Evaluate for noncompliance by direct question, pill counts, or determining whether the prescription has been refilled. Many patients do not understand the importance of their medication regimen. Eighty percent of newly diagnosed hypertensive patients do not have symptoms. Help the patient to understand that the medications will ultimately prevent complications (heart disease, cerebral vascular disease, retinal changes, and renal disease) 20 to 30 years later. Compliance can be enhanced with convenient medication regimens, single daily dosing, personal attention, and feedback given to the patient by his or her health-care providers, minimizing expense (antihypertension

medication may cost $25 to $80 per month), education about therapy, and the avoidance of adverse effects. Patients may experience adverse effects from the medications, which, combined with the expense, increases the likelihood of noncompliance. Medical personnel have always assumed that antihypertensive medications are associated with a high rate of adverse reactions, but statistically this appears to be untrue. The most common complaints include sleepiness, fatigue, self-assessed depression, and sexual complaints (impotence and decreased sexual desire).

Impotence is often seen with increasing age, but it is more often a function of a disease process such as diabetes, hypertension, or cardiovascular disease than age itself. Other drugs the patient may be taking, such as anticholinergics, antihistamines, and cimetidine, may be responsible for male impotence. See Chapter 47 for additional information on drugs that effect sexual function.

If noncompliance is suspected, a program of drugs suitable for once-daily administration is developed and the patient is given a daily clinic or office appointment for 5 days. By week's end, pressure is nearly always lowered, and both the patient and physician can see the results that the patient will achieve with home therapy.

- Encourage the patient to keep appointments for checkups so that his or her progress can be monitored. If the patient is experiencing adverse effects from one drug, alternate medications can be tried. Often, this is a trial-and-error period. It may be as long as a year before the patient's blood pressure is well controlled with a minimum of adverse effects. Because tolerance may develop from these medications, the patient must continually, for the rest of his or her life, see the physician on a regular basis.
- Evaluate sleeping habits, as several antihypertensives may cause sleep disorders, including clonidine, methyldopa, and the beta-adrenergic blockers propranolol and nadolol. Patients who experience sleep disturbances—ranging from insomnia to nightmares and sleepwalking—may be helped by taking their medication early in the day instead of at night.
- Teach the patient to monitor and chart his or her blood pressure at home, which may often improve compliance. The patient is then an active participant in the treatment.
- Evaluate all other evaluation criteria before the patient is discharged from the hospital, clinic, or physician's office. All previously taught material is reviewed and updated if necessary to ensure that the patient's and family's knowledge base remains accurate.

The more the patient and family know about the treatment regimen, the more likely they are to comply with the program. Hypertension treatment is for a lifetime. Treatment is designed to lower blood pressure to an acceptable level, determined by the physician. Patients are encouraged to return to and maintain a normal weight, to reduce their intake of sodium, and to practice stress reduction techniques. Some patients may be able to control their blood pressure using these therapies alone, but others need to take one or more medications. Any cessation of medication allows the blood pressure to return to pretreatment levels. There is no doubt that the effective control of blood pressure and the prevention of complications enables the patient to live a longer and more satisfying life.

The bibliography for this chapter can be found in Appendix B, which begins on page 1054.

CHAPTER REVIEW QUESTIONS*

1. ACE inhibitors are drugs of choice in a patient with a myocardial infarction because their action is to:
   a. Increase SVR.
   b. Increase PAOP.
   c. Reduce or control remodeling of the left ventricle.
   d. Decrease cardiac output.

2. A common adverse effect of _____ is hair growth, particularly on the face, arms, and back.
   a. Captopril.
   b. Verapamil.
   c. Minoxidil.
   d. Prazosin.

3. John, a patient with hypertension, is 5'6" and weighs 280 pounds. The drugs of choice for treating John are:
   a. Diuretics, ACE inhibitors.
   b. Beta-adrenergic blockers.
   c. Ganglionic blockers, calcium channel blockers.
   d. Serotonin receptor blockers, diuretics.

*See Appendix A, which starts on page 1051, for answers.

4. Which of the following is *correct* regarding methyldopa administration and other concurrent drug use?
   a. The effects of methyldopa are increased when given with amphetamines.
   b. Verapamil may potentiate the effects of methyldopa.
   c. A hyperglycemia effect is seen with methyldopa and tolbutamide.
   d. Use of methyldopa and propranolol results in paradoxic hypotension.

5. Which of the following drugs is metabolized to cyanide if the dose is above 10 μg/min for 10 minutes?
   a. Hydralazine (Apresoline).
   b. Diazoxide (Hyperstat).
   c. Nitroprusside (Nipride).
   d. Methyldopa (Aldomet).

6. Which of the following effects is seen with calcium channel blockade?
   a. Relief of coronary spasm.
   b. Increased afterload.
   c. Stimulation of renin release.
   d. Promotion of reflex tachycardia.

BUILDING YOUR CRITICAL THINKING SKILLS

HYPERTENSION

Patient 1

Jane, a 42-year-old woman, is complaining of a dry hacking cough that is becoming more annoying. She has a temperature of 99.8°F.

Focus of Inquiry: Ampicillin 250 mg qid is ordered for 10 days. After 10 days, the cough is still there, and according to Jane it is worse.

Analysis and Synthesis: Recall that some drugs, particularly ACE inhibitors, may cause a cough that is dry and hacking. Examine the patient's drug history. She is receiving captopril to treat her hypertension. Captopril was started about 4 weeks ago, when her blood pressure was not being controlled on verapamil (Calan).

New Supposition: The cough is most likely due to the captopril.

Resolution: Because the newer ACE inhibitors are less likely to cause a cough, the physician changes Jane from captopril to spirapril (Renormax).

Patient 2

John, a 65-year-old man, has very severe hypertension. His blood pressure is 218/135 mm Hg.

Focus of Inquiry: John is placed on a nitroprusside (Nipride) drip at 5 μg/kg per min. His blood pressure after 4 hours is 200/120 mm Hg. He is now experiencing increasing difficulty in breathing.

Analysis and Synthesis: Recall that nitroprusside is contraindicated in patients with underlying lung disease. Examine John's history. John was diagnosed 1 month ago as having emphysema, but did not tell the admitting physician.

New Supposition: The difficulty in breathing is most likely associated with increased intrapulmonic shunting of blood.

Resolution: Nitroprusside is discontinued and a nitroglycerin drip is started. The respiratory difficulty subsides.

CHAPTER 31

Antidysrhythmic Medications

Merrily A. Kuhn, RNC, PhD

CHAPTER OUTLINE

TABLES

KEY TERMS

Dysrhythmia
Coupled premature
  ventricular contractions
Effective refractory period

Ejection fraction
Proarrhythmic effects
R-on-T phenomenon
Torsades de pointes

LEARNING OBJECTIVES

After reading this chapter, the student will be able to:

1. Identify medications commonly used as antidysrhythmics.
2. Differentiate among antidysrhythmics as to mechanism of action, route of administration, pharmacokinetics, adverse effects, contraindications and precautions, and interactions.
3. Identify specific areas to assess in the patient requiring antidysrhythmics to formulate appropriate patient outcomes.
4. Plan the nursing interventions necessary to administer antidysrhythmics and choose appropriate teaching strategies to achieve patient compliance.
5. Evaluate the patient at various stages of treatment to gauge nursing interventions.

Dysrhythmia is a disorder of heart rate and rhythm. Dysrhythmias occur in approximately 90% to 95% of all patients experiencing a myocardial infarction. Table 31–1 reviews acute myocardial infarction. Dysrhythmias also present in patients with ischemic heart disease and cause a significant increase in mortality. Appropriate antidysrhythmic therapy in these patients substantially reduces mortality.

The Cardiac Dysrhythmia Suppression Trial (CAST) (1989) demonstrated that dysrhythmias require treatment either for alleviating symptoms or for prolonging survival. However, the CAST study showed a definite *proarrhythmic* (causing or worsening a cardiac dysrhythmia) risk for several drugs in the period following myocardial infarction. The CAST findings have resulted in greater caution in prescribing antidysrhythmic drugs. Individual

patient care is paramount, and the benefit versus risk requires evaluation with each patient.

Ejection fraction (the amount of blood ejected with each beat—normally 70 mL or 70%) is the primary determinant of treatment. When ejection fraction falls to 40%, there is a dramatic increase in the likelihood that dysrhythmia may become life threatening. Ventricular dysrhythmias such as *premature ventricular contractions* (PVCs) are frequently observed in patients without ischemic heart disease and may not require treatment unless the patient is symptomatic. More complex PVCs—*coupled* (2 in a row) or *R-on-T phenomenon* (QRS occurs on the T wave, which may precipitate ventricular tachycardia or fibrillation)— and ventricular tachycardia are usually treated even if the patient is asymptomatic.

Atrial disturbances such as atrial fibrillation and flutter

Table 31–1. MYOCARDIAL INFARCTION

Definition: Myocardial infarction (MI) is the necrosis of the cardiac muscle caused by lack of adequate blood supply to the myocardium.

Types: The majority of myocardial infarctions occur in the left ventricle. They may occur at different depths of the heart muscle, such as non-Q wave (subendocardial), Q wave (transmural), and in different areas of the left ventricle, including the anterior, posterior, lateral, inferior, apical, and septal areas.

Etiology: Most often MIs result from the rupture of lipid deposits (atheromas) within the intima (inner lining of the artery wall) of the coronary arteries. The ruptured lipid exposes a rough endothelial lining that then attracts sticky platelets and other clotting components. Sudden occlusions may also occur owing to spasm. Within 3–6 hours after the cessation of blood flow to the distal portion of the heart muscle, that portion of the muscle becomes necrotic.

Symptoms: The primary symptom in men is sudden, sharp retrosternal pain often described as "crushing," with radiation to the arms, throat, jaw, and back. Women often complain of more vague symptoms such as shoulder, back, or chest discomfort. Pallor, gastrointestinal disturbances, profuse perspiration, intense anxiety, hypotension, and cardiac rhythm disturbances may also be present. The pain is not relieved with rest or nitroglycerin and may last for hours.

Management: Differentiate between Q (transmural) and non-Q (subendocardial) wave infarction. Immediate care is to stabilize the cardiac rhythm, to prevent further circulatory impairment, and to keep the hypoperfused area from evolving into a total infarct. Numerous methods are being used today to prevent or limit infarct size, including thrombolytics such as streptokinase, tissue plasminogen activators, or similar products; nitrates; and beta-blockers. Precutaneous transluminal angioplasty, coronary artery bypass surgery, and intra-aortic balloon pumping may also be used in selected patients.

Patients who infarct are placed on bed rest, given oxygen, monitored for dysrhythmias, and given antidysrhythmics, analgesics, and antianxiety drugs as needed.

In secondary care, rehabilitation is started, which includes education about the reduction of risk factors, exercise testing, and prescription.

PROARRHYTHMIC EFFECT

Virtually all antidysrhythmics have been reported to have proarrhythmic effects varying from 5% to 15%. Proarrhythmic effects can be caused by three mechanisms. The first is through prolongation of the action potential and QT intervals, which often occurs in group Ia and III drugs. This becomes a particular problem when antidysrhythmics are combined with diuretics or when bradycardia is present. The second mechanism is by widening the QRS interval, which may actually terminate in ventricular fibrillation (VF). This often happens with group Ic drugs. The third mechanism is when the patient's original rhythm was paroxysmal and becomes incessant, which can occur with the group Ia or Ic drugs.

GROUP I ANTIDYSRHYTHMICS

The group I antidysrhythmics are classified as group Ia, Ib, Ic, and miscellaneous.

GROUP Ia ANTIDYSRHYTHMICS

Group Ia drugs—**quinidine** (as quinidine sulfate, gluconate, or polygalacturonate), **procainamide hydrochloride (Pronestyl)**, and **disopyramide (Norpace)**—act by depressing Na^+ conductance, slowing the action potential upstroke in phase zero, resulting in a slowing of conduction velocity and a decrease in membrane responsiveness. These drugs also prolong action potential duration and increase *effective refractory period* (the time frame after cardiac contraction during which the heart is unable to respond, or would respond abnormally, to another cardiac impulse) in Purkinje fibers. By decreasing automaticity and prolonging the effective refractory period, these drugs are effective in disturbances of either increased automaticity or reentry. The group Ia antidysrhythmics are featured in Table 31–3.

Uses

Group Ia drugs are effective in suppressing dysrhythmias caused by mechanisms of either atrial or ventricular origin: atrial fibrillation (AF), premature ventricular contractions (PVCs), and ventricular tachycardia (VT). They tend to have little effect on the sinoatrial (SA) node and therefore are not used in disturbances of SA nodal function, such as sinus tachycardia. Response rate to ventricular dysrhythmias is only about 50% to 70% for quinidine and disopyramide and may be higher for procainamide. A successful antidysrhythmic response to one group Ia drug, however, does not guarantee response to another group Ia drug.

Contraindications and Precautions

The group Ia drugs are contraindicated in patients with hypersensitivity and in those with complete atrioventricular (AV) block and conduction defects, as there is normal

are generally not life threatening. They may, however, cause significant symptomatology, such as palpitations, dizziness and light-headedness, decreased cardiac output secondary to the loss of atrial contraction, and embolic phenomena, and may exacerbate preexisting heart failure. These rhythm disturbances usually require treatment even if they are asymptomatic. Antidysrhythmic therapy, in these patients, decreases morbidity and mortality associated with cardiac dysrhythmias.

Several major groups of antidysrhythmic medications have been developed. Table 31–2 summarizes the classification of antidysrhythmics. Each group works by a different mechanism to suppress dysrhythmias, as shown in Figure 31–1. Table 31–2 also reviews the generalized action of each type of antidysrhythmic, including several investigational drugs. Antidysrhythmic drugs are reviewed in detail in Tables 31–3 to 31–5. Table 31–6 features the commonly observed dysrhythmias and the medications used to treat them.

Table 31–2. CLASSIFICATION AND MECHANISM OF ACTION OF ANTIDYSRHYTHMICS

Group	Mechanism of Action	Currently Approved Drugs	Investigational Agents
Ia	Depress Na$^+$ conductance, increase action potential duration, decrease membrane responsiveness. Prolong QRS interval.	Quinidine, procainamide, disopyramide	Aprindine, pirmenol, acecainide hydrochloride, cifenline succinate
Ib	Natural blockade, increase K$^+$ conductance, decrease action potential duration and effective refractory period. Do not significantly alter ECG levels.	Lidocaine, phenytoin, mexiletine, tocainide	Pirmenol, aprindine
Ic	Natural blockade, marked depression of phase 0 through profound slowing of conduction. Have a slight effect on conduction. Prolong PR and QRS intervals.	Flecainide, propafenone	Lorcainide
Miscellaneous I	Has local anesthetic properties. Interferes with fast inward depolarizing current carried by sodium ions.	Moricizine	
II	Interfere with Na$^+$ conductance (closes the slow Na$^+$ channel), depress cell membrane, decrease automaticity, and increase effective refractory period of the AV node. Have little effect on conduction. Slow the exit of K$^+$ out of the cell.	Propranolol, acebutolol, esmolol	Practolol
III	Interfere with norepinephrine, increase action potential duration and effective refractory period. Prolong repolarization.	Amiodarone, bretylium, ibutilide, sotalol	
IV	Ca^{++} antagonist, increase AV nodal effective refractory period.	Verapamil, bepridil	Gallopamil, tiapamil
Unclassed	Opens K$^+$ channels.	Adenosine	

slowing through the AV node with these drugs that can result in complete heart block and asystole. These drugs are contraindicated in myasthenia gravis because of their anticholinergic effects. Group Ia drugs are given cautiously with renal and hepatic dysfunction, as the kidney and liver are the organs of biotransformation and elimination and, as drugs accumulate, dysrhythmias may actually be precipitated. Safety in pregnancy (category C), lactation, and children has not been established.

Electrocardiographic Effects

Observed electrocardiogram (ECG) changes are similar for all group Ia antidysrhythmics. Because these drugs increase effective refractory period in Purkinje fiber cells, there is a resulting prolongation of the QRS complex and QT interval in the ECG. This effect can be used to monitor therapy. A 25% to 50% increase in either QRS complex or QT interval over baseline is a reason to discontinue therapy. Therapy is stopped because the increase in the vulnerable period of the ventricles can lead to the development of a ventricular tachycardia known as torsades de pointes. *Torsades de pointes*, depicted in Figure 31–2, is a combination of ventricular tachycardia and ventricular fibrillation, usually at a rate of 100 to 300 beats per minute. The lengthening QT interval changes more consistently as a function of drug concentration than does the widening of the QRS complex. Therefore, this is the preferable parameter to monitor.

○ **Quinidine,** available as quinidine sulfate (Cin-Quin, Quinora, Quinidex Extentabs), quinidine gluconate (Du-

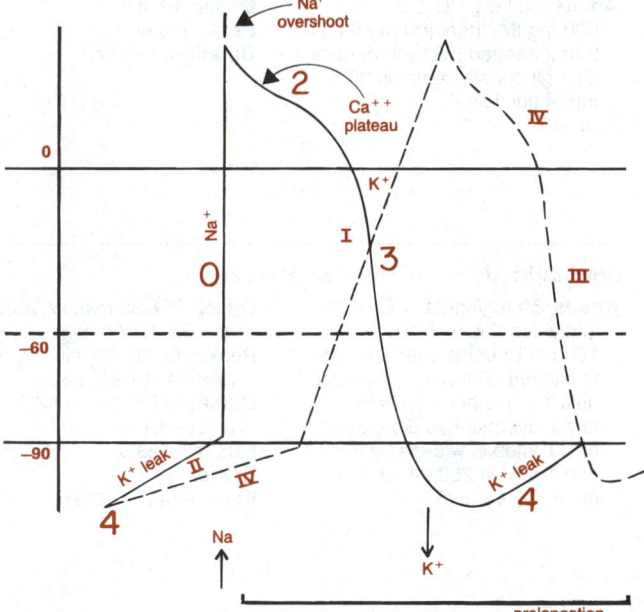

Figure 31–1. All of the antidysrhythmic drugs have an effect on the action potential curve. Phase 0 is depolarization—Na$^+$ influx; phase I overshoot; phase 2 slow period that forms a plateau—K$^+$ efflux and Ca^{++} influx; phase 3 is the rapid phase of K$^+$ efflux; and phase 4 is repolarization where Na$^+$ effluxes and K$^+$ influxes through the Na$^+$-K$^+$-ATPase pump. The group I antidysrhytmias depress phase 0; group II antidysrhythmias depress phase 4; group III antidysrhythmics produce a prolongation of phase 3; and the group IV antidysrhythmics depress phase 4 and lengthen phase 1 and 2 of repolarization. Many antidysrhythmics prolong the action potential duration. The effective refractory period (ERP) is also prolonged with the group I drugs.

Table 31–3. GROUP Ia AND MISCELLANEOUS GROUP I ANTIDYSRHYTHMIC DRUGS

DRUG NAME/ROUTE AND DOSAGE	PHARMACOKINETICS/ DYNAMICS	NURSING IMPLICATIONS
GROUP Ia ANTIDYSRHYTHMICS*		
quinidine sulfate (Cin-Quin) (Quinora)—83% quinidine base		
Adults: 200–400 mg PO q 4–6 hr.	**Onset:** 30 min **Peak:** 1–3 hr **Duration:** 6–12 hr **½L:** 6–7 hr **PB:** 80%–90% **B:** liver **E:** urine (10%–50%)	For all antidysrhythmics: **ASSESSMENT:** Monitor pulse, blood pressure, and ECG (including QT) frequently. Assess for pregnancy (category C). **INTERVENTION:** Tablets may be crushed and capsules opened and mixed with food or fluids. Do not break, crush, or chew extended-release tablets. Use infusion pump to ensure accurate IV dosage of quinidine gluconate. Monitor plasma levels and intake and output. **Patient Teaching**—Tell patient to take medication around the clock, as prescribed, even if feeling better; and to take a missed dose as soon as possible if remembered within 2 hr (4 hr for extended-release tablets). **EVALUATION:** Cardiac dysrhythmias should subside without detrimental adverse effects. Evaluate for prodysrhythmic effect. Report all new dysrhythmics to physician.
quinidine sulfate sustained-release (Quinidex Extentabs)		
Adults: 300–600 mg PO q 8–12 hr.	**Peak:** 3–5 hr	Same as above.
quinidine gluconate (Duraquin) (Quinaglute Dura-Tabs) (Quinalan)—62% quinidine base		
Adults: 324 mg PO q 6–8 hr; 600 mg IM, then 400 mg IM q 2 hr if needed (324 mg of quinidine gluconate contains 200 mg of quinidine).	**Onset:** 10 min **Peak:** 3–4 hr **Duration:** 6–8 hr	Same as for all antidysrhythmics plus: **ASSESSMENT:** Assess for pregnancy (category C). **INTERVENTION:** Take with meals to minimize GI upset. Continuously monitor apical pulse, blood pressure, and ECG for changes. Avoid excessive citrus fruit intake, which changes urine pH and decreases excretion of quinidine. Whole tablet may appear in stool. **EVALUATION:** Notify physician if ringing in ears, visual disturbances, dizziness, or headache occur.
procainimide hydrochloride (Pronestyl)		
Adults: 50 mg/kg/day PO or IM in divided doses q 3–6 hr. Or, 100 mg IV bolus over 5 min not to exceed 50 mg/min, then drip until 1 g has been administered, dysrhythmia disappears, or QT interval widens by 50%; drip 1 g IV in 250 mL at 1–3 mg/min (see text).	**Onset:** PO, 30 min; IV, immediate; IM, 10–30 min **Peak:** PO, 60–90 min; IV, 25–60 min; IM, 15–60 min **Duration:** PO, IV, or IM 3–4 hr **½L:** 2.5–4.7 hr **PB:** 14%–23% **B:** liver **E:** urine (40%–70%)	Same as for all antidysrhythmics plus: **ASSESSMENT:** Patient should remain supine throughout IV administration. Assess CBC and antinuclear antibody (ANA). Assess for pregnancy (category C). **INTERVENTION:** Administer on empty stomach with full glass of water for faster absorption. If GI irritation occurs, may be administered with or immediately after meals. Slight yellow color of solution will not alter potency; do not use if markedly discolored or if precipitate is present. Because total loading dose can cause severe hypotension, it is usually administered as series of small injections. One safe method is to give 100 mg over 5 min, not to exceed 50 mg/min, and repeat until one of the following occurs: dysrhythmia remits, symptomatic hypotension occurs, QT widens by 50% of baseline, or 1 g is administered. After a total dose of 1 g is administered, procainimide should be discontinued as it will not be effective. When converting from IV to oral dose regimen, 3–4 hr should elapse between last IV dose and administration of first oral dose. Nonabsorbable wax core may appear in stool. When administering IV procainamide, discontinue if QT lengthens by 50%, PR intervals become prolonged above 0.20 sec, or if blood pressure drops 15 mm Hg.

Table 31–3. GROUP Ia AND MISCELLANEOUS GROUP I ANTIDYSRHYTHMIC DRUGS, *Continued*

DRUG NAME/ROUTE AND DOSAGE	PHARMACOKINETICS/ DYNAMICS	NURSING IMPLICATIONS
procainimide hydrochloride (Pronestyl)		**EVALUATION:** Notify physician immediately if signs of drug-induced lupus syndrome (fever, chills, joint pain or swelling, pain with breathing, skin rash), leukopenia (sore throat, mouth, or gums), or thrombocytopenia (unusual bleeding or bruising) occur.
procainimide hydrochloride sustained-release (Procan SR) (Pronestyl-SR)		
Adults: 500–1000 mg PO q 6 hr. Tablet remains intact as it is passed through the GI system; however, the active contents have been absorbed.	**Onset:** NA **Peak:** 1–2 hr **Duration:** 6 hr	Same as above (excluding IV information).
MISCELLANEOUS GROUP I ANTIDYSRHYTHMICS		
moricizine hydrochloride (Ethmozine)		
Adults: 600–900 mg PO per day divided in 3 equal doses.	**Onset:** 2 hr **Peak:** 0.5–2 hr **Duration:** 10–24 hr **½L:** 1.5–3.5 hr **PB:** 95% **B:** liver **E:** urine, feces	Same as for all antidysrhythmics plus: **ASSESSMENT:** Assess K^+ and Mg^{++} and return to normal before therapy begins. Hospitalization required when starting this medication. Assess for pregnancy (category B). **INTERVENTION:** When dysrhythmias are controlled, symptoms can often be controlled on q-12-hr dosing.

*Excludes quinidine polygalacturonate and disopyramide.
NA = not available.

raquin, Quinaglute Dura-Tabs, Quinalan), and quinidine polygalacturonate (Cardioquin), is the prototype of group Ia drugs. It has a direct action on the cell membrane. Quinidine also has an indirect anticholinergic effect that inhibits vagal action on the SA and AV nodes. The sinus node may accelerate, provoking a dangerous sinus tachycardia. If quinidine is to be administered to persons in atrial flutter or atrial fibrillation, digoxin or verapamil is administered first to slow conduction at the AV node. Quinidine inhibits cation exchange (sodium influx and

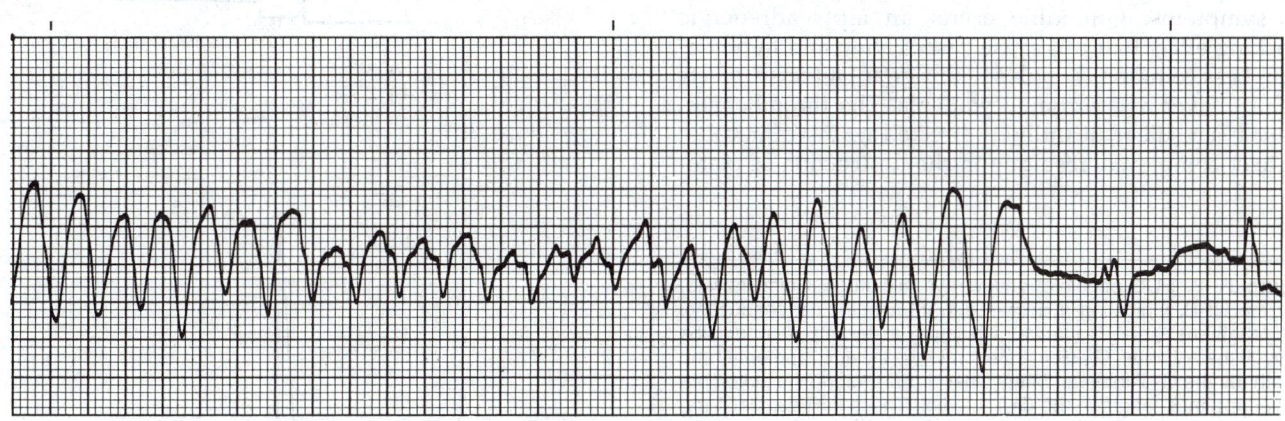

Figure 31–2. Torsades de pointes variation of ventricular tachycardia converting spontaneously to sinus rhythm. Torsades de pointes is a combination of ventricular tachycardia and ventricular fibrillation, usually at a rate of 100 to 300 beats/minute. Torsades de pointes is treated with beta-adrenergic blockers, isoproterenol, atropine, or by the insertion of a pacemaker. (From: Brown, K: Mastering Dysrhythmias. FA Davis, 1986, with permission.)

potassium efflux) and causes a decrease in the rate of depolarization. Through this mechanism, automaticity in ectopic sites in the atria, AV junction, and Purkinje fibers is suppressed or abolished. Ectopic tissue is more sensitive than normal pacemaker tissue, and thus the SA node is permitted to reestablish control over the cardiac impulse formation in the heart. Quinidine slows conduction velocity in all tissues, and a widened QRS and prolonged PR interval can be seen on the ECG, as shown in Figure 31–3. Because quinidine prolongs the effective refractory period of atrial and ventricular fibers, this effect probably exerts an antifibrillatory action by converting a unidirectional block to a bidirectional block, which thereby abolishes the reentry type of dysrhythmias. Quinidine dilates resistance and capacitance vessels by blocking alpha-adrenergic receptors in the smooth muscle of peripheral tissue, which may result in hypotension. Quinidine has not been shown to reduce sudden death or to prolong survival. Despite newly reported adverse effects, quinidine still has a place in therapy.

Each salt form of quinidine contains a different percentage of a base amount of quinidine: quinidine sulfate contains an 83% quinidine base; quinidine gluconate, a 62% quinidine base; and quinidine polygalacturonate, a 60% quinidine base. Therefore, careful dosage calculation may be required.

CONTRAINDICATIONS AND PRECAUTIONS Quinidine is contraindicated in digitalis toxicity manifested by dysrhythmias or AV conduction disorders because they may be worsened. In patients with heart failure, the dosage is lowered because of liver engorgement. Quinidine is also given cautiously to patients with potassium imbalance, as the effect of quinidine is enhanced by potassium or reduced if hypokalemia is present.

ADVERSE EFFECTS The most common adverse effects observed with quinidine are gastrointestinal (GI) complaints, including nausea, vomiting, and diarrhea, which can become very severe. Quinidine, as with other cinchona alkaloids (e.g., quinine), can cause cinchonism, which can manifest as tinnitus, vertigo, visual disturbances, hearing loss, confusion, delirium, psychosis, and GI symptoms. Quinidine exerts an alpha-adrenergic blocking effect that can cause vasodilation and hypotension. Less common though still important adverse effects include fever and thrombocytopenia. The thrombocytopenia is a result of an antibody directed against quinidine-platelet complexes, resulting in the destruction of plate-

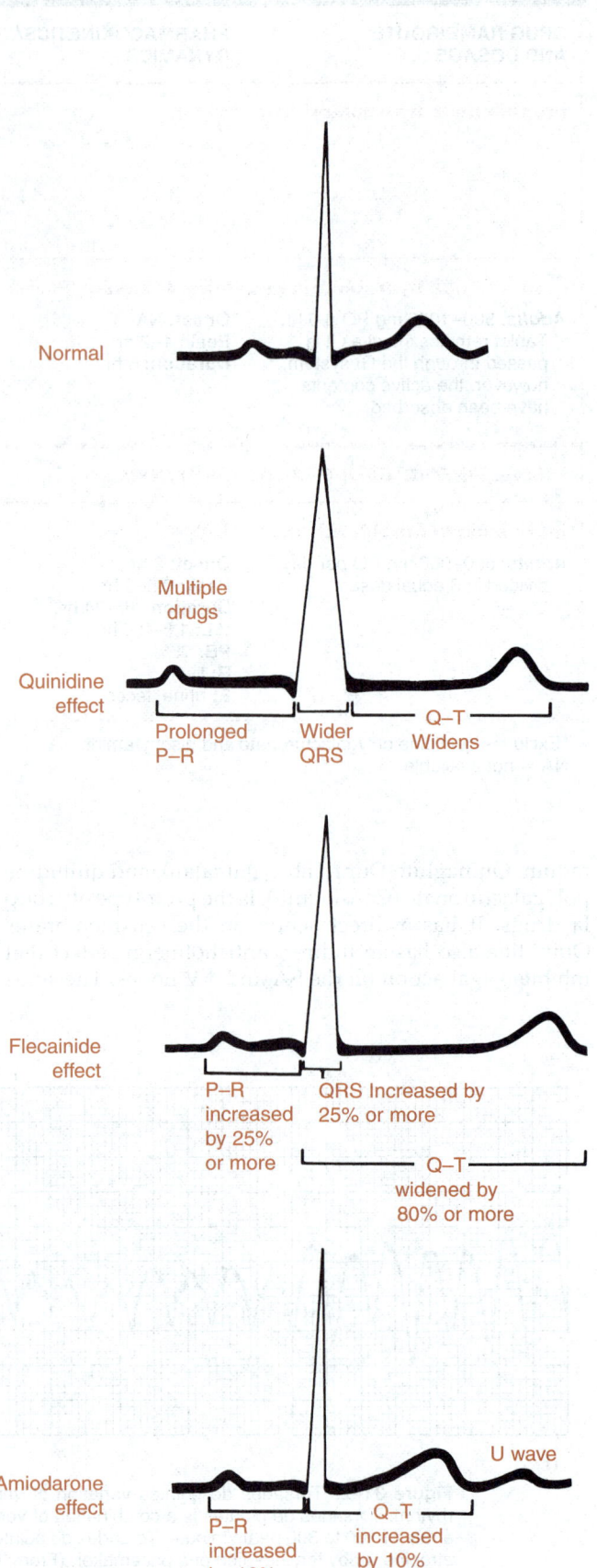

Figure 31–3. ECG effects of antidysrhythmic drugs. Quinidine widens the QRS, indicating a decrease in intraventricular conduction, and lengthens the P–R interval, indicating a slowing of conduction through the AV node. Quinidine also prolongs the action potential and lengthens the Q–T interval. Many other drugs prolong the action potential and thus lengthen the Q–T interval. These include: disopyramide, bepridil, tricyclic antidepressants, the phenothiazines, erythromycin, probucol, and the thiazides. Flecainide may increase the P–R and QRS intervals by 25% or more. The Q–T interval also widens by about 8%, but it is mostly due to the widened QRS. Amiodarone reduces the sinus rate by 15%–20% and increases the P–R and Q–T intervals by as much as 10%. In addition, U waves may appear, as well as changes in the contour of the T wave.

lets. An asthmalike respiratory insufficiency and hepatitis reaction are other quinidine hypersensitivity reactions. Patients on long-term therapy should have periodic complete blood counts (CBCs) performed. A systemic lupus erythematosis (ESL)-like syndrome can also occur.

Dysrhythmias may develop from use of quinidine and include sinus arrest, SA block, and AV block. These are most likely due to slowed conduction through the heart and may even lead to asystole. The anticholinergic effects of quinidine on the AV node can precipitate tachycardias, particularly atrial fibrillation and atrial flutter. Ventricular dysrhythmias such as PVCs, VT, and VF may also occur. "Quinidine syncope" is due to rapid ventricular tachycardia and fibrillation (torsades de pointes). The result can be sudden death, and the risk increases with higher doses and quinidine toxicity.

INTERACTIONS The hepatic elimination of quinidine is inhibited by cimetidine (Tagamet) administration, resulting in an increase in serum levels. Quinidine serum levels may be reduced by concurrent use of barbiturates, hydantoins, nifedipine (Procardia, Adalat), rifampin, and sucralfate (Carafate). Concurrent quinidine and coumarin anticoagulants may reduce prothrombin levels. Quinidine may potentiate neuromuscular blocking agents.

Quinidine can interact with other drugs such as digoxin (see Chapter 29), raising the serum levels of digoxin two to three times. Secondary to its hypotensive effects, quinidine has the potential to increase the antihypertensive effects of drugs such as nitroglycerin, reserpine, and other antihypertensives.

THERAPEUTIC BLOOD LEVELS Blood levels of quinidine relate to both therapeutic efficacy and toxicity and can be used to assess the appropriateness of a dosage regimen or significance of a drug interaction. Available assays differ substantially in their ability to measure quinidine specifically in serum. Nonspecific assays measuring quinidine metabolites as quinidine will have a higher therapeutic range (usually 2 to 6 μg/mL) than specific assays measuring only quinidine. A therapeutic range for these assays is 1 to 4 μg/mL. It is therefore important to know the specificity of the assay used before interpreting serum quinidine levels.

○ **Procainamide hydrochloride** (Pronestyl, Procan) has the same indications as quinidine. However, the effect achieved is not always identical. Quinidine is frequently preferred for prolonged oral therapy because of the high incidence of drug-induced lupus erythmatosus associated with long-term administration of procainamide.

Intravenous procainamide is preferred for terminating supraventricular or ventricular dysrhythmias. It is often the drug of choice when the dysrhythmia is resistant to lidocaine. Procainamide slows conduction in accessory pathways and is useful for acute termination of tachydysrhythmias associated with Wolff-Parkinson-White (WPW) syndrome.

PHARMACOKINETICS Procainamide is metabolized in the liver to an equipotent metabolite, N-acetylprocainamide (NAPA). This metabolic process is genetically determined, with patients classified as rapid or slow acetylators. Rapid acetylators produce larger quantities of NAPA. The average half-life of procainamide is 3 to 4 hours. The active metabolite NAPA is excreted renally (50%) and has a half-life of 6 hours. Procainamide is used carefully, with dosage carefully titrated in patients with hepatic and renal insufficiency because of delayed elimination of procainamide and accumulation of NAPA.

CONTRAINDICATIONS AND PRECAUTIONS Procainamide is used with caution in patients with digitalis intoxication because of additive effects on slowing AV conduction and precipitation of ventricular asystole or fibrillation. Procainamide is a myocardial depressant and is used with caution in patients with heart failure.

ADVERSE EFFECTS Gastrointestinal adverse effects occur, but less often than with quinidine. Maculopapular rashes may occur and necessitate discontinuation of the drug. Agranulocytosis has occurred rarely with procainamide therapy and can be fatal. Frequent CBCs are required during therapy to monitor for this adverse effect, the presence of which requires discontinuation of procainamide treatment.

At least 50% of patients on procainamide therapy develop a positive antinuclear antibody (ANA) titer within 2 to 18 months and may develop a syndrome resembling SLE. A positive ANA titer is nonspecific for the diagnosis of procainamide-induced SLE, which must be diagnosed on the basis of the time course of reaction along with symptomatology (fever, myalgias, arthralgia, and pleuritic chest pain). This reaction occurs at a higher frequency in patients who are slow acetylators of procainamide. It is almost always reversible on discontinuation of the drug. However, the development of lupus erythmatosus in 25% to 30% of patients limits the long-term usefulness of procainamide.

When procainamide is administered IV, hypotension, sometimes marked, may occur because of the peripheral vasodilating effect. In addition, widening of the QRS and prolongation of the PR interval suggests toxicity. The QT interval is measured periodically; if it widens by 50% above baseline, procainamide is discontinued to prevent torsades de pointes.

INTERACTIONS Patients with hypersensitivity to procaine will have cross-sensitivity to procainamide. The addition of other antidysrhythmics can cause an additive cardiac effect or even toxic effects. Procainamide enhances the effects of anticholinergics. Concurrent thiazides and antihypertensives may potentiate hypotensive effects. Concurrent cimetidine reduces renal clearance of procainamide. Alcohol may increase hepatic metabolism of procainamide.

THERAPEUTIC BLOOD LEVELS The therapeutic blood concentration for procainamide is between 4 and 8 μg/mL. Frequently, the active metabolite NAPA is measured as well. If this is done, a combined procainamide plus NAPA concentration of 10 to 30 μg/mL is considered therapeutic. Tough levels are more valuable than peak levels. Blood is drawn for the assay 2 hours after administration of the drug.

○ **Disopyramide phosphate** (Norpace) is similar to but chemically unrelated to procainamide and quinidine. Disopyramide affects several phases of the action potential: It prolongs the action duration and refractory period (phases 2 and 3), decreases diastolic depolarization (phase 4), and decreases the excitation velocity (phase 0). Disopyramide has an anticholinergic effect and a significant negative inotropic effect and, in contrast to quinidine and procainamide, it causes peripheral vasoconstriction. Because of these effects, disopyramide is not frequently prescribed. However, because of the marked negative inotropic effect, disopyramide is used in the therapy of hypertrophic obstructive cardiomyopathy.

Selection of Group Ia Antidysrhythmics

Quinidine is reasonably effective in suppressing ventricular premature systolic and recurrent ventricular tachycardia. About one-third of all patients suffer GI complications, which often subside. Therefore, long-term tolerance is generally excellent.

Procainamide is effective against supraventricular tachycardia and ventricular dysrhythmias and is appropriate for short-term use. Because of its serious side effects, long-term therapy is not appropriate.

Disopyramide is particularily appropriate for patients unable to tolerate quinidine because of its GI side effects. On the other hand, disopyramide is particularly unsuitable when there is myocardial depression or when the cholinergic side effects are likely to be troublesome.

GROUP Ib ANTIDYSRHYTHMICS

Group Ib antidysrhythmic drugs include **lidocaine *(Xylocaine)*, mexiletine *(Mexitil)*, phenytoin *(Dilantin)*,** and **tocainide *(Tonocard)*.** Lidocaine and mexiletine are featured in Table 31–4. These drugs depress the phase 4 slope of the action potential and increase the ventricular fibrillation threshold (see Fig. 31–1). In Purkinje fibers, they decrease action potential duration, effective refractory period, and automaticity. They also reduce membrane responsiveness in Purkinje fibers. They have little effect on the duration of the effective refractory period in the AV node. This, however, may vary from drug to drug within this group.

Unlike the group Ia antidysrhythmics, group Ib medications do not decrease conduction velocity and may, at times, actually increase the speed of propagation, which may assist in preventing reentry dysrhythmias. Group Ib medications have no effect on speed of AV conduction and therefore lack the potential for causing heart blocks that group Ia drugs have.

The effects of group Ib drugs on the PR interval can vary depending on the relationship between the direct effects, which slow conduction, and the indirect vagolytic effects, which increase conduction through the AV node.

Uses

Group Ib antidysrhythmic medications are most effective when used to treat or control both acute and chronic ventricular dysrhythmias, including premature ventricular contractions and ventricular tachycardia. Group Ib antidysrhythmics are generally ineffective in treating dysrhythmias of atrial origin.

○ **Lidocaine** (Xylocaine), is often the drug of first choice for treating ventricular dysrhythmias associated with acute myocardial infarction (MI) and cardiac surgery. Lidocaine can be administered both in and out of the hospital to control ventricular premature beats and ventricular tachycardia.

Lidocaine acts as a local anesthetic on the heart. It depresses excessive automaticity of ectopic pacemakers in the His-Purkinje system. Thus, it is very effective in suppressing the premature ventricular contractions that often arise from hypoxia or ischemic cells. Lidocaine has little or no effect on the ECG and therefore has little potential for causing heart block, cardiac asystole, or ventricular ectopic rhythms. Unlike quinidine and procainamide, lidocaine has some effect on the effective refractory period in the AV node or Purkinje fibers. This effect may prevent reentrant types of dysrhythmias.

CONTRAINDICATIONS AND PRECAUTIONS Lidocaine is contraindicated in patients who are sensitive to this compound or similar drugs and who have bradycardia and severe degrees of heart block without an artificial pacemaker. Lidocaine is also contraindicated in Wolff-Parkinson-White and Stokes-Adams syndromes. The elimination of lidocaine is reduced in patients with heart failure and hepatic disease, and the drug is used with caution in these patients. Lidocaine is used cautiously in patients with a genetic predisposition to malignant hyperthermia, and its use in pregnancy (category B) and children has not been established.

ADVERSE EFFECTS Lidocaine distributes well into the central nervous system (CNS), but serious long-term adverse effects are uncommon. Because of its anesthetic properties, it can cause significant CNS adverse effects, which are usually brief and dose related. These include mild disturbances such as paresthesias, numbness, agitation, and disorientation. More severe adverse effects include hallucinations, muscle twitching, seizures, mental confusion, and respiratory arrest. The milder adverse effects usually, but not always, precede the more serious effects and frequently disappear with a reduction in dosage. Adverse effects are also more commonly noted in patients with serum concentrations above 5.0 μg/mL. If serious adverse effects such as seizures are observed, lidocaine is discontinued. To control seizures, diazepam (Valium) can be administered intravenously; however, drug-induced seizures tend to be refractory to treatment. With very high serum concentrations, heart block can occur. In contrast to the group Ia drugs, lidocaine does not have anticholinergic effects and causes only negligible changes in the normal ECG.

INTERACTIONS Drugs reducing hepatic blood flow, such as propranolol (Inderal), decrease lidocaine's elimination and increase serum concentrations. Cimetidine (Tagamet) reduces hepatic blood flow in addition to inhibiting lidocaine metabolism. Concurrent succinylcholine may enhance neuromuscular blockade by impairing transmission of impulses at the motor nerve terminal. Concurrent procainamide may produce additive neurologic effects. Concurrent tocainide, because of similar pharmacologic properties, may cause an increased incidence of adverse reactions.

DOSAGE To achieve rapid therapeutic serum concentrations, lidocaine therapy is initiated with a loading dose, and a simultaneous intravenous infusion is started to maintain therapeutic concentrations. The loading dose required, which is given at a rate of 25 to 50 mg/min, is between 50 and 100 mg and depends on weight (1 mg/kg). More rapid administration increases the risk of seizures. The loading dose is reduced in patients with heart failure. Its onset of action is rapid (90 seconds); however, it is rapidly distributed from blood to tissues, resulting in a decline in plasma concentration such that subtherapeutic concentrations may be reached 15 minutes after the initial loading dose. This can cause reappearance of the dysrhythmias, which then require treatment with a subsequent loading dose. Usually half of the initial loading dose is given at this time. No more than 200 to 300 mg are given per hour.

The infusion is administered using a rate-controlling pump, and the rate is titrated to 1 to 4 mg/min, most frequently 2 mg/min. Patients with heart failure or renal or liver disease usually require lower infusion rates, that is, 1 to 2 mg/min. The infusion is terminated as soon as the cardiac rhythm is stable by just turning off the IV.

If lidocaine does not appear to be working, assess the potassium level. Lidocaine works preferentially on the ischemic myocardium and is most effective in the presence of a high external potassium level; therefore, hypokalemia should be corrected.

○ **Mexiletine hydrochloride** (Mexitil) is structurally similar to lidocaine and is available only in oral form. Mexiletine depresses phase zero and decreases the effective refractory period of the Purkinje fibers. Therefore, it depresses automaticity in ventricles but has little effect on atrial tissue and does not depress sinus node function.

USES Mexiletine is used for the treatment of documented, life-threatening, ventricular dysrhythmias such as sustained ventricular tachycardia in the acute phase of an MI. Because of its proarrhythmic effect, mexiletine is not recommended for lesser dysrhythmias.

CONTRAINDICATIONS AND PRECAUTIONS Mexiletine is contraindicated in patients with cardiogenic shock, bradycardia, and hypotension, and in patients with known hypersensitivity to local anesthetics of the amide type (mexiletine is chemically related to the amide anesthetics).

The drug is used with caution in patients with hepatic disease, as the liver is where it is biotransformed. Safety in pregnancy (category C) and in children has not been determined.

ADVERSE EFFECTS The most common adverse effects of mexiletine include GI symptoms such as nausea, vomiting, indigestion, and unpleasant taste in the mouth; CNS symptoms such as confusion, dizziness, light-headedness, and tremor; and cardiovascular symptoms including hypotension, sinus bradycardia, and palpitations. The hypotension that occurs may be reversed by atropine. Rash, dyspnea, nonspecific edema, and abnormal liver function tests also may occur. Adverse effects are dose related.

INTERACTIONS Phenytoin, rifampin, and phenobarbital and other enzyme inducers taken concurrently with mexiletine may lower serum levels of mexiletine and decrease its effectiveness. Cimetidine can increase or decrease mexiletine plasma levels, so careful monitoring of mexiletine is important. Marked changes in pH affect excretion, so urinary pH should be 5 to 8 (in acidic urine, mexiletine renal clearance may be increased; in alkaline urine, decreased). Antacids and narcotics may slow absorption.

○ **Phenytoin** (Dilantin), a group Ib antidysrhythmic used infrequently, depresses spontaneous depolarization in ventricular tissue. Phenytoin has a mild negative inotropic effect and a peripheral vasodilator action. Phenytoin is indicated in the management of ventricular dysrhythmias with digitalis intoxication because it enhances conduction time through the AV node, which is usually depressed in patients with digoxin intoxication and hypokalemia. Phenytoin has few effects on the ECG. It can, however, shorten the QT interval. Phenytoin is discussed in more detail in Chapter 20.

○ **Tocainide** (Tonocard) is a group Ib antidysrhythmic with electrophysiologic properties similar to lidocaine. Tocainide produces dose-dependent reductions in sodium and potassium conductance, thus decreasing excitability of cells.

USES Tocainide is primarily used to prevent or treat ventricular ectopy and tachycardia. However, because of the severe adverse effects—blood dyscrasias and pulmonary fibrosis—it is used only with caution when other drugs have failed to be effective. Tocainide may be beneficial to patients refractory to group Ia drugs. Responsiveness to lidocaine is a fairly accurate method of selecting patients for therapy as many physicians consider tocainide the oral equivalent of lidocaine.

GROUP Ic ANTIDYSRHYTHMICS

The group Ic drugs—**flecainide acetate (Tambocor)** and **propafenone (Rythmol)**—depress sinus node automaticity and prolong conduction in the atria, AV node, ventricle, accessory pathways, and the His-Purkinje system. These drugs are used only in patients who have life-threatening ventricular dysrhythmias that are not effectively managed with other less toxic drugs. The group Ic drugs are featured in Table 31–4.

○ **Flecainide acetate** (Tambocor) has local anesthetic properties like the group I antidysrhythmics. Flecainide may either increase or decrease ejection fraction with usual therapeutic doses.

USES Flecainide, because of its proarrhythmic effect, is used only for paroxysmal atrial fibrillation/flutter and supraventricular tachycardias. Flecainide is also used in treating reentrant tachycardias involving the AV node or accessory pathways, illustrated in Figure 31–4. It should not be used in patients who have ischemic heart disorder.

CONTRAINDICATIONS AND PRECAUTIONS Flecainide is contraindicated in hypersensitive patients and in those with cardiogenic shock or heart block without the presence of a pacemaker.

Because of its negative inotropic effect, flecainide is given cautiously in patients with heart failure. All group Ic drugs are used with extreme caution in persons with sick sinus syndrome because of the possible slowing of the PR interval. Hypokalemia and hyperkalemia may alter the effects of flecainide, so potassium needs to be

Table 31–4. GROUP Ib AND Ic ANTIDYSRHYTHMIC DRUGS

DRUG NAME/ROUTE AND DOSAGE	PHARMACOKINETICS/ DYNAMICS	NURSING IMPLICATIONS
GROUP IB ANTIDYSRHYTHMICS*		
lidocaine hydrochloride (Xylocaine) *Adults:* 50–100 mg IV bolus (1 mg/kg), followed by a 1–4 mg/min infusion or 20–50 mg/kg per min. *IM*–100–150 mg, dependent on weight. *Children:* 1 mg/kg IV bolus followed by infusion of 30 mg/kg per min	**Onset:** IV, 10–90 sec; IM, 5–15 min **Peak:** IV, minutes; IM, 20–30 min **Duration:** IV, 15 min; IM, 60–90 min **½L:** distribution 10 min; elimination 1.5–2 hr **PB:** 40%–80% **B:** liver **E:** urine (10%)	Same as for all antidysrhythmics plus: **ASSESSMENT:** Monitor ECG for excessive slowing or prolongation of PR interval, blood pressure, respiratory status at onset and frequently during infusion. Assess for pregnancy (category B). **INTERVENTION:** Administer boluses over 1–2 minutes. Mixing 1 g in 250 mL of D_5W makes a 0.4% solution; each mL = 4 mg of lidocaine. Solution is stable for 24 hr. Use infusion pump or microdrip system. Administer IM dosage in deltoid muscle. Use only 10% solution for IM administration. **EVALUATION:** Evaluate serum levels periodically. If ineffective, evaluate and return serum K^+ to normal.
mexiletine hydrochloride (Mexitil) *Adults: Initial dose*–200 mg PO q 8 hr. *Maintenance dose*–200–400 mg q 8 hr or 450 mg PO q 12 hr.	**Onset:** 0.5–2 hr **Peak:** 2–3 hr **Duration:** 8–12 hr **½L:** 10–12 hr **PB:** 50%–60% **B:** liver **E:** urine (10% unchanged)	Same as for all antidysrhythmics plus: **ASSESSMENT:** Assess for pregnancy (category C). **INTERVENTION:** Administer with food or antacid to decrease GI irritation. Maintain urine pH near normal. **Patient Teaching**—Tell patient to not skip or double up on doses and to use all heavy equipment cautiously because of dizziness. **EVALUATION:** If tiredness, yellowing of skin or eyes or sore throat persist, notify physician.
GROUP 1C ANTIDYSRHYTHMICS		
flecainide acetate (Tambocor) **paroxysmal supraventricular tachycardia** *Adults: Initial dose*–50 mg PO q 12 hr; increase 50 mg PO every 4 days. *Maintenance dose*–100–200 mg PO q 12 hr. Reduce dose in renal impairment. **sustained ventricular tachycardia** *Adults: Initial dose*–100 mg PO 12 hr; increase by 50 mg bid q 4 days. *Maintenance dose*–100–200 mg PO q 12 hr. Reduce dosage in renal impairment. Maximum dosage 400 mg/day.	**Onset:** 0.5–1 hr **Peak:** 3 hr (1–6 hr) **Duration:** 12–15 hr **½L:** 12–27 hr (increased in congestive heart failure) **PB:** 40% **B:** liver (50%) **E:** urine (30% unchanged); steady states are reached in 3–5 days	Same as for all antidysrhythmics plus: **ASSESSMENT:** Assess blood pressure and presence of heart failure during therapy. Retinal and eye exam are needed periodically during therapy. Assess for pregnancy (category C). **INTERVENTION:** May be administered with meals to reduce GI irritation. Optimal effect may not be seen for 2–3 days after start of administration. Maintain serum K^+ levels. **EVALUATION:** If neurologic signs (dizziness, visual disturbances, headache, increased fatigue) or weight gain occur, report these to physician. Flecainide is proarrhythmic and worsens or causes new dysrhythmias. Evaluate ECG frequently.
propafenone hydrochloride (Rythmol) *Adults:* 150 mg PO q 8 hr, up to 450 mg/day; increase as needed q 3–4 days to 225 mg q 8 hr to 675 mg/day. Maximum dose is 900 mg/day.	**Onset:** 0.5 hr **Peak:** 2–3 hr **Duration:** 3–5 hr **½L:** 2–10 hr **PB:** 90%–95% **B:** extensively, liver (90%) **E:** <1% urine	Same as above plus: **EVALUATION:** Notify physician of fever, sore throat, chills.

*Excludes phenytoin and tocainide.

normalized. The Ic group drugs are given cautiously to patients with liver impairment as these drugs are extensively biotransformed in the liver and to patients with renal dysfunction, as elimination may be impaired. Safe use in pregnancy (category C), lactation, and children is unknown.

ADVERSE EFFECTS   Because of the adverse effects, the physician starts flecainide in the hospital. Flecainide can aggravate existing dysrhythmias or precipitate new ones. Flecainide crosses the blood-brain barrier and may cause neurologic symptoms such as dizziness, headache, fatigue, and tremor. Additional cardiovascular adverse effects include palpitations, chest pain, edema, AV blocks, and bradycardias. Altered taste sensation and other mild GI symptoms have been reported. Flecainide also has numerous effects on the ECG. The PR, QRS, and QT intervals can all be prolonged from 8% to a maximum of 150% (See Fig. 31–3). If second- or third-degree AV block or right bundle branch block associated with left hemiblock occurs, flecainide is discontinued unless a ventricular pacing wire is in place.

INTERACTIONS   Flecainide may increase plasma digoxin levels 15% to 25%. Concurrent propranolol increases both flecainide and propranolol serum levels and

has an additive negative inotropic effect. Both disopyramide and verapamil have negative inotropic effects, and administration with flecainide is not recommended. Urinary pH should be 5 to 7, as alkalinization decreases excretion and acidification increases excretion of flecainide. Also, dosage of flecainide is reduced with patients taking cimetidine.

○ **Propafenone**   (Rythmol), which acts like the other group Ic drugs, also possesses weak beta-blocking properties (1/40 of propranolol) and slight calcium antagonist properties (1/100 of verapamil). Propafenone also increases the refractory period and decreases conduction velocity. There is no significant effect on the QT interval, but there is a dose-dependent prolongation of the PR interval and QRS duration. Propafenone increases pulmonary capillary wedge pressure and systemic and pulmonary vascular resistance. Propafenone may also slow the heart rate and mildly depress cardiac output.

USES   Because of its proarrhythmic effects, propafenone is used only for documented life-threatening ventricular dysrhythmias and paroxysmal supraventricular tachycardia (PSVT) including atrial fibrillation that has not responded to other drugs. Ventricular ectopy may be suppressed by 74% with propafenone.

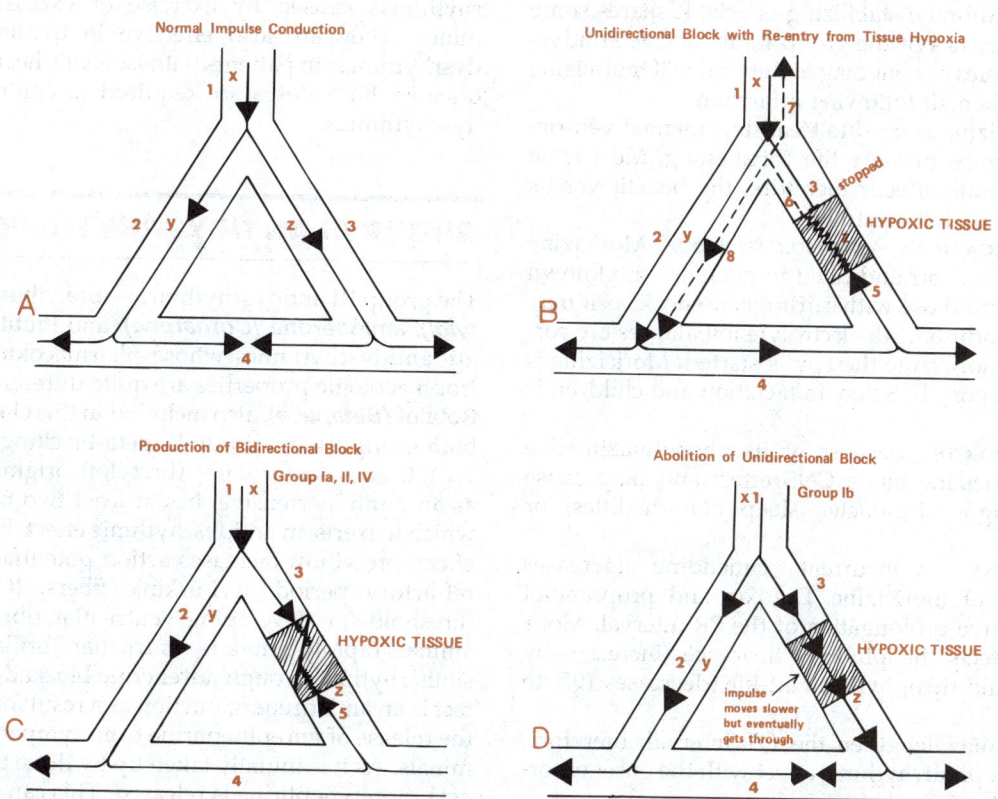

Figure 31–4. The effect of antidysrhythmic drugs on re-entry. (A) represents normal conduction through the Purkinje fiber. Impulse 1, starting in x fiber, spreads through branches y and z and with impulse 2 and 3 activates the ventricular tissue in 4. In (B), an area of tissue ischemia is present in branch z. Again, impulse 1 begins in fiber x; as it traverses down fiber z, it is blocked. Meanwhile, impulse 2 moves quickly down fiber y and activates the ventricular muscle in area 4. Since no opposing impulse arrived in the ventricular muscles, the impulse travels through z and re-enters fibers x and y, thereby causing another beat to occur. The beat that occurs may cause a re-entry supraventricular tachycardia or may be a premature ventricular contraction. In (C), groups Ia, II, and IV drugs increase the refractory time in the "sick" tissue so that it is unable to accept either impulse 3 originally, or impulse 5 for re-entry. This produces a bidirectional block. In (D), group Ib drugs enhance conduction in the "sick" tissue of fiber z, thereby allowing impulse 3 to traverse the sick tissue the first time, which abolishes the unidirectional block.

ADVERSE EFFECTS Propafenone frequently causes GI complaints of nausea, vomiting, and an unusual metallic taste in the mouth. Neurologic effects include dizziness and visual disturbances. Both the GI and neurologic side effects resolve with dosage reduction or discontinuation of therapy. Propafenone has proarrhythmic effects, so patients need to be monitored closely during early therapy. Propafenone may also exacerbate heart failure, particularly in patients with an ejection fraction below 50%; and, less frequently, exacerbate AV block and bundle branch block because of the delayed cardiac conduction. Safe use in pregnancy, (category C), lactation, and children has not been established.

INTERACTIONS Patients taking concurrent digoxin, warfarin, metoprolol, or lidocaine must be monitored for symptoms of drug interactions, particularly for proarrhythmic effects.

MISCELLANEOUS GROUP I ANTIDYSRHYTHMICS

○ **Moricizine hydrochloride** *(Ethmozine),* a miscellaneous group I drug that is a phenothiazine derivative, was developed as an antidysrhythmic drug in 1970 in the Soviet Union. It has potent local anesthetic activity and myocardial membrane stabilizing effects. It shares some of the characteristics of the group Ia, Ib, and Ic antidysrhythmics. Studies are ongoing to determine if moricizine has a possible benefit following infarction.

USES Moricizine is used to treat documented ventricular dysrhythmias that are life threatening. Moricizine has proarrhythmic effects; therefore, the benefit versus risk ratio is evaluated carefully.

CONTRAINDICATIONS AND PRECAUTIONS Moricizine hydrochloride is contraindicated in patients with known sensitivity and in those with cardiogenic shock, as it may worsen this condition. All electrolyte imbalances are corrected before moricizine therapy is started. Moricizine is pregnancy category B. Safety in lactation and children is unknown.

ADVERSE EFFECTS Because of its phenothiazine-like structure, moricizine has a CNS effect and may cause dizziness, fatigue, headache, sleep abnormalities, or nervousness.

INTERACTIONS Concurrent cimetidine increases plasma levels of moricizine. Digoxin and propranolol cause an additive prolongation of the PR interval. Moricizine also affects theophylline clearance (increases by 44% to 66%) and theophylline half-life (decreases 19% to 33%).

Moricizine may lengthen the QT interval; therefore, there may be a proarrhythmic effect with the onset of torsades de pointes.

GROUP II ANTIDYSRHYTHMICS

Group II antidysrhythmics are drugs that exert beta-blockade. Most of the antidysrhythmic effects are adequately explained by this activity. These effects include a blocking of sympathetic stimulation at the sinus node, which decreases resting heart rate only slightly, but reduces exercise-induced tachycardia substantially. Beta-blockade also reduces automaticity in Purkinje fibers. An important effect responsible for their major uses as antidysrhythmic agents is an increase in the effective refractory period of the AV node. Many beta-blockers available in the United States are used to treat dysrhythmias. These include **propranolol** *(Inderal),* **metoprolol** *(Lopressor),* **pindolol** *(Visken),* **atenolol** *(Tenormin),* **nadolol** *(Corgard),* **timolol** *(Blocadren),* and **esmolol hydrochloride** *(Brevibloc).* These drugs are discussed in detail in Chapter 17.

USES

Beta-blockers are used effectively to slow ventricular rate in patients with supraventricular tachyarrhythmias such as atrial fibrillation, atrial flutter, or PSVT. Digitalis glycosides and propranolol can be an effective combination when either fails to control ventricular rate alone. This is a result of digitalis exerting a vagal effect on the AV node, while propranolol decreases sympathetic activity. Beta-blockers can also be used to treat and prevent recurrent tachydysrhythmias resulting from activating accessory bundles, as occurs in Wolff-Parkinson-White syndrome.

Beta-blockers can also be used in ventricular dysrhythmias caused by exercise or excessive catecholamines. They are also effective in treating ventricular dysrhythmias in patients with ischemic heart disease. Frequently, high doses are required to control ventricular dysrhythmias.

GROUP III ANTIDYSRHYTHMICS

The group III antidysrhythmics—**bretylium tosylate** *(Bretylol),* **amiodarone** *(Cordarone),* and **ibutilide** *(Covert)*—are antidysrhythmics whose pharmacokinetic and electrophysiologic properties are quite different (Table 31–5). **Sotalol** *(Betapace),* also included in this classification, has both group III and group II (beta-blocking) properties.

○ **Bretylium tosylate** (Bretylol), originally developed as an antihypertensive, has at least two mechanisms by which it exerts an antidysrhythmic effect. First, by a direct effect, bretylium increases action potential duration and refractory period in Purkinje fibers. It increases the threshold for developing ventricular fibrillation and in animals rapidly converts ventricular fibrillation to normal sinus rhythm through adrenergic blockade. A second effect is an antiadrenergic action as a result of its preventing the release of norepinephrine from sympathetic nerve terminals. As it is initially taken up by these terminals, however, norepinephrine is released. This can cause an initial increase in blood pressure, increased dysrhythmia, and vomiting over the first 30 minutes of therapy. These effects can be avoided by infusing the dose over 8 to 10 minutes if the clinical situation permits this slow infusion. Hemodynamics remain within normal ranges.

USES Bretylium is used for the prophylaxis and treatment of life-threatening ventricular dysrhythmias unresponsive to lidocaine and procainamide. Bretylium is a second-line drug after lidocaine for advanced life support

TABLE 31-5. GROUP III AND UNCLASSED ANTIDYSRHYTHMIC DRUGS

DRUG NAME/ROUTE AND DOSAGE	PHARMACOKINETICS/ DYNAMICS	NURSING IMPLICATIONS
CLASS III ANTIDYSRHYTHMICS*		
bretylium tosylate (Bretylol)		
in emergency situation **Adults:** 5–10 mg/kg IV bolus, undiluted, rapidly. If ventricular fibrillation continues, administer 10 mg/kg and repeat as necessary. Or, 5–10 mg/kg IM undiluted, give again in 1–2 hr, then q 6–8 hr.	**Onset:** 15 min (antifibrillatory effects within minutes) **Peak:** 2–3 hr **Duration:** 6–8 hr **½L:** 5–10 hr **PB:** negligible **B:** not biotransformed **E:** urine (70%–80% unchanged)	Same as for all antidysrhythmics plus: **INTERVENTION:** For short-term use only. Keep patient in supine position. Observe closely for hypotension. Reduce dose gradually and discontinue over 3–5 days if clinical status allows. Do not administer more than 5 mL in one site for IM; rotate sites. Reduce dose in renal failure.
amiodarone (Cordarone)		
Adults: Initial dose–800–1600 mg PO daily for 1–3 weeks, then tapered to 600–800 mg/day. Maintenance dose–400 mg PO in divided doses.	**Onset:** 2–3 days (up to 1–3 wk) **Peak:** 3–7 hr **Duration:** weeks to months **½L:** initial biphasic elimination 2.5–10 days, slower terminal elimination phase 26–107 days **PB:** 96% **B:** liver **E:** bile; steady state occurs in weeks to months	Same as for all antidysrhythmics plus: **ASSESSMENT:** Assess baseline thyroid, liver, and lung and neurologic function. Effects may not be seen for 1–3 wk. Assess for pregnancy (category C). **INTERVENTION:** Gradually all other antidysrhythmics are reduced. Give with food. Monitor K$^+$ level closely. Monitor ECG (amiodarone prolongs PR, QRS, and QT intervals). **Patient Teaching**—Warn patient to protect skin from sun exposure. **EVALUATION:** Obtain chest x-ray film periodically. Report increasing fatigue, dyspnea, cough, or pleuritic pain to physician.
ibutilide (Covert)		
Under 60 kg–1 mg IV over 10 min. Over 60 kg–0.1 mg/kg over 10 min. If rhythm has not terminated, wait 10 min and repeat same dose.	**Onset:** rapid **Peak:** NA **Duration:** NA **½L:** 2–12 hr **PB:** 40% **B:** liver **E:** urine (82%), feces (19%)	Same as for all antidysrhythmics plus: **ASSESSMENT:** Assess baseline rhythm. Assess for pregnancy (category C). **INTERVENTION:** Monitor patient carefully during administration. **EVALUATION:** Evaluate for dysrhythmia and QT prolongation.
UNCLASSED ANTIDYSRHYTHMICS		
adenosine (Adenocard)		
Adults: 6 mg IV push over 1–2 sec; if needed, after 1–2 min, 12 mg may be administered and repeated once.	**Onset:** immediate **Peak:** seconds **Duration:** 1–2 min **½L:** <10 sec **PB:** No **B:** in RBC to AMP **E:** as ADP	**ASSESSMENT:** Assess heart rate and rhythm. Assess for pregnancy (category C). **INTERVENTION:** Administer rapid IV bolus as proximal as possible in IV line and follow by a rapid saline flush. **Patient Teaching**—If possible teach patients they may experience feeling of impending doom and/or have out-of-body experience during therapy. They may also experience acute, but fleeting, chest pain. **EVALUATION:** Evaluate for presence of heart block. Notify physician.

*Excludes sotalol.
NA = not available; RBC = red blood cells; AMP = adenosine monophosphate; ADP = adenosine diphosphate.

during cardiopulmonary resuscitation (CPR). Bretylium should be used only in critical care units where equipment and personnel to maintain constant cardiac and blood pressure monitoring are available.

CONTRAINDICATIONS AND PRECAUTIONS Currently, there are no contraindications to the administration of bretylium. Caution is used in patients with renal failure because of delayed renal excretion of bretylium. Caution is advised in administering bretylium to patients with fixed cardiac output such as occurs in aortic stenosis, pulmonary hypertension, and postural hypotension, because severe hypotension may result from a decrease in peripheral resistance without a compensatory increase in cardiac output. Safety in pregnancy (category C) and in children has not been established.

ADVERSE EFFECTS Hypotension, caused by the inhibition of norepinephrine release at nerve terminals, occurs in a high percentage of patients receiving bretylium. Hypotension can be severe enough to warrant discontinuation of bretylium. In some cases, blood pressure may need to be maintained with an infusion of dopamine (Intropin). Rapid intravenous administration can cause nausea and vomiting (3%) and neurologic symptoms such as vertigo and light-headedness, as well as transient hypertension and proarrhythmic effect from the initial release of norepinephrine.

INTERACTIONS Bretylium is used with caution in patients on digitalis glycosides, as bretylium may aggravate digitalis-induced dysrhythmias. The pressor effect of catecholamines is enhanced with concurrent bretylium.

○ **Amiodarone** (Cordarone), an iodinated benzofuran derivative, is a unique antidysrhythmic drug that exerts a noncompetitive blockade on both alpha- and beta-adrenergic receptors. It also antagonizes the chronotropic and inotropic effects of glucagon. Amiodarone is a potent smooth muscle relaxant and produces marked coronary and peripheral vasodilation. Amiodarone increases the cardiac refractory period and thus reduces automaticity. The sinus rate is reduced by 15% to 20%; the PR and QT intervals are increased by 10%. U waves and a change in T-wave contour may also occur (see Fig. 31–3). These changes do not require discontinuation of amiodarone but may be associated with aggravation of dysrhythmias, so close monitoring is important. Amiodarone is a potent proarrhythmic drug that is highly toxic, so maximal efforts should be made to use alternate antidysrhythmic agents before initiating amiodarone therapy.

USES Amiodarone is effective in controlling ventricular dysrhythmias in patients who are resistant to most other antidysrhythmic medications. Amiodarone suppresses life-threatening ventricular dysrhythmias refractory to other drugs, but its severe toxicity makes it a drug of last resort. Most patients have extensive diagnostic workups before being placed on amiodarone.

CONTRAINDICATIONS AND PRECAUTIONS Amiodarone is contraindicated in patients with bradycardia and severe sinus node dysfunction. Amiodarone is administered cautiously to patients with pulmonary disease, as pulmonary toxicity (interstitial pneumonitis/alveolitis) can occur. Frequent chest radiographs and pulmonary function studies are performed.

Amiodarone, a potent proarrhythmic drug, can aggravate serious dysrhythmias and lead to bradycardia or sinus arrest. Amiodarone is also given cautiously to patients with liver disease because it may cause altered liver enzymes. Frequent serum glutamic-oxaloacetic transaminase (SGOT) and serum glutamate pyruvate transaminase (SGPT) are obtained during therapy. Persistent elevations may necessitate reducing the dose. Use in pregnancy (category D) and in children has not been established.

ADVERSE EFFECTS Amiodarone has significant adverse effects and can be highly toxic, even fatal. The most com-

mon adverse effects include corneal microdeposits, which occur in virtually all adults treated for more than 6 months. These deposits, however, rarely interfere with vision, and are usually dose related. Mild GI effects, including nausea and vomiting, have been noticed. Amiodarone contains iodine (37% by weight), and both hypothyroidism and hyperthyroidism have been reported; therefore, thyroid studies should be done at the onset of therapy and frequently during therapy. Amiodarone has also been associated with bluish-gray skin discoloration in *almost all* patients. The effect may be due to cutaneous deposits of the drug. Photosensitivity also occurs at a relatively high frequency (10%).

▼ **CLINICAL ALERT**

A serious complication that occurs with the use of amiodarone is pulmonary infiltrates and fibrosis (4% to 9%). This is an irreversible and often fatal adverse effect. Abnormal liver function tests and nonspecific hepatic disorders, including hepatitis, also occur.

INTERACTIONS Amiodarone has several significant drug interactions. It inhibits the renal excretion of digoxin, thereby increasing serum digoxin concentrations. It also increases serum concentrations of quinidine and procainamide. Amiodarone potentiates the anticoagulant effect of warfarin. These effects may be caused by an inhibition of renal and hepatic clearance processes by amiodarone and its major metabolite desethylamiodarone. The combination of amiodarone with beta-adrenergic blockers can potentiate effects on the sinus or AV node, producing sinus bradycardia, sinus arrest, or AV block disturbances. During surgery, amiodarone can induce hypotension and atropine-resistant sinus bradycardia. These effects may be additive with those of the anesthetic agents used.

○ **Ibutilide** (Covert) is used for rapid conversion of recent onset atrial fibrillation/flutter. Like other class III drugs, it can cause prolongation of the QT interval and cause life-threatening dysrhythmias. Thus, the patient is monitored while the drug is administered. Safety in pregnancy (category C), lactation, and children under age 18 has not been studied.

○ **Sotalol** (Betapace) has both group II (beta-blocking) and group III properties. Sotalol prolongs the refractory period of the AV node and increases action potential duration in Purkinje fibers and ventricular muscle. Sotalol also decreases automaticity in the SA node and other ectopic pacemakers. Sotalol decreases heart rate and increases the PR and QT intervals.

USES Sotalol is used to treat life-threatening ventricular dysrhythmias. Sotalol appears to be more effective than other currently available drugs in treating sustained PSVTs and suppressing both multifocal and coupled PVCs.

CONTRAINDICATIONS AND PRECAUTIONS Sotalol is contraindicated in patients with asthma, heart failure, or cardiogenic shock, as all may be worsened. It is also contraindicated in patients with second- or third-degree heart block (unless pacemaker is in place) or prolonged QT intervals, as these also are worsened.

ADVERSE EFFECTS Because of the many adverse effects, sotalol is administered only under closely monitored conditions. Hypokalemia and hypomagnesemia may increase sotalol's proarrhythmic effect. Sotalol may precipitate bradycardia, because it decreases conduction through the SA node; torsades de pointes and ventricular dysrhythmias; and congestive heart failure and hypotension. GI symptoms often include nausea, vomiting, and diarrhea.

GROUP IV ANTIDYSRHYTHMICS

Verapamil *(Isoptin, Calan)* and **diltiazem** *(Cardizem)*, group IV antidysrhythmics (calcium channel blocking agents), inhibit the transmembrane flow of calcium ions. Other calcium channel blockers are also used to treat angina and hypertension and are discussed as a group in detail in Chapter 32.

ACTION

Calcium plays a major role in both mechanical and electrical capabilities in the heart. Mechanically, it affects the vascular smooth muscle tone of the coronary arteries and peripheral arteries as well as the contractility of the heart muscle itself. Electrically, calcium is needed for conduction through the SA and AV nodes and "slow cells" in the conduction system. The calcium antagonist (calcium channel blocker) exerts its major antidysrhythmic effect by slowing conduction and increasing the effective refractory period through the AV node, thus reducing the ventricular rate due to atrial flutter and atrial fibrillation. Calcium channel blockers also interfere with reentry of impulses at the AV node and are therefore helpful in restoring normal sinus rhythms in patients with paroxysmal supraventricular tachycardia and Wolff-Parkinson-White syndrome. About 60% to 80% of patients with supraventricular tachycardia convert to normal sinus rhythm within 10 minutes after intravenous administration.

○ **Verapamil** (Isoptin, Calan), a synthetic derivative of papaverine, blocks the slow calcium channel and has a slight nonspecific sympathetic depressant effect. Verapamil is effective in treating supraventricular tachycardias including atrial fibrillation, atrial flutter, and paroxysmal supraventricular tachycardia, including those associated with accessory bypass tracts such as Wolff-Parkinson-White and Lown-Ganong-Levine syndromes. Verapamil is often used as a first-line drug for atrial fibrillation rather than digoxin or quinidine.

Verapamil is highly effective when given intravenously in terminating an attack of AV nodal–resistant tachycardia and may prevent this dysrhythmia when given orally. Verapamil is not effective in treating ventricular dysrhythmias.

○ **Diltiazem** (Cardizem) inhibits calcium ion influx during membrane depolarization. It slows conduction and prolongs refractoriness through the AV node. Therefore, diltiazem is an excellent drug to control paroxysmal supraventricular tachycardia, AV nodal reentry tachycardia, Wolff-Parkinson-White syndrome in atrial flutter or fibrillation. If an accessory pathway is present, it could provoke increased conduction along the pathway, resulting in rapid ventricular response.

UNCLASSED ANTIDYSRHYTHMICS

Adenosine *(Adenocard),* a naturally occurring nucleoside found in all body cells, is an unclassed antidysrhythmic.

○ **Adenosine** (Adenocard), through an enyzymatic activity, inhibits the effects of catecholamine stimulation. Adenosine is released as a byproduct of adenosine triphosphate (ATP) catabolism. Adenosine plays a primary role in regulating coronary blood flow in response to changing metabolic needs. In the face of decreased blood supply to the myocardium or increased oxygen consumption, adenosine release induces coronary vasodilatation and restores the myocardial supply/demand ratio.

Adenosine release is proportional to the degree of myocardial ischemia to attain an adequate hyperemic response. Indeed, if the ischemia persists longer than 30 seconds, adenosine production escalates even further. When sufficiently high levels are reached in SA and AV nodal regions, a sinus bradycardia or AV block can occur secondarily. Sinus bradycardia or AV block decrease the ventricular rate and further reduce myocardial oxygen consumption. Circulation adenosine also limits the release of norepinephrine, an action that has been described as cardioprotective (Thompson, 1994).

USES Adenosine is unrelated to other antidysrhythmics. Adenosine effectively slows conduction through the AV node. Thus, it is effective in restoring normal sinus rhythm (NSR) in patients with PSVT or AV nodal reentry tachycardias and can interrupt reentry pathways such as the Kent bundles in Wolff-Parkinson-White syndrome. Adenosine can also restore NSR in patients with SVT about 60% of the time. Adenosine is often used first to break and treat SVT because of its extremely short half-life. It is ineffective in treating ventricular dysrhythmias, as their mechanism of action is unaffected by AV slowing. If adenosine is ineffective, other drugs, such as calcium channel blockers and digoxin, are administered with no possibility of interaction.

Adenosine is also used as a pharmacologic stress test when standard stress testing is not possible. Although dipyridamole (Persantine) has been used for this purpose, adenosine is becoming an acceptable alternative.

Pharmacologic stress testing is a valuable tool for exposing occult coronary artery disease in that group of individuals who are unable or unwilling to exercise. A negative adenosine thallium imaging (ATI) may avoid the need for invasive studies in individuals who previously carried a high index of suspicion.

Prior to thallium imaging, adenosine is infused via an

infusion pump at a rate of 0.14 mg/kg per minute. This dose has been determined to induce the ideal hyperemic response with tolerable hemodynamic results. If there are no untoward effects in the first 3 minutes, thallium 201 is then injected into another intravenous access. The line is flushed immediately with 10 mL of normal saline solution. The adenosine infusion continues for an additional 3 minutes if the patient response remains favorable. Adenosine is best administered antecubitally; more proximal boluses/infusion may incur a more profound response.

Like dipyridamole, adenosine may induce a "coronary steal" effect. With coronary steal, it is postulated that the myocardium supplied by a severely stenosed vessel is actually perfused more by collateral vessels originating from an adjacent, less stenosed or normal vessel. When the individual is pharmacologically stressed, the more proximally stenosed vessel may vasodilate, with little or no vasodilatation in the peripheral arterioles. This variability in vasodilatation decreases the perfusion pressure to the collateral beds, resulting in diminished flow and ischemia as blood is shunted away from the myocardium it usually supplies (Thompson, 1994).

Adenosine appears to have several distinct advantages over dipyridamole. The action of adenosine is direct rather than indirect like dipyridamole. Dipyridamole blocks the cellular uptake of adenosine, inducing both coronary and peripheral vasodilation. Variable response rates and submaximal coronary vasodilation have been reported following the administration of dipyridamole; this has not been reported with adenosine.

CONTRAINDICATIONS AND PRECAUTIONS Adenosine is contraindicated in patients with second- or third-degree heart block, as it can worsen these conditions. It is used cautiously in patients with asthma, as bronchospasm may occur. Safety in pregnancy (category C), lactation, and children has not been established.

ADVERSE EFFECTS The most common adverse effects of adenosine include facial flushing, dyspnea, and nausea. These effects are transient owing to the drug's short half-life. The usual IV bolus dose of 6 to 12 mg does not have systemic hemodynamic effects. However, when larger doses are administered, hypotension results from a decrease in peripheral resistance. Immediately after adenosine is administered, some patients experience severe chest pain and report a feeling of impending doom. Patients may also talk about a sudden-death episode or an out-of-body experience. Adenosine can be administered to patients who have renal or hepatic dysfunction because it is not dependent on the kidney or liver for elimination or metabolism.

INTERACTIONS Several drug-drug interactions occur. The methylxanthines, such as caffeine and theophylline, competitively antagonize the therapeutic effect of adenosine. A patient taking theophylline concurrently may require higher doses of adenosine, or adenosine may not be effective. Concurrent dipyridamole potentiates administration by blocking nucleoside transport and may result in a profound bradycardia. Concurrent carbamazepine may cause a higher degree of heart block to form.

DOSAGE Because of adenosine's short half-life, it must be administered rapidly by IV bolus and immediately followed by a saline flush. If it is not administered rapidly enough, the drug does not reach the myocardium in a sufficient dose to cause a therapeutic effect.

CARDIAC GLYCOSIDES

The cardiac (digitalis) glycosides (e.g., digoxin, digitoxin) are currently used to treat or control dysrhythmias either alone or in conjunction with other antidysrhythmics. They are used to slow the ventricular rate in atrial flutter and fibrillation and in atrial tachycardias. Digitalis acts by means of vagal stimulation on the AV node to slow conduction; therefore, fewer impulses get through to the ventricles. This effect can be obviated through sympathetic stimulation such as exercise, thus limiting the usefulness of the cardiac glycosides in therapy of chronic atrial fibrillation. The cardiac glycosides are discussed in detail in Chapter 29.

ANTIDYSRHYTHMIC DRUGS FOR BRADYDYSRHYTHMIAS

Atropine sulfate, a potent vagolytic, can be used acutely in IV doses of 0.4 to 1 mg every 1 to 2 hours as needed to treat or control bradydysrhythmias. Atropine increases sinus rate and AV node conduction velocity and decreases the effective refractory period of the AV node by decreasing vagal tone. Likewise, isoproterenol (Isuprel), a beta-adrenergic agonist, can also be used for such dysrhythmias in doses of 1 to 2 mg diluted in 500 mL of D_5W infused slowly with continual monitoring of the electrocardiogram. Isoproterenol increases myocardial oxygen demand and can aggravate ischemia and cause ventricular dysrhythmias. Isoproterenol increases the rate of the idioventricular pacemakers and therefore should not be used unless absolutely necessary in patients with acute myocardial infarctions. Dysrhythmias that are slow can result from sinus bradycardia, SA block, or AV block. Atropine and isoproterenol are used as temporary measures prior to pacing for patients with complete AV block.

ANTIDYSRHYTHMICS FOR SUPRAVENTRICULAR TACHYCARDIAS

Adenosine, digoxin, calcium channel blockers, and beta-adrenergic blockers are generally first-line therapy for treatment and prevention of PSVT and to control PAT (paraxysmal atrial tachycardia). Other drugs, such as quinidine, procainamide, and propafenone are also used alone or in combination. Flecainide and amiodarone are also effective, but because of their adverse effects are used only when all other pharmacology therapy has failed. Catheter ablation procedures are increasing in popularity to permanently control these dysrhythmias.

COMBINATION THERAPY

Combining antidysrhythmic drugs adds to the antidysrhythmic potency while minimizing adverse effects, but may increase the risk of proarrhythmia. An example of effective combination drug therapy is the Ia and Ib drugs, such as mexiletine and quinidine or mexiletine and procainamide. Other useful combinations include quinidine and procainamide, quinidine and propranolol, and quinidine and verapamil. Table 31–6 reviews commonly observed dysrrhythmias and the medications used to treat them.

USING THE NURSING PROCESS

ASSESSMENT

- Obtain a thorough nursing history to develop the data base needed to prepare the nursing care plans. Table 31–7 summarizes the nursing process for patients requiring antidysrhythmics.
- Perform thorough physical and psychologic nursing assessments frequently to evaluate possible critical changes when the patient requiring antidysrhythmic medications is acutely ill. Particularly, assess cardiac rhythm, including rate, regularity, quality, and character of all pulses; the presence of chest pain; electrocardiogram changes such as PR, QT, and QRS intervals and dysrhythmias; neurologic symptoms; urinary output; skin color, temperature, and signs of edema; abnormal respiration, including crackles; and an increased level of anxiety. With frequent assessments, problems are identified quickly and corrective measures instituted before the presenting symptoms cause further deterioration.

- Obtain the patient and family's past history of coronary artery disease. Also, associated risk factors—hypertension, cigarette smoking, obesity, lifestyle, diabetes, stress level, personality type, and cholesterol—are examined. These factors may need to be modified during the intervention phase of the nursing process.

- Assess laboratory tests, as ordered, to determine acid-base balance, electrolyte levels, and blood drug levels. Blood for routine serum drug levels is drawn approximately 30 minutes after the drug is given for a peak level and 30 minutes to immediately before the next dose for a trough level. Any abnormalities must be corrected, as most antidysrhythmics are less effective in the presence of acid-base or electrolyte disturbances, especially a potassium imbalance.

Table 31–6. DYSRHYTHMIAS AND THEIR USUAL MEDICATION TREATMENT

Type of Dysrhythmia	Drugs of Choice	Drug Action
Bradycardias, SA block, SA arrest	Atropine, isoproterenol	Increase sinus rate and AV conduction, enhance automaticity
Supraventricular tachycardia (SVT), paroxysmal atrial tachycardia (PAT), atrial tachycardia, sinus tachycardia	Adenosine, verapamil, cardiac glycosides, propranolol, quinidine, disopyramide, procainamide, edrophonium, moricizine	Depress automaticity and slow conduction velocity; depress SA nodal automaticity and AV nodal conduction
Atrial flutter, atrial fibrillation	Calcium channel blockers, cardiac glycosides, beta-blockers, quinidine, disopyramide, flecainide, propafenone	Prolong AV nodal conduction time and refractoriness
Premature atrial contraction (PAC)	Quinidine, procainamide, disopyramide	Depress automaticity, have local anesthetic properties
Premature ventricular contraction (PVC)	Lidocaine for emergencies, procainamide, quinidine, tocainide, disopyramide, mexiletine	Depress automaticity, have local anesthetic properties
Ventricular tachycardia (VT)	Lidocaine, bretylium, procainimide, amiodarone, flecainide, sotalol, and other group Ic drugs	Depress automaticity and excitability
Ventricular fibrillation (VF)	Lidocaine, procainamide, flecainide, bretylium, amiodarone	Depress automaticity and excitability
First-, second- and third-degree AV block	Atropine, isoproterenol	Only of temporary use to speed SA rate
Wolff-Parkinson-White (WPW) Syndrome	moricizine, propanfenone	Increase anterograde and retrograde refractiveness. Fast Na$^+$ channel blocker

Table 31–7. NURSING PROCESS FOR PATIENT REQUIRING ANTIDYSRHYTHMICS

Assessment

Assess vital signs. Document presence of pulsus alternans, bigeminal pulse, or pulse deficit.

Assess type of dysrhythmia present; note cardiac rhythm, regularity of beats, presence of extra heart beats; dropped beats, presence of chest pain, ECG changes.

Palpate pulses noting rate, regularity, amplitude (full/thready), and symmetry.

Ascertain lifestyle, e.g., exercise, daily activities, and level of stress. Note presence of risk factors, e.g., smoking, obesity, diabetes, personality type, and cholesterol.

Assess sleep pattern, noting presence of long-standing problems.

Assess laboratory findings, e.g., acid-base balance, electrolyte and serum drug levels.

Nursing Diagnosis: Decreased Cardiac Output

RELATED TO: Altered electrical conduction.

AS EVIDENCED BY: Weight gain, fatigue, respiratory embarrassment and possible dysrhythmias.

Desired Outcomes/Evaluation Criteria

Maintains/achieves adequate cardiac output as evidenced by absence of signs/symptoms of decompensation. Observed decreased frequency of dysrhythmia(s). Participates in activities that reduce myocardial workload.

Nursing Actions	Rationale
Provide calm/quiet environment. Review reasons for limitations of activities during acute phase.	Reduces stimulation and release of stress-related catecholamines, which cause/aggravate dysrhythmias and vasoconstriction and increase myocardial workload.
Demonstrate/encourage use of stress management behaviors, e.g., relaxation techniques, guided imagery, slow/deep breathing.	Promotes patient participation, exerting some sense of control in a potentially very stressful situation.
Investigate complaints of chest pain, documenting location, duration, intensity, relieving/aggravating factors.	Reasons for chest pain are variable, dependent on underlying cause of dysrhythmias, but may indicate ischemia due to decreased myocardial perfusion or increased oxygen demand.
Administer antidysrhythmias according to type, e.g., atrial, ventricular, SA/AV node dysfunction.	Treatment depends on kind of dysrhythmia present.
Administer supplemental oxygen as indicated.	Increases amount of oxygen available for myocardial uptake, which decreases irritability caused by hypoxia.
Be prepared for/initiate cardiopulmonary resuscitation as indicated.	Development of life-threatening arrhythmias requires prompt intervention to prevent ischemic damage/death.

Nursing Diagnosis: Knowledge Deficit

RELATED TO: Lack of information/understanding of medical condition/therapy needs.

AS EVIDENCED BY: Questions, statement of concern, failure to improve and/or development of preventable complications.

Desired Outcomes/Evaluation Criteria

Verbalizes understanding of disease and treatment regimen, desired action, and possible adverse side effects.

Nursing Actions	Rationale
Review normal cardiac function/electrical conduction.	Provides a knowledge base to understand individual variations and reasons for therapeutic interventions.
Explain/reinforce specific dysrhythmia problem and therapeutic measures to patient/significant other.	Ongoing/updated information can decrease anxiety associated with the unknown and prepare patient to make necessary lifestyle adaptations.
Identify adverse effects/complications of specific dysrhythmias, e.g., fatigue, dependent edema, progressing changes in mentation, vertigo.	Dysrhythmias may decrease cardiac output as manifested by symptoms of developing cardiac failure/altered cerebral perfusion.
Provide instructions (verbal and written) regarding medications including desired action, dosage and usage particulars, expected side effects, and possible adverse reactions/interactions with other prescribed/OTC drugs or substances.	Information necessary for patient to make informed choices and to manage medication regimen.
Stress importance of routine follow-up, periodic laboratory evaluations.	Evaluates therapeutic needs/effectiveness and provides for early detection of developing complications.

NURSING DIAGNOSIS

- Typical nursing diagnoses for a patient requiring antidysrhythmic medications include Decreased Cardiac Output, Noncompliance with Drug Therapy, and Knowledge Deficit (see Table 31–7).

PLANNING AND INTERVENTION

- The goals of nursing intervention for a patient requiring antidysrhythmics in the acute situation are included in Table 31–7. These goals change as the patient progresses toward discharge from the acute-care unit.

Nursing Responsibilities

- Administer the antidysrhythmics as ordered. The nurse must know all the information featured in the Nursing Implications column in Tables 31–3, 31–4, and 31–5.

All intravenous antidysrhythmics are potentially dangerous drugs and therefore are administered through infusion or volumetric pumps using microdrip tubing (depending on local hospital policy and procedure). The dosage is carefully titrated to control dysrhythmias while minimizing the adverse effects of the drug.

No other medications are added to the IV bottle containing the antidysrhythmic or to the IV line. This prevents deterioration and precipitation of drugs. All these medications are best run piggyback on a keep-open IV line. In case there is a reaction to the medication, the keep-open IV can then be turned on.

Each medication is adequately diluted and administered according to its own special directions (see package inserts for specific directions). Most medications are normally diluted in dextrose and water to avoid the extra sodium in normal saline solution, which may cause excessive fluid accumulation in patients with heart failure. However, when mixing phenytoin, dilute only with special diluent or normal saline and use it immediately.

Patient Teaching

- Teach the patient and family about the medical and nursing regimens. Patient education is the responsibility of the nurse educator and is of primary importance. It has been demonstrated to decrease readmission to the hospital because of noncompliance. The patient and family are involved in the development of the health teaching plan.
- The patient going home on antidysrhythmics is taught how to administer the medications safely at home (Table 31–8).

During future clinic or office visits, check the patient's blood pressure. Patients often complain of orthostatic hypotension, dizziness, and light-headedness. The dosage may have to be reduced to eliminate these symptoms. During prolonged therapy (months to years), the patient

---

Table 31–8. PATIENT TEACHING INFORMATION—ANTIDYSRHYTHMICS

Dear Patient:

This drug has been prescribed for you. This is what you should know about your drug to get the most from your therapy.

☐ 1. Antidysrhythmics are taken to regulate your heart rhythm.

☐ 2. Antidysrhythmic drugs may have to be taken for the rest of your life.

☐ 3. Quinidine, procainamide hydrochloride (Pronestyl), propranolol (Inderal), and phenytoin (Dilantin) are taken with meals.

☐ 4. Do not take your antidysrrhythmics concurrently with [fill in appropriate drugs].

☐ 5. Always check with your doctor or pharmacist before taking other drugs because interactions may occur. Drugs known to cause interactions include over-the-counter products for nasal congestion, allergy, pain, or obesity. Drugs of abuse such as marijuana may raise blood pressure and stimulate heart activity and thus increase abnormal heart rhythm.

☐ 6. If you forget to take your antidysrhythmic, do not take the forgotten dose. *Do not* try to catch up by taking two doses at the same time.

☐ 7. Do not stop taking your drug unless directed by your doctor.

☐ 8. If you have any side effects from your drug, call your doctor. Side effects from taking antidysrhythmics include low blood pressure, light-headedness, gastrointestinal distress, changes in rate or rhythm of the heart, and often blurred vision. Keep a written log of the effects that are noted and the time of day, such as in the morning upon awaking, with meals, or with activity.

☐ 9. Weigh yourself weekly. A gain of 1–2 lb a week may be a sign of increased water. Call your doctor if this occurs.

☐ 10. Check your feet and ankles for swelling. If this occurs, call your doctor.

☐ 11. Limit your coffee, tea, or cola drinks, as caffeine may cause an increase in abnormal heart rhythm.

☐ 12. Store these drugs in a tight, light-resistant bottle to prevent breakdown of drug.

---

should have periodic CBC, serum electrolytes, and blood chemistry studies to determine whether any adverse effects are occurring. Renal and hepatic function are also checked. The patient must understand the importance of taking the medication as ordered to control his or her dysrhythmias and the importance of diet and exercise modifications.

EVALUATION

- Evaluate the effectiveness of antidysrhythmics based on a predetermined list of outcome evaluation criteria developed on an individual basis through discussions involving the nurse, patient, and family (see Table 31–7).

It is extremely important to work with the patient and family to ensure their complete cooperation and support. Once patients understand the importance of their continued medical treatment, most usually are compliant. The fact that the patient is often recovering from an MI, a life-threatening event, also increases compliance. Patients must understand and recognize the adverse effects of their medication and the need to report these and other unusual signs to their physician.

- Continually evaluate the cardiac rhythm of patients who are placed on new antidysrhythmic drugs. It is particularly important to monitor the group Ic drugs. Aggravation of dysrhythmias often occurs without symptoms, goes unrecognized by the patient, and is exposed only by monitoring, exercise testing, or invasive electrophysiologic testing. As a side effect, antidysrhythmic drugs can aggravate and even cause dysrhythmias. The incidence of this proarrhythmic effect ranges from 3% to 15%. The two major mechanisms are facilitations of seen reentry circuits and the production of triggered activity due to early depolarizations.

All other evaluation criteria are assessed and evaluated before the patient is discharged. All previously taught material is reviewed and updated if necessary to ensure that the patient's understanding remains accurate. The nurse stresses the importance of continued medical care. Antidysrhythmic medications should enable the patient to live a more active life.

The bibliography for this chapter can be found in Appendix B, which begins on page 1054.

CHAPTER REVIEW QUESTIONS*

1. Which of the following statements is *correct* regarding the use of antidysrhythmic agents?
   a. The new antidysrhythmic drugs have few side effects or toxic reactions.
   b. All of the antidysrhythmic medications act by similar mechanisms.
   c. Atrial dysrhythmias are not life threatening, but usually require therapy.
   d. Treatment of ventricular dysrhythmias does not affect mortality rate.

2. Procainamide (Pronestyl) is contraindicated in the following patient condition:
   a. Wolff-Parkinson-White syndrome.
   b. Myasthenia gravis.
   c. Parkinson's disease.
   d. Acute myocardial infarction.

3. Which of the following statements is *correct* regarding verapamil, a group IV antidysrhythmic drug?
   a. It is used to treat supraventricular dysrhythmias.
   b. It increases conduction through the heart.
   c. It is used to treat AV nodal blocks.
   d. The drug can be given intravenously with propranolol.

4. The group II antidysrhythmic agents are useful in treating:
   a. Reentrant tachycardias involving AV node or accessory pathways.
   b. Life-threatening ventricular dysrhythmias resistant to lidocaine.
   c. Ventricular dysrhythmias caused by exercise or excessive catecholamines.
   d. Ventricular dysrhythmias that arise from conduction delays.

5. Torsades de pointes can be treated with:
   a. Lidocaine.
   b. Bretylium.
   c. Propranolol.
   d. Quinidine.

6. The following should be monitored for patients on procainamide therapy:
   a. Antinuclear antibodies.
   b. Epstein-Barr.
   c. Indirect Coombs'.
   d. Protein electrophoresis.

*See Appendix A, which begins on page 1051, for answers.

CHAPTER 32

Coronary Vasodilators and Peripheral Vasodilators

Merrily A. Kuhn, RNC, PhD

CHAPTER OUTLINE

KEY TERMS

Arteriosclerosis
Atherosclerosis
Intermittent claudication
Raynaud's disease

Refractory angina
Variant or mixed angina
Vasospasm

LEARNING OBJECTIVES

After reading this chapter, the student will be able to:

1. Identify medications commonly used as both coronary and peripheral vasodilators.
2. Differentiate among the vasodilator agents as to mechanism of action, route of administration, pharmacokinetics, adverse effects, contraindications and precautions, and interactions.
3. Identify specific areas to assess in the patient requiring vasodilators to formulate appropriate patient outcomes.
4. Plan the nursing interventions necessary to administer vasodilators and choose appropriate teaching strategies to gain patient compliance.
5. Evaluate the patient at various stages of treatment to gauge nursing interventions.

The patency and diameter of the vessels can be reduced by the development of *arteriosclerosis* (hardening of the arteries; a condition characterized by thickened arterial walls and a loss of elasticity) and *atherosclerosis* (a condition characterized by the deposition of cholesterol-containing plaque on the inner surface of arterial walls). As these conditions progress, less blood is delivered to the muscle tissue and symptoms develop. In the heart, when blood flow is reduced below demand, angina pectoris develops or, if blood flow is stopped totally to a portion of the heart, a myocardial infarction (MI) occurs. When blood flow is reduced in the blood vessels of the periphery, patients experience pain on activity and cool extremities; symptoms may progress to gangrene. This chapter first reviews the coronary vasodilators—the nitrates—and later the peripheral vasodilators.

Angina pectoris is a disease state characterized by sudden chest pain caused by an imbalance between myocardial oxygen demand and supply. The heart muscle, unlike any other organ in the body, receives its blood flow during diastole (80%). Therefore, if diastole is shortened, as with sinus tachycardia, the heart muscle experiences reduced blood flow and less coronary perfusion.

Coronary vasodilators are part of a general program designed to alleviate symptoms and reduce risk factors that predispose to coronary artery disease. Drug therapy for angina is based on reducing myocardial oxygen requirements and/or increasing blood flow to ischemic myocardium.

Classic angina is managed acutely with short-acting nitroglycerin products (sublingual, transmucosal, or spray), whereas long-term prophylaxis is achieved with oral or topical nitrates, beta-adrenergic blockers (discussed in detail in Chapter 17), and calcium channel blocking agents (discussed later in this chapter). *Variant* or *mixed angina* (Prinzmetal's angina; vasospastic angina) is a form of angina pectoris in which the attacks occur at rest and in which the ST segment is elevated. Variant angina, thought to be due to coronary *vasospasm* (a sudden spasm, or constriction, of a blood vessel), is best treated with calcium channel blocking agents. IV nitroglycerin may alleviate symptoms of *refractory angina* (angina pectoris that does not respond to usual therapy) and improve blood flow to ischemic tissue early in a myocardial infarction.

CORONARY VASODILATORS

The coronary vasodilators—the nitrates—reduce cardiac oxygen demand and increase blood flow through collateral coronary vessels.

NITRATES

The nitrates include **nitroglycerin (Nitrostat, Nitro-bid, and others), isosorbide dinitrate (Isordil),** and **isosorbide mononitrate (ISMO, Monoket, Imdur).**

Action

Nitrates work by directly relaxing smooth muscle through cyclic guanosine monophosphate. This causes generalized dilatation that is nonspecific and affects all smooth muscle in the body, including smooth muscle in the bronchus, heart, and biliary and gastrointestinal tracts. Nitrates redistribute blood flow along collateral channels from the epicardium to the endocardial regions of the heart. Nitrates relieve spasm of both angiographically normal and diseased arteries. In addition to the spasmolytic effect, nitrates have antiplatelet and antithrombotic effects that contribute to maintaining flow in these vessels after acute MI. Nitrates also redistribute regional flow from nonischemic to ischemic regions. Nitrates, including their dosages, pharmacokinetics, and nursing implications, are featured in Table 32–1.

The major systemic action of nitrates is a reduction in venous tone, leading to pooling of blood in peripheral veins, decreasing venous return, and reducing venous volume and myocardial tension (preload). The reduction in preload, and thus the lowered stroke volume, results in a decrease in myocardial oxygen demand and a reduction in pulmonary artery obstructive pressure (PAOP or PAWP). This is believed to be the most beneficial action of nitrates in patients with angina. Because of this effect, blood pressure falls and may precipitate reflex tachycardia; therefore, blood pressure and pulse are used to monitor therapy. At higher doses, nitrates also cause moderate decrease in systemic vascular resistance (SVR), which reduces arterial blood pressure and ventricular outflow resistance (afterload). Patients with depressed cardiac index due to elevated left ventricular filling pressures and SVR, such as in heart failure (HF), are likely to have an improved cardiac index.

A secondary mechanism of nitrate action involves the release of prostacyclin (PGI_2) and nitric oxide from the endothelium. When the endothelium is damaged, as with ischemia, PGI_2 release is reduced. This contributes to aggregation of platelets and the release of vasoactive substances such as thromboxane A_2 and serotonin, both of which cause vasospasm. It is currently being suggested that nitroglycerin stimulates prostacyclin (prostaglandin) release, which inhibits platelet aggregation and relaxes smooth muscle, thus reducing vasospasm.

Uses

Nitrates are used in the acute treatment of acute anginal attacks, accelerated or unstable angina, and the long-term prophylactic management of angina pectoris. The pain of unstable angina may last 15 to 20 minutes and often must be relieved with narcotics. Nitrates are also used in the treatment of both acute and chronic HF. In treating moderate-to-severe HF, nitrates are frequently combined with other drugs such as hydralazine, dopamine, or dobutamine, all of which decrease outflow resistance. IV nitroglycerin is used in critical-care units for managing severe chest pain, decreasing myocardial oxygen demand, and thus improving left ventricular function. Nitroglycerin is used to decrease ischemic injury, limit MI size, decrease infarction-related complications, and decrease morbidity. It also has the potential for decreasing mortality and improving survival following MI. Prolonged administration of nitrates after acute MI might further limit remodeling and preserve left ventricular (LV) function. Nitrates are also used to control blood pressure elevation associated with surgical procedures of the heart or in patients with current angina or MI.

Nitrates are helpful in treating other diseases. Topical application, which causes cutaneous dilatation, has been used to control the symptoms of *Raynaud's disease* (a primary or idiopathic vasospastic disorder characterized by recurring attacks of diminished blood supply to the fingers and/or toes). Topical applications have also been used to improve healing of atrophic ulcers. Nitrates can also relieve esophageal spasms.

Contraindications and Precautions

Nitrates are contraindicated in patients with hypersensitivity to nitrates, in patients with severe anemias because tissue oxygenation would be reduced, and in those with head trauma or cerebral hemorrhage because nitrates may increase intracranial pressure. IV nitroglycerin is contraindicated in patients with severe hypotension and hypovolemia because shock may ensue.

Nitrates are given cautiously to patients with ventricular outflow obstruction, such as in idiopathic hypertrophic subaortic stenosis (IHSS), and with ballooned mitral valve syndrome ("floppy valve syndrome") because angina may be aggravated in these patients due to reduction in preload, or the decrease in preload may increase outflow obstruction. Nitrates are also given cautiously to patients with a history of (1) uncontrolled hypertension, as the blood pressure may need to be maintained at a higher level to maintain organ perfusion;

Table 32–1. CORONARY VASODILATORS: NITRATES

DRUG NAME/ROUTE AND DOSAGE	PHARMACOKINETICS/ DYNAMICS	NURSING IMPLICATIONS
all nitrates		**ASSESSMENT:** Assess baseline cardiac function, heart rate, blood pressure. Assess for pregnancy (category C). **INTERVENTION:** Avoid alcohol concurrently. A tolerance to nitrates may occur. Nitrates do not alter ECG patterns. **Patient Teaching—**Tell patient that all nitrates should stay in original bottle to preserve potency. Caution patient to not change from one brand to another without consulting with physician; products may not be equally effective. See Table 32–6 for additional patient teaching. **EVALUATION:** Report severe headache, dizziness, flushing, blurred vision, or dry mouth to physician. Symptoms should be controlled.

NITRATES FOR ACUTE THERAPY

nitroglycerin tablets (Nitrostat) *Adults:* 0.3–0.6 mg SL (1/100–1/200 gr) PRN (3 consecutive doses maximum).	**Onset:** 1–3 min **Peak:** 3–5 min **Duration:** 30–60 min **½L:** 4 min **PB:** 60% **B:** liver **E:** liver	Same as for all nitrates plus: **ASSESSMENT:** Assess blood pressure, heart rate often. Know blood pressure and heart rate ranges. **INTERVENTION:** Dry mouth decreases absorption; maintain moist mouth. Tablets should cause a slight headache. Patients should sit or lie down to decrease side effects of hypotension. Patients should take no more than 3 tablets per attack, at 5-min intervals. Pain must be relieved in that time (15 min); otherwise, the patient should seek medical help. **Patient Teaching—**Tell patient that all nitrates should stay in original bottle to preserve potency. Discard all bottles with drug 6 mo after opening owing to lack of potency.
nitroglycerin IV (Nitro-Bid IV) (Tridil) *Adults:* 5–100 μg/min continuous IV. Dilute 25–50 mg in a D₅W or NS glass bottle. The nitroglycerin concentration should not exceed 400 μg/mL. *Low-dose therapy*–5–50 μg/min = preload reduction. *High-dose therapy*–50–100 μg/min = balanced effect on preload and afterload.	**Onset:** 1–2 min **Peak:** 1–3 min **Duration:** 3–5 min	Same as for all nitrates plus: **ASSESSMENT:** Assess level of consciousness; alcohol diluent may cause alcohol intoxication. **INTERVENTION:** Mix in a D₅W or NS glass bottle only. Use proper tubing as recommended by manufacturer. Titrate dosage to desired hemodynamic function. Closely monitor heart rate, blood pressure, and wedge pressure. Patients with low wedge pressure or right ventricular infarction are likely to be sensitive to the hypotensive effects of nitrates. Titrate infusion upward q 3–5 min following blood pressure and pulse measurement. When low-dose therapy is used, titrate up by 10–20 μg; and when high-dose therapy, titrate up by 20–50 μg. Titration is continued until desired decline in systolic blood pressure and/or relief of chest pain is obtained.

NITRATES FOR CHRONIC THERAPY

nitroglycerin sustained-release (Nitroglyn) (Nitro-Bid) (Nitrospan) and many others *Adults:* 2.5–6.5 mg PO q 8–12 hr. Swallow tablet or capsule whole.	**Onset:** 20–45 min **Peak:** NA **Duration:** 3–8 hr	Same as for all nitrates plus: **INTERVENTION:** Take on an empty stomach with a full glass of water. Swallow whole, do not chew. Monitor blood pressure closely.

Continued on the following page

Table 32–1. CORONARY VASODILATORS: NITRATES, *Continued*

DRUG NAME/ROUTE AND DOSAGE	PHARMACOKINETICS/ DYNAMICS	NURSING IMPLICATIONS
nitroglycerin ointment (Nitro-Bid) (Nitrol)		
Adults: 1" to 5" (7.5–75 mg) topically q 3–4 hr. Rotate application sites.	**Onset:** 30–60 min **Duration:** 2–12 hr, particularly useful for prevention	Same as for all nitrates plus: **INTERVENTION:** Measure correct amount of ointment on application paper. Do not touch or rub medication into your hands or into patient's skin. Medication may precipitate a headache. The applicator paper may be covered with plastic wrap for better absorption. Wash medication from hands after application. Keep tube tightly closed.
nitroglycerin transdermal patches (Minitran) (Nitrodisc) (Nitro-Dur) (Transderm-Nitro)		
Adults: Apply patch once daily to skin site free of hair (release rate 0.1–0.8 mg/hr).	**Onset:** 30–60 min **Duration:** 18–24 hr	Same as for all nitrates plus: **INTERVENTION:** Remove patch before defibrillation to avoid arcing. Rotate sites. Wash skin when patch is removed. Remove patch for 8–12 hr each day to prevent drug tolerance. Use caution when discarding to prevent toxicity to others.
isosorbide dinitrate (Isordil) (Sorbitrate)		
Adults: 2.5–10 mg SL or chewable tablet PRN. *Initial dose*–5–20 mg *Maintenance dose*–10–40 mg q 6 hr for oral tablets.	**Onset:** SL, chewable tab, 2–5 min; PO, 20–40 min **Duration:** SL, 1–3 hr; chewable tab, 0.5–2 hr; PO, 4–6 hr	Same as for all nitrates plus: **INTERVENTION:** Do not crush or chew sublingual or oral tablets.

SL = sublingual; NA = not available.

(2) carotid disease, because a higher blood pressure is needed to maintain cerebral perfusion; and (3) renal and hepatic dysfunction, because the drug is excreted in the urine and biotransformed in the liver. Use with caution in patients with diuretic-induced fluid depletion or in patients with low blood pressure (<90 mm Hg systolic). In addition, give cautiously to patients with constrictive pericarditis and tamponade. Safety in pregnancy (category C), lactation, and children has not been established.

Adverse Effects

In general, the adverse effects experienced from nitrates include flushing, pounding or pulsating headache (in up to 50% of cases), nausea, and vomiting. The headache may be treated with Tylenol. Cerebral vasodilation increases intracranial pressure and, in conjunction with the fall in systemic blood pressure, decreases blood flow to the brain. Patients between ages 18 and 59 are more likely to complain of flushing than older patients, perhaps because of more sensitive autonomic nervous systems. In patients with normal cardiac function, nitrates can cause hypotension and reflex tachycardia. In patients not on beta-adrenergic blockers, an increase in heart rate by 10 beats per minute can be used to assess adequate vasodilation. If the tachycardia is symptomatic or leads to compromises in myocardial oxygen demand, the administration of a beta-adrenergic blocker counteracts this adverse effect. Nitrates are usually withheld and dosage reduced if hy-

potension is symptomatic or if systolic blood pressure falls below 90 to 100 mm Hg. These symptoms are all related to the generalized systemic vasodilation. Tolerance to some of these adverse effects, particularly the headache, can develop.

Interactions

Nitrates interact with alcohol, which enhances the hypotensive effects related to vasodilation. Patients are instructed to drink alcohol only in moderation (1 to 2 oz per day of liquor or its equivalent in beer or wine). Nitrates also interact with other drugs, such as antihypertensives, calcium channel blockers, and beta-adrenergic blockers, enhancing the hypotensive effects. Patients may need to have antihypertensive drug dosage reduced. Aspirin increases nitrate serum levels. Nitrates also interfere with the laboratory determination of serum cholesterol.

Nitrate Tolerance

Nitrate tolerance appears to develop with sustained and chronic use. Even IV nitrates can produce tolerance with continual IV administration; therefore, interrupted infusions causing fluctuating nitrate blood concentrations are recommended. This fluctuation of blood level can be achieved by having a nitrate-free period of about 8 to 12 hours per day. For most people, this is best achieved by applying patches or ointment in the morning and removing the medication at bedtime. A patient who has nocturnal angina may prefer to apply the medication in the late afternoon or early evening and remove it the next morning. If beta-adrenergic blockers or calcium channel blockers are also prescribed, the dosing schedule can be arranged so that the peak coverage with the oral drugs occurs during the nitrate-free interval. Tolerance can be minimized by using the lowest effective dose, infrequent dosing, short-term preparations, and dosing that allows an adequate nitrate-free interval.

Nitrate tolerance may be associated with direct or indirect mechanisms. Direct mechanisms involve the reduction of the sulfhydryl group. Nitrates produce venodilation by producing nitric oxide (NO), which is an endothelial-derived relaxation factor. With continued dosing of nitrates, the sulfhydryl groups, which are required to produce NO, are depleted. Thus, venodilation does not occur.

An indirect mechanism is neurohormonal activation. For example, in HF levels of both renin and norepinephrine increase. This neurohumoral activation may contribute to the development of nitrate tolerance. Another indirect mechanism is through the expansion of intravascular volume. Nonvascular mechanisms of tolerance may also exist.

Nitrates for Acute Therapy

○ **Nitroglycerin tablets** (Nitrostat) are used sublingually for the rapid relief of anginal pain. The generally accepted maximum dosage is three consecutive doses at 5 to 10-minute intervals. If the patient continues to experience the same intensity of pain with no relief, consult the physician immediately because of the potential for MI.

Nitroglycerin can also be used prophylactically to prevent anginal attacks. The patient is instructed to take a nitroglycerin tablet before any activity—mild to moderate exercise or sexual activity—previously known to cause angina. This technique often prevents angina from occurring by producing adequate vasodilation and decreasing myocardial oxygen demand.

○ **Nitroglycerin IV** (Tridil, Nitro-Bid IV) is used to treat acute unstable angina, acute HF, and hypertension associated with surgical procedures, and to produce controlled hypotension during surgical procedures and in MI. Titration is performed carefully according to patient tolerance, therapeutic response, and hemodynamic trends. Continuous monitoring of hemodynamic parameters—arterial pressure, pulmonary artery pressures (PAP), and PAOP—is extremely important and must be done throughout intravenous nitroglycerin administration. It is important to maintain adequate blood and coronary perfusion pressures. During angina, the nitroglycerin is started low and is titrated up to relieve pain, as long as hypotension does not develop.

In acute MI the greatest benefit from nitroglycerin occurs when it is administered within 4 hours after the onset of pain. However, it can also produce positive effects when given within 8 hours following the onset of symptoms. Positive effects include a decrease in episodes of

---

Table 32–2. PROTOCOL FOR LOW-DOSE INTRAVENOUS NITROGLYCERIN IN ACUTE MYOCARDIAL INFARCTION

1. Intravenous infusion set (standard or special) with infusion pump.
2. Start at 5 μg/min; titrate upward by 5–10 μg/min every 5–10 min to the desired endpoint or a maximum of 200 μg/min.
3. Lower mean blood pressure (BP) by 10% in normotensive and 30% in hypertensive patients, but not below 80 mm Hg.
4. Reassess if systolic BP < 90 mmHg or mean BP < 80 mmHg, or diastolic BP increases >15 mmHg, or heart rate increases >20% or drops <50 beats per minute.
5. Maintain infusion for at least 24 hr, preferably 48 hr.
6. Stop if hypotension; when safe, restart at 5 μg/min.
7. To stop, titrate down by 5–10 μg/min every 5–10 min.
8. Average dose range 30–140 μg/min.

Source: Singh, B, et al: Cardiovascular Pharmacology and Therapeutics. Churchill Livingstone, New York, 1994, p 453, with permission.

---

anginal pain, ventricular ectopic beats, and left ventricular failure. A protocol for administering low-dose IV nitroglycerin during acute MI is presented in Table 32–2.

Nitroglycerin IV is mixed either with D_5W or 0.9% sodium chloride solutions with dilutions ranging from 25 to 500 μg/mL. Infusion concentrations are based on the patient's fluid requirements. Dosage varies widely from 5 to 800 μg/min and thus requires careful titration in a given patient.

Nitroglycerin IV is absorbed by plastic and polyvinyl chloride (PVC) tubing. Therefore, glass bottles and non-PVC tubing are sometimes used. Infusion pumps may fail to occlude the non-PVC infusion sets completely, so great care is taken when administering nitroglycerin by this method.

Other Nitrates for Acute Therapy

○ **Nitroglycerin translingual** (Nitrolingual) is a metered aerosol spray that is available for acute relief or prophylaxis of angina due to coronary artery disease. Nitrolingual is used in a fashion similar to nitroglycerin tablets. At the onset of an acute attack, one or two metered doses (0.4 mg/spray) are sprayed into the oral mucosa. Like the nitroglycerin tablets, no more than three metered doses are recommended within 15 minutes. If chest pain persists and does not change, the patient should seek medical attention. Nitrolingual can also be used prophylactically 5 to 10 minutes prior to any activity known to cause angina. The canister is not shaken, the spray is not inhaled, and swallowing immediately after administration is avoided.

Nitrates for Chronic Therapy

○ **Nitroglycerin sustained-release** (Nitro-Bid, many others) is a capsule or tablet (2.5 to 6.5 mg) swallowed whole and administered every 8 to 12 hours.

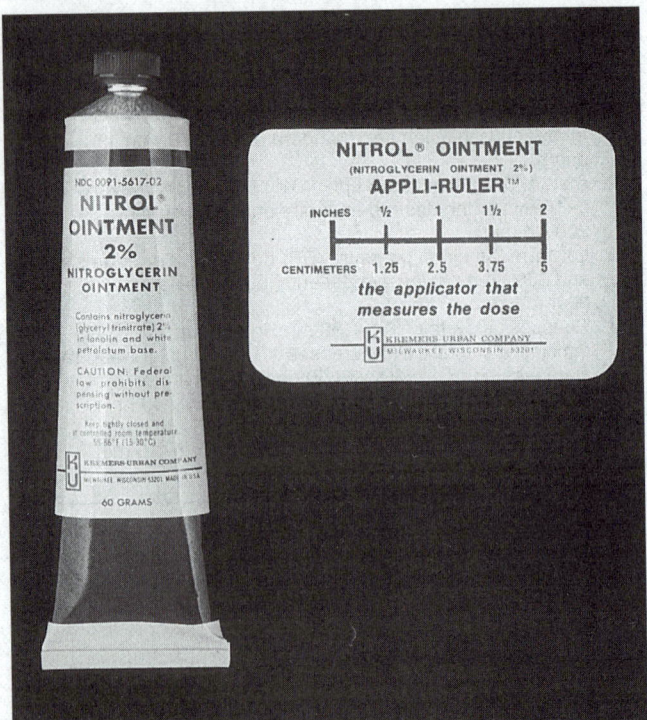

Figure 32–1. Tube of nitroglycerin paste and the special application paper. The correct amount of paste is squeezed onto the paper and then applied to the patient's skin. Clear plastic wrap is applied over the papers to enhance absorption. (Courtesy of Parke-Davis, Division of Warner-Lambert Co, Morris Plains, NJ, and Kremers-Urban Co, Milwaukee, WI)

○ **Nitroglycerin ointment** (Nitro-Bid, Nitrol, Nitrong) contains 2% nitroglycerin in a lanolin base. The ointment is squeezed onto specially marked paper that comes with the tube, as shown in Figure 32–1. The paper, not the fingers, is used to spread the ointment, and the paper is applied to the skin. Further discussion of administration is found in the Nursing Process section of this chapter. The medication can be applied anywhere on the body surface, but the skin should be clean, dry, and hairless. The tube is kept tightly closed and stored in a cool place.

Nitroglycerin ointment dosage is usually titrated by therapeutic response and blood pressure response. It is particularly beneficial in preventing nocturnal angina. When treatment is terminated, dosage is gradually reduced to prevent sudden withdrawal reactions.

○ **Nitroglycerin transdermal patches** (Nitrodisc, Nitro-Dur, Transderm-Nitro, and others) are pockets of medication containing nitroglycerin, glycerin, water, polyvinyl alcohol, and several other ingredients, surrounded by a bandage. The transdermal patches permit the timed release of nitroglycerin over 12 to 24 hours. After the foil cover is removed, the patch resembles an electrocardiogram (ECG) electrode or a round Band-Aid. The patch is applied to the skin, and can be worn during bathing, showering, and swimming.

Transdermal patches are available in several doses, ranging from 9 to 187.5 mg of nitroglycerin. Patches are applied only once daily to any nonhairy area of the body.

Several manufacturers market patches, and each product contains a different amount of nitroglycerin. The release rate of nitroglycerin in milligrams per 24 hours ranges from 2.5 to 15. Patients must be assessed carefully when alternating different manufacturers' products. If a patient is changed from the nitroglycerin ointment containing 12.5 mg nitroglycerin per inch, the smallest dose size of the patch should be used, and the dose appropriately titrated.

○ **Isosorbide dinitrate** (Isordil, Sorbitrate), like nitroglycerin, is available as sublingual and chewable tablets, oral tablets, and sustained-release tablets. Isosorbide is one of the most frequently used long-acting nitrates.

The sublingual and chewable forms are used to treat acute anginal attacks. The oral tablet is used to prevent or decrease the number of anginal attacks. It can also be used as a part of the treatment of HF, where it acts by reducing resistance to cardiac pumping action.

Other Nitrates

○ **Nitroglycerin transmucosal** (Nitrogard) is available for buccal application for both acute and long-term control of angina pectoris. In this form, the nitroglycerin is impregnated in an inert cellulose polymer matrix. The tablet, similar in size to sublingual nitroglycerin, is placed in the buccal cavity between the upper lip and gum, or between the cheek and gum. A gel forms that makes the tablet adhere to the mucosal surface, and the drug diffuses into the systemic circulation. Onset of effect occurs in 2 to 4 minutes. Absorption continues while the tablet remains intact (1 to 6 hours). Nitroglycerin serum levels fall rapidly after the tablet is dissolved. Tolerance to this form of nitroglycerin has not been reported, possibly because of the nitrate-free interval at night.

○ **Isosorbide dinitrate, sustained release** (Isordil Tembids, Sorbitrate SA, Dilatrate-SR) is given in 40-mg oral doses every 6 to 12 hours. The tablets are not chewed or crushed because this eliminates the sustained-release action.

○ **Isosorbide mononitrate** (ISMO, Monoket, Imdur) is used prophylactically in patients with chronic stable angina. Isosorbide mononitrate is the major metabolite of isosorbide dinitrate. The dosing is two times daily, with the first dose in the morning and the second dose 7 hours later. This regimen provides a drug-free interval to prevent tolerance. Imdur is an extended-release formulation that is administered once daily, usually in the morning. Isosorbide mononitrate offers no advantage over other isosorbide products.

OTHER DRUGS USED TO TREAT ANGINA PECTORIS

Other groups of drugs are used in conjunction with vasodilators, or alone, to control anginal attacks. These include the beta-adrenergic blockers and the calcium channel blockers.

BETA-ADRENERGIC BLOCKERS

The beta-adrenergic blockers such as propranolol (Inderal), metoprolol tartrate (Lopressor), and nadolol (Corgard), all discussed in Chapter 17, cause the heart to be more resistant to the effects of catecholamines. This effect decreases the heart rate and the oxygen needs of the myocardium. Beta-adrenergic blockers also decrease the force of cardiac contraction, which also decreases myocardial oxygen needs. Patients usually have an increased tolerance to exercise and report a decrease in the number and severity of their anginal attacks.

CALCIUM CHANNEL BLOCKERS

Calcium channel blockers, or calcium antagonists, are also available to treat angina. These drugs are also used to treat hypertension and dysrhythmias and are mentioned briefly in Chapters 30 and 31. Calcium channel blockers are a heterogeneous group of compounds with differing structures, mechanisms of actions, and therapeutic effects. Because of their inherent differences, agents are selected to meet specific needs of patients. Three distinct groups of calcium channel blockers are available: the phenylalkylamines (verapamil), the dihydropyridines (nifedipine, nicardipine hydrochloride, nimodipine, felodipine, isradipine, amlopidine, and nisoldipine) and the benzothiazapines (diltiazem). Table 32–3 features selected calcium channel blockers. Calcium channel blockers are probably as effective as nitrates and may even be preferred to beta-adrenergic blockers in managing variant, unstable, or vasospastic angina.

Action

All calcium channel blockers have different pharmacologic effects while sharing the ability to competitively block the slow-channel influx of calcium into active cells. The effects of calcium channel blockers are greatest in cells that depend on intracellular influx of calcium for activation. These are mainly vascular smooth muscle cells and cardiac tissue; however, other areas containing smooth muscle cells such as the respiratory and gastrointestinal tracts are also affected. Figure 32–2 reviews the properties of calcium channel blockers.

Cardiac tissue is rapidly depolarized by the rapid influx of sodium ions. This depolarization action is quickly followed by a slow inward current of calcium, which contributes to the plateau phase of the action potential and links myocardial excitation to contraction and controls energy storage and utilization. Most cardiac conducting cells depend on both fast sodium and slow calcium channels. However, the pacer cells of the sinoatrial (SA) and proximal atrioventricular (AV) nodes are depolarized primarily by the calcium current. By inhibiting calcium entry into cardiac and smooth muscle cells of the coronary and systemic beds, peripheral arteries and arterioles dilate. Specific effects of selected calcium channel blockers are included in Table 32–4.

Calcium channel blockers inhibit the voltage-dependent calcium channels. This results in alteration in the inotropic state of the myocardium, in the automaticity of the nodal tissues, and in the tone of vascular smooth muscle. The calcium channel blockers possess short-lasting renal effects: they increase urinary flow rate and urinary sodium excretion. This renal effect may explain the lack of relative sodium and water retention and may contribute to the antihypertensive effect of these drugs.

Uses

The calcium channel blockers have different pharmacologic action, so their uses differ. The antianginal effects of calcium antagonists are explained by their ability to dilate coronary arteries, prevent vasospasm in the coronary arteries, and dilate peripheral arteries. In addition, they decrease myocardial oxygen demand by decreasing afterload, decreasing heart rate, and through their negative inotropic effect; and redistribute blood flow to ischemic areas by increasing coronary blood flow. Calcium antagonists also have a direct cellular anti-ischemic effect.

Recent studies demonstrate that calcium channel blockers retard plaque formation of existing lesions and may even prevent the development of new lesions, and in some cases induce lesion remission. Longer follow-up and further trials are required to assess the appropriate means of widespread clinical application of these agents in coronary artery disease, to determine the optimal timing for their introduction, and to define their mechanisms of action in influencing the natural history of atherosclerosis.

In addition to their use as antidysrhythmic and antianginal drugs, calcium channel blockers are used to treat hypertension, hypertensive emergencies, cerebral vascular spasm, cluster headaches, MI, menstrual cramps, and premature labor. Calcium channel blockers are also used to increase the fibrillation threshold, to control exercise-induced asthma, and to improve the neurologic deficits that are caused by spasm following subarachnoid hemorrhage associated with ruptured congenital aneurysm; they are also used as prophylaxis for sudden death. Diltiazem is being investigated for use in the prevention of reinfarction of non-Q-wave MI.

Calcium channel blockers may also reduce cardiac events after MI. Patients in a large Danish study were 33% less likely to have another MI when taking calcium channel blockers. Proper patient selection is important. Patients placed on calcium channel blockers should have no symptoms of HF because the calcium blockade may further reduce the inotropic state.

Pharmacokinetics

The calcium channel blockers are about 90% absorbed after oral administration. All have a rapid onset of action (20 to 30 minutes) and take 0.5 to 3 hours to reach peak serum levels. All are well bound to plasma proteins. This class of drug is subject to extensive hepatic first-pass effect, and most drugs are converted to different metabolites (e.g., verapamil to norverapamil; diltiazem to desacetyl diltiazem). Half-lives vary from 2 to 7 hours. Only a small amount of drug is excreted unchanged in the urine.

Table 32–3. CORONARY VASODILATORS: CALCIUM CHANNEL BLOCKERS

DRUG NAME/ROUTE AND DOSAGE	PHARMACOKINETICS/ DYNAMICS	NURSING IMPLICATIONS
all calcium channel blockers		**ASSESSMENT:** Establish baseline data—vital signs, ECG, hepatic and renal function. Assess for pregnancy (category C). **INTERVENTION:** If hypotension occurs, tell patient to stay recumbent for 1 hr after taking drug. Know pulse limits; if high or irregular, notify physician. Food delays absorption and decreases plasma concentrations; however, administer sustained-release (SR) forms with food. **EVALUATION:** Notify physician of shortness of breath, swelling of feet, pronounced dizziness, constipation, nausea, and irregular heart beat. Decrease drugs gradually.
PHENYLALKYLAMINES		
verapamil (Calan) (Isoptin) **verapamil sustained-release** (Calan SR) (Isoptin-SR) (Verelan)		
angina *Adults:* 40–120 mg PO tid, up to 480 mg/day. **dysrhythmias** *Adults:* 240–480 mg/day in divided doses; 5–10 mg IV bolus over 2 min (in older patient 3 min), repeat 10 mg in 30 min. *Children under 1 yr:* 0.1–0.3 mg/kg IV bolus over 2 min, repeat in 30 min if no response. *Children 1–15 yr:* 0.1–0.3 mg/kg over 2 min, repeat in 30 min if no response. Do not exceed 5 mg. **hypertension** *Adults:* 240–480 mg/day in divided doses; SR 120–240 mg in AM with food.	**Onset:** PO, 30 min; IV, 1–3 min **Peak:** PO, 1–2 hr; IV, 3–5 min; SR, 6 hr **Duration:** PO, 4–8 hr; IV, 1–6 hr, SR, 24 hr **½L:** 3–7 hr **PB:** 83%–92% **B:** liver **E:** unchanged urine (3–4%)	Same as for all calcium channel blockers plus: **INTERVENTION:** Administer IV bolus doses over 2 min with continuous ECG and blood pressure (BP) monitoring. Repeat in 30 min if no response. Protect IV solution from light.
DIHYDROPYRIDINES		
nifedipine (Adalat) (Procardia) **nifedipine-sustained release** (Adalat CC) (Procardia XL)		
Adults: 10 mg (capsule) PO tid, increase q 7 days to maximum of 120 mg/day; or 30–120 mg (SR tablet) PO once daily.	**Onset:** 20 min **Peak:** 0.5 hr, 6 hr for SR **Duration:** 2.5–3 hr; SR, 24 hr **½L:** 2–5 hr **PB:** 92%–98% **B:** liver **E:** urine (unchanged 1%–2%)	Same as for all calcium channel blockers plus: **INTERVENTION:** Short acting drugs should not be used for long term therapy.
nicardipine (Cardene) (Cardene SR) (Cardene IV)		
angina *Adults:* 20–40 mg (immediate-release [IR] capsule) PO tid. **hypertension** *Adults:* 20–40 mg (IR capsule) PO tid; or 30–60 mg (SR capsule) PO bid. **IV use** *Adults:* 0.5–2.2 mg/hr titrated according to patient response.	**Onset:** PO, 20 min **Peak:** PO, 0.5–2 hr; SR, 2–6 hr **Duration:** PO, 8 hr; SR, up to 12 hr **½L:** 2–4 hr **PB:** 95% **B:** liver **E:** urine (unchanged 1%)	Same as for all calcium channel blockers plus: **INTERVENTION:** Protect IV ampules from light until use. Diluted solution is stable for 24 hr at room temperature. *Transfer to oral antihypertensive agent*—If patient is to receive an oral antihypertensive other than nicardipine, initiate therapy upon discontinuation of IV nicardipine therapy; if oral nicardipine is to be used, administer first dose 1 hr prior to discontinuation of infusion.

Table 32–3. CORONARY VASODILATORS: CALCIUM CHANNEL BLOCKERS, *Continued*

DRUG NAME/ROUTE AND DOSAGE	PHARMACOKINETICS/ DYNAMICS	NURSING IMPLICATIONS
nimodipine (Nimotop)		
Adults: 60 mg PO q 4 hr for 21 days. Begin therapy within 96 hr of subarachnoid hemorrhage. May be drawn out of capsule and injected down nasogastric (NG) tube; flush with 30 ml of NS.	**Onset:** within 30 min **Peak:** 1 hr **Duration:** 3–4 hr **½L:** 1–2 hr **PB:** 95% **B:** NA **E:** less than 1% urine	Same as for all calcium channel blockers plus: **INTERVENTION:** If patient cannot swallow capsule, withdraw fluid from capsule and inject down NG tube. Flush with 30 mL of NS.
amlodipine besylate (Norvasc)		
Adults: 5–10 mg qd. ***Elderly:*** 2.5 mg qd.	**Onset:** slow (not used in acute BP reduction) **Peak:** 6–9 hr **Duration:** 7.6–24 hr **½L:** 35–50 hr **PB:** 98% **B:** liver **E:** urine	Same as for all calcium channel blockers plus: **INTERVENTION:** Monitor BP and pulse prior to and periodically throughout therapy.
BENZOTHIAZINES		
diltiazem (Cardizem) **diltiazem sustained-release** (Cardizem CD) (Cardizem SR) (Dilacor-XR)		
Adults: 30–120 mg PO 3–4 times daily, 60–120 mg (SR capsules) PO bid or 180–360 mg (CD or XR capsules) PO once daily. Or, 0.25 mg/kg IV bolus over 2 min, may repeat in 15 min with 0.35 mg/kg dose. May follow with continuous infusion at 10 mg/hr (range 5–15 mg/hr). Do not give longer than 24 hr or at rate >15 mg/hr.	**Onset:** PO, 30–60 min; SR or XR, 2 hr; IV bolus, 3 min **Peak:** PO, 2–3 hr; SR, 6–11 hr; XR, 10–14 hr; IV bolus, 2–7 min (drug action) **Duration:** PO, 6–8 hr; SR, 12 hr; XR, 24 hr; IV bolus, 1–3 hr; IV infusion, up to 10 hr **½L:** 3–6 hr; SR 5–7 hr **PB:** 70%–80% **B:** liver **E:** urine (2%–4%)	Same as for all calcium channel blockers plus: **INTERVENTION:** For IV drip mix—125 mg in 100 mL, 250 mg in 250 mL, or 500 mg in 250 mL, which gives final concentration of 1 mg/mL, 0.83 mg/mL, or 0.45 mg/mL, respectively. Administer 20-mg bolus over 2 min; then start 10-mg drip, titrated to desired heart rate, and transfer to oral agent as soon as possible. **EVALUATION:** If dizziness and hypotension occur during IV administration, give volume or put patient in modified Trendelenburg.
OTHER CALCIUM CHANNEL BLOCKERS		
bepridil hydrochloride (Vascor)		
Adults: 200 mg PO once daily. May increase to 300 mg day, then to 400 mg daily no more often than every 10 days.	**Onset:** 60 min **Peak:** 2–3 hr (blood levels); 8 days (clinical effect) **D:** NA **½L:** 24 hr **PB:** 99% **B:** liver **E:** urine, feces	Same as for all calcium channel blockers plus: **INTERVENTION:** Monitor QT interval and complete blood count periodically.

NA = not available.

Contraindications and Precautions

The calcium channel blockers are contraindicated in patients hypersensitive to them. Because of their negative inotropic and peripheral vasodilation effects, calcium channel blockers are given cautiously to patients who are hypotensive. Close observation is especially recommended for patients already taking medications that are known to lower blood pressure, such as beta-adrenergic blockers or nitrates. Calcium channel blockers are given cautiously to patients with hepatic and renal dysfunction, because biotransformation and excretion occur in the liver and kidneys. Because the first-pass effect of drugs in this class is high, liver dysfunction allows more drug to circulate, thus increasing the likelihood of side or toxic effects.

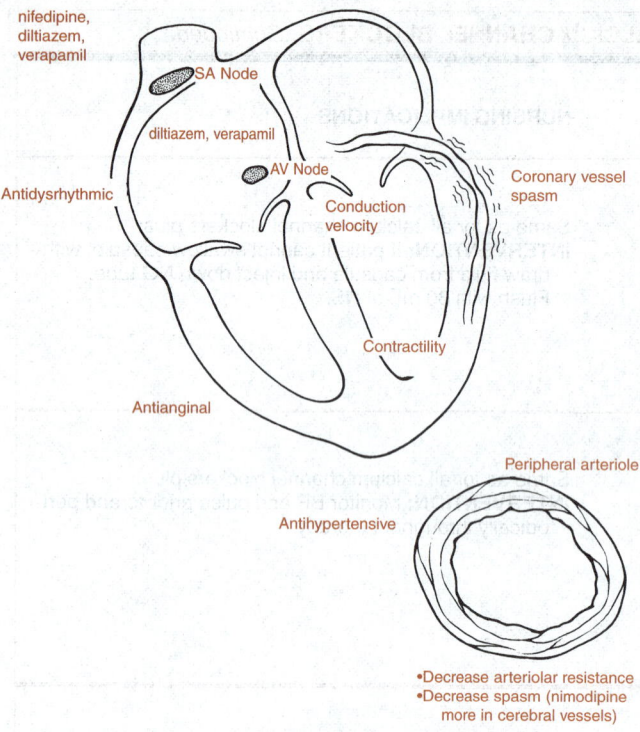

Figure 32–2. Properties of calcium channel antagonists. Calcium antagonists have multiple effects within the heart and periphery.

The elderly patient may experience a greater hypotensive effect than that seen with younger patients. This is probably due to age-related changes in drug disposition. Use during pregnancy (category C) and lactation only when clearly indicated. Safety in children has not been established.

Adverse Effects

Calcium channel blockers do not generally cause serious side effects and rarely require discontinuation of therapy due to side effects. Central nervous system (CNS) effects, which are most common, are related to vasodilation in the brain and include dizziness, light-headedness, and headache. Some changes in bowel habits (either diarrhea or constipation) also occur. Constipation is particularly common with verapamil. Most patients complain of peripheral edema and flushing, both caused by the peripheral vasodilation. Shoe size often goes up a half size. Blood pressure is monitored, as hypotension may also occur.

Interactions

There are many interactions that occur with the calcium channel blockers. Verapamil interacts with beta-adrenergic blockers as they both have negative inotropic and chronotropic effects. This interaction may be beneficial, but it could also be detrimental to cardiac function. Cimetidine and ranitidine may increase the bioavailability of calcium channel blockers because of decreased hepatic first-pass metabolism. Digoxin levels may increase with calcium channel blocker therapy; therefore, digoxin levels must be monitored closely. Concurrent quinidine may lead to hypotension, bradycardia, or AV block and may increase serum quinidine levels. Additional interactions may occur between verapamil and barbiturates, calcium salts, hydantoins, rifampin, vitamin D, cyclosporine, lithium, prazosin, and theophylline. A low-fat meal slows the rate but not extent of absorption; therefore, calcium channel blockers are administered without regard to meals. See drug literature for more specific information.

Phenylalkylamines

The phenylalkylamines are represented by **verapamil (Calan, Isoptin)**, sustained-release verapamil **(Calan SR, Isoptin SR)**, and **controlled-release verapamil (Covera HS)**.

○ **Verapamil** has the most pronounced effect on AV node conduction and is the drug of choice for patients with supraventricular tachycardias with or without anginal symptoms. About 60% to 80% of patients with supraventricular tachycardia convert to normal sinus rhythm within 10 minutes after receiving verapamil. In addition, verapamil is being studied for use in exercise-induced asthma, manic depression, and recumbent nocturnal leg cramps. Recent research indicates that verapamil has an additive or synergistic immunosuppressive effect when used concurrently with cyclosporine in pa-

Table 32–4. RELATIVE EFFECTS OF CALCIUM CHANNEL BLOCKING AGENTS ON VARIOUS CARDIOVASCULAR FUNCTIONS

Function	Nifedipine	Verapamil	Diltiazem
Vascular smooth muscle contraction	0 −	− −	−
Peripheral arterioles	− − −	− −	−
Coronary artery vasodilator effects	+ + +	+ +	+ + +
Myocardial contractility	−	−	
Antidysrhythmic properties	0	+ + +	+ +
Heart rate	+	−	0 −
AV node conduction	+ −	+ +	+
Cardiac output	+ +	+ −	0+

+ − = neither positive nor negative effect; 0 = no effect; + = mild positive effect; + + = moderate positive effect; + + + = great positive effect; − = mild negative effect; − − = moderate negative effect; − − − = great negative effect.

tients with renal transplantation. The concurrent use of these two drugs may permit the lowering of the cyclosporine dose by one-third to one-half.

Verapamil also reduces the left ventricular mass in elderly patients with hypertension. The reduced ventricular mass improves early diastolic filling of the left ventricle and does not reduce cardiac output or ejection fraction. All of the sustained-release or controlled-released products are used only to treat hypertension. Covera HS is administered at bedtime so it is peaking when the pressure rises the most, upon arising.

Dihydropyridines

The dihydropyridines all have similar actions and side effects. The prototype drug of this group is **nifedipine (Procardia, Adalat).** Other drugs in this group include **nicardipine hydrochloride (Cardene), nimodipine (Nimotop), amlodipine (Norvasc), felodipine (Plendil), isradipine (DynaCirc),** and **nisoldipine (Sular).** Many dihydropyridines are available, but in general, there is no benefit in the use of one over another.

○ **Nifedipine** (Procardia, Procardia XL, Adalat) Adalat CC is the most potent peripheral vasodilator, but it has little effect on the SA and AV nodes. It is used in patients with angina along with coexisting sinus bradycardia, as well as cerebral spasm. Research has proved that patients receiving immediate-release nifedipine have a 60% higher risk of having an MI. The long acting products are not associated with this problem. Because of this finding, it is no longer approved for treatment of hypertension, hypertensive crisis, acute MI, and some forms of unstable/chronic stable angina. Nifedipine may be used for prophylaxis of migraine headache. Nifedipine, although not approved, is also used to treat primary pulmonary hypertension and asthma, to decrease uterine contractions in premature labor, to reduce symptoms of cardiomyopathy and Raynaud's syndrome, and to relieve severe pain caused by obstruction of the bile duct or urinary tract.

INTERACTIONS In addition to the general interactions of all calcium channel blockers, nifedipine also may interact with high doses of fentanyl during coronary artery surgery, resulting in severe hypotension or increased fluid volume requirements. Concurrent administration of nifedipine and antihypertensives or quinidine can cause acute hypotension. Theophylline levels may increase when this drug is given concurrently with nifedipine; theophylline dosages may need to be reduced.

○ **Nicardipine hydrochloride** (Cardene) is similar in action to nifedipine. Specifically, nicardipine decreases His-Purkinje conduction and has a mixed effect on the AV node. It increases the heart rate, improves cardiac output, and decreases peripheral vascular resistance.

Nicardipine is currently recommended for treatment of effort-associated chronic stable angina, either alone or with beta-adrenergic blockers. It is also used for the management of essential hypertension, either alone or with other antihypertensives.

○ **Nimodipine** (Nimotop) improves neurologic deficits that are caused by spasm following subarachnoid

hemorrhage (SAH) from rupture of congenital intracranial aneurysms in patients who are in good neurologic condition postictus. Nimodipine has a greater effect on cerebral arteries than the other calcium channel blockers, possibly because it is highly fat soluble, which allows it to cross the blood-brain barrier more readily. Nimodipine is usually started on admission of a patient with SAH and continued for 21 days.

Nimodipine acts like a gasket to tighten up some of the "doors" on brain cells. Aging causes the doors to loosen, allowing more Ca^{2+} to leak into the cell and interfering with cellular function of learning and memory recall. Normally Ca^{2+} rushes into the cells, allowing a charge to move through the cell. But if the door leaks, Ca^{2+} dribbles in and the ability to build excitement and a rapid current of energy in the cell is reduced. Nimodipine is being studied for its usefulness in improving the learning and memory recall in healthy people over age 65 and in improving memory in patients with Alzheimer's disease and various other dementias.

○ **Amlodipine** (Norvasc) is used in combination or alone for the treatment of hypertension, chronic stable angina, and vasospastic angina.

Other Dihydropyridines

○ **Felodipine** (Plendil) is similar to nifedipine but more vascularly selective. It is indicated for the treatment of hypertension and may be used alone or in combination with other antihypertensive agents. It combines well with beta-adrenergic blockers and diuretics. Felodipine is also used to improve the exercise time for 10 to 12 hours in patients with angina pectoris. Felodipine is also being studied in the treatment of HF.

○ **Isradipine** (DynaCirc) is used to manage mild to moderate hypertension. Research indicates that isradipine is as good as hydrochlorothiazide and diltiazem combined and is superior to propranolol alone and prazosin alone. Its ability to control blood pressure may be related to the postdose natriuresis and diuresis that occur. Isradipine is also used to treat effort-associated angina. It is being studied for its antiatherogenic effects.

○ **Nisoldipine** (Sular) is available as an oral extended-release formulation for hypertension. It is five to ten times as potent a vasodilator as nifedipine, with little effect on contractility.

Benzothiazines

Diltiazem (Cardizem) is the only drug in the benzothiazine group.

○ **Diltiazem** (Cardizem) is used orally to manage variant angina, to reduce anginal attacks, and to improve exercise performance. In the parenteral form, it is used to treat atrial fibrillation/flutter or paroxysmal supraventricular tachycardias. Diltiazem is also being studied to prevent reinfarction in non-Q-wave infarction.

CONTRAINDICATIONS AND PRECAUTIONS Diltiazem is contraindicated in patients with sick sinus syndrome, except in those with a functional ventricular pacemaker in place. It is also contraindicated in patients with second- or third-degree heart block.

Other Calcium Channel Blockers

○ **Bepridil hydrochloride** *(Vascor)*, a combined sodium and calcium channel blocker, is used primarily for its antianginal effects. Bepridil, along with other still-investigational products (lidoflazine, prenylamine, flunarizine), constitutes a new class of calcium channel blockers.

▼ **CLINICAL ALERT**

Bepridil has a proarrhythmic effect, which may worsen conduction abnormalities and prolong the QT interval. Thus, bepridil is reserved for patients who have failed to respond optimally to, or are intolerant of, other antianginals.

CONTRAINDICATIONS AND PRECAUTIONS Bepridil is contraindicated in patients with history of serious ventricular dysrhythmias, second- or third-degree heart block, or sick sinus syndrome, as these conditions may worsen. It is also contraindicated in hypotension and HF, as it is a dilator and has negative inotropic activity. Electrolyte disturbances, particularly K^+ and Ca^{++}, are corrected before administrating bepridil, as low K^+ may predispose the patient to the development of torsades de pointes.

ADVERSE EFFECTS Heart failure may develop because of the negative inotropic effects. CNS adverse effects such as dizziness and nervousness may occur, possibly because of the drug's dilatory effect in the brain. Agranulocytosis may also occur; therefore, blood work must be performed routinely during maintenance therapy.

INTERACTIONS Bepridil increases digoxin levels up to 30%, increasing the risk of digitalis toxicity. Digoxin dosage may need to be reduced, and serum levels are monitored. Other drugs that prolong the QT interval (e.g., quinidine, procainamide, digoxin, and tricyclic antidepressants) may exacerbate risk of conduction abnormalities. Diuretics that cause hypokalemia may increase the risk of torsades de pointes.

Selection of Calcium Antagonists

The role of calcium antagonists in stable effort angina and vasospastic angina is well established. In the patient with stable effort angina, two of the prototype calcium antagonists, nifedipine and diltiazem, are equally effective in improving anginal symptoms and exercise tolerance. Compared with beta-adrenergic blockers, diltiazem (120 to 360 mg/day) is as effective as propranolol (200 to 320 mg/day); higher, less well-tolerated doses of the calcium antagonist are more effective. At best, nifedipine is as effective as propranolol. The combinations of each of these calcium antagonists with a beta-adrenergic blocker are about equally effective in prolonging exercise time and

are more effective than calcium antagonist monotherapy. The combination of nifedipine or diltiazem and a beta-adrenergic blocker is better tolerated than verapamil and a beta-adrenergic blocker.

Nifedipine and diltiazem are equally effective in the treatment of vasospastic angina and can be safely combined with conventional antianginal therapy, including a beta-adrenergic blocker or isosorbide dinitrate. Because the pathophysiology of unstable angina is more heterogeneous than that of stable effort angina or vasospastic angina and involves coronary thrombus formation, platelet activation, and coronary vasospasm, the role of calcium antagonists as anti-ischemic agents in unstable angina is more limited. Nifedipine and diltiazem are effective in reducing anginal symptoms in unstable angina. However, their effect on clinical outcome such as death, MI, or need for revascularization is unknown except for nifedipine, which may increase mortality and recurrent angina when used as monotherapy.

USING THE NURSING PROCESS— CORONARY VASODILATORS

ASSESSMENT

- Obtain a thorough history to develop the database needed for preparation of the nursing care plan, which is summarized in Table 32–5. A family history of coronary artery disease or any other vascular disease is obtained. If the patient has been or is currently taking coronary vasodilators, it is important to learn how and when they are taken, how many are being taken per day, how they are stored, and whether the patient experiences any side effects. The nursing history is particularly important for patients with angina pectoris because much of the nursing care is aimed at educating the patient about the condition and ways to prevent anginal attacks.
- Assess the pain and assist the patient in differentiating it from gastrointestinal discomfort or from more serious cardiac conditions. Assist the patient in describing the pain, its duration, precipitating causes, and relief mechanisms to differentiate it from other diseases that produce chest pain. The pain is usually related to physical exertion or emotion such as anger or sexual arousal and may be accompanied by nausea, diaphoresis, and dyspnea.
- Assess the patient's occupation and the amount of physical and psychologic stress to which he or she is exposed. Lifestyle, hobbies, exercise habits, and eating habits are also assessed, because these may need to be modified during the intervention phase.
- Assess whether the patient is physically able to measure the ointment or apply and remove the patches. Patients with physical challenges, such as arthritis, may not be able to manage their medication application.
- Assist with the collection of blood for studies to determine the presence of myocardial damage (creati-

Table 32–5. NURSING PROCESS FOR PATIENT REQUIRING CORONARY VASODILATORS

Assessment

Assess history of past/present illness, including number of pain attacks per day, pain history, precipitating factors, and how patient currently seeks relief from pain.

Assess drug use (OTC, prescription, street drugs, smoking, caffeine).

Assess emotional and psychologic significance of illness.

Assess lifestyle factors, e.g., current level of activity, eating habits.

Nursing Diagnosis: Pain

RELATED TO: Decreased myocardial blood flow, increased cardiac workload/oxygen consumption.

AS EVIDENCED BY: Verbal complaints, grimacing, muscle tension, restlessness, narrowed focus.

Desired Outcomes/Evaluation Criteria

Verbalizes relief of pain. Reports anginal episodes decreased in frequency, duration and severity.

Nursing Actions	Rationale
Place patient at complete rest during anginal episodes.	Reduces myocardial oxygen demand to minimize risk of tissue injury/necrosis
Monitor vital signs every 5 min during anginal attack.	Blood pressure may rise initially due to sympathetic stimulation, then fall if cardiac output is compromised.
Stay with patient experiencing pain or appearing anxious.	Anxiety increases the release of catecholamines, which increases the myocardial workload and can intensify/prolong ischemic attack. Presence of nurse can reduce feelings of fear and helplessness.
Administer antianginal medications promptly, e.g., nitroglycerin.	Rapid vasodilator used to prevent as well as abort anginal attacks.
Administer long-acting medications (Nitro-Dur).	Reduces frequency and severity of attack by producing prolonged/continuous vasodilation.
Administer beta-blockers (Tenormin).	Reduces angina by decreasing heart rate and systolic blood pressure.
Provide supplemental oxygen as indicated.	May increase oxygen available for myocardial uptake/reversal of ischemia.

Nursing Diagnosis: Knowledge Deficit

RELATED TO: Lack of exposure, inaccurate/misinterpretation of information.

AS EVIDENCED BY: Questions, request for information, statement of concern, inaccurate followthrough of instructions.

Desired Outcomes/Evaluation Criteria

Participates in learning process. Verbalizes understanding of condition/disease process and treatment. Participates in treatment regimen and initiates necessary lifestyle changes.

Nursing Actions	Rationale
Review pathophysiology of condition. Stress need for preventing anginal attacks and progression of atherosclerotic process.	Therapeutic management reduces likelihood of myocardial infarction.
Encourage avoidance of factors/situations that may precipitate anginal episode, e.g., emotional stress, physical exertion, ingestion of large/heavy meal, exposure to extremes in temperature.	May reduce incidence/severity of ischemic episodes.
Review importance of weight control, cessation of smoking, dietary changes, exercise. Encourage patient to follow prescribed reconditioning program, caution to avoid exhaustion.	Knowledge of the significance of risk factors provides patient with opportunity to make needed changes. Fear of triggering attacks may cause patient to avoid participation in activity that has been prescribed to increase myocardial strength and form collateral circulation.
Discuss impact of illness on desired lifestyle and activities, including work, driving, sexual activity, and hobbies.	May be reluctant to resume/continue usual activities because of fear of anginal attack/death.
Demonstrate/encourage patient to monitor own pulse during activities.	Allows patient to identify how activities can be modified to avoid increased cardiac stress.
Discuss steps to take when anginal attacks occur, e.g., cessation of activity, administration of PRN medication, use of relaxation techniques.	Being prepared for an event takes away the fear that patient will not know what to do if attack occurs. Promotes sense of control.
Discuss proper times, doses, and medications for control/prevention of anginal attacks.	Angina is complicated illness that often requires use of many drugs given to decrease myocardial workload and control the occurrence of attacks.

Continued on the following page

Table 32–5. NURSING PROCESS FOR PATIENT REQUIRING CORONARY VASODILATORS, *Continued*

Nursing Actions	Rationale
Review ways to deal with possible side effects, e.g., headache, dizziness, (hypotension).	Reduces risk of injury, may enhance cooperation with therapeutic regimen.
Identify symptoms to be reported to physician, e.g., increase in frequency/ duration of attacks, changes in response to medications.	Knowledge of expectations can avoid undue concern for insignificant reasons or delay in treatment of important symptoms.
Stress importance of not discontinuing drug without physician's knowledge.	Sudden cessation may result in rebound ischemic pain.

Other Suggested Nursing Diagnoses: Impaired, Adjustment, Decreased Cardiac Output, and Anxiety.

nine phosphokinase [CPK], serum glutamic-oxaloz-etic transaminase [SGOT], lactate dehydrogenase [LDH]) and with ECGs to determine the presence of changes indicative of angina. Prepare patient for stress tests, as needed, to determine how much work he or she can perform. The patient may also have additional diagnostic studies ordered, such as echocardiograms, radioimmune assay studies, and angiograms.

NURSING DIAGNOSIS

- Typical nursing diagnoses for a patient requiring coronary vasodilators include Pain, Decreased Cardiac Output, Knowledge Deficit, Impaired Adjustment, and Anxiety.

INTERVENTION

The goals of the nursing intervention are primarily to educate the patient and to reduce the number and severity of symptoms.

Nursing Responsibilities

- During an acute anginal attack, record the type of pain, its radiation, its precipitating factors, its duration, and how long before relief was obtained.
- Provide the patient who has acute angina with a supply of nitroglycerin tablets at the bedside, to be restocked as necessary. When transferring medication from stock, make sure hands are dry, as moisture hastens deterioration of the drug. Transfer into an amber-colored bottle. The patient is told to notify the nurse whenever a tablet is taken so the nurse can assess the patient's physical condition and chart administration.
- Mix IV nitroglycerin to the correct concentration. The solution is made by mixing nitroglycerin in either D_5W or normal saline (NS) solution in a concentration of 25 to 500 μg/mL. After determining whether to use low-dose (5 to 50 μg/min) or high-dose (50 to 100

μg/min) therapy, titrate the medication upward every 3 to 5 minutes, after assessing blood pressure and pulse. Low-dose therapy is used for preload reduction and is titrated by increments of 10 to 20 μg. High-dose therapy has a balanced effect on preload and afterload and is titrated by increments of 20 to 50 μg. The dose is titrated to achieve a specific end result: a reduction and/or elimination of chest pain, a change in the ECG, or a lowering of blood pressure. Know the hemodynamic parameter ranges that the patient is to be kept within during therapy.

If a sudden decrease in filling pressure in the left ventricle occurs following a large decline in systolic pressure (defined by a 30 to 40-mm Hg drop in blood pressure within 5 minutes), temporarily stop the nitroglycerin infusion. Monitor blood pressure every 2 to 3 minutes. When the blood pressure recovers, the nitroglycerin is restarted at half the previous rate. The greatest hemodynamic changes are usually seen initially and up to 1 hour after relief of chest pain.

When a patient is ready to be weaned from IV nitroglycerin, the rate of titration is often left to the discretion of the nurse. The average weaning interval is 5 to 10 μg every 15 minutes. A blood pressure and pulse check are performed before each change. Any return of chest pain or rebound hypertension prohibits weaning, and the physician is consulted. When weaning is complete, the effect of nitroglycerin remains for 30 to 60 minutes.

Patient Teaching

- Teach the patient about coronary vasodilators and the importance of proper administration, as presented in Table 32–6.
- Teach the patient about the need to have a 12-hour no-nitrate time to prevent nitrate tolerance. The patches and paste must be removed after 12 hours of wearing. If the patient experiences chest pain during the day, the nitrate is used during the day and removed at night. Conversely, if the chest pain occurs at night, the nitrate is removed during the day. Nitroglycerin degrades when exposed to light, air, or moisture. It is stored in a tightly closed amber-colored

Table 32–6. PATIENT TEACHING INFORMATION—CORONARY VASODILATORS

Dear Patient:

This drug has been prescribed for you. This is what you should know about your drug to get the most from your therapy.

- ☐ 1. Nitrates are used to prevent or treat angina pectoris (chest pain of effect).
- ☐ 2. Coronary vasodilators (nitrates) may be taken for the rest of your life.
- ☐ 3. Several forms of nitrates are available. The following instructions include specific directions for each form of nitrate.

SHORT-ACTING PRODUCTS

Take short-acting coronary vasodilators at the first sign of pain.

Place nitroglycerin tablet under the tongue, let it dissolve, and hold saliva in the mouth for 1–2 min before swallowing. When pain is relieved, the remaining tablet is expelled from mouth.

You may take a total of 3 nitroglycerin tablets (1 tablet every 5 min) for any single attack of chest pain. If the pain is *not* relieved, you should *immediately* seek medical attention, as you may be having a heart attack.

Sit 15–20 min after taking the tablet to prevent dizziness or faintness and to help relieve the discomfort.

You may take nitroglycerin 3–5 min before beginning any activity known to trigger an attack, such as exercise or sexual intercourse. The vasodilating effects are usually sufficient to prevent chest pain during the activity.

Medications should be kept in their original container because they lose their potency when exposed to heat, light, moisture, or other organic and inorganic materials such as cotton or paper. Note the expiration date on the bottle and refill as needed. If the medication is stored tightly closed in its original container, it is stable for approximately 5 months.

Nitroglycerin, translingual—At the onset of an attack or 10–15 min prior to an activity known to cause angina, spray 1–2 metered doses into the mouth. *Do not inhale spray.* Take no more than three metered doses in 15 min.

LONG-ACTING PRODUCTS

Take long-acting coronary vasodilators at the correct prescribed time intervals to keep a constant blood level. These products will not relieve acute anginal attacks.

Generally, long-acting medications can be taken with or between meals (pentaerythritol tetranitrate should be taken only between meals). Tablets or capsules are swallowed whole and not crushed or opened.

Nitropaste—When using nitroglycerin paste, squeeze the paste onto the special application paper supplied by the manufacturer and use the paper, not the fingers, to spread the ointment. Apply the special medicated paper to the skin, but do not rub into the skin. The medication can be applied anywhere on the body surface. Always remove the old paper and wash and dry the skin before the new dose is applied. Sites are rotated to help prevent skin irritation. Plastic wrap may also be applied over the special paper to prevent staining of the clothes and to increase absorption. If plastic wrap is used, skin irritation may occur. Remove paper for 12 hours each day. Consult with your physician about the best time for removal.

The paste is kept tightly closed and stored in a cool place.

Nitro Patches—Apply patch once daily to clean, dry skin. Remove old patch and wash skin with soap and water to remove nitroglycerin. Wear patch for only 12 hours a day.

Nitroglycerin, transmucosal—Place tablet between cheek and gum after eating. A glue forms that holds tablet in place. Tongue movement may dislodge tablet. Drinking hot fluids may increase dissolution of tablet. Remove tablet at bedtime.

- ☐ 4. Do not take coronary vasodilators with alcohol because of the possibility of lowering your blood pressure.
- ☐ 5. Always check with your physician or pharmacist before taking other medications because interaction between drugs may occur.
- ☐ 6. If a dose is forgotten, no attempt should be made to catch up.
- ☐ 7. Do not suddenly stop coronary vasodilators without the physician's permission because of the possibility of a rebound in the number and severity of the attacks. If you are to discontinue taking coronary vasodilators, the dosage will be gradually reduced.
- ☐ 8. If you experience side effects such as dizziness or faintness, recovery is speeded if the head is lowered and deep breathing is started. Also, a mild headache is common; but if it is severe and lasts longer than 15–20 min, the physician should be notified. The dose may have to be altered.
- ☐ 9. Nitroglycerin is not habit-forming, and you can take as many tablets or capsules as needed during the day within reason. However, any change in the number or severity of anginal attacks should be reported to your physician.
- ☐ 10. Carry the medication with you at all times.
- ☐ 11. Carry a medication information card to indicate that you are taking coronary vasodilators.
- ☐ 12. Inform your dentist and any other physician that you are taking coronary vasodilators.
- ☐ 13. Tell your family where the medication is kept in case you need it urgently.

container away from heat. Counsel the patient to refill supplies for periods of no longer than 5 months. Also tell the patient to keep a supply of nitroglycerin tablets nearby at all times. The medication is best carried in a jacket pocket or handbag in the original container.

- Nitrate failure may occur because of increasing severity of angina, loss of potency of tablets, incorrect route of administration, dry mucous membranes, arterial hypoxemia, and noncompliance. If nitrate tolerance develops, investigate the cause and intervene appropriately.

EVALUATION

- Establish evaluation criteria, based on the goals that both the nurse and the patient have developed previously (see Table 32–5).

When the patient first returns home after the initial diagnosis, it is important to have him or her keep a written record of anginal attacks. This record should include the following: predisposing factors, the time of day, the number of attacks per day, how relief was sought, and the adverse effects, if any, encountered from the coronary vasodilators. This chart is reviewed by the physician and nurse at frequent intervals to evaluate the success or failure of the prescribed treatment regimen.

- Discuss potential adverse effects of coronary vasodilators with the patient. The most common adverse effects include flushing, hypotension, and headache. Flushing often subsides in 3 to 5 minutes. Patients in their 30s are more likely to report severe flushing than older patients. Hypotension and its resulting dizziness or faintness can be alleviated by sitting or lying down when the medication is taken and then for an additional 15 to 20 minutes. Headache may subside spontaneously in 3 to 5 minutes, or it may persist. One common reason for noncompliance is a persistent, severe, and long-lasting headache. The intensity of headaches can be decreased by having the physician reduce the dose.

  Overcompliance, taking more than the prescribed number of tablets a day, is rarely a problem with coronary vasodilators because of the headaches that are experienced. Make sure the patient understands that he or she may not take more than three short-acting nitroglycerin tablets for any anginal attack. If the pain still persists at the same intensity, the patient must seek immediate medical attention.

- Evaluate the effectiveness of nitroglycerin paste or patches by taking a baseline pulse and blood pressure reading and then repeating both 1 hour after medication administration. An effective dose decreases the blood pressure by 10 mm Hg or increases the pulse rate by 10 beats compared with resting values.

- Review and update all general points of health teaching with the patient to ensure that his or her knowledge base remains accurate.

Both pharmacologic and surgical treatments are effective in controlling symptoms in patients with unstable angina pectoris.

PERIPHERAL VASODILATORS

Peripheral vasodilators are similar to the coronary vasodilators in that they increase the diameter of the blood vessel and are used to dilate blood vessels in the periphery or the cerebral circulation, or both, in arteries and veins. Peripheral vasodilators are used to treat tissue ischemia in the specific vascular beds of the skin, skeletal muscles, and CNS. They are used primarily to reduce the vasospasm that occurs in disorders like Raynaud's disease and, with limited value, in peripheral vascular disease or cerebral vascular disease.

Peripheral vasodilators act to dilate blood vessels in several ways. First, they act directly on and have a nonspecific relaxant effect on the vascular smooth muscle wall, resulting in dilation. This effect is independent of

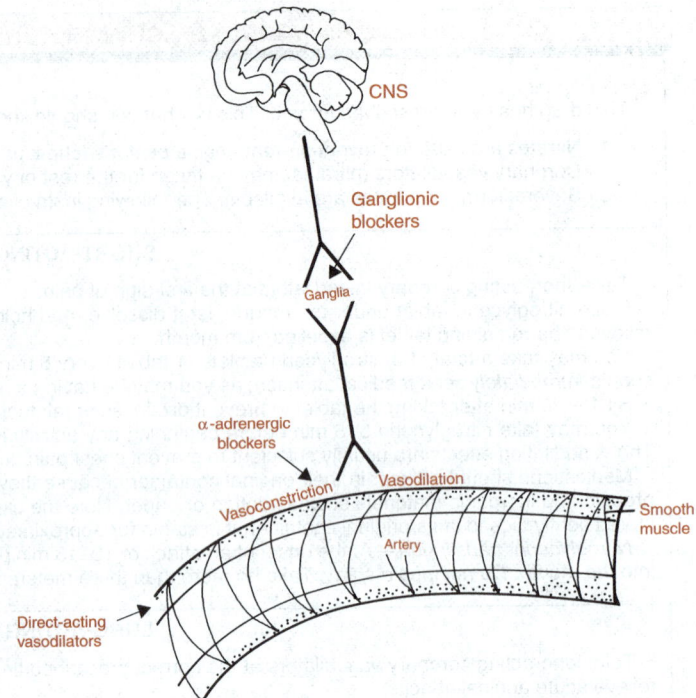

Figure 32–3. Sites of action of peripheral vasodilators.

the sympathetic nervous system. They are not potent vasodilators when given orally, and their efficacy in peripheral vascular disease has not been established. Second, they can stimulate beta-adrenergic receptors, which results in sympathetically medicated relaxation of the smooth muscle surrounding vessels. Third, they can block alpha-adrenergic stimulation, which causes vasoconstriction. The relative sites of action are shown in Figure 32–3. Several medication groups are used as peripheral vasodilators, including the following:

1. direct-acting vasodilators, including papaverine (Cerespan, Pavabid), ethaverine hydrochloride (Ethaquin, Ethatab), cyclandelate (Cyclospasmol), nicotinyl alcohol or tartrate (Roniacol), and isoxsuprine hydrochloride (Vasodilan)

2. sympathetic blocking agents: alpha-adrenergic blockers including phenoxybenzamine (Dibenzyline), reviewed in Chapter 17; and reserpine, guanethidine monosulfate (Ismelin), methyldopa (Aldomet), and prazosin hydrochloride (Minipress), reviewed in Chapter 30

3. calcium channel blockers, including nifedipine (Procardia), reviewed earlier in this chapter

Much controversy surrounds the usefulness of these classes of drugs. There is little evidence that indicates these drugs are effective in treating chronic occlusive vascular diseases. The use of vasodilator drugs in reversing or delaying the deleterious effects of acute or chronic obstruction is questionable. Peripheral vasodilators, by decreasing blood pressure (because this is one of the major determinants of flow in collateral vessels), can actually reduce flow in these areas. Furthermore, studies show

Table 32–7. DIRECT-ACTING PERIPHERAL VASODILATORS

DRUG NAME/ROUTE AND DOSAGE	PHARMACOKINETICS/ DYNAMICS	NURSING IMPLICATIONS
papaverine (Cerespan) (Pavabid) and many others		
Adults: 100–300 mg PO 3–5 times daily (tablets cannot be crushed) or 150–300 mg PO (timed-released) q 8–12 hr (poorly and erratically absorbed); 30–120 mg IM or IV (slowly over 2 min) q 3 hr. **impotence** **Adults:** 30 mg by intracavernosal injection with 0.5–1 mg phentolamine or 60 mg alone. Do not exceed 3 times/wk.	**Onset:** PO, 15–30 min; IV, immediate **Peak:** PO, 1–2 hr **Duration:** PO, 3–6 hr; ER, 8–12 hr; IM or IV, 3 hr; intracavernosal, up to 4 hr **½L:** 6 hr **PB:** 90% **B:** liver **E:** urine	**ASSESSMENT:** Assess vital signs closely during therapy. Obtain baseline liver studies and monitor frequently. Assess for pregnancy (category C). **INTERVENTION:** May be accompanied by a feeling of warmth in extremities. IV administration is incompatible with Ringer's lactate solution—precipitate forms. With intracavernosal injection, erection should not last longer than 4 hr. **Patient Teaching**—Caution patient to make position changes slowly to reduce the possibility of orthostatic hypotension; and to limit alcohol intake because of the additive vasodilation effect. Tell patient to not miss a dose, but if dose is missed to *not* double dose next time. **EVALUATION:** Notify physician if flushing, headache, sweating, skin rash, or abdominal pain becomes pronounced.

that these drugs decrease flow to ischemic areas distal to the vascular occlusions. Therefore, use in occlusive disorders is highly questionable. Some evidence, however, suggests that these drugs may be of modest benefit in patients with vasospastic disease such as Raynaud's disease.

DIRECT-ACTING VASODILATORS

The direct-acting vasodilators—**papaverine (Cerespan, Pavabid), ethaverine hydrochloride (Ethaquin, Ethatab), cyclandelate (Cyclospasmol), nicotinyl alcohol or tartrate (Roniacol),** and **isoxsuprine hydrochloride (Vasodilan)**—act directly on the walls of the smooth muscle to cause vasodilation. The efficiency of these medications administered orally in treating peripheral vascular disease has not yet been established in well-controlled clinical studies.

○ **Papaverine** (Cerespan, Pavabid) is an alkaloid derived from opium that lacks the tolerance, habituation, and analgesic effect seen with narcotics. Although papaverine has been used for many years to relieve a number of conditions such as cerebral and peripheral ischemia associated with arterial spasm, senile dementia, and cerebral ischemia, and to produce vasodilation in some radiologic procedures, there is insufficient objective evidence of any therapeutic value. Papaverine, however, does have some value in treating male impotence. Papaverine is reviewed in Table 32–7.

Other Direct-Acting Vasodilators

○ **Cyclandelate** (Cyclospasmol) exerts a papaverine-like action on the peripheral vascular smooth muscle by a direct action. It is considered "possibly effective" by the FDA in increasing peripheral circulation of the extremities and digits and elevates the skin temperature of the extremities. It is used as adjunctive therapy in arteriosclerosis obliterans, *intermittent claudication* (a peripheral vascular disease characterized by progressive weakness and pain in the lower leg during walking), thrombophlebitis, nocturnal leg cramps, Raynaud's disease, and cerebral vascular disease in some patients.

SYMPATHETIC BLOCKING AGENTS

The medications in this group block the sympathetic vasoconstrictor impulses, either through alpha-adrenergic blockade or by blocking the impulse at the ganglion. This allows beta-adrenergic stimulation to occur unopposed, producing vasodilation, as shown in Figure 32–4.

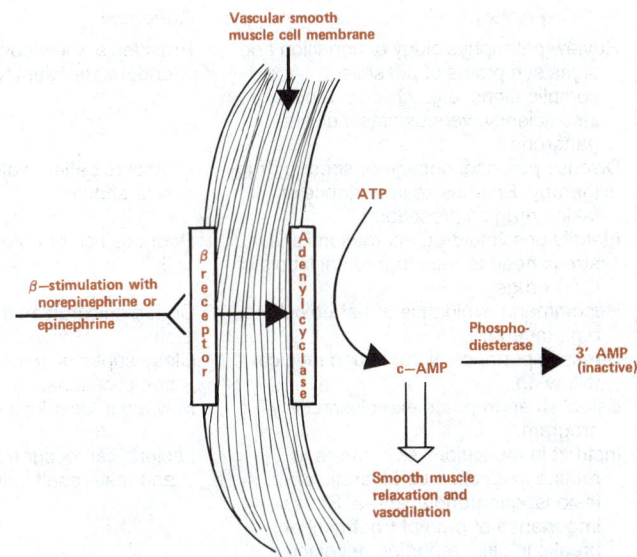

Figure 32–4. Norepinephrine or epinephrine stimulates the beta receptor on the outside surface of the smooth muscle cell membrane. This activates adenylcyclase, which converts adenosine triphosphate (ATP) to cyclic adenosine monophosphate (cAMP), causing the muscle to relax and produce vasodilation.

TABLE 32–8. NURSING PROCESS FOR PATIENT REQUIRING PERIPHERAL VASODILATORS

Assessment

Assess extremities/digits, noting color, temperature, sensations, pulses.
Assess characteristics of pain/discomfort.
Assess lifestyle, including type of work (sedentary/active) and type of leisure activities, smoking.
Assess history of recent injury to the extremity, presence of hypertension, hypercholesterol levels, diabetes, renal disease, and/or cardiac disease.
Assess laboratory results, e.g., clotting, hyperlipidemia studies, ECGs, Doppler and vascular studies.

Nursing Diagnosis: Tissue Perfusion Decreased, peripheral

RELATED TO: Decreased blood flow.
AS EVIDENCED BY: Tissue edema, diminished peripheral pulses, slow/diminished capillary refill, intermittent skin color changes, pallor/erythema, and trophic skin changes, complaints of pain.

Desired Outcomes/Evaluation Criteria

Demonstrates improved perfusion as evidenced by peripheral pulses present/equal, skin color and temperature normal, absence of edema. Engages in behaviors/actions to enhance tissue perfusion. Displays increasing ability to participate in desired activity.

Nursing Actions

Promote restriction/cessation of activity or bed rest during acute phase according to individual needs.
Protect from injury, e.g., refrain from activities using sharp implements, requiring fine motor function, or involving heat/cold (drinking coffee), testing temperature of bath water with hand.
Administer vasodilators, e.g., Cyclospasmol, Ethaquin, Roniacol; or alpha-adrenergic blockers, e.g., Dibenzyline.
Monitor effects of medications/treatments.

Assist patient to identify precipitating factors or situations, e.g., smoking, exposure to cold, and problem-solving solutions.

Rationale

Reduces oxygen and nutrient demands of affected extremity. Minimizes the possibility of dislodging thrombus (if present) and creating emboli.

Sensation is often diminished during attack or chronically in advanced disease. Lack of awareness when sensation is diminished can lead to situations in which the affected body parts are at increased risk for injury.

Although site/mechanism of action varies, intended results are reduction of vasoconstriction, relaxation of vasospasm, a more even blood flow/narrowing of pulse pressure, and elevation of skin temperature.

Improvement may be gradual, requiring several months. Individual responses to prescribed therapies may not be adequate to control disease or may produce untoward side effects, indicating need for change in regimen.
Vasoconstriction is to be limited as it may lead to tissue damage and gangrene.

Nursing Diagnosis: Knowlege Deficit

RELATED TO: Lack of exposure, unfamiliarity with information resources, lack of recall.
AS EVIDENCED BY: Request for information, verbalization of problem, inaccurate follow-through of instruction, development of preventable complications.

Desired Outcomes/Evaluation Criteria

Verbalizes understanding of disease process, treatment regimen, and limitations. Identifies signs/symptoms requiring medical evaluation. Correctly performs therapeutic procedure(s) and explains reasons for actions.

Nursing Actions

Review pathophysiology of condition and signs/symptoms of possible complications, e.g., chronic venous insufficiency, venous stasis ulcers, gangrene.
Discuss purpose, dosage of specific drug therapy. Emphasize importance of taking drug as prescribed.
Identify possible drug interactions and stress need to read ingredient labels of OTC drugs.
Recommend avoidance of beta-blockers, e.g., Inderal.
Stress importance of continued medical follow-up.
Establish appropriate exercise/activity program.
Instruct in meticulous skin care and routine inspection for ulcerations, lesions, gangrenous areas. Stress importance of prompt treatment of breaks in skin, reporting developing lesions/ulcers or changes in skin color.
Discuss importance of proper nutrition, vitamins, restriction of cholesterol.

Rationale

Provides a knowledge base from which patient can make informed choices and understand/identify health-care needs.

Promotes patient safety by reducing risk of inadequate therapeutic response/deleterious side effects.

Reduces risk of untoward reactions and possible complications.

Contraindicated as they worsen vasospasm.

Close supervision of therapeutic response/needs is necessary to reduce risk of complications.
May aid in developing collateral circulation, enhances venous return.

Lesions can occur from pinpoint size to those involving the entire fingertip, for example, and may result in infection or serious tissue damage or loss.

A well-balanced diet, including adequate protein and hydration, is necessary for proper healing and tissue regeneration. Lowering of cholesterol levels may reduce development or progression of atherosclerosis, which can also impair circulation.

Other Suggested Nursing Diagnosis: Impaired Physical Mobility, Chronic Pain, and Anxiety.

Alpha-Adrenergic Blockers

The alpha-adrenergic blocker **phenoxybenzamine (Dibenzyline)** acts selectively on the alpha receptor sites to block the response of the sympathetic nervous stimulation caused by circulating catecholamines. Because alpha receptors are more abundant in skin vessels than in the skeletal muscle vessels, blood flow to the skin is increased. These drugs are most effective in treating Raynaud's disease and have little effect in treating chronic occlusive peripheral vascular disease. Phenoxybenzamine is featured in Chapter 17.

USING THE NURSING PROCESS— PERIPHERAL VASODILATORS

ASSESSMENT

- Develop a thorough nursing history to determine the database, as presented in Table 32–8. Patients with peripheral vascular diseases require lifelong care. Their symptoms can be relieved temporarily but cannot be cured. Determine whether the patient has a history of hypertension, hypercholesterolemia, diabetes, renal disease, and/or cardiac disease. These underlying conditions may contribute to the development of peripheral vascular disease and need to be treated. Also assess for recent injury to extremities, which may worsen the current problem.
- Assess the patient's current smoking habits (including the use of marijuana). Smoking causes further vasoconstriction in the periphery, worsening peripheral vascular disease. If the patient is still smoking, work with him or her during the intervention phase to reduce the smoking habit or to stop it permanently.
- Assess the patient for objective and subjective symptoms of peripheral vascular disease. In addition, the patient's symptoms of pain are assessed. Intermittent claudication may be experienced by patients with Buerger's disease (thromboangiitis obliterans). Persistent pain or rest pain is experienced if an embolism or thrombosis is present.
- Assess the patient's occupation and leisure activities. It is important to assess whether the patient leads an active or sedentary lifestyle. Also, if the patient exercises, determine how often, of what type, and what difficulties are experienced during exercise.
- Assist with the collection of laboratory data such as clotting studies, hyperlipidemia studies, ECGs, Doppler studies, and vascular studies.

NURSING DIAGNOSIS

- Typical nursing diagnoses for a patient requiring medication for peripheral vascular disease include Chronic Pain, Anxiety, Knowledge Deficit, Decreased Peripheral Tissue Perfusion, and Impaired Physical Mobility (see Table 32–8).

PLANNING AND INTERVENTION

- Establish the goals of nursing intervention from the nursing diagnoses. The goals of nursing intervention

Table 32–9. PATIENT TEACHING INFORMATION— PERIPHERAL VASODILATORS

Dear Patient:

This drug has been prescribed for you. This is what you should know about your drug to get the most from your therapy.

- ☐ 1. Peripheral vasodilators are taken to reduce spasm or to improve circulation to your legs or arms.
- ☐ 2. You will most likely take your vasodilator for the rest of your life.
- ☐ 3. Note when your drug is taken in relationship to meals: cyclandelate (Cyclospasmol) is taken with food to prevent gastric irritation; nicotinyl alcohol or tartrate (Roniacol) is taken before meals to increase absorption.
- ☐ 4. If you forget your medication until your next dose, skip it; do *not* try to catch up.
- ☐ 5. Do not omit or stop taking your medication without your physician's approval.
- ☐ 6. The side effects of your medication are _____. If these occur, notify your physician.
- ☐ 7. Change body positions slowly to reduce the possibility of orthostatic hypotension.
- ☐ 8. Limit your alcohol intake because of the additive vasodilation effect.
- ☐ 9. Do not expose yourself to cold, as most peripheral vasodilators are accompanied by a feeling of warmth in the extremities.
- ☐ 10. Avoid hot showers and hot tubs because of the additive vasodilation they cause.
- ☐ 11. Store all medications in tight, light-resistant containers.

in caring for a patient requiring peripheral vasodilators are included in Table 32–8.

Patient Teaching

- Teach the patient the information presented in Table 32–9, because patients self-medicate at home. Because no specific therapy is available to cure these diseases, supportive treatment is directed at removing all the risk factors, including tobacco use, trauma from chemical substances, and exposure to extremes in temperature. Surgery may be indicated to produce permanent vasodilation. Medications do reduce the symptoms and may prevent further deterioration. The patient is taught what symptoms to report to the physician immediately, such as rest pain, change in color of extremities, or ulcer formation.

EVALUATION

- Evaluate the effectiveness of peripheral vasodilators based on a predetermined list of outcome evaluation criteria.
- Teach the patient to recognize the side effects of the medications. Many of the medications may cause flushing of the skin and hypotension. If an unusual symptom is noted, the patient is encouraged to call the physician. The patient is encouraged to keep the extremities warm and not subject them to any unnecessary chill. The patient is also taught to change body positions slowly to prevent orthostatic hypotension.
- Evaluate the patient's knowledge about all previously taught material to ensure that his or her knowledge base remains accurate.

The bibliography for this chapter can be found in Appendix B, which begins on page 1054.

CHAPTER REVIEW QUESTIONS*

1. As a class of drugs, nitrates have the following action:
   a. Constriction of collateral cardiac blood vessels.
   b. Reduction in systemic venous tone.
   c. Relaxation of skeletal muscle tissue.
   d. Constriction of cerebral blood vessels.

2. Which of the following descriptions is *correct* regarding the pharmacokinetics of calcium channel blockers?
   a. Readily absorbed via the oral route.
   b. Dependent on lipids for drug binding.
   c. Estimated half-life of 2 hours.
   d. Extensive first-pass metabolism.

3. When instructing the patient about use of nitroglycerin translingual (Nitrolingual) for relief of chest pain, the following is stressed:
   a. Inhale deeply after administration of translingual spray.

   b. Shake canister well before using translingual spray.
   c. Swallow immediately after administration of the spray.
   d. Spray 1 or 2 metered doses into the oral mucosa.

4. Diltiazem is contraindicated in patients with the following condition:
   a. Cerebral vascular spasm.
   b. Variant angina.
   c. Asthma.
   d. Sick sinus syndrome.

5. After weaning a patient from intravenous nitroglycerin, the effect remains for:
   a. 30 to 60 minutes.
   b. 24 hours.
   c. 2 to 4 hours.
   d. 12 hours.

*See Appendix A, which begins on page 1051, for answers.

CHAPTER 33

Antihyperlipidemic Agents

Kenneth A. Kellick, PharmD

CHAPTER OUTLINE

TABLES

BOX

KEY TERMS

Cholesterol   Rhabdomyolysis
Hyperlipidemia   Triglycerides
Lipoproteins

LEARNING OBJECTIVES

After reading this chapter, the student will be able to:

1. Identify medications that have an effect on hyperlipidemia.
2. Differentiate among the medications as to mechanism of action, routes of administration, pharmacokinetics, adverse effects, contraindications and precautions, and interactions.
3. Determine the specific areas in which patient-focused care by the nurse can influence and improve patient outcomes.
4. Plan the nursing interventions necessary to administer medications and choose appropriate teaching strategies to gain patient compliance.
5. Evaluate the patient at various stages of treatment to gauge nursing interventions.

*H*yperlipidemia is a disorder characterized by increased concentrations of lipids (cholesterol and/or triglycerides) in the blood. *Cholesterol* is a waxy substance produced in animal livers that is used for bile acid, sterol, and cell wall synthesis. Endogenous cholesterol is metabolized in the liver to bile acids and excreted from the biliary tract into the small intestine. *Triglycerides* are fats that consist of three molecules of fatty acid bound with one molecule of glycerol; they are the most common fat stored in humans. Elevated serum levels of cholesterol and triglycerides contribute to the development of atherosclerosis, the most common form of arteriosclerosis. Atherosclerosis is thought to contribute to hypertension, myocardial infarction, cerebrovascular accidents, and coronary artery disease (CAD). Research indicates that controlling lipid blood levels with diet and/or drug therapy may slow or prevent the onset and progression of atherosclerosis and may decrease CAD end points such as myocardial infarction and angina.

Antihyperlipidemic agents, or lipid-lowering agents, are used to lower high serum lipid levels to target values. To understand how these drugs act, the relationship between cholesterol concentrations and the lipoprotein complexes that transport cholesterol and triglycerides must be examined. Goals for cholesterol, low-density lipoproteins, and triglycerides are included in Table 33–1.

LIPOPROTEINS AND THEIR INFLUENCE ON CORONARY ARTERY DISEASE

Because lipids are not water soluble, they cannot dissolve directly in plasma. To move in the bloodstream, lipid compounds bind to plasma proteins such as albumin and globulin, which act as carriers. These protein and lipid (cholesterol, triglycerides, phospholipids) complexes are called *lipoproteins*. All lipoproteins are spherical structures that contain a core of neutral lipids (cholesterol esters and

Table 33–1. BLOOD CHOLESTEROL, LDL, AND TRIGLYCERIDE LEVELS	
Measurement (mg/dL)	Risk
Cholesterol	
<200	Low
201–239	Borderline/moderate
>240	High
LDL	
<130	Low
131–159	Borderline/moderate
>160	High
Triglycerides	
150–200	Low
200–400	Borderline/moderate
400–1000	High
>1000	Very high

triglycerides) and a surface coat of more polar lipids (unesterified cholesterol and phospholipids) and apolipoproteins. The surface coat serves as an interface between the aqueous plasma and the inner nonpolar lipid core. Based on physiochemical properties, there are five major classes of lipoproteins: chylomicrons, very low density lipoproteins (VLDL), intermediate-density lipoproteins (IDL), low-density lipoproteins (LDL), and high-density lipoproteins (HDL).

Each class of lipoprotein is composed of differing percentages of lipids and protein and is named based on their density ratio. The greater the ratio of lipids to proteins, the lower the density.

Chylomicrons In the digestive tract, triglycerides are split into monoglycerides and fatty acids. These products pass through the intestinal wall and are resynthesized into molecules of triglycerides called chylomicrons. Chylomicrons are produced in the small intestine and consist of 85% to 95% triglycerides, 3% to 5% cholesterol, and 1% protein. Chylomicrons are the largest and least dense of the lipoproteins. Chylomicrons are cleared from the bloodstream by the enzyme lipoprotein lipase after 12 to 24 hours, forming chylomicron remnants. These chylomicron remnants are then transformed by the liver into VLDL, which is the precursor of IDL and eventually LDL.

Very Low Density Lipoproteins Triglycerides are synthesized mainly from carbohydrates in the liver and are transported to the adipose and other peripheral tissues in the form of VLDLs. VLDLs, also referred to as pre-beta-lipoproteins, contain 64% to 80% triglycerides, 7% to 14% cholesterol, and 7% protein. High levels of VLDL may be atherogenic. Patients with very high levels are also at risk of developing pancreatitis.

Low-density Lipoproteins LDLs are produced by the action of hepatic lipase on VLDL remnants. LDLs contain a relatively low percentage of triglycerides (7% to 10%), a very high percentage of cholesterol (40% to 50%), and a moderate level of protein (21%). The LDLs are the major carrier of cholesterol in the blood and are therefore considered the most harmful of the lipoproteins. Patients with high serum LDL levels are at high risk for developing atherosclerosis.

Intermediate-density Lipoproteins IDL or broad alpha-lipoproteins, are formed as VLDLs lose their triglycerides. IDLs consist of 30% cholesterol. Like VLDLs, they also tend to be atherogenic. In normally healthy persons, IDLs are not found in significant amounts.

High-density Lipoproteins HDLs or alpha-lipoproteins, contain about 50% protein with smaller concentrations of lipids: 17% to 20% cholesterol and 1% to 7% triglycerides. HDLs are the smallest and most dense. HDL appears to be beneficial, as its primary function is to transport cholesterol away from peripheral tissues to the liver, where it is metabolized and then excreted. HDL, therefore, plays an important role in preventing atherosclerosis. The higher the HDL level, the lower the risk for developing CAD. HDL can be raised by exercise and estrogen replacement in postmenopausal women. Causes of low HDL include cigarette smoking, obesity, androgenic and related steroids, beta-adrenergic blocking agents, diuretics, phenytoin, hypertriglyceridemia, and genetic factors.

MANAGEMENT OF HYPERLIPIDEMIA

There are three common treatment classifications: isolated hypercholesterolemia, combined hypercholesterolemia and hypertriglyceridemia, and isolated hypertriglyceridemia. The diagnosis depends on serum cholesterol and triglyceride levels and lipoprotein fractionation. Therapy aims at modifying CAD risk factors, managing primary causes of elevated lipids, and lowering cholesterol and/or triglyceride levels by hygienic and/or pharmacologic means. Diet modification is the first line of therapy. Drug therapy is used only after dietary measures have been tried.

LIPID GOALS AND RISK FACTORS

The National Cholesterol Educational Panel (NCEP) recommends cholesterol screening for all adults over the age of 20 with at least a nonfasting cholesterol and HDL. A total cholesterol from a nonfasting sample of less than 200 mg/dL and an HDL cholesterol of greater than 35 mg/dL for men and over 45 mg/dL for women are considered desirable. To determine initial CAD risk, divide the total cholesterol by the HDL cholesterol. If the quotient is less than 4.5, the patient is at lower risk for development of CAD. If a patient has nonfasting cholesterol above 240 mg/dL, a 12 to 14 hour fasting lipid profile should be done to calculate the LDL cholesterol. The treatment plan is then based primarily on the LDL goal.

The target LDL is based on the accumulation of the CAD risk factors and/or presence of known CAD or other atherosclerotic vascular disease (AVD). The NCEP has assigned a point score for the following CAD risk factors:

risk factors worth 1 point each—age in males (≥45 years), age in females (≥55 years), family history of premature CAD, smoking (>10 cigarettes per day), hypertension, low HDL cholesterol (<35 mg/dL), and diabetes mellitus

risk factor worth minus 1 point—high HDL cholesterol (≥60 mg/dL)

If the patient does not already have some form of atherosclerotic vascular disease (e.g., myocardial infarction, coronary angioplasty, coronary bypass surgery, angina, or symptomatic peripheral vascular disease) and the risk factor point score totals two or more, the patient is at high risk for the future development of CAD. The addition of definitely diagnosed left ventricular hypertrophy (LVH) further increases the chance of developing AVD. The target LDL cholesterol levels for diet or drug therapy are as follows:

≤100 mg/dL in patients with CAD or AVD

<130 mg/dL in patients with two or more CAD risk factors

<160 mg/dL in patients with less than two CAD risk factors

Normal triglyceride values are between 150 and 200 mg/dL. Triglycerides are measured with a fasting blood sample. Triglycerides cannot be accurately measured postprandially (after a meal) because some patients take up to 12 hours to fully clear chylomicrons from their serum. Therapy aims to restore serum triglyceride values to within the normal range (see Table 33–1).

Risk factors must be identified and corrected when possible. Modifiable risk factors include low HDL cholesterol, smoking, diabetes mellitus, and hypertension. Data support tight diabetic control, systolic and diastolic blood pressure management, and smoking cessation to reduce the risk of CAD. There is some controversy about whether raising HDL reduces the risk of developing CAD or if the risk calculation should be based on only baseline HDL. Exercise, especially running and swimming, has been shown to elevate HDL cholesterol and decrease LDL cholesterol. Thus, an exercise program is instituted when appropriate.

Primary causes of hyperlipidemia, such as hypothyroidism, uncontrolled diabetes, nephrotic syndrome, hepatitis, and exogenous corticosteroids, should also be considered. Additionally, excess alcohol ingestion can exacerbate hypertriglyceridemia. Young adults should follow stringent diet and exercise regimens and avoid drug therapy unless there is a strong family history for early CAD.

DIET THERAPY

Diet is the cornerstone of treatment for managing elevated blood lipids. Patients with hyperlipidemia may be referred to a clinical dietitian or nutritionist for an evaluation of the patient's current eating patterns so changes can be made in the diet that will improve blood lipid levels. The American Heart Association (AHA) recommends a Step I diet as the first intervention, followed by a Step II diet if the first step is unsuccessful (Table 33–2).

While the AHA recommends fat intake as a percent of total calories, a more simple approach is to assign a daily

Table 33–2. DIETARY THERAPY

Dietary Component	Percent Calories*	
	Step I	Step II
Saturated fat†	8–10%	<7%
Polyunsaturated fat‡	Up to 10%	Up to 10%
Monounsaturated fat§	Up to 15%	Up to 15%
Total fat	≤30%	≤30%
Carbohydrates	55% or more	55% or more
Protein	About 15%	About 15%
Cholesterol	<300 mg/day	<200 mg/day

*Total calories: As required to achieve desired weight.
†Saturated fat is found primarily in foods of animal origin, in dairy products, and in some plant products (cocoa butter, palm oil, coconut).
‡Polyunsaturated fat (omega 6 in vegetable oils and omega 3 in fish oils) is a good substitute for saturated fat because it lowers total and LDL cholesterol.
§Monounsaturated fat found in olive oil lowers LDL and either maintains or raises HDL.

calorie requirement (based on height, weight, and frame size) and then use the following formula:

$$\text{Daily fat intake (g)} = \frac{\text{Daily calorie intake (kcal/day)} \times 30\%}{9 \text{ kcal/g of fat}}$$

Using this formula, on an 1800 kcal/day diet, the maximum daily amount of fat that can be ingested is 60 grams.

In patients with isolated hypercholesterolemia, the total daily fat intake should fall between 55 and 65 grams. In patients with hypertriglyceridemia, a lower fat intake is usually recommended. Other diet modifications include reducing intake of concentrated sweets and moderating use of alcohol and salt. If dietary therapy is unsuccessful after a 6-month trial, drug therapy is instituted.

DRUG THERAPY

The primary antihyperlipidemic agents—bile acid sequestrants (colestipol and cholestyramine), 3-hydroxy-3-methylglutaryl coenzyme A (HMG-CoA) reductase inhibitors (lovastatin, pravastatin, simvastatin, and fluvastatin), fibric acid derivatives (clofibrate and gemfibrozil), and nicotinic acid (niacin, vitamin B₃)—affect the lipoprotein fractions in different ways. They are not uniformly effective in reducing serum cholesterol and LDL, which is required to decrease the risk of heart disease. The bile acid sequestrants, niacin, and HMG-CoA reductase inhibitors are used to reduce cholesterol levels. The fibric acid derivatives lower triglycerides more than cholesterol. In cases where the triglycerides are elevated over 300 mg/dL, in the presence of normal or elevated cholesterol, therapy is aimed at lowering the triglycerides first. Drugs that primarily lower cholesterol may raise the triglyceride levels if they are not normalized first. Combination therapy may give added results. For example, a bile acid sequestrant in combination with an HMG-CoA reductase inhibitor is effective in lowering the serum lipids of patients with familial hypercholesterolemia. Non-

Initial Drug Therapy for Hyperlipidemia

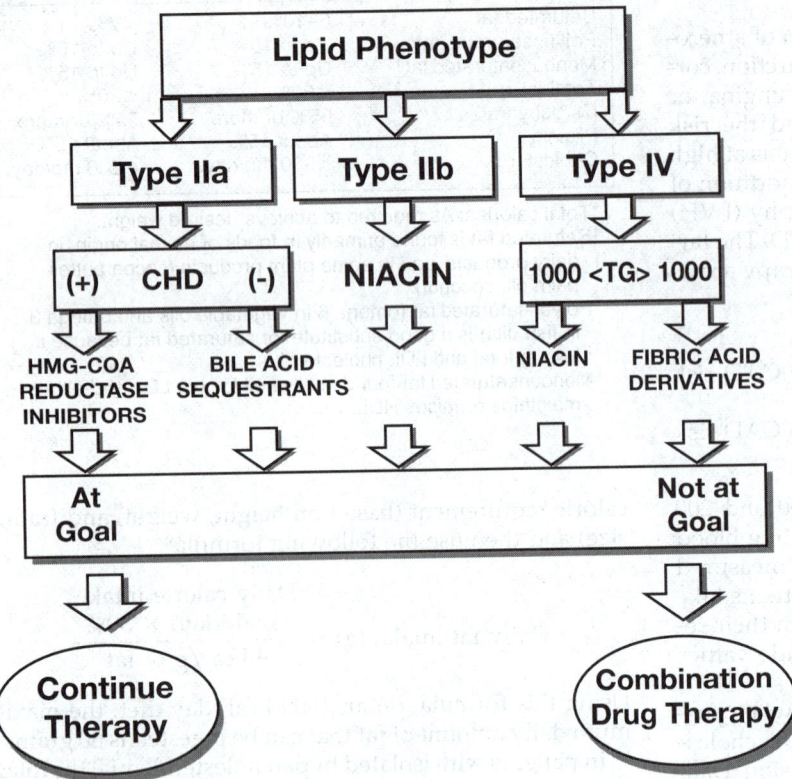

Figure 33–1. Initial drug therapy for hyperlipidemias.

pharmacologic therapies (e.g., diet, weight reduction, and exercise) are continued throughout drug therapy.

A typical decision plan for drug therapy is shown in Figure 33–1. Patients are treated according to their phenotype: IIa, isolated hypercholesterolemia; IIb, combined hypercholesterolemia and hypertriglyceridemia; and IV, isolated hypertriglyceridemia. For phenotypes IIa and IIb, an additional decision point is cardiac status. Patients with known cardiac disorders require the most aggressive therapy.

BILE ACID SEQUESTRANTS

The bile acid sequestrants—**colestipol (Colestid)** and **cholestyramine (Questran, Prevalite Powder)**—are anionic exchange resins that bind bile acids in the small intestine to form an insoluble complex that is excreted in the feces (Fig. 33–2). This leads to decreased enterohepatic cycling of the bile acids, preventing their absorption. As a result, the liver must synthesize new bile acid from cholesterol, which decreases LDL cholesterol levels 10% to 20%. A decrease in LDL is apparent in 4 to 7 days, and the decline in cholesterol is evident by 1 month. No significant increase in HDL occurs, but a 5% to 20% rise in serum triglyceride levels may occur during the first weeks of therapy. Therefore, bile acid sequestrants are not administered to patients with triglyceride levels above 400 mg/dL.

Cholestyramine is available as tablets or powder, and colestipol is available as tablets or granules. Tablets are swallowed whole, not cut, chewed, or crushed. The powder and granules are mixed in liquids, soups, cereals, or pulpy fruits such as applesauce or crushed pineapple. These drugs are featured in Table 33–3.

USES

Because of their efficacy the bile acid sequestrants are often used as first-line drugs in the treatment of hypercholesterolemia in adults. Children who have severe familial hyperlipidemia (FH) are usually treated with only one of these products.

CONTRAINDICATIONS AND PRECAUTIONS

The bile acid sequestrants are used cautiously in patients with bowel obstruction or severe constipation because of

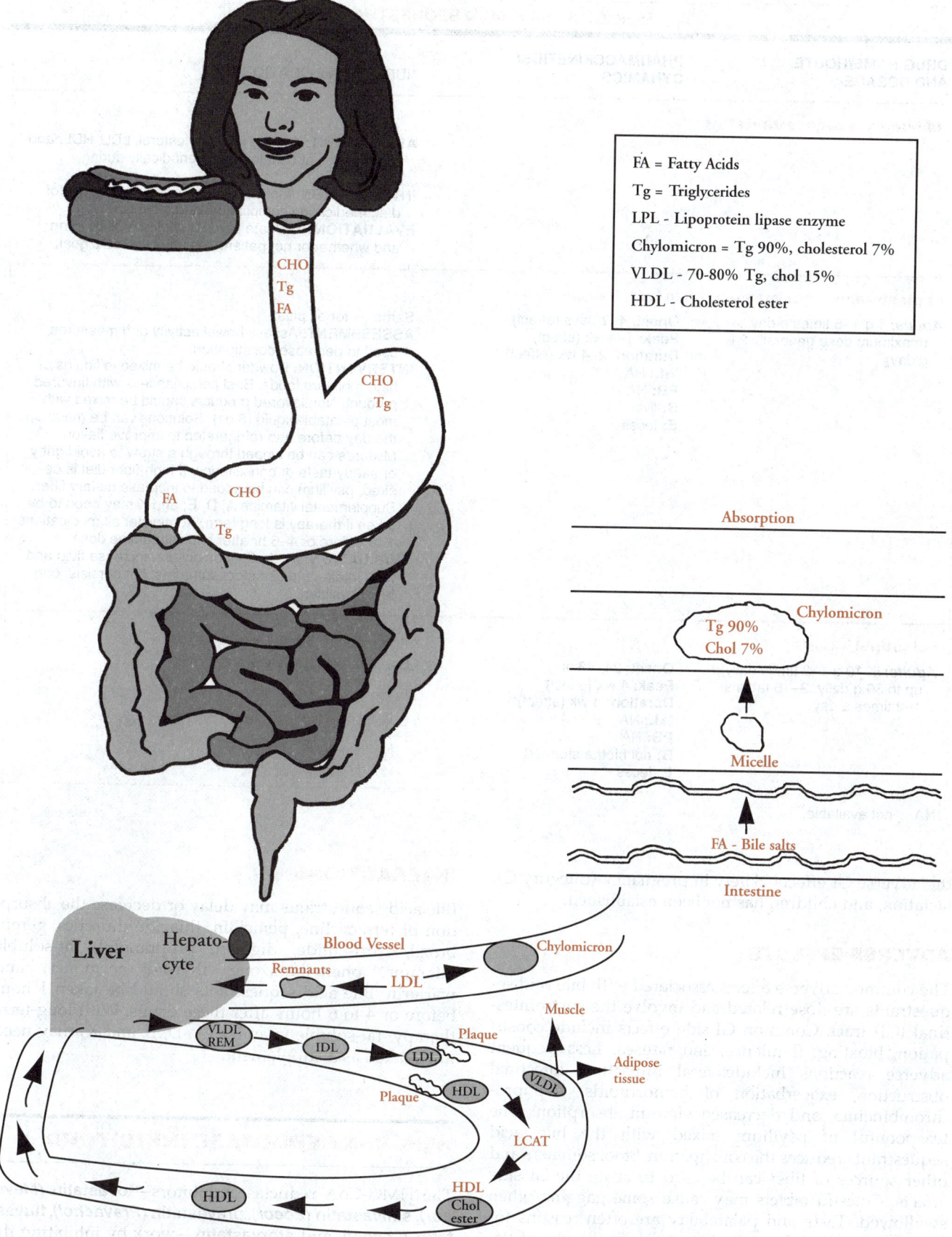

FA = Fatty Acids

Tg = Triglycerides

LPL - Lipoprotein lipase enzyme

Chylomicron = Tg 90%, cholesterol 7%

VLDL - 70-80% Tg, chol 15%

HDL - Cholesterol ester

Figure 33–2. Mechanism of action of bile acid sequestrants (cholestyramine and colestipol). These drugs combine with bile salts and prevent emulsification and absorption of both cholesterol and triglycerides.

Table 33–3. BILE ACID SEQUESTRANTS

DRUG NAME/ROUTE AND DOSAGE	PHARMACOKINETICS/ DYNAMICS	NURSING IMPLICATIONS
all bile acid sequestrants		**ASSESSMENT:** Assess total cholesterol, LDL, HDL, and triglycerides at baseline and periodically during therapy. **INTERVENTION:** Instruct patient on the importance of diet, medication compliance, and exercise. **EVALUATION:** Evaluate percent cholesterol lowering and whether or not patient has achieved LDL goal.
cholestyramine: (Questran, Questran Light, Prevalite Powder) ***Adults:*** 4 g 1–6 times a day. (maximum dose generally 24 g/day).	**Onset:** 4–7 days (effect) **Peak:** 1–4 wk (effect) **Duration:** 2–4 wk (effect) **½L:** NA **PB:** NA **B:** liver **E:** feces	Same as for all plus: **ASSESSMENT:** Assess bowel activity and measures used to decrease constipation. **INTERVENTION:** Powder should be mixed in liquids or high-moisture foods. Best compliance is with flavored product. Nonflavored products should be mixed with most palatable liquid (8 oz). Solutions can be made up the day before and refrigerated to improve flavor. Mixtures can be sipped through a straw to avoid gritty or sandy taste or consistency. If high-fiber diet is desired, psyllium can be added to increase dietary fiber. Supplemental vitamins A, D, E, and K may need to be taken if therapy is long term. Administer all medications 1 hr before or 4–6 hr after cholestyramine dose. **EVALUATION:** If constipation occurs, increase fluid and fiber intake and use stool softeners. If it persists, contact physician.
colestipol (Colestid) ***Adults:*** 5–10 g 1–2 times daily, up to 30 g daily; 2–16 tablets 1–2 times a day.	**Onset:** 24–48 hr **Peak:** 4 wk (effect) **Duration:** 4 wk (effect) **½L:** NA **PB:** NA **B:** not biotransformed **E:** feces	Same as for cholestyramine.

NA = not available.

the adverse GI effects. Safety in pregnancy (category C), lactation, and children has not been established.

ADVERSE EFFECTS

The common adverse effects associated with bile acid sequestrants are dose related and involve the gastrointestinal (GI) tract. Common GI side effects include constipation, bloating, flatulence, and nausea. Less frequent adverse reactions include fecal impaction, intestinal obstruction, exacerbation of hemorrhoids, hypoprothrombinemia, and decreased vitamin absorption. One teaspoonful of psyllium mixed with the bile acid sequestrants reduces the constipation. Stool softeners and other sources of fiber can be used to abate the GI side effects. Colestid tablets may cause some gagging when swallowed. Taste and palatability are often reasons for noncompliance and can be improved by the use of flavored products or mixing the bile acid sequestrant with various juices.

INTERACTIONS

Bile acid sequestrants may delay or decrease the absorption of tetracycline, penicillin, thiazide diuretics, gemfibrozil, furosemide, digoxin, propranolol, fat-soluble vitamins, phenylbutazone, thyroid hormones, and warfarin. Bile acid sequestrants should be taken 1 hour before or 4 to 6 hours after these drugs. With long-term therapy, fat-soluble vitamins (A, D, E, and K) may need to be taken as a supplement.

HMG-CoA REDUCTASE INHIBITORS

The HMG-CoA reductase inhibitors—**lovastatin (Mevacor)**, **simvastatin (Zocor)**, **pravastatin (Pravachol)**, **fluvastatin (Lescol)**, and **atorvastatin**—work by inhibiting the rate-limiting enzyme, HMG-CoA reductase, in the cholesterol biosynthesis pathway. This results in the re-

Table 33–4. HMG-CoA REDUCTASE INHIBITORS

DRUG NAME/ROUTE AND DOSAGE	PHARMACOKINETICS/ DYNAMICS	NURSING IMPLICATIONS
lovastatin (Mevacor)		
Adults: 20 mg/day PO with evening meal. Maximum dose 80 mg daily. Dose may be administered bid for slightly increased efficacy.	**Onset:** 3–7 days (initial action) **Peak:** 2–4 hr **Duration:** 24 hr **½L:** 1.5–2 hr **PB:** 95%–98% **B:** liver **E:** 10% urine, 83% feces	**ASSESSMENT:** Assess total cholesterol, LDL, HDL, and triglycerides at baseline and periodically during therapy. Assess baseline lab values—CPK, renal and hepatic studies. Assess for pregnancy (category X). **INTERVENTION:** Instruct patient on the importance of diet, medication compliance, and exercise. Take with meals to increase bioavailability. **EVALUATION:** Evaluate percent cholesterol lowering and whether patient has achieved LDL goal. Evaluate for symptoms of myopathy (prolonged muscle pain or weakness, visual difficulties) and notify physician if these occur.
simvastatin (Zocor)		
Adults: 5–10 mg/day PO as single dose in evening. Maximum dose 40 mg daily. **Elderly:** 5 mg daily.	**Onset:** 1 hr **Peak:** 1.3–2.4 hr **Duration:** NA **½L:** 15.6 hrs **PB:** 95% **B:** liver **E:** 13% urine, 60% feces	Same as for lovastatin.
pravastatin (Pravachol)		
Adults: 10–20 mg/day PO as single dose in evening. Maximum dose 40 mg daily. **Elderly:** 10 mg hs.	**Onset:** 1 hr (1 wk for effect) **Peak:** 1–1.5 hr (4 wk for effect) **Duration:** 48 hr **½L:** 77 hr **PB:** 43%–48% **B:** liver **E:** 20% urine, 70% feces	Same as for lovastatin.
fluvastatin (Lescol)		
Adults: 20–40 mg/day PO as single dose in evening. Dose may be administered bid for slightly increased efficacy.	**Onset:** 3–7 days (effect) **Peak:** 0.5–1 hr (level); 6 wk (effect) **Duration:** 3–4 hr (level); 4–6 wk (effect) **½L:** 1.2 hr **PB:** >98% **B:** liver **E:** 5% urine, 90% feces	Same as for lovastatin.
atorvastatin (Lipitor)		
Adults: 5–10 mg/day PO as single dose in evening. Maximum dose 80 mg daily.	**Onset:** 3–7 days (effect) **Peak:** 2–4 wk (effect) **Duration:** 2–6 wk (effect) **½L:** 13–18 hr **PB:** NA **B:** liver **E:** feces	Same as for lovastatin.

NA = not available.

duction of endogenous cholesterol production, which in turn upregulates LDL receptor activity and increases the clearance of LDL from the plasma. These drugs lower LDL cholesterol 18% to 45%, decrease plasma triglycerides 7% to 22%, and raise HDL cholesterol 5% to 8%. These drugs are featured in Table 33–4.

Lovastatin and simvastatin are lipophilic, cross the blood-brain barrier, and have a long half-life. Fluvastatin and pravastatin are hydrophilic, do not cross the blood-brain barrier, and have short plasma half-lives. Pharmacokinetic information is found in Table 33–4.

USES

These drugs are used to control lipid serum levels in primary hypercholesterolemia. Clinical studies show that monotherapy with HMG-CoA reductase inhibitors or in combination with other antilhyperlipidemic agents can slow the progression of atherosclerosis (Waters, 1994). Decreased total mortality and mortality due to CAD-related death has been demonstrated in other studies.

CONTRAINDICATIONS AND PRECAUTIONS

The HMG-CoA reductase inhibitors are contraindicated in patients with active liver disease or unexplained persistent elevated liver function tests and in pregnancy (category X). These agents are used cautiously in patients with liver dysfunction or in those who consume large quantities of alcohol. The HMG-CoA reductase inhibitors may increase serum transaminases up to three times the upper limit of normal. Safety in lactation and children has not been established.

ADVERSE EFFECTS

The most common adverse effects are the GI complaints: dyspepsia, flatulence, abdominal pain, constipation, and diarrhea. Elevation of hepatic enzymes occurs in 1 to 2% of patients. Myopathy occurs uncommonly, although the incidence increases in patients taking cyclosporine, erythromycin, gemfibrozil, or niacin concurrently, especially with lovastatin. Myopathy may last weeks to months after discontinuing the offending drug. Slit-lamp examinations are no longer recommended to rule out lens opacities when these drugs are administered. Central nervous system side effects that may occur include insomnia, headache, and fatigue.

INTERACTIONS

There are numerous interactions attributed to the HMG-CoA reductase inhibitors. Lovastatin and simvastatin are metabolized by the cytochrome P-450 enzyme system in the liver and may compete for metabolism with drugs such as quinidine, warfarin, erythromycin, and cyclosporine. Elevated levels of the HMG-CoA reductase inhibitors can result in myopathy and possibly rhabdomyolysis. *Rhabdomyolysis* is an acute, sometimes fatal disease, characterized by destruction of muscular tissue. Gemfibrozil and lovastatin, simvastatin, or pravastatin (but not fluvastatin) have caused myopathy and rhabdomyolysis. Although many physicians use the combination, it should be approached with caution. Bile acid sequestrants given concurrently with HMG-CoA reductase inhibitors may inhibit the absorption of the bile acid sequestrant, but usually not the overall clinical effectiveness.

▼ CLINICAL ALERT

Patients started on HMG-CoA reductase inhibitors are taught the signs and symptoms of myopathy. They should contact their provider if any unusual muscle aches

persist for more than 24 hours. The drug can be stopped and then restarted after symptoms subside. Creatinine phosphokinase (CPK) levels assist in the diagnosis of myopathies, but are often normal despite symptoms.

FIBRIC ACID DERIVATIVES

The fibric acid derivatives—**clofibrate** *(Atromid-S)* and **gemfibrozil** *(Lopid)*—lower serum triglyceride and VLDL levels. Clofibrate appears to accelerate the catabolism of VLDL to LDL and to decrease hepatic synthesis of VLDL. Gemfibrozil inhibits peripheral lipolysis and decreases the hepatic extraction of free fatty acids, resulting in a reduction in hepatic triglyceride production. Fibric acid derivatives lower triglycerides 20% to 50% and increase HDL cholesterol 10% to 15%. In addition, if LDL levels are elevated, they decrease slightly. Gemfibrozil is featured in Table 33–5.

USES

Clofibrate is indicated for patients with type III hyperlipidemia (primary dysbetalipoproteinemia) who do not respond to diet therapy. Both clofibrate and gemfibrozil may be used for hypertriglyceridemia (types IV and V hyperlipidemia) in patients who present a risk of pancreatitis and who do not respond to diet therapy.

CONTRAINDICATIONS AND PRECAUTIONS

Gemfibrozil and clofibrate are contraindicated in renal and hepatic dysfunction and primary biliary cirrhosis, because already elevated cholesterol levels from these conditions may increase. These drugs are also contraindicated in pregnancy and lactation. The fibric acid derivatives are used cautiously in history of jaundice, hepatic disease, peptic ulcer disease, gout, and peripheral vascular disease.

ADVERSE EFFECTS

Gastrointestinal side effects such as abdominal pain, dyspepsia, and diarrhea are common in patients receiving fibric acid derivatives. Fatigue, eczema, vertigo, and headache may also occur. Fibrates can cause cholelithiasis, particularly in patients with a history of gallstones. In patients taking clofibrate, the risk of developing cholelithiasis and cholecystitis requiring surgery is doubled. In clinical trials, clofibrate caused an increased incidence of gallbladder disease, cardiac dysrhythmias, noncardiac-related deaths, and total mortality. Thus, clofibrate is rarely used today. Myopathy has been reported with gemfibrozil monotherapy.

INTERACTIONS

Because of the high risk of myositis and renal failure, fibric acid derivative and HMG-CoA reductase inhibitor

Table 33–5. FIBRIC ACID DERIVATIVES AND NIACIN

DRUG NAME/ROUTE AND DOSAGE	PHARMACOKINETICS/ DYNAMICS	NURSING IMPLICATIONS
FIBRIC ACID DERIVATIVES		
gemfibrozil (Lopid)		
Adults: 600 mg bid.	**Onset:** 2–5 days (effect) **Peak:** 2–4 wk (effect) **Duration:** 2–6 wk (effect) **½L:** 1.5 hr **PB:** 95% **B:** liver **E:** urine 70%, feces 6%	**ASSESSMENT:** Assess total cholesterol, LDL, HDL, and triglycerides at baseline and periodically during therapy. Assess prothrombin time, GI symptoms, liver function studies, and muscle tone periodically. Assess for pregnancy (category B). **INTERVENTION:** Instruct patient on importance of diet, medication compliance, and exercise. Administer 30 min before meals. **Patient Teaching**—Warn patient to observe caution while performing activities requiring alertness because drug may cause dizziness or blurred vision. **EVALUATION:** Evaluate percent cholesterol lowering and whether patient has achieved LDL goal. Notify physician if continued stomach or epigastric pain, diarrhea, nausea, or vomiting occurs.
NIACIN		
nicotinic acid (vitamin B$_3$) (Niacor) (Nicobid) (Nicolar) (Slo-Niacin)		
Adults: 1–8 g/day PO (IR) given with meals in divided doses or 1.3 g/day PO (SR) given with meals in divided doses.	**Onset:** several hours (triglyceride levels); several days (cholesterol levels) **Peak:** 45 min (serum levels) **Duration:** 2–6 wk (effect) **½L:** 20–30 min **PB:** NA **B:** liver **E:** urine	Same as for all plus: **ASSESSMENT:** Assess baseline liver function tests, glucose, and uric acid. Assess for pregnancy (category B). **INTERVENTION:** Take with meals, increase doses slowly, or pretreat with 325 mg aspirin given 30 min before dose to prevent flushing. **EVALUATION:** Evaluate liver function tests; if hepatic transaminases greater than 3 times upper limit of normal on two serial samples, consult physician.

NA = not available.

combinations should be avoided unless patients are under the care of experts. Concurrent clofibrate and warfarin can increase prothrombin time and cause fatal hemorrhage. Concurrent gemfibrozil and warfarin may result in increased anticoagulation. In combination with several sulfonylureas, clofibrate has caused hypoglycemia. Clofibrate significantly interacts with several drugs, resulting in hypoglycemia when added to sulfonylureas.

OTHER ANTIHYPERLIPIDEMIC AGENTS

Other antihyperlipidemic agents include **nicotinic acid (niacin, vitamin B$_3$)** and **fish oils.**

○ **Nicotinic acid** (NicoBid, Niacor, Nicolar, Slo-Niacin, and others), the acid form of niacin, appears to inhibit VLDL production in the liver, resulting in lowered VLDL levels and therefore lower LDL levels. Niacin can lower LDL cholesterol levels 15% to 30%, raise HDL cholesterol levels 15% to 40%, and reduce serum triglycerides 25% to 50%. Nicotinic acid is featured in Table 33–5.

USES   Because of its effects on various lipoprotein classes, nicotinic acid is useful in mixed dyslipidemias. Niacin is not commonly used alone, but in combination with other antihyperlipidemics including the bile acid sequestrants, HMG-CoA reductase inhibitors, and fibric acid derivatives. Niacin has been shown to improve the clinical outcome of patients with known CAD.

Nicotinic acid is available as sustained-release (SR) and immediate-release (IR) tablets or capsules. Giving 3.0 grams of IR niacin can have the same effect on LDL that occurs with 1.5 grams of the SR product. This suggests a potency difference between the two dosage forms. In addition, there are definite pharmacokinetic differences between the various SR products. Additional pharmacokinetic information is found in Table 33–5.

CONTRAINDICATIONS AND PRECAUTIONS   There may be an increased risk of hepatotoxicity with the sustained-release niacin product. Nicotinic acid is contraindicated in renal and hepatic dysfunction, active peptic ulcer disease, hypotension, pregnancy, and lactation. It is used cautiously in history of jaundice, hepatic disease, diabetes, and gout. Because both diabetes and gout can generally be managed despite concomitant niacin therapy, cautious use of this drug rather than avoidance in patients with these diseases is suggested. Patients with non-insulin-dependent diabetes mellitus often develop a glucose intolerance syndrome when niacin is administered. There may be more frequent gouty attacks, although this is not a contraindication to use of nicotinic acid.

ADVERSE EFFECTS Frequent adverse effects are noted with niacin. About 15 to 60 minutes after a dose, prostaglandin-mediated effects, including cutaneous flushing and a sensation of warmth (especially of the face and upper body) and pruritus, can emerge. Taking nicotinic acid on a full stomach or administering 325 mg of aspirin 30 minutes before the nicotinic acid dose may help ameliorate the cutaneous flushing. Pruritus can be managed with diphenhydramine (Benadryl). Dyspepsia, rash, dry skin, and acanthosis nigricans have been reported. Dizziness may also occur, and patients should change body positions slowly.

Niacin can cause drug-induced hepatitis. This is manifested by the severe elevation of the hepatic transaminases (serum aspartate and alanine transferinase, or AST and ALT respectively, to levels greater than three times the upper limit of normal on two serial samples. The SR formulations commonly cause mild elevations of the transaminases and less commonly chemical hepatitis. Drug-induced hepatitis is rare with IR niacin, so experts often recommend it as the only formulation that should be used clinically. However, SR niacin is better tolerated and lowers LDL cholesterol levels more than IR niacin. Hepatotoxicity can be minimized by using only one brand of SR niacin and by regular monitoring of the transaminase levels.

INTERACTIONS Niacin, when given concurrently with some HMG-CoA reductase inhibitors, can increase the incidence of myositis. The reported incidence of myopathy is 2% when niacin is given in combination with lovastatin. Niacin-associated myopathy has not been reported in combination with pravastatin, simvastatin, or fluvastatin.

○ **Fish oils** contain omega-3 fatty acids, which are thought to reduce the incidence or progression of ischemic heart disease. The mechanism of action is unknown, but omega-3 fatty acid fish oils may be effective in lowering VLDL levels, lowering serum triglycerides (up to 50%), and may slightly increase HDL levels. The action is due to two ingredients: eicosapentaenoic acid (EPA) and docosahexaenoic (DHA) acid.

Fish oils are considered a second-line agent and used as an adjunct in management of severe hypertriglyceridemia in patients inadequately responsive to a low-fat diet, niacin, and/or gemfibrozil. The side effects are mild and predominantly related to taste and odor. Some diabetic patients may experience exacerbation of their disease.

USING THE NURSING PROCESS

The positive relationship between cholesterol level and risk of coronary heart disease has led most researchers and health professionals to conclude that the cholesterol level of the U.S. population is too high. Cholesterol levels above 200 mg/dL have been demonstrated to increase risk of CAD.

Nurses are often frontline educators for people in the moderate- to high-risk category. Nurses must (1) understand the importance of cholesterol as a cardiovascular risk factor, (2) be familiar with cholesterol-lowering approaches, and (3) be able to teach and counsel patients and their families about lowering cholesterol. This education is multifaceted and includes diet, weight loss, exercise, and drug therapy. The approach is always individualized, based on the patient's risk factors.

ASSESSMENT

- Obtain a thorough nursing history to develop the database. The information obtained is included in Table 33–6.
- Rule out underlying causes of the disease. Hyperlipidemia that is secondary to hypothyroidism, diabetes, or liver disease does not respond well to therapies until the primary problems are addressed.
- Assess any potential for cardiac disease and review CAD risk factors. The presence of two or more risk factors may change the assignment of risk category, which will affect the treatment plan.
- Obtain and assess laboratory data for clinical trends. Cholesterol screening facilitates the assignment to a relative-risk group. Patients with borderline to high total cholesterol levels should be further evaluated by a 12-hour fasting lipid profile. Therefore, the nurse must be familiar with the tests included in a 12-hour fasting lipid profile. The 12-hour fast is imperative, as it takes that time for chylomicrons to clear from the circulation.
- If the patient requires diet or drug therapy, the nurse assists in defining a treatment goal. Based on the presence or absence of risk factors, an LDL goal is defined. Once a patient has had nutritional instruction from a dietitian, the nurse's role in maintaining compliance begins. The nurse also plays a role in encouraging exercise regimens and identifying psychosocial barriers. Once maximum dietary interventions have been achieved, pharmacotherapy is considered.

NURSING DIAGNOSIS

- Establish the nursing diagnoses to plan, implement, and evaluate nursing care. Typical nursing diagnoses for a patient receiving antihyperlipidemic agents include Knowledge Deficit, Altered Nutrition, Non-compliance, and Impaired Adjustment (see Table 33–6).

PLANNING AND INTERVENTION

- Plan the nursing-care goals from the nursing diagnosis. The goals of nursing intervention for the patient who requires antihyperlipidemic medications are included in Table 33–6. Because hyperlipoproteinemia is often familial, other family members are

Table 33–6. NURSING PROCESS FOR PATIENT REQUIRING ANTIHYPERLIPIDEMIC AGENTS

Assessment

Assess current dietary patterns, including amounts and types of food eaten.
Assess current weight and percent of body fat.
Assess lifestyle patterns, e.g., amount of physical/leisure activity and amount of stress.
Assess patient and family history of smoking, diabetes, hypothyroidism, and diseases such as angina, myocardial infarction, peripheral vascular disease, and hypertension.

Nursing Diagnosis: Knowledge Deficit

RELATED TO: Lack of exposure to or unfamiliarity with resources, information misinterpretation.
AS EVIDENCED BY: Questions, statement of misconceptions, inaccurate follow-through on instruction, development of preventable complications.

Desired Outcomes/Evaluation Criteria

Verbalizes understanding of condition/disease process and therapeutic regimen. Initiates necessary lifestyle changes.

Nursing Actions	Rationale
Discuss normal pathophysiology of cardiovascular system and information about patient variance.	Becoming knowledgeable about disease process and expectations can facilitate adherence to prescribed treatment regimen.
Provide information about drug action, administration, and side effects.	Understanding how the drug works can help patient to realize importance of taking it as prescribed.
Discuss side effects that need to be reported to the physician, e.g., bleeding gums. Stress importance of follow-through care and motivation.	Promotes opportunity for patient to assume control over own treatment and seek help in timely manner.
Review dietary restrictions and assist patient to plan a low-fat, low-cholesterol diet, including the use of fiber sources. Refer for dietary consultation if indicated.	Patients may believe they can continue to eat as they please as long as they take their medication. However, adherence to diet can reduce level of serum cholesterol significantly. In addition, reducing body weight decreases cardiac workload.
Encourage development of an exercise/activity program.	Supports weight loss/maintenance, improves muscle tone and feelings of general well being.
Encourage supplementation of vitamins A, D, K, and E.	Antilipidemics impair absorption of fat-soluble vitamins.
Discuss need to stop smoking and assist with plan for cessation.	Smoking increases vasoconstriction, impairs gas exchange.
Identify other cardiac risk factors that may be present and problem-solve solutions, e.g., stress management.	Promotes general/cardiovascular wellness.

Nursing Diagnosis: Impaired Adjustment

RELATED TO: Disability requiring alterations in lifestyle.
AS EVIDENCED BY: Weight gain, hypercholesterolemia/hypertriglyceridemia.

Desired Outcomes/Evaluation Criteria

Initiates lifestyle changes that permit adaptation to new life situation.

Nursing Actions	Rationale
Discuss identified changes that must to be made to achieve reduction of cholesterol/arteriosclerosis. Assist patient to develop a plan of action to meet needs.	Lack of symptoms, cost of drug therapy, presence of side effects, e.g., nausea/constipation. Thinking about how changes can be accomplished, with as little impact on lifestyle as possible, helps patient to cooperate with treatment regimen.
Encourage expression of feelings and acknowledge realities of difficulty of making required lifestyle changes.	Promotes awareness and acceptance of feelings and identifies areas of need.

encouraged to have regular physical examinations and blood tests. Dietary restrictions of cholesterol may be beneficial to the whole family and are encouraged by the nurse.

Patient Teaching

• Teach the patient and family about the hazards of smoking. There is clear evidence in the literature that smokers have a greater incidence of coronary artery disease and a higher mortality. Smoking reduction is highly recommended and supported. Stress that patients who stop smoking often have a reduction in serum lipid levels that may prolong their lives and prevent further complications from coronary artery, cerebral, or peripheral vascular disease. Although risk factors carry the same point score, not all risk factors are equal when defining aggressiveness of

---

Table 33–7. PATIENT TEACHING INFORMATION—ANTIHYPERLIPIDEMIC AGENTS

Dear Patient:

This drug has been ordered for you. This is what you should know about your drug to get the most from your therapy.

☐ 1. Antihyperlipidemic drugs are taken to reduce blood cholesterol and/or triglyceride levels.

☐ 2. Antihyperlipidemic drugs are taken until your high lipid level is lowered, or possibly for the rest of your life.

☐ 3. When taking cholestyramine (Questran) or colestipol, mix the dry powder with fluids before taking. Any liquid—water, fruit juice, carbonated drinks—and even soft fruits like applesauce can be used. When mixing, drop the powder onto liquid and allow it to stand for about 2 minutes, then stir until it is well mixed. After taking the drug, rinse the glass with liquid and drink this as well, to ensure that the entire dose is received.

☐ 4. Antihyperlipidemic powders (colestipol or cholestyramine) are generally separated from other drugs by taking them 1 hour before or 4 hours after other drugs.

☐ 5. Many antihyperlipidemic agents are to be taken with meals, although some are taken at bedtime without regard to food.

☐ 6. Interactions may occur between antihyperlipidemic agents and other drugs. Always check with your pharmacist or physician before adding another drug or taking over-the-counter products.

☐ 7. Do not skip a dose; however, if a dose is forgotten, do *not* double the dose to catch up.

☐ 8. The side effects of your particular drug may include constipation. Please eat a high-bulk, high-fiber diet to avoid constipation.

☐ 9. Antihyperlipidemic agents may take 1 to 3 months before they begin to lower serum lipid levels. Your physician will order frequent blood tests to check your blood lipid levels. It is also important that you continue to be on a low-cholesterol diet as ordered by your physician.

☐ 10. Your physician may order vitamins to prevent vitamin deficiencies. Take these as ordered.

☐ 11. Store your drugs in a tight, light-resistant container.

☐ 12. Do not stop or change your dose without consulting your physician.

---

unsaturated fats such as olive oil is recommended, although the fat supplied by olive oil must be included in the total daily allowance. Polyunsaturated oils such as soybean, sunflower, safflower, or canola oils are preferred over oils higher in saturated fats. Moderate exercise and a low-cholesterol and low-saturated-fat diet are keys to the nondrug approaches to hyperlipidemia. Additional patient teaching information is found in Table 33–7.

EVALUATION

- Evauate the effectiveness of antihyperlipidemic medications by a predetermined list of evaluation outcome criteria. These evaluation criteria are developed on an individual basis through discussion among the nurse, patient, and family. The information from the database, obtained in the original assessment, is used to formulate the criteria for evaluation. Typical outcome evaluation criteria are included in Table 33–6.

- Work with the patient and family to ensure their assistance and support. Most patients, once they understand the importance of their continued medical treatment, usually are compliant. The fact that they may have previously had a life-threatening coronary or cerebral event may also improve their compliance. The primary reason for noncompliance is usually forgetting the medication (see Chapter 2). Noncompliance with the rest of the treatment regimen can also occur. This might include not altering or modifying diet, smoking, or lifestyle.

- Evaluate the side effects of the medications. If the patient notes any unusual symptoms, such as myositis, visual changes, or GI upset, they should be reported to the physician or nurse. Typical issues are helping the patient cope with niacin-induced flushing and constipation caused by the bile acid sequestrants.

  Encourage the patient to discuss side effects with the physician who prescribed the drug before stopping the drug and giving up on controlling his or her blood cholesterol. The patient should also be aware that a number of drugs are available and that the side effects of drug therapy need to be manageable.

- Evaluate the patient's understanding of the therapy. The patient needs a realistic view of the therapy, including an understanding that treatment may be lifelong. Caution the patient that the drug(s) will lower cholesterol for only as long as he or she takes the medication and follows a low-fat diet. Stress the importance of continued medical care and continued reduction of risk factors.

- All other evaluation criteria are assessed and evaluated before the patient leaves the health care environment. All previously taught material is reviewed and updated with patient and family, if necessary, to ensure that the patient's knowledge base remains accurate.

The bibliography for this chapter can be found in Appendix B, which begins on page 1054.

---

therapy. Most experts suggest that diabetics and patients with strong family history deserve more aggressive therapy than those without these denominators. Stress that a reasonable approach to all underlying risk factors should be taken, with the understanding that it is still possible that despite all the numbers being right, the patient may still have a coronary event.

- Ensure that the patient has adequate knowledge about the medications and treatment program. Most patients who require lipid-lowering agents self-administer these medications at home. It is important to include dietary teaching in the education program. Many patients think they can eat whatever they like while taking their antihyperlipidemic agent.

- Diet therapy involves several basic diet modifications: reducing total fat, eating more fiber, and decreasing intake of concentrated sweets. Alcohol ingestion in moderation is generally permitted. Teach patients to read food labels for fat content. The new food labels make this simple. Cooking with mono-

CHAPTER REVIEW QUESTIONS*

1. Which of the following compounds contains the largest proportion of lipids?
   a. Low-density lipoproteins (LDL).
   b. High-density lipoproteins (HDL).
   c. Very low density lipoproteins (VLDL).
   d. Intermediate-density lipoproteins (IDL).

2. Cholestyramine (Questran) is a type of antihyperlipidemic agent that:
   a. Combines with bile salts, forming a complex that is excreted in the feces.
   b. Reduces triglyceride levels by inhibiting hepatic synthesis.
   c. Inhibits cholesterol biosynthesis, decreasing total plasma concentration.
   d. Reduces synthesis of VLDL and LDL and increases levels of HDL.

3. Which of the following drugs is used as an adjunct in mixed dyslipidemias?
   a. Colestipol.
   b. Lovastatin.
   c. Nicotinic acid.
   d. Gemfibrozil.

4. Which of the following is *correct* regarding diet?
   a. Dietary intervention should continue even after pharmacologic intervention.
   b. Calorie counting is essential for a low-fat, low-cholesterol diet.
   c. Fat counting is essential for a low-fat, low-cholesterol diet.
   d. All of the above.

5. To reduce unwanted effects related to nicotinic acid therapy, the nurse advises the patient to take which of the following 30 minutes before each dose?
   a. Scopolamine.
   b. Aspirin.
   c. Acetaminophen.
   d. Baking soda in water.

*See Appendix A, which begins on page 1051, for answers.

BUILDING YOUR CRITICAL THINKING SKILLS

HYPERLIPIDEMIA

Case Study 1: Hypertriglyceridemia in males

A 66-year-old man has a history of coronary artery disease, non-insulin and hyerlipidemia. On a routine visit to the clinic he is found to have the following: total cholesterol 258 mg/dL, triglycerides 740 mg/dL, HDL 24 mg/dL; and serum glucose 202 mg/dL. He relates symptoms of frequent urination, thirst, and hunger. The patient is diagnosed with non-insulin-dependent diabetes mellitus (NIDDM).

1. Why is the patient's tryglyceride level elevated?
2. What other data should the nurse collect?

3. What would the nurse include in the patient's plan of care relating to his NIDDM and history of hyperlipidemia?

Case Study 2: Hypertriglyceridemia in females

A 23-year-old white woman comes to the clinic for a routine examination. She has no risk factors for coronary artery disease. Her weight is 190 pounds, and a 24-hour diet recall shows that she is in relative compliance with an AHA Step I diet, with a caloric intake of 1200 kcal/24 hr.

1. What should be the focus of nursing intervention in this patient?
2. What should be included in the patient's plan of care?

UNIT 8

DRUGS AFFECTING THE BLOOD

UNIT OUTLINE

CHAPTER 34

Blood, Blood Components, and Artificial Blood

Merrily A. Kuhn, RNC, PhD

CHAPTER OUTLINE

KEY TERMS

Autologous blood
 transfusion
Autotransfusion
Erythroblastosis fetalis

Human leucocyte antigen
Plasma expanders
Plasmapheresis
Sensitizing lymphocytes

LEARNING OBJECTIVES

After reading this chapter, the student will be able to:

1. Identify blood, blood components, and artificial blood that are commonly administered intravenously.
2. Differentiate among blood and blood components as to mechanism of action, adverse effects, contraindications, and interactions.
3. Identify specific areas to assess in the patient requiring blood, blood components, and artifical blood to formulate appropriate patient outcomes.
4. Plan the nursing interventions necessary to administer blood, blood components, and artificial blood.
5. Evaluate the patient at various stages of treatment to measure effectiveness of nursing interventions.

Hypovolemia develops when there is a loss of fluid volume secondary to blood loss from hemorrhage, burns, surgery, sepsis, or other trauma. An individual can tolerate the gradual loss of up to approximately 25% (1.5 liters of a total body blood volume of 5 to 6 liters) of total blood volume. However, if the loss is sudden, only approximately 10% loss is tolerated before symptoms develop. To support vital functions, blood volume must be replaced. This can be done with plasma expanders, blood, blood components, or artificial blood. *Plasma expanders*, substances not obtained from blood that can expand a patient's blood volume, are discussed fully in Chapter 67.

BLOOD AND ITS COMPONENTS

Blood and its components, featured in Table 34–1, are physiologic substances rather than pharmacologic substances. Blood is produced by the human body and donated by an individual for his or her own later use or for someone else's use. In an *autologous blood transfusion*, blood that has been previously collected from a patient is saved and administered to the same person at a later date or it is collected from a patient during surgery. *Autotransfusion* is a method of returning the patient's own extravasated blood to the circulation: blood is collected during an operation and is tranfused immediately into the circulation of the patient, using specialized equipment. Blood is a living tissue that must be carefully preserved and stored to ensure safe and efficient use. Blood is administered as either a blood component or a blood derivative.

Blood components include red blood cells (RBCs), white blood cells (WBCs), platelets, and plasma. RBCs, WBCs, and platelets are all removed from whole blood through centrifugation or gravitational sedimentation. These products may be given fresh or frozen for use at a later time. All fresh products carry the risk of transmitting infections. Blood derivatives include plasma protein products such as albumin and plasma protein fraction, clotting factors such as fibrinogen, and immunoglobulins. Some derivatives are heat-treated to decrease the transmission of diseases such as hepatitis A, B, or C. Derivatives can be assayed and standardized.

COLLECTION AND SCREENING

Blood Donation and Preservation

As blood is donated by an individual, it enters a sterile plastic collection bag containing 50 mL of a preservative anticoagulant. The preservatives used include citrate phosphate dextrose adenine solution (CPDA-1), which allows storage of blood for 35 days, and allows for synthesis of greater levels of adenosine triphosphate in the transfused blood. The preservative contains citric acid, which prevents clotting by combining with the free calcium in the blood. Patients who receive multiple blood transfusions may need supplemental calcium to assist clotting and to prevent tetany. Patients also need to have their acid-base balance assessed for acidosis because of the accumulation of citric acid and high levels of potassium that leak out of the dying red cells.

Preserved blood with CPDA-1 can be stored at 1° to 6°C for up to 35 days. After 35 days, the RBCs begin to die. (Lifetime for an RBC in the body is 120 days.) Whole blood and its derivatives can be frozen for use at a later time.

▼ **CLINICAL ALERT**

Once blood has been thawed, frozen RBCs are outdated after 24 hours, and plasma is outdated after 2 hours.

The donated blood has the ABO group and Rh factor identified. In addition, blood is tested for hepatitis A, B, and C; syphilis; and human immunodeficiency virus (HIV). Any blood found to be contaminated with any of these diseases is destroyed. Donated blood is then labeled. Information typically found on labels is presented in Table 34–2.

Blood Classification Systems

Blood is classified or typed into four major groups—A (41%), B (9%), AB (3%), and O (47%)—using the ABO system. The RBCs are classified on the basis of either the presence or absence of the specific A or B antigen called *agglutinogens* on their surface. For example, individuals with the A antigen on the surface of their RBCs have type A blood. The individuals in each group have in their sera the corresponding antibody, also referred to as an *agglutinin*, to the RBC antigens they lack. Thus, group A individuals have in their blood serum anti-B agglutinins. If an RBC has antigen B on its surface, it is type B blood and also has anti-A agglutinins. If both antigens are present, it is type AB blood and has neither anti-A nor anti-B agglutinins; if neither antigen is present, it is blood type O and both anti-A and anti-B agglutinins are present.

Another system used to classify blood is the Rh system. It is typically used jointly with the ABO system. Individuals are either Rh negative or Rh positive, depending on whether the Rh_0 (D) antigen is absent or present. Rh antibodies may be produced in the blood after an immunizing event. The event may be a transfusion of Rh-positive blood to a person with Rh-negative blood. This may also occur with the diffusion of blood from an Rh-positive baby to an Rh-negative mother during delivery or miscarriage. The first transfusion event merely causes immunization; only if a second event takes place is there a problem.

When an Rh-negative mother gives birth to her first Rh-positive child, she may become sensitized to Rh antigen absorbed following placental bleeding. Any successive pregnancy with an Rh-positive baby may cause her to produce Rh antibodies, which cross the placenta and destroy fetal red blood cells, causing fetal anemia and even death. This condition, known as *erythroblastosis fetalis* (hemolytic disease of the newborn) is preventable. This process can be prevented by administering Rh_0 (D) immune globulin (RhoGAM) intramuscularly to the mother during the second or third trimester of pregnancy or within 72 hours after delivery of her first Rh-positive child. RhoGAM is a short-acting antibody preparation that coats the fetal RBCs that may have entered the mother's circulation and prevents long-term antibody production.

Type O (Rh⁻) blood, referred to as the universal donor blood, can be administered to all blood types, as it contains no antigens. Type AB (Rh⁺) is known as the universal recipient and can receive all types. Transfusion of blood containing new antigens (e.g., type A blood into a type O recipient) causes formation of antibodies to the new antigen. This is why people can receive only one type of blood unless they receive type O (Rh⁻).

▼ **CLINICAL ALERT**

To minimize the possibility of a transfusion reaction, particularly hemolysis, cross-matching and typing are done prior to transfusion. Typing determines whether or not the blood groups of donor and recipient are matched. In cross-matching, the blood of both donor and recipient are mixed together to determine whether an immune reaction (agglutination or clumping) takes place. If no such reaction occurs, they are considered compatible and the patient can be transfused with this blood. A full cross-match takes about 1 hour to complete. If blood is needed quickly, type-specific cells, matched to the patients ABO and Rh, can be made available in 10 to 20 minutes, but may trigger some minor incompatibilities. In a true emergency, type O (Rh⁻) packed cells may be administered without a cross and type.

Infections Transmitted through Blood

When blood donated by one individual is given to another, there exists the possibility of transmitting certain

Table 34–1. BLOOD PRODUCTS

BLOOD OR BLOOD COMPONENTS (VOLUME)	SHELF LIFE	GENERAL INDICATION	COMPATIBILITY	NURSING CONSIDERATIONS
for all blood products				Obtain baseline vital signs before beginning any blood product. Note expiration date, blood group, and Rh factor to ensure their accuracy. Hang blood products piggyback with normal saline (NS) solution, through special blood tubing with a filter. Monitor drip rate: starts at 20 gtt/min for first 10 min; if no reactions, increase to 50–70 gtt/min. Monitor vital signs and patient for reactions. At conclusion of infusion, again take vital signs and record.
citrated whole human blood USP (500 mL)	35 days	Major blood loss, over 250 mL	Requires ABO to be identical	Transfusion time should not exceed 4 hr; each unit should raise the HCT by 3%.
red blood cells (RBCs, adenine saline added; leukocyte-poor RBCs; frozen-thawed RBCs) (180–330 mL)	Up to 3 yr	Blood loss, anemias	Requires ABO compatibility	May have 50–100 mL of NS added to reduce viscosity. Each unit should raise the HCT by 3% and hemoglobin by 1g/dL. Check HCT not more than 24 hr after infusion.
platelets (random donor, single donor) (30–300 mL)	48 hr (cannot be cooled)	Clotting disorders	Desirable but not required	Administer within 10 min–4 hr. One unit random platelets should raise the platelet count by 5–10,000/μL. Monitor platelet count 1 hr after transfusion. One unit of single-donor platelets should raise the platelet count by 30,000–60,000/μl. Do not use microaggregate filter.
white blood cells (220 mL)	24 hr	Low WBC count, depressed marrow function	Requires ABO compatibility	Administer slowly for 45–90 min, then increase rate and finish transfusion within 4 hr. Before administering WBCs, an HLA match or a tissue match is obtained. Do not use microaggregate filter.
normal human plasma usp (fresh/frozen) (200–220 mL)	Fresh: 35–40 days; frozen: 12 mo; thawed: use within 24 hr	Blood loss, bleeding disorders, anticoagulant overdose, thrombotic thrombocytopenic purpura	Requires ABO compatibility	Monitor coagulation factors—PT, PTT, or other specific assays—within 2–4 hr of transfusion.
human serum albumin 5% usp (Albuminar 5%, Albutein 5%, Buminate 5%, Plasbumin 5%) (50 mL, 250 mL, 500 mL, 1000 mL)	3–5 yr	Low blood volume, shock, reduction of cerebral edema, burns, hypoproteinemia	Not required	Monitor blood volume and cardiac and renal function closely.

Table 34–1. BLOOD PRODUCTS, *Continued*

BLOOD OR BLOOD COMPONENTS (VOLUME)	SHELF LIFE	GENERAL INDICATION	COMPATIBILITY	NURSING CONSIDERATIONS
human serum albumin 25% usp (Albuminar 25%, Albutein 25%, Buminate 25%, Plasbumin 25%) (10 mL, 20 mL, 50 mL , 100 mL)	3–5 yr	Low blood volume, shock, reduction of cerebral edema, burns, hypoprotein-emia, exchange transfusions in eryth-roblastosis fetalis, cardiopulmonary by-pass, renal dialysis, nephrosis, hepatic disease	Not required	Monitor blood volume and cardiac and renal function closely.
plasma protein fraction, human usp (Plasmanate, Plasma-Plex, Plasmatein) (Varies)	3–5 yr	Similar to albumin 5%	Not required	Monitor blood volume and cardiac and renal function closely. Ready for use. Does not need type and cross.
coagulation factors (Fibrinogen; Factor VIII; Factors II, VII, IX, X) (10–30 mL)	Frozen: 12 mo	Clotting disorders, he-mophilia A or B	Not required	Monitor clotting studies. Evaluate bleeding.
cryoprecipitate (10–20 mL)	1 yr	Disseminated intravas-cular coagulation, hemophilia	Not required	Administer within 3 min. One unit raises the fibrin count by 5–10 mg/dL.
immunoglobulins (gamma globulin, hepatitis B globulin) (Varies)	3–5 yr	Disease prophylaxis	Not required	Administer IM or IV.

PT = prothrombin time; PTT = partial thromboplastin time.

infections. Would-be blood donors are screened carefully with a thorough history to prevent this occurrence; however, donors may have a lack of knowledge or may deliberately falsify their answers to the questions.

Infections that can be transmitted include hepatitis A, B, and C; malaria; syphilis; and other infections such as Epstein-Barr virus, herpes simplex, HIV, toxoplasmosis, infectious mononucleosis, and cytomegalovirus. Hepatitis A, B, and C transmission have all been greatly reduced since the specific HB$_s$Ag testing of donor blood. The incidence of hepatitis A and B is thought to occur in about 5% of all blood transfusions.

According to officials from the Centers for Disease Control (CDC) the risk of contracting HIV through a blood transfusion is remote, but is five times higher than previously believed. This higher incidence is thought to result because many donors do not develop antibodies until at least 2 months and maybe as long as 5 to 8 years after being infected with the virus. In 1984 the risk was about 1 in 2600; subsequent screening of all blood donations for antibodies to the virus is expected to reduce that threat to 1 in 200,000 by the mid-1990s.

The risk of contracting viral infections from blood has

Table 34–2. LABEL ON DONATED BLOOD

The following information appears on all donated blood packaging:

- Proper name of the component (including an indication of any qualification or modification)
- Method by which the component was prepared (for example, from units of whole blood or by hemapheresis methods)
- Temperature range at which the component should be stored
- Preservatives and anticoagulant used in the preparation of the blood component
- Contents or volume (standard contents, that is as prepared according to this circular, is assumed unless otherwise indicated on the label or in circular supplements)
- Collection date (optional)
- Collection and processing location
- Expiration date (and time if applicable), which varies with the method of preparation (open or closed system) and the preservatives and anticoagulant used. When the expiration time is not indicated, the product expires at midnight of that date
- Donation (unit) number
- Blood grouping
- Special handling information, as required; statements regarding recipient identification, infectious disease risk, and prescription drugs

prompted many people to donate their own blood for their own later use (autologous blood transfusion). Special laboratories have been developed around the United States that process and store an individual's blood for up to 3 years for a fee. At the end of 3 years, the individual is required to redonate.

Plasmapheresis

Plasmapheresis is the removal of plasma from withdrawn blood by centrifugation, which separates the cellular elements from the plasma, and the suspension of the cellular elements in a physiologic solution that is then reinfused into the donor. This technique takes about 2 hours. After donating whole blood, an individual must wait 56 days before donating again. This is the approximate time it takes the body to replace the blood cells. When plasmapheresis is used, the donor is able to donate blood every 72 hours because the cells are returned. Usually plasmapheresis donors are called to donate about once a month.

WHOLE BLOOD

Whole blood is used to restore an acute loss of blood volume (greater than 25%). Minor losses can be managed by other means. Whole fresh blood is still used in exchange transfusion treatment of newborn infants with erythroblastosis fetalis, in ABO incompatibilities, and occasionally in Reye's syndrome and sickle-cell crisis. Stored whole blood has a low pH and calcium level, high potassium and ammonia levels, and low glucose and 2,3-diphosphoglycerate (2,3-DPG) levels. After 24 hours of storage, platelets and granulocytes present in a unit of whole blood are no longer viable. During storage, there is a change in RBC metabolism, as well as hemoglobin structure and function. Ultimately this leads to reduced survival time of transfused RBCs and decreased hemoglobin function. Because of the time required to process and test donated blood, fresh whole blood less than 24 hours old is generally not available. In most cases, specific blood components are used.

BLOOD COMPONENTS

Blood components are obtained by centrifuging whole blood, which separates the cells from the plasma. The cells can then be expressed from the plastic blood pack to a smaller satellite pack. The packed cells contain RBCs, WBCs, and platelets in a volume of about 50 to 250 mL. These cells can further be separated through centrifuging into RBCs in a volume of about 220 mL and into platelets in a volume of about 50 mL. Packed cells contain less potassium, ammonia, and citrate and a smaller volume than whole blood.

RED BLOOD CELLS

RBCs are used specifically when the oxygen-carrying capacity of an individual must be improved. This can be due to blood loss or the patient's inability to produce sufficient RBCs as in aplastic, hemolytic, and sickle-cell anemias and also in anemias associated with leukemias and lymphomas. Packed RBCs are often administered, along with sodium chloride solutions, to patients who have lost less than 1000 mL of their total blood volume. Red blood cells should not be transfused for volume expansion, in place of a hematinic, to enhance wound healing, or to improve general well-being.

RBCs are available in four products: fresh, frozen, leukocyte-removed, and saline-washed. Fresh RBCs are stored like whole blood and may contain platelet and leukocyte debris and products of RBC metabolism. Packed RBCs, mixed with a glycerin and water solution to prevent cell damage from crystallization and low temperatures, can be frozen and stored for 3 years. The glycerin and water solution is removed from the cells by the laboratory before the RBCs are administered to patients. When multiple units of packed cells are needed, after the sixth unit, one or two units of fresh frozen plasma are administered for every two units of packed cells to provide blood clotting components. The RBCs have a 24-hour shelf life after the solution is removed as an open system is created. The use of frozen RBCs can reduce febrile reactions and tissue antigen sensitization because approximately 98% of the *sensitizing lymphocytes* (WBCs, which may activate the body's immune system) are removed through this process. Frozen RBCs also contain no platelets and no plasma. Once the frozen RBCs have been prepared by the laboratory, they must be used within 24 hours.

Leukocyte-removed RBCs, also called buffy coat poor concentrate, have 70% of the leukocytes removed. Saline-washed RBCs have 90% of the leukocytes and platelets removed through washing with saline 24 hours prior to transfusion, and 20% of the RBCs are also lost. All other plasma debris is present. Units prepared by filtration or washing are outdated in 24 hours, as the closed system has been entered. These RBC products are used in persons who have had previous reaction to regular red cells. Type O (Rh$^-$) packed cells can be used in an emergency.

PLATELETS

Platelets are administered to patients with thrombocytopenia. Platelets are less likely to be effective in conditions with increased platelet destruction such as disseminated intravascular coagulation (DIC) because the consumptive process occurs more quickly than platelets can be replaced through transfusion. Platelets share the RBCs' A and B antigens, but typing is often not performed prior to platelet transfusion. Platelets do not contain the Rh(D) antigen that RBCs carry. A small number of RBCs may sensitize an Rh-negative female; therefore, Rh-negative females during their childbearing years should receive Rh$_0$ (D) immune globulin (RhoGAM) after receiving platelets from a positive donor. Platelets are not transfused to patients with immune thrombocytopenia purpura (except in life-threatening bleeding), prophylactically with a massive blood transfusion, or prophylactically following cardiopulmonary bypass.

Platelets share the *human leukocyte antigen* (HLA) histocompatability antigens with WBCs and other tissues. These highly immunogenic antigens are primarily responsible for isosensitization to platelets in the multiple-transfused patient. After 10 to 15 transfusions of random donor platelets, most patients are sensitized, and the life span of the transfused platelet is significantly reduced. Because large numbers of platelets may need to be transfused in persons with thrombocytopenia, an HLA-matched donor may be used.

Platelets are prepared from whole blood within 4 hours of its collection. Platelets are stored at 20° to 24°C with gentle agitation to supply oxygen and facilitate gas exchange. To maintain optimal posttransfusion viability and function, maximal storage time today is 48 hours.

If a patient's platelet count falls below $20,000/mm^3$ (normal 200,000 to $400,000/mm^3$), he or she is likely to bleed spontaneously and must then be treated with platelet-rich plasma or concentrated platelets. A patient under treatment for a neoplastic disease may also have a fall in platelet count. If it falls to even 10% of normal, an average adult male may need 6 to 10 units of platelets to prevent further bleeding. Because of fragility of the platelets, special administration sets are used with a specially designed platelet filter. If special sets are not available, a filter with a pore size of at least 170 μm prevents excess filtration of platelets prior to circulation. After 10 units of packed cells have been transfused, platelets are usually given unit for unit with packed cells.

WHITE BLOOD CELLS

WBCs are used in patients with a low leukocyte or granulocyte count, such as those with primary or secondary leukopenia, to combat infection. WBCs are used until the marrow returns to normal function. WBCs are not appropriate therapy if marrow function is not expected to return.

WBCs are extremely fragile and must be used within 6 hours of their donation. WBCs are also matched using the ABO system because they also contain RBCs. An HLA match (tissue match) may also be performed before the administration of WBCs to decrease the possibility of allergic reactions.

PLASMA

Plasma is the cell-free portion of blood and constitutes 60% of the total blood volume. Plasma contains blood proteins, electrolytes, coagulation factors, and antibodies. The coagulation factors vary in stability: V is stable for ten days; VIII is stable for only 2 days, and then decreases by 30% over time; and VII, IX, X, XI, XII, and fibrinogen remain relatively stable. Two types of plasma are available: fresh and frozen-thawed.

Both fresh and frozen-thawed plasma contain all clotting factors except platelets. Fresh plasma can be stored for 35 to 40 days. Frozen-thawed plasma can be stored for 1 year. Plasma is separated within 4 hours and frozen within 6 hours. Frozen plasma takes 45 minutes to thaw, and once reconstituted is used within 24 hours. Both types of plasma are used for acute volume loss, to control bleeding, in thrombotic thrombocytopenic purpura, and in anticoagulant overdose. Fresh or frozen-thawed plasma should not be used for volume expansion, as a nutritional supplement, prophylactically with a massive blood transfusion, or prophylactically following cardiopulmonary bypass.

BLOOD DERIVATIVES

Blood derivatives are obtained from pooled human plasma. Available blood derivatives include plasma protein products, coagulation factors, and immunoglobulins.

PLASMA PROTEIN PRODUCTS

Plasma protein products include **albumin** *(Albuminar)* and **plasma protein fraction** *(Plasmanate)*. Plasma protein products are considered free of the danger of homologous serum hepatitis and HIV because they are heat-treated for 10 hours at 60°C. No cross-matching is required. Because these products contain no cellular elements, there is no risk of sensitization with repeated infusion.

Plasma protein products are contraindicated in patients with a history of allergic reaction to albumin because they all contain albumin; in severe anemia because plasma volume becomes even more dilute; and in cardiac failure because the increased volume can worsen failure. In chronic nephrosis, infused plasma protein products are promptly lost by damaged nephrons and thus do not relieve edema or hypoproteinemia. Safe use in pregnancy has not been established.

During administration, blood pressure is carefully monitored to assess for hypertension from the returning fluid volume into the vascular space. Also, when large doses of these products are administered, blood products are given to combat the anemia that can result. Plasma protein products are also used cautiously in patients with hepatic or renal failure because of the possible added protein load.

Large doses of plasma protein products can cause the cardiovascular system to develop fluid overload, resulting in hypertension and pulmonary edema. Hypotension can also result following rapid infusion or in patients on cardiopulmonary bypass. Allergic reactions can also occur resulting in fever, chills, flushing, urticaria, back pain, headache, rash, nausea, vomiting, and febrile reaction. If these symptoms occur, the infusion is discontinued and antihistamines are administered.

○ **Albumin** (Albuminar, Albutein, Buminate, Plasbumin) is administered to patients to increase or maintain their colloid osmotic pressure, to restore albumin levels

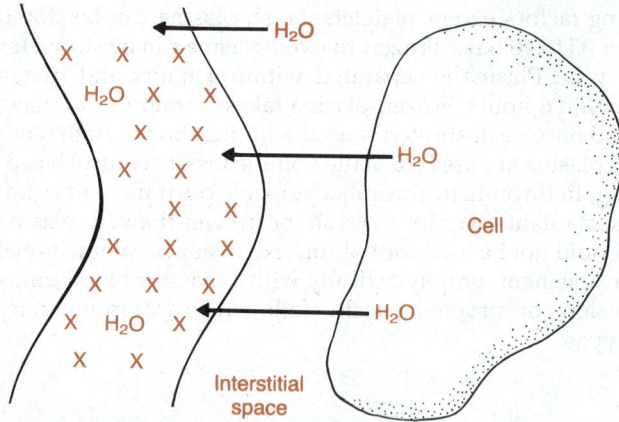

Figure 34–1. Colloid properties of plasma expanders. Plasma expanders (XX) exert a high colloid oncotic pressure in the vascular system and thus pull fluid from the interstitial space and the cell into the vascular system to dilute the solute.

to normal, and to decrease cerebral or peripheral edema. The high-molecular-weight albumin pulls fluid into the circulatory system by osmosis and equalizes pressure on both sides of the vessel wall, as shown in Figure 34–1. In addition, albumin is a carrier of intermediate metabolites in the transport and exchange of tissue products. Albumin comprises about 50% to 60% of the plasma proteins and provides approximately 85% of the colloid osmotic pressure. Albumin also has the ability to bind bilirubin in the circulation; thus, it is often used as an adjunct to exchange transfusion in an infant with erythroblastosis fetalis. It binds with the bilirubin, which helps reduce hyperbilirubinemia and decrease jaundice.

Albumin contains 96% albumin and 4% globulins. It remains stable and can be stored for long periods at room temperature. Albumin is available in 50-mL vials of both 5% and 25% solutions and has a shelf life of 3 to 5 years. Most commonly, a 5% solution is used undiluted and administered at a rate of 2 to 4 mL/min. In children, the rate is 0.25 to 0.5 the adult rate. In patients with a low cardiac reserve, it is given at a rate of 1 mL/min to prevent pulmonary edema. Because albumin in the 5% concentration provides additional fluid for plasma volume expansion, the rate of infusion should be slow enough to prevent too rapid expansion of the plasma volume. A 5% albumin solution is used in patients with shock and burns to restore vascular volume and in hypoproteinemia to replace lost protein. Five percent albumin is osmotically equivalent to an equal volume of citrated plasma. However, if edema is present or a large amount of albumin is lost, 25% albumin is the better product because of the greater protein concentration. Twenty-five percent albumin is osmotically equivalent to five times the volume of citrated plasma.

The 25% albumin solution is commonly used in patients with hypoproteinemia with or without edema to restore protein levels. Twenty-five percent albumin is equal to 2 U (500 mL) of fresh or frozen-thawed plasma, or 25% albumin with 100 mL of normal saline is equal to 500 mL of plasma, which is also equal to two pints of whole blood. The suggested rate of administration is 2 mL/min. A more rapid administration may precipitate circulatory or pulmonary problems. The 25% albumin solution is also administered to patients with hepatic cirrhosis, nephrosis, burns, and shock to restore protein levels and vascular volume. In these states, the rate of administration may vary from 2 to 4 mL/min very rapidly.

○ **Plasma protein fraction** (Plasmanate) is a 5% solution of human plasma proteins (at least 83% albumin, no more than 17% globulin, and no more than 17% of total proteins as gamma globulin) in sodium chloride injection (130 to 160 mEq/sodium). Plasma protein fraction (PPF) has the same indications as 5% albumin. PPF is administered to adults at a rate of 5 to 8 mL/min (1000 to 1500 mL total volume) and to children at 33 mL/kg at a rate of 5 to 10 mL/min.

CLOTTING FACTORS

The coagulation (clotting) factors or fractions can be removed from the plasma in approximate volumes of 10 to 30 mL per pint of blood. The coagulation factors separated are factors X, IX (Christmas factor), VIII (antihemophilic factor), VII, II, and I (fibrinogen). These can be administered to individuals with hemophilia A or B to control bleeding episodes. Coagulation factors for hemophilia—antihemophilic products—include **cryoprecipitate, antihemophilic factor *(Factor VIII, AHF)*, factor IX complex *(Konyne-HT, Profilnine Heat-Treated, Proplex T)*,** and **anti-inhibitor coagulant complex *(Autoplex T, Feiba VH Immuno).***

○ **Cryoprecipitate** contains factors I (fibrinogen, 250 mg) and VIII (100 mg). It results when plasma is frozen and then thawed to 4°C. Cryoprecipitate is used specifically to treat hemophilia and von Willebrand's disease (both hereditary bleeding disorders). Cryoprecipitate is frozen for up to 12 months. After thawing, it must be used within 4 to 6 hours. Cryoprecipitate is totally administered in 3 minutes. Cryoprecipitate carries the same risk of hepatitis and HIV infection as whole blood.

○ **Antihemophilic factor** (Factor VIII, AHF, Hemophil M, Koate, Monoclate), a protein found in normal plasma, is necessary for clot formation. When infused and for the next 9 to 15 hours, it can correct the coagulation deficits in patients with classic hemophilia A. It is used to correct or prevent bleeding episodes or when surgery is needed.

Antihemophilic factor is contraindicated in persons hypersensitive to mouse protein. It contains high levels of blood group antibodies, and when frequent doses are needed, intravascular hemolysis may result. Safety during pregnancy (category C) has not been established. Adverse effects include allergic reactions—hives, fever, urticaria, chills, nausea, and wheezing.

Antihemophilic factor is administered between 2 and 10 mL/min, depending on the severity of the problem. Pulse rate is monitored closely; if it rises more than 10 to 15 beats per minute, the infusion is reduced or discontinued.

○ **Factor IX complex** (Konyne-HT, Profilnine Heat-Treated, Proplex T) restores factor IX levels to patients with a deficiency, such as in those with hemophilia B or

Christmas disease. It is used to prevent or control bleeding and when surgery is indicated in these patients. Dosage varies depending on the severity of the patient's problem.

❍ **Anti-inhibitor coagulant complex** (Autoplex T, Feiba VH Immuno) contains varying amounts of clotting factor precursors, activated clotting factors, and factors of the kinin-generating system. It is used to control hemorrhage in hemophilia A patients. Anti-inhibitor coagulant complex is standardized by its ability to correct the clotting time of factor VIII–deficient plasma or factor VIII–deficient plasma containing inhibitors to factor VIII. Dosage depends on the existing level of inhibitor, whether or not the patient responds to infusions of antihemophilic factor (with increased inhibitor levels), and the severity of the bleeding episode.

IMMUNOGLOBULINS

The immunoglobulins (IgA, IgD, IgE, IgG, IgM) produced by the immune system to prevent certain infections can also be removed from the plasma and administered. Immunoglobulin concentrations (gamma globulin—IgG) are used to prevent hepatitis A in individuals who have been previously exposed. $Rh_0(D)$ immune globulin (RhoGAM) is used in Rh-negative females who abort, have a tubal pregnancy, delivered an Rh-positive child, or who have been given platelets, granulocytes, or Rh-positive blood.

❍ **IVIG** (Gamimune-N, Gammar-IV, Sandoglobulin, Venoglobulin-I) contains different subclasses of IgG and varying amounts of IgA, but no IgM. The half-life is about 30 to 40 days. Intravenous immune globulin can replace missing antibodies and decrease infection in primary immune deficiency and chronic lymphocytic leukemia, increase platelets in idiopathic thrombocytopenic purpura, and prevent complications in Kawasaki syndrome.

ARTIFICIAL BLOOD

Artificial blood, a perflurocarbon emulsion, has been developed to carry oxygen at high O_2 partial pressures in a physically dissolved form that is not chemically combined, as with hemoglobin. To make the product safe in the body, the perflurocarbon emulsion is emulsified with yolk phospholipids and a variety of salts are added. A test dose is administered first to determine allergy.

❍ **Intravascular perflurocarbon emulsion 20%** (Fluosol DA) is approved for intracoronary administration only during percutaneous transluminal coronary angioplasty (PTCA). It is often transfused prior to balloon inflation and continued momentarily after balloon deflation to carry O_2 to the distal myocardium. Perfusion rates are usually greater than 120 mL/min. Patients must inspire a high percentage (80% to 100%) of O_2 for this product to be effective. Intravascular perfluorocarbon emulsion can provide as much as 50% of the O_2 needed by the tissues at a given time. Per flurocarbons are also being placed in the lung to enhance O_2 transport in both infants and adults with severe lung disease.

Intravascular perfluorocarbon emulsion is contraindicated in patients with hypersensitivity or critical stenosis in the PTCA distal to the treated lesion. It is used cautiously in asplenic patients. Use in pregnancy (category B) only if need outweighs risk. The primary route of excretion is the lung. Therefore, side effects include pulmonary edema, chest pain or tightness, respiratory distress, and dysrhythmia. Vascular system half-life is about 8 hours, but traces can be found in the liver and spleen for about 141 days.

▼ **CLINICAL ALERT**

Intravascular perfluorocarbon emulsion is administered not more than once in 6 months. Administration is a complex technique usually performed by specially trained personnel. A test dose of 0.5 mL is injected into a peripheral vein, and the patient is observed for 10 minutes. If no untoward reaction occurs, 60 to 90 mL/min is infused before and after PTCA.

ADMINISTRATION OF BLOOD PRODUCTS IN THE HOME

It is becoming increasingly common for whole blood, blood components, or plasma expanders to be administered in the home setting. Reasons for this include a reduction in cost and an increase in patient comfort. Procedures for administering blood products in the home are the same as those used in a clinical setting. Refer to the *Delivering Home Health Care* box for general procedures for administering blood products in the home.

USING THE NURSING PROCESS

ASSESSMENT

- Develop a thorough nursing history to develop the database needed for preparation of a nursing-care plan (Table 34–3).
- Assess laboratory tests such as hematocrit (HCT) and hemoglobin levels. Other tests are performed based on the patient's diagnosis.
- Obtain baseline laboratory data such as hematocrit when administering plasma expanders (all products lower HCT by increasing plasma volume). Type and cross-match for blood or blood products before beginning administration.
- Assess whether the patient has had previous blood products. Prior transfusion increases the risk of allergic reaction to certain blood products. Prior transfusions have been shown to increase the survival of persons having renal homographs, whereas prior transfusion decreases the survival of persons having bone marrow transplantation.

Table 34–3. NURSING PROCESS FOR PATIENT REQUIRING BLOOD PRODUCTS

Assessment

Assess precipitating factor(s) and duration of blood loss (e.g., trauma with rapid blood loss or chronic subacute gastric bleed).
Assess previous transfusion/reaction history.
Assess current vital signs, hemodynamic pressures, and urinary output.

Nursing Diagnosis: Fluid Volume Deficit, actual

RELATED TO: active loss.
AS EVIDENCED BY: Hypotension, tachycardia, decreased venous filling, confusion.

Desired Outcomes/Evaluation Criteria

Displays improvement of hemodynamic parameters and urine output of >0.5 mL/kg per hr.

Nursing Actions	Rationale
Begin/maintain IV therapy replacement of blood product. Observe drip rate q 15–30 min.	Replaces losses, expanding circulating volume. Ensures accuracy of infusion rate, preventing complications, e.g., too rapid infusion.
Monitor vital signs/hemodynamic parameters q 30–60 min as indicated. Record I/O and urine specific gravity as necessary.	As volume is replaced, parameters should stabilize/return to near normal baseline. Increasing circulating volume should improve renal perfusion and urinary output, decreasing specific gravity.
Monitor laboratory studies as indicated, e.g., Hgb/HCT, electrolytes, calcium, acid-base balance.	Reflects effectiveness of therapy and additional needs. Calcium may be required to promote clotting and prevent tetany in presence of multiple transfusions. Potassium level may rise when stored blood is transfused.
Auscultate breath sounds for development of crackles (rales).	The major risk of volume expansion is pulmonary edema. Volume and rate of replacement are limited by the patient's cardiac competency.

Nursing Diagnosis: Knowledge Deficit

RELATED TO: Unfamiliarity with therapeutic interventions.
AS EVIDENCED BY: Questions, statements of concern.

Desired Outcomes/Evaluation Criteria

Verbalizes understanding of reasons for use of blood products.

Nursing Actions	Rationale
Inform the patient about need for and safety of blood products. Obtain consent for administration of blood as appropriate.	Patient often has unspoken fears about what is happening; accurate information and opportunity to discuss these fears promotes understanding and may enhance cooperation with therapy.

Nursing Diagnosis: Anxiety (specify level)

RELATED TO: Change in health status, perceived threat of death.
AS EVIDENCED BY: Increased tension, apprehension, expressed concerns.

Desired Outcomes/Evaluation Criteria

Verbalizes awareness of feelings. Reports anxiety reduced to manageable level.

Nursing Actions	Rationale
Visit patient hourly. Encourage verbalization of fears and concerns.	Provides assurance that staff is available for help. Identifies problem areas, realities of illness and treatment.
Monitor vital signs. Provide information about physical condition and use of blood products.	Changes in vital signs suggest degree of anxiety. Knowledge can reduce anxiety and thereby enhance coping with situation.

Other Suggested Nursing Diagnosis: Risk for Injury.

The theory that blood transfusions result in immunosuppression is gaining support. Researchers have found that cancer patients receiving homologous transfusions have a 70% greater reoccurrence rate than patients who did not receive homologous transfusions. However, it appears that autologous blood transfusions may not affect the immune system. In patients having hip replacement, the postoperative infection rate is higher in patients receiving homologous transfusions. Patients who received no blood or their own blood had no infections. Therefore, it becomes important to assess and determine the real need for transfusion.

- Assess the patient carefully to determine his or her fluid needs. Several categories of fluid therapy are available for clinical use. These include blood products, plasma expanders (often referred to as colloids), and balanced salt solutions (referred to as crystalloids). Plasma expanders and balanced salt solutions are discussed fully in Chapters 67 and 12, respectively. The most important rule to follow in any patient is to restore vascular volume and RBC mass.

- Obtain baseline hemodynamic data. The volume and rate of fluid administration are initially guided by arterial pressure, central venous pressure (CVP), heart rate, HCT, and cardiac output. The volume and rate of fluid replacement are limited by the patient's cardiac competency, especially in older patients with hypertension or ischemic heart disease. The major risk of volume expansion with any IV fluid is pulmonary edema. Therefore, a thorough and continuous respiratory assessment is performed.

- Assess the patient's and family's anxiety level. Blood therapy is a routine part of nursing. However, it may be a traumatic event for the patient and family. Often, to the patient and family, the administration of blood may erroneously indicate serious illness or impending death. The nurse shares with the patient and family the reason for and purpose of the therapy and helps them recognize and allay their fears. Table 34–4 presents some patient teaching information for the patient receiving blood products.
- Assess for signs and symptoms of transfusion reactions. The nurse must understand the reason for blood therapy in the patient, the presenting symptoms of the condition, and the type of fluid used. Table 34–5 features the various types of transfusion re-

Table 34–5. TRANSFUSION REACTIONS

Type	Etiology	Prevention	Presenting Symptom	R$_x$
Hemolytic	ABO-incompatible blood causing microclots due to hemolyzing of donor RBCs	Check temperature and stay with patient 15–30 min. Use antigen-negative blood. Avoid clerical errors	Fever, chills, flushing, pain in back and legs, decreased BP, tightness in chest, bleeding, vomiting, tachycardia, hemoglobinemia, hemoglobinuria	Stop transfusion. Send urine to lab, check for bleeding and hemorrhage, check urinary output q 1 hr, dialysis, fluids, diuretics, osmotic diuretics.
Allergic	Antibodies react with allergins in donor blood or substances in blood	Prophylactic antihistamines, washed RBCs, premedicate with diphenhydramine	Mild: hives, pruritus, chills, nausea, vomiting Severe: wheezing, bronchospasm, anaphylaxis	Stop transfusion. Administer antihistamines, epinephrine; if severe, steroids.
Febrile	Sensitized to WBCs, platelets, or antigens— those previously transfused or multiparas	Saline-washed or frozen RBCs or micro aggregate filtered blood, antipyretics	Increased temperature (1°C), headache, chills, back pain, tachycardia; generally occurs within 15 min	Stop transfusion. Give IV steroids.
Circulatory Overload	Too much or too fast volume in young/elderly or in renal or CV disease	Packed cells rather than whole blood, diuretics, careful monitoring of infusion rate	Increased CVP, increased PAOP, increased neck veins, dyspnea, cough, crackles	Stop transfusion. Place upright with feet dependent, apply tourniquets, diuretics, digitalis.
Anaphylactoid Reaction	Plasma protein incompatibility due to IgA deficiency and antibody development from previous transfusions and/or pregnancy	Washed RBCs, or deglycerolized RBCs from which IgA have been removed	Coughing, respiratory distress, decreased BP, nausea, vomiting, shock	Stop transfusion. Give epinephrine, oxygen, fluids, steroids.
Noncardiac Pulmonary Edema	HLA or antileukocyte, or platelet antibodies	Washed cells	Increased CVP, increased PAOP, increased neck veins, dyspnea, cough, crackles	Stop transfusion. Place upright with feet dependent, apply tourniquets, diuretics, digitalis.
Transmission of Infectious Diseases	Viruses causing hepatitis A, B, C; HIV; CMV; malaria	Use heat-treated products. Use hepatitis B vaccine. Washed cells for persons susceptible to CMV	Acute symptoms of infecting disease	Treat disease appropriately.

BP = blood pressure; CV = cardiovascular; PAOP = pulmonary artery obstructive pressure; HIV = human immunodeficiency virus (AIDS); CMV = cytomegalovirus.

actions and their causes, presenting symptoms, prevention, and treatment.

NURSING DIAGNOSIS

- Establish the nursing diagnoses, which form the basis for the nursing care, based on the information obtained during the assessment. Typical nursing diagnoses in the patient requiring blood products include Actual Fluid Volume Deficit, Knowledge Deficit, and Anxiety (see Table 34–3).

PLANNING AND INTERVENTION

- Develop the plan for the nursing intervention from the nursing diagnoses. The goals of nursing intervention are designed so that the patient goals or outcome criteria are achieved during the nursing intervention.
- Follow the guidelines established by the hospital for administering blood and blood components. Nursing intervention includes obtaining baseline temperature, pulse, respirations, and blood pressure before starting the infusion. Note the expiration date on the blood and return the blood to the blood bank if it is outdated. Carefully compare the blood group and Rh factor with those of the patient to ensure accuracy. The actual starting of the blood infusion may or may not be part of the nurse's responsibility. This is determined by the employer. CDC mandates that when drawing or administering blood the nurse and/or physician wear gloves. Blood is always administered through Y-type blood tubing with a filter (170-μm filter), which has been flushed with normal saline (NS). If a problem develops, the blood can be turned off and NS solution turned on, and the IV site is not lost. Dextrose solutions are not used because they tend to cause clumping of the RBCs. The tubing is changed after each unit of blood to prevent clogging of the filter. Blood is never given or combined with drugs in an IV line.
- Administer the appropriate solution as ordered. The solution is determined based on the following: the patient's presenting history and current symptoms, what volume (blood or plasma) has been lost, the approximate amount of the loss, and the cause of the loss.

  When the primary circulatory problem is hypovolemia, therapy is directed toward restoration of blood volume. Because colloid solutions expand vascular volume with far less fluid infusion than crystalloid solutions, hemodynamic resuscitation is likely to be accomplished more rapidly with colloids. Crystalloids equilibrate across the vascular membrane such that only $\frac{1}{10}$ to $\frac{1}{4}$ of the solution remains in the plasma at the end of infusion. Crystalloids also dilute plasma proteins and consequently reduce colloid osmotic pressure. Decreases in blood colloid osmotic pressure allow for filtration of fluid from the vascular space into the interstitial space, further potentiating the volume deficit. Also, as colloid osmotic pressure

is reduced, the patient is at increased risk for developing pulmonary edema. When colloids are used, colloid osmotic pressure is maintained, requiring less fluid for resuscitation. The possibility of pulmonary edema is also reduced.

  A single unit of whole blood yields RBCs, plasma, platelets, WBCs, clotting components, and protein. Because few patients require all these blood constituents, the transfusion of whole blood is an exception rather than the rule. The goal is always to restore fluid volume and RBC mass. Blood components are then administered as needed.

- Monitor the drip rate closely. Blood is usually started at 20 gtt per minute for the first 10 minutes. If no reactions are noted, the flow can be increased to 50 to 70 gtt per minute. During the infusion, vital signs are monitored every 0.5 to 1 hour. Be alert for signs of reactions, including backache, change in vital signs, urticaria, chills and fever, headache, flushing, chest pain, and suddenly developing shock. If a reaction occurs, the nurse follows institutional policy. Usually the remaining blood, a sample of blood from the patient, and a urine specimen are sent to the laboratory for examination. Reactions (hemolytic, bacterial, overload, and anaphylactic) can occur during administration and also up to 96 hours after a transfusion (see Table 34–5).
- Administer whole blood and all types of red cells as previously discussed, but other components and derivatives have specific administration techniques. Platelets and cryoprecipitate are administered quickly, within 10 minutes and 3 minutes, respectively. WBCs are run slowly over at least a 2-hour period through a standard blood filter. (Micropore or microaggregate filters should *not* be used). Patients are often premedicated with acetaminophen and antihistamines to reduce the incidence and severity of reactions. WBCs are best not administered concurrently with amphotericin B (Fungizone) because of the increased risk of pulmonary complications. It is best to separate the infusions as far apart as possible. Other ''do nots'' when transfusing blood are as follows:
  - Do not use any solution other than 0.9% sodium chloride solution (NS) to prime a blood administration set, to flush the IV line, or to dilute the blood product.
  - Do not add drugs to blood components or infuse drugs and blood through the same blood administration set.
  - Do not store any blood component on a nursing unit or in an unmonitored refrigerator.
  - Do not keep blood out of the transfusion service's refrigerator for longer than 30 minutes before starting the transfusion.
  - Do not transfuse any blood component without using the appropriate blood filter.
  - Do not use the same blood filter longer than 4 hours.
  - Do not transfuse a unit of blood over a period longer than 4 hours.

○ Do not vent plastic bags.
○ Never add solution containing calcium (Ringer's lactate) to blood components containing citrate.
- During an acute bleeding episode, therapy is aimed at maintaining the following:
  1. blood volume at 100% normal.
  2. hemoglobin at least 8 g/dL and HCT 24%.
  3. total serum protein at least 60% of normal.
  4. plasma coagulant factors above 35% of normal (except factor VIII, which should be at least 50% of normal).
  5. platelets above 25% (50,000) of normal.

In the patient with acute bleeding, the nurse and physician work closely together to improve the patient's chance for survival. Fluid management needed to maintain these criteria is featured in Table 34–6.

If multiple units of blood are needed quickly, the blood may need to be warmed to 37°C prior to infusion to prevent ventricular fibrillation. Several specific types of blood warmers are available. Each type has its own instructions, which must be followed. Using a microwave oven to warm blood or immersing blood in hot water is not acceptable because of the risk of hemolysis. Once the blood is warmed, it must be administered more slowly.

Table 34–6. ACUTE BLEED MANAGEMENT

Blood Loss	Fluids
20% or less (slowly)	Crystalloids (e.g., balanced solutions)
20%–50%	Nonprotein plasma expanders, red cells
Over 50% (slowly) or over 20% (acutely)	Whole blood or PPF and fresh or frozen plasma
80% or more	As above. For every 5 units of blood give 1–2 units fresh frozen plasma, 1 or 2 units platelets to prevent hemodilution of clotting factors and bleeding.

PPF = plasma protein fraction.

EVALUATION

- Evaluate the effectiveness of the blood or blood products. Fluid administration is continued until either the clinical and hemodynamic signs of hypovolemia are reversed or until the safe limit of volume expansion has been reached. Restoration of mental alert-

---

DELIVERING HOME HEALTH CARE

Administration of Blood Components

Blood components must be administered within 30 minutes after removal from the blood bank's refrigerator to ensure that the transfused product is fresh, uncoagulated, and free of any toxic breakdown products. Refrigeration in the home refrigerator will not prevent deterioration.

Before the administration of blood components, do the following:
- Ask the patient and caregiver(s) if they understand the procedure and why it is being performed. Make sure that consent to the procedure is or has been obtained.
- Assess the patient's allergy history and determine any previous reactions to blood products.
- Gather baseline data about the patient's blood studies and vital signs.
- Assess the patient for adequacy of venous access.
- Have the patient void before the procedure.
- Make the patient comfortable in bed or in a reclining chair.
- Check the label on the blood bag and compare the information with the physician's order and patient information. Confirm the patient's identity with at least one other person and check the bag for leaks.

To administer, perform the following:
- Determine the drip rate per minute and time for completion of transfusion.
- Infuse about 60 mL of normal saline solution through the tubing before and after the transfusion.
- After selecting an appropriate site, perform the venipuncture using aseptic technique.
- Administer the blood or blood component slowly for the first 15 minutes.

During administration, perform the following:
- Assess and record vital signs carefully during the first 15 minutes.
- While the blood component is infusing, check the drip rate every 15 minutes and monitor vital signs every hour.
- Assess the infusion site for infiltration.
- Assess the patient for signs of transfusion reactions, including hemolysis (possible blood-type incompatibility), allergic reaction, bacterial contamination, circulatory overload, air embolism, febrile reaction, and viral hepatitis. If reactions occur, stop the transfusion and administer corrective measures. Follow the health-care agency's protocols for emergency action. Stay with the patient until the situation is resolved.
- If more than one unit is to be administered, change the blood tubing and filter.

After the transfusion, do the following:
- Remove the IV canula or needle and ensure that it is intact.
- Document the procedure. Make sure that documentation includes the patient's baseline vital signs, the signature of the person(s) who identified the patient and the blood product, the blood product administered, the time the transfusion was started and completed, the total volume of fluid transfused (listing the starter solution separately), the patient's response to the transfusion, and any nursing intervention performed after an adverse response.

ness, warm skin, urine flow greater than 0.5 mL/kg per hour, normal blood pressure, and hemodynamic stability are appropriate findings indicating effective volume expansion.

- To determine if the blood was effective, evaluate laboratory tests. A unit of packed RBCs should raise the hematocrit by about 3 g; a unit of platelets should raise the platelet count by 5,000 to 10,000 mL; a unit of fibrinogen should raise the fibrinogen count by 10 to 20 μm. If these counts do not increase, further investigation is needed.
- Evaluate the patient for the regular complications of IV therapy such as infiltration, extravasation, thrombosis, thrombophlebitis, pain at the administration site, fluid overload, respiratory complications, and pyrogenic reactions to blood.
- Evaluate the IV site and drip rate hourly or more often, if necessary. IV tubing and dressings must be changed according to institutional policies.
- Evaluate for complications. Two major complications of blood administration are microembolism, which

filters help to prevent, and hypocalcemia. Hypocalcemia is a possibility after infusion of multiple units of packed cells. Banked blood contains an anticoagulant that, when it comes in contact with the patient's blood, mobilizes the patient's bound calcium, causing hypocalcemia. Therefore, the patient is evaluated for signs of hypocalcemia (Chvostek's and Trousseau's signs, bronchospasm, tetany, and seizures).

- Evaluate other nursing-care problems that the patient may have. The blood may have been administered after surgery, trauma, or a medical emergency. In these cases, the patient is usually acutely ill and needs additional emotional support as well as physical nursing care.

The nurse evaluates the effectiveness of treatment by a return to normal homeostasis. This is evaluated through qualitative, quantitative, and laboratory findings.

The bibliography for this chapter can be found in Appendix B, which begins on page 1054.

CHAPTER REVIEW QUESTIONS*

1. Which of the following statements is correct with regard to whole blood or its derivatives?
   a. Platelets do not contain the Rh(D) antigen that red cells carry.
   b. White cells must be given within 48 hours after donation.
   c. Whole blood is used to restore a blood loss of greater than 500 mol.
   d. Packed cells contain only red cells in a volume of 250 mL.

2. In caring for the patient receiving a blood transfusion, the nurse:
   a. Administers the blood concurrently with a dextrose solution to prevent clumping of red blood cells.
   b. Monitors the patient at least every 2 hours for signs of a reaction to the blood transfusion.
   c. Administers the blood using a single tubing with a 170-μm filter.
   d. Compares the blood group and Rh factor on the label with those of the patient.

3. Donated blood is labeled with all of the following information *except* the:
   a. Proper name of the component.
   b. Method by which the component was prepared.
   c. Temperature range for storage.
   d. Type of antibodies present.

4. Plasmapheresis is a donor technique with the advantage of:
   a. Allowing persons to donate every 72 hours if necessary.
   b. Patients retaining their own plasma, platelets, and white blood cells.
   c. Taking only 1 hour for the process to be completed.
   d. Returning the plasma and destroying the red cells.

5. Albumin is separated from plasma and is administered to:
   a. Facilitate oxygen binding capacity.
   b. Bind bilirubin in circulation to reduce jaundice.
   c. Reduce osmotic pressure within the vessel wall.
   d. Facilitate red blood cell production.

*See Appendix A, which begins on page 1051, for answers.

CHAPTER 35

Drugs Affecting Coagulation

Merrily A. Kuhn, RNC, PhD

CHAPTER OUTLINE

KEY TERMS

Aggregation
Angioplasty
Anticoagulants

Fibrinolysis
Hemostasis
Thrombocytopenia

LEARNING OBJECTIVES

After reading this chapter, the student will be able to:

1. Identify medications that affect coagulation.
2. Differentiate among the medications as to mechanism of action, routes of administration, pharmacokinetics, adverse effects, contraindications and precautions, and interactions.
3. Identify specific areas to assess in the patient who requires various medications affecting coagulation to formulate appropriate patient outcomes.
4. Plan the appropriate nursing interventions necessary to administer various medications that affect coagulation and choose teaching strategies to gain patient compliance.
5. Evaluate the patient at various stages of treatment to measure nursing interventions.

Medications that affect coagulation may act in several ways. They may prevent or retard clotting (anticoagulants, antiplatelet agents), hasten clotting (hemostatics, sclerosing agents), dissolve the clot (thrombolytic agents), or prevent the dissolution of the clot (antifibrinolytics). Each drug group is discussed individually.

HEMOSTASIS

Hemostasis is the termination of bleeding by the complex coagulation process of the body. It consists of vasoconstriction, platelet *aggregation* (a clustering or coming together of substances), and thrombin and fibrin synthesis. Injury to the vascular system results in leakage of blood from the system. To prevent or mitigate this loss, the body initiates three sequential steps. First, vasoconstriction in the injured vessel occurs as a reflex response to prevent increased blood loss. Second, a plug forms from platelets and appears at the site of injury to prevent further blood loss. This platelet plug occurs because the break in the continuity of the endothelial lining of the vessel exposes collagen, a fibrous protein, to which platelets adhere. As the platelets clump together (a process known as platelet adhesion), adenosine diphosphate (ADP) is released from the injured site, which causes the surface of the platelets to become very sticky, thus further aiding the formation of the platelet plug. The plug is very unstable and needs the addition of fibrin to stabilize it.

The third step occurs when blood coagulates as a result of a complex series of biochemical reactions and interac-

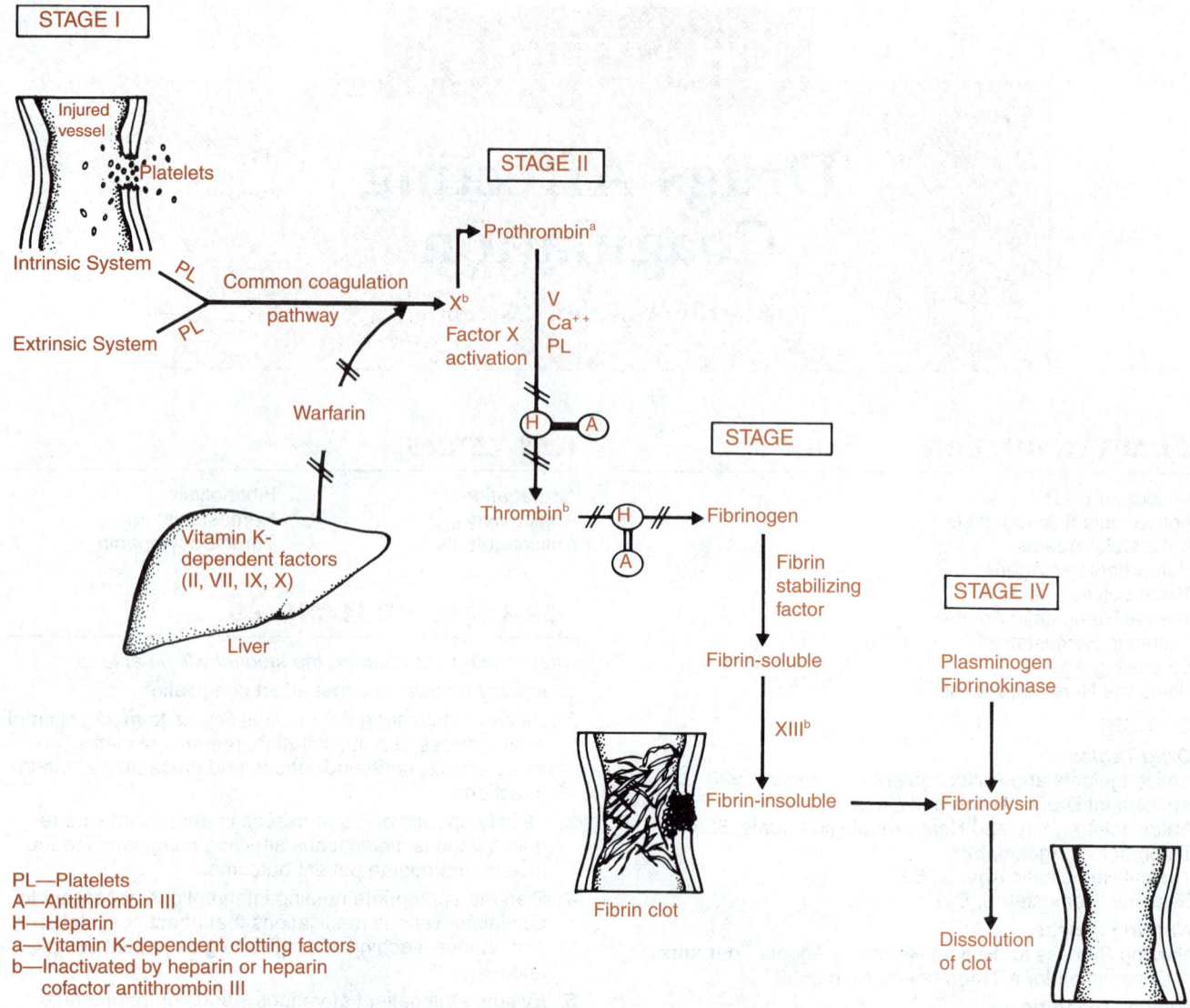

PL—Platelets
A—Antithrombin III
H—Heparin
a—Vitamin K-dependent clotting factors
b—Inactivated by heparin or heparin
cofactor antithrombin III

Figure 35–1. Schematic representation of the blood coagulation mechanism. The intrinsic system activates XII→XIIa, XI→XIa, IX→XIa, X→Xa, which are all found in blood; the extrinsic system is activated by release of tissue thromboplastin, a factor not found in circulating blood, and then activates VII→VIIa and joins to activate IX→1Xa and X→Xa. Activation of the intrinsic system takes several minutes to achieve a clot, whereas the extrinsic system takes only several seconds. From the activation of the extrinsic/intrinsic system the common pathway is entered. Stage II ultimately creates thrombin and stage III fibrin. Stage IV is clot dissolution.

tions, which are not totally understood and identified. Several well-defined proteins are involved in clotting, and the remaining factors are identified by Roman numerals. Several factors are identified by more than one name. The clotting process has four stages: the formation of an active prothrombin-converting substance (thromboplastin) (stage I); the conversion of prothrombin to thrombin by thromboplastin (stage II); and the conversion of fibrinogen to fibrin by thrombin (stage III). Stage IV is the resolution stage in which the clot begins to break up and dissolve. Figure 35–1 illustrates the four stages. The clotting process (hemostasis) or cascade can be activated by either an intrinsic or extrinsic system.

The intrinsic system is activated by the introduction or presence of a surface other than the natural endothelium of the blood vessel, as when a needle is placed into a vein

for the administration of IV fluids. All of the protein factors necessary for coagulation are present in circulating blood. When the intrinsic system is activated, factors V, VIII, IX, X, XI, and XII are needed. The extrinsic system is activated as a result of injury, as when one receives a cut or scratch. Coagulation is activated by release of tissue thromboplastin, a factor that is not normally found in circulating blood. As thromboplastin formation occurs, factors V, VII, and X must be present. In addition, calcium (factor IV) is necessary regardless of the system that is activated. As stage II of clotting begins, prothrombin, synthesized in the liver only in the presence of vitamin K, is converted to thrombin in the presence of calcium and factor V.

When thrombin becomes available in the blood, stage III of clotting begins. Thrombin acts as a catalyst that pro-

Table 35–1. DYSFUNCTIONS OF HEMOSTASIS

	Arterial	Venous
Names	White thrombi	Red thrombi
Clotting Pathway	Intrinsic	Extrinsic
Description	Large platelet head, small fibrin tail	Large fibrin head, small platelet tail
Associated With	ASHD plaques Hypertension Turbulent blood flow	Trauma to venous system Stasis

ASHD = arteriosclerotic heart disease.

motes the conversion of fibrinogen, also synthesized in the liver in the presence of calcium (factor IV), to fibrin, the gel-like substance that then traps other elements in the blood (calcium and platelets), forming the clot. Calcium is involved in the clotting process during all three stages. As the clot is formed, it may undergo either organization, the conversion of the clot to fibrous tissue, or resolution, the dissolution of the clot. Dysfunctions of hemostasis are summarized in Table 35–1.

The fourth stage begins with dissolution. This stage begins when plasminogen and fibrinokinases, which must be present in the blood, are converted to fibrinolysin (plasmin) through an enzymatic process. This process occurs spontaneously and can be accelerated by the thrombolytic agents, such as streptokinase, urokinase, or tissue plasminogen activator (t-PA). The fibrin in the clot is broken down into smaller fragments by plasmin in a process called *fibrinolysis*.

ANTICOAGULANTS

Anticoagulants are drugs or substances that prevent or retard blood coagulation. Anticoagulants do *not* dissolve a clot that is already present, and their use is always prophylactic. Anticoagulants are generally classified as either parenteral (heparin) or oral (coumarin and indanedione derivatives). Drugs in both groups are used to treat venous conditions such as deep-vein thrombosis and pulmonary embolism. Arterial conditions such as coronary artery disease, rheumatic heart disease, atrial fibrillation alone or in combination with valve disease, atrial fibrillation before and after cardioversion, thromboembolic complications of prosthetic devices such as cardiac valves, and cerebral vascular disorders are also treated with anticoagulants. Arterial disorders, however, usually are more responsive to antiplatelet agents. Anticoagulants can also be used prophylactically to treat patients on bed rest for prolonged periods, those who have had major surgeries, and those with a history of previous clotting disorders. Anticoagulants are featured in Table 35–2.

CONTRAINDICATIONS AND PRECAUTIONS

Anticoagulants are contraindicated in patients with hypersensitivity and in those with uncontrolled bleeding, open wounds, or severe hepatic or renal disease. Anticoagulants are given cautiously to patients with hypertension, as there may be a precipitous fall in blood pressure; mild hepatic or renal disease because the liver and kidney are the organs of these drugs' biotransformation and elimination; and to menstruating women or to patients immediately postpartum or after surgery because bleeding may result. Anticoagulants are also contraindicated in patients with a threatened abortion, cerebrovascular hemorrhage, blood dyscrasias, precordial effusion, and subacute bacterial endocarditis, because these conditions may result in bleeding. Oral anticoagulants are used cautiously in patients with diseases that predispose them to bleeding, such as ulcerative diseases of the gastrointestinal (GI) tract or alcoholism.

PARENTERAL ANTICOAGULANTS

The parenteral anticoagulants include **heparin** and the low-molecular-weight heparins—**enoxaparin sodium (Lovenox)** and **dalteparin sodium (Fragmin)**. Antithrombin III (ATnativ), produced from human plasma, is a major coagulation inhibitor in blood.

○ **Heparin** was first isolated in 1916. It can be extracted from many body cells, but the organs richest in heparin are the intestine and the mast cells in the lung. Free heparin is rarely found circulating in the bloodstream unless there has been massive damage to the pulmonary mast cells. However, free heparin can appear in anaphylactic shock because heparin and histamine are bound together within the mast cell. As histamine is liberated, heparin is freed also. The heparin that is administered as an anticoagulant is a natural product derived from either beef or pig lung tissue or from the mucosal linings of pig intestine.

ACTION Heparin acts in the first three steps of the clotting cascade by combining with and activating antithrombin III–thrombin complex to prevent the ultimate formation of fibrinogen to fibrin in stage III of the clotting cascade. (See Fig. 35–1 for sites of action of heparin.)

USES Heparin is used when a rapid anticoagulant is needed and in all the conditions described earlier. Heparin also may be used during blood transfusions, hemodialysis, and extracorporeal circulation during open heart surgery to prevent blood clotting. Heparin is generally the first anticoagulant used because of its rapid action; after several days, the patient can be placed on oral anticoagulants. Low-dose heparin is also used to prevent thromboembolism in high-risk patients after surgery. Heparin is used together with antifibrinolytics to reduce the incidence of myocardial infarction (MI).

Heparin can be used safely during pregnancy (category C) because it does not cross the placenta. Therefore, pregnant women requiring anticoagulants must stay in the hospital and receive heparin, rather than going home on an oral anticoagulant such as warfarin sodium (Coumadin).

Table 35–2. ANTICOAGULANTS AND ANTICOAGULANT ANTAGONISTS

DRUG NAME/ROUTE AND DOSAGE	PHARMACOKINETICS/ DYNAMICS	NURSING IMPLICATIONS
ANTICOAGULANTS		
all anticoagulants		**ASSESSMENT:** Frequent blood tests must be performed to assess clotting time (APTT for heparin, PT for warfarin sodium). Carefully assess all bodily secretions and orifices for bleeding. Antagonists should be on hand. **INTERVENTION:** A flow sheet containing clotting times, time of medication administration, and route used should be kept on patient's chart. **Patient Teaching—** Teach patients about evaluating urine for blood. Warn patient to not take any medications without approval of physician or nurse. **EVALUATION:** Evaluate for bleeding—mucous membranes and urine, stool for occult blood, platelets, complete blood counts. Keep PT/APPT about 1.2–2.5 the control.
ANTICOAGULANTS: PARENTERAL		
heparin ***Adults:*** *Therapeutic dosage–* 8000–20,000 U SC q 8–12 hr; 5000–10,000 U IV bolus q 4–6 hr (50–100 U/kg); 5000–20,000 U IV infusion (0.5 U/kg per min). *Prophylaxis–*5000 U q 8–12 hr or by weight: initial bolus 80 U/kg IV push, and maintenance 18 U/kg per hr. Dose may also be adjusted /PTT: PTT below 35 sec 80 U/kg bolus; PTT 36–70 sec 40 U/kg bolus; PTT 71–90 seconds reduce by 2 U/hr; PTT above 90 sec, hold for 1 hr, then reduce by 3 U/hr. ***Children:*** Initially, 50 U/kg IV infusion, then 50–100 U/kg q 4 hr for maintenance, or 20,000 u/m² per day IV infusion. **clearing heparin lock** ***Adults:*** 10–100 U/ml IV.	**Onset:** SC, 20–60 min; IV, 2–3 min **Peak:** SC, 2 hr; IV, 5–10 min **Duration:** SC, 8–12 hr; IV, 2–6 hr **½L:** 30–180 min (dose dependent) **PB:** highly **B:** liver **E:** urine (50% unchanged)	Same as for all plus: **ASSESSMENT:** Obtain accurate PTT or APTT; there must be at least 4–6 hr after last IV dose and 12–24 hr after last SC dose. Assess for pregnancy (category C). **INTERVENTION:** Carefully administer other IM or SC medication near time of next heparin administration so clotting time is almost back to normal. This prevents prolonged bleeding at site. Continuous IV infusions of heparin are administered through infusion pumps and microdrip regulators. Avoid IM injection as clotting studies are always elevated with continuous drip. Follow special SC technique (in Planning and Intervention section). Older patients are started on smaller doses. Oral anticoagulants are started 3–5 days prior to discontinuing heparin.
enoxaparin sodium (Lovenox) ***Adults:*** 30 mg SC bid started within 24 hr of hip/knee surgery.	**Onset:** 1–2 hr **Peak:** 3–5 hr. **Duration:** 12 hr **½L:** 4.5 hr **PB:** NA **B:** liver **E:** urine	Same as for all plus: **ASSESSMENT:** Assess for signs of bleeding. Assess for pork allergy previous reaction to heparin, and for renal disease. Assess for pregnancy (category B). **INTERVENTION:** Administer SC, with patient lying down, deep into anterolateral/posterolateral abdominal wall. Alternate sites. Pinch skin fold, insert needle the entire length, and hold skin fold during entire injection. Not for IM administration. Do not mix with other drugs.
dalteparin sodium (Fragmin) ***Adults:*** 2500 IU deep SC 1–2 hr before surgery, then once daily for 5–10 days.	**Onset:** rapid **Peak:** 4 hr **Duration:** up to 24 hr **½L:** 2.1–2.3 hr **PB:** NA **B:** NA **E:** NA	Same as for all plus: **ASSESSMENT:** Assess complete blood count, platelet count, and stools for occult blood throughout therapy. Assess for signs of bleeding. Assess for pregnancy (category B). **INTERVENTION:** Special monitoring of clotting times (APPT) is not necessary. Dalteparin cannot be used in-

Table 35–2. ANTICOAGULANTS AND ANTICOAGULANT ANTAGONISTS, *Continued*

DRUG NAME/ROUTE AND DOSAGE	PHARMACOKINETICS/ DYNAMICS	NURSING IMPLICATIONS

ANTICOAGULANTS: PARENTERAL

		terchangeably (unit for unit) with heparin or enoxaparin. Administer deep SC into abdominal wall inferior and lateral to umbilicus, upper outer side of thigh, or upper outer quadrant of buttock. Rotate injection sites. **Patient Teaching**—Advise patient to report any sign of bleeding. Instruct patient not to take any NSAIDs (aspirin, ketoprofen, or ibuprofen) during therapy.

ANTICOAGULANTS: ORAL

warfarin sodium (Coumadin) (Panwarfin) (Sofarin)		
Adults: Initial dose–10–15 mg/day PO, IV, or IM for 3–5 days. *Maintenance dose*–2–15 mg daily based on PT.	**Onset:** 2–12 hr **Peak:** 1.5–3 days **Duration:** 2–5 days **½L:** 1–2.5 days **PB:** 99% **B:** liver **E:** urine, feces	Same as for all plus: **ASSESSMENT:** Assess hepatic and renal function and PT. Assess for pregnancy (category unknown). **INTERVENTION: Patient Teaching**—Patient should not consume large quantities of vitamin K–rich foods (green leafy vegetables, cauliflower, tomatoes, fish, liver, cheese, egg yolks, and fats from red meats). Caution patient to avoid excessive alcohol intake because of its effect on liver and tendency to cause increased bleeding. Inform patient that when traveling to hot climate from cold one, dose of medication may need to be reduced. Patients are encouraged to use soft toothbrush to prevent gum injury, and shaving is done with electric razor to avoid scraping skin. Patients should carry identification card or wear jewelry that states medication that is being taken and physician's name and telephone number. Medications are stored in tight, moisture-resistant container. Patient will need to take 3–5 days before PT rises. **EVALUATION:** Urine may turn red-orange on standing.

ANTICOAGULANT ANTAGONISTS

protamine sulfate		
Adults: 10–50 mg IV, given in 1–3 min, not to exceed 20 mg/min or 50 mg in 10 min (1 mg neutralizes 90 U heparin derived from lung and 115 U derived from intestinal mucosa).	**Onset:** 30–60 sec **Peak:** 5–10 min **Duration:** 2 hr **½L:** NA **PB:** NA **B:** partially by liver **E:** NA	**ASSESSMENT:** Assess bleeding and clotting studies before and during therapy. Assess vital signs closely until all signs of bleeding have passed. Assess closely for allergic reactions. Assess for pregnancy (category C). **INTERVENTION:** Dose is titrated according to clotting studies. Diluents for IV are only 0.9% sodium chloride, 5% dextrose, 5% dextrose in 0.9% sodium chloride. IV solutions are used immediately and not stored. **EVALUATION:** For rebleed evaluate heparin rebound, which may necessitate more protamine.

phytonadione (vitamin K₁) (AquaMEPHYTON) (Konakion) (Mephyton)		
hypoprothrombinemia secondary to oral anticoagulants *Adults:* 2.5–10 mg PO, SC, IV, or IM based on PT, repeated in 12–24 hr after oral dose or 6–8 hr after parenteral dose. **hemorrhagic disease of the newborn** *Neonates:* 0.5–1 mg within 1 hr of birth. 1–5 mg may be given 12–24 hr before delivery.	**Onset:** PO, slowly; IV, rapid; IM, 1–2 hours. **Peak:** PO, 6–12 hr; IV, 15 min; IM, 3–6 hr. **Duration:** IV, 3–6 hr **½L:** NA **PB:** NA **B:** liver **E:** NA	**ASSESSMENT:** Assess baseline clotting studies. Assess for pregnancy (category unknown). **INTERVENTION:** Konakion contains a phenol derivative and is administered only IM. Encourage vitamin K–rich foods. IV use—Severe reactions and fatalities have occurred immediately after IV injection. This is primarily due to anaphylaxis with fast rate of administration. When IV administration is used, inject at rate not exceeding 1 mg/min. **EVALUATION:** Bleeding should decrease.

NA = not available.

Heparin is also used as a flush to keep arterial pressure monitoring lines open. Its use increases the probability of maintaining patency of these lines (American Association of Critical Care Nurses, 1993).

PHARMACOKINETICS Because of its large molecular size and polarity, heparin has poor penetration into the central nervous system (CNS) and into breast milk and cannot cross the placental barrier. It is extensively bound to plasma proteins. Researchers suggest that the mast cells in the lungs may be able to absorb heparin and act as a storage depot.

Heparin is biotransformed in the liver by a heparin-inactivating enzyme called heparinase, and inactive metabolites are excreted in the urine. A patient with renal or hepatic disease may experience a longer anticoagulant effect.

ADVERSE EFFECTS The most common and serious adverse effect of heparin is hemorrhage (10%). If a patient experiences bleeding, the drug is discontinued and the patient is monitored. The effects should dissipate in several hours. If severe bleeding occurs, the direct antagonist of its action, protamine sulfate, can be used.

▼ CLINICAL ALERT

Heparin-induced thrombosis or white clot syndrome (WCS) is the most serious adverse reaction (Kuc, 1993). It may affect as many as 10% of patients. WCS generally occurs 2 or more days after initiation of heparin therapy if the patient has been on heparin before. In those new to heparin therapy, it may take 10 to 15 days to appear. WCS is associated with a progressively falling platelet count (*thrombocytopenia*) to less than 100,000/mm³ (normal 200,000 to 400,0000/mm³); increasing resistance to anticoagulation effects of heparin; and thromboembolism. The thrombocytopenia is generally reversible after withdrawal of heparin, but it may take several days for the platelets to return to normal. Thrombocytopenia occurs in about 15% of patients receiving bovine heparin and 6% of patients receiving porcine heparin. Platelet antibody formation (IgG) secondary to heparin is probably responsible for the thromboembolism that ensues. These complications may result in limb amputation (21%) and a high mortality rate (29%).

Less common adverse effects include fever, chills, and rash from a hypersensitivity reaction; burning sensation at the injection site; and rhinitis. Osteoporosis has been reported in patients taking heparin for longer than 6 months because heparin potentiates parathyroid hormone activity, which results in bone resorption.

Heparin therapy should be withdrawn gradually, and an alternate therapy should be introduced during the time when a primary predisposing condition exists (Singh et al., 1994). Abrupt withdrawal of heparin can lead to a rebound embolization. In a patient with unstable angina it can lead to reactivation of severe angina.

INTERACTIONS Several interactions occur with heparin. Drugs that increase the risk of bleeding when taken concurrently with heparin include oral anticoagulants, aspirin, cephalosporins, and penicillin. These drugs can prolong bleeding time or cause GI hemorrhage. Concurrent nitroglycerin may cause heparin resistance because of changes in antithrombin III induced by nitroglycerin. False elevations of transaminases (serum aspartate and alamine, or AST and ALT, respectively) may occur.

DOSAGE Heparin may be administered subcutaneously, by IV bolus, or IV drip. It should not be given IM, as muscular hematomas result. The best site for the subcutaneous (SC) dose is above the iliac crest or in the abdominal fat layer. After withdrawal of the needle, light pressure is applied but no massage. This prevents damage and bleeding of the sensitive subcutaneous tissues. The dosage is tailored to the patient's weight.

○ **Enoxaparin sodium** (*Lovenox*) is a low-molecular-weight heparin. It consists of fragments of standard heparin that bind to antithrombin III (see Table 35–2). Because these fragments are too short to bind to other components of the clotting cascade, they lose their extensive anticoagulant effects. Thus, enoxaparin is very effective in preventing thrombosis and has fewer bleeding complications. It is indicated for the prevention of deep-vein thrombosis following hip replacement surgery.

Low-molecular-weight heparin has a long half-life, which allows for once-a-day dosing. And, there is no need to do blood monitoring. Adverse effects are the same as for heparin.

INTERACTIONS Enoxaparin is used cautiously with other anticoagulants and platelet inhibitors, as bleeding may ensue. It can cause asymptomatic increases in both AST and ALT.

○ **Dalteparin sodium** (*Fragmin*) is a low-molecular-weight heparin with antithrombotic properties. It is used prophylactically to prevent deep-vein thrombosis in patients undergoing abdominal surgery who are at risk for thromboembolic complications.

○ **Antithrombin III** (*ATnativ*) acts as an anticoagulant by inhibiting thrombin. Antithrombin III is indicated in patients with a hereditary or acquired deficiency of antithrombin III (AT-III). It has also been used as an adjunct to heparin in patients with heparin resistance. Antithrombin III is useful in preventing thrombosis following surgery, during labor and delivery (pregnancy category C), and in the postpartum period in patients with AT-III deficiency. Safety in children has not been established.

A rebound hypercoagulability may occur if antithrombin III is withdrawn abruptly. If withdrawal is necessary, an alternative anticoagulant is administered.

Antithrombin III is administered IV with an initial dose and then maintenance dose every 24 hours until the patient is stabilized. Antithrombin III levels are drawn twice daily until the levels are stable. Dosage is individualized for each patient.

ORAL ANTICOAGULANTS

The oral anticoagulants include the coumarin derivative—**warfarin sodium** (*Coumadin*) and the indanedione derivative—**anisindione** (*Miradon*).

Action

Warfarin and indanedione derivatives have only one main pharmacologic effect: inhibition of the blood clotting mechanism by interfering with the hepatic synthesis of vitamin K–dependent clotting factors, including factors II (prothrombin), VII, IX, and X. These derivatives compete with vitamin K, making it unavailable for synthesis of the clotting factors. (See Fig. 35–1 for site of action.) Therefore, vitamin K is an antagonist for both the coumarin and indanedione derivatives. The dose of coumarin is computed on the basis of the prothrombin time and INR's. (See the Nursing Process section for an explanation of laboratory tests.)

Uses

In addition to the uses already discussed, the warfarin and indanedione products are used for prophylaxis and long-term anticoagulation to protect against sudden thromboembolic phenomena, as an adjunct in treatment of coronary occlusion, and to prevent recurrent transient ischemic attacks. These products have several advantages: they are relatively inexpensive, are available for oral use, and need to be given only once a day to maintain their therapeutic effect.

The effectiveness of low-dose warfarin (1 mg/day) in preventing postoperative thromboembolism is currently being evaluated. This dose causes few, if any, bleeding problems.

Pharmacokinetics

Unlike heparin, these products do cross the placenta and enter breast milk. Research is being conducted to determine their effect on the neonate. More information can be found in Table 35–2.

Contraindications and Precautions

In addition to the contraindications and precautions for all anticoagulants, oral anticoagulants are also contraindicated in pregnancy (category X) because they may cause fatal hemorrhage, spontaneous abortions, and fetal deformities.

Adverse Effects

The most significant adverse effect is hemorrhage. Consequently, oral anticoagulant therapy is closely monitored with coagulation tests and monitoring of clinical signs of bleeding, which include ecchymoses, hematuria, uterine bleeding, melena, hematoma, gingival bleeding, hemoptysis, and hematemesis. Treatment of hemorrhage involves discontinuation of the drug and administration of vitamin K. Severe bleeding episodes are treated with fresh frozen plasma, whole blood, or plasma concentrates of vitamin K–dependent clotting factors. If oral coagulant therapy is to be reinstituted, higher-than-normal doses may be needed until the vitamin K is eliminated from the body. This may take up to several weeks.

Other common adverse effects include anorexia, nausea, vomiting, and dermatitis. Less common adverse effects are hepatitis, jaundice, and increased menstrual flow. Tissue necrosis has also been reported with warfarin therapy.

Interactions

Many interactions occur with oral anticoagulants, which can either potentiate or inhibit their effect. Drugs can potentiate the effect of warfarin by displacing it from its protein-binding sites, inhibiting its metabolic breakdown, or decreasing the amount of vitamin K–producing bacteria in the gut. Protein-binding interactions occur with drugs such as chloral hydrate, loop diuretics, and nalidixic acid. If these drugs are administered with oral anticoagulants, the patient is monitored closely for bleeding episodes for the first 5 to 10 days of concurrent therapy. Because hepatic metabolism increases as more free drug is made available to be metabolized, often a new steady state is reached and an enhanced effect should no longer be observed.

Drugs that inhibit hepatic metabolism of warfarin and cause increased effectiveness and response include phenylbutazone, cimetidine, metronidazole, chloramphenicol, lovastatin, propafenone, quinidine, trimethoprim/sulfamethoxazole, and amiodarone. The dosage of oral anticoagulants may need to be reduced if one of these drugs is added to a patient's therapy.

Most oral anti-infective drugs can destroy intestinal bacteria that produce vitamin K, thereby rendering the patient hypoprothrombinemic. This can result in an increased effect of oral anticoagulants. These interactions take on an added significance if the interacting drug has an effect of its own on the hemostatic system or can cause GI bleeding. This is particularly important when salicylates, steroids, indomethacin, phenylbutazone, antimetabolics, quinidine, or potassium products are used in a patient taking oral anticoagulants.

Several drugs can decrease responsiveness to oral anticoagulants. These include enzyme inducers (e.g., barbiturates, phenytoin, rifampin), which increase the metabolism of oral anticoagulants and decrease plasma concentrations. Cholestyramine and aluminum hydroxide reduce oral anticoagulant absorption. Estrogen products, oral contraceptives, laxatives, vitamin C, antihistamines, and chronic alcohol abuse can also decrease anticoagulant activity.

Ingestion of large quantities of food high in vitamin K may antagonize the anticoagulant effect of warfarin, as vitamin K is its antidote. Foods rich in vitamin K include leafy green vegetables (cabbage, collards, mustard greens, spinach), beans, cheese, fish, milk, pork, rice, turnips, and yogurt.

○ **Warfarin sodium** (Coumadin, Panwarfin, Sofarin, and others) are almost always given once a day. A standard dosage, however, cannot be determined because dosage is individually titrated to the amount required to increase the prothrombin time (PT) 1.3 to 1.5 times normal and the International Normalized Ratio (INR) to 2–3 for prevention of thromboembolism and 1.5 to 2 times normal in patients with prosthetic heart valves or recurrent systemic embolization. Additional information is found in Table 35–2.

○ **Anisindione** (Miradon) is similar in all respects to the coumarin products. However, it is potentially more dangerous, so it is reserved for patients who cannot tolerate warfarin. Anisindione has been reported to cause dermatitis, but it may also cause agranulocytosis, jaundice, nephropathy, diarrhea, and fever.

ANTICOAGULANT ANTAGONISTS

On occasion, heparin and the coumarin and indanedione anticoagulants may cause excessive bleeding. When this occurs, an antagonist that interferes with the anticoagulating effect is administered. The antagonist of heparin, including the low-molecular-weight heparins, is **protamine sulfate.** The antagonist for the oral anticoagulants is vitamin K₁—**phytonadione (AquaMEPHYTON, Konakion, Mephyton).** If bleeding is severe, blood or component therapy may also be indicated. The anticoagulant antagonists are featured in Table 35–2.

○ **Protamine sulfate** is a purified mixture of simple proteins obtained from the sperm of salmon and other fish. When used alone, it has an anticoagulant effect. However, protamine in vitro complexes with heparin to form an inactive complex, which inactivates the anticoagulant effects of both drugs. Heparin's effect of inhibiting platelet aggregation, though, will persist. Each milligram of protamine sulfate neutralizes about 90 units of heparin derived from lung tissue and 115 units of heparin derived from intestinal mucosa. The amount given should equal the amount of heparin overdose minus the heparin that was already metabolized.

Protamine sulfate is contraindicated in hemorrhage not induced by heparin and is given cautiously to patients with cardiovascular disease and to those with allergies to fish. Safety in pregnancy (category C), lactation, and children has not been established. Adverse effects include hypotension, nausea and vomiting, and anaphylaxis.

○ **Phytonadione** (vitamin K₁, AquaMEPHYTON, Konakion, Mephyton) antagonizes the effects of coumarin and indanedione anticoagulants within the liver, which promotes the hepatic synthesis of prothrombin and other clotting factors.

Phytonadione is routinely administered to newborns at birth to prevent hemorrhage. Prothrombin levels in the newborn are often normal at birth but begin to decline until about 6 days after birth, when the liver begins to form its own prothrombin.

Phytonadione is effective only in bleeding disorders that result from a low prothrombin concentration. It may be administered before surgery to persons with deficient prothrombin levels or given to persons with hypoprothrombinemia secondary to overdoses of drugs (salicylates, quinine, sulfonamides, arsenicals, and barbiturates) or secondary to conditions limiting absorption or synthesis of vitamin K (obstructive jaundice, sprue, ulcerative colitis, celiac disease, and regional enteritis). Prothrombin levels are evaluated often.

Phytonadione is contraindicated in patients with known sensitivity. It is also contraindicated in patients with hypoprothrombinemia caused by hepatocellular damage, as liver function may be further depressed. Safety in pregnancy (category C), lactation, and children has not been established.

ANTIPLATELET AGENTS

Platelets are involved with the intrinsic pathway of the clotting cascade. Antiplatelet agents interfere with the platelets' ability to adhere to each other when they are exposed to collagen. These drugs are believed to interfere

Table 35–3. ANTIPLATELET DRUGS: ACTION AND USES

DRUG	ACTION	USES
Aspirin	Inhibits formation of thromboxane A by platelets.	Angina, unstable angina, post MI, prosthetic heart valves, post coronary bypass surgery
dipyridamole (Persantine)	Increases platelet cyclic AMP levels.	Prosthetic heart valves, peripheral vascular disease
prostacyclin (Ilopost)	Increases platelet cyclic AMP levels.	Congenital heart disease (patent ductus arteriosis)
ticlopidine (Ticlid)	Alters reactivity of platelets by blocking Willebrand factor and fibrinogen with platelets. Shortens platelet survival.	Unstable angina, post MI, post PTCA, recent transient ischemic attack or ischemic stroke, prevent reoccurence lesion of coronary stents
sulfinpyrazone (Anturane)	Inhibits platelet cyclooxygenase and platelete adhesion.	Prosthetic heart valves
Dextran 70	Alters platelet surface membrane, inhibits Willebrand factor.	Immediately before and after placement of intracoronary stents
abciximab (ReoPro)	Decreases platelet aggregation by binding to receptors on platelet surfaces.	MI following PTCA

with the release of adenosine diphosphate (ADP), thus retarding platelet aggregation. Drugs in this group include salicylates (Chapter 19), **dipyridamole (Persantine)**, **ticlopidine (Ticlid)**, **sulfinpyrazone (Anturane)**, **Dextran 70, Dextran 75,** and **abciximab (ReoPro)**. All these medications are currently being studied for use in preventing thromboembolism in patients with history of venous and arterial thrombosis; in patients who have recently suffered myocardial infarction, cerebral infarction, or embolus; and in persons who have had prosthetic heart valve replacements. Prosthetic valves, particularly the ball and disk valves, increase the risk of thromboembolism. These thrombi, if they break off and migrate, may cause damage in the brain, heart, kidney, and other organs. Table 35–3 reviews the action of the various antiplatelet agents and their uses.

○ **Salicylates** have long been known to alter blood coagulability by decreasing blood clotting factor VII. Recent research has suggested that low doses of aspirin (one baby aspirin daily) can prevent venous thrombus by inhibiting platelet aggregation.

○ **Dipyridamole** (Persantine) is an antiplatelet agent thought to work best in patients with peripheral vascular disease. Dipyridamole is used with warfarin anticoagulants to prevent postoperative thromboembolism complications of cardiac valve replacement. More information on dipyridamole can be found in Table 35–4.

Dipyridamole is also used as an alternate to exercise

Table 35–4. ANTIPLATELET AGENTS AND HEMORRHEOLOGIC AGENTS

DRUG NAME/ROUTE AND DOSAGE	PHARMACOKINETICS/ DYNAMICS	NURSING IMPLICATIONS
ANTIPLATELET AGENTS		
dipyridamole (Persantine) *Adults:* 75–100 mg PO qid	**Onset:** rapid **Peak:** 75 min **Duration:** 4–6 hr **½L:** 40 min–10 hr **PB:** highly **B:** liver **E:** bile, kidney	**ASSESSMENT:** Asses blood pressure prior to and during therapy. Dipyridamole may decrease blood pressure. Assess for pregnancy (category B). **INTERVENTION: Patient Teaching—**Warn patient to change body position slowly to avoid dizziness. **EVALUATION:** Report dizziness, rash, or pruritis to physician.
ticlopidine hydrochloride (Ticlid) *Adults:* 250 mg PO bid with food	**Onset:** 1–2 hr **Peak:** 2 hr **Duration:** 4–5 days **½L:** 12.6 hr **PB:** 98% **B:** liver **E:** bile, urine (63%), feces (23%)	**ASSESSMENT:** Assess complete blood count before and during therapy (q 3 mo). Assess for pregnancy (category B). **INTERVENTION:** Take with meals. Aspirin potentiates ticlopidine. **Patient Teaching—**Instruct patient to *not* take aspirin or OTC drugs containing aspirin. **EVALUATION:** Report fever, chills, sore throat, and rash to physician.
abciximab (ReoPro) *Adults:* 250 μg/kg IV bolus 10–60 before PTCA, followed by 10 μg/min continuous infusion for 12 hr	**Onset:** within min **Peak:** 2 hr **Duration:** 24–48 hr **½L:** 30 min **PB:** NA **B:** bound to platelet receptors for up to 10 days **E:** NA	**ASSESSMENT:** Assess for current bleeding, platelet count, and pregnancy (category C). **INTERVENTION:** Provide gentle nursing care. Protect skin from injury. Document and monitor all vascular punctures. **EVALUATION:** Evaluate for hypersensitivity reactions. Evaluate for nausea, vomiting, and hypotension. Report all to physician.
HEMORRHEOLOGIC AGENTS		
pentoxifylline (Trental) *Adults:* 400 mg PO 3 times/day with meals	**Onset:** 2–4 wk (effect) **Peak:** 8 wk (effect) **Duration:** NA **½L:** 0.4–1.6 hr **PB:** NA **B:** liver **E:** urine (4%), feces	**ASSESSMENT:** Assess peripheral pulses and distance walked at onset of therapy and periodically. Assess cognitive power and memory. Assess for pregnancy (category C). **INTERVENTION:** Administer with meals to reduce nausea and vomiting. **EVALUATION:** If exercise pain continues or worsens, notify physician.

OTC = over the counter; NA = not available.

testing for the detection and evaluation of coronary artery disease. Dipyridamole produces coronary artery dilation, an action similar to that of exercise-induced vasodilation. Dipyridamole increases the level of myocardial adenosine, a potent coronary artery dilator. Dipyridamole is followed by injection of a contrast material (thallium; technetium 99 M) to see whether or not the myocardium is perfused. If the area is underperfused, this identifies significant coronary artery disease. Dipyridamole is used to assess known or suspected coronary artery disease (CAD); to determine prognosis for CAD before or after infarction; to evaluate therapy for CAD: bypass grafting, balloon angioplasty, thrombolytic drug therapy; to evaluate exercise tolerance; and to assess work capacity related to activities of daily living and employment (Marchiondo, 1994). An *angioplasty* is a procedure in which an artery that is narrowed because of the deposition of placques is catheterized and stretched from within in an attempt to improve blood flow.

○ **Ticlopidine hydrochloride** (Ticlid), a platelet aggregation inhibitor, interferes with platelet membrane function by inhibiting ADP-induced platelet fibrinogen binding. The effects are irreversible for the life of the platelet.

Ticlopidine is used to reduce the risk of thrombotic stroke in persons who have experienced stroke precursors. It is also used to prevent thrombotic activity in stents placed in the coronary vessels. Side effects include life-threatening neutropenia and bleeding disorders, so patients must be monitored closely. Bioavailability is increased by food, so ticlopidine is taken with meals. Additional information is found in Table 35–4.

○ **Sulfinpyrazone** (*Anturane*) is a potent uricosuric agent indicated for use in gouty arthritis. It also has antithrombotic and platelet inhibitor effects. Several studies are being conducted to determine the effectiveness of sulfinpyrazone in decreasing the frequency of systemic embolization in patients with mitral valve disease and decreasing the incidence of sudden cardiac death after MI. Sulfinpyrazone is featured in Chapter 56.

○ **Dextran 70** and **Dextran 75** are high-molecular-weight glucose polymers used as plasma expanders. These products coat the surface of erythrocytes and platelets, and the intimal surface of the blood vessel. Therefore, platelet aggregation may be decreased. These products are discussed more thoroughly in Chapter 68.

○ **Abciximab** (ReoPro) binds to receptors on platelet surfaces, resulting in decreased platelet aggregation. It is used in conjunction with heparin and aspirin to prevent myocardial ischemia following percutaneous transluminal coronary angioplasty (PTCA) in patients at high risk for reclosure of the affected artery. Most frequent adverse effects are hypotension, bradycardia, and bleeding. Hypersensitivity reactions may also occur. Risk of bleeding is increased by concurrent anticoagulants, thrombolytics, nonsteroidal anti-inflammatory drugs, and other antiplatelet agents.

HEMORHEOLOGIC AGENT

○ **Pentoxifylline** (*Trental)* is a trisubstituted xanthine derivative for the treatment of intermittent claudication associated with chronic occlusive peripheral arterial disease. Pentoxifylline produces dose-related hemorheologic effects, lowering blood viscosity by reducing red blood cell and platelet aggregation and improving erythrocyte flexibility. This increases blood flow to the affected microcirculation and enhances tissue oxygenation. The exact mechanism of action is unknown. Pentoxifylline increases cellular adenosine triphosphate (ATP) content, therefore affecting the red blood cells. It also stimulates prostacyclin formation and release, ultimately increasing platelet cAMP, thereby reducing platelet aggregation. Pentoxifylline also increases blood fibrinolytic activity, thus reducing fibrinogen concentration. Tissue perfusion and oxygenation are improved through a mild vasodilator effect. Pentoxifylline is reviewed in Table 35–4.

THROMBOLYTIC AGENTS

Thrombolytic agents, also referred to as fibrinolytics, dissolve clots through activation of the endogenous fibrinolytic system. Three generations of products are available as thrombolytic agents. These preparations assist the conversion of plasma proteins and plasminogen to plasmin (fibrinolysin), which, in turn, digests the fibrin threads, resulting in clot lysis. The thrombus is dissolved rather than having its extension prevented, as with anticoagulants. Several of these products alter stage IV of clotting, and consequently, bleeding is more difficult to control than the bleeding secondary to anticoagulants. These drugs are featured in Table 35–5.

The first generation products include **streptokinase (Kabikinase, Streptase)** and **urokinase (Abbokinase)**; the second generation products include recombinant **alteplase (tissue plasminogen activator, t-PA or TPA; Activase)**, **anistreplase (anisolated plasminogen–streptokinase activator complex, APSAC; Eminase)**, and **prourokinase (scu-PA)**; and the third generation products include synergic combinations (t-PA and scu-PA), hybrids, chimerics, and fibrin-antibody conjugated scu-PA and TPA. Each drug produces clot lysis in its own way and is discussed later. Figure 35–2 compares the action of these products.

USES

All these agents are used in various forms of thromboembolic disease such as phlebothrombosis, pulmonary embolism, thrombophlebitis, and arterial thrombosis (as in arteriovenous cannulae occlusions and acute MI, thromboembolic cerebral vascular accident) to promote the lysis and dissolution of existing fibrin clots and restore normal blood-flow patterns. These medications are used within 6 hours after embolization.

▼ CLINICAL ALERT

Despite their widespread use, the thrombolytics have significant limitations. Resistance to reperfusion occurs in 25% of patients. Stable coronary patency is not uniformly produced, and therefore acute coronary reocclusion oc-

Table 35–5. THROMBOLYTIC AGENTS

DRUG NAME/ROUTE AND DOSAGE	PHARMACOKINETICS/ DYNAMICS	NURSING IMPLICATIONS
streptokinase (Streptase) (Kabikinase)		
deep-vein thrombosis and pulmonary embolism *Adults:* Loading dose–250,000 IU IV over 30 min. *Maintenance dose*–100,000 IU/hr for 24–72 hr. **coronary thrombosis** *Adults:* 20,000 IU IV bolus, then 2000 IU/min for 60 min maintenance. **acute myocardial infarction** *Adults:* 1.5 million U IV infusion over 1 hr.	**Onset:** immediate **Peak:** rapid **Duration:** 12–24 hr **½L:** biphasic 23 min, 83 min. **PB:** NA **B:** antibodies and reticuloendothelial system **E:** NA	**ASSESSMENT:** Assess laboratory values prior to and every 4 hr during therapy, including TT, APTT, PTT, hematocrit, CK-MBs, fibrinogen, and platelet count. Have typed and cross-matched blood available. Assess carefully for bleeding during therapy. Assess for pregnancy (category C). **INTERVENTION:** Maintain continuous ECG monitoring and ST monitoring if available. Assess for chest pain. Handle patient as little as possible during therapy. IM injections, venipunctures, and arterial sticks should not be performed during therapy unless absolutely necessary. IV catheters that infiltrate are left in place during therapy. Follow specific reconstitution procedures. Direct flow of diluent against side of vial. Avoid shaking and agitation of solution. Use solution within 24 hr of preparation. If it must be stored, store at 2°–4°C. Use filters during IV administration. Monitor closely and treat other problems (reperfusion angina or dysrhythmia when given for acute MI as they occur). **EVALUATION:** Evaluate for allergic or febrile reactions. If they occur, decrease dose and call physician.
urokinase (Abbokinase)		
pulmonary embolism *Adults:* Loading dose–4400 IU/kg IV at a rate of 90 mL/hr. *Maintenance dose*–4400 IU/kg per hr at a rate of 15 mL/hr. **coronary artery occlusion** *Adults:* 6000 IU/min for up to 2 hr (or 500,000 units total). **occluded iv catheter** *Adults:* 5000 IU instilled, wait 5–10 min and aspirate. If not open, cap and allow urokinase to remain 30–60 min before next attempt to aspirate.	**Onset:** immediate **Peak:** rapid **Duration:** 12–24 hr **½L:** 20 min or less **PB:** NA **B:** liver **E:** NA	Same as for streptokinase except: **ASSESSMENT:** Assess for pregnancy (category B).
alteplase (Activase)		
accelerated-dose tpa *Adults:* 100 mg in 100 mL diluent over 90 min: 15 mg as bolus over 1–2 min, 50 mg over 30 min, 35 mg over 60 min, or per institutional policy. **accelerated-dose tpa by weight** *Adults:* 100 mg in 100 mL diluent over 90 min: 15 mg as a bolus over 1–2 min, 0.75 mg/kg over 30 min (not >50 mg), 0.50 mg/kg over 60 min (not >35 mg). Total dose, = 15 + 1.25 mg/kg (not to exceed 100 mg) or per institutional policy. **standard-dose tpa** *Adults:* 100 mg in 100 mL diluent over 3 hr: 6–10 mg as bolus over 1–2 min; 50–54 mg over 1st hr, 20 mg over 2nd hr, 20 mg over 3rd hr, or per institutional policy.	**Onset:** immediate **Peak:** 5–10 min **Duration:** 3 hr **½L:** biphasic: 8 min and 1.3 hr **PB:** NA **B:** liver **E:** urine	Same as for streptokinase. **INTERVENTION:** Reconstitute with 18 g needle. Administer within 8 hr of mixing. Assess for pregnancy (category C).

Continued on the following page

Table 35–5. THROMBOLYTIC AGENTS, *Continued*

DRUG NAME/ROUTE AND DOSAGE	PHARMACOKINETICS/ DYNAMICS	NURSING IMPLICATIONS
alteplase (Activase)		
cva **Adults:** 20–100 mg as bolus over 1–2 min peripherally and 50 mg over 30–60 min.		
anistreplase (Eminase) (APSAC) **Adults:** 30 units IV over 2–5 min	**Onset:** immediate **Peak:** 2 hr **Duration:** 12–24 hr **½L:** 70–120 min **PB:** NA **B:** desacetylated in blood or thrombus to plasminogen streptokinase complex; complex is later eliminated via antibodies and through the reticuloendothelial system **E:** NA	Same as for alteplase except: **ASSESSMENT:** Assess for pregnancy (category C).

CK-MB = Isoenzyme of CK for cardiac damage.
NA = not available.

curs in 5% to 25% of patients. The time from injection to reprofusion may be 45 minutes or longer. And, significant bleeding such as intracerebral bleeds may occur.

CONTRAINDICATIONS AND PRECAUTIONS

Contraindications include recent major surgery (within 10 days), serious GI bleeding, organ biopsy, or obstetric delivery; severe uncontrolled arterial hypertension (systolic blood pressure of 200 mm Hg or more or diastolic pressure of 110 mm Hg or more); and recent serious trauma. Minor contraindications include recent minor trauma, including cardiopulmonary resuscitation, high likelihood of left heart thrombus (e.g., mitral stenosis with atrial fibrillation), infectious endocarditis, pregnancy, cerebrovascular accident (within 2 months), diabetic hemorrhagic retinopathy, and hemostatic defects, including those associated with severe hepatic or renal disease. Safety in pregnancy (category C), lactation, and children has not been established. Patients over age 75 are at higher risk of bleeding due to cerebrovascular disease.

ADVERSE EFFECTS

The major adverse effect of the thrombolytic agents is bleeding. Bleeding may occur at invaded or disturbed skin sites, or internally from many organ sites including the brain. Should uncontrolled bleeding occur, these products are discontinued. If necessary, blood loss and

reversal of bleeding tendency can be effectively managed with whole blood (fresh is preferable), packed red cells, platelets, clotting factor such as cryoprecipitate and fibrinogen, or fresh-frozen plasma; a target fibrinogen level of 18 per liter is desirable. Although the effectiveness of

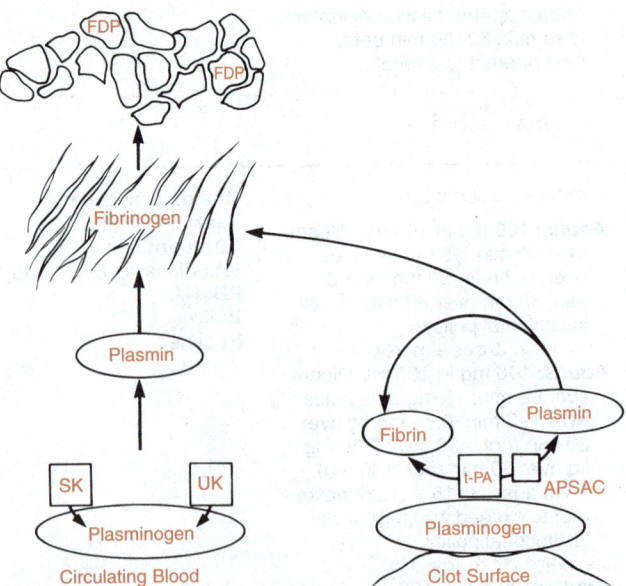

Figure 35–2. A schematic representation of the action of streptokinase (SK), urokinase (UK), and anistreplase (APSAC), which affect the exogenous circulating plasmin; and tissue plasminogen activator (t-PA), which affects only fibrin-bound plasmin.

aminocaproic acid (Amicar) as an antidote has not been documented, it may be used in an emergency. A febrile reaction can also occur after drug administration with streptokinase (33%) as it is a foreign protein. Symptomatic treatment is usually sufficient to relieve discomfort. Allergic reaction, such as serum sickness with streptokinase, can also occur.

▼ **CLINICAL ALERT**

Dysrhythmias occurring after thrombolytic therapy include ventricular tachycardia, sinus bradycardia, premature ventricular contractions, supraventricular tachycardia, and ventricular fibrillation. These drugs are arrhythmogenic, and the dysrhythmias are treated with appropriate antidysrhythmic medications.

The rate of reocclusion (defined as rethrombosis of an infarct-associated artery after successful thrombolysis) ranges from 9% to 45%. Risk factors for reocclusion include high-grade residual stenosis, vasospasm, residual thrombus after fibrinolysis, and exposed injured vessel wall. Ischemia from reocclusion is most likely to occur within the first 24 hours after thrombolysis. Nurses often play a critical role in preventing reocclusion (see Nursing Process section).

INTERACTIONS

Anticoagulant therapy may increase the risk of hemorrhage. Also, drugs affecting platelet function (indomethacin, phenylbutazone, and sulfinpyrazone) are avoided.

○ **Streptokinase** (Kabikinase, Streptase) is not fibrin selective and thereby creates a systemic lytic state. Streptokinase acts with plasminogen to produce an activator complex that converts plasminogen to the proteolytic enzyme plasmin and thus dissolves clots. Streptokinase is derived from bacteria protein. This causes significant antigenicity, creating the potential for allergic responses, including anaphylaxis. Because it is a foreign protein, streptokinase has the ability to cause resistance due to the development of antibodies. Therapy can be administered again if needed within 24 hours. After the second dose within the first 24 hours, streptokinase cannot be repeated for 3 to 6 months, until the antibodies are gone. Dilution and infusion rates for IV doses are presented in Table 35–5.

Streptokinase is administered IV to dissolve clots in the coronary arteries that are less than 6 hours old. Large trials of streptokinase have found that streptokinase administered within 3 to 4 hours of the onset of pain reduces muscle damage and improves the ejection fraction. A reduction of mortality of 50% is achieved when streptokinase is administered within 1 hour. But if streptokinase is not administered until 3 to 6 hours after onset of pain, only the 30-day mortality is reduced with no increase in muscle survival. Streptokinase may also prevent recurrence of infarction.

○ **Urokinase** (Abbokinase) is a nonantigenic protein secreted by the human kidneys and excreted in the urine.

This protein promotes thrombolysis through a direct action on the fibrinolytic system to convert plasminogen into the proteolytic enzyme plasmin. Plasmin then degrades the fibrin clot as well as fibrinogen and other plasma proteins. Urokinase causes a systemic lytic state. The advantage over streptokinase is its lack of antigenicity and antibodies formation. The increase in fibrinolytic activity usually disappears within a few hours after discontinuation of the medication, but may persist for up to 12 to 24 hours. Urokinase is approved for use in the lysis of acute massive pulmonary emboli and for lysis of emboli accompanied by unstable hemodynamics (i.e., failure to maintain blood pressure without supportive measures) in adults. It is effective and can be used to restore patency to occluded IV catheters. Urokinase therapy is initiated as soon as possible. This drug is considerably more expensive than streptokinase; however, urokinase may be useful in patients who require a thrombolytic agent but have high concentrations of streptokinase antibodies. Additional information is presented in Table 35–5.

○ **Alteplase** (Activase, t-PA or TPA) is a protease enzyme purified from uterine tissue and a human melanoma cell line. Alteplase is now produced by genetic recombinant techniques, which provides a large quantity of highly purified material. Because it is a natural protein, it is not associated with antibody formation or with allergic reaction. Alteplase is identical to the natural activator generated locally by endothelial cells of the vessel wall as part of the normal physiologic mechanism for digesting fibrin clots. Recombinant alteplase activates fibrin-bound plasminogen to plasmin. It is selective in that recombinant alteplase acts on new clots. It must actually act on the clot to be activated. The circulation half-life is 3 to 5 minutes. This is an advantage for the patient who may require immediate surgery after thrombolysis. Alteplase given with heparin to patients with indwelling coronary catheters appears to be more effective than IV streptokinase, but it is not necessarily safer for the treatment of coronary artery thrombosis. Altephase is also being administered to patients with unstable angina to reduce the coronary stenosis caused by thrombus. When administered in ischemic stroke, symptoms are unchanged in 24 hours, but there is improvement of clinical outcome in 3 months. Additional information is presented in Table 35–5.

○ **Anistreplase** (Eminase), also known as APSAC, is an acylated inactive complex of streptokinase and human lys-plasminogen. After injection, the acyl group is slowly hydrolyzed away, producing an activation that converts plasminogen to plasmin. Unlike the other thrombolytics available, APSAC is administered as a bolus over 3 to 5 minutes. APSAC appears to be as effective as IV streptokinase for common thrombosis but is much more expensive, and there is no evidence yet that it is safer. Additional information is presented in Table 35–5.

TOPICAL HEMOSTATIC AGENTS

Topical hemostatic agents are preparations used to control capillary bleeding. They are designed to control oozing from minute vessels during surgery or, in an emer-

Table 35–6. TOPICAL HEMOSTATIC AGENTS

NAME	FORM	COMPLETELY ABSORBED BY BODY	COMMENTS
Absorbable gelatin sponge USP/BP (Gelfoam)	Gelatin sponge or cone	4–6 weeks	Can be applied dry, but is often moistened with isotonic saline or thrombin solution. Used in oral and dental surgeries and open prostatic surgery. Does not produce excessive scar formation.
Absorbable gelatin film (Gelfilm)	Thin film sheet	8–14 days	Used in neuro, thoracic, and ocular surgery.
Oxidized cellulose USP/BP (Oxycel)	Surgical gauze or cotton	2–7 days	Causes artificial clot to form when it is buried in tissues. Used in dental and oral surgery and surgery of liver, spleen, pancreas, thyroid, and prostate. It should not be used in bone fractures or as surface dressing on skin.
Thrombin USP (Thrombinar)	Powder	Not available	Acts as catalyst for conversion of fibrinogen to fibrin. Valuble in affixing skin transplants and as aid in hemostasis whenever oozing capillaries are accessible.
Thromboplastin (Thrombokinase)	Powder	Not available	—
Microfibrillar collagen hemostat (Avitene)	Fibrous or nonwoven web	About 84 days	Fibrous form is applied directly to source of bleeding; nonwoven web is applied as small squares to bleeding areas. Used for hemostatis in surgical procedures.

gency, to combat bleeding from sources other than arteries or veins. These preparations are not directly active in the clotting process, but do stop bleeding. They are either absorbable gelatin sponges or films, sterile dry preparations (fibrous microfibrillar collagen hemostat, thrombin, thromboplastin), specially treated surgical gauze or cotton (oxidized cellulose), or nonwoven web (microfibrillar collagen hemostat). All are placed directly on the bleeding area. These preparations either arrest bleeding by forming an artificial clot or provide the mechanical matrix that facilitates clot formation. They are absorbed by the body after varying time periods. Table 35–6 provides more detailed product information.

SYSTEMIC HEMOSTATICS

Systemic hemostatics, also refered to as antifibrinolytics, inhibit the resolution of the clot by inhibiting the breakdown of fibrin. These products control rapid loss of blood. Systemic hemostatics include **aminocaproic acid (Amicar)**, **tranexamic acid (Cyklokapron)**, and **aprotinin (Trasylol)**. These drugs are featured in Table 35–7.

○ **Aminocaproic acid** (Amicar), an antifibrinolytic, is administered orally or intravenously in patients with hemorrhage caused by overactivity of stage IV clot resolution or with excessive bleeding from systemic hyperfibrinolysis and urinary fibrinolysis, as an antidote in patients receiving an overdose of thrombolytic agents such as streptokinase and urokinase, and in patients with hemophilia when fibrin formation is deficient. These patients often require other additional emergency measures.

Aminocaproic acid is contraindicated in severe renal impairment and in the presence of active intravascular clotting process. It is used with caution in patients with cardiac and hepatic dysfunction. Adverse effects are generally mild and include nausea, cramping, diarrhea, dizziness, and malaise. Additional information is presented in Table 35–7.

○ **Tranexamic acid** (Cyklokapron), a synthetic antifibrinolytic agent similar to aminocaproic acid, is designed for concurrent use with coagulation factors to prevent hemorrhage in hemophiliacs undergoing dental extractions. Tranexamic acid competitively inhibits fibrinolysis by saturating lysine binding sites where plasminogen and plasmin bind to fibrinogen and fibrin.

Tranexamic acid is contraindicated in subarachnoid

Table 35–7. SYSTEMIC HEMOSTATICS

DRUG NAME/ROUTE AND DOSAGE	PHARMACOKINETICS/ DYNAMICS	NURSING IMPLICATIONS
aminocaproic acid (Amicar)		
Adults: 5 g PO in first hr, then 1–1.25 g/hr for 8 hr or until bleeding is controlled; 4–5 g in 250 mL IV in first hr followed by 1 g/hr for 8 hr or until bleeding is controlled. Maximum of 30 g/24 hr.	**Onset:** IV, immediate **Peak:** PO and IV, 2 hr **Duration:** PO and IV, 3 hr **½L:** 12 hr **PB:** NA **B:** very little **E:** urine (unchanged)	**ASSESSMENT:** Assess baseline bleeding and clotting studies. Assess routinely for clot. Assess for pregnancy (category unknown). **INTERVENTION:** Monitor pulse, blood pressure, respiratory rate. Monitor for bleeding q 15 min. Monitor intake and output. **EVALUATION:** If thrombosis occurs, aminocaproic acid may need to be discontinued.
tranexamic acid (Cyklokapron)		
before dental surgery ***Adults:*** 10 mg/kg IV. **after surgery** ***Adults:*** 25 mg/kg PO 3–4 times daily for 2–8 days; reduce dose with renal impairment.	**Onset:** 1–2 hr **Peak:** 3 hr **Duration:** 7–17 hr **½L:** 2 hr **PB:** 3% to plasminogen **B:** very little **E:** urine (95% unchanged)	**ASSESSMENT:** Assess bleeding and clotting studies. Assess for pregnancy (category B). **INTERVENTION:** IV tranexamic acid can be mixed with most IV solutions. Do not mix with blood or solutions containing penicillin. Administer IV no faster than 1 mL/min. **EVALUATION:** Evaluate for bleeding.
aprotinin (Trasylol)		
Adults: 1 mL test dose IV. *Loading dose*–200 mL. *Pump prime dose*–200 mL. *Continuous infusion*–50 mL/hr.	**Onset:** rapid **Peak:** NA **Duration:** 10 hr **½L:** 150 min **PB:** NA **B:** lysosomal enzyme **E:** urine	**ASSESSMENT:** Assess for previous allergic reaction. Assess for pregnancy (category B). **INTERVENTION:** Administer 1-mL test dose IV at least 10 min before loading dose. In supine position, administer loading dose in 20–30 min after induction of anesthesia, but before sternotomy. Pump prime dose is added to heart/lung machine. **EVALUATION:** Evaluate for allergic reaction and for further bleeding. Evaluate vital signs.

NA = not available.

hemorrhage because it may aggravate cerebral edema. It is used cautiously in persons with renal dysfunction, as the drug is eliminated in the kidneys.

The most common adverse effects are nausea, vomiting, and diarrhea, all of which usually disappear as the dose is reduced. Patients may complain of visual abnormalities, including abnormalities in color vision. Additional information is found in Table 35–7.

○ **Aprotinin** (Trasylol), a natural proteinase inhibitor, is approved to reduce perioperative blood loss and the need for blood transfusions in patients undergoing repeat coronary artery bypass grafts. Because of possible severe allergic reactions and kidney toxicity, the drug's use in primary bypass surgery is limited to patients whose aspirin therapy, clotting-bleeding disorders, or when transfusion is unavailable or unacceptable because of religious beliefs. Additional information is presented in Table 35–7.

CONTRAINDICATIONS AND PRECAUTIONS Aprotinin should not be administered to patients with known hypersensitivity to the drug. In patients previously treated with the drug, special caution is recommended, including administering an IV antihistamine before the loading dose. Use in pregnancy (category B) only if clearly indicated. Safety in children has not been established.

ADVERSE EFFECTS The most common adverse events are complications that can occur after open heart surgery, such as atrial fibrillation, MI, and heart failure; it is unknown whether these events were drug related.

INTERACTIONS Because of its antifibrinolytic activity, aprotinin may inhibit the effects of fibrinolytic agents. It may also block the hypotensive effect of captopril (Capoten). When given with heparin, aprotinin has been found to prolong clotting times.

SCLEROSING AGENTS

Sclerosing agents—**sodium tetradecyl sulfate (Sotradecol), 50% dextrose,** and **morrhuate sodium (CMC)**—are used to treat small, uncomplicated varicose veins of the lower extremities and bleeding esophageal varices. These products are injected into the vein and cause irritation of the lining of the vessel, tending to clot the blood forming a thrombus. Fibrous tissue develops within the vein, resulting in obliteration of the vein. Sclerosing agents are injected into the bleeding varices under visual examination. The procedure is repeated several times over several weeks until all the varicosities are obliterated.

Table 35–8. NURSING PROCESS FOR PATIENT REQUIRING AGENTS THAT AFFECT COAGULATION FOR A THROMBOEMBOLISM

Assessment

Assess color, pulses, pain and tenderness, cramping and pain.
Assess lifestyle, including type of work (sedentary/active) and type of leisure activities, smoking.
Assess history of recent injury to the extremity, hypertension, hypercholesterol levels, diabetes, renal disease, and/or cardiac disease.
Assess respiratory rate and depth, use of accessory muscles, pursed-lip breathing.
Auscultate lungs for areas of decreased/absent breath sounds and the presence of adventitious sounds, e.g., crackles.
Assess for generalized duskiness and cyanosis in warm tissues such as earlobes, lips, tongue, and buccal membranes.

Nursing Diagnosis: Tissue Perfusion, decreased

RELATED TO: Decreased blood flow.
AS EVIDENCED BY: Tissue edema, diminished peripheral pulses, slow/diminished capillary refill, skin color changes, pallor, erythema.

Desired Outcomes/Evaluation Criteria

Demonstrates improved perfusion as evidenced by peripheral pulses present/equal, skin color and temperature normal, absence of edema. Engages in behaviors/actions to enhance tissue perfusion. Reports/displays increasing tolerance to activity.

Nursing Actions	Rationale
Promote bedrest during acute phase.	Reduces oxygen and nutrient demands on affected extremity and minimizes possibility of dislodging thrombus and creating emboli.
Elevate legs when in bed or chair. Periodically elevate feet and lower legs above heart level.	Reduces tissue swelling and rapidly empties superficial and tibial veins, preventing overdistention and thereby increasing venous return.
Initiate/encourage active or passive exercises while in bed (e.g., flex/extend/rotate foot periodically). Assist with gradual resumption of ambulation.	These measures are designed to increase venous return from lower extremities, reduce venous stasis, and improve general muscle tone/strength.
Caution patient to avoid crossing legs and hyperflexion at knee.	Physical restriction of circulation impairs blood flow and increases venous stasis in pelvic, popliteal, and leg vessels.
Administer anticoagulation, e.g., heparin and/or coumarin derivatives.	Heparin is preferred initially because of its prompt, predictable antagonistic action on thrombin formation and its prevention of further clot formation. Coumadin, which blocks formation of prothrombin from vitamin K, may be used for long-term/postdischarge therapy.
Review coagulation studies, CBC as indicated.	Monitors effectiveness of anticoagulant therapy and risk factors, e.g., hemoconcentration and dehydration, which potentiate clot formation.

Nursing Diagnosis: Knowledge Deficit

RELATED TO: Lack of exposure/unfamiliarity with information resources, lack of recall.
AS EVIDENCED BY: Request for information, verbalization of concerns, inaccurate follow-through of instructions, development of preventable complications.

Desired Outcomes/Evaluation Criteria

Verbalizes understanding of disease process, treatment regimen, and limitations. Identifies signs/symptoms requiring medical evaluation. Correctly performs therapeutic procedure(s) and explains reasons for actions.

Nursing Actions	Rationale
Review pathophysiology of condition and signs/symptoms of possible complications (e.g., pulmonary emboli, chronic venous insufficiency, venous stasis ulcers).	Provides a knowledge base from which patient can make informed choices and understand/identify health-care needs.
Discuss purpose, dosage of anticoagulant. Emphasize importance of taking drug as prescribed.	Promotes patient safety by maintaining serum anticoagulation levels within the narrow therapeutic range, reducing risk of inadequate therapeutic response/deleterious side effect.
Discuss possible drug interactions (e.g., salicylates, alcohol, barbiturates, vitamin K). Stress need to read ingredient labels of OTC drugs and avoidance of foods high in vitamin K (e.g., green leafy vegetables).	Reduces risk of inadequate drug effect, untoward reactions, and possible complications.
Identify untoward anticoagulant effects requiring medical attention (e.g., bleeding from mucous membranes, bruising with little or no trauma, development of petechiae).	Early detection of deleterious effects of therapy allows for timely intervention, prevention of serious complications.
Stress importance of medical follow-up/laboratory testing.	Encourages patient participation. Close supervision of anticoagulant therapy is necessary to maintain therapeutic effectiveness, prevent complications.
Recommend appropriate safety precautions (e.g., use of soft toothbrush, electric razors; avoidance of forceful blowing of nose, walking barefoot).	Reduces risk of traumatic injury, bleeding.

Other Suggested Nursing Diagnoses: Pain, Impaired, Gas Exchange, and Risk for Injury.

The products are contraindicated in patients sensitive to any component of these drugs, acute superficial thrombophlebitis, uncontrolled diabetes, and significant valvular or deep-vein incompetence. Safe use in pregnancy has not been established.

USING THE NURSING PROCESS

ASSESSMENT

- Obtain a thorough past and recent nursing history to develop the database. The information that is obtained is included in Table 35–8. Generally, patients are hospitalized when they first require anticoagulants and then continue their therapy at home.
- Assess the nutritional habits of the patient, as dietary counseling is done when the patient is discharged on oral anticoagulants. Also, the nurse must understand that 50% of human vitamin K is synthesized by bacterial flora in the GI tract. When a patient is allowed nothing by mouth and is taking antibiotics, the amount of vitamin K decreases because it cannot be synthesized. Therefore, people who are not eating for long periods need supplemental vitamin K. Also, to absorb vitamin K, bile must be present. If obstructive jaundice is present, bile salts cannot move into the intestine and vitamin K absorption is reduced.
- Obtain a drug profile to determine whether the patient is currently taking any drugs that will interfere with the drugs that affect coagulation.
- Preform frequent blood tests to assess clotting time. Table 35–9 features frequently used clotting studies. In addition, hematocrit, fibrinogen concentration, and platelet counts are done.

Results may be reported in terms of an International Normalized Ratio (INR). A prothrombin time (PT) of 1.3 to 1.5, for example, equals an INR of 2 to 3. INR was developed because of differences in oral anticoagulant test reagents; it provides a standardized basis for reporting PT values (Catania, 1994). The patient must understand the importance of these clotting tests because medication dosage is regulated by their results. During the first several days, laboratory tests may be needed daily. The frequency of the tests may then be reduced to weekly for about a month, and then monthly, until the medication can be discontinued. Drug administration generally does not begin until after the laboratory results are received.

If the patient is being placed on thrombolytic agents, the thrombin time (TT) and activated partial thromboplastin time (APTT) should be less than twice the normal control times before therapy is started. It is important to draw the first APTT 2 to 3 hours after the thrombolytic drug is completed. Also heparin and/or coumarin products need to be discontinued.

NURSING DIAGNOSIS

- Establish the nursing diagnoses, which become the basis for nursing care and nursing evaluation. Typical nursing diagnoses for the patient who requires medications that affect blood coagulation include Impaired Tissue Integrity, Pain, Anxiety, Risk for Injury, and Knowledge Deficit (see Table 35–8).

PLANNING AND INTERVENTION

- Develop the goals of nursing intervention from the nursing diagnoses (see Table 35–8).

Anticoagulants

- Perform clotting studies when administering parenteral anticoagulants. With heparin, clotting studies are usually performed before the next dose is administered every 6 to 12 hours during early therapy and once daily when stable. When heparin is being given prophylactically (5000 units every 12 hours), clotting studies are not necessary. All body secretions are also examined to detect bleeding. Other medications that must be administered parenterally (IM or SC) are best scheduled near the time of the next heparin administration so that the clotting time is almost back to normal. This prevents prolonged bleeding at the site.

When heparin is administered SC, the best location is the abdomen. The medication is administered deep SC using a 25- or 26-gauge, ½- or ⅝-inch needle. The technique is as follows: Cleanse skin with alcohol (do not rub, however, because tissue may be traumatized) and allow it to dry. Bunch up fat, insert needle at 90°, do not withdraw plunger, inject medication slowly. Still holding the bunch of fat, withdraw the needle in same direction; apply pressure, but do *not* rub. A "belly chart" is kept either in the patient's room or in the chart so all injections can

Table 35–9. TESTS OF BLOOD COAGULATION			
Test	Normal Value	Therapeutic Value	Medications Monitored
Prothrombin time (PT)	11–12 sec	15–25 sec	Coumarin derivatives
International Normalized Ratio INR	1–2 IV	2–3 IV	Coumarin derivatives
Partial thromboplastin time (PTT)	60–90 sec	90–180 sec	Heparin
Lee-White clotting time (LWCT) (done on whole blood)	9–14 min	20–30 min	Heparin
Activated partial thromboplastin time (APTT)	24–36 sec	48–60 sec	Heparin
Activated clotting time (ACT)	80–135 sec	3 min	Heparin
Thrombin time (TT)	10–15 sec	20–25 sec	Heparin

be charted. Injections are not made within 2 inches of the umbilicus or on a scar.

When administering heparin intravenously, a heparin lock is most commonly used. The trap is flushed with a saline-heparin solution (usually 10 to 100 units of heparin in 1 mL of saline) before and after the heparin is injected. Always aspirate before flushing to ensure that the needle is still properly placed in the vein. Heparin locks can safely be left in place for 48 to 72 hours.

When continuous IV infusions of heparin are administered, infusion pumps and microdrip regulators are used to carefully titrate the dose. Flow sheets, containing clotting times, the time of medication administration, and the route used, are kept on the patient's chart. IM injection should be avoided in this patient because the continuous heparin drip elevates the clotting levels continually.

Today, in most patients with venous thromboembolism, heparin therapy is shortened from 10 days to 5 days to shorten hospital stay. Warfarin is started on the first day of heparin therapy and continued for several months.

Heparin has been used as a flush to clear central lines such as subclavian lines. Today, nursing research indicates that central lines can be kept patent in patients with a normal saline flush only.

- Have a supply of the antagonist for heparin—protamine sulfate—always available. If a medication error is made and the patient is given too much heparin, the protamine is used carefully for the first 4 hours after a dose.
- To obtain an accurate PT or INR, at least 4 to 6 hours must elapse after the last IV dose and 12 to 24 hours after the last SC dose. To initiate oral anticoagulant therapy, patients are often started above maintenance dosage levels—typically 10 mg/day for 2 to 4 days. Daily PT and INRS are taken prior to subsequent dosing until stabilization is achieved within therapeutic range. After stabilization, PT and INRS can be performed every 1 to 4 weeks. Any additions or deletions of concomitant medications require a PT or INR to be done after 48 hours.

Thrombolytic Agents

- Administer thrombolytics promptly. When the nurse is administering a thrombolytic enzyme (streptokinase, urokinase, recombinant alteplase, anistreplase), it is generally an acute emergency in which clot dissolution is required to preserve organ or limb function. Acute necrosis begins in about 15 minutes and continues until all tissue becomes necrotic, about 4 to 6 hours. Reperfusion must be preformed before irreversible necrosis occurs. There is evidence that early reperfusion limits necrosis. Patient selection is most important, and the nurse is often in a position to assist with early detection of vascular occlusion. Figure 35–3 includes an algorithm for MI treatment. Before thrombolytics are begun, two to three IV lines (14 to 16 gauge) are started—the first for IV fluids, the second for the thrombolytic, and the third for heparin. The third may be a heparin lock. No IV sites are established during thrombolytic therapy because of the risk of bleeding. Avoid sites that cannot be compressed, such as the jugular and subclavian veins.

Candidates for thrombolytic therapy include (1) patients with acute, massive, or severe life-threatening pulmonary embolism when two-thirds or more of a main branch of the pulmonary artery is obstructed and is accompanied by acute right-sided heart failure with or without shock and unstable circulatory status and (2) those with evolving MI with chest pain for at least 30 minutes but less than 4 hours, ST elevation of at least 0.1 mV in two leads, and no relief of pain with nitroglycerin.

Generally, the potential benefits should outweigh the dangers, such as the increased risk of bleeding. Patients with both anterior and inferior MI are candidates as thrombolysis tends to preserve left ventricular function and improve ejection fraction. Patients should generally be no more than 75 years of age, but it is important to assess the elderly patient's functional and physiologic status as opposed to chronologic age. Studies are currently in progress to determine survival benefits in the older patient. Thrombolytics are generally administered within 6 hours of the onset of chest pain. Studies are currently in progress to determine the potential benefit of late reperfusion.

- Mix thrombolytic agents carefully according to manufacturer's directions found in the package inserts. These agents are administered through microdrip tubing with an automatic IV control pump, and a filter is used.
- Administer heparin as ordered. Heparin is generally started within the first hour of streptokinase and t-PA therapy. Heparin (5000 units IV bolus followed by an IV infusion of 800 to 1000 units per hour) is regulated to maintain the PTT 1½ to 2 times normal (60 to 90 seconds). PTTs are not drawn during thrombolytic therapy as excessive PTT may occur because of the continued thrombolytic activities. PTTs are generally drawn at least 2 hours after thrombolytic therapy is completed and then every 6 hours. If the PTT is beyond 100 seconds, the heparin infusion is discontinued briefly and/or reduced until the PTT returns to the correct range. If the PTT is below 50 seconds, heparin is rebolused and the infusion increased. PTTs are repeated in 2 to 3 hours after high and low levels are obtained.
- Administer antiplatelet agents (e.g., aspirin and dipyridamole) to help decrease reocclusion by decreasing platelet activation and aggregation. These agents are often started during thrombolytic therapy and continued for 6 months or more.
- Monitor for signs and symptoms of reocclusion—return of electrocardiogram (ECG) changes (ST elevation), chest pain, anxiety, and dysrhythmias. When these symptoms return, they are treated as a medical emergency. If spasm is present, nitroglycerin or calcium channel blockers may be administered. Thrombolytic agents can be readministered, but streptokinase can be administered only within 24 hours and not after that for 6 to 8 months. If noninvasive med-

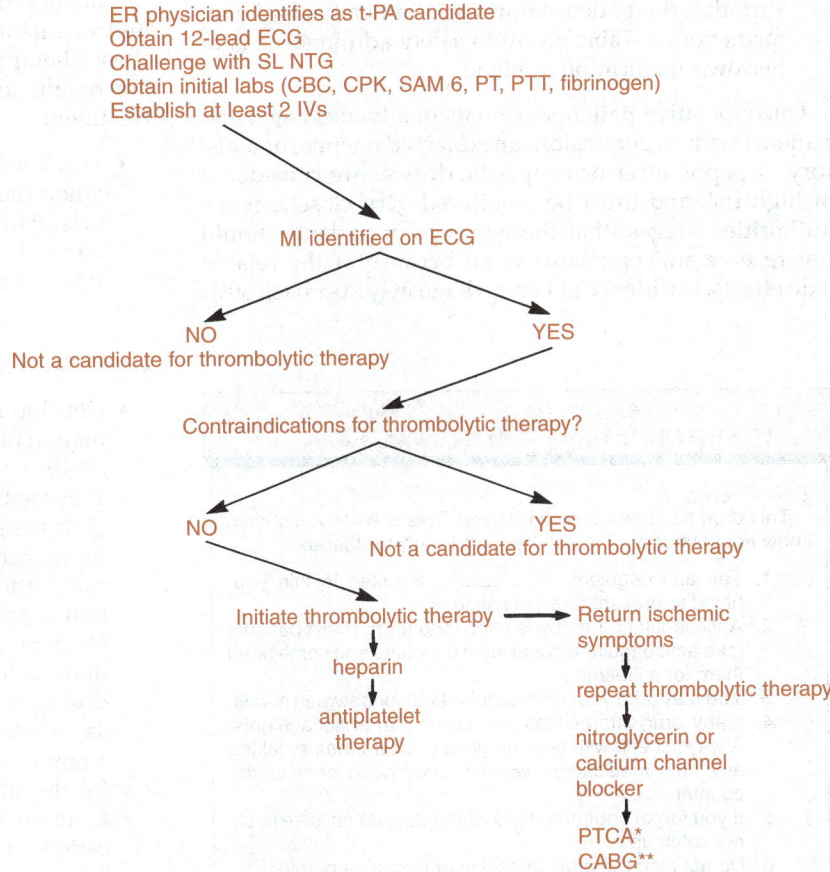

t-PA Administration Algorithm

Patient arrives in ER with
severe chest pain, 6 hr of onset

ER physician identifies as t-PA candidate
Obtain 12-lead ECG
Challenge with SL NTG
Obtain initial labs (CBC, CPK, SAM 6, PT, PTT, fibrinogen)
Establish at least 2 IVs

MI identified on ECG

NO   YES
Not a candidate for thrombolytic therapy

Contraindications for thrombolytic therapy?

NO   YES
                        Not a candidate for thrombolytic therapy

Initiate thrombolytic therapy ──────▶ Return ischemic
                                        symptoms
        heparin
                                        repeat thrombolytic therapy
        antiplatelet
        therapy   nitroglycerin or
                                        calcium channel
                                        blocker

                                        PTCA*
                                        CABG**

*PTCA—percutaneous transluminal coronary angioplasty
**CABG—coronary artery bypass graft

Figure 35–3. Myocardial infarction treatment algorithm.

ical intervention is unsuccessful, emergency PTCA or bypass surgery may be undertaken.

The National Conference of Antithrombotic Therapy, cosponsored by the American College of Chest Physicians and National Institutes of Health–National Heart, Lung, and Blood Institute, recently suggested antithrombotic therapy for various conditions. They suggest that a patient with a diagnosis of an anterior transmural MI should receive full doses of heparin followed by coumarin therapy for 1 to 3 months. After an anterior MI, patients are at high risk for embolic complications because there is an associated incidence of developing mural thrombus (33%). When mural thrombus is present in anterior MI and anticoagulants are not administered, the risk of stroke or embolism ranges from 20% to 43%. In comparison to MIs at other locations, anterior MI carries double the risk of stroke.

Patients who survive an MI and have atrial fibrillation, previous systemic embolism, or congestive heart failure should also receive full doses of heparin followed by coumarin for at least 3 months. Patients with uncomplicated MI should receive aspirin for an unknown duration. Patients with unstable angina should receive 325 mg of aspirin daily for 2 years.

Patient Teaching

- Teach the patient about his or her clotting disorder, which may be idiopathic or due to a determined cause. It is important to teach the patient about the causative factors so action can be taken to prevent recurrence. Deep-vein thrombosis with pulmonary emboli may be related to venous stasis, wearing of garters or panty girdles, varicose veins, trauma, or prolonged immobilization. The patient and family should know and understand these factors and how to prevent recurrence. Clotting disorders such as pulmonary embolism or cerebral vascular diseases may be life threatening.

Several centers are studying self-managed oral anticoagulation. After proper education, patients are sent home with a portable machine to monitor their own PT. From the PT, they then adjust their own warfarin dose.

- Teach the patient about anticoagulant therapy. Ensure that the patient knows and understands the information in Table 35–10 to safely administer his or her own medication at home.

Uncooperative patients, patients of advanced age, and patients with hypertension, unexplained anemia, or a history of peptic ulcer or neoplastic disease are considered at high risk and must be monitored very closely. Some authorities suggest that these groups of patients should not receive anticoagulants at all because of the related side effects. (Incidence of hemorrhage may approach 50%,

whereas in the normal population it ranges from 7% to 15%.) The physician weighs the benefits of therapy against the risk of adverse or serious reactions. Relatives are encouraged to check frequently for undercompliance and overcompliance.

Statistics show that 10% of all patients on long-term anticoagulants bleed at some time during the course of their therapy. However, fatalities are rare. Patients are taught to go to the emergency room for definitive treatment.

- Teach information about food and drug interactions when the patient is going home on coumarin products. Patients need to know the natural sources of vitamin K and to limit the intake of foods rich in vitamin K.

EVALUATION

- Develop the evaluation outcome criteria from information obtained in the original assessment (see Table 35–8).
- Work with the patient and family to ensure their complete assistance and support. Most patients, once they understand the importance of their continued medical treatment, are compliant. The primary reason for noncompliance is forgetting to take the medication. Overcompliance is occasionally a problem in the elderly or emotionally ill patient, who may use overdosing on anticoagulants to create a bleeding episode as an attention-getting mechanism. In these patients, a family member usually must assume responsibility for the administration of the medication.
- Evaluate the patient for adverse effects of the medications. The patient is taught to call the physician if he or she notes any unusual symptoms. The adverse effect most often experienced is bleeding—of the gums or nasal mucosa, into the urine, under the skin when lightly bruised, and/or in the GI tract. The actual incidence of bleeding associated with careful follow-up is estimated to be 4% or less. The physician evaluates the situation and decides whether the patient is to withhold medication, have a clotting study performed, take a dose of vitamin K, or come in to be further evaluated. Oral anticoagulation generally provides maximum benefit at a minimum risk.
- Evaluate the effectiveness of thrombolytics. Monitoring the ST segment after administration is the newest method of monitoring for either a patent or reoccluded vessel. The ST segment should return to normal or at least partially resolve within 3 hours after thrombolytic administration. If the ST segment is less than 30% resolved, cardiac cathertization is undertaken to determine what additional therapies are indicated (PTCA or bypass surgery).
- Evaluate for hemorrhage, the major adverse effect of thrombolytic therapy. Its incidence can be reduced by careful selection of patients and avoidance of unnecessary invasive procedure. More than 70% of the bleeding episodes occur at vascular puncture sites. Most patients with bleeding can be managed with in-

---

Table 35–10. PATIENT TEACHING INFORMATION—ANTICOAGULANTS

Dear Patient:

This drug has been ordered for you. This is what you should know about your drug to get the most from your therapy.

- [ ] 1. The anticoagulant _____ is taken to thin your blood to prevent further clotting.
- [ ] 2. Anticoagulant therapy is often long term. (Most patients take anticoagulants for at least 6 months and some need them for a lifetime.)
- [ ] 3. You may take your anticoagulant with or between meals.
- [ ] 4. Many drug interactions can occur with anticoagulants. Always check with your druggist or doctor before taking any new medication, whether prescribed or over the counter.
- [ ] 5. If you forget your drug for a whole day, *do not* take it. *Do not* catch up.
- [ ] 6. Do not stop the drug without your doctor's approval.
- [ ] 7. If you note any bleeding from the gums, contact your doctor. Use a soft toothbrush to prevent gum injury.
- [ ] 8. If you note any dark brown, orange, or red urine; dark or tarry stools; slight bruising resulting in large black and blue areas; nose bleeds; excessive menstrual flow; or prolonged oozing from any injury, report these to your doctor.
- [ ] 9. Shave with an electric razor to avoid scraping your skin.
- [ ] 10. Do not eat large amounts of foods rich in vitamin K, such as green leafy vegetables (cabbage, spinach, kale, lettuce, cauliflower), tomatoes, fish, liver, cheese, egg yolks, and fats from red meats. Avoid alcohol intake because of its effect on the liver. Drinking even 2 or 3 oz of liquor may increase your tendency to bleed. If you require nutritional supplements such as Ensure, Vital, or Nutramigen, you may have difficulty with coumarin product regulation because of their high vitamin K content. Consult your doctor.
- [ ] 11. When traveling to a hot climate from a cold one, the dose of your drug may need to be reduced. Consult with the doctor before traveling to any area where a change in climate is expected.
- [ ] 12. Carry an identification card or wear jewelry that states the drug you are taking and the doctor's name and telephone number.
- [ ] 13. Always inform all other doctors and dentists that you are taking anticoagulants before any treatments are started.
- [ ] 14. Store anticoagulants in a tight, moisture-resistant container, as they can lose their potency when exposed to air.

terruption of thrombolytic and anticoagulant therapy, volume replacement, and manual pressure applied to the bleeding vessel.

- Evaluate for anticoagulation and for signs and symptoms of reocclusion during the post-thrombolysis period. If reocclusion occurs, prompt diagnosis, reporting, and intervention will prevent reinfarction.

The more the patient and family are involved with health-care planning, the more likely they are to comply.

Stress the importance of continued medical care. All other evaluation criteria are also assessed and evaluated before the patient leaves the health-care facility. All previously taught material is reviewed and updated, if necessary, to ensure that the patient's knowledge base remains accurate.

The bibliography for this chapter can be found in Appendix B, which begins on page 1054.

CHAPTER REVIEW QUESTIONS*

1. In the clotting process, stage II is represented by:
   a. Resolution of clot formation.
   b. Formation of active thromboplastin.
   c. Conversion of fibrinogen to fibrin.
   d. Conversion of prothrombin to thrombin.

2. Anticoagulant agents are used to:
   a. Stimulate fibrinolysis.
   b. Dissolve existing clots.
   c. Retard the clotting process.
   d. Dissolve clotting factors.

3. In the human body, the highest concentration of heparin can be found in the:
   a. Brain.
   b. Pancreas.
   c. Liver.
   d. Lungs.

4. Which of the following is correct regarding recombinant alteplase (Activase)?

*See Appendix A, which begins on page 1051, for answers.

   a. As a synthetic protein, it is associated with antibody formation and allergic reactions.
   b. It is identical to natural activators, produced by vessel wall cells, which digest fibrin clots.
   c. It has a long half-life and is contraindicated in patients requiring immediate surgery.
   d. It is an inexpensive thrombolytic agent that is safer to use clinically than streptokinase.

5. Topical hemostatic agents are used to:
   a. Stimulate platelet aggregation.
   b. Control arterial bleeding.
   c. Interfere in the clotting cascade.
   d. Control capillary bleeding.

6. Protamine sulfate is contraindicated in patients who are allergic to:
   a. Penicillin.
   b. Aspirin.
   c. Citrus fruits.
   d. Fish.

BUILDING YOUR CRITICAL THINKING SKILLS

ORAL ANTICOAGULANTS

A 65-year-old patient underwent a mitral valve replacement 3 months ago and is currently at home and stable. She has been receiving warfarin sodium (Coumadin) 5 mg daily, 6 days a week. The patient comes in for a routine follow-up visit, at which time her prothrombin time (PT) is evaluated. Last month her PT was 22 seconds with a control of 12 seconds. This visit her PT is 44 seconds with a control of 12 seconds. There has been no change in the dosage, and the patient states she has been compliant in taking her medication as prescribed.

1. What is the cause of the increased PT level?
2. What data should the nurse collect to determine the cause of the elevated PT?
3. What nursing interventions are necessary for this patient?

UNIT 9

DRUGS AFFECTING THE URINARY SYSTEM

UNIT OUTLINE

CHAPTER 36

Overview of the Anatomy and Physiology of the Urinary System

Merrily A. Kuhn, RNC, PhD

CHAPTER OUTLINE

Glomerular Filtration
Tubular Reabsorption and Secretion
Other Functions of the Kidney

KEY TERMS

Filtrate
Glomerular filtration rate

Glomerulus
Prostaglandins

LEARNING OBJECTIVES

After reading this chapter, the student will be able to:

1. Identify the functions of the various parts of the nephron.
2. Identify the functions of the kidney that contribute to homeostasis.
3. Identify the areas in the nephron where diuretics have their action.

The kidneys are the major excretory organs and are largely responsible for maintaining the homeostasis of plasma and tissue fluid. The kidneys have regulatory, excretory, and secretory functions, as shown in Figure 36–1. The kidney is located retroperitoneally in the abdominal cavity. The outer portion of the kidney is the cortex. The inner portion, the medulla, consists of 6 to 12 cone-shaped masses known as renal pyramids. The free ends of each pyramid form the renal papillae, which open into the renal pelvis. The renal pelvis collects urine from all the renal pyramids, as shown in Figure 36–2.

The nephron is the functional unit of the kidney; each kidney contains approximately million nephrons. As shown in Figure 36–3, the nephron contains a glomerulus (housed within Bowman's capsule), a proximal tube, a loop of Henle, a distal tube, and a collecting duct. The function of the nephron is to filter blood, excrete waste products (e.g., urea, uric acid, creatinine) into the urine, and reabsorb essential nutrients. Urine formation involves glomerular filtration and tubular reabsorption and secretion.

GLOMERULAR FILTRATION

The filtration of blood occurs at the *glomerulus,* a network of capillaries that derive from an afferent arteriole (see Fig. 36–3). *Glomerular filtration rate* (GFR) is the rate of filtrate formation. The average GFR is about 125 mL/min per 1.73 m². Approximately 180 liters of *filtrate* are formed in Bowman's capsules each day. As the result of tubular reabsorption, only about 1 to 2 liters a day is actually excreted as urine. The rate of blood flow through the glomerulus is regulated by the afferent and efferent glomerular arterioles. Alterations in blood flow, such as the decrease in blood pressure or blood volume that occurs in a shock state, can dramatically reduce renal function. The nephron continues to function with up to a 50% reduction in blood flow, but filtrate production decreases after that.

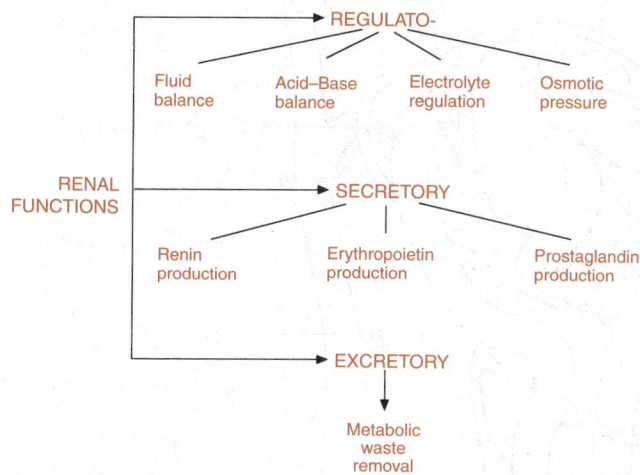

Figure 36–1. Schematic representation of general renal functions.

TUBULAR REABSORPTION AND SECRETION

The final composition of the urine is quite different from the glomerular filtrate. The glomeruli merely act as a filter. The permeability of the capillary membrane determines the composition of the filtrate. Physiologically important substances such as water, glucose, electrolytes, as well as waste products like urea, creatinine, and uric acid are initially found in the filtrate. In the renal tubule, reabsorption and secretion determine the composition of urine.

Substances are reabsorbed completely into the peritubular capillary until normal serum ranges are obtained. Once the threshold level (normal plasma range) is exceeded, the substance is no longer absorbed, but instead is excreted in the urine. For example, when the threshold level of glucose is reached (100 mg/100 mL) and the glomerular filtration rate is 100 mL, approximately 100 mg of glucose is delivered to the glomerular filtrate each minute. Under normal circumstances, all the glucose is reabsorbed into the blood from the proximal tubule. If the serum glucose rises to 200 mg, the glomerular filtration rate also rises until there is more glucose in the filtrate. The excess glucose remains in the filtrate and brings water with it. This results in the clinical condition known as glycosuria.

Another function of the tubule is to reabsorb water. If plasma osmolarity increases, water is reabsorbed to decrease the osmolarity back to normal. The modification of the chemical composition of the filtrate involves primarily the active, selective reabsorption of solutes. Water moves by osmosis out of both the proximal convoluted tubule and the collecting ducts. Electrolytes like K^+ or HCO_3^- move by passive transport from areas of high concentration to areas of low concentration without the expenditure of energy. Approximately 65% of the filtrate is reabsorbed in the proximal convoluted tubule. Sodium and chloride are actively pumped out of the tubule and are followed by water. This component of water reabsorption is termed obligatory reabsorption.

The glomerular filtrate may retain a high concentration of solutes. To compensate for the high osmolarity, water is lost from the body, resulting in an osmotic diuresis. Glycosuria is a representative situation in which osmotic diuresis occurs. The diuretics, which impair the reabsorption of sodium and chloride, cause a similar effect.

URINARY DILUTION AND CONCENTRATION

Filtrate leaving the proximal tubule has a similar osmolality to plasma (i.e., isotonic) as it enters the loop of Henle. However, depending on the needs of the individual, elimination of excess water (hypervolemia, which creates a hypotonic urine) may be essential under certain conditions, whereas conservation of water (hypovolemia, which creates a hypertonic urine) may be needed in other conditions. The countercurrent mechanism enables the nephron to accomplish this task.

The countercurrent mechanism alters urine osmolality as a result of membrane permeability differences within the loop of Henle, the distal convoluted tubule, and the collecting duct. The descending loop of Henle is perme-

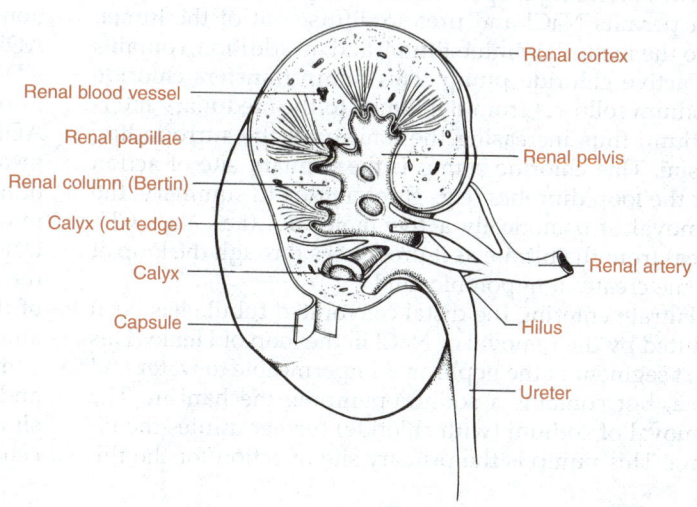

Figure 36–2. Anatomy of the internal structures of the kidney.

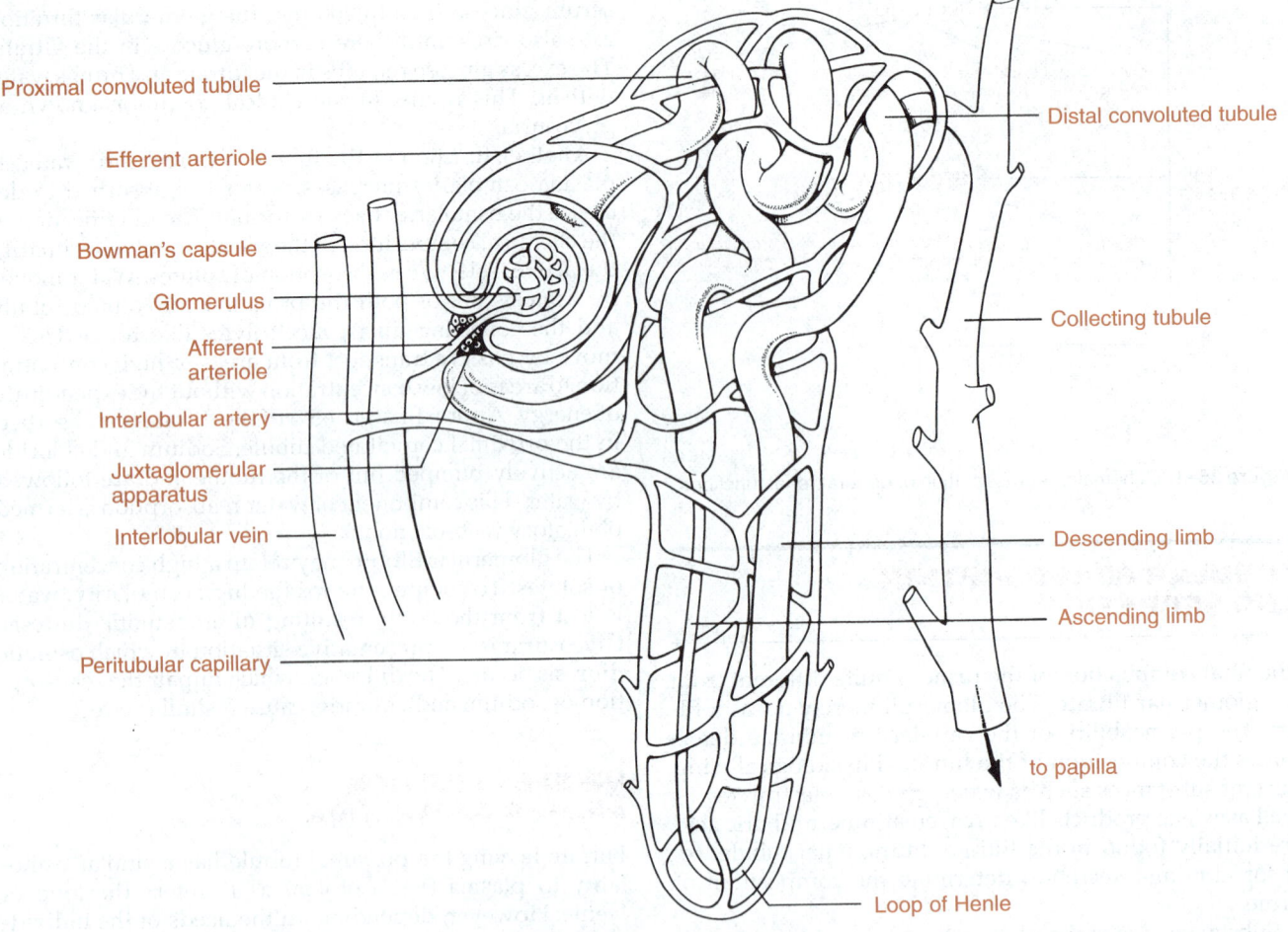

Figure 36–3. Anatomy of the nephron.

able to water but not to sodium chloride (NaCl) or urea. As the nephron progresses deeper into the renal medulla, the tonicity of the surrounding tissue increases, which draws water out of the tubular lumen. The removal of water without solute increases the concentration of NaCl and urea within the lumen. In the loop of Henle, sodium and chloride can move either into or out of the filtrate.

The ascending loop of Henle is impermeable to water, but permits NaCl and urea to diffuse out of the lumen into the medullary interstitium, and, in addition, contains an active chloride pump. This pump transfers chloride (sodium follows) from the lumen to the medullary interstitium, thus increasing the tonicity of the surrounding tissue. This chloride pump is the primary site of action for the loop diuretics (e.g., furosemide). In summary, the removal of osmotically active molecules (i.e., Na$^+$, Cl$^-$, urea) from the filtrate as it progresses through the loop of Henle creates a hypotonic fluid.

Filtrate entering the distal convoluted tubule has been diluted by the removal of NaCl in the loop of Henle. This next segment of the nephron is impermeable to water and urea, but contains a sodium-pumping mechanism. The removal of sodium (with chloride) further dilutes the filtrate. This pump is the primary site of action for the thi-

azide diuretics (e.g., hydrochlorothiazide). Farther along the distal convoluted tubule is the area where aldosterone mediates the exchange of sodium for potassium. The osmolality of the filtrate is not altered here because the segment is permeable. Antagonism of aldosterone is another mechanism of diuretic action to induce a mild diuresis.

In the cortical collecting duct, the presence or absence of antidiuretic hormone (ADH) determines the concentration of the urine. The posterior pituitary gland releases ADH as blood pressure falls. The presence or absence of ADH allows the cortical and medullary collecting ducts to either increase or decrease their water permeability. ADH also enhances the medullary collecting ducts' permeability to urea. The net effect of ADH is the removal of only water from the filtrate and the movement of urea into the medullary interstitium. This results in a concentrated urine. The increased osmolality of the interstitium then causes extraction of water from the descending limb of the loop of Henle. If ADH is not present in sufficient amounts, the urine remains dilute.

In summary, isotonic filtrate leaves the proximal tubule and enters the descending limb of the loop of Henle, shown in Figure 36–4, where water is extracted. The ascending limb of the loop of Henle removes solutes with-

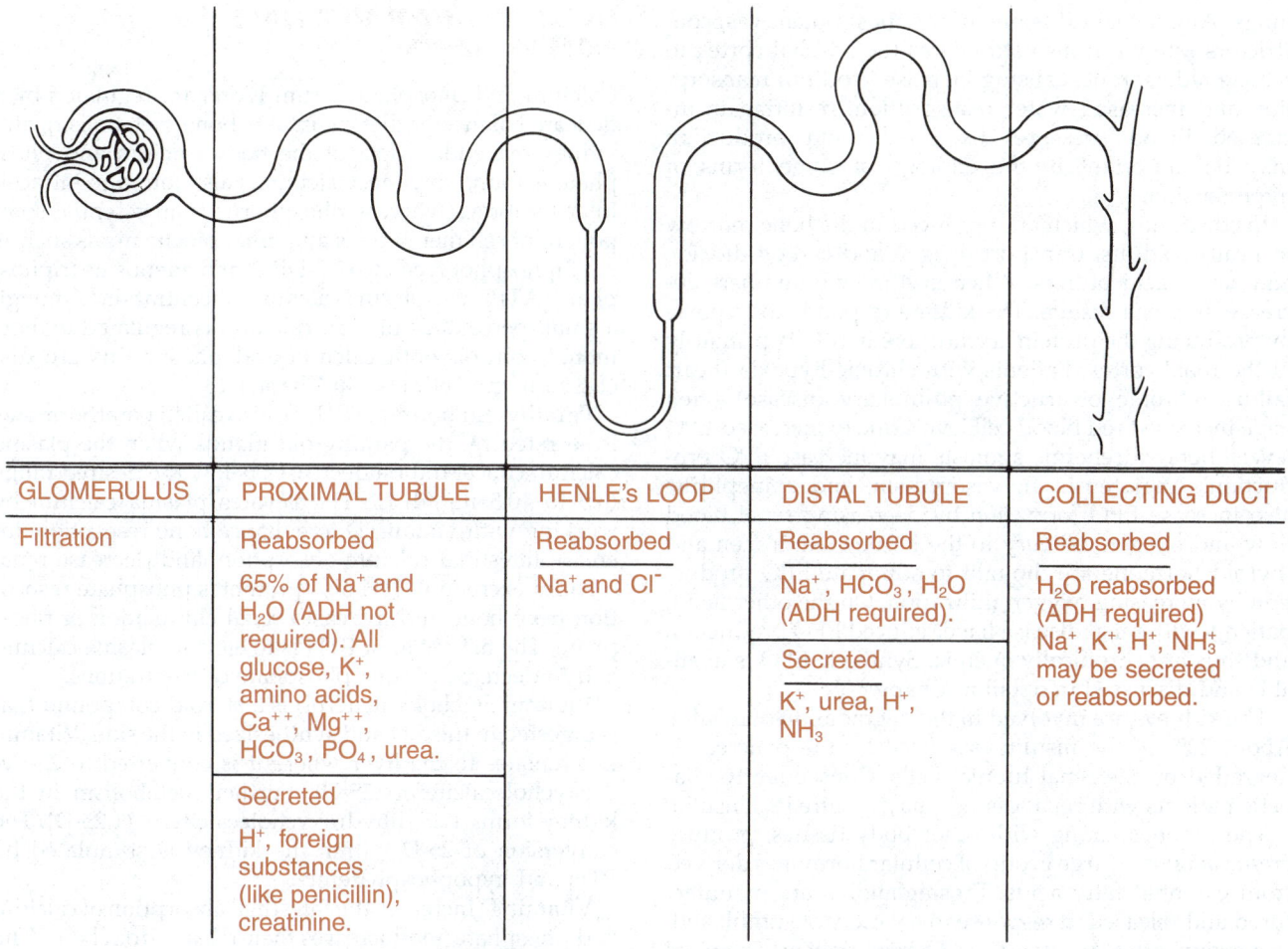

GLOMERULUS	PROXIMAL TUBULE	HENLE's LOOP	DISTAL TUBULE	COLLECTING DUCT
Filtration	Reabsorbed 65% of Na^+ and H_2O (ADH not required). All glucose, K^+, amino acids, Ca^{++}, Mg^{++}, HCO_3, PO_4, urea.	Reabsorbed Na^+ and Cl^-	Reabsorbed Na^+, HCO_3, H_2O (ADH required). Secreted K^+, urea, H^+, NH_3	Reabsorbed H_2O reabsorbed (ADH required) Na^+, K^+, H^+, NH_3^+ may be secreted or reabsorbed.
	Secreted H^+, foreign substances (like penicillin), creatinine.			

Figure 36–4. Tubular reabsorption and secretion along the nephron.

out water, creating a hypotonic filtrate. The presence or absence of ADH determines the fate of the hypotonic filtrate. If ADH is present, a concentrated urine is excreted, whereas in the absence of ADH, a dilute urine is eliminated.

ACID-BASE BALANCE

Hydrogen ion secretion from the tubule cell and bicarbonate reabsorption from the tubule lumen occur in both the proximal and distal tubule and are dependent on the intracellular production of free hydrogen ions. Carbonic acid is freely formed from the waste CO_2 found in the blood. The hydration of carbon dioxide forms carbonic acid, which dissociates into hydrogen and bicarbonate ions, according to the following equation:

$$CO_2 + H_2O \rightleftarrows H_2CO_3 \rightleftarrows H^+ + HCO_3^-$$

Both hydrogen and bicarbonate ions are continuously generated in the tubular cells. In exchange for sodium ions, the hydrogen ions are transferred into the filtrate. These positively charged hydrogen ions diffuse into the tubule not only because of their higher intracellular concentration, but also because of the electrical gradient caused by the simultaneous active transport of positively charged sodium ions from the tubule lumen.

Most of the hydrogen ions that enter the filtrate combine with filtered bicarbonate ions to form carbonic acid, which is then converted in the tubule lumen to carbon dioxide and water. The residual hydrogen ions that remain in the filtrate are finally excreted in the urine as free hydrogen ions (H^+) or in combination with a phosphate ($HPO_4 + H^+ = H_2PO_4^-$) or ammonia ($H^+ + NH_3 = NH_4^+$) buffer.

OTHER FUNCTIONS OF THE KIDNEY

SECRETORY FUNCTIONS

The kidneys secrete renin and are involved in the production of erythropoietin and some prostaglandins. When blood pressure is low, the juxtaglomerular cells secrete renin. Renin is an enzyme that converts angiotensinogen, a circulating plasma protein, to angiotensin I, which is subsequently converted to angiotensin II by an enzyme found almost entirely in the small vessels of the lungs. Angiotensin II is one of the most potent vasoconstrictors known. It also stimulates the adrenal cortex to secrete aldosterone, causing increased sodium reabsorption and increased water reabsorption, resulting in increased blood pressure. Excessive renin production may be important in the etiology of some forms of hypertension.

Erythrocytes, which are produced in the bone marrow in healthy adults, transport oxygen and carbon dioxide and act as acid buffers. When erythrocyte numbers decrease, hypoxia results. The kidney responds to hypoxia by producing the protein erythropoietin (EPO), primarily in the renal cortex. Patients with chronic hypoxia (heart failure, chronic obstructive pulmonary disease) often have increased red blood cell levels due to increased EPO levels. Beta$_2$-adrenergic agonists may increase EPO production. Angiotensin II, vasopressin, and epinephrine also increase EPO formation by decreasing renal blood flow and oxygen delivery to the kidney. Androgen and thyroid hormone are thought to stimulate EPO production by increasing oxygen utilization. On the other hand, patients with renal disease have reduced EPO production and thus are chronically anemic. Synthetic EPO is available and discussed in detail in Chapter 38.

The kidneys are involved in the degradation of insulin. About 20% of the insulin produced by the pancreas is degraded by the renal tubular cells. Consequently, diabetic patients with renal disease may require less insulin.

The kidneys, along with other body tissues, produce *prostaglandins*, a large group of cellular hormones derived from essential fatty acids. Prostaglandins are manufactured and released in response to a variety of stimuli and, as a group, affect virtually every organ system. The renal medulla produces PGA$_2$ and PGE$_2$, which are potent vasodilators. In the kidney, prostaglandins play a role in the regulation of renal blood flow, renin release, and sodium reabsorption (see Chapter 48 for other activities of prostaglandins).

CALCIUM AND PHOSPHATE HOMEOSTASIS

Calcium and phosphate serum levels are regulated by a delicate balance of dietary intake, bone metabolism, and kidney excretion. Most of the body calcium and phosphate is found in bone. Calcium is also found in intracellular locations, whereas phosphorus is an essential component of cell membranes and other biochemicals such as 2,3-diphosphoglycerate (2,3-DPG) and adenosine triphosphate (ATP). The plasma calcium concentration, although a small percentage of total calcium, is regulated by hormonal control. Both calcium and phosphorus are discussed in greater detail in Chapter 13.

Parathyroid hormone (PTH), also called parathormone, is secreted by the parathyroid glands when the plasma calcium concentration decreases below the desired range (8.5 to 10.5 mg/dL). PTH elevates plasma calcium by working with vitamin D to enhance bone resorption, increase intestinal calcium absorption, and decrease renal calcium excretion. PTH also promotes phosphate resorption from bone and increases renal elimination of phosphate. The net result of PTH is to elevate plasma calcium and to decrease plasma phosphate concentrations.

Vitamin D (cholecalciferol) is a steroid compound that is ingested in the diet and synthesized in the skin. Vitamin D circulates to the liver where it is converted to 25-hydroxycholecalciferol (25-D). Further metabolism in the kidney forms 1,25-dihydroxycholecalciferol (1,25-D). The conversion of 25-D within the kidney is stimulated by PTH and hypophosphatemia.

Vitamin D increases the intestinal absorption of calcium and phosphate and increases their release from bone. The action of vitamin D on bone depends on the presence of PTH. Vitamin D is discussed in greater detail in Chapter 13.

The bibliography for this chapter can be found in Appendix B, which begins on page 1054.

CHAPTER REVIEW QUESTIONS*

1. The kidney maintains acid-base homeostasis by:
   a. Keeping extracellular pH within the range of 7.0 to 7.70.
   b. Controlling bicarbonate concentration by renal H$^+$ excretion.
   c. Forming ammonia in the cells of the proximal tubule.
   d. Secreting H$^+$ ions into the proximal tubule in exchange for ammonium ions.

2. As ADH is decreased, assessment findings include:
   a. Hemoconcentration and a dilute urine.
   b. Hemodilution and a concentrated urine.
   c. Hypocalcemia and hypophosphanemia.
   d. Hypotension.

*See Appendix A, which begins on page 1051, for answers.

3. Assessment findings in a patient experiencing a decrease in erythropoietin include:
   a. Increases in red blood cell production.
   b. Chronic anemia.
   c. A higher requirement for insulin.
   d. Excessive renin production.

4. Patients with renal disease and diabetes mellitus may require:
   a. More insulin.
   b. Less insulin.
   c. Longer-acting insulin.
   d. No insulin.

CHAPTER 37

Diuretics

Merrily A. Kuhn, RNC, PhD

CHAPTER OUTLINE

KEY TERMS

Aquaretic
Ascites
Azotemia
Cirrhosis
Diuretic resistance
Hepatic encephalopathy
Hydrostatic pressure
Hypoalbuminemia
Interstitial volume

Kaluretic
Nephrolithiasis
Nephrotic syndrome
Oliguria
Oncotic pressure
Peripheral edema
Pitting edema
Pulmonary edema

LEARNING OBJECTIVES

After reading this chapter, the student will be able to:

1. Differentiate among the diuretics based on site, mechanism of action, and relative potency.
2. Identify pharmacokinetics, pharmacodynamics, contraindications and precautions, adverse reactions, and interactions related to the various diuretics.
3. Discuss the various medical conditions in which diuretics have been shown to have beneficial effects.
4. Identify specific areas of assessment in the patient requiring diuretic therapy to formulate patient outcomes.
5. Plan appropriate nursing interventions and patient teaching for diuretic therapy.
6. Evaluate therapeutic response and revise assessment, diagnoses, and nursing interventions accordingly.

Drugs that increase the rate of urine formation are termed diuretics. The two major effects of a diuretic are to cause a net loss of water from the body and to increase the urine output. This generally results in a negative fluid balance where reduction of edematous fluid occurs and extracellular volume is normalized.

The various types of diuretics—carbonic anhydrase inhibitors, osmotic diuretics, thiazide and thiazide-like diuretics, loop diuretics, potassium-sparing diuretics, and aquaretics—act in different parts of the renal tubule. The carbonic anhydrase inhibitors and the osmotic diuretics act on the proximal tubule. Thiazide diuretics act primarily in the distal tubule, which is sensitive to antidiuretic hormone (ADH). The loop diuretics act in the loop of Henle. Two potassium-sparing diuretics—the aldosterone antagonist spironolactone and the sodium blocker amiloride—act in the collecting tubule. Aquaretics work by interfering with the effect of ADH at the collecting ducts. Figure 37–1 illustrates the sites of action of various diuretics.

Diuretics are used most commonly in the treatment of edema, hypertension, heart failure, and renal failure. Recently, diuretics have also been studied for use in management of bronchoconstriction, near drowning, hyperparathyroidism, hirsutism, chronic macula edema, and Reye's syndrome.

The publisher gratefully acknowledges the contribution of Kenneth A. Kellick, Pharm D. to the third edition.

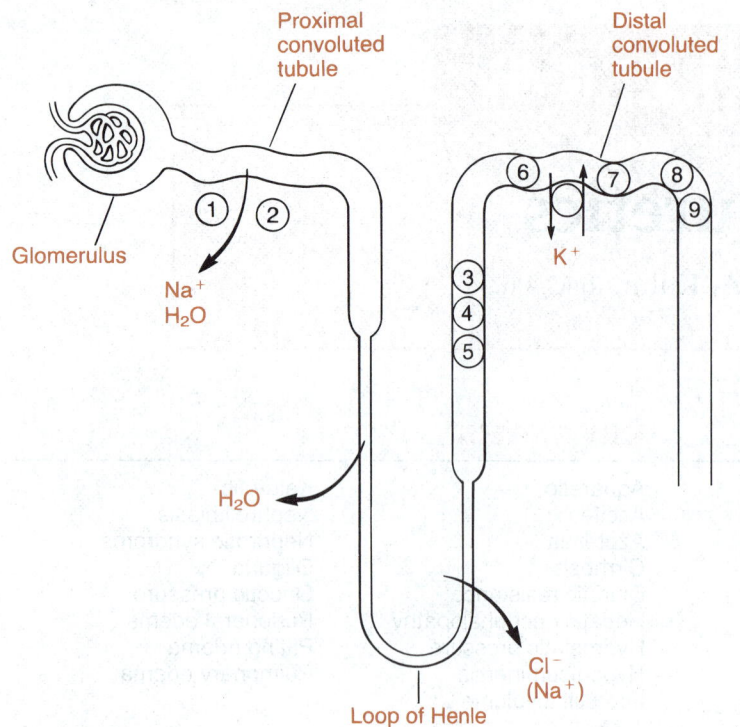

Proximal convoluted tubule

Distal convoluted tubule

Glomerulus

Na^+
H_2O

K^+

H_2O

Cl^-
(Na^+)

Loop of Henle

1. Mannitol
2. Acetazolamide
3. Furosemide
4. Ethacrynic Acid
5. Bumetanide
6. Thiazides
7. Triamterene
8. Amiloride
9. Spironolactone

Figure 37–1. Sites of action of diuretics. The primary site of action is presented. Many of these drugs have multiple sites of action.

CONTRAINDICATIONS AND PRECAUTIONS

All diuretics are contraindicated in patients with hypersensitivity to the product. Diuretics are also contraindicated in patients with anuria renal failures and patients with severe fluid and electrolyte disturbances or at least until these problems have been corrected. Safety in pregnancy, varies among groups (B or C) and in children under 12 has not been established.

ADVERSE EFFECTS OF DIURETIC THERAPY

Diuretic therapy can result in a number of adverse effects. Diuretic use can result in a reduction in serum potassium (K^+) from 5% to 50%. The degree of hypokalemia depends on the type, the dose, and the duration of use. Hypokalemia can lead to diarrhea, vomiting, and anorexia. Corrective measures are taken to return the potassium level to normal limits. Patients who are concurrently receiving digitalis glycosides may experience myocardial irritability as the potassium levels fall. As K^+ levels fall to 3.5 mEq/L or less, the likelihood of dysrhythmia increases. In diuretic therapy, potassium levels are monitored and dietary intake of K^+ is increased or K^+ supplements are administered.

Diuretic therapy can also lead to hyponatremia, which may be particularly dangerous to the elderly patient. If uncorrected, hyponatremia can lead to neurologic dysfunction and death. Rapid correction of hyponatremia should be avoided. Hyponatremia may need to be treated by discontinuing the diuretics.

Chronic administration of diuretics can lead to hypomagnesemia, which can lead to dysrhythmia and cellular K^+ depletion. The body may not respond to K^+ repletion until Mg^{2+} levels are returned to normal. The diuretic may need to be discontinued.

Metabolic alkalosis often results from chronic therapy because of volume contraction and a net loss of acid. Metabolic alkalosis always must be corrected, particularly in the cardiac patient, because of the increased likelihood of coronary spasm and myocardial ischemia.

Recent clinical trials, particularly the Multiple Risk Factor Intervention Trial (MRFIT), raise serious concerns about the safety of diuretics. For example, thiazide diuretics have been demonstrated to increase cholesterol and triglycerides levels. (Indapamide [Lozol], a thiazide derivative, appears to have a lesser impact.) A lower dose usually causes less hyperlipidemia and does not compromise blood pressure control.

TOXICITY IN DIURETIC THERAPY

Diuretics can cause certain toxic effects on body systems, especially the renal, hematologic, and endocrine systems. *Nephrolithiasis* (the presence of calculi in the kidney) is associated with the use of diuretics. It may be due to volume depletion and resultant concentration of urine. Thiazides and loop diuretics can cause acute interstitial nephritis. The duration of diuretic therapy prior to the onset of nephritis is highly variable.

▼ CLINICAL ALERT

Loop diuretics can produce transient or permanent deafness. Patients with renal failure are at a greater risk of developing this complication. Toxicity can be minimized by using divided doses whenever possible and by slow, continuous infusion rather than a large, rapidly administered bolus.

Administration of diuretics occasionally results in idiosyncratic hematologic reactions, which are reversible with drug discontinuation. For example, bone marrow suppression and macrocytic anemia can occur after administration of triamterene (Dyrenium). Another diuretic group, the thiazides, can cause reversible neutropenia and thrombocytopenia.

The aldosterone antagonist spironolactone (Aldactone) has been associated with endocrine dysfunction, including gynecomastia, impotence, diminished libido, and menstrual disturbances. These are probably a consequence of the antiandrogen effects of spironolactone. This property has been used to treat hirsutism in females (Singh et al., 1994).

CARBONIC ANHYDRASE INHIBITORS

The brush border of the proximal tubular epithelium is rich in carbonic anhydrase (CA), an enzyme that catalyzes the reaction between H_2O and CO_2 to form carbonic acid. Following administration of carbonic anyhdrase inhibitors (CAIs), hydrogen ion secretion in the proximal tubule is inhibited.

The urine becomes alkaline, and the overall effect is reduction of bicarbonate reabsorption by 80%, which ultimately leads to a metabolic acidosis. CAIs also decrease the rate of aqueous humor formation in the eye by inhibiting CA, resulting in a reduction in intraocular pressure (IOP). The carbonic anhydrase inhibitors include **acetazolamide (Diamox)** and **methazolamide (Neptazane)**.

USES

Because of the tolerance that develops rapidly to CAIs, these drugs have limited usefulness as diuretics. Today, they are mainly used for the adjunctive treatment of chronic simple (open-angle) glaucoma and secondary glaucoma. Acetazolamide is also used for the prevention and treatment of acute mountain sickness and as an adjunct in the treatment of heart failure and drug-induced edema. Carbonic anhydrase inhibitors can be used as second-line antiseizure agents, either because of the effect of the metabolic acidosis or some unknown direct effect on the central nervous system.

CONTRAINDICATIONS AND PRECAUTIONS

Carbonic anyhdrase inhibitors are also contraindicated in patients with severe pulmonary obstruction because the resulting acidotic state would increase the respiratory rate. Carbonic anyhdrase inhibitors are not used in patients with chronic noncongestive angle-closure glau-

coma. Organic closure of the angle may occur. Although the symptoms are masked by the lowered IOP, the use of CAIs causes worsening of this particular type of glaucoma.

Carbonic anyhdrase inhibitors are used with caution in patients with respiratory acidosis or emphysema because the CAI may aggravate or worsen the acidosis. Because the CAIs are chemically related to the sulfonamides, cross-sensitivity may be experienced.

ADVERSE EFFECTS

Adverse effects of these agents are relatively rare and are usually seen only with high doses. Certain patients may exhibit hypersensitivity reactions, including fever, rash, or bone marrow suppression. Patients may also experience gastrointestinal (GI) complaints such as nausea, vomiting, anorexia, and constipation. Some patients may experience transient myopia resulting from reduced IOP.

INTERACTIONS

Because CAIs may induce hypokalemia, digitalis toxicity may occur in patients receiving cardiac glycosides. Combined therapy with salicylates may result in severe metabolic acidosis, which increases the potential for salicylate toxicity. Acetazolamide with cyclosporine may have increased nephrotoxicity and neurotoxicity.

○ **Acetazolamide** (Diamox) is administered to patients with chronic simple glaucoma and to treat mountain sickness. It is also used as adjunctive therapy to treating congestive heart failure and drug-induced edema. Because acetazolamide does not prevent the life-threatening complications of pulmonary and cerebral edema, it should not be used routinely as a substitute for gradual ascent to higher elevations. Additional information is presented in Table 37–1.

○ **Methazolamide** (Neptazane) is administered orally for glaucoma in a dosage of 50 to 100 mg two or three times daily.

OSMOTIC DIURETICS

Osmotic diuretics include **mannitol (Osmitrol)**, **glucose**, **urea (Ureaphil)**, and **glycerin (Osmoglyn)**. Osmotic diuretics work in the kidney by drawing water from extravascular spaces into the tubular lumen. Osmotic diuretics share the following characteristics: (1) they are freely filtered by the glomerulus, (2) they remain in the tubular lumen in high concentration because of the limited reabsorption by the renal tubule, and (3) they are pharmacologically inactive. When administered intravenously, they cause a shift of free water from the extravascular space into the blood vessels.

USES

The main use for osmotic diuretics, primarily mannitol, is for the relief of *oliguria* (a condition of diminished urine

Table 37–1. DIURETICS: CARBONIC ANHYDRASE INHIBITORS, OSMOTIC DIURETICS, AND THIAZIDE AND THIAZIDE-LIKE DIURETICS

DRUG NAME/ROUTE AND DOSAGE	PHARMACOKINETICS/ DYNAMICS	NURSING IMPLICATIONS
CARBONIC ANHYDRASE INHIBITORS		
acetazolamide (Diamox)		
Adults: 250 mg–1 g/day PO or IV; or 500 mg q 12–24 hr sustained-release (SR) formulation. **Children:** 5–10 mg/kg per 6 hr IM or IV; or 10–15 mg/kg per day PO (individual doses).	**Onset:** PO, 1.5 hr; SR, 2 hr; IV, 2 min **Peak:** PO, 2–4 hr; SR, 8–12 hr; IV, 15 min **Duration:** PO, 8–12 hr; SR, 18–24 hr; IV, 4–5 hr **½L:** 2.4–5.8 hr **PB:** NA **B:** excreted unchanged **E:** kidneys	**ASSESSMENT:** Assess level of motor function during therapy. Assess GI side effects of therapy. **INTERVENTION:** IV administration is preferred because the alkaline solution IM is painful. **Patient Teaching—** Instruct patient not to drive or operate machinery while taking these diuretics. Instruct patient to take with food if GI upset occurs. Tell patient to not stop taking drug unless instructed to do so. Caution patient to avoid prolonged exposure to sun as photosensitivity may occur. **EVALUATION:** Evaluate therapy frequently for efficacy. Evaluate for sore throat, fever, unexplained bleeding or bruising, tingling or tremor, or rash and report to physician.
OSMOTIC DIURETICS		
mannitol (Osmitrol)		
acute renal failure **Adults:** 50–100 g IV as 5%–25% solution. **oliguria** **Adults:** 300–400 mg/kg IV as 20%–25% solution; up to 100 g of 15%–20% solution. **increased intracranial pressure** **Adults:** 1.5–2.0 g/kg IV as 15%–25% solution over 30–60 min. **increased intraocular pressure** **Adults:** 1.5–2.0 g/kg IV as 20%–25% solution over 30 min, 1–1.5 hr before surgery.	**Onset:** 30–60 min **Peak:** 1–3 hr **Duration:** 6–8 hr **½L:** 100 min **PB:** NA **B:** 7%–10% **E:** 90% kidneys	**ASSESSMENT:** Assess for fluid rebound. Assess IV sites (very irritating on infiltration). Assess intake and output—if less than 30 mL/hr, assess for circulatory overload. Assess daily weight. Assess baseline electrolyte levels. Assess for pregnancy (category C). **INTERVENTION:** Use large venous sites and monitor patency. Do not administer through same IV set as blood or blood products. Administer reconstituted solutions within 48 hr. Provide good mouth care and provide ice chips frequently. If crystals form in IV bottle, warm it in hot water bath and shake vigorously. Allow to return to room temperature before administering. Do not administer solutions with crystals. Administer through an in-line IV filter (5 μm). Store mannitol at 59°–86°F. Do *not* give free mannitol with blood. **EVALUATION:** Evaluate therapy frequently for efficacy.
THIAZIDE DIURETICS		
hydrochlorothiazide (Esidrix) (HydroDiuril)		
edema **Adults:** *Initial dose*–25 mg PO daily. *Maintenance dose*–25–100 mg PO daily; larger doses in refractory patients only may go to 200 mg. **hypertension** **Adults:** *Initial dose*–12.5–25 mg PO daily. *Maintenance dose*–25–100 PO mg daily. **Children 6 mo–2 yr:** 12.5–37.5 mg PO daily in 2 divided doses. **Children 2–12 yr:** 37.5–100 mg daily PO in 2 doses. **Children under 6 mo:** 3.3 mg/kg per day PO in 2 doses.	**Onset:** 2 hr **Peak:** 4–6 hr **Duration:** 6–12 hr **½L:** 5.6–14.8 hr **PB:** NA **B:** 5% liver **E:** kidneys	**ASSESSMENT:** Assess serum electrolytes, uric acid, and blood glucose. Weigh daily and record. Assess cardiac activity carefully for dysrhythmias when on digitalis. Assess mood swings when on lithium. Assess for pregnancy (category B). **INTERVENTION:** Provide patient with diet counseling regarding foods high in potassium and sodium. Hyperglycemia may affect diabetes mellitus. Dose of hypoglycemic agent may need to be adjusted. **Patient Teaching—**Advise patient to take with food to avoid GI upset. Instruct patient to administer early in day to avoid sleep disruption; best not to administer after 3 PM. **EVALUATION:** Monitor therapy for efficacy. Renal insufficiency may increase after long-term thiazide therapy. Evaluate weight pattern and input and output. Notify physician of muscle cramps, nausea, vomiting, diarrhea, or dizziness.

Table 37–1. DIURETICS: CARBONIC ANHYDRASE INHIBITORS, OSMOTIC DIURETICS, AND THIAZIDE AND THIAZIDE-LIKE DIURETICS, *Continued*

DRUG NAME/ROUTE AND DOSAGE	PHARMACOKINETICS/ DYNAMICS	NURSING IMPLICATIONS
chlorothiazide (Diuril) and others *Adults:* 0.5–2.0 g/day PO or IV. *Children under 6 mo:* 33 mg/kg per day PO or IV in 2 doses. *Children over 6 mo:* 22 mg/kg per day PO or IV in 2 doses.	**Onset:** PO, 1–2 hr; IV, 15 min **Peak:** PO, 4 hr; IV, 90 min **Duration:** PO, 6–12 hr; IV, 2 hr **½L:** 1–2 hr **PB:** NA **B:** unchanged **E:** kidneys	Same as for hydrochlorothiazide plus: **INTERVENTION:** More effective when administering 250 mg q 6–12 hr than one large dose daily.
bendroflumethiazide (Naturetin) **edema** *Adults:* Initial dose—5 mg PO daily. *Maintenance dose*—2.5–5 mg PO daily, up to 20 mg/day. **hypertension** *Adults:* Initial dose—5–20 mg PO daily. *Maintenance dose*—2.5–15 mg PO daily.	**Onset:** 2 hr **Peak:** 4 hr **Duration:** 6–12 hr **½L:** 3.0–3.9 hr **PB:** NA **B:** unchanged **E:** kidneys	Same as for hydrochlorothiazide.
THIAZIDE-LIKE DIURETICS		
metolazone (Diulo) (Zaroxolyn) **hypertension** *Adults:* 2.5–5.0 mg PO daily; Mykrox—0.5–1.0 mg PO daily. **edema of cardiac disease** *Adults:* 5–10 mg PO daily. **edema of renal disease** *Adults:* 5–20 mg PO daily.	**Onset:** 1 hr **Peak:** 2 hr (Mykrox); 8 hr (other products) **Duration:** 12–24 hr **½L:** 14 hr **PB:** 33% **B:** 10%–20% liver **E:** kidneys	Same as for hydrochlorothiazide.
chlorthalidone (Hygroton) **edema** *Adults:* Initial dose—50–100 mg PO daily. *Maintenance dose*—50–200 mg PO daily. **hypertension** *Adults:* Initial dose—25 mg PO daily. *Maintenance dose*—25–100 mg PO daily.	**Onset:** 2 hr **Peak:** 2–6 hr **Duration:** 24–72 hr **½L:** 54 hr **PB:** 90% to RBC **B:** NA **E:** kidneys	Same as for hydrochlorothiazide.

NA = not available; RBCs = red blood cells.

formation). The early use of osmotic diuretics protects the kidney by ensuring adequate flow of relatively dilute urine. These agents are also used to reduce the pressure and volume of cerebrospinal fluid in patients with elevated intracranial pressure (ICP). Osmotics are used for short-term reduction of increased IOP, particularly preoperatively and postoperatively in patients requiring ocular surgery and in patients with acute glaucoma.

PHARMACOKINETICS

The osmotic diuretics are absorbed, following intravenous administration, either into the extracellular fluid or total body water. Mannitol is only slightly metabolized by the liver, with the balance being excreted unchanged in the urine. Glycerin is largely metabolized by the liver (80%), with the remainder metabolized by the kidney.

Neither urea nor isosorbide are metabolized to any great extent, and both are excreted unchanged by the kidney.

CONTRAINDICATIONS AND PRECAUTIONS

Osmotic diuretics are contraindicated in dehydration, or active intracranial bleeding, as rapid expansion of the extracellular fluid (ECF) may further compromise these patients. This ability to quickly increase ECF limits the use of osmotic diuretics in patients with cardiac decompensation.

ADVERSE EFFECTS

The most common adverse effects are transient volume expansion, hyponatremia, and hypokalemia. These are all due to the rapid expansion of the extracellular fluid, which dilutes ionic concentrations of sodium and potassium. Hypernatremia may occur following administration of mannitol in hypertonic solution. Headache and confusion may occur as a result of rapidly changing intracranial pressure.

INTERACTIONS

The osmotic diuretics have few drug-drug interactions. Urea is known to increase the excretion of lithium, which may decrease the effectiveness of lithium therapy in bipolar disorder.

○ **Mannitol** is an alcohol that has a renal clearance approximating the glomerular filtration rate. Mannitol increases the intraluminal osmolarity, which in turn lowers the concentration of sodium in the tubular fluid and the rate of sodium reabsorption. This abnormal concentration gradient also causes an increased flux of sodium from the peritubular fluid into the tubular fluid. The major segments affected are the proximal tubule and the thick ascending limb. The net result is an increased rate of urine flow. The increasing osmolality of plasma fluid in cerebrospinal fluid (CSF) may be drawn from the CSF back into plasma. The increasing osmolality of plasma can also draw fluid into plasma from ocular tumors. Additional information is presented in Table 37–1.

○ **Glucose** is freely filtered into the kidney and is reabsorbed from the proximal tubule by active transport. If serum glucose concentrations increase, the reabsorptive capacity is diminished and glucose spills into the urine. For this reason there is diuresis associated with hyperglycemia in poorly controlled diabetes.

○ **Urea** (Ureaphil) is indicated to reduce ICP and IOP. Adult dosage is 1.0 to 1.5 g/kg daily as a 30% solution by slow IV infusion, not to exceed 120 g/day. Pediatric dosage is 0.5 to 1.5 g/kg by slow IV infusion.

○ **Glycerin** (Glyrol, Osmoglyn) is used to treat acute attacks of glaucoma and to reduce pressure prior to ocular surgery. It is administered in doses of 1.0 to 1.5 g/kg orally 1 to 1.5 hours before surgery.

THIAZIDE DIURETICS

The thiazide diuretics were developed for clinical use in the 1950s. Thiazides are known to act directly on the kidney and increase the excretion of sodium chloride, water, and potassium. This class of drugs works exclusively in the distal tubule, inhibiting sodium absorption by a mechanism that is not well understood.

Thiazides also have an antihypertensive action by decreasing peripheral resistance. During initial therapy, cardiac output decreases and blood volume diminishes. With chronic therapy, cardiac output normalizes but peripheral vascular resistance falls, which may be due to the inhibition of the intracellular sodium-potassium pump.

The thiazide diuretics include the following: **hydrochlorothiazide (Esidrix, HydroDiuril), bendroflumethiazide (Naturetin), methychlothiazide (Enduron), polythiazide (Renese), metolazone (Diulo, Zaroxolyn), chlorthalidone (Hygroton)** and **indapamide (Lozol).** At maximal therapeutic dosages, all thiazides are approximately equal in diuretic efficacy, but metolazone may be more effective in patients with impaired renal function. Several thiazides are featured in Table 37–1.

USES

Thiazides are used as adjunctive therapy to manage hypertension, heart failure, hepatic cirrhosis, and edema of early renal disease and secondary to estrogen therapy. Thiazides work best when the urinary output is greater than 30 mL/hr. Thiazides may be used as monotherapy or in combination with other drugs to reduce blood pressure in patients with relatively normal renal function. They are also often used in combination with other antihypertensive drugs because they tend to potentiate these drugs by one-third to one-half and may help reverse the fluid retention that occurs with some antihypertensives. However, the full therapeutic antihypertensive effect may take up to 1 month, so that a common error in step therapy (described in Chapter 30) is going on to the next step too soon. Thiazide diuretics may be the initial agent of choice in salt-sensitive patients such as the elderly, African-Americans, some diabetic patients, and the obese.

As renal function decreases, the thiazides have diminished efficacy, probably because of impaired delivery of the drug to the active site. The thiazides also have a decreased ability to produce diuresis due to alterations in functioning of the nephrons.

Thiazides are the primary drugs available to reduce urinary volume in patients with nephrogenic diabetes insipidus and may do so by 30% to 50%.

PHARMACOKINETICS

The thiazides are well absorbed following oral ingestion, and a diuretic effect is initiated within 1 hour and a peak effect in 2 to 4 hours. These agents are distributed throughout extracellular fluid. All of the thiazides are primarily excreted by the kidneys, with only minor hepatic metabolism. The half-life varies from 1 to 25 hours, depending on the product. Administration for 3 to 4 weeks is generally required to obtain optimal therapeutic effect.

The primary difference between the thiazides is their duration of action. Chlorothiazide (Diuril) and hydrochlorothiazide (Esidrix) are short acting; Bendroflumethiazide (Naturetin) is intermediate acting; and methyclothiazide (Enduron) and polythiazide (Renese) are long acting (24 hours or more). The long-acting products cause the loss of more potassium.

CONTRAINDICATIONS AND PRECAUTIONS

Thiazides are administered cautiously to patients with impaired renal function because these agents may precipitate *azotemia* (the presence of excessive concentrations of urea in the blood). When a patient experiences a rising blood urea nitrogen (BUN) level, therapy is discontinued. When creatinine clearance falls below 40 to 50 mL per minute, the kidney is unresponsive to thiazides and a loop diuretic is more effective.

ADVERSE EFFECTS

Hypersensitivity reactions such as dermatitis, photosensitivity, bone marrow suppression, and vasculitis have been reported. Patients are encouraged to use sunscreens and wear protective clothing. Patients may also complain of dizziness, weakness, fatigue, and orthostatic hypotension; these symptoms generally disappear with continued therapy. Leg cramps, often associated with electrolyte imbalances, may also occur.

A primary concern of thiazide therapy is the electrolyte disturbances—hypokalemia, hypomagnesemia, hyponatremia, and hypochloremia—that may result (discussed previously). Hypercalcemia can also occur in patients receiving the thiazides due to an increased protein-bound fraction of calcium. This elevation of calcium levels rarely causes symptoms.

Thiazides increase fasting blood glucose levels and decrease glucose tolerance during long-term therapy. Thiazide-induced glucose intolerance is sometimes attributed to potassium loss. Generally, the effect on blood glucose is not clinically important except in patients with diabetes. These patients may require some alteration in their drug regimens and may be at risk for hyperglycemic hyperosmolar nonketotic coma.

The thiazides may also cause an elevation of BUN or prerenal azotemia. The prerenal azotemia is related to a decrease in renal blood flow and glomerular filtration rate due to the reduction in blood volume. Prerenal azotemia is reversible when the thiazides are discontinued.

Hyperuricemia may develop because of decreased secretion of uric acid by the tubular cells and/or increased renal reabsorption of uric acid. The increased uric acid level rarely causes symptoms unless the patient has a hereditary predisposition to gout or has chronic renal fail-

ure. Patients may continue to take the thiazides if they take colchicine, another uricosuric agent, or allopurinol.

Thiazides may also elevate serum cholesterol, triglyceride, and low-density lipoprotein (LDL) cholesterol levels. The rationale for this elevation is not clearly understood, but obesity, glucose intolerance, and hyperuricemia have been suggested. Combinations of thiazides and potassium-sparing diuretics do not appear to have this effect on lipids. A concurrent lipid-lowering diet may be beneficial.

Thiazides may also induce an allergic interstitial nephritis, resulting in a decrease in renal function. A link has been made between the use of thiazide diuretics and the development of gallstones, particularly in women. Thiazides have also been reported to reduce libido and to cause impotence.

INTERACTIONS

Thiazides may increase serum lithium levels by reducing renal excretion of lithium. It is thought that volume depletion secondary to thiazides increases proximal tubular reabsorption of sodium (and lithium). When thiazides are added to the therapy of patients who are stabilized on lithium, the patients are monitored closely for signs of lithium intoxication such as tremors and GI disturbances. Lithium serum concentrations are also monitored during thiazide treatment.

Thiazides may induce hypokalemia and potentiate digitalis toxicity in patients taking cardiac glycosides. Anion-exchange resins (cholestyramine, colestipol) may bind thiazides, thus preventing their absorption.

Other drug interactions occur with thiazides. Thiazides may increase the incidence of hypersensitivity reactions to allopurinol; may increase the effects of anesthetics, nondepolarizing muscle relaxants, and vitamin D; decrease the anticoagulant effect of anticoagulants; and may enhance electrolyte loss with amphotericin B and corticosteroids.

Nonsteroidal anti-inflammatory drugs (NSAIDs) may cause fluid retention, which can blunt the antihypertensive effect of thiazides. Careful monitoring of blood pressure is done when NSAIDs are added to thiazides. Conversely, thiazides are useful in relieving NSAID-induced edema.

○ **Chlorothiazide** (Diuril and others) is used to treat edema and hypertension in adults. Additional information is presented in Table 37–1.

○ **Hydrochlorothiazide** (Esidrix, HydroDiuril, and others) is used to treat both edema and hypertension. Additional information is presented in Table 37–1.

○ **Bendroflumethiazide** (Naturetin) also is used to treat edema and hypertension. Additional information is presented in Table 37–1.

○ **Methyclothiazide** (Enduron) is a long-acting thiazide diuretic used to treat both edema and hypertension. In adults the oral dose for treating edema ranges between 2.5 and 10 mg once daily; for hypertension the adult dose is 2.5 to 5 mg once daily. If blood pressure is not controlled at a satisfactory level in 8 to 12 weeks with 5 mg, another antihypertensive drug is added.

○ **Polythiazide** (Renese) is a long-acting thiazide diuretic used to treat edema and hypertension. To treat edema, the daily dose is 1 to 4 mg. To treat hypertension, the daily dose is 2 to 4 mg.

THIAZIDE-LIKE DIURETICS

The thiazide-like diuretics—**metolazone (Zaroxolyn)**, **chlorthalidone (Hygroton)**, and **indapamide (Lozol)**—are similar in all respects to the thiazide diuretics.

○ **Metolazone** (Zaroxolyn) is used to treat (1) hypertension and (2) edema secondary to heart failure, hepatic disease, or renal disease. Mykrox, compounded in a different way, is used to treat mild to moderate hypertension. An important additional property of metolazone is that it appears to be effective even in patients with reduced renal function; thus it resembles the loop diuretics. Metolazone has a duration of action of 24 hours and can be used in conjunction with loop diuretics. See Table 37–1 for dosages, pharmacokinetics, and nursing implications.

○ **Chlorthalidone** (Hygroton) is a long-acting thiazide-like diuretic that is used to treat edema and hypertension. See Table 37–1 for dosages, pharmacokinetics, and nursing implications.

○ **Indapamide** (Lozol) is a long-acting thiazide-like diuretic primarily used to treat hypertension and edema of heart failure. Indapamide may decrease lipid levels and blood sugar. The initial dose is 2.5 mg/day. If response is not satisfactory after 1 week, the dose can be increased to 5 mg/day. In general, doses above 5 mg do not provide any additional effects on blood pressure or on heart failure.

LOOP DIURETICS

Loop diuretics, also known as high-ceiling diuretics because they block a substantial portion of the loop function, have a diuretic action far superior to other agents. A particular advantage of loop diuretics is that increasing the dose exerts an increasing diuresis before the "ceiling" is reached. They inhibit electrolyte reabsorption in the thick ascending limb of the loop of Henle. These drugs tend to produce a short-lived increase in renal blood flow without increasing filtration rate. There may also be a minor effect on the distal collecting tubule. They work best when the urinary output is less than 30 mL/hr. The loop diuretics include **furosemide (Lasix)**, **torsemide (Demadox)**, **ethacrynic acid (Edecrin)**, and **bumetanide (Bumex)**. The loop diuretics are featured in Table 37–2.

USES

The loop diuretics are used primarily to treat edema associated with heart failure, hepatic or renal disease, and nephrotic syndrome. These drugs can be administered intravenously when rapid diuresis is necessary, such as in acute pulmonary edema. The loop diuretics promote venodilation and reduce preload and afterload.

The loop diuretics, particularly furosemide, are used concurrently with other drugs to control hypertension. They are reserved for hypertensive patients with fluid retention refractory to thiazides or for patients with impaired renal function. Because they have a different site of action, the loop diuretics may be effective for such patients when thiazides are not. Furosemide is also used with mannitol to manage cerebral edema. The loop diuretics are also used for the short-term management of *ascites* (an abnormal collection of fluid in the abdominal cavity) due to malignancies, lymphedema, nephrogenic diabetes insipidus, and hypercalcemia. In the oliguric patient, the loop diuretics are used for diagnosis and prophylaxis of acute renal failure. Excessive diuresis should be avoided because of the danger of precipitating shock.

PHARMACOKINETICS

The loop diuretics are absorbed rapidly from the GI tract, and their onset of action occurs within 1 hour after oral ingestion. Food slows the rate of absorption but does not alter the total amount absorbed. (Torsemide absorption is not affected by food.) Absorption is also slowed in patients with congestive heart failure. In patients with severe edema of the GI tract, absorption may be erratic and intravenous administration may be required. When given intravenously, the onset of diuresis may be as fast as 10 minutes. All of the loop diuretics are greater than 90% protein bound. The duration of action ranges from 2 hours for intravenous administration to 4 to 6 hours after oral administration. The loop diuretics are primarily excreted by the kidney via glomerular filtration and tubular secretion.

Because of declining renal function with aging and certain diseases such as heart failure, altered pharmacokinetics may occur. Patients with the nephrotic syndrome or cirrhosis often require higher doses of loop diuretics. The hypoalbuminuria accompanying these conditions causes decreased protein binding and thus less drug reaches the kidney.

CONTRAINDICATIONS AND PRECAUTIONS

Bumetanide is also contraindicated in patients with hepatic coma or severe electrolyte depletion because sudden alteration in electrolyte balance may precipitate hepatic encephalopathy, and bumetanide may worsen electrolyte depletion.

The loop diuretics are administered cautiously to the elderly and to patients with cardiovascular disease because the diuresis may induce an acute hypotensive episode along with hemoconcentration that could lead to thromboembolic episodes. The loop diuretics are also administered cautiously to cardiac patients receiving digitalis glycosides. The diuresis and the associated loss of potassium may precipitate digitalis toxicity and dysrhythmias.

Table 37–2. LOOP DIURETICS

DRUG NAME/ROUTE AND DOSAGE	PHARMACOKINETICS/ DYNAMICS	NURSING IMPLICATIONS
furosemide (Lasix)		
edema *Adults:* 20–80 mg PO daily or on alternate days, increased by 20–40 mg to maximum dose of 600 mg/daily; or 20–40 mg IV given slowly over 1–2 min, not to exceed 4 mg/min, then increase by 20 mg after 2 hr up to 1 g/da. **hypertension** *Adults:* Initial dose 20–40 mg daily, reduce dose as blood pressure falls. *Infants and Children:* 2 mg/kg PO; increase 1–2 mg/kg at 6 to 8 hr intervals; maximum dose 6 mg/kg. **acute pulmonary edema** *Adults:* 40 mg IV; if no response, double the dose. *Infants and Children:* 1 mg/kg IV; increase by 1 mg/kg after 2 hr.	**Onset:** PO, within 60 min; IV, within 5 min **Peak:** PO, 60–120 min; IV, 30 min **Duration:** PO, 6–8 hr; IV, 2 hr **½L:** 20 hr **PB:** 96%–98% **B:** 30%–40% liver **E:** kidneys	**ASSESSMENT:** Assess baseline urinary output and fluid balances. Assess for alkalosis and electrolyte imbalance. Assess daily weight and report rapid weight changes. Assess for development of orthostatic hypotension. Assess for pregnancy (category C). **INTERVENTION:** Weigh, measure input and output daily. Administer furosemide no faster than 4 mg/min. Do not use discolored solutions. If furosemide is added to a second diuretic, the other drug may need to be reduced by 50% to prevent falls in blood pressure. **Patient Teaching**—Instruct patient to take with meals to avoid GI upset. Teach patient to administer early in day so sleep is not interrupted. Do not administer after 3 PM. Instruct patient regarding over-the-counter drug use, especially sodium-containing products. Instruct patient in foods high in K+ to increase intake. **EVALUATION:** Evaluate therapy for efficacy. Evaluate lithium and digitalis levels for toxicity. Evaluate diabetics for hyperglycemia, glycosuria, and electrolyte disturbances. Evaluate coagulation studies.
ethacrynic acid (Edecrin)		
Adults: 50–200 mg PO or IV daily or on alternate days; adjust dose in 25–50 mg increments. *Pediatric:* 25 mg/day PO; or 0.5–1.0 mg/kg IV given slowly over several min up to 100 mg.	**Onset:** PO, within 30 min; IV, within 5 min **Peak:** PO, 120 min; IV, 15–30 min **Duration:** PO, 6–8 hr; IV, 2 hr **½L:** 60 min **PB:** 95% **B:** liver **E:** 30%–45% bile, 55%–65% kidneys	Same as for furosemide except: **ASSESSMENT:** Assess for pregnancy (category B). **INTERVENTION:** Use PO or IV forms. IM causes pain and local irritation. If IV solution is hazy or opalescent, do not use.
bumetanide (Bumex)		
Adults: 0.5–2.0 mg/day PO (up to maximum dose of 10 mg/day); or 0.5–1.0 mg IV over 1–2 min (up to a maximum daily dose of 10 mg).	**Onset:** PO, 30–60 min; IV, within minutes **Peak:** PO, 60–120 min; IV, 15–45 min **Duration:** PO, 4–6 hr; IV 2–3 hr **½L:** 60–90 min **PB:** 94%–96% **B:** 45% liver **E:** kidneys	Same as for furosemide.
torsemide (Demadox)		
heart failure *Adults:* 10–20 mg IV or PO daily, double until effect is reached or maximum of 200 mg. **cirrhosis** *Adults:* 5–10 mg IV or PO daily. **renal failure** *Adults:* 20 mg IV or PO daily. **hypertension** *Adults:* 5 mg/day PO or IV; may be increased to 10 mg after 4–6 weeks.	**Onset:** IV, 10 min; PO, 60 min **Peak:** IV, 60 min; PO, 60–120 min **Duration:** IV, 6–8 hr **½L:** 210 min **PB:** >99% **B:** hepatic (80%) **E:** urine (20%)	Same as for furosemide plus: **ASSESSMENT:** Assess for pregnancy (category B). **INTERVENTION:** Oral and IV dosing have the same therapeutic equivalence, so patients can be switched without any changes in dose. Administer IV slowly over 2 min.

ADVERSE EFFECTS

The major complication associated with loop diuretic therapy is the development of fluid and electrolyte imbalances as previously discussed. Loss of sodium and chloride as well as potassium occurs secondary to the potent effects of these diuretics within the loop of Henle. Certain patients may experience abnormal glucose tolerance while on these agents.

Hypersensitivity reactions may occur and present as GI disturbances, skin rashes, and hepatic dysfunction.

▼ CLINICAL ALERT

Rapid intravenous administration of large doses of loop diuretics may induce transient but rarely permanent deafness. The manufacturer of furosemide recommends infusing large doses at a rate no greater than 4 mg per minute. However, smaller doses of 20 to 40 mg may be pushed over 1 to 2 minutes.

Photosensitivity may also occur. Patients must be taught to wear protective clothing and to use sunscreens until tolerance can be determined.

INTERACTIONS

The NSAIDs may reduce sodium and water excretion and the antihypertensive effects caused by loop diuretics. These effects are due to the inhibition of prostaglandins. Probenecid may also decrease the effectiveness of the loop diuretics.

▼ CLINICAL ALERT

Patients who receive concurrent therapy with loop diuretics and aminoglycoside antibiotics may experience additive ototoxicity from these agents. Hearing ability and vestibular function are monitored closely in patients who receive this combination. Patients with renal failure appear to be at greater risk for this drug interaction.

Loop diuretics commonly cause excessive loss of potassium, leading to hypokalemia. The toxic effect of digitalis is potentiated by hypokalemia; therefore, serum electrolyte levels should be monitored in patients who receive loop diuretics and digitalis glycosides.

Concurrent administration of cisplatin may increase the potential for ototoxicity. Loop diuretics may increase levels of lithium. Serum lithium levels are monitored carefully to avoid toxicity. Loop diuretics may increase the hypoprothrombinemic effect of warfarin. Loop diuretics may increase the activity of anticoagulants and theophylline. Care is taken if these products are administered together.

○ **Furosemide** (Lasix) was the first loop diuretic to be released. It is the preferred loop diuretic because it causes fewer GI effects, is more convenient for intravenous use, has a broader dose-response curve, is less ototoxic, and is available in an oral solution.

Oral furosemide is usually effective in patients with heart failure who do not respond to the thiazides. It is also effective in treating edema of renal disease as it is effective even when glomerular filtration is greatly reduced. Dosage is individualized. Some patients may need daily doses, whereas others may benefit with alternate-day dosing.

○ **Torsemide** (Demadox) appears to be more potent than furosemide; however, at high doses it may be equipotent. Doses of 10 to 20 mg of torsemide may be equivalent to 40 mg of furosemide. Furosemide, however, tends to accumulate whereas torsemide is eliminated by additional hepatic metabolism. Torsemide is used to treat advanced chronic renal failure, heart failure, ascites, hypertension, and edema.

○ **Ethacrynic acid** (Edecrin) is a short-acting diuretic with short onset and duration of action. To treat edema, ethacrynic acid may be given orally or on alternate days. The chloruretic effect of ethacrynic acid may cause bicarbonate retention and metabolic alkalosis. Chloride can be administered to correct this condition.

○ **Bumetanide** (Bumex) can be used when the patient has hypersensitivity to furosemide. The striking difference between furosemide and bumetanide is the much greater bioavailability and potency of bumetanide, allowing the use of smaller doses. The average dose of 40 to 80 mg of furosemide is equivalent to 1 to 2 mg of bumetanide. The incidence of side effects and the therapeutic effectiveness of the two drugs are similar.

POTASSIUM-SPARING DIURETICS

The potassium-sparing diuretics are divided into two major subsets: the aldosterone antagonists and the direct-acting type, both featured in Table 37–3. **Spironolactane (Aldactone)** is the only aldosterone antagonist available in the United States. The direct-acting potassium-sparing diuretics are **triamterene (Dyrenium)** and **amiloride (Midamor)**.

USES

The potassium-sparing diuretics are most commonly used to counteract potassium loss induced by other diuretics. They may be given concurrently with thiazides to increase the serum potassium level. They are most useful in patients with increased renal mineralocorticoid activity or primary or secondary aldosteronism. These abnormalities may occur in hepatic cirrhosis, heart failure, renal artery stenosis, Cushing's syndrome, and during chronic prednisone use. When used for increased mineralocortical activity, the potassium-sparing diuretics are usually given alone. Potassium-sparing diuretics counter the tendency for increased potassium secretion in these patients.

CONTRAINDICATIONS AND PRECAUTIONS

The drugs are contraindicated in patients with hyperkalemia because they cause decreased potassium excretion and may lead to toxicity.

Table 37–3. POTASSIUM-SPARING DIURETICS

DRUG NAME/ROUTE AND DOSAGE	PHARMACOKINETICS/ DYNAMICS	NURSING IMPLICATIONS
spironolactone (Aldactone) and others		
hyperaldosteronism *Adults:* 100–400 mg PO daily **edema** *Adults:* 25–200 mg daily *Pediatric:* 3.3 mg/kg/day **hypertension** *Adults:* 50–100 mg daily **hypokalemia** *Adults:* 25–100 mg daily **hirsutism** *Adults:* 50–200 mg from day 4–21 of menstrual cycle.	**Onset:** 24–48 hr **Peak:** 48–72 hr **Duration:** 48–72 hr **½L:** 20 hr (10–35 hr canrenone)' **PB:** 98% **B:** liver, to canrenone and other active metabolites **E:** urine and bile	**ASSESSMENT:** Assess baseline potassium level. Assess blood pressure regularly during therapy. Assess intake and output and weight. **INTERVENTION:** Weigh daily. Record intake and output. Store drug in dark container away from light. **Patient Teaching**—Teach patient to avoid potassium supplements. Counsel patient regarding foods high in potassium. Caution patient to rise slowly to avoid orthostatic hypotension. Warn patient to avoid excessive, strenuous exercise. **EVALUATION:** Evaluate therapy for efficacy. If GI cramping, diarrhea, headache, skin rash, or breast enlargement occur, notify physician.
amiloride (Midamor)		
edema *Adults:* 5–20 mg/day PO	**Onset:** 2 hr **Peak:** 6–10 hr **Duration:** 24 hr **½L:** 6–9 hr **PB:** 23% **B:** minimal **E:** urine (50% unchanged)	Same as for spironolactone plus: **ASSESSMENT:** Assess for pregnancy (category B). **INTERVENTION:** Give with food to avoid GI upset.
triamterene (Dyrenium) *Adults:* 200–300 mg PO daily	**Onset:** 2–4 hr **Peak:** 6–8 hr **Duration:** 12–16 hr **½L:** 3 hr **PB:** 50%–67% **B:** liver 95% to hydroxytriamterene sulfate **E:** kidneys (21% unchanged)	Same as for spironolactone plus: **ASSESSMENT:** Assess for pregnancy (category B). **INTERVENTION:** Take with meals to avoid GI upset. Protect skin from sun. **EVALUATION:** Notify physician of fever, sore throat, nausea, or dry mouth.

ALDOSTERONE ANTAGONISTS

The aldosterone antagonist—spironolactone (Aldactone)—binds to the aldosterone receptors in the distal tubules and collecting ducts. This blocks the reabsorption of sodium and promotes the retention of potassium. An aldosterone antagonist is effective only in the presence of the mineralocorticoid (aldosterone), and its action can be overcome in the face of increasing amounts of the hormone.

○ **Spironolactone** (Aldactone) is effective in lowering both systolic and diastolic blood pressure in both hyperaldosteronism and essential hypertension. Additionally, spironolactone interferes with testosterone synthesis, which may permit a relative increase in estrogen activity; this action may be responsible for endocrine dysfunctions that are occasionally seen during therapy.

Spironolactone is the logical therapy for patients who develop hypertension in the presence of primary mineralocorticoid levels. It is also chosen when diabetes or gout may be present or when there is fear of their precipitation or when it is important to avoid potassium or magnesium loss and thiazide combinations are contraindicated. Spironolactone has antihypertensive activity but does cause more troublesome adverse effects. Because of its androgenic properties, spironolactone has been used for the unapproved therapy of hirsutism.

ADVERSE EFFECTS Spironolactone is associated with estrogenic effects (e.g., gynecomastia). Spironolactone may also produce central nervous system (CNS) symptoms such as drowsiness, ataxia, and mental confusion.

INTERACTIONS The pharmacologic effect of these drugs is to enhance sodium excretion and decrease potassium secretion. As a result, patients receiving angiotensin converting enzyme (ACE) inhibitors or potassium supplements with these drugs may develop hyperkalemia. Ingestion of large amounts of potassium-rich foods, listed in Table 37–4, may also lead to hyperkalemia. Hyperkalemia may induce CNS depression, dysrhythmias, and other effects. These interactions are especially significant in patients with renal failure, who have an inability to excrete excess potassium. In addition, concurrent aspirin use may decrease the diuretic response to spironolactone.

Table 37–4. FOODS THAT CONTAIN HIGH AMOUNTS OF POTASSIUM OR SODIUM		
High-Potassium Foods		
Avocados	Lima beans	Rhubarb
Apricots	Navy beans	Spinach
Bananas	Nuts	Squash
Cantaloupe	Oranges	Sunflower seeds
Dried fruits	Prunes	Tomatoes
Grapefruit	Raisins	
High-Sodium Foods		
Barbecue sauce	Canned spaghetti	Parmesan cheese
Butter, margarine	sauce	Pickles
Buttermilk	Catsup	Potato salad
Most cheeses	Cured meats	Pretzels, potato
Canned chili	Dry soup mixes	chips
Canned seafood	Macaroni and	
Canned soups	cheese	

DIRECT-ACTING POTASSIUM-SPARING DIURETICS

The direct-acting potassium-sparing diuretics—triamterene (Dyrenium) and amiloride (Midamor)—interfere with transport mechanisms in the distal tubule. These compounds impair the exchange of sodium and potassium at the same site as spironolactone, but do not compete with aldosterone. Both of these drugs have their duration of action increased with multiple doses and prolonged therapy. The net effects are a potassium-sparing diuresis and mild alkalinization of the urine.

○ **Triamterene** (Dyrenium) is a pteridine derivative that is chemically related to folic acid. Triamterene is not an effective antihypertensive agent when used alone, but is often used in combination with other diuretics and antihypertensive agents.

Triamterene elicits minor problems such as nausea, vomiting, leg cramps, and dizziness in certain patients. The major concern is the development of hyperkalemia when triamterene is prescribed for patients with impaired renal function. This situation may be made worse if patients are also given potassium supplements. Triamterene-containing kidney stones have also been reported. Triamterene, as a weak folic acid antagonist, may cause the development of megaloblastic anemias.

○ **Amiloride** (Midamor) has a mild diuretic effect similar to that of spironolactone and, like triamterene, is a pteridine compound. Amiloride is primarily used to treat hypertension or edema associated with congestive heart failure and to assist in restoring normal serum potassium levels in patients with hypokalemia. Amiloride is usually administered in combination with other diuretics, such as the thiazides or loop diuretics. Amiloride has a more rapid onset of action than spironolactone. The development of hyperkalemia, as discussed under triamterene, is also a concern during amiloride therapy.

AQUARETICS

An *aquaretic* is an agent that increases renal water excretion out of proportion to solute concentrations. This causes an increase in free water clearance. A drug in this class is **demeclocycline (DMC)** which works by interfering with the effect of antidiuretic hormone at the collecting ducts. Aquaretics are used as treatments for the water retention and hyponatremia associated with the syndrome of inappropriate antidiuretic hormone secretion (SIADH), cirrhosis, and psychogenic polydipsia.

○ **Demeclocycline** (DMC) has been used in the treatment of SIADH. Demeclocycline decreases the responsiveness to ADH. This is probably the result of decreased cyclic AMP formation and effect. Other tetracyclines have not been demonstrated to be as effective as demeclocycline. Patients with liver disease may develop azotemia and nephrotoxicity. Photosensitive reactions have been reported when patients are exposed to sunlight.

NONPRESCRIPTION DIURETICS

Nonprescription diuretics are used to alleviate menstrual discomfort. When taken 4 to 6 days before the onset of menses, they may help relieve symptoms related to water retention including temporary weight gain, bloating, puffiness, painful breasts, cramps, and tension. The most frequently used products are pamabrom (Fluidex with Pamabrom) and combinations of ammonium chloride and caffeine (Aqua-Ban).

Pamabrom is a theophylline derivative and has weak diuretic properties when taken alone. It is often combined with analgesics and antihistamines for relief of symptoms associated with menses or premenstrual syndrome.

Ammonium chloride is an acid-forming salt that has limited value in terms of diuresis. It is often used in combination with caffeine for adjunctive effects. Large doses may cause GI irritation and CNS toxicity. Ammonium chloride is contraindicated for individuals with impaired renal or hepatic function. Metabolic acidosis may occur with large doses of ammonium chloride.

Caffeine promotes diuresis by inhibiting reabsorption of both sodium and chloride. It may alleviate the mental and physical fatigue associated with fluid retention. Doses above 100 mg may cause GI irritation. The calculation of total caffeine intake should include drinking coffee, tea, or caffeine-containing soft drinks, as well as eating chocolate or taking other caffeine-containing products.

CLINICAL USES OF DIURETICS

HEART FAILURE

The primary manifestation of heart failure (HF) relieved by diuretics is edema. In addition, a fall in peripheral vascular resistance (PVR) occurs as a result of an increase in venous capacitance. Edema is a result of the early compensating mechanisms in HF. As stroke volume decreases, antidiuretic hormone (ADH) is stimulated, causing increased renal tubular water retention and reabsorption. Due to vasoconstriction (an attempt to increase blood pressure), the glomerular filtration rate falls. Subsequently, renin is released, which causes a rise in aldosterone levels and an increase in PVR. This causes more fluid retention and increased plasma volume. Eventually this "leaks" out of the intravascular space, causing increased *interstitial volume* (referring to the volume of fluid in the space between cells) and edema. The severity of peripheral edema is determined by the degree the skin is able to rebound from finger pressure. *Pitting edema* (usually of the skin of the extremities, that when pressed firmly with a finger willl maintain the depression produced by the finger) results from a loss of elasticity and is found in advanced failure.

In early heart failure, the symptoms may be controlled with a no-salt-added diet prior to diuretic therapy. Sodium restriction is required when more advanced disease is present. The less potent diuretics—amiloride, triamterene, spironolactone, or the thiazides—are often selected first. When more severe symptomatology occurs, therapy with more potent agents, such as the loop diuretics, may be considered. As adjuncts to the diuretics, other drugs such as vasodilators, nifedipine, or ACE inhibitors can be considered.

In severe HF, therapy with the thiazides may cause a dilutional hyponatremia. Excess sodium is excreted, while the patient often continues to take in excess free water, especially when thirsty. Furosemide rarely causes hyponatremia in this setting. Combinations of ACE inhibitors with furosemide may prevent or reverse the hyponatremia of severe HF. If cardiac decompensation is associated with an acute myocardial infarction (MI), then intravenous loop diuretics are the agents of choice.

In advanced HF, patients often become refractory to diuretic therapy. These patients generally present with volume overload and pulmonary and peripheral edema with or without ascites, as shown in Figure 37–2. In addition, portal vein congestion impairs hepatic metabolism of some drugs. Furosemide is usually administered first, and metolazone may be added. Short courses of intravenous acetazolamide may be advantageous. Oral or intra-

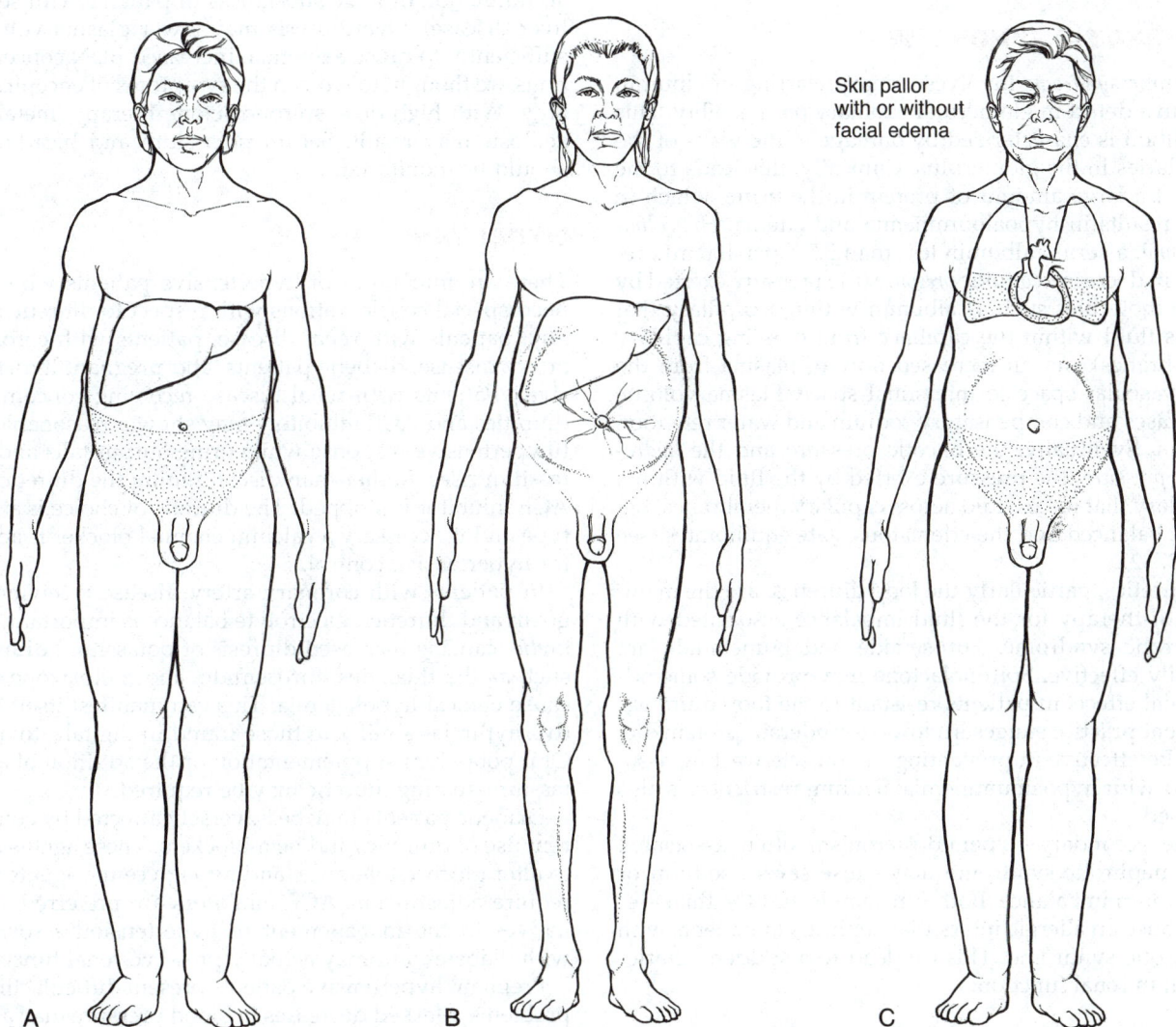

Skin pallor with or without facial edema

Figure 37–2. Comparison of the different forms of edema. (A), Cardiac edema may be peripheral as with RHF or in the lungs with LHF. (B), Liver edema is primarily found in the form of ascites. (C) Renal edema may be peripheral but also occurs in the face—Potter's face.

venous nitrates or other vasodilators have been used in conjunction with diuretics to treat severe HF.

The major complication with diuretic use in HF is hypokalemia and metabolic alkalosis. This often predisposes patients to life-threatening dysrhythmias, especially when digoxin is used. Volume depletion due to overdiuresis may also present problems.

ACUTE PULMONARY EDEMA

Pulmonary edema is an effusion of the fluid from the pulmonary capillaries into the interstitial spaces and eventually into the alveolar spaces. Most commonly it is caused by systolic heart failure, coronary artery disease, or cardiomyopathy. The aim of therapy is to remove the cause of cardiac decompensation and to decrease the workload on the heart. Measures include oxygen, nitrates or nitroprusside, dobutamine, diuretics, and digoxin. The diuretics of choice are the intravenous loop-type diuretics given to rapidly establish a diuresis, reduce blood volume, and reduce preload. Injections are still given slowly, despite the immediacy of the situation.

NEPHROTIC SYNDROME

Nephrotic syndrome involves urinary wasting of albumin due to a defect in glomerular capillary permeability. This condition is characterized by damage to the walls of the capillaries in the glomerulus. Clinically, this leads to the loss of a large amount of protein in the urine, which in turn results in hypoalbuminemia and edema. *Hypoalbuminemia*, a serum albumin less than 3.5 g per 100 mL, results in decreased *oncotic pressure* (the pressure exerted by large molecules such as albumin within a capillary that keeps fluid within the capillary from crossing capillary membranes) and an increased flow of plasma from the intravascular space to interstitial space. Plasma volume decreases and compensatory sodium and water retention occurs. Eventually, the oncotic pressure and the *hydrostatic pressure* (the pressure exerted by the fluid within a capillary that forces fluid across capillary membranes) become balanced and the edematous state equilibrates (see Fig. 37–2).

Diuretics, particularly the loop diuretics, are the mainstay of therapy for the fluid imbalance associated with nephrotic syndrome. Furosemide and bumetanide are equally effective. Spironolactone may provide some additional effects in patients resistant to the loop diuretics. Current practice suggests a low- to moderate-protein diet may be effective in preventing the muscle wasting associated with hypoalbuminemia. Sodium restriction is also advised.

The secondary hyperaldosteronism often associated with nephrotic syndrome may cause severe sodium or potassium imbalance. Both furosemide and the thiazides can cause an allergic interstitial nephritis in patients with nephrotic syndrome. This can lead to a sudden deterioration in renal function.

CIRRHOSIS

Cirrhosis is a chronic liver disease characterized by loss of functioning liver cells and increased resistance to the flow of blood through the liver. The disease leads to hepatic venous outflow obstruction. This in turn increases internal hepatic venous hydrostatic pressures and leads to movement of plasma to the lymphatic systems in the liver. As conditions worsen, protein-containing fluid leaks from the lymph into the peritoneal cavity, causing ascites. Plasma volume decreases and compensatory sodium and water retention further worsen the edematous state (see Fig. 37–2). In cirrhosis, albumin synthesis may decrease, leading to decreased plasma volume. In addition, portal hypertension causes splanchnic venous pooling. This, coupled with the vasodilation associated with nephrotic syndrome, also decreases the volume of the extracellular fluid.

In patients with cirrhosis, levels of circulating aldosterone are very frequently elevated. For this reason, spironolactone is often the diuretic of choice. Spironolactone is generally effective in reducing the volume of ascitic fluid. Small doses of furosemide may also be given to augment the diuretic action.

Patients with cirrhosis also may develop *hepatic encephalopathy* (abnormal function of the brain caused by the accumulation of toxic substances in patients with severe liver disease). Overdiuresis may lower plasma volumes sufficiently to cause azotemia. Increased BUN concentrations are thought to worsen the symptoms of encephalopathy. With high-dose spironolactone therapy, metabolic acidosis may result. Serum potassium and bicarbonate should be monitored.

HYPERTENSION

There are four types of hypertensive patients who may need special considerations with respect to diuretic therapy: patients with renal disease, patients with coronary artery disease, diabetic patients, and pregnant hypertensives. Patients with renal disease receiving concomitant diuretics and ACE inhibitors may show a reasonable antihypertensive response while urine output falls and potassium rises. Rather than discontinuing the diuretic, the ACE inhibitor is stopped. The diuretic of choice is a loop type and if necessary a calcium channel blocker is added for hypertensive control.

In patients with coronary artery disease receiving digoxin and diuretics, electrolyte balance is important. *Kaluretic* (causing increased diuresis of potassium) diuretics such as the thiazides, furosemide, and metolazone may cause clinical hypokalemia. This can manifest itself with dysrhythmias similar to those found in digitalis toxicity. Oral potassium supplementation or the addition of a potassium-sparing diuretic may be required.

Diabetic patients may be adversely affected by concurrent use of diuretics and beta-blockers. These agents tend to alter glucose tolerance, and hypoglycemic agents may require adjustments. ACE inhibitors are preferred alternatives in the management of hypertension associated with diabetes and may actually preserve renal function.

Pregnant hypertensive patients present difficult clinical problems. Marked decreases in blood pressure may affect uterine blood flow and result in decreased placental and fetal perfusion. Vasodilators such as hydralazine are often the preferred agents.

The Veterans Affairs Cooperative Study concluded that

low-dose thiazides should be used in the stepped care of hypertension and that the addition of a second agent would offer more benefit than increasing the dose of the diuretic. The research effort also showed no differences between African-American and Caucasian populations in response to drug therapy (Materson et al., 1990).

Malignant hypertension is a clinical emergency requiring immediate attention. The aim is to reduce diastolic blood pressure by 30% to 40%, but not below normotensive levels. Rapid-acting vasodilators such as diazoxide (Hyperstat), nitroprusside (Nipride), enalapril (Vasotec), or labetalol (Normodyne) are given. Furosemide is given to rapidly increase the excretion of sodium as the other agents quickly decrease the pressure. This protects the patient from the complications of brain encephalopathy and heart failure.

ACUTE RENAL FAILURE

The first principle of management in acute renal failure is to correct all specifically treatable causes of decreasing renal function. These include obstructive uropathy, glomerulonephritis, and renal vascular/interstitial disease. Attempts should be made in establishing a urine output. Diuretics may improve the urine output in most cases; however, there is no evidence that they will decrease overall mortality. Small to large doses of furosemide IV should be tried. Furosemide in doses large enough to improve renal function (60 to 100 mg) is also associated with a high incidence of ototoxicity when given rapidly IV. If no response occurs, mannitol is indicated. If patients remain oliguric after reasonable attempts at diuretic therapy, therapy with dopamine (3 to 5 mg/kg per minute) may increase renal blood flow and facilitate the diuretic response. Bumetanide has been used in patients sensitive to or nonresponsive to furosemide. Torsemide may be considered if the patient is refractory to conventional diuretic and vasodilator therapy, but should not be considered a first-line agent.

CHRONIC RENAL FAILURE

In chronic renal failure, diuretic therapy is used to present and treat heart failure. Furosemide is the diuretic of choice, although furosemide-metolazone combinations may be synergistic. In this situation, large furosemide doses are not uncommon. Metolazone may be beneficial in patients with chronic hyperkalemia, because of its significant kaluretic properties.

DISORDERS OF CALCIUM METABOLISM

Loop diuretics cause a dynamic excretion of calcium in the urine. Furosemide has been shown to inhibit calcium reabsorption in the thick ascending limb. The mechanism of this calcuria is similar to that of the loop diuretics in preventing the reabsorption of sodium. Treatment of hypercalcemia involves hourly infusions of 200 to 300 mL per hour of normal saline. When the patient is fully hydrated, oral or intravenous furosemide (40 to 160 mg/day) is administered. As rapid diuresis occurs, water, sodium, potassium, and magnesium must be closely monitored and replaced as required. Calcium levels have dropped as much as 3 mg/dL following use of this treatment. Other therapies for hypercalcemia include oral phosphates, mithramycin, calcitonin, etidronate, and gallium.

THERAPEUTIC DILEMMAS

In general, pharmacotherapy aims at single-drug dosing to minimize adverse reactions and drug interactions. The principle of dosing each agent individually is sound in theoretical clinical practice. Because diuretics augment other types of antihypertensive agents, this combination of therapeutic agents is accepted. Low doses of diuretics can be found in combination with methyldopa, reserpine, hydralazine, beta-blockers, clonidine, prazosin, and ACE inhibitors. Synergy can be achieved when one or more individual agents of different mechanisms are combined in a fixed-dosage tablet formation. These fixed combinations offer a great deal of convenience to the patient, and the single tablet is usually less expensive than the individual ingredients taken separately. As long as the patient is managed appropriately, these combinations are useful. In complicated cases, each agent is dosed separately.

Chronic diuretic administration can also lead to leveling off of the diuretic effect, or *diuretic resistance*. In the face of a shrunken intravascular volume, the part of the tubular system not affected by the diuretic reacts by reabsorbing more sodium. It is important to evaluate compliance with the dietary salt restrictions, electrolyte disturbances that must be corrected, and concomitant drug therapy which may ameliorate the diuretic effect. An ACE inhibitor drug may have to be added to thiazide or loop diuretics to augment the effect. Other causes of apparent diuretic resistance include excessive circulating catecholamines (frequently seen in HF and corrected by increased inotropic support); the interference of drugs such as NSAIDs; the activation of the renin-angiotensin-aldosterone system (often seen in HF and corrected by ACE inhibitors); and the incorrect use of diuretics. Incorrect diuretic uses include combining two drugs in the same group, using the thiazides when glomerular filtration rate is low, excessive dosing, and poor patient compliance.

DIURETIC-NUTRIENT INTERACTIONS

Dietary modifications may be important, depending on whether a potassium-sparing or potassium-wasting agent is selected. The selection of potassium-rich foods such as fruit and fruit juices (see Table 37–4) is essential when thiazide or loop diuretics are administered. Conversely, excess intake of these types of foods with concomitant spironolactone, amiloride, triamterene, or ACE inhibitor therapy can lead to hyperkalemia.

Because most of these patients are on salt restrictions, monitoring food sources is important. The patient should avoid adding salt to food during preparation and be instructed how to read food labels in a grocery store. The use of potassium salt substitutes may be desired; however, in large quantities these may interact with potassium-sparing diuretics or ACE inhibitors.

Caffeine promotes diuresis by inhibiting reabsorption of both sodium and chloride. It may alleviate the mental and physical fatigue associated with fluid retention.

Doses above 100 mg cause GI irritation. Total intake is considered when drinking coffee, tea, or caffeine-containing soft drinks, as well as when eating chocolate or taking other caffeine-containing products.

USING THE NURSING PROCESS

ASSESSMENT

- Develop a thorough nursing history. Multiple symptoms indicating the need for diuretic therapy may be present and are elicited during both the history and the physical assessment. Typical information to assess is featured in Table 37–5. The patient's self-consciousness may be evident during discussions of urinary patterns and changes. The following specific questions are asked:
    1. Is there any change in amount, color, or odor of the urine?
    2. Is there any change in urinary pattern-dysuria, frequency, hesitation, incontinence?
    3. Do you wake during the night to void?
    4. Do you notice any unusual swelling or puffiness of the hands or feet or around the eyes?
    5. Has there been an unexplained weight change?
    6. Are shoes, rings, or wristwatches too tight? Terminology and phrasing are directed to the patient's educational and knowledge level.
- Assess medication history of drugs currently taken, including nonprescription drugs.
- Establish a baseline assessment in each area to evaluate effectiveness of therapy and to monitor any potential detrimental effects. Physical assessment of patients requiring diuretic therapy includes several areas: neurologic, cardiovascular, respiratory, renal, skin, and nutrition. Each area is assessed to detect preexisting or potential problems that may compromise diuretic therapy.
- Assess for known electrolyte imbalances, hepatic or renal dysfunction, diabetes history, pregnancy and lactation, as well as a history of drug allergies, such as an allergy to sulfonamides (loop diuretics are related to sulfonamides) and specific allergic symptoms. Once the patient has been placed on diuretic therapy, be alert to signs of electrolyte imbalance.

Hypokalemia is a potentially life-threatening condition. Because potassium is necessary for proper neuromuscular and cardiac function, patients with hypokalemia may exhibit cardiac dysrhythmias, muscle weakness and cramps, abdominal distention, and mental status changes such as confusion, apathy, drowsiness, and irritability. Family members often notice changes in the patient's mental status, so be alert to any of their statements that reflect such changes. Patients with underlying cardiac disease who are receiving digitalis glycoside and thiazide therapy run an increased risk of developing digitalis toxicity from potassium depletion. Also, patients with ischemic heart disease, HF treated with digitalis glycosides, or hypertension with left ventricle hypertrophy are at higher risk for developing dysrhythmias. Using a potassium- and magnesium-retaining diuretic, or cotherapy with an ACE inhibitor or calcium channel blocker, may be beneficial for these patients. When ACE inhibitors are used, potassium supplements should be avoided. Encouraging the consumption of foods rich in potassium and low in sodium may be appropriate if potassium supplements are not prescribed. If, however, potassium-sparing diuretics or oral potassium supplementation are part of the patient's medication profile, excessive use of foods abundant in potassium may be detrimental.

NURSING DIAGNOSIS

- Determine nursing diagnoses for the patient requiring diuretic therapy based on the information gained during the history and physical assessment. Typical nursing diagnoses for the patient requiring diuretic therapy include Knowledge Deficit, Fluid Volume Excess, Fluid Volume Deficit, and Electrolyte Disturbance (see Table 37–5).

PLANNING AND INTERVENTION

- Determine nursing goals derived from the nursing diagnoses, which direct the plan of care for patients receiving diuretic therapy (see Table 37–5). In all cases, the plan of care is individually tailored to the needs of each patient. Cooperation cannot be achieved if patients do not see the total picture in regard to therapy. An empathetic nurse can help establish a relationship that encourages the patient to ask questions about treatment.
- Ensure that the patient and family members have some understanding of the underlying pathology. Diuretics are usually part of long-term therapy, and often this is difficult for both the patient and family to accept. Unfortunately, the overnight cure is rarely available. Table 37–6 reviews the numerous conditions that can be treated with diuretics and the usual choice of agents. Cost effectiveness is also important to consider. The newer therapies for hypertension or congestive therapy include the ACE inhibitors and calcium channel blockers. Patients who must pay for their own medications may not be compliant to the newer drugs because of increased cost, but may receive reasonable benefits from the less expensive diuretics.

The use of diuretics in cardiac, hepatic, or renal disease affects a number of body systems. Decreased muscle tone and generalized weakness may be observed along with signs and symptoms of dehydration. Any number of electrolyte imbalances may occur and must be carefully assessed in each patient. Dietary adjustments also must be made to compensate for electrolyte imbalances. Sodium restrictions often accompany diuretic therapy to improve diuresis and decrease high blood pressure. Planning and teaching include potassium replacement and limitations on sodium intake. (Foods that contain high amounts of potassium and sodium are listed in Table 37–4.)

Table 37–5. NURSING PROCESS FOR PATIENT REQUIRING DIURETIC THERAPY

Assessment

Auscultate breath sounds, note presence of cough
Assess for jugular venous distention, hepatojugular reflux, S3.
Palpate abdomen for hepatomegaly, hepatic pulsations, ascites, splenomegaly.
Assess dependent, generalized, or periorbital edema.
Assess weight, note recent changes.
Assess dietary intake of potassium and sodium.

Nursing Diagnosis: Knowledge Deficit	**Desired Outcomes/Evaluation Criteria**
RELATED TO: Unfamiliarity with information resources/ misinterpretation. **AS EVIDENCED BY:** Questions, request for information, inaccurate follow-through of instructions, development of preventable complications.	Verbalizes understanding of illness/condition and treatment. Identifies signs/symptoms or side effects requiring medical attention.

Nursing Actions	**Rationale**
Review pathophysiology of condition and need for diuretic therapy.	Provides opportunity for patient/significant other (SO) to ask questions, clarify misconceptions, and make informed choices.
Discuss medications, dosage, schedule, and side effects.	Understanding function of the medication in own terms can help patient to manage own regimen; promotes sense of control.
Stress importance of follow-up and reporting of side effects.	Provides for timely intervention to prevent occurrence of drug-related complications.
Discuss importance of sodium limitation, signs/symptoms of imbalance. Provide list of foods high in sodium that are to be avoided/limited. Encourage reading of labels on food and drug packages.	Dietary intake of sodium above 3 g daily will offset diuretic effect.
Recommend taking diuretic early in morning.	Provides adequate time for drug effect before bedtime to prevent/limit interruption of sleep.
Suggest patient weigh self regularly.	Documents changes in fluid overload/edema in response to therapy.
Encourage discussion of situation and treatment and how it affects lifestyle.	Provides insight about how patient/SO view condition and are coping with needed changes.

Nursing Diagnosis: Fluid Volume Excess	**Desired Outcomes/Evaluation Criteria**
RELATED TO: Altered glomerular filtration, increased ADH production, excess intake or retention of sodium/water. **AS EVIDENCED BY:** Orthopnea, S3 heart sound, oliguria, edema, weight gain, hypertension, respiratory distress.	Demonstrates stabilized fluid volume with balanced intake and output, breath sounds clear/clearing, vital signs within acceptable range, stable weight, and absence of edema.

Nursing Actions	**Rationale**
Calculate 24-hour intake and output balance. Compare with weight.	Aids in identifying therapeutic needs/effectiveness and potential complications. Diuretic therapy may result in sudden/excessive fluid loss (circulating hypovolemia) even though edema/ascites.
Maintain chair or bed rest in semi-Fowler's position.	Recumbency increases glomerular filtration and decreases production of ADH, thereby enhancing diuresis.
Establish fluid intake schedule, incorporating beverage preferences when possible. Give frequent mouth care.	Involving patient in therapy regimen may enhance sense of control and cooperation with restrictions.
Monitor laboratory studies, e.g., Hgb/HCT, electrolytes.	Evaluates response to therapy and identifies additional therapeutic needs to prevent complications.

Other Suggested Nursing Diagnoses: Fluid Volume Deficit and Electrolyte Disturbance.

• Monitor for decreased muscle tone and generalized weakness, along with signs of dehydration. Hypokalemia (decreased serum potassium level) is a potentially life-threatening condition. Replacement of potassium can be accomplished by increasing the dietary intake of potassium-rich foods. Foods especially high in potassium content include bananas, oranges, orange juice, and dried fruits. One 6-inch banana or one 8-ounce glass of orange juice contains 25 to 50 mEq of potassium, which is one-third to one-half more than the minimum daily requirement (MDR).

• Understand when and how to administer diuretics. Most diuretics are administered with meals to avoid GI upset. All diuretics are best given in the morning as soon as the patient wakes up. At times, patients may be able to take diuretics on alternate days or several times per week rather than on a daily basis.

Table 37–6. DISEASE AND CHOICE OF DIURETIC

Disease	First Choice	Second Choice
Heart failure	Thiazide	Loop
Acute pulmonary edema	Loop	
Cirrhosis	Spironolactone	Thiazide
Nephrotic syndrome	Thiazide	Loop
Hypertension	Thiazide	Loop
Hypercalcemia	Loop	
Acute renal failure	Loop	
Nephrogenic diabetes insipidus	Thiazide	
Syndrome of inappropriate antidiuretic hormone	Loop	

Patient Teaching

• Develop a teaching plan geared to the patient's knowledge level and level of understanding. Table 37–7 presents patient teaching information for diuretics.

   Patients should understand the function of their medication in their own terms (a diuretic or a "fluid pill") and its clinical use in the body. Patients are also taught the appropriate dosage and schedule to ensure their compliance with the therapeutic regimen. Signs and symptoms of potential problems are

Table 37–7. PATIENT TEACHING INFORMATION— DIURETICS

Dear Patient:
   The drug that has been ordered for you is called a *diuretic*, or a fluid pill. This drug helps to reduce the amount of fluid in your body by causing the kidneys to pass a large amount of water and salt from your blood. Removing this fluid helps to decrease the work on your heart and to decrease the edema, or swelling, in your body. This is what you need to know about this drug:

☐ 1. The name of your drug is _____ .
☐ 2. Diuretics may be needed for the rest of your life.
☐ 3. Change positions slowly to avoid dizziness.
☐ 4. Limit the amount of sodium that you take in. (High-sodium foods are listed in Table 37–4).
☐ 5. You may need to replace potassium in your body. Be guided by instructions from your nurse or physician. (High-potassium foods are listed in Table 37–4.)
☐ 6. Always check with your physician or pharmacist about possible interactions between nonprescription drugs and diuretics.
☐ 7. Do not take this drug after 3 P.M. unless otherwise directed by your doctor. If you do, you will be awake during the night to go to the bathroom.
☐ 8. Do not stop taking this drug without checking with your physician or nurse.
☐ 9. Be aware of signs of dehydration, such as increased thirst or dry, scaly skin, and report these to the nurse or physician.
☐ 10. Report signs of potassium loss, such as muscle weakness or irritability, to the nurse or physician.
☐ 11. Check your weight daily and record it. If you lose or gain more than 3 pounds in 1 day, report it to the nurse or physician.
☐ 12. Store your medication in a tight, light-resistant container.

also vital parts of patient education. Patients are taught how to avoid orthostatic hypotension. Patients should change positions, from lying down to sitting to standing, slowly. Patients are taught to limit their alcohol intake as alcohol also acts as a mild diuretic. During warm weather, patients must be careful to avoid strenuous exercise and heavy sweating to prevent the possibility of fluid and electrolyte imbalances.

EVALUATION

• Evaluate the patient at all steps of the intervention. Guidelines for evaluation of the patient receiving diuretic therapy are included in Table 37–5. As a general rule, these criteria include the following: (1) an informed client and family who understand the disease process and both the medical and nursing regimens, (2) a reduction in uncomfortable symptoms due to medication compliance, (3) dietary controls, and (4) minimum side effects related to diuretic therapy.

• Evaluate the patient's compliance with therapy. Diuretics are used in conditions that present with a variety of clinical manifestations; therefore, both the patient and the nurse must be aware of the underlying pathology. Because many of these conditions are chronic problems, the patient may have to make major lifestyle adjustments. The patient needs a clear understanding of the consequences of any action that he or she may take or refuse to take. Compliance may become a problem if the patient expects an overnight cure.

   During therapy of edematous states, excessive diuresis may occur. The result is a reduction in venous pressure and ventricular filling so that cardiac output drops and tissues become underperfused. Overdiuresis is most frequently seen during hospital admissions when a rigid policy of regular administration of diuretics is carried out. Excessive diuresis is most commonly seen when intravenous loop diuretics are used. It may be necessary to cautiously administer a fluid challenge with a saline solution or a colloid preparation while checking the patient's cardiovascular status. If the resting heart rate falls, renal function improves, and blood pressure stabilizes, the ventricular filling pressure has been inadequate.

• Evaluate for diuretic resistance. Diuretic resistance may be caused by compensatory mechanisms resulting from a decreased intravascular volume, hormonal changes, incorrect drug or dose selection, drug interactions, or patient noncompliance. In the face of a shrunken intravascular volume, the part of the tubular system not affected by the diuretic reacts by reabsorbing more sodium. It is important to evaluate the following: Is there compliance with the dietary salt restriction? Is the optimal agent being used? Is complete bed rest required? Is the optimal dose being used? Are there any electrolyte disturbances that must be corrected? Has the general cardiovascular status been made optimal by judicious use of unloading or inotropic drugs? To achieve ideal metabolic hormonal status, an ACE inhibitor may have to be added to thiazide or loop diuretic therapy. Sometimes fewer drugs work better.

Other causes of apparent diuretic resistance include excessive circulating catecholamines (frequently seen in HF and corrected by increased inotropic support); the interference of drugs such as the NSAIDs; the activation of the renin-angiotensin-aldosterone system (often seen in congestive heart failure and corrected by ACE inhibitors); and the incorrect use of diuretics. Incorrect use of diuretics may include use of two drugs in the same group, use of thiazides when the glomerular filtration rate is low, excessive dosing, and poor patient compliance.

• Evaluate the goals of the patient for therapy. In ideal diuretic therapy, the patient's urine output increases, electrolyte imbalances are corrected, and edema decreases. If all of these goals are not possible, realistic goals must be set within the limits of the illness by the patient and the family. The nurse provides the encouragement to help the patient overcome anxieties and to make lifestyle adjustments.

The bibliography for this chapter can be found in Appendix B, which begins on page 1054.

CHAPTER REVIEW QUESTIONS*

1. Patients receiving aldosterone antagonists are assessed for:
   a. Bone marrow suppression.
   b. Ototoxicity.
   c. Nephrotoxicity.
   d. Endocrine dysfunction.

2. Fluid accumulates in the interstitial space when there exists:
   a. Increased intravascular oncotic pressure.
   b. Decreased intravascular hydrostatic pressure.
   c. Altered capillary permeability.
   d. Reduced volume of sodium in interstitial space.

3. When treating patients who have ascities but no evidence of peripheral edema, the maximum extra diuresis that should be induced is:
   a. 900 mL/day.
   b. 2000 mL/day.
   c. 1500 mL/day.
   d. 1200 mL/day.

4. Thiazide diuretics acting in the distal tubule have been associated with:
   a. Metabolic alkalosis.
   b. Nephrotoxicity when administered with aminoglycosides.
   c. Decreased lithium levels leading to ineffectiveness of lithium.
   d. Hypercholesterolemia and triglyceridemia.

5. Loop diuretics:
   a. Can safely be administered quickly by bolus.
   b. May produce transient and even permanent deafness.
   c. May cause impotence, gynecomastia, and diminished libido.
   d. Improve acute interstital nephritis.

*See Appendix A, which begins on page 1051, for answers.

BUILDING YOUR CRITICAL THINKING SKILLS

DIURETIC TOXICITY

A 75-year-old man with a history of hypertension and insulin-dependent diabetes mellitus is admitted to the emergency room with a blood pressure of 195/110. He is given 200 mg of furosemide (Lasix) IV to reduce the blood pressure. Shortly thereafter, the patient appears uninterested in his surroundings and misinterprets questions. The wife relates the patient has an infected toe, for which he is receiving "some antibiotic."

1. What is the relevancy of the patient's behavior related to this drug therapy?
2. What other assessments should the nurse make for this patient?
3. What implication could the type of antibiotic have for this patient's case?

CHAPTER 38

Drug Therapy for the Patient with Renal Disease

Merrily A. Kuhn, RNC, PhD

CHAPTER OUTLINE

Acute Renal Failure
Chronic Renal Failure
Acid-Base Balance
Miscellaneous Problems
Dialysis
Drug Dosing in Renal Failure
Using the Nursing Process

TABLES

Drug Tables
Hemopoietic Agents, 569

Nursing Process
Nursing Process for Patient with Renal Disease, 573

BOXES

Delivering Home Health Care, 575
Building Your Critical Thinking Skills, 577

KEY TERMS

Acute renal failure
Chronic ambulatory
 peritoneal dialysis (CAPD)
Continuous cycling
 peritoneal dialysis
 (CCPD)
Dialysis
Erythropoiesis

Kaluretic
Manual peritoneal dialysis
Oliguria
Osteitis fibrosa
Osteomalacia
Osteoporosis
Uremic frost

LEARNING OBJECTIVES

After reading this chapter, the student will be able to:

1. Understand how to assess for hyperkalemia of renal failure.
2. Understand the use of diuretics and vasoactive substances in ameliorating the excretory and cardiovascular aberrations associated with renal failure.
3. Understand the role of the kidney in regulation of acid-base balance and procedure to treat acid-base abnormalities.
4. Discuss the use of various agents to control calcium, potassium, and phosphate imbalances in renal failure.

The kidney is responsible for regulation of fluid and electrolyte balance, maintainance of homeostasis, and elimination of most drugs. In renal failure, which can be either acute or chronic, the kidneys are unable to properly excrete wastes, concentrate urine, and conserve electrolytes. This chapter focuses on the clinical problems associated with renal failure—oliguria, hypertension, electrolyte imbalances, anemia, hyperuricemia, and acid-base disturbances—and the drug regimens used to modify these situations. Dialysis and drug dosage adjustments in patients with renal disease are also discussed.

The publisher gratefully acknowledges the contribution of Kenneth A. Kellick, Pharm D to the third edition.

ACUTE RENAL FAILURE

Acute renal failure, loosely described as the sudden onset of renal dysfunction, is categorized as prerenal, postrenal, and intrarenal or acute tubular necrosis (ATN). (See a medical-surgical nursing text for more detailed discussion of acute renal failure.) Acute renal failure may begin in minutes to hours of the precipitating event (e.g., trauma, obstruction of the urinary tract, hypovolemia) and may last for days, weeks, or months. Renal function may return to normal or chronic renal failure may follow. Precise measurements of urine output, blood urea nitrogen (BUN), serum creatinine, and other waste products are obtained throughout acute renal failure.

OLIGURIA

The goal of initial therapy for *oliguria* (a condition of diminished urine formation) associated with renal failure is to increase urine flow. If volume depletion is suspected, a fluid challenge with 500 to 1000 mL of 0.9% sodium chloride may be administered intravenously over 30 to 60 minutes. If unsuccessful, an osmotic diuretic such as mannitol may be given. Osmotic diuretics increase the osmolarity of the glomerular filtrate, drawing more water into the nephron, thereby increasing the urine flow. Mannitol may be particularly effective because it easily passes through the glomerulus of the nephron but is not reabsorbed into the interstitial tissues. The use of mannitol is discussed in greater detail in Chapter 37.

Large doses of a loop diuretic, such as furosemide (Lasix), are often used in the treatment of acute renal failure. Doses may need to be slowly increased every hour until the furosemide threshold for the patient has been established. (This is the minimum number of milligrams of the drug necessary to produce an adequate urinary response.) If patients are not responsive to furosemide, concurrent administration of metolazone (Zaroxolyn, Diulo) may be of value.

CARDIOVASCULAR STATUS

The patient with acute renal failure may demonstrate signs of hypotension or shock. In this situation, the use of a vasopressor such as dopamine may be indicated. Dopamine is an endogenous catecholamine precursor of norepinephrine. It acts on alpha, beta, and dopaminergic receptors. In the lower dosage ranges, such as 1 to 2 $\mu g/kg$ per minute, dopamine dilates the renal and mesenteric vessels, producing a corresponding increase in glomerular filtration rate (GFR). Because of profound cardiotonic effects, dopamine is given only in emergency situations or in intensive care monitoring environments.

Often in acute renal failure, maximal cardiac output is insufficient to improve the clinical picture. The administration of cardiotonic agents such as digoxin, dobutamine, amrinone, or milrinone may be warranted to improve the hemodynamic status and thus increase GFR. Digoxin must be administered cautiously because it is primarily excreted by the kidney and toxicity may develop rapidly.

HYPERKALEMIA

Hyperkalemia often accompanies acute renal failure and is managed in several ways. Sodium bicarbonate is used to treat renal tubular and metabolic acidosis, but is also an accepted therapy for treating hyperkalemia. Using bolus injections of 50 mL (44.6 mEq) of sodium bicarbonate in patients who are not volume overloaded is a rapid method of lowering serum potassium. Using an intravenous solution containing dextrose and regular insulin also ameliorates hyperkalemia. The drawback with both of these methods is that the potassium is merely driven intracellularly. It can reemerge at any time, causing the problem again. The most efficacious method of treating hyperkalemia is by using sodium polystyrene sulfonate (Kayexalate). Sodium polystyrene sulfonate is a cation-exchange resin that exchanges sodium for potassium in the lumen of the intestine or colon. It is administered orally or rectally. See Chapter 53 for more information.

▼ **CLINICAL ALERT**

Hypernatremia may be a complication of sodium polystyrene sulfonate use, particularly in patients with severe renal failure (renal function that is only 10% of normal; a creatinine clearance <10 mL/min).

GLOMERULONEPHRITIS

One of the etiologic factors of acute renal failure may be glomerulonephritis. This is often a rapidly progressing pathology involving degeneration of the subcellular fabric of the glomerulus. Glomerulonephritis may result from an autoimmune process or an infectious process. Drug treatment of glomerulonephritis may require large doses of glucocorticoids, such as methylprednisolone (Solu-Medrol) or prednisone. Immunosuppression therapy with cyclophosphamide (Cytoxan) or azathioprine (Imuran) is also used, pending the findings of renal biopsy. In addition, appropriate antibiotic therapy with drugs such as trimethoprim/sulfamethoxazole (Septra, Bactrim), ampicillin, or a fluoroquinolone such as ciprofloxacin (Cipro) or floxacin (Floxin) may be necessary.

CHRONIC RENAL FAILURE

Many of the clinical management problems mentioned in the context of acute renal failure become intensified in the setting of chronic renal failure (CRF). Prolonged injury and stress cause hypertrophy of previously healthy nephrons in an attempt to normalize the patient's fluid and electrolyte balance. In patients with diabetic nephropathy, multiple myeloma, amyloidosis, and malignant hypertension, the kidney remains hypertrophied. In patients with other pathologies, the kidneys shrink and become smaller. The previously discussed use of diuretics, sodium polystyrene sulfonate, and anti-infectives also play a role in the therapy of the patient with chronic renal failure.

HYPERTENSION

Hypertension may be the cause or result of chronic renal failure. Currently, angiotensin converting enzyme (ACE) inhibitors and calcium channel blockers are the preferred agents. There is postulated to be a calcium channel receptor in the kidney that may improve GFR in response to therapy with the calcium channel blockers. The calcium channel blockers include diltiazem, verapamil, isradipine, amlodipine, felodipine, nifedipine, and nicardipine. In those patients with decreased renal perfusion secondary to bilateral renal artery disease, the ACE inhibitors may decrease glomerular filtration rate, so careful assessment of BUN, creatinine, and proteinurea are made. Sodium restriction (2 g/day) may also play an important role in the management of hypertension associated with chronic renal failure.

CALCIUM AND PHOSPHATE METABOLISM

The autoregulation of serum calcium and phosphate is greatly affected during renal dysfunction. As serum phosphate rises due to decreased excretion, calcium phosphate crystals begin to precipitate in soft tissue. This causes a biphasic effect on calcium metabolism. Mobile calcium stores in the epiphysis of long bones are shifted to increase serum calcium at the same time there is increased excretion of renal phosphate. Normally, the kidney converts 25-hydroxyvitamin D into 1,25-hydroxyvitamin D, which increases gastrointestinal (GI) absorption, thereby increasing serum calcium. As renal failure progresses, 1,25-hydroxyvitamin D levels fall and serum phosphate levels continue to rise, both of which reduce serum Ca^{2+} and lead to a secondary hyperparathyroidism. Continued resorption of bone leads to *osteomalacia* (adult rickets; a condition caused by vitamin D deficiency and is characterized by soft brittle bones, bone deformities, bone pain, and weakness), *osteoporosis* (a condition of reduced bone mass sufficient to interfere with the support function of the bone), or *osteitis fibrosa* (a condition resulting from hyperparathyroidism and characterized by decalcification and softening of the bone, nephrolithiasis, increased serum calcium, and decreased serum phosphorus).

Early therapy is aimed at reducing the absorption of phosphate from the GI tract. Aluminum-containing antacids bind with phosphate, creating a nonabsorbable complex. Products containing aluminum hydroxide include Amphojel, Basaljel, AlternaGEL, and Alu-Caps. The usual dose is 30 to 60 mL or one to three capsules before meals. Once the phosphate has been lowered to acceptable levels (5 to 6 mg/dL), calcium carbonate (650-mg tablets) calcium acetate products (Phos-Ex, PhosLo) may be used in an attempt at normalizing the serum calcium. Excess aluminum hydroxide ingestion has lead to increased serum aluminum levels and a syndrome called "dialysis dementia." Central nervous system (CNS) depression and lethargy are typical symptoms. If these measures are unsuccessful, therapy with exogenous vitamin D may be useful. There are currently four vitamin D products available: vitamin D_2 (ergocalciferol); 25 (OH)-D_3 (calcifediol, Calderol); dihydrotachysterol (DHT, Hytakerol); and 1,25(OH)$_2$-D_3 (calcitriol, Rocaltrol). These products are discussed in greater detail in Chapter 13. Calcitrol and DHT are approved for the hyperparathyroidism of renal failure and are generally administered as one dose daily.

ANEMIA

Anemia, (generally normocytic and normochromic) is a common occurrence in acute and chronic renal failure. Erythrocyte survival time is shortened, and blood shunting and GI bleeding contribute to the decrease in hemoglobin. Transfusions are generally not indicated, owing to the possibility of volume overload. If required, the newly

developed superpacked products (e.g., packed red cells or platelet packs) are selected. Androgens, iron, folic acid, and B vitamins are also used to combat the anemia of renal failure. Epoetin alfa (EPO, Epogen, Procrit) may be administered to stimulate *erythropoiesis* (the formation of red blood cells).

○ **Epoetin alfa** *(EPO, Epogen, Procrit)* is an amino acid glycoprotein manufactured by recombinant DNA technology that contains the identical amino acid sequence and the same biologic effects as endogenous erythropoietin. Erythropoietin is a hormone that stimulates red blood cell production. In the kidney, where it is produced, it triggers the division and differentiation of committed erythroid precursors in the bone marrow. Erythropoietin production is normally regulated by the level of tissue oxygenation. Anemia and hypoxia usually increase erythropoietin production, which incites erythropoiesis. Erythropoietin plasma levels normally range from 0.01 to 0.03 units per milliliter, but increase 100 to 1000 times during the anemia of hypoxia.

USES In patients with end stage renal disease (ESRD) and CRF, epoetin alfa stimulates erythropoiesis. Epoetin alfa is also used to treat the anemia associated with zidovudine therapy (or other antiviral therapy) in HIV-infected patients and with cancer patients undergoing chemotherapy. Epoetin alfa is also being used to increase the procurement of autologous blood in patients about to undergo elective surgery. It increases the amount of autologous blood collected and decreases the need for homologous blood transfusions. It takes 2 to 6 weeks after initiation of therapy before a clinically significant increase in hematocrit is observed. Therefore, this agent is not intended for patients who require immediate correction of severe anemia and is not a substitute for emergency transfusions. Epoetin alfa is also given to elevate or maintain the red blood cell counts and decrease the need for transfusions. Patients who receive this medication should be normotensive, have a serum ferritin of 100 ng/mL or more, and a transferrin saturation of >20%.

Patients on epoetin alfa show an improvement in appetite, cold tolerance, sexual function, daily activities, sleep habits and decreased daytime napping, skin color, hair thickness, fingernail growth, fingernail hardness, and taste of food. Use of epoetin alfa improves the quality of life and provides a feeling of well-being to the patients.

CONTRAINDICATIONS AND PRECAUTIONS Epoetin alfa is contraindicated in patients with uncontrolled hypertension and known hypersensitivity to mammalian cell derived protein or albumin (human). Patients may not respond to therapy for a number of different reasons. The most common reasons include (1) iron deficiencies, (2) underlying infections or malignant/inflammatory processes, (3) other hematologic problems such as thalassemia or myelodysplastic disorders, (4) occult blood loss, (5) folic acid or B_{12} deficiencies, (6) hemolysis, or (7) aluminum intoxication from antacid therapy. Patients currently using hemodialysis may require increased anticoagulation with heparin to prevent clotting of their vascular access or the artificial kidney.

Safety in pregnancy (category C) has not been established. Use in pregnancy only if the potential benefit justifies the potential risk to the fetus. Exercise caution during lactation. Safety and efficacy have not been established in children.

ADVERSE EFFECTS Most common adverse effects include hypertension due to the increase in hematocrit, headache, arthralgia, nausea, edema, fatigue, diarrhea, vomiting, and chest pain. Most patients with CRF experience these symptoms, but because they are so fatigued often do not notice them. As the hematocrit and thus activity level improves, these symptoms may become more pronouned. Regular blood pressure monitoring is important. Hypertension is a common problem in patients with CRF, and it can be aggravated following erythropoietin administration. Antihypertensive and/or dietary restrictions may be necessary.

▼ CLINICAL ALERT

The adverse effects in patients with HIV or in those on cancer chemotherapy are consistent with progression of HIV or cancer. Thus, it may be difficult to distinguish among the adverse effects of the drugs and the underlying pathology.

DOSAGE Doses vary among patients, from 50 to 100 U/kg IV three times weekly. (See Table 38–1 for dosing information.) The desired hematocrit is 30% to 33%. As the hematocrit approaches or exceeds 36%, the dose of epoetin alfa is reduced or withheld. Except in those patients with transfusional iron overload, it is recommended that prophylactic supplementation with ferrous sulfate (325 mg three times a day) or regular iron dextran injections be provided to maximize the effect of the drug.

Table 38–2 reviews monitoring guidelines during epoetin alfa therapy. Hematocrits are monitored twice weekly during the initial dosing phase and during any period of dosage adjustment.

ACID-BASE BALANCE

The homeostatic mechanisms regulate acid-base balance. The metabolic component is well balanced with respiratory mechanisms. The major factor in the metabolic control of pH is renal function. Acid-base abnormalities—metabolic alkalosis, metabolic acidosis, respiratory alkalosis, and respiratory acidosis—are treated appropriately. See a medical-surgical text for further discussion.

MISCELLANEOUS PROBLEMS

Gastrointestinal bleeding may be a problem in the patient with uremia (toxic condition in which nitrogenous substances such as urea are retained in the blood instead of being eliminated). Gastritis due to an altered mucosal lining is not uncommon, and bleeding may also reflect altered platelet function. Acute therapy with an H_2 antagonist (e.g., cimetidine [Tagamet] or famotidine [Pepsid]) or sucralfate (Carafate) is suggested if these symptoms

occur. H_2 antagonists require dosage adjustments in renal failure; caution is advised.

Hyperuricemia (abnormal amount of uric acid in the urine) is a common sequela of acute renal failure. Uric acid is a breakdown product of protein metabolism via the enzyme xanthine oxidase. Hyperuricemia often accompanies the administration of cytotoxic therapy owing to rapid cell lysis. Intraluminary sludging is often a common cause of acute renal failure. Therapy includes alkalinization of the urine with sodium bicarbonate or acetazolamide (Diamox). Allopurinol (Zyloprim), a xanthine oxidase inhibitor, may be necessary to decrease the production of uric acid. Initial dosage is 600 mg/day for several days, followed by maintenance doses of 300 mg/day.

▼ CLINICAL ALERT

Nonsteroidal anti-inflammatory drugs (NSAIDs) such as ibuprofen (Motrin, Advil), naproxen (Naprosyn, Ansaid), sulindac (Clinoril), and diclofenac (Voltaren) are avoided in patients with severe renal failure. These agents can cause abrupt and sustained reductions in renal plasma flow and GFR and inhibit vasodilatory prostaglandin release and thus reduce renal hemodynamics. If NSAIDs are used in this patient population, caution is advised and the nurse assesses for abdominal pain, blood in stool, and nausea.

DIALYSIS

Dialysis is the process by which small molecules are passed through a semipermeable membrane, leaving the large molecules behind. The two distinct methods of dialysis are hemodialysis and peritoneal dialysis. In hemodialysis, arterial blood is passed across an artificial membrane and the uremic toxins and excess electrolytes are collected in the dialysate as the blood is recirculated to a vein, as depicted in Figure 38–1. In peritoneal dialysis, the dialysate is infused directly into the peritoneal cavity, and the abdominal viscera acts as the semipermeable membrane (Fig. 38–2). There are several techniques used for peritoneal dialysis. *Manual peritoneal dialysis* refers to the use of a Y tubing attached to the patient's peritoneal catheter. One end of the tubing enters the dialysis solution, and the other ends in a collection device. The fluid is infused and is allowed to dwell in the abdomen for generally 30 minutes, then it is drained. With *chronic ambulatory peritoneal dialysis (CAPD)*, the patient performs the exchanges himself or herself at home, three to four times a day. Generally, three of the exchanges use a 1.5% glucose solution; for the last one, a 4.25% glucose solution is selected. These exchanges are performed each and every day, 7 days a week, usually before breakfast, lunch, dinner, and bedtime. The exchanges may include small amounts of heparin (500 IU per liter) to prevent clotting of the catheter. In *continuous cycling peritoneal dialysis (CCPD)*, the patient is connected to an automated machine and is given three exchanges (dwell time, 3 hours) at night. When the patient wakes in

Table 38–1. HEMOPOIETIC AGENTS

DRUG NAME/ROUTE AND DOSAGE	PHARMACOKINETICS/ DYNAMICS	NURSING IMPLICATIONS
erythropoietin (Epogen) (Procrit)		

chronic renal failure Target hematocrit (Hct) = 30%–33%. ***Starting Dose:*** 50–100 U/kg SC or IV 3 times/wk. When Hct increases >4 points per 2 wk or reaches 30%–33%, reduce initial dose by about 25 U/kg 3 times/wk. ***Maintenance Dose:*** Individualize to maintain Hct within target range. Increase or decrease dose by 25 U/kg 3 times/wk as necessary (dose increases should not be more frequent than once/mo unless clinically indicated). ***Hct Approaching or Exceeding 36%:*** Withhold epoetin until Hct decreases to target range of 30%–33%. Reduce dose by about 25 U/kg 3 times/wk on reinitiation of therapy. ***Delayed or Diminished Response:*** Increase dose by 25 U/kg 3 times/wk in presence of adequate iron (further increase of 25 U/kg 3 times/wk may be made at 4 to 6-wk intervals until desired response is attained.) ***Rapid Response (>4-point increase in 2-wk period):*** Immediately decrease dose by 25 μ/kg 3 times/wk. **cancer patients on chemotherapy** ***Initial dose:*** 150 U/kg SC 3 times/wk. Monitor Hct weekly. If Hct does not improve after 8 wk, increase dose to 300 U/kg SC 3 times/wk. If patients do not respond, it is unlikely they will respond to higher doses. If Hct exceeds 40% withhold dose until it falls to 36%, then maintain dose to maintain Hct. **hiv-infected patients taking zidovudine (azt)** If serum EPO levels are >500 mU/mL, consider other therapy. ***Initial Dose:*** If patients are receiving dose of <4200 mg AZT/wk, and serum EPO levels are <500 mU/mL, administer EPO 100 U/kg IV or SC 3 times/wk for 8 wk. If response is not satisfactory, increase dose 50–100 U/kg 3 times/wk and evaluate results in 4–8 wk. Maximum suggested doses are 300 U/kg 3 times/wk. ***Maintenance Dose:*** After effective dose has been achieved, titrate dose to accommodate changes in AZT doses. Maintain Hct between 36% and 40% by dose adjustments or discontinuations.	**Onset:** 1 wk **Peak:** 5–24 hr (SC) **Duration:** NA **½L:** 4–13 hr **PB:** NA **B:** NA **E:** NA	**ASSESSMENT:** Assess blood pressure and Hct frequently, weekly at first, then every 2–6 wk when Hct has stabilized. Antihypertensive therapy may have to be increased during therapy. **INTERVENTION:** Administer IV or SC after dialysis 3 times/wk. Use in AIDS anemia may be more frequent. Do not shake bottle. Keep vial refrigerated at all times. Discard all partially used vials. Use only 1 dose per vial and do not reenter vial. Discard unused portion. If diminished response occurs, check iron stores and consider other underlying causes. **Patient Teaching**—Patients may be taught to administer their own injections at home. Patients on peritoneal dialysis are taught to administer SC, while patients on hemodialysis may use either SC or IV route. **EVALUATION:** Evaluate for increased blood pressure; report to physician.

NA = not available.

Table 38–2. SUGGESTED MONITORING AND LABORATORY TESTING DURING EPOETIN THERAPY			
Laboratory Test	During Initial Phase	During Maintenance Phase	Following Dose Adjustment
Hematocrit	2 times/wk	2–4 times/mo	2 times/wk for 2–6 mo
CBC with differential	Regularly	Per routine*	Per routine*
Platelet count	Regularly	Per routine*	Per routine*
Blood pressure	3 times/wk	3 times/wk	Per routine*
BUN	Regularly	Per routine*	Per routine*
Creatinine	Regularly	Per routine*	Per routine*
Potassium	Regularly	Per routine*	Per routine*
Iron stores	Prior to therapy and monthly	Per routine*	Per routine*

*Follow local routines for monitoring or as indicated.

the morning, the last exchange (4.25% glucose) is made. It is left in the peritoneal cavity throughout the day, freeing the patient so that normal daily activities can be performed.

While both peritoneal dialysis and hemodialysis use exchange fluids, the major difference between the two is the glucose content of the peritoneal solutions. In hemodialysis, an ultrafiltration system produces a positive pressure within the blood path or another system produces a low-pressure gradient around the blood path in the dialysis fluid (negative pressure). Peritoneal solutions need a minimum concentration of about 1.5% glucose to cause the small molecular particles (urea, potassium) to move from within the peritoneal circulation across a membrane into the dialysate. The larger the glucose content, the greater the osmotic gradient, and the more waste products can be removed.

As shown in Table 38–3, the dialysis solutions available in the United States contain glucose concentrations of 1.5%, 2.5%, and 4.25%. The pH of the solutions is about 5.5 to prevent caramelization of the sugar during the sterilization processes. The normal blood pH is 7.4, so the difference in acidity may cause some discomfort as the dialysate is first infused. The solutions contain no potassium; however, this may be added extemporaneously to offset hypokalemia. The sodium content is generally less than 140 mEq/liter, which apparently prevents a potential hypernatremia by pulling off some free sodium with water. Calcium content is generally about 3.5 mEq/liter to promote positive calcium balance. Magnesium content varies between 0.5 and 1.5 mEq/liter. Dialysis solutions with 0.5 mEq of magnesium per liter may be used to treat patients with hypermagnesemia or patients who cannot tolerate the aluminum hydroxide suspensions. With this low magnesium concentration in the dialysate, conventional magnesium/aluminum hydroxide anatacids can be administered without fear of magnesium toxicity. Finally, the solutions are generally buffered with lactate, which is converted in the liver to bicarbonate.

Most patients tolerate dialysis well. Occasionally patients with abdominal adhesions or fistulas do not tolerate peritoneal dialysis and must be hemodialyzed. Peritonitis is a common sequela to CAPD or CCPD and is generally treated by the inclusion of a cephalosporin or aminoglycoside into the dialysate. The factors involved in deciding which patient is qualified for which dialysis technique are complicated and beyond the scope of this review.

Patients undergoing hemodialysis have an altered im-

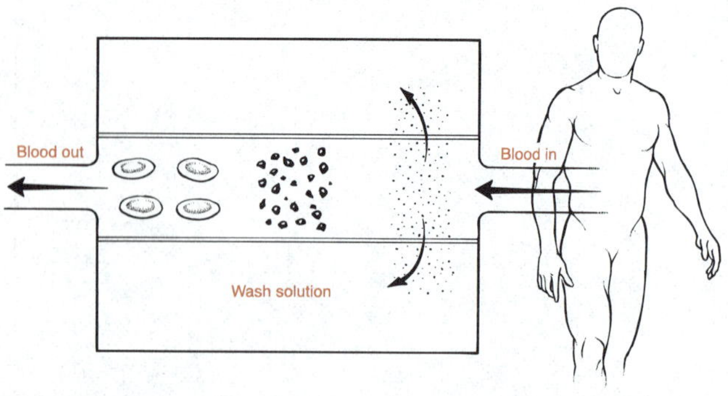

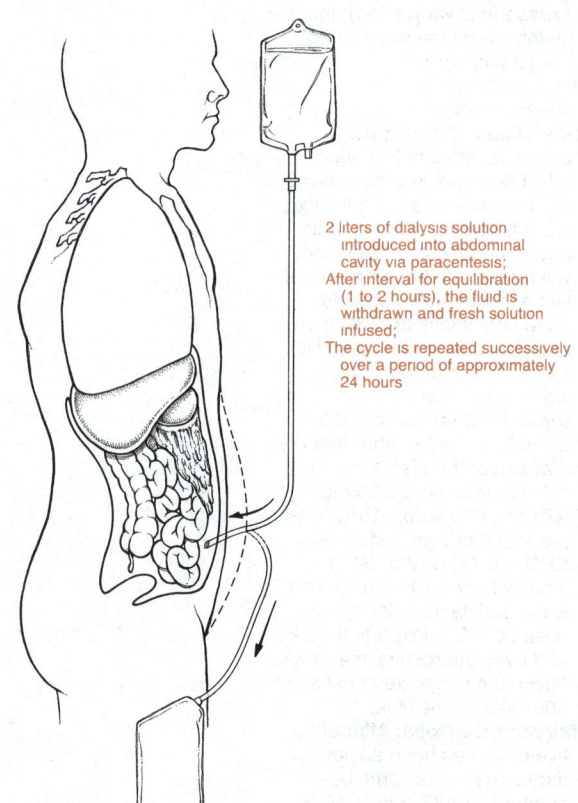

2 liters of dialysis solution introduced into abdominal cavity via paracentesis; After interval for equilibration (1 to 2 hours), the fluid is withdrawn and fresh solution infused; The cycle is repeated successively over a period of approximately 24 hours

Figure 38–2. Peritoneal dialysis. A diagram of a typical peritoneal dialysis setup for CAPD or CCPD.

Blood out

Blood in

Wash solution

Figure 38–1. Hemodialysis. A schematic diagram of the inner workings and mechanisms of some hemodialysis machines.

Table 38–3. CONTENTS OF REPRESENTATIVE DIALYSIS SOLUTIONS

Solution	Glucose (g/L)	Na (mEq/L)	Ca (mEq/L)	Mg (mEq/L)	Cl (mEq/L)	Lactate	Osmolarity (mOsm/L)
Dianeal with 1.5% dextrose	15	141	3.5	1.5	101	45	364
Impersol LM with 1.5% dextrose	15	132	3.5	0.5	96	40	346
Impersol with 2.5% dextrose	25	132	3.5	0.5	96	40	396
Dianeal with 4.25% dextrose	42.5	141	3.5	1.5	101	45	503

mune system and are at risk for hepatitis B infection. Two recombinant hepatitis vaccines are available. (Refer to Chapter 59 for more information.)

In addition to the treatment of acute or chronic renal failure, dialysis is often used to treat drug intoxication. Depending on their metabolism, structure, and pharmacokinetics, many drugs are suitable for dialysis in the face of an acute overdose. Agents such as phenobarbital, chloral hydrate, salicylates, methanol, and others respond to various methods of dialysis. The individual literature is consulted in each and every case of poisoning.

DRUG DOSING IN RENAL FAILURE

The kidney and liver are the two routes of elimination for most drugs. During renal failure, many of the drugs elim-inated by the kidney require a decrease in dose or an increase in dosing interval to prevent drug toxicity. As a patient's creatinine clearance (CrCl) falls below 50 mL per minute, it is necessary to know which drugs may require such dosage modification and to what extent. For example, a drug like digoxin has a narrow therapeutic index, and a patient with renal failure may quickly develop digitalis toxicity. In Table 38–4 alterations in dosing interval are given for some of the drugs, and decreases in the actual dose administered are listed for others. Thus, a 60-kg patient with an estimated CrCl of less than 10 mL per minute who might normally receive 80 mg of gentamicin every 8 hours for infection might receive 80 mg of gentamicin every 24 hours.

Many of these dosage alterations can be confirmed by serum drug samples. The use of steady-state or peak/trough levels is an important tool for the prescriber to use in monitoring the drug therapy of a renal failure patient.

Table 38–4. DOSAGE ADJUSTMENT GUIDES FOR SELECTED PHARMACEUTICALS IN RENAL FAILURE

Drug	Method of Dose Adjustment	Dose Adjustment in Renal Failure by CrCl >50 mL/min	10–50 mL/min	<10 mL/min	Dialysis	Toxicity
Aminoglycosides						
Amikacin	Dose	↓ 60%–90%	↓ 30%–70%	↓ 20%–30%	H, P	All are ototoxic
Gentamicin	Interval	q 12 hr	q 12–18 hr	q 24 hr		and nephrotoxic
Tobramycin						
Ace Inhibitors						
Captopril	Dose	Unchanged	Unchanged	↓ 50% for CrCl	H	
Enalapril				<30 mL		
Lisinopril						
Fosinopril	Dose and interval	Unchanged	Unchanged	Unchanged	H	
Benazepril	Dose	Unchanged	5 mg q 24 h	5 mg q 24 h	H	
Ramipril	Dose	Unchanged	1.25 mg q 24 hr	1.25 mg q 24 hr	H	
Cardiac Agents and Cardiac Glycosides						
Amrinone	Dose and interval	Unchanged	Unchanged	Unchanged	?	
Digoxin	Dose	Unchanged	↓ 25%–75%	↓ 10%–25%	No	↑ Level with
	Interval	q 24 hr	q 36 hr	q 48 hr		quinidine
Dopamine	Dose and interval	Unchanged	Unchanged	Unchanged	?	
Dobutamine	Dose and interval	Unchanged	Unchanged	Unchanged	?	
Nitrates	Dose and interval	Unchanged	Unchanged	Unchanged	?	
H₂ Antagonists						
Cimetidine	Dose	Unchanged	↓ 75%	↓ 50%	No	
Ranitidine	Dose	Unchanged	↓ 75%	↓ 50%	H	
Famotidine	Interval	Unchanged	Unchanged	q 36–48 hr	?	
Nizatidine	Interval	Unchanged	q 48 hr	q 72 hr	?	

Dose: Dose is adjusted in renal failure with adjustment given as percentage; e.g., ↓ 50% = new adjusted dose is 50% (0.5) times normal dose.
Interval: Dosing interval is adjusted in renal failure with adjustment given as interval in hours; e.g., q 8 hr = every 8 hours.
H = removed by hemodialysis; P = removed by peritoneal dialysis.

USING THE NURSING PROCESS

Table 38–5 suggests assessment data that must be collected and shows how to apply other steps of the nursing process for the patient with renal disease.

ASSESSMENT

- Assess for signs of deteriorating renal function. These can vary from easily identifiable markers, such as hematuria, to vague symptoms. If any of the signs are present, take a careful history to substantiate the objective information.

Changes in urination may proceed or be coincident with renal dysfunction. Normally 1200 to 1500 mL of urine is produced every day and voided in 4 to 6 intervals throughout the day. The normal process of micturition is painless and effortless.

Classically, oliguria is described with kidney disorders. Some patients, however, may exhibit an increase in urinary frequency or urgency or even polyuria. Manifestations of abnormal pathology—urinary hesitancy, dysuria, burning on urination, or incontinence—may be exhibited. Chemically detectable abnormalities such as proteinuria and hematuria may also be found. Hematuria may indicate acute glomerulonephritis, renal tuberculosis, or cancer of the genitourinary tract. (Nonrenal causes of hematuria are ruled out.) Blood may be visible to the eye or detected microscopically.

Genitourinary pain does not always develop in renal disease. It may be a dull ache in the costovertebral angle, back pain, or lower abdominal soreness. Flank (the side between the ribs and ileum) pain which radiates is often called renal colic. A stinging sensation at the urethral meatus can occur in urethritis. Prostatic inflammations can cause severe pain in the scrotal region.

Gastrointestinal complaints may accompany other symptoms of urinary dysfunction. The kidneys are in close proximity to other intestinal organs. Symptoms of nausea, vomiting, diarrhea, and paralytic ileus may occur, but are not mutually exclusive of renal disease.

- Obtain a current and past history. The following are important points to consider during the dialogue with the patient: chief complaint, what motivated the patient to seek help; past history of other renal problems, urinary tract infections (UTIs) in the patient or other family members; and occupational or environmental hazards (chemicals, and so on). Also obtain the following information. Does the patient have any predisposing factors (i.e., diabetes, hypertension, smoking history, previous hospitalization for UTI or previous antibiotic therapy)? Does the patient exhibit any classic urinary tract symptoms? If so, when did they start and how often do they occur? Symptoms can include the following: nocturia, dysuria, hesitancy, straining, changes in urine color, incontinence, stress incontinence, urgency incontinence, hematuria, fever chills, passage of stones. If pain is present, where is it located, is it sharp or dull, how long does it last, what brings it on, what relieves it, and is it related to voiding?

- Perform a general physical exam to assess the size and mobility of the kidneys. Placing one hand below the level of the ribs and the other hand anterior to the kidney, ask the patient to inhale deeply and push the anterior hand forward. The size and location of the kidney may be felt between both hands. More importantly is the diagnosis of pain or tenderness on palpation. Pressing on the costovertebral angle, determine the location and level of pain or discomfort. See Table 38–5.

Nervous disorders such as coarse muscular twitches, tics, and cramps may be present. The patient may suffer from tactile abnormalities, peripheral neuropathies, and other various motor disorders as a result of poor kidney function. If present, seizures are dealt with appropriately (see Chapter 20 for treatment of seizure disorders).

- Assess the patient's general appearance. Malnutrition leading to tissue wasting is often common in uremia. The sclerae and the skin may be discolored, often to a yellow-brown. *Uremic frost* is characterized by the presence of topical yellow-white crystals which come from the excess urea contained in sweat. Patients with uremic frost may very often complain of mild to severe pruritis.

- Auscultate the chest for fluid changes in the lungs because many of these patients have underlying cardiac or pulmonary problems. Crackles or rhonchi are appropriately noted in addition to any suggestion of dyspnea or orthopnea. Screening for abnormal heart sounds or a pericardial friction rub is also performed.

- Obtain a clear, concise dietary history to discover early GI manifestations of renal failure. Symptoms of stomatitis, unpleasant tastes, halitosis, anorexia, nausea, and vomiting are documented. More severe symptoms may include coffee-ground emesis or heme-positive stools as signs of active GI bleeding. Proper dietary counseling as to nitrogen and sodium intake is essential to chronic maintenance of these patients.

- Assess daily weights to determine if the patient is retaining fluids. Often, edema is insidious and weight gain may be the first symptom (the usual rule is 1 kg of weight gain equals one liter of fluid). Monitoring fluid intake and output is often an underrated tool for assessment. Any patient who shows discrepancies between intake and output is assessed further to determine if renal function has been compromised. This is especially important if, for some reason, blood flow to the kidneys may have been affected (e.g., by hemorrhage or dehydration).

- Record both supine and standing blood pressures routinely in these patients. Extra fluid can cause an increase in blood pressure when the patient assumes a supine position. Also, if the patient is receiving antihypertensive drugs, he or she may be susceptible to orthostasis.

- Assist with diagnostic testing. These include tests such as calculated creatinine clearance (based on a serum creatinine level) and blood urea nitrogen (BUN) to assess renal function. Radiographic examinations are used to determine the size, shape, and position of the kidneys and to disclose any deviations

Table 38–5. NURSING PROCESS FOR PATIENT WITH RENAL DISEASE

Assessment

Assess history of past and present illness.
Assess heart rate, blood pressure and central venous pressure (CVP) (if available).
Assess fluid intake/output, current weight, and pattern of weight gain/loss.
Ascertain dietary intake, especially in relation to sodium.
Assess general appearance, presence of nervous disorders.
Assess effectiveness of individual/family coping mechanisms.
Identify behaviors indicative of failure to follow treatment program.

Nursing Diagnosis: Fluid Volume Excess

RELATED TO: Compromised regulatory mechanism (renal failure) with retention of water.

AS EVIDENCED BY: Intake greater than output, oliguria, changes in urine specific gravity, generalized tissue edema, weight gain.

Desired Outcomes/Evaluation Criteria

Displays appropriate urinary output with special gravity/laboratory studies near normal, stable weight, and absence of edema.

Nursing Actions	Rationale
Monitor heart rate, blood pressure (supine and standing), and CVP.	Tachycardia and hypertension can occur because of failure of the kidneys to excrete urine, excessive fluid resuscitation, and/or changes in the reninantiotensin system. Orthostatic hypotension and tachycardia can occur if hypovolemia develops in response to excessive diuretic-induced fluid losses.
Record accurate intake and output. Calculate 24-hour balance.	Necessary for determining renal function and fluid replacement needs and reducing risk of fluid overload.
Monitor urine specific gravity.	Measures kidney's ability to concentrate urine.
Weigh daily on the same scale.	Daily weight is best monitor of fluid status, although muscle wasting may affect accuracy.
Note presence/degree of edema.	Useful in noting progression/resolution of fluid imbalance and effectiveness of therapy.
Observe for dry mucous membranes, thirst, dulled sensorium, peripheral vasoconstriction.	Indicators of fluid and electrolyte imbalances, e.g., dehydration or sodium depletion.
Explain dietary modifications, i.e., sodium, potassium, protein, fluid.	Restrictions are based on severity of condition to prevent worsening or failure/dangerous accumulation of waste products.
Plan oral fluid replacement, spacing desired beverages and varying choices.	Helps avoid periods without fluids, minimizing boredom with limited choices and reducing sense of deprivation and thirst.
Provide hard candy or saliva substitute as appropriate.	Use in relieving discomfort associated with dryness of mouth and may help limit desire for additional fluids.
Administer diuretics (furosemide, mannitol); antihypertensives (clinidine, methyldopa).	Given to flush the tubular lumen, reduce hyperkalemia, and promote adequate urine volume. May be given to treat hypertension by counteracting effects of decreased renal blood flow and/or circulating volume overload.
Monitor laboratory studies, e.g., BUN, creatinine, urine sodium and creatinine, serum sodium/potassium, hemoglobin/hematocrit (HGB/Hct), chest x-ray films.	Assess progression and management of renal dysfunction/failure and need for additional therapies.

Nursing Diagnosis: Knowledge Deficit

RELATED TO: Cognitive limitation, lack of exposure/recall, information misinterpretation.

AS EVIDENCED BY: Questions/request for information, statement of concern, inaccurate follow-through of instructions/development of preventable complications.

Desired Outcomes/Evaluation Criteria

Verbalizes understanding of condition/disease process and treatment. Correctly performs necessary procedures and explains reasons for the actions.

Nursing Actions	Rationale
Review disease process/prognosis and future expectations.	Provides knowledge base on which patient can make informed choices. Prevents serious complications, e.g., reduces risk of bone demineralization/fractures and tetany, osteodystrophy, hypermagnesemia.
Discuss drug therapy, including use of calcium supplements, phosphate binders (with meals), and avoidance of magnesium antiacids.	Allows patient to schedule medication and still maintain usual activities, adequate sleep.
Identify peak action time of diuretics.	
Review dietary restrictions, including sodium, phosphorus, (e.g., milk products, poultry, peanuts) and magnesium (e.g., whole grain products, legumes).	Sodium potentiates fluid retention, increasing edema, hypertension, and risk of cardiac complications. Retention of phosphorus stimulates the parathyroid glands to shift calcium from bones, and accumulation of magnesium can impair neuromuscular function and mentation.
Instruct in home monitoring of BP, including scheduling rest period before taking pressure, using same arm/position.	Incidence of hypertension is increased in CRF, often requiring management with antihypertensive drugs, necessitating close observation of treatment effects.

Other Suggested Nursing Diagnoses: Noncompliance, Fear, and Pain in the kidney or urinary tract. Before the patient receives any x-ray, a cathartic may need to be administered. This eliminates the fecal material and gas from the colon so that there are no obstacles to visualizing the kidneys.

- Monitor laboratory values. Although a 24-hour creatinine clearance is one of the best indicators of renal function, collection may not always be possible or feasible. Assessment of the creatinine clearance may be made by nomogram or by equation. The BUN level is another measure of renal function, increasing as the kidneys are unable to secrete nitrogenous byproducts. However, this number is often vague in its clinical significance, and creatinine clearances remain the most valuable indicator of renal status. A CrCl of 30 mL/min may be broadly classified as moderate renal failure, whereas a CrCl of 10 mL/min or less is termed severe renal failure. Accurate estimation or determination of creatinine clearance is essential for establishing dosages for various drugs in the patient with renal failure.

  A routine urinalysis is invaluable. Gross appraisal of color, clarity, and odor is documented. Using commercially available lab dipsticks, determine the presence of proteinuria, red blood cells, glucosuria, and ketonuria. A measurement of urine acidity and specific gravity may be helpful. In addition, sodium/potassium excretion values often provide valuable information.

  Urine samples to be sent for microbiologic testing are obtained from the patient by the clean-catch midstream technique. Consult the appropriate texts for this technique. A 24-hour urine collection may be required for more quantitative analyses. The patient voids early in the morning before beginning the collection. Contents of all voidings for the next 24 hours are collected and transferred to a light-resistant container usually stored in the refrigerator.

  Serum electrolytes, bicarbonate, and hemoglobin values are also obtained.

NURSING DIAGNOSIS

- Typical nursing diagnoses for a patient with renal disease include Knowledge Deficit, Pain (acute or chronic), Fear, Fluid Volume Excess, Impaired Adjustment, and Noncompliance (see Table 38–5).

PLANNING AND INTERVENTION

- Ensure that both the patient and family can demonstrate their understanding of the implications of renal disease. If the renal condition is a chronic one, both must understand that this means a modification in lifestyle.
- Educate the patient about his or her disease process. Many barriers to patient education exist, including preformed ideas of disease processes, educational level and capacity of the patient, reading ability, language barriers, motivation, and previous compliance. Psychologic depression with the underlying realiza-

tion that the problem will not disappear after a routine course of drug therapy needs to be addressed with patients. In this setting, education is not a matter of one 30- to 60-minute intervention session, but may need repeat encounters. The professional nurse plans educational goals for each patient; assesses the patient's knowledge; establishes a teaching plan using formalized sessions; periodically evaluates the patient's response and reevaluates the teaching plan; and finally, provides ongoing patient support and follow-up. See the *Delivering Home Health Care* box.

Diet

- Understand the dietary and fluid restrictions of the patient. Early in therapy, sodium and fluids may require moderate restriction. As the patient gradually loses more renal function, diet is severely modified in relation to sodium, potassium, protein, and fluid intake.

  Salt restrictions often pose the biggest problem because the average American diet is too high in salt. Salting food before it is even tasted is a common habit. By removing the salt shaker from the table and using herbs or spices for flavoring, salt intake can be drastically reduced. Common salt substitutes, while advisable, are used in small quantities as they are high in potassium content.

  An accurate way for the patient to measure fluid restrictions is as follows: If the patient is restricted to 1 liter of fluid, he or she should use a quart container as a measuring device, and every time the patient consumes any fluid, the same amount of water must be placed in the container. When the container is full, the patient has used up the allotted fluid intake allowance. The nurse must be sure that the patient understands that all fluids must be considered when measuring intake, including soups, ice cubes, and the liquid used to take medications. Using hard candy or a saliva substitute instead of drinking fluids can help to relieve mouth dryness.

Medications

- Educate the patient regarding his or her medications. The patient who is receiving aluminum hydroxide gel should remember to take it along with meals. The phosphate-binding effect is best when it is taken with food. The liquid preparations are superior because they have a larger surface area. If the tablets are used, they are chewed well before swallowing. Aluminum-containing antacids are constipating, and a stool softener or additional bulk-type laxative may be necessary to relieve this uncomfortable side effect. The antacid may be left at the bedside to be taken as "dessert."

  Patients taking diuretics at home are instructed not to take them in the evening. The peak action of the drug should not be during the night if the patient is to have a restful sleep. If these are taken for hyper-

DELIVERING HOME HEALTH CARE

Administration of Home Dialysis

Patients with chronic renal failure can be maintained for many years on peritoneal dialysis at home. But to prevent complications that would necessitate readmission to the hospital, patients and their caregivers need to be taught about the procedure and equipment and how to solve problems when various situations arise.

The best place to teach the procedure is in the patient's home with his or her own equipment. In many cases, a nurse educated about dialysis goes with a home health nurse to the patient's home.

Before starting dialysis, do the following:
- Ask the patient and significant others what they know about dialysis. (The teaching plan is based on their level of knowledge.)
- Gather baseline data about vital signs, blood studies, and any complications that were experienced during dialysis while in the hospital.
- Explain all the equipment.
- Explain how to mix the dialysate solutions and how they are to be obtained. (Patients may need assistance from other professionals to determine who will pay for the equipment and supplies.)
- Assist the family in creating an area of a room that is set aside for the dialysis procedure and all the needed equipment.
- Obtain and record the patient's weight, temperature, blood pressure, pulse, respiratory rate, and abdominal girth.
- Assess the patient's abdomen for bowel distension; urinary bladder distention, empty bladder; and abdominal skin integrity for signs of local infection.

To perform dialysis, do the following:
- Determine the number of dialysis bags to be used.
- Set up equipment and walk through procedure with family.
- Know the dwell times.
- Prepare peritoneal catheter-inserting site.

During dialysis, do the following:
- Monitor all equipment. Teach the patient and family common problems and how to solve them.

- Monitor patient response. Teach patient what he or she would expect to experience, common deviations from the norm, and how to correct them.
- Prime the patient's abdomen with fluid.

   ◦ Check priming solutions for sterility; warm to body temperature.
   ◦ Prime the inflow tubing with dialysate.
   ◦ Assess patient carefully for respiratory distress and abdominal discomfort.
   ◦ Accurately measure amount of fluid instilled.

- Place the patient in a 45° position.
- Apply dressing.
- Check composition of dialysate on label with physician order, giving particular attention to the concentration of potassium and glucose.
- Check dialysis machine and temperature of dialysate, which should approximate body temperature.
- Monitor outflow phase. Ensure that (1) all clamps from the patient to the outflow bottle are released, (2) dialysis tubing is free of kinks, and (3) the inflow clamping mechanism is activated. Observe the ease and speed of outflow drainage.

After dialysis, do the following:
- Remove the needles from the catheter. Show the patient how to dress insertion sites. Discuss what to do if bleeding occurs and/or does not stop.
- Teach the patient how to properly dispose of the needles in a safety container.
- Document the procedure using established guidelines.
- Calculate inflow and outflow volumes at the end of each outflow cycle. Add amount of inflow fluid remaining and amount of fluid in outflow bottle to obtain total fluid volume, then subtract initial dialysate volume from sum of inflow and outflow volumes.
- Determine and record on log sheet the duration for each phase.
- Ask the patient questions about different steps in the procedure to assess understanding.

tension alone or with other medications, their effect is greatest in the morning, at the ebb of the diurnal cycle. Even if the diuretic is a potassium-losing (kaluretic) diuretic, the patient's dietary intake of potassium may have to be limited because of renal failure. For example, orange juice, bananas, dried fruits, and other rich sources of K$^+$ are avoided. Potassium-sparing diuretics are usually not indicated for the patient with renal failure. Electrocardiogram (ECG) changes are prevalent with both hyperkalemia and hypokalemia.

If the patient is on daily antihypertensive therapy, it might be helpful to devise a chart to record blood pressure and medication. By helping the patient to establish a routine, there is less chance of forgetting

a dose. Also, by having the time for each dose written down, the patient has a tangible way to check the administration. Similar results can be achieved or augmented by use of specially divided pill boxes available from most pharmacies. These contain either daily time divisions or day-by-day separators. High-tech alarm pill boxes are also available.

Both the family and the patient are given instruction on how to take a blood pressure. Automatic blood pressure reading and recording devices are now available at nominal cost to the patient. Patients should practice under the supervision of the nurse until they feel competent. Patients should use the same device from one reading to another to establish consistency.

Care during Hemodialysis

- Monitor the patient's diet during dialysis. This is extremely important. Protein usually is restricted to minimize uremia. Supplemental vitamins, as ordered, are encouraged. Patients who are taking medications such as digoxin should have routine serum levels to prevent toxicity.
- Support the patient during hemodialysis. Common problems that are dealt with may include difficulty in holding a job, financial problems, impotence, and depression. Support the patient and the family by letting them know that feelings of anger and despair are normal.

Care during Peritoneal Dialysis

- Verify the required doctor's orders and the signing of patient consents. The peritoneal solutions to be used are double-checked against the order to verify accuracy. Many of the solutions have similar names but dissimilar contents.
- Ensure that the patient is made as comfortable as possible after catheter insertion. The patient and family are informed of the progress of the dialysis treatment. Aseptic technique is used when adding or emptying exchange containers. Blood pressure and pulse are monitored every 15 minutes during the first exchange and every hour thereafter. The patient's temperature is taken at regular intervals (generally every 4 hours), particularly after catheter removal.
- Keep exact records of the patient's fluid balance during treatment. Detailed records of the exchanges and the patient's vital signs are maintained. Particular attention is paid to changes in weight.
- Monitor the patient for possible complications of dialysis, including peritonitis, bleeding, respiratory difficulties, abdominal pain, leakage around the catheter site, constipation, and low serum albumin.
- Assist in the appropriate training courses if CAPD is administered. Patient training includes basic pathophysiology of the kidney, measurement of vital signs, catheter care, and universal precautions.
- Provide or coordinate dietary instructions.

EVALUATION

- Evaluate the urine. The nurse and patient are observant of any changes in urine characteristics or quantity. Any changes that are related to specific medications are explained at the time the patient is given the medication. Table 38–6 provides a listing of drugs that may color the urine. Any blood or unusual odor to the urine is also reported. Explaining to the patient that accurate reporting is tantamount to a good treatment plan.
- Evaluate for signs of fluid retention. If the patient is on diuretic therapy, edema should decrease. If renal disease is worsening, edema increases. Does the patient notice tight rings, tight shoes, swollen ankles, or difficulty breathing? The patient should also know

Table 38–6. DRUGS THAT COLOR URINE

Drug	Color
Amitriptyline	Blue-green
Cascara	Brown (acid urine)
	Pink (alkaline urine)
Chlorzoxazone	Red-purple, orange
Indomethacin	Green
Levodopa	Red-tinged
Methocarbamol	Brown, black
Methyldopa	Red, brown-black
Nitrofurantoin	Brown or rust yellow
Phenazopyridine	Orange, red
Phenolphthalein	Orange, rust (acid urine)
	Pink, red, purple (alkaline urine)
Phenothiazines	Pink, purple, orange, rust
Phenytoin	Pink, red, red-brown
Primaquine	Rust yellow, brown
Quinine	Brown
Riboflavin	Yellow
Rifampin	Red-orange
Senna	Yellow-brown (acid urine)
	Yellow-pink (alkaline urine)
Sulfonamides	Rust yellow, brown
Triamterene	Blue, green

what to expect so he or she can give accurate information and seek appropriate medical intervention while symptoms are mild.
- Evaluate for personality changes. The psychologic implications of renal disease are often the most frustrating for the patient, family, and nurse. Some people undergo an almost complete personality change. They become easily irritated and lack the ability to remember details and to concentrate. The exhibited symptoms are not always consistent with uremia, but may generally improve as the creatinine clearance improves or after the patient has undergone dialysis.
- Evaluate patients for the desired effects of their medications. Diuretics produce diuresis and weight loss.
- Evaluate the patient's compliance with the treatment regimen. Patients are cautioned not to discontinue their medications as soon as they are feeling better and not to take their medications as needed for symptomatic relief.

Cost is often a barrier to proper compliance. If patients do not belong to prescription plans, a reevaluation of therapy may be needed. The use of less costly, but equally effective, generic medications may be possible in some instances.

If the patient has a chronic condition, compliance may be poor because he or she sees no reason to adhere to the restrictions. Make the patient aware of the consequences if he or she does not comply with the prescribed regimen. Help the patient and family set realistic goals. As the patient begins to respond to treatment and feel better, he or she may decide that a modification in lifestyle is not the threat it may first have seemed.

The bibliography for this chapter can be found in Appendix B, which begins on page 1054.

CHAPTER REVIEW QUESTIONS*

1. Of the following values, which represents a normal creatinine clearance for women?
   a. 86 mL/min.
   b. 102 mL/min.
   c. 140 mL/min.
   d. 167 mL/min.

2. Patients with renal failure may need dosage adjustments of which medications?
   a. Aminoglycoside antibiotics.
   b. ACE inhibitors.
   c. Dopamine.
   d. Nitrates.

3. In a patient with chronic renal failure, the regulation of serum calcium and phosphate is altered. As a result of this dysfunction, the nurse may assess:
   a. Hypothyroidism.
   b. Hypoparathyroidism.
   c. Secondary hyperparathyroidism.
   d. Primary hyperthyroidism.

4. Which statement is *not* true of epoetin alfa?
   a. Epoetin alfa has the same biologic effects as endogenous erythropoietin.
   b. Epoetin alfa is used to treat the anemia associated with cancer chemotherapy.
   c. Epoetin alfa can safely be used during pregnancy and lactation.
   d. Some adverse effects include headache and a rapid rise in hematocrit.

5. In peritoneal dialysis, excess urea and waste products can be removed by:
   a. Increasing the concentration of glucose in dialysate.
   b. Decreasing the concentration of sodium in dialysate.
   c. Adding potassium to the peritoneal dialysate.
   d. Decreasing the nitrogen-containing products in dialysate.

*See Appendix A, which begins on page 1051, for answers.

BUILDING YOUR CRITICAL THINKING SKILLS

PERITONEAL DIALYSIS

A 35-year-old woman has been on home peritoneal dialysis twice a week for 4 months. Recent laboratory studies indicate her serum creatinine continues to rise. Further assessment reveals the patient has begun taking over-the-counter ibuprofen (Motrin) 400 mg three times daily for worsening arthritis.

1. What effect could the Motrin have on serum creatinine in this patient?
2. Should the patient's frequency of dialysis be increased given the information about her use of Motrin?
3. What teaching and monitoring needs to be done for this patient?

UNIT 10

DRUGS AFFECTING THE RESPIRATORY SYSTEM

UNIT OUTLINE

CHAPTER 39

Overview of the Functional Anatomy of the Respiratory System

Robert W. Hirnle, MS, RRT

KEY TERMS

Airway resistance
Alveoli
Bronchioles
Bronchospasm
Carina
Chemoreceptors
Compliance
Cyclic 3′,5′-AMP
Cyclic 3′,5′-GMP
Diaphragm
External intercostals

Larynx
Mucociliary escalator
Muscarinic receptors
Obstructive breathing
  disorders
Pharynx
Restrictive breathing
  disorders
Surfactant
Ventilation

LEARNING OBJECTIVES

After reading this chapter, the student will be able to:

1. Name the major structures of the respiratory system, and describe the primary functions of those structures of the upper and lower airways.
2. Describe several mechanisms that protect the airways against trauma, obstruction, and infection.
3. Explain the autonomic control of bronchial smooth muscle.
4. Describe the roles played by the nervous system, the circulatory system, and musculature in breathing.
5. Explain factors that affect normal breathing.
6. Compare and contrast obstructive and restrictive respiratory disorders.

Breathing is an essential life function. For breathing to occur properly, the respiratory system, which consists of the upper airway, lower airway, lung parenchyma, and extrapulmonary structures, must operate efficiently. Figure 39–1 shows the anatomy of the pulmonary system.

The airways and the lungs provide the route for oxygen to enter the blood. These structures also regulate the removal of the body's primary metabolic waste product, carbon dioxide, from the blood. To accomplish gas ex-

change, the respiratory system is assisted by the neural, musculoskeletal, and circulatory systems.

THE UPPER AIRWAY

The upper airway consists of the nose, mouth, and throat (larynx). These structures condition the air we breathe

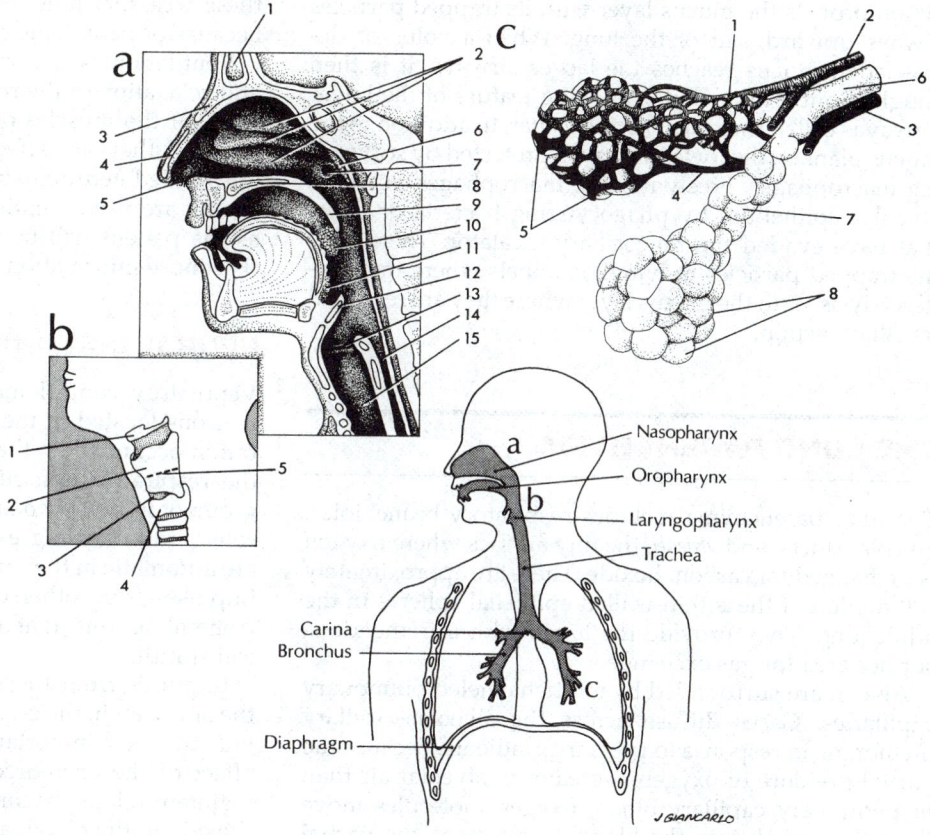

Figure 39–1. Anatomic landmarks of the pulmonary system. (A), 1. Frontal bone and sinuses; 2. turbinates; 3. bony structure to upper third of nose; 4. cartilaginous structure to lower two-thirds of nose; 5. vibrissae and nasal vestibule; 6. pharyngeal tonsils ("the adenoids"); 7. eustachian tube stoma (taurus tubarus); 8. hard palate; 9. soft palate; 10. faucial tonsils ("the tonsils"); 11. lingual tonsils; 12. epiglottis; 13. vocal cords; 14. esophagus; and 15. trachea. (B), 1. Hyoid bone; 2. thyroid cartilage; 3. cricothyroid membrane; 4. cricoid cartilage; and 5. area of vocal cords. (C), 1. Pulmonary venule; 2. small pulmonary vein; 3. small pulmonary artery; 4. pulmonary arteriole; 5. pulmonary capillaries; 6. terminal respiratory bronchiole; 7. alveolar duct; and 8. alveolar sacs. (From Shapiro, B, et al: Applications of Respiratory Care, ed 3. Year Book Medical Publishers, Chicago, 1985, with permission.)

and help protect the lung from harmful substances. The mouth and the nose provide the primary passageway for air to enter the respiratory system. In addition, these cavities filter, warm, and humidify incoming air, and help to prevent aspiration of foreign bodies into the lower airway and to control germ growth.

Immediately beneath the nasal passages lies the *pharynx*, the common connection between the nose, mouth, and throat. Lymphoid tissues of the adenoids and tonsils in the upper portions of the pharynx trap bacteria, thereby helping to prevent respiratory infections. The epiglottis, a leaf-shaped structure at the junction of the esophagus and the pharynx, protects the airway by closing the pharynx during swallowing.

The *larynx* demarcates the juncture of the upper and lower airways. In addition to its primary function as the organ of speech, the larynx also protects the lower airway from aspiration. Complex neural reflexes cause the larynx to close tightly when food or liquids enter the oropharynx.

Any solid or liquid substances that manage to enter the larynx trigger the cough reflex. A cough results from sudden release of this pressure, and the offending material is expelled. Because it is essential for maintaining airway patency and sterility, an effective cough reflex is the most important defense mechanism of the respiratory tract.

THE LOWER AIRWAY

The lower airway is composed of the trachea, the bronchi and their many branches, and the gas exchange portion of the lung. The primary function of the lower airway is to provide a means for air to reach the lung parenchyma. Extrapulmonary portions of the respiratory system include those structures or systems that allow the mechanical act of breathing to take place.

The trachea branches at the *carina* to become the two primary bronchi. These large airways are supported by cartilage, so they are relatively rigid. The bronchi branch in a treelike fashion, giving rise to successively smaller and more numerous bronchi. *Bronchioles*, the smallest branches of the lower airways, have no cartilage to support them, but are held open by subatmospheric pressure and smooth muscle tone. This system provides for very low airway resistance, making normal breathing in the healthy individual practically effortless. After numerous generations of branching, the conducting airways ultimately blend into the lung parenchyma, where gas exchange occurs.

As air travels through the conducting air passageways, it is further cleansed and conditioned. The larger airways are lined with a ciliated epithelial cell layer that secretes sticky mucus. These mucous secretions trap most of the dust and bacteria that get past the upper airways. Ciliary action propels the mucus layer with its trapped particles always upward, out of the lung. When a bolus of debris-laden mucus reaches the larger airways, it is then coughed out. This unique cleansing feature of the lower airway is called the *mucociliary escalator.* In addition to the mucus blanket, the lower airway is protected by scavenging macrophages. Freely moving macrophages clean the alveolar epithelium by phagocytizing bacteria or dusts that have evaded the mucociliary escalator. They carry the trapped particles to lymph channels where they undergo lysis, or to the mucus layer where they are removed by ciliary action.

THE LUNG PARENCHYMA

The lung parenchyma includes respiratory bronchioles, alveolar ducts, and *alveoli,* the tiny air sacs where oxygen is exchanged for carbon dioxide. There are approximately 300 million of these thin-walled epithelial spheres in the adult lung. They provide the lungs with a tremendous surface area for gas exchange.

Alveoli are surrounded by multichanneled pulmonary capillaries. Gases diffuse across the alveolar-capillary membrane in response to pressure gradients. Because the partial pressure of oxygen is greater in alveolar air than in pulmonary capillary blood, oxygen molecules move from the alveoli into the blood. Conversely, the partial pressure of carbon dioxide is lower in the alveoli and higher in the pulmonary capillary blood. Thus, carbon dioxide diffuses from the blood to the alveoli.

The lung parenchyma is very elastic and has a tendency to collapse. Surface tension exerted by the fluid lining the alveoli, which is necessary for the diffusion of gases, adds to this tendency. *Surfactant,* a phospholipid produced by specialized alveolar cells, reduces surface tension and helps prevent alveolar collapse.

EXTRAPULMONARY PORTIONS OF THE RESPIRATORY SYSTEM

The airways and lungs are directly responsible for gas exchange. However, these structures are passive and depend on coordinated efforts of muscles, nerves, and the circulatory system for complete functioning.

RESPIRATORY MUSCLES

For gas exchange to occur, air must move in and out of the lungs. This is accomplished by breathing, or *ventilation.* The primary muscles of ventilation are the *diaphragm* (dome-shaped muscle dividing abdominal and thoracic cavities) and the *external intercostals* (muscles that pull the ribs upward and outward during inspiration). In addition, healthy individuals use muscles of the neck and upper chest during heavy exercise to increase the efficiency of breathing. People with chronic lung disease also use these accessory muscles as part of their regular breathing because of pathologic changes in the lungs and chest.

Ventilation is accomplished by alternate contraction and relaxation of the respiratory muscles.

All of the muscles of ventilation are skeletal muscles. As such they are affected by skeletal muscle relaxants (also called neuromuscular blocking agents). When these agents are used, ventilatory support must be provided, as the patient will be unable to breathe spontaneously. (For more information on these agents, see Chapter 22.)

NEURAL CONTROL OF VENTILATION

Ventilatory control mechanisms arise from specialized neurons located in the medulla of the brain stem. Inspiration occurs when these neurons discharge impulses to the respiratory muscles, signaling them to contract. A group of inhibitory neurons turn off the "inspiratory neurons," thus causing exhalation. The medullary neurons are automatic in their function, but they are influenced by impulses from other centers in the brain and from peripheral neurons that are sensitive to chemical and physical stimuli.

Impulses from the *chemoreceptors* (neurons located in the aortic arch, the carotid arteries, and the medulla) provide the most important influence on ventilation. The net effect of the chemoreceptors is to adjust ventilation to maintain relatively constant levels of oxygen and carbon dioxide in the blood, as well as to regulate blood pH.

These neural control mechanisms can be influenced by different drugs. Respiratory neurons in the brain stem can be depressed by alcohol, barbiturates, and narcotics; they can be stimulated by the methylxanthines (such as theophylline), analeptic agents, and certain hormones. The central and peripheral chemoreceptors can be either stimulated or depressed by oxygen or carbon dioxide therapy. They are also affected by agents that alter the acid-base balance of the blood.

CIRCULATION AND RESPIRATION

Adequate blood flow is the final element essential for effective respiration. The capillaries of the pulmonary circulation are well suited for gas exchange. They are narrow and thin-walled, with many channels. This maximizes the surface area available for diffusion and provides for optimal gas exchange.

FACTORS AFFECTING BREATHING

Normal breathing is almost effortless. Lung tissue stretches readily, allowing for easy inspiration. Airways remain open by a dynamic balance of pressures and smooth muscle tone. However, any malfunction of the respiratory system can greatly increase the work of breathing. For some individuals with severe lung disease, breathing becomes an exhausting activity that can ultimately lead to respiratory failure.

NORMAL BREATHING

The work required for normal breathing depends on the lungs' ability to stretch and the patency of the airways.

Compliance   The ease with which the lung is stretched is described by the term *compliance*. The healthy lung is very compliant, able to accept large volumes of air with minimal effort. Lung parenchyma is made of relatively inelastic fibers, interwoven to form a matrix of highly elastic tissue, much the same as stiff nylon threads are woven to form a pliable stocking. The lung remains compliant so long as nothing damages this delicate matrix.

Bronchial Smooth Muscle Tone   Caliber of the small airways is primarily controlled by the autonomic nervous system (ANS). The two components of the ANS, the sympathetic nervous system (SNS) and the parasympathetic nervous system (PNS), exert opposing effects on bronchial smooth muscle. The effects of these two systems are the result of biochemical changes that occur at specific receptors, as shown in Figure 39–2.

Stimulation of the *muscarinic receptors* (cholinergic receptors that may also be activated by muscarine) of the PNS results in constriction of bronchial smooth muscle. Neural impulses from the PNS activate an enzyme, guanylate cyclase, which catalyzes the formation of cyclic 3′,5′-guanosine monophosphate (*cyclic 3′,5′-GMP*). This substance causes the smooth muscle fibers to contract, increasing *airway resistance*.

The muscarinic receptors are opposed in their action by the adrenergic beta$_2$ receptors of the SNS. Beta$_2$ stimulation causes bronchial dilation. SNS activity increases circulating levels of epinephrine and other catecholamines, which are released from the adrenal gland. These substances stimulate beta$_2$ receptors in bronchial smooth muscle and trigger the activation of adenylate cyclase. This enzyme catalyzes the production of cyclic 3′,5′-adenosine monophosphate (*cyclic 3′,5′-AMP*) from the high-energy compound adenosine triphosphate (ATP). Cyclic 3′,5′-AMP relaxes bronchial smooth muscle, thus increasing airway lumen size and maintaining low airway resistance.

Bronchial constriction caused by muscarinic (PNS) stimulation is countered by the relaxing effects of beta$_2$ (SNS) activity. The antagonism of these receptors creates a balance, which results in bronchial smooth muscle tone. Other receptors (e.g., alpha, prostaglandin, purinergic) found in bronchial smooth muscle may also play a part in normal airway control.

FACTORS THAT HINDER BREATHING

Any process that decreases lung compliance or airway patency makes breathing more difficult. Breathing problems are generally categorized as either restrictive or obstructive in nature. Either type of problem has the potential for profoundly decreasing gas exchange.

Restrictive Breathing Disorders   Any condition that prevents full expansion of the lungs is called a *restrictive disorder*. Breathing can be restricted by diseases that directly affect the lungs' compliance. Common conditions such as pneumonia inflame and stiffen lung tissue. Less commonly, respiratory distress syndromes cause surfactant loss, which leads to alveolar collapse. Either circumstance can seriously limit blood oxygenation and cause a dramatic increase in the work of breathing.

Problems with chest expansion can also impair breathing, even when the lungs themselves are healthy. Obesity, abdominal gas or fluid, pregnancy, incisional pain, or a tight postoperative binder can decrease chest expansion, which in turn limits lung expansion. The same is true of respiratory muscle weakness, which can be caused by general debilitation, overwork (perhaps caused by underlying respiratory disease), or neuromuscular diseases such as polio or myasthenia gravis.

Various pharmacologic agents are used to treat restrictive breathing disorders. Except in the case of surfactant deficiency, the causes of breathing restriction are nonrespiratory in origin, so these agents are discussed elsewhere.

Obstructive Breathing Disorders   Those conditions that decrease the movement of air through the airways are called *obstructive disorders*. Effective gas exchange occurs only when air flows unimpeded through the conducting airways, as this is the only route to the alveoli. Any degree of airway obstruction can greatly increase airway resistance, which in turn increases the work of breathing. The primary goal of respiratory pharmacology is to counteract airway obstruction and minimize airway resistance.

Physical obstructions such as tumors or aspirated foreign bodies are obvious causes of increased airway resistance. More commonly, airway obstruction results

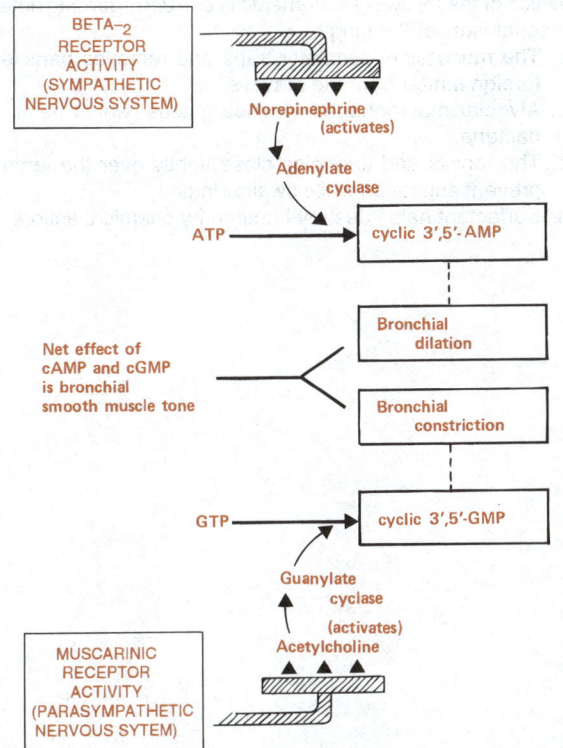

Figure 39–2. Autonomic control of bronchial smooth muscle.

from excessive mucus production, edematous inflamed tissue, or bronchial smooth muscle spasm.

Excessive mucus production is a clinical feature of several diseases, most notably chronic bronchitis, cystic fibrosis, and asthma. Airway irritation, inflammation, or pathologic epithelium changes cause hypersecretion of mucous glands. Mucus can fill small airways, fostering bacteria growth and leading to possible airway collapse.

Airway edema occurs in the diseases just mentioned and in many other disorders. Inflammation initiated by disease, allergy, physical trauma, or chemical irritation promotes leakage of fluids from capillaries into surrounding tissues, causing them to swell. The swollen bronchial epithelium decreases airway lumen size as tissue edema increases. As with excessive mucus, airway edema can result in complete airway obstruction.

Bronchospasm is a complex process that occurs primarily in asthma but is often encountered in bronchitis, emphysema, and several other diseases. Bronchospasm constricts the smallest airways, severely limiting airflow. An alteration in autonomic smooth muscle control is the most important factor in bronchospasm, although other receptors probably play a significant role. Allergy, infection, exercise, or physical stimuli such as cold air or inhaled dusts can cause bronchospasm by triggering the release of chemical mediators (e.g., histamine) from mast cells and basophils. These mediators may hyperstimulate PNS receptors, inhibit (or completely block) beta$_2$ receptors, or stimulate bronchial alpha receptors. This upsets the precise balance of sympathetic and parasympathetic influences on bronchial smooth muscle, and the result is bronchial constriction.

The bibliography for this chapter can be found in Appendix B, which begins on page 1054.

CHAPTER REVIEW QUESTIONS*

1. Which statement is *correct* regarding neurologic control of bronchial smooth muscle?
   a. Parasympathetic stimulation causes bronchial smooth muscle relaxation.
   b. The autonomic nervous system stimulates bronchial smooth muscle to produce surfactant.
   c. Sympathetic stimulation promotes bronchial constriction.
   d. Bronchial smooth muscle tone is maintained by a balance of sympathetic and parasympathetic stimulation.

2. Which of the following statements is *correct* concerning airway resistance?
   a. Increased mucus production can cause decreased airway resistance.
   b. Bronchospasm and edema can increase airway resistance.
   c. High airway resistance reduces work of breathing.
   d. When airway lumen size increases, so does airway resistance.

*See Appendix A, which beings on page, 1051 for answers.

3. Bronchioles are kept open primarily by:
   a. Intrathoracic pressure and smooth muscle tone.
   b. Surfactant.
   c. Pulmonary capillaries.
   d. Cartilage.

4. A lung that has high compliance:
   a. Is easy to stretch.
   b. Has narrow airways.
   c. Is less effective at gas exchange than a lung with low compliance.
   d. Is very difficult to inflate.

5. Which of the following statements is *correct* regarding defense mechanisms of the lung?
   a. The mucociliary escalator traps and removes particles of foreign matter from the airways.
   b. Alveolar macrophages produce mucus, which helps trap bacteria.
   c. The tonsils and adenoids close tightly over the larynx to prevent aspiration while swallowing.
   d. Surfactant helps destroy bacteria by chemical action.

CHAPTER 40

Agents Used to Treat Bronchial Obstruction

Robert W. Hirnle, MS, RRT

CHAPTER OUTLINE

TABLES

BOXES

KEY TERMS

Bronchodilators
Bronchospasm
Expectorant
Methylxanthine

Mucokinesis
Mucolytic
Sympathomimetics

LEARNING OBJECTIVES

After reading this chapter, the student will be able to:

1. Describe the primary causes of bronchial obstruction.
2. Given a list of physical symptoms, identify appropriate medications for treating specific causes of bronchial obstruction.
3. Describe the mechanisms of action, routes of administration, pharmacokinetics, adverse effects, contraindications and precautions, and interactions of agents used to treat bronchial obstruction.
4. Gather and use relevant assessment data pertaining to bronchial obstruction for the purpose of formulating appropriate patient outcomes.
5. Plan nursing intervention needed to administer medications to treat bronchial obstruction and choose appropriate teaching strategies for gaining patient compliance.
6. Evaluate patient response at various stages of treatment to measure the effectiveness of nursing interventions.

Bronchial obstruction makes breathing very difficult and interferes with gas exchange. Patients with asthma, chronic obstructive pulmonary disease (COPD), cystic fibrosis, and a variety of other respiratory disorders often experience bronchial obstruction. This problem can be caused by airway inflammation, bronchospasm, or excessive mucous secretions. Inhaled corticosteroids, antiasthmatic agents, bronchodilators, and mucokinetic agents are used to counteract the causes of airway obstruction.

ANTI-INFLAMMATORY AGENTS: INHALED CORTICOSTEROIDS

Chemical or physical irritants, allergy, and infection cause airway inflammation. Chemical mediators such as histamine that are released from injured tissues cause airways to swell with edema. These mediators also act as irritants, which can provoke bronchial smooth muscle spasm and stimulate production of thick, viscous mucus. These effects all greatly decrease airflow through the air passages to the alveoli. Inflammation is a hallmark of chronic bronchitis and is considered the most significant problem in the treatment of asthma. In recent years, the primary approach to asthma management has centered on the aggressive use of anti-inflammatory agents, particularly aerosolized corticosteroids. These agents are highly effective in helping to control both acute and chronic airway inflammation. Some patients require large, long-term doses of oral or intravenous prednisone or methylprednisolone to control asthma symptoms or to relieve exacerbations of COPD. However, chronic use of systemic corticosteroids causes a host of severe adverse effects.

Fortunately, many patients are able to decrease airway inflammation with the use of locally acting aerosolized corticosteroids. **Beclomethasone (Beclovent, Vanceril, Vancenase AQ**—as a nasal spray), **betamethasone (Valisone), triamcinolone acetonide (Azmacort),** and **flunisolide (AeroBid)** are examples of corticosteroids that are available as aerosol medications. These inhaled agents are discussed here; for a complete discussion of the use and effects of systemic corticosteroids, see Chapter 44.

ACTION

Inhaled steroids act locally to suppress the inflammatory response in the lung. Their precise mechanism of action is unknown, but they evidently decrease both the release and effects of inflammatory mediators from injured tissues. Aerosolized steroids decrease airway edema by stabilizing capillary membranes, making them less prone to leakage. Inhaled steroids potentiate sympathomimetic bronchodilating agents by increasing beta receptor responsiveness to their effects. Finally, steroids promote *mucokinesis* (mobilization of mucus) by improving mucociliary activity and by altering mucous gland function to increase the water content of airway secretions.

USES

Inhaled corticosteroids are indicated for use by patients with asthma, chronic bronchitis, COPD, cystic fibrosis, or any lung disease characterized by chronic or acute inflammation.

PHARMACOKINETICS

Corticosteroids available in metered-dose inhalers are almost exclusively local in their actions. Absorption across the alveolar capillary membrane is minimal at recommended doses, as are systemic effects. Because small amounts of the drug are swallowed with each treatment, systemic absorption and toxicity may occur over time in the heaviest users.

CONTRAINDICATIONS AND PRECAUTIONS

Patients with known or suspected hypersensitivity to the propellants used in metered-dose inhalers should not use

these agents. Use with caution in the patient with active respiratory infection or with known bacterial colonization because corticosteroid use can promote infection. Patients who have received long-term oral steroid therapy for breathing problems must gradually be weaned from systemic therapy to allow the patient's suppressed adrenal cortex to resume normal function.

▼ **CLINICAL ALERT**

Inhaled corticosteroids are maintenance drugs. They are not useful in acute exacerbations of asthma and may actually aggravate symptoms. These agents are not bronchodilators: they are ineffective against acute bronchospasm. Severe exacerbations of either asthma or COPD may require additional dosing with systemically administered corticosteroids, because inhaled steroids alone may be insufficient to maintain airway patency.

Use of inhaled steroids at doses higher than recommended may lead to systemic absorption. This can cause the systemic side effects described in Chapter 44.

ADVERSE EFFECTS

If the use of long-term oral steroids is discontinued abruptly in favor of using inhaled drugs exclusively, the resulting adrenal insufficiency can cause death. Side effects from inhaled steroids are generally minor. Most common complaints include oropharyngeal irritation and coldlike symptoms. Sore throat, sinusitis, and oral fungal infections can occur, but are usually avoidable by thorough mouth rinsing after each dose. Some patients experience diarrhea, nausea and vomiting, and stomach upset. Headache, fever, dizziness, angioedema, rash, urticaria, and paradoxic bronchospasm occur rarely.

INTERACTIONS

Inhaled steroids have no significant interactions when they are administered within the therapeutic dosage range.

Inhaled corticosteroids are presented in Table 40–1.

ANTIASTHMATIC AGENTS

Antiasthmatic agents such as **cromolyn sodium (Intal)** and **nedocromil sodium (Tilade)** are similar to inhaled steroids in that their function is to limit inflammation. Unlike inhaled corticosteroids, which decrease signs and symptoms of established inflammation, these agents prevent airway inflammation from occurring. Irritants

Table 40–1. INHALED CORTICOSTEROIDS

DRUG NAME/ROUTE AND DOSAGE	PHARMACOKINETICS/ DYNAMICS	NURSING IMPLICATIONS
beclomethasone (Vanceril, Beclovent, Vancenase AQ)		
Adults: 336 μg/day (1–2 puffs 4 times daily; dosage may be higher initially, not to exceed 20 inhalations daily) by MDI; 1 mg (or 5 200-μg Rotacaps) daily by oral dry powder inhaler; 100 μg per nostril 3–4 times daily (12 sprays daily maximum) by nasal MDI. ***Children:*** Half adult dose.	**Onset:** very gradual (maintenance drug) **Peak:** NA **Duration:** used for long-term effects **½L:** not absorbed (local) **PB:** 87% **B:** locally by tissues **E:** feces	**ASSESSMENT:** Assess for bronchospasm (do not use if present). Check for sore throat and signs of oral candidiasis. Monitor sputum color and viscosity; change can indicate infection. Assess breath sounds regularly to determine several of wheezing and to follow patient progress. Check for presence and character of cough: harsh, burning cough may indicate steroid-induced tracheitis. Watch for new signs of systemic absorption in long-term user. Observe for signs of adrenal crisis if MDI is used to replace systemic steroid therapy. Assess for other adverse effects: rhinitis, nausea and vomiting, diarrhea, GI upset, menstrual disturbances, and palpitations. **INTERVENTION:** When patient is changing from systemic to aerosol regimen, administer both forms gradually as ordered until complete transition to aerosol is made. At first signs of adrenal crisis, inform physician and administer systemic steroid therapy as ordered. Use bronchodilators (if ordered) 15 min prior to aerosol inhaler to promote aerosol distribution and to minimize potentially toxic effects of propellants. Do not use in acute asthma attack. **Patient Teaching**—Instruct patient to rinse mouth thoroughly to avoid *Candida* overgrowth; to take this drug regularly (not on PRN basis; to *not* use during acute wheezing; to not exceed recommended dose; and to clean inhaler daily. **EVALUATION:** Effectiveness is demonstrated by increase in comfort in patient's breathing (decreased burning in chest, less harsh coughing), and by decrease in number and severity of wheezing attacks. Same as for beclomethasone.
triamcinolone acetonide (Azmacort)		
Adults: 800 μg/day (1–2 puffs qid), not to exceed 20 inhalations daily) by MDI; 110 μg per nostril (2 sprays each nostril bid by nasal MDI. ***Children:*** 1–2 puffs 3–4 times daily (12 puffs maximum).		Same as beclomethasone. **INTERVENTION:** Used for prophylactic therapy or chronic control.
flunisolide (AeroBid, Nasalide)		
Adults: 2 puffs bid (250 μg per puff, not to exceed 4 puffs bid) by MDI; 2 sprays per nostril bid (25 μg per puff, not to exceed 8 sprays per nostril daily) by nasal MDI. ***Children:*** 2 puffs bid (1000 μg daily maximum) by MDI; 1 spray per nostril tid or 2 sprays bid (4 sprays per nostril daily maximum) by nasal MDI.		Same as for beclomethasone.

NA = not available.

or allergens cause mast cells to break down, or degranulate, during acute episodes of asthma. Histamine and other mediators are spilled into the airways, causing airway edema, bronchospasm, and excess mucus production.

ACTION

When mast cells are irritated by allergens or other stimuli, the membrane becomes more permeable and more susceptible to degranulation. Cromolyn sodium and nedocromil sodium alter mast cell membrane permeability to calcium ions, decreasing the membrane's sensitivity to irritants. By stabilizing the membrane, these drugs help prevent mast cell degranulation and its resultant asthmatic symptoms. In addition, nedocromil diminishes the inflammatory effects of a variety of mediators, and while it is not an antitussive, decreases coughing by reducing airway sensitivity.

USES

Particularly effective for the allergic asthmatic patient, these drugs can reduce both the frequency and intensity of asthma attacks. These agents are also available as nasal sprays and eyedrops and are highly effective against hay fever symptoms.

PHARMACOKINETICS

Cromolyn and nedocromil are effective only when administered by inhalation. They are locally acting agents that are absorbed by the respiratory mucosa. Because of these drugs' poor absorption characteristics, only a fraction of each dose absorbs into the mast cell membranes, so efficacy is not immediately evident. Therapeutic effects become noticeable gradually, after a period of 3 weeks or more of daily dosing. Because of their very limited ability to cross cell membranes, systemic absorption of these drugs is negligible.

CONTRAINDICATIONS AND PRECAUTIONS

Both cromolyn and nedocromil sodium are contraindicated for use in patients with hypersensitivity to their ingredients. The metered-dose inhaler is used with caution in patients with cardiac dysrhythmias, as fluorocarbon propellants may have cardiotoxic effects. Patients with impaired renal or hepatic function may receive lowered dosages.

Cromolyn and nedocromil are prophylactic agents: they do not reverse bronchospasm and can actually provoke it. These drugs are contraindicated in acute asthma attacks.

ADVERSE EFFECTS

Side effects from antiasthmatic agents are mild and relatively rare. Most commonly reported reactions include

Table 40–2. ANTIASTHMA PROPHYLACTIC AGENTS		
DRUG NAME/ROUTE AND DOSAGE	**PHARMACOKINETICS/ DYNAMICS**	**NURSING IMPLICATIONS**
sodium cromolyn (Intal, Nasalcrom)		
Adults and Children: 20 mg qid by SpinHaler or as nebulizer solution; 2 puffs qid (800 μg per puff) by MDI	**Onset:** 2–4 wk **Peak:** 30 min–1 hr **Duration:** used as maintenance drug for long-term effects **½L:** NA **PB:** acts locally in lung **B:** excreted unchanged **E:** urine, bile	**ASSESSMENT:** Record frequency and severity of asthma attacks. Monitor pulmonary function before beginning cromolyn therapy. Assess breath sounds periodically. Check for dry throat and hoarseness. Assess for reflex bronchospasm after treatment. **INTERVENTION:** Instruct patient in use of SpinHaler. **Patient Teaching**—Instruct patient to not swallow capsules (they are ineffective if swallowed). Advise patient to take drug 2–4 wk as ordered before expecting results. Tell patient to rinse mouth after administration of drug to prevent dry throat. Warn patient against taking during asthma attack as cromolyn can aggravate symptoms. Tell patient to use bronchodilator (as ordered) 20–30 min prior to cromolyn to maximize cromolyn inhalation. **EVALUATION:** Effectiveness of this drug is demonstrated by eventual (within 4 wk) decrease in number and intensity of asthma attacks. It is also demonstrated by reduction in need for other asthma medications.
nedocromil (Tilade)		
Adults and Children: 2 puffs (2 mg per puff) qid by MDI	**Onset:** gradual, over weeks **Peak:** 90 min **Duration:** same as cromolyn **½L:** 3.3 hr **PB:** 89% **B:** not **E:** urine-unchanged	Same as for cromolyn. **Patient Teaching**—Use regularly, even when no symptoms are present.

NA = not available.

dry mouth, irritated throat, cough, unpleasant taste, and headache. Very infrequently patients report rash, urticaria, erythema, allergy, parotitis, and bronchospasm.

INTERACTIONS

Neither cromolyn nor nedocromil interacts significantly with any drug. Antiasthmatic drugs are described in Table 40–2.

LEUKOTRIENE RECEPTOR ANTAGONIST

The leukotriene receptor antagonist zafirlukast (aerolate) is the first of a new group of drugs to control asthma. This group treats the cause of the disease as opposed to Rxing the symptoms, as other groups of drugs.

BRONCHODILATING AGENTS

Sudden hyperresponsiveness of the small airways to stimuli (e.g., allergy, exercise, infection) that results in abrupt narrowing of the airways is called *bronchospasm*. Malfunction of autonomic muscle control mechanisms is thought to play a central role in this process. *Bronchodilators* are administered to counteract bronchospasm. Major categories of bronchodilators include sympathomimetics, methylxanthines, and anticholinergics.

SYMPATHOMIMETIC BRONCHODILATORS

Sympathomimetics are agents that mimic the effects of the sympathetic (adrenergic) nervous system. Sympathomimetic bronchodilators can be classified as either catecholamines or noncatecholamines. Commonly prescribed catecholamines include **epinephrine *(Primatene Mist)*** and **isoproterenol *(Isuprel)***. The noncatecholamine sympathomimetics used for bronchospasm include **metaproterenol (Alupent)**, **albuterol *(Proventil, Ventolin)***, and **salmeterol (Serevent)**. Combination products are also available to improve control of bronchospasm **(ipratropium bromide/albuterol sulfate [Combivent])**.

Action

All sympathomimetics stimulate beta$_2$ receptors to increase production of cyclic adenosine monophosphate (AMP). Cyclic AMP relaxes bronchial smooth muscle, thus reducing airway resistance and improving airflow. Catecholamines such as epinephrine and isoproterenol are not selective in their adrenergic receptor activity (affecting both alpha and beta receptors) and thus cause sig-

nificant cardiovascular side effects. Noncatecholamine, preferential beta$_2$ stimulants, such as metaproterenol, albuterol, and salmeterol, are longer lasting and evoke less severe side effects.

Pharmacokinetics

Because of differences in their susceptibility to specific metabolic enzymes, catecholamines and noncatecholamines vary in their duration of effects. Catecholamine bronchodilators are readily degraded by monoamine oxidase (MAO) and catechol-ortho-methyltransferase (COMT), which are plentiful in the liver and in bronchial smooth muscle. Their susceptibility to these enzymes severely limits the duration of action of bronchodilators like epinephrine or isuprel, thus limiting their clinical effectiveness. This enzyme susceptibility also makes oral catecholamine preparations ineffective, as they are deactivated by first-pass effects of the liver.

Because of differences in their molecular structures, noncatecholamine sympathomimetic agents possess characteristics that make them clinically superior to catecholamines. The chemical nucleus of these agents makes them far more resistant to degradation by COMT, so their duration of action is substantially longer. They are also effective as oral preparations. Molecular structural differences also make these agents more beta$_2$ specific than their catecholamine counterparts.

Contraindications and Precautions

The use of sympathomimetics is contraindicated for anyone with known hypersensitivity to any of the ingredients in these medications. Sympathomimetics are used with caution in patients with cardiovascular disease because they can increase myocardial oxygen demand. Catecholamines are not recommended for patients with active dysrhythmias and are contraindicated for patients with tachydysrhythmias. They can exacerbate the symptoms of hyperthyroidism. Because of their ability to stimulate the liver to increase glucose synthesis, sympathomimetics are used cautiously in the diabetic patient. Safety or some agents has not been established in children under age 12.

Adverse Effects

The major adverse effects associated with sympathomimetics are caused by their ability to stimulate the cardiovascular and central nervous systems. All sympathomimetics can cause tachycardia, palpitations, and increased blood pressure. In susceptible patients they have the potential to exacerbate hypertension, precipitate angina attacks, cause or aggravate dysrhythmias, or extend an acute myocardial infarction. Anxiety, agitation, restlessness, hyperactive reflexes, insomnia, irritability, and tremors are common central nervous system (CNS) effects. Paradoxic or rebound bronchospasm can occur. Occasionally sympathomimetics may cause nausea and urinary retention. Because of their superior receptor

Table 40–3. SYMPATHOMIMETIC BRONCHODILATORS

DRUG NAME/ROUTE AND DOSAGE	PHARMACOKINETICS/ DYNAMICS	NURSING IMPLICATIONS
epinephrine (Adrenalin) *Adults:* 0.2–0.5 mg q 2 hr of 1:1000 solution SC; 0.5 mg q 4 hr PRN of 1:200 suspension IM; 1–2 puffs with 1 min between puffs (0.1–0.2 mg per puff) q 4 hr MDI *Children:* 0.01 mg/kg, max 0.5 mg q 4 hr of 1:1000 solution SC; 0.02–0.025 mg/kg q 4 hr PRN of 1:200 suspension IM	**Onset:** 1–10 min **Peak:** 10–20 min **Duration:** 1–1.5 hr **½L:** NA **PB:** NA **B:** liver, neuron ends **E:** urine, breast milk	**ASSESSMENT:** Monitor heart rate and blood pressure always, ECG PRN; check urinary output in shock patients, and blood glucose in diabetic patients. Assess for overdose or hypersensitivity (dysrhythmias, chest pain, hypertension or hypotension, headache, nervousness). Assess breath sounds. Check for drug interactions. **INTERVENTION:** Check dose and route carefully. Administer two doses as ordered, with 2nd dose 20–30 min after initial dose. Avoid gluteal IM injection to prevent abscess. **Patient Teaching**—Discourage overuse of inhalers. Tell patient not to use with antihistamines or decongestants unless directed by physician to prevent potentiation of effects. **EVALUATION:** Increased air movement, decreased wheezing, and relief of dyspnea indicate drug effectiveness.
isoproterenol (Isuprel) *Adults:* Up to 2.5 mg q 3–4 hr by inhalation; 1–4 puffs q 3–4 hr *Children:* Up to 1.25 mg q 3–4 hr by inhalation; 1–4 puffs q 3–4 hr (80–131 µg per puff)	**Onset:** 1–10 min **Peak:** 10–20 min **Duration:** 1–2 hr **½L:** NA **PB:** NA **B:** tissue reuptake **E:** urine	Same as for epinephrine plus: **INTERVENTION:** Use oxygen to treat hypoxemia as needed. If heart rate increases by 20%, discontinue treatment and notify physician of hypersensitivity.
metaproterenol (Alupent) *Adults:* 20 mg PO 3–4 times daily; 10–15 mg 3–4 times daily by inhalation (0.2–0.3 mL of 5% solution); 2–3 puffs q 3–4 hr by MDI (650 µg per puff) *Children:* 10 mg 3–4 times daily (6–9 yr and <27 kg) PO; 20 mg 3–4 times daily (>9 yr and >27 kg) PO; 3–4 times daily by inhalation; 2–3 puffs q 3–4 hr by MDI	**Onset:** 1–15 min **Peak:** 0.5–1 hr **Duration:** 1–5 hr **½L:** NA **PB:** NA **B:** liver **E:** urine	Same as for epinephrine.
albuterol (Ventolin) *Adults and Children over 12:* 2–4 mg PO 3–4 times daily; extended release tabs, 4 mg bid; 2.5 mg q 4–6 hr by inhalation; 2 puffs q 4–6 hr (90 µg per puff) by MDI; 1 Rotacap q 4–6 hr by Rotahaler (inhaled powder)	**Onset:** 5–15 min inhaled, 30 min PO **Peak:** ½–2 hr **Duration:** 3–6 hr (up to 12 hr extended tabs) **½L:** approx 4 hr **PB:** NA **B:** liver **E:** urine	Same as for epinephrine plus: **INTERVENTION:** Avoid contact with eyes. Take oral preparations with meals to avoid gastric irritation. Not recommended for children under age 12.
salmeterol xinafoate (Serevent) *Adults and Children >12 years:* 2 puffs (21 µg/puff) bid	**Onset:** 30+ min **Peak:** NA **Duration:** 12 hr **½L:** NA **PB:** NA **B:** NA **E:** NA	Same as for epinephrine plus: **INTERVENTION:** Do not administer this drug as treatment for acute asthma attack (rapid onset, short-acting bronchodilator is required). **Patient Teaching**—Instruct the patient to take this drug regularly as ordered for chronic asthma maintenance. Because of its slow onset of action, Serevent is inappropriate and potentially dangerous to use during acute bronchospastic episodes. Not recommended for children under age 12.

SC = subcutaneous; NA = not available.

selectivity, noncatecholamine bronchodilators generally elicit fewer and less severe adverse effects than catecholamines.

▼ **CLINICAL ALERT**

Patients commonly experience nervousness and tremors when first using sympathomimetic bronchodilators. These effects are generally benign and usually subside over time as the patient develops tolerance.

Interactions

Sympathomimetics are antagonized by beta-blocking agents such as propranolol. Concomitant use of these drugs results in diminished effects of both agents. Sympathomimetics can potentiate both the therapeutic and adverse effects of other bronchodilator agents, especially theophylline. Antidepressants such as MAO inhibitors and some tricyclic compounds, as well as thyroid hormone, decongestants, and some antihistamines, can potentiate the cardiovascular effects of sympathomimetics.

Sympathomimetic bronchodilators are summarized in Table 40–3.

METHYLXANTHINE AGENTS

Methylxanthines are xanthine derivatives that act as smooth muscle relaxants and are used as bronchodilators. The methylxanthine bronchodilators include **aminophylline (Truphylline), dyphylline (Dilor), theophylline (Uniphyl, Theo-Dur,** and many others), and **oxtriphylline (Choledyl)**.

○ **Theophylline** is a compound closely related to caffeine. Its adverse effects profile and narrow margin of safety have diminished theophylline's popularity, but it is still widely prescribed.

Dosing must be individualized and carefully monitored. Theophylline's narrow safety margin, the many preparations and concentrations that are available, and the many factors that affect serum levels make it a drug that must be administered with relative precision.

ACTION Theophylline's mechanism of action is poorly understood. It indirectly increases cyclic AMP (CAMP) in bronchial smooth muscle by inhibiting phosphodiesterase, the enzyme that destroys CAMP. Additionally, theophylline affects intracellular calcium channels and adenosine receptors, which appear to play a role in regulating bronchial smooth muscle tone. A combination of actions seems likely. Theophylline derivatives (e.g. aminophylline, dyphylline) are similar in all practical respects to theophylline, except with regard to dosages.

USES Theophylline is used as a maintenance drug by asthmatics to control mild to moderate bronchospasm. It is also prescribed for patients with COPD and cystic fibrosis. In addition to counteracting bronchospasm, theophylline promotes diaphragm strength and improves pulmonary blood flow.

CONTRAINDICATIONS AND PRECAUTIONS Theophylline is contraindicated in patients with uncontrolled cardiac dysrhythmias and is given with caution to patients with any cardiovascular disease. Because it can cause seizures, theophylline is administered to patients with seizure disorders only if their bronchospasm is unresponsive to other treatment approaches and only with extreme caution. Theophylline exacerbates symptoms of hyperthyroidism, so patients with this condition should not receive the drug. Finally, theophylline increases gastric acid secretion, which can worsen preexisting conditions such as esophageal reflux or ulcers.

PHARMACOKINETICS Oral theophylline is generally well absorbed from the gastrointestinal (GI) tract. Its rate of absorption depends on the preparation, with popular sustained-release (SR) products absorbing more slowly than shorter-acting forms. Because of its variable absorption rate, peak serum theophylline levels vary depending on the type of preparation taken. Oral aminophylline reaches peak blood levels in 1 to 2 hours, while SR products can take up to 15 hours to reach peak serum levels. By contrast, intravenous infusion of aminophylline allows blood levels of drug to be readily predictable and controllable.

Theophylline does not seem to enter adipose tissue, so dosages must be calculated on the basis of lean body weight. It can cross the placenta and enter breast milk, where concentrations are about half those of serum concentrations.

Several factors can affect serum theophylline levels. Clearance of the drug occurs more rapidly in smokers; young children metabolize the drug faster than adults. Conversely, theophylline metabolism is slowed by a variety of pharmacologic agents (as discussed later) and by a number of pathologic conditions. Patients with hepatic failure, heart failure (HF), viral illnesses, or pneumonia have a prolonged serum half-life of theophylline. Neonates and elderly patients also have a slower rate of theophylline clearance. It is particularly difficult to maintain a consistent serum theophylline level in young children with lung disease complicated by viral illness.

Cardiovascular collapse can occur when aminophylline is infused too rapidly. For this reason aminophylline must be administered no faster than 25 mg/min in concentrations no stronger than 25 mg/mL.

Because theophylline toxicity can be life threatening and because so many factors can affect the rate of metabolism of this drug, strict guidelines concerning its administration have been established. These dosage recommendations, listed in Table 40–4, should be carefully followed. To ensure patient safety, frequent regular monitoring of serum theophylline levels is necessary.

ADVERSE EFFECTS Adverse effects associated with theophylline products are very similar to those seen with sympathomimetics. In general, however, toxic reactions caused by theophylline are much more severe, so great caution must be exercised in its administration. When serum levels are maintained within the therapeutic range of 8 to 20 μg/mL, serious adverse reactions are rare. Potentially dangerous toxic effects appear quickly when serum levels exceed 20 μg/mL.

Patients receiving theophylline complain most frequently of caffeinelike symptoms, such as nervousness, insomnia, jitteriness, headache, frequent urination, and palpitations. These can be very mild, appearing

Table 40–4. METHYLXANTHINE BRONCHODILATORS: THEOPHYLLINE PREPARATIONS

DRUG NAME/ROUTE AND DOSAGE	PHARMACOKINETICS/ DYNAMICS	NURSING IMPLICATIONS
theophylline anhydrous (Uniphyl, Theo-Dur)		
Adults: 3–6 mg/kg PO initially, 100–300 mg q 6 hr maintenance; or, up to 900 mg/day PO sustained release (SR) tabs once or twice daily *Children:* 3–6 mg/kg PO initially then 50–100 mg q 6 hr maintenance; or, up to 500 mg/day PO SR tabs taken twice daily	**Onset:** within 1 hour **Peak:** depends on peak serum levels **Duration:** 4–15 hr, depending on preparation **½L:** varies with age and preparation used (approx 3 hr in young children, 8 hr adults) **PB:** 50% (avg) **B:** liver **E:** urine	**ASSESSMENT:** Monitor heart rate and blood pressure. Monitor ECG in patients with cardiac problems. Assess serum levels often. Observe for toxicity (signs/symptoms include nausea, tachycardia, insomnia, dysrhythmias, seizures, restlessness). Assess for interactions. Assess breath sounds for decreased wheezing and improved aeration. Check for factors that could affect drug clearance and therefore dosage (e.g., smoking, viral illness). Many dosages and preparations require extra care in administration; check orders carefully. Monitor patient response to SR preparations: assess whether relief is continuous. **INTERVENTION:** Adjust dose as ordered if patient smokes (smokers need up to 100% larger than usual dose), if interacting drugs are part of regimen, or if serum level is outside therapeutic range of 8–20 µg/mL. If signs of toxicity appear, hold dosage and inform physician. (**ALERT!** Do not give if seizures or dysrhythmias occur!) Give drug around the clock as ordered. Do not crush SR tablets, as this will release full dose immediately. **EVALUATION:** Relief of dyspnea, improved air distribution, and improved quality of breath sounds indicate successful drug therapy.
aminophylline (Truphylline)		
Adults: *Loading*–5.6 mg/kg over 30 min. 0.2–0.9 mg/kg per hr by continuous IV infusion as determined by serum level; or 500 mg PO followed by 250–500 mg q 6–8 hr *Children:* *Loading*–6 mg/kg over 20 min. *Maintenance*–1 mg/kg per hr by continuous IV infusion as determined by serum level; 7.5 mg/kg followed by 3–6 theophylline mg/kg PO q 6–8 hr	**Onset:** 15–60 min **Peak:** same as theophylline **Duration:** 6–12 hr, depending on preparation **½L:** same as theophylline **PB:** same as theophylline **B:** liver **E:** urine	**ASSESSMENT:** Same as for theophylline plus: Monitor IV infusion rate frequently. **INTERVENTION:** Same as for theophylline plus: Keep infusion rate slower than 25 mg/min (intermittent dosing), 0.3–1.2 mg/kg per hr (continuous infusion). Do not mix aminophylline with other drugs in IV solution owing to incompatibilities. Flush main IV line before administering drug by infusion. **EVALUATION:** Same as theophylline.
dyphylline (Dilor)		
Adults: 15 mg/kg q 6 hr up to qid (up to 800 mg/dose) PO *Children:* 4.4–6.6 mg/kg per day in divided doses (up to 15 mg/kg q 6 hr) PO	**Onset:** within 1 hr **Peak:** 1 hr **Duration:** short **½L:** 2 hr **PB:** NA **B:** liver **E:** urine	**ASSESSMENT:** Same as for theophylline plus: Assess need for more frequent or larger doses (because of shorter duration and lower potency than other theophylline products). Observe closely for signs of toxicity, especially as serum levels are not available. **INTERVENTION:** If signs of hypersensitivity or toxicity appear, stop use of drug at once and notify physician. **EVALUATION:** Same as aminophylline.
oxtriphylline (Choledyl)		
Adults: 200 mg qid or 400–600 mg sustained release tabs q 12 hr *Children:* 3.6 mg/kg qid PO	**Onset:** slow and variable; otherwise same as theophylline	Same as for theophylline.

NA = not available.

METHYLXANTHINE BRONCHODILATORS: THEOPHYLLINE PREPARATIONS

even when the patient's serum level is relatively low. Mild symptoms usually disappear in a short period. These same symptoms may be the first indication of serious toxicity, however, so they must be carefully monitored.

As serum levels increase, adverse effects become more severe; with concentrations of 15 to 25 $\mu g/mL$, severe nausea, vomiting, and anorexia occur. Tachycardia is common. More intense CNS effects, such as agitation, tremors, and anxiety, also appear when serum levels are within this range. When serum levels exceed 30 $\mu g/mL$, dangerous cardiac effects commonly occur. Atrial and ventricular dysrhythmias, including ventricular fibrillation, can occur suddenly with fatal results. Although seizures can occur at lower serum levels, they are most common when serum levels exceed 40 $\mu g/mL$. Seizures caused by theophylline toxicity are usually refractory to treatment and can be fatal.

Because of the potentially lethal nature of theophylline's adverse effects, it is essential that patient response to therapy be monitored closely and that serum levels be monitored regularly. It is also vital to remember that a wide variety of conditions can affect theophylline metabolism. When any of these conditions are present, the nurse must be extra vigilant in monitoring the patient for drug reactions.

INTERACTIONS Metabolism of theophylline is accelerated by tobacco or marijuana smoking, as well as by several drugs. These agents decrease serum half-life significantly, making it necessary to increase dosing in these patients by up to 50% above the usual dose.

Several enzyme-inducing drugs also increase metabolism of theophylline. These include phenytoin, rifampin, barbiturates, and carbamazepine. These agents shorten theophylline's duration of action, much like smoking.

Drugs that slow theophylline's rate of metabolism include allopurinol, beta-adrenergic blockers, and cimetidine. Antibiotics, notably erythromycin, clindamycin, troleandomycin, and lincomycin, also decrease the clearance of theophylline. Patients receiving these drugs with theophylline are thus at greater risk of developing toxic reactions from elevated serum levels.

Because there are so many drugs that are incompatible in solution with theophylline, this drug should not be mixed with other medications.

Sympathomimetic agents, anticholinergics, cardiac glycosides, and theophylline are mutually potentiating. When combined, each one enhances both therapeutic and adverse effects of the others. Theophylline also enhances the effectiveness of some diuretic agents and decreases the therapeutic effects of lithium.

Beverages and foods that contain caffeine may accentuate some of the stimulatory effects of theophylline preparations. Patients who use these together report diuretic effects and nervousness. A full stomach slows theophylline's rate of absorption, but does not change the total amount absorbed.

Theophylline preparations are described in Table 40–4.

○ **Leukotriene Receptor Antagonist Zafirvukast** (Accolate) blocks leukutrienes which are activated in asthma and cause broncho-constriction and inflamma-

tion. Zafirvukast is recommended for maintenance treatment of chronic asthma. It is relatively well tolerated, with only a few patients experiencing gastrointestinal disturbances and mild headache. The usual dosage is 20 mg BID, 1 hour before or 2 hours after meals in persons over 12 years of age.

ANTICHOLINERGIC AGENTS

In some patients bronchospasm is caused less by adrenergic dysfunction than by excessive parasympathetic influence on the bronchioles. Sympathomimetic agents and theophylline have limited effect on this process, so these drugs provide limited relief for such patients. When bronchospasm is unresponsive to these agents, aerosolized anticholinergic agents such as **ipratropium bromide (Atrovent)** may be useful. Inhaled anticholinergic drugs decrease activity of the parasympathetic nervous system on bronchial smooth muscle.

○ **Ipratropium bromide** (Atrovent) is chemically related to atropine, another anticholinergic agent.

ACTION Chronic airway inflammation and irritation can increase vagal tone, stimulating production of acetylcholine, which in turn activates cyclic 3',5'-guanosine monophosphate (cyclic GMP). This biochemical mediator promotes mast cell degranulation, increases mucus production, and is a powerful bronchoconstrictor. Ipratropium competitively antagonizes acetylcholine. By preventing acetylcholine from occupying its receptors, ipratropium inhibits cyclic GMP production and its negative airway effects.

USES Ipratropium helps control bronchospasm in patients with chronic bronchitis, COPD, and selected cases of asthma. It is used as an adjunct along with other bronchodilators and is especially helpful for those who are unresponsive to sympathomimetic agents. Generally, this agent is well tolerated by nearly all patients because its actions are almost exclusively local.

CONTRAINDICATIONS AND PRECAUTIONS Use of ipratropium is contraindicated in patients hypersensitive to it or to atropine or to the propellants or preservatives used in the product. Ipratropium is used with caution by the patient with narrow-angle glaucoma, as it can affect pupillary size. Because it can increase heart rate, it is used cautiously by patients with acute hemorrhage, tachycardia caused by cardiac insufficiency, or any cardiac disease. Because its anticholinergic effects include urinary retention, ipratropium is also used cautiously by the patient with prostate hypertrophy, bladder-neck obstruction, or any chronic renal disease. It can aggravate thyrotoxicosis.

ADVERSE EFFECTS The most common reactions include dry mouth, nausea and GI upset, and cough. Rarely patients experience nervousness, headache, drowsiness, and even confusion. Blurred vision can occur, especially if this product is inadvertently sprayed into the eyes. Ipratropium can contribute to mucus plugging in severely dehydrated patients.

INTERACTIONS There are no documented drug interactions with ipratropium bromide. Ipratropium bromide is described in Table 40–5.

Table 40–5. ANTICHOLINERGIC BRONCHODILATOR

DRUG NAME/ROUTE AND DOSAGE	PHARMACOKINETICS/ DYNAMICS	NURSING IMPLICATIONS
ipratroprium bromide (Atrovent)		
Adults: 2 puffs (20 μg per puff) 3–4 times daily (160 μg maximum) by MDI; 1–2 mL (250–500 μg) q 4–6 hr of solution for inhalation by nebulizer ***Children:*** Half adult dose	**Onset:** within 15 min **Peak:** 1–2 hr **Duration:** 4–6 hr **½L:** 2 hr **PB:** does not absorb **B:** by local tissue **E:** feces	**ASSESSMENT:** Assess breath sounds for wheezing and aeration. Check for hypersensitivity and overdose (cough, headache, GI upset/nausea, irritated throat, mucus plugging, tachycardia, or tremor). **INTERVENTION: Patient Teaching**—Instruct patient to not use this drug alone against acute bronchospasm, but to administer with sympathomimetic bronchodilator as ordered for more rapid reversal of symptoms. Warn patient to avoid spraying MDI into eyes to prevent blurred vision. Caution patient against mixing with cromolyn (if also ordered) to prevent precipitate. **EVALUATION:** Increased air movement, decreased wheezing, and relief of dyspnea indicate drug effectiveness.

MUCOKINETIC AGENTS

One of the most common problems of the respiratory patient is obstruction of bronchial tubes by mucus. Like bronchospasm or inflammation, mucus in the airways hinders airflow and can limit gas exchange and greatly increase the work of breathing. It also promotes bacterial growth, predisposing the patient to respiratory infections.

This problem is especially serious for the patient with thick, viscous mucus who cannot cough effectively. Patients with COPD, bronchiectasis, cystic fibrosis, and pneumonia can have copious amounts of mucus. Control of airway secretions depends on the patient's clinical circumstances. The most effective means for mobilizing mucus from airways is a strong cough. Moist, fluid secretions are easiest to mobilize. The simplest and most reliable means of rehydrating thick, dried secretions is an adequate fluid intake. If this is impracticable, rehydration may require the use of water or saline aerosols as wetting agents. Delivered via large-volume nebulizer, they are usually sufficient to promote secretion mobility.

When mucus is very thick and wetting agents are unable to loosen it, an aerosolized *mucolytic* (an agent that dissolves mucus) may be used. **Acetylcysteine (Mucomyst)** and the proteolytic enzyme **Dornase alfa (*rhDNAse; Pulmozyme*)** help break up thick secretions. *Expectorants,* such as **guaifenesin (Robitussin)** and various iodide preparations, help produce thinner secretions that are more easily expectorated.

ACTION

Acetylcysteine helps dissolve mucus by breaking strong disulfide bonds in mucoprotein molecules, replacing them with weaker sulfhydryl bonds. Proteolytic enzymes lyse DNA strands in thick, purulent secretions, such as

those generated by chronic airway infection. Expectorants stimulate mucous glands to secrete thinner, less viscous mucus. All of these drugs make removal of mucus easier, although they increase mucus volume.

USES

Mucolytics and proteolytic enzymes are used to control thick, difficult-to-expectorate secretions. Proteolytics have been used with greatest success by patients with chronically infected lungs, such as those with cystic fibrosis or bronchiectasis. By making their thick, bacteria-laden mucus easier to expectorate, aerosolized enzymes help reduce the frequency of acute respiratory infections in these patients. Expectorants are used to make mucus expectoration easier.

CONTRAINDICATIONS AND PRECAUTIONS

Mucolytics are to be used with caution by asthmatic patients; they should not use proteolytic enzymes, because of the elevated potential for generating allergy. Patients with hypersensitivity to any of these substances (including expectorants) should not use them. Patients with thyroid problems should not receive iodide expectorants because of their ability to further alter thyroid function.

ADVERSE EFFECTS

Mucolytics and proteolytic enzymes may precipitate bronchospasm in some patients, so they are usually administered with a bronchodilator. Oral irritation, sore throat, cough, nausea and vomiting, and headache have been reported with the use of these agents. Expectorants may cause nausea, headache, and allergic response. In addition, iodide preparations can cause parotitis, thyroid enlargement, or rash.

Table 40–6. MUCOKINETIC AGENTS: EXPECTORANTS, MUCOLYTIC, AND PROTEOLYTIC ENZYMES

DRUG NAME/ROUTE AND DOSAGE	PHARMACOKINETICS/ DYNAMICS	NURSING IMPLICATIONS
EXPECTORANTS		
guaifenesin (many cough products) **Adults:** 200–400 mg q 4 hr **Children (6–7 yr):** 100–200 mg q 4 hr (1200 mg daily maximum) **Children (2–5 yr):** 50–100 mg q 4 hr (600 mg daily maximum)	**Onset:** rapid (<30 min) **Peak:** NA **Duration:** 4–6 hrs **½L:** NA **PB:** NA **B:** liver **E:** urine	**ASSESSMENT:** Assess character of cough and sputum. Watch for hypersensitivity and for adverse effects (GI upset, nausea, vomiting). **INTERVENTION: Patient Teaching**—Instruct patient to avoid drinking fluids for 30 min after taking cough medications to promote demulcent effects. Tell patient to not chew capsules, but to swallow them whole. Advise patient to seek medical help if cough persists for more than wk or is accompanied by fever, headache, or rash. **EVALUATION:** The effectiveness of this drug is demonstrated by increased sputum clearance.
iodide preparations (various products) **Adults:** 300–600 mg qid of saturated solution of potassium iodide; or, 60 mg qid of iodinated glycerol **Children:** Half adult dose	**Onset:** NA **Peak:** NA **Duration:** NA **½L:** NA **PB:** NA **B:** NA **E:** urine and breast milk	**ASSESSMENT:** Same as for guaifenesin. **INTERVENTION:** Administer with fruit juice or milk to disguise bitter taste. (Give drug with whole glass after meals to minimize gastric irritation.) Advise patient to discontinue if rash or other sign of sensitivity appears. **EVALUATION:** Same as guaifenesin.
MUCOLYTIC		
acetylcysteine (Mucomyst) **Adults and Children:** 3–5 mL of 20% solution (or 6–10 mL of 10% solution) 3 or 4 times daily by aerosol; 140 mg/kg followed by 70 mg/kg q 4 hr for 17 doses orally (for acetaminophen OD)	**Onset:** rapid **Peak:** 1–2 hr **Duration:** brief **½L:** 6.25 hr **PB:** 50% **B:** local-acting, small amounts metabolized by liver **E:** in respiratory mucus and in urine	**ASSESSMENT:** Assess character of cough (Is it productive? Is sputum thick and viscous? How much sputum is produced? Does patient have difficulty raising sputum?) Check for sensitivity (wheezing, nausea). **INTERVENTION:** Have patient rinse mouth after therapy to prevent oropharyngeal irritation. When 25% of drug remains in nebulizer, dilute with equal amount of normal saline solution to minimize drug reconcentration. Promote adequate fluid intake to help decrease sputum viscosity. Be prepared to suction airways if patient has ineffective cough. Inform physician and consider recommending concurrent bronchodilator if wheezing occurs. Store unused drug for up to 4 days in refrigerator; discard after 4 days. Administer orally as ordered for acetaminophen poisoning or as loosening agent for inspissated intestinal contents in cystic fibrosis. **EVALUATION:** Effectiveness of this drug is demonstrated by increased sputum productivity and decreased sputum viscosity.
PROTEOLYTIC ENZYME		
dornase alfa (Pulmozyme) (rhDNAse) **Adults and Children (>5 yrs):** 2.5 mL once or twice daily (2.5–5.0 mg)	**Onset:** 15 min **Peak:** NA **Duration:** NA **½L:** NA **PB:** NA **B:** NA **E:** NA	**ASSESSMENT:** Assess character of cough and sputum: most effective for thick, purulent, difficult to raise sputum. Watch for signs and symptoms of hypersensitivity (wheezing, stridor, harsh cough, sore throat). Assess for pregnancy category B. **INTERVENTION:** Have patient rinse.

NA = not available.

Table 40-7. SIGNS OF BRONCHIAL OBSTRUCTION

Sign	Degree of Obstruction		
	Mild	*Moderate*	*Severe*
Breath sounds	Wheezing on auscultation	Wheezing may be audible without stethoscope	All breath sounds greatly diminished
Use of accessory muscles	Minimal	Marked	Maximal
Dyspnea	Mild	Moderate	Severe
Respiratory pattern	Slightly elevated	Elevated rate, prolonged exhalation	Elevated rate, prolonged exhalation
Heart rate and pulse	Slightly elevated, strong pulse	Tachycardia, usually accompanied by bounding pulse	Tachycardia; pulse may be weak, thready
Mental status	Alert, may be anxious	Alert, often anxious and irritable	May be somnolent, disoriented

INTERACTIONS

Taken orally, acetylcysteine can be used to alter the metabolic pathway of acetaminophen, acting as an effective antidote for acetaminophen overdose. Iodide expectorants may alter radioactive iodine tests.

Mucolytics, proteolytic enzymes, and expectorants play relatively minor roles in the treatment of bronchial obstruction. Table 40-6 describes key features of these drugs.

USING THE NURSING PROCESS

The nurse assesses the causes and the extent of bronchial obstruction, as well as the effects of therapeutic intervention. Often bronchial obstruction occurs suddenly, and prompt treatment is necessary. The nurse must recognize the primary signs and symptoms of bronchial obstruction, presented in Table 40-7, so that proper therapy can be initiated. Relevant assessment data are featured in Table 40-8.

ASSESSMENT

- Recognize major indicators of respiratory distress, notably use of accessory muscles, tachypnea, tachycardia, anxiety, diaphoresis, and prolonged expiration. Cyanosis may or may not be present. The patient often assumes an upright posture to maximize breathing comfort. Generally, respiratory distress reflects the degree of bronchial obstruction present.
- Auscultate breath sounds to confirm airway obstruction. Bronchospasm and airway inflammation cause wheezing, high-pitched musical sounds heard more commonly during exhalation. Loud wheezing indicates mild to moderate bronchospasm, while quieter, higher-pitched wheezes indicate a more severe degree of airway obstruction. Wheezing patients often describe their chests as feeling "tight." Excessive mucus in the airways causes rumbling or gurgling sounds, usually accompanied by a moist or productive cough.
- Assess relevant laboratory data. Elevated white blood cell count usually confirms the presence of infection, the specific cause of which is determined through sputum culture. Arterial blood gases (ABGs) indicate whether obstruction is impeding oxygenation or ventilation. Pulmonary function measurements that indicate airflow obstruction include decreased vital capacity, prolonged exhalation time, and decreased peak flow rate.

NURSING DIAGNOSIS

Suggested nursing diagnoses for the patient who requires agents to counter airway obstruction include Ineffective Breathing Pattern, Ineffective Airway Clearance, and Impaired Gas Exchange (see Table 40-8).

PLANNING AND INTERVENTION

- The effectiveness of medications delivered by inhalation depends on the proper use of aerosol delivery devices, shown in Figure 40-1. Delivery of medications by aerosol is generally safe, convenient, and simple to administer. It makes self-medication simple. It has the advantage of providing for rapid onset of drug action and limits systemic side effects. Conversely, aerosol delivery is imprecise, requires patient cooperation and coordination, and holds the potential for abuse because of ready availability.

Become familiar with the various types of aerosol delivery systems available and assess patient suitability. Metered-dose inhalers (MDIs) are compact, portable, gas-powered canisters that have gained wide usage. They are convenient and appropriate for most people, but weakened patients may find them difficult to operate. Small-volume nebulizers are easier for patients to use, but are less portable and require an external gas source. Powdered drug delivery

Table 40–8. NURSING PROCESS FOR PATIENT WITH BRONCHIAL OBSTRUCTION

Assessment

Assess respiratory pattern; note use of accessory muscles, pursed lip breathing, tachypnea, diaphoresis, and prolonged exhalation. Auscultate breath sounds.
Assess history of seasonal allergies.
Assess respiratory status in presence of increasing anxiety.
Assess history for presence of hypertension, angina, arrhythmias, thyroid dysfunction, narrow-angle glaucoma, diabetes.

Nursing Diagnoses: Ineffective Airway Clearance, Impaired Gas Exchange, Ineffective Breathing Pattern	Desired Outcomes/Evaluation Criteria
RELATED TO: Bronchial obstruction, increased sputum volume and viscosity, altered oxygenation status. **AS EVIDENCED BY:** Difficulty in expectorating secretions, presence of crackles and/or wheezes, dyspnea, changes in rate or depth of respirations, restlessness	Demonstrates improved ventilation and adequate oxygenation with ABGs within patient's normal ranges and absence of symptoms of respiratory distress.

Nursing Actions/Evaluation Criteria	Rationale
Maintain airway, elevate head of bed or position patient appropriately. Provide airway assistance or suctioning as needed.	Promotes adequate ventilation.
Encourage deep breathing, use of pursed lip coughing exercises; splint chest/incision while coughing.	Promotes passage of air through breathing, narrowed airways. Splinting maximizes effort while minimizing discomfort associated with cough.
Increase fluid intake within nonproscribed expectoration.	Liquefies secretions and facilitates limits.
Administer medications as indicated, e.g. theophylline, albuterol, cromolyn.	Respiratory medications promote airflow and help open narrowed airways.
Schedule/carefully time administration of intermittent drugs with aerosol therapy.	Provides for more sustained drug effects, maximizing effectiveness and minimizing potentiation of side effects.
Administer supplemental oxygen as indicated.	Provides additional oxygen for cellular uptake, relief of dyspnea.
Review laboratory findings, e.g., ABGs, pulmonary function tests.	Identifies therapeutic needs, evaluates effectiveness of therapy.

Other Suggested Nursing Diagnoses: Knowledge Deficit, Anxiety, Impaired Home Management Maintenance, and Activity Intolerance.

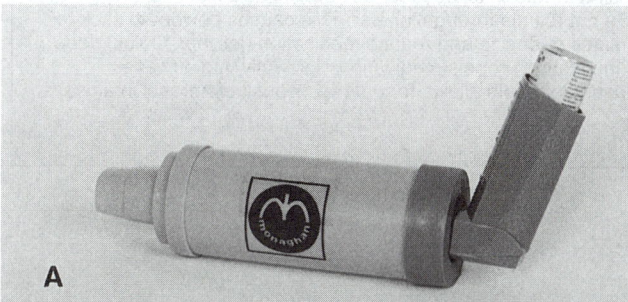

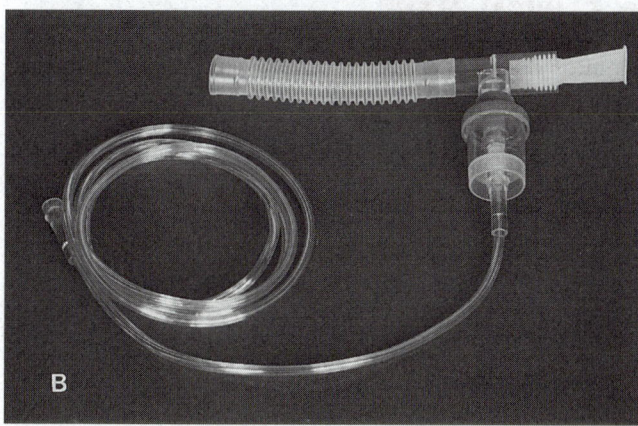

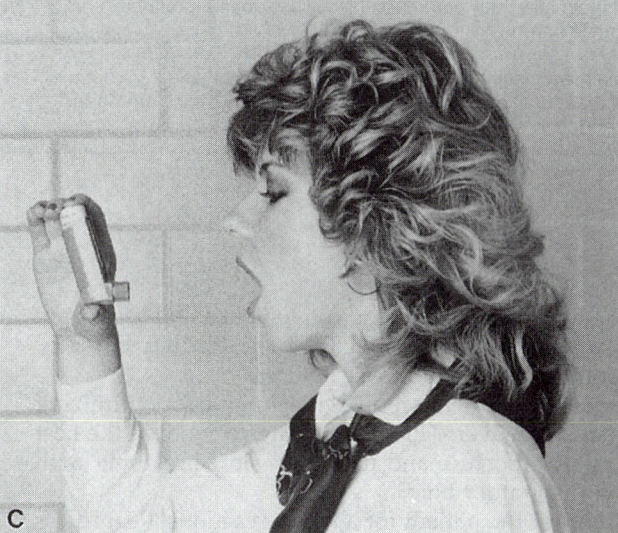

Figure 40–1. Delivery systems for aerosol medications. (A) Metered dose inhaler (with spacer). (B) Small-volume nebulizer. (C) Proper use of metered dose inhaler. (A and B from Hess, D: Aerosolized drug delivery: Technical aspects. In Kacmarek, RM, and Stoller, JK (eds): Current Respiratory Care. BC Decker, Toronto, 1988, p 58, with permission. C from Petty, TL, and Nett, LM: Enjoying Life with Emphysema, ed 2. Lea & Febiger, Philadelphia, 1987, p 45, with permission.)

Table 40–9. AEROSOL MEDICATION DELIVERY SYSTEMS: INSTRUCTING THE PATIENT

Instructions for Patient	Remarks/Rationale
I. General Rules for Use of All Types of Aerosol Medication Delivery Systems	
• Sit upright, using good posture.	Good posture allows patient to take deepest breath.
• Keep chin level or slightly upward.	This provides more direct route for medication to enter airways.
• Hold nebulizer upright an inch from mouth; open mouth wide.	This ideally minimizes deposition of drug in mouth.
• Exhale fully.	This allows for deeper inspiration.
• Inspire deeply and slowly until lungs are full.	Steady inspiratory flow enhances even distribution of medication in airways.
• Hold breath for several seconds.	This promotes maximum deposit and absorption of medication.
• Clean mouthpiece thoroughly after each use.	This minimizes infection risk and helps ensure optimal nebulizer function.
II. Special Instructions for Use of Metered-Dose Inhaler (MDI)	
• Shake cartridge before each activation.	This disperses medication thoroughly throughout the propellant and ensures uniform dosage delivery.
• Begin deep inspiration through mouth, and depress cartridge fully.	Puff of medication must be delivered at beginning of inspiration to ensure deposit of aerosol in distal airways. Full depression of cartridge ensures delivery of full dose. Coordination of effort is essential for optimal effectiveness.
• Wait 1–2 minutes between inhalations.	This allows any reflex bronchial narrowing from first puff to subside. Also minimizes risk of adverse reaction to propellant.
• Take only as many puffs as prescribed.	This helps prevent overdose.
IF PATIENT USES SPACER (AEROSOL CHAMBER):	
• Shake canister well just before attaching it to spacer.	Use of aerosol spacer simplifies administration of metered-dose aerosol medication. MDI is not easy to shake once it is attached.
• Exhale into room while pressing canister once to spray medication into spacer.	Aerosol is momentarily suspended in chamber.
• Inhale deeply from spacer mouthpiece and hold inspiration for several seconds.	The chamber reduces need for close coordination of activation of manual efforts and inhalation. More aerosol is available for deposit in distal airways and less will be swallowed.
III. If Nebulizer Is Powered by Oxygen or by Compressor	
• Use fingertip regulator or tip nebulizer on its side to deliver medication only on inspiration.	This prevents wasting of medication.
• Turn on compressor, or, if using oxygen from wall outlet, adjust flow meter to 5–7 liter/min.	Sufficient flow is needed to provide adequate aerosolization of medication.
IV. If Patient is Using Inhaler for Use with Powdered Medications	
• Insert capsule into inhaler and break it according to manufacturer's directions. Keep inhaler upright.	Holding inhaler improperly can cause medication to spill.
• Hyperextend neck.	This allows patient to keep inhaler upright and provides more direct route to airways for powder.
• Exhale fully into room, then place lips around mouthpiece and inhale sharply.	Do not exhale through inhaler: This causes powder to stick to sides of device and reduce medication delivery. Quick, deep inspiration propels medication more fully into airways.
• Maintain inspiration for 3–4 seconds, then exhale into room. Repeat until capsule is empty. Several inhalations are often needed to empty capsule.	Inspiratory hold allows for optimal deposit of aerosol in airways.

systems are as small and convenient as MDIs and are gaining in popularity. Table 40–9 discusses key points in operating these devices.

• Assist the patient on proper technique for optimizing aerosol delivery. Ensure that the patient has the best possible posture and uses deep slow breathing with an inspiratory hold.

• Monitor the patient for adverse reactions. Regardless of type, all bronchodilators can cause a substantial increase in heart rate. If the pulse rises significantly, an alternative medication may be needed. Monitor the electrocardiogram (ECG) in patients with known cardiovascular problems who need bronchodilator therapy.

▼ **CLINICAL ALERT**

Monitor the patient receiving theophylline carefully for signs of toxicity. Nausea, nervousness, tremor, headache, and tachycardia may indicate blood levels higher than 20 μg/mL. If the patient exhibits these signs, and if the theophylline level exceeds this range, withhold the next dose and notify the physician.

• Bronchodilators are often used in combination, making the patient more susceptible to adverse effects. Note the development of all adverse effects and make

Table 40–10. PATIENT TEACHING—AGENTS USED TO TREAT BRONCHIAL OBSTRUCTION

Dear Patient:

This medication has been prescribed for you. This is what you must know in order to get the most from your therapy.

☐ 1. Bronchodilators are generally taken by adults for their entire lifetime. Children who take these drugs often outgrow the need for them before reaching adulthood.

☐ 2. Take your pulse before and after using your bronchodilator. If your pulse rises by more than 20–30 beats per minute, tell your physician.

☐ 3. Taking theophylline with meals may minimize stomach upset. Other bronchodilators can be taken with or without food.

☐ 4. If you are taking prescribed beta-blockers or calcium channel blockers, consult your physician if wheezing worsens.

☐ 5. Do not use over-the-counter medications for breathing relief unless specifically authorized by your physician. These medications have many undesirable side effects.

☐ 6. Stick to your dosage schedule. If you miss one dose of bronchodilator, do not double the next dose. Instead, take the missed dose and readjust your dosing schedule accordingly.

☐ 7. Do not stop taking your bronchodilator without authorization from your physician.

☐ 8. The side effects of most bronchodilators include increased heart rate, palpitations, nervousness, tremors, and sweating.

☐ 9. If you must mix drugs, be sure to mix them precisely according to your prescription.

☐ 10. Liquid mixtures of bronchodilators should be stored in the refrigerator.

☐ 11. Drink plenty of fluids to keep mucus easy to expectorate.

☐ 12. Inhaled steroids or cromolyn sodium are not bronchodilators. They should *not* be used during an acute attack of wheezing. They can aggravate your symptoms.

☐ 13. Use your bronchodilators strictly as prescribed. Use long-acting medications (such as Serevent) only as maintenance drugs and not for acute attacks of wheezing.

recommendations based on these observations concerning drug combinations and dosing schedules.

Patient Teaching

The teaching plan, presented in Table 40–10, should also include the following:

- Note any changes in breathing pattern (such as tightness in the chest, increasing dyspnea, pain) as possible signs of exacerbation.
- Be aware of common side effects and identify signs that indicate toxicity.
- Because MDIs are so convenient to use, and because many patients experience few obvious adverse effects from them, the potential for abuse exists.

EVALUATION

Effectiveness of therapy is gauged by the extent to which the patient's breathing is improved.

- Evaluate for decreased use of accessory muscles, decreased wheezing and improved aeration, improved comfort, increased ease of expectoration, and decreased anxiety.
- Evaluate compliance with the medication regimen by noting frequency of prescription refilling. MDIs usually contain a 3- to 4-week supply of medication.
- Evaluate objective indicators of improved breathing. ABG values should be with the patient's normal baseline limits, and spirometric data should improve.
- Evaluate for toxicity when bronchodilators are used. Note tachycardia, palpitations, nervousness, tremors, or nausea.

The bibliography for this chapter can be found in Appendix B, which begins on page 1054.

CHAPTER REVIEW QUESTIONS*

1. An asthmatic patient complains of frequent oral thrush infections. She states that she never had these infections before starting to take AeroBid, an inhaled corticosteroid. She expresses reluctance to continue taking this drug. Which of the following is the most appropriate action for the nurse to take?
   a. Inform the patient to stop taking the AeroBid until the thrush infection clears.
   b. Reinforce the importance of continuing the AeroBid and remind her of the need to rinse the mouth after each treatment.
   c. Tell the patient to decrease her AeroBid dosage and increase her bronchodilator dosage until the infection clears.
   d. Reassure her that the thrush infection is coincidental and is not related to the AeroBid.

2. Elena Ricardo is a 15-year-old asthma patient who presents to your hospital's emergency department with a severe asthma attack. Which of the following bronchodilators is *least* appropriate to administer in this situation?
   a. Albuterol.
   b. Metaproterenol.
   c. Salmeterol.
   d. Isoproterenol.

3. As a nurse in the pulmonary clinic, you instruct patients on proper medication use. Mr. Kingman, a patient you instructed last week on the use of Tilade (nedocromil) states that he doesn't want to continue taking the drug because it has made no difference in his asthma symptoms. Which of the following responses is most appropriate?
   a. Reassure him that the drug is appropriate based on the findings of his physician and ask him to be patient.
   b. Explain to him that this drug relieves symptoms for only a certain percentage of asthmatics who take it and that he may be one who cannot benefit from it.
   c. Remind him that this agent requires a few weeks of administration before any results can be expected.

*See Appendix A, which begins on page 1051, for answers.

   d. Accept his decision and reaffirm his right to refuse all medications.

4. Mrs. Keller has a very moist cough. Upon auscultation you determine that she has coarse rumbles. Her cough is occasionally productive of thick secretions, which she finds difficult to raise. Which of the following drugs would be most helpful for her?
   a. Beclomethasone.
   b. Metaproterenol.
   c. Cromalyn sodium.
   d. Acetylcysteine.

5. Mr. Keenes, a 33-year-old patient with asthma, complains of anxiety and shakiness, nausea, and palpitations after taking Theo-Dur (an extended-release theophylline preparation). Which of the following actions is *least* appropriate for the nurse to take?
   a. Check the appropriateness of Mr. Keenes' dosage.
   b. Ask the physician to authorize a check of Mr. Keenes' serum theophylline level.
   c. Reassure Mr. Keenes that these effects are normal and that they will disappear after a few doses.
   d. Review the importance of swallowing (not chewing) extended-release products.

6. Your patient with a nagging cough cannot control it with lozenges alone, so her physician orders an expectorant containing guaifenesin. As the nurse you instruct her to:
   a. Monitor her pulse closely, and observe for tremors and nervousness.
   b. Withhold fluids for 30 minutes after taking guaifenesin.
   c. Chew capsules thoroughly before swallowing.
   d. Contact her physician if the cough persists longer than 3 weeks.

7. When administering a metered-dose inhaler to a patient, it is most important for the nurse to ensure that the patient:
   a. Lies in a semi-Fowler's position.
   b. Holds the chin in a downward position.
   c. Holds breath for several seconds after inspiring the medication.
   d. Places the lips firmly around the nebulizer mouthpiece.

BUILDING YOUR CRITICAL THINKING SKILLS

METERED DOSE INHALERS

Case Study 1: Atrovent vs. Albuterol

A 64-year-old patient is admitted to the emergency department with severe dyspnea caused by an exacerbation of his chronic obstructive pulmonary disease (COPD). On auscultation the nurse hears moderate wheezing. The patient reports that he used his albuterol metered-dose inhaler (MDI) "dozens of time" in the hours preceding his coming to the hospital. Albuterol is administered with minimal effect.

1. What pathophysiologic mechanisms could be causing the patient to have bronchospasm?
2. What factors could be contributing to the lack of therapeutic effect for albuterol MDI?
3. What course of action should be taken to relieve the patient's bronchospasm?
4. What nursing interventions would assist the patient's breathing?

Case Study 2: Alupent

A 20-year-old female student has a history of lifelong asthma. She has remained generally free from wheezing for most of the year and experienced only one or two self-limiting asthma attacks during allergy season. This past year, however, she has had several severe attacks, and has noticed that she now has a slight chronic wheeze. For several years she has used a metaproterenol (Alupent) inhaler for relief from episodic bronchospasm. Although the drug seems to be effective against acute bronchospasm, it does not seem to control her persistent wheezing. She asks if there are any stronger bronchodilators available.

1. What could be the cause of the patient's persistent wheezing?
2. What additional data could be gathered at this time?
3. What additional therapies might be considered for this patient and why?

CHAPTER 41

Miscellaneous Respiratory Agents

Robert W. Hirnle, MS, RRT

CHAPTER OUTLINE

Antirhinitis Agents
Antitussive Agents
Lung Fluid Replacement Therapy
Oxygen Therapy

TABLES

Drug Tables
Common Antihistamines, 603
Common Decongestants, 604
Common Antitussives, 608

Nursing Process
Nursing Process for Patient Requiring Antirhinitis
    Medications, 606
Nursing Process for Patient Requiring Antitussives, 610

Patient Teaching
Patient Teaching—Antihistamines and Decongestants, 607
Patient Teaching—Antitussives, 611

BOXES

Delivering Home Health Care, 612
Building Your Critical Thinking Skills, 613

KEY TERMS

antihistamine   protease inhibitor
antitussive   rhinitis
decongestant   surfactant

LEARNING OBJECTIVES

After reading this chapter, the student will be able to:
1. Differentiate the various mechanisms of action, routes of administration, pharmacokinetics, adverse effects, contraindications, and interactions among medications that affect the respiratory system.
2. Categorize drugs as antihistamines, decongestants, or antitussives.
3. Formulate appropriate nursing diagnoses by identifying specific areas to assess in the patient who requires respiratory medications.
4. Plan the nursing interventions necessary to administer respiratory system medications and choose appropriate teaching strategies to gain patient compliance.
5. Evaluate the patient at appropriate intervals during treatment to determine appropriateness of nursing interventions.

A variety of drugs affect respiration. In addition to those that relieve bronchial obstruction (discussed in the previous chapter), agents such as antihistamines and decongestants are used to reduce the discomfort of rhinitis. Antitussives relieve the torment of a wracking cough. Growing in importance are agents that replace vital components of lung fluid. These include enzyme-replacing agents, which are being used to help prevent a genetically based form of emphysema, and surfactants, which have profoundly altered the course of respiratory problems in premature infants and possibly in adults.

ANTIRHINITIS AGENTS

Rhinitis, or inflammation of the nasal passages, is caused by allergies, infections, and chemical or physical irritants.

Swollen nasal membranes produce extra mucous and serous fluid, and the victim is often tormented by severe nasal itching. Tissue edema swells the epithelium, making breathing through the nose uncomfortable or difficult. The sufferer of rhinitis endures constant sneezing, sniffing, and dripping. *Antihistamines* help relieve symptoms of rhinitis caused by allergy, while *decongestants* provide relief for nonallergic rhinitis.

ANTIHISTAMINES

Histamine is one of many naturally occurring chemical mediators found throughout the body's tissues and organs. These mediators are stored primarily in basophils and mast cells of the skin, gut, and respiratory system. Tissue injury releases these chemicals, triggering the inflammatory response. Vasodilation, hyperemia, and increased capillary permeability create the edema and discomfort associated with inflammation.

Antihistamines commonly in use include **brompheniramine *(Dimetane)*, clemastine *(Tavist, Travist-1, Travist-D, azelastine HCL [Astelin])* chlorpheniramine *(Chlor-Trimeton)*, diphenhydramine *(Benadryl)*,** and the newest group of nonsedating antihistamines—**terfenadine *(Seldane)*, astemizole *(Hismanal)*, loratadine *(Claritin)*, cetirizine hydrochloride *(Zyrtec)*,** and **fexofenadine *(Allegra)*** Table 41–1 features selected antihistamines.

Action

Antihistamines are agents that compete with histamine for space on histaminic receptors. These agents do not inhibit the release of histamine, but they do antagonize most of its effects. Antihistamines decrease capillary permeability and reverse the vasodilation present at the site of inflammation. They help prevent further extravasation of fluid from the blood vessels and so reverse tissue edema.

Uses

Antihistamines are commonly used to treat the irritating symptoms of allergic rhinitis (hay fever), sinusitis, and conjunctivitis. They are found alone or combined with other medications as remedies for coughs and colds. These agents are highly effective in relieving the itchy, swollen mucous membranes of the eyes, nose, and throat.

Table 41–1. COMMON ANTIHISTAMINES

DRUG NAME/ROUTE AND DOSAGE	PHARMACOKINETICS/ DYNAMICS	NURSING IMPLICATIONS
brompheniramine maleate (Dimetane)		
Adults: 4 mg q 4–6 hr PRN (24 mg daily maximum); extended release (ER), 8–12 mg q 8–12 hr PRN PO *Children:* 2 mg q 4–6 hr PRN (12 mg daily maximum); ER, 8–12 mg q 12 hr PRN	**Onset:** 15–60 min **Peak:** 3–9 hr **Duration:** 4–25 hr **½L:** 12–35 hr **PB:** NA **B:** liver **E:** urine	**ASSESSMENT:** Obtain medications history to assess for potential interactions. Assess for contraindications (glaucoma, urinary retention, prostatic hypertrophy, peptic ulcer, 3rd trimester pregnancy). Assess for adverse effects (sedation, dry mouth and throat, difficulty raising phlegm). **INTERVENTION:** Recommend antihistamine use for relief of allergic rhinitis or the common cold. Recommend use at bedtime to reduce effects of daytime drowsiness. Encourage fluid intake to keep secretions moist. **Patient Teaching**—Instruct the patient to avoid alcohol and other CNS depressants that can potentiate antihistamine effects and to avoid driving or operating machinery until CNS effects are known. Tell patient to expect drowsiness to become less prominent with repeated doses. Warn patient to discontinue use of drug at least 72 hr in advance of prescribed allergy testing. Tell patient to discontinue drug and notify health care provider if visual changes, weakness, fatigue, palpitations, irritability, confusion, or urinary retention occur. **EVALUATION:** Effectiveness of this drug is evidenced by alleviation of allergy or cold symptoms. If no improvement is seen, another antihistamine can be tried. Symptoms persisting beyond 5–7 days may require fuller evaluation.
clemastine fumarate (Tavist, Travist-1, Travist-D)		
Adults: 1.34 mg and 2.68 mg twice daily PO tablets; 10–20 mL (1–2 mg) twice daily (6 mg daily maximum) PO syrup *Children:* half adult dose	**Onset:** 15–60 min **Peak:** 2–4 hr **Duration:** 10–12 hr **½L:** NA **PB:** NA **B:** liver **E:** urine	Same as for all antihistamines.
terfenadine (Seldane)		
Adults: 60 mg PO twice daily *Children 6–12 yr:* 30–60 mg PO twice daily *Children 3–6 yr:* 15 mg PO twice daily	**Onset:** 1–2 hr **Peak:** 3–6 hr **Duration:** NA **½L:** 16–24 hr **PB:** 97% **B:** liver and GI tract **E:** feces and urine	Same as for all antihistamines plus: **ASSESSMENT:** Same as for all antihistamines. Plus, terfenadine generally causes less drowsiness than other antihistamines. **INTERVENTION:** Avoid use with erythromycin antibiotics and other drugs that prolong the QT interval.

NA = not available.

Table 41–2. COMMON DECONGESTANTS

DRUG NAME/ROUTE AND DOSAGE	PHARMACOKINETICS/ DYNAMICS	NURSING IMPLICATIONS
phenylephrine hydrochloride (Neo-Synephrine) *Adults:* 0.5%, 2–3 gtt/spray, q 4 hr by nasal drops or spray *Children 6–12 yr:* 0.25%, 2–3 gtt/spray, q 4 hr by nasal drops or spray	**Onset:** 1–2 min **Peak:** 5–10 min **Duration:** ½–4 hr **½L:** NA **PB:** NA **B:** liver **E:** urine	**ASSESSMENT:** Assess patient's history for possible contraindications to decongestant use. Obtain medication history to determine possible drug interactions. Assess pregnancy status: Decongestants should not be used during pregnancy. **INTERVENTION:** Recommend topical spray decongestant for short-term therapy (less than 3 consecutive days) for nasal congestion caused by allergy. Recommend oral decongestants for long-term therapy, such as treatment of cold symptoms. To minimize systemic absorption when administering topical decongestant sprays, apply medication with the patient in upright position. Administer drops to nostrils with head tilted back. Following instillation of drops, have patient remain in head-tilted position for a few minutes. Encourage self-care measures, hydration, and humidification. **Patient Teaching**—Instruct the patient to identify symptoms that are relieved by decongestants. Caution patient to avoid using topical decongestants for more than a few days; these agents can be habit-forming. Tell patient to rinse nasal droppers and spray bottle tips after each use to minimize potential for bacterial contamination. Advise patient to use oral preparations for long-term therapy. Caution patient against using dencongestants with caffeinated beverages, as they can cause nervousness, tremors, or insomnia. Warn patient to discontinue use if symptoms of toxicity appear (headache, nausea, vomiting, heart irregularity, extreme nervousness, confusion, delirium, or muscle tremors). Advise patient against using decongestants for more than 5–7 days without medical supervision. Warn patient that prolonged use of topical preparations can cause rebound congestion. Advise patient to administer to children only those preparations specifically designated for children. **EVALUATION:** Topical decongestants should provide relief within minutes; oral preparations should relieve symptoms within an hour. If patient experiences systemic adverse reactions, review proper administration and dosage of decongestant. With continued adverse effects, discontinue use and consult health care provider.
phenylpropanolamine hydrochloride (Triaminic) (Contac) (many others) *Adults:* 25 mg PO q 4 hr; slow release, 75 mg PO q 12 hr (maximum 150 mg daily) *Children 6–12 yr:* 12.5 mg PO q 4 hr (maximum 75 mg daily) *Children 2–6 yr:* 6.25 mg q 4 hr PO	**Onset:** 15–30 min **Peak:** 1–2 hr **Duration:** 3 hr (12–16 hr ER) **½L:** 3–4 hr **PB:** NA **B:** liver **E:** urine	Same as for all decongestants.
pseudoephedrine hydrochloride (Sudafed) (various others) *Adults:* 60 mg PO q 4–6 hr; ER, 120 mg q 12 hr (maximum 240 mg daily) *Children 6–12 yr:* 30 mg PO q 4–6 hr (maximum 120 mg daily) *Children 2–6 yr:* 15 mg liquid q 4–6 hr (maximum 60 mg daily)	**Onset:** 15–30 min **Peak:** ½–1 hr **Duration:** 4–6 hr (8–12 hr ER) **½L:** NA **PB:** NA **B:** liver **E:** urine	Same as for all decongestants.

Table 41–2. COMMON DECONGESTANTS, *Continued*		
DRUG NAME/ROUTE AND DOSAGE	**PHARMACOKINETICS/ DYNAMICS**	**NURSING IMPLICATIONS**
oxymetazoline hydrochloride (Afrin spray) (Dristan extended spray)		
Adults: 2–3 gtt/spray each nostril morning and bedtime or q 8–12 hr of 0.5% spray ***Children 6–12 yr:*** same as adults ***Children 2–6 yr:*** 2–3 gtt/spray each nostril morning and bedtime or q 8–12 hr of 0.25%	**Onset:** 1–2 min **Peak:** 5–10 min **Duration:** up to 12 hr ½L: NA PB: NA B: NA E: NA	Same as for all decongestants.

NA = not available.

Their anticholinergic effects make them strong drying agents and antipruritics. Because of their action on central histaminic receptors, some antihistamines are used to treat motion sickness and are sold as over-the-counter (OTC) sedatives. They are vital in the reversal of anaphylactic shock.

Contraindications and Precautions

Antihistamines are contraindicated in patients with known sensitivity to their ingredients. Because of their anticholinergic activity, antihistamines are not to be used by patients with prostatic hypertrophy, narrow-angle glaucoma, hyperthyroidism, peptic ulcer disease, and cardiac dysrhythmias. They cause thick secretions, so they are used with caution by patients with bronchial asthma. Antihistamines can cause sensitivity to sunlight, so patients are advised to protect themselves from the sun. Their safe use during pregnancy has not been established.

Adverse Effects

Common adverse effects of antihistamines include drowsiness, dry mouth, and headache. Less often they can cause blurred vision, urinary retention, nausea, and gastrointestinal (GI) upset. Additional adverse effects include dizziness and hypotension. They can also cause hyperexcitability in children.

The nonsedating antihistamine group (excluding cetirizine hydrochloride and fexofenadine) may cause cardiovascular effects, including lethal dysrhythmias, by lengthening the QT interval. It is important to take a drug history to eliminate the concurrent use of the nonsedating antihistamine with other drugs that lengthen the QT interval (e.g., some antidysrhythmics, erythromycins, and ketoconazole). Seizures may also occur with the drugs in this group. Adverse effects are more common and accentuated in patients over age 60.

Interactions

Monoamine oxidase (MAO) inhibitors may prolong or potentiate the anticholinergic (drying) and central nervous system (CNS) effect of antihistamines. Concurrent use with CNS depressants or alcohol potentiates sedative effects. Allergen skin tests may be negated by antihistamines: Do not use them for at least 72 hours prior to such tests.

DECONGESTANTS

Nonallergic rhinitis resembles the allergic symptoms of hay fever without the familiar irritating itchiness. Common decongestants include **phenylephrine hydrochloride** *(Neo-Synephrine)*, **phenylpropanolamine hydrochloride** *(Triaminic, Contac)*, **pseudoephedrine hydrochloride** *(Sudafed)*, and **oxymetazoline hydrochloride** *(Afrin, Dristan extended sprays)*. These drugs are featured in Table 41–2.

Action

Decongestants stimulate alpha-adrenergic receptors in nasal arterioles, restricting blood flow. Vasoconstriction further reduces leakage of fluid from capillaries into the tissues. This decreases pressure on lymph vessels; once reopened, lymph drainage removes accumulated fluid and tissues return to normal.

Uses

Decongestants are used to treat the stuffiness and drippy nose associated with the common cold, flu, or nonallergic sinusitis.

Contraindications and Precautions

Decongestants are contraindicated in patients who are sensitive to adrenergic amines. They are not used by severely hypertensive patients, those with advanced coronary artery disease, nursing mothers, or persons using MAO inhibitor antidepressants. Decongestants can aggravate hyperthyroidism, diabetes, glaucoma, prostatic hypertrophy, and insomnia. Tachyphylaxis occurs commonly.

Adverse Effects

Decongestants can cause excessive dryness of mucous membranes. Topical administration can cause sneezing and mucosal stinging. Rebound congestion is relatively common, which limits the usefulness of these drugs in many people. Because they are adrenergics, decongestants may stimulate the cardiovascular system, causing palpitations, hypertension, and tachycardia. CNS effects commonly include restlessness, tremor, anxiety, insomnia, and dizziness. Nausea, appetite loss, and urinary retention are additional adverse reactions.

Interactions

MAO inhibitors and tricyclic antidepressants can increase the sympathomimetic activity of decongestants. Concurrent use with beta-blockers may decrease effects of both drugs. Use with digitalis glycosides may precipitate dysrhythmias. Decongestants also decrease the effects of many antihypertensive agents.

USING THE NURSING PROCESS

Assessment of Patient Requiring Antirhinitis Medications

Allergies and the common cold share several symptoms, including nasal congestion, rhinorrhea (drippy nose), and sneezing. The patient with these symptoms who also complains of itching eyes and nasal passages is likely to be experiencing an allergy and will benefit from antihistamine therapy. The patient who has no indication of allergy will respond best to decongestants. Typical assessment data to collect appear in Table 41–3.

Nursing Diagnosis

Possible nursing diagnoses for the patient requiring antirhinitis therapy include the following: Ineffective Airway clearance; Risk for Injury (related to antihistamine-induced drowsiness); Altered Oral Mucous Membrane (related to drying effects of medications); and Pain (see Table 41–3).

Planning and Intervention

- Monitor the patient on antihistamine therapy for sedative effects.
- Promote hydration and alleviation of dry mouth by ensuring adequate fluid intake.
- Observe for anxiety, restlessness, insomnia, and agitation in the patient taking decongestants. Withhold medication and inform physician if symptoms become severe.

Table 41–3. NURSING PROCESS FOR PATIENT REQUIRING ANTIRHINITIS MEDICATIONS

Assessment

Assess onset of rhinorrhea, nasal stuffiness, sneezing, cough, myalgia, and characteristics/location of discomforts.
Assess frequency and effectiveness of cough effort.
Assess concurrent health problems (e.g., heart disease, asthma, narrow angle glaucoma, urinary retention, pregnancy or lactation, diabetes) and drug use (e.g., MAO inhibitors, CNS depressants, tricyclic antidepressants, adrenergic medications, or digitalis preparations).
Assess previous use of antihistamines/decongestants and any adverse reactions. Determine present self-medication and length of use.
Assess knowledge regarding OTC medications and self-care practices for specific cold symptoms.

Nursing Diagnosis: Impaired Airway Clearance and Pain	Desired Outcomes/Evaluation Criteria
RELATED TO: Excessive secretions and inflammation of nasal passages. **AS EVIDENCED BY:** Complaints of difficulty breathing, itchy nasal passages, and stuffy nose; noisy respirations; cough; possibly sore throat.	Demonstrates improved clearing of nasal secretions; reports alleviation of localized discomfort.

Nursing Actions	Rationale
Recommend an effective antihistamine and/or decongestant as appropriate.	Use of antihistamines can dry secretions and decrease itchiness of allergic rhinitis; decongestants can relieve nasal stuffiness. Use unless contraindicated by preexisting medical conditions or concommitant drug use.
Encourage adequate hydration with oral intake of 2–3 liters per day, use of room humidifier.	Adequate hydration and use of warm fluids help counteract drying side effects of drugs by keeping secretions loose and facilitating expectoration.
Recommend abstention from smoking.	Smoking can decrease clearance mechanisms and may aggravate nasal congestion.
Note complaints of persistent or worsening congestion.	May indicate misuse or overuse of topical nasal decongestant.
Recommend a safe and effective analgesic for myalgia associated with allergy.	OTC analgesics (e.g., acetaminophen, aspirin) are usually effective in relieving myalgia.

- Assess for urinary retention or difficulty in urination.

Patient Teaching

- Stress the importance of avoiding alcohol and other CNS depressants while on antihistamine therapy to minimize the danger of additive effects.
- Suggest caffeinated beverages to help counter antihistamine-induced drowsiness.

▼ **CLINICAL ALERT**

Antihistamines cause severe drowsiness in many patients. Warn the patient to avoid driving, operating machinery, and all potentially dangerous activities until the sedative effect of antihistamines is controlled.

- Suggest hard candy, lozenges, chewing gum, or ice chips for dry mouth.
- Caution against concurrent use of OTC medications because adrenergics may potentiate the adverse effects of decongestants.
- Suggest antihistamines be taken with food or milk to minimize nausea, except for astemizole, which should be taken on an empty stomach.
- Report any adverse cardiovascular effects such as palpitations or tachycardia. Patient teaching measures concerning antirhinitis medications are listed in Table 41–4.

Evaluation

Successful antihistamine or decongestant therapy is demonstrated by a decrease in the symptoms of rhinitis with an absence of adverse effects.

- Evaluate for reduced nasal stuffiness, increased comfort with nasal breathing, reduction of nasal secretions, and less sneezing.
- Evaluate for adverse cardiovascular and CNS effects.

ANTITUSSIVE AGENTS

The cough reflex is a protective mechanism that helps remove sputum from the airways. Physical irritants (such as heat, cold, or dryness), chemical irritants (noxious gases, aspirated liquids, histamine, and so on), and mechanical irritants (such as dusts and foreign bodies) stimulate impulses that are relayed to the cough center in the medulla and then to the respiratory muscles. The resultant forceful expulsion of air helps propel mucus and any trapped irritants out of the airways.

A cough that produces mucus is useful. However, a nonproductive cough is simply an annoyance. It can cause pain in the postsurgical patient and disrupts sleep and comfort in all patients.

Antitussives are agents that decrease the intensity and frequency of coughing episodes. "Cough medicines" are among the most commonly used types of medication. Dozens of prescription and nonprescription antitussive preparations are available in the United States and Canada. **Codeine** and **hydrocodone** are important narcotic antitussives, while **benzonatate (*Tessalon Perles*), dextromethorphan,** and **diphenhydramine *(Benylin)*** are the

---

Table 41–4. PATIENT TEACHING— ANTIHISTAMINES AND DECONGESTANTS

Dear Patient:
This drug has been prescribed for you. This is what you should know about your medication to get the most from your therapy.

If you are taking an antihistamine:

☐ 1. Antihistamines cause drowsiness, so driving or operating machinery can be dangerous. If these activities cannot be avoided, please exercise extra caution.
☐ 2. Check with your physician before using any OTC medications. Do not drink alcoholic beverages because they compound the drowsiness caused by antihistamines.
☐ 3. Coffee or caffeinated beverages may help counteract drowsiness caused by antihistamines.
☐ 4. Antihistamines can dry your mouth. Drinking fluids, chewing gum, and sucking hard candies can help relieve oral dryness.
☐ 5. Notify your physician if unusual symptoms such as nervousness, difficulty with urination, or dizziness occur.
☐ 6. If your antihistamine becomes less effective at relieving allergy symptoms, inform your physician. Another antihistamine may be prescribed in its place.
☐ 7. Inform your physician if drowsiness becomes intolerable. Another antihistamine that causes less drowsiness may be prescribed in its place.
☐ 8. Headaches may occur, but they are usually resolved with a mild analgesic. If they are severe or persistent, consult your physician.
☐ 9. Be sure not to exceed your prescribed dosage. Dangerous side effects can occur if you take too much of some antihistamines.
☐ 10. Be sure to closely follow any dietary instructions about whether or not to take with food. A full or empty stomach can affect the way antihistamines work.
☐ 11. Stop taking this drug 3 days before any scheduled allergy testing sessions. This helps ensure that test results will be accurate.
☐ 12. Some antihistamines make you sensitive to sun. Use a sunscreen to avoid sunburn.

If you are taking a decongestant:

☐ 1. Use topical decongestants (nasal sprays or nose drops) only for acute episodes of rhinitis and for no longer than 3 to 5 days.
☐ 2. Nasal stuffiness may worsen with chronic use of decongestants. If this happens, avoiding their use for several days may allow the nose to regain its responsiveness to these drugs.
☐ 3. Don't use decongestants too often. Nervousness, insomnia, or restlessness may occur with excessive use.
☐ 4. To avoid insomnia, do not take decongestants within 2 hours of bedtime.
☐ 5. Consult your physician before taking any OTC drugs for colds if you are already taking drugs for your breathing.

Table 41–5. COMMON ANTITUSSIVES

DRUG NAME/ROUTE AND DOSAGE	PHARMACOKINETICS/ DYNAMICS	NURSING IMPLICATIONS
NARCOTIC ANTITUSSIVE AGENTS		
codeine, codeine phosphate, codeine sulfate (many products)		
Adults: 10–20 mg PO q 3–4 hr (maximum 120 mg daily) **Children 6–12 yr:** 5–10 mg PO q 4–6 hr (maximum 60 mg daily) **Children 2–6 yr:** 1.5–5.0 q 4–6 hr PO (maximum 30 mg daily)	**Onset:** less than 30 min **Peak:** 1–1.5 hr **Duration:** 4–6 hr **½L:** 3 hr **PB:** 30%–35% **B:** liver **E:** urine, feces	**ASSESSMENT:** Check cough and secretions to ensure that they are mobile. Check for nausea, vomiting, or abdominal pain before administering. Check for bowel function. Assess history for hypersensitivity, contraindications (including asthma, pregnancy), or potential interactions. Although addiction potential is mild, assess for excessive use. Assess for adverse effects (respiratory depression, hypotension, bradycardia, sedation, confusion, constipation, headache). **INTERVENTION: Patient Teaching**—Inform patient of sedative effects, and caution against operating automobiles or machinery. Ensure adequate hydration to assist in raising mucus. Instruct patient to avoid alcohol and other depressants. **EVALUATION:** Effectiveness of this drug as a cough suppressant is evaluated in terms of decreased intensity and frequency of cough.
hydrocodone (Hycodan) (Hycomine)		
Adults: 5–10 mg 3 or 4 times daily PO **Children 2–12 yr:** 2.5 mg PO 3 or 4 times daily **Children 1–2 yr:** 1.25 mg PO 3 or 4 times daily	**Onset:** rapid **Peak:** 30–90 min **Duration:** 4–8 hr **½L:** 4 hr **PB:** 30%–35% **B:** liver **E:** urine, feces	Same as for codeine.
NON-NARCOTIC ANTITUSSIVE AGENTS		
benzonatate (Tessalon Perles)		
Adults: 100 mg PO 3 times daily (maximum 600 mg daily) **Children:** 8 mg/kg per day PO in 3–6 doses	**Onset:** 15–20 min **Peak:** NA **Duration:** 3–8 hr **½L:** NA **PB:** NA **B:** NA **E:** NA	**ASSESSMENT:** Same as for codeine, except addiction potential is low. **INTERVENTION:** Instruct patient to swallow drug rapidly to avoid local anesthetic effect on tongue and throat. **EVALUATION:** Same as for all antitussives.
dextromethorphan (Robitussin DM) (many others)		
Adults: 15–30 mg PO 3 or 4 times daily PO **Children 6–12 yr:** 5–10 mg PO q 4 hr **Children 2–6 yr:** 2.5–5.0 PO mg q 4 hr	**Onset:** 15–30 min **Peak:** 1–2 hr **Duration:** 3–6 hr **½L:** NA **PB:** NA **B:** liver **E:** NA	**ASSESSMENT:** Check cough and secretions to ensure they are mobile. **INTERVENTION:** Same as for codeine, plus do not take water for 30 min to optimize antitussive effect. **EVALUATION:** Same as for codeine.
diphenhydramine hydrochloride (Benylin)		
Adults: 25–50 mg and id or QID **Children:** 12.5 mg and id or QID	**Onset:** 15–60 min **Peak:** 1–2 hr **Duration:** 4–8 hr **½L:** 2.4–9.3 hr **PB:** 80%–85% **B:** liver **E:** urine	Same as for all, plus: **Patient Teaching:** Use sunscreen to protect against photosensitivity.

NA = not available.

primary non-narcotic antitussives available. These antitussive agents are described in Table 41–5.

ACTION

Centrally acting antitussives (which include the narcotic preparations) modify the cough reflex by suppressing the cough center's stimulation threshold, making it less responsive to incoming impulses from the irritant receptors. Peripherally acting antitussives decrease the irritant receptors' sensitivity to stimulation.

USES

Antitussives are indicated for control of disruptive, harsh nonproductive cough.

CONTRAINDICATIONS AND PRECAUTIONS

Antitussives are contraindicated for use by patients with hypersensitivity to any ingredient contained in the various preparations. Narcotic preparations must be used with caution by patients with head trauma, severe renal or liver disease, hypothyroidism, or adrenal insufficiency. In addition to these precautions, use non-narcotic preparations cautiously in patients with hypotension, seizure disorders, glaucoma, or prostatic hypertrophy. Safe use during pregnancy has not been established. Observe age-specific dosing recommendations on each antitussive product.

ADVERSE EFFECTS

Narcotic antitussives commonly cause sedation, drowsiness, and constipation. Nausea, vomiting, blurred vision, sweating and flushing, and psychologic or physical dependence are also potential problems caused by narcotic antitussives. The most serious adverse effects of narcotic overdose include hypotension, bradycardia, and respiratory depression.

Adverse effects of nonnarcotic antitussives vary depending on the type of preparation. Like the narcotic agents, antihistamine cough preparations (e.g., diphenhydramine) cause drowsiness, blurred vision, dizziness, and headache. In addition, they cause dry mouth, palpitations, thickened respiratory mucus, anorexia, urinary retention or frequency, dysuria, diarrhea, and skin photosensitivity. Benzonatate preparations can cause similar CNS and gastrointestinal (GI) effects, but additionally can cause nasal congestion, burning eyes, and pruritic skin eruptions.

INTERACTIONS

Narcotic cough suppressants (as well as antihistamine agents) are potentiated by monoamine oxidase (MAO) inhibitors, alcohol, anticholinergics, sedatives, and tranquilizers. Narcotic effects are reversed by narcotic antagonists.

▼ **CLINICAL ALERT**

Patients using MAO inhibitor antidepressants should not use dextromethorphan-containing preparations, because this combination can cause coma, hypotension, hyperpyrexia, and death.

USING THE NURSING PROCESS

Assessment of Patient with Cough

- Assess cough productivity. Does the patient raise sputum? Or is the cough dry?
- Assess cough frequency. Are coughing sessions brief and self-limiting? Or are coughing episodes repeated and lengthy? Is the patient tired and short of breath afterwards?

▼ **CLINICAL ALERT**

Narcotic antitussives may become habit-forming. Patients who request narcotic-containing antitussives frequently, or who express a need for them when their cough is well controlled, may be at risk for development of dependence on these agents. Closely assess the patient's need for antitussives, and explore their reasons for requesting them.

- Assess whether the cough disrupts sleep patterns. Does it cause pain or discomfort? See Table 41–6 for other suggested assessment data to collect.

Nursing Diagnosis

Possible nursing diagnoses for the patient who requires antitussive therapy include Ineffective Airway Clearance and Pain (see Table 41–6).

Planning and Intervention

Once the patient is comfortable, plan the patient's schedule to allow for additional rest as needed.

- Group together procedures and disturb the sleep-deprived patient as seldom as possible to provide for longer periods of uninterrupted sleep.
- Because codeine-containing preparations cause constipation, initiate preventive measures as needed.
- Encourage fluids to the patient with a dry hacking cough to promote thin, easily expectorated secretions.

Table 41–6. NURSING PROCESS FOR PATIENT REQUIRING ANTITUSSIVES

Assessment

Assess cough for quality and frequency (including time of day); note whether productive or nonproductive, as well as amount and consistency of sputum.
Assess complaints of pain, disruption of sleep associated with coughing.
Assess level of knowledge regarding treatment regimen.

Nursing Diagnosis: Pain	**Desired Outcomes**
RELATED TO: Mucosal irritation caused by dry, hacking, nonproductive cough. AS EVIDENCED BY: Complaints, guarding behavior.	Reports pain is relieved or minimized.

Nursing Actions	**Rationale**
Administer narcotic antitussive (e.g., codeine preparation) or non-narcotic antitussive (e.g., diphenhydramine). Provide room humidification. Encourage increased fluid intake.	These drugs decrease the force and frequency of nonproductive coughing, and they promote comfort. Soothes dry mucosa and thins secretions to aid expectoration.
Promote use of hard candy, throat lozenges, and cough drops as indicated.	These exert a local soothing effect on the throat, decreasing irritating tickle, dryness, and discomfort.

Nursing Diagnosis: Sleep Pattern Disturbance	**Desired Outcomes/Evaluation Criteria**
RELATED TO: Consistent or recurrent cough. AS EVIDENCED BY: Interrupted sleep, irritability; verbalization of being poorly rested.	Reports improvement in sleep/rest pattern with increased sense of well-being and feeling rested.

Nursing Actions	**Rationale**
Administer medications as ordered hs. Provide comfort measures (e.g., back rub, warm bath).	Promotes suppression of cough to allow for increased length/quality of sleep. Promotes relaxation and improves quality of rest.
Encourage adequate balance between rest and activity. Provide for uninterrupted periods of sleep/rest.	Conserves energy, prevents undue fatigue, promotes general well-being.

- Consider antihistamines or decongestants if the cough appears to be caused by allergy or postnasal drips.
- Encourage use of hard candy (as appropriate) to help keep throat moist.

Patient Teaching

The teaching plan includes the following:

- Do not drink liquids for half an hour after taking cough syrup or using a lozenge, to maximize locally soothing effects.
- Because some cough medicines cause drowsiness, be aware of the danger in driving or operating machinery.
- Do not exceed recommended dosages of cough medicines, as they have the potential for abuse.
- Because narcotic side effects are potentiated by alcohol, do not drink alcoholic beverages while using these cough preparations.
- Use a vaporizer as tolerated to help decrease coughing.

Patient teaching information is summarized in Table 41–7.

Evaluation

- Evaluate frequency and intensity of the patient's cough. A decrease in both with an increase in patient comfort indicates antitussive success.
- Evaluate the frequency of the patient's requests for cough medicine. Excessive need may indicate abuse.

LUNG FLUID REPLACEMENT THERAPY

Traditional treatment for emphysema and for infant respiratory distress syndrome has been primarily limited to supportive measures. Recent advances in pharmacology have contributed greatly to improving morbidity from

Table 41–7. PATIENT TEACHING—ANTITUSSIVES

Dear Patient:
This drug has been prescribed for you. This is what you should know about your medication to get the most from your therapy.

☐ 1. Antitussives are used for the harsh, irritating, nonproductive cough. If your cough produces sputum, you should not take antitussives unless the cough disrupts sleep patterns.
☐ 2. Antitussive therapy is normally of short duration. When the cough diminishes in intensity and frequency, antitussive therapy should be discontinued. If a harsh cough persists for several days, seek medical advice.
☐ 3. Take no liquids or food for one-half hour after taking an antitussive. This allows the medication to soothe the inflamed tissues of the throat.
☐ 4. If the antitussive contains a narcotic or antihistamine, do not consume alcohol during the course of therapy. Use barbiturates only as directed by your physician.
☐ 5. Do not exceed single-dose or 24-hour prescribed dosage of the antitussive.
☐ 6. Major side effects include drowsiness, decreased coordination, constipation, and potential for abuse.
☐ 7. Use caution when driving or operating machinery, as many antitussives may diminish alertness.
☐ 8. Keep antitussives away from children.

these diseases. Although quite dissimilar, these disorders share one common feature: some cases of each disease are caused by deficiencies of specific lung fluid components. Some patients with emphysema genetically lack an enzyme-inhibiting protein. Infants born prematurely and adults with adult respiratory distress syndrome (ARDS) are deficient in surfactant. Replacement of these substances is growing in importance.

PROTEASE INHIBITOR: PROLASTIN

Lung damage caused by uninhibited proteolytic enzyme action can cause emphysema. This disease is characterized by alveolar wall destruction and severe airway obstruction. The vast majority of the millions of Americans with this disease develop it after a long history of cigarette smoking. However, a small but significant percentage of emphysema patients have never smoked. Their lung dysfunction is caused by lack of alpha-1 proteinase (also called alpha-1 antitrypsin, or *protease inhibitor*).

Neutrophils in the lungs regularly release proteases as part of the inflammatory response. Although these enzymes are useful in helping to neutralize bacteria and clear the lung of debris, they can also damage the lung itself. Ordinarily, lung fluid contains alpha-1 antiprotease, which protects lung tissues by inhibiting the actions of these proteases. Without this protein, the lung is subject to the caustic, destructive effects of protease.

○ **Alpha-1 proteinase inhibitor** (Prolastin) is derived from human plasma. It is used for chronic replacement therapy by those emphysema patients who have a genetic deficiency of natural alpha-1 antiprotease. Prolastin is supplied in single-dose vials. It is packaged as a powder that is reconstituted with sterile water and administered intravenously. A weekly dose of 60 milligrams per kilogram of body weight is typical. Treatment is usually lifelong, beginning in early adulthood. Because the drug is a plasma product, the possibility of viral transmission exists.

SURFACTANT

Surfactant is a naturally occurring phospholipid that reduces the work of breathing by decreasing alveolar surface tension. Sufficient quantities develop in the fetal lung around the 34th week of gestation. Infants born prior to this gestational age often lack enough of this important substance to keep the alveoli open and develop respiratory distress syndrome. This disorder makes the infant's lungs extremely stiff and difficult to ventilate. Very often this leads to respiratory failure, which may be fatal.

Surfactant replacement therapy can prevent and/or decrease the severity of respiratory distress syndrome and its complications. Surfactant is placed into the lung via endotracheal tube into the infant's airways. The intubated infant is placed in specific positions to ensure distribution of the fluid throughout all regions of the lung.

There are several exogenous surfactants, such as Survanta (derived from animal sources) and Exosurf (synthetic). Results of surfactant replacement have been encouraging, but some risks are associated with its use. Complications such as pulmonary hemorrhage and apnea have occasionally been noted. Also, the rapid reversal of hypoxemia that occurs with successful surfactant instillation can itself pose a potential risk to the infant. Unless the infant's supplemental oxygen is monitored closely, the resultant elevation of blood oxygen levels can expose the infant to possible toxic effects of hyperoxia, including eye damage. The long-term effects of surfactant replacement therapy are unknown.

OXYGEN THERAPY

Oxygen therapy provides tissues with sufficient oxygen to carry on metabolic processes. It is used to treat patients with decreased cardiac output, reduced blood-oxygen carrying capacity, or decreased partial pressure of oxygen in arterial blood. It is also used when the patient has increased oxygen demands. Emphysema, cor pulmonale, and acute pulmonary edema are conditions that typically require oxygen therapy. In some cases, it may be necessary for oxygen therapy to be administered at home (see Delivering Home Health Care box).

The bibliography for this chapter can be found in Appendix B, which begins on page 1054.

DELIVERING HOME HEALTH CARE

Oxygen Delivery Systems

TYPES OF OXYGEN DELIVERY SYSTEMS

High-pressure cylinders

Advantages:
• Appropriate for occasional or low-volume oxygen user.
• Widespread availability.

Disadvantages:
• Bulky, heavy cylinders are cumbersome to manage.
• High pressure poses safety hazard.
• Frequent use requires frequent delivery.

Liquid oxygen

Advantages:
• Stores large amount of oxygen in small space.
• Can be used to refill portable units.

Disadvantages:
• Oxygen evaporates when not in use.
• Extremely low temperature poses safety hazard (may cause burns).

Oxygen concentrator

Advantages:
• Provides continuous supply for high-volume user (most cost-effective option for continuous user).
• Eliminates need for oxygen delivery.

Disadvantages:
• Requires continuous electrical power to operate.
• Not useful for patient requiring high concentrations of oxygen. Limited output provides only low to medium concentrations.

SAFETY CONSIDERATIONS AND PATIENT TEACHING

• Absolutely no smoking near oxygen systems.
• Follow prescribed dose precisely; do not exceed prescribed flow rate.
• If using cylinders or liquid systems, reorder when tank is ¼ full.
• Handle cylinders and liquid tanks with extreme care.
• If traveling by plane, arrange with airline to provide in-flight oxygen. Arrange with vendor to have oxygen.

CHAPTER REVIEW QUESTIONS*

1. Mr. Klein, an operator of heavy bulldozing equipment, has severe hay fever allergy symptoms. He asks you which antihistamine would allow him to breathe comfortably and to remain awake and alert on the job. Which of the following agents would you recommend as most appropriate?
   a. Terfenadine (Seldane).
   b. Diphenhydramine (Benadryl).
   c. Chlorpheniramine (Chlor-Trimeton).
   d. Broimpheniramine (Dimetane).

2. Your patient is scheduled to begin allergy tests next week. Which of the following drugs should the patient be sure to avoid for at least 72 hours before the test?
   a. Nasal decongestants.
   b. Non-narcotic antitussives.
   c. Antihistamines.
   d. Caffeine.

*See Appendix A, which begins on page 1051, for answers.

3. Which of the following statements is *not* true about narcotic antitussive agents?
   a. Narcotic antitussive agents commonly cause sedation, drowsiness, and constipation.
   b. Narcotic antitussive agents do not cause psychologic or physical dependency.
   c. The most serious adverse effects caused by overdose of narcotic antitussive agents include hypotension, bradycardia, and respiratory depression.
   d. Narcotic antitussive agents are potentiated by MAO inhibitors and alcohol.

4. Coma, hypotension, hyperpyrexia, and death can occur when patients taking monoamine oxidase (MAO) inhibitors combine it with:
   a. Terfenadine.
   b. Dextromethorphan.
   c. Oxymetazoline.
   d. Oxygen therapy.

BUILDING YOUR CRITICAL THINKING SKILLS

ANTITUSSIVE/DECONGESTANTS

Case Study 1: Diphenhydramine (Benylin)

A 75-year-old patient develops a case of bronchitis following a mastectomy. Her harsh, rasping cough disrupts her sleep and causes her great discomfort. At times her airways are so sensitive that deep breathing triggers a coughing fit. Diphenhydramine (Benylin) cough syrup is ordered. However, after 2 days there is little relief from her coughing and she indicates that the medication has made her airways feel "tighter and drier" than before.

1. Why might Benylin not be an appropriate medication for this patient?
2. What other drugs could be used; what is the rationale for their use?

Case Study 2: Pseudoephedrine

A 48-year-old man with chronic hypertension comes to the clinic for a checkup. He indicates that he hasn't felt as well as usual lately, and wonders whether his medication (propranolol) is still effective. Assessment reveals a blood pressure significantly higher than on previous visits. He also notes that he has had a bout of severe rhinitis and nasal itching caused by seasonal allergies, which he has been treating with psuedoephedrine, an over-the-counter decongestant.

1. What could be the role of psuedoephedrine in this patient's symptoms?
2. What alternative course of action could be taken for this patient?
3. What teaching is indicated for this patient?

DRUGS AFFECTING THE ENDOCRINE SYSTEM

CHAPTER 42

Overview of the Anatomy and Physiology of the Endocrine System

Merrily A. Kuhn, RNC, PhD

CHAPTER OUTLINE

Hormones
Biorhythms

KEY TERMS

Circadian
Hormones

Negative feedback
mechanism

LEARNING OBJECTIVES

After reading this chapter, the student will be able to:

1. Identify all glands of the endocrine system and the specific hormones they secrete.
2. Describe the functions of the various endocrine hormones.
3. Explain the regulatory functions of the endocrine system.
4. Describe the feedback loops within the endocrine system.

The endocrine system is one of the body's control systems (the nervous system is the other) and produces hormones that regulate aspects of metabolism. These may be grouped into four broad categories: (1) fluid balance and pH, (2) growth and development, (3) reproduction, and (4) energy production and utilization.

The endocrine system consists of ductless glands that synthesize hormones and release them directly into the bloodstream for transport to their target organs or target tissues. (Exocrine glands, such as the pancreas with its digestive enzymes, have ducts to carry their secretions to an epithelial surface.) The endocrine glands, shown in Figure 42–1, include the pituitary, thyroid, parathyroids, pancreas (both an exocrine and endocrine gland), adrenals, ovaries, and testes. Hormone synthesis is not exclusive to endocrine glands. Estrogen, for example, can be formed from testosterone and androstenedione in ovary, brain, adipocytes, and hair follicles.

Table 42–1 reviews the endocrine glands, the hormones they produce, and their functions. Table 42–2 describes their hypofunctions and hyperfunctions.

HORMONES

Hormones are chemicals secreted by one group of cells that exert physiologic effects on other cells. The quantity of hormones in the body is normally very small compared with the quantity of other substances such as electrolytes. Structurally, hormones are either steroids, proteins or small peptides, or amines.

Compounds classified as steroids are complex molecules containing carbon atoms in interlocking rings. These include gonadal and adrenocortical hormones, sterols, bile acids, and vitamin D. Steroid hormones are synthesized from cholesterol and work directly inside a target cell by binding to intracellular receptors. Ultimately, steroid hormones stimulate the transcription of deoxyribonucleic acid (DNA) to initiate the synthesis of proteins, which may be structural proteins, secretions, or enzymes for the cell's functions.

Protein (insulin, parathyroid hormone, growth hormone, glucagon) and peptide (antidiuretic hormone

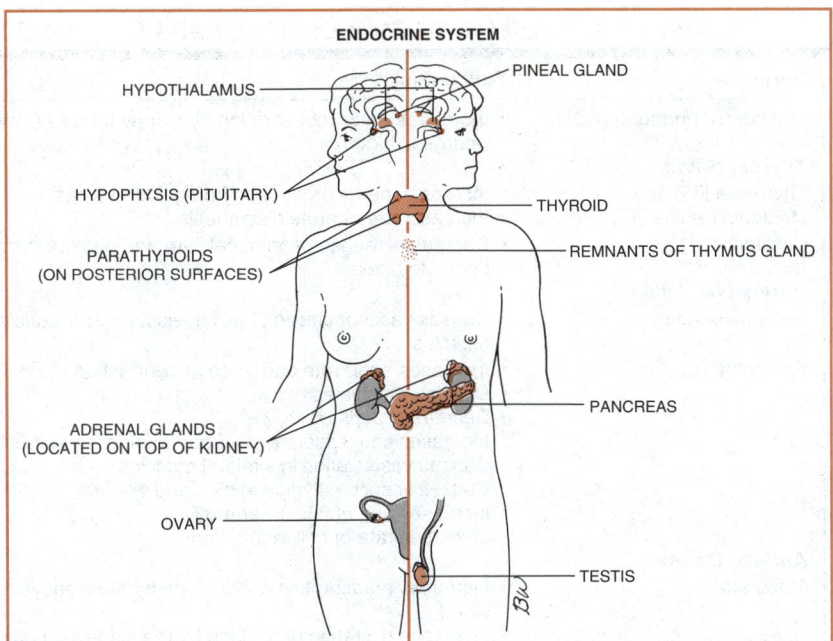

Figure 42–1. The endocrine glands, which secrete hormones directly into the bloodstream. (From Taber's Cyclopedic Medical Dictionary, ed 17. FA Davis, Philadelphia, 1993, p 640, with permission.)

Table 42–1. SUMMARY OF ENDOCRINE GLANDS AND HORMONES THEY PRODUCE

Hormone	Function(s)	Regulation of Secretion
Anterior Pituitary Gland		
Growth hormone (GH)	• Increases rate of mitosis • Increases amino acid transport into cells • Increases rate of protein synthesis • Increases use of fats for energy	• GHRH (hypothalamus) stimulates secretion • GHIH—somatostatin (hypothalamus) inhibits secretion
Thyroid-stimulating hormone (TSH)	• Increases secretion of thyroxine and T_3 by thyroid gland	• TRH (hypothalamus)
Adrenocorticotropic hormone (ACTH)	• Increases secretion of cortisol by adrenal cortex	• CRH (hypothalamus)
Prolactin	• Stimulates milk production by mammary glands	• PRH (hypothalamus) stimulates secretion • PIH (hypothalamus) inhibits secretion
Follicle-stimulating hormone (FSH)	**IN WOMEN:** • Initiates growth of ova in ovarian follicles • Increases secretion of estrogen by follicle cells	• GnRH (hypothalamus)
	IN MEN: • Initiates sperm production in testes	• GnRH (hypothalamus)
Luteinizing hormone (LH) (ICSH)	**IN WOMEN:** • Causes ovulation • Causes ruptured ovarian follicle to become corpus luteum • Increases secretion of progesterone by corpus luteum	• GnRH (hypothalamus)
	IN MEN: • Increases secretion of testosterone by interstitial cells of testes	• GnRH (hypothalamus)
Posterior Pituitary Gland		
Oxytocin	• Promotes contraction of myometrium of uterus (labor) • Promotes release of milk from mammary glands	• Nerve impulses from hypothalamus, the result of stretching of cervix or stimulation of nipple • Secretion from placenta at the end of stimulus gestation unknown

Continued on the following page

Table 42–1. SUMMARY OF ENDOCRINE GLANDS AND HORMONES THEY PRODUCE, *Continued*

Hormone	Function(s)	Regulation of Secretion
Antidiuretic hormone (ADH)	• Increases water reabsorption by kidney tubules (water returns to blood)	• Decreased water content in body (alcohol inhibits secretion)
Thyroid Gland		
Thyroxine (T_4) and triiodothyronine (T_3)	• Increase energy production from all food types • Increase rate of protein synthesis	• TSH (anterior pituitary)
Calcitonin	• Decreases reabsorption of calcium and phosphate from bones to blood	• Hypercalcemia
Adrenal Medulla		
Norepinephrine	• Causes vasoconstriction in skin, viscera, and skeletal muscles	
Epinephrine	• Increases heart rate and force of contraction • Dilates bronchioles • Decreases peristalsis • Increases conversion of glycogen to glucose in the liver • Causes vasodilation in skeletal muscles • Causes vasoconstriction in skin and viscera • Increases use of fats for energy • Increases rate of cell respiration	• Sympathetic impulses from the hypothalamus in stress situations
Adrenal Cortex		
Aldosterone	• Increases reabsorption of Na^+ ions by the kidneys to the blood • Increases excretion of K^+ ions by the kidneys in urine	• Low blood Na^+ level • Low blood volume or blood pressure • High blood K^+ level
Cortisol	• Increases use of fats and excess amino acids for energy • Decreases use of glucose for energy (except for brain) • Increases conversion of glucose to glycogen in liver • Anti-inflammatory effect: stabilizes lysosomes and blocks effects of histamine	• ACTH (anterior pituitary) during physiologic stress
Testes		

Testosterone	• Promotes maturation of sperm
	• Initiates development of secondary sex characteristics:
	   —growth of reproductive organs
	   —growth of larynx
	   —growth of facial and body hair
	   —increased protein synthesis, especially in skeletal muscles
		• LH (anterior pituitary)

Inhibin	• Decreases secretion of FSH to maintain constant rate of spermatogenesis	• Spermatogenesis
Ovaries		

Estrogen	• Promotes maturation of ovarian follicles
	• Promotes growth of blood vessels in endometrium
	• Initiates development of secondary sex characteristics:
	   —growth of uterus and other reproductive organs
	   —growth of mammary ducts and fat deposition in breasts
	   —broadening of pelvic bone
	   —subcutaneous fat deposition in hips and thighs
		• FSH (anterior pituitary)

Progesterone	• Promotes further growth of blood vessels in endometrium and storage of nutrients • Inhibits contractions of myometrium	• LH (anterior pituitary)
Parathyroid Glands		
Parathyroid Hormone (PTH)	• Increases reabsorption of calcium and phosphate from bone to blood • Increases absorption of calcium and phosphate by small intestine • Increases reabsorption of calcium and excretion of phosphate by kidneys	• Hypocalcemia
Pancreas		
Glucagon	• Increases conversion of glycogen to glucose in liver • Increases use of excess amino acids and of fats for energy	• Hypoglycemia
Insulin	• Increases glucose transport into cells and use of glucose for energy production • Increases conversion of excess glucose to glycogen in liver and muscles • Increases amino acid and fatty acid transport into cells and their use in synthesis reactions	• Hyperglycemia

Source: Adapted from Scanlon, and Sanders, FA Davis, Philadelphia, with permission.

Table 42–2. ENDOCRINE HYPOFUNCTIONS AND HYPERFUNCTIONS

Gland	Hormone	Dysfunction	
		Hyposecretion	Hypersecretion
Pituitary ADENOHYPOPHYSIS	Somatotropin, or growth hormone (GH)	Dwarfism	Giantism, acromegaly
	Thyrotropin, or thyroid-stimulating hormone (TSH)	Hyperthyroidism	Hypothyroidism
	Corticotropin, or adrenocorticotropic hormone (ACTH)	Addison's disease	Cushing's disease
	Follicle-stimulating hormone (FSH)	Anovulation, aspermatogenesis	Primary gonadal failure
	Luteinizing hormone (LH)		Primary gonadal failure
	Prolactin, or luteotropic hormone (LTH)		Amenorrhea, galactorrhea
NEUROHYPOPHYSIS	Antidiuretic hormone (ADH)	Diabetes insipidus	Syndrome of inappropriate ADH
Thyroid	Thyroxine, triiodothyronine	Cretinism, myxedema, hypothyroidism	Graves' disease, hyperthyroidism, thyrotoxicosis
	Calcitonin	Increased Ca	Decreased Ca
Parathyroid	Parathormone	Decreased Ca	Increased Ca
Pancreas	Insulin	Diabetes mellitus, ketoacidosis, hyperglycemia, hyperosmolar nonketotic coma (HHNK)	Hypoglycemia, insulin shock
Adrenals CORTEX	Mineralocorticoids (aldosterone)	Addison's disease	Hyperaldosteronism
	Glucocorticoids (cortisol)	Addison's disease, acute adrenal crisis	Cushing's syndrome
	Sex hormones (androgens, estrogens, progestins)		Adrenogenital syndrome
MEDULLA	Epinephrine, norepinephrine		Pheochromocytoma
Gonads OVARIES	Estrogen	Sexual dysfunction, infertility	Sexual dysfunction, precocious puberty
TESTES	Testosterone	Delayed male puberty, male hypogonadism	Hirsutism in women, genetic female pseudohermaphroditism

[ADH] and oxytocin) hormones bind with specific receptors on the cell membrane, activating the conversion of adenosine triphosphate (ATP) into cyclic adenosine 3',5'-monophosphate (cAMP). Cyclic AMP interacts with the enzymes in the target cell to bring about that cell's characteristic response to the hormone.

Hormones are deactivated in the liver, and the end products are excreted by the kidneys. Hepatic and renal disease may decrease the rate at which hormones are metabolized and excreted, thereby prolonging hormone function.

FEEDBACK RELATIONSHIPS

The distinguishing characteristic of the endocrine system is the feedback control of hormone production. In most instances, the control is through a *negative feedback mechanism*, which is defined as a control system in which a stimulus initiates a response that reverses or reduces the stimulus, thereby decreasing or stopping the response until the stimulus reoccurs. Figure 42–2 illustrates feedback systems. As an example, as blood glucose rises, insulin is secreted. The blood sugar then falls as insulin carries glucose into the cell for use and storage. Insulin secretion is then decreased. The main factor in this mechanism is the degree of activity of the target organ.

All hormones are under feedback control, some by cations (calcium on parathyroid hormone), some by metabolites (glucose on insulin and glucagon), some by other hormones (somatostatin on insulin and glucagon), and some by osmolality or extracellular fluid volume (ADH, aldosterone).

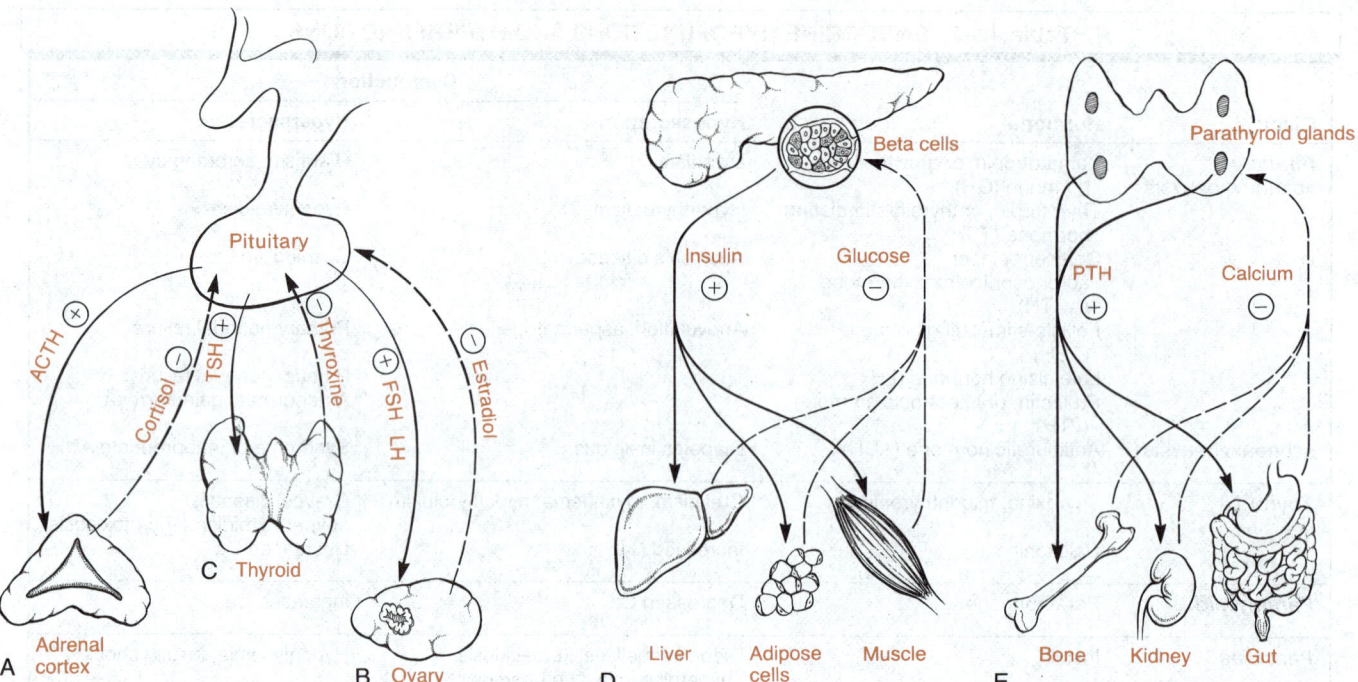

Figure 42–2. A diagrammatic representation of several feedback systems. (A), (B), and (C) represent the feedback control in which the hormonal product of the target gland acts on the release of the corresponding pituitary hormone. (D) and (E) illustrate feedback control in which the metabolic substance controlled by the hormone acts directly upon its release. Solid lines indicate direct control; dotted lines indicate feedback mechanisms. (A) Corticotropin-releasing hormone (CRH) stimulates the pituitary to release ACTH. ACTH stimulates the adrenal cortex to secrete cortisol. The effect of cortisol inhibits the secretion of CRH by the hypothalamus. (B) Gonadotropin-releasing hormone (GNRH) stimulates the pituitary to release follicle-stimulating hormone (FSH) and luteinizing hormone (LH). FSH and LH stimulate the ovaries to to release estradiol. Estradiol feeds back to the hypothalamic-pituitary axis and inhibits GNRH-FSH/LH release. (C) Thyrotropic-releasing hormone (TRH) stimulates the pituitary to release thyroid-stimulating hormone (TSH). TSH stimulates the thyroid to secrete thyroxine. The effect of thyroxine returns to the hypothalamic-pituitary axis and inhibits TRH/TSH release. (D) Insulin release is controlled by glucose in the blood. If glucose increases, insulin is secreted. If glucose decreases, insulin secretion is inhibited. (E) The parathyroid glands regulate serum calcium. A drop in serum calcium stimulates parathormone (PTH) secretion. Conversely, an increase in calcium shuts off PTH production.

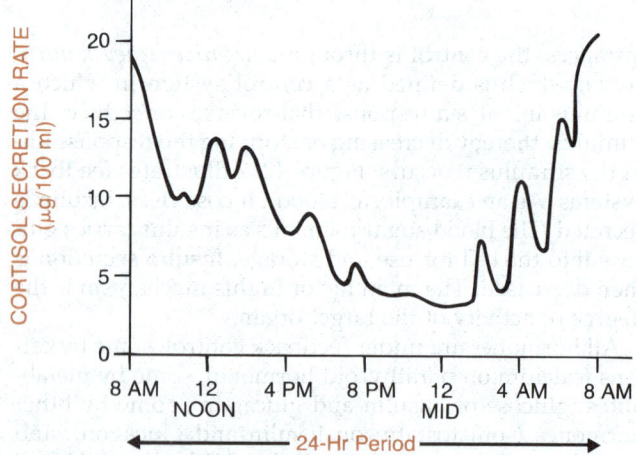

Figure 42–3. The circadian rhythm of cortisol. Cortisol peaks daily at approximately 8:00 AM and troughs daily at approximately midnight. Its production is on a day/night cycle.

BIORHYTHMS

The endocrine glands produce hormones in rhythms that can vary from hours (luteinizing hormone and testosterone) to a day (*circadian* rhythm of cortisol, depicted in Figure 42–3) to weeks (menstrual cycle) or even longer, such as seasonal variation of thyroxine. These cycles are regulated by sleep-associated alterations, light-dark cycles, and environmental factors. The mechanisms by which these rhythms operate and the physiologic ramifications of the rhythms are currently being researched.

The bibliography for this chapter can be found in Appendix B, which begins on page 1054.

CHAPTER REVIEW QUESTIONS*

1. A polypeptide hormone synthesized by the anterior pituitary gland is:
   a. Oxytocin
   b. Thyrotropin
   c. Prolactin
   d. Pituitary

2. Which statement is *correct* regarding the regulation of the endocrine system?
   a. Neuroregulation operates on a positive feedback principle.
   b. Endocrine glands secrete a limited amount of hormone when stimulated.
   c. When the target organ responds strongly, endocrine activity is suppressed.
   d. The main factor in neuroregulation is the strength of the regulating hormone.

3. Somatostatin, secreted by the hypothalamus and the delta cells of the pancreas, has the following action:
   a. Inhibition of insulin secretion.
   b. Stimulation of glucagon synthesis.

*See Appendix A, which begins on page 1051, for answers.

c. Inhibition of growth hormone.
d. Stimulation of insulin/glucagon modulates the activity.

4. Feedback loops in the endocrine system are under the control of:
   a. Metabolites, cation, or fluid volume.
   b. Hypothalamus and posterior pituitary.
   c. Circadian rhythms.
   d. Hormones only.

5. Antidiuretic hormone (ADH), or vasopressin, is released from the posterior pituitary and controls:
   a. Decreased blood pressure.
   b. Expansion of atrial stretch receptors.
   c. Decreased osmotic pressure.
   d. Water balance.

CHAPTER 43

Anterior and Posterior Pituitary Hormones

Merrily A. Kuhn, RNC, PhD

KEY TERMS

Craniopharyngioma	Neurogenic diabetes
Diabetogenic effect	insipidus
Growth hormone	Somatomedins
Ketogenic effect	

LEARNING OBJECTIVES

After reading this chapter, the student will be able to:

1. Identify those medications commonly used as pituitary drugs.
2. Differentiate among the pituitary drugs as to mechanisms of action, routes of administration, pharmacokinetics, adverse effects, contraindications and precautions, and interactions.
3. Identify specific areas to assess in the patient requiring pituitary drugs to formulate appropriate patient outcomes.
4. Plan the nursing interventions necessary to administer pituitary drugs and choose appropriate teaching strategies to gain patient compliance.
5. Evaluate the patient at various stages of treatment to gauge patient outcomes.

Many medications are used to treat dysfunction of the pituitary. Those discussed in this chapter are growth hormone (GH), secreted from the anterior pituitary; and antidiuretic hormone (ADH), secreted from the posterior pituitary. Other anterior pituitary hormones are discussed in other chapters: adrenocorticotropic hormone (ACTH), Chapter 44; and thyroid-stimulating hormone (TSH), Chapter 46. Figure 43–1 identifies the pituitary hormones, their target organs, and their specific actions.

ANTERIOR PITUITARY HORMONES

Growth hormone (GH), also known as somatotropin or somatotropic hormone (STH), is a polypeptide (protein) that has growth-promoting and anabolic properties. Growth hormone secretion is regulated by two hormones from the hypothalamus: growth hormone releasing hormone stimulates the secretion of GH, and growth hormone inhibiting hormone or somatostatin suppresses the secretion of GH. Growth hormone is available as **somatrem (Protropin)** and **somatropin (Nutropin, Humatrope).** Somatostatin is available as **octreotide acetate (Sandostatin),** a long-acting octapeptide that mimicks the action of the natural hormone. These drugs are featured in Table 43–1.

GROWTH HORMONE

Action

Growth hormone has no specific target gland; rather, many tissues are affected, leading to increased cellular and organ size and increased rates of growth. Specifically, it facilitates transport of amino acids across cell mem-

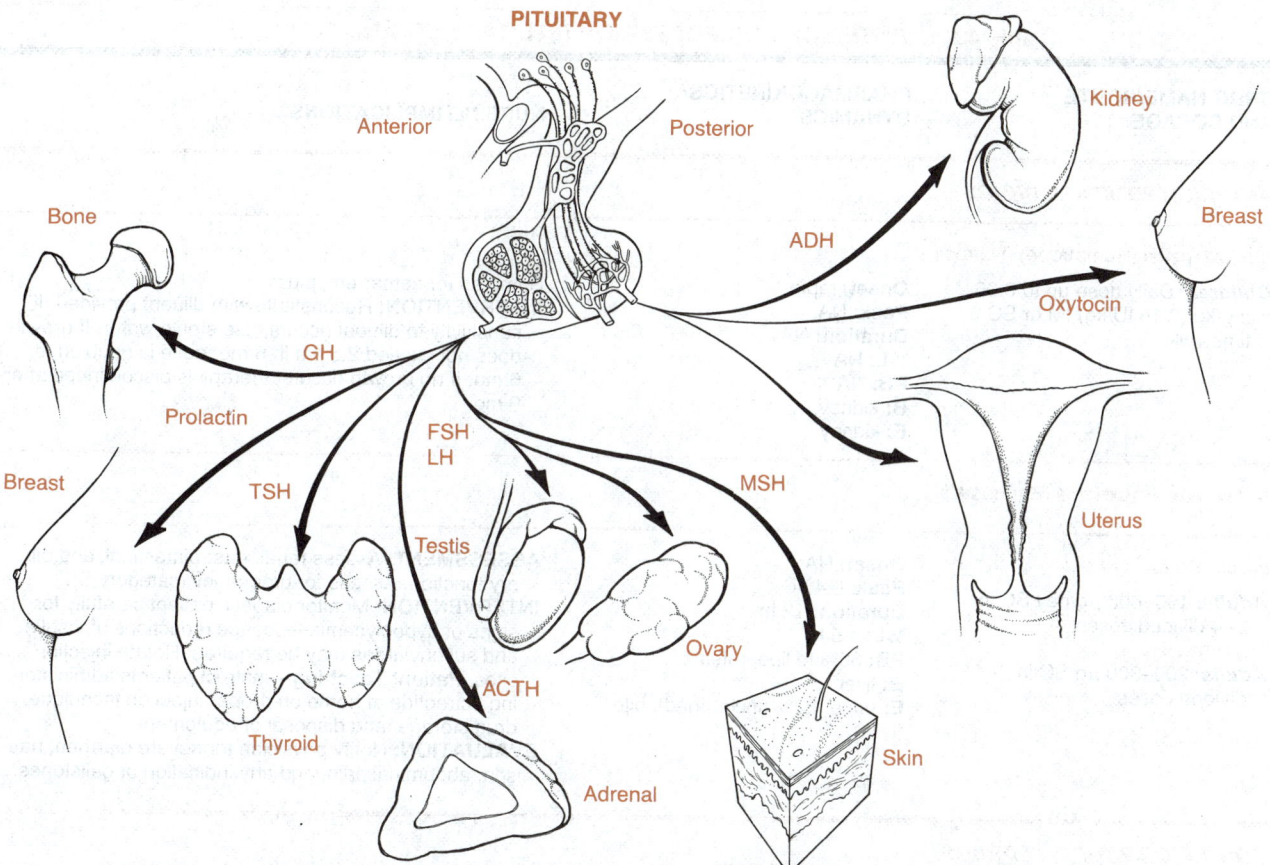

Figure 43–1. A summary of the pituitary hormones and the target organs involved with each hormone. The anterior pituitary hormones include the following: growth hormone (GH), which controls body growth and metabolism; prolactin, which controls breast growth and milk production; thyroid-stimulating hormone (TSH), which regulates the thyroid gland; follicle-stimulating hormone (FSH) and luteinizing hormone (LH), which affect function of the gonads; corticotropin, or adrenocorticotropic hormone (ACTH), which regulates the adrenal cortex; and melanocyte-stimulating hormone (MSH), which controls pigmentation. The posterior pituitary hormones include antidiuretic hormone (ADH), which affects water balance in the body; and oxytocin, which affects the breast and uterus.

Table 43–1. ANTERIOR AND POSTERIOR PITUITARY DRUGS		
DRUG NAME/ROUTE AND DOSAGE	**PHARMACOKINETICS/ DYNAMICS**	**NURSING IMPLICATIONS**
ANTERIOR PITUITARY DRUGS		
somatrem (Protropin) *Children:* Individualized maximum daily dose 0.1 mg/kg (0.26 IU/kg) IM or SC 3 times/ wk.	**Onset:** rapid **Peak:** NA **Duration:** NA **½L:** NA **PB:** NA **B:** kidney **E:** kidney	**ASSESSMENT:** Establish true pituitary deficiency. Assess glucose at onset and periodically. Assess thyroid function and treat as needed. Assess benzyl alcohol sensitivity. Assess for pregnancy (category unknown). **INTERVENTION:** Reconstitute with sterile bacteriostatic water for injection only. Do not shake. Solution should be clear with no particles. Inject into muscle or SC tissue. **EVALUATION:** Evaluate growth every 6 mo or more often.

Continued on the following page

Table 43–1. ANTERIOR AND POSTERIOR PITUITARY DRUGS, *Continued*

DRUG NAME/ROUTE AND DOSAGE	PHARMACOKINETICS/ DYNAMICS	NURSING IMPLICATIONS
ANTERIOR PITUITARY DRUGS		
somatropin (Humatrope) (Nutropin) ***Children:*** Daily dose up to 0.06 mg/kg (0.16 IU/kg) IM or SC 3 times/wk.	**Onset:** rapid **Peak:** NA **Duration:** NA **½L:** NA **PB:** NA **B:** kidney **E:** kidney	Same as for somatrem, plus: **INTERVENTION:** Reconstitute with diluent provided. If sensitivity to diluent occurs, use sterile water. If growth does not exceed 2.5 cm in 6 mo, dose is doubled for 6 mo. If no growth occurs, therapy is discontinued after 6 mo.
octreotide acetate (Sandostatin)		
carcinoid tumors ***Adults:*** 100–600 µg/day SC in 2–4 divided doses. **VI pomas** ***Adults:*** 200–300 µg SC in 2–4 divided doses.	**Onset:** NA **Peak:** 0.4 hr **Duration:** 12 hr **½L:** 1.5 hr **PB:** 65% to lipoproteins **B:** liver **E:** urine (32% unchanged), bile	**ASSESSMENT:** Assess renal, gastrointestinal, and biliary function. Assess for pregnancy (category B). **INTERVENTION:** Monitor diabetic patient carefully for signs of hypoglycemia—dosage reductions of insulin and sulfonylureas may be required. Rotate injection sites. **Patient Teaching**—Instruct patients administering octreotide at home on proper injection technique, drug storage, and disposal of equipment. **EVALUATION:** Notify physician for severe diarrhea, nausea, abdominal pain, and any indication of gallstones.
POSTERIOR PITUITARY DRUGS		
lypressin (Diapid) ***Adults and Children:*** 1–2 sprays in each nostril qid; do not use more than 3 sprays per nostril for any one dose.	**Onset:** quickly **Peak:** 30–120 min **Duration:** 3–8 hr **½L:** 15 min **PB:** NA **B:** kidney, liver **E:** urine	**ASSESSMENT:** Assess urinary output and weight at onset and periodically. Assess for presence of cardiac disease or respiratory infection. Assess for pregnancy (category unknown). **INTERVENTION:** Drug should not be inhaled. Allergic rhinitis or upper respiratory infections may affect absorption. Hold bottle upright, and patient should be in a vertical position with head upright. Do not use more than 3 sprays per nostril. **EVALUATION:** If unusual drowsiness, headache, shortness of breath, nausea, or severe nasal congestion occur, call physician.
desmopressin acetate (DDAVP) (Stimate)		
diabetes insipidus ***Adults:*** 10–40 µg/day intranasally in divided doses. ***Children 3 mo–12 yr:*** 5–30 µg/day intranasally. **hemophilia a and von willebrand's disease** ***Adults:*** 0.3 µg/kg IV dilute in normal saline. 10 kg or less—10 mL. More than 10 kg—50 mL slowly over 30 min. Administer 30 min prior to surgery. **primary nocturnal enuresis** ***Children over 6 yr:*** 0.2 mL (2 µg) intranasally at bedtime with adjustments up to 40 µg if needed; half of dose is placed in each nostril. PO, 0.05 mg bid daily. Dose range 0.1–1.2 mg divided in 2–3 doses per day.	**Onset:** 30 min **Peak:** 90–120 min **Duration:** 8–20 hr **½L:** biphasic 7.8/75.5 min **PB:** NA **B:** kidney, liver **E:** urine	Same as for lypressin except: **ASSESSMENT:** Assess for pregnancy (category B). **INTERVENTION:** Administer IV drip slowly over 15–30 min. Use for noctural enuresis for 4–8 wk only. Restrict fluid after dinner to decrease urine production.

SC = subcutaneous; NA = not available.

branes, thereby stimulating a protein-building cycle. This increases nitrogen balance and decreases urea production. GH also decreases the transport of glucose into the cells and decreases glucose utilization, which can result in what is known as the *diabetogenic effect* of growth hormone; that is, it may cause diabetes mellitus. GH also facilitates the release of free fatty acids from adipose tissues, leading to an increased fat storage in the liver and an increased availability of fatty acids for energy needs. This latter effect is referred to as the *ketogenic effect* (or lipolytic effect) of growth hormone, as it results from fat lipolysis and leads to the conversion of fatty acids to ketone bodies. Many of these actions are mediated by substances called *somatomedins* that are synthesized in the liver (and possibly in the kidney, muscle, and other tissues). Somatomedins, under the regulation of growth hormone, promote growth of cartilage and bone. Somatomedin levels increase with age up to the second decade of life. In children, growth hormone is essential to stimulate linear bone growth.

Although levels of GH are high in the neonate, it does not appear to be a requisite for either fetal or neonatal growth. After 2 to 4 weeks, this level decreases, with increases occurring after activity, during sleep, and during adolescence and pregnancy. Stress, emotional excitement, and hypoglycemia also can increase the secretion of GH. Secretion of GH is suppressed by glucocorticoid drugs.

Uses

Presently, the sole medical use for GH, or somatotropin, is to stimulate linear growth in patients with documented growth failure caused by a deficiency of endogenous GH, a condition called pituitary dwarfism. To have a therapeutic effect, the drug must be administered before the closure of the bone epiphyses. Epiphyseal closure, occurring during adolescence and sooner in females than males, varies considerably from individual to individual and is usually determined by radiographic examination of the hands and wrists. In terms of attainment of a normal adult height, the best results are obtained when the hormone administration is begun in early childhood.

▼ **CLINICAL ALERT**

The use of growth hormone (GH) raises many ethical questions. For example, should GH be prescribed for children with genetic short stature in the normal range; persons who consider a short stature to be a functional handicap; or for children whose parents focus on athletic or business advantage for a taller child? These questions and other ethical considerations need to be addressed.

Human growth hormone is also being touted as the latest miracle cure for the aging process. Some researchers claim it develops stronger muscles and bones, improves vision, and restores vitality and sexual prowess. However, at dosage levels needed to achieve antiaging effects, GH causes some serious adverse effects. These include carpal tunnel syndrome, male breast enlargement, risk of grotesque enlargement of facial features, and possibly

cancer. This is the reason that manufacturers restrict the use of GH to hormone-deficient children.

○ **Somatrem** (Protropin) **and somatropin** (Nutropin, Humatrope, Saizen) are both produced in bacteria through recombinant DNA technology. Somatropin has the same amino acid sequence as endogenous growth hormone, while somatrem has an extra methionine group.

CONTRAINDICATIONS AND PRECAUTIONS Somatrem and somatropin are contraindicated in children with closed epiphyses. Both are also contraindicated in patients who exibit evidence of underlying intracranial tumor because tumor growth rate may increase. These products are administered only under the supervision of physicians experienced in the diagnosis and treatment of patients with pituitary hormone deficiency. Caution is advised in patients with diabetes because a state of insulin resistance resulting in hyperglycemia may develop. Safety in pregnancy (category C) and lactation has not been established, so caution is exercised. Thyroid function is monitored throughout therapy owing to the possible developments of hypothyroidism.

ADVERSE EFFECTS A common adverse effect in about 30% of patients is the development of antibodies to somatrem. (This effect is not as pronounced with somatropin.) In general, these antibodies do not interfere with the growth response. In patients who are not responding to GH, antibody levels should be measured.

INTERACTIONS Concurrent corticosteriods may inhibit the growth-promoting effect of GH.

DOSAGE Dosage is individualized. If growth does not exceed 2.5 cm in a 6-month period, dosage may be doubled for the next 6 months. If no growth occurs, therapy is discontinued after 6 months.

GROWTH HORMONE INHIBITING HORMONE

○ **Octreotide acetate** (Sandostatin) is a potent inhibitor of GH and suppresses secretion of serotonin, gastrin, glucagon, insulin, and vasoactive intestinal peptide to result in a reduction in the volume of gastric and intestinal secretions.

USES Octreotide acetate is used to reduce GH levels in patients with acromegaly (too much GH), to treat the symptoms of metastatic carcinoid tumors, and to help control diarrhea in patients with vasoactive intestinal peptide tumors.

CONTRAINDICATIONS AND PRECAUTIONS Octreotide acetate is contraindicated in patients with hypersensitivity.

▼ **CLINICAL ALERT**

Octreotide acetate is administered cautiously to patients with previous biliary tract problems as there is an increase in stone formation. Patients are monitored for stone formation throughout therapy.

Octreotide acetate is used during pregnancy (category B) and lactation only if clearly needed. It is safe to use in children. Diabetic patients must be monitored closely and may require a change in their insulin dosage. Monitor closely for dysrhythmias, bradycardias, and prolongation of the QT interval.

ADVERSE EFFECTS The most common adverse effects include diarrhea, nausea, gallstone formation and abdominal discomfort. These symptoms may be dose dependent. Central nervous system (CNS) side effects include headache, dizziness, and fatigue. Hypoglycemia or hyperglycemia may also occur and are of particular problem to the diabetic.

POSTERIOR PITUITARY HORMONES

ANTIDIURETIC HORMONE

The posterior pituitary releases antidiuretic hormone (ADH), which functions to conserve water. Because pharmacologic amounts (much larger than those required for antidiuretic effect) of ADH also serve to cause widespread vasoconstriction, its synonymous name is vasopressin. In response to certain physiologic parameters within the body, ADH can either be inhibited, leading to diabetes insipidus, or released, leading to syndrome of inappropriate antidiuretic hormone (SIADH).

Available vasopressin derivatives include **vasopressin (Pitressin Synthetic)**, which is rarely used; **lypressin (Diapid)**; and **desmopressin (DDAVP, Stimate)**, which is used most commonly. Lypressin and desmopressin, synthetic analogs of vasopressin, are both available as nasal sprays, which make dosing extremely easy (see Table 43–1).

Action

Vasopressin is synthesized in the hypothalamus in the supraoptic nuclei. It is stored in the posterior pituitary to be released as needed, as the rate of hypothalamic synthesis and transport are too slow to meet immediate needs for water conservation. The primary stimuli for secretion of vasopressin are an increase in plasma osmolality as detected by osmoreceptors in the supraoptic nuclei and a decreased blood volume as detected by baroreceptors in the heart. Hemorrhage and circulatory shock probably are the most potent stimuli for release of vasopressin. Vasopressin secretion is also stimulated by pain; anxiety; and certain drugs such as nicotine, barbiturates (in large doses), chlorpropamide (Diabinese), and the tricyclic antidepressants. Other drugs inhibit vasopressin release, including alcohol, phenytoin (Dilantin), glucocorticoids, chlorpromazine (Thorazine), and reserpine (Serpasil).

In physiologic doses, vasopressin acts in the kidneys in the distal tubules and collecting ducts to increase the cellular permeability to water, thus increasing the amounts of water reabsorbed by the kidney and decreasing urine output.

In larger doses, vasopressin stimulates smooth muscle contraction, especially in small arterioles. This vasoconstriction causes decreased blood flow to the splanchnic, coronary, gastrointestinal, pancreatic, skin, and muscular systems. Direct administration of vasopressin into the superior mesenteric artery constricts the gastroduodenal, superior mesenteric, and splenic arteries. It is important to remember, though, that the amount of vasopressin necessary to promote water conservation is seldom large enough to cause this widespread pressor effect.

In similarly large doses, vasopressin also increases peristaltic activity of the large bowel and contraction of the smooth muscle of the gallbladder and urinary bladder. Some oxytocic activity may also occur, causing uterine contractions.

As with other hormones, the action and adverse effects of exogenous vasopressin are the same as those of the endogenous hormone.

○ **Vasopressin** (Pitressin Synthetic), **lypressin** (Diapid), **and desmopressin** (DDAVP, Stimate) are used primarily in the control of neurogenic or central diabetes insipidus. *Neurogenic diabetes insipidus* is a disorder of water metabolism that results from a partial or complete deficiency in the production and secretion of vasopressin from the neurohypophysis (main portion of the posterior lobe of the pituitary gland). Vasopressin injection (Pitressin) is also used as an intravenous or intra-arterial infusion via the superior mesenteric artery in the emergency management of massive gastrointestinal bleeding. Intravenous and intra-arterial infusion have been found to be equally effective; therefore, the intravenous route is preferred. Vasopressin (Pitressin) is also used to relieve postoperative intestinal gaseous distention and to dispel gas shadows appearing before abdominal roentgenography. Vasopressin (Pitressin) decreases portal blood pressure and reduces blood loss.

Desmopressin is used alone or adjunctive to behavorial conditions to control primary nocturnal enuresis. Some researchers have suggested that nocturnal production of vasopressin may be low in some enuretic children. Up to the age of 6, children do not require any therapy for nocturnal enuresis, which usually stops spontaneously in about 15% of cases each year after that. With desmopressin therapy, water intoxication, convulsion, and coma can occur. Because of this and the high incidence of spontaneous resolution, this drug should be used cautiously in children. Desmopressin is also used to control bleeding when factor VIII levels are reduced and to maintain hemostasis during surgery and postoperatively in patients with hemophilia A and von Willebrand's disease.

Pharmacokinetics and dosage for lypressin and desmopressin appear in Table 43–1.

CONTRAINDICATIONS AND PRECAUTIONS Lypressin and desmopressin are contraindicated in hypersensitive patients. Use only when clearly needed during pregnancy (Lypressin, category unknown; desmopressin, category B). Use cautiously in patients with angina as the vasoconstrictor properties may precipitate hypertension and angina. Use the nasal spray cautiously in patients who have nasal blockage, congestion, or severe atrophic rhinitis as absorption may be compromised.

ADVERSE EFFECTS Adverse effects of vasopressin are usually mild with small dosages. The most common side effects are headache, rhinitis, nausea, mild abdominal cramps, and slight elevation of blood pressure. All are related to the change in body water volume. When the nasal spray is used, rhinitis and gastric irritation may occur from the postnasal drip. Local erythema and burning pain can also occur.

INTERACTIONS Drugs that potentiate ADH also potentiate lypressin and desmopressin. These include vasopressors, carbamazepine, and chlorpropamide.

USING THE NURSING PROCESS

- Obtain a thorough nursing history to establish the database. Tables 43–2 and 43–3 summarize the nursing process for patients requiring somatotropic hormones and for patients requiring antidiuretic drugs, respectively.

ASSESSMENT

Patients Requiring Growth Hormone

- Assess growth patterns of the child. Repeated physical examination of the child yields important information relative to growth patterns.
- Obtain and monitor plasma levels of growth hormone, which are detected by immunoassay.

Two important points in relation to diagnostic testing are made. First, almost one-half of the children with growth hormone deficiency have deficiencies of other tropic hormones (TSH, ACTH); therefore, careful evaluation for other hormone deficiencies is necessary. (See Chapters 44 and 46 for information on testing related to adrenal and thyroid hormones.) Second, careful assessment is performed for any signs and symptoms of *craniopharyngioma* (a tumor of the pituitary gland, which is the most common pituitary tumor in children and the most common cause of prepubertal hypopituitarism). This may include skull radiography and computerized axial tomography. It is important to question the parents about any history of nausea, vomiting, headache, loss of vision, or increase in head circumference—all indications of increased intracranial pressure.

Patients Requiring Antidiuretic Hormone

- Assess for the signs and symptoms of diabetes insipidus, which can be either sudden or insidious in onset. Signs of dehydration such as dry skin and mu-

Table 43–2. NURSING PROCESS FOR PATIENT REQUIRING SOMATOTROPIC HORMONES

Assessment

Assess linear bone growth, weight and height comparisons.
Assess plasma levels of growth hormone (by immunoassay) and radiograph for bone age to determine epiphyseal closure.
Assess effect of condition on child's self-esteem.
Assess concomitant/previous use of glucocorticoids, thyroid preparations.
Assess family history for presence of diabetes mellitus.

Nursing Diagnosis: Altered Growth and Development	Desired Outcomes/Evaluation Criteria
RELATED TO: Deficiency of growth hormone. AS EVIDENCED BY: Altered physical growth.	Verbalizes understanding of developmental deviation and plans for interventions.

Nursing Actions	Rationale
Administer somatotropin as ordered.	Used to stimulate linear growth in patients documented to have growth failure caused by a deficiency of endogenous GH or pituitary dwarfism.
Discuss administration, safety factors, and possible adverse side effects with both parents and child.	Understanding of the pituitary function and need for continued therapy and monitoring helps the family to cooperate with treatment regimen.
Request parent to accurately measure and record height at regular intervals.	Indicator of success of treatment or need to alter or discontinue therapy.
Discuss importance of annual elevation of bone age.	Monitors the effectiveness of therapy and determines epiphyseal closure.

Nursing Diagnosis: Body Image/Self-Esteem Disturbance	Desired Outcomes/Evaluation Criteria
RELATED TO: Failure to develop at an expected rate, size; is smaller than peers. AS EVIDENCED BY: Depression.	Verbalizes increased sense of self-esteem in relation to individual situation. Demonstrates adaptation to changes as evidenced by setting of realistic goals and active participations in play and relationships.

Nursing Actions	Rationale
Discuss child/parent perceptions of condition/threat to self.	Provides base on which to decide appropriate interventions. Identifies depth of concern.
Stress need to avoid comparing self with others. Active-listen to expressions of concern. Use I-messages to provide information and give positive feedback.	Helps patient to focus on own concerns and abilities. Conveys sense of caring, support, promoting belief in patient's own ability to manage situation.
Support patient's need to progress at own rate.	Adaptation to change depends on its significance to individual, how disruptive it is, and degree and length of debility.

Other Suggested Nursing Diagnosis: Knowledge Deficit.

**Table 43–3. NURSING PROCESS FOR PATIENT REQUIRING ANTIDIURETIC DRUGS
(VASOPRESSIN, LYPRESSIN, DESMOPRESSIN)**

Assessment

Assess history of cardiovascular disease, hypertension.
Assess presence of irritability and general weakness.
Assess accurate baseline measurement of body weight.
Assess serum and urine osmolality and results of water deprivation test.

Nursing Diagnosis: Fluid Volume Deficit	**Desired Outcomes/Evaluation Criteria**
RELATED TO: Failure of regulatory mechanisms. **AS EVIDENCED BY:** Large urinary output, dehydration, and weight loss.	Demonstrates improved fluid balance as evidenced by individually appropriate urinary output, stable vital signs and weight, moist mucous membranes, good skin turgor.

Nursing Actions	**Rationale**
Provides information relating to condition and treatment.	Provides for early assessment and intervention to prevent serious complications, death.
Record intake, output, and specific gravity. Calculate 24-hr fluid balance.	Useful for identifying therapy needs and effectiveness.
Observe for excessive thirst, poor skin turgor, dry skin/mucous membranes.	Signs of dehydration indicating need for prompt intervention/changes in therapy.
Administer vasopressin, lypressin, or desmopressin acetate as ordered, e.g., by injection, subcutaneous, or intranasal administration.	Antidiuretic effect promotes water reabsorption and more appropriate rate urine output.
Review laboratory studies, e.g., urine/serum sodium, potassium, osmolality.	Rapid depletion of electrolytes may occur in diabetes insipidus requiring prompt intervention.

Nursing Diagnosis: Knowledge Deficit	**Desired Outcomes/Evaluation Criteria**
RELATED TO: Lack of exposure/unfamiliarity with information resources, misinterpretation. **AS EVIDENCED BY:** Questions, statement of concern, inaccurate follow-through of instructions/development of preventable complications.	Verbalizes understanding of condition and treatment needs. Correctly performs necessary procedures and explains reasons for the actions.

Nursing Actions	**Rationale**
Provide information about antidiuretic drugs, including action, use, adverse effects, and interactions.	Understanding of medication and treatment regimen allows patient to make informed choices and participate knowledgeably in treatment.
Review side effects of antidiuretic drugs.	Helps patient to recognize problems that might indicate onset of water intoxication (e.g., nausea, vomiting, confusion, drowsiness, and headaches) or hypovolemia (e.g., weight loss, dizziness, and light-headedness).
Demonstrate correct preparation and administration technique. Discuss site rotation.	Maximizes therapeutic effect and avoids problems of lipodystrophy.
Instruct patient to contact physician if nasal congestion occurs, e.g., allergic rhinitis, upper respiratory infection.	Can impair absorption of drug when administered intranasally, possibly requiring an increase in dosage.
Show patient how to monitor intake, output, and specific gravity. Stress importance of adequate fluid replacement.	Promotes sense of control, accurate measure to prevent development of untoward complications.
Encourage wearing of a medical identification bracelet.	Identifies problem immediately in case of an emergency situation, avoiding possibility of complications.
Discuss necessity of abstaining from alcohol and reading of over-the-counter (OTC) drug labels.	Alcohol may alter therapeutic response to drug even in smaller amounts as may be found in OTC products.
Review need for further medical follow-up.	Provides opportunity to identify problems and adjust therapy if needed.

Other Suggested Nursing Diagnosis: Chronic Confusion.

cous membranes, irritability, and weakness are noted on physical examination.

• Accurately measure and monitor body weight, which is a reflection of water losses in diabetes insipidus.
• Obtain and monitor other laboratory tests. Measurements of serum and urine osmolality and serum so-

dium are used in assessing the patient for diabetes insipidus. Other laboratory tests are used to determine whether the patient can produce endogenous antidiuretic hormone and whether the kidneys are responsive to it.

• Assist the patient with diagnostic tests such as the

water deprivation test. (See a medical-surgical nursing text for more information.)

NURSING DIAGNOSIS

- Typical nursing diagnoses for patients with growth (somatotropic) hormone deficiency include Altered Growth and Development, Body Image/Self-Esteem Disturbance, and Knowledge Deficit (see Table 43–2). Suggested nursing diagnoses for patients with neurogenic diabetes insipidus include Fluid Volume Deficit, Knowledge Deficit, and Chronic Confusion (see Table 43–3).

INTERVENTION

- Identify specific information related to drug administration, patient safety, and patient teaching. These points can be found in the Nursing Implications column in Table 43–1. When administering anterior pituitary drugs (antidiuretic hormone) the family is taught how to administer them and what to monitor for effectiveness. Because diabetes insipidus can occur secondary to neurologic injuries (head trauma, brain surgery), affecting levels of consciousness, certain patients may be unable to monitor their own signs and symptoms. For these patients, it is vital to obtain accurate body weights, intake and output measurements, and urine specific gravities.

Patient Teaching

- Educate the child requiring growth hormone and the parents as well. Complex explanations are, of course, unsuitable for the young child, but the parents are educated about pituitary function and the need for growth hormone. Parents should understand the need for continued therapy with somatropin and should be aware of the possibility of adverse effects. Specific teaching points are listed in Table 43–4.
- Educate the patient requiring antidiuretic drugs (vasopressin, lypressin, desmopressin) about the disease process (diabetes insipidus), the medication, and the possible occurrence of adverse effects. Patients taking antidiuretic hormone are taught to avoid alcohol because it can alter therapeutic response. Information for the nurse to use in the teaching plan is included in Table 43–5.

EVALUATION

- Determine the effectiveness of the nursing interventions and achievement of goals. This evaluation is based on the goals for nursing intervention determined by the nurse, patient, and family (see Tables 43–2 and 43–3).

Patients Requiring Growth Hormone

- Evaluate growth rates. These should average about 7 cm (2.8 in) per year. An annual evaluation of bone

age is necessary to monitor the effectiveness of therapy and to determine epiphyseal closure.
- Know and monitor for the adverse effects of somatotropin.
- Evaluate the patient's and family's understanding of adverse effects. In particular, emphasize to the patient those side effects that require immediate medical attention.

Table 43–4. PATIENT TEACHING INFORMATION—SOMATOTROPIC HORMONES

Dear Patient:
   This drug has been prescribed for you/your child. This is what you should know about the drug to get the most from therapy.

☐ 1. Somatotropin is taken to help your growth.
☐ 2. Drugs will be taken until you are 5 feet tall or until your bones stop growing.
☐ 3. Reconstitute (mix) somatotropin with sterile water. Gently roll the vial between your hands. Do not shake. Inject deep into muscle.
☐ 4. Drugs are administered by a shot in your muscle.
☐ 5. Drugs are usually given 3 times per week, and 48 hours should pass between shots.
☐ 6. Drugs must be given as prescribed; do not stop the drug without first consulting with your doctor.
☐ 7. If side effects occur, consult with your doctor. These might include less than expected growth rates, tiredness, and infection.
☐ 8. You should not give a shot in the same place 2 times in a row. Keep a record of the sites. This will help to decrease soreness at the sites.
☐ 9. Record your (child's) height regularly.
☐ 10. Test your (child's) urine for glucose regularly.

Table 43–5. PATIENT TEACHING INFORMATION—ANTIDIURETIC DRUGS (LYPRESSIN, DESMOPRESSIN)

Dear Patient:
   This drug has been prescribed for you. This is what you should know about your drug to get the most from your therapy.

☐ 1. Antidiuretic hormone is taken to _____.
☐ 2. Antidiuretic drugs will often be taken indefinitely.
☐ 3. Antidiuretic drugs are generally taken at the following times:
    a. Desmopressin in the morning and evening.
    b. Lypressin 4 times a day.
☐ 4. Lypressin and desmopressin are taken by spraying the solutions into one or both nostrils. *Do not inhale* the drugs. The head may be tilted back slightly while a short spray is given. Pinching the nose for a few seconds afterward may help. Practice is necessary. If nasal congestion is present, a decongestant should be given first.
☐ 5. Do not drink much alcohol (beer, wine, whiskey) as these can change your response to antidiuretic drugs. Also, some liquid medicines are mixed with alcohol (cough syrups). Do not take these medicines.
☐ 6. Do not stop taking antidiuretic drugs without first talking to your doctor.
☐ 7. Call your doctor if you begin to experience side effects of _____.
☐ 8. If you experience increased urination or thirst, notify your doctor; your dosage may need to be altered.

Patients Requiring Antidiuretic Hormone

- Evaluate the patient for polyuria, nocturia, or increased thirst. Ask the patient to briefly review medication schedules and, if the patient has not obtained a medication card or necklace, take time to reinforce the importance of this type of identification.
- Evaluate for the adverse effects of the antidiuretic hormone drugs.
- Evaluate the patient's knowledge and understanding of adverse effects, especially those that, should they occur, require medical attention. Adverse effects of ADH drugs occur with greater frequency when larger doses are used. A worsening of polyuria or signs of

dehydration are reported immediately, as they indicate a need for alteration in dosage.
- Evaluate patient compliance. Most patients taking these pituitary drugs comply with their medication regimens because the drugs alleviate their symptomatology.

Stress the need for medical follow-up care and periodically review all previously taught information with the patient and family to ensure that the patient's knowledge remains accurate and current.

The bibliography for this chapter can be found in Appendix B, which begins on page 1054.

CHAPTER REVIEW QUESTIONS*

1. The ketogenic effect (lipolytic effect) of growth hormone leads to:
   a. Excess low-density lipids in the plasma.
   b. Reduction of fat storage in the liver.
   c. Conversion of fatty acids to ketone bodies.
   d. Decreased availability of fatty acids for energy.

2. In large doses, the following effect may occur with vasopressin therapy:
   a. Inhibition of peristaltic activity in the large bowel.
   b. Dilation of the superior mesenteric artery.
   c. Increased blood flow to the splanchnic system.
   d. Contraction of smooth muscle in arterioles.

3. Vasopressin is synthesized in the:
   a. Posterior pituitary.
   b. Anterior pituitary.

   c. Hypothalamus.
   d. Thymus.

4. The secretion of growth hormone is suppressed by:
   a. Stress.
   b. Emotional excitement.
   c. Hypoglycemic agents.
   d. Glucocorticoid drugs.

5. When giving lypressin or desmopressin, the patient is taught the drug is:
   a. Contraindicated in massive gastrointestinal bleeding.
   b. Recommended for long-term treatment of diabetes mellitus.
   c. Never inhaled when nasal spray is used.
   d. Used to decrease the permeability of the distal tubules to water.

*See Appendix A, which begins on page 1051, for answers.

CHAPTER 44

Adrenocortical Drugs: Mineralocorticoids and Glucocorticoids

Merrily A. Kuhn, RNC, PhD

CHAPTER OUTLINE

Mineralocorticoids
Glucocorticoids
Using the Nursing Process

TABLES

Drug Tables
Adrenocortical Drugs: Mineralocorticoids and
    Glucocorticoids, 633
Adrenal Steroid Inhibitors, 640

Nursing Process
Nursing Process for Patient Requiring Adrenocortical Drugs
    (Glucocorticoids), 641

Patient Teaching
Patient Teaching Information—Adrenocortical Drugs, 643

BOXES

Building Your Critical Thinking Skills, 644

KEY TERMS

Bradykinins
Glucocorticoids
Gluconeogenesis
Interleukin
Lipogenesis
Lipolysis
Mineralocorticoid
Prostaglandins
Pulse therapy

LEARNING OBJECTIVES

After reading this chapter, the student will be able to:

1. Identify those medications commonly used as adreno-cortical drugs.
2. Differentiate among the adrenocortical drugs as to mechanisms of action, routes of administration, pharmacokinetics, adverse effects, contraindications and precautions, and interactions.
3. Identify specific areas to assess in the patient requiring adrenocortical drugs to formulate appropriate patient outcomes.
4. Plan the nursing interventions necessary to administer adrenocortical drugs and choose appropriate teaching strategies to gain patient compliance.
5. Evaluate the patient at various stages of treatment to measure the effectiveness of nursing interventions.

The adrenal gland is composed of both a medulla and a cortex. The medulla secretes the sympathetic amines epinephrine and norepinephrine (see Chapter 17). The adrenal cortex produces corticosteroids, including mineralocorticoids such as aldosterone, glucocorticoids such as cortisol (referred to pharmaceutically as hydrocortisone), and gonadal hormones (androgens, estrogens, and progestins). The focus of this chapter is the mineralocorticoids and glucocorticoids. The gonadal hormones are discussed in Chapter 47.

Corticosteroids are synthesized in the adrenal cortex from cholesterol and are not stored in appreciable amounts. They regulate water and electrolyte balance (mineralocorticoid effect) and carbohydrate, protein, and fat metabolism (glucocorticoid effect). Many corticosteroids have both mineralocorticoid and glucocorticoid effects, but the effect that predominates varies for each hormone. This is also true of the pharmaceutical corticosteroids.

The adrenal cortex is stimulated by corticotropin, or adrenocorticotropic hormone (ACTH), produced in the adenohypophysis (anterior pituitary). The ACTH-secreting cells of the anterior pituitary are, in turn, regulated by corticotropin-releasing hormones (CRH) from the hypothalamus. When glucocorticoids are needed (such as during stress), ACTH stimulates the adrenal gland, and within minutes glucocorticoids are released. Secretion of ACTH is inhibited by a negative feedback effect of glu-

631

cocorticoids. Stress (e.g., trauma, anxiety, severe infection, hypoglycemia, and surgery) is one of the most potent stimulators of ACTH production. If the adrenal cortex must be stimulated, corticotropin (ACTH) is commercially available for intravenous, intramuscular, or subcutaneous administration.

MINERALOCORTICOIDS

Mineralocorticoid is a term applied to corticosteroids that have their major effects on water and electrolyte balance. Aldosterone is the prototypic drug in this group; but its use is limited by its high cost, limited availability, and requirement of parenteral administration. The only product that is available today is synthetic **fludrocortisone (Florinef)**, featured in Table 44–1.

O **Fludrocortisone** (Florinef) has mineralocorticoid activity and also has a modest glucocorticoid effect. However, it is used only for its mineralocorticoid effects.

ACTION Fludrocortisone acts primarily on the kidney's distal tubules, enhancing the reabsorption of sodium and chloride ions and the excretion of potassium and hydrogen ions. By extension, these compounds then help to maintain cardiac output and blood pressure by maintaining extracellular fluid volumes.

USES Fludrocortisone is used in replacement therapy for treatment of primary and secondary adrenocortical insufficiency and for treatment of salt-losing adrenogenital syndrome. It is also used in some patients with renal failure to assist with potassium balance.

CONTRAINDICATIONS AND PRECAUTIONS Fludrocortisone is contraindicated in patients hypersensitive to this product and in patients with hypertension, heart failure, and cardiac disease because it may increase sodium and water retention, worsening these conditions. Safety in pregnancy (category C) and in children has not been established.

ADVERSE EFFECTS The major adverse effect of fludrocortisone is sodium retention and subsequent water retention. In certain individuals, this increase in blood volume could lead to increases in blood pressure. These effects are dose related and are generally not problematic at replacement levels.

Hypokalemia, secondary to the potassium loss associated with the sodium-retaining activity of the mineralocorticoids, can also occur. It generally can be avoided by encouraging the patient to maintain a diet high in potassium-rich foods.

Frontal and occipital headaches, probably caused by the sodium and water retention, have been reported. Arthralgias and hypersensitivity reactions are less common adverse effects of mineralocorticoid therapy.

GLUCOCORTICOIDS

Glucocorticoids are those corticosteroids that have the most pronounced effect on carbohydrate, protein, and fat metabolism. Through their action, glucocorticoids inhibit inflammation, allergic reactions, and stress. And, although glucocorticoids may be administered only for their anti-inflammatory effects, catabolic effects of these drugs also occur. This explains many of the adverse effects that occur with glucocorticoid therapy.

Numerous synthetic analogs of cortisol (hydrocortisone) have been developed. The significant differences between the synthetic analogs and the natural parent compounds, cortisol and cortisone, are as follows: (1) the synthetics have a greater anti-inflammatory potency, (2) the synthetic analogs often have a longer duration of action, and (3) the sodium-retaining potential of the natural glucocorticoids is lessened or eliminated.

The glucocorticoids are classified as short-acting—**cortisone acetate (Cortone)** and **hydrocortisone (Cortef, Hydrocortone)**; intermediate-acting—**prednisone (Deltasone, Meticorten)**, **prednisolone (Prelone, Delta-Cortef)**, **triamcinolone (Aristocort, Kenacort)**, and **methylprednisolone (Medrol)**; long-acting—**dexamethasone (Decadron, Dexone)** and **betamethasone (Celestone)**. Selected glucocorticoids are featured in Table 44–1.

ACTION

Glucocorticoids exert three important therapeutic actions: anti-inflammatory, anti-allergic, and antistress. Glucocorticoids inhibit the inflammatory response by inhibiting local edema formation (probably by decreasing capillary permeability and dilation), fibroblast proliferation, and deposition of fibrin and collagen. Glucocorticoids suppress signs of inflammation, such as heat and redness, by preventing synthesis or release of vasodilator substances such as *bradykinins* (polypeptide kinin hormones produced in the blood that act as a potent vasodilator, promote smooth muscle contraction, and produce pain when nociceptors are stimulated), *prostaglandins* (large group of cellular hormones derived from essential fatty acids that inhibit the migration of macrophages and leukocytes toward areas of inflammation), and histamine. Cortisol also functions to stabilize the lysosomal membranes within the cells and prevents the release of hydrolyzing enzymes. Glucocorticoids also have an inhibitory effect on fibroblast formation and other substances (e.g., fibrin and collagen) that take part in the late healing phase. This interference helps to prevent scar tissue formation that may damage delicate structures like the eye.

Anti-allergic actions of glucocorticoids are similar to their anti-inflammatory actions. Immediate hypersensitivity reactions are suppressed by the interference of histamine release. Delayed hypersensitivity reactions are suppressed by decreasing activity of cellular mediators of immune reactions such as macrophages, monocytes, and T and B lymphocytes. Glucocorticoids also suppress or prevent cell-mediated immune reactions by reducing the concentration of leukocytes, monocytes, and eosinophils; by inhibiting synthesis of *interleukin* (a member of a group of hormones known as lymphokines that are produced by lymphocytes and that regulate the immune system); and by decreasing the binding of immunoglobulins to cell surface receptors.

Glucocorticoids improve cardiovascular function by several mechanisms. First, the natural hormones have a

Table 44–1. ADRENOCORTICAL DRUGS: MINERALOCORTICOIDS AND GLUCOCORTICOIDS

DRUG NAME/ROUTE AND DOSAGE	PHARMACOKINETICS/ DYNAMICS*	NURSING IMPLICATIONS
MINERALOCORTICOIDS		
fludrocortisone (Florinef)		
Adults: 0.01–0.2 mg/24 hr PO	**Onset:** Rapid **Peak:** 1.7 hr **Duration:** 24–48 hr **½L:** 3.5 hr (Drug); 18–36 hr (Metabolite) **PB:** yes **B:** liver **E:** urine	**ASSESSMENT:** Assess blood pressure and weight at onset and periodically. Assess for pregnancy (category C). **INTERVENTION: Patient Teaching**—Instruct patient to monitor salt intake to avoid edema, weight gain, and hypertension; and to eat potassium-rich foods. Tell patient to store drug in airtight, light-resistant containers. Instruct patient to take missed dose as soon as possible and to not double the dose next time. **EVALUATION:** Notify physician if persistent dizziness, headache, or weight gain occurs.
GLUCOCORTICOIDS		
all glucocorticoids		
	PB: yes **B:** liver **E:** urine	**ASSESSMENT:** Assess for signs of adrenal insufficiency throughout therapy. Obtain baseline CBC, electrolytes, eye exams, vital signs, and weight. Obtain tuberculin test before long-term therapy. **INTERVENTION:** Obtain an order for parenteral form if patient unable to take PO. Weigh patient regularly, and check urine for glucosuria. Wearing gloves, apply topical drugs sparingly and massage into area thoroughly and gently. Apply occlusive dressing only if ordered. Inject IM deeply into dorsal gluteal or ventrogluteal of buttock. Rotate injection sites and record. Dilute IV solutions according to package direction. **Patient Teaching**—Tell patient to take antacids as prescribed, to avoid aspirin, and to take oral drugs with food. Teach patient at what time of day drug is to be taken. Teach patient that dose must be increased with physiologic stress and that physician should be consulted. Caution patient to never discontinue drug abruptly without checking with physician. Instruct patient to carry identification card or wear a bracelet or necklace if on long-term therapy. Tell patient to store drug in dry, tightly closed container and to protect it from light. **EVALUATION:** Disease symptoms should lessen. Notify physician if unusual weight gain, swelling of lower extremities, vomiting, GI distress, prolonged sore throat, fever, or cold occur.
hydrocortisone sodium succinate (Solu-Cortef)		
Adults: 100–500 mg IM or IV at 2-, 4-, or 6-hr intervals	**Onset:** Rapid **Peak:** NA **Duration:** 1–1.5 day **½L:** 8–12 hr	Same as for all plus: **ASSESSMENT:** Assess for pregnancy (category unknown).
cortisone acetate (Cortone)		
Adults: 25–300 mg/day PO; or 20–300 mg/24 hr IM in 4 divided doses (also ophthalamic drop)	**Onset:** PO, rapid; IM, slow **Peak:** PO, 2 hr; IM, 20–48 hr **Duration:** 1.25–1.5 days **½L:** 8–12 hr	Same as for all plus: **ASSESSMENT:** Assess for pregnancy (category C).

Continued on the following page

Table 44–1. ADRENOCORTICAL DRUGS: MINERALOCORTICOIDS AND GLUCOCORTICOIDS, *Continued*

DRUG NAME/ROUTE AND DOSAGE	PHARMACOKINETICS/ DYNAMICS*	NURSING IMPLICATIONS
prednisone (Deltasone) (Meticorten)		
Adults: 5–60 mg/24 hr PO in 1–3 doses *Pediatric:* 0.14–2 mg/kg per 24 hr PO	**Onset:** hours **Peak:** NA **Duration:** 1.25–1.5 days **½L:** 18–36 hr	Same as for all plus: **ASSESSMENT:** Assess for pregnancy (category unknown). **INTERVENTION:** Monitor for liver dysfunction.
prednisolone (Delta-Cortef) (Prelone)		
Adults: 5–60 mg/24 hr PO in 1–4 doses *Pediatric:* 0.14–2 mg/kg per 24 hr PO in 3 doses **multiple sclerosis** *Adults:* 200 mg/day IM or IV for 1 wk followed by 80 mg every other day for 1 mo	**Onset:** 1 hr **Peak:** 1–2 hr **Duration:** 1.25–1.5 days **½L:** 18–36 hr	Same as for all plus: **ASSESSMENT:** Assess for pregnancy (category unknown). **INTERVENTION:** May be used daily or for alternative day therapy.
methylprednisolone (Medrol)†		
Adults: 4–48 mg PO in 2–4 divided doses *Pediatric:* 0.117 mg/kg per 24 hr PO in 3 doses	**Onset:** hours **Peak:** 1–2 hr **Duration:** 1.25–1.5 days **½L:** 18–36 hr	Same as for all plus: **ASSESSMENT:** Assess for pregnancy (category unknown).
triamcinolone (Aristocort) (Kenalog)†		
Adults: 4–60 mg/24 hr PO *Pediatric:* 0.117–1.66 mg/kg per day PO	**Onset:** NA **Peak:** 1–2 hr **Duration:** 2.25 days **½L:** 18–36 hr	Same as for all plus: **ASSESSMENT:** Assess for pregnancy (category unknown). Available in both tablets and syrup.
betamethasone (Celestone)†		
Adults: 0.6–7.2 mg/24 hr PO; or 0.5–9 mg/day IM, intra-articularly, or intrasynovially *Pediatric:* 17.5–200 μg/kg per day PO in 3 doses	**Onset:** rapid **Peak:** 1–2 hr **Duration:** 3.25 days **½L:** 36–54 hr.	Same as for all plus: **ASSESSMENT:** Assess for pregnancy (category unknown).
dexamethasone (Decadron) (Hexadrol)‡		
Adults: 0.75–9.0 mg/24 hr PO in 2–4 doses *Pediatric:* 23–333 μg/kg per day PO in 3–4 doses	**Onset:** NA **Peak:** 1–2 hr **Duration:** 2.75 days **½L:** 36–54 hr	Same as for all plus: **ASSESSMENT:** Assess for pregnancy (category unknown).

*For all glucocorticoids: Onset of action, peak, and duration depend on dose being administered and condition being treated.

†Little sodium retention.

‡No sodium retention.

NA = not available.

salt- and water-retaining effect, which can prevent hypovolemia in patients with adrenocortical insufficiency and improve cardiovascular performance. Second, glucocorticoids increase the responsiveness of the heart, blood vessels, and other tissues to circulating catecholamines such as epinephrine and norepinephrine. The improved cardiovascular function increases cardiac output and local perfusion pressure.

In terms of carbohydrate metabolism, the glucocorticoids exert an effect opposite to that of insulin; that is, they stimulate *gluconeogenesis* (formation of glucose from noncarbohydrate sources such as protein or fat), decrease utilization of glucose by many body cells, and promote glucose storage as glycogen.

The increase in glucose production is at the expense of protein stores, and protein catabolism occurs with high, nonphysiologic levels of glucocorticoids. The increase in protein catabolism leads to poor wound healing, muscle wasting, and scanty hair growth.

Fat (or lipid) metabolism is also affected by exogenous glucocorticoid therapy. These drugs enhance the breakdown of triglycerides in the body's fat deposits to fatty acids (*lipolysis*). Glucocorticoids also indirectly increase the formation of fat and its storage in adipose tissue (*li-*

Table 44–2. ACTIVITY CONTINUUM OF ADRENOCORTICOIDS

Activity	Products	Half-Life	Uses
Highest mineralocorticoid activity, no glucocorticoid activity	Fludrocortisone	3.5 hr	Replacement in Addison's disease
Equal mineralocorticoid and glucocorticoid activities	Cortisone, cortisol, hydrocortisone	8–12 hr	Replacement in adrenocortical insufficiency, anti-inflammatory, immunosuppression
	Prednisone, prednisolone, methylprednisolone	18–36 hr	Autoimmune disorders, anti-inflammatory, immunosuppression
Highest glucocorticoid activity, no mineralocorticoid activity	Dexamethasone, betamethasone	36–54 hr	Increased intracranial pressure, anti-inflammatory

pogenesis) as a result of the action of insulin released from the pancreas. The subsequent rise in blood sugar is secondary to the effects of glucocorticoids on carbohydrate metabolism. The fat distribution changes are discussed later in this chapter.

Central nervous system and emotional functioning is, in part, maintained by the glucocorticoids. Exogenous glucocorticoid administration has been shown to increase brain excitability.

Corticosteroid drugs exert pharmacologic actions that are on a continuum, presented in Table 44–2, with sodium retention and anti-inflammatory actions being on opposing ends. Many drugs have both glucocorticoid and mineralocorticoid activity.

USES

Aside from their use in replacement therapy for adrenocortical insufficiency (Addison's disease), glucocorticoid drugs are most often used for their anti-inflammatory effects to treat a variety of disorders such as rheumatic fever, osteoarthritis, rheumatoid arthritis, nephrotic syndrome, inflammatory bowel disease, chronic obstructive pulmonary disease, and collagen diseases. Glucocorticoids may cause a rapid and marked reduction in symptoms but do not alter the course of the disease. Glucocorticoids are used for their antilymphocytic effect to treat leukemias, lymphomas, myelomas, and multiple sclerosis. Glucocorticoids are also used to reduce or prevent cerebral edema associated with neoplasms, neurosurgery, and trauma. Glucocorticoids suppress the inflammatory response and relieve hypersensitivity reactions in patients with asthma, bee stings, hay fever, contact and exfoliative dermatitis, ulcerative colitis, and vasculitis. Glucocorticoids are commonly used to decrease ocular inflammatory processes. Glucocorticoids are also combined with other immunosuppressants to prevent or manage transplant rejection.

Glucocorticoids are also used to suppress adrenocortical hyperfunction in patients with adrenogenital syndrome. Glucocorticoids increase calcium excretion and are used for treatment of hypercalcemia in patients with cancer with bone metastases such as breast cancer, multiple myeloma, and vitamin D intoxication.

ROUTES OF ADMINISTRATION

Glucocorticoids may be administered via a variety of different routes, depending on the desired use. Most can be given orally, intramuscularly, and intravenously. The intravenous route allows a faster onset of action and is preferred in emergencies.

Local administration of glucocorticoids may be preferred over systemic routes. The advantage of local administration is that it avoids much of the systemic adverse effects. Topical administration, for example, is a mainstay of much dermatologic therapy.

▼ CLINICAL ALERT

Systemic absorption may occur with topical application of glucocorticoids and can cause hypothalamic-pituitary-adrenal (HPA) suppression if the agent is used long term.

Other adverse effects can also occur when glucocorticoids are applied over a large area of body surface, especially if the skin is more permeable such as when inflamed, and if occlusive dressings are used. When intralesional injections of glucocorticoids are used in treating severe forms of skin disorders such as acne, systemic absorption may occur.

Intra-articular injections of glucocorticoids are a useful form of local therapy for patients with inflammatory joint problems. Rectal administration via enemas or foams for the treatment of inflammatory bowel disorders is another example of local use.

Glucocorticoids may also be administered to the respiratory tract via inhalation. Beclomethasone (Vanceril) and other glucocorticoids are used via this route in the treatment of asthma that does not respond to conventional therapy with bronchodilators (see Chapter 40). Again, it must be noted that when this route of administration is properly used, systemic adverse effects are minimal; however, abuse or overuse may in fact cause some HPA suppression.

PHARMACOKINETICS

Glucocorticoids are highly protein bound to corticosteroid-binding globulin or transcortin- and corticosteroid-binding albumin. It is the unbound, or free, fraction of cortisol that is pharmacologically active. These products are distributed to all body tissues. Glucocorticoids are metabolized by the liver and excreted in the urine. Biologic half-life varies with the specific drug and ranges from 8 to 54 hours (see Table 44–2).

CONTRAINDICATIONS AND PRECAUTIONS

Glucocorticoids are contraindicated in systemic infection and active or arrested tuberculosis as these conditions may worsen with glucocorticoid therapy. Before patients are started on long-term therapy, a tuberculosis test is always done to determine the presence of inactive disease. Patients with inactive disease are usually given prophylactic isoniazid (INH).

Because of their effects on numerous body systems and because they interfere with the inflammatory response, glucocorticoids must be given cautiously to patients who have certain disease conditions (active or latent peptic ulcer disease, diverticulitis, ocular herpes simplex, hypertension, osteoporosis, and chronic active hepatitis B), which may be exacerbated.

Patients should not be immunized when taking glucocorticoids acutely as the antibody response is decreased. Mothers should not breast feed while receiving glucocorticoids. In children, growth and development need to be monitored closely if chronic use is required.

ADVERSE EFFECTS

The occurrence of adverse effects from glucocorticoid administration is related to the alterations in physiologic function of the adrenal hormones. Generally, the pharmacologic doses of glucocorticoids cause adverse effects, not the physiologic or replacement doses; and the occurrence of adverse effects is related to the amounts of the medications used and the duration of therapy. The adrenal cortex generally produces about 20 to 30 mg (total) of glucocorticoids per day and in acute stress situations can produce ten times as much. Pharmacologic doses of glucocorticoids are usually greater than 30 mg per day.

Chronic glucocorticoid treatment suppresses HPA activity and leads to adrenocortical atrophy. This can result in acute adrenocortical insufficiency—indicated by syncope, general muscular weakness, nausea, anorexia, and hypotension—espsecially when patients are abruptly withdrawn from long-term therapy. Supplemental amounts of glucocorticoids are administered to alleviate the symptoms of insufficiency and to prevent vasomotor collapse. These additional glucocorticoids are withdrawn gradually over a period of several days until the maintenance dose is reached. HPA responsiveness may take many months to return to normal.

The catabolic effect of glucocorticoids on protein metabolism leads to many changes. Steroid myopathy (muscle weakness) involving all extremities, but especially the lower extremities, can occur. Myopathy is mainly a result of negative nitrogen balance, which develops despite the fact that these drugs increase the patient's appetite. Triamcinolone, a synthetic glucocorticoid, is reported to neither stimulate appetite nor lead to weight gain (unlike other steroids) and thus may be more likely to cause muscle wasting. Protein catabolism may also appear as osteoporosis, largely due to wasting of the bone matrix from calcium depletion (most noticeable in the vertebrae). Decreased calcium absorption by the GI tract combined with enhanced renal excretion of calcium is also involved.

Some studies indicate that the risk of osteoporosis is most pronounced in patients with certain predisposing factors, such as decreased calcium intake, immobility, and menopause. The protein component of skin and vascular walls is also affected. The patient on long-term glucocorticoid therapy may bruise readily, related to capillary fragility; and have a very "thin," delicate skin, related to decreased protein. Wound healing is also decreased by glucocorticoids as they decrease fibroblast proliferation and collagen deposition.

In children, the skeletal system may be markedly affected, and a decrease in growth rate is often noted, as glucocorticoids impair cell division and increase bone demineralization. After steroid therapy is discontinued, most children experience a growth spurt, although large doses given for long periods may cause irreversible growth retardation.

The hematopoietic system also suffers from the protein catabolism induced by nonphysiologic doses of glucocorticoids. Eosinophils and lymphocytes decrease in numbers. Although lymphoid tissue may atrophy, reduction of antibody production usually does not occur unless large amounts of corticosteroids are used over long periods of time. Nevertheless, delayed hypersensitivity responses may be altered. For example, skin sensitivity to tuberculin, as in the Mantoux test, may be lost. In addition, neutrophils may increase. A moderately high white blood cell count of 10,000 to 15,000/mm^3 may result from steroid use.

Another effect to consider is that although patients on glucocorticoids are more susceptible to infection, the anti-inflammatory action of the medications tends to hide, or mask, the more common signs of inflammation such as fever, redness, swelling, and pain.

Carbohydrate metabolism is profoundly affected by the use of exogenous glucocorticoid therapy. In fact, the normal physiologic role of these hormones is to provide for glucose production during periods of decreased carbohydrate intake. As glucose synthesis is increased, glucose utilization is decreased at the same time. This may lead to an increase in blood glucose, sometimes referred to as adrenal diabetes or steroid-induced diabetes.

Fat metabolism is affected as well. Redistribution of fat stores occurs. This results in the typical cushingoid appearance of patients on long-term therapy: a cervicodorsal fat pad (buffalo hump), obesity of the torso, moon face, and decreased fat deposits in the extremities, as shown in Figure 44–1. These changes can occur with doses of 25 mg/day of prednisone or its equivalent for 2 weeks. Glucocorticoid therapy is also associated with hyperlipidemia, most notably increases in triglycerides.

Significant changes in fluid and electrolyte balance can occur when either mineralocorticoids or glucocorticoids with pronounced mineralocorticoid activity, such as hydrocortisone, are used. Sodium retention and the subsequent water retention may be great enough to produce hypertension in some patients. Potassium-depleting effects can lead to hypokalemia.

Currently, it is believed that glucocorticoids are ulcerogenic. Evidence exists that gastric mucus production is decreased and mucosal cell renewal is affected. These factors alter the mucosal defense mechanisms and potentiate

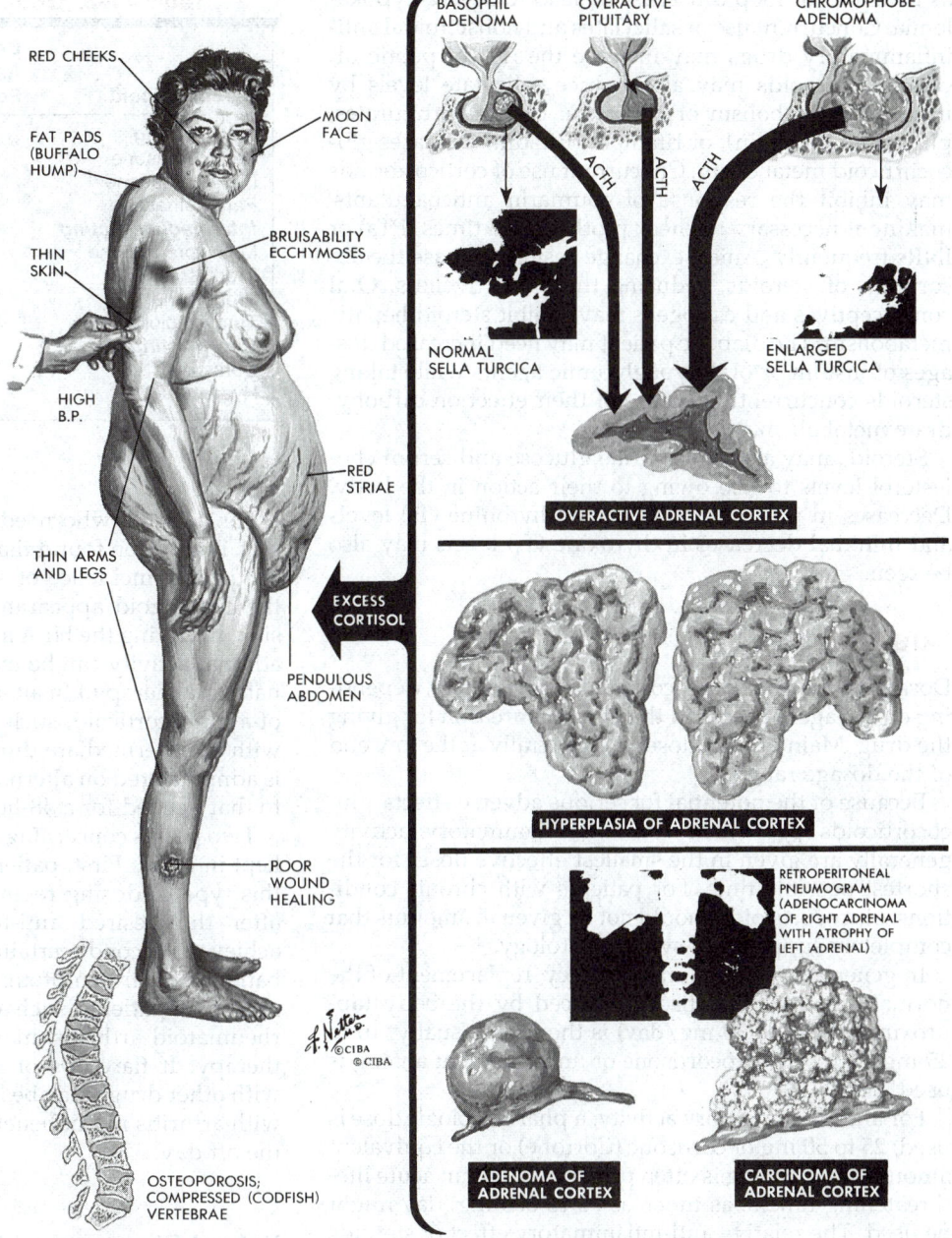

Figure 44–1. Cushingoid appearance often seen in patients on long-term steroid therapy due to excessive cortisol. (*Source*: Ciba Collection Endocrine System Vol. 4 p. 85, 1965, with permission.)

the development of gastric ulcers, especially when other factors, such as aspirin intake, are introduced. In addition, the anti-inflammatory effects of the glucocorticoids may hide the symptoms of ulceration, and perforation can occur with few symptoms. Another, although less common, adverse effect on the GI system is pancreatitis. The mechanisms by which glucocorticoids cause this is unknown; again, the clinical signs and symptoms may be masked by the medications.

Increases in intraocular pressure can occur with either ocular or systemic use of glucocorticoids. Glaucoma may occur in high-risk patients, such as those genetically predisposed or those with diabetes. Cataracts can also develop from long-term use of these agents.

Lastly, central nervous system and psychiatric disturbances can occur. As noted previously, glucocorticoids do

cause an increase in brain excitability. Cases of spontaneous seizure activity have been noted with large doses. Psychiatric reactions are usually reversible, but vary widely. Some evidence suggests that they are less common with the use of the more potent synthetic analogs. Many researchers feel that these reactions are most common in individuals who have a history of personality disorders. Changes that may occur include insomnia; nervousness; euphoria; and depression, sometimes suicidal in severity.

INTERACTIONS

Corticosteroids can interact with a number of other drugs. The concurrent use of potassium-depleting diuretics such as thiazides or loop diuretics can lead to severe hypokalemia. Concurrent use of salicylates and nonsteroidal anti-inflammatory drugs may increase the risk of peptic ulceration. Steroids may also reduce salicylate levels by increased metabolism or clearance. Use of barbiturates, phenytoin (Dilantin), or rifampin (Rifadin) increases glucocorticoid metabolism. Concurrent use of corticosteroids may inhibit the response of coumarin anticoagulants, making it necessary to check prothrombin times (PTs) or INRs frequently. Anion exchange resins decrease the absorption of steroids, reducing their effectiveness. Oral contraceptives and estrogens may inhibit steroid hepatic metabolism. The diabetic patient may need increased dosages of insulin or oral hypoglycemic agents while taking steroids concurrently because of their effect on carbohydrate metabolism.

Steroids may also cause urine glucose and serum cholesterol levels to rise owing to their action in the body. Decreases in potassium and triiodothyronine (T_3) levels and minimal decreases in thyroxine (T_4) levels may also be seen.

DOSAGE

Dosages of various glucocorticoids vary widely, depending on the agent used and the particular reason for giving the drug. Maintenance doses are generally at the low end of the dosage range.

Because of the potential for serious adverse effects, glucocorticoids prescribed for anti-inflammatory activity generally are given in the smallest effective doses for the shortest possible time. For patients with chronic conditions, glucocorticoids should not be given in amounts that completely suppress all symptomatology.

In general, in adrenal insufficiency, replacement of the normal amount of cortisol produced by the body (approximately 20 to 30 mg/day) is the goal. Usually, 10 to 25 mg/day of hydrocortisone or an equivalent analog is used.

For anti-inflammatory activity, a pharmacologic dose is used; 25 to 50 mg of cortisone (Cortone) or the equivalent amount of an analog is often prescribed. For an acute life-threatening illness, as much as 75 to 300 mg/day might be used. The relative anti-inflammatory effect of steroids is based on hydrocortisone, which is given a value of 1, as presented in Table 44–3.

Frequently, glucocorticoid therapy is adjusted to mimic, as closely as possible, the normal diurnal pattern of cortisol secretion in the body. Cortisol secretion is highest in the early morning (6 to 9 AM) and lowest later in the day (9 PM to 12 midnight). Therefore, replacements may be administered in divided doses, with two-thirds given in the morning and one-third given in the early afternoon. Or, the entire daily dose might be administered early in the morning (7 to 8 AM). If the entire dose is administered in the morning, the adrenal gland may be suppressed. If suppression of gland activity is not desired, the entire dose may be administered in the early afternoon. This allows the gland to function normally and also gives the patient a second peak of hormone to manage his or her current symptoms.

Table 44–3. GLUCOCORTICOID POTENCY

Glucocorticoid	Comparative Anti-Inflammatory Potency	Approximate Equivalent Dose (mg)
Long-Acting		
Betamethasone	25	0.6–0.75
Dexamethasone	20–30	0.75
Paramethasone	10	2
Intermediate-Acting		
Methylpredisolone	5	4
Prednisolone	4	5
Prednisone	4	5
Triamcinolone	5	4
Short-Acting		
Cortisone	0.8	25
Hydrocortisone	1	20

For patients who need long-term glucocorticoid therapy, it has been found that alternate-day therapy helps to reduce the incidence of some adverse effects, especially the cushingoid appearance and adrenocortical suppression, by giving the HPA axis a chance to recover. (Normal adrenal activity can be minimally suppressed with alternate-day therapy.) In alternate-day therapy, a single dose of a glucocorticoid, such as prednisone or prednisolone, with an intermediate duration of action (24 to 36 hours) is administered on alternate mornings in an amount equal to that needed for a 48-hour period.

Two points concerning alternate-day therapy should be kept in mind. First, patients are not initially treated with this type of dosing regimen. It is used for maintenance after the desired anti-inflammatory action has been achieved. Second, certain patients may have an exacerbation of their symptoms on the "off" day. For this reason, some patients, such as those with ulcerative colitis or rheumatoid arthritis, may be unsuited for alternate-day therapy. If flare-ups of symptoms do occur, treatment with other drugs may be helpful. For example, the patient with arthritis might benefit from the use of analgesics on the off day.

Natural Glucocorticoids

○ **Hydrocortisone** (Cortef, Hydrocortone) is the principal natural glucocorticoid secreted by the adrenal cortex. It is administered in oral doses for replacement therapy and for other conditions. In acute situations, it is not a preferred drug because of its slow onset of action. When needed, hydrocortisone is also administered via the intramuscular, intra-articular, intralesional, topical, and ophthalmic routes. Hydrocortisone is metabolized to cortisone.

○ **Hydrocortisone sodium succinate** (Solu-Cortef), an ester of hydrocortisone and water-soluble salt, is one of the most commonly administered parenteral glucocorticoids. It is primarily used to treat adrenocortical insufficiency and severe inflammation (see Table 44–1).

○ **Cortisone** (Cortone) is usually the drug of choice for replacement therapy in patients with adrenocortical insufficiency. It has both glucocorticoid and mineralocorticoid properties (see Table 44–1).

Synthetic Glucocorticoids

The synthetic glucocorticoids are more potent than cortisone and hydrocortisone, generally have fewer adverse effects, and have a longer duration of action. For example, prednisone and prednisolone are four to five times more potent than cortisone and hydrocortisone. The long duration of action of these potent synthetic products can cause suppression of the HPA axis, which can be beneficial or detrimental. Alternate-day dosing of intermediate-acting products like prednisone, prednisolone, and methylprednisolone can be used if HPA axis suppression is not required.

○ **Prednisone** (Deltasone, Meticorten, and others) is the most commonly administered synthetic oral glucocorticoid. It is primarily used for its anti-inflammatory or immunosuppressant effects (see Table 44–1).

○ **Prednisolone** (Prelone, Delta-Cortef, and others) is used primarily as an anti-inflammatory or immunosuppressant agent (see Table 44–1).

○ **Prednisolone acetate** (Key-Pred 25, Predcor 50), the synthetic acetate salt of prednisolone, is used for its anti-inflammatory or immunosuppressant effects. It is administered intramuscularly, intra-articularly, intralesionally, topically, or ophthalmically.

○ **Prednisolone sodium phosphate** (Hydeltrasol, Predicort-RP, Pediapred) is a water-soluble, rapid-acting, short-duration product used for its anti-inflammatory or immunosuppressant effects. It can be injected intramuscularly, intravenously, intralesionally, intra-articularly, or into soft tissue. Pediapred is a liquid product free of alcohol, sugar, and dye that is very palatable. It is especially useful in children who require long-term, high-dose steroids for chronic inflammatory disease.

○ **Methylprednisolone** (Medrol) is an oral agent used primarily as an anti-inflammatory or immunosuppressant agent. It is not used alone in adrenocortical insufficiency because it has minimal mineralocorticoid activity. A 21 Dosepak, designed for 1 week of therapy, is available for acute inflammatory conditions. A large first dose is taken, and each of the next days a smaller dose is consumed. The patient is taught to follow the manufacturer's directions (see Table 44–1).

○ **Methylprednisolone acetate** (Depo-Medrol), the acetate salt of methylprednisolone, is used for its anti-inflammatory properties. It has a low solubility and, therefore, a sustained effect. Methylprednisolone acetate can be given through the intra-articular, intralesional, and topical routes.

○ **Methylprednisolone sodium succinate** (Solu-Medrol) is used with prednisone and prednisolone in *pulse therapy* (administration of intermittent high doses of a drug) for patients with severe lupus nephritis or incapacitating rheumatoid arthritis. If pulse therapy is effective, the patient has a temporary remission. Methylprednisolone sodium succinate is given either intramuscularly or intravenously.

○ **Triamcinolone** (Aristocort, Kenacort) is used primarily as an anti-inflammatory or immunosuppressant drug. It has minimal mineralocorticoid activity, so it is not used alone to treat adrenocortical insufficiency (see Table 44–1).

○ **Triamcinolone diacetate** (Aristocort Forte) is administered intramuscularly, intra-articularly, or intrasynovially (into the joints).

○ **Betamethasone** (Celestone) has potent anti-inflammatory and immunosuppressant properties. It has minimal mineralocorticoid activity, so it is not used alone to treat adrenocortical insufficiency. It may be administered orally or injected into inflamed joints or bursas (see Table 44–1).

○ **Beclomethasone dipropionate** (Vanceril, Beclovent) is used to control bronchial asthma in patients requiring chronic treatment with corticosteroids in conjunction with other therapies. The use of an inhaler makes it possible to provide effective local steroid activity with minimal systemic effect. Beclomethasone dipropionate is discussed in more detail in Chapter 40.

○ **Dexamethasone** (Decadron, Hexadrol) is used systemically and locally for a wide variety of acute and chronic inflammatory, allergic, hematologic, neoplastic, and autoimmune diseases. Dexamethasone is also useful in the acute early management of cerebral edema and septic shock. Dexamethasone is used as a diagnostic aid to test for Cushing's syndrome and depression (see Table 44–1).

○ **Dexamethasone phosphate** (Decadrol, Dexone), a salt of dexamethasone, is available for intramuscular or intravenous use or it can be injected into joints.

Topical Glucocorticoids

Topical glucocorticoids are available as creams, ointments, gels, aerosols, lotions, solutions, and drug-impregnated tape. They are used to treat numerous inflammatory and proliferative skin diseases. The numerous preparations available have similar action and can cause similar adverse effects. These products are reviewed in Chapter 65.

ADRENAL STEROID INHIBITORS

The adrenal steroid inhibitors—**trilostane *(Modrastane)*, aminoglutethimide *(Cytadren)*,** and **RU-486 *(mifepristone)*—are used to control the symptoms of Cushing's syndrome.

○ **Trilostane** (Modrastane) **and aminoglutethimide** (Cytadren) control the symptoms of Cushing's syndrome, but do not cure the disease process. Trilostane reversibly lowers elevated circulation levels of glucocorticoids by inhibiting the enzyme system essential for their production in the adrenal gland. Aminoglutethimide inhibits the enzymatic conversion of cholesterol to delta[5]-pregnenolone, again reducing synthesis of all the adrenal hormones. Aminoglutethimide is also being used to palliate postmenopausal women with advanced breast carcinomas and in patients with advanced prostate carcinoma. More information on these drugs is presented in Table 44–4.

Table 44–4. ADRENAL STEROID INHIBITORS

DRUG NAME/ROUTE AND DOSAGE	PHARMACOKINETICS/ DYNAMICS	NURSING IMPLICATIONS
trilostane (Modrastane) **Adults:** 30 mg PO qid, up to 480 mg/day.	**Onset:** several days **Peak:** NA **Duration:** NA **½L:** NA **PB:** yes **B:** liver **E:** urine	**ASSESSMENT:** Assess steroid level, cause of underlying disease. Assess for pregnancy (category X). **INTERVENTION:** Monitor blood pressure often. If severe stress present, patient may need supplemental corticosteroids. Frequently monitor urine and plasma hormones and electrolyte levels. If response is not noted in 2 wk, therapy is discontinued. **Patient Teaching—** Warn patient that drug does not cure underlying disease process.
aminoglutethimide (Cytadren) **Adults:** 250 mg PO qid; increase q 1–2 wk by 250 mg.	**Onset:** rapid **Peak:** 4–6 hr **Duration:** 6–8 hr **½L:** 11–16 hr **PB:** minimal **B:** liver **E:** urine (50% unchanged)	**ASSESSMENT:** Same as above except assess for pregnancy (category D). **INTERVENTION: Patient Teaching—**Warn patient that drug may cause dizziness and to observe caution while driving or performing tasks requiring alertness. **EVALUATION:** Notify physician of pronounced nausea (should subside within 1st or 2nd wk of therapy), loss of appetite, faintness, headache, and rash.

NA = not available.

○ **RU-486** (mifeprostone), the anti-progesterone drug used in Europe to induce abortion and soon to become available in the United States, produces its antiglucocorticoid effect by blocking cortisol secretion.

USING THE NURSING PROCESS

Table 44–5 suggests assessment data that must be collected and shows how to apply other steps of the nursing process to the patient requiring adrenal corticosteroids.

ASSESSMENT

- Obtain a careful nursing history to establish the database. One very important component of the history is to identify whether or not the patient is currently taking any type of corticosteroid and the condition for which he or she is taking it. It is equally important to know if the patient has taken corticosteroids at any time within the past year.
- Assess for a current and past history of GI upset, ulcers, or epigastric pain.
- Assess the patient for any GI complaints 1 to 3 hours after meals; and for nausea, vomiting, bloody stools, hematemesis, and coffee-ground vomitus during therapy.
- Obtain baseline laboratory data before the patient begins long-term glucocorticoid therapy. This data includes an electrocardiogram (ECG), chest and spinal x-ray films, glucose tolerance test, Mantoux test for tuberculosis, complete blood count (CBC), and tests

for fluids and electrolyte balance. Measurement of ocular pressure is also performed.
- Obtain record baseline blood pressure (BP) and body weight.
- Perform a physical examination. The physical examination of the patient with suspected adrenal cortical dysfunction may reveal some typical changes in physical appearance related to either an increase or decrease in production of the hormones of the adrenal cortex. Table 44–6 summarizes the metabolic effects of adrenocortical dysfunction.
- Assess diet, nutrition history, and history of weight control. A nutrition consultation is often necessary, and baseline data is important. Also, a discussion of emotional stability is important. Often the patient on glucocorticoids has frequent mood swings, and it is important to determine pretreatment patterns.
- Assess carefully before and during therapy for signs of delayed wound healing, infection, and fever. Typical signs and symptoms may be nominal or absent.

NURSING DIAGNOSIS

- Typical nursing diagnoses for a patient requiring adrenocortical drugs (glucocorticoids) include the following: Knowledge Deficit, Fluid Volume Deficit, Altered Nutrition, Impaired Adjustment, Altered Thought Processes, and Body Image Disturbance (see Table 44–5).

INTERVENTION

- Develop the goals for nursing interventions from the list of nursing diagnoses. (Typical goals are included in Table 44–5.)

Table 44–5. NURSING PROCESS FOR PATIENT REQUIRING ADRENOCORTICAL DRUGS (GLUCOCORTICOIDS)

Assessment

Assess current/past drug history.
Assess dietary/nutritional and weight control history.
Assess baseline laboratory data, e.g., ECG, chest and spinal x-ray films, glucose-tolerance test, Mantoux, CBC, fluid and electrolyte balance, and ocular pressure.
Assess BP, body weight, and HPA axis function.
Assess for muscle weakness/wasting, redistribution of fat deposits, changes in hair growth, presence of edema.

Nursing Diagnosis: Knowledge Deficit

RELATED TO: Information misinterpretation, unfamiliarity with resources.
AS EVIDENCED BY: Questions, statement of concern, inaccurate follow-through of instruction/development of preventable complications.

Desired Outcomes/Evaluate Criteria

Verbalizes understanding of condition/disease process, administration and side effects of steroid therapy.
Initiates necessary lifestyle changes and participates in treatment regimen.

Nursing Actions	Rationale
Review pathophysiology of disease process/condition and therapeutic regimen.	Understanding of need for therapy helps patient to make informed decisions and cooperate with therapy.
Provide information about hormone replacement therapy (adrenal drugs) and necessity of adherence to drug schedule.	Promotes effective therapy, reducing risk of adverse effects.
Stress need to wear identification bracelet and to carry emergency drugs, e.g., IM or IV dexamethasone sodium.	Assists with prompt appropriate intervention in case of emergency and prevents abrupt withdrawal from drug.
Define and problem-solve ways to limit or control stressors, e.g., infection, dental work, personal/family crises, increased activity.	Dosage of glucocortocoids may need to be adjusted (double or tripled) during periods of stress.
Stress importance of avoiding exposure to infection or trauma/irritation of skin that may result in dermal injury.	Suppression of the inflammatory response increases risk of infection and possibility of progression to life-threatening situation.
Discuss necessity of regular medical checkup.	Facilitates control of chronic condition and prevention of complications.
Recommend limiting use of caffeine and alcohol, products containing aspirin.	Increasing secretion of gastric acid, irritation of gastric mucosa potentiates risk of GI bleed.

Nursing Diagnosis: Altered Nutrition, Less Than Body Requirements

RELATED TO: Glucocorticoid deficiency; abnormal fat, protein, and carbohydrate metabolism.

Desired Outcomes/Evaluation Criteria

Reports relief of nausea and vomiting. Demonstrates stable weight or weight gain toward desired goal with absence of presenting signs and normalization of laboratory values.

Nursing Actions	Rationale
Auscultate bowel sounds and assess for abdominal pain, nausea, or vomiting.	Cortisol deficit can cause GI symptoms, affecting ingestion and absorption of nutrients.
Monitor dietary intake and weigh daily.	Aids in identifying nutritional needs and effectiveness of therapy.
Increase sodium in diet, e.g., meats, fish, poultry, milk, eggs.	May help to prevent/correct hyponatremia.
Administer medications, e.g., glucocorticoids;	Corrects hypoglycemia, provides energy source for cellular function. Stimulates gluconeogenesis, decreases utilization of glucose, and promotes glucose storage as glycogen.
androgens.	May be useful in debilitated or malnourished patient to improve appetite, foster a positive nitrogen balance.
IV glucose as indicated. Perform fingerstick glucose testing as indicated.	Provides fluid replacement when needed. Evaluates serum glucose level and therapy needs.

Other Suggested Nursing Diagnoses: Fluid Volume Deficit, Impaired Adjustment, Altered Thought Processes, and Body Image Disturbance.

Table 44–6. SUMMARY OF METABOLIC EFFECTS OF ADRENAL CORTEX DYSFUNCTION

	Hyperfunction (Cushing's Syndrome)	Hypofunction (Addison's Disease)
Carbohydrate	Hyperglycemia	Hypoglycemia
Protein	Protein wasting affecting skin, skeletal muscles, bone matrix, and so on; scanty hair growth, ecchymosis, poor wound healing, muscle weakness.	—
Fat	Redistribution of fat deposits, obesity of torso, cervicodorsal fat pad, moon face.	—
Fluid and Electrolyte	Sodium retention, potassium loss, edema, hypertension.	Sodium loss, potassium retention, hypovolemia, hypotension, muscle weakness.

Nursing Responsibilities—Administration

Safe administration of adrenocortical drugs depends on the nurse knowing specific information related to administration, patient safety, and patient teaching. This information is summarized in the drug tables in the Nursing Implications column.

- Monitor the adverse effects. Patients receiving glucocorticoids for inflammation are those most likely to experience adverse effects that result from the intensification of the basic functions of the hormones in the body (see Table 44–6). Although not all of these effects are preventable, careful nursing interventions are invaluable in detecting and managing these patient problems.
- Teach patients to take the medications exactly as prescribed. This is especially important to emphasize for patients who are on alternate-day therapy. Extra doses of medications are never taken, nor is the dosage altered in any way; and medications are never stopped without first checking with the physician. Patients need to understand the ramifications of long-term therapy. Patients who have been on long-term therapy (the equivalent of greater than 20 mg of hydrocortisone per day for longer than 1 to 2 weeks) are never abruptly withdrawn from corticosteroids. Rather, the physician tapers the dose gradually. A reduction of 5 to 10 mg every 3 to 7 days, as tolerated, is usually employed.
- Monitor laboratory data. Regular measurements of serum glucose levels are performed. Known diabetic patients frequently must have their insulin or oral hypoglycemic therapy altered to assist them in adapting to increases in blood glucose.
- Perform skin testing for infectious diseases such as tuberculosis before instituting glucocorticoid therapy. If a patient has inactive or encapsulated tuberculosis, glucocorticoid administration may cause the tuberculosis to become active. Patients with encapsulated tuberculosis may need concurrent administration of prophylactic antituberculosis therapy, usually isoniazid (INH), during glucocorticoid therapy.
- Monitor all wounds. The anti-inflammatory effects of the glucocorticoids may cause a delay in wound healing. This is particularly important in patients who undergo surgical procedures while on glucocorticoid therapy. Use meticulously sterile technique when dressing wounds and handling tubes and catheters. Also, white blood cell counts are performed routinely on patients receiving large doses and/or long-term therapy.
- Monitor for psychologic changes. Glucocorticoid administration can cause psychologic disturbances in some patients. Be alert to subtle changes in behavior such as restlessness, insomnia, and nightmares, as these may precede more serious disturbances.
- Teach the patient about well-defined emergency indicators and what action they should take. For example, the patient with Addison's disease who is subjected to stress must increase the dosage of corticosteroids according to the physician's guidelines. The occurrence of a sudden weight gain, weakness or undue fatigue, change in sleep patterns, black or tarry stools, injuries, or infections are reported to the physician.

Patient Teaching

- Teach the patient information concerning adrenocortical drugs that is included in Table 44–7. Patients who have adrenocortical insufficiency are taught that they need to increase corticosteroid dosage when subjected to physiologic stress. They should follow their physician's guidelines in these instances.
- Teach the patient to carry a card or wear a bracelet or necklace identifying his or her condition. This measure could prove lifesaving.
- Teach patients to take corticosteroids with food or at mealtimes. Administration of the medications in the morning mimics the normal diurnal secretion of cortisol, which is highest in the early morning. The entire dosage may be administered at 4 PM. This provides a second daily peak of steroid level, thus protecting the patient late in the day.
- If antacids or H_2 inhibitors are prescribed to decrease stomach irritation, instruct the patient to take them faithfully.
- Teach the patient to restrict his or her intake of caffeine and alcohol. These substances increase gastric secretions, which can lead to the development of a peptic ulcer. Also teach the patient to avoid excessive use of aspirin or aspirin-containing compounds because the additional gastric irritation may initiate ulcer development.

Table 44–7. PATIENT TEACHING INFORMATION— ADRENOCORTICAL DRUGS

Dear Patient:

This drug has been prescribed for you. This is what you should know about your drug to get the most from your therapy.

Adrenal drugs are used for many conditions. They are being used for you to _____ .

☐ 1. Adrenal drugs (corticosteroids) are to be taken exactly as prescribed.

☐ 2. Extra doses of medication are *never* to be taken, nor should you change your dose in any way. *Exception:* Patients who have adrenocortical insufficiency must increase corticosteroid dosage when subjected to physiologic stress; you should follow your doctor's instructions for times of stress.

☐ 3. Corticosteroids are taken with food to avoid stomach upset.

☐ 4. If your physician prescribes it, be sure to faithfully take your antacid or antiulcer drug while you are taking corticosteroids.

☐ 5. Check with your physician or pharmacist before taking other drugs. Generally, you should not take aspirin or aspirin-containing drugs.

☐ 6. You should not drink much coffee, tea, or alcohol while taking corticosteroids (one cup of coffee or tea per day; one or two beers, five glasses of wine or shots of whiskey per week).

☐ 7. *Never* stop taking your corticosteroids without first talking to your physician. IMPORTANT: If you have been taking corticosteroids for longer than 1–2 weeks, you *must not* stop taking them abruptly; your physician will taper you off.

☐ 8. If you experience side effects from corticosteroids, check with your physician. Common side effects include swelling of feet and hands, weight gain, nausea, and vomiting.

☐ 9. If you have an injury that does not heal or if you develop an infection, call your physician.

☐ 10. Have your blood pressure checked every week, as corticosteroids may increase it.

☐ 11. If you are taking corticosteroids for a long period of time, you should wear a bracelet or carry a card with this information on it.

☐ 12. Store your corticosteroids in a light-resistant, tightly closed bottle.

- Test the stools for occult blood at regular intervals to detect a bleeding ulcer.
- Teach the patient that sodium and potassium levels may need to be monitored. Dietary sodium restriction or potassium supplementation may be needed. The patient should follow his or her physician's orders in this regard.
- Teach patients to have regular tonometry testing, as increases in intraocular pressure can occur.
- Stress the need for continued medical follow-up, and periodically review the teaching with the patient in order to ensure that the patient's knowledge is accurate, complete, and up to date.

EVALUATION

- Determine the effectiveness of the adrenocortical medications. This evaluation is based on outcomes determined by the nurse and patient.
- Evaluate the patient's understanding of the adverse effects of the adrenal corticosteroids. Sodium retention, potassium loss, hypertension, muscle wasting, and peptic ulceration can occur with long-term use.

Most patients requiring adrenal corticosteroids comply with their medication regimen because they note improvements in their symptomatology. Occasionally, a few "overcomply," rationalizing that if some amount of corticosteroid makes them feel better, taking more will cause greater improvement. Patients on alternate-day therapy may need a great deal of encouragement and support to stay on their medication schedule.

The cushingoid appearance, caused by long-term glucocorticoid use, can be very disturbing to patients and may interfere with compliance for some. The knowledge that the cushingoid changes reverse themselves on discontinuance of therapy may be helpful.

The bibliography for this chapter can be found in Appendix B, which begins on page 1054.

CHAPTER REVIEW QUESTIONS*

1. An agent used for maintenance therapy for patients with salt-losing adrenogenital syndrome is:
   a. Fludrocortisone
   b. Prednisolone
   c. Dexamethasone.
   d. Beclomethasone dipropionate.

2. Glucocorticoid regulation is mediated by:
   a. Somatotropin.
   b. Renin.
   c. Sodium levels.
   d. Corticotropin.

3. Patients who are on long-term glucocorticoid therapy may take on the cushingoid appearance, typified by the following characteristic:

*See Appendix A, which begins on page 1051, for answers.

   a. Fat deposits in extremities.
   b. Cervicodorsal fat pad.
   c. Clubbing of fingernails.
   d. Exophthalamos.

4. When patients are abruptly withdrawn from long-term glucocorticoid therapy, acute adrenal insufficiency may occur. One indicator of this life-threatening complication is:
   a. Syncope
   b. Palpitations
   c. Hypertension
   d. Shortness of breath.

5. Glucocorticoids exert an anti-inflammatory response by:
   a. Increasing capillary permeability and dilation.
   b. Stimulating fibroblast proliferation.
   c. Preventing the release of bradykinins and prostaglandins.
   d. Promoting movement of neutrophils to the site of injury.

BUILDING YOUR CRITICAL THINKING SKILLS

GLUCOCORTICOID THERAPY

A patient with an 8-year history of multiple sclerosis (MS) is admitted to the emergency department with severe fatigue and severe dehydration. He had an acute exacerbation of his MS 1 month ago, for which he was treated with prednisolone. He has felt very good since this episode.

Currently, his serum glucose is 66 mg/dL, and serum potassium 6.5 mEq/dL.

1. How might this patient's drug therapy be related to his symptoms?
2. What other data should the nurse assess?
3. What teaching is indicated for this patient?

Antidiabetic Agents

Christine M. Bellari, MS, RN

KEY TERMS

Diabetes mellitus
Dawn phenomenon
Disulfiram-like reaction
Exogenous insulin
Glucogenesis
Glycogenolysis
Gluconeogenesis
Glycosylated hemoglobin
Glycosuria
Hyperglycemic
    hyperosmolar nonketotic
    coma

Insulin resistance
Ketoacidosis
Ketosis
Lipoatrophy
Lipohypertrophy
Neuropathy
Normoglycemia
Somogyi effect

LEARNING OBJECTIVES

After reading this chapter, the student will be able to:

1. Identify those medications commonly used in the treatment of diabetes mellitus.
2. Differentiate between insulin and oral antidiabetic agents as to the mechanism of action, route of administration, pharmacokinetics, contraindications and precautions, adverse effects, and interactions.
3. Identify specific areas to assess in the patient requiring antidiabetic agents to formulate appropriate patient outcomes.
4. Plan the nursing interventions necessary to administer antidiabetic medications and choose appropriate teaching strategies to gain patient compliance.
5. Evaluate the diabetic patient at various stages of treatment to measure the effectiveness of nursing interventions.

*D*iabetes mellitus is a disease characterized by an absolute or relative deficiency of insulin, resulting in an elevated level of sugar in the blood. This leads to abnormalities of carbohydrate, protein, and fat metabolism and to eventual complications of the eye, kidney, blood vessels, and nervous system. More than 14 million Americans have diabetes, and the overall incidence is increasing each year. Diabetes, along with its complications, is a major cause of morbidity and mortality in the United States.

There are two major types of diabetes, type I and type II. Type I, or insulin-dependent diabetes mellitus (IDDM),

is characterized by an absolute deficiency of insulin, abrupt onset of symptoms, and proneness to *ketosis* (abnormally high concentration of ketone bodies in the blood). Without insulin, fats are broken down rapidly to be used as the body's energy source. The fragments of fatty acid metabolism are called ketones, and the accumulation of ketones can cause death. This type of diabetes most commonly occurs in youth, but may occur at any age.

Type II, or non-insulin-dependent diabetes mellitus (NIDDM), frequently occurs without any symptoms. The individual is able to produce some insulin and therefore is not prone to ketosis. In many cases, the individual produces an above-normal amount of insulin, and the hyperglycemia is due to the body cells being resistant to the insulin. Type II diabetes is most frequently seen after the age of 40, but may occur at any age. Usually, the individual has a family history of diabetes and is overweight. For a more detailed comparison of type I and type II diabetes, refer to Table 45–1.

There is no known cure for diabetes. However, it can be controlled, primarily with diet modification, exercise, and, if necessary, insulin and/or oral antidiabetic agents.

The major goals of management are to accomplish the following: restore cellular utilization of glucose, prevent ketosis, abolish symptoms indicative of hyperglycemia, attain normal growth and development for a child, and maintain the blood glucose at a near-normal level without frequent episodes of hypoglycemia. Normalization of blood glucose levels is desired in an effort to prevent, postpone, or reverse the chronic complications of diabetes.

INSULIN

Insulin is classified biochemically as a protein, composed of 51 amino acids and having a molecular weight of 6000 daltons. It is composed of two amino acid chains—chain A (acidic) and chain B (basic)—linked together by two disulfide bridges. Both of these chains are formed from a single-chain precursor, namely, proinsulin. In the final step of insulin synthesis, which occurs in the islets of Langerhans in the pancreas, proinsulin is converted to insulin.

ACTION

Insulin plays an important role in carbohydrate, protein, and fat metabolism. Most of the body's cells require insulin to allow the entry of glucose. The major cells in which insulin plays a significant role include liver, muscle, and adipocyte cells. The brain requires a constant supply of glucose to function. However, insulin is not required for glucose to enter the brain.

One of the most important functions of insulin is to facilitate the conversion of glucose to glycogen in the liver. This glycogen is then converted to glucose when the body is in a fasting state to provide cell nourishment and to prevent hypoglycemia. Insulin also promotes fatty acid synthesis in the liver. These fatty acids are then transported to the adipocyte cells for storage. Additionally, insulin decreases the rate of *gluconeogenesis* (the formation of glucose from noncarbohydrate sources such as protein and fat) in the liver.

In the muscle, insulin transports glucose to be used as energy after a meal if the individual is exercising. However, if the individual is sedentary, the glucose is converted to glycogen for later use. Insulin also stimulates the uptake of amino acids and conversion to protein in the muscle.

In the adipocyte cell, insulin allows glucose to enter and be converted to free fatty acids. It inhibits hormone-sensitive lipase and therefore decreases the amount of fatty acids released in the blood. Lastly, insulin forms a substance that binds with the fatty acids to form triglycerides, the storage form of fat in the adipocyte cells.

In the absence of insulin, there is an underutilization of glucose, as it is no longer readily transported into the cells. Protein synthesis ceases and wasting of the muscle cells begin. Large amounts of amino acids are released into the plasma. Because gluconeogenesis is no longer suppressed, these amino acids are converted to glucose. This combination of effects leads to hyperglycemia, resulting in *glycosuria* (sugar in the urine). In the absence of

Table 45–1. DIABETES MELLITUS

Definition
A chronic disorder of carbohydrate metabolism, resulting from the overproduction and underutilization of glucose due to the lack of or inactivity of insulin.

Types
Only major types are listed.
Type I, or Insulin-Dependent Diabetes Mellitus (IDDM): Individual has an absolute deficiency of insulin from the beta cells of the pancreas.
Type II, or Non-Insulin-Dependent Diabetes Mellitus (NIDDM): Individual has a relative lack of insulin or a resistance to its effect.

Etiologies

Type I (IDDM)	Type II (NIDDM)
More frequently found in HLA types B8, BW15, DW3, and DW4. Viral insult may trigger beta cell damage, possibly via an autoimmune reaction. Islet cell antibodies can frequently be found.	Serum insulin levels may be depressed, normal, or elevated. Inability to utilize insulin may be due to fewer receptor sites, increased circulating insulin antibodies, or receptor defects that impair insulin binding to cells of the body. Often related to obesity or stress.
Onset most commonly before the age of 20, but can occur in the adult.	Onset after the age of 40 with gradual onset.

Objective Symptoms	Type I	Type II
Elevated blood glucose	x	x
Glycosuria	x	x
Polyuria	x	x
Ketonuria	x	
Weight loss	x	x
Susceptibility to infection	x	x
Poor wound healing	x	x

Subjective Symptoms	Type I	Type II
Fatigue	x	x
Thirst	x	x
Hunger	x	x
Blurred vision	x	x
Dry, itchy skin	x	x

Management	Type I	Type II
Insulin	x	x
Diet management	x	x
Oral antidiabetics		x
Urine and/or blood testing	x	x
Weight loss		x
Exercise program	x	x
Patient education	x	x

insulin, there is an increase in the metabolism of fat stores to free fatty acids and glycerol. These fragments of fatty acid metabolism are referred to collectively as "ketone bodies" and consist of acetone, beta-hydroxybutyric acid, and acetoacetic acid. Their presence in large quantities in the body fluids is called ketosis, and because two of the three compounds are acids, the term ketoacidosis also applies. *Ketoacidosis* is characterized by an abnormally low blood pH caused by the buildup of acidic ketone bodies, leading to acidosis, coma, and death.

Additionally, the lack of insulin increases the amount of stored triglycerides in the liver, resulting in a fatty liver. The excess of fatty acids in the liver promotes conversion of some of the fatty acids into phospholipids and cholesterol. Along with triglycerides, these substances are discharged into the blood stream as lipoproteins. This can lead to rapid development of atherosclerosis. Biochemically, insulin works by binding with receptors on the cell membrane. This activates a second messenger, guanidine monophosphate (cyclic GMP), which serves to activate the cell's metabolic processes to utilize glucose as a source of energy.

USES

Insulin therapy is indicated in the treatment of all patients with type I (insulin-dependent) diabetes. It is also used for the type II (non-insulin-dependent) diabetic patient who is pregnant or for the gestational diabetic patient, to achieve diabetic control. Insulin may be used for the type II diabetic patient during periods of stress, surgery, or infection. Insulin may also be used for the type II diabetic individual who has failed to achieve glycemic control by following a diet, exercise regimen, and oral hypoglycemic therapy.

TYPES OF INSULIN

Insulin is available for parenteral administration from animal (beef or pork pancreas), recombinant DNA, and semisynthetic sources. The insulin obtained from beef pancreas differs from human insulin by three amino acids, whereas the insulin obtained from a pig differs by only one amino acid. As a result of this difference, diabetics taking beef and pork insulin form some insulin-blocking antibodies that delay the activity of *exogenous insulin*, which is the insulin produced outside the body and administered by injection. Products from animal sources are either standard or purified. Standard insulins contain no more than 25 parts per million (ppm) of proinsulin, the major contaminant (tends to promote adverse reactions); and purified insulins contain no more than 10 ppm of proinsulin. A biosynthetic human insulin, developed through recombinant DNA technology, and a semisynthetic human insulin, created by altering the amino acid structure in pork insulin to the structure of human insulin, are also available.

The purified pork and human insulins are more costly and are generally equal to each other in price. Because human insulin causes less antibody formation than the purified pork insulin, it is the insulin of choice for individuals with special needs. Human insulin is recommended for patients using insulin intermittently because these individuals are more likely to develop an insulin allergy and/or increased antibody formation if they require insulin therapy at a later time. Patients who fall into this category include individuals with gestational diabetes, those with type II diabetes who need close regulation during surgery or during an infectious process, and nondiabetic individuals who are receiving parenteral nutrition. A pregnant woman with type I diabetes should be given human insulin because the insulin antibodies that may form are passed to the fetus. Some diabetologists believe that all newly diagnosed diabetic patients should be started on human insulin.

INSULIN PREPARATIONS

Although the pharmacologic action of all types of insulin is the same, different preparations have been developed with varying onsets, peaks, and durations of action to allow for individualized control. These are divided into rapid-acting insulins (Regular, Semilente, Insulin Lispro), intermediate-acting insulins (NPH, Lente), and long-acting insulin (Ultralente). Mixtures of rapid-acting insulin with intermediate-acting insulin is also available. The insulin utilized for the premade mixtures are NPH and regular insulin.

Regular insulin was the first insulin preparation available. Insulins with longer onset, peak, and duration were created by adding a protein such as protamine or globin or by the addition of zinc to regular insulin. Recently, a rapid-acting analog was developed by reversing amino acids on the insulin B chain. It is important to note that the onset, peak, and duration of the different types of insulin have been derived through many laboratory studies and that the diabetic patients chosen for the study were often volunteers who were in optimal health. In any patient these times can be altered by an individual's metabolism and diabetic pathology. Refer to Table 45–2 for dosage; onset, peak, and duration; and nursing implications of the various types of insulin.

Rapid-Acting Insulins

The rapid-acting insulins include **regular insulin *(Humulin R, Novolin R, Iletin I, Novolin R PenFill, Regular Purified Iletin II, Velosulin BR*, and *Regular U-500)*, insulin lispro *(Humalog)*,** and **Semilente insulin *(Semilente Iletin I)*.** Rapid or short-acting insulins have the quickest onset, peak, and duration of activity. Depending on the type of rapid-acting insulin the patient is on, he or she must eat within 15 minutes to ½ hour to prevent a hypoglycemic reaction.

Regular insulin is a clear solution without any added modifying agent, and thus it is the only insulin that can be used intravenously and used with the insulin pump. A buffered insulin, Velosulin BR, is used especially for pump therapy because the buffering may lessen the chance of catheter obstruction. Regular insulin is also given subcutaneously to regulate the blood glucose. The dosage of regular insulin to be given can be determined by a sliding scale dependent on blood glucose levels or may be a set dosage. Regular insulin may be used in combination with intermediate- or long-acting insulins to obtain better diabetic control.

Table 45–2. INSULINS

DRUG NAME/ROUTE AND DOSAGE	PHARMACOKINETICS/ DYNAMICS	NURSING IMPLICATIONS
all insulins	**PB:** not bound **B:** mainly in liver, kidney, and muscle tissue (lesser extent) **E:** kidney	**ASSESSMENT:** Obtain baseline and periodic assessments of blood glucose levels; blood cell counts; potassium, triglyceride, and cholesterol levels. Assess glycosylated hemoglobin (Hb A_{1C}) level. If patient has DKA, monitor ECG and assess for cardiac dysrhythmias. Assess the patient's present knowledge of diabetes and basics of care including meal pattern, hyperglycemia, hypoglycemia, role of exercise, blood glucose monitoring and/or urine testing, and skin and foot care. If patient is on insulin therapy, assess injection technique. Assess injection sites for lipohypertrophy. If patient is on pump therapy, assess abdomen for abscesses at catheter insertion site. Assess insulin injection sites for local or delayed allergy. Continually assess for hyperglycemia and hypoglycemia. **INTERVENTION:** Only regular insulin can be administered by IV route. Dosage is always expressed in USP units. Use only syringes calibrated for particular concentration of insulin. Because no syringes are made for U-500 insulin, it must be administered with U-100 syringe. Dosage adjustments may be required if you interchange different insulin sources. Avoid interchanging. Switching from separate injections to prepared mixture may alter patient response. Monitor blood glucoses closely. Administer insulin as ordered. Double check type and dosage with another nurse before administration. When administering insulin intravenously, do not mix insulin with any other medication in IV bag. Some insulin adheres to IV bottle as well as IV tubing. Flush 50 mL of solution through tubing to minimize further adherence. IV pumps or controllers should be used to safely monitor intermittent or continuous insulin infusions. Serum potassium levels must be monitored. Give patients their insulin and meals on time. **Patient Teaching**—Educate patient according to needs determined through needs assessment. If mixing insulins, advise patient not to alter order of mixing or to change model or brand of syringe or needle without permission of physician. **EVALUATION:** Evaluate patient's blood glucose level and urinary glucose and ketones. Evaluate patient's knowledge of diabetes and basics of treatment. Evaluate all technical skills that will be performed in home setting. Evaluate patient's desire to adhere to prescribed regimen, using verbal and nonverbal cues. Determine if there is need for follow-up care at home.

RAPID-ACTING INSULINS

regular insulin (Humalin R) (Novolin R) (Regular Iletin I) (Novolin R PenFill) (Regular Purified Iletin II) (Velosulin BR) (Humulin RU-500)		
May be given subcutaneously (SC), IV, or in insulin pump. Dosage is individualized according to patient's blood glucose values. When given SC, give 15–30 min before meals (ac).	**Onset:** 0.5–1 hr **Peak:** 2–5 hr **Duration:** 6–8 hr **½L:** NA	Same as for all.
insulin lispro (Humalog) (Humalog cartridge)		
SC route only: Give ≤15 min ac.	**Onset:** within 15 min **Peak:** 30–90 min **Duration:** 300 min **½L:** NA	Same as for all.

Table 45–2. INSULINS, *Continued*

DRUG NAME/ROUTE AND DOSAGE	PHARMACOKINETICS/ DYNAMICS	NURSING IMPLICATIONS
RAPID-ACTING INSULINS		
Semilente insulin (Semilente Iletin I)		
SC route only: Give 15–30 min ac breakfast and supper. Dosage is individualized.	**Onset:** 1–1.5 hr **Peak:** 5–10 hr **Duration:** 12–16 hr **½L:** NA	Same as for all.
INTERMEDIATE-ACTING INSULINS		
NPH insulin (Humulin N) (Novolin N) (NPH Iletin I) (NPH Iletin II Purified) (Novolin N PenFill)		
SC route only: Usually given 15–30 min ac breakfast and supper. Dosage is individualized.	**Onset:** 1–1.5 hr **Peak:** 4–12 hr **Duration:** 24 hr **½L:** NA	Same as for all.
Lente insulin (Humulin L) (Novolin L) (Lente Iletin I) (Lente Iletin II)		
SC route only: Usually given 15–30 min ac breakfast and supper. Dosage is individualized.	**Onset:** 1–2.5 hr **Peak:** 7–15 hr **Duration:** 24 hr **½L:** NA	Same as for all.
insulin mixtures (Humulin 70/30) (Novolin 70/30) (Humulin 50/50) (Novolin 70/30 PenFill)		
SC route only: Usually given 15–30 min ac breakfast and supper. Dosage is individualized.	**Onset:** 0.5 hr **Peak:** 4–8 hr **Duration:** 24 hr **½L:** NA	Same as for all.
LONG-ACTING INSULINS		
Ultralente insulin (Humulin U)		
SC route only: Usually given 15–30 min before breakfast. Dosage is individualized.	**Onset:** 4–8 hr **Peak:** 10–30 hr **Duration:** >36 hr **½Life:** NA	Same as for all.

DKA = diabetic ketoacidosis; NA = not available.

Insulin lispro has the quickest onset, peak, and duration of any of the available insulins. Because of its ultra-rapid-acting activity, the patient must eat within 15 minutes of taking this insulin and must use an inter-mediate- or long-acting insulin as well to achieve diabetic control. Insulin lispro is given subcutaneously.

Semilente insulin is a prompt acting zinc suspension. It may be used in combination with Lente or Ultralente insulin to achieve optimal control for the patient with diabetes.

Intermediate-Acting Insulins

Intermediate-acting insulins include **NPH insulin *(Humu-lin N, Novolin N, NPH Iletin I and II, Novolin N PenFill)*** and **Lente insulin *(Humulin L, Novolin L, Lente Iletin I and II).*** Intermediate-acting insulins are commonly administered once or twice daily before breakfast and/or supper to achieve diabetic control. The most likely time for an insulin reaction to occur in a patient taking an intermediate-acting insulin in the morning is before supper, whereas the most likely time for a reaction to occur in a patient taking an intermediate-acting insulin before supper is around midnight. Afternoon and evening snacks incorporated into the meal plan can help prevent these reactions. Both NPH and Lente insulin are often mixed with a rapid-acting insulin because it takes several hours for these intermediate-acting insulins to have a measurable effect. Both insulin combinations—NPH regular; and Lente and Semilente—are stable mixtures.

Long-Acting Insulins

Ultralente insulin *(Humulin U, Novolin U)* is the only long-acting insulin available. This insulin is frequently combined with a rapid-acting insulin to provide control throughout the day and night. At low doses, Ultralente insulin mimics physiologic insulin release by supplying a basal level of insulin to suppress *glycogenolysis* (the conversion of glycogen to glucose) and *gluconeogenesis*. Then, regular insulin is added before meals to cover the intake.

▼ **CLINICAL ALERT**

Insulin reactions for the patient taking Ultralente insulin may occur during the night. This may be dangerous because the patient may not waken. Irritability, nightmares, and diaphoresis during the night may signal a hypoglycemic reaction.

Concentration of Insulin

Insulin is available in the United States in two different concentrations: U-100 and U-500. The U-500 insulin is used for the occasional person who is insulin resistant and requires more than 300 units (U) of insulin per day. The concentration indicates how many units of insulin are contained in each cubic centimeter (cc) or milliliter (mL). For example, U-100 insulin provides the patient with 100 units of insulin per milliliter. Because U-500 insulin is used infrequently, the only syringe available is the U-100 insulin syringe. Care must be taken to draw up the correct amount. The correct amount to draw up can be determined proportionately. For example, if the patient requires 200 units of U-500 insulin the nurse draws up 40 units of the U-500 insulin in the U-100 syringe. U-500 insulin requires a prescription for purchase.

Pharmacokinetics

Insulin must be given parenterally to avoid enzymatic destruction in the intestine. A variety of factors may affect absorption. These factors include the following: the site of injection, the depth of the injection, the presence of *lipohypertrophy* (accumulation of fatty tissue at the site of the insulin injection), increased blood flow to the injection site through massage or exercise, and diminished peripheral circulation.

Some sites where insulin is given absorb more rapidly than others. The order of absorption speed for injection sites from highest to lowest is the abdomen, arm, buttock, and thigh, respectively. The depth of the injection is also an important consideration. Intravenous administration is the most direct way in which to administer insulin, followed by intramuscular injection, then subcutaneous administration. Lipohypertrophy at the injection site may cause erratic absorption; therefore, it is essential that insulin injection sites be systematically rotated so this condition does not occur. A problem with the development of lipohypertrophy is that patients continue to inject in these sites as many report less pain than at other sites. With the purer preparations of insulin available today, this condition does not occur as frequently as it did in the past.

Massaging the site immediately after injection increases the blood flow to the area and, therefore, speeds up absorption. If an individual exercises, the absorption of insulin is quicker if it is injected into an area that is heavily exercised. For example, if an individual jogs, insulin injected into the legs absorbs more rapidly than insulin injected into the arms or abdomen. Insulin lispro has the quickest onset of all insulins, and an individual must eat within 15 minutes of injecting the insulin. Decreased blood flow due to decreased cardiac output or atherosclerosis may decrease absorption.

Insulin does not bind significantly with plasma proteins. Primarily, it circulates in the blood and lymph as a free hormone.

The plasma half-life of insulin injected intravenously is less than 9 minutes in humans. However, as a result of antibody binding, the half-life may be extended up to 13 hours. Insulin is primarily metabolized in the liver and to a lesser extent in the kidneys and muscle tissue.

In the kidney, insulin is filtered at the glomerulus and is 98% reabsorbed in the proximal tubule. About 40% of the reabsorbed insulin returns to the venous blood, and 60% is metabolized in cells lining the proximal tubule. In patients without renal impairment, less than 2% of the filtered insulin dose is excreted unchanged in the urine.

Commonly, as a result of vascular insufficiency, the patient with diabetes experiences renal dysfunction. Renal damage reduces the amount of insulin required as there will no longer be excretion of normal quantities of the drug. Severe impairment of renal function appears to affect the rate of disappearance of circulating insulin to a greater extent than hepatic disease.

Contraindications and Precautions

Administration of rapid-acting insulin is contraindicated if the blood glucose level is below 70 mg/dL or if the signs of hypoglycemia are present. Regular insulin is the only insulin that may be given intravenously, because it does not have a modifying agent.

Adverse Effects

The most common adverse effects of insulin therapy include hypoglycemia, lipoatrophy, delayed local reactions at the injection site, systemic allergic reactions, and insulin resistance.

The most serious adverse effect of insulin therapy is hypoglycemia. The patient is carefully monitored to avoid this and taught the symptoms of hypoglycemia to facilitate early recognition. Hypoglycemic reactions often can be avoided by carefully balancing dietary intake, meal times, exercise, and insulin dosage. If the patient is aware of the symptoms, he or she may notice early signs of hypoglycemia: weakness, hunger, tachycardia, the development of a cool clammy sweat, and inner trembling. These manifestations are the result of epinephrine release as the body tries to elevate blood glucose levels through normal compensatory mechanisms. As hypoglycemia worsens, headache, blurred vision, diplopia, mental confusion, incoherent speech, unconsciousness, and convulsions may result owing to the lack of glucose to the brain. If hypoglycemia occurs while the patient is asleep, he or she may awaken with a nightmare and notice a cool, clammy, profuse sweat.

Some individuals do not feel the sensation of hypoglycemia. These individuals include patients who have had diabetes for many years in whom the lack of sensation is due to *neuropathy* (chronic complication of diabetes that affects the nervous system, resulting in diminished peripheral sensation, diarrhea, and impotence); patients taking beta-blockers; and patients whose blood sugar is dropping very slowly. It is important to assess whether the patient can feel the warning symptoms of hypoglycemia. If they are unable to tell when the blood sugar drops, a plan that includes frequent blood glucose testing should be developed.

Because the brain depends on a constant supply of glucose to function, rapid treatment of hypoglycemia is essential to prevent brain damage. Ten to fifteen grams of a fast-acting carbohydrate such as one-half or three-fourths of a cup of regular soda pop or two or three sugar cubes can be administered if the patient is able to tolerate food or fluid. Otherwise, glucagon or IV dextrose is given to patients who are unconscious.

Insulin *lipoatrophy* is a benign condition in which a loss of subcutaneous fat occurs at the injection site. The cause of this problem is unknown, and lipoatrophy does not occur frequently since the development of the more purified insulins. The immune response to insulin contaminants is thought to be involved. The treatment for lipoatrophy involves injecting a purer insulin into the depressed area to allow the reaccumulation of the fatty tissue.

Insulin-induced lipohypertrophy results from repeated injections in the same spot. Avoidance of these areas for future injection may result in the disappearance of this extra tissue. The patient must also be taught a systematic method of site rotation.

Delayed localized reactions can occur in patients receiving insulin, especially in those receiving insulin for the first time. Lesions, which are reddened and itchy, appear 3 to 6 hours after an injection. These lesions are often preceded by a stinging or burning sensation at the time of injection. Delayed localized reactions are self-limiting and usually disappear in a few days to a few weeks. No treatment is indicated. However, switching to a purer form of insulin may resolve the problem.

A systemic insulin allergy or true insulin allergy is a rare occurrence. This complication begins as an immediate reaction at the injection site and quickly spreads all over the body. Anaphylactic shock may occur. This situation is more common in patients with a history of interrupted insulin therapy. The manifestations of insulin allergy are usually seen 1 to 2 weeks after the resumption of insulin therapy. Because the patient seems to be allergic to the insulin molecule itself, desensitization is the only effective treatment.

In *insulin resistance* the individual requires more than 200 units of insulin per day. A history of intermittent insulin use is common in these patients. Switching from beef or beef-pork mixtures to purified pork or human insulin is often helpful. It is important to note that insulin resistance may abruptly cease and the patient may become hypoglycemic from the large doses of insulin. Patients must be monitored closely.

Interactions

Many medications affect blood glucose levels by promoting either hyperglycemia or hypoglycemia. Refer to Table 45–3 for a listing of these medications.

Some medications antagonize the effect of insulin. Epinephrine antagonizes the effect of insulin by mobilizing glycogen to increase the blood glucose level. Glucocorticoids increase hepatic *glucogenesis* (formation of glucose from glycogen) and gluconeogenesis. Thiazide diuretics and, to a lesser extent, furosemide and ethacrynic acid also elevate the blood glucose, possibly through potassium depletion or inhibition of insulin secretion. Calcium channel blockers, diazoxide, and phenytoin inhibit insulin secretion. Lithium salts may also decrease insulin secretion.

Some medications have been found to augment the effect of insulin and, therefore, cause hypoglycemia. Fenfluramine (Pondimin) increases the uptake of glucose by the muscles and may have intrinsic hypoglycemic activity. Monoamine oxidase inhibitors and alcohol use can cause hypoglycemia because they inhibit hepatic gluconeogenesis. Concurrent use of insulin with oral antidiabetic agents in the treatment of type II diabetes decreases the blood glucose level.

Beta-adrenergic blocking agents may cause hyperglycemia through inhibition of insulin secretion or hypoglycemia through inhibition of glycogenolysis. These medications also mask some of the warning symptoms of hypoglycemia and prolong the period of hypoglycemia

Table 45–3. MEDICATIONS THAT AFFECT BLOOD GLUCOSE

Hypoglycemia	Hyperglycemia
Alcohol	ACTH
Allopurinol*	Albuterol
Anabolic steroids	Amphetamines
Beta-blockers	Asparaginase
Chloramphenicol*	Beta-blockers
Clofibrate*	Calcium channel blockers
Disopyramide	Carbonic anhydrase inhibitors
Fenfluramine	Decongestants (i.e., Sudafed)
Guanethidine	Diazoxide
H₂ inhibitors	Epinephrine
Isoniazid	Estrogens
Oral anticoagulants*	Furosemide
MAO inhibitors	Glucagon
Oxyphenbutazone*	Glucocorticoids
Oxytetracycline	Glycerol
Phenylbutazone*	Lithium salts
Salicylates*	Marijuana
Sulfonamides*	Nicotinic acid
	Oral contraceptives
	Pentamidine
	Phenytoin
	Rifampin
	Ritodrine
	Terbutaline
	Thyroid Hormones

*These medications interact with the sulfonylurea agents only.

by blocking gluconeogenesis. Pentamidine, a common therapy for pneumocystic pneumonia, can cause hypoglycemia. It is believed that pentamidine is cytoxic to the beta cell and that inappropriate insulin release may occur during its use. Continued beta-cell damage may lead to hyperglycemia and eventually to insulin-dependent diabetes mellitus.

Some medications may contain varying amounts of hidden dextrose. Often, the sugar base is an attempt to make the medication more palatable. The sugar content may be classified as an inactive ingredient and thus is not listed on the label. It is also important to avoid diluting medications with a dextrose solution, to avoid the hyperglycemic effect.

INSULIN THERAPY

Determining the Initial Dosage

Several methods can be used to determine the initial amount of insulin necessary for the patient with diabetes. Many physicians start with an average dose of an intermediate-acting insulin for the individual being treated. The initial dosage range is usually 15 to 30 U of insulin per day, or 0.5 units/kg per day. The obese patient requires the greater amount. The dosage is then adjusted to meet the patient's individualized insulin requirement. Sometimes patients are hospitalized and are given a rapid-acting insulin on a sliding scale according to blood glucose elevations. This provides the physician with an idea of the patient's daily insulin requirement. Traditionally, most patients with diabetes were managed on one injection of an intermediate-acting insulin before breakfast. This abolished the problem of ketosis and the symptoms of hyperglycemia during the day, but did not control hyperglycemia during the night. Research through the Diabetes Control and Complications Trial indicates that intensive therapy or maintaining the blood glucose levels as close to that of a nondiabetic as possible effectively delays the onset and slows the progression of diabetic retinopathy, nephropathy, and neuropathy in patients with insulin-dependent diabetes mellitus (Nathan et al., 1993). Today's management is to maintain a blood glucose as close to that of the nondiabetic as possible, without undue risks of hypoglycemia. This may include a regimen of self blood glucose monitoring, administration of split and mixed insulin dosages, intensified insulin therapy using the insulin pump or multiple injections of regular insulin daily combined with an intermediate- or long-acting insulin. To achieve this requires collaboration between the physician and patient and the motivation and commitment of both parties.

General Insulin Dosing

Once the amount of daily insulin requirements is determined, intermediate-acting insulin is initiated. Usually a single dose of the intermediate-acting insulin does not provide optimal control. The individual may achieve adequate control during the day but be hyperglycemic at night. Therefore, one daily injection is often limited to the

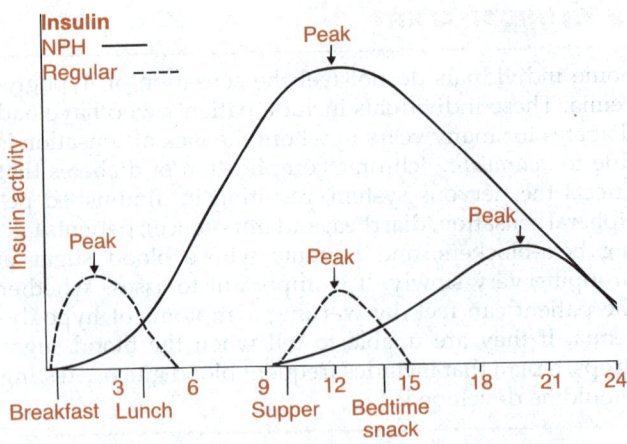

Figure 45–1. Time and activity of split and mixed dosages of insulin.

type II patient with advanced age and other chronic complications who requires insulin. In this case, advancing age and health status diminishes the value of strict control of blood glucose levels in preventing or delaying complications of diabetes. Also, this patient may be at a greater risk for hypoglycemia.

Most patients begin control with one-half to two-thirds of the intermediate-acting insulin dose given before breakfast and the rest given before supper. Blood glucose levels are then taken before breakfast, 2 hours after breakfast, before supper, and at bedtime to assess the results of the intermediate-acting insulin and to determine if rapid-acting insulin is necessary at both or either of those times. For example, if the blood glucose level is elevated before supper, it indicates that the morning's intermediate-acting insulin dosage must be increased. However, if the blood glucose level is elevated 2 hours after breakfast, rapid-acting insulin is indicated along with the morning's intermediate-acting insulin. Refer to Figure 45–1 for a pictorial diagram of the course of action for this split and mixed insulin regimen. If control is not achieved on the two injections of mixed insulin, another option is to use a three-dose regimen. With this regimen, the patient is given an intermediate- and rapid-acting insulin prior to breakfast, a rapid-acting insulin prior to supper, and an intermediate- and rapid-acting insulin at bedtime. This regimen is recommended to avoid the dawn phenomenon and Somogyi effect. The *dawn phenomenon* is an early morning rise in blood glucose as a result of normal counterregulatory hormone production, and the *Somogyi effect* is a situation in which the person experiences rebound hyperglycemia caused by excessive insulin administration.

Intensified Insulin Therapy

Intensified insulin therapy is designed to enable the patient with diabetes to achieve a daily blood glucose profile that mimics a physiologically normal glucose profile (*normoglycemia*). This has only been made possible through the development of self blood glucose monitoring devices. The patient usually has to monitor his or her blood sugar four times daily and adjust his or her own insulin dosage according to a scale provided by the physician.

Intensified insulin therapy is indicated for the pregnant diabetic patient for whom normoglycemia is essential to prevent fetal morbidity and mortality. It is also indicated for the highly motivated individuals with type I diabetes who desire to reduce their blood glucose, glycosylated hemoglobin, and lipid levels to possibly prevent, postpone, or reverse the chronic complications of diabetes. The *glycosylated hemoglobin* is a test that measures a person's diabetic control over a 3- to 8-week time period. Some patients believe that intensified insulin therapy promotes a flexibility in lifestyle that they did not previously have, especially with meal timing. Two forms of intensified therapy exist: continuous subcutaneous insulin infusion via the insulin pump and multiple injections of regular and intermediate- or long-acting insulin daily.

The insulin pump, shown in Figure 45–2, consists of a small programmable battery-operated box, about the size of a calculator. Insulin is delivered to the body through a plastic catheter that is attached to a fine needle placed subcutaneously in the abdomen.

A basal dose or continuous small pulsations of regular insulin is given over a 24-hour period. This amount is supplemented by a bolus dosage of regular insulin that is given approximately 30 minutes before each meal. The bolus dosage depends on the blood glucose reading at the time, taking into account the size of the meal to be ingested and anticipated exercise. Generally, the patient uses a sliding scale. It must be noted that this is an open-loop system in which frequent blood glucose monitoring is an essential requirement for pump use. Patients must demonstrate ability and willingness to adhere to the intense regimen. They must be reliable and competent.

Regular insulin is the only insulin that may be used in the insulin pump. Velosulin R is buffered insulin made especially for pump therapy. It is thought that the buffering may prevent clogging of the tubing. The most common problems with pump therapy are the acute effects of hyperglycemia and hypoglycemia. If the catheter is blocked or if it malfunctions, an individual may experience hyperglycemia and diabetic ketoacidosis in a short period, because there is no intermediate- or long-acting insulin circulating in the bloodstream. An alarm system indicates when the pump is malfunctioning; however, to check the system the patient must remove the needle from his or her skin, program a bolus dose, and then assume that the same insulin is then being delivered in the subcutaneous tissue.

Additionally, many patients do not experience the less severe symptoms of hypoglycemia and therefore may have severe reactions. There also have been some catheter-related problems such as blocking by aggregated insulin and abscesses at the site of needle injection. Lastly, some patients find the pump troublesome owing to cosmetic appearance and the constant external reminder that they have diabetes.

Another method of achieving tight control of blood glucose levels is through multiple or bolus injections of regular insulin or insulin lispro before meals plus a basal dose of an intermediate-acting or long-acting insulin, usually at bedtime. The benefits of this type of approach are similar to those achieved through pump therapy. The patient is able to have tight control of his or her blood glucose levels and have flexibility in meal timing and size. Blood glucose monitoring is mandatory for this system because the bolus amount of insulin that is taken before meals depends on the blood glucose level.

The patient using multiple daily injections of insulin is not as likely to develop ketoacidosis as the patient using the insulin pump as there is some long- or intermediate-acting insulin circulating in the bloodstream. However, similar to the individual using the insulin pump, the patient may have insulin reactions.

The patient, physician, and diabetes nurse/educator must discuss the pros and cons of both systems and determine which system would best fit into the patient's lifestyle, if intensified insulin therapy is desired.

Factors That Alter Insulin Requirements

Regardless of the diabetic regimen the patient is following, it must be recognized that numerous factors can affect insulin requirements. Initially, if the patient begins

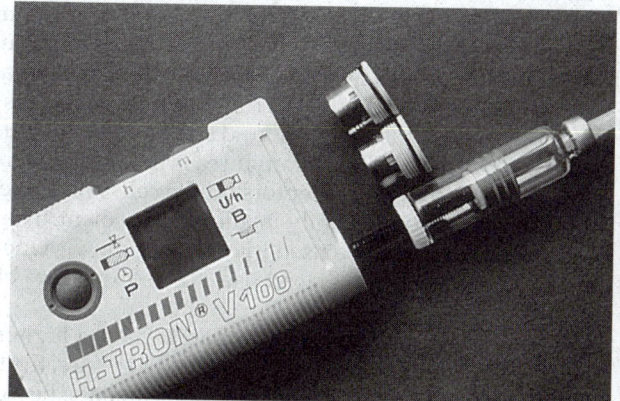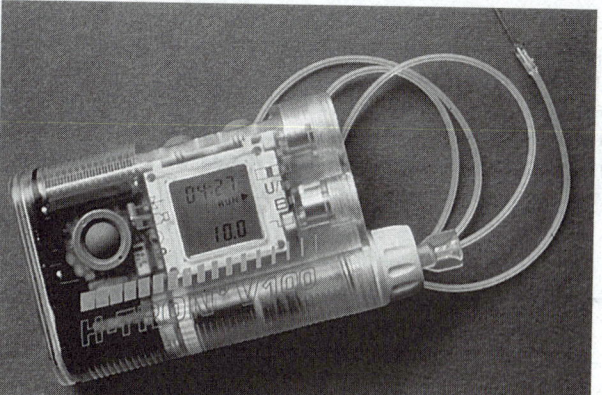

Figure 45–2. Insulin infusion pump. (Courtesy of Disetronic Medical Systems, Plymouth, Minn.)

insulin therapy in the hospital setting, the dosage will most likely have to be altered once he or she returns to his or her normal surroundings and activity level. Fluctuations in food intake may necessitate adjustments in insulin dosage. Stress, either physiologic or emotional, causes the release of epinephrine, which elevates blood glucose levels. This is especially common when the patient develops an infection. Other hormones including glucagon, cortisol, and growth hormone can elevate blood glucose levels. Exercise lowers blood glucose by oxidizing carbohydrates after facilitating their transport into cells. A good daily exercise program can decrease the amount of insulin a patient must take. However, sporadic, unplanned exercise can result in episodes of hypoglycemia. The amount of insulin prescribed for a patient can vary on different days if the schedule is very erratic in terms of exercise.

Any individual requiring more than 200 units of insulin per day is said to be insulin resistant. Insulin resistance may be due to insulin antagonists or to circulating antibodies that inactivate the insulin. It may also be due to an inadequate number of insulin receptors. The relative number of insulin receptors can be increased by weight reduction. Insulin resistance may also be related to the intermittent use of insulin. For this reason, once insulin therapy is begun it generally is continued, even if the dosage requirements are small. This is especially true in the type I diabetic patient who experiences a "honeymoon" phase after initial diagnosis. The insulin requirement may drop tremendously as there is partial restoration of the beta cells. However, this does not last and within a few weeks or several months, the patient requires insulin again.

If it is known that therapy will be intermittent, such as in a woman with gestational diabetes or a type II diabetic patient experiencing an infection or undergoing surgery, a human form of insulin is used.

When a patient's insulin requirements seem to be steadily increasing without an apparent cause (e.g., infection) and fluctuations between hypoglycemia and hyperglycemia occur, the Somogyi effect should be suspected. This asymptomatic phenomenon is a rebound hyperglycemia, directly resulting from the hormonal response to hypoglycemia, induced by excessive insulin administration. Hypoglycemia is overcompensated for by a slow prolonged release of glucose from the liver. When the patient's blood sugar level is again tested, it is high. Thus, the physician prescribes more insulin, which only contributes to more severe hypoglycemia. Usually, rebound hyperglycemia occurs 6 to 12 hours after periods of hypoglycemia. Blood samples drawn around 4:00 or 5:00 AM often reflect this hypoglycemia. A decrease in insulin dosage will control the rebound hyperglycemia.

ORAL ANTIDIABETIC AGENTS

Oral antidiabetic agents are indicated for the type II diabetic patient when diet and exercise fail to control hyper-

glycemia. These agents are useful to patients who can produce some of their own insulin. The oral antidiabetic agents currently available in the United States are classified as sulfonylureas, biguanides, and alpha-glucosidase inhibitors.

SULFONYLUREAS

The sulfonylureas are divided into two groups: first generation and second generation. The first generation agents, released in the late 1950s, include **chlorpropamide (Diabinese)**, **tolazamide (Tolinase)**, **tolbutamide (Orinase)**, and **acetohexamide (Dymelor)**. The second generation agents were released in 1984. These include **glyburide (Diabeta, Micronase)** and **glipizide (Glucotrol)**. Two new formulations of these products, **micronized glyburide (Glynase Prestab)** and **glipizide extended release (Glucotrol XL)**, are also available. The second generation agent **glimepiride (Amaryl)** was released in 1996.

Action

The exact mechanism by which sulfonylureas work is not completely understood. Initially, these agents stimulate the beta cells of the pancreas to produce insulin. However, this effect tends to last for only 2 to 3 weeks after initiation of therapy. The sulfonylureas also have been found to suppress hepatic glucose production, which accounts for lower blood glucose levels found in individuals taking these medications. Also, the sulfonylureas are thought to lower the blood glucose by increasing the number of insulin receptors on the cell and may influence events within the cell after glucose has been transferred inside.

Uses

Sulfonylureas may be used in the treatment of the type II or non-insulin-dependent diabetic. They are to be used only after therapy with diet and exercise fail. These agents may be tried as sole treatment of a type II diabetic patient on less than 30 units of daily insulin. Additionally, they may also be used concurrently with insulin in the treatment of a type II diabetic who requires a large amount of insulin. The patient who may benefit from combination therapy typically weighs over 300 pounds, requires 300 or more units of insulin daily, and still has a blood glucose above 300 mg/dL. The sulfonylurea is thought to increase the number of insulin receptors on the cells and therefore decrease the patient's daily insulin requirement. The sulfonylureas may also be used in combination with metformin (Glucophage) or acarbose to reduce the blood glucose.

The second generation sulfonylureas have a higher potency than the first generation agents. Therefore, the therapeutic effective dose is lower for these agents; however, this has no clinical relevance. Also, these agents have fewer drug interactions and adverse reactions than the first generation agents. For this reason the second generation agents are gradually replacing the first generation agents.

Pharmacokinetics

The sulfonylureas are administered orally and are rapidly absorbed from the GI tract, with the exception of tolazamide (Tolinase), which is absorbed at a slower rate. Glipizide (Glucotrol) is the only oral antidiabetic agent that must be taken on an empty stomach. Food delays absorption of glipizide by approximately 40 minutes. The extended-release glipizide preparation may be taken with a meal and must be swallowed whole. It is not to be chewed, divided, or crushed. The micronized glyburide formulation allows for a more complete GI absorption than glyburide.

Once absorbed, the sulfonylureas are widely distributed throughout the body. Chlorpropamide (Diabinese) and tolbutamide (Orinase) have been found to be excreted in breast milk. All of the oral antidiabetic agents are highly bound to plasma proteins, which accounts for their differences in duration of action. The first generation agents have ionic binding, and the second generation agents have nonionic binding. Therefore, the second generation agents are thought to have fewer displacement reactions from other ionic binding drugs and therefore should have fewer drug interactions.

All of the sulfonylureas are metabolized in the liver. Acetohexamide (Dymelor) is reduced to an active metabolite that has about three times the half-life of the parent drug. Glipizide and tolbutamide are metabolized to inactive metabolites. Tolazamide is metabolized to a mildly active metabolite and glyburide is metabolized to several compounds, one of which may be weakly active. Because of the metabolism in the liver, individuals with hepatic dysfunction are monitored carefully for hypoglycemia as the action of the drug may be prolonged.

Most of the sulfonylureas are eliminated from the body through the kidneys. Therefore, individuals with impaired renal function may have a prolonged effect of the drug. This is especially true with chlorpropamide, which has a long duration, and with acetohexamide, whose metabolites are active. Glyburide is excreted in bile in addition to urine, and glimepride is excreted in the feces and urine.

Contraindications and Precautions

Sulfonylureas are contraindicated for use in the type I insulin-dependent diabetic patient, because they do not work for these patients and the individuals may develop ketoacidosis. They are also contraindicated for the type II diabetic patient when the diabetes is complicated by fever, severe infections, severe trauma, or major surgery. Precise blood glucose control, which may be achieved only through insulin therapy, is necessary in the preceding situations. Sulfonylureas are not indicated for the pregnant diabetic patient; strict control is necessary during pregnancy to prevent fetal abnormalities, and fetal mortality and sulfonylureas do not provide the strict control that is needed. Chlorpropamide and tolbutamide have been found in breast milk, and it is assumed that other oral agents may be passed to the infant by this route. Therefore, sulfonylureas are not recommended for the lactating woman as hypoglycemia of the nursing infant may occur.

▼ **CLINICAL ALERT**

The extended-release preparation glipizide (Glucotrol XL) should not be used in patients with severe GI narrowing. Rare reports of obstructive symptoms have occurred in patients taking this type of preparation, which does not change in size or shape.

Sulfonylureas are contraindicated in patients with severe hepatic or renal disease because of prolonged metabolism and excretion. Caution is advised for patients who have a history of allergy to sulfa medications as cross-sensitivity may occur. Cross-sensitivity may occur in individuals allergic to tartrazine; however, the incidence of this is low. Often people who are allergic to aspirin have this sensitivity.

Patients with thyroid or endocrine disorders may be difficult to control with oral antidiabetic agents and, therefore, may benefit from insulin therapy.

▼ **CLINICAL ALERT**

Sulfonylureas are used with caution in geriatric patients and patients with renal insufficiency. These patients may be more sensitive to the effects of sulfonylureas because of the medications' prolonged metabolism and excretion. This is especially true with chlorpropamide (Diabinese), which has a long duration. For these patients, dosage is initiated at a lower level and adjusted very cautiously. Additionally, hypoglycemia is more difficult to recognize in the elderly and causes more neurologic symptoms.

Adverse Effects

One of the major adverse effects of the sulfonylureas is hypoglycemia. This occurs most frequently in the elderly, debilitated, or malnourished individual. It may also occur in a patient with impaired renal or hepatic function because of delayed metabolism or excretion of the drug. Hypoglycemic episodes may occur if a meal is omitted or if exercise is performed erratically. Therefore, it is emphasized that the patient taking these oral antidiabetic agents must follow a regular meal pattern and exercise regimen.

The hypoglycemia that occurs from sulfonylureas requires treatment over a period of days owing to the prolonged action of the medication.

Gastrointestinal disturbances may occur with any of the sulfonylureas, especially at the beginning of therapy. Divided dosages may resolve this problem.

Chlorpropamide and tolbutamide interact with alcohol, causing a *disulfirim-like* reaction. The patient will notice flushing, warmth, and palpations 5 to 10 minutes after consuming alcohol while being on this medication. The effect is self-limiting and lasts only 30 minutes to several hours. This reaction may occur with other sulfonylureas but to a lesser extent, especially with the second-generation oral antidiabetic agents.

▼ **CLINICAL ALERT**

Inappropriate antidiuretic hormone (ADH) secretion may occur when a patient is taking chlorpropamide or, to a lesser extent, tolbutamide. Both drugs may stimulate ADH release from the hypothalamus and potentiate its effect in water excretion, leading to a drop in serum sodium levels. Prompt medical attention is necessary if the patient complains of headache, lethargy, and swelling, early signs of this syndrome, which may progress to stupor, seizures, and coma.

All of the other sulfonylureas possess a mild diuretic effect.

Hematologic conditions (leukopenia, agranulocytosis, thrombocytopenia, pancytopenia, and hemolytic anemia) have been reported rarely in patients taking sulfonylureas. Cutaneous manifestations such as photosensitivity and rashes may also occur. Hepatic manifestations such as elevated serum alkaline phosphatase levels and cholestatic jaundice are infrequent adverse effects. These conditions can be reversed by discontinuation of the drugs.

Package inserts today indicate that there is a higher incidence of cardiovascular disease in patients taking sulfonylureas, based on a previous study. However, the study from which the information was obtained had many flaws, and the American Diabetes Association has withdrawn its endorsement of the study. The physician, pharmacist, or nurse should discuss the study with the patient before initiating sulfonylurea therapy.

Some patients do not respond to sulfonylureas when therapy is initiated. This is called primary failure. Other patients respond to the sulfonylureas for a while, then lose their responsiveness to the drug and experience a rise in blood sugar levels. This condition is called secondary failure, and has an annual occurrence rate of about 10%. In many cases, this is due to the patient's failure to adhere to the prescribed diet.

Interactions

The same medications that interact with insulin (refer to the section on interactions with insulin) can also affect the function of the sulfonylureas. Some medications interact only with the sulfonylureas, altering diabetic control. Salicylates and other nonsteroidal anti-inflammatory agents may displace sulfonylureas from protein-binding sites, resulting in enhanced hypoglycemic activity. Anabolic steroids inhibit the metabolism of the sulfonylureas. Allopurinol, chloramphenicol, and dicumarol inhibit the metabolism of the oral agents, giving them an increased half-life.

The sulfonylureas may enhance the metabolism of digoxin by microsomal enzyme induction. There have also been reports that H_2 inhibitors may potentiate the hypoglycemic effect of the sulfonylureas.

With regard to laboratory test values, the only interaction that may occur is a false urine test for albumin when a patient is taking tolbutamide.

Table 45–3 provides a listing of medications that interact with the sulfonylureas and insulin to raise or lower the blood glucose levels. See Table 45–4 for dosages, pharmacokinetics/dynamics, and nursing implications of the sulfonylureas.

BIGUANIDES

The only biguanide available in the United States is **metformin hydrochloride (Glucophage).** For years metformin has been used successfully in Canada and several European countries. However, it took until 1995 to be introduced in the United States owing to problems phenformin, another biguanide, caused with lactic acidosis in the 1960s.

○ **Metformin** (Glucophage) differs in several pharmacologic ways from the sulfonylureas. It works primarily in lowering plasma glucose levels by improving insulin sensitivity. Therefore, glucose production in the liver is reduced and glucose utilization in the skeletal muscle is increased. Metformin does not increase insulin secretion and therefore does not cause hypoglycemia when used alone or cause hyperinsulinemia. In contrast to other antidiabetic agents, metformin does not cause weight gain. Initially, it is associated with weight loss. Metformin has demonstrated slight improvements in plasma lipid levels.

USES Metformin is indicated for patients with type II diabetes mellitus as an adjunct to diet and exercise when the patient cannot be controlled on diet or exercise alone. It may also be used concurrently with a sulfonylurea when diet, exercise, metformin alone, or a sulfonylurea alone do not result in adequate glycemic control.

PHARMACOKINETICS Metformin is slowly and incompletely absorbed from the small intestine. The extent of absorption is proportionally reduced at higher dosages. Food decreases the extent and slightly delays absorption. Metformin is distributed rapidly and does not undergo metabolism. It is excreted unchanged in the urine. There are no metabolites. See Table 45–4 for dosage, pharmacokinetics/dynamics, and nursing implications.

CONTRAINDICATIONS AND PRECAUTIONS Metformin should be withheld for 48 hours before and after in patients undergoing radiographic studies involving par-

Table 45–4. ORAL ANTIDIABETIC AGENTS

DRUG NAME/ROUTE AND DOSAGE	PHARMACOKINETICS/ DYNAMICS	NURSING IMPLICATIONS
SULFONYLUREAS		
all sulfonylureas		**ASSESSMENT:** Obtain baseline and periodic assessments of blood glucose levels, blood cell counts; glycosylated hemoglobin levels; and liver function tests, especially bilirubin, cholesterol, AST, and ALT. Before initiation of treatment, assess whether the patient has any allergies to sulfonylureas. Ask the patient if he or she is taking any other medications and determine if they interact with sulfonylureas. If female patient is of childbearing age, ask if she is planning pregnancy in near future. Assess patient's present knowledge of diabetes care including meal pattern, role of exercise, medication, hypoglycemia, blood glucose or urine testing, and skin and foot care. **INTERVENTION:** Provide sulfonylureas 30 min before breakfast with exception of Glucotrol XL, which is to be taken with food. If divided doses are ordered, administer 2nd dosage ½ hr before supper. Continually assess for hypoglycemia. Monitor blood and urine glucose levels. If patient complains of GI upset, inquire whether divided dosages may be used. **Patient Teaching**—Educate patient according to needs assessment. Instruct patient to keep medication away from heat and direct light. **EVALUATION:** Evaluate patient's blood and urinary glucose levels. Evaluate patient's knowledge of diabetes and basics of treatment. Evaluate all technical skills that will be used in home setting. Evaluate patient's desire to adhere to prescribed regimen, using verbal and nonverbal cues.
FIRST-GENERATION SULFONYLUREAS		
chlorpropamide (Diabinese) (Apo-Chlorpropamide)		
Adults: 100–200 mg/day PO; dosage may be increased by 50–125 mg at 1-wk intervals until diabetic control is achieved. Maximum: 750 mg/day.	**Onset:** 1 hr **Peak:** 3–6 hr **Duration:** up to 60 hr **½L:** 35 hr **PB:** very highly bound **B:** liver **E:** kidney	Same as for all sulfonylureas plus: **ASSESSMENT:** Assess for pregnancy (category C).
tolazamide (Tolinase) (Ronase)		
Adults: 100–250 mg/day PO until diabetic control is reached; when more than 500 mg is required, dosage should be divided and given before morning and evening meals. Maximum: 1g/day.	**Onset:** 4–6 hr **Peak:** 4–10 hr **Duration:** 12–24 hr **½L:** 7 hr **PB:** very highly bound **B:** liver **E:** kidney	Same as for all sulfonylureas plus: **ASSESSMENT:** Assess for pregnancy (category C).
tolbutamide (Orinase) (Oramide)		
Adults: 0.5 g PO 1–2 times/day until diabetic control is reached. Maximum: 3 g/day.	**Onset:** 1 hr **Peak:** 3–5 hr **Duration:** 6–12 hr **½L:** 4–5 hr **PB:** 95% **B:** liver **E:** kidney	Same as for all sulfonylureas plus: **ASSESSMENT:** Assess for pregnancy (category C).

Continued on the following page

Table 45–4. ORAL ANTIDIABETIC AGENTS, *Continued*

DRUG NAME/ROUTE AND DOSAGE	PHARMACOKINETICS/ DYNAMICS	NURSING IMPLICATIONS
FIRST-GENERATION SULFONYLUREAS		
acetohexamide (Dymelor)		
Adults: 250 mg PO once/day; adjust gradually until diabetic control is achieved. Maximum: 1.5 g/day. If 1.5 g/day is required, dosage should be divided and given before morning and evening meals.	**Onset:** 1 hr **Peak:** 2–4 hr **Duration:** 12–24 hr **½L:** Parent, 1.5 hr; metabolite, 6 hr **PB:** very highly bound **B:** liver **E:** kidney	Same as for all sulfonylureas plus: **ASSESSMENT:** Assess for pregnancy (category C).
SECOND-GENERATION SULFONYLUREAS		
glyburide (Micronase) (Diabeta)		
Adults: 2.5–5 mg PO daily (elderly, 1.25 mg); increase dosage 2.5 mg/wk if necessary to achieve diabetic control. When 10 mg or more per day is required, dosage should be divided and given before morning and evening meals. Maximum: 20 mg/day.	**Onset:** 2–4 hr **Peak:** 6 hr **Duration:** 24 hr **½L:** 10 hr **PB:** 99% **B:** liver **E:** kidney and bile	Same as for all sulfonylureas plus: **ASSESSMENT:** Assess for pregnancy (category B).
micronized glyburide (Glynase Prestab)		
Adults: 1.5–3 mg PO. Maximum: 12 mg.	**Onset:** 1 hr **Peak:** 2–3 hr **Duration:** 24 hr **½L:** 1.5–1.8 hr **BP:** 99% **B:** liver **L:** kidney and bile	Same as for all sulfonylureas plus: **ASSESSMENT:** Assess for pregnancy (category B).
glipizide (Glucotrol)		
Adults: 5 mg PO daily (elderly, 2.5 mg) increase by 2.5–5 mg/wk to achieve diabetic control. If dosage reaches ≥15 mg/day, divide dose at breakfast and supper. Maximum: 40 mg daily.	**Onset:** 1–1.5 hr **Peak:** 1–3 hr **Duration:** 10–24 hr **½L:** 2.1–3.6 hr **PB:** 92%–99% **B:** liver **E:** kidney	Same as for all sulfonylureas plus: **ASSESSMENT:** Assess for pregnancy (category C).
glipizide extended release (Glucotrol XL)		
Adults: 5 mg/day PO given with breakfast (same starting dose for geriatric patients). After 3-mo trial may be increased to 10 mg if control was inadequate. Maximum: 20 mg/day.	**Onset:** 2–3 hr **Peak:** 6–12 hr **Duration:** 24 hr **½L:** NA **PB:** very highly bound **B:** liver **E:** kidney	Same as above.
glimapiride (Amaryl)		
Adults: 1–2 mg PO qd with breakfast. Patients more sensitive to hypoglycemia (i.e., impaired renal function) begin with 1 mg. Usual maintenance dose is 1–4 mg qd. Maximum: 8 mg/d.	**Onset:** 1 hr **Peak:** 2–3 hr **Duration:** 24 hr **½L:** NA **PB:** >99.5% **B:** liver **E:** kidney and feces	Same as for all sulfonylureas plus assess for pregnancy (category C).

Table 45–4. ORAL ANTIDIABETIC AGENTS, *Continued*

DRUG NAME/ROUTE AND DOSAGE	PHARMACOKINETICS/ DYNAMICS	NURSING IMPLICATIONS

BIGUANIDES

metformin hydrochloride (Glucophage)

Adults: Generally, clinical responses are not seen at doses below 1500 mg/day PO. However, lower starting dose is recommended to minimize GI complaints.

500-mg tablets

Adults: 1 tablet bid with morning and evening meals. Increase by one tablet/wk in divided doses up to 2000 mg. Maximum: 2550 mg tid with meals.

850-mg tablets

Adults: 1 tablet PO with morning meal, increase in increments of one tablet every other wk, given in divided doses up to 2550 mg/day.

Onset:
Peak: 2–3.3 hr
Duration: 17.6 hr
½L: 6.2 hr
PB: negligible
M: does not undergo hepatic metabolism or biliary excretion
E: kidney

ASSESSMENT: Obtain baseline and periodic assessments of blood glucose and glycosylated hemoglobin. Assess renal function before initiating therapy and annually, and more frequently for patients at high risk for renal dysfunction. Assess if patient is hypersensitive to metformin prior to initiating therapy. Assess if patient is currently using any cationic drugs. Assess vitamin B_{12} level. Assess patient's knowledge of diabetes and basics of treatment. If woman is of childbearing age, assess if she is planning pregnancy in near future.

INTERVENTION: Provide metformin PO with breakfast and supper if ordered. Withhold metformin 48 hr prior to and for 48 hr after patient undergoes any radiographic study that involves parenteral administration of iodinated contrast materials. Restart medication when renal function is verified as normal. Discontinue metformin for any surgical procedure; it should not be restarted until oral intake and renal function return to normal. **Patient Teaching**—Instruct patient regarding diabetes and basics of treatment based on needs determined through needs assessment. Instruct patient to call physician if unusual fatigue, unusual muscle pain, difficulty breathing, stomach discomfort, dizziness, light-headedness, or irregular heartbeat occurs. These symptoms may indicate onset of lactic acidosis, which is often subtle.

EVALUATION: Evaluate patient's blood and urinary glucose levels and glycosylated hemoglobin level. Evaluate patient's knowledge of diabetes and basics of treatment as well as ability to perform technical skills such as self blood glucose testing and urine testing. Evaluate patient's desire to adhere to therapeutic regimen through verbal and nonverbal cues.

ALPHA-GLUCOSIDASE INHIBITORS

acarbose (Precose)

Adults: 25 mg PO tid at start of each main meal. Evaluate at 4- to 8-week intervals. Maximum dosage: 100 mg tid; if patient has body weight <60 kg, should not receive >50 mg tid.

Onset: NA
Peak: NA
Duration: NA
½L: NA
PB: NA
B: GI tract
E: feces

ASSESSMENT: Obtain baseline and periodic assessments of blood glucose levels (especially 1 hr pc), glycosylated hemoglobin, and serum transaminase levels. Assess for inflammatory bowel disease, colonic irritation, partial intestinal obstruction or any condition that may cause obstruction, disorder of gas formation, and disorders of digestion or absorption (all contraindications).

INTERVENTION: Provide acarbose with first bite of each meal. Assess for GI complaints, pain, cramping, and flatulence. **Patient Teaching**—Instruct patient regarding diabetes and basics of management based on needs determined through needs assessment. Instruct regarding causes, symptoms, and treatment of hypoglycemia if patient is taking sulfonylurea in conjunction with this medication. Instruct patient regarding correct time to take acarbose and inform him or her regarding usual side effects of abdominal discomfort and flatulence. If symptoms do not subside with time or worsen, instruct patient to call physician.

EVALUATION: Evaluate patient's blood and urinary glucose levels as well as glycosylated hemoglobin. Evaluate patient's knowledge of diabetes, basics of treatment, and desire to adhere to regimen using verbal and nonverbal cues.

AST = serum aspartate aminotransferase; ALT = serum alanine aminotransferase; NA = not available.

enteral administration of iodinated contrast materials. Use of such products may result in acute alterations in renal function. Renal function should be reviewed and found to be normal prior to reinstating metformin. Metformin is contraindicated for anyone hypersensitive to metformin and contraindicated in individuals with acute or chronic metabolic acidosis, including diabetic keto-acidosis.

▼ **CLINICAL ALERT**

Metformin is contraindicated in patients with renal or hepatic dysfunction. Lactic acidosis may occur, resulting from the buildup of metformin in the blood.

Use of medications that may affect renal function or cause hemodynamic changes such as cationic drugs (amiloride, digoxin, morphine, procainamide, quinidine, quinine, ranitidine, triamterene, trimethoprim, vancomycin) that are eliminated by tubular secretion should be used with caution. Metformin should be discontinued if the patient develops acute congestive heart failure, cardiovascular collapse, an acute myocardial infarction (MI), or any other condition characterized by hypoxemia. This may result in lactic acidosis.

Metformin therapy should be discontinued for any surgical procedure and should not be restarted until oral intake and renal function return to normal. Alcohol potentiates the effects of metformin on lactate metabolism. Patients should be warned against excessive alcohol intake. Metformin is not used during pregnancy as normoglycemia is essential in preventing fetal mortality and morbidity and metformin does not provide the tight control that is needed.

ADVERSE EFFECTS   Lactic acidosis is a major adverse effect associated with metformin. This condition occurs rarely in patients without any predisposing factors (renal impairment, cardiopulmonary insufficiency, hepatic disease, alcoholism, and active infection). Hypoglycemia is a possibility, but because the action of the drug occurs in peripheral tissues, not in the pancreas, it is unlikely. The most frequent side effects are gastrointestinal and include nausea, vomiting, metallic or bitter taste, abdominal discomfort, bloating, anorexia, and diarrhea. These effects tend to occur within the first few weeks of therapy and are generally mild and transient. Beginning therapy with low doses and gradually increasing the dose is usually effective in minimizing the GI side effects. Because significant diarrhea and vomiting may cause dehydration and prerenal azotemia, metformin should be temporarily discontinued. Nonspecific GI symptoms should not be attributed to therapy unless illness or lactic acidosis has been excluded.

INTERACTIONS   Some pharmacokinetic studies have indicated that interactions occur between metformin and compounds that share the same excretion pathway. Administration of medications that cause hyperglycemia could lead to a loss of control (see Table 45–3).

ALPHA-GLUCOSIDASE INHIBITORS

Alpha-glucosidase inhibitors have a nonsystemic mechanism of action that is different from either the sulfonylureas or biguanides. The only member of this new drug classification is **Acarbose (Precose)**.

○ **Acarbose**   (Precose) works by inhibiting the action of pancreatic alpha-amalyse and membrane-bound intestinal alpha-glucoside hydrolase enzymes. This inhibition causes a delay in the digestion of carbohydrates and thus slows the absorption of glucose in the small intestine. This lowers glycosylated hemoglobin and postprandial hyperglycemia in the non-insulin-dependent diabetic patient.

USES   Acarbose is used for the management of type II or non-insulin dependent diabetes mellitus when exercise and diet therapy fail to achieve glycemic control. It may be used alone or in combination with a sulfonylurea if either agent alone with diet and exercise does not adequately control blood glucose levels.

PHARMACOKINETICS   Less than 2% of an oral dose of acarbose is absorbed as an active drug, and approximately 35% of an inactive metabolite is absorbed. An average of 51% of the oral dose is excreted as an unabsorbed drug. Because acarbose works locally in the GI tract, this low systemic bioavailability is desirable. Acarbose is metabolized exclusively in the GI tract primarily by intestinal bacteria and to a lesser extent by digestive enzymes.

The fraction of acarbose that is absorbed is excreted as an intact drug in the kidney, whereas the primary route of excretion is the feces. Refer to Table 45–4 for dosage, pharmacokinetics/dynamics, and nursing implications.

CONTRAINDICATIONS AND PRECAUTIONS   Acarbose is contraindicated in patients with known hypersensitivity to the medication as well as those with ketoacidosis or cirrhosis. Acarbose is also contraindicated in patients with inflammatory bowel disease, colonic irritation, partial intestinal obstruction or proneness to intestinal obstruction, or chronic intestinal diseases with marked disorders of digestion or absorption, and in those who have conditions that may worsen as a result of increased gas formation in the intestines. Acarbose may worsen all these conditions.

Because of its mechanism of action, acarbose alone should not cause hypoglycemia. However, if acarbose is used in combination with a sulfonylurea, additional lowering of the blood glucose may result, causing hypoglycemia.

▼ **CLINICAL ALERT**

Oral glucose, dextrose whose absorption is not inhibited by acarbose, should be used to treat mild to moderate hypoglycemia instead of sucrose or cane sugar when a patient is taking a sulfonylurea and acarbose. The absorption of sucrose is inhibited by acarbose. For severe hypoglycemia, IV glucose or a glucagon injection may be required.

Acarbose is not recommended for patients with renal impairment as the plasma concentrations of acarbose increases relative to the degree of renal impairment.

The safety of acarbose for use in pregnancy has not been established. However, because literature strongly suggests that elevated blood glucose levels are associated with congenital anomalies as well as increased neonatal morbidity and mortality, most authorities recommend that insulin be used during pregnancy and blood glucose levels be as close to that of a nondiabetic person as possible. Acarbose is not recommended for nursing mothers as some of the medication was found present in lactating rats.

In the event of stress, trauma, fever, or surgery, a temporary loss of glycemic control may occur and insulin therapy may be temporarily necessary.

ADVERSE EFFECTS Most adverse effects from acarbose are gastrointestinal, resulting from its mode of action. Carbohydrates not digested in the small intestine are naturally metabolized by bacteria in the large intestine. The fermentation of undigested carbohydrates may cause abdominal pain, diarrhea, or flatulence. Abdominal pain and diarrhea disappear over time if this was not a problem prior to therapy. If it was, the abdominal pain and diarrhea return to the prior pattern. The intensity of the flatulence tends to abate over time.

An elevated serum transaminase level has been noted in clinical trials in which many of the patients received more than 100 mg tid and most were under 60 kg. These elevations were asymptomatic, reversible, more common in females, and in general were not associated with other evidence of liver dysfunction. Small reductions in hematocrit have occurred in patients treated with acarbose. Low plasma vitamin B₆ levels have also occurred. However, these are thought to be of no clinical significance.

INTERACTIONS Studies have shown that acarbose does not interact with digoxin, nifidepine, propranolol, or rantidine. It does not interfere with the sulfonylurea glyburide in diabetic patients. However, administration of any medication that may cause hyperglycemia may lead to a loss of control.

USING THE NURSING PROCESS

The diagnosis of diabetes is often a crisis for the patient. The individual is suddenly faced with a chronic illness that alters his or her lifestyle. It is a condition in which the patient must take control to successfully manage. The physician, nurse, dietitian, and other members of the health-care team provide care when the patient is hospitalized and acutely ill. However, once the patient is out of the controlled hospital environment, the health-care professionals become mere consultants in helping the patient achieve diabetic control. The patient is the one who must follow the prescribed meal pattern, omitting foods that previously were enjoyed and eating at designated times whether hungry or not. The patient must also monitor blood and/or urinary glucose levels; balance exercise and medication with meal patterns; inject insulin; know the causes, symptoms, and treatment of hyperglycemia and hypoglycemia; and take meticulous care of the skin and feet. The patient must know how to manage diabetes during illness and travel. This requires tremendous motivation and commitment. Therefore, major concerns are focused not only on the nursing care such as maintaining appropriate fluid balance and nutrition, but on education of the patient to be the manager of his or her disease.

ASSESSMENT

- Review the patient's medical history and laboratory blood and urine values before initiating the nursing assessment. Assessment of the blood glucose determines what type of diabetic control the patient is currently in, assessment of the presence of ketones in the urine will determine if the client is in ketoacidosis, and assessment of the glycosylated hemoglobin level can determine whether the patient has been in control prior to the clinic visit or admission.

- If the patient is in a life-threatening situation, such as diabetic ketoacidosis or *hyperglycemic hyperosmolar nonketotic coma* (a situation that may occur with type II diabetics that is characterized by very high blood glucose levels, osmotic diuresis, and coma without the presence of high levels of ketone bodies), assessment is basic and it is necessary to intervene and care for the patient. Wait until the patient is physically stable and able to answer questions to do a complete educational assessment.

- If the patient is hospitalized, assess blood glucose values daily. These levels can be determined by venous blood samples and analyzed in a laboratory. Self blood glucose monitoring equipment is also being used in clinics and on hospital units, as well as in the home setting. The self-monitoring products provide a blood glucose value within 2 to 3 minutes and allow prompt regulation of blood glucose levels. Often a sliding scale of regular insulin is used to lower the blood glucose level. The amount of regular insulin the patient receives depends upon the results of the blood test.

- For a stable patient, during the initial assessment, determine who manages the patient's diabetes. Generally, it is the patient. However, if the patient is a child, the parent/guardian is involved. Take growth and development into consideration.

- If age and cognitive level permit, assess the child and the parent separately and then together to obtain a complete management picture. With the elderly patient, children are often involved. Assess both parties. Regardless of age assess family involvement and support. Develop a nonthreatening, trusting relationship in which the patient feels free to discuss previous diabetes management if any, as well as fears and concerns. Do not make the patient feel that he or she was erroneous in his or her management. Point out positive aspects of the past regimen.

- Assess daily routines, meal times, dietary preferences, and previous medical management. Ask open-ended questions to allow the patient to explain situations. A patient may be asked if he or she follows a 1200 ADA diet and the patient may say yes. However, if open-ended questions are asked and the patient's daily routine is explored, the nurse may find that the patient consumes all of the calories at suppertime.

- Assess the patient's knowledge of the antidiabetic medication he or she is receiving. Sometimes patients taking a sulfonylurea stop the therapy because of shakiness and dizziness if a meal is missed. Frequently, these patients are unaware of the meal plan and the importance of eating on time. If the patient is taking insulin, assess the measurement and injection technique by having the patient draw up and inject the dosage at least once while in the hospital. In the clinic setting, this may be done after a fasting blood sugar is drawn on a routine visit. Assess the pattern of insulin site rotation by inquiring about the method and then inspecting the sites for lipohypertrophy.

- Assess self-monitoring practices at home such as blood and urinary glucose and ketone testing. If the patient does this, assess the technique using the equipment the patient uses at home as well as the patient's use of the results. Assess how the patient feels when he or she is experiencing hyperglycemia or hypoglycemia and what action the patient takes if these situations occur. Inquire how the patient cares for his or her skin and feet and how he or she feels about having diabetes.

- Assess the patient's anxiety level. This is important because learning is less productive when a patient is highly anxious. Learning may not take place despite excellent teaching. Because of the anxiety of diagnosis and the large volume of information the patient must learn in order to control diabetes, only survival information is provided during a newly diagnosed diabetic patient's hospitalization. This information is expanded over time through outpatient education, future clinic visits using one-one consultations, or diabetes classes. For the housebound individual, the community health nurse continues the education in the home setting.

- Assess literacy as well as cognitive functioning. Many patients are unable to read or understand the literature available regarding diabetes. By assessing the patient's reading level, appropriate literature that will be understood can be used in education. A film, slide and tape presentation, or videotape can be used for the illiterate individual. For children it is important to use material that is appropriate for their level of growth and development.

- Assess the patient for physical limitations, especially in the areas of physical dexterity, visual impairment, and sensory defects. Often, the diabetic patient who has been out of control cannot see the written literature or the numbers on an insulin syringe owing to the osmotic changes in the eye as a result of glucose fluctuation. The changes generally stabilize in about 5 weeks. However, it is frustrating for the patient because his or her vision is too poor to draw up the insulin dosage or read any material about the condition. Modifications in management may be necessary for the individual with poor vision or poor fine motor coordination. These problems most frequently occur in the elderly patient who suffers from other medical conditions and in the patient who has had diabetes for many years. These modifications may include using prefilled insulin syringes, having a community health nurse monitor blood or urinary glucose levels, or using a Meals on Wheels service.

- Assess cultural and religious preferences. The Jewish patient may prefer not to use pork insulin or consume pork in the diet owing to dietary codes. Protein sources other than meat are explored for the vegetarian patient. Holiday feasting in any culture or religion has social significance that makes traditions difficult to change.

- Assess the client's financial situation and medical insurance. The cost of changes in diet, medications, syringes, self blood glucose monitoring equipment, urine testing equipment, and frequent physician visits can impose a financial burden on the patient, especially if he or she is on a fixed income. Low-income individuals may subsist on a high-carbohydrate diet because that is all they can afford. They may also try to test their urine or blood with a reagent strip cut in half or thirds to economize and thus obtain inaccurate results. Food stamps, Medicare and Medicaid eligibility, and other financial assistance should be explored.

NURSING DIAGNOSIS

Nursing diagnoses may relate to physical or psychologic findings. Suggested nursing diagnoses for the patient with diabetes taking insulin and/or an oral agent include the following: Fluid Volume Deficit; Altered Nutrition, Less than Body Requirements; Altered Nutrition, More than Body Requirements; Knowledge Deficit; Noncompliance; Risk for Infection; Risk for Injury; Pain; and Noncompliance. Table 45–5 summarizes the nursing process.

INTERVENTION

Many of the following interventions are performed by the nurse if the patient is hospitalized and acutely ill. As the patient recovers, these interventions are taught to the patient so he or she can manage the diabetes at home.

Meal Pattern

Dietary management is of the utmost importance in achieving control of diabetes. The patient must follow a meal pattern. The physician prescribes a specific calorie value American Diabetes Association (ADA) diet, based upon individual need. The diet generally ranges from

Table 45–5. NURSING PROCESS FOR THE INSULIN-DEPENDENT DIABETIC PATIENT

Assessment

Assess duration/intensity of present symptoms, e.g., vomiting, excessive urination.
Assess peripheral pulses, capillary refill, skin turgor, and mucous membranes.
Assess usual dietary pattern and intake.
Assess drug history.

Nursing Diagnosis: Fluid Volume Deficit

RELATED TO: Failure of regulatory mechanisms, osmotic diuresis, excessive gastric losses (diarrhea, vomiting), restricted intake.
AS EVIDENCED BY: Increased urine output, dilute urine, weakness, thirst, dry skin/mucous membranes, hypotension.

Desired Outcomes/Evaluation Criteria

Demonstrates adequate hydration as evidenced by stable vital signs, palpable peripheral pulses, good skin turgor and capillary refill, individually appropriate urinary output, and electrolyte levels within normal range.

Nursing Actions	Rationale
Monitor vital signs, note orthostatic changes; changes in respiratory pattern (e.g., Kussmaul respirations, periods of apnea, use of accessory muscles, presence of acetone breath, cyanosis).	Hypovolemia may be manifested by hypotension and tachycardia. Lungs remove carbonic acid through respirations, producing a compensatory respiratory alkalosis for ketoacidosis.
Measure intake and output, note specific gravity. Obtain weight daily.	Provides ongoing estimate of volume replacement needs, kidney function, and effectiveness of therapy.
Maintain fluid intake of at least 2500 mL/day within cardiac tolerance.	Maintains hydration/circulating volume.
Review laboratory studies, e.g., Hg/HCT, serum osmolality, electrolytes, BUN/Cr.	Useful in evaluating level of hydration, effectiveness of therapy, and additional needs.

Nursing Diagnosis: Knowledge Deficit

RELATED TO: Lack of exposure/recall, information misinterpretation, unfamiliarity with information resources.
AS EVIDENCED BY: Questions, statement of concern, inaccurate follow-through of instructions, development of preventable complications.

Desired Outcomes/Evaluation Criteria

Verbalizes understanding of disease process. Identifies relationship of signs/symptoms to the disease process and correlates symptoms with causative factors. Correctly performs necessary procedures and explains reasons for the actions. Initiates necessary lifestyle changes and participates in treatment regimen.

Nursing Actions	Rationale
Discuss normal blood glucose level and compare with patient's, type of diabetes mellitus patient has, relationship between insulin deficiency and high glucose level.	Provides knowledge base on which patient can make informed lifestyle choices.
Discuss acute and chronic complications of the disease.	Awareness helps patient to be more consistent with care and may prevent/delay onset of complications.
Demonstrate fingerstick testing.	Self-monitoring of blood glucose (SMBG) four or more times a day allows flexibility in self-care, promotes tighter control of serum levels, and may prevent/delay development of long-term complications.
Review medication regimen, including onset, peak, and duration of prescribed insulin.	Understanding all aspects of drug usage promotes proper use.
Review self-administration of insulin and care of equipment. Have patient demonstrate procedure.	Identifies understanding and correctness of procedure or potential problems so that alternate solutions can be found if necessary.
Discuss factors that play a part in diabetic control, e.g., exercise, stress, surgery. Review sick-day rules.	Promotes diabetic control and can greatly reduce occurrence of ketoacidosis.
Identify symptoms of hypoglycemia, e.g., weakness, dizziness, lethargy, hunger, irritability, diaphoresis, pallor, tachycardia, tremors, headache, changes in mentation, and explain causes.	May promote early detection and treatment, preventing occurrence.
Review signs/symptoms requiring medical evaluation.	Prompt intervention may prevent development of more serious/life-threatening complications.
Identify community resources, e.g., American Diabetic Association, VNA, weight loss/stop smoking clinic, and contact person/diabetic instructor.	Continued support is usually necessary to sustain lifestyle changes and promote well-being.

Other Suggested Nursing Diagnoses: Altered Nutrition, Less than Body Requirements; Altered Nutrition, More than Body Requirements; Risk for Injury; Pain; and Noncompliance.

1000 to 3000 calories and is arranged around a system of exchanges determined by the number of calories prescribed. The exchanges include starches, proteins, fats, vegetables, and fruits. The patient receives 60% carbohydrate, 20% protein, and 20% fat. In some cases, the patient is taught to make meal choices based on counting carbohydrates and balancing insulin on the usual amount of carbohydrates the individual consumes at each meal.

- In the hospital setting, ensure that the patient receives meals on time and that the entire meal is consumed. Collaborate with the dietitian to help the patient understand the system of exchanges and the dietary guidelines.
- Teach the patient that eating the food at the prescribed time is important for diabetic control. Lunch is consumed 4 to 5 hours after breakfast, and supper is consumed 5 to 6 hours after lunch. An evening snack is necessary for the patient receiving oral antidiabetic agents or insulin therapy to prevent hypoglycemia during the night. Midmorning and midafternoon snacks may also be incorporated into the meal plan.
- In collaboration with the dietitian, discuss the use of alcohol with the patient. Because alcohol can block gluconeogenesis and thus induce a hypoglycemic reaction in individuals taking insulin or oral antidiabetic agents, ingesting alcohol is discouraged unless the patient is well controlled. Teach the patient that if a drink is desired on occasion, it must be taken immediately before or with a meal to prevent a hypoglycemic reaction. Alcohol also contains additional carbohydrates. If alcohol consumption is a regular occurrence, it is incorporated into the meal pattern.
- Discuss dining out guidelines.

Blood Glucose Monitoring

Blood glucose monitoring may be used in the hospital setting to help the diabetic patient regain control. This procedure is performed on the nursing unit by a nurse or laboratory technician, depending on hospital policy. A capillary blood glucose reading is obtained within 2 to 3 minutes. The result usually differs from a venous sample analyzed in the laboratory by 10%. The capillary blood glucose tests using self glucose monitoring equipment are simple to perform and provide more information about diabetic control than a urine test. The products used vary, so it is crucial to read the information packet and follow the procedure precisely. For most products, a small drop of blood is required, taken from the outer aspect of the finger by a lancet. The blood is dropped on a reagent paper, timed for a specific amount of time, wiped off, timed again, and then the results are read by comparing the strip to a color chart. The results are as good as the technique of the individual performing the test. Some institutions prefer to use a meter such as the one shown in Figure 45–3 to perform the reading. The procedure is gen-

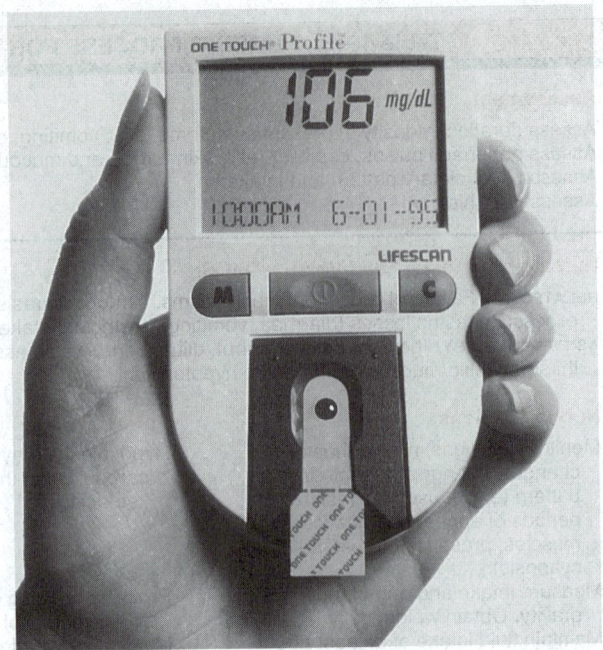

Figure 45–3. LifeScan ONE TOUCH Profile Diabetes Tracking System. (Courtesy of Lifescan Inc., Milpitis, Calif.)

erally the same for the meter readings as for visual readings, with the exception that an electronic eye reads the blood glucose level with the meter and gives a digital value instead of the individual's visual interpretation. With some meters the blood does not have to be wiped off the strip prior to insertion to obtain a blood glucose reading. Once again, it must be stressed that proper technique and care of the equipment is necessary to obtain accurate results.

- Teach the patient how to use self blood glucose monitoring, if this is included in the regimen.
- Demonstrate several visual and meter methods and allow the patient to decide which product is preferred.
- Assist the patient in receiving insurance coverage for these products.

In the hospital, record the blood glucose/urinary ketone reading on a flow sheet and instruct the patient to do the same thing when at home. Such a record allows all pertinent information regarding diabetic control to be located in the same place.

Urine Testing

The nurse or laboratory technician may test the patient's urine for glucose and ketone bodies during the hospitalization. The nurse can compare the urine tests with the blood tests to determine the approximate renal threshold. This record can be used as a reference guideline for the patient who tests urine at home.

Urine is routinely tested before meals and at bedtime.

Ketonuria without glycosuria usually indicates starvation rather than poor diabetic control.

- Record urine tests in percentages (1/10%, 1/4%, 1/2%, and so on), because readings of 1+, 2+, 3+, and so on, do not always correspond to the same amount of glycosuria when different testing agents are used and, therefore, may lead to misinterpretation of results.
- Teach the type II non-insulin-dependent diabetic patient to test for glucose in the urine.
- Teach the type I insulin-dependent diabetic to test for glucose and ketones in the urine. Even if the type I diabetic patient uses self blood glucose monitoring, advise to test for ketones if the blood glucose reading exceeds 250 mg/dL.
- Assist the patient in choosing the appropriate method for urine testing.
- In the hospital, record the urine glucose ketone on a flow sheet and instruct the patient to do the same thing at home.

Insulin Administration

In providing the patient with insulin, it is the nurse's responsibility to draw up the correct type and dosage of insulin. It is recommended that another nurse double-check the type and amount of insulin before the first nurse administers the insulin to the patient.

The exact technique for insulin injection may vary slightly from institution to institution, but the goal remains the same. Subcutaneous (SC) insulin is injected between the fat and muscle layer to ensure proper absorption. This may be accomplished by lightly pinching a large fold of skin and inserting the needle at a 90-degree angle.

Hypodermic syringes for insulin injection are either disposable or reusable. The syringes are calibrated to hold 100 units of insulin per milliliter. Several types of insulin syringes are designed to aid the individual receiving a small volume of insulin. These syringes are calibrated to contain 50 units per 1/2 mL, 30 units per 1/3 mL, and 25 units per 1/4 mL. The decreased diameter of these syringes with the calibrations farther apart permits easier reading and more accurate measurement of insulin. Patients receiving 50 or more units of insulin must use the 100 unit per 1 mL syringe.

- Inspect the insulin vial before drawing up the insulin.
- Roll intermediate- and long-acting insulins. They should appear uniformly cloudy after mixing.
- Do not shake. Do not use the vials if insulin material remains at the bottom of the bottle, if clumps are floating in the insulin after mixing, or if particles on the bottom or wall of the bottle have a frosted appearance.
- Check the expiration date of the insulin.
- Be accurate in drawing up the number of units that the physician has prescribed. Avoidance of bubbles is important. The volume of the bubble can easily displace a few units of insulin, which can make a substantial difference in dosage.

- Assess the patient's ability to draw up and inject insulin accurately. Various aids are commercially available to help the patient draw up and administer insulin. Magnifying glasses are available that clip directly on the insulin syringe and enlarge the numbers so visually impaired patients can see them.

Injection aids that can be used with standard syringes may be a help to some patients. Using these aids, a standard syringe is filled with insulin and placed in the device. The device is placed against the desired site and a button is pushed or the device is pressed against the skin to release a spring mechanism that pushes the needle automatically into the skin. All the patient has to do is push the plunger to inject the insulin. Some devices even push the plunger.

Injection pens are also available. A cartridge containing insulin is stored in a device about the size of a ballpoint pen. A disposable needle is used at one end of the pen, and there is a push button or turn knob on the other end. The pen is held and the needle is inserted into the skin like an ordinary injection. These pens are convenient as the patient does not have to carry syringes and bottles of insulin to give the prescribed dose. The pens also have audible clicks and enlarged numbers that help the visually impaired patient determine how much insulin is being injected. An example of this type of device is the Novo 1.5 Insulin Delivery Pen, shown in Figure 45–4. For individuals who dislike injecting insulin or fear needles, no-needle injectors or jet injectors are an alternative. These injectors deliver a tiny stream of insulin under pressure directly through the skin. Often there is little or no sensation at the time of the injection. There are differences in insulin absorption and distribution when jet injectors are used compared to the traditional syringe that should be taken into consideration. Jet injection results in a greater decrease in plasma glucose than an equal amount of insulin administered by syringe. Also the duration of insulin action appears shorter. An example of a no-needle injector is the Medi-Jector EZ. Another injection aid is the Button Infuser. This device is inserted subcutaneously into the abdomen and taped so doses of insulin can be inserted through the opening at the top. The device must be changed every 2 or 3 days.

- If mixing two different types of insulin, follow guidelines for mixing presented in Table 45–6.
- If the desired insulins may be mixed, instruct the patient to draw up the insulins the same way each time. Air should be added to each vial, then the proper amount of rapid-acting insulin drawn into the syringe, followed by the proper amount of intermediate-acting insulin. This prevents contamination of the rapid-acting by the intermediate-acting insulin.
- If the patient is unable to safely draw up two different types of insulin in the same syringe, alternatives are available. A family member can be taught to prefill the syringes with the designated amount of insulin, so that the patient will have a week's supply for injection.
- Instruct the patient that the prefilled syringes should be stored in the refrigerator and gently rotated before

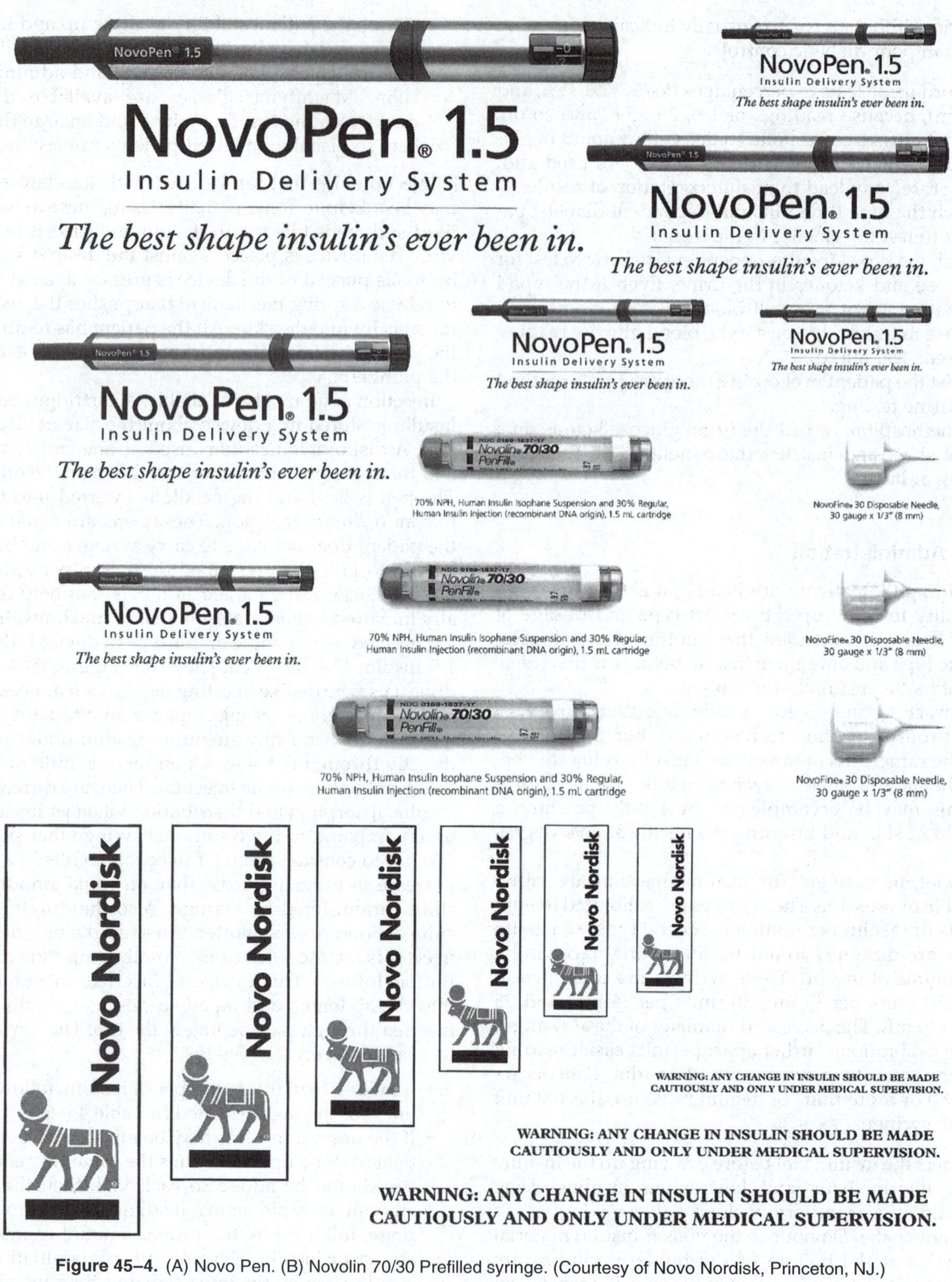

NovoPen® 1.5
Insulin Delivery System

The best shape insulin's ever been in.

NovoPen® 1.5
Insulin Delivery System
The best shape insulin's ever been in.

NovoPen® 1.5
Insulin Delivery System
The best shape insulin's ever been in.

NovoPen® 1.5
Insulin Delivery System
The best shape insulin's ever been in.

NovoPen® 1.5
Insulin Delivery System
The best shape insulin's ever been in.

NovoPen® 1.5
Insulin Delivery System
The best shape insulin's ever been in.

NDC 0169-1837-17
Novolin® 70/30
PenFill®
70% NPH, Human Insulin Isophane Suspension and 30% Regular,
Human Insulin Injection (recombinant DNA origin), 1.5 mL cartridge

NovoFine® 30 Disposable Needle,
30 gauge x 1/3" (8 mm)

NDC 0169-1837-17
Novolin® 70/30
PenFill®
70% NPH, Human Insulin Isophane Suspension and 30% Regular,
Human Insulin Injection (recombinant DNA origin), 1.5 mL cartridge

NovoFine® 30 Disposable Needle,
30 gauge x 1/3" (8 mm)

NDC 0169-1837-17
Novolin® 70/30
PenFill®
70% NPH, Human Insulin Isophane Suspension and 30% Regular,
Human Insulin Injection (recombinant DNA origin), 1.5 mL cartridge

NovoFine® 30 Disposable Needle,
30 gauge x 1/3" (8 mm)

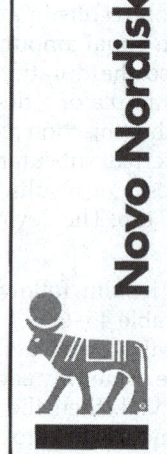 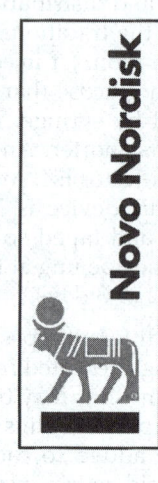 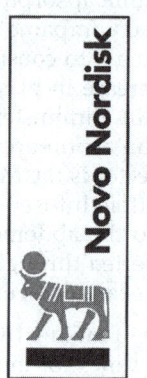 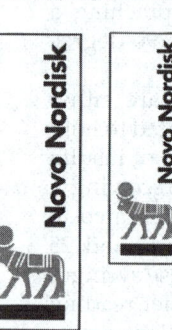 

WARNING: ANY CHANGE IN INSULIN SHOULD BE MADE CAUTIOUSLY AND ONLY UNDER MEDICAL SUPERVISION.

WARNING: ANY CHANGE IN INSULIN SHOULD BE MADE CAUTIOUSLY AND ONLY UNDER MEDICAL SUPERVISION.

WARNING: ANY CHANGE IN INSULIN SHOULD BE MADE CAUTIOUSLY AND ONLY UNDER MEDICAL SUPERVISION.

Figure 45–4. (A) Novo Pen. (B) Novolin 70/30 Prefilled syringe. (Courtesy of Novo Nordisk, Princeton, NJ.)

Table 45–6. GUIDELINES FOR MIXING TWO TYPES OF INSULIN IN SAME SYRINGE

1. Patients who are well controlled on a particular mixed-insulin regimen should maintain their standard procedure for preparing their insulin doses. Use the same procedure each time you prepare an insulin mixture.
2. Use of commercially available premixed insulins is preferred to extemporaneous mixing by the patient if the insulin ratio is appropriate to the patient's insulin requirements. Mix insulins produced by the same manufacturer only.
3. Semilente, Lente, and Ultralente insulins may be combined in any ratio desired. They are stable when mixed.
4. NPH regular mixtures are stable mixtures.
5. Mixing of regular and Lente insulins are not recommended unless the patient is already adequately controlled on these mixtures. On mixing, the zinc binds with the regular insulin and delays its onset. The patient should standardize the interval between mixing and injection.
6. Formulations of buffered insulins (all brands of NPH, Velosulin) should not be mixed with any Lente family insulin. The phosphate buffer will precipitate the zinc from one suspension converting the extended insulin to a regular line insulin.
7. There is no rationale for mixing animal source insulin with human insulin.
8. Insulin formulations may change; therefore, the manufacturer should be consulted if its recommendations appear to conflict with the American Diabetes Association guidelines.

injection. Several mixtures of NPH and regular insulin are commercially available in a 70/30 ratio (70% NPH and 30% regular) or a 50/50 ratio (50% NPH and 50% regular). These premixed insulins are desirable for individuals who can fill the syringe but cannot master the technique of mixing, but who happen to require a mixed dose.

In addition to instructing the patient on insulin injection technique, instruct the patient regarding injection site rotation to prevent lipohypertrophy. As mentioned previously, lipohypertrophy is an adverse reaction to insulin therapy that occurs when insulin is injected frequently into the same area.

- In the hospital, follow a site rotation pattern.
- Teach the patient to systematically rotate injection sites using areas of the upper arms, back, abdomen, and buttocks.
- Teach the patient to avoid areas around old scars, varicosities, and the immediate area around the navel. One method that may be used is to choose a general area and select sites one inch or two fingers apart. Then, after approximately 15 days of using one area, instruct the patient to choose a different site. See Figure 45–5 for injection sites. Other systems have been developed that have the patient change injection sites from area to area. When using this system, instruct the patient not to return to the previously used site too soon.
- Instruct the patient to use the abdomen as the only

site when consistent control is desired. The abdomen is generally a large enough area to accommodate a month's worth of injections, and injecting into this one area eliminates the different absorption rates of the various sites.

- The insulin you are using for the patient does not need to be refrigerated, but it must be protected from extremes of temperature. Freezing or excessive heat can affect the potency of the insulin. Insulin products remain stable at room temperature (68° to 75°) for 1 month with a very small loss of potency.
- Instruct the patient to leave the bottle he or she is using at room temperature and to refrigerate other bottles. When traveling, insulin can be protected from extremes of temperature by carrying it in a vacuum bottle.

Exercise

- Assess the patient's general exercise regimen.
- Stress that planned exercise is helpful in lowering the blood glucose level, increasing cardiovascular fitness, increasing circulation, and promoting a feeling of well-being.
- Explain that exercise is done preferably after a meal and not at a time when a meal is due because of the risk of hypoglycemia. If the patient wishes to exercise before a meal, have the patient test his or her blood sugar; if it is low normal, the patient should eat two peanut butter crackers or half of a sandwich and half a cup of milk, the amount of food depending on the amount of exercise that is planned.
- Teach the patient that if the blood sugar level is greater than 250 mg/dL or if spilling ketones, not to exercise as exercise elevates the blood sugar when the person is in poor control.

Oral Antidiabetic Agents

- Administer the oral antidiabetic agent that is prescribed for the patient. At the time of administration, identify the medication, describe its use, and the time of administration.

Management of Hyperglycemia and Hypoglycemia

In caring for the diabetic, it is essential to have knowledge of the causes, symptoms, and treatment of hyperglycemia and hypoglycemia as well as the acute complications of ketoacidosis and hyperglycemic hyperosmolar nonketotic coma. Table 45–7 compares these disorders. The patient must be taught how to recognize when diabetes is out of control and to take appropriate action.

Hyperglycemia

- Assess the cause of hyperglycemia, so that it may be treated. For example, if an infection has elevated the

Injection Sites

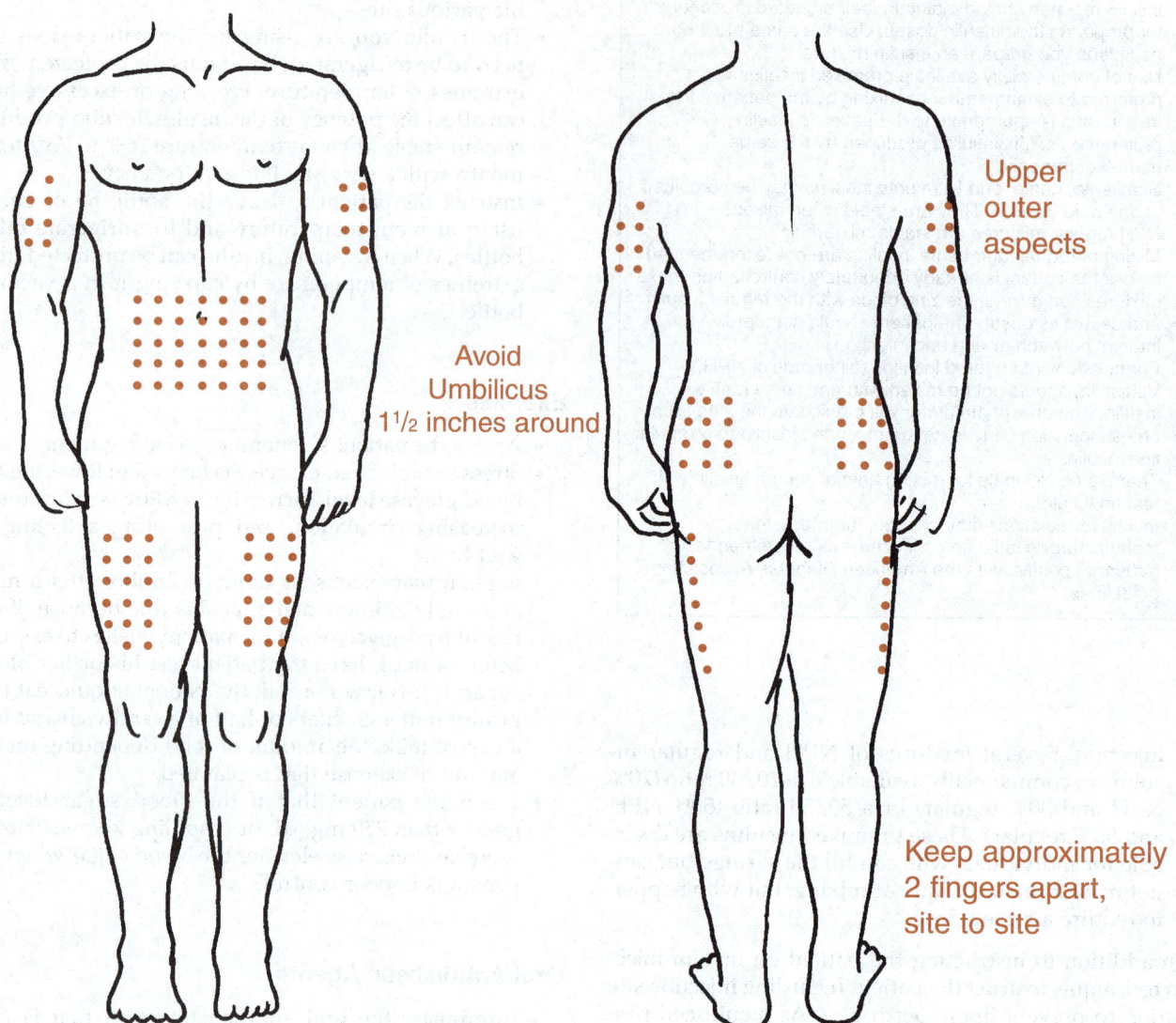

Avoid
Umbilicus
1½ inches around

Upper
outer
aspects

Keep approximately
2 fingers apart,
site to site

Figure 45–5. Insulin injection sites. (Redrawn with permission of Deborah G. Smith, Diabetes Clinical Specialist, Buffalo, NY, 1985.)

blood sugar level, the infection must be treated, rather than just increasing the insulin dosage.

- Test the blood glucose levels at specific intervals and administer regular insulin based on a sliding scale coverage as ordered.
- Provide sliding scale insulin coverage along with or instead of the usual insulin dosage. An order for sliding scale coverage may resemble the following, based on blood glucose values:

180 mg/dL	No insulin
180–240 mg/dL	10 units of regular insulin
240–400 mg/dL	20 units of regular insulin
400 mg/dL	Call physician

- Test the urine for ketones before meals and at bedtime when the blood sugar is tested.

- If an individual has a daily insulin order and is on sliding scale coverage, follow both orders.

Ketoacidosis

If the patient is admitted to the hospital with ketoacidosis, treatment consists of hydration and insulin therapy. Continuous low-dose infusion of regular insulin is the preferred treatment in managing ketoacidosis, as IV delivery of insulin rapidly establishes effective blood glucose levels that can be maintained or altered quickly. An IV bolus of 0.1 unit per kilogram of body weight is often given, followed by an infusion of 5 to 10 units per hour or 0.1 unit per kilogram per hour. The insulin infusion is kept separate from the fluids being used to replace volume. An insulin concentration of 1 U/10 mL may be obtained

Table 45–7. COMPARISON OF HYPOGLYCEMIA, KETOACIDOSIS, AND HYPERGLYCEMIC HYPEROSMOLAR NONKETOTIC COMA (HHNK)

	Hypoglycemia	Ketoacidosis	HHNK
Diabetes Type	Either	IDDM, usually young	NIDDM, usually over age 50
Onset	Rapid: minutes to hours	Slow: hours to days (usually <2 days)	Insidious (>5 days), then rapid
Causes	Delayed or skipped meal; increased exercise without additional food; too much insulin; Somogyi effect; gastroenteritis	Undetected diabetes; stress (physical or emotional); illness or infection; excessive food intake; inadequate insulin or dosage errors; drugs such as thiazides or corticosteroids; reduced exercise	May be first indication of diabetes; usually adult onset with enough insulin production to prevent ketosis; steroid therapy; stress states; hyperalimentation; dialysis, especially with solutions high in dextrose; pancreatic disease
Signs and Symptoms			
NEUROLOGIC	Weak, light-headed, drowsy, trembly, headache, numbness of the mouth and tongue, anxious, memory loss, seizures, primitive reflexes (Babinski present)	Early: irritable, tired, headache, weakness; progressively more listless, decreased sensation until coma. No focal symptoms; hyporeflexia	Focal symptoms (aphasia, homonymous hemianopsia, hemiparesis, hemisensory defects, unilateral hyperreflexia and Babinski, hallucinations and psychic disturbances)
RESPIRATORY	Bradypnea; in shock, respiratory rate may increase	Kussmaul respiration (deep and rapid); sweet (acetone) odor to breath	Increased respiratory rate; no Kussmaul respirations or sweet odor to breath
CARDIOVASCULAR	Increased blood pressure and heart rate	Lower blood pressure, especially orthostatic; weak, rapid pulse	Lower blood pressure; weak, rapid pulse
RENAL	Asymptomatic	Early: great increase in urine output; later, as shock develops: oliguria or anuria	Great increase in urine output, causing massive dehydration and hyperosmolarity; progresses to decreased output as shock develops
GASTROINTESTINAL	Nausea, hunger, stomachache, vomiting	Nausea and vomiting, thirst, abdominal cramping, decreased bowel sounds, acute abdomen symptoms, weight loss	Nausea and vomiting, thirst, hunger, less acute abdomen symptoms
SKIN	Diaphoretic, cold, clammy, pale; circumoral pallor	Hot, flushed, and dry; low body temperature	Flushed, very dry; elevated body temperature
MUCOUS MEMBRANES	Normal	Very dry	Extremely dry
Clinical Data			
BLOOD SUGAR LEVEL	Below 60 mg/dL or when sudden drop occurs (e.g., a drop from 400 mg/dL to 200 mg/dL)	Above 200 mg/dL; usually 400–800 mg/dL, sometimes higher	Usually >600 mg/dL; up to 3000 mg/dL
URINE GLUCOSE LEVEL	Negative	2% or higher	2% or higher
URINE KETONE BODIES	Negative	Positive	Negative
OTHER LABORATORY TESTS	Essentially normal, except for low blood sugar levels	Falling pH (below 7.3); increased BUN and serum creatine; increased Hct, Hbg, and total protein; initially increased, normal, or decreased K^+; normal or decreased Na^+; increased WBC, SGOT, SGPT, and LDH; increased osmolarity, <350 mOsm/kg	Normal or decreased pH due to lactic acidosis, not ketosis; increased BUN; increased, normal, or decreased K^+; normal or decreased Na^+; increased WBC; serum osmolarity increased, >350 mOsm/kg
TREATMENT	Validate blood sugar level; administer 10–15 g fast-acting carbohydrate, followed by slow-acting carbohydrate. If patient is unable to swallow, give glucagon, 0.5–1.0 mg (IV, IM, or SC); repeat in 15 min, if needed. If no response, give 25–50 mL 50% dextrose; follow with slow-acting carbohydrate meal when patient is alert.	Validate blood sugar level; monitor blood sugar, urine glucose, and acetone levels; hydration, first with normal saline, then dextrose solution as blood sugar level approaches 250 mg/dL; give regular insulin, IV or SC. Monitor vital signs and urine output; give K^+ supplements, if needed, after insulin is administered and when urine output is adequate.	Hydration; give small doses of regular insulin; very sensitive to insulin, blood sugar level may drop suddenly with only small amounts of insulin; give K^+ supplements.

BUN = blood urea nitrogen; WBC = white blood count; SGOT = serum glutamic-oxaloacetic transaminase; serum glutamic = pyruvic transaminase; LDH = lactic dehydrogenase.

by adding 50 units of regular insulin to 500 mL of normal saline. If the blood glucose is unchanged after 2 hours, the infusion rate is doubled. Insulin adheres to glass and plastic IV bottles and IV tubing. The problem can be minimized by flushing the tubing with the insulin preparation before connecting it to the patient. This is not a major problem when the patient's blood sugars are monitored closely and insulin adjustments can be made.

If the patient is in shock, poor peripheral perfusion prevents adequate absorption when the insulin is administered subcutaneously. Observe for rebound hypoglycemia when the shock is reversed and the insulin absorbed. Rehydration, as well as insulin administration, lowers serum potassium. Hypokalemia, as well as hyperkalemia, can have a detrimental effect on the cardiovascular and respiratory status. Monitor serum potassium values and the electrocardiogram (ECG). Potassium is given only in the presence of adequate urine output.

Hyperglycemic Hyperosmolar Nonketotic Coma

Hyperglycemic hyperosmolar nonketotic coma (HHNK) is a metabolic disorder that may occur in the diagnosed or undiagnosed type II diabetic patient. The mortality rate is 50% to 70%. In HHNK, the patient's blood sugar level becomes elevated. Because the type II diabetic patient produces some insulin, ketosis is prevented. Therefore, the blood glucose level rises dramatically, often above 1000 mg/dL. The osmotic pull of the serum glucose is great, which causes profound dehydration in the body's cells and tissues and a fluid shift in the bloodstream. This fluid is rapidly eliminated by the kidney. The treatment of HHNK focuses on hydration to reverse shock and small doses of insulin to counteract hyperglycemia.

The emergency room nurse must be especially aware of this condition, as many patients are admitted to the hospital to rule out a stroke when it is really HHNK. Prompt determination of the blood glucose level is therefore imperative.

Hypoglycemia

Hypoglycemia is a medical emergency and must be treated promptly to avoid brain damage. The nurse must be alert to recognize hypoglycemic symptoms and initiate prompt treatment. Hypoglycemic reactions most likely occur when the patient's insulin dose is peaking.

Illness

When the diabetic patient becomes ill, control is more difficult. Provide the patient guidelines to follow when illness occurs.

- Insulin is not omitted.
- Suggest liquid carbohydrates such as carbonated beverages or fruit juices if the patient is unable to eat regular meals to fulfill daily caloric needs.
- Test the blood or urine glucose levels at least four times a day to detect hyperglycemia.
- Test the urine for the presence of ketones.

- Instruct the patient to notify the physician if the illness progresses past 2 days or if vomiting or diarrhea occurs.
- Instruct the patient to notify the physician immediately when signs of infection are present. Infection is more common among patients with diabetes, and healing occurs more slowly than among nondiabetic persons. Infections cause blood glucose levels to rise and, if untreated, can cause diabetic ketoacidosis.
- Encourage a good program of skin care to lessen the incidence of local infection.

Foot Care

Often as a result of neuropathy, which is a chronic complication affecting the nervous system, the patient loses the ability to feel discomfort or pain in the feet and legs. Therefore, if the patient develops an injury, he or she does not recognize it; the injury then worsens and the blood glucose goes out of control.

- Teach the patient with diabetes about proper foot care.
- Encourage the patient to wear slippers at home as well as in the hospital.
- Teach the patient how to inspect the feet and perform care of the feet at home.

Management of the Pregnant Woman with Diabetes

The nurse often cares for the pregnant diabetic patient in the hospital or a clinic. Teaching is extremely important in this situation because strict diabetic control is necessary in pregnancy to prevent abnormalities and mortality of the fetus. For a known diabetic individual, this requires self blood glucose monitoring and mixed and split doses of insulin or insulin pump therapy. It is recommended that the blood glucose level remain around 100 mg/dL.

Oral antidiabetic agents are not recommended during pregnancy because they do not control the blood sugar levels as precisely as insulin therapy. The insulin that is used is human insulin; the insulin antibodies from beef or pork insulin are passed to the fetus.

Generally, during the first trimester of pregnancy, the patient who previously received insulin requires the same amount or the dose may have to be decreased. Nausea and vomiting during early pregnancy may make the meal pattern more difficult to follow and the diabetes more difficult to control. As the pregnancy progresses, the patient requires increasing amounts of insulin because the placenta produces hormones (cortisol, human placental lactogen, estrogens, progesterones, and prolactin) that elevate blood glucose levels. Research indicates that there is also insulin resistance on a cellular level.

This situation often produces a glucose intolerance, commonly referred to as gestational diabetes, in some pregnant women. This type of diabetes generally begins in the 26th to 28th week of pregnancy, when the hormones are elevated, and frequently disappears as soon as the baby is born. The woman may have to take insulin during this period, like the woman who has had diabetes prior to conception. Normoglycemia is a goal for the gestational diabetic patient as well as the pregnant woman with preexisting diabetes.

Traditionally, women with diabetes were hospitalized during the last trimester of pregnancy to achieve strict control of the blood glucose levels. Today, with self blood glucose monitoring, the woman can monitor her blood glucose levels and adjust her insulin dosage according to her physician's specified guidelines. Blood glucose testing is generally done before breakfast and 2 hours after each meal.

During the postpartum period, the mother's insulin requirement returns to her prepregnancy level. Frequently, the infant of a diabetic mother is large for gestational age. The infant is placed in a special care nursery and monitored for hypoglycemia, which frequently occurs.

Management of the Patient Having Surgery

The major goals for good management of the diabetic patient during surgery are prevention of diabetic ketoacidosis and prevention of severe fluid loss and hypoglycemia, especially during the period of anesthesia.

Specific orders for the patient undergoing a surgical procedure must be obtained before the day of surgery. If the patient is managed on an oral antidiabetic agent, it is generally discontinued 24 hours before surgery except for chlorpropamide, which may have to be stopped 48 hours before surgery. The patient may then be placed on a low dose of an intermediate-acting insulin, or blood glucoses are covered with regular insulin on a sliding scale. For the patient who was on insulin therapy, he or she should have his or her blood glucose monitored every 2 to 3 hours during the perioperative period and receive insulin coverage subcutaneously or intravenously. Generally, IV insulin therapy is the preferred route of administration owing to fluid shifts during the operative period and different absorption rates of the insulin given SC. Previously, half of the usual daily dose of intermediate-acting insulin was given subcutaneously on the morning of surgery and one or two liters of 5% glucose and water was given during the surgical procedure. Every 4 to 6 hours after the initial insulin dosage was administered, additional regular insulin could be given depending on the degree of hyperglycemia. With the availability of the self blood glucose monitoring equipment and more precise management trends, this traditional method is usually reserved for outpatient surgeries. The individual would take the remaining intermediate-acting insulin prior to the meal he or she was ready to consume after surgery.

Regardless of the specific medical management of the diabetic patient undergoing surgery, it is imperative to make frequent assessments of diabetic control and monitor continually for hyperglycemia and hypoglycemia. It is also important to strive to prevent infection as infection further compromises diabetic control.

Patient Teaching

A thorough assessment of each patient with diabetes is essential to develop an individualized teaching plan.

- Assess the patient's knowledge of diabetes and its management, psychomotor skills such as insulin administration and urine testing, psychologic factors such as stress and anxiety, physical limitations such as arthritis and retinopathy, sociologic factors, support system, and economic factors.
- Assess motivation and what diabetes means to the individual.

Teaching is essential because the patient must learn how to manage the condition in order to live a long, productive life. Through assessment determine the appropriate method and materials to be used for instruction and the rate at which the information is to be delivered.

- Determine if survival or very basic information is all that the patient can comprehend or if a more detailed explanation of the disease process is necessary.
- Teach the patient what he or she needs to know. The teaching plan, therefore, differs according to whether the patient's diabetes is controlled by diet alone, diet and oral antidiabetic agents, or diet and insulin therapy.
- If the patient is solely on dietary management, instruct regarding the physiology of diabetes and treatment of hyperglycemia, dietary management, urine or blood glucose testing, exercise, and foot and skin care. Advise the patient to call for further instruction if the treatment routine changes.
- If the patient is managed on diet and oral antidiabetic agents, teach all of the previously stated information. In addition, teach the type, dosage, and action of the oral antidiabetic agent; causes, symptoms, and treatment of hypoglycemia if on a sulfonylurea; and travel and sick day management. Do not teach about insulin therapy unless it is going to be used within a few days. Encourage the patient to attend follow-up classes if he or she does not respond to the oral antidiabetic agents and insulin therapy is warranted.
- Teach the patient who is on dietary management and insulin therapy all of the previously stated information except the information regarding oral agents unless the patient is on combination therapy. In addition teach the type, dosage, and action of the insulin; drawing up and injection technique; site rotation; and storage of insulin.

All patients should understand the basic function of the pancreas in terms of insulin production. It is important for the patient to understand the function of insulin in lowering the blood glucose by transporting it into the cell to provide energy. Pamphlets and visual aids are helpful in explaining what is occurring in the body. Understanding how the body functions allows the patient to understand the symptoms of the disease and why they occur.

The teaching plan must be specific, as shown in Table 45–8. Minor changes in technique, which are well within acceptable nursing practice, can be confusing for the

Table 45–8. PATIENT TEACHING INFORMATION FOR THE DIABETIC PATIENT TAKING INSULIN

Dear Patient:

This drug has been prescribed for you. This is what you should know about your drug to get the most from your therapy:

☐ 1. Insulin is a medication that will lower your blood sugar level. It takes the sugar from your bloodstream and brings it into the muscle cells in your body to give you energy. The insulin you are taking will make up for the insulin your body is not able to produce.

☐ 2. You will be taking insulin for the rest of your life.* The dosage and the times you administer the insulin may change over the course of time.

☐ 3. The amount of insulin you will be taking depends on your doctor's orders. Obtain the correct vial of insulin and insulin syringe. Rotate the vial slowly between the palms of your hands to mix the solution thoroughly. Do not shake the vial. Take the insulin syringe and, using sterile technique, measure an amount of air equal to the amount of insulin you need and inject it into the vial. Turn the vial upside down and withdraw the correct number of units of insulin from the vial. Inject the insulin under the skin in a place that is ½″ away from the previous place that you have used in the past 30 days. Follow the injection pattern of site rotation that you learned in the hospital. If you are using 2 types of insulin, draw the insulin up in the same order each day.

☐ 4. Many prescription and nonprescription medications may raise or lower your blood sugar level. Before taking any over-the-counter medications (i.e., cold and cough preparations, laxatives, antacids, and other medications you can get without a prescription), consult with your physician, pharmacist, or diabetes nurse/educator about medications that do not contain sugar. If you are placed on any prescription medications, ask your doctor about the medication's effect on your blood sugar level.

☐ 5. If you forget to take your insulin, your blood sugar level will go up. Take the usual dosage of insulin if you remember and it is 2 hours or less after the scheduled dosage was omitted. If more time elapses, consult your doctor to obtain the amount of insulin you should take. If you can't remember whether you took your insulin or not, do not take it.

☐ 6. Do not stop taking your insulin. High blood sugar levels, diabetic ketoacidosis, and even death can result from not taking your medication.

☐ 7. Your insulin dosage may change over time. You may be given a specific dosage by your doctor, or you may adjust your insulin dosage according to a scale based on your blood glucose monitoring results. *Do not* adjust your insulin dosage without your doctor's advice.

☐ 8. You should not drink alcoholic beverages (beer, wine, whiskey) as they may lower your blood sugar level and cause an insulin reaction. If you have an occasional drink, it should be consumed before a meal. If you plan to drink alcoholic beverages on a regular basis, contact your doctor and dietitian to incorporate them into your meal pattern.

☐ 9. If you take too much insulin, skip or delay a meal, or exercise too hard, you may develop low blood sugar, which is a side effect of the medication. You will suddenly feel tired, dizzy, shaky, nervous, weak, and irritable and will break out into a cold-clammy sweat. Immediately, take 2 sugar cubes, half a cup of orange juice, or half a cup of sweetened soft drink to reverse these symptoms. It is important that your family learn how to give you glucagon in case you pass out and are unable to eat or drink. Wear a Medical Alert bracelet so emergency care can be given if you are unconscious. Another side effect of insulin therapy is a painless hardened area or lump in the skin area where you inject your insulin. Contact your doctor or nurse to review site rotation with you. If you notice any reddened areas around the insulin injection site, notify your doctor. Generally if the reddened areas occur several hours after the injection, this problem will disappear on its own. If it occurs within 1 hour of the injection, this could be an insulin allergy that requires prompt medical attention.

☐ 10. Insulin may be stored at room temperature for up to 1 month. However, it must be protected from extremes of temperature, which can alter its potency. It is stable in the refrigerator for 3 months. Do not use your intermediate- or long-acting insulin if the insulin material remains at the bottom of the bottle after mixing or if particles on the bottom or wall of the bottle give it a frosted appearance.

*The type II diabetic patient may not require insulin for the rest of his or her life, and this must be discussed.

patient who is trying to learn. Because there are various insulin syringes available as well as urine and blood testing products, be consistent in using the same product. Make sure to communicate with other nurses about what products the patient is using. For education materials, publications, and additional information on diabetes, contact one or more of the organizations listed in Table 45–9.

Diabetes teaching should proceed slowly and begin with simple instruction before the presentation of complex information. Teaching must focus on individual need. For example, if an individual is highly anxious regarding insulin therapy with numerous questions, and blood glucose testing was to be taught that day, switch the agenda and discuss insulin therapy. Otherwise, the patient will not listen to the discussion on blood glucose testing.

Teaching that occurs in the hospital is reinforced and expanded in follow-up classes after discharge. Generally,

after discharge the patient is less anxious and has questions based on problems that arose while at home. The classes also provide support in allowing the patient to feel that he or she is not alone with this disease. Family members and friends should be encouraged to take part in diabetes instruction.

The patient with type II non-insulin-dependent diabetes, on diet alone or receiving oral agents, may have a more lax attitude than the diabetic patient receiving insulin. Sometimes the patient feels that the diabetes is less serious or that he or she has "just a touch" of diabetes. Stress that control is as important for this person as for the person on insulin. The individual's weight may increase over time from poor dietary adherence, and the diet and oral antidiabetic agents may fail. The individual then may be placed on insulin. In this case, it is essential to explain that insulin is not a lifelong sentence. Inform the patient that weight reduction brings the blood glucose levels back to normal and, although the patient still has

Table 45–9. RESOURCES FOR INFORMATION REGARDING DIABETES

Organizations

American Association of Diabetes Educators
444 North Michigan Avenue
Suite 1240
Chicago, IL 60611
1-312-644-2233

American Diabetes Association
National Service
1660 Duke St.
Alexandria, VA 22314
1-800-232-3472

Canadian Diabetes Association
National Office
15 Toronto St.
Suite 1001
Toronto, ON M5C2E3
1-416-363-3373

Juvenile Diabetes Foundation
120 Wall Street
19th Floor
New York, NY 10005
1-800-223-1138

National Diabetes Information Clearinghouse
9000 Rockville Pike
Building 31 Room 9 A52
Bethesda, MD 20892
1-301-496-5383

diabetes, insulin or even oral antidiabetic agents may no longer be required.

The changes in diet and lifestyle are often more difficult for the elderly patient with diabetes. The elderly patient may live alone and find it difficult to prepare three meals daily and may forget to take his or her medication. Elderly patients may also have other health problems, such as arthritis, poor vision, or poor motor coordination, which affect how well they are able to accomplish new tasks. Also, the added expense that diabetes imposes can be stressful for the elderly patient who is on a fixed income. The nurse can assist the elderly patient by seeing if he or she is eligible to receive Meals on Wheels (if the patient is unable to cook) and arranging for a community health nurse or nurse's aide to help with care.

EVALUATION

During the evaluation phase of the nursing process, the patient is evaluated to determine the effectiveness of the interventions. Evaluation of the patient's knowledge of and compliance with the treatment plan is essential. Evaluation is an ongoing process, and it is important to update the teaching plan frequently.

- Evaluate the patient's knowledge base by having the patient verbalize knowledge or demonstrate a technique previously taught.

- Evaluate objective data such as blood glucose values, urine testing, and glucosylated hemoglobin tests to evaluate diabetic control. These objective data are important because, even though the patient may be able to verbalize knowledge of the diabetes regimen and demonstrate techniques appropriately, compliance may not occur. The patient's urine test record is a valuable reflection of diabetic control. Glycosuria is to be avoided, and evidence of its existence may indicate failure to adhere to the diabetic regimen, underlying infection, or a need to increase diabetic medication. Blood glucose levels are important to evaluate the effectiveness of the diabetes regimen. The timing of these tests is just as important as the actual results. All of the blood sugars are done to ascertain that the blood glucose levels are close to the levels of the individual without diabetes. Generally, when a person is on insulin therapy, the fasting blood sugar is done to determine whether the intermediate-acting insulin given the day before is still effective. Blood sugar samples taken before lunch are used to evaluate the need for, or effectiveness, of the rapid-acting insulin given before breakfast. Blood sugar samples drawn in the evening (8:00 to 9:00 PM) are used to determine the need or effectiveness of rapid-acting insulin given before supper. Samples drawn during the night might indicate the need for giving a dose or adjusting a dose of intermediate-acting insulin before supper. A laboratory test that is helpful in evaluating diabetic control over a long period is the glycosylated hemoglobin level. This test reflects the mean blood glucose level over a period of 3 to 8 weeks. This test avoids the problem of evaluating the patient who adheres to the recommended diet for 2 to 3 days before the physician's visit so that he or she appears to be well controlled. It also can aid in determining if the extremely elevated blood glucose levels that prompted a hospitalization were part of a singular event such as an infection or if the elevated levels have been occurring for a while. The normal glycosylated hemoglobin level for the well-controlled patient is 8% or less. Certain conditions such as hemolytic anemia, severe hemorrhage, and pregnancy can invalidate the results obtained for this test.

Improper diabetic control, leading to diabetic ketoacidosis, HHNK coma, or insulin shock (all previously discussed), can be very dangerous. Every diabetic patient has fluctuations of blood glucose levels, but severe fluctuations must be detected and treated promptly. It is important for the nurse to realize that poor diabetic control is not always the result of noncompliance. An infection or differing metabolic demands can create severe problems in maintaining control.

Following prompt treatment, assessment of the underlying causes is important in preventing recurrent episodes of hypoglycemia or hyperglycemia. Modifications in medication, diet, or exercise may be necessary.

The bibliography for this chapter can be found in Appendix B, which begins on page 1054.

DELIVERING HOME HEALTH CARE

Insulin Administration

In many cases, patients with type II diabetes are placed on insulin therapy at home rather than being hospitalized when oral antidiabetic agents stop working. This is more realistic in the management of the diabetes, as individuals can continue with their usual activities, which in turn influence insulin requirements. If able, the individual usually attends outpatient classes for initial instruction.

Initially, the nurse may have to administer the first few doses of insulin until the patient or caregiver can do it. Before administration, the insulin bottle that is in use should be left out of the refrigerator; this will decrease local irritation at the injection site. The extra bottle should remain in the refrigerator because of a possible loss of potency.

Before the administration of insulin, do the following:
• Assess the patient's history and determine if he or she has ever received insulin before.
• Assess the patient's allergy history.
• Ask the patient and caregiver if they understand the procedure and why it is being performed.
• Assess what the patient learned in classes and determine what he or she can do to help with the injection, such as draw up and/or inject the insulin with verbal prompting.
• Gather data regarding the patient's blood glucose level. This may be done with a self glucose monitoring device, if available.
• Have the patient sit in a chair near a table.
• Check the insulin's expiration date. If out of date, or if any clumping, frosting, or precipitation is present, discard.

To administer, perform the following:
• Wipe the insulin bottle with 70% isopropyl alcohol.
• Roll the vial(s) in the palms of the hands.
• Inject air equal to the dose of insulin.
• Invert the bottle and withdraw the correct dosage in the syringe.
• Inspect fluid for air bubbles, flick forefinger against the syringe to allow the bubbles to escape.
• If mixing insulins follow guidelines presented in Table 45–6.
• If prefilling syringes, inform the patient that they are stable in the refrigerator for up to 3 weeks. If possible, the syringes should be stored in a vertical position with the needle pointing upward so the suspended insulin particles do not clog the needle. The predrawn syringe should be rolled between the hands before administration.
• Select an appropriate injection site.
• Inject the insulin.

After the insulin injection, do the following:
• Do not recap the syringe or bend or break the needle.
• Place the syringe in a puncture-resistant disposal container or use a needle clipping device, which retains the clipped needle in an inaccessible compartment.
• In areas with container-recycling programs, placement of containers with the used syringes with materials to be recycled is prohibited. Consult local trash-disposal authorities to determine the appropriate disposal of such containers.
• Inspect the injection site for irritation.
• Review diabetes management. Focus especially on the causes, symptoms, and treatment of hypoglycemia.

CHAPTER REVIEW QUESTIONS*

1. Jason Black receives a mixture of NPH and regular insulin at 7:30 AM. Of the following times, when should the nurse be especially alert to the potential for a hypoglycemic reaction?
   a. Before lunch.
   b. At midnight.
   c. Before bedtime.
   d. After supper.

2. Ann Morris, a 40-year-old patient, is receiving 36 units of NPH insulin and 10 units of regular insulin at 8 AM. She is receiving 20 units of NPH insulin and 8 units of regular insulin at 4 PM. Her blood glucose levels have been elevated at 3 PM every day. What insulin adjustment is needed?
   a. Her morning regular insulin dosage should be increased.
   b. Her morning NPH insulin suspension dosage should be increased.
   c. Her afternoon regular insulin dosage should be increased.
   d. Her afternoon NPH insulin dosage should be increased.

3. When teaching a patient about the signs and symptoms of hypoglycemia, the nurse includes the following sign:

   a. Sweating.
   b. Polyuria.
   c. Polydipsia.
   d. Fruity breath.

4. Which of the following statements from your patient with diabetes indicates a need for further education?
   a. It is important to accurately draw up the correct dosages of insulin.
   b. I will inject the insulin at a 90-degree angle.
   c. I should carry some form of sugar with me in case I feel like I am having an insulin reaction.
   d. When I anticipate that I will be exercising more than usual, I realize that I will need more insulin.

5. Patient teaching for a patient taking chlorpropamide (Diabinese) includes which of the following?
   a. Report weight gain, headache, and feelings of lethargy promptly.
   b. Take the medication with an antacid.
   c. Sporadic meal times are allowed with this agent.
   d. Hypoglycemic episodes do not require treatment when taking this agent.

*See Appendix A, which begins on page 1051, for answers.

INSULIN

A 12-year-old girl has had insulin-dependent diabetes mellitus for the past 6 years. She recently started having insulin reactions leading to unconsciousness at school every day around 2:30 PM. Paramedics called to the scene have treated her with glucagon. This time the patient was brought to the emergency department and given glucagon. Her mother tells the nurse this rarely occurs at home on weekends or days off of school. The patient routinely takes 16 units of NPH and 10 units of regular insulin every morning and 10 units of NPH and 5 units of regular insulin every day before supper. She follows her 2000-calorie ADA diet.

1. What are the possible causes for this patient's hypoglycemic reactions?
2. What additional data should be gathered?
3. How could the nurse most effectively intervene for this patient's problems?

CHAPTER 46

Thyroid and Parathyroid Agents

Merrily A. Kuhn, RNC, PhD

KEY TERMS

Carpopedal spasm   Euthyroid
Chvostek's sign   Trousseau's sign

LEARNING OBJECTIVES

After reading this chapter, the student will be able to:

1. Identify those medications used in thyroid and parathyroid disorders.
2. Differentiate among the thyroid and parathyroid medications as to mechanism of action, route of administration, pharmacokinetics, adverse effects, contraindications and precautions, and interactions.
3. Identify specific areas to assess in the patient requiring thyroid or parathyroid medications to formulate appropriate patient outcomes.
4. Plan the nursing interventions necessary to administer thyroid or parathyroid medications and choose appropriate teaching strategies to gain patient compliance.
5. Evaluate the patient at various stages of treatment to determine the effectiveness of nursing interventions.

Thyroid and parathyroid agents include the thyroid hormones; thyroid hormone antagonists that inhibit the synthesis of thyroid hormones; and antihypocalcemic agents and antihypercalcemic agents that are used to treat calcium and vitamin D imbalances. The parathyroid glands play an important role in calcium and phosphate metabolism by means of parathyroid hormone and its cofactor, vitamin D.

THYROID HORMONES

Three hormones are produced by the thyroid gland: thyroxine (T_4), triiodothyronine (T_3), and thyrocalcitonin in response to thyroid-stimulating hormone (TSH), secreted by the anterior pituitary, which is in turn stimulated by thyrotropin-releasing hormone (TRH), secreted by the hy-

pothalamus. The storage and secretion of these hormones depends on circulating thyroid and iodine levels. The ratio of T_4 to T_3 is normally about 4:1, with T_3 being the more potent form of thyroid hormone. T_4 is converted to T_3 by peripheral tissues. Both of these hormones function to control the metabolic rate of tissues by accelerating chemical reactions, oxygen consumption, and heat production. Thyrocalcitonin or calcitonin regulates calcium levels by opposing parathyroid hormone. Thyrocalcitonin, released in response to a high serum calcium, exerts its effects on bone, preventing resorption by decreasing osteoclastic activity; on the gastrointestinal (GI) tract, decreasing absorption of calcium; and on the renal tubule, increasing calcium excretion.

Normal daily production of thyroxine is about 70 to 90 μg and triiodothyronine, 15 to 30 μg. In the presence of adequate iodide substrate, the thyroid stores more T_4 than T_3 and releases about 1% of its stores daily. Both T_3

Table 46–1. THYROID HORMONES

DRUG NAME/ROUTE AND DOSAGE	PHARMACOKINETICS/ DYNAMICS	NURSING IMPLICATIONS
levothyroxine (Synthroid) (Levothroid) and others (T_4)		
Adults: Initial dose–0.2–0.5 mg IV as a solution containing 0.1 mg/mL. Maintenance dose–25–200 μg PO daily **Pediatric:** 0–6 mo, 8–10 μg/kg PO; 6–12 mo, 6–8 μg/kg; 1–5 yr, 5–6 μg/kg; 6–12 yr, 4–5 μg/kg; over 12 yr, 2–3 μg/kg	For all thyroid hormones: **Onset:** slow **Peak:** 1–2 wk **Duration:** 3 wk **½L:** 2–7 days **PB:** 99% **B:** liver and kidney **E:** bile, urine	For all thyroid hormones: **ASSESSMENT:** Assess baseline thyroid studies and weight. Assess for thyrotoxicosis, acute myocardial infarction uncomplicated by hypothyroidism, hypersensitivity (contraindications), and for cardiac disease, hypertension, and angina (cautious use). **INTERVENTION:** This medication should not be taken for weight loss. **Patient Teaching**—Advise patient to carry a Medic Alert card. Tell patient to check pulse rate: if above 100 beats per minute, to consult physician before taking medication. Caution patient to not decrease this medication without physician approval and to not change between products, as bioavailability may be different. Advise patient that some products contain tartrazine yellow dye, which may cause bronchial asthma and other allergic reactions. Tell patient to protect drug from light and to store it in dry, tightly closed container. **EVALUATION:** Notify physician of severe headache, diarrhea, excessive sweating, heat intolerance, or chest pain.
liothyronine (Cytomel and others) (T_3)		
Adults: Initial dose–25 μg (PO da ↑ dose by 12.5–25 μg every 1–2 wk Maintenance dose–25–75 PO μg/da **Pediatric:** 5–50 μg PO da		

and T_4 are transported in the serum bound to protein thyroxine-binding globulin produced in the liver, which stores T_3 and T_4 for up to several months. This long-term storage helps to explain why patients do not exhibit symptoms of hypothyroidism until several months after thyroid production has ceased.

Iodine is the major component of T_3 and T_4. In the United States and Canada, the average daily iodine intake is 200 to 500 μg. The average daily requirements range from 100 to 300 μg. Iodine is found in iodized salt, iodine-rich foods such as shellfish, and foods such as milk that have been stabilized with iodine. The GI tract reduces two-thirds of the iodine, and it enters the circulation as iodide. The remaining one-third is taken up by the thyroid. The ratio between iodide in the thyroid gland to that in the serum is referred to as the T/S ratio. The normal T/S ratio is 20:1, but if the gland is hyperactive, the T/S ratio may be as high as 250:1; if the gland is hypoactive, the T/S ratio may be as low as 10:1.

Thyroid hormones are available as natural or synthetic products. The natural products are derived from beef or pork. Synthetic forms of thyroid hormone exert the same physiologic effects as T_3 and T_4 and vary from the natural compounds in their potency, in the ratio of T_3 and T_4 contained within them, or both. The thyroid hormones available today include **levothyroxine** (T_4, *Levothroid, Synthroid*), **liothyronine** (T_3, *Cytomel, Triostat*), **thyroid dessicated** *(thyroid USP, Armour Thyroid)*, and **thyro-**

globulin *(Proloid)*. Levothyroxine and liothyronine are featured in Table 46–1.

ACTION

The principal action of thyroid hormones is to increase the metabolic rate of body tissues. Thyroid hormones increase the rate and depth of respiration; strengthen the rate and force of contraction of the heart; increase heat production; accelerate the metabolism of foodstuffs for energy; increase metabolic activity of all body tissues; increase growth, appetite, and weight; regulate female sex function; increase activity of the cellular enzyme systems; increase the rate of protein synthesis and catabolism; regulate growth in children; stimulate lipid synthesis, mobilization, and degradation; lower the concentration of cholesterol in plasma; and maintain nervous system development and cerebration.

USES

Thyroid hormones are used to replace deficient hormone in cases of inadequate thyroid production and to treat simple goiter. The pituitary hormone, thyrotropin, is used primarily in the diagnosis of hypothyroidism and to enhance radioactive iodine uptake in the treatment of metastatic thyroid carcinoma.

CONTRAINDICATIONS AND PRECAUTIONS

Use of thyroid hormones is contraindicated in patients with diagnosed thyrotoxicosis and acute myocardial infarction uncomplicated by hypothyroidism (as these conditions may be worsened) and where hypersensitivity exists. Thyroid hormones are used with great caution in patients with cardiac disease, including coronary artery disease and hypertension, as these drugs increase the metabolic demands on the heart. These products are not administered to persons with uncorrected adrenal insufficiency, as thyroid agents increase tissue demand for adrenal hormones. This increased demand may precipitate an acute adrenal crisis.

ADVERSE EFFECTS

The adverse effects of these drugs are primarily due to overdosage and are essentially the occurrence of the signs and symptoms of hyperthyroidism The onset of tachycardia is often an early sign of overdosage; consequently, patients are taught to monitor their pulse rates, particularly during initial therapy. The occurrence of anginal pain or symptoms of heart failure is usually related to the increased cardiac workload resulting from the increase in metabolism. The elderly patient is especially at risk for these adverse effects. In addition, patients may experience increased blood pressure and dysrhythmias.

Sweating and intolerance to heat may develop. Diarrhea and abdominal cramping may occur, and weight loss may ensue related to the increased metabolic rate. Adverse effects relating to the central nervous system (CNS) include tremors, headache, nervousness, and sleep disturbances; these are all related to the increased metabolic rate.

▼ CLINICAL ALERT

Long-term use of levothyroxine is associated with decreases in bone density in the hip and spine in women. This loss can be minimized by using the minimum dose to achieve the desired effects and by monitoring of bone density.

The occurrence of any adverse effect is reported immediately to the physician. Reduction of the dosage of the thyroid drug usually resolves the problem.

INTERACTIONS

The use of thyroid hormones concurrently with other drugs can lead to various interactions. Aspirin may compete for protein binding of T_3 and T_4. Patients who are hyperthyroid should not be given aspirin as this releases more T_3 and T_4 into circulation. Cholestyramine (Questran) decreases the effects by interfering with absorption of thyroid.

Thyroid hormone can also alter the effects of other drugs. Concurrent use tends to increase the effects of oral anticoagulants (by enhanced metabolism of clotting factors); decreases the effects of beta-blockers (because their effects are modified as the patient goes from a hypothyroid state to normal); and estrogens may decrease the response of thyroid hormones. The therapeutic effectiveness of digitalis products may be decreased, with possible exacerbations of cardiac dysrhythmias or heart failure. Numerous drugs have a tendency to interfere with accurate testing of T_3, T_4, and serum TSH levels, as presented in Table 46–2.

Table 46–2. EFFECTS OF SELECTED DRUGS ON THYROID FUNCTION TESTS

	Serum T_4	T_3 Uptake Resin	Free Thyroxine Index (FTI)	Serum T_3	Serum TSH
Antithyroid (PTU, methimazole)	▼	▼	▼	▼	0
Asparaginase	▼	▲	0	▼	0
Barbiturates	▼	0/△	▼	0	0
Contraceptives, oral	▲	▼	0	▲	0
Corticosteroids	0/▼	▲	0	▼	▼
Diazepam	▼	—	▽	—	—
Estrogens	▲	▼	0/△	▲	0
Heparin (IV)	▼	0/▲	▲	0	—
Insulin	▲	—	—	—	—
Lithium carbonate	0/▼	0/▼	0/▼	0/▼	0/▲
Methadone	▲	▼	0	▲	0
Nitroprusside	▼	—	—	—	—
Phenytoin	▼	0/△	▼	0/▲	0/▲
Propranolol	0/▼	0/▲	▼	▼	0
Salicylates (large doses)	▼	0/△	0	▼	—
Sulfonylureas	▼	0	0	—	—
Thiazides	0	—	—	▲	—

Source: Adapted from Med Lett Drugs Ther 23:30–32, 1981, with permission from the Medical Letter, Inc.; modified in 1996.
▲ Increased
△ Slightly increased
▼ Decreased
▽ Slightly decreased
0 No effect
— No data

DOSAGE

Generally, patients are started on small doses of thyroid hormones and gradually given increasing doses until the signs and symptoms of hypofunction disappear. This may take up to 6 weeks, depending on the product used. In the treatment of simple goiter, complete response may not occur for several months. Full therapeutic doses are not begun initially; this could impose a severe strain on the cardiovascular system because of cardiac stimulation.

Therapeutic equivalents include 60 to 65 mg of thyroid USP; 65 mg of thyroglobulin; or 0.1 mg of levothyroxine. Dosage is presented in Table 46–1.

○ **Levothyroxine** (Levothroid, Synthroid, and many others), a synthetic form of T_4, available in parenteral and oral forms and is used to treat primary hypothyroidism and congenital hypothyroidism in infants and children. Some products contain tartrazine yellow dye, which can cause bronchial asthma and other allergic reactions in susceptible persons.

○ **Liothyronine** (Cytomel, Triostat), a synthetic form of T_3, is used to treat hypothyroidism and in the T_3 suppression test to differentiate hyperthyroidism from euthryoidism (normal thyroid function status) in patients with borderline to high values in the ^{131}I thyroid uptake test.

○ **Thyroid desiccated USP** (Thyroid) is used to treat hypothyroidism and to suppress excessive thyrotropin hormone in patients with simple goiter or chronic lymphocytic thyroiditis. It is a natural product derived from domesticated animals such as pigs, sheep, and cattle, with the active hormones available in their natural state and ratio.

○ **Thyroglobulin** (Proloid), obtained from hog thyroid glands, is used primarily for replacement in hypothyroidism. It has no clinical advantage over thyroid USP. It contains T_4 and T_3 in an approximate ratio of 2.5:1.

THYROID HORMONE ANTAGONISTS

The thyroid hormone antagonists—**propylthiouracil (PTU)**, **methimazole (Tapazole)**, and **sodium iodide (I-131)**—inhibit the synthesis of thyroid hormones. Table 46–3 features these agents. Propylthiouracil also partially inhibits the peripheral conversion of T_3 to T_4.

Table 46–3. THYROID HORMONE ANTAGONISTS

DRUG NAME/ROUTE AND DOSAGE	PHARMACOKINETICS/ DYNAMICS	NURSING IMPLICATIONS
prophlthiouracil (PTU)		
Adults: Initial dose–300–450 mg/day PO divided q 8 hr. Maintenance dose–100–150 mg/day **Pediatric:** Initial dose–6–10 yr, 50–150 mg/day PO; ≥10 yr, 150–300 mg/day PO	Onset: 10–21 days Peak: 6–10 wk Duration: weeks ½L: 1–2 hr PB: 75%–80% B: liver E: urine	For all thyroid hormone antagonists: ASSESSMENT: Assess baseline vital signs and weight. Assess for pregnancy (category D) or contraindications. INTERVENTION: Patient Teaching—Advise patient to carry card indentifying condition and drug therapy. Tell patient to take medication at regularly spaced intervals (e.g., q 8 hr) and to take medication with food to minimize gastric distress. Tell patient to protect drug from light and to store it in dry, tightly closed container. EVALUATION: Notify physician if fever, sore throat, unusual bleeding or bruising occur.
methimazole (Tapazole)		
Adults: Initial dose–15–60 mg PO in 3 equal doses Maintenance dose–5–15 mg/day in divided doses **Pediatric:** Initial dose–0.4 mg/kg per day PO in divided doses Maintenance dose–half initial dose	Onset: 1 week Peak: 4–10 wk Duration: weeks ½L: 5–13 hr PB: 0% B: liver E: urine, 10% unchanged	Same as for all.
strong iodine solution (Lugol's solution)		
Adults: 2–6 drops PO tid for 10 days prior to surgery	Onset: 24–48 hr Peak: 10–15 days Duration: 6 wk ½L: NA PB: highly B: NA E: NA	INTERVENTION: Patient Teaching—Caution patient to avoid use of OTC cough and cold remedies containing iodides and to limit intake of iodine-rich dietary products. Tell patient to dilute liquids in milk or fruit juice and to take medication after meals. EVALUATION: Notify physician of fever, rash, metallic taste, swelling of throat, sore gums and teeth, and severe GI distress.

NA = not available; OTC = over the counter.

USES

The thyroid hormone antagonists are used to treat hyperthyroidism. They are also used, along with certain iodides, to bring the patient to an *euthyroid* (normal thyroid function) state before thyroid surgery and in conjunction with radioactive iodine therapy to hasten recovery and to control the signs and symptoms of hyperthyroidism until the radioactive iodine therapy becomes effective.

CONTRAINDICATIONS AND PRECAUTIONS

All drugs are contraindicated in persons hypersensitive to them. Use of antithyroid drugs is generally contraindicated during pregnancy (category D), as they cross the placental barrier and can cause hypothyroidism in the fetus. All are excreted partly in breast milk, and mothers on this therapy should bottle-feed their infants. These drugs are given cautiously in persons with hematologic diseases such as agranulocytosis, leukopenia, and thrombocytopenia, as these conditions may be worsened. It is important to monitor the complete blood count (CBC) for at least the first 3 months of therapy.

ADVERSE EFFECTS

Adverse effects of propylthiouracil and methimazole, similar for both drugs, are relatively rare and include arthralgias, nausea and vomiting, headache, abnormal hair loss, hyper pigmentation, and paresthesias. Severe skin rashes may necessitate switching to another antithyroid drug; milder rashes may be treated symptomatically with antihistamines.

▼ CLINICAL ALERT

The most serious adverse effects occurs in about 1 in 500 patients. Agranulocytosis may develop during the first few months of therapy. It is vital, therefore, that the patient understand the importance of reporting the onset of a fever or any sign of infection, especially a sore throat, immediately. If laboratory tests confirm the presence of agranulocytosis or granulocytopenia, the drug is discontinued and recovery usually occurs. Thrombocytopenia and hypoprothrombinemia, with subsequent bleeding, can also occur with antithyroid therapy. The nurse teaches the importance of regular observation for petechiae, ecchymosis, or other unexplained bleeding. Prothrombin time or International neutral ratio (INR) may be monitored regularly, along with cell counts. Patients are also directed to avoid the excessive use of aspirin or aspirin-containing compounds. The use of anticoagulants or drugs that might suppress cell counts is undertaken only with close medical supervision.

With continued antithyroid therapy, clinical manifestations of goitrogenic hypothyroidism may appear. To prevent this, thyroid hormone may be added to the treatment regimen once the patient has reached an euthyroid state. Because hypothyroidism may occur very insidiously, the nurse alerts the patient to watch for such signs and symptoms as intolerance to cold, increased weight gain, goiter, and decreased cardiac rate.

INTERACTIONS

The concomitant use of thyroid hormone antagonist with heparin or oral anticoagulants may enhance the anticoagulant effects.

Dosages of all medications are found in Table 46–3.

OTHER DRUGS TO TREAT HYPERTHYROIDISM

○ **Propranolol** (Inderal) is commonly used in the treatment of thyroid storm or crisis to minimize manifestations of catecholamine activity by decreasing heart rate and metabolic activity (Chapter 17). Thyroid crisis can be fatal because of excessive cardiac stimulation. In these instances, intravenous propranolol can protect the heart from stimulation. Propranolol administered before and after radioactive iodine controls the symptomatology associated with this cardiac stimulation. Propranolol must be used cautiously in the patient with hyperthyroidism who exhibits indications of systolic heart failure.

DRUGS FOR PARATHYROID DYSFUNCTION

The parathyroid glands secrete parathyroid hormone (PTH), also known as parathormone, a principal regulator of calcium and phosphate metabolism. Parathormone af-

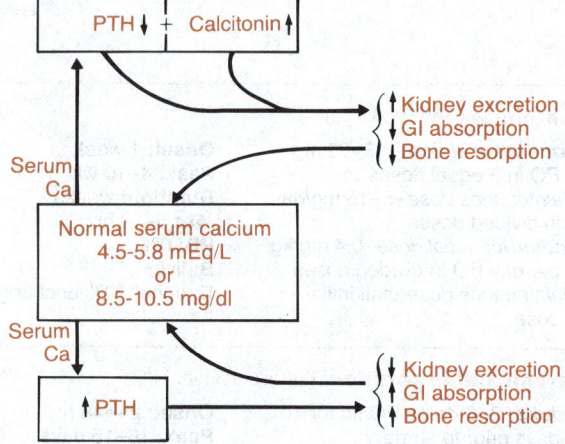

Figure 46–1. Regulation of serum calcium. Normal serum calcium is regulated by PTH and calcitonin. As serum calcium rises, PTH is inhibited by calcitonin. In turn, the kidney excretes more calcium, the GI system absorbs less, and there is a reduction in bone resorption. As serum calcium falls, PTH is secreted, and in turn, raises the calcium level by decreasing the amount of calcium lost in the kidney, increasing the amount absorbed in the GI tract and increasing bone resorption.

fects bone, causing bone resorption of calcium; the kidney, increasing the excretion of phosphate and decreasing the excretion of calcium and magnesium; and the GI tract, promoting calcium absorption. Vitamin D, an essential cofactor for PTH, also affects calcium absorption, as it facilitates the transfer of calcium from the intestinal lumen into the cells. In effect, PTH serves to increase serum calcium concentration and to decrease serum phosphate concentration, as shown in Figure 46–1. Disruptions in calcium and phospate regulation from parathyroid dysfunction can result in hypocalcemia or hypercalcemia.

ANTIHYPOCALCEMIC AGENTS

Hypocalcemia results from numerous causes, including parathyroid hypofunction, vitamin D deficiency, pancreatitis, renal failure, massive blood transfusion, alcoholism, chemotherapy, chronic liver disease, and osteoporosis. Regardless of the cause, however, treatment is necessary to prevent complications such as convulsions, tetany, laryngospasm, respiratory spasms, and other muscle spasms. The initial treatment of severe symptomatic hypocalcemia is intravenous infusion of a rapidly available calcium product, such as calcium gluconate. This is followed by oral calcium salts (calcium gluconate, 9%; calcium carbonate, 40%). Vitamin D may also be administered. More information on calcium imbalance is found in Chapter 12.

ANTIHYPERCALCEMIC AGENTS

Antihypercalcemic drugs lower serum calcium levels in patients with a variety of conditions, such as hyperparathyroidism, malignancies, vitamin D intoxication, and milk-alkali syndrome, that lead to hypercalcemia. Several drugs are available to lower serum calcium levels. Plicamycin (Mithracin), an antineoplastic agent, lowers serum calcium levels in patients who have hypercalcemia associated with malignancies (see Chapter 55). Furosemide (Lasix), a diuretic, reduces the serum calcium concentration by increasing calcium excretion (see Chapter 37). Furosemide is often administered with large amounts of 0.9% sodium chloride infusion. **Calcitonin (Calcimar, Cibacalcin),** discussed briefly here, and etidronate disodium, discussed in Chapter 12, are also used.

○ **Calcitonin-salmon** (Calcimar) or calcitonin-human (Cibacalcin) is obtained from salmon, derived from pigs, or manufactured synthetically. Salmon calcitonin lasts longer and is more potent than calcitonin derived from pigs. It also prevents bone resorption of calcium. Human calcitonin, a synthetic hormone, is also available and may be used when patients have developed resistance to salmon or pig calcitonin. Calcitonin is generally antagonistic to PTH. Calcitonin is used in patients with Paget's disease and postmenopausal osteoporosis and as an adjunct to chemotherapy and anabolic steroids to treat multiple myeloma.

Calcitonin-salmon is available as a nasal spray (Miacalcin). The usual dose is 200 IU per day. Patients should receive supplemental calcium carbonate 1.5 g/day and adequate supply of vitamin D.

USING THE NURSING PROCESS

ASSESSMENT

Thyroid Disease

Assessment of the patient with possible thyroid dysfunction can be a difficult problem because the signs and symptoms of hypothyroidism and hyperthyroidism often appear insidiously and over long periods. This is especially true in hypothyroidism. In addition, the signs and symptoms often vary in intensity from patient to patient and from time to time.

- Obtain a careful health history to establish a database, as presented in Table 46–4 and begin the nursing-care plan.
- Determine whether the patient has been treated for any thyroid disease in the past. Patients being treated for hypothyroidism may, if their medication regimen is not well controlled, exhibit indications of hyperthyroidism. Likewise, the patient who has been treated for hyperthyroidism may go on to develop hypofunction of the thyroid gland. To illustrate, after antithyroid therapy, 5% to 10% of patients develop hypothyroid conditions; after surgical intervention, 15% to 20%; and after radioactive iodine therapy, 30% to 50% of patients eventually develop hypothyroidism.
- Assess current weight and recent pattern of weight loss or gain.
- Assess level of nutrition and dietary intake as teaching may be necessary.
- Assess and obtain laboratory tests to measure thyroid function. Direct measurement of thyroid function can be done by assessing the gland's uptake of radioactive ^{131}I (RAIU test). T_3, T_4, and TSH can be measured directly by radioimmunoassay. It is important to note that many of these tests may be interfered with by the use of common drugs (see Table 46–2). The resin T_3 uptake test (RT$_3$U) measures the degree to which thyroid-binding globulin is saturated, thus indirectly indicating the level of circulating hormone.

Parathyroid Disease

Assessment of the patient with hypoparathyroidism or hyperparathyroidism depends on the nurse's ability to assess the effects of either increased or decreased serum calcium levels on the body systems. As with many other endocrine disorders, signs and symptoms of parathyroid dysfunction can be variable from patient to patient; chronicity of the disorders may also determine the degree of symptomatology. Table 46–5 summarizes the nursing process for patients requiring antihypercalcemic or antihypocalcemic drugs.

- Obtain a thorough health history. Identify some factors that relate to the cause and course of parathyroid dysfunction. A history of previous neck surgery (for example, thyroidectomy) is noted, as inadvertent removal of the parathyroids is a cause of parathyroid insufficiency.

Table 46–4. NURSING PROCESS FOR PATIENT REQUIRING THYROID/ANTITHYROID DRUGS

Assessment

Assess onset and duration of symptoms/illness, recent stress situations (emotional/physical).
Assess family history of thyroid problems.
Assess history for hypothyroidism, recent partial thyroidectomy, use of thyroid/antithyroid drugs, premature withdrawal of antithyroid drugs.
Assess recent weight loss and amount.

Nursing Diagnosis: Decreased Cardiac Output

RELATED TO: Decreased venous return, vasodilation, and tachycardia.

Desired Outcomes/Evaluation Criteria

Maintains adequate cardiac output for tissue needs as evidenced by stable vital signs, palpable peripheral pulses, good capillary refill, usual mentation, and absence of arrhythmias.

Nursing Actions	Rationale
Monitor vital signs, obtain blood pressure lying/sitting and standing, if able.	General/orthostatic hypotension may occur as a result of excessive peripheral vasodilation and decreased circulating volume. Pulse is typically elevated, and even at rest, tachycardia may be noted.
Investigate complaints of chest pain/angina.	May reflect increased myocardial oxygen demands/ischemia.
Monitor temperature, provide cool environment, limit bed linens/clothes, administer tepid sponge baths.	Fever may occur as a result of excessive thyroid levels and can aggravate diuresis and dehydration and cause increased peripheral vasodilation, venous pooling, and hypotension.
Record intake/output. Note urine specific gravity. Weigh daily.	Significant fluid losses can lead to profound dehydration, concentrated urine, and weight loss.
Observe signs/symptoms of severe thirst, dry mucous membranes, weak/thready pulse, poor capillary refill, decreased urine output, and hypotension.	Rapid dehydration can occur, which reduces circulating volume and compromises cardiac output.
Administer thyroid hormone, sodium iodine IV or supersaturated potassium iodide (SSKI) by mouth, beta-blockers (Inderal, Tenormin).	Blocks thyroid hormone synthesis and inhibits peripheral conversion of T_4 to T_3. Temporarily acts to prevent release of thyroid hormone into circulation by increasing the amount of thyroid hormone stored within the gland. Given to control thyrotoxic effects of tachycardia, tremors, and nervousness and is first drug of choice for acute storm.
Monitor patient response to administration of thyroid, Proloid, Synthroid, and so on.	Initial treatment of a hypothyroid state can cause tachycardia, increasing cardiac workload with possibility of resultant cardiac decompensation.

Nursing Diagnosis: Fatigue

RELATED TO: Hypermetabolic state with increased energy requirements; irritability of CNS; altered body chemistry.
AS EVIDENCED BY: Verbalization of overwhelming lack of energy to maintain usual routine, decreased performance, emotional lability/irritability; nervousness, impaired ability to concentrate.

Desired Outcomes/Evaluation Criteria

Verbalizes increase in level of energy. Displays improved ability to participate in desired activities.

Nursing Actions	Rationale
Provide quiet environment: cool room, decreased sensory stimuli, quiet music.	Reduces stimuli that potentiate hyperactivity insomnia, promotes rest.
Encourage patient to restrict activity and rest in bed as much as possible.	Helps to counteract effects of increased metabolism.
Assist with self-care activities.	Conserves energy, prevents undue fatigue.
Provide routine comfort measures (e.g., judicious touch/massage, cool showers) and diversional activities that are calming.	May decrease nervous energy, promoting relaxation. Allows for use of nervous energy in constructive manner and may reduce anxiety.
Discuss with significant other (SO) reasons for fatigue and emotional lability.	Understanding that behavior is physically based may enhance coping with current situation and encourage SO to respond more positively and provide support for patient.

Other Suggested Nursing Diagnoses: Altered Nutrition, Less than Body Requirements; and Knowledge Deficit.

• Obtain diagnostic tests such as serum calcium, inorganic phosphorus levels and urinary calcium excretion. Radiologic examinations of the skeletal system give an indication of bone status in the face of excessive parathyroid activity, with osteoporosis, pathologic fractures, and skeletal deformities appearing in severe cases. PTH can be measured directly by radioimmunoassay.

• Assess for symptoms of hypocalcemia such as nervousness and irritability, muscle cramps, paresthesias,

Table 46–5. NURSING PROCESS FOR PATIENT REQUIRING ANTIHYPERCALCEMIC/ANTIHYPOCALCEMIC DRUGS

Assessment

Assess previous history of neck surgery (e.g., thyroidectomy), alcohol abuse (pancreatitis, chronic liver disease), renal failure, osteoporosis, chemotherapy, massive blood transfusions.
Assess laboratory studies, e.g., serum calcium and inorganic phosphorus levels and assessment of urinary calcium excretion.
Assess nutritional history.
Assess skeletal system for indication of bone status (osteoporosis, pathologic fractures, and skeletal deformities).

Nursing Diagnosis: Risk for Injury

RELATED TO: Increased nervous and muscular excitability/tetany (hypoparathyroidism).

Desired Outcomes/Evaluation Criteria

Verbalizes understanding of individual factors that contribute to possibility of tetany/convulsions. Reports absence of muscle spasms/tetany.

Nursing Actions	**Rationale**
Administer medications to gain optimal effect, e.g., IV, IM, or orally.	Severity of symptoms dictates choice of route to provide adequate availability of drug.
Give calcium salts slowly when using IV method.	This drug is highly irritating to veins, may cause thrombosis; too rapid administration can cause cardiac arrest.
Give Rocaltrol, Ergocalciferol, or Drisdol.	Vitamin D products increase absorption of calcium.
Encourage use of antacids as appropriate.	Aluminum hydroxide gel binds phosphate and decreases intestinal absorption.
Observe for complaints of renal colic.	May have stone formation if too much calcium accumulates.
Identify signs/symptoms that must be reported to health-care provider, e.g., anorexia, nausea and vomiting, diarrhea, polyuria, polydipsia, headache, muscle cramps/spasms.	Indicators of hypercalcemia, which requires alteration/discontinuation of therapy.
Monitor laboratory results of serum/urine calcium, inorganic phosphorus, PTH levels.	Evaluates therapeutic needs/effectiveness.

Nursing Diagnosis: Deficit Fluid Volume

RELATED TO: Excessive losses from vomiting, diarrhea, and polyuria (hyperparathyroidism).

Desired Outcomes/Evaluation Criteria

Maintains fluid balance and is free of signs of dehydration.

Nursing Actions	**Rationale**
Promote oral intake.	Route of choice for fluid replacement if possible.
Measure intake/output. Observe mucous membranes, skin turgor, and capillary refill.	Reflects effectiveness of therapy/therapeutic needs.
Administer glucose, isotonic IV fluids, electrolytes. Give inorganic phosphate.	Replacement necessary to provide adequate hydration, promote calciuria. Reduces calcium levels when hypercalcemia is life threatening.
Monitor blood pressure, note complaints of dizziness with changes in position.	Administration of phosphate may potentiate hypotension if present.
Review serial serum calcium levels.	Decreasing level indicates dehydration is being corrected/renal clearance of calcium is progressing.

Other Suggested Nursing Diagnoses: Urinary Retention and Knowledge Deficit

---

and tetany as evidenced by *carpopedal spasms* (involuntary contraction of the muscles of the wrists and ankles as seen in tetany).

• Observe for latent tetany by inducing *Chvostek's sign* (a sign of tetany characterized by facial muscle spasm in response to tapping those muscles) and *Trousseau's sign* (a sign of tetany characterized by facial muscle spasm in response to pressure applied to that muscle).

NURSING DIAGNOSIS

• Typical nursing diagnoses for the patient requiring thyroid or parathyroid drugs include Knowledge Deficit, Risk for Injury, Altered Nutrition, and Fatigue (see Tables 46–4 and 46–5).

PLANNING AND INTERVENTION

• Determine the goals for the nursing interventions from the nursing diagnoses. Typical goals when caring for patients requiring thyroid or parathyroid medications are included in Tables 46–4 and 46–5.

Nursing Responsibilities

• Understand specific information related to administration guidelines, patient safety, and patient teaching. These are summarized in Tables 46–1 and 46–3 in the Nursing Implications column.
• Focus on educating the patient about the disease process, the medications being taken, and the potential occurrence of adverse effects.

Table 46–6. PATIENT TEACHING INFORMATION—THYROID DRUGS

Dear Patient:

This drug has been ordered for you. This is what you should know about your drug to get the most from it:

☐ 1. Thyroid drugs replace the hormones in your body and bring your blood levels back to normal.
☐ 2. Thyroid drugs are generally taken for the rest of your life. Most are slow acting and full effect may not be felt for a few weeks.
☐ 3. Take your thyroid drugs exactly as ordered.
☐ 4. Check your pulse; if it is greater than 100 beats per minute, don't take your drug for that day.
☐ 5. Take your thyroid drug in the morning on an empty stomach.
☐ 6. Do not use more than 2 aspirin per day while taking thyroid drugs.
☐ 7. If you forget a day's dose, do not try to make it up.
☐ 8. Do not stop your thyroid drug without first asking your doctor.
☐ 9. Notify your doctor if you have any adverse effects. Some common side effects are skin rash, headache, chest pain, increased nervousness, or increased pulse rate.
☐ 10. Carry a medication card or other similar identification.
☐ 11. Store your thyroid drug in a light-resistant, dry, tightly closed container.

A concept mentioned earlier in this chapter deserves reemphasis. In treatment of hypothyroidism, replacement hormones are introduced gradually because of the increase in the overall metabolism they cause. Once a maintenance dose is established, patients are taught that they will need thyroid replacement forever. Although missing medication for one or two days may not lead to the re-

Table 46–7. PATIENT TEACHING INFORMATION—ANTITHYROID DRUGS

Dear Patient:

This drug has been ordered for you. This is what you should know about your drug to get the most from it:

☐ 1. Antithyroid drugs, such as _____, are ordered to reduce the level of thyroid hormone in your body.
☐ 2. Antithyroid drugs are taken for different lengths of time; your doctor will tell you how long you will need to take this drug.
☐ 3. Take your drugs exactly as ordered.
☐ 4. Antithyroid drugs should be taken with food. *Exceptions:* Liquid iodides are diluted in milk or fruit juice and taken after meals.
☐ 5. Avoid the use of over-the-counter cough and cold remedies that contain iodides. Ask your pharmacist if you have any questions about which over-the-counter drugs you may take.
☐ 6. Limit your intake of iodine-rich foods, such as iodized salt and seafood.
☐ 7. Do not stop taking your antithyroid drug without consulting with your doctor.
☐ 8. Report any adverse effects to your doctor. Some adverse effects are skin rash, unexplained bleeding, sore throat, and fever. If you are taking iodides, adverse effects may include runny nose, headache, increased salivation, and a brassy taste in your mouth.
☐ 9. Carry a medication card or other similar identification.
☐ 10. Store your drugs in a light-resistant, tightly closed container.

Table 46–8. PATIENT TEACHING INFORMATION—ANTIHYPOCALCEMIC DRUGS

Dear Patient:

This drug has been ordered for you. This is what you should know about your drug to get the most from it:

☐ 1. Antihypocalcemic drugs, such as _____, are ordered to elevate your serum calcium level.
☐ 2. Antihypocalcemic drugs are taken for an indefinite amount of time; your doctor will tell you how long you will need to take this drug.
☐ 3. Take your drugs daily, exactly as directed.
☐ 4. Take your drugs 1 to 1.5 hours after meals; you may take them with milk.
☐ 5. Avoid use of mineral oil as a laxative, because it decreases vitamin D absorption. Vitamin D is needed to work with your drug.
☐ 6. Avoid eating too much spinach, rhubarb, bran, or whole-grain cereals, because they decrease calcium absorption.
☐ 7. Eat more foods that have calcium in them. Good dietary sources of calcium are milk products, dark green leafy vegetables, clams, oysters, sardines, and orange juice with calcium.
☐ 8. Do not stop your drug without first consulting your doctor.
☐ 9. Report adverse effects to your doctor. Some of these effects are loss of appetite, constipation, nausea, vomiting, increased urination, thirst, and flank pain.
☐ 10. Carry a medication card or other similar identification.
☐ 11. Store your drugs in a light-resistant, tightly closed container.

currence of symptoms, discontinuance of the drug certainly will.

Patient Teaching

• Teach patients about their drugs (Tables 46–6, 46–7, 46–8, and 46–9).

Table 46–9. PATIENT TEACHING INFORMATION—ANTIHYPERCALCEMIC DRUGS

Dear Patient:

This drug has been ordered for you. This is what you should know about your drug to get the most from it:

☐ 1. Antihypercalcemic drugs, such as _____, are ordered to reduce your blood level of calcium.
☐ 2. Antihypercalcemic drugs are taken for varying lengths of time; your doctor will tell you how long you will need to take this drug.
☐ 3. Calcitonin is taken in subcutaneous injections (shots).
    a. Be sure to rotate injection sites to minimize inflammation.
    b. Do not inject more than 0.5 mL of solution; check label for mixing instructions.
☐ 4. Take your etidronate disodium (Didronel) on an empty stomach (approximately 2 hours before meals). Take with a full glass of water to reduce stomach upset.
☐ 5. If your doctor wants you to eat less food that contains calcium, you should not eat as many leafy green vegetables and dairy products.
☐ 6. Do not stop taking your drugs without asking your doctor.
☐ 7. Report signs of low calcium levels to your doctor. These signs include headache, numbness or tingling, nausea or vomiting, diarrhea or constipation, and abdominal pain.
☐ 8. Carry a medication card or other similar identification.
☐ 9. Refrigerate reconstituted calcitonin.

- Teach the importance of carrying a Medic Alert card or other similar identification.
- Teach patients not to change from one brand of this drug to another without consulting their pharmacist or physician. Products from different manufacturers may not be equally effective.

EVALUATION

- Determine the effectiveness of the nursing interventions. Generally, evaluation criteria are included in Tables 46–4 and 46–5.
- Ensure that the patient fully understands the potential for adverse effects of the medications.

- Ensure that patients follow their therapy program. Because treatment for thyroid and parathyroid disorders can cause the opposite disorder to occur, the nurse ensures that patients are familiar with symptoms of both hypofunction and hyperfunction of these organs.
- Continuously stress the need for regular medical follow-up and periodically review all previous teaching with the patient, adding or revising information to keep the patient's knowledge current and accurate.

The bibliography for this chapter can be found in Appendix B, which begins on page 1054.

CHAPTER REVIEW QUESTIONS *

1. A function of the thyroid hormones (T_3 and T_4) is to:
   a. Decelerate chemical reactions.
   b. Increase oxygen consumption.
   c. Impede heat production.
   d. Act as enzymes.

2. Iodides are used as antithyroid drugs for:
   a. Increasing the vascularity of the thyroid gland.
   b. Decreasing the quantity of bound thyroid.
   c. Inhibiting the release of T_3 and T_4 into circulation.
   d. Binding the TSH for thyroid inhibition.

3. An action of the antithyroid medication propylthiouracil (PTU) is to:
   a. Block TSH production.
   b. Reduce serum calcitonin levels.
   c. Inhibit peripheral conversion of T_3 and T_4.
   d. Block release of TRH.

4. Vitamin D derivatives elevate serum calcium by:
   a. Stimulating the kidney to reduce excretion.
   b. Inducing parathyroid hormone production.
   c. Stimulating calcium absorption in the intestine.
   d. Inducing the production of calcitonin by the thyroid.

5. Thyroid hormones are contraindicated for individuals with:
   a. Adrenal insufficiency.
   b. Lithium therapy.
   c. Lymphocytic thyroiditis.
   d. Metastatic cancer.

6. The following is correct regarding thyroid drugs:
   a. Thyroglobulin (Proloid) is obtained from beef sources.
   b. Thyroid USP (Thyroid) may be given intravenously for myxedema.
   c. Thyroid hormones may be used to treat simple goiter.
   d. Liothyronine (Cytomel) is obtained from pork sources.

*See Appendix A, which begins on page 1051, for answers.

DRUGS AFFECTING SEXUALITY AND THE REPRODUCTIVE SYSTEM

UNIT OUTLINE

CHAPTER 47

Male Hormones and Female Hormones

Merrily A. Kuhn, RNC, PhD

CHAPTER OUTLINE

KEY TERMS

Azoospermia
Cryptorchidism
Endometriosis
Eunuchism
Hypogonadism

Priapism
Proptosis
Spermatogenesis
Thermogenic

LEARNING OBJECTIVES

After reading this chapter, the student will be able to:

1. Identify those medications commonly used as male and female hormones and those used to treat disorders of the reproductive systems.
2. Differentiate among the male and female hormones as to mechanisms of action, route of administration, pharmacokinetics, adverse effects, contraindications and precautions, and interactions.
3. Identify specific areas to assess in the patient requiring male or female hormones to formulate appropriate patient outcomes.
4. Plan the nursing intervention necessary to administer male and female hormones and choose appropriate teaching strategies to gain patient compliance.
5. Evaluate the patient at various stages to determine the effectiveness of nursing interventions.

Both male and female hormones are discussed. Male hormones, both as androgenic and anabolic therapies; and female hormones as related to their variety of uses, including that of contraception are reviewed. This chapter also reviews other medications that in some manner affect the female reproductive system such as those drugs used to treat infertility, premenstrual syndrome, and menopause.

MALE HORMONES

ANDROGENS

Testosterone, the principal androgen and male sex hormone, is synthesized in the greatest amounts in the male testes by the interstitial cells of Leydig in response to stimulation by the gonadotropic hormones (interstitial cell–stimulating hormone) of the adenohypophysis. A negative feedback system involving the hypothalamus, the anterior pituitary, and the testes controls hormone secretion. Cholesterol is the common precursor for the biosynthesis of the androgens.

The androgenic steroids available today include short-acting testosterone—**testosterone in aqueous suspension (Testosdro)** and long-acting testosterone—**testosterone propionate (Testex), testosterone enanthate (Andro L. A. 200), testosterone cyprionate (Depotest, Duratest), testosterone transdermal system (Testoderm), methyltestosterone (Android, Oreton Methyl, Metandren),** and **fluoxymesterone (Halotestin).**

Action

In most body tissues, with the exception of skeletal muscle and bone marrow, testosterone is converted to dihydrotestosterone (DHT), the active form of the hormone. At the cellular level, DHT binds to cytoplasmic protein receptors and increases protein synthesis.

In the male fetus, testosterone is necessary for the differentiation, growth, and development of the male sexual organs. During puberty, testosterone is necessary for the development of the primary sex characteristics of the male, causing increased growth of the penis, scrotum, and testes. The male secondary sex characteristics are also influenced by the action of testosterone: male pattern of hair growth, enlargement of the larynx leading to a deepening of the voice, increased thickness of the skin, and increased activity of the sebaceous glands.

In women, androgens are responsible for the growth of pubic hair and for stimulation of libido. They also act as estrogen precursors, particularly after menopause. Excessive production of androgens leads to masculinizing effects such as acne, hirsutism, hoarseness, menstrual irregularities, permanent deepening of the voice, and clitoral enlargement.

Testosterone also has anabolic activity. By increasing the rate of amino acid transfer into the cells, a positive nitrogen balance is achieved, an increase in musculature occurs, and an increase in bone thickness and calcium deposition leads to greater length and size of the bones. In the presence of testosterone, basal metabolic rate and red blood cell production are both increased. Finally, testosterone has some salt- and water-retaining properties, causing men to have a greater blood and extracellular fluid volume than women. Large doses of androgens may suppress *spermatogenesis* (formation of mature functional spermatozoa) through feedback inhibition of pituitary follicle-stimulating hormone.

Uses

Testosterone and similar compounds are administered for their androgenic properties or for their anabolic properties. Although several anabolic steroids with minimal androgenic properties have been developed, it is important to remember that all of these drugs have both effects to some extent. Androgens may be used to replace androgen deficiencies in states of *hypogonadism* or decreased testosterone production.

The longer-acting esters of testosterone, testosterone cypionate (Depo-Testosterone), and testosterone enanthate (Delatestryl) are usually preferred for therapy; they must be administered intramuscularly, on a regular basis, until the sexual characteristics have developed. Following this, one of the shorter-acting oral preparations, such as fluoxymesterone (Halotestin) or methyltestosterone (Metandren), can be substituted. The postpubertal male may be treated with the oral androgen preparations or a testosterone skin patch (worn for 22 to 24 hr/day) as replacement therapy. In the adult male, replacement of testosterone should supply approximately 10 mg/day. All products must be administered on a lifelong basis, with dosages adjusted to the individual.

Administration of exogenous testosterone to boys with undescended testes (*cryptorchidism*) may prompt descent of these organs into the scrotum. Human chorionic gonadotropin, a natural polypeptide hormone produced by the human placenta, can also be used for this purpose.

Several disorders in the female are often treated by androgen administration. In *endometriosis*, a condition in which ectopic endometrial tissue implants occur, androgens antagonize the effects of estrogen and cause suppression of gonadotropin secretion. Endometriosis can be treated with a synthetic androgen, danazol (Danocrine). Danazol has mild androgenic properties and causes pituitary suppression of follicle-stimulating hormone (FSH) and luteinizing hormone (LH), leading to an ovulation, amenorrhea, and involution of endometrial implants. However, danazol is very expensive to use. For most patients, the use of progestins or combined oral contraceptives is just as effective, with the added advantage of having no androgenic effects. Danazol is also used to partially or completely relieve the breast pain, tenderness, and nodularity in women with fibrocystic breasts.

Androgens may also be used in the palliative therapy of metastatic breast malignancies in postmenopausal women. Testolactone (Teslac) has little androgenic activity in therapeutic doses and has been found to be effective in the treatment of some patients with estrogen-responsive tumors. However, masculinizing side effects occur frequently at the dosages needed to interfere with tumor growth. In the treatment of breast cancer, many clinicians prefer to use the shorter-acting oral preparations rather than the sustained-acting parenteral preparations. In this way, should adverse effects occur, the drug can be withdrawn quickly. Tamoxifen (Nolvadex), an estrogen antagonist that causes no distressing masculinizing effects, is an alternative to androgen therapy.

Anabolic steroids also are used in the treatment of mild to moderate aplastic and hemolytic anemias, as well as those anemias associated with chronic renal failure, lymphoma, and leukemia. It is believed that androgens stimulate the production of erythropoietin by the kidney, leading to an increase in red blood cell production.

Pharmacokinetics

Synthetic forms of the hormone vary somewhat in their potencies, durations of action, and absorption following oral administration.

Contraindications and Precautions

Conditions in which androgen use is contraindicated include pregnancy and lactation, because the use of androgens may lead to precocious puberty in males and masculinization in females; carcinoma of the prostate or male breast, which may be stimulated by androgens; hepatic disease, which may be exacerbated (see Adverse Effects); prostatic hypertrophy, which is increased; and coronary artery disease, because of the retention of fluids and alteration of cholesterol levels.

Androgens are given cautiously to patients who have experienced allergic reactions during previous androgen therapy and to elderly males because their risk of developing prostatic hypertrophy and prostatic carcinoma is increased.

Adverse Effects

The occurrence of adverse effects is related to dosage and length of administration. Given at replacement doses to men with hypogonadism, adverse effects are usually minimal.

In both sexes nausea, vomiting, gastric irritation, and diarrhea may occur with the administration of oral preparations. The use of buccal tablets may irritate the oral mucosa, and stomatitis can occur. Local inflammation and induration can follow administration of intramuscular preparations. Inflammation at the site of pellet implantation can also occur, in severe cases causing skin sloughing and subsequent loss of the pellets.

In both sexes sleeplessness and excitation may occur, as may changes in libido. Psychotic symptoms, including hallucinations, delusions, and manic episodes, have been reported when large doses are used.

Sodium and water retention may occur, leading to edema, especially in the elderly patient or in the patient with cardiovascular disease. This occurs most often with larger doses of androgens and can usually be controlled with dietary salt restriction or diuretic therapy.

Allergic reactions to testosterone or its salts are rather rare, but may range from urticaria to frank anaphylaxis. For this reason, it is important to ascertain in the medical history whether the patient has ever experienced an allergic reaction to previous androgen therapy. Some of these products contain tartrazine, which may cause allergic-type reactions in susceptible person.

In both sexes, hepatic dysfunction can occur during androgen therapy. Cholestatic hepatitis has been noted and tends to occur in greater frequency with larger doses. Patients need to understand the importance of reporting such signs and symptoms as darkened urine, pruritus, and color changes in the skin and sclera. Liver tests (bilirubin, lactic dehydrogenase [LDH], serum glutamic-oxaloacetic transaminase [SGOT], alkaline phosphatase) are monitored regularly, and increases in these levels may warrant termination of therapy. Hepatic carcinoma has developed in some patients on prolonged (1 to 7 years) therapy.

Androgen therapy may alter serum cholesterol levels; therefore, patients with coronary artery disease are monitored carefully, and cholesterol levels are determined periodically during therapy. Androgen therapy may alter the results of diagnostic tests. Creatinine levels may increase as well as T_3 uptake. Excretion of 17-ketosteroids and the production of clotting factors II, V, VII, and X may be decreased.

In boys being treated with androgens, determinations of bone maturation are vital to prevent early epiphyseal closure prompted by androgens. In addition, signs and symptoms of precocious puberty may occur, including phallic enlargement and growth of facial and body hair. *Priapism* (persistent abnormal erection of the penis) may occur in the initial stages of therapy, but usually subsides with continued treatment.

Adult males being treated with androgens may de-velop breast tenderness and, occasionally, gynecomastia. Impotence and *azoospermia* (absence of spermatozoa in the semen) may also develop, as prolonged androgen therapy tends to inhibit gonadotropin secretion.

Women requiring androgen therapy, especially those receiving it for disseminated breast cancer, tend to develop virilizing effects: hoarseness, or deepening of the voice, and changes in libido. Growth of facial hair, acne, baldness, decreased breast size, and menstrual irregularities can occur. Unfortunately, some of the masculinizing changes may be permanent and will not reverse with the discontinuation of therapy. The benefits of androgen therapy as opposed to adverse effects must be carefully weighed.

Another adverse effect of androgen therapy that occurs most often in women with breast cancer and bone metastases is hypercalcemia. Therefore, the onset of the representative symptoms of nausea, vomiting, anorexia, constipation, polyuria, and muscle weakness are reported immediately. Generally, these symptoms necessitate termination of androgen therapy.

Interactions

Androgens can interact with other medications. Sensitivity to oral anticoagulants is increased, as are the hypoglycemic effects of insulin and the oral hypoglycemic agents. Concomitant use of androgens with adrenal corticosteroids may tend to enhance the occurrence of edema, as both have a tendency to cause water retention.

Selected androgenic and anabolic steroids are featured in Tables 47–1 and 47–2.

ANDROGENIC STEROIDS

○ **Testosterone** (Andro 100) and **testosterone propionate** (Testex) are used primarily for their androgenic effects to treat *eunuchism* (a condition characterized by the absence of testes and male hormone) and male climacteric symptoms. Testosterone is used to treat breast cancer in postmenopausal women and breast engorgement in postpartum women.

○ **Testosterone enanthate** (Delatestryl) and **testosterone cypionate** (Depo-Testosterone) are long acting and are used for the same purposes as testosterone. In addition, testosterone enanthate is used to treat oligospermia (insufficient sperm in the semen).

○ **Testosterone transdermal system** (Testoderm, Androderm) used for primary hypogonadism, is a patch that is applied to the scrotal skin. Scrotal skin is at least five times more permeable to testosterone and other androgens and steroids than any other skin site. The patch is worn for 22 to 24 hr per day and changed daily. If desired serum levels are not attained after 6 to 8 weeks, another product should be used.

○ **Methyltestosterone** (Metandren) is used for the same purposes as testosterone. In addition, methyltestosterone is also used to treat postpubertal cryptorchidism. Oral and buccal products are available.

○ **Fluoxymesterone** (Halotestin) is used primarily to treat hypogonadism and impotence caused by testicular

Table 47–1. ANDROGENIC STEROIDS AND ANABOLIC HORMONE INHIBITORS

DRUG NAME/ROUTE AND DOSAGE	PHARMACOKINETICS/ DYNAMICS	NURSING IMPLICATIONS
ANDROGENIC STEROIDS		
	Onset: rapid **Peak:** NA **PB:** 98% **B:** liver **E:** urine, as 17-ketosteroids, feces	**all androgenic steroids** **ASSESSMENT:** Obtain baseline weight and blood pressure. **INTERVENTION:** *Oral:* Take shortly before or with meals. Protect from light. Store in dry, tightly closed containers. Take with food to decrease GI upset. *IM:* Inject deeply into gluteal muscles. Rotate injection sites. Shake vials to disperse medication evenly. Store at room temperature. Warming or shaking vial redissolves crystals that may have formed. *Buccal:* Place under tongue or between gums and cheek. Change location with each dose. Do not chew or swallow. Do not eat, drink, or smoke until tablet is absorbed. *All routes:* Check weight. **EVALUATION:** Report weight gain, nausea, vomiting, priapism, or jaundice to physician.
short-acting testosterone (Andro 100)		
androgen replacement *Adults:* 25–50 mg IM 2–3 times per wk **palliation of mammary cancer** *Adults:* 50–100 mg IM 3 times per wk **delayed puberty** 25 mg IM 2–3 times per wk for 4–6 mo		
testosterone propionate (Testex)		
Adults: 25–100 mg IM 2–4 times per wk **postpartum breast engorgement** *Adults:* 25–50 mg/day IM for 3–4 days	Same as above ½L: 10–100 min	Same as for all.
long-acting testosterone enanthate (Delatestryl)		
androgen replacement *Adults:* 50–400 mg IM q 1–6 wk	Same as above **Duration:** 2–4 wk ½L: 10–100 min	Same as for all.
testosterone cypionate (Depo-Testosterone)		
palliation breast cancer in women *Adults:* 50–400 mg IM q 4–6 wk	Same as above **Duration:** 2–4 wk ½L: 8 days PB: 98% B: liver E: urine	Same as for all.
methyltestosterone		
Adults: 10–40 mg/day PO in divided doses; or 5–25 mg/day buccal administration	Same as above ½L: 2.5–3.0 hr	Same as for all.

Continued on the following page

Table 47–1. ANDROGENIC STEROIDS AND ANABOLIC HORMONE INHIBITORS, *Continued*

DRUG NAME/ROUTE AND DOSAGE	PHARMACOKINETICS/DYNAMICS	NURSING IMPLICATIONS
ANABOLIC HORMONE INHIBITORS		
finasteride (Proscar) *Adults:* 5 mg PO once daily	**Onset:** 30 min **Peak:** 1–2 hr (blood level); 8 hr (effect on 5-alpha-dihydrotestosterone); 6 mo (effect on prostatic symptoms) **Duration:** 2 wk **½L:** 6 hr **PB:** 90% **B:** liver **E:** urine (39%), feces (57%)	**ASSESSMENT:** Assess sexual function before therapy. **INTERVENTION:** A pregnant woman should not handle crushed tablet of finasteride because it may cause abnormalities in male fetus. A male receiving finasteride should not expose his female sex partner to finasteride if she is pregnant or could become pregnant. Volume of ejaculate may be reduced during therapy. Tablet may be taken with or without food. **EVALUATION:** Report impotence and decreased libido to physician.

NA = not available.

deficiency. It can also be used in women to treat postpartum breast engorgement and as a palliative treatment for breast cancer. Daily doses range from 5 to 20 mg/day.

○ **Danazol** (Danocrine) is a synthetic androgen that, like other androgens, suppresses the pituitary-ovarian axis by inhibiting the output of pituitary gonadotropins. Danazol also depresses the output of FSH and LH. Danazol is primarily used in women to treat endometriosis (400 mg twice daily for 3 to 6 months) and fibrocystic breast disease (100 to 400 mg/day). If a favorable response occurs, the dose is decreased by 50% at 1 to 3 month intervals.

ANDROGEN HORMONE INHIBITOR

○ **Finasteride** (Proscar), a synthetic compound, competitively and specifically inhibits the steroid 5-alpha-reductase, an intercellular enzyme that normally converts testosterone to the potent androgen 5-alpha DHT. The development of the prostate gland depends on levels of DHT. By inhibiting DHT production, finasteride reduces prostatic tissue, and thus the symptoms of benign prostatic hyperplasia (BPH) are reduced. It may be necessary to administer finasteride for 6 months before a satisfactory response is obtained.

Table 47–2. ANABOLIC STEROIDS

DRUG NAME/ROUTE AND DOSAGE	PHARMACOKINETICS/DYNAMICS	NURSING IMPLICATIONS
nandrolone decanoate (Deca-Durbonin and others) *Females:* 50–100 mg/wk IM.	**Onset:** NA **Peak:** 1–2 days **Duration:** NA	all anabolic steroids **ASSESSMENT:** Baseline blood glucose should be obtained in diabetic patients and checked periodically during therapy. **INTERVENTION:** Administer deep IM, gluteal muscle preferred. **Patient Teaching**—Tell patient to take with food, may cause GI upset. **EVALUATION:** Notify physician if nausea, vomiting, change in skin color, or ankle swelling occur.
oxandrolone (Oxandrin) *Adults:* 2.5–20.0 mg/day PO in divided doses; 2–4 wk of therapy is usually adequate. *Children 2–13 yr:* 0.1–0.25 mg/kg per day PO.	**Onset:** NA **Peak:** 1–2 days **Duration:** 9 hr	Same as for all.
oxymetholone (Anadrol) *Adults:* 1–5 mg/kg PO. Administer for at least 3–6 mo. Continued maintenance with aplastic anemia is usually necessary.	**Onset:** 3–6 mo **Peak:** NA **Duration:** NA	Same as for all.

NA = not available.

ANABOLIC STEROIDS

The anabolic steroids—**nandrolone decanoate *(Deca-Durabolin)*, oxandrolone *(Anavar)*, oxymetholone *(Anadrol)*, stanozolol *(Winstrol)*, and nandrolone phenpropionate *(Durabolin)*—**reverse catabolic processes and promote bodybuilding processes. These products can be used in patients who are underweight due to a recent illness, in patients with senile or illness-produced osteoporosis, in patients with certain types of anemias, and in women with metastatic breast cancer. Anabolic steroids are used in many debilitating diseases to improve appetite, foster a positive nitrogen balance, cause weight gain, and promote a feeling of well-being. These drugs may be used in patients recovering from extensive surgery, burns, trauma, or infection and in emaciated, debilitated patients. In these instances, it has been found that beneficial effects of the anabolic steroids are related to an adequate dietary intake of calories and protein by the patient. Although there are no adequate clinical trials proving efficacy, use of anabolic agents as adjunctive or supportive therapy in such conditions, particularly in terminal patients, may be helpful. Anabolic steroids are also used by athletes to improve athletic performance.

The use of anabolic steroids to improve athletic performance is "contrary to the ethical principles of athletic competition and is deplored" according to the American College of Sports Medicine. Even with conflicting reports of the actual effects and benefits of steroid use from numerous studies, many male and female athletes, bodybuilders, and others who desire a bigger, more muscled appearance for aesthetic reasons or who are employed in jobs where quick, bold action is often necessary (e.g., law enforcement, firefighting, lifeguarding, bar bouncing) feel that the use of anabolic androgenic steroids is beneficial. The increase in muscular strength and size, heightened aggressive tendencies, enhanced energy levels, and the ability to train more intensively attract many people to abuse steroids.

Steroid abusers usually use "stacking" or "pyramiding" techniques during a steroid "cycle." During a typical 12-week cycle, an individual may begin with low doses of one steroid. As the cycle progresses, additional steroids are "stacked" and doses are increased. During approximately the fifth to the seventh weeks, the use of these drugs peak. During this peak, megadoses of steroids are being used. After the seventh week, abusers gradually reverse the pyramid and stacking procedure. When the 12-week cycle is completed, abusers observe a 4- to 8-week drug-free period called a "drug holiday." Usually this drug holiday occurs just prior to a competition to avoid steroid use detection through testing. During this time it is common for the newly acquired size and weight to decrease. Thus, it is usual for abusers to lengthen a cycle and shorten the drug holiday.

Because oral anabolic androgenic steroid agents are relatively ineffective, abusers tend to take megadoses to achieve the desired effect. Many times, dosages exceed normal therapeutic levels by 100 times. Steroid abusers risk the development of many serious side effects, which are documented in the medical literature. Subjective side effects reported to some degree in nearly all of the various

studies include increased or decreased libido, headache, dizziness, muscle spasm, nausea, irritability, aggression, euphoria, edema, acne, skin rash, urethritis, increased urine output, male pattern baldness, and excessive hair growth.

▼ **CLINICAL ALERT**

Men and women who use anabolic steroids are at risk of altered liver function tests, hepatitis, liver tumors and cancer, decreased libido, and altered hair growth. Men are also prone to decreased testicular size, prostate enlargement and cancer, decreased spermatogenesis, sterility, and impotence. Women risk the following side effects: a reduction in breast size, increase in and darkening of facial and body hair, thinning of scalp hair, menstrual irregularities, deeper voice, wider shoulders, and enlarged clitoris. Retention of salt and water, increased low-density lipoprotein (LDL) and decreased high-density lipoprotein (HDL) levels, and hypertension are side effects of steroid use that are readily recognized as a precursor to the development of cardiomyopathy, myocardial infarction, and cerebral vascular accident in both men and women.

Aggressive training regimens without resting the body predispose the steroid user to injury. Recent medical literature cites cases of avascular necrosis of the femoral heads, as well as muscle, tendon, and ligament tears as a result of steroid abuse.

▼ **CLINICAL ALERT**

Because of the potential for abuse, all of the androgenic steroids have been classified as schedule III controlled substances (C III).

○ **Nandrolone decanoate** (Deca-Durabolin) is primarily used to treat refractory anemia and to build tissue.
○ **Oxandrolone** (Anavar) is used to promote weight gain after chronic infection, trauma, or other causes of weight loss; and to offset bone pain of osteoporosis.
○ **Oxymetholone** (Anadrol) is used to treat anemias caused by deficient red cells, acquired or congenital aplastic anemia, myelofibrosis, and myelotoxic drugs.
○ **Stanozolol** (Winstrol) is used to treat hereditary angioedema. Two to six milligrams per day is administered orally in divided doses. After a response, the dose is decreased every 1 to 3 months to a maintenance dose of 2 mg/day.
○ **Nandrolone phenpropionate** (Durabolin) is used primarily to control metastatic breast cancer. It is administered intramuscularly in doses of 50 to 100 mg/week.

COMBINATION ESTROGEN AND ANDROGEN PRODUCTS

Combination estrogen and androgen steroids are available in various combinations. These products are indicated for moderate to severe vasomotor symptoms associated with menopause. Several combinations are available in intramuscular forms (Depotestogen, Duratestrine, and others with 2 mg estradiol cypionate and 50 mg testosterone/mL) and oral forms (Premarin with methyltestosterone, Estratest with varying doses of estrogen and methyltestosterone).

USING THE NURSING PROCESS

ASSESSMENT

- Obtain a detailed history to develop the database (Table 47–3).

Table 47–3. NURSING PROCESS FOR PATIENT REQUIRING ANDROGENS

Assessment

Assess developmental level, noting excessive growth of long bones, high-pitched voice, poor musculature, absence of male pattern hair growth, and small external genitalia in late teens.
Assess libido (may be decreased), note problem with impotence and presence of sterility.
Assess drug history.
Assess findings of diagnostic tests of endocrine function.

Nursing Diagnosis: Sexual Dysfunction	**Desired Outcomes/Evaluation Criteria**
RELATED TO: Altered body function.	Verbalizes understanding of disease and effect on sexual functioning. Reports improvement and expresses satisfaction with sexual functioning. Develops normal pubescent growth.
AS EVIDENCED BY: Change in physical appearance, decreased libido, impotence, inability to achieve desired satisfaction, failure to develop at puberty.	

Nursing Actions	**Rationale**
Provide information about reasons for lack of growth, inability to function sexually. Discuss how drugs can be expected to correct the problem.	Understanding of condition and treatment provides opportunity for patient to make informed choices and cooperate with treatment.
Determine degree of impairment according to patient's perception.	Provides base for identification of individual interventions.
Encourage expression of feelings and concerns about lack of development, lack of ability to perform, father a child.	The teenager in need of male hormone treatment has concerns about his appearance and if he will grow up "normal." The adult male may feel embarassed about his virility and question his ability to function as a man.
Active-listen to patient concerns and assist with problem solving.	Provides opportunity for patient to be actively involved in planning and maintain a sense of control.
Note onset of conditions such as priapism, reduced ejaculatory volume, impotence.	Reduction of dosage/temporary drug holiday may reverse or control these problems when they are the result of drug side effects.

Nursing Diagnosis: Knowledge Deficit	**Desired Outcomes/Evaluation Criteria**
RELATED TO: Information misinterpretation, unfamiliarity with information resources.	Verbalizes understanding of condition/illness and treatment regimen. Correctly performs necessary procedures and explains reasons for the actions.
AS EVIDENCED BY: Questions, statement of concern, inaccurate follow-through of instructions or development of preventable complications.	

Nursing Actions	**Rationale**
Provide information about pathophysiology of condition and reasons for treatment.	Understanding will help patient to make informed decisions and cooperate with treatment regimen.
Discuss administration of drug, possible side effects.	Facilitates safety and prompt identification of undesired side effects.
Discuss and demonstrate rotation of injection sites.	Drug absorption is slow, and inflammation or abscess may occur.
Demonstrate proper placement of buccal tablets when used.	Use of four possible locations reduces chance of mucosal ulceration.
Take oral medications with food.	Minimizes GI upset.
Stress importance of regular checkup with health-care provider.	Early identification of damaging side-effects or premature epiphyseal closure provides opportunity to reassess comparison of risks versus benefits of continued medication.
Recommend daily weighing and observance for swelling, changes in fit of jewelry/clothing.	Fluid retention may occur requiring medical evaluation.
Review signs/symptoms of vomiting, lethargy, constipation, muscle weakness, increased urinary output.	Early detection and prompt intervention may prevent serious side effects, e.g., hypercalcemia and renal calculi may develop, especially in the bedfast patient.

- Assessment of the patient requiring male sex hormones for either their androgenic or their anabolic properties can be complex. The nurse should also be alert to the possibility of ergogenic, or performance-enhancing, abuse in clients. Indications of such use include the following: rapid muscle and weight gain, as much as 20% to 30% increase over a period of 4 to 8 weeks; puffiness or bloating in the upper body, particularly in the face; severe acne, especially if the onset is rapid; spotty or blotchy skin; purple or red spots on the body; unexplained darkening of the skin; persistent bad breath; unexplained aggressiveness and other behavioral changes.
- Assess endocrine function. Hypogonadism may be suspected when a male has not reached puberty at the expected age. Because variances in developmental rates are normal, it is not uncommon to wait until the patient is in his late teens to carefully assess his endocrine function.
- Obtain a sexual history. Often men come for a medical examination because of complaints of decreased libido and impotence. Patients are often confused and embarrassed about their lack of desire or their lack of arousal even though desire is present.

Important factors that affect sexual function include the individual's self-worth or self-esteem, his general health and age, his partner's ability and interest, and the environment. It is also important to take a drug history. Many drugs can affect sexuality or sexual functioning. Table 47–4 features selected drugs and their possible sexual side effects.

- Obtain diagnostic tests to determine whether the hypogonadal state is primary (due to testicular dysfunction) or secondary (due to pituitary disorders).
- Assess nutritional status, including body weights, both past and current; serum protein determinations to give a picture of nitrogen and protein balance; and a complete blood count for patients requiring anabolic steroids. The physical examination may show a patient who is underweight to varying degrees and weak, with a poor appetite and poor food intake.

NURSING DIAGNOSIS

- Develop the nursing diagnoses. Typical nursing diagnoses for a patient requiring androgen replacement include Knowledge Deficit, Sexual Dysfunction, Self-Esteem Disturbance, and Body Image Disturbance.

INTERVENTION

- Determine the patient goals (see Table 47–3).

Nursing Responsibilities when Administering Male Hormones

The safe administration of androgenic medications depends on the nurse being familiar with specific information related to drug administration, patient safety, and patient teaching. This information can be found in the Nursing Implications column in Tables 47–1 and 47–2.

- Administer all IM injections deep IM, preferably in the gluteal muscle. Give patients on self-administra-

Table 47–4. SELECTED DRUGS AFFECTING SEXUAL FUNCTION

Drug	Possible Sexual Dysfunctions							
	A	B	C	D	E	F	G	H
Methyldopa (Aldomet)	x	x	x*	x	x	x		
Omeprazole (Prilosec)	x							
Sertraline (Zoloft)		x	x		x	x		
Verapamil (Calan)		x						
Barbiturates	x	x						
Clonidine (Catapres)	x	x			x	x		
Digoxin	x	x						
Phenytoin (Dilantin)	x	x						
Estrogen	x							x
Haloperidol (Haldol)		x	x					
Propranolol (Inderal)	x	x					x	
Lithium (Eskalith)	x	x	x*		x			
Prazosin (Minipress)		x						
Phenobarbital	x							x
Fluphenazine (Prolixin)	x	x	x*					
Fluoxetine (Prozac)					x	x		x
Atenolol (Tenormin)		x					x	
Thiazide diuretics			x					
Nifedipine (Adalat)			x*					
Diazepam (Valium)	x	x	x*	x	x	x		x
Alprazolam (Xanax)	x		x		x			

This is not a complete list, but does identify some commonly administered drugs.
*Impairs orgasm in women.
A = decreased sexual drive; B = impotence; C = impaired orgasm; D = hormonal alterations; E = erection or lubrication difficulties; F = delayed or no ejaculation; G = increased sexual drive; H = priapism.

tion of androgen medications instructions that are clear and simple.

- Teach the importance of high-quality nutrition as part of their therapy. The nurse may need to request the assistance of the dietitian to assist the patient and family in planning dietary modifications. General information concerning male hormones that the nurse educator includes in the teaching plan is found in Table 47–5.

EVALUATION

- Determine the effectiveness of the nursing interventions. Typical patient outcome criteria are included in Table 47–3.
- Evaluate the patient for the occurrence of adverse effects.
- Evaluate for noncompliance. Changes in body image in both men and women may possibly lead to noncompliance with medication regimens. Patients need a great deal of support and encouragement from their families and the nurse during this therapy.
- Continually stress to the patient the need for regular medical follow-up.
- Periodically review teaching with the patient to ensure that the patient's information remains current and accurate.

FEMALE HORMONES

ESTROGENS AND PROGESTOGENS

The estrogens are formed in the ovary from androstenedione, an androgen precursor, where it is converted to testosterone, which in turn is converted to estrogen. Estrogens are also produced in much smaller amounts in the adrenals and testes and in some peripheral tissues.

Six estrogens are secreted by the ovary; however, only three are present in significant quantities: about 100 to 600 μg per day of 17-beta-estradiol (the most potent and the major product), estrone (about one-half as potent as estradiol), and estriol (the weakest estrogen). Progesterone is the naturally occurring hormone and is also produced by direct secretion from the ovary. Progesterone has a *thermogenic* effect (an effect that produces heat, thereby raising body temperature) and may affect basal body temperature. Several estrogens and progestogens are featured in Table 47–6.

Secretion of the ovarian hormones is regulated by the gonadotropic hormones of the anterior pituitary; production of the gonadotropins is in turn regulated by the plasma levels of estrogen and progesterone. The normal female menstrual cycle is featured in Figure 47–1.

Action

Development of the sexual organs of the female and development of the secondary sex characteristics (growth of axillary and pubic hair, and pigmentation of the nipples and genitals) are regulated by the presence of estrogen. In addition, estrogen in varying concentrations gives rise to many of the characteristics of the normal menstrual cycle: proliferation of vaginal and uterine mucosa, increased cervical secretions, and breast fullness. Increasing amounts of estrogen inhibit FSH released by the pituitary, which again contributes to the cyclic nature of the female reproductive system.

Estrogens are also involved with (1) shaping the skeleton by conserving calcium and phosphorus and encouraging bone formation, (2) maintenance of tone and elasticity of the urogenital structures, and (3) changes in the epiphyses of the long bones that allow for the pubertal growth spurt and its termination.

The net effects of progesterone in the female are to prepare the uterus for pregnancy and the breasts for lactation. Thus, the uterine endometrium becomes secretory, cervical secretions become viscid, and the acini of the mammary glands proliferate. Progesterone is a requisite for the maintenance of pregnancy; it has also been shown to decrease uterine contractility, thus preventing spontaneous abortion. Progesterone also suppresses T-lymphocyte activity, preventing immunologic rejection of the fetus by the mother's body. In addition, progesterone influences the menstrual cycle; the declining levels of progesterone give rise to the onset of menses.

Although not as potent as the androgens in terms of anabolic effects, the estrogens do cause some salt, water, and nitrogen retention. At the cellular level, similarly to

Table 47–6. FEMALE HORMONES

ESTROGENS*

DRUG NAME/ROUTE AND DOSAGE	PHARMACOKINETICS/ DYNAMICS	NURSING IMPLICATIONS
conjugated estrogens (Premarin) Administer cyclically, PO 3 wk on/1wk off or daily. **female castration, primary ovarian failure, vasomotor symptoms** 0.625–1.25 mg/day PO. **atrophic vaginitis** 0.3–1.25 mg/day; intravaginal cream 2–4 times/day. **female hypogonadism** 2.5–7.5 mg/day PO for 20 days followed by rest period of 10 days. **osteoporosis** 0.625–1.25 mg/day PO. **mammary carcinoma** 10 mg PO tid for 3 mo. **prostatic cancer** 1.25–2.5 mg PO tid. **abnormal uterine bleeding** 25 mg IV or IM, may repeat in 6–12 hr.	For all estrogens: **Onset:** rapid **Peak:** NA **Duration:** NA **½L:** NA **PB:** 80% **B:** liver **E:** bile, urine	For all estrogens and progestins: **ASSESSMENT:** Practice regular breast self-examination. Obtain regular Pap test and pelvic examinations. Assess blood pressure regularly. Assess for pregnancy (category X). **INTERVENTION:** Teach patient not to smoke during therapy. Obtain Pap smears every 6–12 mo and do breast self-exam monthly. *PO:* Take after meals. Protect from light. Store in dry, tightly closed container. *IM:* Inject deeply into gluteal muscles. Rotate injection sites and record. Shake vial to ensure uniform dispersion. *Intravaginal:* Administer at bedtime to enhance absorption. Use a sanitary napkin to protect clothing. *Patch:* Apply to clean, dry skin over trunk, preferably the abdomen. Rotate sites. Apply the system immediately after opening pouch. Press firmly in place with palm of hand for about 10 sec. **EVALUATION:** Notify physician if pain in calf occurs, suspected pregnancy, lumps in breast, or severe headaches.
estradiol, transdermal (Estraderm) 0.05 mg/24 hr skin patch; 0.10 mg/24 hr applied 2 times per wk.	Same as for all plus: **Duration:** 3–4 days	Same as for all.
estradiol cypionate (Depo-Estradiol) **vasomotor symptoms** 1–5 mg IM q 3–4 wk. **female hypogonadism** 1.5–2 mg/mo IM.	Same as for all plus: **Duration:** 3–4 days	Same as for all.

PROGESTINS

hydroxyprogesterone caproate (Delalutin) (Hylutin) **amenorrhea** 375 mg IM.	**Duration:** 9–17 days	**ASSESSMENT:** Same as for estrogen. **INTERVENTION:** Same as for estrogen plus: If GI upset occurs, take with food. **Patient Teaching—** Teach patient not to smoke during therapy. Instruct patient to obtain Pap smears every 6–12 mo and self-examine breasts monthly. **EVALUATION:** Same as for estrogen.
medroxyprogesterone acetate (Provera) (Amen) (Curretab) **amenorrhea** 2.5–10.0 mg PO qd for 5–10 days.	**Duration:** prolonged and variable	Same as for all.

Continued on the following page

Table 47–6. FEMALE HORMONES, *Continued*

ESTROGENS*

DRUG NAME/ROUTE AND DOSAGE	PHARMACOKINETICS/ DYNAMICS	NURSING IMPLICATIONS
norethindrone (Norlutin)		
amenorrhea, abnormal uterine bleeding 5–20 mg PO starting day 5 ending day 25. **endometriosis** 5–10 mg/day PO for 14 days; increase by maximum of 2.5–5 mg/day q 2 wk until maximum of 30 mg/day.		Same as for all.
norethindrone acetate (Norlutate)		
amenorrhea 2.5–10 mg PO qd; start day 5, end day 25.		Same as for all.
progesterone (Gesterol 50)		
amenorrhea 5–10 mg IM qd; start day 5, end day 25. **uterine bleeding** 5–10 mg/day IM for 6 doses; discontinue when menstrual flow begins.		Same as for all.

CONTRACEPTIVE IMPLANT

levonorgestrel (Norplant System) 6 capsules (each containing 36 mg of levonorgestrel) implanted subdermally in midportion of upper arm during first 7 days of menses.	**Onset:** NA **Peak:** NA **Duration:** 5–14 days after removal **½L:** NA **PB:** NA **B:** liver **E:** NA	**ASSESSMENT:** Assess for pregnancy and PID before insertion. **INTERVENTION:** Ensure patient understands insertion and removal technique. **EVALUATION:** Evaluate any abnormal bleeding and report to doctor.
38 mg progesterone (Progestasert) T-shaped unit inserted into uterus; releases 65 μg/day. Effective for 1 yr.	**Onset:** NA **Peak:** NA **Duration:** 1 yr **½L:** NA **PB:** NA **B:** NA **E:** NA	**ASSESSMENT:** Assess for pregnancy, sexual history, and current sexual practices. **INTERVENTION:** Teach importance of remaining in a monogamous relationship; teach about yearly replacement. **EVALUATION:** Evaluate for signs of abnormal bleeding and report to doctor.

*Doses of estrogen are not equivalent: 1 mg diethylstilbesterol = 0.5 mg estradiol = 5 mg conjugated or esterified estrogen = 0.8 mg mestranol.

NA = not available.

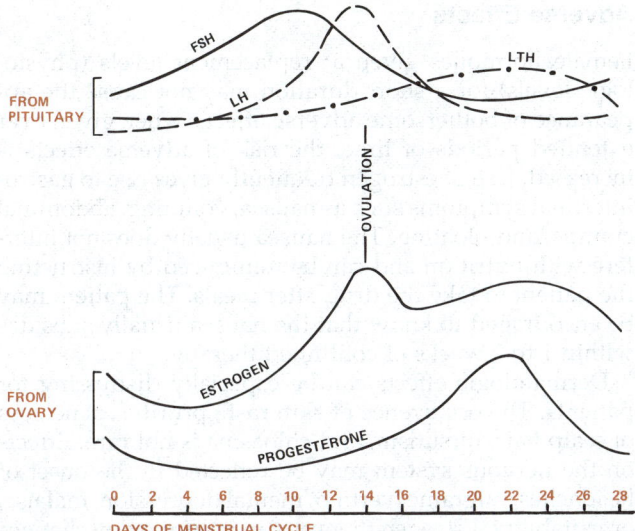

Figure 47–1. Relative relationship of gonadotropins, female hormones, to the menstrual cycle. Beginning at day 1 (onset of menses), FSH stimulates follicular growth in the ovary; within 6 days, estrogen levels begin to rise and continue to do so until ovulation; at ovulation, a rise in FSH and LH secretion occurs, leading to an increase in progesterone secretion by the corpus luteum, which reaches its maximum at about the 22nd day (of a 28-day cycle); the corpus letueum then begins to involute, leading to a decrease in the secretion of estrogen and progesterone, which in turn leads to the onset of menses and the beginning of another cycle. (Adapted from Guyton, AC: Textbook of Medical Physiology, ed 8. WB Saunders, Philadelphia, 1990, with permission.)

the androgens, estrogens and progesterone are bound to cytoplasmic receptor proteins with an end result of an increased protein synthesis.

Uses

Estrogens and progestogens are used clinically to treat hormonal deficiency states that may result from a failure of ovarian development, as in hypopituitarism, or from declining ovarian function, as in menopause. Combinations of estrogens and progestins (synthetic progesterone-like drugs) are more widely used as contraceptive agents: administration of these agents suppresses levels of FSH and LH, thus leading to an anovulatory state. (Oral contraceptives are discussed later in this chapter.) Estrogen, most commonly diethylstilbestrol, is also used as a postcoital, or morning after, pill. This method of contraception is recommended only for isolated incidents of unprotected intercourse, and treatment must commence within 72 hours of intercourse. Dysmenorrhea, endometriosis, and dysfunctional uterine bleeding are three other indications for the combined use of estrogens and progestogens. Most of the agents used therapeutically are synthetic or naturally occurring analogs of endogenous hormones. Estrogens, progesterone, and progestins are available in a variety of preparations for oral, parenteral, or topical administration.

Estrogens are used in the pharmacologic management of menopause and are effective in controlling both hot flushes due to vasomotor instability and atrophic vaginitis. For women requiring long-term therapy with estro-

gens, cyclic therapy with progestin is usually recommended to avoid continuous stimulation of the breasts and uterus (discussed later in the chapter).

▼ CLINICAL ALERT

This combination therapy reduces the incidence of endometrial hyperplasia, which can occur with estrogen therapy alone.

▼ CLINICAL ALERT

Conjugated estrogens are particularly effective in preventing osteoporosis, including loss of height and dowager's hump, both in women who have undergone oophorectomy before natural menopause and in women who have had a natural menopause. Estrogens inhibit bone resorption. The addition of progestin appears to be even more beneficial by not only inhibiting bone resorption, but also adding to bone mass. This therapy is best started before significant bone loss. In addition to drug therapy, weight-bearing exercise and calcium supplements are encouraged.

Statistics today say that 40% of women will suffer at least one spinal fracture by age 80 and 20% to 25% will break a hip. Estrogen therapy can reduce the risk by 90% of spinal fractures and by 60% of hip fractures. Estrogen therapy is continued from menopause for the next 10 to 20 years to obtain these results.

The 20-Year Nurses Health Study—its 116,470 participants makes it one of the largest studies to date—concludes that estrogen use cuts the risk of major coronary disease and fatal cardiovascular disease in half. Heart disease kills 600,000 women yearly, twice as many as cancer. Estrogen alone increases plasma levels of HDL and decreases LDL, which promotes atherosclerosis. Unfortunately, a dilemma exists: when progesterone is added, it increases LDL and decreases HDL. Long-term studies are ongoing.

Progestin by itself or in combination with estrogen is used as a contraceptive. In the single-agent minipills, the progestins do not reliably block ovulation; they probably exert their contraceptive action through their effects on the endometrium and cervical mucus, causing these to be unfavorable for sperm transport and implantation. The minipills are taken once daily for all 28 days of the menstrual cycle. When taken as directed, these drugs offer approximately 97% protection from pregnancy. The progestin minipills do have a higher incidence of breakthrough bleeding and spotting. However, they do not cause the more serious toxicities associated with the use of estrogen.

Oral progestins are used with success in the treatment of endometriosis and premenstrual syndrome (PMS). Long-term use results in regression of endometrial growths, giving symptomatic relief in about 80% of cases and a return of fertility in about 50%. Progestins also are useful in the palliative treatment of endometrial carcinomas.

Pharmacokinetics

The administration of exogenous estrogens or progestins causes the same physiologic responses as the endogenous hormones. Synthetic versions of these hormones vary in duration and intensity of action.

Natural estrogens and their esters are metabolized by the liver too rapidly to be effective orally. Nonsteroidal estrogens may be administered orally but are also metabolized rapidly, and frequent (usually daily) administration is required. Aqueous or oil suspensions of estrogen are administered parenterally; absorption takes place over a period of days. Subcutaneous implantation of estrogen-containing pellets allows for absorption over a period of months. Absorption through skin and mucous membranes is also good and, in fact, can give rise to systemic effects.

Estrogens circulate in the blood bound to globulin and albumin (80%). The greatest concentration of estrogen appears in fat deposits. Estrogens are metabolized by the liver and are excreted primarily into the urine. Excretion of estrogens averages 25 to 100 μg at midcycle, 5 to 10 μg after menopause, and about 30 mg during the later stages of pregnancy.

Progestins are rapidly metabolized by the liver and excreted primarily into the urine; small amounts are stored in fat tissue. Synthetic progestins may be administered orally as well as parenterally.

Contraindications and Precautions

Estrogens and progestins are contraindicated during pregnancy (category X), because of an increased incidence of the fetus developing vaginal or cervical cancer in later years.

▼ CLINICAL ALERT

Estrogen and progestin therapy is generally contraindicated in the patient who has a history of thromboembolic disease, genital or mammary malignancies, hepatic dysfunction, or hypertension, as estrogen is associated with an increased incidence or worsening of these conditions.

Because of the increased incidence of thromboembolism occurring in women who smoke, smoking may either be a contraindication or a caution. Because estrogens are metabolized by the liver, the function of that organ should be unimpaired.

▼ CLINICAL ALERT

Estrogens may increase the risk of endometrial carcinoma, but the risk depends on dose and duration of therapy. There is also a twofold to threefold increase in the risk of gallbladder disease, so patients with preexisting gallbladder disease should not take estrogens.

Adverse Effects

Female hormones given at replacement levels (physiologic levels) for a short duration may not cause the appearance of bothersome adverse effects; when given over extended periods of time, the risk of adverse effects is increased. Use of estrogen frequently gives rise to gastrointestinal symptoms such as nausea, vomiting, abdominal cramps, and bloating. The nausea usually does not interfere with nutrition and can be minimized by instructing the patient to take the drug after meals. The patient may be encouraged to know that the nausea usually subsides within 1 to 2 weeks of continued therapy.

Dermatologic effects can be especially distressing for patients. The occurrence of skin rash, pruritus, acne, loss of scalp hair, hirsutism, and chloasma is not rare. Effects on the nervous system may be reflected in the onset of headaches, migraine, vertigo, mental depression, malaise, or irritability. Estrogen therapy can induce many changes in the metabolic function of the body. Edema and sodium retention can occur, leading in some instances to hypertension. Blood glucose levels may increase, a factor of special concern in the care of the diabetic patient. The occurrence of cholestatic jaundice reflects estrogen's effects on the biliary system. Endocrine changes are reflected in the possible occurrence of breakthrough bleeding and spotting, breast enlargement, increased cervical mucus production, and changes in menstrual flow. (In males, gynecomastia, testicular atrophy, feminization, and reversible impotence can occur with estrogen administration.)

Perhaps the most serious adverse effects of estrogen therapy are related to its effect on the vascular system. The occurrence of thromboembolism in women and men receiving estrogen therapy is well documented. Men who receive estrogen therapy are at the same increased risk. The higher the dose of estrogen, the higher the risk. The risk of thromboembolic disorders related to estrogen increases with age beginning at about 30 years and increasing even more after 40 years of age. In addition, even women who discontinue long-term estrogen use also have a higher incidence of thromboembolic complications. Women who use estrogen-containing oral contraceptives for 5 years or more have a tenfold increase in the risk of death from thromboembolic disorders in contrast to women who have not used these products. Peripheral thrombophlebitis is not the only concern, however, as the incidence of cerebral and coronary thromboses also increases.

Progestin administration also can cause adverse effects, most of which are similar to those caused by estrogen. In fact, when the two hormones are used in combination, as in the oral contraceptives, it is not always possible to tell which effects are due to which hormone.

▼ CLINICAL ALERT

When progestins are administered during pregnancy, masculinization and birth defects can occur.

Eye changes can occur suddenly with progestin therapy; the nurse should inform the patient to immediately report such changes as loss of vision, diplopia, or *proptosis* (downward displacement of the eyeball in exophthalmic goiter or in inflammatory conditions of the orbit). Medication should be withheld until these can be investigated.

Interactions

The effects of estrogen may be decreased by the concurrent use of antibiotics, and anticonvulsant drugs like phenytoin, primidone, and barbiturates, as hepatic breakdown is enhanced. Women taking oral contraceptives concurrently with these products must use another method of birth control for that cycle, as they may not have full protection. Estrogens can alter the effectiveness of many drugs. They decrease the effect of oral anticoagulants, through increasing the action of selected clotting factors; anticonvulsants, by depressing breakdown of anticonvulsant; and antidiabetic drugs, by decreasing glucose tolerance. Conversely, estrogen increases the effects of tricyclic antidepressants by decreasing hepatic breakdown. Selected estrogens and progestines are featured in Table 47–6.

Estrogen-Only Agents

○ **Conjugated estrogens** (Premarin), a product of three estrogens obtained from horse urine, is used to relieve the vasomotor symptoms of menopause and to treat atrophic vaginitis, kraurosis vulvae, female hypogonadism, surgical castration, primary ovarian failure, postpartum breast engorgement, and abnormal uterine bleeding from hormone imbalance.

○ **Transdermal estradiol** (Estraderm, Climara) is available as a patch in two dosage forms. The patches, applied once or twice weekly, may minimize the problems and maximize the benefits of hormone replacement because the hormone is released in small amounts continually for the time it is worn.

○ **Estradiol cypionate** (Depo-Estradiol) is a long-lasting preparation administered intramuscularly every 3 to 4 weeks for primary ovarian failure, surgical castration, or menopausal symptoms.

○ **Ethinyl estradiol** (Estinyl, Feminone), a synthetic oral estrogen, is administered in a 21-day cycle for menopausal symptoms. For female hypogonadism, ethinyl estradiol is administered 0.05 mg three times a day for 2 weeks per month. It is followed by 2 weeks of progesterone therapy. This series is continued for 3 to 6 months, followed by 2 months off therapy.

○ **Quinestrol** (Estrovis), a long-acting synthetic estrogen, is used to treat female hypogonadism, primary ovarian failure, atrophic vaginitis, and kraurosis vulvae; and to relieve menopausal symptoms. For all conditions, quinestrol is administered orally 100 μg/day for 7 days, then no drug for 7 days, followed by a maintenance dosage of 100 to 200 μg/week.

Progestin-Only Agents

○ **Medroxyprogesterone** (Provera, Amen, Curretab) is a synthetic progestin that can be administered orally to treat amenorrhea or abnormal uterine bleeding caused by

hormonal imbalance, and it is used in menopause. It is available in IM form as a contraceptive.

○ **Hydroxyprogesterone caproate** (Delalutin) is a long-acting synthetic progestin administered intramuscularly to treat amenorrhea and abnormal uterine bleeding caused by hormonal imbalance.

○ **Norethindrone** (Norlutin) and **norethindrone acetate** (Norlutate), which is twice as potent, are synthetic products that are administered orally to treat amenorrhea, abnormal uterine bleeding caused by hormonal imbalance, and endometriosis.

○ **Progesterone** (Gesterol 50), a natural progestin product, is available for intramuscular injection to treat amenorrhea, abnormal uterine bleeding caused by hormonal imbalance, and premenstrual syndrome. It is also available as an intrauterine contraceptive device (Progestasert), inserted once yearly. For premenstrual syndrome, progesterone is available as a suppository, inserted either rectally or vaginally, once or twice daily.

○ **Norplant subdermal implants** (Norplant System) are six flexible closed capsules composed of 36 mg of progestin available for subdermal implantation. The system allows for a slow diffusion of levonorgestrel over 5 years. Levonorgestrel is also available as a 2-rod implant which provides 3 years of contraception. After removal, plasma levels are no longer detectable after 5 to 14 days. The pregnancy rate is less than 1/100 women through 5 years.

ACTION Progestin decreases ovulation; if ovulation does occur, the mucus is thick and scanty, which prevents sperm migration. The constant low level of progestin further suppresses endometrial development and growth and suppresses progesterone secretion during the luteal phase. Following removal, the endometrium returns to normal and can support pregnancy.

ADVERSE EFFECTS The adverse effects are similar to oral contraceptives. Women who weigh more than 150 pounds have a higher pregnancy rate of 11% over 5 years. The recent introduction of more porous capsules, which release the hormone into the bloodstream more quickly, appears to reduce this percentage.

○ **Progestasert,** an intrauterine system, is a T-shaped unit that releases 65 μg/progesterone per day for 1 year. The mechanism is local, not systemic. Progesterone suppresses proliferation of endometrial tissue, therefore implantation of the egg is prevented. This system is used in women who have had at least one child, are in a stable monogamous relationship, and have no history of pelvic inflammatory disease (PID).

CONTRAINDICATIONS AND PRECAUTIONS Pregnancy, PID, multiple sexual partners, sexually transmitted disease, postpartum endometritis, uterine or cervical cancer, vaginal infection, IV drug abuse, or conditions associated with increased susceptibility to infections are all contraindications. The implant is used cautiously in persons prone to develop subacute bacterial endocarditis as the incidence of infection is increased.

ADVERSE EFFECTS Adverse effects include infection, spontaneous abortion, perforation of the uterus or cervix, intermenstrual spotting, and backaches. Neurovascular episodes including bradycardia and syncope secondary to insertion have also been reported. Some of these adverse effects can lead to loss of fertility, partial or total removal of reproductive organs, hormonal imbalance, or death.

○ **Megestrol acetate** (Megace) is a progestin that is used in the palliative treatment of carcinoma of the breast or endometrium (see chapter 55 for more information).

Selected progestins are featured in Table 47–6.

PREMENSTRUAL SYNDROME

Premenstrual syndrome (PMS) affects 9 to 12 million (30% to 40%) of all women in the United States. PMS may occur in any menstruating woman, but the incidence increases in those over age 30. PMS has been implicated in work absenteeism, criminal behavior, marital discord, and billions of dollars worth of business loss.

The etiology remains obscure, but symptoms generally begin about 7 to 10 days before the onset of menses and resolve within 24 hours after menstruation begins. The typical symptoms reported include mood swings, abdominal bloating, irritability, depression, crying, food cravings, and sleep disorders.

Several drugs for the relief of the symptoms of PMS are being studied, including alprazolam (Xanax) (Chapter 25) and danazol (Danocrine, a synthetic androgen discussed previously). Diuretics are also used in the treatment of PMS to relieve symptoms related to fluid retention. Another method of treating PMS is the use of progesterone, which is able to control both the physical and emotional symptoms of the worst cases of PMS. About 90% of patients who have tried progesterone find relief. One theory why progesterone works is that some women have too much estrogen and too little progesterone.

Research is ongoing to find other treatments for PMS. Diet therapy may be helpful in some women. Eating carbohydrate-rich, low-protein meals during the second half of the menstrual cycle helps some women.

CONTRACEPTION

Since the relationship between coitus and pregnancy became known, efforts have been made to limit the number of pregnancies. Various methods of contraception are currently available. Table 47–7 compares the therapeutic effectiveness and adverse effects of the various methods. A brief overview of oral contraceptives, vaginal spermicides, and intrauterine devices follows. For a more detailed review, please see an obstetrical nursing text.

ORAL CONTRACEPTIVES

Oral contraceptives, featured in Table 47–8, are highly effective in preventing pregnancy. They have different actions dependent on the product being used. The combination oral contraceptives inhibit ovulation through a negative feedback effect on the hypothalamus. The cervical mucous thickens, rendering it unfavorable to penetration by sperm. In addition, the endometrial lining is unfavorable for implantation. The progestin-only minipills do not inhibit ovulation, but cause the formation of a thick cervical mucous that is relatively impenetrable to sperm.

The oral contraceptives are available in low-, medium-, or high-estrogen doses, as presented in Table 47–9. The preparation chosen should closely mimic the balance of the patient's endogenous hormones or minimize problems with her specific hormone sensitivities. For example, a woman with symptoms of estrogen sensitivity (vomiting, fluid retention, increased menstrual flow) is given

Table 47–7. EFFECTIVENESS AND ADVERSE EFFECTS OF VARIOUS METHODS OF CONTRACEPTION			
Method	**% Theoretical Effectiveness**	**% Use Effectiveness**	**Adverse Effects**
Oral contraceptives: Fixed ratio (estrogen and progestin)	100	97–98	Nausea, edema, increased weight gain, fatigue, leukorrhea, thromboembolic disorders, increased incidence of gallbladder disease, teratogenesis in pregnancy.
Minipill (progestin only)	99	96–97.5	
Intrauterine devices: Progestasert system	96–99	90–94	Dysmenorrhea, alterations in menstrual flow, pelvic inflammatory disease. Infection, perforation of uterus or cervix, PID, loss of fertility, prolonged menstrual flow.
	100	99	
Copper T 380 A (Paragard)	100	99	Cervical irritation, may be difficult to fit.
Medroxyprogesterone acetate (Depo-Provera)	100	99	Menstrual irregularities, headache, weight gain. Need injection q 3 mo.
Condom	97	80–97	None.
Diaphragm	97	80	Possible allergies to rubber or irritation from spermicides.
Cervical cap with spermicide	90	82	Cervical irritation, may be difficult to fit.
Spermicidal foams	97	70–72	Local irritation.
Rhythm	95	70–75	None.
Subdermal progestin implant (Norplant)	100	99	Irregular, decreased, prolonged menses, local reaction, headache, acne.

Table 47–8. ORAL CONTRACEPTIVES

DRUG NAME/ROUTE AND DOSAGE	PHARMACOKINETICS/ DYNAMICS	NURSING IMPLICATIONS
		all oral contraceptives **ASSESSMENT:** Assess blood pressure, weight, pregnancy status, and liver function before starting oral contraceptives. **INTERVENTION:** Take as directed. For missed table information, see text. Women who smoke more than 15 cigarettes/day and are over 35 have marked CV complications. **EVALUATION:** If breakthrough bleeding occurs 2nd mo, notify physician.
PROGESTINS		
norethindrone (Micronor) **norgestrel** (Ovrette) 0.35 mg PO qd (norethindrone), 0.075 mg PO qd (norgestrel)	**Onset:** rapid **Peak:** 0.5–4.0 hr **Duration:** NA **½L:** 5–45 hr **PB:** to albumin **B:** liver **E:** bile, urine	Same as for all.
COMBINATIONS		
norethindrone/mestranol (Norinyl) (Ortho Novum) (Ortho Novum 2) Progestin/estrogen 1 mg/50 μg PO qd (Norinyl); 1 mg/50 μg, 1 mg/35 μg (Ortho Novum); 2 mg/100 μg (Ortho Novum 2).	Same as above	Same as for all.
norethindrone/ethinyl estradiol (Loestrin) (Norlestrin) 1.5 mg/30 μg PO qd (Loestrin); 1 mg/50 μg, 5mg/75 μg PO qd (Norlestrin)	Same as above	Same as for all.
medroxyprogesterone acetate (Depo-Provera) 150 mg IM q 3 mo	**Onset:** slow **Peak:** 3 wk **Duration:** 3 mo **½L:** 50 days **PB:** NA **B:** NA **E:** NA	Same as for all plus: **ASSESSMENT:** Assess for pregnancy at time of first injection. **INTERVENTION:** Inject deep IM into gluteal or deltoid muscle. **Patient Teaching**—Unpredictable bleeding or spotting may occur at first. Eventually amenorrhea occurs. Injection is needed q 3 mo. **EVALUATION:** Report leg pain, chest pain, headache, or visual changes to doctor.

CV = cardiovascular; NA = not available.

low-dose estrogen products. Patients with androgen sensitivity (oily skin and scalp, acne) or progestin sensitivity (depression, noncyclic weight gain) are given a product low in both androgenic and progestational activities.

Types of Oral Contraceptives

Several types of oral contraceptives are available: monophasic, biphasic, triphasic and estrophasic products. These products are graphically represented in Figure 47–2.

Monophasic Oral Contraceptive Products The monophasic oral contraceptive products are the most common and provide a fixed dose of estrogen and progestin throughout a 21-day cycle.

Biphasic Oral Contraceptive Products The biphasic oral contraceptive products, introduced in 1982, simulate a woman's normal hormonal pattern. Low-dose estrogen

Table 47–9. ESTROGEN CONTENT OF SELECTED BIRTH CONTROL PILLS	
Brand Name	
High Estrogen	
Enovid 5	
Medium Estrogen	Ovral*
Norinyl 1 + 50	
Ortho-Novum 1/50	
Low Estrogen	Ortho Novum 10/11‡‡
Loestrin 1/20†	Tri-Levlen‡
Loestrin 1.5/30†	Tri-Norinyl‡
Norinyl 1 + 35†	
Ortho Novum 7/7/7	

*In high doses, is being used as "morning after" pill.
†Monophasic.
‡Triphasic.
‡‡Biphosic.

(35 μg) is kept constant throughout the cycle, while the progestin is increased (0.5 to 1.0 mg) from day 11 through day 21. The biphasic pill is intended to reduce total steroid exposure while alleviating problems with breakthrough bleeding and spotting common with lower-dose pills.

The benefits of decreasing progestin include a possible reduction in hypertension, pelvic congestion, depression, fatigue, headache, and HDL levels. However, there may also be a loss of some noncontraceptive benefits of progestins such as protection against pelvic inflammatory disease, less dysmenorrhea and menstrual blood loss, and protection against endometrial cancer and fibrocystic breast disease.

Triphasic Oral Contraceptive Products   The triphasic products approximate the normal female cycle even more closely. Both low-dose estrogen and progestin change in a low-higher-low pattern. Estrogen is constant, while progestin rises at midcycle and falls before the onset of bleeding. The triphasic pill reduces the total steroid exposure while providing greater protection at midcycle. Breakthrough bleeding is also reduced. The triphasic products

are available in a 28-day cycle with 7 inert tablets or in a 21-day cycle with the inert pills omitted.

Estrophasic Products   The estrophasic products (Estrostep) combines gradual estrogen intake and steady progestin intake.

Adverse Effects

During the 1970s, many studies reported an increased risk of disease or death among women using oral contraceptives. This created widespread controversy and resulted in modification of the formulation of oral contraceptives. Results of later studies suggest that women who use oral contraceptives have dramatically fewer risks with the newer formulations than with earlier preparations. Recent reports also suggest that there is a protective effect; users are half as likely to develop ovarian and endometrial cancer as women who have never used oral contraceptives.

A recent study of 918 women suggests that oral contraceptive use during the early and late fertile years is associated with an increased risk of breast cancer, and is associated with more recent use in older women (more than 46 years of age). Similar investigations are needed before clinical recommendations can be established (Rookus and Leeuwen, 1994).

The primary risk factors involved in complications of oral contraceptive use appear to be (1) the estrogen dose, (2) the age of the woman, (3) tobacco smoking, and (4) the duration of therapy. The more risk factors that are present for coronary artery disease (hypertension, hypercholesterolemina, obesity, diabetes), the greater the risk.

Women using oral contraceptives who smoke 15 or more cigarettes a day have a fivefold to tenfold increase in the risk of having a fatal myocardial infarction (MI) in comparison with women taking oral contraceptives who do not smoke.

Clotting disorders such as pulmonary embolism, retinal vein thrombosis, and thrombophlebitis have occurred more frequently in women using oral contraceptives. There is also an increase in certain blood factors associated with coagulation, an increase in platelet count with changes in electrophoretic mobility of platelets, and an

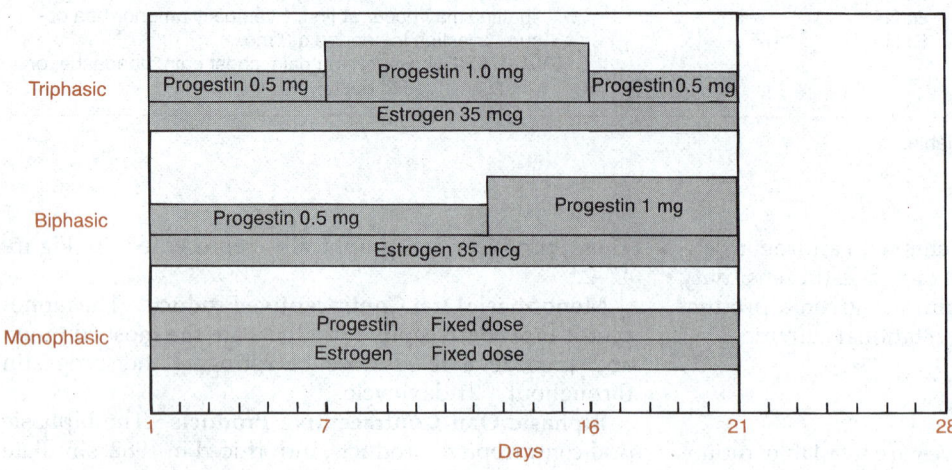

Figure 47–2. The three types of oral contraceptives. Monophasic products contain fixed amounts of estrogen and progestin throughout the 21-day cycle. Biphasic products contain a fixed low dose of estrogen (35 μg) and progestin that increases from 0.5 mg to 1 mg at day 11. The triphasic products also contain a fixed dose of estrogen (35 μg) and progestin in a low-high-low pattern.

increase in vascular lesions and venous stasis. The estimated risk of hemorrhagic stroke is two times greater, and the risk of thrombotic stroke is ten times greater. The risk continues for 9 years after discontinuing oral contraceptives if they have been taken 5 years or more and the user is over 40 years of age.

If a woman develops deep-vein thrombosis while taking oral contraceptives, the contraceptives are stopped and never restarted. Also, caution is used when oral contraceptives are used after any surgical procedure, as the incidence of deep-vein thrombosis is almost twice that of nonusers.

Hypertension has been observed in about 5% of all contraceptive users. Although the increase in blood pressure is usually gradual, it may be quite severe. Generally, the hypertension is reversible within several months of discontinuation of medications. These effects probably result from the retention of sodium and water secondary to the increased circulating concentration of renin and angiotensin.

Various ocular conditions have also been reported, including corneal sensitivity, retinal thrombosis, optic neuritis, diplopia, and others. Women wearing contact lenses may experience intolerance to their lenses due to a change in corneal curvature; they are encouraged to have periodic eye exams.

Many other minor disturbances have been attributed to oral contraceptives. Some symptoms, including depression of mood, easy fatigue, and lack of initiative, have been attributed to progestin tablets. An increase in female-initiated sexual activity that is said to be present at the time of ovulation is suppressed or absent in women using oral contraceptives. The triphasic contraceptives may decrease this side effect.

Women frequently complain of mild side effects including nausea, occasional vomiting, dizziness, headache, discomfort in the breasts, and weight gain. These symptoms are all found in early pregnancy and are the direct result of estrogen in the preparation. Usually these symptoms are present during the first or second cycle and then disappear. Irregular menstrual bleeding, so-called breakthrough bleeding, is also more frequent at first. It appears to be less troublesome with preparations containing larger amounts of estrogen.

Oral contraceptives also may cause intolerance to carbohydrates, resulting in elevations of blood glucose and insulin. If notable alteration in blood sugar occurs, oral contraceptives are discontinued. Oral contraceptives may also alter lipoprotein levels.

Interactions

Oral contraceptives may interact with other drugs through various mechanisms. Table 47–10 features drugs that reduce the efficacy of oral contraceptives. Spotting or bleeding that takes place between menstrual periods may be a sign that the contraceptive is not working well enough to inhibit ovulation. It is likely that current knowledge of these types of interactions is far from comprehensive and that other drugs, not yet identified, can enter into such interactions.

SPERMICIDES

Vaginal spermicides containing nonoxynol 9, such as creams (Conceptrol), gels (Gynol II, Koromex Gel), foams (Delfen foam), and suppositories (Encare), are available for topical vaginal application. All these products are inexpensive, easy to use, and available over the counter. These products are applied minutes to 1 hour before coitus and then reapplied before each ejaculation. Douching is avoided for the next 6 to 8 hours. Manufacturers of vaginal spermicides are currently conducting studies to determine their exact effectivenss.

INTRAUTERINE DEVICES

Only one intrauterine device (IUD) remains on the market in the United States today—the Progestasert system (previously discussed). This device contains progesterone and must be replaced annually. IUDs prevent implantation of the blastocyst by altering the biochemical milieu of the endometrium. Progesterone may also inhibit the metabolism, capacitation, and swimming speed of sperm. IUDs are not recommended as a contraceptive method until a woman has completed her family.

SUBDERMAL IMPLANTS

Norplant subdermal implants (previously discussed) prevent pregnancy for 5 years, and the levonorgestral system provides 3 years of protection.

ANTIPROGESTERONE AGENTS

○ **RU 486** or mifepristone, first released in France, produces an abortion without the dual hazards of surgery and anesthesia. Mifepristone is an antiprogesterone agent that causes the uterine lining to slough, eliminating the pregnancy (the embryo is about the size of a pea at this time). Mifepristone is 96% effective, but only within the first 3 weeks following a missed menstrual period.

Mifepristone is being studied as a contraceptive with once weekly administration; as a treatment for endometriosis by suppressing hormone production and thus controlling pain and discomfort; as a treatment for breast cancer by removing progesterone as a stimulus for tumor growth (15% to 20% of tumor growth could be controlled); and as a labor enhancer by causing the cervix to soften, open, and dilate, facilitating a natural vaginal delivery.

The FDA has recently recommended the use of mifepristone along with mesoprostal (Cytotec) (Chapter 57) to terminate pregnancy through 49 days gestation or a com-

Table 47-10. DRUG INTERACTIONS OF ORAL CONTRACEPTIVES

Interacting Drug	Interaction	Management
Antibiotics and Antibacterials rifampin, griseofulvin, penicillins, tetracycline (and probably most others)	Decreased pharmacologic effect of oral contraceptives (OCs).	May lead to contraceptive failure. Use alternative birth control method.
Anticonvulsants barbiturates, hydantoins	Anticonvulsants induce estrogen metabolism by hepatic microsomal enzymes.	Use of this combination must be carefully assessed with respect to possible failure of contraception and, in some cases, also to increased incidence of seizures (combined OCs may cause fluid retention, which may precipitate seizures in epileptics; OC-induced exacerbations of epilepsy have been reported). The combination may also cause an increase in serum phenytoin concentrations, which could lead to enhanced phenytoin toxicity. Three possible methods of management are: (1) change to a nonhormonal method of contraception, (2) change the antiseizure drug from phenytoin to sodium valproate (which does not seem to affect contraceptive efficacy), or (3) increase the OC dosage by prescribing two types of OC preparations simultaneously to bring the total estrogen dosage up to 80 μg/day although this may be undesirable because of the increased risk of side effects, which cannot as yet be quantified. Where possible, it would be better to advise alternative methods of contraception.
Analgesics acetaminophen, salicylates	Data suggest increased clearance of analgesics from plasma.	Clinical significance of this interaction has not been established, but women taking OCs may require larger doses of the analgesic than those used by women not taking OC steroids.
Anticoagulants	Oral contraceptives increase the synthesis of specific blood coagulation factors; this may impair the efficacy of anticoagulant therapy.	No patient who requires anticoagulants should take OCs.
Antidiabetic Agents Oral products	Both an impairment of glucose tolerance with development of overt diabetes mellitus and an increase in insulin requirements have been reported in women taking OCs.	The use of other methods of contraception may be required for some diabetics. If this is not practical, the patient should be carefully monitored for decreased diabetic control; existing antidiabetic treatment may have to be modified. The risk of cardiovascular complications and microangiopathic changes in diabetic patients is increased when OCs are used.
Hypnotics, Sedatives Diazepam, phenothiazines	Hepatic metabolism of these products may be decreased.	Monitor for increased or toxic effects of these drugs.

Source: Adapted from D'Arcy, PF: Drug interactions with oral contraceptives. Drug Intell Clin Pharm 20(5):353–361, 1986. Modified in 1996.

bination of mesoprostal and methotrexate (Rheumatrex) (Chapter 55).

MALE CONTRACEPTION

The availability of safe, effective, and reversible male contraceptive methods is an important goal in expanding the choices available to couples for family planning. Studies are ongoing to assess the contraception efficiency of weekly injections of testosterone enanthate (Delatestryl 200 mg/wk for 12 months) to induce azoospermia in previously fertile men. In general, about half the men become azoospermic within 120 days. After the injections are dis-

continued, fertility returns in approximately 3.7 months. Weekly depot testosterone enanthate injection may join the ranks of contraceptive techniques in the future.

FEMALE MENOPAUSE

Menopause is the cessation of cyclic function of the ovaries. The follicles are depleted and no longer function. At the beginning of menopause (perimenopause), there is a decreasing frequency of ovulation, associated with irregular menses and variable periods of amenorrhea. Several years before there is a change in menses, women often begin to report insomnia, mood changes, headaches, joint pains, fatigue, unusual skin sensitivities, memory loss, night sweats, vaginal dryness, lack of sexual desire, and pain during intercourse. Although the list is long, one woman will not experience all of them. Estrogen production now begins to decline, which precipitates signs and changes of hormone deficit in the estrogen-dependent organs such as the pituitary, uterus, cervix, vagina, and breasts. The endometrium atrophies, and vaginal epithelium becomes thin and fails to become keratinized due to its lack of glycogen.

Perimenopausal treatment with estrogen relieves hot flushes and vaginal dryness in most women, prevents genitourinary atrophy, and decreases the risk of osteoporosis and cardiovascular disease. About 40% of women taking HRT (hormonal replacement therapy) do not have control of signs and changes of menopause, particularly by hot flashes, and will need to have their HRT monitored closely. A negative effect of long-term unopposed estrogen is an increase in endometrial hyperplasia and about an eightfold increase in the incidence of endometrial cancer. Also, estrogen replacement may add a small increase in risk of breast cancer for some women.

Because of the increased risk of cancer, estrogen is recommended along with progesterone. The usual routine is estrogen (Premarin is the most commonly used drug) for days 1 to 25 of the month or every day with progesterone added for days 15 to 25. This combination results in the build up and sloughing of the uterine wall so menses still occurs.

Two products combining conjugated estrogens (Premarin) with medroxyprogesterone acetate (Cycrin) are combined in one package as tablets (Prempro, Premphase). With Prempro, both tablets are taken daily continuously; with Premphase, the estrogen is taken daily, but the progestin is taken sequentially on days 15 through 28 of each 28-day cycle.

Women without a uterus may take unopposed estrogen. Estraderm and Vivelle are estrogen patches. Estraderm is changed weekly whereas Virelle is changed twice a month.

In a study of postmenopausal women who developed breast cancer, postmenopausal hormone replacement therapy did not negatively affect cancer diagnosis and prognosis, and the women who took hormone replacement, if their cancer returned, did better. (Bonnier et al., 1995)

Many other body changes occur, including the development of postmenopausal osteoporosis. Estrogen replacement begun at menopause and continued for 5 to 7 years appears to have little effect on the development of osteoporosis. It appears that starting estrogen at about age 70 seems to have the greatest effect on bone mineralization (Felson et al., 1994). But women need to keep in mind the other benefits of estrogen therapy (relief of menopausal symptoms and the reduction of heart disease risk) and its drawbacks (higher risk for breast cancer). The addition of progestin to the estrogen may precipitate menstrual-like bleeding. Several drugs are available to increase bone density, decrease bone loss, and improve bone strength: aledronate (Fosamax), calcitonin fluoride, boron, and etidronate (Didronel). More detail can be found in Chapter 46.

USING THE NURSING PROCESS

ASSESSMENT

Assessment of the patient requiring female hormones or other drugs affecting the female reproductive system can be very complex, depending on individual circumstances. Information the nurse needs to obtain is featured in Table 47–11.

- Obtain diagnostic tests to determine the specific cause of decreased ovarian function. Urinary levels of estrogens and progesterone and their metabolites can be measured. Radioimmunoassays are also used to measure levels of ovarian hormones. In primary ovarian insufficiency, the levels are low.

  Blood and urine measurements of the gonadotropic hormones are also useful in determining whether the hypogonadal state is due to a primary or secondary ovarian insufficiency. Low levels of the gonadotropins are characteristic of secondary insufficiency, whereas high gonadotropin levels are consistent with primary ovarian dysfunction. (Because low gonadotropin levels may be indicative of widespread pituitary dysfunction, this finding should be followed up with a thorough assessment of pituitary function.)

- Assess ovarian function indirectly by assessing for the effects of the hormones. Vaginal epithelium may be examined for the estrogenic effect, cornification of the epithelial cells. Endometrial tissue may be examined for secretory changes characteristic of progesterone stimulation. Endocervical mucus also reflects hormonal influences. Women may experience an estrogen or progestin excess or deficit. Table 47–12 features common signs associated with these hormonal disturbances.

- Assess menstrual function and ovarian dysfunction, as well as dysmenorrhea, dysfunctional bleeding, or menopausal symptoms.

- Assess medications history, because disruption of the menstrual cycle can be due to pharmacologic influences. Specific questions to ask include age at menarche, interval and duration of menstrual periods, amount of flow, occurrence of pain, and dates of onset of the last period or last two periods.

As menopause approaches, the menstrual cycles come closer together. Women often experience hot flushes and excessive perspiration due primarily to hypothalamic imbalances induced by decreased release of ovarian steroids. Hormonal therapy may be helpful in alleviating these symptoms.

- Obtain a recent sexual history as well as a recent drug history to look for drugs that might decrease the efficacy of oral contraceptives. The reasons for using

---

Table 47–11. NURSING PROCESS FOR PATIENT REQUIRING FEMALE HORMONES

Assessment

Assess history of menstrual function, including presence of dysmenorrhea, dysfunctional bleeding or menopausal symptoms, PMS. Note history of other endocrine and genitourinary problems.

Assess previous/current medications patient is taking, including oral contraceptives and OTC/street drugs, use of tobacco. Assess exercise habits.

Assess laboratory studies, e.g., urinary levels of estrogens and progesterone and their metabolites; blood and urine measurements of the gonadotropic hormones.

Assess vaginal epithelium for estrogenic effect, cornification of epithelial cells, secretory changes characteristic of progesterone stimulation of endometrial tissue, and hormone influences on endocervical mucus.

Assess radioimmunoassay reports that measure levels of ovarian hormones.

Nursing Diagnosis: Knowledge Deficit

RELATED TO: Information misinterpretation, unfamiliarity with information resources.

AS EVIDENCED BY: Questions, statement of concern, inaccurate follow-through of instructions, development of preventable complications.

Desired Outcomes/Evaluation Criteria

Verbalizes understanding of condition/disease process and need for treatment. Identifies relationship of signs/symptoms to the disease process. Participates in treatment regimen.

Nursing Actions	**Rationale**
Provide information about condition/disease and treatment regimen.	Understanding helps patient to make informed choices and participate in treatment.
Discuss action, use, dose, storage, and side effects of hormones.	Promotes correct use of medications to maximize effectiveness and minimize adverse reactions.
Discuss ways to minimize GI upset, reduce discomfort, and improve sexual relations.	Although transient side effects may disappear with continued use of estrogen, simple measures may reduce others, e.g., taking drug with meals, use of mild antidiarrheal drugs, use of a vaginal lubricant.
Instruct patient to monitor for significant side effects, e.g., fluid retention, increased blood pressure, vaginal candidiasis, thromboembolism, jaundice, or depression.	Early identification allows for appropriate intervention to avoid complications.
Recommend cessation of smoking.	Smoking increases risk of thromboembolic side effects of these drugs.
Stress importance of routine follow-up.	Because of increased risk of thromboembolic and cardiovascular problems, checkups may detect early signs and promote preventive actions.
Discuss necessity of contacting physician if taking oral contraceptives and pregnancy is suspected.	Estrogen and progesterones can cause fetal abnormalities, and medication must be discontinued.

Nursing Diagnosis: Sexual Dysfunction

RELATED TO: Altered body structure/function, illness, fear of pregnancy.

Desired Outcomes/Evaluation Criteria

Verbalizes understanding of individual reasons for sexual difficulties/changes that have occurred. Follows treatment regimen. Identifies and uses appropriate method of contraception.

Nursing Actions	**Rationale**
Provide privacy and have patient describe problem(s) in own words.	Promotes identification and clarification of problems and defines interventions.
Discuss pathophysiology of condition/illness, e.g., menopause, hypogonadism, avoidance of pregnancy.	Promotes understanding and informed choices.
Encourage open discussion with significant other.	Clarifies problems and provides opportunity to resolve misunderstandings/improve the relationship.

Other Suggested Nursing Diagnoses: Altered Sexual Patterns, Body Image Disturbance, and Self-Esteem Disturbance.

---

this birth control method are discussed. Also, it is important to determine how well the patient will comply with therapy.

- Obtain baseline weight and blood pressure and perform eye exams—particularly for contact lens wearers. These items must be reassessed periodically during therapy.
- Assess current smoking history. If the patient smokes, it is important to do health teaching during the intervention phase to help her quit. There is an increased

incidence of complications in women on estrogen therapy who continue to smoke.

NURSING DIAGNOSIS

- Establish the nursing diagnoses. Typical nursing diagnoses for patients requiring estrogen and progestogens include the following: Knowledge Deficit, Altered Sexual Patterns, Sexual Dysfunction, Body Image Disturbance, and Self-Esteem Disturbance.

Table 47–12. SIGNS OF ESTROGEN/PROGESTIN EXCESS AND DEFICIT

Sign	Estrogen Excess	Progestin Excess	Estrogen Deficit	Progestin Deficit
Abnormal distention	x	—	—	—
Breast tenderness	x	x	—	—
Cystic breasts	x	—	—	—
Dysmenorrhea	x	—	—	x
Edema	x	—	—	—
Hypermenorrhea	x	—	—	x
Increased breast size	x	x	—	—
Migraine headache	x	—	—	—
Nervousness	x	—	x	—
Uterine cramping	x	—	—	—
Weight gain	x	x	—	—
Change in libido	—	x	—	—
Depression	—	x	—	—
Fatigue	—	x	—	—
Hypomenorrhea	—	x	x	—
Vaginal infection	—	x	—	—
Amenorrhea	—	—	x	x
Cystocele, rectocele	—	—	x	—
Irritability	x	—	x	—
Decreased breast size	—	—	—	x
Weight loss	—	—	—	x

INTERVENTION

- Develop the list of goals for nursing interventions from the list of nursing diagnoses (see Table 47–11).

Nursing Responsibilities when Administering Female Hormones

- Encourage all patients taking estrogen, progestins, or oral contraceptives to practice preventive health measures. Regular gynecologic examinations with Pap tests are important.
- Ensure that the patient understands how to practice breast self-examination and encourage this practice on a monthly basis.
- Monitor body weight and blood pressure regularly.
- Assist the patient in selecting the form of medication that is best. Estrogen is available in many forms such as pills, patches, creams, and gels. The administration route and dosage will depend on symptoms, medical history, and contraindications.

Patient Teaching

- Teach patients about the use of oral contraceptives, as presented in Table 47–13. Additional information may include the recommended use of additional methods of birth control during the first week of the initial cycle and instructions for dealing with missed pills. The following serves as a guideline only:
  One omitted pill: The missed tablet can be taken as soon as remembered or taken the next day with the regular dose (double up).
  Two consecutive omitted pills: Use another contraceptive method for the next 7 days, then take 2 tablets daily for 2 days, and resume regular schedule.
  Three consecutive omitted pills: The cycle should be resumed 7 days after the last tablet was taken; an-

other method of contraception should be used during this period and for 7 days into the cycle.

If pregnancy is suspected, the woman should contact her physician. Estrogen and progesterones can cause fetal abnormalities and, therefore, must be discontinued.

Table 47–13. PATIENT TEACHING INFORMATION—FEMALE HORMONES

Dear Patient:
  This drug has been prescribed for you. This is what you should know about your drug to get the most from your therapy.
  Female hormones are used for several reasons. For you they are being used for _____.

- ☐ 1. Female hormones are taken for an indefinite time; your doctor will tell you what is best for you.
- ☐ 2. Take your drugs exactly as ordered.
- ☐ 3. Do not take female hormones if you have a history of blood clots, stroke, cancer (breast or genitalia), or liver disease.
- ☐ 4. Do not take female hormones if you are pregnant or breast-feeding.
- ☐ 5. Take oral female hormones after meals to decrease feeling "sick to your stomach."
- ☐ 6. Do not stop taking your female hormones without first checking with your doctor.
- ☐ 7. Report any side effects to your doctor. Two are weight gain and jaundice (yellowing of skin or eyeball).
- ☐ 8. Immediately report any pain, redness, or swelling in your legs; these could be signs of a blood clot.
- ☐ 9. Immediately report sudden partial or complete loss of vision, double vision, or migraine. *Do not* continue to take your drugs until you talk with your physician.
- ☐ 10. Check your weight weekly at the same time of day. Report a gain/loss of weight of more than _____ pounds per week.
- ☐ 11. Practice regular breast self-examination and have regular PAP exams.
- ☐ 12. Stop smoking.
- ☐ 13. Carry a Medic Alert card or other similar identification.
- ☐ 14. Store your drugs in tightly closed containers.

- Teach the female patient about other methods of contraception and emphasize the importance of safe sex not only to prevent an unwanted pregnancy but also to prevent sexually transmitted diseases including HIV. This teaching includes the use of condoms—both male and female—and diaphragms.

EVALUATION

- Determine the effectiveness of the nursing interventions. The expected outcomes for patients requiring drugs affecting the female reproductive system are included in Table 47–11.

     The patient using female hormones for contraception should be expected to have an understanding of her reproductive cycle, the function of oral contraceptives within that cycle, side effects and potential risks associated with them, and the necessity for consistent use to achieve maximum effectiveness.

- Understand and monitor for the adverse effects of these drugs. The nurse determines that the patient understands them as well. Adverse effects of the estrogens and progestins include nausea, vomiting, diarrhea, skin rashes, irregular menstrual bleeding, and headache.

Compliance with medication regimens depends somewhat on the circumstances that initiate therapy. For example, patients taking fertility drugs are usually very conscientious about their medication, as it reflects yet another in a series of interventions designed to achieve pregnancy. Once pregnant, the patient is cautioned about taking all medications. (Refer to a maternal text for more information.) Compliance by patients taking oral contraceptives is related to the strength of their desire to avoid pregnancy and to their feelings regarding pregnancy or a termination of pregnancy should it result.

A large number of unplanned pregnancies continue to occur in the adolescent population. Studies of unmarried sexually active adolescents initiating use of oral contraceptives have found predictors of compliance to include white race, age (over 18 years), history of prior contraceptive use, older sexual partner, and satisfaction with the pill. Additional predictors of compliance include having a private suburban health-care provider, married parents, and suburban residence. Much health teaching is required to gain compliance in the nonwhite, young group.

Throughout, the nurse stresses the need for continuous medical follow-up and should periodically review teaching with the patient to ensure that the patient's information is accurate and up to date.

GONADOTROPIN-RELEASING HORMONES

Products that affect gonadotropin-releasing hormone (GnRH) include the following: **gonadorelin acetate (Lu-**

trepulse); **leuprolide acetate (Lupron)** which stimulates the release of GnRH; and **nafareline acetate (Synarel)** and **histrelin acetate (Supprelin)**, which are GnRH agonists that decrease or control GnRH release. Gonadotropin acetate is used to stimulate ovulation in women with primary hypothalamic amenorrhea. Nafarelin acetate is a potent agonistic analog of GnRH. Within 2 to 4 weeks of the start of administration, LH and FSH production are reduced. Thus nafarelin is used to reduce the size and decrease the pain associated with endometriosis lesions. Histrelin acetate is also a GnRH releasing hormone agonist that is used to reduce the biochemical and clinical manifestations of central precocious puberty. After therapy for 3 months, there is a decrease in FSH and LH production.

These drugs should be administered only by physicians familiar with their use. Patients are monitored closely with ovarian ultrasound and pelvic exams at regular intervals.

Pharmacokinetics and dosages are presented in Table 47–14.

Adverse effects include hot flushes, edema, vaginal dryness, multiple gastrointestinal complaints, and headaches.

○ **Gonadorelin acetate** (Lutrepulse), a synthetic product identical to GnRH, is administered IV in a pulsatile fashion to approximate the natural hormonal secretion of GnRH, which in turn causes the release of LH and FSH.

CONTRAINDICATIONS AND PRECAUTIONS Contraindications include (1) any condition that could be exacerbated by pregnancy and (2) sensitivity to this product. Ovarian cysts, hormone dependent tumors, or any condition that may worsen is also a contraindication. Multiple pregnancies (12%) are a possibility, but can be minimized by careful attention to recommended doses.

ADVERSE EFFECTS Adverse effects occur in approximately 10% of all treated patients. Ovarian hypersecretion (sudden ovarian enlargement) with ascites or pleural effusion may necessitate temporary interruption of therapy.

○ **Nafarelin acetate** (Synarel) is administered by nasal spray.

CONTRAINDICATIONS AND PRECAUTIONS Nafarelin acetate is contraindicated in hypersensitivity and undiagnosed abnormal vaginal bleeding, pregnancy, and lactation. Use cautiously use in patients with a strong family history of osteoporosis, chronic alcohol or tobacco use, and other risk factors that are known to decrease bone mineralization. Bone density may decrease during use.

ADVERSE EFFECTS Nasal irritation may also occur, as nafarelin acetate is administered by nasal spray. If rhinitis occurs a decongestant may be ordered, but should not be used for at least 30 minutes after the nafarelin acetate dose.

○ **Histrelin acetate** (Supprelin) is administered as a subcutaneous injection on a daily basis for precocious puberty in girls before eight and in boys before 9.5.

CONTRAINDICATIONS AND PRECAUTIONS Histrelin acetate is contraindicated in known hypersensitivity, pregnancy (category X), and lactation.

Table 47–14. GONADOTROPIN-RELEASING HORMONES

DRUG NAME/ROUTE AND DOSAGE	PHARMACOKINETICS/ DYNAMICS	NURSING IMPLICATIONS
gonadorelin acetate (Lutrepulse)		
Lutrepulse Pump–2.5–20 μL IV q 90 min for 21 days.	**Onset:** immediate **Peak:** NA **Duration:** NA **½L:** 2–40 min **PB:** NA **B:** hepatic **E:** urine	**ASSESSMENT:** Thorough history is needed; assess for pregnancy (category B). **INTERVENTION:** Maintain sterility at pump site. Change IV site and cannula q 48 hr.
nafarelin acetate (Synarel)		
endometriosis *Adults:* 1 spray (200 μg) into 1 nostril in AM and other nostril in PM. Start treatment between days 2 to 4 of menstrual cycle, for 6 mo.	**Onset:** rapid **Peak:** 10–40 min **Duration:** NA **½L:** 3 hr; 85.5 hr (metabolites) **PB:** 80% **B:** liver **E:** urine, feces	**ASSESSMENT:** Assess for pregnancy (category X) and rhinitis. Monitor for bone loss. **INTERVENTION:** Administer by nasal spray. **EVALUATION:** Notify physician if irregular menses persists.
histrelin acetate (Supprelin)		
Adults: 10 μg/kg SC daily.	**Onset:** NA **Peak:** NA **Duration:** NA **½L:** NA **PB:** NA **B:** liver **E:** urine	**ASSESSMENT:** Assess baseline information such as height and weight and other endocrine function and dysfunction. Assess for pregnancy (category X). **INTERVENTION:** Teach importance of complying with daily injection to be given at about same time each day. Store medication in refrigerator and protect from light. Allow to reach room temperature before administration. Rotate injection sites. **EVALUATION:** Report rash, urticaria, irregular heart beat, difficulty in swallowing to doctor. Evaluate q 3 mo for effectiveness.
leuprolide acetate (Lupron)		
IV–0.3 mg/kg q 4 wk as single dose; *IM*–3.75 mg/kg q 4 wk.	**Onset:** NA **Peak:** NA **Duration:** NA **½L:** 3 hr–12 wk depending on product **PB:** NA **B:** NA **E:** urine	Same as above.

NA = not available.

FERTILITY MEDICATIONS

Infertility is generally defined as the inability to conceive after 1 year or more of unprotected, regular sexual intercourse. About 10% to 15% of American couples are estimated to be involuntarily infertile. Depending on the etiology of the infertility problem, medications may be prescribed to bring hormone levels to normal or to enhance ovarian function—the so-called fertility drugs. Several drugs are currently used to stimulate ovulation in the anovulatory infertile woman. These drugs are featured in Table 47–15. Three are gonadotropins: **human chorionic gonadotropin, or *HCG (Follutein)*,** prepared from the urine of pregnant women; **menotropins**—human menopausal gonadotropin, or **HMG *(Humegon, Pergonal)*;** and **urofollitropin *(Metrodin)*,** a preparation of FSH and LH extracted from the urine of postmenopausal women. Chorionic gonadotropin is secreted by the placenta during pregnancy and functions to sustain the corpus luteum. The fourth drug is **clomiphene *(Clomid)*,** which is often classified as an antiestrogen but has weak estrogenic properties as well.

The use of menotropins and urofollitropin stimulates growth and maturation of ovarian follicles owing to the FSH and LH activities. Clomiphene competes for estrogen-binding sites, leaving fewer receptors available for endogenous estrogen attachment. This interferes with the normal feedback mechanism, and the body (hypothalamus) interprets this as a low level of estrogen. Conse-

Table 47–15. FERTILITY DRUGS

DRUG NAME/ROUTE AND DOSAGE	PHARMACOKINETICS/ DYNAMICS	NURSING IMPLICATIONS
clomiphene (Clomid) 50 mg/day PO for 5 days starting on 5th day of cycle; if ovulation does not occur, increase to 100 mg/day for 5 days.	**Onset:** rapid **Peak:** NA **Duration:** 6 wk **½L:** 5 days **PB:** NA **B:** liver **E:** feces	**ASSESSMENT:** A pelvic exam is done to determine ovarian size. Endometrial biopsy may be obtained. Assess for pregnancy (category unknown). **INTERVENTION:** Take exactly as prescribed for 5 consecutive days. Do not administer if history of ovarian cysts exists. **Patient Teaching—**Instruct patient that properly timed coitus is important. **EVALUATION:** Report any visual changes, bloating, abdominal pain, persistent hot flushes at once.
HUMAN MENOPAUSAL GONADOTROPIN (HMG)		
menotropins (Pergonal) **Females:** 75–150 IU IM qd for 9–12 days. **Males:** 1 amp IM 3 times per week	**Onset:** NA **Peak:** NA **Duration:** NA **½L:** FSH, 70 hr; LH, 4 hr **PB:** NA **B:** NA **E:** NA	**ASSESSMENT:** Same as above. **INTERVENTION:** *Females*—Administer 7th to 14th day of cycle. Dose is dependent on estradiol levels and follicle size as determined by ultrasound. *Males*—Pretreat with 5000 IV of HCG 3 times per wk for 4–6 mo. If after 6 mo there is still no sperm, start menotropins. Administer deep IM. Prepare by diluting with 1–2 mL of sterile normal saline solution. Administer immediately after preparation. Do not administer if history of ovarian cysts exists. Couple should have intercourse every other day starting with last day of therapy.
urofollitropin (Metrodin) 75 IU/day IM for 7–12 days plus 2 more courses	**Onset:** NA **Peak:** NA **Duration:** NA **½L:** NA **PB:** NA **B:** NA **E:** NA	**ASSESSMENT:** Assess for pregnancy (category X). **INTERVENTION:** Administer for 7–12 days. Dose depends on estradiol levels and follicle size as determined by ultrasound. Couple should have intercourse daily starting with last day of therapy. Dissolve amp in 1–2 mL saline and administer immediately. Discard unused medication. Protect from light.
human chorionic gonadotropins (HCG, Follutein) **Males:** 500–5000 U IM 2–3 times/wk **Females:** Single dose of 10000 U IM	**Onset:** NA **Peak:** 2 hr **Duration:** 3–4 days **½L:** 23 hr **PB:** NA **B:** NA **E:** NA	**ASSESSMENT:** Assess for pregnancy (category C). **INTERVENTION:** Administer at optimal estrogen levels to stimulate ovulation. Administer deep IM. Reconstitute with diluent supplied by manufacturer. Stable for 1–3 months after reconstitution under refrigeration.

NA = not available.

quently, there is an increased secretion of gonadotropins. Clomiphene is most effective in women who have adequate amounts of estrogen and follicular function, but who lack effective stimulation from the pituitary gonadotropins.

In many treatment regimens for infertility, clomiphene is employed initially, particularly when inadequate gonadotropic stimulation exists. Most women who respond to clomiphene ovulate after the first course of therapy. Generally, no more than three courses of therapy are recommended if there is no response to the drug.

If ovulation still has not occurred, HCG can be administered in conjunction with the clomiphene during that cycle. HCG is given at midcycle to induce ovulation within approximately 18 to 48 hours. If this therapy, too, proves ineffective, menotropins can be administered during the next cycle. FSH and LH are administered intramuscularly for 9 to 12 days. Then chorionic gonadotropin is given until optimal estrogen levels have been reached. Two to five such treatment cycles may be required for success. A 90% ovulation rate and a 50% to 70% pregnancy rate have been attained. The use of menotropins necessitates almost daily ultrasound to determine follicle size and to strictly monitor estradiol levels.

Therapy with fertility drugs is not without problems. The most common reactions to clomiphene administration include hot flushes, breast discomfort, headache, nausea and vomiting, abdominal distention, and pain related to ovarian enlargement. Visual disturbances such as blurred vision, sparkling visual sensations, ghosting, and photophobia can also occur.

The use of chorionic gonadotropin and menotropins is associated with an increased risk of thromboembolic disease. Headache, irritability, and restlessness can occur when HCG is administered to pregnant women. Both drugs can also induce the ovarian hyperstimulation discussed in relation to clomiphene.

The possibility of multiple births increases with the use of the fertility drugs. Clomiphene administration is associated with a 10% chance of multiple births (usually twins); use of menotropins and HCG is associated with a 5% chance of having three or more babies.

USING THE NURSING PROCESS

ASSESSMENT

- Assess all of the information listed in the section on female hormones, along with further specialized testing. Disorders that are at least partly amenable to drug therapy include unfavorable cervical mucus, anovulation, luteal phase defect, and endometriosis. Because infertility can be due to factors affecting the male as well as the female, both partners are assessed.
- Obtain a thorough sexual history (including, but not limited to, frequency of intercourse, timing in relation to ovulation, and use of contraceptives) from both partners. Assessment of the male includes an endocrine evaluation and semen analysis. Assessment of the female includes the previously mentioned tests of ovarian function as well as regular measurements of basal body temperature (progesterone has a thermogenic effect), endometrial biopsy, and the tubal insufflation or Rubin test. Endoscopic procedures such as culdoscopy or laparoscopy may also be used.

NURSING DIAGNOSIS

- Establish the nursing diagnoses. Typical nursing diagnoses for the woman requiring fertility medica-

tions include Altered Family Process and Body Image Disturbance.

INTERVENTION

- Plan the nursing interventions. For the infertile patient electing use of ovulatory medications, the nurse must again emphasize the teaching aspects of care, giving the client and her partner necessary information about the drugs she is taking and the expected results.
- Provide psychologic support for these clients. The process of diagnosis and treatment for infertility can be a long, frustrating one in which the anticipated outcome (pregnancy) cannot be guaranteed.
- Teach the patient proper administration times. The timing of administration of the fertility drugs is crucial to their successful use. Following drug administration, couples should be directed to have intercourse within 12 to 18 hours and daily for the next 2 days.

EVALUATION

- Develop evaluation criteria. Although the patient may feel that the only successful outcome of treatment with fertility drugs is a pregnancy, that cannot be guaranteed. Criteria should include a patient who is knowledgeable about her therapy and her drugs and who experiences minimal side effects.

The nurse should make certain that the patient is aware of side effects to anticipate. Adverse effects of the fertility drugs include nausea and vomiting, headache, and ovarian enlargement. The ovarian enlargement that can occur with clomiphene use can pose serious problems. The hyperstimulated ovaries are enlarged, fragile, and often cystic. Strenuous physical activity, a pelvic examination, or intercourse can, at this time, cause rupture of ovarian cysts. Symptoms of enlargement to caution the patient about include (1) unilateral pelvic discomfort aggravated by walking and/or (2) abdominal distention. Should these occur, the nurse encourages the patient to minimize her activity, avoid intercourse, and notify her physician. Other indicators of distress include sudden weight gain, abdominal pain, vaginal bleeding, and dyspnea.

The bibliography for this chapter can be found in Appendix B, which begins on page 1054.

CHAPTER REVIEW QUESTIONS

1. Androgen therapy is contraindicated in which of the following conditions?
   a. Postpartum breast engorgement.
   b. Endometriosis
   c. Cancer of the prostate gland
   d. Metastatic breast cancer.

2. Estrogen preparations increase the effect of which of the following drugs when used in combination?
   a. Hydrocortisone
   b. Phenytoin
   c. Tetracycline
   d. Rifampin

3. Which of the following signs indicates the need to discontinue oral contraceptives?
   a. Nausea and vomiting
   b. Upper-quadrant abdominal pain
   c. Headache with eyestrain
   d. Pain and tenderness in the calf

4. An advantage of triphasic oral contraceptive products is:
   a. Reduced risk of vascular effects
   b. Reduced breakthrough bleeding
   c. Increased protection in the early cycle
   d. Increased resistance to infection

*See Appendix A, which begins on page 1051, for answers.

5. Progestin-only agents used for contraception are referred to as minipills. The progestins exert their contraceptive action by:
   a. Altering cervical mucus
   b. Causing delayed ovulation
   c. Blocking ovulation
   d. Interfering with androstenedione

6. Women taking androgenic therapy for cancer of the breast should be observed for signs of:
   a. Hypercalcemia
   b. Hypokalemia
   c. Hyponatremia
   d. Hypermagnesemia

CHAPTER 48

Drugs Used in Pregnancy, Labor and Delivery, and Abortion

Patricia Robin McCartney, RNC, PhD

CHAPTER OUTLINE

Introduction to Drug Use During Pregnancy and Lactation
Drugs Used For Maternal Conditions
Drugs Used For Pain Management in Labor and Delivery
Drugs That Affect Uterine Activity

TABLES

Drug Tables
Magnesium Sulfate, 720
Tocolytics, 723
Oxytocics, 726
Nursing Process
Nursing Process for the Pregnant or Lactating Mother
    Requiring Medication, 719

BOXES

Delivering Home Health Care, 729
Building Your Critical Thinking Skills, 730

KEY TERMS

Abortifacient	Teratogen
Oxytocic	Tocolytic

LEARNING OBJECTIVES

After reading this chapter, the student will be able to:

1. Describe alterations in pharmacokinetics during pregnancy.
2. Identify mechanisms that affect transfer of drugs to the fetus during pregnancy and to the infant during lactation.
3. Outline guidelines for safe drug administration during pregnancy and lactation.
4. Apply the nursing process to pregnant and lactating mothers receiving medication.
5. Discuss drugs used during pregnancy for maternal conditions.
6. Discuss drugs used for pain management during labor and delivery.
7. Discuss drugs used to suppress uterine activity.
8. Discuss drugs used to stimulate uterine activity.

The use of drugs by both pregnant women and women of childbearing age is common. Increasingly, drugs are a component of therapy in conditions associated with pregnancy. This chapter will summarize essential elements to consider for safe administration of drugs during pregnancy and refer the reader to sections of this text where drugs are discussed in more depth. Both prescription and over-the-counter (OTC) drugs are discussed. Substance abuse is addressed in Chapter 67, for detailed obstetric protocols see specialty resources.

Paramount to the administration of drugs during pregnancy and lactation is the recognition of the presence of two patients. The benefits versus risks for both mother and fetus or infant are considered. Maternal physiologic stability is necessary for fetal survival, and the mother has the right to relief of symptoms and treatment that is necessary for her health. Collaboration and consultation among health-care providers for the best interests of the mother and the fetus or infant are essential.

A framework for safe administration of drugs during pregnancy starts with a discussion of the effect of pregnancy on pharmacokinetics, the placental transfer of drugs, the effect of drugs on the fetus, and the breastmilk transfer of drugs, and concludes with both guidelines for administration of drugs during pregnancy and a nursing-care plan.

INTRODUCTION TO DRUG USE DURING PREGNANCY AND LACTATION

EFFECT OF PREGNANCY ON PHARMACOKINETICS

Hormone changes and physiologic adaptations of pregnancy alter pharmacokinetic variables of absorption, distribution, metabolism, and excretion, which may necessitate modifications in drug administration during pregnancy.

During pregnancy, increased production of progesterone decreases gastrointestinal motility and prolongs gastric emptying time while increased production of estrogen stimulates gastric secretion of hydrochloric acid and causes gastric pH changes. Although this suggests altered drug absorption of orally administered drugs, clinical evidence has not supported this conclusion. The oral route may be limited in pregnancy with nausea and vomiting occurring during early pregnancy or during labor. Pulmonary absorption of inhaled drugs is thought to be enhanced due to increased pulmonary blood flow and increased tidal volume.

As pregnancy advances, there is a progressive and substantial increase in total body water, with the greatest portion of the increase occurring in the extracellular fluid. Plasma volume increases by 50%, causing hemodilution of plasma albumin and potential alteration in drug distribution. Endocrine hormones compete for the protein-binding sites available. The combination of hemodilution, expanded volume of distribution, and reduced protein-binding sites may decrease the serum concentration of drugs. Drugs with low lipid solubility that remain highly bound to plasma protein are widely distributed within this increased volume. A larger portion of unbound or free drug may be available to leave the vascular bed and enter the placental circulation.

Circulating steroid hormones are believed to stimulate metabolizing enzymes in the liver, but also are suspected to compete with drugs for these enzyme sites. The placenta and fetal liver do contribute to drug metabolism.

Hepatic blood flow is unchanged during pregnancy, so drugs dependent on hepatic blood flow for clearance are eliminated at the same rate as in the nonpregnant woman. As pregnancy progresses, there is a substantial increase in renal plasma blood flow, glomerular filtration, and creatinine clearance, resulting in a more rapid renal excretion of drugs.

Despite physiologic alterations, most medication dosages are unchanged during pregnancy. Serum concentrations of some drugs used during pregnancy are monitored to maintain therapeutic levels. Drugs with a long half-life may require a loading dose to achieve therapeutic serum levels, especially in drugs with a large volume of distribution (which may result in a longer half-life). A higher concentration of the unbound fraction of a drug may promote pharmacologic effects at a subtherapeutic level.

PLACENTAL TRANSFER OF DRUGS

The placenta actually functions more like a conduit than a barrier as nearly all medications can and do transfer from maternal to fetal circulation in the placenta. Most drug transfer is accomplished by diffusion along a concentration gradient. A small amount of drugs are transferred by active transport or facilitated diffusion. Variables that affect transfer include chemical properties of the drug, acid-base status, concentration gradient, and placental blood flow.

Physicochemical properties of the drug that influence placental transfer include molecular weight, degree of ionization, lipid solubility, and capacity for plasma protein and tissue binding. Substances with a molecular weight less than 600 (e.g., warfarin sodium) cross the placenta easily, substances with a molecular weight between 600 and 1000 cross more slowly, and substances with a molecular weight greater than 1000 (e.g., heparin) do not cross the placenta. The more highly ionized a drug molecule is, the less likely it is to cross the placenta. Lipid-soluble drugs cross the placenta more easily. Drugs that are highly bound to maternal plasma protein or tissue do not cross the placenta into the fetus, and drugs that are highly bound to fetal plasma protein or tissue remain concentrated in the fetus. Because fetal pH is slightly lower than maternal, drugs that have an alkaline pH can accumulate in the fetus. This effect is more pronounced with fetal acidosis.

The rate of drug transfer across the placenta is affected by blood flow. Uterine circulation—and consequent placental, umbilical, and fetal circulation—depend on optimum blood volume and pressure in the mother. Any condition that renders the mother hypertensive, hypotensive, or hypovolemic reduces uterine blood flow. Uterine blood flow is reduced when the mother lies supine, because the gravid uterus compresses circulation in the vena cava and aorta. Uterine contractions of labor reduce placental circulation. The rate of drug transfer is decreased at these times of decreased blood flow and may result in an accumulation of drugs in the fetus. Transfer occurs across a thin layer of trophoblastic tissue. Any damage to this tissue can result in direct mixture of maternal and fetal blood and concomitant drugs.

EFFECT OF DRUGS ON FETUS

Once a drug enters the fetal circulation, factors that mediate the effect on the fetus include fetal pharmacokinetics, properties of the specific drug, and the fetal gestational age. These factors influence whether the drug is a potential *teratogen*, an agent that causes fetal harm.

Fetal plasma protein-binding capacity is lower than maternal, resulting in more free drug available for tissue binding and tissue-specific accumulation. The central nervous system (CNS) is especially vulnerable as permeability of the fetal blood-brain barrier is greater than maternal. Fetal hepatic and renal biotransformation and excretion capacity is lower than maternal and is further reduced if placental circulation is compromised.

Factors that determine degree of fetal effect include

drug properties, dose, duration of exposure, and time of exposure. The degree of teratogenicity varies with fetal gestational age at the time of exposure. The first trimester is a critical period of organogenesis, and insult at this time can cause spontaneous abortion or gross structural defects identifiable prenatally or at birth. Exposure during the second and third trimester can cause more subtle, delayed, or long-term defects that may not manifest until several years after birth.

BREASTMILK TRANSFER OF DRUGS

Studies on drug transfer into breastmilk are limited, but most drugs absorbed by the mother are believed to pass into breastmilk to some extent. Transfer is accomplished largely by diffusion and minimally by facilitated diffusion or active transport. Variables that determine the transfer and concentration of drugs include physicochemical properties of the drug, mammary gland blood flow, and breastmilk secretion.

Mammary blood flow determines the distribution of drugs to the breast. The sucking infant stimulates the release of milk from the mammary gland, so the infant should not be fed at the time of peak maternal serum levels. Administration of drugs prior to feeding increases the chance of transfer into breastmilk, whereas administration after a feeding or before the infant's longest sleep period decreases the chance of transfer. Secretion of breastmilk requires secretion of the hormone prolactin from the anterior pituitary and is affected by drugs. Exogenous estrogen and progesterone suppress prolactin secretion, as the placental estrogen and progesterone did during pregnancy. Further information on estrogen and progesterone can be found in Chapter 47. Nonpharmacologic methods of suppressing lactation have largely replaced lactation suppression drugs.

GUIDELINES FOR DRUG ADMINISTRATION DURING PREGNANCY AND LACTATION

Ethical concerns limit human research on drug administration during pregnancy. Most reported studies either use animal models or are retrospective human studies that are confounded by the maternal condition originally requiring medication and/or the administration of multiple medications. More studies are needed to determine the effective dosage of drugs during pregnancy. The Federal Drug Administration (FDA) has defined five potential fetal risk categories to improve drug labeling, as presented in Table 48–1; however, authorities are cautious and disagree regarding research interpretations and recommendations. Many manufacturers have not labeled their products with a pregnancy risk category. Detailed teratogenicity is provided by Briggs et al. (1994) and TERIS (Teratogen Information System), a computerized database of teratogen research. A number of drugs and their respective risks during pregnancy or lactation are summarized in Table 48–2 and Table 48–3.

General principles for administration of medication during pregnancy and lactation include the following:

Table 48–1. FDA FETAL RISK CATEGORIES FOR DRUGS USED DURING PREGNANCY

Category A: Controlled human studies fail to demonstrate fetal risk.

Category B: Animal studies fail to demonstrate fetal risk and there are no controlled human studies, or animal studies demonstrate fetal risk and controlled human studies fail to demonstrate fetal risk.

Category C: Animal studies demonstrate fetal risk and there are no controlled human studies to rule out fetal risk, or there are no animal or human studies. Benefit justifies risk.

Category D: Controlled human studies demonstrate fetal risk. Benefit justifies risk. Use in life-threatening situation.

Category X: Controlled human studies demonstrate fetal risk. Risk outweighs benefit. Use in pregnant or potentially pregnant women is contraindicated.

1. Assess women of childbearing age for pregnancy prior to drug therapy.
2. Use medication only when clearly indicated.
3. Use nonpharmacologic alternatives when possible.
4. The risk-versus-benefit ratio should justify the use of a particular medication.
5. Delay medication until after the first trimester when possible.
6. Use the minimum therapeutic dose for as short a duration as possible.
7. Monitor serum levels with long-term use.
8. Monitor mother, fetus, and infant for toxic effects.
9. Use as few medications as possible to reduce interactions and synergistic toxic effects.
10. Avoid use of combination products.

Table 48–2. DRUG USE DURING PREGNANCY

Safely Used Drugs	Cautiously Used Drugs	Contraindicated Drugs
Acetaminophen	Acyclovir	ACE Inhibitors
Bisacodyl	Antihistamines	Aminopterin
Cephalosporins	Antithyroids	Androgens
Docusate sodium	Antitussives	Coumadin derivatives
Heparin	Aspirin	and warfarin
Immune globulins	Atropine	Chloramphenicol
Insulin	Barbiturates	Estrogens
Maalox	Clindamycin	Ibuprofen
Penicillins	Chlorpromazine	Indomethacin
	Decongestants	Iodide
	Diazepam	Isotretinoin lithium
	Digitalis	Live vaccines
	Erythromycin	Methotrexate
	Expectorants	Podophyllin
	Gentamicin	Progestins
	Glucocorticoids	Radioiodine
	Inactive vaccines	Ribavirin
	Isoniazid	Streptomycin
	Metronidazole	Sulfonylureas
	Propranolol	Tetracycline
	Propylthiouracil	Thiazide diuretics
	Rifampin	Valproic acid
	Sulfonamides	
	Theophylline	

Table 48–3. DRUG USE DURING LACTATION		
Safely Used Drugs	**Cautiously Used Drugs**	**Contraindicated Drugs**
Bisacodyl	Acetaminophen	Bromides
Cephalosporins	Acyclovir	Chloramphenicol
Digitalis	Aminoglycosides	Cimetidine
Docusate sodium	Ampicillin	Diazepam
Epinephrine	Aspirin	Ergotamine
Heparin	Atropine	Estrogen
Insulin	Barbiturates	Furosemide
Methyldopa	Casanthranol	Indomethacin
Milk of Magnesia	Cascara	Iodide
Phenothiazines	Chlorpromazine	Isoniazid
Propranolol	Clindamycin	Methadone
	Codeine	Methotrexate
	Coumadin derivatives and warfarin	Metronidazole
	Erythromycin	Propylthiouracil
	Gentamicin	Sulfonylureas
	Hydralazine	Tetracycline
	Ibuprofen	
	Magnesium sulfate	
	Meperidine hydrochloride	
	Methylergonovine	
	Morphine	
	Oxycodone	
	Phenytoin	
	Prednisone	
	Senna	
	Sulfonamides	
	Thiazide diuretics	

Table 48–4 provides a nursing-care plan for drug administration during pregnancy and lactation.

DRUGS USED FOR MATERNAL CONDITIONS

Drugs are used during pregnancy and lactation for a number of conditions existing prior to pregnancy or arising during pregnancy. Table 48–5 summarizes drugs of choice.

PREGNANCY-INDUCED HYPERTENSION

Pregnancy-induced hypertension (PIH) consists of both preeclampsia (hypertension, edema, and proteinuria) and eclampsia (preeclampsia with convulsions). Maternal and fetal mortality is significant with PIH, and the only known cure is delivery of the fetus.

Hypertension occurring during pregnancy may be a chronic problem or induced by pregnancy. In either case, the antihypertensive most widely used for long-term control is methyldopa (Aldomet); and for marked hypertension or hypertensive crisis, hydralazine (Apresoline). These drugs lower blood pressure without reducing placental perfusion. More information on these antihypertensive drugs is found in Chapter 30.

Seizure prophylaxis is accomplished with the administration of magnesium sulfate ($MgSO_4$), phenytoin, or aspirin. Phenytoin is a well-tolerated alternative to magnesium sulfate. The intravenous administration of phenytoin involves a loading dose, followed by a maintenance dose, and the monitoring of serum phenytoin levels. Recently, low-dose aspirin (60 to 150 mg per day) taken during the second and third trimester has been shown to reduce the risks of PIH with no maternal or neonatal adverse effects. Aspirin selectively inhibits the synthesis of the vasoactive prostaglandin thromboxane A_2, thereby reducing the occurrence of vasoconstriction.

○ **Magnesium sulfate** is the standard drug of choice for seizure prophylaxis in PIH (see Table 48–6). It is given intravenously and less frequently intramuscularly for immediate stabilization and maintenance. Maintenance therapy with oral magnesium sulfate has been reported. This anticonvulsant acts as a CNS and muscular depressant by producing peripheral neuromuscular blockade. Magnesium sulfate secondarily relaxes smooth muscle and decreases blood pressure; however, it is not classified as an antihypertensive agent. The smooth muscle relaxation also decreases uterine contractions, often necessitating oxytocin administration for labor progress.

Administration protocols differ in method, dosage, and target serum magnesium level. The intravenous route is preferred as the intramuscular route is associated with pain and uneven serum levels. Magnesium sulfate is diluted in a physiologic solution and administered with an infusion controller into a primary intravenous infusion as close to the venipuncture site as possible.

Side effects include flushing, burning at infusion site, sweating, thirst, weakness, slurred speech, visual blurring, headache, nausea, confusion, sedation, and hypotension. Hypotensive episodes reduce placental perfusion and can cause fetal hypoxia. Diminished deep-tendon reflexes and respiratory depression indicate approaching toxicity. A serum level greater than 4 mEq/liter is associated with toxicity. Pulmonary edema can develop in the presence of an increased intravascular volume. Magnesium sulfate readily crosses the placenta and results in a fetal serum concentration similar to the maternal serum concentration. Fetal effects include fetal heart rate changes, and neonatal effects include hypotonia and respiratory depression.

▼ CLINICAL ALERT

Concurrent use of magnesium sulfate with neuromuscular blocking agents may result in severe potentiation of neuromuscular blockade. Administration with digitalis glycosides may cause cardiac conduction changes and heart block. Use cautiously in patients with impaired renal function. The antidote for magnesium toxicity is calcium gluconate: 1 gram of a 5% to 10% solution is given intravenously over 1 to 2 minutes.

Using the Nursing Process in Pregnancy-Induced Hypertension

Assessment

- Assess vital signs, breath sounds, fluid intake, urinary output, edema, and deep-tendon reflexes hourly.

Table 48–4. NURSING PROCESS FOR THE PREGNANT OR LACTATING MOTHER REQUIRING MEDICATION

Assessment

Assess obstetric history including expected delivery date, previous pregnancies, and outcomes. If potentially pregnant, note last menstrual period.
Assess maternal, fetal, or infant status.
Assess indication for drug therapy.
Assess knowledge level, anxiety, and support systems.

Nursing Diagnosis: Risk for Maternal, Fetal, or Infant Injury	**Desired Outcomes/Evaluation Criteria**
RELATED TO: Adverse effects of drug therapy.	Therapeutic effect is achieved with minimal adverse effects to mother, fetus, or infant.
AS EVIDENCED BY: Signs of adverse effects or toxicity.	

Nursing Actions	**Rationale**
Identify drug FDA category and adapt drug administration to pregnancy protocols.	Some drugs are known teratogens or are contraindicated during pregnancy or lactation (see Tables 48–1, 48–2, 48–3).
Identify and monitor drug's desired effect; adverse effects; signs of toxicity in mother, fetus, or infant.	Early recognition of unfavorable effects allows for dose adjustments to reverse side effects or prevent toxicity.
Incorporate alternative nonpharmacologic actions for condition requiring medication.	Nonpharmacologic methods complement drug's effect and reduce dose or duration of therapy.
Inform infant care provider of maternal drug therapy.	Prenatal or infant drug exposure data needed for optimum infant care.
If toxic drug is necessary, discontinue breast-feeding and assist mother to pump breasts at regular intervals.	Pumping maintains milk production for future resumption of breast-feeding.
Schedule drugs to be taken after breast-feeding or at night. Avoid long-acting preparations.	Drugs taken after breast-feeding or during the infant's longest sleep period ensure least amount of drug present in milk at next feeding.

Nursing Diagnosis: Knowledge Deficit	**Desired Outcomes/Evaluation Criteria**
RELATED TO: Unfamiliarity with drug therapy.	Mother refrains from using unapproved drugs. Attends to teaching; verbalizes understanding of drug, therapeutic indication, adverse effects. Follows drug regimen correctly.
AS EVIDENCED BY: Inappropriate use, statements of misconception, questions, failure to report adverse effects.	

Nursing Actions	**Rationale**
Assess knowledge and readiness to learn about therapeutic drug use and risks during pregnancy (or if anticipating pregnancy).	Data provide baseline for individualized teaching.
Advise mother to inform all care providers of pregnancy or lactation and drugs she has taken, including OTC. No drugs should be taken without care-provider approval. Dosages should not be changed without care-provider approval.	Database necessary for optimum care.
Teach indication for drug (benefits) and adverse effects (risks). Provide written instructions and vary instructional format. Advise whom to call with questions.	Knowledge facilitates compliance with drug therapy. Written information can be reviewed frequently.

Other Suggested Nursing Diagnoses: Anxiety and Ineffective Individual or Family Coping.

- Weigh patient daily.
- Identify indicators of impending eclampsia including hyperreflexia, visual changes, headache, and epigastric pain.
- Measure urine specific gravity and protein.
- Monitor fetal heart rate and uterine activity.
- With magnesium sulfate, assess for toxicity including sedation level, weakness, respiratory depression, serum Mg level, and continuous cardiac monitoring.
- Assess the mother's knowledge level and anxiety.

Nursing Diagnosis

Typical nursing diagnoses for the patient requiring medication for PIH include Knowledge Deficit related to unfamiliarity with magnesium sulfate therapy and Risk for Maternal-Fetal Injury related to adverse effects of magnesium sulfate.

Intervention

- Maintain bed rest in lateral position.
- Maintain seizure precautions.

Table 48–5. DRUGS OF CHOICE DURING PREGNANCY

Drug Category	Drug of Choice
Analgesic/Antipyretic	Acetaminophen
Antacid	Aluminum hydroxide and magnesium hydroxide
Antiarrhythmic	Lidocaine
Antibiotic	Penicillin G
	Ampicillin
	Cephalosporins
	Erythromycin
Anticoagulant	Heparin
Anticonvulsant	Phenobarbital
PIH prophylaxis	Magnesium sulfate
Seizure arrest	Diazepam
Antidiabetic	Insulin
Antifungal	Miconazole (topical)
Antihypertensive	
(Chronic)	Methyldopa
(Acute, PIH)	Hydralazine
Antithyroid	Propylthiouracil
Antitrichomonal	Metronidazole (after 1st trimester)
Antituberculin	Isoniazid
Bronchodilator	Theophylline
Cardiac glycoside	Digitalis
Diuretic	Furosemide
HIV Antiviral	Zidovudine
Steroid	Prednisone
Stool softener	Docusate sodium
Thyroid supplement	Levothyroxine
Vasopressor	Ephedrine

- Keep nothing by mouth (NPO) status with parenteral fluids held at 100 to 125 cc/hr.
- Insert indwelling urinary catheter.
- Place emergency medications including the antidote calcium gluconate at the bedside.

- Stop infusion with symptoms of toxicity, including a respiratory rate below 12 per minute, urine output less than 100 mL per 4 hours, diminished deep-tendon reflexes, and serum Mg levels greater than 8 mg/dL.
- Alert neonatal personnel to assess the neonate for side effects.
- Provide emotional support and teaching.

Evaluation

Desired outcomes of successful therapy include the following:

- The mother receiving magnesium sulfate for seizure prophylaxis will display fewer symptoms of impending eclampsia.
- The eclamptic mother will display no further seizure activity.
- The mother and fetus will experience minimal adverse effects of magnesium sulfate.
- The mother will verbalize an understanding of magnesium sulfate therapy and cope effectively.

RH ISOIMMUNIZATION PROPHYLAXIS

Rho(D) immune globulin (RhoGAM) is administered to the Rho(D) negative woman who is unsensitized (negative antibody titer) and has been potentially exposed to Rh positive blood (antigen). Because isoimmunization of the Rh negative pregnant woman can occur anytime after 8 to 10 weeks' gestation, Rh immune globulin is administered after spontaneous or induced abortion, ectopic pregnancy, amniocentesis, chorionic villous sampling, trauma or feto-maternal hemorrhage, at 28 weeks' gestation, and after delivery of an Rh positive newborn with a negative antibody titer (direct Coombs). Immune glob-

Table 48–6. MAGNESIUM SULFATE

DRUG NAME/ROUTE AND DOSAGE	PHARMACOKINETICS/DYNAMICS	NURSING IMPLICATIONS
magnesium sulfate		
therapeutic serum level: 4–8 mg/dL *Loading Dose*–4–6 g/100 mL solution infused IV over 20–30 min. *Maintenance Dose*–1–3 g/hr. *IM*–1–5 g as 25%–50% solution q 4 hr.	**Onset:** IV, immediate; IM, 1 hr **Peak:** NA **Duration:** IV, 30 min; IM, 3–4 hr **½L:** NA **PB:** NA **B:** not biotransformed **E:** renal	**ASSESSMENT:** Daily weight, I/O, urine protein (PIH) and SG, edema, BP, RR; symptoms of pulmonary edema, uterine activity, and cervical changes (PTL); FHR, serum Mg levels, DTR, neurologic side effects. Assess for pregnancy (category A—PO; category D—IM/IV). **INTERVENTION:** Provide safety in presence of altered neurologic status, strict bed rest in lateral recumbent position, seizure precautions (PIH). Cautious fluid administration, NPO. Continuous cardiac monitoring with intravenous infusion. Keep calcium gluconate (antidote) available. Maintain therapeutic serum level of 1.5–2.5 mEq. **EVALUATION:** Patient demonstrates absence of convulsions or symptoms of impending convulsions (PIH). Patient demonstrates reduction and cessation of uterine contractions, absence of significant cervical change (PTL).

NA = not available; SG = specific gravity; BP = blood pressure; RR = respiratory rate; PTL = preterm labor; FHR = fetal heart rate; DTR = deep-tendon reflexes.

ulin is given to the pregnant and nonpregnant woman following a mismatched blood transfusion. For more information on how maternal sensitization occurs, consult an obstetrics textbook.

Rh immune globulin provides temporary (3 to 6 months) passive antibody protection by causing lysis of fetal Rh positive blood cells in the maternal circulation, effectively suppressing the development of maternal antibodies. Maternal antibodies could cross the placenta and hemolyze fetal positive red blood cells in a subsequent pregnancy. Prophylaxis must be repeated with each pregnancy.

The blood type and Rh factor of women of childbearing age is assessed to identify possible candidates for Rh immune globulin. If the woman is Rh negative, the antibody titer (indirect Coombs) is measured. The woman is given information describing the need for Rh immune globulin to protect future pregnancies and is instructed to carry identification of her Rh factor and immune globulin administration.

See Chapter 59 for information on immune globulin dosage and administration.

DRUGS USED FOR PAIN MANAGEMENT IN LABOR AND DELIVERY

Pharmacologic pain relief during labor and delivery is intended to decrease maternal discomfort and minimize adverse effects on the fetus and the progress of labor. Analgesics and anesthetics complement but do not replace nonpharmacologic methods of pain relief.

ANALGESICS

Systemic analgesics used during labor include meperidine hydrochloride (Demerol), nalbuphine (Nubain), butorphanol (Stadol), and morphine sulfate. The most common maternal side effects include nausea and vomiting, mild respiratory depression, transient CNS depression, postural hypotension, and urinary retention. Analgesics given before the onset of active labor decrease uterine activity. Analgesics readily cross the placenta and may cause fetal heart rate changes. Analgesics are not administered if delivery is expected to be less than 2 hours away because neonatal respiratory depression is possible. A narcotic antagonist such as naloxone hydrochloride (Narcan) should be available. Maternal vital signs, fetal heart rate, and cervical changes are assessed prior to analgesic administration, and maternal vital signs and fetal heart rate are assessed following administration. See Chapter 18 for more information on analgesics and narcotic antagonists.

ANESTHETICS

Anesthetics used during labor and delivery include local, regional, and general. A rapid-onset, short-acting anesthetic such as lidocaine hydrochloride (Xylocaine) is ad-

ministered by local infiltration at the time of delivery for pain relief during perineal repair.

Regional anesthetics used for active labor and delivery include pudendal block, paracervical block, subarachnoid block (spinal), and epidural block (lumbar and caudal). These anesthetics decrease uterine activity if given before active labor is established. Anesthetics also decrease the mother's urge to push, necessitating forceps or vacuum assistance with delivery. The pudendal and paracervical blocks are infrequently used, whereas the subarachnoid and the epidural are the most commonly used regional blocks.

Spinal anesthesia is used for delivery, whereas epidural anesthesia can be given continually from establishment of active labor on through delivery. Anesthetic agents used include lidocaine (Xylocaine) and the longer-acting bupivacaine (Marcaine). Epidural narcotic analgesics (fentanyl, butorphenol, morphine) have been used in combination with anesthetics to enhance pain relief while minimizing the sympathetic blockade of anesthetics. Combination analgesic and anesthetic are used for labor, delivery, and cesarean section. Epidural analgesics are used postoperatively with cesarean section. With pregnancy, vasodilation occurring with epidural and spinal regional blocks can cause maternal hypotension, reduce placental perfusion, and cause fetal hypoxia. Fluid volume deficit is corrected prior to anesthesia, and lateral uterine displacement is used to facilitate placental perfusion. Other side effects significant with pregnancy include labor and postpartum urinary retention and postpartum uterine atony.

General anesthetics are rarely used for uncomplicated vaginal deliveries but are used for cesarean deliveries. See chapter 21 for detailed information on anesthesia.

DRUGS THAT AFFECT UTERINE ACTIVITY

As labor begins, uterine muscle activity involves phasic contractions that constrict the upper fundal portion and change the cervix. These contractions are assessed in terms of frequency, strength, duration, and resting tone (relaxation between contractions) by gently placing the fingertips on the fundus. Cervical changes that facilitate labor are assessed in terms of progressive softening (effacement) and progressive opening (dilation) by vaginal examination. Following delivery, uterine muscle activity accomplishes involution, or contractions that reduce the size of the uterus and provide hemostasis at the placental site. Involution is assessed by palpating uterine tone, identifying fundal height, and evaluating vaginal bleeding (lochia).

When necessary, uterine muscle activity can be pharmacologically suppressed (such as in preterm labor) or stimulated (such as in pregnancy termination, labor induction or augmentation, or postpartum hemorrhage control). Medications that relax (suppress) the uterine muscle are classified as *tocolytics*. Drugs that stimulate contractions of the uterine muscle are classified as *oxytocics*.

TOCOLYTICS

Because preterm birth is a major factor in neonatal morbidity and mortality, efforts are taken, when appropriate, to suppress uterine activity and allow the fetus to mature in utero. Preterm labor consists of uterine activity, occurring after 20 weeks gestation but before 36 weeks gestation, resulting in significant cervical change. This uterine activity ranges from subtle, as manifested by backache, abdominal or pelvic cramping or pressure, or cervical discharge, to palpable uterine contractions at a rate greater than four to six an hour. Significant cervical change is greater than 2 to 4 cm dilation and 80% effacement.

Conservative therapy including bed rest, hydration, and sedation suppresses uterine activity in some cases. Pharmacologic tocolysis is most effective when treatment is begun as soon as the diagnosis of preterm labor is made and is not appropriate once progression to active labor has occurred. Rupture of the amniotic membranes, commonly occurring with preterm labor, adds an increased risk of infection, contraindicating tocolysis. Other contraindications to tocolysis include situations in which the prolongation of pregnancy is hazardous to either the mother or the fetus. The selection and management of candidates for tocolysis require ongoing perinatal and neonatal consultation on an individual basis. Agency protocols based on national standards are necessary.

Agents currently used for tocolysis include betasympathomimetics—**ritodrine hydrochloride *(Yutopar)*** and **terbutaline sulfate *(Brethine, Bricanyl)*—**and **magnesium sulfate.** Prostaglandin inhibitors (indomethacin) and calcium channel blockers (nifedipine) may also be used. Magnesium sulfate is an effective tocolytic, especially when betasympathomimetics are contraindicated. More than one pharmacologic agent is often necessary as uterine receptors desensitize and breakthrough activity occurs. Stabilization, or initial suppression of uterine activity, is achieved with intravenous titration of betasympathomimetics or magnesium sulfate until contractions cease. The intravenous infusion is then titrated down to the lowest possible dose that will accomplish absence of contractions and is continued for 12 to 24 hours. An oral maintenance therapy of a tocolytic is then initiated and continued until fetal maturity or until medical judgment dictates discontinuing the drug. A significant number of women break through the oral maintenance regime and have a reoccurrence of preterm labor, requiring restabilization. A continuous low-dose subcutaneous infusion of betasympathomimetics (terbutaline sulfate) has been shown to be a safe and effective therapy when oral tocolysis fails. Whereas stabilization treatment is confined to the hospital, maintenance therapy is initiated in the hospital and may be continued in the home setting with a program of home uterine monitoring (see Home Health Care box).

○ **Betasympathomimetics** (ritodrine hydrochloride and terbutaline sulfate) used for tocolysis are chosen for their intended effect on the beta$_2$ receptors that cause smooth muscle relaxation in the uterus. A full discussion of the physiologic action and pharmacokinetics of betasympathomimetics is found in Chapter 17. Ritodrine hydrochloride is approved by the FDA for use in preterm labor. Although tocolysis is an unlabeled use of terbutaline sulfate, it is widely used because it is as effective as ritodrine and less costly.

DOSAGE Betasympathomimetics are administered intravenously for stabilization, by oral or continual subcutaneous infusion for maintenance, and subcutaneously for short-acting rapid tocolysis. Intravenous infusions are accomplished with a controlled infusion of a dilute solution of drug, piggybacked into a primary infusion, as close to the venipuncture site as possible. Administration of betasympathomimetics for tocolysis is summarized in Table 48–7.

ADVERSE EFFECTS The cardiovascular effects of the betasympathomimetics can result in maternal and fetal tachycardia, palpitations, a widening of the maternal pulse pressure, and maternal hypotension. Additional cardiovascular effects include arrhythmias and palpitations. Possible metabolic disturbances include hyperglycemia, ketoacidosis, hypokalemia, glucosuria, and ketonuria.

▼ **CLINICAL ALERT**

Sodium and fluid retention create a danger of iatrogenic fluid overload. Pulmonary edema has been reported with concurrent use of corticosteroids to enhance pulmonary lung maturity.

Nausea, vomiting, ileus, and diarrhea can occur. Headache, sweating, drowsiness, or agitation and restlessness also can occur. Neonatal effects include hypoglycemia and ileus. The antidote is propranolol, 1 mg, given over 1 minute.

CONTRAINDICATIONS AND PRECAUTIONS Betasympathomimetics are contraindicated in women with a history of cardiac, renal, or hepatic disease; migraines, hyperthyroidism, asthma, hypertension. Pregnancy factors contraindicating betasympathomimetics include pregnancy-induced hypertension, active labor, infection, rupture of membranes, fetal distress, or a gestation of less than 20 weeks. They are used very cautiously with diabetes.

○ **Magnesium sulfate** is effective in arresting preterm labor at therapeutic serum levels of 5 to 8 mg/dL. The administration is similar to that for seizure prophylaxis in pregnancy-induced hypertension, with a loading and maintenance intravenous infusion. Successful intravenous stabilization of preterm labor is followed with maintenance oral magnesium gluconate at 280 mg every 6 hours. A full discussion of magnesium sulfate during pregnancy is found in the section of this chapter on pregnancy-induced hypertension, and administration is summarized in Table 48–6.

Using the Nursing Process in Labor Suppression

Assessment

- Initial assessment includes obstetric history, gestational age, uterine activity, cervical change, any va-

Table 48–7. TOCOLYTICS

DRUG NAME/ROUTE AND DOSAGE	PHARMACOKINETICS/ DYNAMICS	NURSING IMPLICATIONS
ritodrine hydrochloride (Yutopar)		
Adults: 50–100 μg/min (.05–.1 mg/min) IV via infusion pump; increase q 10–20 min in increments of 50 μg (.05 mg) until contractions stop, then continue 12–24 hr. Maximum dose 350 μg/min (.35 mg/min). Or, 10 mg PO 30–60 min before IV infusion discontinued; then q 2 hr for 24 hr. *Maintenance Dose*–10–20 mg PO q 4–6 hr until term. Maximum dose 120 mg/day. Short term rapid relaxation: 0.25 mg SC into upper arm, repeated q 1–6 hr.	**Onset:** PO, 30–60 min; IV, 5 min (at effective dose) **Peak:** PO, 20–60 min; IV, 60 min **Duration:** NA ½**L:** PO (2 phases), 1.3 and 12–20 hr; IV (3 phases), 6–9 min, 1.5–2.5 hr, 15–17 hr **PB:** 32% **B:** hepatic **E:** renal; crosses placenta	**ASSESSMENT:** Assess uterine contractions, cervical changes, cervical discharge, FHR, BP, RR, symptoms of pulmonary edema, apical pulse, baseline ECG, serum glucose and potassium, CBC, daily weight, I/O, edema, urine glucose and ketones. Assess for pregnancy (category B). **INTERVENTION:** Strict bed rest in lateral recumbent position, cautious fluid administration, NPO. Continuous cardiac monitoring with intravenous infusion. Give oral preparations with food to avoid GI upset. Keep propranolol (antidote) available. **EVALUATION:** Patient demonstrates cessation of uterine contractions and absence of significant cervical change.
terbutaline sulfate (Brethine) (Bricanyl)		
Adults: 10 μg/min (.01 mg/min) IV via infusion pump initially, increasing by 5 μg (.005 mg) q 10–20 min until contractions cease. Maximum dose 80 μg/min (.08 mg/min). Or, 2.5–5 mg PO q 4–6 hr or 250 μg (.25 mg) SC q 1–6 hr. *SC Pump:* 0.5–0.1 mg/hr basal rate; 0.25 mg bolus dose.	**Onset:** PO, 30 min; IV and SC, within 15 min **Peak:** PO, within 1–2 hr; IV or SC, 0.5–1 hr **Duration:** PO, 4–8 hr; IV or SC, 1.5–4 hr ½**L:** NA **PB:** NA **B:** hepatic, partially **E:** renal; crosses placenta	Same as for ritodrine.

NA = not available; FHR = fetal heart rate; BP = blood pressure; RR = respiratory rate.

ginal discharge suggesting infection or rupture of the membranes, and fetal status.

- During stabilization, continuous electronic monitoring of fetal heart rate and uterine activity is needed, as well as manual abdominal palpation for uterine contractions. During maintenance, assessment is intermittent.
- Obtain cervical cultures to rule out infection, complete blood counts (CBC's) to monitor for infection. Perform vaginal exams as infrequently as possible.
- Identify contraindications to either betasympathomimetics or magnesium sulfate. Baseline and ongoing assessments necessary to identify drug toxicity include maternal vital signs and manifestations of pulmonary edema including dyspnea, tachycardia, rales, rhonchi, or cough. Cardiac rhythm is assessed during stabilization with continuous monitoring and during maintenance with auscultation of apical pulse.
- With betasympathomimetics, residual side effects can persist 12 to 24 hours after termination of the drug; therefore assessment is continued for this period of time. Hydration is assessed very cautiously, to maintain optimum vascular volume yet prevent the hazard of iatrogenic fluid overload. Daily weight and strict intake and output are measured. Serum levels of glucose and potassium, urine glucose and ketones,

and a baseline electrocardiogram (ECG) are indicated with betasympathomimetic therapy.
- With magnesium sulfate, obtain serum levels of magnesium and urine specific gravity. Assess deep-tendon reflexes, respiratory status, and neurologic status.
- Assess the mother's anxiety and knowledge level regarding preterm labor and tocolytic therapy. Assess home environment and situational supports necessary for planning home maintenance therapy.

Nursing Diagnosis

- Typical nursing diagnoses for the patient requiring tocolytics include the following: Knowledge Deficit related to unfamiliarity with tocolysis; Anxiety related to preterm labor, possibility of preterm delivery, and side effects of tocolytics; Risk for Maternal-Fetal Injury related to side effects of tocolytics; Pain related to procedures and side effects of tocolytics; and Activity Intolerance related to preterm uterine contractions.

Intervention

- Identify uterine activity, cervical changes, and maternal-fetal responses with each change in dose or tocolytic agent, according to agency protocol.

- The development of unacceptable side effects may dictate stopping the drug and administering the antidote (propranolol for betasympathomimetics, calcium gluconate for magnesium sulfate).
- Betasympathomimetics are held when maternal pulse is greater than 120, fetal heart rate is greater than 180, systolic blood pressure is less than 90 or diastolic less than 40, with symptoms of respiratory distress, or in the presence of cardiac rhythm changes.
- Magnesium sulfate is held when serum magnesium levels are greater than 8 mg/dL, deep-tendon reflexes are diminished, respiratory rate is less than 12, or the urinary output is less than 100 cc per 4 hours.
- Maintain strict bed rest to keep pressure off the cervix and to reduce physical activity, which can increase uterine activity. The left lateral recumbent position relieves vena caval compression and promotes utero-placental circulation. Further safety precautions may be needed if magnesium sulfate has altered the neurologic status.
- Maintain NPO status during stabilization. Oral maintenance betasympathomimetics are taken with food to reduce gastrointestinal (GI) upset.
- Provide emotional support and encourage the mother to verbalize her fears as anxiety can stimulate further uterine activity. Provide information on the status of both mother and fetus, and allow the mother choices.
- Teach symptoms of preterm labor, tocolytic drugs, procedures, and activity restrictions. Prior to discharge, teach uterine activity monitoring by self-palpation or electronic monitor. Teach how to assess own pulse.
- Provide comfort measures, relaxation techniques, and diversional activities while on bed rest during hospital stabilization.
- Plan for discharge by assessing household help needed to maintain activity restrictions and addressing family's concerns regarding financing of home therapy.

Evaluation

Desired outcomes of successful therapy include the following:

- Reduction and cessation of uterine contractions and cervical change until fetal maturity.
- Minimal effects of therapy on the mother and fetus.
- The mother will verbalize an understanding of the drug and cope with the therapy.

OXYTOCICS

Oxytocics are drugs with the pharmacologic properties of the posterior pituitary hormone oxytocin, which stimulates contractions of the uterine muscle. These drugs are used as *abortifacients* (drugs that cause abortion of pregnancy) for elective or therapeutic termination of pregnancy during the second trimester, to induce (initiate) or augment (improve) labor contractions, and to control postpartum hemorrhage caused by uterine atony. The

oxytocics include prostaglandins, synthetic oxytocin, and the ergot alkaloids. The prostaglandins are used as abortifacients and to control postpartum hemorrhage due to uterine atony. However, they are approved for ripening the cervix in anticipation of stimulating labor. Oxytocin (Pitocin), a synthetic posterior pituitary hormone, is used to induce or augment labor during the near term and to control hemorrhage following an abortion. Oxytocin and the ergot alkaloids are used to manage postpartum hemorrhage related to uterine atony.

○ **Prostaglandins** stimulate uterine contraction and cervical change at any stage of pregnancy, as well as stimulate uterine contraction in the postpartum period. Uterine sensitivity to prostaglandins increases toward term. Prostaglandin stimulates smooth muscle contraction of the GI and respiratory tracts in addition to the uterus, causing uncomfortable side effects during administration.

Prostaglandins are used for elective or therapeutic termination of pregnancy during the second trimester, incomplete and missed abortions, termination of pregnancy for fetal death during the third trimester, cervical preparation for the induction of labor in the presence of a viable fetus, and for control of postpartum hemorrhage caused by uterine atony.

Prostaglandin termination of pregnancy during the second trimester may result in a retained placenta and necessitate additional oxytocic drugs or surgical intervention. Delivery of a fetus with signs of life may be possible. Other agents may be used prior to or concurrent with prostaglandins to facilitate cervical dilation and uterine contraction. *Laminaria* (dried Japanese seaweed), Lamicel (hydrogenous magnesium sulfate), and Dilapan (hydrophilic polyacryloniprile) are osmotic dilators inserted into the cervix 10 to 24 hours before induction to soften and dilate the cervix. Prostaglandins used as abortifacients include **dinoprost tromethamine (PGF$_2$)** (intra-amniotic), **dinoprostone (PGE$_2$)** (intravaginal, endocervical), and **carboprost tromethamine (Hemabate)** (intramuscular). Both endocervical prostaglandin E$_2$ (dinoprostone) gel (Prepidil) and intravaginal inserts (Cervidil) are used for cervical preparation or ripening in the presence of a viable fetus. The prostaglandin used for postpartum hemorrhage is carboprost tromethamine (intramyometrial, intramuscular).

Using the Nursing Process in Pregnancy Termination

Assessment

- Assess knowledge level regarding prostaglandin and the termination procedure.
- Obtain informed consent.
- Assess emotional status regarding termination of pregnancy.
- Review the history to screen for any contraindications or risk factors requiring precautions with prostaglandins.
- Assess and document gestational age.
- In nonelective terminations, confirm fetal death.
- During administration of the drug, monitor for pain, GI and respiratory side effects, and hydration.

- Assess vital signs and vaginal bleeding to monitor blood loss.
- Monitor progress through assessment of uterine contractions, cervical changes, and fetal descent.

Nursing Diagnosis

- Typical nursing diagnoses for the patient requiring abortifacients include Knowledge Deficit related to unfamiliarity with the medication and abortion procedure, Pain related to uterine contractions and side effects of prostaglandin, and Anxiety related to termination of pregnancy.

Intervention

- Encourage verbalizations of grief and loss. Offer emotional support and privacy, especially during drug administration.
- Give information on drugs and procedures, follow-up, and contraception.
- Provide comfort measures, including temperature support, antipyretics, analgesics, antidiarrheals, and antiemetics. Guide use of relaxation techniques.
- Because the woman is usually NPO, administer intravenous fluids.
- Inform woman of progress.
- Save all tissue passed for examination.

Evaluation

With successful therapy, the woman will do the following:

- Achieve delivery of the complete products of conception without excessive blood loss.
- Experience as little discomfort and side effects of prostaglandin administration as possible.
- Verbalize knowledge and feelings related to the procedure.

○ **Oxytocin** (Pitocin) produces the same effects as endogenous oxytocin, which is a hormone from the posterior pituitary that stimulates the smooth muscle of the uterus by increasing intracellular calcium. The resulting muscle activity produces phasic contractions. As pregnancy progresses the uterus is progressively more responsive to the effects of oxytocin. In early pregnancy the uterus is not responsive to exogenous oxytocin. Although it does not appear that endogenous oxytocin alone actually causes labor to begin, it is certain that exogenous oxytocin can facilitate labor.

Administration of exogenous synthetic oxytocin is used to induce (initiate) labor contractions and to augment (improve) existing labor contractions. Induction of labor is initiated to achieve a vaginal delivery only when there is a maternal or fetal medical indication and is not done for elective or convenience indications.

Oxytocin may also be given for a contraction stress test (CST) to evaluate uteroplacental reserve during pregnancy, during the third stage of labor, and the postpartal period to enhance uterine contraction and therefore decrease postpartal bleeding, or to stimulate uterine contraction following a spontaneous or elective abortion. Endogenous oxytocin plays a role in lactation by stimulating muscles that eject milk downward into the mammary sinuses, where it is available for the suckling infant. This effect is referred to a as "milk ejection" or "milk letdown."

DOSAGE Individual agency protocols based on professional guidelines must be established for the administration of oxytocin (Pitocin). A slow intravenous infusion is the route of choice as dosage can be adjusted precisely. Intravenous administration is accomplished with a primary intravenous line of a physiologic electrolyte solution and a secondary line of oxytocin on a controlled infusion pump, connected as close as possible to the primary venipuncture site. With this method, the drug infusion can be quickly stopped and cleared at the infusion site if toxic reactions occur. See Table 48–8 for specific dosage.

The CST evaluates the ability of the placenta to meet fetal oxygen needs during contractions and, therefore, whether or not the pregnancy can safely be continued and/or whether the fetus can safely tolerate labor. The rate is gradually increased until three contractions within a 10-minute period are produced. Continuous electronic monitoring of the fetal heart rate and uterine contractions is performed before, during, and after the infusion. An abnormal fetal heart pattern is indicative of low placental oxygen reserve and is termed a positive test.

To stimulate uterine contraction following a missed abortion or with postpartum hemorrhage, a dose of 10 units is administered intravenously at a rate of 20 to 40 milliunits per minute. For control of postpartal hemorrhage, the oxytocin is administered following the delivery of the infant and preferably the placenta. A dilute intravenous infusion is recommended as bolus oxytocin is associated with pronounced hypotension. An alternative dose of 3 to 10 units of oxytocin can be administered intramuscularly for control of postpartum hemorrhage.

PHARMACOKINETICS The onset of action of intravenous oxytocin is almost immediate and subsides within 1 hour. The plasma half-life of intravenous oxytocin is 1 to 6 minutes, with the shorter interval occurring in late pregnancy and during lactation. The onset of action of an intramuscular injection of oxytocin is 3 to 5 minutes and persists for up to 2 to 3 hours. Oxytocin has a low protein binding, is rapidly metabolized in the liver and kidney, and is excreted by the kidney. Because the intravenous route has such a short duration of action and rapid metabolism and excretion, a constant infusion is necessary to maintain a stable blood level.

CONTRAINDICATIONS AND PRECAUTIONS Oxytocin is used with caution in cardiovascular, hypertensive, or renal disease. It is contraindicated for induction with cephalopelvic disproportion (CPD), unfavorable fetal positions, and placental hemorrhaging. Oxytocin is used cautiously with previous cesarean birth or preterm birth. If delivery is not imminent, oxytocin is contraindicated with fetal distress.

ADVERSE EFFECTS The adverse effects of oxytocin are dose related and may manifest in both the mother and the fetus. The fetal effect is usually related to the degree of uterine activity. To maintain effective oxygenation to the uterine muscle, the placenta, and fetus, it is essential that uterine contractions remain no longer in duration than 60 seconds and no closer together than 2 minutes,

Table 48–8. OXYTOCICS

DRUG NAME/ROUTE AND DOSAGE	PHARMACOKINETICS/DYNAMICS	NURSING IMPLICATIONS
oxytocin (Pitocin)		
labor induction or augmentation **Adults:** 1–2 milliunit (mU)/min IV via infusion pump; increase by 1–2 mU/min q 30–60 min until desired labor pattern established. **postabortion or postpartum hemorrhage** **Adults:** IV rate of 20–40 mU/min (maximum concentration 40 mU/1000 mL); 3–10 units IM after delivery of placenta.	**Onset:** IV, immediate; IM, 3–5 min **Peak:** NA **Duration:** IV, 1 hr; IM, 2–3 hr **½L:** 1–6 min **PB:** low **B:** hepatic, renal **E:** renal; does not cross placenta. Minimal excretion in breastmilk	**ASSESSMENT:** Labor–obstetric history, obtain baseline data, VS, FHR, contractions, status of membranes. Assess fluid status. Postpartum—uterine tone, vaginal bleeding, hypovolemia. Assess for pregnancy (category unknown). **INTERVENTION:** Labor—Explain need for induction or augmentation. Use infusion control pump. Monitor I/O, position patient on left side, apply continuous fetal monitoring, evaluate contractions and uterine resting tone. Document maternal VS, FHR, uterine contractions with dose increments. Postpartum—Massage uterus. **EVALUATION:** Labor—labor progress and delivery without adverse effects. Postpartum—contracted uterus, absence of excessive bleeding.
PROSTAGLANDINS		
dinoprost tromethamine (PGF$_2$) (Prostin F2 Alpha)		
pregnancy termination **Adults:** 40 mg intra-amniotic injection.	**Onset:** 1 min **Peak:** mean abortion effect 20–24 hr **Duration:** NA **½L:** in amniotic fluid, 3–6 hr; plasma <1 min **PB:** NA **B:** lungs, liver, kidneys **E:** primarily renal, 5% in feces	**ASSESSMENT:** In abortion, ascertain gestational wk. Monitor temperature. Monitor uterine contractions and tone. Assess for pregnancy (category X). **INTERVENTION:** Store prostaglandins in refrigerator. With abortions, premedicate with antiemetic and antidiarrheal. Administer antipyretic, provide warmth as needed. Provide pain relief and emotional support. **EVALUATION:** Save all tissue passed for examination. Evaluate for uterine response and bleeding.
dinoprostone (PGE$_2$) (Prostin E2)		
pregnancy termination **Adults:** Initially, 20 mg intravaginal suppository, then q 3–5 hr until delivery; maximum dose 240 mg.	**Onset:** within 10 min **Peak:** mean abortion time—15–17 hr **Duration:** 2–3 hr **½L:** NA **PB:** NA **B:** lungs, liver, kidneys **E:** primarily renal	Same as for dinoprost tromethamine plus: **INTERVENTION:** Use gloves with unwrapped suppository to prevent skin absorption. Warm to room temperature before use. Lubricate with water-soluble gel and insert into posterior vaginal fornix. Patient should remain supine for 1 hr after.
dinoprostone (PGE$_2$) (Prepidil)		
preinduction cervical ripening **Adults:** 0.5 mg gel endocervically q 6 hr, max 3 doses.	Same as above except: **Onset:** rapidly absorbed **Peak:** 30 min–1 hr **Duration:** NA	**ASSESSMENT:** Monitor FHR, uterine activity, labor progress. **INTERVENTION:** Bring to room temperature before use. Use gloves to prevent skin absorption. Keep supine for 30 min–1 hr after insertion. **EVALUATION:** Progressive cervical changes.
dinoprostone (PGE$_2$) (Cervidil)		
preinduction cervical ripening **Adults:** Single dose 10 mg controlled-release vaginal insert inserted into posterior vaginal fornix.	Same as above except: **Onset:** NA **Peak:** NA **Duration:** over 12 hr	**ASSESSMENT:** Same as dinoprost endocervical gel. Monitor continuously. **INTERVENTION:** Keep supine 2 hr after insertion. Remove after onset of active labor, hyperstimulation, or 12 hr. Oxytocin may be administered 30 min after removal. There is no need for previous warming of product.

Table 48–8. OXYTOCICS, *Continued*

DRUG NAME/ROUTE AND DOSAGE	PHARMACOKINETICS/ DYNAMICS	NURSING IMPLICATIONS
carboprost tromethamine (Prostin/15M) (Hemabate) (15 Mehtyl PGF₂)		
abortion **Adults:** Initially , 250 µg IM, then 250 µg q 1.5–3.5 hr, as needed. Maximum dose 12 mg. **postpartum hemorrhage** **Adults:** 250 µg IM, intramyo-metrial, transvaginally q 15–90 min, max 5 doses.	**Onset:** NA **Peak:** 30 min **Duration:** NA **½L:** NA **B:** enzymatic deactivation in tissues **E:** primarily renal	For abortion—Same as for dinoprost tromethamine. For hemorrhage— **ASSESSMENT:** Uterine contraction, VS, hemorrhage. Assess for pregnancy (category C). **INTERVENTION:** Store in refrigerator. **EVALUATION:** Contracted uterus, normal vaginal bleeding.
ERGOT ALKALOIDS		
ergonovine maleate (Ergotrate, Ergometrine) **methylergonovine maleate** (Methergine, Methylergometrine)		
Adults: 0.2–0.4 mg PO 2–4 times daily; 0.2 mg IM q 2–4 hr; or 0.2 mg over 1 min IV.	**Onset:** PO, 10 min; IM, 2–8 min; IV, immediate **Peak:** NA **Duration:** PO, 3 hr; IM, 3 hr; IV, 45 min **½L:** PO, 2 hr **PB:** NA **B:** hepatic **E:** renal	**ASSESSMENT:** Assess VS, vaginal bleeding, fundal height. Assess for pregnancy (category C). **INTERVENTION:** Monitor VS, vaginal bleeding, fundal height. Explain need for drug. Forewarn that uterine cramping will occur. Offer analgesics. **EVALUATION:** Decrease in vaginal bleeding, contracted uterus, VS within normal limits.

NA = not available; VS = vital signs; FHR = fetal heart rate.

with adequate relaxation of the myometrium between contractions. Oxytocin can induce contractions that are hypertonic (too strong), tetanic (too long), or too close together, and can increase the uterine resting tone. This hyperstimulation disrupts the oxygen supply to the uterine muscle, placenta, and fetus.

▼ **CLINICAL ALERT**

Uterine hyperstimulation can lead to uterine pain, placental separation, uterine rupture, and fetal distress. Infusion should be stopped at the first sign of uterine hyperstimulation or fetal distress. Concomitant use with other oxytocics can potentiate uterine hyperstimulation. The antidote is a tocolytic such as terbutaline sulfate. Discontinuing an intravenous infusion lowers the plasma concentration quickly.

Tumultuous and rapid labor and delivery can cause maternal genital trauma and neonatal trauma.

Maternal hypertension or hypotension can occur with oxytocic use. Nausea, vomiting, and anaphylaxis can also occur. Cardiac arrhythmias, premature ventricular contractions, and palpitations have been reported. Oxytocin has antidiuretic properties and, when given in large amounts, may lead to fluid retention and water intoxication as evidenced by symptoms of oliguria, edema, con-fusion, drowsiness, headache, nausea and vomiting, and tachycardia.

INTERACTIONS   Severe hypertension has been reported when oxytocin is given with a vasopressor or a regional block anesthesia and vasoconstrictor combination. Hypotension may result when oxytocin is used in conjunction with cyclopropane. Enflurane, halothane, and possibly isoflurane relax uterine muscle and antagonize the uterine response to oxytocin. Magnesium sulfate use for PIH also antagonizes stimulation of the uterine muscle. Use of oxytocin with other oxytocics could cause uterine hyperstimulation.

Using the Nursing Process in Labor Induction and Augmentation

Assessment

- Gather a thorough nursing history including an obstetrical history and the expected delivery date.
- Assess baseline maternal vital signs, fetal heart rate, and uterine contraction pattern. Continual electronic monitoring of fetal heart rate patterns and correlation with uterine contraction patterns is the national standard.
- Determine the status of the membranes, cervical changes, and fetal descent to evaluate the progress of labor.
- Monitor the hydration status of the mother, particularly for symptoms of water intoxication.

- Evaluate the knowledge level and emotional status of the mother regarding the procedure. Continually assess the mother's comfort level.

Nursing Diagnosis

- Typical nursing diagnoses for the patient requiring oxytocics for labor induction or augmentation include Knowledge Deficit related to unfamiliarity with the induction procedure; Pain related to uterine contractions; Altered Tissue Perfusion related to vascular constriction of the uterus, placenta, and consequently fetal circulation; and Risk for Maternal Injury related to antidiuretic effects of oxytocin.

Intervention

- Provide information regarding the indication for induction; the induction procedure, drugs, and equipment; and information regarding her progress in labor.
- Offer comfort measures and help with relaxation. Analgesics are provided as appropriate.
- Follow individual agency protocols outlining the responsibilities of the nurse and the physician. Document maternal status, fetal status, and labor progress with each change in the infusion dosage.
- Position the mother on her left side to relieve vena cava compression and facilitate uterine circulation.
- Facilitate emptying bladder.
- If a toxic reaction occurs, stop the oxytocin infusion, increase the primary infusion rate, give oxygen by tight face mask, and notify physician. In this situation, the side-lying position not only facilitates circulation, but also decreases contraction intensity. A tocolytic such as terbutaline sulfate may be given as an antidote.

Evaluation

Desired outcomes for successful therapy include the following:

- effective uterine contractions
- absence of signs of maternal or fetal distress
- verbalization of an understanding of the treatment
- effective coping with the procedure
- delivery of a healthy baby

○ **Ergot alkaloids,** derived from a fungus affecting rye grain, increase the force and frequency of uterine contractions. In large doses ergot alkaloids increase the resting muscle tonus and result in sustained tonic contractions. These drugs are not used to induce or augment labor, or prior to placental delivery, because of the risk of nonphasic, sustained contractions. They are used to treat postpartum hemorrhage resulting from uterine atony. The sensitivity of the uterus to these drugs increases as the pregnancy progresses toward term. Ergots have pronounced vasoconstrictive effects.

DOSAGE Ergonovine maleate (Ergotrate), a natural ergot preparation, and methylergonovine maleate (Methergine), a synthetic ergot, are administered intramuscularly, orally, and rarely, intravenously. See Table 48–8 for dosage. The intravenous route is hazardous as these drugs are powerful vasoconstrictors; it is reserved for cases of life-threatening uterine bleeding.

PHARMACOKINETICS The onset of uterine contractions occurs 5 to 15 minutes after oral administration, 2 to 5 minutes after intramuscular administration, and immediately after intravenous administration. The drug effects continue for approximately 3 hours after oral and intramuscular administration and 45 minutes after intravenous administration. The half-life of methylergonovine maleate is 0.5 to 2 hours. Metabolism of ergonovine maleate occurs in the liver with excretion by the kidney.

CONTRAINDICATIONS AND PRECAUTIONS Ergot alkaloids are contraindicated in women with a history of hypersensitivity to ergot, hepatic or renal impairment, hypertension, cardiovascular disease, or PIH. Ergots are contraindicated in pregnancy before the delivery of the placenta.

ADVERSE EFFECTS Women frequently complain of discomfort from the uterine contractions this drug causes. Uterine hyperstimulation may occur. An allergic reaction is manifested by itching and shortness of breath. Headache and confusion have been reported. Additional side effects reported include nausea, vomiting, and diarrhea from smooth muscle contraction in the GI tract. Pain in the arms, legs, and lower back has also been reported with the use of ergot alkaloids.

▼ **CLINICAL ALERT**

Vasoconstrictive effects can cause hypertension and coronary vasospasm. The concomitant use of ergot alkaloid with vasopressors or vasoconstrictors may result in severe hypertension.

Using the Nursing Process in Postpartum Hemorrhage

Assessment

- Review the mother's history for contraindications to these drugs.
- Assess maternal vital signs prior to administration to identify hypertension, which contraindicates ergots, and assess throughout therapy to monitor hypovolemia.
- Assess the mother frequently to determine effectiveness of drug (ergots, oxytocin, or prostaglandins) in controlling hemorrhage and to identify the development of side effects. Assess uterine tone and fundal height. Assess vaginal bleeding for amount and presence of clots.
- Assess bladder distention, which impedes uterine contraction.
- Assess pain from uterine contractions.
- Assess the woman's knowledge level regarding the medication.

Nursing Diagnosis

- Typical nursing diagnoses for the patient requiring medication for postpartum hemorrhage include Pain related to stimulation of uterine contractions, Altered Tissue Perfusion related to uterine blood loss or hypertensive side effects of ergot alkaloids, and Knowledge Deficit related to unfamiliarity with oxytocic drugs.

Intervention

- Explain that the drug may cause uterine cramping and discomfort. Offer comfort measures and analgesics for uterine cramping.
- Empty the bladder, catheterizing if necessary.
- Perform uterine massage abdominally to promote contraction.
- Establish an intravenous fluid line for fluid replacement.

Evaluation

Desired outcomes for successful therapy are that the mother will do the following:

- Achieve effective uterine contraction, involution, and vaginal bleeding within normal limits.
- Exhibit vital signs within normal limits and minimal side effects of therapy.
- Verbalize an understanding of the treatment and cope effectively.

The bibliography for this chapter can be found in Appendix B, which begins on page 1054.

DELIVERING HOME HEALTH CARE

Administration of Terbutaline

Mothers at risk for preterm labor may be stabilized in the acute-care setting and then treated at home with a continuous subcutaneous transfusion of terbutaline sulfate (Brethine). Although the transfusion is designed to be self-administered, the home health nurse will validate correct administration. Home treatment is more comfortable for the family and more cost effective for the health-care system.

Before the administration of terbutaline, do the following:

- Assess the mother's knowledge of preterm labor, uterine activity monitoring (self-palpation or uterine monitor), terbutaline tocolysis, and infusion equipment including pump, supplies, dose, and settings.
- Obtain a baseline assessment of uterine activity, fetal status, maternal blood pressure, heart rate, respiratory rate and lung sounds, CNS, CBC, lytes, glucose, I/O, weight.
- Verify physician orders.
- Assemble pump, prefilled syringes, and prime tubing.
- Review settings and manufacturer's guidelines.
- Prepare site (thigh, abdomen, upper arm) with povidone solution, wipe with alcohol. Maintain and reinforce asepsis.

To administer, do the following:

- Insert needle subcutaneously into prepared site and tape to skin.
- Administer low continuous basal rate to reduce uterine irritability.
- Program intermittent bolus doses to coincide with periods of uterine activity.
- Guide mother in self-administration of additional bolus doses at times of uterine activity.

During administration, do the following:

- Continue to monitor uterine activity, fetal status, maternal blood pressure, heart rate, respiratory rate, and lung sounds.
- Encourage verbalization of feelings regarding pregnancy, treatment, and activity restrictions. Assess coping strategies and support system.

After the administration of terbutaline, do the following:

- Review danger signs, indications to call care provider, methods of obtaining supplies, and telephone numbers.
- Reinforce activity restrictions.
- Document procedure and mother's response.

CHAPTER REVIEW QUESTIONS*

1. Which of the following is correct regarding drug distribution and excretion during pregnancy?
   a. Pharmacologic drug effects are increased as a result of an increase in plasma albumin.
   b. The increase in intracellular fluid volume increases the potential for toxic drug effects.
   c. Increased elimination reduces drug plasma concentrations.
   d. Drug half-life is prolonged due to the increase in hepatic circulation.

2. The variables that determine the transfer of drugs across the placenta include all of the following *except:*
   a. Gestational age.
   b. Physiochemical characteristics.
   c. Placental blood flow.
   d. Physiochemical properties.

3. The antihypertensive of choice for long-term control during pregnancy is:
   a. Captopril.
   b. Hydralazine.
   c. Methyldopa.
   d. Propranolol.

*See Appendix A, which begins on page 1051, for answers.

4. Methergine is contraindicated:
   a. Before the delivery of the placenta.
   b. If uterine pain is present.
   c. In breastfeeding women.
   d. With hypotension.

5. With regard to phenytoin administration during pregnancy, it is usually necessary to:
   a. Discontinue the medication.
   b. Increase the daily dosage.
   c. Reduce the daily dosage.
   d. Maintain the prepregnant dosage.

BUILDING YOUR CRITICAL THINKING SKILLS

MAGNESIUM SULFATE TOXICITY

A pregnant woman (G_1P_0) is hospitalized at 36-weeks' gestation for treatment of preeclampsia and has been receiving magnesium sulfate 2 gm/hr for 18 hours. Currently, her BP is 138/92 in the left lateral position, pulse 92/min, respiratory rate 10/min. She is somnolent and has slurred speech.

1. What could be occurring with the magnesium sulfate that would cause this woman's symptoms?
2. What other assessments should be made?
3. What nursing measures are appropriate for this patient?

UNIT 13

DRUGS AFFECTING THE GASTROINTESTINAL SYSTEM

UNIT OUTLINE

CHAPTER 49

Overview of the Anatomy and Physiology of the Digestive System

Merrily A. Kuhn, RNC, PhD

CHAPTER OUTLINE

Alimentary Canal
Biliary System
Pancreas

LEARNING OBJECTIVES

After reading this chapter, the student will be able to:

1. Identify the major parts of the gastrointestinal system and name the specific secretions and hormones they produce and require for function.
2. Describe the movement of food from the mouth to the anus and the transformation of food within the digestive system.

The digestive system consists of the digestive tract or alimentary canal, the biliary system, and the pancreas. This chapter briefly reviews each section of the digestive system.

ALIMENTARY CANAL

The *alimentary canal*, which extends from the mouth to the anus and is open at both ends, includes the mouth, esophagus, stomach, small intestine, and colon. The alimentary canal has four primary functions: it (1) moves ingested food through the system, (2) secretes electrolytes and enzymes for chemical digestion, (3) absorbs the end products of digestion into the blood, as shown in Figure 49–1, and (4) eliminates the indigestible residues.

MOUTH AND ESOPHAGUS

The first stage of digestion is chewing *(mastication)*, which exposes a larger surface area of food to digestive en-

zymes. It is controlled by the fifth cranial nerve. During mastication, solid and semisolid food is mixed thoroughly with saliva, which lubricates and softens food so it may be swallowed. The saliva contains the enzyme amylase (ptyalin), produced by the parotid glands, which begins the breakdown or hydrolysis of starches. Table 49–1 summarizes the digestive secretions of the alimentary canal and accessory organs.

The food is now a mass called a *bolus* and may be swallowed. The esophagus has mucus-secreting glands along its length, which further lubricate the bolus and protect the esophageal mucous membrane from damage from partially chewed food.

STOMACH

The stomach is a muscular, distensible pouch capable of holding 1500–2000 mL. The stomach functions to (1) store large quantities of food directly after a meal; (2) mix the bolus with gastric secretions like pepsin, mucus, and hydrochloric acid to form a semisolid mixture called *chyme;* (3) begin protein digestion; and (4) regulate delivery of chyme to the intestine.

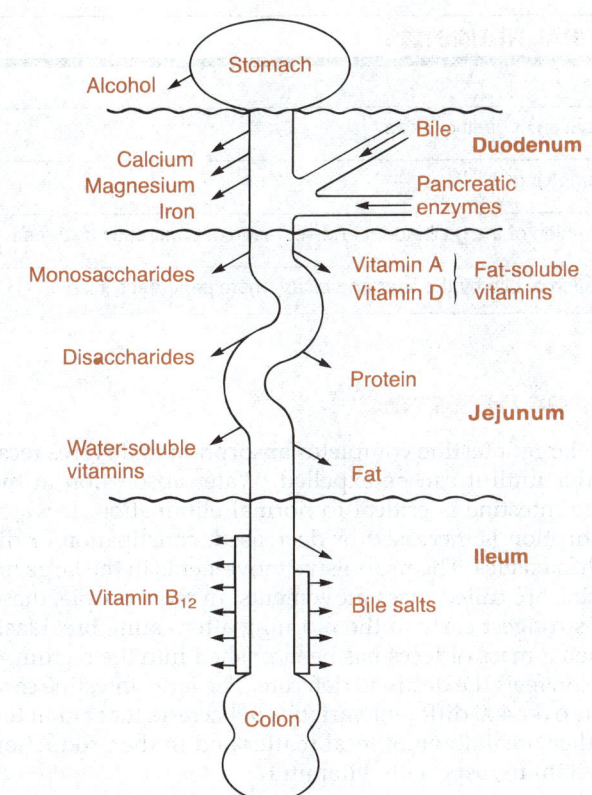

Figure 49–1. The sites of absorption of end products of digestion within the gastrointestinal system.

stimulates further motility and secretion in the stomach. Table 49–2 lists gastrointestinal hormones.

The gastric glands contain four different types of cells: mucous neck cells, chief cells, parietal cells, and oxyntic cells. The mucous neck cells produce mucus identical to that produced by the pyloric and cardiac glands. The chief cells produce the digestive enzyme pepsin that begins protein digestion. The parietal cells produce intrinsic factor, necessary for absorption of vitamin B_{12} in the small intestine. The parietal cells also produce hydrochloric acid, which provides the medium in which pepsin works. The pyloric and a few cardiac glands (found in cardiac portion of the stomach) produce mucus, which protects the gastric mucosa. The pyloric glands also produce pepsinogen and gastrin. Pepsinogen is converted into pepsin in the presence of gastric acid or pepsin itself.

The pyloric sphincter allows chyme to exit the stomach slowly, at a rate of approximately 10 to 15 mL per minute, depending on the volume and degree of fluidity of the chyme and the small intestine's receptivity to it. As the highly acidic chyme moves into the duodenum, enterogastrone, a hormone produced in the small intestine, is secreted and absorbed into the blood. Enterogastrone helps regulate the rate at which the stomach empties. If the duodenum is receiving a highly acidic chyme, enterogastrone inhibits gastric emptying, thereby protecting the duodenal walls and ensuring the alkaline pH necessary for intestinal enzymes. At the same time, the duodenum activates the enterogastric reflex to slow down peristalsis in the stomach. This action prevents the duodenum from becoming too full. The enterogastric reflex is also activated if the pH of the chyme falls below 3.5 to 4, if there is distention of the duodenum, if there is excessive protein breakdown or hypotonicity or hypertonicity of the chyme, or if there is irritation of the mucosa. Activation of this reflex when the chyme is either hypotonic or hy-

Partial digestion of food in the stomach begins when the stomach secretes gastric juice in response to the sight, smell, or taste of food. Then, stimulated by the presence of food in the stomach, the gastric mucosa secretes the hormone gastrin. Gastrin is absorbed into the blood and

Table 49–1. DAILY SECRETIONS OF THE DIGESTIVE SYSTEM

Source	Secretion	Enzyme	Digests	Daily Volume (mL)	pH
Mouth	Saliva	Ptyalin	Starches	1200	6.0–7.0
Gastric secretions	Mucus Hydrochloric acid	Pepsin Gastric lipase	Proteins Fats	2000	1.0–3.5
Intestinal secretions	Small intestine: Mucus (Brunner's gland)			3000 50	7.8–8.0 8.0–8.9
		Peptidases Maltase Lactase, sucrase, isomaltase	Proteins Starches Starches and carbohydrates		
	Large intestine: Mucus			60	7.5–8.0
Pancreatic secretions		Trypsin Chymotrypsin Carboxypeptidase Nucleases Lipase Amylase	Proteins Proteins Proteins Nucleic acids Fats Starches	1200	8.0–8.3
Liver	Bile		Fats	700	7.8

Table 49–2. GASTROINTESTINAL HORMONES

Hormone	Source	Action
Gastrin	Mucosa of stomach	Stimulates production of gastric juices
Enterogastrone	Small intestine	Inhibits gastric emptying
Cholecystokinin	Duodenum	Stimulates contraction of the gallbladder and secretion of pancreatic enzymes
Secretin	Duodenum	Stimulates secretion of bile by the liver and bicarbonate pancreatic juice

pertonic prevents the body from developing water and electrolyte disturbances.

After all food has left the stomach, the pH falls to 2.0 or lower, inhibiting gastric secretions. This prevents the emptying of large quantities of hydrochloric acid and pepsin into the duodenum.

SMALL INTESTINE

The small intestine is composed of the duodenum, jejunum, and ileum. Chyme enters the small intestine and is pushed along slowly, with regular peristaltic waves occurring at the rate of about 11 per minute. These contractions "chop" and rotate the chyme to better expose it to the intestinal secretions and the many microvilli in the intestinal wall where absorption occurs. The microvilli are one cell thick, and proteins and carbohydrates are absorbed directly into the vascular system inside each villus. Fats are absorbed into a fingerlike projection of the lymphatic system, the lacteal. The villi cells replace themselves every 36 to 48 hours and receive their nutrients directly from food in the intestines.

Mucus is produced in large quantities by both the Brunner's glands, located only in the duodenum, and the goblet cells, found extensively in the intestinal mucosa, to protect the wall of the small intestine from breakdown by the strongly acidic chyme. In the presence of anxiety, fear, and stress, the Brunner's glands are strongly inhibited by the sympathetic nervous system. When this inhibition occurs, the duodenum is left unprotected from the gastric secretions.

Small tubular glands called crypts of Lieberkühn are found in the intestinal mucosa and secrete about 2000 mL of alkaline secretions daily. These secretions contain peptidases for splitting small peptides into amino acids; and four additional enzymes for splitting disaccharides into monosaccharides—sucrase, maltase, isomaltase, and lactase. When digestion is complete, the following transformations have occurred: carbohydrates have been converted to disaccharides and monosaccharides; proteins have become amino acids; and fats have been converted to fatty acids and glycerol. The end products are absorbed along with electrolytes by both passive diffusion and active transport, while water is absorbed by osmosis.

The ileocecal valve allows the chyme to enter the large intestine at a rate of only 4 mL per peristaltic wave, for a total of about 750 mL per day. This delay further facilitates absorption in the terminal ileum.

LARGE INTESTINE

The large intestine completes absorption and stores fecal matter until it can be expelled. Water absorption in the large intestine is critical to normal elimination. If water absorption is increased or decreased, constipation or diarrhea ensues. The propulsive movements in the large intestine are called mass movements. In most people, these are strongest early in the morning after eating breakfast. When a mass of feces has been pushed into the rectum, a person feels the desire to defecate. The large intestine contains over 400 different varieties of bacteria that aid in the further breakdown of fecal matter and in the production of vitamins, especially vitamin K.

NERVE CONTROL OF THE ALIMENTARY CANAL

The autonomic nervous system, acting through both the parasympathetic and sympathetic divisions, controls the functioning of the alimentary tract. The parasympathetic nervous system, primarily through the vagus nerve, is responsible for swallowing, gastric secretion, intestinal motility, and defecation. Any psychologic stimulation of the parasympathetic nervous system, as with aggression, anger, resentment, and prolonged worry, increases activity of the alimentary canal and possibly results in digestive disturbances such as indigestion and diarrhea.

In general, the sympathetic nervous system slows or stops completely all gastrointestinal tract function. Therefore, any stimulation of the sympathetic nervous system, such as fear or excitement, can alter function of the gastrointestinal tract.

BILIARY SYSTEM

The biliary system is composed of the liver and gallbladder, both of which contribute to the digestion of fats.

LIVER

The liver, the largest gland in the body, performs more than 500 individual functions. The liver's only digestive function is to form bile. The hepatic duct transports bile to the gallbladder, which rests directly beneath the liver, for storage. Bile salts emulsify fats, which facilitate their digestion and are required for efficient absorption of fatty acids and fat-soluble vitamins. Most of the bile salts secreted in bile are reabsorbed by the intestines and then resecreted by the liver over and over again.

The liver receives all of the venous blood from the intestinal tract by way of the portal vein. This means that the liver has the first opportunity to absorb nutrients and drugs from the blood after the blood leaves the intestines.

The liver's role in metabolism includes (1) the biotransformation of carbohydrates, fats, and proteins and (2) the storage of vitamins. In carbohydrate metabolism, the liver synthesizes and stores glycogen (which helps regulate blood sugar), converts galactose and fructose to glucose, takes part in gluconeogenesis, and forms many intermediate products of carbohydrate metabolism. In fat metabolism, the liver converts fatty acids to acetoacetic acid; forms lipoproteins, cholesterol, and phospholipids; and converts large quantities of carbohydrates and proteins to fats. The liver is also active in *deamination* (removal of an amino group from an amino acid with the consequent formation of ammonia or urea) and the formation of plasma proteins. The liver stores vitamins A, D, and B_{12}, as well as iron in the form of ferritin. Ferritin is released by the liver when iron stores in the body reach a low level.

The liver synthesizes cholesterol, and the clotting factors fibrinogen, prothrombin (II), and Factors V, VII, VIII, IX, and X. Vitamin K, normally absorbed only in the presence of bile salts in the small intestine, is needed by the liver to synthesize prothrombin and clotting factors VII, IX, and X. The Kupffer cells are the macrophages of the liver and remove bacteria and toxins from the blood. The liver inactivates and excretes thyroxine, estrogens, progesterone, testosterone, and other hormones such as aldosterone and the glucocorticoids.

The liver is the chief organ of biotransformation of drugs. The hepatocytes of the liver are capable of inactivating and excreting many different drugs and excreting them into the bile. Drug metabolism can be depressed in starvation, obstructive jaundice, hepatic disease, severe cardiovascular disease, and immaturity, which all depress the microsomal drug metabolizing system. Drug metabolism can also be stimulated by substances, such as certain central nervous system depressants, xanthines, pesticides, food preservatives, and dyes that activate the microsomal drug-metabolizing enzymes (see Chapter 4 for more information).

The liver has long been recognized as the major site of drug biotransformation. A protein known as cytochrome P-450 has been identified as having paramount importance for the deactivation and detoxification of medications and other substances. Recent research has found that when cytochrome P-450 detoxifies and biotransforms some substances that are relatively benign, other substances that may be toxic or even carcinogenic are released. As an example, benzpyrene, found in city smog, cigarette smoke, and charcoal-cooked foods, although not a toxic substance itself, yields substances that ultimately can act as carcinogens in the body after biotransformation. Cytochrome P-450 is also responsible for the serious and sometimes fatal liver and kidney injuries that are produced by an overdose (10 g or more) of acetaminophen (Tylenol). (Refer to Chapter 18 for more information on acetaminophen.)

GALLBLADDER

The gallbladder collects and concentrates bile produced in the liver and stores it until it is needed for digestion. The gallbladder is capable of holding about 45 mL of concentrated bile. Gallbladder bile is about 10 times more concentrated than unconcentrated hepatic bile. At intervals, the gallbladder contracts and empties the bile into the common bile duct, which carries the bile to the relaxed sphincter of Oddi and into the duodenum. The normal stimulus for contraction of the gallbladder is the acid chyme in the duodenum; however, the strongest stimulus is the presence of fatty foods in the chyme. This contraction is mediated by the hormone cholecystokinin.

PANCREAS

The pancreas is both an endocrine and exocrine gland. As an endocrine gland, it secretes insulin and glucagon, which, in conjunction with other hormones, helps regulate carbohydrate metabolism (see Chapter 42). As an exocrine gland, the pancreas produces digestive juice that is transported via ducts to the common bile duct and into the duodenum. Digestive juice contains trypsin, chymotrypsin, and carboxypeptidases, which digest proteins; nucleases (ribonuclease and deoxyribonuclease), which digest nucleic acid; lipase, which digests fats; and amylase, which digests starches. It is important that the proteolytic enzymes of the pancreatic juice not become activated until they have been secreted into the intestine, because the trypsin and other enzymes would digest the pancreas itself. The same cells that secrete the proteolytic enzymes simultaneously secrete another substance called trypsin inhibitor. This substance is stored in the glandular cells surrounding the enzyme granules, and it prevents activation of trypsin both in the cells and in the ducts of the pancreas. When the pancreas becomes severely damaged, large quantities of pancreatic secretions become pooled in these damaged areas and may overwhelm trypsin inhibitor. The pancreatic secretion then becomes rapidly activated and begins to literally digest the entire pancreas. This is called acute pancreatitis.

Pancreatic secretions are also high in bicarbonate and low in chloride. As sodium bicarbonate enters the duodenum, it reacts with hydrochloric acid to form NaCl and carbonic acid. The carbonic acid is a weak acid, which creates carbon dioxide. The carbon dioxide is absorbed into body fluids, leaving a neutral sodium solution behind. This reaction neutralizes the acidic stomach contents and consequently protects the intestinal mucosa. The change in pH is also necessary for the activation of pancreatic enzymes.

The bibliography for this chapter can be found in Appendix B, which begins on page 1054.

CHAPTER REVIEW QUESTIONS*

1. Salvia contains large amounts of:
   a. Amylase.
   b. Phosphate.
   c. HCl.
   d. E. coli.

2. Digestion within the small intestine depends on:
   a. Peptidases for splitting neutral fats into fatty acids.
   b. Lipase for splitting peptides into amino acids.
   c. Lactase for splitting starch into disaccharides.
   d. Bacteria for splitting food byproducts.

3. The primary role of cytochrome P-450, within the liver, is to:
   a. Stimulate steroid release as a stress response.
   b. Deactivate and detoxify medications and other substances.

c. Produce fibrinogen, prothrombin, and Factor V.
d. Deaminate amino acids, forming urea.

4. Intrinsic factor is produced by:
   a. Villi in the small intestine.
   b. Kupffer cells in the liver.
   c. Parietal cells in the stomach.
   d. Goblet cells in the duodenum.

5. The normal pH of gastric secretions is:
   a. 1.0 to 3.5.
   b. 4.5 to 6.0.
   c. 7.8 to 8.0.
   d. 8.0 to 8.3.

*See Appendix A, which begins on page 1051, for answers

CHAPTER 50

Drugs Used to Treat Gastric Acidity

Merrily A. Kuhn, RNC, PhD

CHAPTER OUTLINE

KEY TERMS

Acid neutralizing capacity
Acid rebound
Duodenal ulcers
Gastric ulcers

Milk-alkali syndrome
Peptic ulcer
Reflux esophagitis
Stress ulcers

LEARNING OBJECTIVES

After reading this chapter, the student will be able to:

1. Identify medications commonly used to treat gastric hyperacidity.
2. Differentiate among the medications to treat gastric hyperacidity as to mechanism of action, route of administration, pharmacokinetics, adverse effects, contraindications and precautions, and interactions.
3. Identify specific areas to assess in the patient requiring medications to treat gastric hyperacidity to formulate appropriate patient outcomes.
4. Plan the nursing interventions necessary to administer medications for gastric hyperacidity and choose appropriate teaching strategies to gain patient compliance.
5. Evaluate the patient at various stages of treatment to measure effectiveness of nursing interventions.

A *peptic ulcer*, illustrated in Figure 50–1, is an erosion in the mucosal lining of the walls of the esophagus, duodenum, or jejunum. The etiology of peptic ulcers is unclear, but may be related to genetic, environmental, infectious, and/or psychologic factors. Peptic ulcer disease can occur in patients of any age, although rarely in children under age 10. It is estimated that approximately 10% to 15% percent of the world's population has peptic ulcers, with about 16 million occurring in the United States. There are over 4 million hospitalizations per year, with about 1.5% of these ending in death.

Ulcers appearing in the stomach or esophagus are called *gastric ulcers*; those appearing within the duodenum are *duodenal ulcers*; and those appearing as a result of severe stress, trauma, sepsis, burns (Curling's ulcers), or head injuries (Cushing's ulcers) are called *stress ulcers*.

Figure 50–2 shows the distribution of peptic ulcers. Approximately 16% of patients admitted to an intensive care unit develop stress ulcers, or stress ulcer syndrome (SUS), any time from 5 hours to 21 days after admission. Mechanical ventilation for more than 5 days has been associated with a 40% incidence of major stress ulcer bleeding. Normal gastric pH is 1.0 to 3.5. Maintenance of a pH above 5 has been shown to prevent stress ulcers, but as pH rises, gram-negative bacteria begin to grow.

For the past 10 years, in both Europe and the United States, more emphasis has been placed on *Helicobacter pylori* as a cause of ulcers. *H. pylori*, a gram-negative bacterium, is present in the gastric antrum of 90% of duodenal ulcers and 80% of gastric ulcers. It lives in the mucosal layers and surface epithelial cells. *H. pylori* can mediate the inflammatory response, and may alter gastric

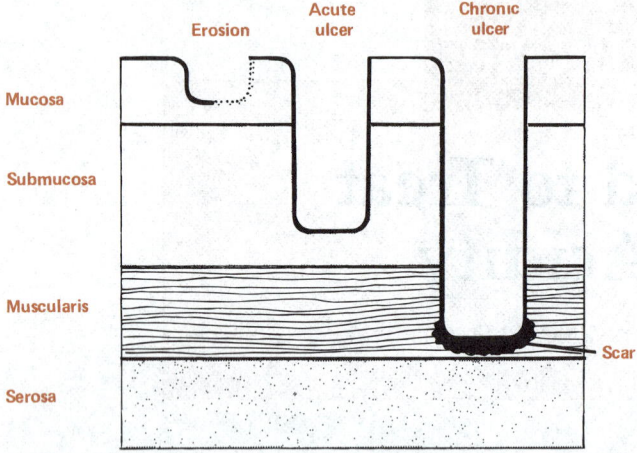

Figure 50–1. Peptic ulcers, illustrating an erosion, acute ulcer, and chronic ulcer. Both acute and chronic ulcers may penetrate the entire stomach wall. (From Price, S, and Wilson L: Pathophysiology, McGraw-Hill, New York, 1978, with permission.)

acid secretion and gastric response to meals and even decrease bicarbonate secretion. The prevalence increases with age and is more common among African-Americans, Hispanics, persons from lower socioeconomic groups, institutionalized persons, and persons traveling to underdeveloped countries. *H. pylori* can be transmitted from person to person via the oral-oral or fecal-oral route. Therefore, ulcers are often found in members of the same family.

Goals of treating peptic ulcers include decreasing symptoms, hastening healing, preventing complications (hemorrhage 15% to 20%, perforation 6% to 10%, and obstruction 5%), and preventing recurrences. These goals can usually be achieved through a combination of avoidance of irritating drugs (e.g., aspirin, nonsteroidal anti-inflammatory drugs [NSAIDs], steroids), avoidance of

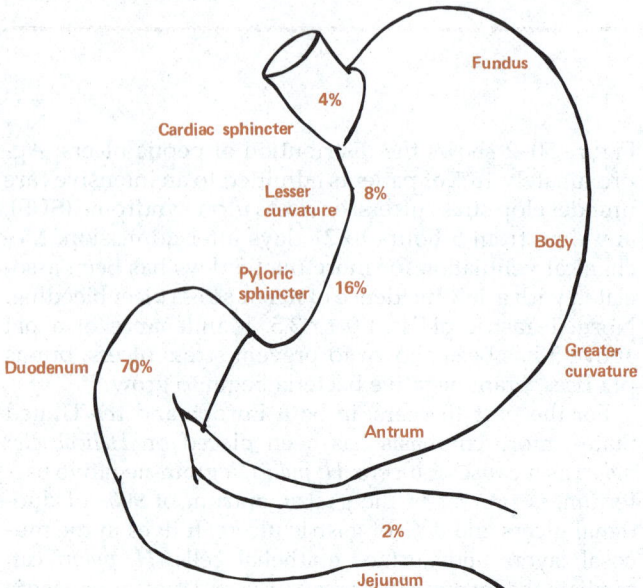

Figure 50–2. The distribution of peptic ulcers.

smoking, control of emotional factors, elimination of *H. pylori* bacteria, and combination drug therapy.

Traditionally, therapy for peptic ulcer has been a combination of products to protect the gastroduodenal mucosa. Within the last few years, there has been an explosion of new products that offer patients many alternatives. Therapeutic agents are aimed today at modifying gastric acidity and reducing *H. pylori*.

The most common medications used to treat peptic ulcers include antacids (aluminum hydroxide, magnesium hydroxide, calcium carbonate); histamine H_2 inhibitors (cimetidine, famotidine, ranitidine, nizatidine); proton pump inhibitors (omeprazole, lansoprazole); mucosal protectants (bismuth salycilate, sucralfate); prostaglandins (misoprostol); and antibiotics to eliminate *H. pylori* (metronidazole, tetracycline, amoxicillin, clarithromycin). Antiulcer drugs are featured in Table 50–1. Gastrointestinal stimulants (metoclopramide, cisapride), which stimulate GI motility and empty the stomach and duodenum more quickly, may also be used. Other medications used to treat patients with hyperacidity include anticholinergics (Chapter 16) and antianxiety medications and hypnotics (Chapter 25).

ANTACIDS

The pH of the gastric contents is 1.0 to 3.5—a very highly acidic medium. The pain and discomfort associated with hyperacidity or hyperchlorhydria are frequent complaints of patients with peptic ulcers.

Antacids are one of the mainstays for the treatment of peptic ulcers because of their ability to effectively reduce acidity at relatively low cost and with low incidence of side effects. Unfortunately, these over-the-counter (OTC) preparations are frequently abused by many consumers who use them habitually and improperly to treat self-diagnosed hyperacidity, heartburn, indigestion, or discomfort resulting from overindulgence in food or alcohol.

ANTACID CLASSIFICATION

There are two general classifications of antacids—systemic and nonsystemic. The systemic antacids are soluble in gastric contents and are capable of being absorbed systemically; therefore, they may alter electrolyte balance and precipitate metabolic alkalosis. The most commonly used systemic antacid is sodium bicarbonate, USP (baking soda).

The nonsystemic antacids, composed of calcium, aluminum, or magnesium, or a combination, neutralize gastric contents but do not cause systemic alkalosis because the products are not absorbed to any significant extent. Magnesium is the best overall antacid whereas aluminum is the weakest antacid. Calcium carbonate has high neutralizing capabilities, followed by magnesium hydroxide and aluminum hydroxide. All three products have a duration of action of 30 minutes in a fasting patient and 2 to 4 hours when there is food in the stomach. Nonsystemic antacids, including their dosages, pharmacokinetics, and nursing implications, are featured in Table 50–2.

Class	Mechanism of Action	Drugs
	Table 50–1. ANTIULCER DRUGS	
Antacids	Convert gastric acid to neutral salts. Raise pH of stomach to 4–5	Aluminum hydroxide Magnesium hydroxide Calcium carbonate
Histamine H_2 Inhibitors	Suppress acid secretion by blocking H_2 receptors on parietal cells	Cimetidine (Tagamet) Famotidine (Pepcid) Nizatidine (Axid) Ranitidine (Zantac)
Proton Pump Inhibitors	Suppress acid secretion by inhibiting H^+, K^+-ATPase, the enzyme that makes gastric acid	Omeprazole (Prilosec) Lansoprazole (Prevacid)
Mucosal Protectants	Form a barrier over the ulcer crater that protects against acid and pepsin Form a barrier over the ulcer crater that protects against acid and pepsin; reduce colonization with *H. pylori*	Sucralfate (Carafate) Bismuth salycilate (Pepto-Bismol)
GI Stimulants	Stimulate upper GI motility and increase rate of gastric emptying without stimulating gastric, biliary, or pancreatic secretions	Metoclopramide (Reglan) Cisapride (Propulsid)
Prostaglandins	Protect against NSAID-induced ulcers by stimulating secretion of mucus and bicarbonate, maintaining submucosal blood flow, and suppressing secretion of gastric acid	Misoprostol (Cytotec)
Antibiotics	Eradicate *H. pylori* infection	Metronidazole (Flagyl) Tetracycline Amoxicillin (Amoxil) Clarithromycin (Biaxin)

ACTION

Antacids interact with gastric secretions, releasing anions that partially neutralize gastric hydrochloric acid and thereby increase the gastric pH. They do not absorb the acid—a popular misconception. Antacid therapy generally raises the pH of the stomach to above 4.0. Pepsin, a proteolytic enzyme, primarily responsible for inflammation, is suppressed with a pH above 3 and inactivated with a pH above 7 to 8. If a patient is bleeding, pH has to be above 6.5 for blood to clot.

Acid-neutralizing capacity (ANC), expressed in mEq/mL, is a primary consideration in selecting an antacid. Milliequivalents of antacid is defined by the mEq of hydrochloride required to keep an antacid suspension at pH 3.0 for 2 hours in vitro. The higher the ANC, the more effective the antacid.

USES

Antacids are effective in treating conditions such as acid indigestion, heartburn, *reflux esophagitis* (inflammation of the esophagus caused by the reflux of acid and pepsin from the stomach into the esophagus), both active and chronic peptic ulcers, and in preventing stress ulcers. Antacids may also be effective in relieving pain from ulcers and are especially effective in binding bile salts that reflux into the stomach.

Aluminum hydroxide antacids (Amphojel, Gelusil) can also be used to treat individuals who are prone to the development of phosphate kidney stones or treatment of hyperphosphatemia associated with chronic renal failure. Aluminum binds with phosphate in the bowel, causing an insoluble precipitate (aluminum phosphate) that is excreted in the feces. Therefore phosphate does not enter the bloodstream. Because phosphate and calcium have an inverse relationship, plasma phosphate levels fall and calcium levels rise. Because a large quantity of phosphate is

found in saliva, antacids are best given after meals. Prolonged use of these antacids can create hypophosphatemia with symptoms of anorexia, malaise, and muscle weakness.

CONTRAINDICATIONS AND PRECAUTIONS

In general, the antacids are contraindicated in individuals with sensitivities to the component's properties. Antacids are contraindicated in patients with renal dysfunction as metal ions may accumulate in the compromised kidney, leading to additional kidney impairment, systemic alkalosis, and fluid and electrolyte imbalance. In particular, increased magnesium ion may create neurologic, cardiovascular, and neuromuscular dysfunction; whereas excessive calcium may result in hypercalcemia, weakness, and mental confusion. Additional symptoms of hypercalcemia include nausea, vomiting, anorexia, weakness, headache, dizziness, and a change in mental status.

Precautions are used when administering aluminum antacids in patients with gastric outlet syndrome as aluminum inhibits smooth muscle contraction and thus inhibits gastric emptying. Patients with cardiovascular and renal disease must be given antacids low in sodium to help prevent the retention of water, which could worsen their condition. Most antacids today have low sodium contents. Sodium content is more a marketing tool than a true chemical hazard today.

ADVERSE EFFECTS

In general, most antacids are nontoxic. The most common complaint from patients is a change in bowel habits. Aluminum and calcium products generally cause constipation, whereas magnesium products attract and retain water, creating an osmotic effect leading to diarrhea. The

Table 50–2. ANTACIDS

DRUG NAME/ROUTE AND DOSAGE	PHARMACOKINETICS/ DYNAMICS	NURSING IMPLICATIONS
all antacids		**ASSESSMENT:** Assess pain, food history. Assess for cardiovascular or renal disease. **INTERVENTION:** Take between meals, 1 hr before or 3 hr after meals, or both. Dosage for acute ulcer treatment is 15–45 mL q 3–6 hr for 2 wk. Dosage for healing stage is 15–30 mL 1–3 hr before meals and at bedtime. Note any changes in bowel habits. If constipation occurs, alternate with other preparations. Given cautiously to patients on low-sodium diet. **Patient Teaching—**Tell patient to chew tablets thoroughly and take with full glass of water and to take other drugs 1 hr before or 2 hr after antacids. **EVALUATION:** Notify physician if continued pain or tarry stools.

CALCIUM COMPOUNDS

calcium carbonate (Alka-Mints) (Chooz) (Amitone) (Tums) (Dicarbosil) (Equilet)		
Adults: 0.5–1.5 g PO (liquid, tablets) every 2–4 hr ANC—10–16	**Onset:** rapid **Duration:** 30–60 min	Same as for all plus: **INTERVENTION: Patient Teaching—**Teach patient about symptoms of milk-alkali syndrome if drug is being used chronically: headache, confusion, nausea, vomiting, distaste for food, abdominal pain, and hypercalcemia.

ALUMINUM COMPOUNDS

aluminum hydroxide gel USP (Amphojel) (Alu-Cap) (Dialume)		
Adults: 5–30 mL PO 3–6 times daily between meals and at bedtime *Children:* 2–5 mL PO every 4–6 hr ANC—8.5–10	**Onset:** rapid **Duration:** 30–60 min (not absorbed)	Same as for all plus: **INTERVENTION:** Aluminum hydroxide interferes with the absorption of phosphates from the intestine, and in the presence of a low-phosphate diet may cause deficiencies. When administering aluminum products continuously through a nasogastric tube, dilute them 1:2 or 1:4 with water.
aluminum carbonate, basic (Basaljel)		
Adults: 10–15 mL PO in water or fruit juice, 2 caps or tabs q 2 hr, up to 12 times/day. To prevent phosphate stones: 2–6 caps or tabs 1 hr pc and hs. Extra strength = 5–15 mL ANC—12	**Onset:** rapid **Duration:** 30–60 min (not absorbed)	Same as above.

MAGNESIUM PRODUCTS

magnesium hydroxide NF (Milk of Magnesia)		
Adults: 650 mg PO (1–2 tablets) qid **laxative** *Children 2–6 yr:* 5–15 mL PO single dose *Children 6–12 yr:* 15–30 mL single dose ANC—14	**Onset:** rapid **Duration:** prolonged	Same as for all plus: **INTERVENTION:** Long-term use is not advisable. Note consistency of stools daily. Tell physician that you are taking magnesium products when other medications are prescribed. Store in tightly covered container.

Table 50–2. ANTACIDS, *Continued*		
DRUG NAME/ROUTE AND DOSAGE	**PHARMACOKINETICS/ DYNAMICS**	**NURSING IMPLICATIONS**
MIXTURES		
aluminum hydroxide and magnesium hydroxide USP (Rulox) (Maalox) (Wingel)		
Adults: 300–600 mg PO suspension, tablets ANC—10–16	**Onset:** rapid	Same as for all.

ANC = acid-neutralizing capacity.

diarrhea can result in an increased risk of potassium depletion and acidosis. This condition can usually be eliminated by using combination products or by alternating aluminum and calcium products with magnesium products during the day. However, calcium products may stimulate rebound gastric acid secretion and are usually not recommended in a patient with ulcer disease.

Many antacids can lead to electrolyte disturbances, such as hypermagnesemia, hypophosphatemia, and hyperphosphatemia. It is important to stress that the use of magnesium-containing antacids can result in hypermagnesemia (5% to 10% absorption) in patients with renal insufficiency or renal failure, due to the decreased clearance. An elevated magnesium may cause central nervous system (CNS) toxicity, which could result in hypotension and respiratory arrest. Therefore, it is recommended that magnesium-containing products be avoided in this subgroup of patients.

Calcium products may promote positive phosphate balance. Sodium bicarbonate and calcium carbonate are implicated as the culprits in the development of the *milk-alkali syndrome* (a syndrome of hypercalcemia, tissue calcification, renal insufficiency, and crystalluria occurring from the chronic administration of sodium bicarbonate with milk or calcium products). Patients at high risk for developing milk-alkali syndrome are those receiving hydrochlorothiazide, which decreases the renal excretion of calcium carbonate, and 0.5 to 10 g of calcium antacids a day. Patients prone to the development of these electrolyte disturbances must have routine electrolyte studies performed.

Rebound hyperacidity may be an adverse effect in some patients receiving calcium carbonate. Many years ago (1973) researchers demonstrated that 2 g of calcium carbonate orally causes significant stimulation of acid secretion and a small increment in serum gastrin. The magnitude of the acid rebound may be as high as one-third the maximal gastric secretory capacity. This is probably mediated by increased serum calcium, although there is no relationship between serum calcium levels and the stimulation of acid secretion. Acid rebound does not seem to be related to significant increases in serum gastrin. Because of the rebound effect, calcium carbonate and all calcium products including milk are recommended less frequently. Renal calculi may also develop in patients receiving calcium carbonate. The patient must be encouraged to drink at least 2 liters of fluid daily to prevent stones from forming.

▼ **CLINICAL ALERT**

Elderly patients particularly are cautioned about continued intake of calcium carbonate (found in Tums). The calcium carbonate neutralizes HCl in the stomach. The HCl levels in the elderly drop by 50%; therefore, the elderly may experience digestive disturbances.

INTERACTIONS

Drug interactions occur because of increased absorption, delayed gastric emptying, renal elimination (change in urinary pH), and formation of insoluble complexes. Since 1977, many reports of drug interactions with antacids have appeared in the literature, but few of them are clinically relevant. Drug interactions are covered in Table 50–3. In general, most drug interactions with antacids can be eliminated if the antacid is separated by at least 2 hours from any other drug. But remind the patient to take antacids within 3 hours of a meal.

▼ **CLINICAL ALERT**

Antacids, because they change the pH of the stomach, are not given concurrently with enteric-coated tablets. The acid-resistant enteric coating is broken down in an alkaline medium, causing the drug to be released in the stomach rather than in the alkaline duodenum. This can irritate the stomach and change the absorption characteristics of the medication.

DOSAGE

Dosage of antacids must be adjusted to achieve a pH of at least 3.5 in the gastric contents. Usually, the manufacturers suggested doses are far too low to effect the neutralization. The production of acid in a patient with a du-

Table 50–3. INTERACTION OF ANTACIDS			
Absorbing/Binding	Increasing pH Decreases Drug Effect/Absorption	Increased Drug Absorption of Basic Drugs	Change in Urine pH Affects Drug Excretion
Tetracycline	Digoxin	Pseudoephedrine	*Increased Drug Excretion*
Quinolones	Phenytoin	Levodopa	Salicylates
Iron products	Chorpromazine		*Decreased Drug Excretion*
Dicumarol	Isoniazid		Quinidine
	H_2 antagonists		Amphetamine
	Ketoconazole		
	Sucralfate		
	Phenothiazines		
	Benzodiazepines		
	NSAIDs		

Interaction can be avoided by separating interacting drug by 2 hours from antacids.

odenal ulcer is 50 to 80 mEq/hour, while acid production is 25 to 40 mEq/hour in a patient with a gastric ulcer. For any antacid to be effective, it must be capable of neutralizing that amount of acid per hour.

Antacids are available as liquid suspensions, chewable tablets, tablets to be swallowed, capsules, and powders. Liquid suspensions are the preparation of choice because of the large surface area covered and quick onset of action, and they are most cost effective. Liquid preparations may not be palatable and may, therefore, decrease the patient's compliance and desire for food and drink. Chewable tablets are another alternative, but they must be thoroughly chewed, as their neutralizing capacity is related to the surface area of the particles. They must be taken with a full glass of water. Also, numerous tablets must be taken to achieve the same neutralizing ability of a liquid. The patient is encouraged to use several different preparations concurrently to avoid "taste fatigue."

SYSTEMIC ANTACIDS

○ **Sodium bicarbonate USP** (baking soda) is the most commonly used systemic antacid. It is rarely prescribed by the physician but is frequently taken by the public because it is readily available in the home. Sodium bicarbonate is also contained in many effervescent OTC drugs such as Alka-Seltzer, Soda Mint, and Instant Metamucil. Sodium bicarbonate readily produces a gastric pH of 8.5. This rapid rise in pH inactivates and overneutralizes the gastric contents. A rapid return of pH to the acidic side occurs, which necessitates retaking sodium bicarbonate at more frequent intervals. As sodium bicarbonate enters the stomach, it combines with hydrochloric acid and liberates water and carbon dioxide. This carbon dioxide may cause gastric distention or may cause the patient to eructate (burp), which seems to relieve distention.

The chronic administration of sodium bicarbonate with milk or calcium products can cause milk-alkali syndrome, resulting in hypercalcemia, tissue calcification (with calcium), renal insufficiency, and crystalluria. Milk-alkali syndrome can also occur when sodium bicarbonate is taken along with or mixed with milk or calcium.

NONSYSTEMIC ANTACIDS

○ **Calcium carbonate,** once regarded as the agent of choice for its long action, insolubility, and low cost, has recently fallen into disfavor and is no longer recommended. Research has indicated that about 10% of the calcium may be absorbed and cause electrolyte disturbances. The metabolic alkalosis is presumed to develop because the net loss of hydrogen ions in the stomach is no longer balanced by the binding of bicarbonate ions in the upper small intestine by unabsorbed calcium. Calcium carbonate is the only antacid that causes *acid rebound* (acid hypersecretion after neutralization of the gastric content). Tums, Rolaids, and Di-Gel are made of calcium and also offer versions that contain calcium carbonate. Calcium-based antacids are a poor source of dietary calcium as only 17% of the calcium is absorbed.

○ **Aluminum products,** the most commonly used group of antacids, vary in their neutralizing ability, and are available as liquids, solid forms, and gels. Aluminum absorbs and temporarily inactivates pepsin, which may contribute to healing of peptic ulcers. Aluminum products also relax gastric smooth muscles and delay gastric emptying, which prolongs their duration of action. Aluminum hydroxide (Amphojel, AlternaGEL, Basaljel Extra Strength), the most common preparation, has demulcent (soothing), absorbent, and astringent properties. The aluminum products commonly cause constipation by binding with bile salts but are generally nontoxic. Aluminum can be combined with sodium carbonate to form dihydroxyaluminum sodium carbonate (Rolaids, Camalox, Gaviscon), which combines the assets of both aluminum and sodium carbonate to neutralize rapidly.

○ **Magnesium products** are found as antacids in combination with carbonate, oxide, hydroxide, trisilicate, or phosphate salts. Because magnesium causes diarrhea (by an osmotic effect), it is often combined with aluminum or calcium products to avoid this side effect. Magnesium hydroxide (Milk of Magnesia) is used mainly as a laxative. It has a rapid onset of action and somewhat prolonged duration of action. Some of the magnesium is absorbed and may cause hypermagnesemia in patients with renal impairment.

Magnesium hydroxide and magnesium oxide have a high neutralizing capacity with a rapid onset of action.

Table 50–4. COMMON ANTACIDS WITH THEIR INGREDIENTS

Name	Aluminum Hydroxide	Magnesium	Other Ingredients	Form*	ANC (mEq)[†]
Amphojel	X			ML	10
Amphojel	X			T	16
Gelusil II	X	X	Simethicone	T	21
Gelusil II	X	X	Simethicone	ML	24
Maalox concentrate	X	X		ML	27.2
Maalox tablets	X	X		T	28
Mylanta	X	X		ML	12.7
Mylanta	X	X		T	11.5
Mylanta II	X	X		ML	25.4
Mylanta II	X	X		T	23
Riopan	X		Magaldrate	T	13.5
Rolaids			Sodium carbonate, dihydroxyaluminum	T	7.5
Tums			Calcium carbonate	T	10
Gaviscon	X		Magnesium trisilicate	T	0.5
Gaviscon	X		Alginic acid	ML	3–4

*Form: T = tablet; ML = liquid.
[†]ANC = acid neutralizing capacity for therapeutic dose of 5 mL or tablet.

These preparations hydrolyze to water and magnesium salts in the stomach after combining with hydrochloric acid. The dose is determined by the number of substitutions with either aluminum or calcium products, which results in normal stools for the patient.

Magnesium carbonate has a high neutralizing capacity; it is similar to the previous preparations, but it liberates carbon dioxide rather than water.

Magnesium phosphate has a neutralizing capacity just below that of magnesium carbonate. Magnesium trisilicate is a poor acid buffer and has a slow onset of action because of its slow solubilization.

○ **Combination products** are used more commonly than single ingredient products. Because each of the antacid ingredients—calcium, aluminum, and magnesium—has an effect on bowel activity, the best antacid is achieved by combining these products into mixtures containing, most commonly, aluminum and magnesium. Other combinations contain calcium carbonate and both aluminum hydroxide and magnesium hydroxide. Antacids may also contain other significant additives, such as magaldrate, simethicone, and alginic acid.

Magaldrate (Riopan), a complex molecule of aluminum hydroxide and magnesium hydroxide, is not absorbed and therefore is unlikely to cause acid-base imbalances.

Simethicone, an antiflatulent and an antifoaming agent (not an antacid), alters the surface tension of the gas bubbles and thus relieves flatulence. The gas bubbles do not disappear, but may form one large gas mass that is potentially more easily eliminated. Simethicone is added to various antacids (Mylanta, Mylanta II, Gelusil, Gelusil II, Gelusil M, and Maalox Plus). In addition, Mylicon (40- and 80-mg chewable tablets) and Silain (50-mg tablets) are available as 40 mg/0.6 mL drops (sugar free), and both contain only simethicone. These medications are taken four times daily, after meals and at bedtime, and as needed for control of flatulence. The efficacy of simethicone with or in combination with antacids at this time is doubtful.

Alginic acid (not an antacid itself) is added to Gaviscon.

It causes a viscous solution to float on top of the gastric contents and protects the esophageal mucosa of patients with esophageal reflux or ulcers or hiatal hernias.

The most common antacid preparations are listed in Table 50–4, with a comparison of their ingredients and neutralizing capacity.

HISTAMINE H₂ ANTAGONISTS

For many years, researchers have tried to develop a drug that would suppress gastric secretions. Finally in the mid-1970s, **cimetidine (Tagamet)**, the first commercially available histamine H_2 receptor antagonist, was placed on the market in the United States. Today additional histamine₂ antagonists including **ranitidine (Zantac), famotidine (Pepcid)**, and **nizatidine (Axid)**, all featured in Table 50–5, are also available. In 1995–1996, all drugs received OTC approval.

ACTION

Histamine stimulates contractions of the smooth muscles of the gastrointestinal (GI) tract. H_2 antagonists occupy the receptor site in the parietal cells and do not allow it to be stimulated by incoming histamine; thus they are called H_2 receptor antagonists. These drugs are potent inhibitors of secretions caused by histamine, muscarinic agonists, and gastrin, inhibiting all phases of gastric acid secretion from the parietal and oxyntic cells, labeled H_2 receptors. Secretions are inhibited during fasting (day and night); those normally produced by food, insulin, and caffeine are also inhibited.

USES

The histamine H_2 antagonists are all effective in alleviating symptoms and preventing complications of peptic ulcer disease (most patients heal within 4 to 6 weeks); they

Table 50–5. HISTAMINE H₂ ANTAGONISTS

DRUG NAME/ROUTE AND DOSAGE	PHARMACOKINETICS/DYNAMICS	NURSING IMPLICATIONS
all histamine H₂ antagonists		**ASSESSMENT:** Check for signs and symptoms of occult bleeding; assess stool color and vital signs daily. Assess for pregnancy (category B); nizatidine is category C. **INTERVENTION:** Antacids are given concurrently but not at same time. Monitor gastric pH whenever possible. A pH of 3.5 or higher is desirable, and for stress ulcers a pH above 7.4 is desirable. Check for reduced dosages in elderly or in patients with reduced renal function. **Patient Teaching**—Advise patients to avoid all products that increase gastric acid secretion, like smoking. **EVALUATION:** Notify physician of diarrhea, dizziness, black tarry stools.
cimetidine (Tagmet)		
active ulcer, duodenal ulcer *Adults:* 300 mg PO 4 times/day, 400 mg bid, or 800 mg hs; or 300 mg/5 mL (liquid). **healed ulcer** *Adults:* 400 mg PO hs. **hypersecretion syndrome** *Adults:* 300 mg PO qid. 300 mg diluted with any IV solution to 1.2–5.0 mg/mL. Administer over 15–30 min. 300 mg IV bolus mixed with 20 mL administered over 5 min.	**Onset:** PO 30 min; IV 10 min **Peak:** PO 1 hr; IV 30 min **Duration:** 4–5 hrs **½L:** 2 hr **PB:** 13%–25% **B:** liver (30%–40% metabolized) **E:** urine (PO, 48% unchanged; IV, 75% unchanged)	Same as for all plus: **INTERVENTION:** Cimetidine can be administered IV by slow bolus or drip every 4–6 hr during the 24–hr period. It is compatible with most IV solutions and can be administered piggyback with insulin, antibiotics, and total parenteral nutrition. Bolus of 300 mg should be diluted with normal saline solution to total volume of 20 mL and given over 5 min. Rapid IV dosing has been associated with dysrhythmia and hypotension. IV drip of 300 mg should be diluted in at least 50 mL of any solution and given over 15–20 min. Cimetidine is given with meals and at bedtime when it is given orally and the patient is eating. If patient is receiving nothing by mouth, medication is spaced at even intervals around the clock. Administer antacids concurrently but not at same time.
ranitidine hydrochloride (Zantac)		
active ulcer *Adults:* 150 mg PO q 12 hr or 300 mg hs. **healed ulcer** *Adults:* 150 mg PO hs. **hypersecretion syndrome, gastroesophageal reflux** *Adults:* 150 mg PO bid up to 6 g/day; 50 mg IV bolus q 6–8 hr, dilute to 20 mL and give over 5 min, 50 mg intermittent IV infusion in 100 mL over 15–20 min; 150 mg continuous IV in 250 mL run at 6.25 mg/hr; 50 mg (2 mL) IM q 6–8 hr.	**Onset:** PO rapid; IV 0.25 hr **Peak:** 1–3 hr **Duration:** 8–12 hr **½L:** 2–3 hr **PB:** 15% **B:** liver (<10%) **E:** urine (PO, 30%–35% unchanged; IV, 68%–79% unchanged)	Same as for all plus: **INTERVENTION:** May be administered before, during, or after meals. Therapy is usually for 4 wk. Administer antacids concurrently but not at same time. Slow IV administration decreases adverse effect of bradycardia. Do not add other drugs to IV bottle. Compatible in most IV solutions. **Patient Teaching**—Caution patient about consuming alcohol as enzyme needed for breaking alcohol down in stomach is reduced by ranitidine.
famotidine (Pepcid)		
active ulcer *Adults:* 40 mg PO hs or 20 mg q 12 hr; or 40 mg/5 mL (liquid). **healed ulcer** *Adults:* 20 mg PO hs. **hypersecretion syndromes** *Adults:* 20 mg PO q 6 hr up to 160 mg/day; 2 mL in 10 mL IV bolus over 2 min; 2 mL IV drip with 100 mL over 15–30 min.	**Onset:** 1 hr **Peak:** 2–4 hr **Duration:** 10–12 hr **½L:** 2.5–3.5 hr **PB:** 15%–20% **B:** liver (30%–35%) **E:** urine (PO, 30% unchanged; IV, 70% unchanged)	Same as for all.

Table 50–5. HISTAMINE H₂ ANTAGONISTS, *Continued*		
DRUG NAME/ROUTE AND DOSAGE	**PHARMACOKINETICS/ DYNAMICS**	**NURSING IMPLICATIONS**
nizatidine (Axid)		
active ulcer *Adults:* 300 mg PO hs or 150 mg bid. **healed ulcer** *Adults:* 150 mg PO at bedtime.	**Onset:** 0.5–1 hr **Peak:** 0.5–3 hr **Duration:** 3–10 hr **½L:** 1–2 hr **PB:** 35% **B:** liver (<18%) **E:** urine 90% (60% unchanged)	Same as for all plus: **INTERVENTION:** Therapy often continued for 1 yr.

also prevent stress ulcers, to reduce the incidence of heartburn, increase healing in gastroesophageal reflux disease, and reduce recurrence of all ulcers. In addition, they are used to treat pathologic hypersecretory disorders such as Zollinger-Ellison syndrome (all but nizatidine) and, in multidrug therapy, to eradicate *H. pylori*. The OTC indications include heartburn, acid indigestion, and sour stomach. Unlabeled uses include the following: prevention of aspiration pneumonitis during anesthesia and surgery; prophylaxis for tinea capitis, herpes virus infection, hirsutism in women, chronic idiopathic urticaria, and acetaminophen overdose by reduction of formation of the toxic intermediate via the cytochrome P-450 oxidase system; and finally, improvement of survival in patients with colorectal cancer. Most of the unlabeled uses have been studied with cimetidine.

Recent research indicates that cimetidine, famotidine, and nizatidine are of limited value in treating or preventing NSAID-induced GI distress or ulcers. Cimetidine has been used in both the United States and other countries in the treatment of upper GI hemorrhage. However, conflicting research is available. Large numbers of publications compared antacids and cimetidine and concluded that patients receiving high doses of antacids bleed less than those who receive cimetidine. Therefore, the routine prescription of cimetidine instead of antacids in all patients admitted to intensive care units does not seem to be justified.

PHARMACOKINETICS

The H₂ inhibitor antagonists are well absorbed by mouth, although absorption may be slowed in the presence of antacids. Therapeutic levels can be achieved after both oral and intravenous bolus or drip infusion (nizatidine is available only in an oral form). Peak action occurs in 30 minutes to 3 hours after administration. Half-life varies between 1 and 3.5 hours. All are distributed to all body tissues. Protein binding ranges from 13% to 35%.

All H₂ inhibitor antagonists are biotransformed in the liver. Most drugs are metabolized in two phases. Phase 1 is mediated through the microsomal enzyme oxidase system of cytochrome P-450 and is accomplished by oxidation, reduction, and hydrolysis; it is the phase in which compounds are made more water soluble. In phase 2,

drugs are eliminated by conjugation. Cimetidine reversibly inhibits microsomal metabolism in either a competitive or noncompetitive manner. This specific action of cimetidine accounts for numerous drug interactions that occur with cimetidine to be discussed later. Approximately 35% to 60% of the oral H₂ inhibitor antagonist drugs are excreted unchanged in the urine, whereas 65% to 79% are found in the urine following intravenous or intramuscular injection. Therefore, a patient with renal disease should have the dosage reduced.

CONTRAINDICATIONS AND PRECAUTIONS

Contraindications include hypersensitivity to the individual agent. There are no adequate studies that demonstrate safety in pregnancy (category B or C), so administer only when benefits outweigh risk. All drugs are given cautiously to nursing women as they all are excreted in breast milk (do not nurse with cimetidine, and exercise caution with ramitidine, mizatidine, and famotidine) and to persons with impaired renal or hepatic function as clearance may be reduced. Cimetidine is given cautiously to patients seriously ill as there may be an increase in reversible CNS effects such as mental confusion, agitation, psychosis, depression, anxiety, and disorientation.

ADVERSE EFFECTS

Many adverse effects occur with H₂ inhibitor antagonists, including endocrine effects, renal and hepatic effects, CNS effects, effects on the immune and cardiovascular systems, and several miscellaneous effects. The adverse effects of cimetidine are discussed first. Ranitidine appears to be a very safe drug with less than 2% of patients complaining of adverse effects.

Cimetidine displaces testosterone from its receptor site and causes gynecomastia in men. Cimetidine may also cause breast pain and breast enlargement in both men and women. These effects are generally dose and duration dependent and usually disappear when treatment is discontinued. Also, prolonged high-dose cimetidine may reduce libido and cause impotence.

Small increases in serum creatinine have been noted but are not usually associated with significant changes in renal function. Acute interstitial nephritis is a rare complication and is thought to be an idiosyncratic reaction to cimetidine. Some patients receiving cimetidine experience an increase in their liver transaminase levels, which return to normal after discontinuation of cimetidine.

Elderly patients in particular with decreased renal or hepatic function may develop confusion, agitation, drowsiness, and even coma after receiving any of the H$_2$ antagonists. Mental changes improve with discontinuation of the drugs.

Histamine and H$_2$ receptors are found in leukocytes and in suppresser T lymphocytes. Therefore, cimetidine may depress the immune system.

The cardiovascular system is also affected, particularly following rapid intravenous administration of cimetidine or ranitidine. Patients may develop bradycardia and sinus and cardiac arrest.

Patients may also experience mild and transient GI symptoms including nausea, diarrhea, and abdominal pain. CNS signs such as dizziness, somnolence, and headache have also been reported. Patients may also complain of rash, myalgia, and arthralgia.

INTERACTIONS

As previously discussed, cimetidine reversibly inhibits hepatic microsomal metabolism of the enzyme oxidase system of cytochrome P-450. Thus, because of these actions, cimetidine decreases the clearance of benzodiazepines, caffeine, beta-blockers, calcium channel blockers, lidocaine, phenytoin, quinidine, metformin, theophylline, and warfarin. Cimetidine also decreases the formation of toxic metabolites from acetaminophen. The effect of cimetidine on drug metabolism can be detected 24 to 48 hours after initiation of its administration and usually disappears 48 hours after cimetidine is discontinued. The doses of the just-named drugs must be adjusted to prevent toxic plasma levels of the associated drug.

If cimetidine is given concurrently by mouth with antacids in a fasting state, cimetidine absorption may be slowed. Therefore, oral cimetidine as well as rantidine and antacids are always separated by 1 hour. Serum digoxin levels may decrease during coadministration with cimetidine.

Cimetidine and ranitidine both inhibit the stomach enzymes that normally help break down alcohol before it gets into the bloodstream. Therefore, patients must be cautioned about the increased effect that 1 or 2 alcoholic beverages may have.

The remaining H$_2$ inhibitor antagonists do not have an effect on the cytochrome P-450 pathway; therefore, they have fewer interactions.

O **Cimetidine** (Tagamet) is administered by mouth, slow IV bolus, or IV drip. Dosing is in Table 50–5.

O **Ranitidine hydrochloride** (Zantac) is a second generation H$_2$ receptor antagonist with a slightly different structure than cimetidine. For this reason, ranitidine lacks some of the adverse effects (the antiandrogenic properties) and drug interactions that are common to cimetidine. Ranitidine is 13 times more potent in inhibiting pentagastrin-stimulated acid secretion and 10 times more potent than cimetidine in inhibiting pepsin secretion. Rani-

tidine hydrochloride inhibits both daytime and nocturnal basal gastric acid secretion, as well as gastric acid secretions stimulated by food and histamine from 3 to 13 hours after a dose (the 13 hours is for nocturnal suppression).

O **Famotidine** (Pepcid) is similar to cimetidine and ranitidine. Its inhibitory effect is also more prolonged than that of cimetidine and it does not seem to have antiandrogenic properties.

O **Nizatidine** (Axid) appears to be as effective as the other H$_2$ inhibitors already discussed.

PROTON PUMP INHIBITORS

O **Omeprazole** *(Prilosec)* and **lansoprazole** *(Prevacid)* are proton pump inhibitors, which suppress gastric acid secretion by specific inhibition of the H$^+$/K$^+$ ATPase enzyme system in the gastric parietal cell. These drugs inhibit secretion of acid by about 50% to 90% and have no effect on gastric emptying. Suppression of gastric acid begins in 1 hour, reaches its maximal effect within 2 hours, and half of the peak effect is still present 24 hours. After use for 1 to 2 weeks, the mean decrease in gastric acidity is about 90%. Additional pharmacokinetics are presented in Table 50–6.

USES The proton pump inhibitors are used with active ulcer disease, erosive esophagitis, and pathologic hypersecretory conditions such as Zollinger-Ellison syndrome.

CONTRAINDICATIONS AND PRECAUTIONS The proton pump inhibitors are contraindicated in patients hypersensitive to its components. Use in pregnancy only if the potential benefit outweighs the risk (omeprazole, pregnancy category C; lansoprazole, pregnancy category B). Safety and efficacy in lactating women and children has not been established. Symptomatic response to therapy does not preclude gastric malignancy.

ADVERSE EFFECTS The proton pump inhibitors are generally well tolerated, and adverse effects occur in fewer than 1% of patients. Most common adverse effects include headache, diarrhea, abdominal pain, and nausea.

▼ **CLINICAL ALERT**

The primary concern about these drugs has been the uncertain long-term effects of the intense acid suppression, which causes an increase in secretion of gastrin. Gastrin has a trophic effect on the gastric mucosa, which may lead to the development of gastric carcinoid tumors and the overgrowth of bacteria, which might lead to infection.

INTERACTIONS Omeprazole inhibits the oxidative metabolism of diazepam, which increases plasma concentration of diazepam while decreasing total body clearance. Omeprazole reduces the plasma clearance of phenytoin and prolongs the elimination of warfarin. Lansoprazole and sucralfate administered concurrently reduce the availability of lansoprazole by 30%. Therefore, separate by at least 30 minutes.

Table 50–6. PROTON PUMP INHIBITORS AND MUCOSAL PROTECTANTS

DRUG NAME/ROUTE AND DOSAGE	PHARMACOKINETICS/ DYNAMICS	NURSING IMPLICATIONS
PROTON PUMP INHIBITORS		
omeprazole (Prilosec)		
Adults: 20 mg PO once daily before a meal. Pathologic hypersecretory conditions may require up to 360 mg daily.	**Onset:** <1 hr **Peak:** 2 hr **Duration:** 72–96 hr **½L:** 0.5–1 hr **PB:** 95% **B:** liver **E:** urine (77%), bile	**ASSESSMENT:** Assess symptoms before and during therapy. Assess for pregnancy (category C). **INTERVENTION:** Take before eating, swallow whole—do not crush or open capsule. Therapy usually continues for 4–8 wk. Do not use as maintenance therapy. Take antacids with drug. **EVALUATION:** Report headache, severe diarrhea to physician.
lansoprazole (Prevacid)		
duodenal ulcer **Adults:** 15 mg PO before meals for 4 wk. **esophagitis** **Adults:** 30 mg PO before meals for 8 wk. May repeat 2 times if needed. **hypersecretion syndrome** **Adults:** 60 mg PO once daily up to 90 mg bid.	**Onset:** rapid **Peak:** 1.7 hr **Duration:** acid-inhibiting effect lasts 24 hr **½L:** 1.5 hr **PB:** 97% **B:** liver **E:** renal	**ASSESSMENT:** Assess symptoms before and during therapy. **INTERVENTION: Patient Teaching**—Instruct patient to take before meals and to not open, chew, or crush capsules. **EVALUATION:** Report headache, severe diarrhea.
MUCOSAL PROTECTANTS		
sucralfate (Carafate)		
Adults: 1 g PO 4 times/day 1 hr ac and hs. Suspension available for oral use.	**Onset:** 30 min **Peak:** NA **Duration:** 6 hr **½L:** 6–20 hr **PB:** NA **B:** liver **E:** stool (90%)	**ASSESSMENT:** Assess symptoms before and during therapy. Assess for pregnancy (category B). **INTERVENTION: Patient Teaching**—Do not administer antacids within 30 min before or after sucralfate. Administer on empty stomach 1 hr before or 2 hr after meal and hs. **EVALUATION:** GI pain symptoms should subside. Monitor for diarrhea, dry mouth, vertigo. Report to physician.

NA = not available.

MUCOSAL PROTECTANTS

○ **Sucralfate** *(Carafate)* (see Table 50–6) exerts its effect through a local, rather than a systemic, action to heal ulcers. Sucralfate forms an ulcer-adherent complex with protein exudates (albumin and fibrinogen) at the ulcer site. This complex covers the ulcer site and protects it against further attack by acid, pepsin, or bile salts. Sucralfate has a negligible acid-neutralizing capacity, but does inhibit pepsin activity in gastric juice by 32%. Sucralfate also blocks the diffusion of gastric acid across the protective barrier and limits proteolytic activity of pepsin. Sucralfate also appears to stimulate synthesis of prostaglandins by the mucosa of the stomach and duodenum. Sucralfate requires an acid environment for optimal effectiveness, so it should not be administered concurrently with an antacid. Several clinical trials have compared cimetidine and sucralfate as to healing rate after 4 to 8 weeks. The relapse rate after 6 to 12 months was significantly lower for patients treated with sucralfate.

USES Sucralfate is indicated for short-term therapy of duodenal ulcers and prophylaxis of stress ulcers. Sucralfate appears to also have a protective effect on spontaneous, aspirin-induced, or NSAID-related gastric microbleeding. Sucralfate is also being used to provide relief for oral ulcers and mucosal pain associated with chemotherapy and radiation. A sucralfate suspension is swished in the mouth for 2 minutes up to six times per day. Sucralfate deposits a pasty protective layer over the mucosa, reduces pain, and promotes healing. Sucralfate may also have a beneficial effect in the treatment of reflux esophagitis and bile reflux gastritis as well as recurrent ulcer following gastric surgery. Sucralfate may also be used to prevent stress ulcers in the critically ill. The fact that the pH is unaffected with sucralfate may offer an advantage as gram-negative bacillus cannot grow in a very acidic medium. Gram-negative bacillus growth may be related to nosocomial infection in the critically ill.

CONTRAINDICATIONS AND PRECAUTIONS There are no known contraindications to sucralfate at this time. Safety and effectiveness in pregnancy (category B), lactation, and children have not been established.

ADVERSE EFFECTS Because it is not a systemic drug, adverse effects of sucralfate are minor. The most frequent adverse effect is constipation. Additional adverse effects include diarrhea, nausea, gastric discomfort, indigestion, dry mouth, rash, dizziness, and vertigo.

INTERACTIONS Cimetidine, quinolones, digoxin, phenytoin, warfarin, ketoconazole, and quinidine may bind in the stomach and have decreased bioavailability. They are given 2 hours before or after sucralfate.

GASTROINTESTINAL STIMULANTS

○ **Metoclopramide** *(Reglan)* and *cisapride* *(Propulsid)* stimulate motility of the upper GI tract and increase the rate of gastric emptying, without stimulating gastric, biliary, or pancreatic secretions. The exact mechanism of action is unknown, but these drugs appear to sensitize tissues to the effects of dopamine. Pharmacokinetic and dosage information is presented in Table 50–7.

USES Metoclopramide and cisapride are used to relieve the symptoms of gastroesophageal reflux. In addition, metoclopramide is used to treat acute and recurrent diabetic gastroparesis and to prevent nausea and vomiting associated with cancer chemotherapy. Metoclopramide is also used to treat nausea and vomiting of pregnancy and labor, gastric ulcer disease, and anorexia nervosa. Metoclopramide is being studied to improve lactation because it elevates serum prolactin levels. Metoclopramide may also enhance absorption of ergotamine products used in migraine headaches. Metoclopramide and aspirin (900 mg) are being studied for the prevention of migraines.

CONTRAINDICATIONS AND PRECAUTIONS Metoclopramide and cisapride are contraindicated in patients with known sensitivity and in patients in whom stimulation of GI motility may be dangerous such as in mechanical obstruction or perforation or GI hemorrhage. In patients with pheochromocytoma, metoclopramide may precipitate hypertensive crisis due to the release of catecholamines from the tumor.

▼ CLINICAL ALERT

Cisapride is metabolized by the cyctochrome 450 system in the liver and may lengthen the QT interval; therefore, great care is taken during the drug history to identify other medications the patient is taking that also can

---

Table 50–7. GASTROINTESTINAL STIMULANTS

DRUG NAME/ROUTE AND DOSAGE	PHARMACOKINETICS/ DYNAMICS	NURSING IMPLICATIONS
metoclopramide (Reglan)		
diabetic gastroparesis 10 mg PO 30 min before meals and bedtime for 2–8 weeks. **gastroesophageal reflux** 10–15 mg PO qid 30 min before meals and hs. **facilitation of intubation of small bowel** 10 mg IV over 1–2 min. **nausea secondary to chemotherapy** 1–2 mg/kg IV over 1–2 min. If over 10 mg, mix with 50 mL and administer in not less than 15 min. Repeat q 2 hr for 2 doses then q 3 hr for 3 doses. **gastric stasis** 10 mg IM 30 min before meals and hs.	**Onset:** PO 30–60 min; IV 1–3; IM 10–15 min **Peak:** PO 60 min; IV immediately **Duration:** 1–2 hr **½L:** 2.5–5 hr **PB:** 30% (weakly bound) **B:** liver (minimal) **E:** urine (80% unchanged), bile (25%)	**ASSESSMENT:** Assess for pregnancy (category B). **INTERVENTION:** Dosage of insulin may require adjustment as food reaches intestine more quickly. Drug may be removed with dialysis. If extrapyramidal symptoms occur, administer 50 mg diphenhydramine IM. **Patient Teaching**—Take medication 30 min before meals and hs. May produce drowsiness and dizziness, so observe caution while operating heavy equipment. **EVALUATION:** Notify physician if involuntary movement of eyes, face, or limbs occurs.
cisapride (Propulsid)		
Adults: 10 mg PO qid up to 20 mg qid if needed.	**Onset:** 30–60 min **Peak:** 1–1.5 hr **Duration:** 8–10 hr **½L:** 6–12 hr **PB:** 98% **B:** liver **E:** urine (10% unchanged)	**ASSESSMENT:** Assess for pregnancy (category C). Obtain any drug history to eliminate any drug interactions. **INTERVENTION:** Administer 15 min before meals and hs. **Patient Teaching**—Caution patient about drinking alcohol because it may cause increased drowsiness. **EVALUATION:** Report severe diarrhea, rash, fever or infection.

lengthen the QT interval (quinidine, propranolol, erythromycin, benzothiapines, ketoconozale, and most nonsedating antihistamines).

Safety in pregnancy (category C), lactation, and children has not been established; metoclopramide is pregnancy category B.

ADVERSE EFFECTS Adverse effects of metoclopramide and cisapride are usually mild and transient. Because these drugs are widely distributed to all tissues, there is a high incidence of CNS effects. These effects include restlessness, drowsiness, extrapyramidal reactions, dizziness, insomnia, and headache. Patients on metoclopramide can also experience Parkinson-like reaction (extrapynomidal symptoms). If this occurs, the drug is stopped. The Parkinson-like reaction is rare with cisapride. Metoclopramide increases the release of prolactin and may cause galactorrhea, reversible amenorrhea, nipple tenderness, and gynecomastia in males. Metoclopramide may also increase bronchospasm in patients with asthma.

INTERACTIONS Metoclopramide interacts with numerous drugs. Anticholinergics and narcotic analgesics antagonize metoclopramide. Alcohol, sedatives, cyclosporine, and tranquilizers have an additive effect. Drug absorption in the stomach may be diminished whereas drug absorption in the small bowel may be accelerated. Cisapride may also increase the absorption of cimetidine and ramitidine when administered concurrently.

PROSTAGLANDINS

Prostaglandins (PGs) are potent inhibitors of gastric acid secretion and have a stabilizing effect on the gastric mucosa. PGE, PGA, and PGI inhibit basal acid secretion by food, histamine, pentagastrin, and cholinergic agents. Two synthetic analogs—PGE_2 and PGE_1—have been developed. Antisecretory effects of these agents last longer than the actual natural product, and they can be given orally. Prostaglandins being studied investigationally today may be more effective than H_2 antagonists or sucralfate in treating peptic ulcers in refractory patients, especially in smokers and patients receiving NSAIDS. The prostaglandins—misoprostol (Cytotec), investigational arbaprostil—used to prevent ulcer formation in patients taking NSAIDs are discussed in Chapter 57.

CHOICE OF DRUG

Initially, the treatment of minor GI complaints such as heartburn and acid indigestion is to remove the offending stimulus. A nondrug approach to managing ulcer disease in smokers is strongly encouraged. Smoking decreases ulcer healing rates and increases the probability of an ulcer recurrence. Cessation of smoking can be highly therapeutic. Also, the presence or absence of pain is not an effective indication of ulcer healing. Some patients experience pain whereas others do not. In addition, symptomatic pain relief does not necessarily imply ulcer healing. Ulcers in the elderly who suffer from achlorhydria may be best treated with nonsystemic agents such as sucralfate.

Because *H. pylori* is the causative agent in most ulcers, the use of antibiotics, Prilosec, and bismuth salycilate are becoming the number one treatment options.

The decision to use one H_2 receptor antagonist rather than another is based on many factors: efficacy, cost, compliance, safety, interactions with other drugs, and the physician's own experience. The efficacy of all H_2 receptor antagonists is similar for the treatment of duodenal ulcer and for maintenance. Omeprazole, at this time, appears to be more effective than ranitidine for the treatment of gastroesophageal reflux and appears to heal ulcers more quickly. However, long-term safety has not been proven, so omeprazole is reserved for short-term therapy only.

If ulcers do not heal after 8–12 weeks of treatment with H_2 antagonists, other causes of symptoms, such as food intolerances, hypersecretion states, cancer, ulcerogenic drugs, Crohn's disease, lymphoma, or noncompliance with therapy, must be considered.

Approximately 60% to 80% of ulcers relapse within 1 year when treated with antacids and H_2 antagonists. When ulcers are treated with antibiotics, prilosec, and bismuth, the one year release rate is only about 14%.

All the H_2 receptor antagonists along with omeprazole decrease gastric acid secretion, which in turn allows for the overgrowth of gram-negative bacteria. These bacteria in turn may be responsible for precipitating pneumonia. Many studies, including a large meta-analysis, have examined the efficacy of sucralfate and H_2 antagonists in the prevention of stress bleeding and the frequency of pulmonary infection. Results demonstrate that sucralfate was significantly more effective than H_2 antagonists in controlling stress bleeding. The analysis also found that there is an increase in pulmonary infections in patients treated with antacids or H_2 antagonists, especially patients with a consistently high gastric pH above 6. The pneumonia rate in patients with high gastric pH was 92% compared with 9% in the patients with a low pH (Tryba, 1991).

The pathophysiology of gastroesopheageal reflux disease (GERD) is multifactorial. After diagnosis, nondrug therapies are also instituted including elevating the head of the bed on blocks, cessation of smoking, and dietary modification including the elimination of caffeine. Drugs that lower the esophageal sphincter tone (theophylline, progesterone, calcium channel blockers) may require dosage adjustments or discontinuation. Antacids may assist with acute pain control of GERD. H_2 antagonists are considered secondary therapy in managing GERD.

USING THE NURSING PROCESS

ASSESSMENT

- Obtain a thorough nursing history to develop the database. Information to be obtained from the patient, which is used to prepare the nursing plan, is included in Table 50–8.

Table 50–8. NURSING PROCESS FOR PATIENT REQUIRING DRUGS TO REDUCE GASTRIC ACIDITY

Assessment

Assess history of current illness, including pain and dietary patterns (types, quantities, and time food is consumed); alcohol, caffeine use; and smoking habits.

Assess medication use (prescription and OTC), including when, how, and amount of antacids taken.

Assess emotional/stress factors (financial, relationship, job related).

Assess laboratory studies, e.g., CBC, electrolytes, BUN, stool specimens, and ECG.

Assess bowel habits (diarrhea/constipation) and relationship to current problems.

Nursing Diagnosis: Pain (Acute)/Chronic

RELATED TO: Physical response, e.g., reflex muscle spasm in the stomach wall, chemical burn of gastric mucosa.

AS EVIDENCED BY: Complaints, abdominal guarding, rigid body posture, facial grimacing, autonomic responses.

Desired Outcomes/Evaluation Criteria

Verbalizes relief of pain. Demonstrates relaxed body posture and is able to sleep/rest appropriately.

Nursing Actions	Rationale
Note complaints of pain, including location, duration, intensity (1–10 scale).	Pain is not always present, but if present, should be compared with previous pain symptoms to assist in diagnosis of etiology/development of complications.
Review factors that aggravate or alleviate pain.	Helpful in establishing diagnosis and treatment needs.
Provide frequent small meals as indicated for individual patient. Identify and limit foods that create discomfort.	Has an acid-neutralizing effect as well as diluting the gastric contents. Small meals prevent distention and release of gastrin.
Administer antacids.	Decreases gastric acidity by absorption or by chemical neutralization. Evaluate type of antacid in regard to total health picture, e.g., sodium restriction.

Nursing Diagnosis: Knowledge Deficit

RELATED TO: Lack of information, unfamiliarity with information resources.

AS EVIDENCED BY: Questions, statement of concern, inaccurate follow-through of instructions/development of preventable complications.

Desired Outcomes/Evaluation Criteria

Verbalizes understanding of illness, cause, treatment, and prognosis. Begins to discuss own role in preventing recurrence. Identifies necessary lifestyle changes and participates in treatment regimen.

Nursing Actions	Rationale
Provide/review information regarding etiology/pathophysiology of illness, cause/effect relationship of lifestyle behaviors, and ways to reduce risk/contributing factors.	Provides knowledge base on which patient can make information choices/decisions about future and control of health problems.
Review drug regimen and possible side effects. Problem-solve solutions to side effects as appropriate	Helpful to patient's understanding of reason for taking drugs, and important symptoms to report to health caregiver. Although dry mouth or photophobia may be annoying, drowsiness/dizziness encountered with initial anticholinergic therapy may increase risk of injury if not anticipated/planned for.
Discuss common side effects, e.g., constipation/diarrhea.	Anticipation of problems and taking appropriate action can prevent untoward complications.
Caution against use of other OTC products/antacids.	Combinations of antacids may potentiate development of milk-alkali syndrome, rebound acidity, sodium retention.
Review signs of electrolyte disturbance for particular drug patient is taking.	Electrolyte imbalance can be a serious side-effect of antacid use, and prompt identification can prevent complications.
Encourage patient to follow diet as prescribed.	Modifications are based on individual needs. Avoiding late-night snacks, eating smaller but more frequent meals each day, eliminating caffeine, limiting milk and dairy products, and eliminating foods that cause problems for the patient have been found to be helpful.
Encourage cessation of smoking. Discuss use of alcohol.	Nicotine increases gastric secretions. Consumption of alcohol on an empty stomach may delay healing, but moderate use with food intake does not seem to aggravate symptoms.
Stress importance of returning for regular medical checkup.	Monitoring for/early identification of developing complications can prevent untoward results (e.g., hypercalcemia).

Other Suggested Nursing Diagnoses: Altered Nutrition, More or Less Than Body Requirements, Diarrhea, Constipation, and Body Image Disturbance.

- Obtain a complete medication history. Determine what medications are taken including prescription and OTC to determine if any of these will cause or aggravate current symptoms. There is evidence that NSAIDs aggravate mucosal damage, delay healing, and/or predispose to bleeding. Therefore, NSAIDs are avoided in patients with peptic ulcer. Determine when and how patients take their medication—with food or between meals on an empty stomach. Determine how long it takes them to use a bottle of antacid. As an example, if a patient says he uses a bottle (12 oz) a week, then he takes less than 2 oz/day, which is less than 15 mL per dose qid. This dose is probably less than effective. Also determine if patients substitute tablets for liquid. Because tablets are less effective than liquids, their dosing, again, may not be adequate.
- Assess eating habits, including the types, quantities, and time food is consumed. There is little evidence that any single dietary factor influences the healing of peptic ulcers, and the so-called ulcer diet consisting of bland soft foods with milk or cream does not affect the rate of healing or recurrence. However, foods, spices, and liquids that provoke or worsen symptoms are avoided, and patients should eat three meals a day that comprise a balanced diet of their choosing. Eating small meals every 2 or 3 hours may minimize variations in intragastric pH, but may not be necessary in patients receiving antiulcer medications. Alteration of dietary pattern may be part of the nursing intervention phase.
- Assess any emotional factors that may contribute to the development of peptic ulcers. The resolution of problems that contribute to emotional distress may reduce the extent and frequency of pain. Reassurance by the nurse can often reduce anxiety and promote compliance with the medical regimen.
- Assess for smoking, as cigarette smoking delays healing and may increase recurrence. In addition, smoking may decrease the effectiveness of cimetidine and other antiulcer medications.
- Assess laboratory data such as complete blood count (CBC), electrocardiogram (ECG), fluid and electrolyte levels, and stool specimens for the presence of melena. Melena is caused by bleeding from a level above the ileocecal valve. A blood urea nitrogen (BUN) is also obtained. Transient elevation of BUN without corresponding increases in serum creatinine concentration occurs regularly in patients with upper GI bleeding and restricted renal perfusion. Lower GI bleeding is usually typified by a normal BUN. Patients may also be prepared for radiographs or endoscopic exam.

NURSING DIAGNOSIS

- Typical nursing diagnoses for a patient requiring medications to reduce gastric acidity include Acute or Chronic Pain, Knowledge Deficit, Altered Nutrition, Diarrhea, and Constipation (see Table 50–8).

PLANNING AND PREVENTION

- Establish the goals of nursing intervention. Typical goals of nursing intervention are included in Table 50–8. These goals can usually be achieved by eliminating precipitating or aggravating factors and administering drug therapy.

Nursing Responsibilities

- Dilute aluminum products either 1:2 or 1:4 with water when administering via nasogastric (NG) tube. Aluminum hydroxide interferes with the absorption of phosphates from the intestine and in the presence of a low-phosphate diet may cause deficiencies.
- Obtain gastric samples to monitor gastric pH as ordered. This procedure is timed so that it does not interfere with medication administration. Proper paper is important to use, one that has a range in increments starting with 0.5, 1, 2, to 7. Gastric pH can change from the area near the mucosal surface to fluid in deep gastric villi. Therefore, it is suggested that trends be measured rather than individual numbers. A sudden increase in pH may mean that the NG tube has migrated from the stomach to the duodenum or the esophagus. Conversely, inability to increase pH above 4 with antacids may be one of the first signs of unrecognized sepsis. A pH above 7.5 is not physiologically possible even with antacid therapy.
- When administering H$_2$ receptor antagonists, administer antacids concurrently but not at the same time.

Patient Teaching

- Teach the patient about his or her medications. The patient requires medications to reduce gastric acidity while in the hospital as well as administration at home. He or she may need them for only a few weeks or months or for a lifetime. The patient is made aware of the general information relevant to safe antacid administration included in Table 50–9.
- Ensure that the patient has an adequate level of knowledge about the disease.
- Review the pain pattern that the patient exhibits and strategies for alleviating some of the discomfort with diet or behavior modification. Patients are also encouraged to follow the diet prescribed for them. Based on recent research, patients with ulcers are cautioned to avoid late-night snacks, as this increases nocturnal gastric secretions; to eat smaller, more frequent meals each day, because this has been shown to decrease gastrin production (although this may not be necessary if the patient is receiving antiulcer medications); to eliminate caffeine, not only in coffee, but also in tea and cola beverages; to limit milk and dairy products because recent evidence has shown that the calcium and protein in milk may even increase gastric secretion (this information may contradict the information the patient believed or was given several years ago); and to eliminate any foods that cause

Table 50–9. PATIENT TEACHING INFORMATION—ANTACIDS

Dear Patient:

This drug has been prescribed for you. This is what you should know about your drug to get the most from your therapy.

☐ 1. Antacids make your stomach less acidic.

☐ 2. You will take antacids until your current medical problem is resolved, that is, pain is relieved and/or ulcer is healed (4–6 weeks).

☐ 3. Shake all liquids well before taking them so they are well mixed. Refrigerating them may make them taste better. Chew tablets well (the smaller the particles, the faster they work) and take with a full glass of water.

☐ 4. Antacid tablets are not equal to liquid. Do not substitute without your doctor's OK.

☐ 5. Carry a small bottle of liquid to have doses available away from home.

☐ 6. Always measure your antacid dose; do not drink from the bottle.

☐ 7. Make sure you take your antacid on time. Antacids are taken 1–3 hours after eating and at bedtime.

☐ 8. In general, the following drugs interact with antacids and are given either 1 hour before or 1–2 hours after the antacids. These include tetracycline and quinolone antibiotics, phenothiazine tranquilizers, cardiac glycosides (lanoxin, digoxin), iron salts, isoniazid (INH), propranolol (Inderal), diazepam (Valium) amphetamines, all enteric-coated tablets (Ecotrin), and salicylates. In addition, antacids help your body rid itself of aspirin products. You may have to increase the amount of aspirin product you take to keep pain and inflammation under control. Talk to your doctor about adjusting your aspirin dose.

☐ 9. Observe the number of bowel movements and what they look like daily; if diarrhea or constipation develops, the antacid preparation may be changed. If stools get loose, substitute aluminum hydroxide products every other dose or so; and if constipation occurs, substitute Milk of Magnesia.

☐ 10. The age of the antacid is important. Aluminum hydroxide gel does not work as well when it is past its expiration date.

☐ 11. It is best not to take other medications within 1–2 hours of your antacid. A general rule is to take all drugs before meals by approximately 1 hour.

☐ 12. Antacids are stored in tight, light-resistant bottles.

---

problems for the patient (e.g., spicy foods, gas-producing vegetables or legumes, or onions).

- Encourage the patient to decrease or, if possible, stop smoking. The nicotine in cigarette and tobacco smoke increases gastric secretions. However, cessation of smoking may cause increased anxiety and tension for the patient, which can also increase gastric secretions.
- Teach the patient about alcohol. Consumption of alcohol on an empty stomach may delay healing and is not recommended, but moderate alcohol intake with meals does not aggravate symptoms or delay healing.
- Teach the patient that when administering calcium preparations, serum calcium levels are measured frequently to assess for hypercalcemia. The nurse and patient understand the symptoms of hypercalcemia, including nausea, vomiting, abdominal pain, poly-

uria, cloudy memory, loss of muscle tone, and muscle and joint pain. In addition, the patient with renal impairment should take calcium carbonate cautiously because of the possible development of renal calculi. All patients are made aware of the symptoms of milk-alkali syndrome (previously discussed) if calcium products and sodium bicarbonate are being used chronically.

Patients are cautioned against using sodium bicarbonate and fizzy-type antacids not prescribed by the physician as an antacid because of the rebound acidity, systemic absorption, and high sodium content.

- Teach the patient the signs and symptoms of occult bleeding, which are increasing fatigue, lightheadedness, dizziness, and a change in the color of the stool.
- Discuss interactions that occur with other medications. The patient should always carry the medication profile card to the physician's office or to the pharmacy when filling a prescription or buying an OTC preparation.
- Identify areas of stress for the patient. Stress, anxiety, and tension may be predisposing factors to ulcer formation. The nurse shares with the patient methods of stress reduction or behavior modification methods that may be beneficial.

EVALUATION

- Evaluate the effectiveness of medications to reduce gastric acidity based on a list of evaluation criteria (see Table 50–8) that have been developed in relation to the goals determined by the nurse, patient, and family.
- Work with the patient and family to ensure their complete assistance and support.
- Teach the patient about potential adverse effects so that a patient taking this medication at home is more likely to report any unusual symptom to the physician or nurse. The most common complaint from patients taking antacids is a change in bowel habits, which can usually be corrected by altering the dose or type of antacid used.
- The physician may wish to evaluate the patient for ulcer healing through endoscopic examinations. The patient and family need to know the importance of this procedure. Also, the patient is encouraged to keep the scheduled clinic or physician visits, even though he or she is feeling better.
- Evaluate all previously taught material with patient and family to ensure that their knowledge base remains accurate.

The more the nurse involves the patient and family with the planning and care, the more likely they are to comply. The nurse must stress the importance of continued medical care.

The bibliography for this chapter can be found in Appendix B, which begins on page 1054.

CHAPTER REVIEW QUESTIONS*

1. As a group, antacids act by:
   a. Reducing gastric acid secretions.
   b. Absorbing gastric acid.
   c. Stimulating an alkaline secretion.
   d. Raising the gastric pH.

2. Jane is receiving multiple drugs (digitalis, tetracycline, propranolol, and a phenothiazine). Which of the following statements is *correct* regarding antacids and drug interactions and is most important to share with Jane?
   a. Antacids increase the absorption of digitalis products.
   b. Antacids decrease the absorption of tetracycline antibiotics.
   c. Aluminum products enhance the absorption of propranolol.
   d. Antacids products increase the absorption of the phenothiazine.

3. Prolonged use of aluminum-containing antacids may cause hypophosphatemia, characterized by:
   a. Increased appetite.
   b. Muscle weakness.
   c. Irritability.
   d. Muscle rigidity.

*See Appendix A, which begins on page 1051, for answers.

4. In addition to their neutralizing ability, aluminum-containing antacids have the following action:
   a. Stimulation of peristalsis.
   b. Increased gastric muscle tone.
   c. Delayed gastric emptying.
   d. Reduced number of parietal cells.

5. Cimetidine acts to reduce gastric irritation by:
   a. Coating the stomach lining with an insoluble protective coating.
   b. Blocking the action of histamine in the parietal cells.
   c. Stimulating the release of histamine, which inhibits gastrin.
   d. Blocking the production of pepsinogen in the chief cells.

6. Which of the following is a nursing action associated with sucralfate (Carafate)?
   a. Administer with meals.
   b. Crush if giving via nasogastric tube.
   c. Give cimetidine 2 hours before or after sucralfate.
   d. Give along with antacids.

7. Kelly, a patient with duodenal ulcer, has taken lansoprazole (Prevacid) for 12 weeks. You approach the physician because:
   a. Long-term safety has not been established.
   b. Multiple drug interaction problems can occur.
   c. There has been a chronic reduction in GI bacteria.
   d. The drug is not being administered with an antacid.

BUILDING YOUR CRITICAL THINKING SKILLS

ANTIULCER DRUGS

A 37-year-old woman with a 6-year history of peptic ulcer disease comes to the emergency room with acute abdominal pain described as intense burning for the last 3 hours. The patient admits to medicating herself with over-the-counter products, including antacids 4 times a day and cimetidine (Tagamet) once a day.

1. What other information should the nurse elicit from this patient?
2. What should the patient receive for her drug therapy and what teaching should the nurse incorporate into the plan of care?

CHAPTER 51

Antiemetic and Emetic Medications

Merrily A. Kuhn, RNC, PhD

CHAPTER OUTLINE

Antiemetics
Emetics

TABLES

Drug Tables
Centrally Acting Antiemetics, 756
Miscellaneous Antiemetics, 758
Emetic Medications, 763

Nursing Process
Nursing Process for Patient Requiring Antiemetic
   Medication, 761

Patient Teaching
Patient Teaching Information—Antiemetics, 762

KEY TERMS

Antiemetics
Chemoreceptor trigger zone
Dystonia

Emetics
Extrapyramidal symptoms

LEARNING OBJECTIVES

After reading this chapter, the student will be able to:

1. Identify those medications commonly used as antiemetic and emetic medications.

2. Differentiate among the antiemetic and emetic medications as to mechanism of action, route of administration, pharmacokinetics, adverse effects, contraindications, and interactions.

3. Identify specific areas to assess in the patient requiring antiemetic and emetic medications to formulate appropriate nursing diagnoses.

4. Plan the nursing interventions necessary to administer antiemetic and emetic medications and choose appropriate teaching strategies to gain patient compliance.

5. Evaluate the patient at various stages of treatment to measure the effectiveness of nursing interventions.

Nausea and vomiting are often symptoms of disease that must be controlled while the disease is being treated. In certain patients, it may become necessary to induce vomiting when poisons and toxins have been ingested. Antiemetics and emetics are both discussed in this chapter.

Nausea, vomiting, and vertigo are not diseases in themselves, but are symptoms of an underlying problem. Nausea and vomiting may occur secondary to excessive food/drink, drugs, radiation, metabolic disorders, trauma, anxiety, tension, fear, surgery, motion, pregnancy, gastrointestinal (GI) disorders, infection, food intolerances, disease states, and the list could go on forever. The mechanism may be psychologic, chemical, or caused by abdominal organ abnormalities or stimulation of vestibular organs.

In general, nausea and vomiting occur after the *che-*

moreceptor trigger zone (CTZ) in the medulla of the brain is stimulated by ascending efferent messages, as shown in Figure 51–1, and in turn stimulates the vomiting center (VC), also in the medulla. Consequently to this stimulation, there is increased activity of central neurotransmitters—dopamine in the CTZ and acetylcholine in the VC—which are the major mediators for the induction of vomiting. Excitatory messages are then transmitted through efferent fibers to the salivary glands and the muscles of the diaphragm, anterior abdominal wall, gastric antrum, duodenum, and vomiting ensues, as depicted in Figure 51–2.

This chapter describes the drugs most commonly used as antiemetics. These agents are reviewed in Tables 51–1 and 51–2. Antihistamines are generally considered the best group of drugs for the alleviation of motion sickness and vestibular-induced vomiting. Dimenhydrinate

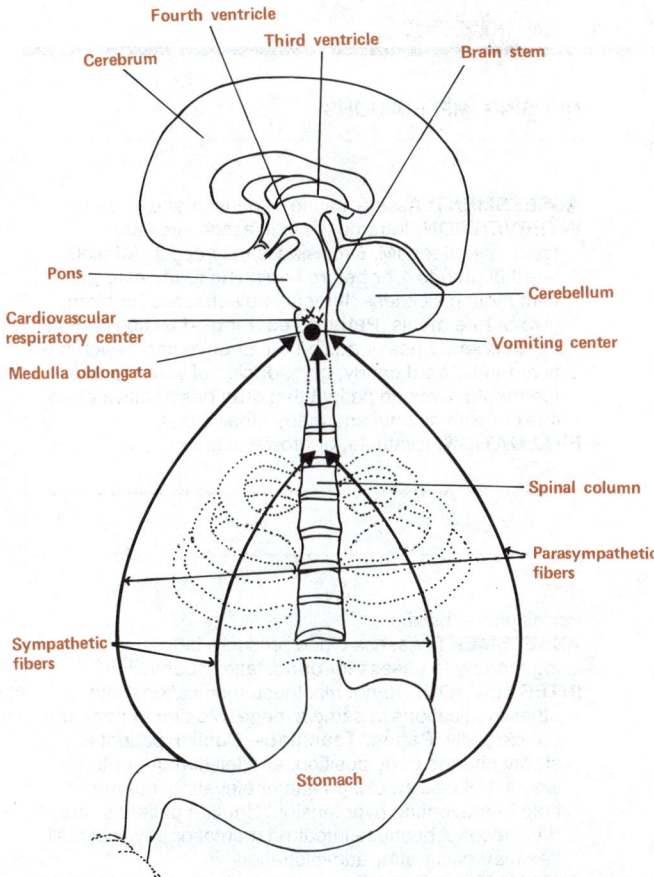

Figure 51–1. Stimuli leave the stomach or other sensory centers, follow the afferent parasympathetic fibers or the sympathetic fibers, and travel via the spinal column to the vomiting center in the medulla oblongata.

(Dramamine), diphenhydramine (Benadryl), and meclizine (Bonine) are sold over the counter (OTC) for the prevention of motion sickness. Antihistamines are also used to modify symptoms of the common cold or allergic rhinitis and are discussed in detail in Chapter 41.

ANTIEMETICS

It is important to understand the cause of the nausea and vomiting and to administer a medication with the correct site of action. In general, antiemetics are more successful in preventing vomiting than in treating it. They are best administered as prophylaxis before actual vomiting has occurred.

TYPES OF ANTIEMETICS

Antiemetics prevent or relieve the symptoms of nausea and vomiting by acting on one or several of the following areas: locally in the stomach; or centrally in the chemoreceptor trigger zone within the vomiting center of the medulla, in the cerebral cortex, or in the aural vestibular apparatus.

Antiemetics may be either locally acting or centrally

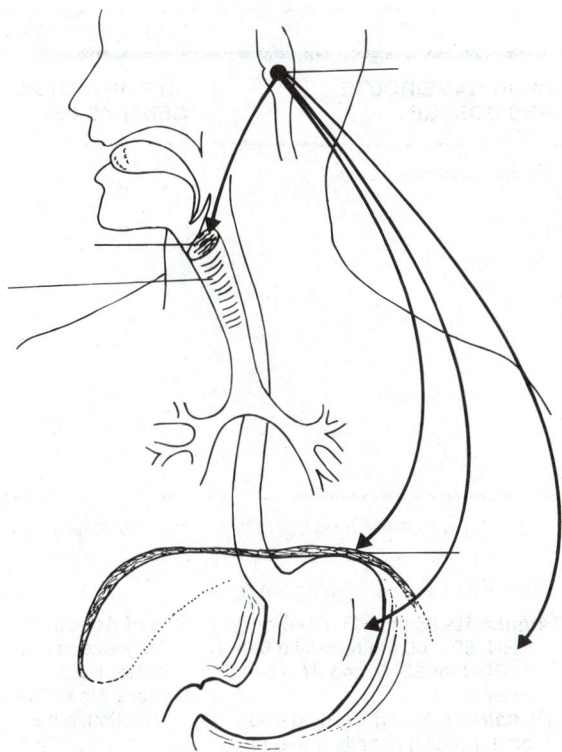

Figure 51–2. Efferent impulses travel to the diaphragm, glottis, stomach, and anterior abdominal muscle, and vomiting occurs.

acting. The locally acting antiemetics soothe the gastric mucosa. The centrally acting drugs include the antidopaminergic agents such as the phenothiazines (e.g., chlorpromazine, promethazine, and metoclopramide); the anticholinergics (scopolamine); the antihistamines (e.g., diphenhydramine, dimenhydrinate, and others) (discussed in Chapter 41); and the miscellaneous agents (e.g., benzquinamide hydrochloride and trimethobenzamide hydrochloride).

Locally Acting Antiemetics

Vomiting caused by local irritation of the gastric mucosa can be treated with locally acting agents. In general, vomiting caused by local irritation is self-limiting: When the stomach rids itself of the irritant, the sensations are relieved. However, an individual with acute or chronic inflammation of the GI tract, such as gastritis or gastroenteritis, may have prolonged symptoms.

Locally acting medications soothe the receptors or reduce the reactivity of the irritants. These are temporary measures that can be used while the patient's GI tract heals. A topical anesthetic, such as viscous lidocaine, raises the threshold of the receptor reactivity to irritants; consequently nausea and vomiting are relieved. Antacids (Chapter 50), adsorbents and demulcents (Chapter 52), and medications that reduce distention (Chapter 55) all act on the stomach mucosa or the receptor centers, or both, to make them less sensitive. These preparations are given between meals. Other protective agents are phosphorated carbohydrate solution (Emetrol) and cola syrup, which are both taken as undiluted liquid. These sub-

Table 51–1. CENTRALLY ACTING ANTIEMETICS

DRUG NAME/ROUTE AND DOSAGE	SITE OF ACTION/ GENERAL USE	NURSING IMPLICATIONS
all antiemetics		**ASSESSMENT:** Assess cause of nausea and vomiting. **INTERVENTION:** Intramuscular injection sites are rotated, give deep IM. Drowsiness may occur. Administered 30 min to 1 hr before beginning to travel to prevent motion sickness. If mealtime nausea is problem, give before meals. **Patient Teaching**—Caution patient to not operate heavy equipment or drive car. Teach patient to use hard candy, gum, or sips of water to moisten mouth. Caution patient that drug has additive effect if taken with alcohol and many other drugs. **EVALUATION:** Evaluate for drowsiness.

ANTIDOPAMINERGIC AGENTS: ALIPHATIC PHENOTHIAZINES

DRUG NAME/ROUTE AND DOSAGE	SITE OF ACTION/ GENERAL USE	NURSING IMPLICATIONS
chlorpromazine (Thorazine) **Adults:** 10–25 mg PO q 4–6 hr PRN; 50–100 mg rectally q 6–8 hr PRN; or 25–50 mg IM q 3–4 hr PRN. **Pediatric:** 0.55 mg/kg PO q 4–6 hr; 1.1 mg/kg rectally q 6–8 hr; or 0.55 mg/kg IM q 6–8 hr. Do not use in patients under 6 mo old.	**Site of Action:** Chemoreceptor trigger zone (CTZ), vomiting center (VC) **General Uses:** Chemotherapy, radiation, other	For all phenothiazines: **ASSESSMENT:** Assess blood pressure before and during therapy to assess for orthostatic hypotension. **INTERVENTION:** Do not mix these medications with other medications in same syringe. Monitor urinary output carefully. **Patient Teaching**—Caution patient to slowly change body position, and tell him or her that wearing elastic stockings and/or elevating feet may help in preventing hypotension. Caution patient to not drink alcohol because impaired mental or physical abilities may occur after administration. **EVALUATION:** Carefully evaluate patient for occurrence of any extrapyramidal adverse effects.
promethazine (Phenergan) **Adults:** 12.5–25 mg IM q 4–6 hr; 12.5–50 mg rectally; or 25–50 mg PO. **Children:** 0.25–0.5 mg/kg q 4–6 hr PO. Do not use in children <2 yr.	**Site of Action:** CTZ (?), labyrinth **General Uses:** Motion sickness, postoperative, chemotherapy, radiation.	Same as for chlorpromazine.
promazine (Sparine) **Adults:** 25–50 mg PO q 4–6 hr; or 50 mg IM q 4–6 hr.	**Site of Action:** Same as for chlorpromazine **General Uses:** Postoperative	Same as above.

ANTIDOPAMINERGIC AGENTS: PIPERAZINE PHENOTHIAZINES

DRUG NAME/ROUTE AND DOSAGE	SITE OF ACTION/ GENERAL USE	NURSING IMPLICATIONS
prochlorperazine (Compazine) **Adults:** 5–10 mg PO or IM 3–4 times/day; 10–30 mg PO (sustained-release tablets) q 12 hr; 25 mg 2 times/day rectally. **Pediatric:** 2.5 mg PO 1–3 times daily; or 0.13 mg/kg IM q 12 hr.	**Site of Action:** CTZ, VC. **General Uses:** Postoperative, chemotherapy, radiation	Same as for all antiemetics plus: **INTERVENTION:** Do not crush or chew sustained-release tablets.
fluphenazine (Permitil) (Prolixin) **Adults:** 0.5–10 mg PO; 12.5–25 mg IM or SC once a month (decanoate); 2.5–25 mg IM or SC q 1–3 weeks (enanthate).	**Site of Action:** CTZ, VC. **General Uses:** Postoperative, chemotherapy, radiation.	Same as above.

Table 51–1. CENTRALLY ACTING ANTIEMETICS, *Continued*

DRUG NAME/ROUTE AND DOSAGE	SITE OF ACTION/ GENERAL USE	NURSING IMPLICATIONS
thiethylperazine (Torecan) *Adults:* 10 mg PO (tablets) 1–2 times/day; 10 mg IM 1–3 times daily; or 10 mg rectally.	**Site of Action:** CTZ, VC. **General Uses:** Postoperative, chemotherapy, radiation	Same as above.
ANTIDOPAMINERGIC AGENTS: MISCELLANEOUS		
metocolopramide (Reglan) *Adults:* 0.75–1 mg/kg IV diluted in 50 mL over 15 min, 30 min before and after chemotherapy as necessary; or 0.5 mg/kg PO 4–6 times/day.	**Site of Action:** CTZ, increases GI motility. **General Uses:** Chemotherapy, gastric stasis due to narcotics, diabetic gastroparesis	Same as above: **INTERVENTION:** If extrapyramidal symptoms occur, treat with 50 mg of diphenhydramine IM.
ANTICHOLINERGICS		
scopolamine (Hyoscine) (Transderm-Scōp) **scopolamine (hyoscine)** *Adults:* 0.2–0.4 mg IM, IV, SC 1 hr preoperatively. **scopolamine (Transderm-Scōp)** *Adults:* 1.5 mg transdermally (delivers 0.5 mg over 3 days). Apply 4 hours before antiemetic effect is desired.	**Site of Action:** CNS, aural vestibular apparatus, CTZ, labyrinth, increased esophageal tone, decreased retrograde motility **General Uses:** Motion sickness	**INTERVENTION:** Observe patient closely for excitement, delirium, and disorientation, which may occur shortly after drug is administered. **Transdermal**—Wash hands before applying patch. Wash site after removing transdermal patch and hands after touching patch. If more than 72 hr of therapy are needed, first patch is removed, area is cleaned, and second patch is applied to new postauricular location.
ANTIHISTAMINES		
dimenhydrinate (Dramamine) *Adults:* 50–100 mg PO q 4–6 hr; or 50 mg IV or IM as needed not to exceed 400 mg in 24 hr. *Children 2–6 yr:* 12.5–25 mg PO q 6–8 hr. *Children 6–12 yr:* 25–50 mg PO q 6–8 hr.	**Site of Action:** VC, CTZ (?), increased gastroesophageal sphincter tone **General Uses:** Motion sickness, vertigo	Same as for all plus: **INTERVENTION:** Administer 30–60 min before activity is to begin. **Patient Teaching**—Advise patient to take care if operating heavy equipment.
diphenhydramine (Benadryl) *Adults:* 25–50 mg PO (tablets); 12.5 mg/mL PO (elixir) 3–4 times/day; or 10–50 mg IV or IM q 4–6 hr. *Pediatric:* 12.5–25 mg PO 3–4 times/day; or 5 mg/kg IV or IM 4 times/day.	**Site of Action:** Same as for dimenhydrinate **General Uses:** Motion sickness, vertigo, chemotherapy, pregnancy	Same as above.
meclizine (Antivert, Bonine) *Adults:* 25–50 mg PO (tablets) 1 hr prior to travel.	**Site of Action:** Labyrinth; CNS; decreased conduction in vestibular/cerebellar pathways **General Uses:** Motion sickness, vertigo, radiation, pregnancy	Same as above.

Table 51–2. MISCELLANEOUS ANTIEMETICS

DRUG NAME/ROUTE AND DOSAGE	PHARMACOKINETICS/ DYNAMICS	NURSING IMPLICATIONS
all miscellaneous antiemetics		
		ASSESSMENT: Assess vital signs, causes of vomiting. Assess for pregnancy (category unknown). **INTERVENTION:** Administer 15 min before vomiting is expected. Inject IM well into the muscle mass. Do not use deltoid unless well developed. Reconstituted solutions are not refrigerated and remain potent for 14 days at room temperature. Moisten mouth with hard candy. **Patient Teaching**—Caution patient about performing activities that require mental alertness. **EVALUATION:** Monitor for drowsiness, a major adverse effect, and cardiovascular effects of hypotension.
benzquinamide hydrochloride (Emete-Con)		
Adults: 50 mg or 0.5–1 mg/kg IM q 3–4 hr; or 25 mg or 0.2–0.4 mg/kg IV over 10 min, then give frequent doses IM. ***Site of Action:*** Chemoreceptor trigger zone (CTZ), vomiting center (VC).	**Onset:** 15 min **Peak:** 30 min **Duration:** 3–4 hr **½L:** 40 min **PB:** 58% **B:** liver **E:** urine (10% unchanged)	Same as for all plus: **INTERVENTION:** Reconstitute in 2.2 mL solution for injection.
diphenidol (Vontrol)		
Adults: 25–50 mg PO q 3–4 hr. ***Children over 6 yr:*** 0.88 mg/kg. ***Site of Action:*** Aural vestibular apparatus, CTZ, labyrinth.	**Onset:** 15 min **Peak:** 1.5–3 hr **Duration:** 3–4 hr **½L:** 4 hr **PB:** NA **B:** liver **E:** urine (90%)	Same as for all plus: **ASSESSMENT:** Assess for allergy to tartrazine.
trimethobenzamide hydrochloride (Tigan)		
Adults: 250 mg PO q 3–4 hr; 100–250 mg rectally 3–4 times/day; 200 mg IM 3–4 times/day; or 200 mg IM or rectally as a single dose before or during surgery. ***Pediatric:*** 4–5 mg/kg PO q 6–8 hr; or 100–200 mg rectally 3–4 times/day. ***Site of Action:*** CTZ.	**Onset:** 10–40 min **Peak:** NA **Duration:** 2–4 hr **½L:** NA **PB:** NA **B:** liver **E:** urine	Same as for all plus: **ASSESSMENT:** Pregnancy (category unknown).
ondansetron hydrochloride (Zofran)		
Adults: 0.15 mg/kg IV over 15 min starting 30 min before administration of chemotherapy and repeat 4 hr and 8 hr later to total of 3 doses; or 32 mg IV as single dose prior to chemotherapy. ***Site of Action:*** Selectively antagonizes serotonin at its receptors located in the CTZ.	**Onset:** immediate **Peak:** immediate **Duration:** 30 hr **½L:** 3.5–5.5 hr **PB:** 73% **B:** liver **E:** urine	Same as for all plus: **ASSESSMENT:** Assess for pregnancy (category B). **INTERVENTION:** Dosage adjustment may be necessary in elderly. Infuse IV over 15 minutes beginning 30 min before start of chemotherapy.
granisetron hydrochloride (Kytril)		
Adults: 1 mg PO 1 hr before chemotherapy and 1 mg 12 hr later; or 10 mg/kg IV over 5 min given 30 min before chemotherapy. ***Site of Action:*** Selectively antagonizes serotonin at its receptors located in the CTZ.	**Onset:** NA **Peak:** NA **Duration:** 30–40 hr **½L:** 4–9 hr **PB:** 65% **B:** liver **E:** urine, feces	Same as for ondansetron.

TABLE 51–2. MISCELLANEOUS ANTIEMETICS, *Continued*

DRUG NAME/ROUTE AND DOSAGE	PHARMACOKINETICS/ DYNAMICS	NURSING IMPLICATIONS
CANNABANOIDS		
dronabinol (Marinol)		
Adults: 5 mg/m^2 PO 1–3 hr prior to chemotherapy, then 2–4 hr after chemo for a total of 4–6 doses/day. Increase dose by 2.5 mg/m^2 increments to max of 15 mg/m^2.	**Onset:** rapid **Peak:** 60–90 min **Duration:** 2–3 hr **½L:** 4 hr (25–36 hr) (extensive first pass effect) **PB:** 97%–99% **B:** liver **E:** feces (50%), urine (10%–15%)	**ASSESSMENT:** Assess vital signs. Assess for hypersensitivity to marijuana or sesame oil. Assess for pregnancy (category B). **INTERVENTION:** Administer 1–3 hr prior to chemotherapy. Patients should remain under control of responsible adult. **Patient Teaching**—Advise patient to avoid alcohol and other CNS depressants; drug may cause drowsiness. Caution patient about driving or other performing activities requiring mental alertness. **EVALUATION:** Behavioral changes may occur. Patient and family should be alert to these.
nabilone (Cesamet)		
Adults: 1–2 mg PO 2 times/day, max daily dose is 6 mg 3 times/day. Administer 1–3 hr before chemotherapy begins.	**Onset:** rapid **Peak:** 60–90 min **Duration:** 2–3 hr **½L:** 2 hr (35 hr) (extensive first-pass effect) **PB:** 95% **B:** liver **E:** bile (65%), urine (20%)	Same as for dronabinol.

NA = not available.

stances are believed to relax GI muscle spasms and thereby permit fewer afferent impulses to reach the vomiting center.

Centrally Acting Antiemetics

The centrally acting antiemetics inhibit or depress the afferent nerve impulses in the brain pathways, consequently preventing nausea and vomiting. Table 51–1 features the various groups of medications used as centrally acting antiemetics, their specific site of action, their common antiemetic dose, their common indications, and nursing implications. Most of these medications, excluding the miscellaneous group, are used for other purposes but possess antiemetic qualities. Only their antiemetic use is reviewed here, as they are discussed fully in other chapters.

CONTRAINDICATIONS AND PRECAUTIONS

Caution is always required with all antiemetics as they mask the symptoms of organic disease or the toxic effects of other drugs. Antiemetics are not recommended for uncomplicated vomiting in children and administered cautiously during pregnancy.

ADVERSE EFFECTS

Antiemetics are not without adverse effects. Most commonly, drowsiness occurs so patients must be cautioned about performing activities that require alertness.

▼ **CLINICAL ALERT**

Patients also must avoid alcohol and other central nervous system (CNS) depressants that could further depress their CNS.

Antidopaminergics

○ **Phenothiazines,** major tranquilizers or antipsychotic agents, act mainly by decreasing the sensitivity to stimulation of the CTZ in the VC to the stimulation by the central neurotransmitter dopamine. This decrease in sensitivity probably accounts for a wide range of effectiveness.

The antiemetic effect of phenothiazines occurs with very low doses. However, because of their relative toxicity, they are administered only when vomiting cannot be controlled by other means or when no more than a few doses will be needed. This approach is important when medicating patients with acute presurgical conditions or neurologic syndromes because the phenothiazine may mask diagnostic symptoms. They are used most commonly to control postoperative nausea and vomiting, radiation sickness, nausea and vomiting from cancer chemotherapy, and the nausea and vomiting secondary to the ingestion of toxins. They have also proved effective in controlling intractable vomiting in patients with terminal uremia. With the exception of promethazine (Phenergan), they are relatively ineffective in treating motion sickness. The aliphatic phenothiazine compounds used as antiemetics include **promethazine *(Phenergan)*,** promazine *(Sparine)*, and **chlorpromazine** *(Thorazine)*. The piperazine phenothiazine compounds that are used include **prochlorperazine** *(Compazine)*, **fluphenazine** *(Prolixin)*, **perphenazine** *(Trilafon)*, and **thiethylperazine** *(Torecan)*. Because of the side effects, these medications are administered with great caution. More information can be found on the phenothiazines in Chapter 27.

○ **Metoclopramide** (Reglan), like the phenothiazines, has an antidopaminergic effect at the CTZ, but also increases GI motility. Metoclopramide is used to combat the nausea and vomiting associated with antineoplastic agents, to reverse the gastric stasis induced by narcotics, and to treat diabetic gastroparesis. Metoclopramide is discussed in detail in Chapter 50.

Anticholinergics

○ **Scopolamine hydrobromide** (Hyoscine) is one of the most effective medications to prevent motion sickness, but it has limited usefulness when administered orally because of side effects of blurred vision and dryness of mouth. It has a very short duration time, so it may be used if only a one-time dose is needed. Repeated doses may have a cumulative effect.

Scopolamine is also available as a skin patch (Transderm-Scōp), which allows for a continuous release of scopolamine for up to 3 days. Transderm-Scōp is applied to a hairless area of the skin behind the ear 3 to 4 hours before the antiemetic effect is required.

Miscellaneous Antiemetics

The miscellaneous antiemetics are specifically designed to be used as antiemetics. Several of these products are available, including **benzquinamide hydrochloride (Emete-Con)**, **diphenidol hydrochloride (Vontrol)**, **trimethobezamide hydrochloride (Tigan)**; the selective serotonin antagonists **ondansetron (Zofran)** and **granisetron hydrochloride (Kytril)**; and the cannabinoids, discussed later in this chapter. All are featured in Table 51–2.

Contraindications and Precautions Contraindications include hypersensitivity to the agent and cardiovascular disease because of the cardiac adverse effects. Safety in pregnancy, lactation, and children has not been established.

Adverse Effects Established adverse effects are similar to those of the aliphatic phenothiazine compounds and include drowsiness, dizziness, dry mouth, orthostatic hypotension, and sometimes excitation and nervousness.

○ **Benzquinamide hydrochloride** (Emete-Con) has antiemetic, antihistaminic, anticholinergic, and antisedative effects and is available for IM and IV administration. Because of this combination of actions, it is thought to depress the VC and inhibit stimuli from entering the CTZ. This unique action increases cardiac output, blood pressure, and respiration, and therefore may be particularly effective in patients with CNS depression.

○ **Diphenidol hydrochloride** (Vontrol) inhibits the vestibular-cerebellar pathways and possibly the CTZ in the medulla. It is an oral, rapid-acting product, best used to combat nausea and vomiting secondary to surgery, radiation, and chemotherapy or for motion sickness and middle ear disease.

CONTRAINDICATIONS AND PRECAUTIONS Diphenidol hydrochloride is contraindicated in persons who have low blood pressure and those with known sensitivity. It is also contraindicated in persons with renal failure and anuria, as 90% is excreted in the urine. It should be administered cautiously to persons with glaucoma or those in whom pyloric stenosis and spasm are present because of its weak peripheral anticholinergic effect. Diphenidol contains tartrazine which may cause allergic reactions.

ADVERSE EFFECTS Adverse effects, in addition to those already discussed, include drowsiness, sleep disturbances, and auditory and visual hallucinations. This drug is, therefore, reserved for hospitalized patients who can be observed.

○ **Trimethobenzamide hydrochloride** (Tigan) has both an antiemetic effect and an antihistaminic effect and is available in parenteral, oral, and rectal doses. Oral and rectal doses, however, are somewhat unpredictable. This drug inhibits activity of the CTZ. It is generally less effective than the phenothiazine antiemetics.

CONTRAINDICATIONS AND PRECAUTIONS Trimethobenzamide is potentiated by CNS medications and the phenothiazines, so it is given cautiously to patients receiving these medications.

ADVERSE EFFECTS Adverse effects are similar to those of the phenothiazine antiemetics, but much less severe. They include allergic reactions, extrapyramidal symptoms, hypotension (parenteral), headache, diarrhea, and blurred vision.

○ **Ondansetron hydrochloride** (Zofran) **and** **granisetron hydrochloride** (Kytril) selectively antagonize serotonin and its receptors located in the CTZ. Both agents are used to prevent and treat nausea and vomiting associated with cancer chemotherapy. Ondansetron hydrochloride is available only in an IV form, which is administered approximately 30 minutes before chemotherapy begins. Dexamethasone (Decadron), a corticosteroid, may be administered to enhance the antiemetic activity. One dose is often effective as its half-life is 5 to 8 hours; thus, it takes 25 to 40 hours to clear from the body.

Granisetron is available in both IV and oral forms. It is infused IV 30 minutes before chemotherapy. Ganisetron has a half-life of 6 hours, so it takes about 30 hours to be eliminated. Oral therapy may also be used with the first dose given 1 hour before chemotherapy and the second dose 12 hours later. Continued therapy has not been found to be helpful.

▼ **CLINICAL ALERT**

CONTRAINDICATIONS AND PRECAUTIONS Both of these drugs are metabolized by the hepatic cytochrome P-450 drug metabolizing enzymes. Therefore, caution is used with liver disease and when other drugs are administered such as phenytoin.

ADVERSE EFFECTS The most common adverse effects include headache, somnolence, constipation, and sedation. Bronchospasm may also occur or worsen, so respiratory assessments are important.

Cannabinoids

Two cannabinoids, both controlled substances, are currently available: **dronabinol *(Marinol)*,** which is the principal psychoactive substance present in *Cannabis sativa* L. (marijuana), and **nabilone *(Cesamet)*,** which is a synthetic cannabinoid. These drugs are featured in Table 51–2. These products are indicated in persons receiving cancer chemotherapy who have not responded to or have developed a tolerance for other antiemetics. Both dronabinol and nabilone are most effective when given with methotrexate and high-dose cisplatin (see Chapter 55). Because these products are related to marijuana, they may alter the mental state and are used only in persons who will be closely supervised.

▼ **CLINICAL ALERT**

Contraindications and Precautions The cannabinoids are contraindicated in nausea and vomiting from any cause other than cancer chemotherapy and in persons hypersensitive to marijuana or to sesame oil.

They are given cautiously to persons with increased blood pressure and heart disease as they may cause transient tachycardia and in large doses may produce orthostatic hypotension. Safety in pregnancy (category B), lactation, and children has not been established. Both drugs are highly abuseable and are not administered to persons with previous psychiatric disorders for whom abuse may become a problem.

Adverse Effects The cannabinoids cause numerous adverse effects within the CNS including drowsiness, a high or heightened awareness, dizziness, muddled thinking, concentration difficulties, depression, and weakness all due to their complex CNS effect.

Interactions The cannabinoids are not administered with alcohol or other CNS depressants like sedatives and hypnotics because of the possible combined effect.

USING THE NURSING PROCESS WITH PATIENT REQUIRING AN ANTIEMETIC

Assessment

- Obtain a thorough nursing history to develop the database. The information to obtain is included in Table 51–3. A thorough drug history is important in ruling out serious causes of nausea and vomiting, such as

---

Table 51–3. NURSING PROCESS FOR PATIENT REQUIRING ANTIEMETIC MEDICATION

Assessment

Assess medication history, including recent change of medication, chemotherapy, current antiemetic therapy.
Assess history of current illness, pregnancy, drug overdose (poisoning), motion sickness.
Assess use/effectiveness of home remedies.

Nursing Diagnosis: Risk for Fluid Volume Deficit	**Desired Outcomes/Evaluation Criteria**
RELATED TO: Excessive losses through vomiting, reduced oral intake/absorption of fluids.	Verbalizes individual risk factors and appropriate interventions. Demonstrates adequacy of fluid balance with moist mucous membranes, good skin turgor, stable vital signs, individually appropriate urinary output.

Nursing Actions	**Rationale**
Record intake and output, including emesis. Measure urine specific gravity.	Useful in evaluation of fluid needs.
Weigh daily as appropriate.	Sensitive indicator of fluid volume shifts.
Evaluate mucous membranes, skin turgor strength/rate of peripheral pulses. Monitor vital signs.	Indicators of additional therapy needs/effectiveness.
Administer antiemetics, e.g., benzquinamide hydrochloride, trimethobenzamide hydrochloride.	Given to eliminate nausea/vomiting.
Evaluate effectiveness of drug.	Prolonged use may result in tolerance requiring increased dosage or change of drug.
Encourage increased oral intake of bland beverages, gelatin, sherbet, etc. in small/frequent amounts.	Replaces losses, small amounts may be retained/absorbed better.
Recommend changing body position slowly as appropriate.	Parenteral administration of antiemetics may result in othostatic hypotension.
Discuss strategies for dealing with unpleasant results of vomiting, e.g., eliminate noise and unpleasant odors; provide clean environment, removing vomitus promptly; provide frequent oral care.	These measures can contribute to lessening of the vomiting reflex.

Other Suggested Nursing Diagnosis: Knowledge Deficit.

side effects of medications. Antiemetics are resorted to only when no other therapy is available, especially in children. When administering an antiemetic, it is important to assist the physician in determining the cause of the vomiting. If the vomiting is associated with motion, there are numerous OTC products available. The patient must be taught how to take the medication for effective use.

A woman in her first trimester of pregnancy or just starting on birth control pills may experience nausea and vomiting early in the morning or with the sight or smell of certain foods. This is usually transient, but the woman still must be assessed for dehydration, fluid and electrolyte derangements, and acid-base imbalances.

Nursing Diagnosis

- Possible nursing diagnoses for a patient requiring antiemetics include Knowledge Deficit and Risk for Fluid Volume Deficit (see Table 51–3).

Planning and Intervention

- Develop the goals of intervention from the nursing diagnoses. Typical goals for the patient requiring antiemetic medication are included in Table 51–3.
- Understand specific information about the antiemetics to ensure their safe administration. This information is summarized in Tables 51–1 and 51–2 in the Nursing Implications column.

Nursing Responsibilities

- Rotate injection sites when administering antiemetics intramuscularly to prevent irritation of the tissues. Because all antiemetics dry mucous membranes, particularly of the mouth, suggest that patients use hard candy or gum to moisten their mouths.

    A nauseated postoperative patient who vomits may need additional treatments, such as insertion of a nasogastric tube or IV therapy. Violent retching could put undue pressure on the suture line, as well as further agitating the patient.
- Monitor results of laboratory reports and report any significant findings to the attending physician. A patient who vomits for any length of time may become dehydrated or develop a fluid, electrolyte, or acid-base imbalance. Obese patients tend to be more nauseated and to vomit postoperatively because their fat cells act as reservoirs for anesthetic drugs, thus slowing the drug's elimination. Also, the longer the duration of anesthesia, the greater the risk of nausea. Nausea secondary to anesthesia generally lasts only 12 to 24 hours. Nausea present after 3 postoperative days is most likely associated with narcotics or an underlying medical problem such as an ileus.

    If the patient has had regional anesthesia with Duramorph or fentanyl, nausea occurs because these drugs activate the emetic center. Naloxone (Narcan),

titrated slowly, may relieve the nausea without reversing the analgesia.

In general, when a patient is taking antiemetics to control the nausea and vomiting that accompany radiation or chemotherapy, many helpful suggestions may be given to the patient and family. These are outlined in Chapter 55.

Patient Teaching

- Teach patients how to take their own antiemetics at home for various conditions. General teaching measures are included in Table 51–4.

Evaluation

- Evaluate the effectiveness of antiemetic medications. This evaluation is based on a list of outcome evaluation criteria that has been developed in relation to the goals determined by the nurse, patient, and family. Typical patient outcome evaluation criteria are included in Table 51–3.
- Work with the patient and family to ensure their complete assistance and support. Patients who understand the importance of their continued medical treatment are usually compliant. The nurse teaches the patient about potential side effects so that a patient taking these medications at home reports any unusual symptoms to the physician or nurse. In general, the side effects of the antiemetics include drowsiness, dizziness, vertigo, and hypotension.

Table 51-4. PATIENT TEACHING INFORMATION—ANTIEMETICS

Dear Patient:
   This drug has been prescribed for you. This is what you should know about your drug to get the most from your therapy.

- ☐ 1. The antiemetic drug _____ has been specifically ordered for you to reduce your nausea and vomiting associated with _____ .
- ☐ 2. Antiemetic drugs will be taken until your current health problem is resolved.
- ☐ 3. Antiemetic medications are taken about 30 to 60 minutes before the activity or the event that may lead to nausea and vomiting.
- ☐ 4. Antiemetics are taken on an empty stomach (at least 2 hours after a meal).
- ☐ 5. Antiemetics react with other medications; therefore, always check with your pharmacist or doctor before taking other medications with your antiemetic.
- ☐ 6. Antiemetic medications may also worsen the effects of alcohol (beer, wine, liquor), some cough or cold medications, or other central nervous system depressants (tranquilizers, sleeping pills); therefore, *do not* take these products together.
- ☐ 7. All antiemetics tend to cause sleepiness or slowed mental or physical abilities, so you should avoid driving a car or operating heavy equipment for several hours after taking these medications.
- ☐ 8. Medications are stored at room temperature away from heat and in light-resistant containers. Suppositories are stored below 77°F, below room temperature.

▼ **CLINICAL ALERT**

Patients who receive parenteral antiemetics should change their body position slowly to prevent the occurrence of orthostatic hypotension. When the phenothiazine group and several miscellaneous antiemetics are administered, the patient may experience *extrapyramidal effects* (see Chapter 27), which include masklike face, tremors, *dystonia* (abnormal muscle tone, usually manifested as spasm of the tongue, face, neck, or back), akathisia (inability to sit still), and tardive dyskinesia (involuntary rhythmic movements of the face). Dosage is decreased or the medication discontinued to prevent these side effects from becoming permanent.

EMETICS

Emetics are agents used to induce vomiting when poisons or toxins that have been ingested are still in the stomach. Before emetics are administered, the substances that were taken *must be known*. For example, emetics are not administered if the individual swallowed a strong acid or alkali such as those found in many household cleansers. The poison may have already burned the throat and esophagus and would do so again were vomiting induced. In all cases, where possible, the local poison control center is notified before any intervention is begun. Emesis is more effective than gastric lavage in removing the substance from the stomach.

Emetics induce vomiting by acting in several locations in the reflex arc. They irritate the stomach and stimulate the VC, promoting vomiting about 15 to 60 minutes after they are ingested by mouth or given subcutaneously (SC). The most common emetics are ipecac syrup, available OTC in the pharmacy, and apomorphine hydrochloride. Both are featured in Table 51–5.

CONTRAINDICATIONS AND PRECAUTIONS

Emetics are contraindicated when strong alkaline, acidic, strychnine, or petroleum distillate poisons have been consumed. Other treatment modalities must be used in these patients, such as nasogastric suction or dialysis. Emetics are further contraindicated for any patient who is not alert. In a comatose, semicomatose, inebriated, or sedated patient, there is increased risk of aspiration if vomiting is induced. Emetics are also contraindicated in patients who have taken CNS stimulants. The emetics cause further CNS stimulation, which may result in convulsion. Nasogastric suction is the best treatment with overdoses of CNS stimulants.

○ **Ipecac syrup** acts on both the stomach and the CTZ and induces vomiting only if medullary centers are responsive. It also has an expectorant action, which lowers sputum viscosity. It is available without a prescription for emergency use.

○ **Apomorphine hydrochloride** stimulates the CTZ to induce vomiting only when medullary centers are responsive. In the CTZ, apomorphine combines with dopamine receptors to produce emesis, thus apomorphine is a dopaminergic agonist. It is also classified as a narcotic, has a mild sedative effect, and may depress the respiratory center. After vomiting occurs, in about 15 minutes

---

Table 51–5. EMETIC MEDICATIONS

DRUG NAME/ROUTE AND DOSAGE	PHARMACOKINETICS/ DYNAMICS	NURSING IMPLICATIONS
ipecac syrup USP **Adults and Children over 1 yr:** 15–30 mL PO. **Children under 1 yr:** 5 mL; repeat dose after 30 min if necessary. **Children:** 1–12 yr: 15 mL.	**Onset:** 20–30 min	**ASSESSMENT:** Assess baseline pulse and rhythm. Assess for pregnancy (category C). **INTERVENTION:** Follow ipecac with 1 glass of lukewarm water. Walking induces emesis more quickly. Obtain pulse 1 hr after administration. If vomiting does not occur, repeat in 20–30 min. If still no vomiting, give activated charcoal or remove through gastric suctioning. If not removed, may induce intestinal bleeding. Ipecac syrup is outdated 1 yr after opening. **EVALUATION:** GI absorption may precipitate convulsions, dysrhythmias, and coma. Notify physician.
apomorphine hydrochloride **Adults:** 2–10 mg SC (IM, IV rarely used). **Infants and Children:** 0.1 mg/kg in 1 dose. **Do not repeat.**	**Onset:** 15–30 min	**ASSESSMENT:** Assess baseline vital signs. Assess for pregnancy (category C). **INTERVENTION:** Administer 1 glass milk or lukewarm water to enhance vomiting. Walking induces vomiting more quickly. Monitor vital signs q 15 min for 2 hr. **EVALUATION:** If prolonged vomiting occurs, administer narcotic antagonist.

after an SC injection, the sedative effects begin and last about 2 hours. If the CNS depression is too great, the narcotic antagonist naloxone hydrochloride (Narcan) must be administered intramuscularly to counteract the CNS depression. Naloxone hydrochloride may also help antagonize the violent and protracted vomiting often seen with the use of apomorphine. The dopaminergic effects result in lacrimation, salivation, nausea, and perspiration.

USING THE NURSING PROCESS WITH PATIENT REQUIRING AN EMETIC

Assessment

- Obtain a thorough nursing history to develop the database. This information should be obtained from the family if the patient is comatose or too young to supply it.
- Determine what was swallowed before evoking emesis to prevent further damage to the mucous membranes during vomiting. The poisoning could be deliberate, as with a drug overdose (see Chapter 6), or accidental, as in the case of a child who has swallowed a medication or an improperly stored household preparation not meant for oral ingestion. In general, the patient is hospitalized for observation for at least 24 hours after the acute poisoning incident.

Nursing Diagnosis

- Possible nursing diagnoses for the patient requiring emetics include Risk for Poisoning and Knowledge Deficit.

Planning and Intervention

- Develop the goals of the nursing intervention from the nursing diagnoses.
- Call the poison control center, physician, or local hospital for immediate advice before instituting treatment. In most cases, emesis is preferred over stomach lavage. However, emetics are never administered in the following cases:
  1. Patients with significant CNS depression who may have lost their gag reflex and there is a risk of aspiration.
  2. Patients at high risk of seizures, as emetics may produce or worsen seizures.
  3. Patients who have ingested petroleum distillates, as there is a potential for lipid droplet aspiration.
  4. Patients who have ingested caustics, as this will expose the already damaged mouth and esophagus to the caustic substance again.
  5. Patients who have ingested drugs with antiemetic activity, as their effectiveness is reduced.
- Give psychologic support to the patient and family during the treatment, and assist them in obtaining further help if needed.
- Counsel the family about placing bottles and jars out of the reach of small children, if such misplacement caused the incident. Suggest safety locks on kitchen cupboards and high, locked cabinets in the garage for outdoor pesticides and fertilizers. Families with small children should keep syrup of ipecac on hand. The parents are instructed not to use it without first checking with the poison control center. Also, parents and guardians are encouraged to learn the current first aid treatment for poisonings and to keep a first aid reference handy. Many old "universal antidotes" have proved useless. Do not use them!

In general, most effects of emetics are enhanced if given on a full stomach. Therefore, they are generally given along with water or milk. Vomiting usually occurs in 30 to 60 minutes. The emetic effect can also be enhanced by walking an adult or bouncing a child.

Evaluation

- Evaluate the effectiveness of the treatment. The medication can be repeated once, but if vomiting does not occur, some other means of emptying the stomach must be used, such as gastric lavage.
- Evaluate for side effects. Because all emetics sedate the patient after the vomiting episode, evaluate the patient's vital signs and the amount of CNS depression. Also, prevent aspiration to reduce the risk of aspiration pneumonia. If the patient is too sedated, particularly when apomorphine is used, a narcotic antagonist may be needed.
- Ensure that the patient understands the treatment regimen. The patient and family are likely to comply with instructions and treatment procedures to the extent that they are involved with the planning of patient care. Stress the importance of continued medical care whenever necessary.
- Evaluate the patient's knowledge base. Review and update all previously taught material with the patient and family, if necessary, to ensure accuracy.

The bibliography for this chapter can be found in Appendix B, which begins on page 1054.

CHAPTER REVIEW QUESTIONS*

1. As a group of drugs, antiemetics:
   a. Are best administered after vomiting occurs.
   b. Act either locally or centrally.
   c. Treat rather than prevent vomiting.
   d. Cause local irritation of gastric muscosa.

2. An extrapyramidal side effect that may occur with administration of high doses of phenothiazine drugs is:
   a. Spasms of the tongue, face, neck, and back.
   b. Drowsiness.
   c. Nasal congestion.
   d. Rebound hypertension.

*See Appendix A, which begins on page 1051, for answers.

3. An example of an antidopaminergic antiemetic is:
   a. Diphenhydramine (Benadryl).
   b. Benzquinamide (Emete-Con).
   c. Promethazine (Phenergan).
   d. Cyclizine (Marezine).

4. In general, antiemetics are contraindicated in the following patient situation:
   a. Glaucoma.
   b. Pregnancy.

c. Gastric ulcers.
d. Metastatic cancer.

5. An example of a cannabinoid antiemetic is:
   a. Dronabinol (Marinol).
   b. Fluphenazine (Protixin).
   c. Diphenidol (Vontrol).
   d. Dimenhydrinate (Dramamine).

CHAPTER 52

Medications for Common Digestive Problems

Merrily A. Kuhn, RNC, PhD

CHAPTER OUTLINE

Digestants
Antidiarrheals
Laxatives
Using the Nursing Process

TABLES

BOXES

KEY TERMS

Achlorhydria
Auerbach's plexus
Diarrhea
Digestants
Hypochlorhydria
Steatorrhea

LEARNING OBJECTIVES

After reading this chapter, the student will be able to:

1. Identify those agents commonly used as digestive system medications.
2. Compare the digestive system medications as to mechanism of action, route of administration, pharmacokinetics, adverse effects, contraindications and precautions, and interactions.
3. Identify specific parameters to assess in the patient requiring digestive system medications to formulate patient outcomes.
4. Plan the nursing interventions necessary to administer digestive system medications, monitor effects, and choose appropriate teaching strategies to gain patient compliance.
5. Evaluate the patient at various stages of treatment to measure the success of nursing interventions.

The gastrointestinal tract is responsible for the digestion of food substances and absorption of nutrients. When maladies affect bowel function, digestion and absorption of nutrients are affected. This chapter discusses the pharmacologic management and nursing interventions for problems of digestion and the bowel, including both diarrhea and constipation. Ulcerative colitis remission drugs are also received.

DIGESTANTS

Carbohydrates, fats, and protein must be broken down by gastric acid and enzymes into their simplest form be-

fore they are available to the body. Products designed to aid digestion are known as *digestants*. Digestants include gastric acidifiers such as hydrochloric acid (as glutamic acid HCl), stomach enzymes such as pepsin, and pancreatic enzymes such as pancrelipase and pancreatin. Combination products are also available. Digestants, including dosages, adverse effects, and nursing implications, are featured in Table 52–1.

GASTRIC ACIDIFIERS

Hydrochloric acid secretion can be diminished (*hypochlorhydria*) or almost completely absent (*achlorhydria*). Achlorhydria is most likely to occur in elderly patients and those with gastric cancer. Pernicious anemia occurs with achlor-

Table 52–1. ORAL DIGESTANTS

DRUG NAME/ROUTE AND DOSAGE	ADVERSE EFFECTS	NURSING IMPLICATIONS
ACIDIFIERS/DIGESTIVE ENZYMES		
glutamic acid hydrochloride (Acidulin)		
Adults: 1–3 340-mg capsules PO tid ac	Metabolic acidosis, fall in bicarbonate, rise in serum chloride	**ASSESSMENT:** Assess for hyperacidity and peptic ulcer (contraindications). **INTERVENTION:** Give with 8 oz water. Monitor lab values closely.
PANCREATIC ENZYMES		
pancrelipase (Cotazym) (Ilozyme) (Ku-Zyme HP) (Pancrease) (Viokase) **pancreatin** (Dizyme)		
Adults: 1–3 tablets or capsules or 1–2 packets with meals or snacks **Pediatric:** 4000–8000 units PO 3 times/day	Anorexia, nausea, vomiting, diarrhea	**ASSESSMENT:** Assess for allergy to pig, ox, or beef protein; and acute pancreatitis (contraindications). **INTERVENTION:** Take with or before meals. Packets may be sprinkled on food, capsules may be opened, or tablets crushed and sprinkled on food. Do not take milk or antacid within 1 hr of pancreatic enzymes. Do not chew capsule contents. Avoid inhalation of powder as it may cause asthma. Do not spill powder on hands as it may cause irritation. Do not change brands as bioequivalency is not equal. Do not take concurrently with antacids.

hydria and leads to peripheral neuritis and possibly death. Surprisingly, patients with hypochlorhydria have more gastric complaints than do those with achlorhydria.

Hydrochloric acid can be administered in capsule form as **glutamic acid hydrochloride (Acidulin),** which provides 1.8 mEq of hydrochloric acid. The capsules release their hydrochloric acid on contact with water and therefore are administered with an 8-ounce glass of water.

PANCREATIC ENZYMES

The pancreatic products include amylase to digest starches, lipase to digest fats, trypsin (a protease) to digest protein, and bicarbonate, which protects the enzymes from denaturation by acid and pepsin. The absence of enzymes causes major digestive disturbances. Replacement therapy may be effective in a variety of conditions: chronic pancreatitis, pancreatectomy, cystic fibrosis, pancreatic duct obstruction, and carcinomas of the pancreas.

The most commonly used pancreatic enzymes are **pancrelipase (Cotazym and others),** extracted only from porcine pancreas, and **pancreatin (Dizymes Tablets and others),** produced from beef, porcine, or vegetable sources. All patients treated with these enzymes must be reminded to eat a well-balanced diet including fat, protein, and starch to avoid indigestion. *Steatorrhea* (fatty stools) is a major finding in pancreatic enzyme deficiency, and this symptom is an important sign of treatment success or failure.

ANTIDIARRHEALS

A common malady, *diarrhea* is an acute or chronic condition of excess water elimination from the bowel. It is difficult to conceive of an older or more universal scourge than diarrhea. When the number of liquid stools approaches 10 per day, perianal irritation causes the patient discomfort. Stools may contain mucus and blood as the diarrhea becomes more severe. Associated with diarrhea is cramping from intermittent spasm of the intestine as well as distention from gas production caused by rapid fermentation occurring in the bowel. Hyperactive bowel sounds are usually present.

Acute diarrhea can result from infection, gastrointestinal (GI) disease, a change in diet, nervousness and anxiety, allergic reaction, intoxication, or as the side effect of a medication. In the United States, the most common causes of brief acute episodes of diarrhea are probably viruses, protozoa, or enterotoxin-producing *Escherichia coli.* Symptoms associated with acute diarrhea often include fever, headache, anorexia, vomiting, malaise, or myalgia and can persist for 1 to 3 days. Diarrhea can be chronic, as part of a malabsorption syndrome, inflammation of the bowel, endocrine dysfunction, or, periodically, certain rare hormone-producing neoplasms. Any episode of diarrhea causes water and electrolyte depletion, which can lead to dehydration and electrolyte imbalance. The very young and the elderly are more likely to develop these symptoms quickly, and the effects may become life threatening because of the body's inability to compensate.

Diarrhea is usually a self-limiting condition. Diagnostic testing is rarely necessary if diarrhea lasts less than 3 days. However, if symptoms persist beyond 3 days, a diagnostic work-up is performed. Diarrhea can be treated with antidiarrheal preparations, which act either locally in the bowel or systemically to decrease the number, consistency, and fluidity of the stool. To date, there is no absolute clinical evidence substantiating antidiarrheals' therapeutic effect in curing the underlying disease causing diarrhea. However, these drugs do reduce the number of stools and therefore reduce the interference with daily activities. Antidiarrheals are useful for (1) symptomatic control of both acute and chronic diarrhea and diarrhea secondary to radiation or GI surgery and (2) reduction of the volume of intestinal discharge in patients with ileostomies and colostomies. If symptoms of acute diarrhea have not improved, or fever persists, or blood or mucus appears in the stool, antidiarrheals are discontinued.

LOCALLY ACTING ANTIDIARRHEALS

Locally acting antidiarrheals act locally on the bowel wall to soothe and reduce irritation of the mucous lining. There are two forms: adsorbents, which may also have a soothing (demulcent) effect on the irritated mucous membrane, and intestinal flora modifiers, which help replace the normal bacterial flora but are of questionable benefit as antidiarrheals. Most of these preparations are over-the-counter (OTC) drugs easily obtainable by the general public and safe, but their effectiveness is debatable; most researchers feel that a patient experiencing diarrhea would improve even if left untreated by these preparations. (Generally, the systemically acting antidiarrheals are more effective than locally acting agents.) Table 52–2 features a sampling of the common locally acting antidiarrheals.

Adsorbents

Adsorbents bind gas, toxins, and irritants and thus inactivate them until they are excreted. Adsorbents contribute to the adhesion of the stool, but do not necessarily stop or control diarrhea. The most commonly used adsorbents not requiring a prescription include kaolin, activated charcoal, bismuth subsalicylate, and attapulgite. All have the advantage of being nontoxic and inexpensive, and some (including bismuth salts and kaolin with pectin) have an additional demulcent effect. Because of the large amounts of adsorbents taken after each loose bowel movement, constipation is often a side effect of these agents.

All of the medications acting as adsorbents have a tendency to also absorb other concurrently administered medications, such as digoxin, quinidine, and antibiotics. Drug interactions are minimized by separating the administration of any drug and the antidiarrheal adsorbent by at least 2 hours.

Adsorbents currently are thought to cause more fluid and electrolyte loss than if the diarrhea were not treated at all. Adsorbents may also give both the patient and medical personnel a false sense of security by increasing the fecal mass. There is little literature to support their effectiveness or use.

○ **Kaolin** (Kapectolin, Kao-Span) is composed of kaolin, a natural aluminum silicate clay that has been used for hundreds of years to treat diarrhea, and attupulgite, which acts as both an adsorbent and a demulcent. Currently, kaolin is not recognized as effective by the FDA.

○ **Activated charcoal,** a powder, is probably the most effective adsorbent of toxins and irritants, but it does not necessarily control diarrhea. It is used mostly as an antidote for certain types of poisonings.

○ **Bismuth subsalicylate** (Pepto-Bismol) is a relatively insoluble compound with adsorbent, demulcent,

---

Table 52–2. LOCALLY ACTING ANTIDIARRHEALS

Medication	Dosage	Type	Comments
Kaolin with pectin (Kaopectate)	60–120 mL after each bowel movement	A, D	Decreases fluidity but total water loss seems unchanged. Given in large doses after each loose bowel movement. Not recognized by FDA as effective.
Kaopectate Concentrate	45–90 mL	A, D	Same as above.
Bismuth subsalicylate (Pepto-Bismol)	30 mL or 2 tabs; dissolved or chewed q ½–1 hr; up to 8 doses	A, As	Contraindicated in people allergic to salicylates or taking coumarin products. Shake well before using. Stools may turn grey-black.
Activated attapulgite (Rheaban)	750 mg/tablet	A	Administer 2 tablets after each bowel movement.
Psyllium (Metamucil, Cillium, Konsyl, and many others)	1 rounded tsp in 8 oz of water 1–3 times daily; drink immediately and follow with 8 oz water	A	Bulk-producing laxative absorbs excess fluid and ultimately controls diarrhea. Comes as plain or flavored. May be more palatable if mixed with milk or juice. Has 14 calories/dose.
Methylcellulose (Cologel, Citrucel)	5–20 mL tid with water	D	Take with full glass of water. Citrucel is less gritty and better tasting. High in calories.

A = adsorbent; D = demulcent; As = astringent.

astringent, and weak antacid properties. It removes gas, toxins (*E. Coli* and *Vibrio cholerae*), bacteria (*H. pylori*), and viruses from the intestinal tract by adsorption. The bismuth salts can be used to treat peptic ulcers, diarrhea, enteritis, dysentery, and ulcerations of the bowel, and sometimes act as a local protectant for the skin. In addition, bismuth is used to prevent travelers' diarrhea: 2 tablets with meals and at bedtime should prevent travelers' diarrhea in most patients.

Bismuth subsalicylate is hydrolyzed to liberate salicylate and is contraindicated in patients allergic to salicylates and in patients taking coumarin products as anticoagulants. A 2-oz dose of bismuth salts can produce the same salicylate blood level as one 5-gr aspirin tablet.

○ **Attapulgite** (Rheaban) is possibly superior to kaolin in its adsorptive abilities for bacteria, viruses, and toxins. Prolonged use of attapulgite may interfere with intestinal adsorption of nutrients, resulting in constipation.

Other Adsorbents

○ **Cholestyramine** (Questran) has a direct affinity for acidic materials such as bile acids and the toxin *Clostridium difficile*. Cholestyramine relieves diarrhea due to excessive bile salts and may be effective for antibiotic-induced pseudomembranous colitis. It is administered most commonly to patients with high cholesterol levels. It is described in more detail in Chapter 33.

Intestinal Flora Modifiers

The bowel is filled with many different bacteria that break down and digest food. Often, in patients receiving antibiotics, many of these bacteria are destroyed, resulting in diarrhea. The growth of normal intestinal flora can be encouraged when the patient ingests *Lactobacillus acidophilus* found in Bacid or Lactinex (both OTC preparations) or acidophilus tablets, sweet acidophilus milk, or unpasteurized yogurt, buttermilk, or cottage cheese. The presence of this bacillus also allows the growth of *E. coli*, another normal bacterium found in the bowel. Well-controlled studies to support the use of these products are needed.

To assist in the treatment of diarrhea, particularly secondary to antibiotic therapy, the diet can also be increased in carbohydrates containing lactose and dextrose—milk, buttermilk, and yogurt, all of which are equally effective in recolonizing the intestine. Recent research has indicated that diet therapy may be more effective than actual ingestion of the *Lactobacillus* organism. When the antibiotics are discontinued, the diarrhea subsides in several days.

○ **Lactinex** (*Lactobacillus acidophilus* and *bulgaricus*) and available as both tablets and granules that can be sprinkled on food or taken with milk. Stools may have a fruity odor.

○ **Bacid** contains *Lactobacillus acidophilus* in sodium carboxymethylcellulose. Bacid may also cause stools to have a fruity odor.

SYSTEMICALLY ACTING ANTIDIARRHEALS

The systemically acting antidiarrheals are much more effective than the locally acting preparations in treating and controlling diarrhea. These agents, featured in Table 52–3, have both antispasmodic and antiperistaltic properties and are available both OTC and with a physician's prescription, depending on the dose. The systemically acting antidiarrheals include the opiates (opium tincture, paregoric, and codeine); synthetic opiate products (diphenoxylate, difenoxin hydrochloride, and loperamide). Another group of medications that can be used in the treatment of diarrhea includes antibiotics, generally used in acute infectious diarrhea (Chapter 58).

Opium Products

Opium products in current general use include **paregoric tincture** and **codeine** (Chapter 18). Opiates, mostly used to control pain, act on the GI system to decrease intestinal motility, reduce the cramping associated with diarrhea, and increase tone of smooth muscles and sphincters in the GI tract. This effect is used advantageously to treat a patient with diarrhea. However, because of their addictive properties, they are rarely used today.

Synthetic Opiates

Three derivatives of the synthetic opiate meperidine (Demerol)—**diphenoxylate hydrochloride (Lomotil)**, **difenoxin hydrochloride (Motofen)**, and **loperamide (Imodium)**—are less addictive than opium products, while still retaining the antidiarrheal effect common to the opiates. These products are available in tablet, capsule, or liquid form. All agents act directly on the intestinal smooth muscle to decrease transit time.

▼ **CLINICAL ALERT**

Synthetic opiates, as well as narcotics, should not be administered in acute diarrhea caused by antibiotics, poisons, infectious organisms (bacteria, parasites, viruses), or exotoxins until the toxic material has been eliminated. Such causative agents may penetrate the intestinal wall if retained. These agents are also not used in patients with antibiotic-induced pseudomembranous colitis because the irritating agent *C. difficile* and its toxins will be retained in the bowel.

○ **Diphenoxylate hydrochloride with atropine** (Lomotil, Logen, Low-Quel, Lonox, and many others) limits peristalsis by inhibiting mucosal receptors, which abolishes the local mucosal peristaltic reflex.

CONTRAINDICATIONS AND PRECAUTIONS Diphenoxylate is contraindicated in patients hypersensitive to its ingredients and in patients with obstructive jaundice, glaucoma (because it contains atropine), or diarrhea associated with pseudomembranous enterocolitis. It is

Table 52–3. SYSTEMICALLY ACTING ANTIDIARRHEALS

DRUG NAME/ROUTE AND DOSAGE	PHARMACOKINETICS/ DYNAMICS	NURSING IMPLICATIONS
diphenoxylate hydrochloride and atropine sulfate (Lomotil and others)		
Adults: 5 mL liquid, 2.5-5 mg tablets qid, PO. **Children 2–5 yr:** 1.5–4.5 mg PO qid. **Children 6–8 yr:** 2.5–5 mg PO qid. **Children 9–12 yr:** 3.5–5 mg PO qid.	**Onset:** 45–60 min **Peak:** 2 hr **Duration:** 3–4 hr **½L:** 3–14 hr **PB:** NA **B:** liver **E:** feces (49%), urine (14%)	**ASSESSMENT:** Determine cause of diarrhea. Assess number and color of stools. Assess fluid and electrolyte balance and daily weights. **INTERVENTION:** Give with sufficient water to allow medication to enter stomach. **EVALUATION:** Notify physician if diarrhea persists.
difenoxin hydrochloride with atropine sulfate (Motofen)		
Adults: 2 tablets PO to start, then 1 tablet after each loose stool q 3–4 hr PRN. Do not exceed 8 tablets in 24 hr.	**Onset:** NA **Peak:** 40–60 min **Duration:** NA **½L:** NA **PB:** NA **B:** liver **E:** urine, feces	Same as above plus: **INTERVENTION:** If relief is not obtained within 48 hours, medication should be discontinued and patient examined to determine cause of diarrhea. **Patient Teaching**—Warn patient to avoid tasks requiring alertness as drug may cause drowsiness. Advise patient to avoid alcohol and to keep medication out of reach of children.
loperamide (Imodium)		
Adults: 4 mg PO initially, then 2 mg after each loose bowel movement, up to 16 mg/day. **Children weighing 20 kg or less:** 1 mg PO tid. **Children weighing 21 kg or more:** 2 mg PO bid–tid.	**Onset:** 1 hr **Peak:** 5 hr **Duration:** 10 hr **½L:** 9.1–14.4 hr **PB:** NA **B:** liver **E:** feces 25%, urine 1.3%	Same as above.

NA = not available.

given cautiously to patients with abnormal liver function studies (as this is site of metabolism), to addicted persons, and to patients with ulcerative colitis. Safety has not been established in pregnancy (category C). Administer with caution to children and nursing mothers. Because diphenoxylate may cause drowsiness, patients are cautioned about driving or performing tasks requiring alertness.

ADVERSE EFFECTS Adverse effects of diphenoxylate include nausea, vomiting, sedation, vertigo. Because it also contains atropine, such adverse effects as dry mouth and blurred vision may occur, although these are rare in the low doses that are used. Diphenoxylate also can contribute to the development of paralytic ileus.

INTERACTIONS Diphenoxylate may potentiate the central nervous system–(CNS)-depressant effects of alcohol, barbiturates, and tranquilizers when given concurrently. The patient taking these products be closely observed. Long-term use has resulted in dependence. Opiate dependence can be by the CNS, as seen with heroin addicts, or by the GI system, as seen with loss of bowel regularity without opiates. There is great potential for serious intoxication in children from as few as six tablets. Parents must keep this medication out of the reach of children.

○ **Difenoxin hydrochloride** (Motofen) is similar to diphenoxylate hydrochloride.

○ **Loperamide hydrochloride** (Imodium) is a synthetic opioid for oral antidiarrheal use. This product has both a direct cholinergic effect and other effects on the neuronal pathways in the intestine, which slow intestinal motility and improve absorption of water and electrolytes.

CONTRAINDICATIONS AND PRECAUTIONS Loperamide hydrochloride is contraindicated in persons hypersensitive to its ingredients. It is used cautiously during pregnancy (category B) and lactation and in children under age 2.

ADVERSE EFFECTS The adverse effects of loperamide hydrochloride are generally minor and self-limiting and include abdominal pain, drowsiness, dry mouth, constipation, GI irritation, nausea and vomiting, and CNS depression. Naloxone (Narcan), a short-acting narcotic antagonist, may be administered to reverse these effects. Because of loperamide hydrochloride's long duration of action, the nurse must closely monitor the patient for at least 24 hours.

Antibiotics

Antibiotic medications used for the specific treatment of acute infectious diarrhea include antibacterial agents and antiprotozoal agents, listed in Table 52–4. It is important to obtain a stool culture to isolate the causative agent before any of these medications is prescribed, especially to the very young and the elderly patient. Often, while waiting for the results of the culture, broad-spectrum antibi-

Table 52–4. COMMON INFECTIOUS CAUSES OF DIARRHEA AND SPECIFIC MEDICATIONS

Type or Causative Organism	Treatment Medication
E. coli	Neomycin Ciprofloxacin Colistin sulfate (Coly-mycin S) Trimethoprim/sulfamethoxazole (Bactrim)
Shigella	Ampicillin Erythromycin
Pseudomonal enterocolitis	Gentamicin Polymyxin B
Coagulase-positive staphylococcal enterocolitis	Vancomycin (Vancocin) Ciprofloxacin
Acute amebic dysentery	Metronidazole (Flagyl) Tetracyclines
Travelers' diarrhea	Fluoroquinolones Doxycycline (Vibramycin) Ampicillin Trimethoprim/sulfamethoxazole (Bactrim)
Salmonellae	Ampicillin
C. difficile	Vancomycin (Vancocin) Metronidazole (Flagyl)

otics such as tetracyclines are prescribed. The most common causes of acute infectious diarrhea include *Salmonella* species, *Shigella* species, *Vibrio parahaemolyticus*, and certain strains of *E. coli*. For short-term diarrhea secondary to *Salmonella*, anti-infectives may not actually be necessary and in fact may increase the amount of time the individual "carries" *Salmonella*; these organisms usually cause a self-limiting infection, which usually clears in several days with fluid and electrolyte replacement. However, more prolonged, systemic, or severe infections call for anti-infective therapy. Appropriate therapy to prevent dehydration and electrolyte imbalance is always undertaken.

Antibiotics (cephalosporins, carbapenems, and others) may actually cause antibiotic-associated colitis (AAC) or pseudomembranous colitis associated with the overgrowth of *C. difficile*. Patients on these antibiotics are monitored closely for frequent, liquid stools. The offending antibiotic is stopped and vancomycin and/or metronidazole (Flagyl) are started. Both help heal the bowel and control *C. difficile*.

Travelers' diarrhea, often associated with ingestion of the food and water in a foreign country, may be caused by certain strains of *E. coli*. It frequently is accompanied by cramps, nausea, vomiting, headache, and fever of several days' duration, which can be relieved by prophylactic antibiotics such as trimethoprim/sulfamethoxazole (Bactrim) once daily (may cause serious skin reaction), doxy-

cycline (Vibramycin) once daily (may cause photosensitivity), ciprofloxacin hydrochloride (Cipro) 500 mg every 12 hours, trimethoprim (Proloprim) alone 200 mg per day, bismuth subsalicylate (Pepto-Bismol) 60 mL four times daily, or a simple antispasmodic and antiperistaltic agent. Many physicians suggest Pepto-Bismol prophylactically. If travelers' diarrhea occurs, therapy for 3 days is usually effective to control symptoms.

Diarrhea sometimes accompanies or results from tube feeding because of the high osmolarity of the feeding. (See Chapter 14 for additional information.) Diarrhea can also be caused by certain drugs containing sorbitol. Large quantities of sorbitol (over 20 g per day) can cause watery stools. Many oral products contain sorbitol, which improves the taste and maintains their suitability for diabetics. Examples of such products include the following: acetaminophen elixir 7.1 g/650 mg, oxtriphylline (Choledyl) 5.8 g/600mg, theophylline/guaifenesin (Elixophyllin-GG) 42 g/600 mg of theophylline, cimetidine (Tagamet) 8.6 g/900 mg, theophylline liquid 76 g/640 mg, and theophylline (Theolair Liquid) 18.4 g/640 mg. If possible, a different form of the drug is used. If that is not possible, stool analysis and calculation of the stool osmotic gap are performed by the laboratories.

$$\text{Osmotic gap} = \text{Stool osmolarity} - 2 \times (\text{stool Na}^+ + \text{K}^+)$$

Readings above 140 mmol/L indicate osmotic diarrhea. Therefore, a low osmotic diet should be administered.

LAXATIVES

Daily bowel movements may not be normal for everyone. Whereas some may evacuate their bowels daily, for others every 2, 3, or even 4 days is normal regularity. Constipation is the occurrence of hard, dry stool that lacks sufficient water to allow it to be passed easily. The majority of laxatives are self-prescribed for treatment of what individuals perceive to be constipation. Some people become neurotically preoccupied with bowel habits and use laxatives habitually. Because laxatives are generally available OTC, laxative abuse is a major health problem.

USES

Laxative, or cathartic, medications available both OTC and by prescription accelerate the passage of feces through the bowel. Their use may be necessary to treat constipation; to prepare patients for diagnostic tests (see Chapter 11); to prevent or decrease colonic absorption of ammonia in patients with hepatic encephalopathy; to hasten the excretion of various parasites or poisons from the intestinal tract; to treat children with congenital or acquired megacolon; to treat geriatric patients with poor muscle tone; to provide fresh stool for parasitologic exam; to empty the bowel before surgery, colonoscopy, or barium enema; and to modify the effluent in patients with an ileostomy or colostomy. Laxatives are also used in patients with congenital decreased bowel activity or in geriatric patients with chronic atonic constipation.

Table 52–5. CLASSIFICATION OF LAXATIVES BY MECHANISM OF ACTION

Contact-Stimulant Laxatives
Cascara sagrada
Senna products

Bulk-Forming Agents
Plantago seed (psyllium seed)
Calcium polycarbophil
Methylcellulose

Fecal Softeners
Docusate sodium (Colace)
Docusate calcium (Surfak)
Docusate potassium (Dialose)

Osmotic/Saline Agents
Magnesium salts
Sodium salts
Potassium salts
Lactulose

Lubricants
Mineral oil

Miscellaneous
Glycerine suppository

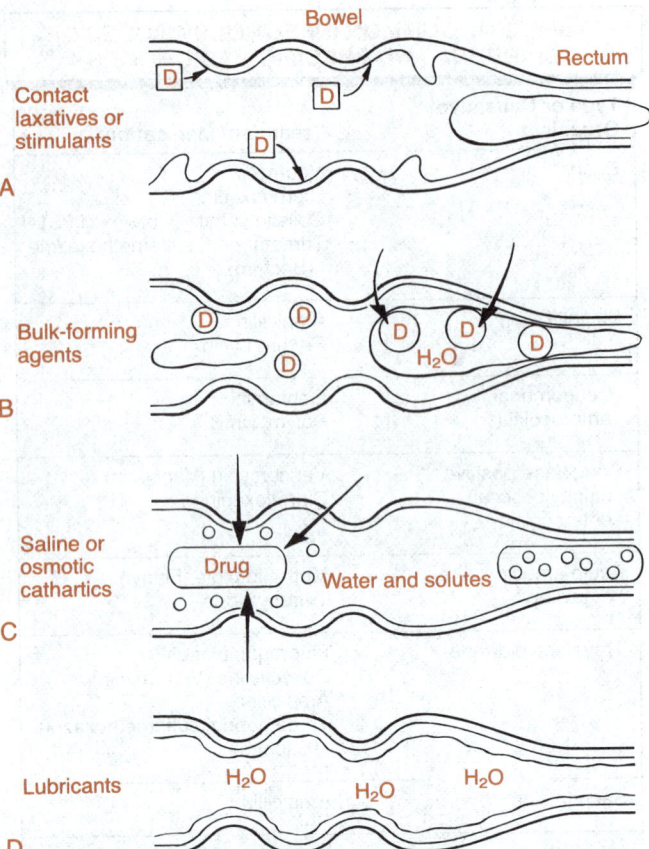

Figure 52–1. Mechanism of action of laxatives. (A) Contact laxatives stimulate the intestinal wall, thus producing an increase in peristalsis. (B) Bulk-forming agents absorb water into the fecal contents, giving more bulk to the stool. (C) Saline or osmotic cathartics are osmotically active and pull solutes and water into the bowel, thus increasing intestinal contents and bulk. (D) Lubricants lubricate and soften the intestinal contents and retard water absorption.

A classification system for laxatives used today is based on the mechanism of action: contact laxatives or stimulants, bulk-forming agents, saline or osmotic cathartics, fecal softeners, lubricants (as mineral oil), and several miscellaneous agents, as listed in Table 52–5 and Fig. 52–1. Each of these groups of medications is discussed individually in the following sections; the medications are featured in Tables 52–6 to 52–10.

ACTION

Laxatives promote bowel evacuation by promoting net fluid accumulation within the bowel lumen by a hydrophilic effect, an osmotic action, and/or a direct action on mucosal cells to decrease absorption and/or enhance secretion of water and electrolytes.

CONTRAINDICATIONS AND PRECAUTIONS

Laxatives are contraindicated in persons hypersensitive to any ingredient; in patients who have acute symptoms of appendicitis, acute abdomen, intestinal obstruction, or undiagnosed abdominal pain; and in patients suspected of having a fecal impaction. Administer laxatives cautiously to persons who may develop fluid and electrolyte imbalances such as the elderly, small children, and persons who are acutely ill. All laxatives are given cautiously to persons with oral and/or rectal fissures. Preparations containing sodium are given cautiously to patients with cardiac or renal diseases because of the possibility of sodium retention. Products containing magnesium or calcium are also administered cautiously to patients with renal disease as these electrolytes may be retained.

ADVERSE EFFECTS

All laxatives are capable of causing excessive bowel activity such as diarrhea, nausea, and vomiting. The frequent stools may cause perianal irritation. Patients may also experience abdominal cramps, bloating, and flatulence.

CONTACT/STIMULANT LAXATIVES

The contact/stimulant laxatives are all obtained from the bark, seed pods, leaves, and roots of a number of plants including cascara or senna. Contact/stimulant laxatives produce an increase in peristalsis when either the laxative itself or its breakdown products come in contact with the wall of the small or large intestine. The contact/stimulant cathartics also release prostaglandins and cause an increase in the mucosal concentration of cyclic 3′,5′-adenosine monophosphate (cAMP), which in turn increases secretion of electrolytes and may contribute to the total cathartic effect. Specifically, **bisacodyl (Dulcolax, Dacodyl)**, **phenolphthalein (Modane)**, and two anthraquinone-containing laxatives, **cascara sagrada** and **senna**,

Table 52–6. CONTACT/STIMULANT LAXATIVES

DRUG NAME/ROUTE AND DOSAGE	ONSET OF ACTION, SITE OF ACTION, TYPE OF STOOL	NURSING IMPLICATIONS
bisacodyl (Dulcolax) (Fleet Bisacodyl) (Theralax) (Dacodyl) (Deficol) and others		
Adults: 5–15 mg PO, up to 30 mg for special procedures; or 10 mg rectally *Children over 6 yr:* 5–10 mg PO or rectally at bedtime or before breakfast *Children under 2 yr:* 5 mg rectally	**Onset:** PO, 6–10 hr; rectal, 15–60 min **Site of Action:** C **Type of Stool:** SS	For all contact/stimulant laxatives: **ASSESSMENT:** Assess history of bowel activity. Assess fluid and electrolyte balance. Assess dietary patterns, fiber, and fluid intake. **INTERVENTION:** Take all with full glass of water or juice. Laxatives are only a temporary measure and should not be used long term in most patients. **Patient Teaching**—Teach patient about proper diet: fiber, fluids, and daily exercise. Caution patient that some products may discolor urine. **EVALUATION:** Notify physician of persistent constipation, rectal bleeding, or signs of fluid and electrolyte imbalance (muscle pain, dizziness, weakness). Enteric-coated products should not be taken within 1 hr of drinking milk or ingesting antacid, because enteric coating will be broken down in stomach and medication may cause gastric irritation. Administer with water only. Do not chew tablets.
cascara sagrada		
Extract (powder and starch added): 325 mg PO *Fluidextract:* 5 mL PO	**Onset:** 6–10 hr **Site of Action:** C **Type of Stool:** SS	Same as for all plus: **INTERVENTION:** Several products contain alcohol. Do not administer to alcoholics taking disulfiram. **Patient Teaching**—Warn patient that cascara changes urine color: acid urine, yellow-brown; alkaline urine, reddish.
phenolphthalein (Modane, Ex-Lax, Feen-a-mint, Correctol)		
Adults: 60–194 mg at bedtime *Children 6–11 yr:* 30–60 mg *Children 2–5 yr:* 15–30 mg	**Onset:** 6–10 hr **Site of Action:** C **Type of Stool:** SS	Same as for all plus: **INTERVENTION: Patient Teaching**—Warn patient of change in color of urine to pink-red, which may last 3–4 days. **EVALUATION:** Report rash to physician.

C = colon; SS = semisoft, semifluid, 6–12 hr.

are believed to stimulate the submucosal and mysenteric plexus (see Table 52–6).

▼ **CLINICAL ALERT**

The contact/stimulant laxatives should not be used regularly for longer than 1 week. Continuous use can produce irritable bowel–like diarrhea that is often severe enough to cause fluid and electrolyte imbalances. This type of laxative is often abused, particulary in the elderly.

Contraindications and Precautions

The anthraquinone-containing product, cascara, should not be given to lactating mothers because this medication is excreted in breast milk. The contact/stimulant laxatives are rarely used in children.

Adverse Effects

The adverse effects of the contact/stimulant laxatives include mild cramping, nausea, vomiting, diarrhea, and even dehydration in certain individuals. Patients receiving biscodyl (Dulcolax) in rectal suppositories may also complain of rectal burning. Phenolphthalein can cause a mild to severe skin rash in susceptible patients, and severe systemic allergic reactions have also been reported.

○ **Bisacodyl** (Dulcolax) is a synthetic contact/stimulant laxative. Because less than 5% is systemically absorbed and it is relatively nontoxic, it is widely used to treat various types of constipation and to evacuate the colon before endoscopy, surgery, and radiologic examinations.

○ **Phenolphthalein** is similar to bisacodyl in its pharmacologic properties, and it acts mainly on the colon. Onset of action is within 6 to 10 hours, with little associated pain or colic. Approximately 15% of this drug is absorbed and resecreted into the bile, which may prolong the cathartic effect for 3 to 4 days. If urine and feces are alkaline, they will turn pink-red. Because of its mild action and pleasant taste, it is found in many OTC products such as Ex-Lax and Feen-A-Mint.

○ **Cascara sagrada,** an anthraquinone cathartic obtained from the bark of the buckthorn tree (*Rhamnus pur-*

Table 52–7. FECAL SOFTENERS

DRUG NAME/ROUTE AND DOSAGE	ONSET OF ACTION, SITE OF ACTION, TYPE OF STOOL	NURSING IMPLICATIONS
docusate calcium (Surfak)		
Adults: 240 mg/day. *Children over 6 yr:* 50–150 mg/day	**Onset:** 24–72 hr **Site of Action:** SM and LG **Type of Stool:** S	For all fecal softeners: **ASSESSMENT:** Assess history of bowel activity. Assess fluid and electrolyte balance. Assess dietary patterns, fiber and fluid intake. **INTERVENTION:** Take all with full glass of water or juice. Laxatives are only temporary measure and should not be used long term in most patients. Add 50–100 mg (5–10 mL of liquid) to a retention or flushing enema. Follow syrup or solution with ½ cup of milk or juice to help mask taste. **Patient Teaching**—Teach patient about proper diet: fiber, fluids, and daily exercise. Caution patient that some products may discolor urine. **EVALUATION:** Notify physician of persistent constipation, rectal bleeding, or signs of fluid and electrolyte imbalance (muscle pain, dizziness, weakness).
docusate potassium (Dialose) (Kasof)		
Adults: 100–300 mg /day *Children over 6 yr:* 100 mg hs	**Onset:** 24–72 hr **Site of Action:** SM and LG **Type of Stool:** S	Same as for all plus: **INTERVENTION:** Several products contain alcohol. Do not administer to alcoholics on disulfiram.
docusate sodium (Colase) (Doss) (Modane Soft)		
Adults: 50–500 mg *Children: 6–12 yr:* 40–120 mg *Children 3–6 yr:* 20–60 mg *Children under 3 yr:* 10–40 mg	**Onset:** 24–72 hr **Site of Action:** SM and LG **Type of Stool:** S	Same as for all.
docusate sodium (Therevac-SB) (283 mg docusate sodium in soap base)		
Adults: 1 enema	**Onset:** Immediate	Same as for all.

SM = small intestine; LG = large intestine; S = soft formed, 1–3 days.

shiana), is one of the most popular cathartics. Cascara sagrada is partially absorbed in the small intestine and reaches the large intestine via the bloodstream and by passage along the GI tract. Cascara sagrada causes propulsive movements of the colon by direct chemical irritation, which evacuates the bowel in approximately 8 hours. The anthraquinone-containing stimulants, absorbed in the small intestine, circulate through the body and are excreted in bile, urine, saliva, colonic mucosa, and in the milk of lactating mothers. Because anthraquinone-containing stimulant laxatives are excreted in the urine, the patient may note a change in urine color; cascara, in particular, may tint acid urine yellow-brown and alkaline urine reddish.

Cascara sagrada is available in three forms: as an extract, as a fluidextract, and as tablets. Cascara sagrada extract is a powder with starch added. Cascara sagrada fluidextract has alcohol added as a preservative, which gives it a very bitter taste. Aromatic cascara fluidextract is treated with magnesium oxide to make it less bitter and more palatable. In addition, flavoring agents, sweeteners, and alcohol (18%) are added. Cascara is also available as 325-mg tablets.

▼ **CLINICAL ALERT**

Patients who abuse alcohol and are taking disulfiram for control should not take Cascara sagrada fluidextract or any other medication with alcohol added.

○ **Senna products** are anthraquinone derivatives, similar to cascara sagrada, but with more potent action. Senna products are converted in the colon to active aglycones, which stimulate *Auerbach's plexus* to induce peristalsis. (Auerbach's plexus is a network of autonomic nerve fibers located in the intestinal wall which, when stimulated, increase peristalsis.) Senna products are available as crude drugs (Black Draught) and standardized senna concentrations (Senokot). The senna products produce bowel evacuation in 6 to 10 hours, which may be accompanied by abdominal pain and colic.

FECAL SOFTENERS

Docusate salts—**docusate sodium** *(Colace)*, **docusate calcium** *(Surfak)*, and **docusate potassium** *(Dialose)*—are

Table 52–8. BULK-FORMING LAXATIVES

DRUG NAME/ROUTE AND DOSAGE	ONSET OF ACTION, SITE OF ACTION, TYPE OF STOOL	NURSING IMPLICATIONS
psyllium hydrophilic mucilloid (Metamucil) (Konsyl) (Fiberall) and many others		
Adults: 7 g or 1 packet or 1 rounded teaspoonful	**Onset:** 12–24 hr **Site of Action:** SM and LG **Type of Stool:** S	For all bulk-forming laxatives: **ASSESSMENT:** Assess history of bowel activity. Assess fluid and electrolyte balance. Assess dietary patterns, fiber and fluid intake. **INTERVENTION:** Take all with full glass of water or juice. Laxatives are only temporary measure and should not be used long term in most patients. All bulk-forming laxatives are slow acting and may need to be repeated for 2–3 days to achieve satisfactory results. Powders are diluted in 1 full glass of water, milk, fruit juice, or other liquid and mixed thoroughly before drinking. Another full glass of liquid should then be consumed. Do not take before bedtime to prevent intestinal obstruction. **Patient Teaching**—Teach patient about proper diet: fiber, fluids, and daily exercise. Caution patient that some products may discolor urine. **EVALUATION:** Notify physician of persistent constipation, rectal bleeding, or signs of fluid and electrolyte imbalance (muscle pain, dizziness, weakness).
calcium polycarbophil (Mitrolan) (FiberCon)		
Adults: 1–4 g/day. Do not exceed 6 g in 24 hr. *Children 6–12 yr:* 500 mg 1–3×/in 24 hr prn. *Children 3–6 yr:* 500 mg bid prn/24 hr. Do not exceed 4 g in 24 hr.	**Onset:** 12–24 hr **Site of Action:** SM and LG **Type of Stool:** S	Same as for all plus: **INTERVENTION:** Space the administration of tablets throughout day to overcome abdominal fullness. Tablets are vanilla or citrus flavored and are chewed thoroughly and followed by 8 oz of water.
methycellulose (Cologel, Citrucel)		
Adults: 1 tbsp in 8 oz cold H₂O, 1–3×/daily. *Children 6 yr and over:* 1 tbsp in 4 oz cold H₂O, 1–3×/daily.	**Onset:** 12–24 hr **Site of Action:** SM and LG **Type of Stool:** S	Same as for all.

SM = small intestine; LG = large intestine; S = soft formed, 1–3 days.

presumed to soften the feces by an emollient action that reduces surface tension, thus permitting penetration of the fecal mass by intestinal fluids (see Table 52–7). These products may also inhibit water absorption in the jejunum and colon. The electrolyte component of docusate—the sodium, calcium, or potassium—is not absorbed from these products. One or two days or more may be needed before a softened fecal bolus reaches the rectum.

❍ **Docusate sodium** (dioctyl sodium sulfosuccinate, Colace) is available as a capsule, tablet, syrup, or solution. Docusate sodium is also available as a disposable enema.

❍ **Docusate calcium** (Surfak) is claimed to be superior to the sodium product. It is indicated in patients when only the prevention of constipation is indicated and no cathartic effect is desired.

❍ **Docusate potassium** (Dialose) is administered to adults and children at bedtime until bowel movements are normal.

BULK-FORMING LAXATIVES

Bulk-producing agents, including natural and semisynthetic cellulose derivatives—**psyllium hydrophilic mucilloid (Metamucil, Konsyl, Fiberall), calcium polycarbophil (Mitrolan, Fibercon),** and **methycellulose (Citrucel)**—are made from agar, natural bran, plantago seed (psyllium seed), and methylcellulose and polycarbophil, which absorb water into the fecal contents and expand, giving more bulk to the stool (see Table 52–8). This increased bulk occurs naturally and promotes peristalsis and natural elimination about 12 to 24 hours after administration, but these drugs may be administered for several consecutive days before they achieve their maximal effect. These laxatives are the least harmful and do not interfere with the absorption of food. They are less likely to be habit-forming than other types of laxatives because of their slower action time and because they evacuate only the descending, sigmoid colon and rectum, rather than emptying the whole bowel as contact/stimulant laxatives do.

Table 52–9. OSMOTIC/SALINE LAXATIVES

DRUG NAME/ROUTE AND DOSAGE	ONSET OF ACTION, SITE OF ACTION, TYPE OF STOOL	NURSING IMPLICATIONS
magnesium hydroxide (Milk of Magnesia) (Magnesia Magma)		
Adults: 15–60 mL/day *Children 6–11 yr:* 15–30 mL *Children 2–5 yr:* 5–15 mL	**Onset:** 0.5–3 hr **Site of Action:** SM and LG **Type of Stool:** W	For all osmotic/saline laxatives: **ASSESSMENT:** Assess history of bowel activity. Assess fluid and electrolyte balance. Assess dietary patterns, fiber and fluid intake. **INTERVENTION:** Laxatives are only temporary measure and should not be used long term in most patients. Take with at least 240 mL of fluid in morning or early afternoon before eating any food or drinking any liquid. Fluid ensures that medication reaches bowel. All liquid preparations are shaken well before being poured. **Patient Teaching**—Teach patient about proper diet: fiber, fluids, and daily exercise. Caution patient that some products may discolor urine. **EVALUATION:** Notify physician of persistent constipation, rectal bleeding, or signs of fluid and electrolyte imbalance (muscle pain, dizziness, weakness).
magnesium citrate solution (Citrate of Magnesia)		
Adults: 240 mL, prn *Children 6–11 yr:* 100 mL *Children 2–5 yr:* 50 mL	**Onset:** 0.5–3 hr **Site of Action:** SM and LG **Type of Stool:** W	Same as for all. **Patient Teaching**—Instruct patient that magnesium citrate tastes bitter and is best served chilled and mixed with cold fruit juice or ice chips.
dibasic sodium phosphate/sodium monophosphate (Phospho-soda Fleet)		
Adults: 20–30 mL *Children 10–11 yr:* 5–15 mL *Children 5–9 yr:* 2.5–10 mL	**Onset:** 0.5–3 hr **Site of Action:** C **Type of Stool:** W	Same as for all. Mix in at least 4g of H_2O.
polyethylene glycol–electrolyte solute (CoLyte, Golytely)		
4 L of solution: 240 mL every 10 minutes	**Onset:** 30–60 min **Site of Action:** SM and LG **Type of Stool:** W	Same as for all.
lactulose (Cephulac) (Chronulac)		
Adults: 15–30 ml PO, 3–4 times/day, up to 60 mL/day *Children:* 2.5–10 mL/day **portal encephalopathy** *Adults:* initially, 30–45 ml PO tid, then reduced so fecal pH remains between 5–5.5	**Onset:** 24–48 hr **Site of Action:** C **Type of Stool:** S	Same as for all plus: **ASSESSMENT:** Assess blood glucose levels in patient with diabetes. **INTERVENTION:** Maintain adequate fluid volume. In elderly, periodically measure electrolytes. May be mixed with fruit juice or milk to increase palatability. *Do not* take other laxatives at same time. **EVALUATION:** Notify physician if diarrhea ensues.

C = colon; SM = small intestine; LG = large intestine; W = watery, 2–6 hr; S = soft formed, 1–3 days.

Some physicians recommend bran or dried fruits rather than bulk-forming laxatives, as they have the same effect. Dietary fiber should be 6 to 10 g per day to prevent or treat constipation.

The bulk-forming laxatives contain sugar, salt, and potassium. This may pose a problem for patients who must restrict their intake of sugar and salt.

Often, the bulk-forming laxatives are combined with other products such as fecal softeners or stimulant laxatives or emulsified with liquid petroleum (Petrogalar, Agoral), cascara, phenolphthalein, or magnesium hydroxide.

The bulk-forming laxatives are generally used in treating chronic, atonic (in the elderly), or spastic constipation. Currently, the bulk-forming laxatives are used to treat patients with diverticulosis and irritable bowel syndrome and to relieve painful defecation in patients with hemorrhoids.

The bulk-forming laxatives are always administered with a full glass of liquid and are followed by 8 oz of water to prevent the likelihood of either esophageal or intestinal obstruction or impaction.

○ **Psyllium hydrophilic mucilloid** (Metamucil, Konsyl, and many others) is a mixture of 50% powdered plan-

Table 52–10. LUBRICANT AND MISCELLANEOUS LAXATIVES

DRUG NAME/ROUTE AND DOSAGE	ONSET OF ACTION, SITE OF ACTION, TYPE OF STOOL	NURSING IMPLICATIONS
all laxatives		
		ASSESSMENT: Assess history of bowel activity. Assess fluid and electrolyte balance. Assess dietary patterns, fiber and fluid intake. **INTERVENTION:** Take all with full glass of water or juice. Laxatives are only temporary measure and should not be used long term in most patients. **Patient Teaching**—Teach patient about proper diet: fiber, fluids, and daily exercise. Caution patient that some products may discolor urine. **EVALUATION:** Notify physician of persistent constipation, rectal bleeding, or signs of fluid and electrolyte imbalance (muscle pain, dizziness, weakness).
LUBRICANT LAXATIVES		
mineral oil (Kondremul) (Petrogalar Plain) (mineral oil) (Oil Enema) (Agoral Plain)		
Adults and Children ≥12 yr: 15–45 mL PO; or 120 mL rectally **Children 2–11 yr:** 5–15 mL PO; or 30–60 mL rectally.	**Onset:** 6–8 hr **Site of Action:** C **Type of Stool:** S	Same as for all plus: **INTERVENTION:** Best administered at bedtime on an empty stomach. Best administered cold or mixed with orange juice, or patient may suck on lemon or orange slice after drinking medication. Prolonged use of lubricants can interfere with absorption of fat-soluble vitamins A, D, E, and K. Mineral oil retention enema should always be followed 30–60 min later with cleansing enema. Should be taken regularly at same time each day to promote normal bowel activity.
MISCELLANEOUS LAXATIVES		
glycerin suppositories		
Adults: 1 suppository rectally. Retain for 15 min. **Children under 6 yr:** slivers rectally	**Onset:** 0.25–0.5 hr **Site of Action:** C **Type of Stool:** S	Same as for all.

C = colon; S = soft formed, 1–3 days.

tago seeds, which swell in the presence of moisture to form an indigestible, jellylike mass, and 50% percent dextrose or a sugar-free variety in a cream-colored powder. It is effective in about 12 to 72 hours and also has a demulcent effect on an inflamed bowel. Psyllium hydrophilic mucilloid can be administered as many as three times a day.

○ **Calcium polycarbophil** (Mitrolan, Fibercon) is recommended for treating both constipation and diarrhea. Its effectiveness as a stool normalizer comes from its ability to bind up to 60 to 100 times its weight of water. This is three times as much as is possible with previously available hydrophilic substances obtained from psyllium seeds.

When calcium polycarbophil is used to manage constipation, it keeps free water from being absorbed out of the intestine, which in turn converts dry, hard, scanty stools into a soft, bulky mass. When calcium polycarbophil is used to manage acute diarrhea that results when water rushes out of the intestine at abnormally rapid rates, this drug binds with excessive fluid. This helps to stop the frequent liquid bowel movements.

Calcium polycarbophil is especially useful for symptomatic relief of GI disorders in which diarrhea and constipation alternate, as in irritable bowel syndrome and diverticulosis.

○ **Methylcellulose** (Citrucel) is a hydrophilic semisynthetic cellulose derivative. Oral preparation swells on contact with water and forms a demulcent nonabsorbable gel that facilitates passage of stool and reflexly stimulates stool. Methylcellulose is also available as 500-mg tablets, which should not be chewed to avoid the risk of esophageal obstruction. These preparations should either be mixed in 8 oz of fluid or followed by 8 oz of fluid.

OSMOTIC/SALINE LAXATIVES

The most rapid-acting and powerful of all laxatives are the osmotic/saline laxatives—**magnesium citrate, sodium phosphate,** and **magnesium hydroxide** *(Milk of Magnesia)* (see Table 52–9). Usually a salt of nonabsorbable anions or cations, they act by increasing the bulk of the intestinal contents. Consequently, peristalsis occurs more quickly than with bulk laxatives. Their cathartic action can occur within 2 to 6 hours after administration. **Polyethylene glycol–electrolyte solution** *(Colyte, Go-LYTELY)* is used prior to GI exams to cleanse the bowel. **Lactulose syrup** *(Cephulac)* increases the number of bowel movements and is used in patients with liver disease.

The greater the concentration of the salt, the greater the osmotic ability once the salt enters the bowel. A hypertonic saline solution causes diffusion of fluid from the plasma into the intestine to dilute the solution to isotonic. The magnesium salts cause an increase in the secretion of cholecystokinin from the duodenum, which is thought to increase secretion and motility of the small intestine and colon and may contribute to the cathartic effect. The greater their concentration, the more likely the osmotic laxatives are to cause nausea. Therefore, a hypertonic saline solution is made isotonic by adding water when administering it. All preparations are accompanied by at least 8 oz of water. The water also assists the laxative to leave the stomach.

Uses

Because of their short action time, the osmotic/saline laxatives are often used to cleanse the entire intestinal tract for diagnostic tests, to flush poisons, or to remove parasites. These laxatives create a liquid stool, but do not rupture the egg capsules of the parasites.

Contraindications and Precautions

The magnesium and potassium salts are contraindicated in renal disease as these electrolytes may be retained. They are given cautiously to a patient with renal disease because of their sodium content. Also, they are given cautiously to patients receiving CNS depressants as there may be a significant decrease in serum calcium which could precipitate more seizure activity.

○ **Magnesium citrate** is flavored and carbonated. It is not very soluble; therefore, relatively large doses need to be administered. Magnesium citrate is more palatable when served chilled.

○ **Sodium phosphate** is readily dissolved in water and has a more agreeable taste than other compounds.

○ **Effervescent sodium phosphate** contains sodium bicarbonate and citric and tartaric acids.

○ **Fleet Phospho-Soda** is a concentrated aqueous solution of sodium biphosphate and sodium phosphate. Fleet Phospho-Soda is also available as a disposable enema unit, but is administered cautiously to persons on a low-sodium diet.

○ **Magnesium hydroxide** (Milk of Magnesia) reacts with hydrochloric acid to form magnesium chloride, which then becomes the laxative.

○ **Polyethylene glycol–electrolyte solution** (Colyte, GoLYTELY) is used prior to GI exams. After oral administration, the solution induces diarrhea within 30 to 60 minutes and rapidly cleanses the bowel, usually within 4 hours. Polyethylene glycol–electrolyte solutions are nonabsorbable solutions that act as osmotic agents. The patient should fast 3 to 4 hours prior to ingestion of the solution. The patient must drink 4 liters of this solution—240 mL every 10 minutes until the 4 liters are consumed. The solution is more palatable when chilled. Only liquids are permitted after ingestion of polyethylene.

○ **Lactulose syrup** (Cephulac) is a synthetic disaccharide analog of lactose consisting of galastose and fructose that increases the daily number of bowel movements. Lactulose is primarily used in patients with hepatic dysfunction to decrease blood ammonia levels and reduce the symptoms of hepatic encephalopathy and renal failure. Lactulose acidifies the colon from a normal pH of 7 to 5. The acidification pulls amononia into the bowel, and thus an osmotic effect occurs.

CONTRAINDICATIONS AND PRECAUTIONS Lactulose is contraindicated in patients on a low-galactose diet, as it contains galactose. It is given cautiously to pregnant women and to patients concurrently receiving neomycin. Neomycin and other nonabsorbable antibiotics may reduce or destroy enough colonic bacteria to interfere with the effective action of lactulose syrup. Lactulose syrup, because of its sugar content, is given to diabetic patients with caution; changes in blood sugar have been noted. Also, elderly patients receiving lactulose syrup for 6 months or longer should have periodic measurements of their serum electrolytes including potassium and chloride as electrolytes may be lost in the stool.

ADVERSE EFFECTS Adverse effects from lactulose syrup include flatulence, intestinal cramps, gas, and belching. Excessive doses may produce diarrhea with hypokalemia and nausea, because of its sweet taste. Because it acts on the colon, there is no interference with absorption of secretion in the small intestine.

LUBRICANT LAXATIVES

The only lubricant laxative available today—**mineral oil**—is used for temporary relief of constipation, to prevent tearing of hemorrhoids or fissures, and to prevent straining at stool for patients with recent surgery or cardiac disease.

○ **Mineral oil** lubricates and softens the intestinal contents and retards water absorption; it takes effect 6 to 8 hours after administration. Mineral oil is minimally absorbed from the intestinal tract, with distribution to the liver, spleen, mesenteric lymph nodes, and intestinal mucosa. Mineral oil is featured in Table 52–10.

ADVERSE EFFECTS The adverse effects of mineral oil include anorexia, nausea, vomiting, and nutritional deficiencies. Also, lipid pneumonia may occur if it is accidentally aspirated. Small children and the elderly are at high-

Table 52–11. COMBINATION LAXATIVES

Name	Mineral Oil	White Phenolphthalium	Docusate Sodium	Casanthranol	Magnesium Hydroxide	Irish Moss	Standardized Senna Concentration	Alcohol
Agoral	X	X						
Haley's M-O	X				X			
Kondremul	X	X				X		
Peri-Colace (Capsules)			X	X				
Peri-Colace Syrup			X	X				
Senokot S				X			X	X

est risk for aspiration. Chronic use may decrease the absorption of vitamins (particularly the fat-soluble vitamins A, D, E, and K), food, and bile salts. Some researchers believe that only the precursor of vitamin A (carotene) is affected, and that natural vitamin A is absorbed in the intestine in the presence of mineral oil.

MISCELLANEOUS LAXATIVES

Glyceric suppositories, the miscellaneous laxative available today, stimulates the rectal mucosa.

○ **Glycerin suppositories** promote peristalsis through local irritation of the mucous membranes of the rectum. Glycerin suppositories are safe for temporary use to reestablish proper bowel habits in patients who have lost the rectal reflex. Glycerin suppositories are often helpful in bowel retraining regimens and in individuals with intermittent constipation. Glycerin suppositories are effective in 15 minutes to 1 hour.

COMBINATION PRODUCTS

The combination products combine ingredients from two or more classes of laxatives. Sufficient evidence is not available to confirm the effectiveness of combination preparations. Several examples are included in Table 52–11.

ULCERATIVE COLITIS REMISSION DRUGS

Two drugs, **mesalamine (Rowasa, Asacol, Pentasa)** and **olsalazine sodium (Dipentum)**, are available to treat and maintain a remission in ulcerative colitis. These drugs are featured in Table 52–12. The exact mechanism of both drugs is unknown, but both are thought to act locally to diminish inflammation by blocking cyclooxygenase and inhibiting colon prostaglandin production in the bowel mucosa.

Table 52–12. ULCERATIVE COLITIS REMISSION DRUGS

DRUG NAME/ROUTE AND DOSAGE	PHARMACOKINETICS/ DYNAMICS	NURSING IMPLICATIONS
mesalamine (Rowasa) (Pentasa) (Asacol)		
Adults: 800 mg PO tid for a total of 2.4 g/day for 6 wk. **Retention enema:** 60 mL units (4 g) usually at bedtime for 3–6 wk. **Rectal Suspension:** 500 mg bid, retain for 1–3 hr; use for 3–21 days. **Rectal Suppository:** 1 suppository bid for 3–6 wk.	**Onset:** PO, slowly; rectal, NA **Peak:** PO, 4–12 hr; rectal, 3–12 days **Duration:** PO, 12–18 hr; rectal, NA **½L:** PO, 12 hr; rectal, 0.5–1.5 hr. **PB:** 44%–80% **B:** liver, gut mucosa **E:** feces, urine	**ASSESSMENT:** Assess for sulfate and salicylate sensitivity. **INTERVENTION:** Enema is retention enema, which should remain in bowel for 8 hr. Swallow tablets whole, do not break outer coating. Intact or partially intact tablet may be found in stool. If this occurs, notify physician. Insert suppository gently into rectum, pointed end first. **EVALUATION:** Report severe abdominal pain and cramps to physician.
olsalazine sodium (Dipentum)		
Adults: 1 g/day PO in 2 divided doses.	**Onset:** NA **Peak:** 1 hr **Duration:** NA **½L:** 0.9 hr **PB:** 99% **B:** liver **E:** urine (1%)	**ASSESSMENT:** Assess for salicylate sensitivity. **INTERVENTION:** Take with food in 2 doses/day. Diarrhea is likely to occur, so contact physician for therapy.

Contraindications and Precautions

Both drugs are contraindicated in persons with salicylate hypersensitivity as they are converted to salicylate. Safety and efficacy in pregnancy (mesalamine, category B; olsalazine, category C), lactation, and children have not been established. Use olsalazine cautiously in renal dysfunction as the drug's metabolism may worsen preexisting renal disease.

O **Mesalamine** (Rowasa) is administered orally or rectally as a suspension enema. Improvement may be seen in 3 to 21 days; however, the usual course of therapy is 3 to 6 weeks.

ADVERSE EFFECTS Mesalamine is generally well tolerated with most adverse effects being mild and transient. The most common adverse effects include abdominal pain/cramps/discomfort, headache, gas and flatulence, eructation, and nausea. Patients are assessed for the development of pancolitis.

O **Olsalazine sodium** (Dipentum) is administered to keep patients with ulcerative colitis in remission. The 6-month relapse rate is approximately 19%.

ADVERSE EFFECTS The most common adverse effect is diarrhea, and in about 6% of patients it necessitates discontinuing the drug. Additional adverse effects include pain and cramps, headache and nausea, and dyspepsia.

USING THE NURSING PROCESS

ASSESSMENT

- Develop a thorough nursing history to create the database. The patient requiring these medications may be acutely ill in the hospital or relatively healthy and self-treating a digestive problem with OTC preparations. Typical information obtained from the patient is included in Table 52–13.

Diarrhea

- If the patient's chief complaint is diarrhea, assess whether he or she traveled recently to areas where hygiene is poor or whether the patient has had altered normal dietary habits. To implement the correct treatment of diarrhea later, it is important to discover the cause of the malady. In general, antidiarrheals are not chosen to treat acute diarrhea associated with organisms that penetrate the intestinal mucosa, such as viruses, *E. coli*, *Salmonella*, or *Shigella*. A nurse who suspects the presence of these organisms always requests a stool sample for culture.
- Assess the character, frequency, and odor of stools (foul-smelling feces indicates a need for increased digestive enzymes); note the number of stools per day; and detect the presence of mucus, blood, or fat. The very young or old must have close assessments to prevent dehydration and electrolyte imbalances. Patients who have chronic diarrhea resulting from reaction to stress, excessive alcohol consumption, or improper dietary habits need counseling during the implementation phase to help them correct the problem.
- Assess personal hygiene patterns.

Constipation

- Assess the possible cause of constipation before planning and starting treatment. This assessment begins with the patient describing, in detail, what he or she perceives as constipation and how much time is spent defecating. Often, by increasing the time allowed for defecating, the patient can avoid constipation.
- Assess dietary patterns and suggest that the patient add fresh fruits, vegetables, and whole grains to the diet to provide bulk; and drink 8 to 10 glasses of water daily to ensure adequate hydration. This may help to regulate bowel activity.
- Assess the amount of daily exercise; increased physical activity can stimulate peristalsis.
- Assess the cardiovascular status of the patient; a patient with cardiovascular impairment is encouraged during the intervention phase to avoid straining at stool, which activates the vagus nerve (Valsalva maneuver) and slows the heart rate. In most instances, laxatives are used only as a temporary measure.
- Assess bowel sounds and determine there is no fecal impaction, nausea and vomiting, abdominal pain, or bowel obstruction before administering cathartics. Cathartics are contraindicated for patients who exhibit these symptoms. If stool is present, but not impacted, insert the rectal suppository alongside the bowel wall, not in the fecal mass.

NURSING DIAGNOSIS

- Determine the nursing diagnosis appropriate for the patient's diagnosis. Typical nursing diagnoses for a patient requiring medications for digestive problems include Diarrhea, Constipation, and Knowledge Deficit (see Table 52–13).

PLANNING AND INTERVENTION

- Develop the goals of nursing intervention from the nursing diagnoses. Typical nursing goals for the patient with digestive problems are included in Table 52–13.
- Encourage the patient to eat a well-balanced diet; dietary modification may be a long-term solution to digestive problems. The addition of fresh fruits and vegetables may prevent constipation, whereas the addition of whole grains and additional bulk (bran, fresh fruits and vegetables, cereal fibers) may prevent diarrhea. Patients should drink sufficient water to prevent dehydration and to soften the stool. Exercise is also important to restore normal bowel activity.

Table 52–13. NURSING PROCESS FOR PATIENT REQUIRING DRUGS FOR DIGESTIVE DISORDERS

Assessment

Assess current complaints of diarrhea, constipation, nausea/vomiting, abdominal pain, frequency of bowel movement, and odor of stool. Auscultate bowel sounds.

Assess history for fecal impaction, bowel obstruction, chronic disease/conditions, cardiovascular impairment.

Assess dietary patterns, noting fluid intake and amount of daily exercise.

Assess medication history; alcohol, laxative, and enema use/abuse; and patient perception of what constipation is.

Assess laboratory studies, e.g., stool specimen.

Nursing Diagnosis: Constipation

RELATED TO: Altered dietary intake, inadequate bulk, chronic use of laxatives/enemas, some medications, changes in level of activity.

AS EVIDENCED BY: Frequency less than usual pattern, hard-formed stool, straining at stool, decreased bowel sounds.

Desired Outcomes/Evaluation Criteria

Reestablishes normal patterns of bowel functioning. Verbalizes understanding of factors and appropriate interventions/solutions related to individual situation.

Demonstrates changes in lifestyle as necessitated by causative/contributing factors.

Nursing Actions	Rationale
Administer laxatives (e.g., Dulcolax, Fleet Enema) as indicated.	Promotes bowel evacuation and relieves constipation.
Remove fecal impaction if present.	Impaction must be removed before regular bowel function can be reestablished.
Discuss use of stool softeners (Surfak), bulk-forming products (Metamucil, Fiberall).	Useful in preventing constipation based on individual need.
Encourage intake of well-balanced diet (including fresh fruits/vegetables), fluid intake of at least 3000 mL/day as tolerated, fiber at least 6–10 g/day.	May be sufficient to correct situation by promoting more normal amount and consistency of stool.
Establish regular exercise program.	Increased activity promotes increased bowel motility and regularity.

Nursing Diagnosis: Diarrhea

RELATED TO: Toxins, contaminants, medications, dietary intake, inflammation/irritation, or malabsorption of bowel.

AS EVIDENCED BY: Abdominal pain, urgency, cramping, increased frequency, loose/liquid stools.

Desired Outcomes/Evaluation Criteria

Reestablishes and maintains normal pattern of bowel functioning. Verbalizes understanding of causative factors and rationale of treatment regimen. Demonstrates appropriate behavior to assist with resolution of causative factors, e.g., proper food preparation and avoidance of irritating foods.

Nursing Actions	Rationale
Administer antidiarrheal (e.g., Paregoric, Lomotil, Imodium) or digestive enzymes (e.g., bile salts and pancreatic enzymes) as indicated.	Slows GI motility, prolonging transit time to reduce frequency of stools; promotes normal digestive process and absorption of fat.
Monitor vital signs as appropriate. Observe mucous membranes, skin turgor.	Indicators of degree of dehydration.
Restrict foods/fluids as indicated.	Promotes intestinal rest and may prevent precipitation of further diarrhea.
Encourage patient to drink fluids (boiled/bottled water if indicated), eat bland food, and get extra rest.	Maintains hydration and helps to regain homeostasis.
Suggest intake of whole grains and additional bulk (e.g., bran, cereal fibers).	Aids in promoting firm, soft stool that is more easily passed.
Stress importance of medical follow-up.	Further evaluation and treatment may be required when diarrhea continues for extended period.
Discuss side effects. Advise patient not to drive and to report untoward reactions.	Dry mouth and drowsiness are expected and depend on dose and individual response. More serious reactions may require change of dose or choice of drug.
Suggest use of ointment, skin barrier preparations.	Provides relief for irritated anal tissue, helps protect skin from excoriation.
Discuss preventive use of antidiarrheal drugs.	May be helpful in preventing diarrhea when traveling in foreign country.

Other Suggested Nursing Diagnosis: Knowledge Deficit.

Diarrhea

- Teach the patient that diarrhea is often a symptom of disease, not a disease in itself. Patients are encouraged not to self-treat immediately because diarrhea can be a defense mechanism to rid the body of a toxin or other causative agent. If treatment is started too early, this normal defense may be hindered.
- Monitor the patient's other drugs. Drug therapy may also precipitate diarrhea. Sorbitol concentration in certain drugs may create an osmotic diarrhea as previously discussed. Antibiotics in general cause diarrhea, but diarrhea is most likely to occur with clindamycin, the aminopenicillins, the cephalosporins, and the aminoglycosides (excluding parenteral gentamicin and tobramycin). Symptoms may occur acutely or take several weeks to occur. As many as 20% of people taking antibiotics develop colitis (and sometimes pseudomembranous colitis) or antibiotic-associated colitis (AAC). The offending antibiotic is discontinued. (Treatment has been discussed previously.) Antidiarrheals are never administered to counteract AAC because they slow the passage of stool through the intestines, prolonging the mucosa's exposure to toxins.
- Teach the patient traveling to a foreign country where travelers' diarrhea is likely to occur to choose hotels and restaurants with good sanitary conditions and to drink only bottled water with no ice cubes unless the restaurant makes ice cubes from boiled water. Salad, cold sandwiches, and uncooked vegetables are avoided. Fruits and vegetables are eaten only after they are peeled or washed in chlorinated water. Buffet-table foods, which may have spent hours away from proper refrigeration, are avoided. If travelers' diarrhea does occur, the individual should rest, keep warm, drink only boiled or bottled water, and eat bland, cooked foods. It is important to avoid dehydration and to provide an easily digestible energy source.

Constipation

- Teach the patient most constipation is due to poor dietary or living conditions; however, a change in bowel habits can also be a symptom of a more serious problem such as bowel obstruction and/or a malignancy. After the physician rules out such organic problems, the patient can be helped to normalize bowel habits.
- Teach the patient what is a normal bowel movement. Often patients believe that they must evacuate the bowel on a daily basis; if they do not have a bowel movement, they take a laxative. The laxative empties their lower bowel, which in turn prevents a normal bowel movement the following day. Instead of the laxative restoring normal regularity, the continued use of cathartics soon makes it difficult for the laxative abuser to ever achieve a natural movement. This dependence can become both physiologic and psychologic. This cycle must be interrupted if normal bowel activity is to return.

- Monitor the patient's other drugs. Constipation may be a side effect of opiates, antacids, phenothiazines, sedatives, multiple vitamin complexes, and tricyclic antidepressants. Patients having constipation secondary to these drugs are encouraged to modify their diet to include extra fluid and bulk. These additions may eliminate the constipation.

Chronic constipation can cause numerous problems for the patient, including hemorrhoids or diverticulosis, and may even predispose an individual to cancer of the colon. Therefore, the nurse encourages the patient to prevent constipation on a daily basis.

Patient Teaching

- Teach the information found in each drug table in the Nursing Implications column. Additional information for patient teaching can be found in Tables 52–14, 52–15, and 52–16.

Patients who have experienced chronic constipation may be placed on a bowel retraining program. The first step of any retraining program is to ensure that the diet is high in fluid and bulk, particularly breakfast. Breakfast should also be consumed at approximately the same time each day. The patient then sits on the toilet or commode for 15 to 30 minutes after the meal. If reflex defecation does not occur, a lubricated glycerin suppository is inserted into the rectum. If defecation still does not occur, a Fleet enema is generally administered. Within a short time, the patient begins to defecate on a regular schedule following breakfast without the use of the suppository or enema. The importance of diet, exercise, and adequate fluids is stressed to each patient.

EVALUATION

- Evaluate the effectiveness of the medications that alter the digestive system. This evaluation is based on a list of outcome evaluation criteria that has been developed in relation to the goals determined by the

---

Table 52–14. PATIENT TEACHING INFORMATION—DIGESTANTS

Dear Patient:
This drug has been prescribed for you. This is what you should know about your drug to get the most from your therapy.

☐ 1. Digestants such as _____ are taken to help in the digestion of food you eat.
☐ 2. Digestants will usually be taken for the rest of your life.
☐ 3. Digestants are taken with meals to make sure that the drug is present when the food enters the stomach and bowels. They are best sprinkled on the food.
☐ 4. Check your stools daily for the presence of fat, an increasing foul smell, or bulky or foamy stool. Both an increase in fat and foul smell may mean that your dose may need to be changed.

Table 52–15. PATIENT TEACHING INFORMATION—ANTIDIARRHEALS
Dear Patient:
This drug has been prescribed for you. This is what you should know about your drug to get the most from your therapy.
☐ 1. Antidiarrheals such as _____ are taken to control diarrhea and reduce the number of stools daily.
☐ 2. Many locally acting antidiarrheals are available as over-the-counter preparations. Do not take them when fever is present or for more than 3 days if the symptoms are not stopped. The diarrhea may mean you have a more serious problem that needs medical attention. Systemically acting antidiarrheals should also not be taken for longer than 2 days if symptoms are not stopped.
☐ 3. During the acute attack, you may be asked to not eat anything for a few days, or to drink a clear liquid or to eat a bland diet and not eat any milk products (ice cream, pudding, and so on), to rest the bowel for a few days.
☐ 4. You may also have other medications such as anti-infectives, antiemetics, digestive enzymes, narcotics or their derivatives, and steroids added to control diarrhea.

Table 52–16. PATIENT TEACHING INFORMATION—LAXATIVES
Dear Patient:
This drug has been prescribed for you. This is what you should know about your drug to get the most from your therapy.
☐ 1. Laxatives such as _____ are taken to soften and make the passage of stool easier.
☐ 2. Take your laxatives either at bedtime or before breakfast to allow for the peak action to occur at a convenient time.
☐ 3. Often, laxatives are best taken with milk or fruit juice. Many types of laxatives must be taken with a full glass of water or liquid.
☐ 4. Enteric-coated tablets are not taken within 1 hour of drinking milk or taking an antacid, because their enteric coating is broken down in the stomach and may lead to stomach upset. Enteric-coated tablets should not be chewed.

nurse, patient, and family. Typical outcome evaluation criteria are included in Table 52–13.

It is extremely important to work with the patient and family to ensure their compliance. Patients who understand the importance of their continued medical treatment are usually compliant. The primary reasons for noncompliance are forgetting to take the medication or disliking the unpleasant side effects.

- Teach the patient about potential common side effects so that a patient who takes medication at home reports any unusual symptoms to the physician or nurse. Patients with renal or hepatic disease must be watched more closely for side effects.
- Evaluate bowel activity frequently. Constipation is often a complication of antidiarrheal medication. Encouraging the patient to drink plenty of liquids may help to prevent constipation.
- Stress the importance of continued medical care. All previously taught material is reviewed and updated with the patient and family, if necessary, to ensure that the patient's knowledge base remains accurate.

The bibliography for this chapter can be found in Appendix B, which begins on page 1054.

CHAPTER REVIEW QUESTIONS*

1. The pancreatic replacement enzyme pancrelipase (Cotazym) is used in the following patient situation:
   a. Pernicious anemia.
   b. Following gallbladder surgery.
   c. Cystic fibrosis.
   d. Hypochlorhydria

2. Jerry is being discharged on Pepto-Bismol to assist with control of his diarrhea. Which of the following is a nursing intervention associated with the administration of this drug?
   a. Withhold other medications for 2 hours after administration.
   b. Give absorbents at least 3 times daily for soothing effect.
   c. Discontinue if a fruity odor is apparent in the stool.
   d. Administer absorbent sparingly because of risk of addiction.

3. Which of the following statements is *correct* regarding diphenoxylate hydrochloride (Lomotil)?
   a. It should be given to patients with infectious diarrhea.
   b. The drug is used to control antibiotic-induced pseudomembranous colitis.

   c. Lomotil is classified as a class III drug.
   d. It contains atropine, causing dry mouth and blurred vision.

4. Patients taking cascara sagrada with Milk of Magnesia should be alert to the following side effect:
   a. Foul smelling urine.
   b. Fruity odor to the breath.
   c. Oily skin.
   d. Reddish or yellow-brown urine.

5. The agent found in over-the-counter products such as Ex-Lax and Feen-A-Mint is:
   a. Senna.
   b. Phenolphthalein.
   c. Castor oil.
   d. Belladonna.

6. Bulk-forming laxatives:
   a. Produce harmful nutritional side effects.
   b. Expand as water is absorbed into the fecal contents.
   c. Empty both the large and small intestines.
   d. Interfere with vitamin A absorption.

*See Appendix A, which begins on page 1051, for answers.

BUILDING YOUR CRITICAL THINKING SKILLS

DIGESTIVE PROBLEMS

Case Study 1: Diarrhea

A 55-year-old man has been treated for acute sinusitis for the last week with a cephalosporin antibiotic. He developed diarrhea 3 days ago that has worsened. He comes to the clinic indicating his stools are watery with shreds of feces.

1. What is the most likely cause of this man's diarrhea?
2. What additional assessments should be made for this patient?
3. What interventions should the nurse anticipate?

CHAPTER 53

Medications Used in Hepatic and Biliary Disease

Merrily A. Kuhn, RNC, PhD

CHAPTER OUTLINE

Medications To Treat Hepatic Cell Necrosis
Medications To Manage Pruritus
Medications To Manage Ascites
Medications To Treat Hepatic Encephalopathy
Medications To Treat Cholelithiasis
Using The Nursing Process

TABLES

Drug Tables
Gallstone Solubilizing Agents, 788

Nursing Process
Nursing Process in Hepatic Disease, 789

KEY TERMS

Ascites
Cholelithiasis
Glutathione

Hepatitic encephalopathy
Lithotripsy

LEARNING OBJECTIVES

After reading this chapter, the student will be able to:

1. Identify medications commonly used to manage hepatic and biliary disease.
2. Differentiate among the various types of medications used to manage hepatic and biliary disease in reference to mechanisms of action, routes of administration, pharmacokinetics, contraindications and precautions, adverse effects, and interactions.
3. Identify specific areas to assess in the patient requiring management of complications of hepatic and biliary disease to formulate appropriate patient outcomes.
4. Plan the nursing interventions necessary to administer medications used in the management of complications of hepatic and biliary disease safely and choose appropriate teaching strategies to gain patient compliance.
5. Evaluate the patient at various stages to measure nursing interventions.

The hepatic and biliary systems, major parts of the digestive system, include the gallbladder and the pancreas (which is also an endocrine gland, producing insulin). See Chapter 49 for a review of the normal functioning of the hepatic and biliary systems in digestion. The patient with any type of hepatic or biliary disease (e.g., cirrhosis or hepatitis) is acutely ill and must be continually observed and evaluated. As most medications used to treat the patient with hepatic or biliary disease are covered elsewhere in this text, only a brief overview is presented. Drug therapy to treat hepatitic cell necrosis, to manage pruritis and ascites, and to treat encephalopathy and cholelithiasis is reviewed in this chapter.

MEDICATIONS TO TREAT HEPATIC CELL NECROSIS

Hepatic cell necrosis can occur secondary to the ingestion of many drugs and poisons. The most common hepatotoxic agent is acetaminophen (large doses). The cytochrome P-450 mixed-function oxidase system, shown in Figure 53–1, normally processes minor amounts of acetaminophen into reactive metabolites that are normally bound to *glutathione* (a tripeptide that normally carries oxygen to the liver and is fundamental for cellular respirations). When large doses of acetaminophen (Tylenol)

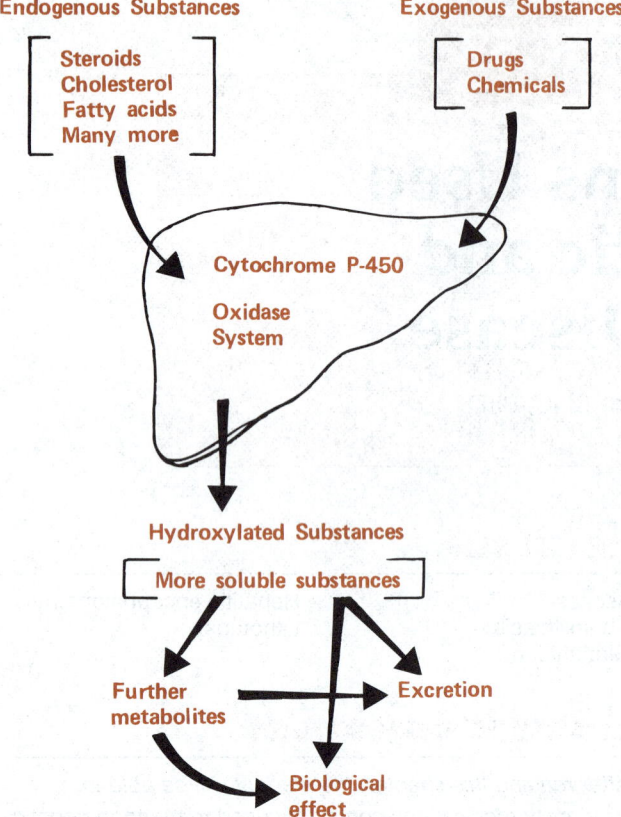

Figure 53–1. The action of cytochrome P-450 in the oxidase system of the liver. Both endogenous and exogenous substances are biotransformed with the help of cytochrome P-450.

are ingested, glutathione is depleted. This allows the active metabolites of acetaminophen to accumulate and bind to hepatocellular proteins, which results in cell death.

It is important to obtain the time and amount of acetaminophen that was ingested. If more than 7.5 g or 140 mg/kg was ingested, it is important to begin prophylactic antidotal therapy with N-acetylcysteine (Mucomyst). N-acetylcysteine is a mucolytic agent that provides additional glutathione and thereby prevents cell injury and necrosis. It is described in Chapter 40.

MEDICATIONS TO MANAGE PRURITUS

Pruritus, often associated with biliary disease, is due to the accumulation of bile salts in the skin. The pruritus associated with hepatic disease can often be alleviated by prolonged administration of the ion-exchange resin **cholestyramine (Questran)**.

○ **Cholestyramine** (Questran) acts by adsorbing and combining with intestinal bile salts to form an insoluble, nonabsorbable complex, which is then excreted in the feces, thus preventing intestinal reabsorption. Since bile salts are excreted, the amount of bile acids deposited in the skin decreases and the pruritus is lessened. The effects

of this medication take place 1 to 3 weeks after initiation of therapy. Continued treatment can control pruritus for years. If the medication is discontinued, pruritus returns in 1 to 2 weeks. Cholestyramine is discussed in detail in Chapter 33.

MEDICATIONS TO MANAGE ASCITES

Ascites (an abnormal collection of fluid in the abdominal cavity) associated with liver disease is due to several factors: increased capillary permeability, portal hypertension, hypoproteinemia due to decreased albumin production in the liver, and sodium retention and hypervolemia secondary to increased aldosterone production. Ascites is a serious complication in patients with cirrhosis, because it indicates that more than 75% of normal liver function has been lost. Maintenance of normal nutrition is compromised due to early satiety. Respiratory function is also compromised by the elevation of the diaphragm. In addition, the presence of fluid within the peritoneal cavity continuously exposes the patient to the possibility of bacterial infection and peritonitis.

Ascites can be lessened through the administration of diuretics or by surgical implantation of shunts. (See a medical surgical nursing text for further information.) Because there is increased aldosterone production and decreased metabolism in the liver, the aldosterone levels increase in the body and promote fluid retention. Therefore, diuretics that are aldosterone antagonists are often helpful in treatment. The drug of choice is **spironolactone (Aldactone)**. When spironolactone, in doses of 100 to 600 mg/day, is combined with a 10 to 20 mEq sodium diet, 70% to 80% of patients have a satisfactory diuresis. If spironolactone is not effective, thiazide diuretics are added. For more information on diuretics, see Chapter 37.

MEDICATIONS TO TREAT HEPATIC ENCEPHALOPATHY

The diagnosis of *hepatic encephalopathy* (abnormal function of the liver caused by the accumulation of toxic substances in patients with severe liver disease) is based on a number of clinical symptoms and laboratory studies. Symptoms range from personality changes, difficulty with mental performance, and confusion to frank coma. The goals of treatment of hepatic encephalopathy are to reverse precipitating or causative factors—including high-protein diet, gastrointestinal (GI) bleeding, infections, fluid and electrolyte balance, and drugs such as sedatives or narcotics—and to decrease the amount of ammonia and other toxins in the brain.

Ammonia is a key intermediate in the excretion of nitrogenous residues from the body. The major sites of ammonia production are the intestine and the kidney. Within the intestine, there are two major substrates for ammonia production: nitrogenous substances, including blood and dietary protein, and urea, which is converted by bacteria in the colon into ammonia. The kidney produces ammonia in the tubular cell by deamidization of glutamine. Ammonia (NH_3) combines with excess hydrogen ion in the renal tubule to form ammonium (NH_4), which is then excreted. The liver is the sole site for conversion of ammonia to urea. Reduced liver function and shunting of blood around the liver due to portal hypertension are the probable causes of ammonia intoxication. As ammonia levels rise, it is postulated that there is a diminished cerebral metabolism of ammonia in the brain (which normally removes small amounts of NH_3 from the blood) or that there is an accumulation of ''false neurotransmitters.'' Both of these hypotheses need to be proved through research and clinical investigation.

In treating hepatic encephalopathy, special enteral and parenteral diets are available (see Chapter 14). Pharmacologic treatment includes the administration of **neomycin (Mycifradin)** or other aminoglycosides, **lactulose (Cephulac)**, and **levodopa (Dopar, L-Dopa, Larodopa)**.

○ **Neomycin** (Mycifradin) is used to reduce the number of colonic bacteria that normally convert urea and amino acids into ammonia and other toxic metabolites. Other aminoglycosides such as kanamycin or paromomycin may also be used. These medications are capable of reaching high antibacterial concentrations in the colon without causing systemic toxicity.

When treating hepatic encephalopathy, neomycin is given only orally or via the nasogastric tube and only 1% to 3% of the dose is absorbed. In a person with normal renal function, this small amount of drug is easily excreted via the kidneys, so no toxicity occurs.

▼ **CLINICAL ALERT**

However, a patient with hepatic disease and resultant encephalopathy may have altered renal function due to the hepatorenal syndrome. The abnormally functioning liver suppresses kidney function through an unknown process. If the patient has altered renal function, the small amount of absorbed neomycin is not excreted and can accumulate. This can lead to further kidney damage. Whether neomycin is used in patients with impaired renal function depends on the treatment goals. Neomycin is discussed in more detail in Chapter 58.

○ **Lactulose** (Cephulac), a synthetic derivative of the sugar lactose, is classified as a nonosmotic cathartic. It is effective in reducing ammonia levels in most patients with portal-systemic encephalopathy, including those not helped by neomycin. Lactulose also improves protein tolerance in patients with advanced hepatic cirrhosis.

Lactulose is administered orally in the form of a syrup. It is not changed or absorbed and reaches the lower digestive tract intact, where the colonic bacterial enzymes convert it to lactic and acetic acids, which lower the colon's pH (from 7 to 5.5). This acidification of the colon's contents converts ammonia to ammonium ion and thus reduces the concentration of ammonia, allowing more ammonia to diffuse from the blood to the colon where the ammonium ion can then be evacuated in the feces. The laxative action of lactulose speeds this evacuation. Refer to Chapter 52 for additional information.

○ **Levodopa** (Dopar, L-Dopa, Larodopa) is given experimentally at this time for liver failure, but it is thought to improve brain function in hepatic encephalopathy. Levodopa is discussed in detail in Chapter 23.

MEDICATIONS TO TREAT CHOLELITHIASIS

Cholelithiasis (the presence of gallstones) affects approximately 10% of the general population in the United States and 20% of those over age 40. Peak occurrence is seen in obese females who are more than 40 years of age. The most common precipitating factors include overconsumption of cholesterol and calories, metabolic as well as genetic factors, inadequate exercise, and medications such as birth control pills. Patients generally complain of fat intolerance and experience nausea and vomiting, which eventually may be complicated with biliary colic and jaundice.

The major constituents of normal bile are water, various inorganic ions, bile salts, cholesterol, lecithin, and conjugated bilirubin. Cholesterol and lecithin are insoluble in water and are rendered soluble in bile water by the action of bile salts. The cholesterol found in bile has no known function. It is assumed to be a by-product of bile salt formation, and its presence is linked to the excretory function of bile. Many bile salt ions join with cholesterol and lecithin molecules to form water-solute complexes. Specific etiology is unknown, but a change in the nature of bile permits low-solubility bile components to precipitate out of the bile. As they do, they form small crystals on the gallbladder mucosal surface that gradually increase in size. Three substances usually precipitate to form gallstones: cholesterol, calcium salt of bilirubin (calcium bilirubinate), and calcium carbonate. Gallstones composed of cholesterol occur when the cholesterol content of the bile becomes greater in proportion to the bile salt and phospholipid content.

In many cases, the presence of stones in the gallbladder produces no symptoms; in fact, many are first discovered in x-ray films of the abdomen taken for reasons unrelated to their presence. The major complication of cholelithiasis is the movement of a stone into the duct system where it obstructs bile flow. Several techniques are available to treat gallstones: surgery, laparoscopic cholecystectomy, *lithotripsy* (the crushing of calculi by sound waves), and several drugs that dissolve gallstones. Regardless of the choice of therapy, patients are encouraged to return to their ideal body weight and consume a high-fiber diet.

Medications used to treat gallstones include **chenodiol (Chenix)**, **monoctanoin (Moctanin)**, and **ursodiol (Actigall)**, all featured in Table 53–1. These agents are used only in selected patients, depending on the components and size of the gallstones. Radiopaque or large calculi are relatively resistant to dissolution by bile acids, as are cholesterol stones containing more than 4% calcium. Some dissolution of stones occurs in 40% to 80% of patients

Table 53–1. GALLSTONE SOLUBILIZING AGENTS

DRUG NAME/ROUTE AND DOSAGE	PHARMACOKINETICS/ DYNAMICS	NURSING IMPLICATIONS
chenodiol (chenodeoxycholic acid) (Chenix)		
Adults: 250 mg PO bid for 2 wk, increased weekly by 250 mg until maximal tolerated dose is reached or dose of 13–16 mg/kg is achieved. **Children:** 15 mg/kg per day has been used although safety and efficacy have not been studied.	**Onset:** slow **Peak:** up to 24 mo **Duration:** NA **½L:** 16 min **PB:** 96% **B:** liver **E:** feces (80%)	**ASSESSMENT:** Assess baseline liver function studies and CBC and periodically during therapy. **INTERVENTION:** Chenodiol should be taken as directed **EVALUATION:** Contact physician if nonspecific abdominal pain and sudden RUQ pain, nausea, or vomiting occur (all associated with gallstone complications).
monoctanoin (Moctanin)		
Adults: 3–5 mL/hr into T-tube daily for 2–10 days.	**Onset:** NA **Peak:** NA **Duration:** NA **½L:** NA **PB:** NA **B:** NA **E:** NA	**ASSESSMENT:** Assess liver and gallbladder function. **INTERVENTION:** Warm to 70° to 80°F before perfusing into T-tube. Perfusion pressure should not exceed 15 cm. Water pump is needed to maintain pressure. **EVALUATION:** If no dissolution occurs in 72 hr, stop therapy. Report difficulty in breathing or severe abdominal pain to physician.
ursodiol (ursodeoxycholic acid) (Actigall) (Urso)		
Adults: 8–10 mg/kg per day PO in 2–3 divided doses with meals.	**Onset:** weeks to months **Peak:** up to 6–12 mo **Duration:** NA **½L:** NA **PB:** highly **B:** liver **E:** bile	**ASSESSMENT:** Assess baseline liver function and SGOT and SGPT. Follow stones by ultrasound q 6 mo. **INTERVENTION:** After complete dissolution of stones, continue for 1–3 mo. Stones may recur in 50% of patients within 5 yr. More common in patients with multiple stones originally. Separate dose by 2 hr from antacids. **EVALUATION:** Report nausea, vomiting, diarrhea, or rash to physician.

NA = not available; CBC = complete blood count; RUQ = right upper quadrant; SGPT = serum glutamate pyruvate transaminase.

within about 2 years. Although 25% to 75% of patients experience recurrences within 5 years, retreatment is usually successful.

O **Chenodiol** (chenodeoxycholic acid, Chenix) is a natural bile salt that decreases cholesterol saturation of bile by decreasing the secretion of cholesterol and perhaps by increasing the secretion of bile salts. Chenodiol is administered for 9 to 12 months. Adverse effects include diarrhea and possible hepatotoxicity from its breakdown products.

O **Monoctanoin** (Moctanin) is a semisynthetic esterified glycerol (vegetable oil) that can be used when stones of calcium bilirubinate and calcium soaps are resistant to dissolution by oral chenodiol. Monoctanoin is administered through a T-tube, nasobiliary catheter, or percutaneous transhepatic catheter. It is considered a contact solvent and is effective only when it is in contact with the stone. Monoctanoin is generally well tolerated if the administration rate is slow (3 to 5 mL per hour). Monoctanoin is continued for 7 to 21 days with diagnostic studies such as T-tube cholangiograms taken every 3 to 4 days to assess the process of dissolution. If the number or size of the stones has not changed in 7 days, treatment is discontinued. The major adverse effects include diarrhea, nausea, and abdominal pain.

O **Ursodiol** (ursodeoxycholic acid, Urso, Actigall) is a naturally occurring bile salt. It suppresses hepatic synthesis and secretion of cholesterol and inhibits intestinal absorption of cholesterol. After repeated dosing steady state is achieved in 3 weeks. Gallstone dissolution with ursodiol requires months of therapy. Ultrasound images of the gall bladder are obtained within 6 months. If partial stone dissolution has not occurred within 12 months, the likelihood of success is greatly reduced.

Urso is also effective when used as treatment for primary biliary cirrhosis characterized by portal inflammation and necrosis of biliary cells resulting in destruction of bile ducts and progressive cholestasis. Patients receiving ultrasound have clear improvement in terms of severity of pruritis, biochemical indicators of hepatitic and immune function, and most histologic features.

USING THE NURSING PROCESS

ASSESSMENT

• Obtain a complete nursing history from the patient or the family. Typical items to be included are fea-

Table 53–2. NURSING PROCESS IN HEPATIC DISEASE

Assessment

Assess history of current illness, medication use (prescription, over-the-counter, alcohol/street drugs).
Assess respiratory status, noting increased respiratory rate, dyspnea.
Ascertain dietary patterns.
Assess exposure to hepatitis or household/commercial cleaning agents that might be hepatotoxic.
Assess laboratory studies, e.g., serum bilirubin, glucose, LDH, SGOT, albumin, total protein, ammonia levels.

Nursing Diagnosis: Excess Fluid Volume

RELATED TO: Compromised regulatory mechanism (e.g., syndrome of inappropriate diuretic hormone, decreased plasma proteins, malnutrition).
AS EVIDENCED BY: Edema/ascites, weight gain; intake greater than output, oliguria, changes in urine specific gravity, dyspnea, pleural effusion, elevated blood pressure.

Desired Outcomes/Evaluation Criteria

Demonstrates appropriate fluid volume with balanced intake and output, stable weight, vital signs within patient's normal range, and absence of edema.

Nursing Actions

Administer diuretics (e.g., spironolactone), potassium, positive inotropic drugs and arterial vasodilators.

Measure intake/output, noting positive balance (intake in excess of output).
Weigh daily and note gain greater than 0.5 kg/day.
Inspect dependent tissues routinely. Measure abdominal girth as indicated.
Monitor blood pressure and central venous pressure. Note jugular/abdominal vein distention.
Auscultate lungs, noting diminished or absent breath sounds and developing adventitious sounds.

Rationale

Used to control edema and ascites, block effects of aldosterone and increase water excretion while sparing potassium.
Serum and cellular potassium are usually depleted because of liver disease as well as urinary losses.
Given to increase cardiac output/improve renal blood flow and function, promoting reduction of fluid volume.
Reflects circulating volume status, developing/resolution of fluid shifts, and response to therapy. Positive balance/weight gain reflect continuing fluid retention.

Useful in monitoring development/resolution of edema/ascites.

Blood pressure elevations are usually associated with excess in circulating volume, but may occur because of fluid shifts out of the vascular space.

Indicative of pulmonary congestion/edema, which may result in consolidation, impaired gas exchange, and respiratory distress.

Nursing Diagnosis: Altered Nutrition, Less Than Body Requirements

RELATED TO: Inadequate diet; inability to process/digest nutrients, anorexia, nausea, abnormal bowel function.
AS EVIDENCED BY: Weight loss, changes in bowel sounds, abdominal cramping, aversion to eating/lack of interest in food.

Desired Outcomes/Evaluation Criteria

Demonstrates increased muscle mass/progressive weight gain toward goal with normalization of laboratory values and free of signs of malnutrition.

Nursing Actions

Record daily intake by calorie count.
Assist and encourage patient to eat; explain reasons for type of diet. Consider individual food preferences in food choices.
Provide mouth care frequently and prior to meals.
Weigh as indicated. Compare changes in fluid status, recent weight history, triceps skin measurement.
Recommend cessation of smoking, as appropriate.
Consult with dietician as indicated.

Rationale

Provides information about intake needs/deficiencies.
Proper diet is vital to recovery. May eat better when preferred foods are included.

Patient is prone to sore and/or bleeding gums and bad taste in mouth, which adds to anorexia.
It may be difficult to use weight as a direct indicator of nutritional status in view of edema/ascites. Triceps skinfold measurement is useful in assessing changes in muscle mass and subcutaneous fat reserves.
Reduces excessive gastric stimulation and risk of irritation/bleeding.

Useful in determining individual needs.

Other Suggested Nursing Diagnoses: Knowledge Deficit and Altered Thought Processes.

tured in Table 53–2. The patient's recent use of cleaning agents such as oven cleaners, toilet cleaners, or commercial cleaners is determined; hepatic injury has been known to occur from the mixing of several commercial cleaners together and from breathing vapors of any or all of them in a poorly ventilated area for a prolonged period. If, as is often the case, an interaction of medications has precipitated the hepatic injury, the causative medication may not be identified when hepatic injury is first diagnosed. Therefore, all medications are stopped immediately while supportive care is instituted. Selected medications that can

Table 53–3. SELECTED MEDICATIONS ADVERSELY AFFECTING THE LIVER

Anesthetics
Halothane

Anti-Inflammatory and Anti-Muscle Spasm Agents
Allopurinol
Colchicine
Gold salts*
Indomethacin*
Phenylbutazone*
Probenecid*

Antimicrobials
Antifungal agents
Chloramphenicol
Erythromycin estolate* (occurs most frequently with estolate, but all salts and bases have been implicated)
Griseofulvin
Isoniazid (INH)
Pyrazinamide (PZA)
Rifampin
Streptomycin
Sulfonamides*
Tetracyclines, IV

Antineoplastics
Azathioprine*
Chlorambucil*
L-Asparaginase†
Mercaptopurine (6-MP)
Methotrexate
Nitrogen mustard

Cardiac Drugs
Chlorothiazide
Methyldopa (Aldomet)
Procainamide (Pronestyl)
Propranolol (Inderal)
Quinidine

Hormones—Derivatives
Contraceptives, oral
Oral hypoglycemics

Tranquilizers, Hypnotics, Pain Medications
Acetaminophen—only when ingested in large amounts
Benzodiazepine derivatives
Phenobarbital
Phenothiazines
Salicylates
Tricyclics

The medications listed in this table have been identified as possibly affecting adversely the functions of or being directly toxic to the liver. The medications marked with an asterisk (*) may affect the liver in some persons through an idiosyncratic reaction that is not entirely understood. The medications marked with a dagger (†) cause liver toxicity in many patients, and persons receiving these preparations must be watched very closely. The nurse must also remember that when the patient has hepatic disease, medications normally biotransformed by the liver will need the dosage modified or the patient will develop toxic effects.

adversely affect liver function are featured in Table 53–3.

- Obtain specimens for laboratory tests as ordered, including lactate dehydrogenase (LDH) and serum glutamic-oxaloacetic transaminase (SGOT), to assess he-

patocellular damage and other laboratory tests to assess liver function. A serum bilirubin (indirect and direct) test is often used in cases of jaundice to determine the presence of an elevated serum bilirubin.

- Assess medication intake. Whenever a patient has any hepatic problem—cirrhosis, hepatitis, or chronic alcoholism—be very alert to the medications prescribed for and administered to the patient. Any medication that is biotransformed in the liver to inactive metabolites is given at lower dosage levels or is withheld altogether.
- Assess the patient for toxic drug effects and report them as soon as they are suspected. Table 53–4 identifies drugs normally excreted by the liver.
- Assess all current symptoms and how they have changed over time such as intolerance to fatty meals,

Table 53–4. SELECTED MEDICATIONS EXCRETED BY THE LIVER

Medication	Site of Excretion*
Antibiotics	
Ampicillin	Renal (hepatic)
Carbenicillin	Renal (hepatic)
Methicillin	Renal (hepatic)
Nafcillin	Hepatic
Oxacillin	Renal (hepatic)
Penicillin	Renal (hepatic)
Tetracycline	Renal (hepatic)
Doxycycline	Renal (hepatic)
Minocycline	Hepatic
Erythromycin	Hepatic
Lincomycin	Hepatic (renal)
Analgesics (Non-Narcotic)	
Acetaminophen (Tylenol)	Hepatic
Acetylsalicylic acid	Renal (hepatic)
Narcotics and Narcotic Antagonists	
Codeine	Hepatic (renal)
Morphine	Hepatic (renal, GI)
Naloxone (Narcan)	Hepatic
Pentazocine (Talwin)	Hepatic (renal)
Central Nervous System Drugs	
BARBITURATES	
Phenobarbital	Hepatic (renal)
Secobarbital	Hepatic
BENZODIAZEPINES	
Diazepam (Valium)	Hepatic (renal, GI)
Haloperidol	Hepatic (renal, GI)
PHENOTHIAZINES	
Chlorpromazine	Hepatic
Cardiovascular Drugs	
ANTIARRHYTHMIC AGENTS	
Lidocaine	Hepatic (renal)
Procainamide	Renal (hepatic)
Propranolol	Hepatic
ANTIHYPERTENSIVE AGENTS	
Hydralazine	Hepatic (renal, GI)
Methyldopa	Renal (hepatic)
DIURETICS	
Ethacrynic acid	Hepatic

Selected medications only; not a complete list.
*First organ is primary organ of excretion. Organ in parentheses is secondary organ of excretion.

change in stool or skin color, or itching. Symptoms of the current condition are assessed, and they are then treated during the intervention phase.

NURSING DIAGNOSIS

- Develop the nursing diagnoses. Typical nursing diagnoses for patients with hepatic and/or biliary disease include Fluid Volume Excess, Altered Nutrition, Altered Thought Processes, and Knowledge Deficit (Table 53–2).

PLANNING AND INTERVENTION

- Determine the goals of nursing intervention, which are included in Table 53–2. Patients with hepatic or biliary diseases are managed with a diet usually high in proteins, carbohydrates, and vitamins. However, a patient in hepatic coma would have a reduced-protein diet to help eliminate the ammonia from the body. Numerous specialized nutritional products, such as Hepatic Aid and HepatAmine, are available. These are discussed in Chapter 14.
- Monitor fluid and electrolyte balance carefully, particularly in the patient with vomiting or diarrhea.

Hepatotoxicity from Other Drugs

- If hepatotoxicity is found to be drug induced, typical nursing goals might include (1) identification of the causative agent if possible and (2) education of the patient to discourage further exposure to or ingestion of the causative agent or a chemically similar agent.
- During the acute phase, all previous medications are stopped and only supportive therapy, such as corticosteroids or exchange transfusions, is used. Both therapies are still controversial but should not be omitted. A few days could be crucial to any patient this acutely ill. Constant nursing supervision includes close monitoring of all body systems, including the neurologic, cardiovascular, renal, respiratory, and GI systems. Any change in these systems signals the need for immediate interventions to prevent further deterioration of the patient's condition.

- Treatment of a patient with drug-induced hepatotoxicity is managed similarly to that of a patient in hepatic coma. If the causative agent or agents have been identified, the patient and family must be educated about the danger of further use of it or similar drugs.

EVALUATION

- Evaluate every nursing intervention to determine if the goals are being achieved. The goals of nursing intervention become the outcome criteria for evaluation (see Table 53–2).
- Evaluate liver function studies to monitor progress. If it becomes necessary to administer supportive medications to the patient during the acute phase, these medications are evaluated closely to prevent further hepatic toxicity. Some drugs remain active until they are biotransformed by the liver's microsomal system; if this system is injured, the medications remain active longer and result in the development of adverse effects or toxic effects. All medications being administered to the patient are reviewed closely to determine if they cause more hepatic damage. When possible, medications that are totally excreted by the kidney are used.
- Evaluate to determine whether the medications being administered are effective. If the medication is ineffective, or adverse or toxic effects are being experienced, the medication is discontinued. Often, patients are discharged from the acute care setting on medications to control chronic symptoms. Patient compliance and knowledge level are evaluated. Adequate knowledge about the disease condition and medications often helps patients comply with their medical and nursing regimen.
- Evaluate symptoms of jaundice, pruritus, hypoprothrombinemia, ascites, and vitamin and iron deficiencies to determine if they are being brought under control. The treatment regimen is then modified as necessary.

The bibliography for this chapter can be found in Appendix B, which begins on page 1054.

CHAPTER REVIEW QUESTIONS*

1. The antidotal therapy for acetaminophen overdose is:
   a. Naloxone (Narcan).
   b. Protamine sulfate.
   c. Vitamin K.
   d. N-acetylcysteine (Mucomyst).

2. Which of the following drugs is an aldosterone antagonist, useful in the management of ascites?
   a. Spironolactone (Aldactone).
   b. Furosemide (Lasix).
   c. Acetazolamide (Diamox).
   d. Ethacrynic acid (Edecrin).

3. Which of the following agents improves protein tolerance in patients with advanced hepatic cirrhosis?
   a. Vitamin K.
   b. Furosemide (Lasix).
   c. Lactulose (Cephulac).
   d. Folic acid.

4. Adverse effects associated with chenodiol (chenodeoxycholic acid) include:
   a. Muscle tremors.
   b. Photosensitivity.
   c. Diarrhea.
   d. Urinary retention.

*See Appendix A, which begins on page 1051, for answers.

UNIT 14

DRUGS AFFECTING THE IMMUNE SYSTEM

UNIT OUTLINE

CHAPTER 54

Overview of the Anatomy and Physiology of the Immune System

Brenda K. Shelton, MS, RN, CCRN, OCN

CHAPTER OUTLINE

KEY TERMS

Allergy
Antigen
Antibodies
Barrier immunity
Bone marrow
Cell-mediated immunity
Chemotactins
Complement
Cross-reaction
Cytokines
Granulocytes
Humoral immunity
Immune competence
Immunity

Immunodeficiency
Immunoglobulins
Inflammation
Leukocytosis
Lymphatic system
Lymphocytes
Macrophage
Monocytes
Neutropenia
Nonspecific immune system
Phagocytic immune
  response
Specific immune response

LEARNING OBJECTIVES

After reading this chapter, the student will be able to:

1. Outline the anatomic structure and physiology of the five immune subsystems of the body.
2. Describe the pathophysiology of granulocyte and lymphocyte deficiencies.

The immune system performs many important integrative functions in assisting the body to recognize and destroy possible foreign substances. In other words, it is responsible for providing *immunity* (the state of being protected against disease). An understanding of the normal physiology and resulting pathophysiology of deficiency or dysfunction in this system assists nurses in identifying and managing individual patient responses to immunologic disorders.

OVERVIEW OF THE IMMUNE SYSTEM

The human immune system is analogous to a "border patrol" for the body. It monitors areas with access to the external environment and destroys potential invading pathogens. The general functions of the immune system are defense, homeostasis, and surveillance. The system is divided into two distinct processes: the nonspecific and

Table 54-1. IMMUNE SYSTEMS OF THE BODY

Component Systems

Barrier immunity (body secretions)
Phagocytic immunity (neutrophils)
Inflammation (complement)
Humoral immunity (B lymphocytes)
Cell-mediated immunity (T lymphocytes)

Characteristics of Components
  General recognition
  Same response to different substances
  No diversity
  No memory
  Selective recognition
  Diverse responses to different substances
  Heterogeneity (a variety of cells and products)
  Memory

Source: Adapted from Allen, MA: Hematology anatomy and physiology. In Wright, J, and Shelton, BK (eds): Desk Reference for Certified Critical Care Nursing Practice. Jones and Bartlett Publishers, Boston, 1993, p 1092. Reprinted with permission.

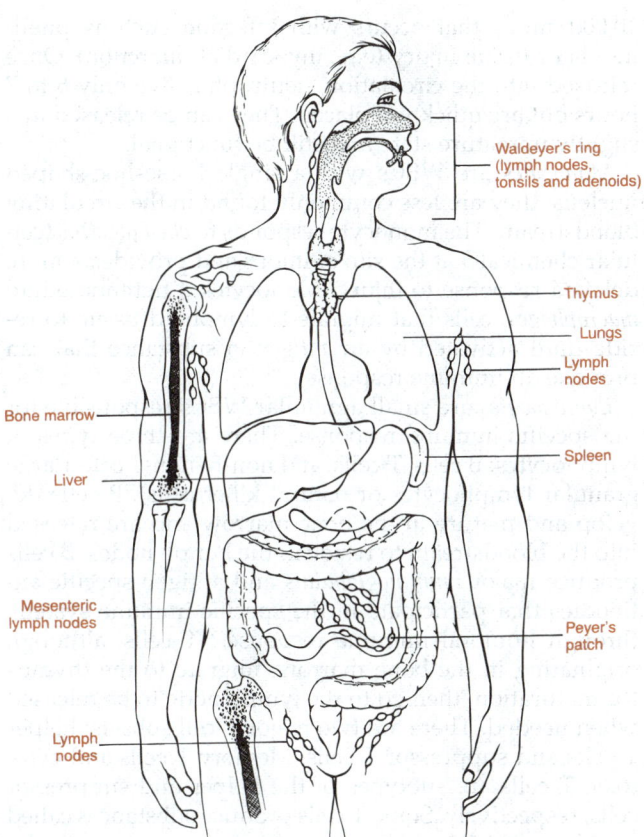

Figure 54-1. The major human lymphoid organs and tissues.

specific immune responses. Within these two categories are subsystems working together to mediate body responses to pathogens: barrier immunity, inflammation, phagocytic immunity, humoral immunity, and cellular immunity, as listed in Table 54-1. These immunologic subsystems are based in hematopoietic tissues, but operate throughout the body and are considered the anatomic immune structures.

The *immune competence* of individuals is based on the intactness and functional ability of the immunologic systems. Underfunctioning or suppression of the immune system by immunosuppressive medications or disease states (e.g., renal failure, hepatic failure, diabetes mellitus) leads to different types of *immunodeficiency* the loss of immune function which has previously been intact. Overfunctioning of the immune system may result in autoimmune disease or atopy (a type of hypersensitivity or allergic reactions). Many internal and external factors contribute to an individual's immune competence. These include age, nutritional status, breaks in the body's external barriers, stress, disease states, and medications. When assessing patients with possible immune disorders, it is important to assess intactness of both the anatomic structures and their immunologic activity.

ANATOMY OF THE IMMUNE SYSTEM

IMMUNE STRUCTURE

The most important structure for the origination and function of the immune system is the *bone marrow,* the hematopoietic organ where all blood cells are produced. Some blood cells are immediately released into the circulation to perform immunologic functions, whereas others rely on the lymphatic system to assist them. The *lym-*

phatic system includes more than 200 lymph nodes scattered throughout the body, lymphatic plexes joining the nodes, and lymph fluid flowing through the lymphatic structures. Immunologic activity also occurs in lymphoid tissues and organs, including the spleen, liver, thymus gland, gastrointestinal (GI) tract, and lungs, as depicted in Figure 54-1. Nonlymphoid body systems such as the microglia of the brain also have cells that express immunologic properties. The core of immune function is carried by immunocompetent cells located in all of these anatomic structures.

IMMUNOCOMPETENT CELLS

The functional units of the immunologic system are the white blood cells (WBCs) and the hematopoietic tissues in which they reside. There are three major immunocompetent cells: granulocytes, monocytes, and lymphocytes. Each of these types of WBCs performs specific functions that then work together to produce an integrated response. All blood cells originate in the red bone marrow of the long bones and axial skeleton.

Granulocytes are multigranulated WBCs produced and stored in the bone marrow to be released in the presence of infection, inflammation, or tissue necrosis. The three subtypes of granulocytes are neutrophils, eosinophils, and basophils. The most prevalent and active is the neutrophil. Rapid proliferation of these cells is apparent in the brisk *leukocytosis* (total WBC elevation greater than

10,000/mm³) that occurs with infection such as pneumonia or tissue injury (e.g., myocardial infarction). Once released into the circulation, neutrophils live only 6 to 7 hours but are quickly replaced. They can be released in a slightly immature state and still be functional.

Monocytes are WBCs with a single horseshoe-shaped nucleus; they are less commonly found in the circulating bloodstream. The monocyte responds to *chemotactins* (cellular chemicals) at the site of injury and provides a more delayed response to injury. Monocytes differentiate into *macrophages*, cells that migrate to lymphoid tissue to reside until activated by an *antigen* (a substance that can provoke an immune response).

Lymphocytes are small agranular WBCs responsible for the specific immune response. There are three types of lymphocytes: B cells, T cells, and non-B–non-T cells (large granular lymphocytes or natural killer cells). B cells develop and mature in the bone marrow and are released into the bloodstream to reside in the lymph nodes. B cells produce major *immunoglobulins* and antigen-specific antibodies that participate in the specific immune system, through humoral immune responses. T cells, although originating in the bone marrow, migrate to the thymus for maturation, then go to the lymph node to be released when needed. There are two major T-cell subsets: helper T cells and suppressor T cells. Memory T cells and cytotoxic T cells are subtypes of the helper and suppressor cells, respectively. Some T cells produce substances called *cytokines*, which produce a specific immune response by recognizing foreign or mutant cells and activating other leukocytes. The T cells are responsible for immune surveillance in the body, called the cellular immune response. Atypical, large granular lymphocytes (natural killer cells) are thought to have a major role in combating cancer; however, their precise cause, production, and mechanism of action is unknown.

The anatomic structures of the immune system work together to provide comprehensive protection against misplaced endogenous antigens, exogenous pathogens, and mutant cells. The methods by which these components function independently and work together constitute the physiology of the immune system.

PHYSIOLOGY OF THE IMMUNE SYSTEM

When the immunologic system is functional, all substances entering the body first filter through the lymphatic channels and local lymph nodes to detect foreign antigens. The antigen activates the lymphocytes within the nodes, producing inflammatory lymph node enlargement and tenderness.

External substances are carried by the lymphatics to the spleen, where they must flow by macrophage-lined channels before reaching the systemic circulation. The spleen recognizes and removes foreign or abnormal proteins, whether they are bacteria or dysfunctional and old red blood cells. Splenic disease such as occurs in splenic in-

Table 54–2. IMMUNOGLOBULINS

IgG. The major immunoglobulin in the blood, IgG constitutes about 75% of the serum immunoglobulin fraction. It is also found in extravascular fluids: lymph, cerebrospinal fluid, synovial fluid, and peritoneal fluid.

IgG is the second immunoglobulin (after IgM) to respond to an antigen in a primary immune response, but it is the major immunoglobulin to respond after reexposure to the antigen (secondary, anamnestic antibody response). After IgG combines with an antigen, the immunoglobulin's Fc portion (stem of the IgG monomer) can bind to the first component of the classical complement pathway; this activates the complement cascade, by which the humoral immune response takes place.

IgM. Found mainly in the blood, IgM constitutes about 10% of the serum immunoglobulin fraction. IgM is the first immunoglobulin to respond to an antigen and the major antibody involved in the primary immune response. It functions like IgG but activates the complement system more effectively, triggering the complement cascade by binding with viral and bacterial antigens.

IgA. This immunoglobulin exists in two types: serum IgA and secretory IgA. Serum IgA accounts for about 10%–15% of the serum immunoglobulin fraction. Secretory IgA, the predominant form, is concentrated in the exocrine secretions, such as colostrum, milk, tears, sweat, and saliva, and in other respiratory, gastrointestinal, and urogenital secretions. At these potential antigen entry sites, it provides specific antibody protection against pathogens.

IgD. This immunoglobulin makes up less than 1% of the serum immunoglobulin fraction. Found on the surface of B cells, it may play a role in their differentiation.

IgE. This immunoglobulin is normally present in only trace amounts. Elevated levels usually appear in allergic disorders and certain parasitic infections. Most IgE-producing cells exist in the respiratory and intestinal mucosa. IgE functions mainly in allergic reactions. When two or more IgE molecules bind to an allergen, mast cells or basophils release histamine, kinins, serotonin, leukotrienes, and neutrophil chemotactic factor. These chemical mediators, in turn, produce the characteristic wheal-and-flare allergic skin reaction, allergic (extrinsic) asthma, and allergic seasonal rhinitis (hay fever).

Source: Used with permission from Hematologic Problems/ Nurse Review, 1990, © Springhouse Corporation.

farction with sickle cell anemia leads to reduced ability to recognize these antigens, particularly those that are disguised by coverings such as the encapsulated tubercular bacteria. The splenic macrophages also participate in the production of the body's major immunoglobulins—IgA, IgD, IgE, IgG, and IgM—responsible for combating common antigens. Table 54–2 features these immunoglobulins. When the spleen is removed or dysfunctional, the liver performs the spleen's normal activities, although less efficiently.

Ingested antigens are normally recognized and destroyed by the macrophages located in the Peyer's patches of the small intestine. If they pass into the systemic circulation, the portal vessels carry them into the liver where Kupffer's cells (liver macrophages) line the sinusoids and remove the antigens. The liver macrophages are also able to produce immunoglobulins.

NONSPECIFIC IMMUNITY

The body is unable to develop specific immunity against all possible antigens, thus the nonspecific immune responses are essential as well. Barrier, phagocytic, and complement immunity form the *nonspecific immune system*, which acts against all foreign proteins in a general cytotoxic manner. These three subsystems are present and functional at birth.

Barrier Immunity

Barrier immunity includes the physical, chemical, mechanical, and microbial barriers that are the first line of protection against the entry of pathogens. All orifices of the body are lined with protective epithelial linings and secretions that provide barriers against bacterial growth. When these barriers are invaded, such as with catheters or vascular access devices, there is potential for microorganisms to enter the opening. The barriers may still prevent the organisms from proliferating or disseminating. For instance, enteric flora that line the GI tract combat exogenous microorganisms, and the acidic pH of the urine inhibits microbial growth. Many therapies performed alter these barriers and expose individuals to pathogenic organism growth. For example, systemic antibiotics destroy the normal flora of the GI, genitourinary, and vaginal areas; alter the pH of oral secretions; and may slow the activity of WBCs, resulting in superinfection with fungi.

Inflammation

If the barrier defenses are breached, organisms can proliferate and destroy normal tissue. This stimulates the body's inflammatory response. *Inflammation* dilutes the pathogens and stimulates the activation of WBCs that destroy the organism or limit the spread of disease. The signs and symptoms of inflammation are edema, erythema, and warmth. Inflammatory responses can be localized and self-limiting or widespread. Other constitutional symptoms of inflammation may include malaise, fatigue, anorexia, weight loss, and lymphadenopathy.

Phagocytic Immunity

Phagocytic Immune Response When microorganisms overcome the barrier defenses of the body, the *phagocytic immune response* is stimulated. Phagocytes are specialized WBCs that destroy foreign particles by engulfment. Bacteria, because they do not contain protective envelopes, are the most susceptible to phagocytic destruction. Both neutrophils and monocytes/macrophages have phagocytic potential. Neutrophils are more likely to act within the bloodstream, and monocytes/macrophages perform their phagocytic activity within the lymphoid tissues. When infection or inflammation occurs, chemicals released at the site of injury attract phagocytes. Phagocytes line the damaged endothelium in a formation called pavementing, which walls off the infection, preventing its spread.

The combination of inflammation and phagocytic immunity produce the inflammatory-immune response. The inflammatory-immune response, depicted in Figure 54–2, begins with vasodilation and capillary permeability as seen with inflammation. The phagocytic response generates many white cell mediators such as bradykinin, histamine, and leukotrienes. These enhance vasodilation, capillary permeability, and clotting. Under normal circumstances, antibody production destroys the pathogens

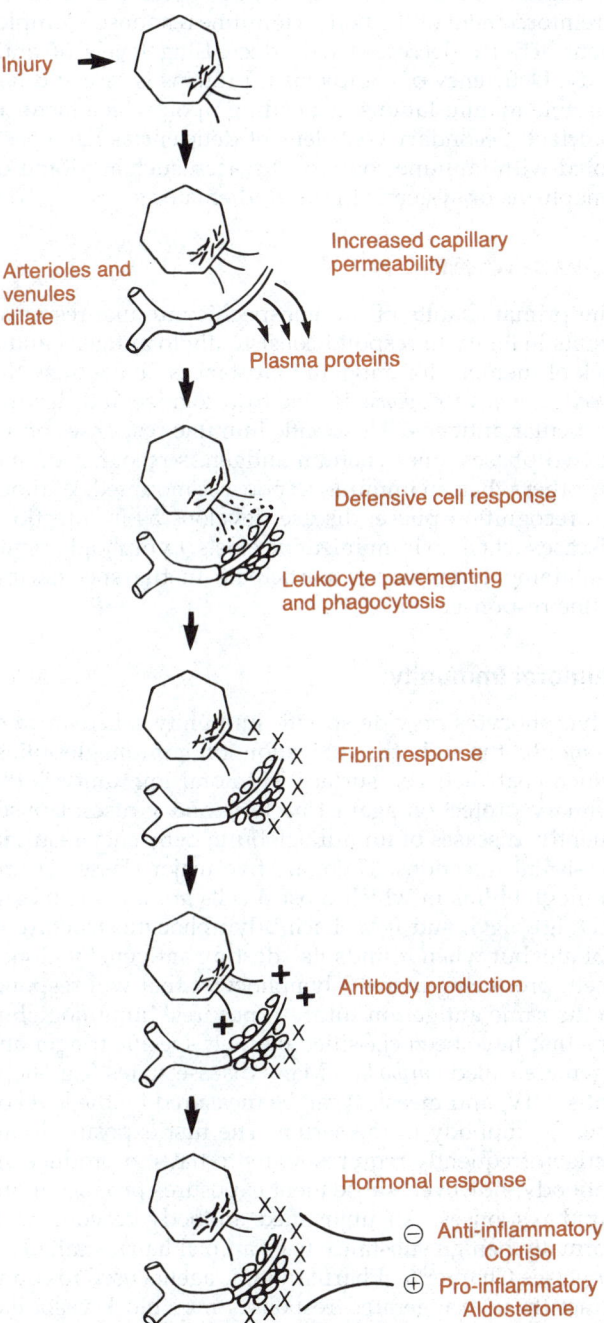

Figure 54–2. The inflammatory-immune reaction is stimulated by injury or infection. The states of this response are always the same; however, the intensity of individual reactions varies from one situation to another, even within the same individual.

and the hormonal phase notes the destruction of the antigen, suppressing the inflammatory reaction. However, inflammatory reactions can become uncontrolled even in the absence of an offending organism, producing disorders such as endometriosis, peritonitis, adult respiratory distress syndrome, or septic shock. Anti-inflammatory medications are used to block this response.

Complement Component *Complement* is a group of over 30 glycoproteins in the serum and on cell surfaces that mediate the inflammatory-immune response. Complement is synthesized by macrophages and circulates in a nonactive state. When activated, complement serves as a reinforcement of the body's immune response. Complement activity decreases with decreasing levels of antibody. Deficiency of complement proteins is rare and has variable manifestations, depending upon which factor is deficient. Secondary complement deficiencies have been noted with immune complex diseases, such as glomerulonephritis or systemic lupus erythematosis.

SPECIFIC IMMUNITY

The primary faults of the nonspecific immune response are its inability to respond consistently to antigens and a lack of memory for antigenic substances. In contrast, the *specific immune response* is able to recognize and destroy particular antigens. All specific immune responses occur in two phases: one when an antigen is recognized, and the other when an immune response is mounted. Without the recognition phase, disease develops as in infectious diseases when no immunization exists. Lymphoid organs containing lymphocytes participate in the specific immune response.

Humoral Immunity

B lymphocytes provide specific immunity called *humoral immunity* through the activation of immunoglobulins, which coat their cell surface. Humoral immunity is the primary protection against bacteria and viruses. Consequently, diseases of immunoglobulin deficiency result in persistent infections. There are five major classes of immunoglobulins in which most B cells are included: IgA, IgD, IgE, IgG, and IgM. Each B lymphocyte structure is unique, but when it finds its "destiny antigen," it clones itself, producing many B lymphocytes that will respond to the same antigen in future exposures. Immunoglobulins that have been classified by their specific trigger antigen are called *antibodies*. Many disease states (e.g., hepatitis, HIV, and measles) can be measured by the level of specific antibody in the serum. The first exposure to an antigen frequently requires hours to days to produce an antibody; however, subsequent exposures produce more rapid responses. An unjustified antibody reaction to a normally benign substance (e.g., animal hair) is called *allergy* (see Chapter 6). Pharmacologic agents used to counteract these exaggerated responses may block vasodilators such as histamine, suppress all inflammatory reactions, or simply treat the physiologic effects of immune reaction.

The tendency for reactivity of substances entering the body depends on several factors. Substances must be large enough to have a complex foreign chemical makeup. Direct systemic routes of entry, large doses of antigen, complex antigen configuration, and accessible receptor sites increase the possibility that a substance will cause a reaction. Certain pathogens resemble normal cells and produce body reactions against themselves. This is called *cross-reaction*. An example of this is the propensity for streptococcus infections to strike myocardial cells, causing rheumatic fever.

Cellular Immunity

Cell-mediated immunity provides protection against infections from intracellular organisms such as viruses, fungi, and protozoa. This form of immunity is mediated by the T lymphocyte and is the primary immune response involved in allograft rejection and the recognition and killing of malignant cells. The immunity conferred by the T cell is thought to last for months to years.

The T cell is considered the conductor of the orchestrated immune response because of its ability to direct other immunocompetent cells. The T lymphocyte has surface receptors (TCRs) that are activated by antigenic substances. When activated, they release substances called cytokines, which effect the action of granulocytes, monocytes, and B lymphocytes. Cytokines released by T cells have been genetically engineered and are now given to patients with cancer to produce WBC growth or an antitumor response. Such cytokines include interferon, interleukin, and colony-stimulating factor (see Chapter 56). The T-cell subsets have identifying surface markers labeled by letters and numbers (i.e., CD4, CD8). The major subtypes of T cells are the T4 (CD4) helper cells and T8 (CD8) suppressor cells. Cellular immunity provides the final monitoring mechanism for invading microorganisms.

LEUKOCYTES AND DISEASE

When pathogens escape recognition and destruction by all of the body's immune systems, infection results. As mentioned earlier, immunodeficiency describes the loss of immune function that has previously been intact. Immunodeficient patients, although at immense risk of infection, do not always have clinical infection. The primary clinical manifestations of deficiency or dysfunction of any of the components of these immune systems are the specific infections that can no longer be counteracted.

The invasion of microorganisms may present as either localized or systemic infection. *Neutropenia* (neutrophil count less than $2500/mm^3$) is a significant side effect of chemotherapy regimens and the most common form of deficient immune function. The absence of neutrophils reduces the body's ability to destroy pathogens or wall off the infection with fibrin, resulting in infections more likely to spread throughout the body, producing septicemia. This decreased ability to produce symptoms and increased propensity to dissemination leads to a high risk and rapid onset of bacterial sepsis.

LEUKOCYTOSIS AND INFECTION

Leukocytosis, excessive leukocytes in the circulating serum, has three major etiological factors: inflammation, infection, and tissue injury or necrosis. The inflammatory-immune response often clinically appears the same as infection and cannot be separated from infection without body cultures to prove the growth of a specific organism. In fact, in as many as 40% of all patients exhibiting septic shock, all body cultures remain negative. Unfortunately, uncontrolled infection, recurrent infection, or overactive inflammatory responses can lead to destruction of normal tissue by phagocytosis.

DEFICIENCY OF LYMPHOCYTES

Lymphocytes are responsible for the specific immune response—making antibodies against intracellular organisms or recognizing and destroying cancer cells. A deficiency of lymphocytes had been an unusual disorder until the advent of the current health problem of human immunodeficiency virus (HIV) infection and acquired immunodeficiency syndrome (AIDS). Outside of HIV infection, lymphocyte dysfunction has occurred with leukemia, Hodgkin's or non-Hodgkin's lymphoma, multiple myeloma, and in transplantation. Lymphocyte disorders are characterized by infection with viruses, intracellular bacteria, and opportunistic organisms.

When B lymphocytes are unable to produce immunoglobulin or produce abnormal immunoglobulin, there is an inability to recognize and respond to common antigens. Once again, an analogy can be made to the lack of border-patrolling police, resulting in increased immigration into the country: the inadequate number of "qualified" lymphocytes are unable to block the passage of resilient pathogens. This permits mutant cells to grow without control or microorganisms to colonize normal tissues, often incorporating their DNA into the host's cells.

HIV has the ability to incorporate itself into the RNA of normal T4 cells, causing replication of the viral DNA with cell multiplication. HIV's progressive occupation of the T4 cells causes decreased T4 counts and a propensity for opportunistic infections that are normally recognized and destroyed by T4 helper cells. Many of the infections associated with HIV are latent organisms residing in the body but not activated and prolific in immunocompetent individuals.

The T cell depends on the thymus for its development; the fact that the thymus atrophies and becomes dysfunctional with age lends support to the notion that cancer and opportunistic microorganisms (e.g., herpes zoster) are more common in the elderly.

The bibliography for this chapter can be found in Appendix B, which begins on page 1054.

CHAPTER REVIEW QUESTIONS*

1. T cells play the following role in the immune response:
   a. Producing antibody-like proteins
   b. Assisting B cells in antibody synthesis
   c. Producing specific antibodies
   d. Inhibiting the humoral response

2. In humans, B cells mature in the:
   a. Immature thymus gland
   b. Liver and pancreas
   c. Epiphyses of long bones
   d. Bone marrow

3. Barrier immunity of the body involves all *except:*
   a. Enteric flora
   b. Respiratory cilia
   c. Lymphocytic cytokines
   d. Acidity of the stomach

4. The most significant risk factor for sepsis is:
   a. Splenectomy
   b. Altered mucous membranes
   c. Leukocytosis
   d. Neutropenia

*See Appendix A, which begins on page 1051, for answers.

CHAPTER 55

Antineoplastic Chemotherapy

Anne Marie Moraca-Sawicki, RN, BSN, MSN

CHAPTER OUTLINE

KEY TERMS

Adjuvant chemotherapy
Alkylating agent
Alopecia
Anaplasia
Antimetabolites
Cachexia
Cell loss
Chemotherapy
Clonal cell
Doubling time
Growth fraction (GF)
Informed refusal
Intra-arterial chemotherapy
   (IAC)
Leukopenia
Metastasis
Mitotic index (MI)
Neoadjuvant therapy
Neoplasm
Pancytopenia
Stem cell theory
Stomatitis

LEARNING OBJECTIVES

After reading this chapter, the student will be able to:

1. Explain what differentiates the growth of a cancerous cell from that of a normal cell.
2. Identify the principles of antineoplastic chemotherapy.
3. Identify medications commonly used as antineoplastic agents.
4. Differentiate among the antineoplastic drugs as to mechanism of action, route of administration, absorption and rate, adverse effects, contraindications, and interactions.
5. Identify specific areas to assess in the patient requiring antineoplastic medications to formulate appropriate patient outcomes.
6. Plan the nursing interventions necessary to administer antineoplastic drugs and choose appropriate teaching strategies to enhance patient compliance.
7. Evaluate the patient at various stages of treatment to measure the effectiveness of nursing interventions.

Approximately 1 million new cases of cancer are diagnosed each year in the United States. About 500,000 cancer deaths occur per year, making cancer second only to cardiovascular disease as a major cause of death. In men, the lung is the most common cancer site. In women, the breast is the most common cancer site. One in nine women will be diagnosed with breast cancer. Figure 55–1 shows cancer incidence and death by site for both men and women.

INTRODUCTION TO CANCER AND ANTINEOPLASTIC CHEMOTHERAPY

The term *neoplasm* comes from the Greek words meaning "new formation" and means any new tissue growth benign or malignant where the growth is uncontrolled or progressive. Malignant neoplasms differ from benign neoplasms in that they generally show a greater degree

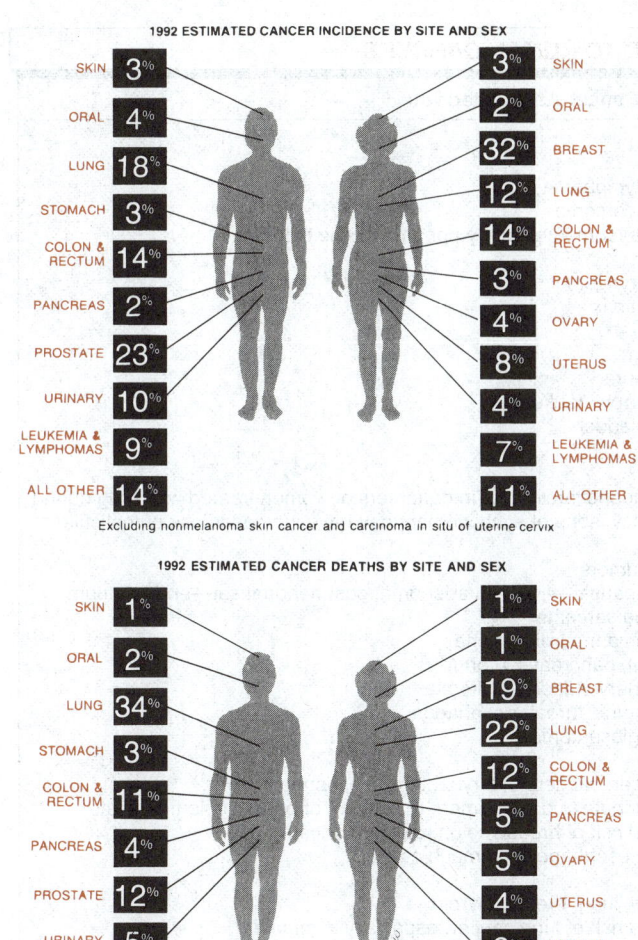

1992 ESTIMATED CANCER INCIDENCE BY SITE AND SEX

	Male		Female	
SKIN	3%		3%	SKIN
ORAL	4%		2%	ORAL
			32%	BREAST
LUNG	18%		12%	LUNG
STOMACH	3%		14%	COLON & RECTUM
COLON & RECTUM	14%		3%	PANCREAS
PANCREAS	2%		4%	OVARY
PROSTATE	23%		8%	UTERUS
URINARY	10%		4%	URINARY
LEUKEMIA & LYMPHOMAS	9%		7%	LEUKEMIA & LYMPHOMAS
ALL OTHER	14%		11%	ALL OTHER

Excluding nonmelanoma skin cancer and carcinoma in situ of uterine cervix

1992 ESTIMATED CANCER DEATHS BY SITE AND SEX

	Male		Female	
SKIN	1%		1%	SKIN
ORAL	2%		1%	ORAL
			19%	BREAST
LUNG	34%		22%	LUNG
STOMACH	3%		12%	COLON & RECTUM
COLON & RECTUM	11%		5%	PANCREAS
PANCREAS	4%		5%	OVARY
PROSTATE	12%		4%	UTERUS
URINARY	5%		3%	URINARY
LEUKEMIA & LYMPHOMAS	9%		9%	LEUKEMIA & LYMPHOMAS
ALL OTHER	19%		19%	ALL OTHER

Cancer Statistics 1992 American Cancer Society New York N Y

Figure 55–1. Cancer incidence and deaths by site and sex—1992 estimates. (Based on Cancer Statistics 1992, American Cancer Society Professional Publication, Atlanta, Ga, 1992.)

of *anaplasia* (loss of cell differentiation) and also have the properties of invasion and *metastasis* (process by which tumor cells are spread to distant parts of the body).

The term "cancer" does not refer to one disease but is used to describe a group of diseases that share the common feature of unrestrained cell growth resulting in tumors that invade and destroy normal tissue. Cancer may arise in any organ or tissue in the body. The cancer process is the end result of a series of complex interactions at the chemical, biochemical, cellular, tissue, organ, and organism levels. Five major categories of factors are implicated as being able to initiate the cancer process. These are viruses such as herpes and Epstein-Barr; chemical carcinogens such as asbestos; physical carcinogens such as chronic irritation, radiation, and radionucleides; nutritional factors such as obesity, high-fat diets, alcohol consumption; and the mechanism of radiation carcinogenesis. Table 55–1 lists factors by category.

Chemotherapy is the use of a drug to weaken or kill an unwanted organism or cell without undue harm to the host (patient). Chemotherapy has been used therapeuti-cally since 1942. Currently, the major classifications of antineoplastic chemotherapeutic agents include alkylating agents, antimetabolites, mitotic inhibitors (*Vinca* alkaloids), antineoplastic antibiotics, hormones and hormone antagonists, radioactive isotopes, orphan or miscellaneous drugs.

Antineoplastic chemotherapeutic drugs have several principal mechanisms by which they act. However, to understand the activity of chemotherapeutic agents, a somewhat detailed knowledge of stem cell theory, cell growth and division (cell cycle), and cell kinetics is necessary.

STEM CELL THEORY

It is possible for many different cell types to undergo malignant change. In some cases, the primary tumor arises from a single cell, described as a *clonal cell*, that is capable of reproducing in kind. According to the *stem cell theory*, only a small number of cells are clonogenic. It is this clonogenic (stem cell) population that has the potential for division and the ability to reproduce the entire tissue from its genetic storehouses. It is believed that neoplastic tumors may arise from a single aberrant stem cell. In some neoplastic tumors, it is possible to prove that all the tumor cells have a common origin, and this supports the theory of a single aberrant stem cell origin. Research indicates a certain percentage of stem cells in a given population are in the resting (G_0) phase. This percentage of stem cells at rest remains constant in tissues. Certain stimuli can encourage the resting cells to enter the cell cycle and begin the division process. For example, a break in the skin causes some at-rest skin stem cells to enter the cell cycle and repair the wound. Once repair is complete, the stimulus ends and the G_0 skin stem cell population returns to its constant level. Thus, normal growth and repair of tissue occur. Normal cells grow logarithmically until they reach critical mass, when their growth rate is altered by hormonal and cellular factors. Cancer cells lack these normal control factors and continue to multiply past the critical mass state, although growth is at a slower-than-logarithmic rate.

Malignant tumors have their own population of stem cells. Although malignant tumors somehow escape normal growth controls, not all malignant cells are involved in division at a given time. This can make antineoplastic therapy difficult, because many drugs do not affect resting cells. Total kill of the stem cell population in solid tumors such as lung cancer is difficult; however, chemotherapy of other tumors such as leukemia has shown that cure is possible. Thorough knowledge of cell kinetics makes it possible to measure tumor growth to evaluate the effectiveness of chemotherapy.

THE CELL CYCLE

The normal cell cycle consists of several distinct phases of biochemical activity. There are essentially five phases in the cell cycle, as shown in Figure 55–2. These phases are the same in both normal and malignant cells.

Following cell division, the daughter cells enter the resting phase (G_0), indicating that the cell is out of the cycle, yet not actively committed to replication. The cell

Table 55–1. FACTORS LINKED TO HUMAN CANCERS

Factor	Type of Cancer Associated with
Viruses	
B-type	Breast
Epstein-Barr	Burkitt's lymphoma
Human immunodeficiency virus	Kaposi's sarcoma
Retrovirus, HTLV-1	Leukemia (some types), Lymphoma (some types)
Hepatitis-B virus	Liver
Herpes simplex type I	Nasopharyngeal
Herpes simplex type II; human papillomavirus	Uterine cervix
Chemical Carcinogens	
Arsenic	Skin, lung
Asbestos	Lung, pleura
Benzene	Bone marrow (leukemia)
Beta-naphthalene	Urinary bladder
Carbon tetrachloride	Liver
Chromium	Lung
Diethylstilbestrol (DES)	Vaginal adenocarcinoma (in daughters of women treated with drug during pregnancy; sons of such women may have increased risk of testicular tumors)
Dioxin	Various tumors
Estrogens	Premenopausal—liver cell adenoma; postmenopausal—endometrium
Phenoxyacetic acids and herbicides	Soft tissue sarcoma
Phenytoin	Lymphoma, neuroblastoma
Polycyclic hydrocarbons (present in tobacco smoke)	Lung, oral, pancreatic, uterine
Rubber industry chemicals	Lung, urinary bladder, leukemia
Smokeless tobacco	Mouth, larynx, throat, esophagus
Vinyl chloride	Liver (angiosarcoma)
Nutritional Factors/Carcinogens	
Alcohol	Oral cancer, cancers of larynx, throat, esophagus, liver
High-fat diet	May contribute to development of cancers of breast, colon, prostate
Obesity	Increased risk of breast, colon, uterine cancers
Salt-cured, smoked, and nitrite-cured foods	Linked to esophageal, stomach cancers
Radiant Energy Carcinogens	
Atomic radiation (bombs)	Leukemia, lung, breast, thyroid
Excessive radon exposure in homes	Increased risk of lung cancer, especially in smokers
Ionizing radiation (radium, x-rays)	Leukemia, bone cancers

thus remains dormant until a biochemical stimulus triggers the onset of the replication process. Once triggered, the cell enters interphase, in which several activities occur. The postmitotic gap 1 (G_1) phase begins with the manufacture of enzymes necessary for DNA synthesis to occur.

During the next phase of the cell cycle—the S phase—actual DNA synthesis occurs. Once the DNA replicates itself, there are two identical molecules, each with one original strand and a newly copied strand from the original. When completed, there are two molecules of DNA, one for each cell, resulting from the division process.

Most cell cycle–specific drugs exert the greatest activity during the S phase of the cell cycle, blocking the DNA replication process. Although the S phase is relatively long, the time spent in this DNA replication phase is only about 10 to 20 hours. Many chemotherapeutic agents affect only dividing cells and only during certain phases of

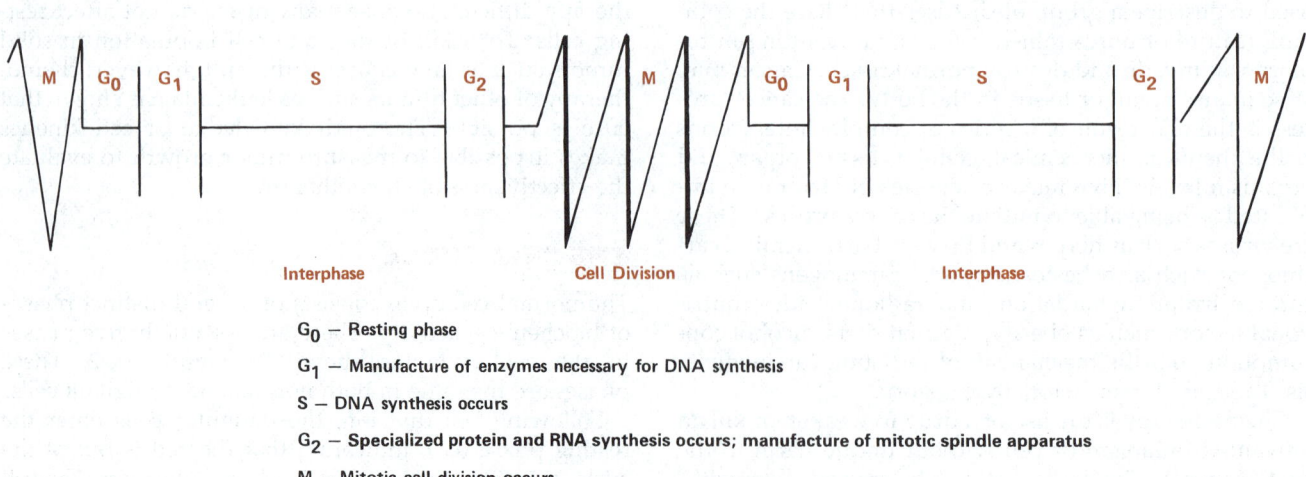

Interphase Cell Division Interphase

G_0 — Resting phase

G_1 — Manufacture of enzymes necessary for DNA synthesis

S — DNA synthesis occurs

G_2 — Specialized protein and RNA synthesis occurs; manufacture of mitotic spindle apparatus

M — Mitotic cell division occurs

Figure 55–2. The cell cycle.

the cell cycle. Thus, the number of tumor cells involved in the cell division process (often referred to as the "growth fraction") is a crucial factor in the effectiveness of drug therapy.

The second gap (G₂) is a short, premitotic phase. Specialized protein and RNA synthesis occur, as well as manufacture of the mitotic spindle apparatus. Also synthesized is a special DNA necessary for cell division to occur. The G₂ phase may take from 2 to 10 hours.

The next phase is the M phase, in which mitosis, the actual cell division process, occurs. This brief phase generally lasts an hour or less. The mitotic phase of the cell cycle has four distinct phases in itself. Following mitosis, the daughter cells differentiate into functioning cells of the parent cell's tissue type. Most cells then enter a resting phase (G₀) and are not actively dividing. A portion of the cells retain proliferative abilities to maintain the necessary number of stem cells.

Cell Cycle–Specific Agents

Antineoplastic agents that affect the cell during only one phase of the cell life cycle are called cell cycle–specific agents. They are sometimes described as cell cycle phase specific, because they act only in a specific phase of the cell cycle. Cell cycle–specific drugs are most often described as being antimetabolic. Each drug of this type works by causing a biochemical blockade of a reaction or reactions occurring in a specific phase of the cell cycle. Most often, these chemical blockades occur because of the drugs' structural similarity to vitamins, coenzymes, or normal cell intermediary products essential for growth and division. The antineoplastic agent is an impostor that the cell takes in to use during the life cycle. Once the antineoplastic agent binds within the cell, the normal metabolic pathway is interrupted, halting growth and division and leading to cell death.

The antineoplastics mercaptopurine, methotrexate, fluorouracil, procarbazine, bleomycin, and vincristine are all examples of cell cycle–specific agents. Many of these drugs are also referred to as being schedule dependent because they produce a greater cell kill when given in multiple, repeated fractions rather than in a single large dose or bolus.

Cell Cycle–Nonspecific Agents

Antineoplastic agents effective in more than one phase of the cell cycle are termed cell cycle–nonspecific agents. These drugs are effective against large tumors where the growth fraction and mitotic index are low. Drugs in this group are the alkylating agents, used to treat hematopoietic tissue malignancies; neuroblastoma; and disseminated carcinomas of the breast, ovaries, testes, and lungs. Drugs belonging to this cell cycle–nonspecific class are not schedule dependent, but are dose dependent. Dose dependency indicates the degree of cell kill is directly proportional to the amount of drug given, so these drugs are typically given in a bolus. Examples of cell cycle–nonspecific class drugs include the alkylating agents melphalan and mechlorethamine; the nitrosoureas carmustine and lomustine; the anthracyclines doxorubicin and daunorubicin; and dacarbazine and cisplatin.

The activities of these drugs do depend on the cell at some point, either attempting division or repair of drug-induced damage. At this point the drug-induced intracellular lethal effects become apparent and cell death ensues. Some drugs in this class, such as nitrogen mustard and the nitrosoureas, have an uncharacteristically nonselective effect on normal and malignant cells, prompting some experts to classify these agents as nonselective, phase-nonspecific drugs.

CELL KINETICS

The study of cell kinetics led to the development of the principles of cancer chemotherapy and enhanced the development of new antineoplastic agents. *Mitotic index (MI)* refers to the fraction of cells in mitosis at a given time. *Growth fraction (GF)* describes the overall number of proliferating neoplastic cells in the system. *Doubling time* is the time required for a tumor cell population to double itself. *Cell loss* refers to the loss of neoplastic cells from the tumor mass.

The most important factor in determining the relative specificity of antineoplastic agents is the growth fraction. In general, neoplastic cells have a higher growth fraction than do normal cells. A higher growth fraction (more cells actively dividing) correlates with a greater cell kill from chemotherapy agents. Unfortunately, certain normal tissue types—the bone marrow, hair follicles, and cells of the gastrointestinal (GI) tract—also have high growth fractions. Thus, these rapidly dividing normal cells suffer the most toxicity during chemotherapy.

PRINCIPLES OF ANTINEOPLASTIC CHEMOTHERAPY

Chemotherapy is no longer a treatment given when all else fails, but is actually the treatment of choice for many malignancies such as inflammatory carcinomas of the breast, acute leukemias, and Hodgkin's disease. Table 55–2 presents related remission rates. Chemotherapy makes normal life expectancy possible in at least ten different malignancies. In advanced cancers, it may be combined with surgery, radiotherapy, hyperthermia or immunotherapy to achieve the highest possible cell kill.

Goals of Antineoplastic Chemotherapy

The ultimate goal of antineoplastic chemotherapy is total cell kill by selective toxicity: The drug destroys cancer cells without irreversibly damaging normal cells. To date, no drug destroys cancer cells only. Several principles make this goal difficult to achieve. First, the presence of a single clonogenic malignant cell may yield sufficient offspring to kill the human host. A second factor is the negligible contribution of host immune mechanisms and defenses in augmenting therapy. If a patient had a 1-kg tumor and you gave a 99.9% effective drug, the patient would still have about 1 g of cancer cells in the body. A way of dealing with this residual body burden of tumor cells is to administer antineoplastic drugs in combination or sequences. Other methods include reductive therapy, adjuvant therapy, and intermittent therapy.

Table 55–2. REMISSION RATES IN SELECTED CHEMOTHERAPY-TREATED TUMORS

Type of Cancer	CR* Rate (%)	10-Year Survival CR (%)	5-Year Survival CR (%)
Acute childhood lymphoblastic leukemia	90	50	70
Acute myelocytic leukemia	60	20	70
Hodgkin's disease	80	—	70
Burkitt's lymphoma	90	60 (for those treated in early stages of disease), 50 (for later stages)	—
Choriocarcinoma	90	90 (cure for those treated in early disease stages), 75 (cure in metastatic stages)	—
Ewing's sarcoma	†	—	66
Ovarian cancer	33	40	—
Wilms' tumor	†	—	80

*Complete remission (CR) is defined as complete regression of all evidence of cancer by physical, radiologic, and biochemical criteria and a return to normal performance status. Remissions are always expressed in terms of duration.

†Chemotherapy is used as part of multidisciplinary treatment approach to this disease. Surgery and/or radiotherapy are used in conjunction with combination chemotherapy.

Combination Chemotherapy Combination chemotherapy, the use of multiple drug therapy, has been highly successful in the treatment of diseases such as lymphocytic leukemia and against certain tumors such as Hodgkin's disease. Although tumor effectiveness is additive, host toxicity need not be, owing to the pairing of drugs with different side effects.

Reductive Therapy Reductive therapy to decrease the body burden of cancer cells may be done before chemotherapy through surgery, radiotherapy, or other therapy. This can increase the effectiveness of chemotherapy.

Adjuvant Chemotherapy *Adjuvant chemotherapy*, the administration of chemotherapy to destroy micrometastasis and to prevent secondary tumors after the removal or destruction of a primary tumor, is employed prior to clinical signs of recurrent disease. It is hoped this therapy will reduce residual tumor burden to levels more likely handled by the host's immunologic mechanisms. Remember that cytotoxic therapy in itself can be immunosuppressive and teratogenic. *Neoadjuvant therapy*—giving chemotherapy to shrink the tumor and then removing the tumor surgically—has been effective in certain types of tumors.

Intermittent Therapy The timing of chemotherapy doses can be critical. Intermittent high-dose (pulse) therapy with cell cycle–specific and cell cycle–nonspecific agents gives better therapeutic results with less toxic side effects than more frequent divided doses. It allows the host to achieve better recovery of normal cells, such as those in bone marrow and the GI tract, during the drug-free interval. Timing drug doses in relation to another drug can allow for cell synchronization to yield greater cell kill with the second drug's administration. However, this principle applies to the normal cells also.

Major Toxicities of Antineoplastic Chemotherapeutic Agents

Rapidly dividing normal cells, such as those in bone marrow, hair follicles, and the GI tract, suffer the most toxicity during chemotherapy, causing bone marrow suppression (neutropenia, thrombocytopenia, anemia); *alopecia* (hair loss); and *stomatitis* (inflammation of the oral mucosa) and

diarrhea, respectively. Other major characteristic side effects of antineoplastic chemotherapy include nausea and vomiting, hyperuricemia, local injury from extravasation of vesicants, embryonic death and fetal malformation, and irreversible sterility in men.

Some antineoplastic drugs cause distinctive and unique toxicities, and agents have been developed to control these toxicities. Dexrazoxane (Zinecard) was developed to reduce the incidence and severity of cardiomyopathy from doxorubicin in women with metastatic breast cancer who have received a cumulative dose of doxorubicin of more than 300 mg/m². Mesna (Mesnex) Table 55–3 is used to prevent ifosfamide-induced hemorrhagic cystitis.

Antianemic Agents

Two drugs that can be used in conjunction with antineoplastics help accelerate bone marrow recovery due to chemotherapy-induced depression are filgrastim (Neupogen) and sargramostim (Leukine, Prokine). For dosages, uses, and nursing implications, refer to Table 55–3. Epoetin (Epogen, erythropoietin, Procrit) is a hormone that is used to manage anemia from chemotherapy in patients with nonmyeloid malignancies. It is discussed in detail in Chapter 38.

○ **Filgrastim** (Neupogen) is used to treat and prevent neutropenia secondary to cancer chemotherapy. Filgrastim is a recombinant-DNA product that is identical to the human neutrophil-stimulating factor. Filgrastim stimulates neutrophil proliferation and development and enhances phagocytic activity.

ADVERSE EFFECTS Adverse effects with filgrastim are leukocytosis; transient hypotension; bone pain; and increased uric acid, lactic dehydrogenase (LDH), and alkaline phosphatase levels.

○ **Sargramostim** (Leukine, Prokine, Leukine Liquid) helps accelerate bone marrow recovery in non-Hodgkin's and Hodgkin's lymphoma and acute lymphoblastic leukemia patients undergoing autologous bone marrow transplant. It is also used to treat and prevent neutropenia secondary to cancer chemotherapy. Sargramostim is a recombinant-DNA product that works by stimulating neutrophil and macrophage proliferation and development.

Table 55–3. ANTIDOTES		
DRUG NAME/ROUTE AND DOSAGE	**USES**	**NURSING IMPLICATIONS**
mesna (Mesnex) Give the equivalent of 20% of the concomitant ifosfamide dose IV at the time of ifosfamide administration and repeat 4 and 8 hr afterward (total dose should equal 60% of ifosfamide dose).	As a prophylactic agent to reduce the incidence of ifosfamide-induced hemorrhagic cystitis	**ASSESSMENT:** Assess urinary elimination, assess for hematuria. **INTERVENTION:** Administer IV bolus in dose equal to 20% of ifosfamide. Maintain fluid balance. Monitor urine for blood. **EVALUATION:** Evaluate for development of bloody urine. Report to doctor immediately.
filgrastim (G-CSF) (Neupogen) 5 μg/kg once daily, SC or IV.	Treat and prevent neutropenia secondary to cancer chemotherapy	**ASSESSMENT:** Assess granulocyte count routinely throughout therapy. **INTERVENTION:** May be administered at home. **Patient Teaching**—Instruct patient on proper injection technique and disposal of syringes. **EVALUATION:** Evaluate for bone pain.
sargramostim (GM-CSF) (Leukine) (Prokine) 250 μg/m² once daily, IV infusion over 2 hr.	Accelerate bone marrow recovery in patients with non-Hodgkin's and Hodgkin's lymphoma and acute lymphoblastic leukemia undergoing autologous bone marrow transplantation; treat and prevent neutropenia secondary to cancer chemotherapy	**ASSESSMENT:** Monitor granulocyte count, CBC. **INTERVENTION:** Reconstitute with 1 mL sterile H_2O for injection without preservatives. Do not shake vial. Monitor patient for hypersensitivity reactions. **EVALUATION:** Evaluate therapeutic response, WBC recovery.

Megakaryocytes and erythrocytes may also be stimulated in certain circumstances.

ADVERSE EFFECTS Adverse effects with sargramostim include leukocytosis; fluid retention; edema; pleural effusion; pericardial effusion; arrhythmias; and dyspnea.

Resistance to Antineoplastic Chemotherapy

The effectiveness of chemotherapy can be diminished by cell resistance. There are three types of resistance:

1. Type I resistance, in which permanently resistant tumor cells cannot be affected by the drug at all.
2. Type II resistance, in which temporarily resistant tumor cells can be affected through a combination of therapies including radiation or surgery.
3. Type III resistance, which occurs when the tumor cells receive less than adequate drug exposure owing to tumor site or local conditions. Once these conditions are overcome by using different administration techniques, this resistance is overcome.

INTRODUCTION TO CHEMOTHERAPEUTIC AGENTS

Chemotherapeutic agents are classified by their probable mode of action (e.g., alkylation, antimetabolic) and the phase of the cell cycle on which they act. Note that dosages for all drugs are given in milligrams per square me-

ter (body surface area) or milligrams per kilogram of body weight. Dosing by body surface area is the most accurate means of dose calculation. To ascertain the patient's surface area, refer to pediatric nomograms (Chapter 7) or adult nomograms, both of which are widely available. Unless otherwise specified, all drug dosages cited are for adults.

All chemotherapy doses are highly individualized and depend on many factors: the patient's level of bone marrow depression, concurrent illnesses, and the presence of adverse effects. All doses of chemotherapy drugs are triple checked by more than one person to help prevent errors, especially when high drug doses are ordered. Any dose outside the normal range is reverified with both the physician and the pharmacist, especially in new protocol situations. Overdoses can cause patient death.

ADMINISTRATION AND HANDLING

Administration

Antineoplastic chemotherapy may be administered orally, intramuscularly, intravenously, intrathecally, by intra-arterial infusion, or by perfusion pump. Chemotherapeutic agents also can be administered directly into the bladder to treat bladder cancer (bladder instillation) or via the portal vein to treat liver metastases. Intracavitary drug administration is used to treat neoplasms in the pleural and peritoneal cavities. Specific nursing measures relative to each type of administration depend on the drug and its properties (e.g., photosensitivity). Actual approaches and interventions relative to nursing goals are detailed later in this chapter.

Handling

There has been increasing concern recently about the handling of antineoplastic drugs. Many antineoplastics are capable of producing mutagenic or carcinogenic effects, in addition to causing direct injury to eyes, skin, or mucous membranes on contact. The handling of antineoplastic drugs is currently considered to be an occupationally hazardous task necessitating specific safety precautions to protect the health and safety of all health-care personnel who may be exposed to these drugs.

Research shows the major hazard in mixing and administering chemotherapeutic agents is from droplet contamination. This results from aerosol exposure of the skin and mucous membranes during drug preparation and administration. Handling these drugs regularly causes low-level exposure that may produce long-term effects.

The National Institutes of Health, National Cancer Institute, Centers for Disease Control and Prevention, Occupational Safety and Health Administration, and the International Agency for Research on Cancer have proposed guidelines for the safe handling of antineoplastic drugs. The basic principles of handling these drugs deal with protective equipment and safety precautions. Mixing and transfer procedures should occur in a class II biological safety cabinet (vertical flow laminar hood); otherwise, a face mask and protective clothing must be worn to protect the preparer from airborne particles or aerosolization of the drug. Oral pipetting is prohibited; pharmacy work and storage areas where chemical carcinogens are present must be posted as such; and materials contaminated by these drugs must be labeled as biohazards and disposed of as such. Additional guidelines and procedures for management of spills or exposure to carcinogenic chemicals are detailed by the manufacturer on the package insert. Owing to the hazards inherent in handling these drugs, they should not be prepared on patient-care units or in poorly ventilated medications rooms. Each institution has definite protocols for handling, preparing, and administering these drugs, and for the disposal of equipment used in handling these drugs. Such protocols should comply with recently published guidelines of the Office of Occupational Medicine, Department of the Occupational Safety and Health Administration (OSHA). Material Safety Data Sheets (MSDSs) must be available to all workers who may come in contact with these drugs. Nurses must remember to use caution not only when handling the drugs and administration materials, but when disposing of patient urine for up to 48 hours after therapy, as most drugs are excreted in the urine. Thus, gloves are worn when any contact with administration materials and urine may occur. Gowns and eye protection are also advised.

ALKYLATING AGENTS

Alkylating agents were derived from the sulfur mustard gases used in the World Wars. They are so named because their primary mode of action is the alkylation of nucleic acids, which results in the inactivation of DNA, thereby halting cell replication processes. Alkylating agents also react with amino, phosphate, and sulfhydryl groups to cause multiple lesions in both dividing and nondividing cells. (This means these drugs are non–cell-cycle dependent.) These agents affect cells in the same way that radiation exposure does and are often referred to as being radiomimetic. Most alkylating agents are similar in effect.

The drugs included in this category are: (1) the nitrogen mustards—**mechlorethamine (nitrogen mustard, NH$_2$), cyclophosphamide (Cytoxan), melphalan (Alkeran),** and **chlorambucil (Leukeran)**; (2) the nitrosoureas—**carmustine (BCNU), lomustine (CCNU), semustine (Methyl CCNU),** and **streptozocin (SZN, Zanosar R)**; (3) the heavy metal compounds—**cisplatin (Platinol, Platinol-AQ)** and **carboplatin (Paraplatin)**; (4) the alkyl sulfonate—**busulfan (Myleran)**; (5) the ethylenimine—**thiotepa (Thioplex)**; and (6) the triazene—**dacarbazine (DTIC-Dome)**. Alkylating agents are used primarily in treatment of hematopoietic tissue malignancies, neuroblastoma, and disseminated carcinomas of the breast, ovaries, testes, and lungs. Selected alkylating agents the dosage, pharmacokinetics, nursing implications are featured in Table 55–4.

PHARMACOKINETICS

The absorption, distribution, metabolization, and excretion of drugs in the alkylating agent class are similar. Busulfan, chlorambucil, cyclophosphamide, lomustine, melphalan, and semustine are all absorbed from the GI tract following oral administration. The other alkylating agents must be administered parenterally. All alkylating agents are widely distributed to body tissues. Carmustine, lomustine, and thiotepa cross the blood-brain barrier. All the alkylating agents except thiotepa and carboplatin are metabolized in the liver and excreted in the urine. Thiotepa is excreted unchanged by the kidneys. Carboplatin is also excreted by the kidneys.

ADVERSE EFFECTS

As a class, the alkylating agents share the common adverse effects of alopecia, bone marrow depression, nausea, and vomiting. These drugs can also cause impaired spermatogenesis in males and amenorrhea in females. All alkylating agents are teratogenic and carcinogenic. Busulfan can also cause an irreversible pulmonary fibrosis, which is also termed "busulfan lung." Cyclophosphamide tablets contain tartrazine which may cause allergic asthmalike reactions in those sensitive to tartrazine.

INTERACTIONS

Most significant drug interactions in this group of drugs occur with cyclophosphamide. Concomitant administration of corticosteroids or chloramphenicol causes reduced activity of cyclophosphamide; therefore, these drugs are used together cautiously. Succinylcholine administration can cause apnea and should be avoided in patients taking cyclophosphamide or thiotepa. Concurrent use of cyclophosphamide and daunorubicin or doxorubicin may in-

Table 55–4. ALKYLATING ANTINEOPLASTIC AGENTS

DRUG NAME/ROUTE AND DOSAGE	USES	NURSING IMPLICATIONS
cyclophosphamide (Cytoxan) **Adults:** 40–50 mg/kg per day IV as single dose, or up to 5 divided doses daily; or 1–5 mg/kg PO qd for 10 days. **Children:** 2–8 mg/kg or 60–250 mg/m^2 PO or IV daily.	Acute lymphocytic leukemia; Hodgkin's disease; lymphosarcoma; many solid tumors; Wilms' tumor; rhabdomyosarcoma; Ewing's sarcoma **Nonneoplastic uses:** Severe rheumatologic conditions; polyarteritis	**ASSESSMENT:** Assess respiratory status, breath sounds. Assess oral cavity for stomatitis. **INTERVENTION:** Monitor CBC, platelets, and liver enzymes. Push fluids and monitor intake. Promote good oral care and bland diet to decrease oral irritation. **EVALUATION:** Determine effectiveness of antinausea and nutritional enhancement actions. Adequate hydration is achieved, cardiopulmonary status is unimpaired. Health teaching is successful.
melphalan (Alkeran) 6 mg PO daily for 2–3 wk; then stop drug 4 wk beore resuming cycle. *Maintenance Dose*–2–4 mg/day. *IV Dose*–16 mg/m^2 q 2 wk for 4 doses, then q 4 wk.	Myeloma; cancer of breast; ovary, and testes; osteogenic sarcoma; malignant melanoma; and reticulum cell sarcoma	**ASSESSMENT:** Assess respiratory status, breath sounds. Assess oral cavity for stomatitis. **INTERVENTION:** Monitor CBC and platelets. Promote good oral care and bland diet to decrease oral irritation. Administer drug on empty stomach as food delays absorption. **EVALUATION:** Same as for mechlorethamine.
chlorambucil (Leukeran) 0.1–0.2 mg/kg day PO for 3–6 wk. *Maintenance Dose*–2–12 mg/day.	Chronic lymphocytic leukemia; Hodgkin's disease; lymphosarcoma; cancer of breast, ovary, or testes	**ASSESSMENT:** Assess respiratory status, breath sounds, oral cavity for stomatitis. **INTERVENTION:** Monitor CBC, platelets, uric acid levels, and nutritional status. **EVALUATION:** Same as for cyclophosphamide.
carmustine (BCNU) 150–200 mg/m^2 q 6 wk or 75–100 mg/m^2 by slow IV infusion daily for 2 days; repeat q 6 wk if WBC above 4000/mm^3 and platelets above 100,000/mm^3.	Primary/secondary CNS tumors; lymphomas; multiple myeloma; malignant melanoma; Hodgkin's disease; GI, breast, bronchogenic, and renal carcinomas	**ASSESSMENT:** Assess respiratory status, breath sounds. **INTERVENTION:** Nausea and vomiting occur approximately 6 hr after administration; give antiemetics. Local vein discomfort and flushed sensation frequently occur after administration; explain to patient. Explain to patient that bone marrow depression occurs 3–6 wk after dose. Monitor CBC. **EVALUATION:** Same as for cyclophosphamide.
thiotepa (Thioplex) 0.3–0.4 mg/kg IV q 1–4 wk or 0.2 mg/kg per day IV for 5 days. *Maintenance Dose*–0.2 mg/kg IV q 1–3 wk. **bladder instillation** 60 mg in 60 mL sterile water q wk for 4 wk. **malignant effusions** 10–15 mg intracavitarily PRN.	Cancer of breast, ovary lungs, or bladder; lymphomas; Hodgkin's disease; control of malignant effusions	**ASSESSMENT:** Assess for hypersensitivity reactions, signs of infection; bleeding; assess oral cavity and nutritional status. **INTERVENTION:** Monitor CBC, platelets, and renal enzymes, as drug used with preexisting renal, heptic, or bone marrow dysfunction. Appropriate health teaching. Monitor for signs of gout. **EVALUATION:** Adequate nutritional status maintained. Health teaching successful.
busulfan (Myleran) 4–8 mg/day PO, up to 8 mg PO qid until WBC drops from 100,000/mm^3 to 20,000/mm^3.	Chronic myelocytic (granulocytic) leukemia	**ASSESSMENT:** Assess respiratory status, breath sounds, hypersensitivity reactions. **INTERVENTION:** Monitor CBC (WBC continues to fall for 2 wk after therapy), platelets, urinary output. Explain side effects of amenorrhea, gynecomastia, and skin changes so patient is prepared if they occur. **EVALUATION:** Same as for cyclophosphamide.
lomustine (CCNU) 130 mg/m^2 PO q 6 wk; reduce dose according to bone marrow depression.	Hodgkin's disease; primary and secondary CNS tumors; gastric, renal, and bronchogenic cancers. Multiple myeloma	**ASSESSMENT:** Assess oral mucosa for lesions, stomatitis. Assess respiratory status.

Continued on the following page

Table 55–4. ALKYLATING ANTINEOPLASTIC AGENTS, *Continued*

DRUG NAME/ROUTE AND DOSAGE	USES	NURSING IMPLICATIONS
lomustine (CCNU), *Continued*		**INTERVENTION:** Give 2–4 hr after meals. Give antiemetic before chemotherapy. Nausea and vomiting occur 2–6 hr after dose. Warn patient that bone marrow depression can occur 4–6 wk after dose; infection and bleeding precautions necessary. Teach appropriate oral care that minimizes trauma to oral tissues. **EVALUATION:** Antinausea and nutritional enhancement actions successful. Health teaching effective. Infection/bleeding precautions successful.
streptozocin (Zanosar) 500 mg/m² IV for 5 consecutive days q 6 wk until maximum benefit or toxicity occurs; maximum single dose 1500 mg/m². Discard reconstituted solutions within 12 hr of dilution.	Pancreatic islet cell cancer, metastatic carcinoid tumor, Hodgkin's disease, colorectal cancer	**ASSESSMENT:** Assess IV site frequently for signs of infiltration. Assess oral cavity for lesions and stomatitis. Assess signs of infection, hypersensitivity reactions, bleeding, dyspnea, ECG changes, chest pain. **INTERVENTION:** Test urine for glycosuria. Avoid extravasation; check vein patency before administering. Tell patient drug often burns on administration and this sensation will pass. Give IV infusion slowly. Store drug in refrigerator. Drug is photosensitive; protect from light. Monitor nutritional status. **EVALUATION:** Antinausea and nutritional enhancement actions successful. No extravasation at sites. Nephrotoxicity avoided.
cisplatin (Platinol) 20 mg/m² IV qid for 5 days; repeat q 3 wk for metastatic testicular cancer; 100 mg/m² IV q 4 wk as adjunct in metastatic ovarian cancer.	Metastatic ovarian or testicular cancer, bladder cancer. Head/neck, cervical cancer, lung cancer	**ASSESSMENT:** Assess for signs of bleeding allergic reaction, infiltration, infection, hearing loss, nausea and vomiting. Assess fluid, electrolyte, nutritional status. **INTERVENTION:** Prehydration and mannitol-induced diuresis may significantly decrease ototoxicity and nephrotoxicity. Do not repeat dose of drug unless WBC above 4000/mm³, BUN less than 25 mg/dL, and creatinine less than 1.5 mg/dL. Metoclopramide is useful in treating nausea and vomiting associated with Platinol. Reconstituted drug stable 24 hr at room temperature. **EVALUATION:** Antinausea and nutritional enhancement actions successful. Nephrotoxicity avoided.
carboplatin (Paraplatin) 300–360 mg/m² IV on day 1 every 4 wk.	Ovarian carcinoma—recurrent. Investigational for: cervical, head and neck, lung, and testicular tumors; and for recurrent leukemia and advanced endometrial cancer	**ASSESSMENT:** Same as for cisplatin. **INTERVENTION:** Do not use any needles that contain aluminum, as reaction may occur. Other interventions as for cisplatin. **EVALUATION:** Evaluate closely for bleeding and infection. Report to doctor immediately.

*Doses of all antineoplastics are highly individualized and depend on many factors, including level of bone marrow depression, illness, nutritional status, and so on. Listed doses are guidelines only.

crease cardiotoxicity. Streptozocin should not be used with other nephrotoxic drugs like aminoglycoside antibiotics, cisplatin, or polymixins. Most alkylating agents antagonize the effects of antigout drugs so increased antigout drugs may be needed.

○ **Cyclophosphamide** (Cytoxan) is the most commonly used drug in the alkylator group and also has the widest spectrum of activity. Cyclophosphamide is not active itself; rather, it requires multistep metabolic activation. The first steps are in the liver, but the final step to the active antineoplastic compound phosphoramide mustard and a side product, acrolein, occurs within target cells. Because tumor cells contain large quantities of the converting enzymes, cyclophosphamide was originally thought to be a tumor-specific antimetabolite. However, this has proved not true, and the phosphoramide mustard is capable of cross-linking DNA in many normal cells, causing considerable toxicity.

ADVERSE EFFECTS The adverse effects of cyclophosphamide are the same as with all alkylating agents. The hematologic toxicity is generally dose limiting. Gonadal suppression and sterility can also occur.

▼ CLINICAL ALERT

Cyclophosphamide can cause cardiotoxicity when given in high doses or when given in combination with doxorubicin (Adriamycin).

Cyclophosphamide is thought to be relatively platelet-sparing, as platelets or thrombocytes are devoid of the enzymes necessary for activation. The side product of activation, acrolein, is thought to cause two unusual urologic toxicities: hemorrhagic cystitis and syndrome of inappropriate antidiuretic hormone (SIADH), also known as water intoxication. Hemorrhagic cystitis is especially common in high-dose intravenous or long-term oral therapy. The patient may develop microscopic or gross hematuria. The best treatment is prevention by hydration and patient education. Patients are told to drink plenty of fluids, empty their bladders frequently, and not to take oral cyclophosphamide at night. The SIADH effect is also more common with high-dose drug therapy. The patient may become water overloaded, hyponatremic, and even develop seizures. The syndrome is reversible and usually treated with only water deprivation.

○ **Carmustine** (BCNU, BiCNU, Biodel, Gliadel), **lo-mustine** (CCNU, CeeNU), and **semustine** (Methyl CCNU), the alkylating nitrosoureas, have the unique ability to cross the blood-brain barrier, a capability linked to their lipid solubility. Thus, they are especially useful against primary and metastatic brain tumors. Alkylating agents are curative only in the treatment of Burkitt's lymphoma. However, long-term remissions have occurred in the treatment of acute lymphoblastic leukemia. Long-term lomustine use increases chance of renal failure. The most significant interaction in this group is with lomustine, which can be potentiated by succinylcholine.

○ **Cisplatin** (Platinol) inhibits DNA synthesis by cross-linking. The drug has an alkylating-like action effective in all phases of the cell cycle and is excreted primarily unchanged in the urine. It is most effective in the treatment of germinal cell neoplasms of the testes, especially when used in combination with bleomycin (Blenoxane) and vinblastine (Velban). Cisplatin also shows antitumor activity against lymphoma, ovarian cancer, bladder cancer, and squamous cell tumors of the head and neck.

ADVERSE EFFECTS   The adverse effects from cisplatin include ototoxicity, and nephrotoxicity. Concomitant administration of aminoglycoside antibiotics causes additive nephrotoxicity. Almost 100% of patients experience nausea and vomiting, which my be severe and protracted. Metoclopramide hydrochloride (Reglan) is especially helpful in relieving cisplatin-induced emesis.

○ **Carboplatin** (Paraplatin) is a platinum coordination compound. It works by producing interstrand DNA cross-links and, to a lesser extent, DNA-protein cross-links. Carboplatin is used for palliative treatment of ovarian cancer recurrent after treatment by other antineoplastic drugs such as cisplatin.

ADVERSE EFFECTS   Additional adverse effects of carboplatin include renal tubular damage, cardiac abnormalities, convulsions, central neuropathy, peripheral neuropathy, impotence and sterility.

ANTIMETABOLITES

The antimetabolites include the following: (1) the folic acid antagonist **methotrexate (MTX, Mexate)**; (2) the pyrimidine antagonists **floxuridine (FUDR), fluorouracil (5-FU),** and **cytarabine (Cytosar, Ara-C)**; (3) the purine antagonists **mercaptopurine (6-MP, Purinethol), thioguanine (6-TG),** and the immunosuppressant **azathioprine (Imuran),** which is covered in Chapter 60. Allopurinol (Zyloprim), an antigout medication, is frequently used in conjunction with thioguanine to prevent the formation of uric acid crystals. Although allopurinol was originally developed as an adjunct for cancer treatment, its primary usage now is in the management of non-neoplastic diseases.

ACTION

Antimetabolites are structurally similar to vitamins, coenzymes, or normal cell intermediary products needed for growth and division of both normal and neoplastic cells. They interfere with the metabolic pathways of dividing cells and exert their greatest effect in the S phase of the cell cycle. A drug-induced block of DNA synthesis occurs when the antimetabolic agent is taken into the cell rather than the necessary nutrient or enzyme. This is the major cause of cell death from antimetabolite therapy. The antimetabolic antineoplastic agents are most effective against rapidly growing tumors. However, these properties also make them highly toxic to rapidly proliferating normal tissues such as the hair and lining of the GI tract.

USES

Antimetabolites are often used in combination to treat acute and chronic leukemia, breast, head, and neck tumors. Colon, ovarian, and bronchogenic carcinomas; trophoblastic tumors; and liver metastases may also be treated by antimetabolites alone or in combination with other agents. Azothioprine is used to suppress rejection following renal transplants and for treatment of severe, active rheumatoid arthritis unresponsive to the other therapy.

PHARMACOKINETICS

The antimetabolite drugs are absorbed, distributed, metabolized, and excreted as follows: Hydroxyurea, mercaptopurine, methotrexate, and thioguanine are well absorbed following oral administration. Cytarabine, floxuridine, and fluorouracil are given parenterally as they are not well absorbed from the GI tract. Fluorouracil is sometimes given orally and topically for the local treatment of some GI tumors. The antimetabolites are all widely distributed in body tissues and fluids, metabolized in the liver, and excreted in the urine. The antimetabolites are effective during the S and G_2 phases of the cell cycle.

ADVERSE EFFECTS

As a group, these drugs share the common adverse effects of myelosuppression (leukopenia, anemia, thrombocytopenia), GI disturbances (nausea, vomiting, stomatitis), renal for hepatitis dysfunction, and alopecia. Mercaptopurine causes fewer GI problems than methotrexate, and thioguanine causes fewer than mercaptopurine.

Table 55–5 features the antimetabolites, and includes dosage and nursing implications for selected agents.

FOLIC ACID ANTAGONISTS

O **Methotrexate** (MTX, Mexate) is the prototype antimetabolite. This B-complex impostor was the first of its class to demonstrate effective antineoplastic activity. Its use in children with acute leukemia during the 1940s induced many remissions.

PHARMACOKINETICS Methotrexate is a potent antimetabolite whose cytotoxic effect is achieved by binding with the enzyme dihydrofolate reductase and blocking conversion of folic acid and dihydrofolate to tetrahydrofolic acid, the active form of folic acid. Tetrahydrofolate is essential for protein synthesis. Methotrexate is cell cycle–specific and arrests DNA synthesis at the G_1-S interphase of the cell cycle. High doses of folic acid analogs like methotrexate can have severe, potentially fatal toxic effects owing to the death of bone marrow and other rapidly proliferating normal cells deprived of tetrahydrofolate. Administration of folic acid cannot reverse the damage to normal cells. This is because the methotrexate-produced enzyme inhibition prevents folic acid from being converted to the necessary active metabolite. Normal cells suffering the toxic effects of methotrexate can be saved by the administration of an antidote called leucovorin (folinic acid, citrovorum factor). This substance provides a tetrahydrofolate derivative that can be used in protein synthesis by the normal cells. The cancer cells are not able to use the leucovorin. Use of this antidote several hours after a massive dose (up to 15 g/m²) of methotrexate has made it possible to kill tumors previously resistant to safe doses of methotrexate (MTX). The toxic effects of methotrexate on normal cells can be greatly diminished with leucovorin administration after the methotrexate has had sufficient time to kill resistant tumor cells, such as is done in osteogenic sarcoma. Thus, the leucovorin is used to "rescue" the normal cells from the toxic effects of methotrexate.

ADVERSE EFFECTS Additional adverse effects include: diarrhea, hyperuricemia, photosensitivity, and pulmonary interstitial infiltrates. Intrathecal administration can cause arachnoiditis within hours after administration.

INTERACTIONS Patients should avoid alcoholic beverages, which can increase hepatoxicity. Concurrent administration of probenecid, tetracyclines, sulfonamides, phenytoin, phenylbutazone, and salicylates can increase methotrexate toxicity and should be avoided if possible. Methotrexate can increase the effect of anticoagulants like warfarin and can decrease the effectiveness of oral digoxin.

PYRIMIDINE ANTAGONISTS

Action The antimetabolite pyrimidine analogs—fluorouracil (5-FU), cytarabine (ara-C, Cytosar), and floxuridine (FUDR)—work by inhibiting pyrimidine synthesis in DNA synthesis. Fluorouracil and cytarabine inhibit thymidylate synthetase to prevent DNA synthesis during the S phase of the cell cycle. Floxuridine is catabolized to fluorouracil and produces the same toxic antimetabolic effects as doses of fluorouracil.

Uses The pyrimidine antagonists are used to treat a variety of solid tumors. Temporary remissions for patients with cancer of the colon, rectum, stomach, and pancreas occur with fluorouracil. Although all antineoplastics are immunosuppressive, cytarabine is especially immunosuppressive, particularly when given via continuous infusion.

O **Fluorouracil** (Adrucil, 5-FU) and **floxuridine** (FUDR) have been in use about 25 years. Biochemical modulation of fluorouracil in combination with leucovorin enhances its clinical activity. This is an example of how research and technology enable therapists to devise more effective cancer treatments, not with new drugs, but with new regimens using existing drugs. Fluorouracil is used to treat bladder, breast, cervical, colon, liver, ovarian, pancreatic, and rectal cancers. Floxuridine is used to treat bile duct, bladder, brain, breast, head and neck, gall bladder, and liver cancers.

ADVERSE EFFECTS Additional adverse effects include: ataxia; vertigo; nystagmus; convulsions; depression; hemiplegia; lethargy; erythema; pruritus; hyperpigmentation (especially in blacks); and malaise.

Because of fluorouracil's narrow margin of safety, the patient's blood count must be carefully monitored for signs of severe bone marrow depression and dangerously low white blood count (WBC). Systemic toxicity of fluorouracil and its derivative floxuridine can also be minimized by injecting the drug directly into the arteries supplying blood to the involved organs (intra-arterial chemotherapy [IAC]). IAC is useful in the treatment of liver metastasis with floxuridine injected into the hepatic artery. Damage to normal cells is greatly reduced because most of the drug is metabolized by the liver before entering the systemic circulation. Suitable patients receiving IAC may have an intra-arterial catheter permanently inserted so they can manage their chemotherapy on an outpatient basis.

INTERACTIONS There are no significant interactions seen with either floxuridine or fluorouracil, although both drugs may potentiate other antineoplastics (may be a desired effect) or increase their toxic effects (not desired).

O **Cytarabine** (cytosine arabinoside, ara-C) works by inhibiting pyrimidine synthesis and is used to treat acute myelocytic and other acute leukemias. Pharmacokinetically, it is well absorbed following parenteral administration, widely distributed to all body tissues, metabolized in the liver, and excreted by the kidneys. Additional adverse effects include megablastosis; reversible hepatoxicity; hyperuricemia; rash; and flulike symptoms. There are no significant interactions with cytarabine.

Table 55–5. ANTIMETABOLITES

DRUG NAME/ROUTE AND DOSAGE	USES	NURSING IMPLICATIONS
methotrexate (MTX) (Mexate)		
antineoplastic 3.3 mg/m² PO, IM, or IV daily 4–6 wk or until remission occurs; doses vary greatly, depending on disease being treated and patient status; high-dose therapy (over 100-mg IV doses) must be followed by leucovorin rescue. **rheumatoid arthritis or psoriasis** 5–15 mg PO/wk in single or 3 divided doses.	Acute leukemia; choriocarcinoma; lymphosarcoma; solid tumors; osteogenic sarcomas; head, neck, lung, breast, and ovarian tumors. Also for severe adult psoriasis and rheumatoid arthritis	**ASSESSMENT:** Assess oral mucosa for lesions, stomatitis. Assess for signs of bleeding, infection, impaired renal function. Assess nutritional status. **INTERVENTION:** Monitor CBC, platelets, and liver and renal enzymes. Effects of drug toxicity increased by salicylates, sulfonamides, phenylbutazone, and PABA. Tell patient to avoid use of self-administered vitamins. If possible, avoid giving with tetracyclines, chloramphenicol, and phenytoin. Patient should abstain from alcohol while on this drug, as it can cause increased hepatotoxicity. Teach appropriate oral care. **EVALUATION:** Same as for cisplatin (see Table 55–4).
floxuridine (FUDR)		
0.1–0.6 mg/kg per day by intra-arterial infusion pump, or 0.4–0.6 mg/kg per day into hepatic artery.	Breast, brain, liver, gallbladder, or bile duct tumors; head and neck tumors	**ASSESSMENT:** Assess for GI toxicity, CNS toxicity, infiltration, nausea, vomiting, stomatitis. **INTERVENTION:** Monitor intake and output, CBC, and renal and hepatic functions. Reconstitute with sterile water and add to 5% dextrose in water or 0.9% sodium chloride solution for IV infusion. Observe and care for arterial line appropriately. Teach appropriate oral care. **EVALUATION:** Antinausea and nutritional enhancement actions successful. Hepatic and renal toxicity avoided. Health teaching successful.
fluorouracil (5-FU)		
Individualize dose, 12.5 mg/kg per day for 3–5 days; smaller doses 1–2 times/wk for maintenance; may also be given intra-arterially or topically.	Cancer of GI tract, breast, uterus, lung, ovary, liver, skin, bladder, and oropharynx; pancreatic cancer	**INTERVENTION:** Monitor CBC and platelets. Drug most effective in mildly toxic range. Give frequent oral care; administer antiemetics before fluorouracil therapy. Stop drug if WBC drops below 3500/mm³ or platelets below 100,000/mm³. **EVALUATION:** Antinausea and nutritional enhancement actions successful. Bone marrow toxicity minimized.
cytarabine (cytosine arabinoside) (Cytosar)		
200 mg/m² qid by continuous IV infusion for 5 days; may also be given SC and intrathecally; intrathecal dose range 10–30 mg/m² up to 3 times/wk.	Acute myelocytic leukemia, lymphocytic leukemia	**INTERVENTION:** Give antiemetics (start before cytarabine), as nausea and vomiting are common with high doses of drug. Good oral hygiene and bland diet should be promoted. Monitor CBC, platelets, and liver enzymes. Store unreconstituted drug in refrigerator. Once mixed, drug is stable for 48 hours in refrigerator. **EVALUATION:** Same as for fluorouracil.
mercaptopurine (6-MP) (Purinethol)		
Adults: 80–100 mg/m² PO qid as single dose, up to 5 mg/kg daily. **Children:** 70 mg/m² qid *Maintenance Dose*—1.5–2.5 mg/kg per day.	Acute lymphoblastic leukemia in children; chronic myelocytic leukemia	**ASSESSMENT:** Observe oral mucosa for lesions, stomatitis. **INTERVENTIONS:** Monitor CBC, platelets, uric acid, and liver enzymes. Push fluids. Give antiemetics as needed. Teach oral care that minimizes trauma to oral tissues. **EVALUATION:** Antinausea and nutritional support actions successful. Bone marrow and hepatic toxicity avoided.
thioguanine (6-TG)		
2 mg/kg per day PO; dose may be increased to 3 mg/kg day if no toxic effects occur.	Acute leukemia; chronic graulocytic leukemia	**ASSESSMENT:** Observe oral mucosa for lesions, stomatitis. **INTERVENTION:** Monitor CBC, platelets, and liver enzymes. Teach appropriate oral care. **EVALUATION:** Same as for mercaptopurine.

PURINE ANTAGONISTS

The antimetabolite purine analogs—mercaptopurine and thioguanine—are useful alone or in combination therapy to treat acute and chronic leukemia. Mercaptopurine was the first clinically effective antipyrine. It remains the most important and widely used drug of this group. In addition to their antileukemic activity, drugs of this class also have immunosuppressive activity. Table 55–5 contains dosage and drug implications.

○ **Mercaptopurine** (6-MP, Purinethol) is a hypoxanthine analog that acts against tumor cells through interference with purine biosynthesis and the interconversions for nucleic acid synthesis. Mercaptopurine is well absorbed after oral administration, distributed widely throughout body tissues, metabolized in the liver, and excreted via the kidneys.

ADVERSE EFFECTS In addition, patients are monitored carefully for signs of bone marrow depression, hepatic necrosis, and hyperuricemia.

INTERACTIONS The only significant interaction with mercaptopurine is with allopurinol, but the interaction is beneficial. Purines are released when cells are destroyed following mercaptopurine administration. Xanthine oxidase converts these excess purines to uric acid, which can lead to precipitation of uric acid crystals and kidney damage. Allopurinol, the antigout medication, is often prescribed to prevent this. Allopurinol inhibits the enzyme xanthine oxidase, preventing crystal formation. This enzyme is needed to break down mercaptopurine, so use of allopurinol can prolong and potentiate mercaptopurine's cytotoxic effects on bone marrow. Patients receiving both allopurinol and mercaptopurine require only one-third to one-fourth of the normally prescribed antimetabolite dose.

○ **Thioguanine** (6-TG, Thioguanine) is an antimetabolite purine antagonist similar to and used to treat the same diseases as mercaptopurine. It is one of the most effective agents against acute granulocytic leukemia, though not very effective against solid tumors. Pharmacokinetically, thioguanine is well absorbed after oral administration, widely distributed to body tissues, metabolized in the liver, and excreted by the kidneys.

INTERACTIONS There are no significant interactions with thioguanine; however, as with mercaptopurine, this drug also causes increased uric acid levels, so concomitant administration of allopurinol is often needed. Unlike mercaptopurine, thioguanine is not affected by allopurinol, so therapeutic doses stay the same.

MITOTIC INHIBITORS

Drugs in this group include the vinca alkaloids—**vincristine (Oncovin), vinblastine (Velban), vindesine sulfate (Eldesine, DAVA)**, and **vinorelbine (Navelbine)**. These drugs are featured in Table 55–6.

ACTION

The vinca alkaloids are derivatives of the plant *Vinca rosea* (periwinkle) and differ structurally from each other. They are cell cycle–specific, active only when the cell is in the mitotic (M) phase of division. Although similar in mode of action and metabolism, they differ strikingly in antitumor spectrum, dose, and toxicity.

USES

The major use of vinca alkaloids are palliative chemotherapy of leukemias, lymphomas, sarcomas, and carcinomas such as breast and testicular tumors. For more detailed lists of cancers treated by vinca alkaloids, their dosage and nursing implications see Table 55–6.

PHARMACOKINETICS

The vinca alkaloids are administered intravenously only. They are widely distributed to body tissues but penetrate the blood-brain barrier poorly. Vincristine and vindesine are metabolized in the liver and eliminated in both the urine and feces. Vinblastine is metabolized extensively by the liver and excreted in bile.

ADVERSE EFFECTS

Adverse effects common with the vinca alkaloids are numbness and tingling of the extremities (paresthesias), loss of deep-tendon reflexes, and ataxia. All the vinca alkaloids can produce tissue necrosis if intravenous infusions containing these agents are allowed to extravasate (infiltrate), as presented (with guidelines for treatment) in Tables 55–7 and 55–8.

INTERACTIONS The vinca alkaloids can interact with methotrexate to increase methotrexate activity.

○ **Vinblastine** (Velban, Velsar) interferes with microtubule assembly by binding to or crystallizing microtubule proteins necessary for the formation of the mitotic spindle. It can also bind to other types of microtubules to affect the function of phagocytes and neurons.

USES Vinblastine is used to treat breast, choriocarcinoma, histiocytosis, Hodgkin's and non-Hodgkin's lymphomas, lymphosarcoma, mycosis fungoides, neuroblastoma, and testicular cancers. In Hodgkin's disease, vinblastine is probably the most effective single drug and is often used in combination chemotherapy.

ADVERSE EFFECTS Unlike vincristine, vinblastine has bone marrow depression as a dose-limiting side effect. Nausea, vomiting, and stomatitis are also frequent. Neurotoxicity has been reported, but is less common with vinblastine. Paresthesias, peripheral neuropathy, numbness, and loss of deep-tendon reflexes can occur. Other adverse effects include tachycardia, pulmonary fibrosis, urinary retention, SIADH, and renal failure.

○ **Vincristine** (Oncovin, Vincasar PFS, Vincrex) has similar chemistry, biologic effects, and mechanism of action to vinblastine. One remarkable feature is the lack of cross-resistance between these two drugs so similar in chemical structure.

USES Vincristine is effective in Hodgkin's disease and other lymphomas. Although somewhat less effective against Hodgkin's disease when used alone, vincristine is considered the drug of choice for combination chemotherapy in states III and IV of the disease. The combina-

Table 55–6. MITOTIC INHIBITORS: VINCA ALKALOIDS

DRUG NAME/ROUTE AND DOSAGE	USES	NURSING IMPLICATIONS
vincristine (VCR) (Oncovin) **Adults:** 0.4–1.4 mg/m² IV per wk. **Children:** 1.5–2 mg/m² IV per wk. Maximum single dose for adults and children is 2 mg. **Children Under 10 kg:** 0.05 mg/kg. **Children Over 10 kg:** 1.5–2 mg/m² IV per wk, not to exceed 2 mg. Not to be used intrathecally.	Acute lymphoblastic leukemia; other leukemias; lymphoma; neuroblastoma; Wilms' tumor; rhabdomyosarcoma; cancer of the testes, lung, or breast; reticulum cell, osteogenic, and other sarcomas	**ASSESSMENT:** Assess oral mucosa. Assess infusion site. **INTERVENTION:** Monitor CBC and platelets. Do frequent neurologic checks. Watch for signs of neurotoxicity. Give drug direct IV or into tubing of running IV after determining that needle is placed in vein. Give antiemetics as needed. Teach good oral care. Monitor for constipation (may be early sign of neurotoxicity.) **EVALUATION:** Antinausea and nutritional support actions are successful. No extravasation at IV sites occurs. Bone marrow and neurotoxicities are avoided.
vinblastine (Velban) (VLB) 0.1 mg/kg or 3.7 mg/m² IV per wk or q 2 wk; dose may be increased to maximum of 0.5 mg/kg or 18.5 mg/m² IV q wk for adults. Not to be used intrathecally.	Hodgkin's and other lymphomas; breast or testicular malignancies; lymphosarcoma; neuroblastoma; mycosis fungoides, choriocarcinoma, and histiocytosis	**ASSESSMENT:** Assess oral mucosa. Assess IV infusion site. **INTERVENTION:** Monitor CBC and platelets. Do frequent neurologic checks. Watch for IV site infiltration—phlebitis, cellulitis, and tissue necrosis can occur if drug extravasates. Monitor for leukopenia, thrombocytopenia, constipation, and urinary retention. Teach good oral care. **EVALUATION:** Same as vincristine.
vindesine sulfate (DAVA) (Eldisine) 3–4 mg/m² IV q 7–14 days; or by continuous IV infusion of 1.2–1.5 mg/m² daily for 5 days q 3 wk.	Acute lymphoblastic leukemia; breast cancer; malignant melanoma; lymphosarcoma; non–small-cell lung cancer	Same as for other vinca alkaloids.
vinorelbine (Navelbine) **Adults:** 30 mg/m² IV given over 20 min once weekly.	Advanced non–small-cell lung cancer, breast and ovarian cancer; Hodgkin's disease; non-Hodgkin's lymphoma	Same as other vinca alkaloids plus: **INTERVENTION:** May increase the risk of mucositis caused by 5-fluorouracil.

Table 55–7. ANTINEOPLASTIC DRUGS DAMAGING TO TISSUES ON EXTRAVASATION

Drug	Effect
Carmustine (BCNU)	Can cause intense pain on infusion.
Dacarbazine (DTIC)	Corrosive to tissues on infiltration.
Dactinomycin (actinomycin D, Cosmegen)	Extravasation can cause phlebitis, severe soft tissue damage.
Daunorubicin (Cerubidine)	Severe cellulitis and tissue sloughage if drug extravasates.
Doxorubicin (Adriamycin, ADRIA)	Severe cellulitis and tissue sloughage if drug extravasates.
Idarubicin (Idamycin)	Very toxic to tissues if infiltrated.
Mechlorethamine/nitrogen mustard (Mustargen)	Corrosive to tissue on contact.
Mithramycin (Mithracin)	Extravasation causes irritation, cellulitis.
Mitomycin (Mutamycin)	Extravasation causes cellulitis, necrosis, tissue sloughage.
Mitoxantrone (Novantrone)	Corrosive to tissues on infiltration.
Vinblastine (Velban) Vincristine (Oncovin) Vindesine (DAVA, Eldisine)	Extravasation can cause irritation, phlebitis, cellulitis, or necrosis.

tion therapy most useful in Hodgkin's disease is the MOPP regimen, which groups vincristine (Oncovin) with mechlorethamine, prednisone, and procarbazine. Vincristine is extremely effective against acute leukemia in children. It shows significant activity against Wilms' tumor, neuroblastoma, melanoma, breast cancer, and osteogenic and other sarcomas.

ADVERSE EFFECTS The major adverse effect of vincristine is neurotoxicity, which limits the maximum single dose to 2 mg. It has the same adverse effects as other vinca alkaloids. Vincristine is bone marrow sparing, which makes it useful in combination with bone marrow–toxic agents. Urinary retention, diplopia, and alopecia can also occur.

○ **Vindesine sulfate** (Eldisine, DAVA) is a semisynthetic alkaloid derivative. It works by producing metaphase arrest during mitosis to prevent cell division.

USES Vindesine it is used to treat acute lymphoblastic leukemia, breast cancer, malignant melanoma, lymphosarcoma, and non–small-cell lung cancer.

ADVERSE EFFECTS Vindesine sulfate shares adverse effects similar to those of the other vinca alkaloids, but has both bone marrow and neurotoxic effects.

○ **Vinorelbine** (Navelbine) is used as a second-line

Table 55–8. GUIDELINES FOR TREATMENT OF EXTRAVASATION OF VESICANT CHEMOTHERAPEUTIC AGENTS

General

If extravasation is suspected, the IV should be discontinued immediately. With needle or catheter still in place, attempt to remove the material from the vein with a syringe fixed to the catheter (remove catheter or needle afterwards).

If ice packs are used, they should be used on and off intermittently for half-hour periods for 18–24 hours.

Topical corticosteroid creams spread in the area of extravasation and covered with gauze may also help reduce cutaneous reactions.

Specific Antidotes

It is generally recognized that 50–100 mg hydrocortisone (Solu-Cortef) or 4–12 mg dexamethasone (Decadron) subcutaneously injected in a series of small punctures in the area of extravasation followed by ice packs for 24 hours is an effective means to deal with most cases (inject with TB or insulin syringe).

Specific antidotes *may* be needed for the following drugs:

Drug	*Specific Antidotes*	*Dose*
Carmustine	Sodium bicarbonate 7%–8.5%	3–5 mL SC
Doxorubicin	Sodium bicarbonate 7%–8.5%	3–5 mL SC
Daunorubicin	Sodium bicarbonate 7%–9.5%	3–5 mL SC
Dactinomycin	Sodium thiosulfate 10% 4 mL plus sterile H_2O 6 mL (to make 10 mL)	3–5 mL SC
Mithramycin	Sodium edetate 150 mg/mL	1 mL SC
Mechlorethamine	Sodium thiosulfate 10% 4 mL plus sterile H_2O 5 mL (to make 10 mL)	3–5 mL SC

Source: Kelly, W: Hamot Medical Center Chemotherapy Information Manual. Hamot Medical Center, Erie, Pa., 1984, with permission.

agent for advanced breast and ovarian cancers and Hodgkin's and non-Hodgkin's lymphomas. Its primary use is to treat advanced non–small-cell lung cancer.

ANTINEOPLASTIC ANTIBIOTICS

Certain antibiotics are useful antineoplastic agents, including the anthracycline antibiotics **daunorubicin (Cerubidine)**, doxorubicin (Adriamycin, Rubex), and idarubicin (Idamycin); bleomycin (Blenoxane); plicamycin (Mithramycin, Mithracin); mitomycin (Mitomycin-C, MTC); mitoxantrone hydrochloride (Novantrone); and dactinomycin (Actinomycin D, Cosmegen). Many of these drugs were originally developed to treat bacterial infections, but were too toxic for that purpose. Most antibiotics affect the function and synthesis of nucleic acids, although cytotoxicity does not always correlate directly with altered DNA functions.

Antibiotics have different types of effects on the cancer cell. For example, dactinomycin combines with deoxyguanine residues to inhibit DNA-directed RNA synthesis. It is useful in the treatment of Wilms' tumor, rhabdomyosarcoma, and methotrexate-resistant choriocarcinoma in women, and in combination therapy for Ewing's sarcoma and testicular tumors. Bone marrow depression, GI disturbances, and local inflammation of parenteral sites are common side effects with this drug. Daunorubicin, doxorubicin, bleomycin, and mitomycin all act as alkylating agents, although the exact mechanism of action is not completely understood with these agents. The antineoplastic antibiotics are featured in Table 55–9.

PHARMACOKINETICS The antineoplastic antibiotics are widely distributed to body tissues following intravenous administration. They are metabolized by the liver, and the inactive metabolites are eliminated in urine and feces.

ANTHRACYCLINE ANTIBIOTICS

Daunorubicin and doxorubicin, although only slightly different in chemical structure, these two drugs display markedly different antitumor activity. Both drugs act by reacting with DNA to form complexes that block DNA-directed RNA and DNA transcription. Both drugs are probably effective during all phases of the cell cycle and therefore are cell cycle–nonspecific. Idarubicin is a synthetic anthracycline for intravenous use.

○ **Daunorubicin** (Cerubidine). The effectiveness is limited to acute nonlymphocytic leukemia (myelogenous, monocytic, and erythroid).

ADVERSE EFFECTS Many of the adverse effects of the antineoplastic antibiotics are similar to the effects produced by the alkylating agents. Adverse effects common to both are myelosuppression, alopecia, and GI disturbances. They are also corrosive to tissue on extravasation. Daunorubicin adverse effects may also cause hepatotoxicity, heart failure (HF), and cardiac dysrhythmias. Cardiotoxicity is one unique, potentially fatal side effect with high doses of either anthracycline. It is a chronic, cumulative, dose-dependent cardiomyopathy that presents like HF. This syndrome is usually rapidly progressive and may be unresponsive to therapy. To lessen the risk of cardiotoxic effects, the maximum cumulative dose of daunorubicin is limited to 550 mg/m². Those who have received other cardiotoxic drugs (i.e., cyclophosphamide) or radiation to the chest or with preexisting cardiomyopathy may be limited to a much lower cumulative dose. Monitoring techniques such as echocardiography can determine if cardiac effects are occurring. Dexrazoxane (Zinecard) is administered with these products to bind the iron which decreases the cardiotoxicity.

INTERACTIONS Daunorubicin should not be mixed with heparin, as a precipitate may form. Daunorubicin can interact with other antineoplastics or radiation to increase their toxicity.

Table 55–9. ANTIBIOTIC ANTINEOPLASTICS

DRUG NAME/ROUTE AND DOSAGE	USES	NURSING IMPLICATIONS
bleomycin (Blenoxane) 10–20 units/m² IV, IM, or SC 1–2 times/wk. Maximum total dose: 300–400 units. **Hodgkin's disease** Follow same dosing schedule; after 50% patient response, give maintenance dose of 1 unit IM or IV daily or 5 units/wk.	Hodgkin's disease; lymphomas; testicular and urinary tract carcinomas; head, esophageal, and neck tumors; skin and cervical cancer; myocosis fungoides, lymphosarcoma.	**ASSESSMENT:** Assess oral mucosa. Assess respiratory status. **INTERVENTION:** Fever generally occurs only on first day of therapy and subsides with acetaminophen. Watch patient for signs of pulmonary fibrosis. Monitor CBC, platelets, uric acid levels, blood gases, and pulmonary function studies. Teach good oral care. **EVALUATION:** Antinausea and nutritional support actions successful. Pulmonary side effects avoided. Health teaching effective.
daunorubicin (Cerubidine) **depending on patient's protocol:** 45–80 mg/m² IV qd on days 1–3 of 3- or 4-wk cycle when used as sole induction agent; in combination chemotherapy, dose is 45 mg/m² IV qd, days 1–3 of first chemotherapy cycle and days 1 and 2 of subsequent cycles. *Maximum Total Lifetime Dose–*450–550 mg/m² owing to cumulative cardiotoxicity.	Acute nonlymphocytic leukemia; acute myeloid leukemia; Ewing's sarcoma; Wilms' tumor; neuroblastoma.	**ASSESSMENT:** Assess oral mucosa. Assess IV infusion site. **INTERVENTION:** Monitor CBC, platelets, cardiac enzymes, and ECG. High resting pulse rate may indicate cardiac side effects. Urine turns red owing to drug, no hematuria; warn patient of this harmless side effect. Inject drug into free-flowing IV. Never give drug IM or SC. Do not mix with heparin; precipitate will form. **EVALUATION:** Same as dactinomycin plus cardiotoxicity, nephrotoxicity, and hepatotoxicity are avoided.
doxorubicin (Adriamycin) 60–75 mg/m² in single or divided doses q 3 wk IV; or 30 mg/m² single daily dose IV, days 1–3 of 28-day cycle. *Maximum Total Lifetime Dose–*550 mg/ms² owing to risk of cardiotoxicity.	Sarcomas; Hodgkin's disease, acute leukemia; breast, genitourinary, thyroid, and lung cancers; neuroblastoma; lymphomas; Wilms' tumor; head, neck, and ovarian tumors.	**ASSESSMENT:** Assess cardiac status with ECG. Assess oral mucosa. Assess IV infusion site. **INTERVENTION:** Monitor CBC, platelets, liver enzymes, ECG, and cardiac enzymes. Observe for signs of cardiac decompensation. Forewarn patient that drug causes red urine (not hematuria). Avoid extravasation—inject into free-flowing IV. Teach patient good oral care. **EVALUATION:** Same as for dactinomycin except cardiotoxicity avoided.
mitomycin (Mutamycin) ***Adults:*** 20 mg/m² IV as single dose; repeat cycle q 6–8 wk. May be given by bladder instillation (20 mg drug per 20 mL diluent) or by intra-arterial administration via hepaticartery.	Gastric, breast, cervical head, and neck carcinoma; malignant melanoma; lung, colon and pancreatic cancers; chronic myleogenous leukemia; bladder and some hepatic tumors.	**ASSESSMENT:** Assess oral mucosa. Assess IV site. **INTERVENTION:** Monitor CBC, platelets, and renal and hepatic enzymes. Take care not to allow drug to infiltrate tissues. Give antiemetics before drug. Stop drug if WBC drops below 4000/mm³ or platelets below 75,000/mm³. **Patient Teaching—**Teach patient bland diet and oral care to help reduce discomfort of stomatitis. **EVALUATION:** Antinausea and nutritional support actions are successful. No extravasation at IV sites occurs. Renal, hepatic, bone marrow and neurotoxicities are avoided. Health teaching is effective.
plicamycin (Mithracin) 25 μg/kg IV daily for 3–4 days for treatment of hypercalcemia secondary to cancer; or 25–50 μg/kg IV daily for 3–8 doses.	Greatest antitumor effect is against disseminated embryonal carcinoma of the testes. Greatest clinical use is in treatment of hypercalcemia of malignancy unresponsive to other therapy.	**ASSESSMENT:** Assess oral mucosa. Assess IV site. **INTERVENTION:** Monitor CBC, platelets, liver and kidney functions, prothrombin bleeding and clotting times, and calcium and potassium levels. Prevent IV infiltration. Infuse over 4 to 6 hr in large-volume dilutions or over 20–30 minutes in small-volume dilutions. Observe patient for signs of hypocalcemia, muscle weakness, and signs of bleeding. Give emetics as needed. **Patient Teaching—**Teach patient oral care. **EVALUATION:** Health teaching is effective. Extravasation at IV sites is avoided. Renal, hepatic, and bone marrow toxicities are avoided.

Continued on the following page

Table 55–9. ANTIBIOTIC ANTINEOPLASTICS, *Continued*

DRUG NAME/ROUTE AND DOSAGE	USES	NURSING IMPLICATIONS
idarubicin hydrochloride (Idamycin)		
12 mg/m^2 by slow IV injection daily for 3 days in combination with cytarabine.	Induction therapy of acute myelocyte leukemia in adults.	**ASSESSMENT:** Obtain baseline ECG. Assess cardiovascular and bone marrow functions. Assess nutritional status. **INTERVENTION:** Administer slowly in free flowing IV. *Never* administer IM/SC. Take precautions when mixing solution. Use gloves and goggles. If skin is exposed, wash thoroughly with soap and water. Do not mix with other drugs. Report infection and bleeding to doctor immediately. **EVALUATION:** Toxic adverse effects avoided. Antinausea and nutritional enhancement actions are effective.

○ **Doxorubicin** (Adriamycin, Rubex).

USES Doxorubicin has a much broader spectrum of activity than daunorubicin and is especially useful in sarcomas; breast, ovarian, cervical, and testicular carcinomas; neuroblastoma; Wilms' tumor; lymphomas; thyroid cancer; and acute leukemia. It is often used in combination against various solid tumors.

ADVERSE EFFECTS The major adverse effects of doxorubicin are the following: leukopenia, thrombocytopenia, cardiac depression, dysrhythmia, cardiomyopathy, hyperpigmentation of skin, hepatotoxicity, and enhancement of cyclophosphamide-induced bladder injury.

INTERACTIONS A significant interaction with doxorubicin occurs with streptozocin, which can cause increased, prolonged levels of doxorubicin in the blood. The doxorubicin dose may need to be adjusted. Doxorubicin can also increase the toxic effects of radiation therapy.

OTHER ANTINEOPLASTIC ANTIBIOTICS

○ **Bleomycin** (Blenoxane) is cell cycle–specific for the mitosis and G$_2$ phases of the cell cycle.

USES Bleomycin is useful in the treatment of squamous cell carcinomas of the head and neck, vulva, vagina, penis, and skin, as well as lymphomas, testicular carcinoma, and mycosis fungoides.

ADVERSE EFFECTS Adverse effects of bleomycin include fever; anaphylaxis; idiosyncratic reaction (hypotension, confusion fever, chills, wheezing); alopecia; and skin and nail changes. Acute pulmonary fibrosis has been reported in 10% of patients, especially those receiving high doses of the drug. This limits the cumulative bleomycin dose to 400 units. Bleomycin produces only minimal bone marrow depression and is useful in combination with bone marrow–toxic agents.

INTERACTIONS Bleomycin may interact with other antineoplastics or radiation therapy to increase their toxicity.

○ **Plicamycin** (Mithracin, Mithramycin).

USES This drug's use is limited almost exclusively to embryonal cell carcinoma of the testes. Plicamycin inhibits osteocytic activity, limiting calcium and phosphorus resorption from the bones. Thus, it can produce a dramatic drop in elevated serum calcium levels and is used to treat hypercalcemias of malignancy unresponsive to other therapies.

PHARMACOKINETICS Plicamycin is widely distributed to body tissues and fluids. It is the only antibiotic antineoplastic drug that crosses the blood-brain barrier in significant amounts.

ADVERSE EFFECTS Adverse effects of plicamycin include bone marrow depression, drowsiness, hepatotoxicity, renal toxicity, and possible decreased serum levels of calcium, potassium, and phosphorus; it is caustic to tissues on extravasation. A unique toxic effect of this drug is a hemorrhagic syndrome, which may initially manifest itself as facial flushing, epistaxis, or hematemesis.

INTERACTIONS Plicamycin may interact with other antineoplastics or radiation therapy to increase their toxic effects.

○ **Mitomycin** (Mitomycin-C, MTC) produces chromosomal aberrations and is teratogenic. It is usually used in combination with fluorouracil or the nitrosoureas against gastric and breast carcinomas.

ADVERSE EFFECTS Mitomycin causes myelosuppression; renal and hepatic damage; nail changes; alopecia; and fever.

INTERACTIONS Mitomycin may interact with the vinca alkaloids and radiation to increase their toxic effects.

This drug is not given if white blood cells drop below 4000/mm^3 or when platelets fall below 75,000/mm^3. Mitomycin is sometimes given topically or by bladder instillation and can also be given intra-arterially via the hepatic artery.

○ **Mitoxantrone hydrochloride** (Novantrone) is used in combination with other drugs for initial therapy of acute nonlymphocytic leukemia in adults (ANLL). Acute nonlymphocytic leukemia is a type of cancer that includes myelogenous, promyelocytic, monocytic, and erythroid leukemias. About 8000 patients in the United States are eligible for treatment with this drug. Because of this relatively limited number of potential patients, this drug is one of the few designated an "orphan drug" under the terms of the Orphan Drug Act, passed by Congress in 1983. It has a cytocidal effect on both proliferating and nonproliferating cells, suggesting lack of cell cycle phase specificity.

ADVERSE EFFECTS   Toxic adverse effects of mitoxantrone are myelosuppression and cardiac problems, including electrocardiogram (ECG) changes, dysrhythmias, chest pain, HF, and tachycardia. Other adverse effects include hepatotoxicity and alopecia.

INTERACTIONS   The only drug interaction with mitoxantrone is with heparin. The two drugs should not be mixed because a precipitate will form.

HORMONES AND HORMONE ANTAGONISTS

Hormones have a wide range of therapeutic uses, but this discussion is limited to their antineoplastic effects. The use of hormones in cancer therapy has the major advantage of not causing bone marrow depression, as do many other cytotoxic agents. The exact mechanism of antitumor action is not completely clear. However, for tumors sensitive to hormonal growth controls, giving opposite sex hormones changes hormonal input to the cell, creating an unfavorable setting for tumor growth. For this to occur, tumor cells must have retained hormone receptors. These receptors are what cause the tumor cell's sensitivity to hormones. Hormonal treatment is most frequently used to treat breast cancer and is also useful in cancer of the endometrium of the uterus and prostatic cancer. Steroids and antisteroid compounds in this class of drugs are (1) the corticosteroids, most notably prednisone; (2) the estrogens; (3) the antiestrogen tamoxifen (Nolvadex) and others; (4) the androgens; and (5) the progestins. Drugs that alter hormone balance include estramustine phosphate (Emcyt), mitotane (Lysodren), and aminoglutethimide (Cytadren). Hormones, hormone antagonists, and drugs that alter hormonal balance are featured in Table 55–10.

CORTICOSTEROIDS

Action   The lympholytic effect of the glucocorticoids is presumed responsible for their therapeutic effect in acute lymphoblastic leukemia, chronic lymphocytic leukemia, and the malignant lymphomas. Prednisone is the most commonly used because it has four to five times the anti-inflammatory effect of cortisol. Prednisone is a component of the MOPP regimen, long considered the most effective means of producing remissions in advanced Hodgkin's disease.

Uses   The corticosteroids are occasionally useful in breast cancer and are a needed replacement hormone after adrenalectomy for metastatic breast cancer. Their anti-inflammatory effects may help reduce some sequelae of neoplastic activity. They help reduce cerebral edema secondary to cranial tumor growth or radiation therapy. Corticosteroids can help the general debility, fever, and anorexia commonly seen in cancer patients, because they produce euphoria that tends to decrease patient perception of these symptoms. Although the patient may feel better, tumor growth may not be significantly inhibited. For additional information see Chapter 44.

ESTROGEN THERAPY

Action and Use   Estrogen therapy is useful for postmenopausal women with metastatic breast carcinoma and in men with metastatic prostate cancer. Tumor regression may not be evident for 6 to 10 weeks in breast carcinoma, but subjective responses in those with prostatic carcinoma are often rapid. Positive estrogen therapy response in breast cancer patients rises with increasing patient age to a high of about 30%. Response rate in prostatic cancer is about 80%. The most commonly used estrogens are diethylstilbestrol (DES), ethinyl estradiol (Estinyl), and the conjugated estrogens (e.g., Premarin), which are more expensive than DES but produce less nausea. For additional information see Chapter 47.

ANTIESTROGEN THERAPY

Hormonal therapy for breast cancer was revolutionized by the discovery that the presence of estrogen-binding receptors in breast cancer tissue was highly correlated with the likelihood of response to endocrine manipulative therapy. An estrogen-dependent cancer needs estrogen for growth. So, if an estrogen impostor is present and taken into the cancer cell instead of the needed hormone, tumor cell growth will be blocked. This occurs when the estrogen antagonist tamoxifen is taken into cancer cells.

O **Tamoxifen**   (Nolvadex) is a synthetic antiestrogen used to treat breast cancer. Action occurs by two mechanisms. First, tamoxifen produces a simple blockade of the estrogen receptors in the cytosol of the cell; and second, the estrogen receptor–tamoxifen complex is translocated to the cell nucleus, where it inhibits messenger RNA synthesis to block nucleic acid synthesis. This competitive inhibitor of estrogen achieves therapeutic effects similar to those of androgen therapy in women with advanced breast cancer, without the masculinizing effects of androgens.

PHARMACOKINETICS   Tamoxifen is well absorbed following oral administration, widely distributed to body tissues, metabolized in the liver, and excreted in the urine.

ADVERSE EFFECTS   Tamoxifen has the minor adverse effects of nausea, vomiting, hot flashes, and occasional vaginal spotting. These reactions rarely require discontinuation of therapy. Bone marrow depression and renal and hepatic toxicity are rare. Some patients have an initial flare of bone pain in metastatic lesions or erythema of skin lesions. Although this can be frightening, these actions may be an indicator of positive response to therapy. They are not indications to discontinue tamoxifen. The major adverse effect is the increased evidence of uterine cancer with use over 5 years. For this reason, if use is continued after 5 years, a hysterotomy is recommended. For dosages see Table 55–10.

ANDROGENS

Androgen therapy produces response in about 20% of women with disseminated breast cancer. Androgens are favored over estrogens in women with premenopausal onset of disease who responded favorably to oophorectomy in the past. It can also be useful to treat early post-

Table 55–10. HORMONES, HORMONE ANTAGONIST, AND DRUGS THAT ALTER HORMONE BALANCE

DRUG NAME/ROUTE AND DOSAGE	USES	NURSING IMPLICATIONS
STEROIDS		
prednisone (Deltasone) (Orasone)		
Cancer therapy: 1–100 mg/day PO.	All steroids: leukemia, lymphoma; breast, ovary and prostate cancers; multiple myeloma	**ASSESSMENT:** Assess patient for mood swings, changes in psychologic status. **INTERVENTION:** All steroids: Monitor electrolytes; patient should have electrolyte levels done regularly during therapy. Observe diabetics carefully, as steroid administration makes diabetes more difficult to manage. Encourage intake of foods high in potassium. Monitor blood pressure. Report any dramatic mood swings to physician. **Patient Teaching**—Instruct patient to avoid aspirin and to take drug with milk or antacid. **EVALUATION:** Health teaching is effective. Serious GI effects are avoided.
ESTROGEN ANTAGONIST		
tamoxifen citrate (Nolvadex)		
Adults: 10–20 mg PO bid.	Advanced premenopausal and postmenopausal breast cancer Possible breast cancer preventative in patients at high risk for the disease	**ASSESSMENT:** Ask patient if she is premenopausal or post-menopausal. **INTERVENTION:** Monitor WBC and platelets. Side effects are generally minor. Short-term therapy causes ovulation in premenopausal women—mechanical contraception is recommended. Appropriate health teaching. **EVALUATION:** Health teaching is effective.
megestrol acetate (Megace) **breast cancer** *Adults:* 40 mg PO qid. **endometrial cancer** *Adults:* 40–320 mg/day PO.	Breast, endometrial carcinomas, renal cell cancers	**ASSESSMENT:** Assess for signs of phlebitis. **INTERVENTION:** All progestins: Encourage low-salt diet. Monitor weight. Caution if hypertension or cardiac disease is present so patient complies with follow-up care needed. Observe for signs of hypercalcemia. Monitor blood pressure. **EVALUATION:** Health teaching is effective. Serious vascular problems are avoided.
ANDROGENS		
fluoxymesterone (Halotestin)		
Adults: 10–40 mg/day PO.	For all androgens: Breast cancer postmenopausal or postcastration (in females)	For all androgens: **ASSESSMENT:** Assess patient for masculinizing effects. **INTERVENTION:** Monitor weight, encourage low-salt diet, and observe for edema. Restrict fluids if necessary. Give antiemetics if needed. Give psychologic support and explain that masculinizing effects abate when drug is discontinued. Monitor blood pressure. **EVALUATION:** Health teaching is effective. Patient's self-image does not suffer unduly from masculinizing effects of drugs.
ANTIANDROGEN		
flutamide (Eulexin)		
Adults: 250 mg PO q 8 hr, in combination with LHRH-agonist such as leuprolide.	Advanced prostate carcinoma	Same as for testosterone.

Continued on the following page

**Table 55–10. HORMONES, HORMONE ANTAGONIST,
AND DRUGS THAT ALTER HORMONE BALANCE,** *Continued*

DRUG NAME/ROUTE AND DOSAGE	USES	NURSING IMPLICATIONS
DRUGS ALTERING HORMONE BALANCE		
mitotane (Lysodren) ***Adults:*** 9–10 g PO qid in 3–4 divided doses.	Inoperable adrenocortical cancer	**ASSESSMENT:** Assess pulmonary and renal functions. **INTERVENTIONS:** Give antiemetics. Monitor liver enzymes, weight. **Patient Teaching**—Warn patient to use care when operating vehicles or doing anything requiring coordination and concentration. **EVALUATION:** Health teaching is effective. Antinausea measures are effective.
aminoglutethimide (Cytadren) ***Adults:*** 1 g/day PO in divided doses (at 6-hr intervals); dose may be increased every 1–2 wk to maximum of 2 g.	Cushing's syndrome, adrenal cancer, hormone-responsive metastatic breast cancer	**ASSESSMENT:** Assess knowledge gaps to determine needed health teaching. **INTERVENTION:** Appropriate health teaching to patient/family since drug produces medical adrenalectomy in inhibiting synthesis of glucocorticoids, mineralocorticoids, and other steroids. Many patients may require hydrocortisone and mineralocorticoid replacement therapy while receiving aminoglutethimide. Monitor blood pressure regularly. Also monitor thyroid studies, CBC. Warn patient that drug can cause drowsiness, orthostatic hypotension. Tell patient to report persistent skin rash (more than 5–8 days in duration). **EVALUATION:** Health teaching is effective.

menopausal women with breast cancer. Fluoxymesterone (Halotestin, Ora-Testryl) is a commonly used synthetic androgen. For additional information see Chapter 47.

PROGESTINS

Progestins are useful in treating carcinomas of the endometrium and in some cases of advanced breast cancer. About 30% of the women with disseminated endometrial cancer respond to progestin therapy, as do some patients with prostatic or renal tumors. Drugs of this type most commonly include hydroxyprogesterone caproate (Delalutin), medroxyprogesterone acetate (Provera), and the synthetic hormone megestrol (Megace). These drugs act by altering the hormonal environment so it is less favorable to tumor growth. For additional information see Chapter 47.

DRUGS ALTERING HORMONE BALANCE

Drugs that produce their therapeutic effect by altering hormone balance include estramustine phosphate, mitotane, and aminogluthimide. These agents are featured in Table 55–10.

PHARMACOKINETICS All drugs are well absorbed after oral administration, metabolized in the liver, and excreted in the urine.

○ **Estramustine phosphate** (Emcyt), or emustine, is used to treat prostatic carcinoma. This drug is especially effective against metastatic prostate cancer in patients resistant to estrogen. It is a combination of nitrogen mustard and a derivative of estradiol, and as such combines hormone therapy with cytotoxic therapy. It was designed to achieve selective transport of the cytotoxic agent to the prostate gland and is one of the most effective drugs used in patients with hormone-resistant prostatic cancer. Estramustine is superior to diethylstilbestrol (DES), producing a longer disease-free interval, better control of pain, higher response rate, and less cardiovascular toxicity than DES. There is no significant difference in overall survival rates between the two drugs.

ADVERSE EFFECTS The most common adverse effects are gynecomastia (due to the estrogenic nature of this compound); fluid retention; nausea; and occasional diarrhea.

There are no significant interactions with estramustine.

○ **Mitotane** (o, p'-DDD, Lysodren) is an adrenocortical suppressant closely related to the insecticide chlorophenothane (DDT). Mitotane is selectively toxic to adrenocortical tissue. Mitotane also hinders the extra-adrenal metabolism of cortisol. Use of this drug is limited to palliation of metastatic or inoperable adrenocortical carcinoma. Because of the action of this drug, adrenal insufficiency can occur; thus, administration of adrenocorticosteroids is necessary.

ADVERSE EFFECTS Adverse effects include hypoadrenalism, dermatitis, visual disturbances, lethargy, and somnolence, all of which abate with decreased dosage of the drug. Nausea and vomiting are generally dose limited, and there is no liver, kidney, or bone marrow toxicity with this drug.

INTERACTIONS Spironolactone should not be taken by patients on mitotane, as it interferes with the adrenal suppression produced by the mitotane.

○ **Aminoglutethimide** (Cytadren), which is not a hormone, alters hormonal balance by suppressing adrenal function in adrenal cancer and Cushing's syndrome. It may also be used to produce medical adrenalectomy in those with metastatic breast cancer.

ADVERSE EFFECTS Adverse effects of aminoglutethimide include adrenal and thyroid hypofunction, especially under stressful conditions, transient *leukopenia*, severe *pancytopenia*, drowsiness, hypotension and tachycardia, nausea, anorexia, morbilliform skin rash, and masculinization and hirsutism in females. Skin rash usually subsides after the first week of therapy. Drowsiness, anorexia, and nausea generally diminish within 2 weeks after therapy begins.

There are no significant interactions with this drug.

RADIOACTIVE ISOTOPES

Some cancers respond to treatment by radioactive isotopes. Theoretically, the radioactive element selectively destroys cancer cells without harm to normal tissues. However, both neoplastic and some normal cells are destroyed by these substances. The radioactive elements used to treat cancer are sodium radiophosphate (^{32}P), and sodium radioiodine (^{131}I), featured in Table 55–11.

All radioactive isotopes emit beta particles that damage both normal and neoplastic cells. Although beta particles travel only short distances, anyone in prolonged close contact with the patient so treated may experience some potentially damaging effects. Thus, patients undergoing such therapy are placed on protective isolation precautions until this hazard is past. Isotope half-life, radioactive materials, OSHA regulations and laws, and drug excretion determine when precautions are no longer necessary. All dosages of radioactive isotopes are highly individualized.

○ **Sodium radiophosphate** (^{32}P) is available as a solution for oral use and in sterile form for injection. Its half-life is 14.3 days. When given orally, about 25% of the drug is excreted unabsorbed in the feces. Renal elimination of the absorbed dose begins rapidly, excreting 25% to 50% in the first 4 to 6 days, then slowing to 1% a day. The isotope concentrates in the bones, regardless of the initial distribution of the drug.

Radioactive phosphate was once the therapy of choice in chronic leukemias because of its affinity for bones. Because of its potentially serious adverse effects, such as an increased risk of leukemia to the patient, and availability of more effective chemotherapeutic agents, current use of sodium radiophosphate is rare. Radioactive phosphate is occasionally used to palliate metastatic bone pain in ovarian cancer.

○ **Sodium radioiodine** (^{131}I) is the most effective of the radioisotopes used in cancer therapy. It has a half-life of 8.8 days and is used to treat well-differentiated follicular and papillary thyroid carcinomas to achieve complete thyroid ablation (destruction) after thyroidectomy. Because iodine is readily absorbed and trapped by thyroid tissue, sodium radioiodine is successful in destroying the neoplastic as well as normal thyroid tissue. Thus, it is also used to treat hyperthyroidism.

PHARMACOKINETICS Sodium radioiodine is absorbed after oral administration and is "trapped" in thyroid tissue wherever it is located within the body. The isotope is excreted mainly in urine, although scant amounts are present in saliva and perspiration. About 80% of the isotope is excreted in 24 to 48 hours.

To achieve adequate uptake of the isotope and optimum benefit from the therapy, patients are deprived of

Table 55–11. RADIOACTIVE ISOTOPES

DRUG NAME/ROUTE AND DOSAGE	USES	NURSING IMPLICATIONS
sodium radioiodine (^{131}I) (sodium iodide I 131) (Iodotope) **sodium radiophosphate** (^{32}P) (sodium phosphate P 32)		
sodium radioiodine 50–150 µCi PO. **sodium radiophosphate** Note: All doses of radioisotopes are highly individualized.	^{131}I: Thyroid cancer ^{32}P: Polycythemia vera, lesions	For all radioisotopes: **ASSESSMENT:** Assess for side effects and ability to cooperate with restrictions due to radioactive isotopes. **INTERVENTION:** Explain to patient/family that patient is on isolation until sufficient quantities of the isotope have been excreted. All urine is collected for 24–48 hours so the amount of radioisotope excreted can be measured. Follow hospital protocol carefully to prevent unnecessary exposure of self, staff, patient visitors to radiation. Carefully explain to patient/family any restriction following discharge; some trace amounts of radioactive elements may be excreted for several days after discharge, so patient should avoid extended close contact with small children/infants for several days. (Example: should not hold infant or small child on lap for extended periods.) **EVALUATION:** Health teaching is effective.

thyroid hormone for several weeks prior to therapy to induce mild hypothyroidism. Most thyroid cancers respond well to this therapy, although two to three courses of treatment several months apart may be needed to achieve total thyroid ablation.

Patients are placed in isolation after drug ingestion, and urine is collected for radioactive assay for 48 hours to determine when sufficient drug amounts are excreted. Once 80% has been excreted (usually 24 to 48 hours), the patient is removed from isolation. It generally takes 7 to 10 days for the rest of the radiation to dissipate. Close contact for extended periods (sleeping in the same bed or holding an infant for an extended period) during that interval is not recommended, as this increases the risk of thyroid cancer to individuals so exposed. Linens and clothing are handled with care, as some of the isotope may be excreted in perspiration.

ADVERSE EFFECTS Adverse effects with this treatment are transient and mild. Patients may experience sensations of fullness in the neck, or transient neck swelling ("radiation mumps"), or may experience a metallic, sweet taste in the mouth. Women experience the latter more frequently than men. There is an increased risk of developing leukemia in later life after this therapy.

INTERACTIONS Lithium carbonate and ^{131}I used together may cause hypothyroidism. Because thyroid ablation (destruction) is the goal in cancer treatment and lifetime thyroid hormone replacement will be necessary, this interaction is more problematic for patients with hyperthyroidism who may receive this therapy.

MISCELLANEOUS ANTINEOPLASTIC AGENTS

Miscellaneous antineoplastic agents include **hydroxyurea (Hydrea)**, **paclitaxel (Taxol)**, **docetaxel (Taxotere)**, **procarbazine (Matulane)**, and **asparaginase (Elspar)**. These drugs are featured in Table 55–12.

○ **Hydroxyurea** (Hydrea) acts as an antimetabolite; but it cannot be assigned to any of the previous subgroups. Hydroxyurea inhibits DNA synthesis through its action on the enzyme ribonucleotide diphosphate reductase and acts specifically in the S phase of the cell cycle.

USES The primary use of hydroxyurea is in busulfan-resistant chronic granulocytic leukemia. Hydroxyurea is sometimes used to treat melanoma and metastatic ovarian cancers and in combination with radiation to treat cancers of the head and neck.

PHARMACOKINETICS Hydroxyurea is well absorbed following oral administration and is widely distributed to body tissues, metabolized in the liver, and excreted via the kidneys.

ADVERSE EFFECTS Bone marrow depression is the major toxic effect and subsides rapidly after the drug is discontinued several days. Adverse effects also include GI disturbances, mild dermatologic reactions, and rarely, stomatitis, alopecia, and neurologic manifestations.

○ **Paclitaxel** (Taxol) is obtained from the bark of the yew tree. Docetaxel (Taxotere) is obtained from the needles. Both are used to treat recurrent ovarian carcinoma.

CONTRAINDICATIONS AND PRECAUTIONS Paclitaxel is contraindicated in patients with a history of hypersensitivity to cyclosporine. Contact of the undiluted concentrate with plasticized polyvinyl chloride (PVC) tubing and equipment is not recommended. When paclitaxel is given following chemotherapy with cisplatin, bone marrow depression is greater than when paclitaxel is given before cisplatin therapy.

ADVERSE EFFECTS Severe hypersensitivity reactions can occur with paclitaxel administration. Other adverse effects are flushing; myalgia; arthralgia; nausea; vomiting; alopecia; bone marrow depression; mild dyspnea; skin reactions; and cardiovascular symptoms, including bradycardia and hypotension during infusion. Monitor patient vital signs carefully the first hour of drug infusion. Ketoconazole *may* inhibit paclitaxel metabolism.

▼ **CLINICAL ALERT**

To minimize adverse effects of paclitaxel, premedicate the patient with dexamethasone 20 mg by mouth both 12 and 6 hours before therapy or diphenhydramine (Benadryl) 50 mg IV 30 to 60 minutes before therapy. The patient must also be premedicated with either cimetidine (Tagamet) 300 mg or ranitidine (Zantac) 50 mg 30 to 60 minutes prior to therapy. During drug infusion observe the patient for signs of anaphylaxis. If the patient develops angioedema or dyspnea needing treatment, discontinue the drug.

○ **Procarbazine** (Matulane), although not an antibiotic, it acts in a similar manner. Procarbazine has a plasma half-life of only 7 minutes. Its greatest clinical use is as a component of the MOPP regimen in treatment of Hodgkin's disease. It may also be used as a single agent to treat lung cancer and brain tumors, as it is a highly lipophilic drug.

ADVERSE EFFECTS Adverse effects of procarbazine include bleeding tendencies, nausea, vomiting, stomatitis, myelosuppression, alopecia, CNS depression, insomnia, confusion, hallucinations, pleural effusion, and MAO-inhibiting effects similar to MAO-inhibiting antidepressants. It can also cause azospermia and cessation of menses with resultant infertility.

INTERACTIONS Procarbazine inhibits monoamine oxidase (MAO) and should be avoided or used with caution in patients receiving sympathomimetics, tricyclic antidepressants, or phenothiazines. (See section on MAO inhibitor drugs in Chapter 25. Patients should limit intake of foods with high tyramine content. A significant interaction can occur if a patient on procarbazine drinks any alcohol-containing beverage, so patients must abstain from alcohol to prevent disulfiram-like reactions.

○ **Asparaginase** (Elspar), also called L-asparaginase, is the first enzyme to be successfully used to treat cancer. This drug was first isolated from the bacterium *Escherichia coli* and is primarily used to treat acute lymphoblastic leukemia, especially in patients beginning to show resistance to other drugs. Its antitumor effect is to deprive tumor cells of the necessary amino acid L-asparagine, causing

Table 55–12. MISCELLANEOUS ANTINEOPLASTIC AGENTS

DRUG NAME/ROUTE AND DOSAGE	USES	NURSING IMPLICATIONS
paclitaxel (Taxol) 135 mg/m³ every 3 wk as 24-hr IV infusion.	Refractory ovarian carcinoma. Paclitaxel is being studied in a variety of other malignancies, including breast cancer.	**ASSESSMENT:** Assess CBC frequently during therapy. May need supplemental blood products. **INTERVENTION:** Premedicate all patients with 20 mg PO dexamethasone 12 and 6 hr before administration; 50 mg IV diphenhydramine 30–60 min before; and 300 mg cimetidine IV 30–60 min before administration. Use gloves and goggles when handling drug. Wash skin or flush mucous membranes if drug contact occurs. Use bottles to mix and administer drug. **EVALUATION:** Report signs of infection, bleeding, and extreme fatigue to physician.
procarbazine (Matulane) 100–150 mg/m² PO for 10 days until WBC drops below 4000/mm³ or platelets drop below 100,000/mm³. *Maintenance Dose*–1–2 mg/kg per day PO when bone marrow recovers.	Hodgkin's disease; non-Hodgkin's lymphoma; bronchogenic carcinoma; multiple myeloma; malignant melanoma; polycythemia vera; and brain tumors.	**ASSESSMENT:** Assess oral mucosa. Assess IV site. **INTERVENTION:** Give antiemetics but no phenothiazines for nausea and vomiting. Monitor CBC, platelets, and liver enzymes. Observe patient for signs of bleeding. **Patient Teaching**—Drug is an MAO inhibitor, so tell patient to avoid alcohol, sedatives, narcotics, tricyclic antidepressants (check with physician before taking any medication). Also, patient should avoid foods with high tyramine content. Warn patient that alcohol intake can produce acute illness (disulfiram-like reaction). Teach patient appropriate oral care. **EVALUATION:** Health teaching of food/fluid restrictions is effective and adverse reactions are avoided. Antinausea interventions are effective. Severe bone marrow depression is avoided.
asparaginase (Elspar) **acute lymphocytic leukemia (in combination therapy):** 1000 IU/kg per day IV infusion for 10 days; administer over 30 min in 0.9% NaCl solution. **as sole induction agent:** 200 IU/kg per day IV for 28 days.	Acute lymphocytic leukemia.	**ASSESSMENT:** Assess oral mucosa for lesions, stomatitis. **INTERVENTION:** Monitor CBC, platelets, renal and pancreatic enzymes, clotting studies, uric acid, glucose, and serum albumin levels. Do not shake vial. Administer clear solutions only. Risk of hypersensitivity increases with each dose. Test dose administration can identify patients at risk. Teach patient oral care. Give antiemetics as needed. **EVALUATION:** Hypersensitivity avoided. Antinausea and nutritional enhancement activities successful. Health teaching effective. Renal, hepatic, and pancreatic toxicities are avoided.

inhibition of protein synthesis and death of the leukemic cells. Asparaginase causes serum asparagine to break into nonfunctional aspartic acid ammonia. Many normal cells are not as sensitive to the effects of this drug enzyme because they synthesize their own supply of asparagine, which tumor cells cannot do. Antitumor effects occur primarily in the G_1 phase of the cell cycle. Tissues of the body usually affected adversely by chemotherapy (GI mucosa, bone marrow, hair follicles) are not affected by asparaginase.

When asparaginase was first introduced, it was believed to be almost nontoxic to normal cells. It is now known that many normal tissues are sensitive to the effects of asparaginase. Toxic effects can result from the impairment of synthesis of secreted proteins such as insulin,

prothrombin, and other clotting factors. The main role of asparaginase is in combination chemotherapy of acute lymphoblastic leukemia when other drugs have failed to induce remission.

PHARMACOKINETICS   Asparaginase is well absorbed after intramuscular injection. It can also be administered intravenously. Metabolization and excretion routes of asparaginase are unknown; only trace amounts are present in the urine.

ADVERSE EFFECTS   Asparaginase is a foreign protein that can cause hypersensitivity and anaphylactic reactions. Skin sensitivity testing and desensitization, if necessary, must be done before administration. Fever, anorexia, nausea, and vomiting are all signs of acute toxic reaction. Elevated blood urea nitrogen (BUN) and ammonia levels can result from the enzyme action of this drug. Liver function is often impaired and can increase the toxicity of other antileukemic drugs. Toxic effects have also been noted in the kidney, pancreas, CNS, and the clotting mechanism. Some patients suffer a temporary decrease in insulin production during treatment, which may be due to toxic effects of L-asparagine on the pancreas.

INTERACTIONS Asparaginase may increase the toxicity of vincristine and prednisone, decrease the action of methotrexate, and increase toxic effects of radiation.

COMBINATION THERAPY

Often, several different drugs are used to treat cancer, as their effect may be stronger together than separately. Table 55–13 lists several common drug combinations used to treat various cancers. Researchers are continually updating combination regimens to devise new, more effective therapies.

NEW AND INVESTIGATIONAL DRUGS

New cancer drugs become available as soon as clinical trials determine their therapeutic value, which can take years. Drugs currently under study (investigational drugs) are expected to be available in the near future, when clinical trials are completed and the Food and Drug Administration (FDA) grants new drug approval. Sometimes when a drug is in the final phase of the study, the FDA grants it investigational new drug (IND) status, so physicians can obtain the IND for their patients. Once drugs are approved for general use, they are closely monitored for several years to determine if any rare or unusual effects occur with their use. Among the drugs under investigation are altretamine (HMM); azacytidine (5-azactydine); iproplatin (CHIP); topotecan; aclacinomycin A; irinotecan (Camptosar); and interferon.

○ **Hexamethylmelamine** (HMM) is a triazene derivative with clinical activity and toxicity resembling those of the alkylating agents. The drug may have some antimetabolite activity. The exact mechanism of its antitumor activity is unknown. Hexamethlmelamine is useful in treating malignant lymphoma, cancer of the ovary, and bronchogenic cancer.

○ **Azacytidine** (5-azactydine) is useful in treatment of cytarabine-resistant acute myelogenous leukemia. It may also be useful in the treatment of melanoma, breast, and colon cancers. Azacytidine acts as an antimetabolite, disrupting the translation of nucleic acid sequences into protein.

○ **Iproplatin** (CHIP) is a second-generation cisplatin derivative with a spectrum of activity similar to that of cisplatin.

○ **Topotecan** is under study for the treatment of lung, colorectal, and ovarian cancers. Bone marrow and GI adverse effects are most common.

○ **Aclacinomycin A** is an investigational anthracycline being used in the treatment of acute leukemias. This drug is a pyrimidine antagonist that produces less cardiotox-

Table 55–13. EXAMPLES OF COMBINATION CHEMOTHERAPY REGIMENS

Type of Cancer	Therapy	Components of Therapy Regimen
Advanced bladder cancer	CMV	Cisplatin, methotrexate, vinblastine
Breast	FAC	5-Fluorouracil, doxorubicin (Adriamycin), cyclophosphamide (Cytoxan)
	CMF	Cyclophosphamide, methotrexate, 5-fluorouracil
	Cooper's Regimen (CVFMP)	Cytoxan, vincristine (Oncovin), 5-fluorouracil, methotrexate, prednisone
Cervical cancer	AMV	Adriamycin, mitomycin, vinblastine
	BM	Bleomycin, mitomycin
Colon (adjuvant therapy)	MOF	Semustine (methyl CCNU), Oncovin, 5-fluorouracil
Hodgkin's disease	MOPP	Mechlorethamine (Mustargen), Oncovin, procarbazine, prednisone
	ABVD	Adriamycin, bleomycin (Blenoxane), vinblastine (Velban), and dacarbazine (DTIC)
	B-DOPA	Bleomycin, dacarbazine, Oncovin, prednisone, Adriamycin
Hodgkin's disease salvage (for patients who relapse)	PVCP	Procarbazine, vinblastine, cyclophosphamide, prednisone
Leukemia	OAP	Oncovin, cytarabine (ara-C), prednisone
	COAP	Cyclophosphamide, Oncovin, ara-C, prednisone
	Ad-OAP	Adriamycin, Oncovin, ara-C, prednisone
	DAT	Daunorubicin, ara-C, thioguanine
Lung (incompletely resected non–small-cell lung cancer)	CAP	Cytoxan, Adriamycin, cisplatin (Platinol)
Multiple myeloma	VBAP	Vincristine, BCNU (carmustine), Adriamycin, prednisone
	VCAP	Vincristine, Cytoxan, Adriamycin, prednisone
Non-Hodgkin's lymphoma	CHOP*	Cytoxan, doxorubicin,* Oncovin, prednisone
	COP	Cytoxan, Oncovin, prednisone
Ovarian carcinoma	VAC	Vincristine, dactinomycin (actinomycin D), cyclophosphamide
Stomach	FAM	5-Fluorouracil, Adriamycin, Mitomycin-C
Testicular carcinoma	BEP	Bleomycin, etoposide, Platinol
Testicular tumors	VB-3	Vinblastine, bleomycin

*The H in this regimen refers to hydroxyldaunorubicin, a chemical synonym for doxorubicin.

icity and mutagenicity than the well-known anthracycline doxorubicin.

○ **Irinotecan** (Camptosar) recently received approval for treatment of colorectal cancer.

○ **Interferon** is a protein that inhibits viruses. Interferon alfa-2a (Roferon-a) and interferon alfa-2b (Intron-a) are now available for cancer therapy, and several other types of interferons are under investigation. Interferons are discussed in detail in Chapter 56.

UNPROVED SUBSTANCES

Unorthodox and unproved methods of cancer treatment abound and often rob patients of time in which conventional therapy could yield a remission or cure. These therapies may include drugs such as Laetrile, diets, energy therapies, shark cartilage, devices, or vitamins. Often, the "therapist" is an expert salesperson who tells the desperate patient there is a cure for cancer that is easy and painless, without the side effects of traditional therapy. Even after therapeutic failure, many are convinced the therapy did not work because of some failure on their part.

Organizations such as the Cancer Control Society and the Committee for Freedom of Choice in Cancer Therapy are clamoring for access to "alternative therapies." About a dozen states allow patients to buy Laetrile or other substances for personal use.

Patients or their families often question nurses about unproved therapies that receive publicity in the lay press. Stress that the best treatment is one that has proved results. Even when comfort and palliation measures are the only alternatives available, it is important for patients to know that care efforts continue even if a cure may not be possible.

Despite the nurse's best efforts, a patient may ultimately choose an unproved therapy. The nurse should not feel a sense of failure if efforts were made to motivate patient compliance. Some people must try everything themselves. The individual has the legal right to choose his or her own therapy, and the health-care team cannot control what will happen.

USING THE NURSING PROCESS

The nurse plays a vitally important role in the care of the patient receiving antineoplastic chemotherapy. Many patients receive chemotherapy as outpatients or take the drugs at home, so nursing implications center mainly on anticipatory care and health teaching. Once the patient is systemically assessed, the information can be put together to help the whole patient—physically and psychologically.

ASSESSMENT

The focus of the assessment and interventions discussed in this chapter is specifically in relation to chemotherapy and the cancer patient.

- A comprehensive nursing history is an essential component of the assessment process. Areas of patient assessment relative to chemotherapy are highlighted in Table 55–14.

- Physical assessment is essential in establishing a pretherapeutic database. Good pretherapy assessment of physical status yields more accurate evaluation of patient response to therapy and assists in recognizing changes that may warn of impending drug toxicity.

- Observation of lesions is important in the objective evaluation of patient response to chemotherapy. Direct, accurate measurement is essential. The nurse may take photographs, map lesions, and record measurements.

- Indirect methods of tumor measurement are more common and may include computed tomography (CT) scans; magnetic resonance imaging; sonograms; and x-ray scans. Positron emission tomography (PET) is the newest, most accurate scanning method to date, producing a unique metabolic portrait of how the tissue or organ is functioning.

- The prechemotherapy laboratory work-up includes as complete a database as possible. Acid and alkaline phosphatase levels, carcinoembryonic antigen (CEA), complete blood count (CBC), electrolytes, and renal, liver, and cardiac enzymes are a few of the chemistry values monitored. Throughout therapy, regular testing is essential, as many drugs have wide dosage ranges, dependent on patient response and toxic effects in the bone marrow, liver, and kidneys. Drug doses are adjusted accordingly. This is why it is imperative for the outpatient to return for regular blood testing throughout therapy.

- Assessment of the patient's sexual status relative to chemotherapy should be made. Some drugs produce libido changes and may temporarily produce physical changes such as gynecomastia in men receiving estrogens. Women on androgen therapy may experience virilization. Patients should be told these effects may occur. Because physical appearance is so strongly linked to sexual desirability, any changes can have a dramatic impact on the patient's self-concept. Assess patient understanding of antineoplastic drugs related to parenthood, as most of these drugs can be teratogenic. Males receiving alkylating agents usually develop sterility. A young male patient should be discreetly counseled about freezing sperm.

- Most drugs used in chemotherapy will be present in breast milk; therefore, nursing of infants is generally not recommended. Likewise, many of these drugs are teratogenic. Therefore, pregnancy can be risky to the fetus. Women should discuss these issues with their oncologist, obstetrician, or fertility specialist. Adults who had chemotherapy for childhood leukemia may have concerns about the possible effects on future offspring.

- Assess hydration and nutritional status. Anorexia and *cachexia* (state of ill health, malnutrition, and wasting) often occur and can be the result of drug toxicity, adverse effects, tumor involvement, emotional stress, or effects of radiation or surgery. Poor nutrition and hydration can lead to poor uptake of antineoplastic drugs by cancer cells, thereby increasing systemic drug toxicity. Also, poor nutritional sta-

Table 55–14. NURSING PROCESS FOR PATIENT RECEIVING ANTINEOPLASTIC CHEMOTHERAPY

Assessment

Assess type of cancer present, length of illness, prognosis, previous chemotherapy.
Assess nutrition/hydration status.
Assess signs/symptoms of chemotherapy/radiation side effects, e.g., stomatitis, edema, hypertension, signs of bone marrow depression.
Assess respiratory status.
Assess cardiac status via ECG/telemetry reading as appropriate.
Assess urinary output.
Assess dental health and oral hygiene; note if lesions are present.
Assess lymph node areas.
Assess knowledge level regarding illness and chemotherapy to determine gaps.

Nursing Diagnosis: Altered Nutrition, Less than Body Requirements

RELATED TO: Consequences of treatment.
AS EVIDENCED BY: Reported inadequate food intake, altered taste sensation, loss of interest in food, loss of weight, sore/inflamed buccal cavity.

Desired Outcomes/Evaluation Criteria

Demonstrates stable weight or progressive weight toward goal with normalization of laboratory values and absence of signs of malnutrition.
Participates in specific interventions to stimulate appetite/increase dietary intake. Antinausea medications are effective.

Nursing Actions

Monitor daily food intake.
Encourage patient to eat high-calorie, nutrient-rich diet with adequate fluid intake.
Provide supplements and frequent/smaller meals spaced throughout day.
Time chemotherapy doses to interfere least with meals.
Administer antiemetic on regular schedule before/during and after administration of antineoplastic agent as appropriate.
Review laboratory studies as indicated, e.g., total lymphocyte count, serum transferrin, and albumin.
Recommend use of viscous lidocaine as appropriate for oral lesions. Refer to dietitian/nutritional support team.

Rationale

Useful in identifying nutritional needs.
Metabolic tissue and fluid needs are increased.

Supplements can play important part in maintaining adequate caloric and protein intake.

Effectiveness of diet adjustment is very individualized in relief of posttherapy nausea. Patients need to experiment to find best solution/combination.
Nausea/vomiting are frequently most disabling and psychologically stressful side effects of chemotherapy.

Helps identify degree of biochemical imbalance/malnutrition and influences choice of dietary interventions.

May be given to relieve oral pain associated with stomatitis to improve oral intake. Provides for specific dietary plan to meet individual needs and reduce problems associated with protein-calorie malnutrition and micronutrient deficiencies.

Nursing Diagnosis: Risk for Altered Oral Mucous Membranes

RELATED TO: Side effects of chemotherapeutic agents (e.g., antimetabolites).

Desired Outcomes/Evaluation Criteria

Displays moist mucous membranes, which are free of inflammation/ulcerations. Verbalizes understanding of causative factors. Demonstrates techniques to maintain/restore integrity of oral mucosa.

Nursing Actions

Inspect oral cavity daily, noting changes in mucous membrane integrity.

Discuss/demonstrate methods of good oral hygiene care with soft toothbrush/toothette, flossing, or cautious use of WaterPik.
Avoid use of commercial mouthwashes, lemon-glycerine swabs.
Suggest use of mouthwash made from warm saline, dilute solution of hydrogen pyroxide, or baking soda and water.
Administer analgesics, topical xylocaine jelly, and/or antimicrobial mouthwash preparation, e.g., nystatin.

Rationale

Range of response extends from mild erythema to severe ulceration, which can be very painful, inhibit oral intake, and be potentially life threatening. Early identification enables prompt treatment.
Good care is critical during treatment to control stomatitis complications, prevent oral trauma, inhibit bacterial growth.

Products containing alcohol or phenol may exacerbate mucous membrane dryness/irritation.
May be soothing to membranes.

Patient is more likely to eat if mouth is free from discomfort/pain.

Nursing Diagnosis: Risk for Impaired Skin/Tissue Integrity

RELATED TO: Effects of chemotherapy, immunologic deficit, altered nutritional state/anemia, or presence of lesions, drug extravasation.

Desired Outcomes/Evaluation Criteria

Identifies interventions appropriate for specific condition.
Participates in techniques to prevent complications/promote healing as appropriate.

Continued on the following page

Table 55–14. NURSING PROCESS FOR PATIENT RECEIVING ANTINEOPLASTIC CHEMOTHERAPY, Continued

Nursing Actions	Rationale
Inspect skin frequently for side effects of cancer therapy, e.g., breakdown, early signs of infection.	Skin reactions may occur with some chemotherapy agents.
Bathe with lukewarm water and mild soap.	Maintains cleanliness without irritating skin.
Encourage patient to avoid scratching and to pat skin dry instead of rubbing.	Helps prevent skin friction/trauma.
Turn/reposition frequently.	Promotes circulation and prevents undue pressure on skin/tissues.
Review expected dermatologic side effects seen with chemotherapy, e.g., rash, hyperpigmentation, alopecia, and peeling of palms with 5-FU.	Anticipatory guidance may help adjustment to/decrease concern if side effects do occur.
Advise patients receiving 5-FU and methotrexate to avoid sun exposure.	Sun can cause exacerbation of burn spotting or can cause red "flash" area with methotrexate, which can exacerbate adverse drug effect.
Report to physician if sunburn is present as he or she may order drug to be withheld.	
Ascertain that IV is infusing well, dilute anticancer drug per protocol.	Reduces risk of tissue irritation/injury.
Instruct patient to notify caregiver promptly of discomfort at IV insertion site.	Development of pain at infusion site needs prompt determination of cause. If owing to drug infiltration/extravasation, prompt intervention to prevent more serious reaction is essential. IV site or flow rate may need changing.
Observe skin/IV and vein for erythema, edema, tenderness, weltlike patches, itching/burning or swelling, soreness, blisters.	Presence of phlebitis, vein flare, or extravasation requires immediate discontinuation of antineoplastic agents and medical intervention.
Wash skin immediately with soap and water if antineoplastic agents are spilled on unprotected skin. Wear gloves, protective eye covering (glasses, goggles) if drawing up drug, starting or discontinuing IV. Dispose of drug-contaminated waste properly.	Dilutes drug to reduce risk of skin irritation/burn. Complies with OSHA safety rules.
Administer appropriate antidote per protocol and physician's orders if extravasation should occur: Hyaluronidase; Sodium bicarbonate; One-sixth molar sodium thiosulfate.	Reduces local tissue damage. Injection of antidotes is a controversial therapy; however, some studies show that it is beneficial. Injected subcutaneously for vincristine. Injected IV and/or into surrounding tissues for carmustine. Injected subcutaneously for nitrogen mustard.
Apply topical ointment, e.g., silver sulfadiazine as ordered.	May be used to prevent infection/facilitate healing if chemical burn occurs.
Apply icepack/warm compresses as ordered.	Controversial intervention depends on type of agent used to restrict blood flow, keeping drug localized, or to enhance dispersion of antidote.

Other Suggested Nursing Diagnoses: Noncompliance (with dietary restrictions); Risk for Fluid Volume Deficit; Impaired Gas Exchange; Fear/Anxiety; or Knowledge Deficit.

tus may prevent normal cells from recovering from chemotherapeutic effects. Insufficient fluid intake can cause increased toxicity to the urinary tract, hemorrhagic cystitis, increased uric acid levels, and obstructive uropathy. Key factors to observe include weight, tissue turgor, complexion, coloring, and condition of mucous membranes, hair, and nails. Inquire about food likes and dislikes and ascertain deficiencies perceived by the patient/family.

- Assess oxygenation status as poor oxygenation may result from tumor growth or extension, concurrent diseases such as emphysema, or the toxic effects of drugs such as bleomycin. Poor oxygenation can result in poor uptake of antineoplastic agents by tumor cells, again leading to increased systemic toxicity and decreased antitumor effect.
- Assess vital signs. Some patients experience pyrexia. If this happens, infection should be ruled out before

chemotherapy. Fever can also result from tumor-produced toxins, other disease processes, or attendant to the use of certain drugs or therapies.

- A waiting period of 4 to 8 weeks between courses of chemotherapy is needed because most chemotherapeutic agents cannot produce adequate tumor cell kill without causing the destruction of many normal cells. Assess the patient for GI effects that can be minimized by the use of pharmacologic agents such as antiemetics. Anticipation of adverse effects and careful monitoring by nursing staff are essential to help prevent/minimize toxic drug effects.
- Assess patient status related to concurrent illnesses that complicate, not rule out, chemotherapy. Active infections, bleeding, and serious illness may be aggravated by chemotherapy. This is due to antineoplastics decreasing immune resistance and affecting the speed of the healing process. Use of certain agents

may aggravate or exacerbate serious emotional illnesses, so it is important to assess psychosocial as well as physical status.

- Assess the patient's lymph nodes. This is important owing to tumor affinity to spread via this route. Observation and palpitation of lymph node areas in the axillary, supraclavicular, sternocleidomastoid, and groin area are essential to assess tumor spread.
- Assess the patient's psychologic status. Assess both patient and family understanding of the illness and its treatment and their anxiety levels.
- Assess patient level of compliance. Because of the seriousness of cancer, most patients comply with therapy despite adverse effects. However, some may decide the adverse effects are more debilitating than their disease symptoms and discontinue therapy. This is the patient's right as long as he or she understands the ramifications of stopping treatment. This concept is referred to as *informed refusal*.

NURSING DIAGNOSIS

The nursing diagnosis is derived from the assessment data. Possible nursing diagnoses relative to chemotherapy are presented in Table 55–14. Individual patient needs may vary according to their level of understanding, therapy schedule, disease stage, and ability to cope with their illness.

INTERVENTION

The nurse needs to consider the patient's feelings and goals in determining long- and short-range goals consistent with the therapeutic objectives of the health team. Nursing interventions associated with assessment data relative to chemotherapy are featured in Table 55–14.

- Lesion-associated interventions include knowledge of radiogram, scan, and test results, and record keeping appropriate to the type of lesion and institutional policies. The nurse is often responsible for direct measurement of visible lesions and documentation by diagrams or photographs. Measurement of lesions is especially important in the use of investigational agents to determine objective remissions, and lesions are often photographed.
- Antineoplastic drugs are capable of causing bone marrow depression, which can place the patient at increased risk of infection. Caution the patient to avoid contact with persons who have contagious illnesses. Patients who have vascular access devices (VADs) in place for home-managed chemotherapy are at risk for developing infections at the exit site or related to septicemia. Proper health teaching regarding VAD care is discussed later in this chapter under health teaching.
- Hydration and nutritional interventions can have a dramatic impact on the patient's overall status. Weigh the patient regularly, as differences of as little as 1 kg may require drug dose recalculation. Fluids are encouraged, forced if necessary, to prevent urinary tract problems and dehydration. Frequent oral care minimizes stomatitis and promotes healing. Encourage the patient to eat soft, bland types of food to decrease the mechanical irritation of chewing and possibility of bleeding gums.
- For patients receiving drugs that cause GI irritation, give drugs with antacids to help decrease gastritis. Nursing interventions related to nausea and vomiting include the use of antiemetics, and the scheduling of drug doses for the least interference with mealtime. Concurrent administration of antiemetics and/or CNS depressants with chemotherapy may decrease nausea and vomiting (refer to Chapter 51 for information on drugs to treat nausea and vomiting). Nabilone or phenothiazines are often used to treat nausea, although cisplatin-related nausea is severe and may require high-dose metoclopramide (Reglan), or lorazepam (Ativan) or dexamethasone (Decadron).
- Patients with nausea-related anorexia are encouraged to eat any way possible, including use of elemental diets and supplements, such as Vivonex (see Chapter 14).
- Stomatitis is a common side effect, especially with the antibiotics and antimetabolites. Interventions include promoting comfort, maintaining adequate hydration and nutritional status, and reducing the chance of bleeding or secondary infections by *Candida, Pseudomonas*, herpes simplex, and *E. coli*. Medicated mouth rinses like nystatin suspension may be ordered for patients with candidiasis. Viscous lidocaine may be ordered to relieve oral pain.
- Interventions to prevent drug infiltration are essential (review Table 55–7 for drugs that damage tissues) and include the following:
  ○ Always test the intravenous line for correct placement before administering a chemotherapeutic drug.
  ○ When inserting a new line, do not probe excessively with the needle, as this may create a tract along which the drug can infiltrate.
  ○ Throughout the infusion of a chemotherapeutic drug, frequently check the site for infiltration and take corrective measures promptly. See Table 55–8 for chemotherapy infiltration antidotes.
- Nursing interventions to alleviate respiratory problems are crucial because respiratory status is an indicator of toxic effects such as pulmonary fibrosis from certain agents such as busulfan, carmustine, melphalan, or bleomycin. Monitor the patient for signs of crackles and rhonchi. Obtain arterial blood gas specimens as ordered, monitor reports closely, and inform the physician of significant changes. Observe skin and nail bed for color changes and for central cyanosis. Oxygen may be administered prior to the chemotherapeutic agent. Encourage the patient to rest for specific intervals during the day.
- Help the patient and family cope with the psychologic impact of cancer by supportive communication techniques and by referrals to appropriate community agencies or therapists, counselor, financial or insurance advisor, or clergyman.
- Drastic mood changes, euphoria, and signs of im-

pending psychosis or depression may be drug related and should be brought to the attention of the physician.

- Maintain an attitude of realistic hope when dealing with the cancer patient and family. Even when cure goals must be changed to comfort goals, it is psychologically uplifting for the patient and family to know that continuing efforts are being made on the patient's behalf.
- Help to allay patient fears, especially those founded in outdated knowledge, misinformation, or just plain fear of the unknown. Be honest explaining drug effects without being too descriptive to highly suggestible patients.
- Parenthood during chemotherapy needs to be discussed with the physician. All chemotherapeutic agents cross the placenta and are capable of producing fetal abnormalities. Most physicians prefer patients wait until chemotherapy is completed to father or bear children. Consultation with the physician is needed to determine the best method of birth control, as birth control pills may not be appropriate owing to their hormonal composition. Some drugs or treatments may impair fertility or increase the risk of birth defects in offspring, so patients may consult fertility specialists when planning parenthood following cancer treatment.

- Anticipatory guidance and health teaching are increasingly important, as so many patients continue chemotherapy at home.
- Vascular access devices (VADs) require specialized health teaching to the person responsible for device care. Tunneled catheters like the Broviac and Hickman are larger and more versatile, have a larger bore, and are made of silicone with a Dacron cuff.

A third type of VAD is the venous access port, which lies completely beneath the skin. It has a catheter attached to a plastic or titanium port. The P.A.S. Port has a top-across lumen, and the Norport SP has a single lumen port that is skin parallel. To deliver medication via these devices, the patient's skin must be punctured and the lumen punctured. Because the device is totally implanted, there are no maintainance costs for dressing or connector changings. The device does need to be flushed at regular intervals.

Table 55–15. PATIENT TEACHING FOR PATIENT TAKING ANTINEOPLASTIC DRUGS AT HOME

Patients taking antineoplastic drugs at home need to know about potentially serious drug adverse effects and which symptoms require prompt medical attention. A card or form with the following information is helpful summary for patients/family. The information below is on the drug procarbazine (Matulane).

Dear Patient:
The drug procarbazine (Matulane) has been prescribed to treat your cancer. This drug works by inhibiting the DNA and RNA and interfering with protein synthesis in cells to cause cell death.

How Long to Take Drug: Follow doctor's orders.

When to Take: At same time each day. Best taken after light meal. Drink extra fluids between meals.

When On Drug, Don't Use: Alcoholic beverages, marijuana, cocaine—serious adverse effects can occur.

Other Food/Fluid Restrictions: Avoid foods with high tyramine content such as homemade breads with lots of yeast, sour cream, strong cheeses, crackers containing cheese, aged game meats, robust red wines, beer.

Possible Drug Side Effects: Decreased white blood cell count (you will be more prone to infections, so avoid contact with sick persons); decreased red blood cell count (anemia); decreased platelets; mouth ulcers; fatigue; dizziness; insomnia.

Other Precautions: Avoid pregnancy if possible. Consult physician before breast-feeding as safety not yet established (drug may pass to milk). Avoid tanning salons, prolonged sunbathing, as drug can cause photophobia, increased risk of sunburn. Avoid driving, piloting, or operating hazardous machinery until you learn how medicine affects you (it can cause dizziness.)

Storage: Keep out of reach of children. Contact Poison Control Center if child ingests any of the drug (see overdose section).

How Supplied: Tablets or capsules.

If You Forget a Dose: Take as soon as you remember but *do not* double up on doses ever.

Possible Interactions with Other Drugs: Amphetamines, anticonvulsants, tricyclic antidepressants, diuretics, guanethidine, levodopa. Always consult with oncologist before taking any new medication, even over-the-counter drugs, while on procarbazine.

Any Life-Threatening Side Effects: None expected.

Contact Physician Right Away If You Experience Any of the Following:

☐ 1. Fever = 102°F with or without shaking chills.
☐ 2. Unusual bleeding, bruising, chest pain.
☐ 3. Extreme weakness/fatigue.
☐ 4. Mouth sores.
☐ 5. Continued vomiting.
☐ 6. Severe headaches.

Overdose/Poisoning Emergency Symptoms—Restlessness, agitation, fever, convulsions, bleeding.
Call ambulance, transport patient to hospital. *Do not induce vomiting.* If patient is unconscious and not breathing, give mouth-to-mouth resuscitation; if no breathing or heartbeat, give cardiopulmonary resuscitation until ambulance arrives.

EVALUATION

It is the evaluation step of the nursing process that determines the effectiveness of interventions and modifies or reformulates nursing diagnoses based on patient responses.

- Patients with anorexia induced by nausea begin to eat better and show weight gain, so this is objective proof of successful nursing intervention.
- If your nursing goal was to improve respiratory status and evaluation after intervention does show improvement, you are remiss not to take the evaluation one step further. Determining which interventions were most helpful in solving patient problems and sharing this information with other members of the health-care team ensure prompt, appropriate intervention on the patient's behalf the next time the problem occurs. Modify interventions when appropriate.
- In the area if health teaching, the nurse has a specific responsibility in evaluating the effectiveness of interventions taken.
- If drug therapy puts the patient at risk for bone marrow depression, have the patient or caregiver explain actions to lower infection risk or bleeding such as reporting signs of fever and any wound redness or swelling to the physician; avoiding contact with ill persons; and avoiding aspirin. Any petechiae or increased tendency to bruising is reported to the physician. Diabetics who take insulin should use extra care when administering injections.
- Evaluate the patient's understanding of potentially serious adverse effects such as the following: endocrinologic effects of hormone therapy; neurologic effects; signs of cardiac toxicity; therapeutic adverse effects such as altered body image or alopecia; neurologic effects such as numbness in fingers or toes; and the possibility of seizures due to certain drugs.
- Evaluate the effectiveness of alopecia-related interventions such as use of a scalp tourniquet and ice caps; or use wigs, hairpieces, scarves, or turbans to disguise and cope with this temporary problem.
- Evaluate the success of discharge planning interventions. If current trends in health-care continue, more patients than ever before will be taught how to manage care in the home. For patients who can continue therapy at home, this will mean less disruption of the family unit and may diminish some of the feelings of loneliness and isolation that occur in hospitalization.

The bibliography for this chapter can be found in Appendix B, which begins on page 1054.

CHAPTER REVIEW QUESTIONS*

1. As a group, the antimetabolites act as antineoplastic agents by:
   a. Interfering with the pathways of dividing cells.
   b. Exerting the greatest effect on the G_1 phase.
   c. Cross-linking RNA replication.
   d. Producing toxic coenzymes.

2. The toxic effects of methotrexate on normal cells can be reduced by the administration of:
   a. Levorphanol.
   b. Cytarabine.
   c. Leucovorin.
   d. Allopurinol.

3. Antineoplastic agents that act by inhibiting pyrimidine synthesis include:
   a. Hydroxyurea.

*See Appendix A, which begins on page 1051, for answers.

   b. Thioguanine.
   c. Cisplatin.
   d. Fluorouracil.

4. A unique adverse effect of the anthracyclines (doxorubicin and daunorubicin) is:
   a. Photosensitivity.
   b. Cardiotoxicity.
   c. Psychosis.
   d. Neurotoxicity.

5. OSHA standards relative to workers exposed to chemotherapeutic drugs include all of the following except:
   a. Use of biologic safety cabinets for safe drug preparation.
   b. Use of gowns, masks, and gloves by those preparing chemotherapeutic solutions.
   c. Proper labeling and disposal of equipment.
   d. Use of special oral pipettes for chemotherapy preparation.

CHAPTER 56

Biotherapy and Biotherapeutic Agents: Biologic Response Modifiers

Brenda K. Shelton, RN, MS, CCRN, OCN

KEY TERMS

Adoptive biotherapy
Antitumor biotherapy
Antitumor vaccines
Attenuated organisms
Autologous
Biologic response modifiers
Biologic therapy
Biotherapy
Complement
Cytokines
Effector cells
Hematopoietic growth
  factors
Immunotherapy
Interferon
Interleukins
Lymphokines
Monoclonal antibodies
Null cells
Optimal biologic dose
  (OBD)
Tumor-associated antigens
Tumor infiltrating
  lymphocytes (TILs)
Tumor necrosis factor
Tumor-specific antigens

LEARNING OBJECTIVES

After reading this chapter, the student will be able to:

1. Identify host antitumor immune mechanisms and discuss methods by which tumors may escape host immune system detection.
2. Describe the antitumor effects of specific biotherapeutic agents and identify which administration routes are used with each drug discussed.
3. List nursing diagnoses appropriate to the patient receiving biologic drugs.
4. Plan interventions essential to the safe administration of biologic drugs and teach the patient/family relevant information about the therapy and its side effects.

T he homeostatic mechanism of immunity is essential for human survival in a world of potentially pathogenic organisms. *Biologic therapy* or *biotherapy*, previously termed *immunotherapy*, is a broad term used to describe the use of agents derived from natural sources that both augment and suppress the body's immune activity. Biotherapeutic agents modify the body's biologic response to malignant cells by interacting with or augmenting normal immune activity against tumors. This chapter discusses basic principles of immune manipulation and biotherapy. It also focuses on the nurse's role in the assessment, planning, intervention, and evaluation of nursing care relative to patients undergoing these therapies.

Hericourt and Richet in 1895 became the first to document tumor immunotherapy in humans, which involved the unsuccessful injection of human melanoma patients with animal antisera. The first successful trial of biologic therapy occurred in the 1970s with the introduction of bacillus Calmette-Guérin (BCG) vaccine in the topical treatment of bladder cancer (Jassak, 1995). Biologic agents licensed or approved for investigational use by the U.S. Food and Drug Administration (FDA) include *interferons* (proteins produced by a cell when exposed to a virus, which acts to interfere with the virus's ability to replicate), *interleukins* (members of a group of hormones known as lymphokines, which are produced by lymphocytes and regulate the immune system; they include interleukin-1 and interleukin-2), *tumor necrosis factor* (cachectin; substance produced by macrophages having a complex role in inflammation, the body's response to tumors, and weight loss associated with cancer), vaccines, and *monoclonal antibodies* (antibodies derived from the fusion of an antibody-producing cell such as a B lymphocyte and another cell such as a cancer cell). Drug delivery via gene transfer technique, depicted in Figure 56–1, is also in the developmental phase.

IMMUNE FUNCTION

The major function of the human immune system is to protect the body from intrinsic and extrinsic foreign biologic and chemical products. This is accomplished through nonspecific and specific immune activities. Granulocytes cause nonspecific immune activities that are responsible for destruction of microbes. Specific immunity is conferred by lymphocytic cell-mediated and humoral immune systems. Cell-mediated immunity induced by T lymphocytes involves the production of *cytokines* (cell killer substances) capable of recognizing and destroying malignant cells, viral particles, and foreign tissue. Humoral immunity creates antibodies (immunoglobulins), which are protein structures capable of recognizing and neutralizing foreign organisms and chemicals. There are four types of cells that are *effector cells* (cells that kill cancer): the killer T cell, the lymphokine-activated killer (LAK) cell, the natural killer (NK) cell, and the macrophage.

Lymphocytes fall into three categories: T cells, B cells, and *null cells* (lymphocytes lacking the marker for both T and B cells). The T cells are classified into three groups: helper cells, killer cells, and suppressor cells. It is the second group, the killer T cells, that are effector cells. The

Figure 56–1. All retroviruses have a common structure (**A**). The Ltr (long terminal repeat) is the promoter region, ψ controls packaging of the viral RNA in the viral particle. Gag and env encode structural proteins that form the "envelop" or outer membrane of the virus. Pol encodes reverse transcriptase, necessary to make DNA from viral RNA.

Construction of the retroviral vector is a complicated process involving several steps. First, the therapeutic gene must be inserted into the viral genome. This is accomplished by replacing retroviral genes (gag, pol, env) with the therapeutic gene (**A**). The therapeutic gene must then be "packaged" into a viral particle that can "infect" the target cell. Packaging takes place in a packaging cell line, which contains a "helper" virus (**B**). The helper virus provides the genes for viral structural genes (gag, env) and the gene for reverse transcriptase (pol) but cannot be packaged because it lacks the ψ region. The therapeutic gene thus becomes part of an infection virion, which is used to infect target cells (**C**). Once in the target cell, the therapeutic gene is reverse transcribed from RNA into DNA by the viral polymerase, then processed by the target cell to produce the therapeutic product. (From Croghan, TW: Advances in Gene Therapy. Hospital Formulary 26(11): 1991, with permission.)

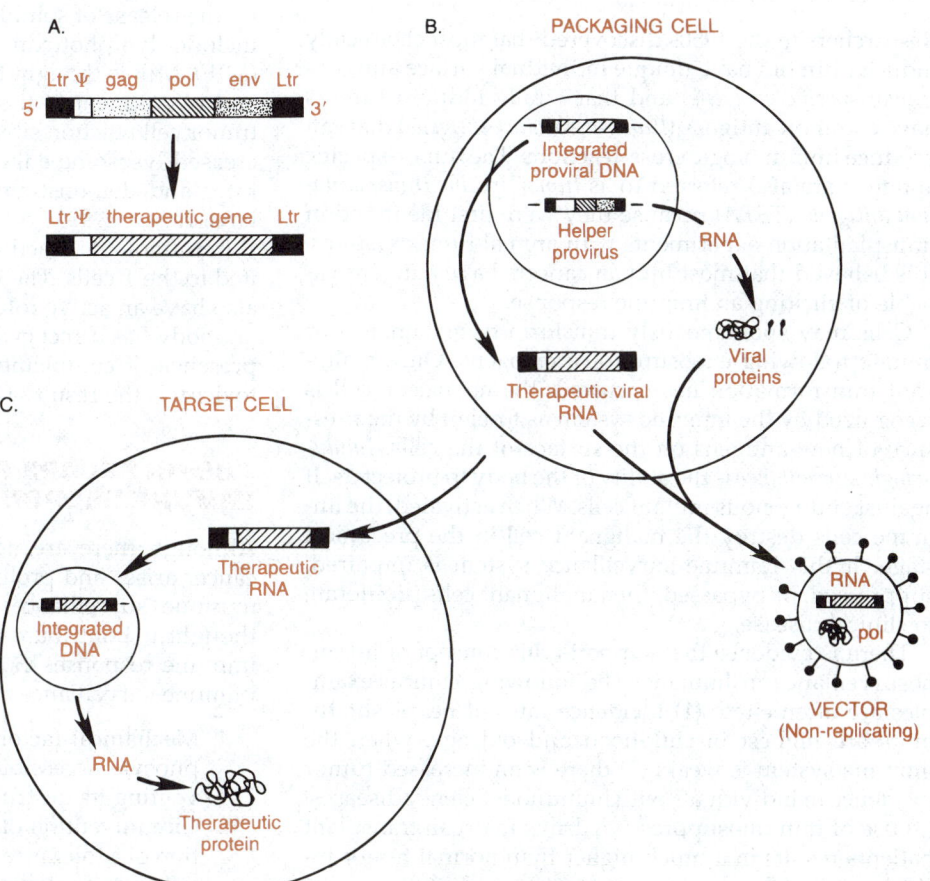

DESIGN OF RETROVIRAL VECTORS

helper T cells secrete substances that stimulate B cells to make antibodies or immunoglobulins. One of these substances is interleukin-2 (also known as T-cell growth factor), which also stimulates the killer T cells to secrete substances such as interferon-gamma.

The LAK and NK cells are included in the null cell population. However, when LAK cells are activated by interleukin-2, they exhibit the same surface markers as do killer T cells. Thus, there is some controversy as to whether LAK cells are truly null cells or if they are just unactivated T cells. Natural killer cells are cells that, without previous exposure to a cancer, are able to kill the cancer without needing nonspecific immune enhancers such as *complement* (a group of glycoproteins in the serum and on cell surfaces that help mediate the inflammatory-immune response) or antibody when stimulated by interferon or interleukin-2.

The macrophage plays a dual role in the immune system's response to foreign cells. First, it recognizes various antigen/antibody complexes and presents these complexes to the T cell. When this T cell comes in contact with the macrophage, it is able to transmit this information to other effector cells. The macrophage is also capable of acting as an effector cell that can secrete substances that can both affect the helper T cells and directly attack cancer cells. Macrophage secretions include interleukin-1 (also called lymphocyte-activating factor) and tumor necrosis factor.

HUMAN IMMUNOLOGIC SURVEILLANCE

Researchers in the 1950s discovered that most chemically induced tumors have unique individual surface antigens (*tumor-specific antigens*) and that virally induced tumors have common antigens (*tumor-associated antigens*) that can produce immunologic cross-reactions. The tumor-specific antigens are also referred to as *tumor-specific transplantation antigens (TSTA)* because they were first identified in transplantation experiments with animal tumor systems. It is believed that most human cancers have antigens capable of eliciting an immune response.

Cells may spontaneously transform to malignancy or mutate following exposure to carcinogens. Once malignant transformation has occurred, the neoplastic cell is recognized by the immune system as foreign by the presence of new antigens on the surface of the cells. *Immunologic surveillance* is the ability of the body to protect itself against endogenous mutant cells. When activated, the immune cells destroy the malignant cell in the preclinical stage. If this immune surveillance system is impaired, suppressed, or bypassed, then malignant cells proliferate to clinical disease.

There is evidence that supports this concept of immunosurveillance in humans. The following clinical examples are often cited: (1) Incidence rates of neoplastic tumors are highest in childhood and old age, when the immune system is weak; (2) there is an increased tumor incidence in individuals with immunodeficiency diseases; (3) use of immunosuppressive drugs in organ transplant patients results in a much higher than normal tumor incidence; and (4) organ recipients who accidentally receive transplanted malignancies develop gross tumor growth due to immunosuppressive drug therapy to prevent organ rejection. Once these drugs are discontinued, the patient's own cells destroy the invading tumor as well as the transplanted organ.

HOST DEFENSE MECHANISMS IN MALIGNANCY

Host defense mechanisms play a role even in clinically evident malignancy. An example of this principle is demonstrated through spontaneous tumor regression that has been reported, especially in patients with small tumor burdens, suggesting that the immune system may be able to deal with certain tumor loads. It has also been shown that cancerous tumors of the breast, bladder, cervix, stomach, and malignant melanoma that are heavily infiltrated by lymphocytes generally have a better prognosis than those without such infiltration. Women with lymphocyte-predominant breast tumors have a well-documented improved prognosis over their counterparts with lymphocyte-depleted cancers. Likewise, patients who demonstrate immunocompetence via an intact cell-mediated immune response at the time of initial treatment will respond better to drug therapy. How successful these mechanisms are can ultimately influence the spread of the tumor, its response to treatment, and the patient's prognosis.

Once T lymphocytes become sensitized by the foreign antigens of tumor cells, the killer T cell response may be initiated. The effects of these sensitized cells are enhanced by the release of soluble factors called *lymphokines*, which include lymphotoxin and migration inhibitory factor (MIF). MIF is thought to be responsible for the activation and recruitment of tissue macrophages at T-lymphocyte tumor cell reaction sites. Activated macrophages have increased lysosome enzyme content and increased mitotic rates and demonstrate more aggressive phagocytic behavior.

Immunologic reactions to malignant cells are not limited to the T cells. The B cells and their humoral products also have an active role. For example, tumor-specific IgM antibody has direct cytotoxic effects on tumor cells in the presence of complement. Antibody-dependent lymphotoxicity is the result of IgG antibodies.

TUMOR ESCAPE FROM HOST IMMUNE RESPONSES

Although there are no definitive mechanisms for how cancer arises and proliferates in the presence of complex immune surveillance mechanisms, several factors are thought to contribute to the escape of tumors from host immune responses. Some escape mechanisms from host immune surveillance are thought to be the following:

1. Mechanical factors, which may interfere with lymphocyte accessibility to the tumor, limiting or preventing its destruction.
2. Circumvention of the immune response by production of a tolerance to the foreign antigen so the tumor antigens go unrecognized as foreign.

3. Drug cytotoxicity, which may decrease tumor antigen production that would sensitize the host to tumor presence.

4. The "sneaking through" phenomenon, in which the tumor does not immunize the host until too large a tumor burden for the immune system to handle is established.

5. The biphasic nature of some antitumor responses may actually foster malignant growth. For example, when a tumor elicits a strong immune response, the tumor may be destroyed; but if a weak immune response is triggered, then the tumor may actually be stimulated.

6. Weakly antigenic tumors may not stimulate sufficient immunologic defense mechanisms. Tumor growth occurs in immunologically privileged sites with poor lymphatic connections.

7. The presence of blocking factors or blocking antibodies can be found in many human tumors. This can occur if antibody or tumor antigen-antibody complexes cover the antigenic sites on the cancer cells, or when large tumor burdens overwhelm the host's immune system with antigen. Some patients exhibit an unblocking ability in their serum, and this is associated with a better prognosis.

BIOTHERAPY IN NEOPLASTIC DISEASE

Certain disease states such as cancer suppress or circumvent the sophisticated survival system of immunity. As knowledge of normal and abnormal immunologic processes increases, so too have hopes for application of an immunologic approach to cancer therapy. Biotherapy is often referred to as the fourth major treatment modality (surgery, chemotherapy, and radiotherapy are the other three).

GOALS

There are three basic goals in anticancer biotherapy. They are as follows: (1) to stimulate immunocompetence in the cancer patient through direct and indirect immune activation; (2) to promote tumor-specific immunity; and (3) as an adjunct to other treatments, to produce tumor regression in the cancer patient.

PRINCIPLES

The basic principles of biotherapy are often used as criteria to determine patient eligibility for this therapy, as not all patients will benefit from this particular treatment. The following considerations are important:

1. **Tumor reduction:** Reduction of tumor body burden is achieved by removing as much of the tumor as possible, as large tumor burdens depress the immune system. Large tumor burdens are less likely to demonstrate an antitumor response with biotherapy because the tumors grow faster than the slow im-

munologic destruction induced by biotherapy agents.

2. **Tumor type:** Patients who derive the most benefit from therapy have disease that has not progressed beyond stage II and are not severely immunosuppressed. Patients with hairy cell leukemia, chronic myelocytic leukemia, malignant melanoma, AIDS-related Kaposi's sarcoma, renal cell carcinoma, superficial bladder cancer, and follicular lymphomas respond best to biotherapy.

3. **Immunocompetence:** Assessment of immune response mechanisms can be done by delayed hypersensitivity skin testing with such agents as purified protein derivative of tuberculin (PPD), mumps vaccine, and *Candida*. There is a better prognosis for patients able to mediate sufficient immune response, as demonstrated by these and other qualitative examinations. Quantitiative assessment of immune function is made by peripheral blood counts, immunoglobulin assays, and bone marrow aspiration.

4. **Treatment scheduling:** Treatment should be timed carefully in relation to surgery, chemotherapy, and radiotherapy, so the patient's immune system can recover from the depressive effects of these modalities. Certain chemotherapeutic agents demonstrate synergistic antitumor activity with biotherapeutic agents.

Unlike traditional chemotherapy in which the philosophy of treatment says that more drug is better, biotherapy is not dosed according to maximal tolerated dose (MTD). Biotherapy may exert its optimal biologic effect at a dose much lower than the maximum tolerated and is hence administered based on the premise of the *optimal biologic dose (OBD)*, defined as "that dose which, with a minimum of side effects, produces the optimal desired responses for the parameters deemed important with respect to a particular biologic agent" (Creekmore et al., 1991). The proposed reasons that biotherapeutic agents can be administered differently than chemotherapeutic agents are the inherent differences seen with naturally occurring biologic products that work by preprogrammed mechanisms of action, receptors, and are similar to human or mammalian genes.

In addition to differences in administration principles, there may also be variability in the techniques used to evaluate efficacy of biotherapeutic agents. With traditional measures of clinical toxicity and tumor responses, clinical trials of biotherapy agents must incorporate measures of bioavailability, pharmacokinetics, biologic effects on immunologic activities, and immunologic assays. It has been proposed that stabilization of disease may be the most accurate goal of biotherapy, not irradication of malignancy as currently used with chemotherapy.

The major advantage of biotherapy is that it does not usually produce life-threatening adverse effects. Most adverse effects are acute in nature and are totally reversible at discontinuation of therapy. The two most commonly experienced adverse effects of biotherapy are fatigue and flulike syndrome. Fatigue is almost universal for patients receiving biotherapy and may significantly alter quality of life. Some patients require counselling, for they mistake therapy-associated fatigue with the fatigue of disease progression. Flulike syndrome includes chills, fever, headache, rhinitis, arthralgias, and myalgias. The most common reason for discontinuation of therapy is severe hypersensitivity reactions (anaphylaxis), which is a rare occurrence.

TYPES OF BIOTHERAPY

No clear classification system of biotherapeutic agents exist, for many are pleomorphic, having multiple immunologic activities against tumors. Early attempts to classify agents used the active and passive deliniations typical of vaccines; however, these are not an accurate reflection of the activities of biologic agents used as antineoplastic therapy. Currently, clinicians group agents as (1) antitumor, (2) adoptive, (3) restorative, (4) cytomod-ulatory, and (5) gene manipulative (Mitchell, 1992; Oncology Nursing Society, and 1995; Jassak, 1995).

Antitumor Biotherapy

In *antitumor biotherapy*, agents that combine active and passive mechanisms to enhance or stimulate the nonspecific and specific host-tumor immune responses of the individual are used. Antitumor biotherapeutic agents include cytokines, vaccines, and monoclonal antibodies. This type of therapy has been used in the treatment of bladder cancer, malignant melanoma, hairy cell leukemia, chronic myelogenous leukemia, mycosis fungoides, AIDS-related Kaposi's sarcoma, renal cell carcinoma, and basal cell carcinoma.

Cytokines Cytokines are cell killer substances modeled after lymphocyte secretions present in normal hu-

Table 56–1. ANTITUMOR CYTOKINES

DRUG NAME/ROUTE AND DOSAGE	PHARMACOKINETICS/ DYNAMICS	NURSING IMPLICATIONS
interferon alpha-2a (Roferon-a) **interferon alpha-2b** (Intron-a) **interferon alpha-n1** (Wellferon) **interferon alpha-n3** (Alferon N) Doses noted are guidelines only: *hairy cell leukemia:* 2–3 million units IV/day. *AIDS-related kaposi's sarcoma:* 30–50 million units IV/day or 3 times/wk. *metastatic malignant melonoma:* 12–50 million units/m² IM 3 times/wk. *adjuvant postoperative for malignant melanoma:* 20 million units/m² IV/day, 5 days/wk for 4 wk, then 10 million units/m² SC 3 times/wk for 48 wk. *chronic myelogenous leukemia:* 2–5 million units/m² per day IM. *condylomata acuminata:* 1 million units injected intralesionally 3 times/wk for 3 wk in patients with <5 lesions. *chronic non-A, non-B/C hepatitis:* 3 million units SC 3 times/ wk for 6 mo. *chronic hepatitis B:* 5–10 million units SC 3 times/wk for 16 wk.	**Onset:** 15–30 min **Peak:** SC or IM, 4–8 hr **Duration:** SC or IM, 16 hr; IV, 4 hr **½L:** SC or IM, 4–9 hr; IV, 2 hr **PB:** NA **B:** liver and bile **E:** urine	**ASSESSMENT:** Assess patient's mental status, mood state, and perception of the goal of therapy. Check solution for clarity and absence of particulate matter. Monitor hepatic transaminases; blood counts for reduced WBCs, RBCs, and platelets; and fluid intake, weight, presence of edema, and blood pressure to determine fluid balance. Assess abdomen for tenderness. Assess for signs and symptoms of congestive heart failure; monitor for cardiac ischemia. Check visual acuity periodically. Monitor thyroid function tests during long-term therapy. Assess home situation, social support, and need for assistance with activities of daily living that are disrupted by profound fatigue. During administration assess for stridor, dyspnea, chest pain indicative of anaphylaxis. Assess for pregnancy (category C). **INTERVENTION:** Prepare reconstituted injection immediately prior to use: Reconstituted solutions are stable refrigerated for up to 1 month; reconstitute interferon powder with diluent provided; swirl mixture—do not shake; may use glass or plastic infusion/injection reservoirs; use small-gauge needle for injection; rotate injection sites. Institute infection-prevention precautions owing to possible granulocytopenia. Administer fluids as ordered for transient hypotension that usually peaks 2 days after therapy initiation. Use narcotics, hypnotics, and sedative cautiously in conjunction with interferon therapy; administer acetominophen for arthralgias, myalgias, fever, and headache as ordered; have emergency equipment and medications available during administration for rare circumstance of anaphylaxis. **Patient Teaching**—Teach patient reconstitution technique for home administration, self-injection technique, and proper needle disposal. Instruct patient to promote rest with intermittent periods of moderate exercise as fatigue-relieving methods. **EVALUATION:** Change IM to SC if platelets are <50,000/mm³. Baseline and periodic eye exams are performed during chronic therapy. Constantly evaluate patient's neurologic status and coping mechanisms.

Continued on the following page

Table 56–1. ANTITUMOR CYTOKINES, *Continued*

DRUG NAME/ROUTE AND DOSAGE	PHARMACOKINETICS/ DYNAMICS	NURSING IMPLICATIONS
interferon-beta (Betaseron)		
relapsing/remitting multiple sclerosis: 0.25 mg (8 million IU) SC every other day.	**Onset:** slow **Peak:** 1–8 hr **Duration:** NA **½L:** 8 min–4.3 hr **PB:** NA **B:** NA **E:** urine	**ASSESSMENT:** Assess patient's mental status, mood state, and perception of the goal of therapy. Check solution for clarity and absence of particulate matter. Assess home situation, social support, and need for assistance with activities of daily living that are disrupted by profound fatigue. Assess baseline neurologic function, motor activity, and strength prior to initiation of therapy. **INTERVENTION:** Provide safe environment owing to dizziness. Prepare reconstituted injection immediately prior to use; reconstitute interferon powder with diluent provided; swirl mixture—do not shake; may use glass or plastic infusion/injection reservoirs; use small-gauge needle for injection; rotate injection sites; institute infection-prevention precautions; administer acetominophen for arthralgias, myalgias, fever, and headache as ordered; have emergency equipment and medications available during administration for rare circumstance of anaphylaxis. **Patient Teaching**—Same as for interferon-alpha plus: Prepare patient for emotional swings associated with therapy and exacerbated by disease process or its limitations on body function. **EVALUATION:** Assess for improvement of motor function and strength indicative of positive response to therapy. Monitor for severe depression and suicidal tendencies that may reflect toxicity of therapy.
interferon-gamma (Actimmune)		
chronic granulomatous disease: >5 m² body area—50 μg/m² SC (1.5 million IU/m²) 3 times/wk. <5 m² body area—1.5 μg/kg SC 3 times/wk. Unlabeled use with malignancies treated with alpha interferon.	**Onset:** NA **Peak:** 4–7 hr **Duration:** NA **½L:** NA **PB:** NA **B:** NA **E:** urine	Same as for interferon-alpha.
aldesleukin (Proleukin) (interleukin-2)		
High Dose: 600,000 units/kg IV over 15 min q 8 hr for 14 doses, followed by 9 days rest and repeated 14 doses. This cycle of 15 days is given monthly for at least 2 mo and continued as tolerated if response is noted. *Lower Moderate Dose:* ranges from 1,000,000–18,000,000 units SC 3 to 7 times/wk (unlabeled use).	**Onset:** IV, 5 min; SC or IM, NA **Peak:** IV, 13 min; SC or IM, NA **Duration:** IV, 180–240 min; SC or IM, NA **½L:** IV, 85 min; SC or IM, NA **PB:** NA **B:** kidneys **E:** urine	**ASSESSMENT:** Assess patient's mental status, mood state, and perception of the goal of therapy. Check solution for clarity and absence of particulate matter. Monitor hepatic transaminases; blood counts for reduced WBCs, RBCs, and platelets; and fluid intake, weight, presence of edema, and blood pressure to determine fluid balance. Assess abdomen for tenderness. Assess for signs and symptoms of congestive heart failure; monitor for cardiac ischemia. Monitor for hypothyroidism during long-term therapy. Assess home situation, social support, and need for assistance with activities of daily living that are disrupted by profound fatigue. Assess injection sites for redness and induration. During administration assess for stridor, dyspnea, and chest pain, which indicate anaphylaxis. Assess for pregnancy (category C). **INTERVENTION:** Use plastic infusion/injection reservoirs; use small-gauge needle for injection; rotate injection sites. Institute infection-prevention precautions owing to possible granulocytopenia. Administer fluids as ordered for transient hypotension that usually peaks 2 days after therapy initiation. Use narcotics, hypnotics, and sedatives cautiously; administer acetominophen or nonsteroidal anti-inflammatory drugs as ordered for arthralgias, myalgias, fever, or headache; *Do not* coadminister corticosteroids—these may abrogate aldesleukin's beneficial immunologic effects. Apply ice or warmth as the patient prefers for injection site irritation.

Continued on the following page

Table 56–1. ANTITUMOR CYTOKINES, *Continued*		
DRUG NAME/ROUTE AND DOSAGE	**PHARMACOKINETICS/ DYNAMICS**	**NURSING IMPLICATIONS**
aldesleukin (Proleukin) (interleukin-2)		Have emergency equipment and medications available during administration for rare circumstance of anaphylaxis. **Patient Teaching**—Teach patient reconstitution technique for home administration, self-injection technique, proper needle disposal. Instruct patient to promote rest with intermittent periods of moderate exercise as fatigue-relieving methods. **EVALUATION:** Change IM to SC if platelets are <50,000/mm³. Baseline and periodic eye exams are performed during chronic therapy. Constantly evaluate neurologic status and coping mechanisms that may reflect severe depression and neurologic impairment.

NA = not available; WBCs = white blood cells; RBC = red blood cells.

man immune responses. Although harvest of human cytokines has been used, most cytokine therapy is genetically engineered. The engineered product is administered to the host with cancer with the goal of enhancing normal immune defense mechanisms. Antitumor cytokines licensed by the FDA as anticancer agents include interferon and interleukin-2, featured in Table 56–1. Tumor necrosis factor is a cytokine commonly used investigationally. Human growth factors (e.g., erythropoietin, granulocyte colony-stimulating factor, granulocyte-macrophage colony-stimulating factor) are termed cytokines in some texts, but do not have antitumor properties and are described as restorative biotherapy in this text.

Vaccines *Antitumor vaccines* are antibodies specifically engineered to destroy particular tumor antigens. The theoretic rationale for vaccine therapy is that vaccines may (1) be tumor specific, (2) create immunity that should be long lived, (3) be relatively nontoxic, and (4) have the potential to prevent cancer in susceptible populations as well as prevent recurrence if given after removal of the primary tumor (Bach et al., 1993). Human cancers associated with viral infections, including hepatitis B with hepatocellular carcinoma, Epstein-Barr virus and HTLV-I viruses with lymphomas, and certain papilloma (wart) viruses with cervical cancer, are theoretically ideal clinical disorders to be treated with vaccine therapy. If immunization against these viruses were possible, it could significantly decrease the incidence of the associated cancers. Use of tumor-specific antigens is also being studied as possible vaccine therapy for cancers such as B-cell lymphoma, which produces a unique tumor-specific immunoglobulin antigen (Pardoll, 1993). A major problem in vaccine therapy is the identification and purification of relevant antigens to be used in preparing potent vaccines. The only currently available antitumor vaccine is bacillus Calmette-Guérin (BCG), featured in Table 56–2.

Monoclonal Antibodies Monoclonal antibodies are antibodies derived from the fusion of an antibody-producing cell such as a B lymphocyte and another cell such as a cancer cell. The hybrid cell is capable of producing a continuous supply of antibody. These antibodies are specific and useful in the identification of antigens on

certain viruses, in blood and tissue typing, and in the diagnosis of infectious diseases or identification of tumor antigens. Monoclonal antibody research has been targeted to generate human antitumor antibodies in cancers such as multiple myeloma, breast, colorectal, malignant melanoma, and lymphomas. Monoclonal antibodies licensed by the FDA are muromonab-CD3 (Orthoclone OKT3) (discussed in Chapter 60) and satumomab pendetide (OncoScint CR/OV), featured in Table 56–3.

Adoptive Biotherapy

Adoptive biotherapy is based on the assumption that tumor-associated antigens exist that can elicit an autologous antitumor response in the host (patient). *Autologous* is a term that relates to products derived from a patient for use by that same patient. In adoptive biotherapy, active antitumor cells are infused into the host with cancer. Cells may originate from the host (tumor vaccines, tumor infiltrating lymphocytes), other humans, or an animal donor (monoclonal antibodies).

One technique of adoptive biotherapy uses autologous tumor cells. Tumor is harvested from the patient, and the lymphocytes within the tumor are cloned and nurtured, then reinfused. Clinical trials using the patient's own genetically altered tumor cells are termed *tumor infiltrating lymphocytes (TILs).*

Another method confers passive immunity by incubating donor lymphocytes with tumor cells from the patient or a cytokine such as interleukin-2 to sensitize the lymphocytes. The sensitized lymphocytes are then reinfused into the patient. It is hoped that the patient's immunologic defense system will accept and use these new immune cells.

Restorative Biotherapy

Restorative biotherapy uses agents that increase the patient's immune response, especially the number of mature, functioning leukocytes. Substances that augment the patient's immune system in this manner are called immunologic stimulants or *hematopoietic growth factors.*

Table 56–2. VACCINES

DRUG NAME/ROUTE AND DOSAGE	PHARMACOKINETICS/ DYNAMICS	NURSING IMPLICATIONS
bacillus Calmette-Guérin (BCG)		
nonspecific anticancer agent **Adults:** *Intradermal*–0.1 mL injected intradermally or by scarification technique weekly (rarely used today) *Intrabladder*–81 mg reconstituted according to manufacturer recommendations instilled intrabladder and retained for 2 hr once a week for 6 wk **Infants and Children:** 0.2–0.3 mL intradermally for one injection	**Onset:** NA **Peak:** NA **Duration:** NA **½L:** NA **PB:** NA **B:** NA **E:** NA	**ASSESSMENT:** Assess patient's perception of goal of therapy, baseline and ongoing skin integrity, and fever patterns and his or her association to treatments. During administration assess for stridor, dyspnea, chest pain indicative of anaphylaxis. Assess for pregnancy (category C). **INTERVENTION:** *Do not* use alcohol to prepare skin as it can kill organisms. Apply antipruritic cream to site if irritated and itchy. Apply cold compress to injection site if painful. Administer acetaminophen as ordered for fever, chills, or other generalized aches; have emergency equipment and medications available during administration for rare circumstance of anaphylaxis. Refrigerate drug and protect it from light. **Patient Teaching—** Remind patient not to scratch or use alcohol-containing lotions on injection sites and to avoid alcohol ingestion. Teach patient or significant other to measure test sites if applicable. Teach reportable symptoms after bladder instillation—severe cramping, hematuria. **EVALUATION:** Read intradermal sites and observe scarification sites periodically for induration or injection. Avoid concomitant administration of isoniazid, which may inhibit BCG multiplication. Evaluate tumor size every 8–12 wk during therapy.

NA = not available.

Growth factors are glycoprotein hormones that enhance the production rate, differentiation, maturation, and functional ability of hematopoietic cells. They are subclassified as lineage restricted (acting on one cell type), or multilineage (affecting more than one cell type). The three hematopietic growth factors that are licensed for management of cancer- or AIDS-therapy–induced bone marrow suppression include: epoetin alfa (erythropoietin), granulocyte colony-stimulating factor (G-CSF), and granulocyte-macrophage colony-stimulating factor (GM-CSF), featured in Table 56–4. Other agents approved for investigational use are macrophage colony-stimulating factor (M-CSF), IL-3 (multi-CSF), and PIXY-321 (GM-CSF and IL-3 together).

Cytomodulatory Biotherapy

Cytomodulatory biotherapy includes agents that cause increased recognition of tumor-associated antigens and histocompatibility (HLA) antigens on the surface of tu-

Table 56–3. MONOCLONAL ANTIBODIES

DRUG NAME/ROUTE AND DOSAGE	PHARMACOKINETICS/ DYNAMICS	NURSING IMPLICATIONS
satumomab penditide (OncoScint)		
	Onset: 5 min **Peak:** NA **Duration:** NA **½L:** NA **PB:** NA **B:** NA **E:** NA	**ASSESSMENT:** Check solution for clarity and absence of particulate matter. During administration assess for stridor, dyspnea, chest pain indicative of anaphylaxis. **INTERVENTION:** Premedicate with acetominophen for fever; have emergency equipment and medications available during administration for rare circumstance of anaphylaxis. **Patient Teaching—**Teach patient reason for administration of drug. Instruct patient to use acetominophen for persistent fever. Teach patient reportable symptoms of delayed allergic reaction—dyspnea, wheezing, chest tightness. **EVALUATION:** Success of monoclonal detection of tumor.

NA = not available.

Table 56–4. HEMATOPOIETIC GROWTH FACTORS

DRUG NAME/ROUTE AND DOSAGE	PHARMACOKINETICS/ DYNAMICS	NURSING IMPLICATIONS
granulocyte colony-stimulating factor (filgrastim) (G-CSF) (Neupogen)		
neutropenia due to antineoplastic chemotherapy, antiretroviral or ganciclovir therapy, myelodysplastic syndrome **Adults:** 5 µg/kg per day SC or IV as a single daily injection. May be increased in increments of 5 µg/kg for each chemotherapy cycle. Administered for up to 2 wk or until the WBC count reaches 10,000 cells/mm³.	**Onset:** NA **Peak:** SC, 8 hr; IV, 2 hr **Duration:** SC, 4 days; IV, 4 days **½L:** 210–230 min **PB:** NA **B:** NA **E:** NA	**ASSESSMENT:** Assess for hypersensitivity to *Escherichia coli* products, evidence of infection, baseline CBC and platelet count. Assess for pregnancy (category C). **INTERVENTION:** Store in refrigerator; use at room temperature; swirl mixture—do not shake; may use glass or plastic infusion/injection reservoirs; use different needles for preparation and injection; use small-gauge needle (25 gauge) to inject SC; rotate injection sites; if dose exceeds >1 mL, consider using two injection sites. Implement infection-prevention precautions until WBC has improved. Implement oral care regimen immediately to reduce risk of severity of stomatitis. Provide antiemetics or small frequent feeding for possible nausea and vomiting. **Patient Teaching**—Teach patient reconstitution technique for home administration, self-injection technique. Advise patient to plan for scarves or wig as needed for adverse effect of alopecia. Instruct patient to report fever, chills, severe bone pain, weakness, and pain at injection site. **EVALUATION:** Monitor CBC with differential for response to treatment.
granulocyte-macrophage colony-stimulating factor (GM-CSF) (sargramostim) (Leukine) (Prokine)		
myeloid reconstitution after autologous bone marrow transplant **Adults:** 250 µg/m² IV over 2–4 hr every day for 21 days, starting several hours after bone marrow reinfusion and not less than 24 hr after last chemotherapy.	**Onset:** Immediate **Peak:** 2 hr **Duration:** 6 hr **½L:** 12–17 min **PB:** NA **B:** NA **E:** NA	**ASSESSMENT:** Assess for evidence of infection. Assess baseline CBC and platelet count. Assess for pregnancy (category C). **INTERVENTION:** Reconstitute with 1 mL sterile water for injection; do not mix with any solution other than sterile water or 0.9% normal saline solution; use within 6 hr of reconstitution; use at room temperature; swirl mixture—do not shake; do not use an in-line filter. Implement infection-prevention precautions until WBC has improved; implement oral care regimen immediately to reduce risk or severity of stomatitis; provide antiemetics or small frequent feeding for possible nausea and vomiting. **Patient Teaching**—Teach patient reconstitution technique for home administration, self-injection technique. Advise patient to plan for scarves or wig as needed for adverse effect of alopecia. Instruct patient to report fever, chills, severe bone pain, weakness, and pain at injection site. **EVALUATION:** Monitor CBC with differential for response to treatment.

NA = not available; HCT = hematocrit; CBC = complete blood count; WBC = white blood count.

mor cells. This category of agents includes natural products such as cyclosporine and tacrolimus used as immunosuppressive agents after solid organ transplantation. These agents exert a variety of immunoproliferative or immunomodulatory functions that are thought to enhance the patient's existing immune defenses. Anticancer agents classed as cytomodulatory include levamisole hydrochloride and retinoids. Levamisole hydrochloride (Ergamisol), featured in Table 56–5, is the only agent currently licensed for use.

Gene Manipulative Biotherapy

Human gene therapy involves a biologic technique to insert a functioning gene into the patient's cells to reverse a defective gene or add functions to an existing cell (Wheeler, 1995). Gene therapy has been used investigationally to correct enzyme deficiencies or augment intrinsic antitumor immune responses. This technology is not yet able to remove dysfunctional genes or limit overproduction of biologic substances. Gene therapy is delivered

Table 56–5. CYTOMODULATORY AGENTS

DRUG NAME/ROUTE AND DOSAGE	PHARMACOKINETICS/ DYNAMICS	NURSING IMPLICATIONS
levamisole hydrochloride (Ergamisol)		
metastatic colorectal cancer	**Onset:** varies	**ASSESSMENT:** Assess CBC, WBC differential, platelets, electrolytes, and hepatic transaminases prior to therapy and periodically during therapy. Assess for elevated phenytoin levels if indicated. During administration assess for stridor, dyspnea, chest pain indicative of anaphylaxis. Assess for pregnancy (category C).
Adults: 50 mg PO q 8 hr for 3 days starting 7–30 days after surgery, then combined with a 5-day fluorouracil (5-FU) regimen beginning 21–34 days postsurgery.	**Peak:** 1.5–2 hr **Duration:** 3–4 hr **½L:** 12–17 min **PB:** NA **B:** liver **E:** urine, feces	
maintenance for postsurgical treatment or with metastatic disease		**INTERVENTION:** Administer antidiarrheal agents as ordered. Implement oral hygiene measures at onset of therapy. Administer acetaminophen as needed for arthralgias, myalgias, fever, or headache. Have emergency equipment and medications available during administration for rare circumstance of anaphylaxis.
Adults: 50 mg PO q 8 hr for 3 days every 2 wk along with fluorouracil (5-FU) given once per week. May be given alone after chemotherapy regimen is complete.		**Patient Teaching—**Teach patient to avoid alcohol; concomitant administration causes disulfiram-like reaction. Advise patient to use birth control as this agent is fetal toxic. Instruct patient to report severe diarrhea with dehydration or stomatitis preventing oral intake.
		EVALUATION: Evaluate tumor size every 8–12 wk during therapy.

NA = not available; CBC = complete blood count; WBC = white blood cell.

by one of two methods: in vivo gene therapy delivers the gene directly to the targeted cell in the body, and ex vivo gene therapy removes cells from the body and returns replacement genes in a retroviral vector. Specific biotherapeutic agents utilized in gene therapy are not clearly identified at this time.

INTERFERONS

The term "interferon" does not refer to a single substance, but rather to an entire class (group) of substances classified as lymphokines. Interferons were first discovered by virologists Alick Isaacs and Jean Lindenmann in 1957, but were not developed until recombinant DNA technology in the mid-1970s enabled cancer researchers to produce large quantities of cloned interferons. Interferon (IFN) was the first biologic response modifier licensed for cancer therapy. The current nomenclature of interferons is based on their antiviral activity, and they are labeled as interferon-alfa, -beta, and -gamma. Each subtype of interferon has a different stimulus or source: (1) Interferon-alpha is produced by leukocytes after exposure to B-cell antigens or foreign protein, (2) interferon-beta is produced by fibroblasts after exposure to viruses or foreign proteins, and (3) interferon-gamma is produced by T lymphocytes after immunologic stimulation by specific antigens or interleukin-2. These differing mechanisms of stimulation result in minor variations in indications.

ACTION

Interferon directly inhibits cell growth by inducing changes in the cell cycle, inhibiting cellular differentiation, and interfering with oncogene expression. It brings the cells from the resting phase (G_0) of the cell cycle into the growth phase (G_1) of the cell cycle, thereby causing them to be killed. It is hoped that the combination of interferon therapy with chemotherapy can result in augmentation of cell kill and enhance response rates against many cancers.

USES

Interferons are primarily used as antitumor agents; however, their antiviral effects are well known, and their use with venereal warts and viral hepatitis are in the investigational stages. Interferons are often administered with chemotherapy for a proposed synergistic antitumor effect.

CONTRAINDICATIONS AND PRECAUTIONS

Interferons are administered cautiously to individuals with hepatic disease or neurologic impairment because the interferons themselves are potentially hepatotoxic and neurotoxic and may worsen these conditions.

ADVERSE EFFECTS

The adverse effects of all subtypes of interferon are proportionate to the dose given, with adverse and toxic effects increasing significantly as the dose increases. Interferon-associated adverse effects can be acute or chronic. Common acute adverse effects include flulike symptoms of fever, chills, mylagia, fatigue, and headache. These effects tend to diminish with continued therapy. The chronic adverse effects are the dose-limiting effects and include lability, chronic fatigue, and depression. Unusual but possibly life-threatening effects are hepatic insufficiency, dysrhythmias, coma, and seizures.

At present, no undesirable interactions with interferons have been identified.

○ **Interferon-alpha** (Roferon-a, Intron-a, Wellferon) is currently available in three commercial formulations. Two are alpha-2 interferons: Roferon-a and Intron-a. Both preparations are different clones of the same interferon. Interferons are subtyped into letters and numbers based on the cloned source. The alpha-2a was called leukocyte-a interferon in earlier nomenclature, and this is now Roferon-a. Alpha-2b was called interferon-alpha2 and is now Intron-a. The only difference in these two preparations is a single amino acid substitution. Although each company claims that this different amino acid makes their product more effective, the literature supports that both substances work equally (Moldawer and Figlin, 1995). Wellferon is the first alpha interferon of lymphoblastoid origin, named alpha n1. All alpha interferons have the same therapeutic activity and adverse effects.

USES Alpha interferons are licensed for the treatment of hairy cell leukemia, myelocytic leukemia, renal cell carcinoma, AIDS-related Kaposi's sarcoma, chronic hepatitis, and as postsurgical adjuvant therapy in malignant melanoma. In hairy cell leukemia, there is a 5% complete response rate, but 80% to 100% of treated patients have long-term remission with interferon-alpha therapy. Other tumors treated with interferon-alpha in combination with other biologic or chemotherapeutic agents have response rates varying from 10% to 60% (Moldawer and Figlin, 1995). The use of interferon-alpha in autologous bone marrow transplantation to induce graft-versus-host response and enhance graft-versus-tumor response is investigational at present.

○ **Interferon-beta** (Betaseron, Avonex) is similar in structure and mechanism of action to interferon-alpha, and they share the same receptor on their cells; however, interferon-beta has proven more effective in the treatment of relapsing-remitting multiple sclerosis. Interferon-beta's ability to inhibit interferon-gamma may be the mechanism by which this biologic agent successfully reduces exacerbation rates and severity in patients with multiple sclerosis (INF-b Multiple Sclerosis Study Group, 1993). Avonex is a nonsynthetic interferon-beta also now available for investigational use in multiple sclerosis. Antibodies to interferon-beta are thought to be responsible for treatment failures.

○ **Interferon-gamma** (Actimmune) is similar in clinical activity to both interferon-alpha and -beta. Interferon-gamma originates in a different cell line, has different cell surface receptors than other interferons, and is a more potent stimulator of macrophages. These differences cause interferon-gamma to have a synergistic effect when given with either of these other interferons. If interferon-alpha and -beta were given together, they would have to compete for the same receptor in order to kill a disease cell.

▼ **CLINICAL ALERT**

Interferon-gamma also shows greater antiproliferative activity than other interferons and is more likely to produce myelosuppression. For unknown reasons, interferon-gamma more often produces hypotension (Moldawer and Figlin, 1995).

USES This subtype of interferon is used to treat chronic granulomatous disease and has modest activity in renal cell carcinoma.

INTERLEUKINS

There are at least twenty-two identified biologically active T-lymphocyte cytokines called interleukins. Interleukins have multiple biologic functions involving immunomodulation. They are responsible for many of the integrated immune activities of the body. Interleukins are designated numerically in the order in which they were identified. Interleukins 1, 2, 3, 4, and 6 have been used in clinical practice; however, only interleukin-2 (aldesleukin, Proleukin) is FDA licensed for use.

○ **Interleukin-2** (aldesleukin, IL-2, Proleukin) is a cytokine secreted by antigen-activated T lymphocytes that enhances lymphokine-activated killer T cells and natural killer cells.

ACTION IL-2 stimulates activated lymphocytes, induces interferon-gamma secretion, and enhances the generation of both LAK cells and natural killer cells. Interleukin-2 regulates its own receptor expression, thereby causing production of more IL-2 via a feedback mechanism. Interleukin-2 also supports the growth of B and T lymphocytes and macrophages. These actions stimulate hematopoiesis, enhance antibody recognition and destruction of foreign proteins, and augment the host anti-tumor responses.

USES Aldesleukin (Proleukin) is FDA-licensed for treatment of metastatic renal cell carcinoma; however, it is used extensively in treatment of malignant melanoma, lymphoma, and colorectal carcinoma. Other potential treatment indications include chronic hepatitis, preoperatively for colorectal cancer, post bone marrow transplantation, and for stabilization of T-helper counts in HIV disease. Some studies in progress combine interleukin-2 with chemotherapeutic agents, LAK cells, or tumor infiltrating lymphocytes.

ADVERSE EFFECTS The adverse effects seen in IL-2 are similar to those seen with interferon and other biologic response modifiers.

▼ **CLINICAL ALERT**

Adverse effects of aldesleukin are dose and schedule related, but may vary greatly from one individual to another. Adverse effects are cumulative during the therapy cycle. More severe effects usually occur in the longer treatment cycles of high-dose therapy, but may not occur at all with the first few days of high-dose therapy.

Acute adverse effects of IL-2 are fever, nausea, vomiting, violent chills, hypotension, and altered mental status.

High doses of IL-2 can cause dyspnea, ventricular dysrhythmias, supraventricular tachycardias, and can even lead to myocardial infarction. Chronic adverse effects of IL-2 therapy are fatigue, anorexia, and depression. Interleukin-2 can also cause arthralgias, myalgias, diarrhea, skin rash, thrombocytopenia, oliguria, and elevated hepatic transaminases.

TUMOR NECROSIS FACTOR

In 1975, Carswell and associates discovered a factor able to induce hemorrhagic necrosis, growth inhibition, or regression in a variety of human and mouse tumors, hence its name tumor necrosis factor (TNF). It was later discovered that the major source of TNF is macrophage cells, and its use has grown since the development of recombinant technology. TNF mediates a number of immunologic events, suggesting that it plays an important role in host response to inflammation as well as tumors.

The exact role of TNF is not completely understood at present; however, several potential actions are suggested. Tumor necrosis factor stimulates macrophage-mediated antitumor activity, endothelial cells, and granulocytes. Research has shown that TNF-induced effector molecules are responsible for the cytotoxic activities of natural cytotoxic (NC) cells that may be important in natural immunity. These cells can cause tumor cell lysis, but also initiate the inflammatory cascade. If in enhancing natural immune functions, the individual's natural immune system is better able to recognize malignant cells as abnormal or different, then the role of TNF will be defined. There also seems to be synergy between TNF and interferon-gamma. As with other biologic response modifiers, the major use of this substance in the future may not be as a single agent, but rather as part of a combination therapy against cancer.

VACCINES

○ **Bacillus Calmette-Guérin** (BCG), a bacterium isolated in 1910 at the Pasteur Institute by Calmette and Guérin, is a live *attenuated organism* (microorganism or cell that has been rendered less capable of producing disease). It was clinically tested in 1921 for use as a tuberculosis vaccine. Its use in cancer therapy did not come until the 1960s, when it became the first anticancer biotherapeutic agent available.

ACTION The exact mechanism by which BCG achieves its antitumor effects is not completely understood, but it is believed to cause a nonspecific immunostimulant effect.

USES Although studied with many different cancers, it has demonstrated significant antitumor activity only in the treatment of bladder cancer. Repeated contact of the bladder mucosa with instilled BCG solution augments the immune system to produce antitumor effects. Prolonged disease-free intervals in bladder cancer patients also occur with intravesical BCG therapy with or without concurrent intradermal BCG.

When intending to administer BCG by injection, do not prepare the skin with alcohol, as this will destroy the live organisms present in the vaccine. The vaccine is protected from light when stored and only the supplied diluent used for reconstitution.

Diluents with chemical preservatives, such as bacteriostatic water or normal saline, are not used to reconstitute BCG vaccine. The number of viable organisms present in each vial varies among suppliers and lots within the same supplier's stock. Because of this biologic variability, doses are commonly listed in acceptable ranges. Bacillus Calmette-Guérin dosage for cancer therapy is 3×10^7 organisms. Adjustments in dose can be made by serial dilutions from the accompanying vial of diluent solution. The only known drug interaction with BCG is with the antitubercular drug isoniazid (INH). INH inhibits multiplication of BCG organisms and should therefore not be used concomitantly.

ADVERSE EFFECTS Side effects seen in BCG therapy depend on the route of administration used. Most patients experience influenza-like symptoms within 12 to 24 hours of therapy, which subside within 48 hours. Intralesional administration of BCG can cause abscess formation. Rarely, a generalized infection can occur following BCG administration. Anaphylaxis and death, although rare, may also occur. Because BCG is a live bacterium, it should not be administered to patients who are severely immunocompromised.

MONOCLONAL ANTIBODIES

○ **Satumomab penditide** (OncoScint) is one of two licensed biologic agents in this class (the other, muromonab-CD3, used to treat acute allograft rejection, is discussed in Chapter 60). When attached to radiolabeled 5 mCi of indium in 111 chloride, satumomab penditide attaches to malignant cells and produces radioluscence. It is used to detect extrahepatic metastases and malignant recurrence in patients with ovarian or colorectal cancer (Oncology Nursing Society, 1995; and Dujulio and Liles, 1995). Its adverse effects are usually minimal and similar to other vaccines. In addition to itching, fever, or chills, rare instances of severe hypersensitivity have occurred.

HEMATOPOIETIC GROWTH FACTORS

Although over ten hematopoietic growth factors have been identified, the only three are in use: **epoetin alfa (Epogen, EPO, erythropoietin, Procrit)**, **granulocyte colony-stimulating factor (G-CSF, filgrastim, Neupogen)**, and **granulocyte-macrophage colony-stimulating factor (GM-CSF, sargramostim, Leukine)** (see Table 56–4). Others currently in clinical trials include macrophage colony-stimulating factor (M-CSF), interleukin-3 (IL-3), stem cell factor (SCF), and a combination of G-CSF and IL-3 called PIXY321 (GM-CSF fusion protein).

ACTION

The hematopoietic growth factors regulate hematopoiesis by stimulating an orderly and specific duplication of bone marrow stem cells into mature leukocytes (white blood cells), erythrocytes (red blood cells), or thrombocytes (platelets). Growth factors act upon immature cells called progenitor cells of a defined target-cell lineage to enhance maturation and differentiation of those cells. This increases the circulating pool of cells and their subsequent activity within the body. Growth factors enhance oxygen-carrying capacity with increased erythrocyte levels, increase the individual's ability to fight infection when leukocytes are affected, and improve clotting functions when platelets are stimulated.

USES

Growth factors have been used in various conditions that are the result of inadequate number or function of the hematopietic cells. The first licensed use for growth factors was the use of erythropoietin in managing renal failure-induced anemia. It is now common to see erythropoietin ordered in patients with anemia caused by chemotherapy, radiation therapy, or antiretroviral therapy. Medication-induced leukopenia is managed with G-CSF or GM-CSF. Criteria used to choose between these two CSFs may include the depth and length of the leukopenia. Growth factors are also used in autologous peripheral blood progenitor cell transplantation (PBPCT) to mobilize commited stem cells and enhance the peripheral circulating pool. These cells are then pheresed and reinfused after marrow-suppressing therapy. The use of growth factors after autologous and allogenic bone marrow transplantation has recently increased, as studies have shown no increase in graft-versus-host disease or relapse of leukocytic malignancies.

CONTRAINDICATIONS AND PRECAUTIONS

The literature still recommends cautious use of growth factors in hematopoietic malignancies owing to the potential stimulation of malignant cell lines. Many investigators do not believe this concern is valid when they are being used for chemotherapy-induced leukopenia. No interactions are known at this time.

○ **Epoetin alfa** (Epogen, EPO, erythropoietin, Procrit) is a recombinant form of the naturally occurring substance that stimulates red blood cell production. Its use has reduced transfusions in many patients with renal disease and in those with chemotherapy-induced or antiretroviral therapy-induced anemia. For more information see Chapter 38.

○ **Granulocyte colony-stimulating factor** (G-CSF, filgrastim, Neupogen) is a lineage-restricted growth factor product of macrophages and endothelial cells. It enhances neutrophil differentiation and margination, reducing the incidence or severity of bacterial infections. It is used to abrogate the effects of drug-induced neutropenia in patients with nonmyeloid malignancies.

CONTRAINDICATIONS AND PRECAUTIONS G-CSF and GM-CSF should not be given to patients with active myeloid malignancy, for their effects on malignant cell growth are unclear.

ADVERSE EFFECTS The most frequent adverse effect of G-CSF is medullary bone pain. Other adverse effects include excessive leukocytosis, and pain and redness at the subcutaneous site.

○ **Granulocyte-macrophage colony-stimulating factor** (GM-CSF, sargramostim, Leukine) is a multilineage hematopoietic stimulant that enhances maturation of both granulocytes and monocytes/macrophages. The reported additional benefit of macrophage stimulation may be in their potential action against fungi. The action of this CSF is similar to G-CSF, but it is used more in those with prolonged bone marrow aplasia, preexisting fungal infection, or bone marrow transplantation.

ADVERSE EFFECTS The most frequent adverse effects are related to the following systems: musculoskeletal (bone pain, myalgias, arthralgias), central nervous (headache), and dermatologic (rash, itching). Other adverse effects include dyspnea, fever, chills, peripheral edema, pericardial effusion, and transient supraventricular tachycardia. A first dose reaction—flushing, hypotension, syncope, weakness—may also occur.

CYTOMODULATORY AGENTS

○ **Levamisole hydrochloride** (Ergamisol) restores immune function, stimulating antibody formation and T-cell activation and proliferation; increases neutrophil mobility; and potentiates monocyte and macrophage functions, including phagocytosis and chemotaxis. Levamisole also inhibits alkaline phosphatase and cholinergic activity. The only current indicated use for levamisole is in combination therapy with 5-fluorouracil (5-FU) to treat Duke's stage C colon cancer. The exact mechanism of synergy in this regimen is unknown.

ADVERSE EFFECTS Adverse effects seen in patients taking levamisole include the following: nausea, vomiting, stomatitis, diarrhea, abdominal pain, agranulocytosis, thrombocytopenia, skin rash, alopecia, dizziness, headache, arthralgias, myalgias, fatigue, fever, and altered sensations of taste.

▼ CLINICAL ALERT

Agranulocytosis is a potentially life-threatening effect. A flulike syndrome may or may not be a predictive prodromal sign of the agranulocytosis, so patients should report such symptoms promptly.

INTERACTIONS Ingestion of alcoholic beverages while on levamisole may result in a disulfram-like reaction. Patients taking levamisole and 5-FU who are also on phenytoin may experience elevated serum phenytoin levels. Such patients should be monitored and phenytoin dosages adjusted relative to serum drug levels.

USING THE NURSING PROCESS

The science of cancer biotherapy is still in the developmental stage. Nursing-care efforts center on educating the patient, family members, and staff members about the immune process, as well as assessing patients prior to and throughout therapy. Planning and implementation of nursing care depend on the results of assessment. Because of the investigational nature of most biotherapy, scrupulous recordkeeping is essential to achieve valid data interpretation. The nurse is also responsible for understanding the method of administration, usual dosages, mechanism of drug action, and potential adverse effects of each drug administered.

ASSESSMENT

Detailed information on the assessment of the cancer patient is included in Chapter 55, Antineoplastic Chemotherapy. Nursing process examples for the patient receiving cancer biotherapy are summarized in Table 56–6.

- During the initial assessment, and with each subsequent visit, carefully assess the patient's psychologic and emotional status. Remember to include the patient's family in the assessment.
- Delayed hypersensitivity skin testing is sometimes a precursor to biotherapy. Prepare and/or administer these agents and assess the resultant skin reactions, as ordered. Careful, accurate descriptions of local reactions including measurements, diagrams, and photographs are essential.
- Assess for adverse effects that are unique to biotherapy rather than chemotherapy: fever and chills, arthralgias, myalgias, and profound fatigue.
- Assess fever patterns and associated symptoms to aid in differentiation between biotherapy toxicity and complications of infection.
- Skin reactions to biotherapeutic drugs are common. Perform regular skin assessments at regular intervals throughout the patient's therapy.
- Assess for the physical limitations and feelings of depression that may have a significant negative impact on the patient's quality of life. Assess the patient's performance status, desired activity level, and importance of these variables to the patient. Biotherapy requires many follow-up visits to the hospital or clinic, reminding patients of their cancer diagnosis.
- Assess insurance coverage for home or outpatient therapy. Reimbursement for biotherapy is inconsistent and may depend on the setting in which it is administered.

NURSING DIAGNOSIS

Following careful assessment of the patient and family, the nurse makes nursing diagnoses centered on the patient's nutritional, psychologic, rest, elimination, and pain status, as well as on objective observational findings. Typical nursing diagnoses for the patient requiring biotherapeutic agents include Altered Thermoregulation, Pain, and Fatigue.

PLANNING AND INTERVENTION

- Schedule biotherapy around other therapy such as radiation treatments, chemotherapy, and/or surgery to maximize immune function and minimize adverse effects.
- Use a biologic agent specific toxicity grading scale to optimize the accuracy of adverse effect observations.
- Use universal precautions to administer biotherapeutic agents. Biotherapeutic agents are not considered biohazards like many other antineoplastic agents (Oncology Nursing Society, 1995).
- Administer biotherapeutic agents via intradermal, scarification, multiple puncture, intralesional, intraabdominal, and intravenous techniques. The nurse does not inject drugs intralesionally or intrapleurally.
- Biotherapeutic drugs may contain live organisms and must be protected from heat.
- When preparing biotherapeutic solutions for injection, use only the diluent provided. Use of other solutions for dilution may be incompatible with the vaccine or render it nonviable. Sterile water and normal saline with preservatives both contain small amounts of alcohol, which can kill the organisms in the BCG vaccine or inactivate cytokines.
- When giving BCG vaccine, alcohol is not used for skin preparation, as its presence on the skin surface can kill vaccine organisms. Acetone is effective for skin preparation.
- When mixing the drugs preparatory to drawing up solutions, do not agitate the vial. Gently roll the vial between the hands to achieve a uniform dilution. Excessive agitation of the vial can damage vaccine organisms.

EVALUATION

- Evaluate patient/family compliance with the therapeutic regimen.
- Evaluate patient/family understanding of health teaching given and coping mechanisms to determine if successful adjustment is being achieved.
- Adverse effects experienced by patients receiving biotherapy are usually limited to flulike symptoms such as fever, chills, or malaise. Patients who are successfully taught about which symptoms require the prompt contacting of their physician will experience less severe sequelae.
- Patients receiving biotherapy for the first time who may have experienced chemotherapy side effects should be reassured that adverse effects can be abrogated.
- Remind outpatients *not* to take aspirin or other over-the-counter medications that may contain aspirin or drink alcoholic beverages during the treatment period, as these substances have immunosuppressive properties.

Table 56–6. NURSING PROCESS FOR PATIENT REQUIRING BIOTHERAPEUTIC AGENTS

Assessment

Assess body temperature every 4 hr.
Assess warmth and flushing of skin.
Assess other body system responses to fever: tachycardia, low mean blood pressure, oliguria, mental status changes.
Assess diaphoresis.
Assess presence of chills.
Assess presence, location, quantity, and quality of pain.
Assess actions that relieve discomfort.
Assess normal sleep, activity, and rest patterns.
Assess severity and extent of activity tolerance.
Assess for evidence of respiratory compromise, weak muscle tone, or cardiovascular signs of exertion with activity.

Nursing Diagnosis: Ineffective Thermoregulation

RELATED TO: Fever.
AS EVIDENCED BY: Elevated temperature, diaphoretic.

Desired Outcomes/Evaluation Criteria

Patient is afebrile, even after biotherapy administration. Discomforts accompanying fever are minimized. Complications of fevers, such as cardiovascular failure, vascular volume depletion, and cognitive dysfunction, are minimized by nursing measures.

Nursing Actions	Rationale
Monitor body temperature throughout therapy, establish a fever pattern associated with biotherapy. Determine the most accurate method of obtaining these temperature based on individual patient variables.	Most biotherapy regimens have established fever pattern that is predictable and can be abrogated with medication. Fevers may also reduce in frequency and severity with prolonged therapy.
Abrogate fever with antipyretics as ordered—usually acetominophen 650 mg before and every 4 hr after intermittent biotherapy doses, or around the clock with continuous biotherapy.	Reducing fever with antipyretics may enhance quality of life.
Premedicate with antipyretics such as acetominophen or nonsteroidal anti-inflammatory agents as ordered.	Fevers may be totally abrogated with antipyretic premedication.
Keep room comfortable temperature. Control environmental or extraneous sources of fever such as warm air from low-air-loss beds, overheating of mechanical ventilator circuits, and so on.	External sources of fever can worsen this already prevalent adverse effect.
Encourage tepid fluids.	Moderate-temperature fluids will neither warm or enhance chills. Fluids are needed to reduce risk of vascular volume depletion.
Administer biotherapy agent on schedule so that fevers do not interfere with sleep cycle.	Biotherapy agents scheduled appropriately should not interfere with rest and sleep.
Monitor for possible cardiovascular changes that may occur with fevers—low diastolic and mean blood pressures, tachycardia, congestive heart failure.	Vasodilation and increased metabolism that occur with biotherapy fevers can increase workload on heart and lead to cardiovascular compromise.
Supply dry sheets after diaphoretic episodes. Retake temperature after diaphoresis.	After diaphoresis, body temperature is usually dropping. Wet sheets enhance chills. Diaphoresis may deplete circulating blood volume and cause orthostasis or hypotension.

Nursing Diagnosis: Pain

RELATED TO: Fever, chills, headache, myalgias, arthralgias, bone pain, injection site tenderness.
AS EVIDENCED BY: Facial expression change in vital signs.

Desired Outcomes/Evaluation Criteria

Patient verbalizes effective measures to control discomforts associated with biotherapy.

Nursing Actions	Rationale
Administer acetaminophen, nonsteroidal anti-inflammatory agent, or more potent anagesic as ordered for biotherapy-related discomfort.	Discomfort is reduced if fever severity is controlled. Many antipyretics also have analgesic properties.
Use blankets (warmed when possible) to maintain comfort during chills associated with fever.	Warm blankets increase patient comfort during chills.

Table 56–6. NURSING PROCESS FOR PATIENT REQUIRING BIOTHERAPEUTIC AGENTS, *Continued*

Nursing Actions	**Rationale**
Encourage patient to find positions of comfort, using pillows and blankets as needed.	Patients often reduce their own discomfort by established positions, reducing weight or stressors to painful area.
Administer cool or warm compresses as helpful to aching areas. Cool compresses may be more helpful for headaches, and warmth may be more helpful for joints.	Topical heat and cold reduce pain in many situations.
Quiet, darkened room may be helpful in abrogating headache.	Reduces the photosensitivity component of headaches and may enhance rest.
Relaxation or mental imagery may reduce discomfort of many symptoms.	Relaxation therapy has been proven to reduce sensation of discomfort and increase tolerance.
Offer diversional therapy such as games or television to take patient's mind off discomfort.	May distract patient from focusing on uncomfortable symptoms.
Moderate activities to tolerance, being careful not to encourage excessive immobility.	Activity management reduces actions that precipitate or worsen discomfort for that individual.

Nursing Diagnosis: Fatigue	**Desired Outcomes/Evaluation Criteria**
RELATED TO: Adverse effects of biotherapy agents. **AS EVIDENCED BY:** Inability to perform daily activities.	Fatigue does not interfere with patient's physical or social activities to extent of negatively influencing quality of life. Patient develops positive coping mechanisms for handling therapy-related fatigue.

Nursing Actions	**Rationale**
Plan biotherapy administration schedules to enhance normal sleep-wake cycles	Uninterrupted sleep may help reduce severity of biotherapy-induced fatigue.
Teach patient to monitor physiologic responses to activity: taking pulse, monitoring respiratory pattern.	This action helps patient to moderate activity level prior to onset of fatigue.
Teach cognitive coping strategies for handling fatigue.	Effective coping strategies help reduce associated depression and help patient to see effect as temporary.
Arrange more stressful activities after prolonged rest periods.	This is time when patient has greatest reserve energy.
Encourage socialization with less physical exertion—e.g., use of wheelchairs or recliners.	Positive recognition of physical limitations without altering socialization demonstrates positive coping mechanisms.
Provide written instructions with all verbal ones.	Patients with fatigue may have difficulty concentrating on instructions or remembering them.
Reinforce that fatigue during biotherapy is common adverse effect and does not indicate possible tumor progression.	Many patients experience fatigue with tumor progression and may misinterpret fatigue as related to tumor rather than treatment.

Other Suggested Nursing Diagnoses: Knowledge Deficit; Decreased Cardiac Output; Risk for Impaired Skin Integrity; Altered Nutrition, less than body requirements; Urinary Elimination, Altered Patterns; Diarrhea; Ineffective Individual Coping; and Altered Thought Processes.

Biotherapy of neoplastic disease is a relatively new modality of cancer treatment with many investigational studies currently underway. Understanding immunity is integral to the understanding of biotherapy and the drugs used to stimulate the immune system in various ways.

The bibliography for this chapter can be found in Appendix B, which begins on page 1054.

CHAPTER REVIEW QUESTIONS*

1. A goal of cancer biotherapy is to:
   a. Produce remission as a single-agent cancer therapy.
   b. Promote tumor-nonspecific immunity.
   c. Stimulate immunocompetence in cancer patients.
   d. Bypass side effects of traditional chemotherapy.

2. Common adverse effects of interferon therapy include:
   a. Flulike symptoms.

*See Appendix A, which begins on page 1051, for answers.

b. Seizures.
c. Peripheral neuropathy.
d. Alopecia.

3. An FDA-licensed indication for the hematopoietic growth factor granulocyte colony-stimulating factor (G-CSF) is:
   a. Adjuvant therapy after resection of renal cell carcinoma.
   b. Metastatic malignant melanoma.
   c. Antineoplastic therapy–induced neutropenia.
   d. Bladder cancer.

4. The nurse administering BCG vaccine by scarification technique should prepare the injection site by:
   a. Thorough cleansing with alcohol prior to injection.

b. Application of heat prior to injection.
c. Application of Xylocaine cream to reduce discomfort.
d. Abrading the skin with the bevel of the needle prior to rubbing vaccine into area.

5. Patients receiving biotherapy may become depressed for all of the following reasons *except:*
   a. The therapy requires frequent hospital visits.
   b. There are many permanent toxicities with this therapy.
   c. Neurologic toxicity alters mental status and perceptions.
   d. Biotherapy-related fatigue may exacerbate depression tendency.

BUILDING YOUR CRITICAL THINKING SKILLS

MONITORING ADVERSE EFFECTS

Patient 1

A 55-year-old white man is admitted for intensive interleukin-2 therapy for metastatic renal cancer of the liver and right iliac crest. He has a family history of coronary artery disease. However, a stress test was normal, as was his admitting ECG. He was a 2 pack/day smoker for 30 years, but quit 1 year ago. He had a cholecystectomy 18 years ago; persistent eczema of the right arm, shoulder, and back; and intermittent bouts with gout for which he did not require medication. Shortly after the IL-2 therapy, his blood work shows an elevated AST and he relates that his eczema and gout are worse.

1. To what might the symptoms reported by this patient be related?
2. How does this patient's past medical history influence the nurse's monitoring of this patient after his IL-2 therapy?
3. What nursing interventions are appropriate for the

symptoms exhibited by this patient after his IL-2 therapy?

Patient 2

A 36-year-old female with premenopausal breast cancer is seen in the clinic for adjuvant chemotherapy after her mastectomy. Currently, she is on her third cycle of cyclophosphamide, adriamycin, and 5-fluorouricil. She required admission to the hospital for her two previous treatments because of neutropenia and fevers related to urinary tract infections. Typically, her neutropenic period lasts only 5 to 7 days. The physician has ordered the client to begin granulocyte colony-stimulating factor (G-CSF) 12 days after this round of chemotherapy.

1. Explain why infections are common approximately 2 weeks after therapy.
2. Why would the physician select G-CSF for this patient, and what is the significance of starting G-CSF at that particular point following post therapy?

CHAPTER 57

Anti-Inflammatory Agents

Merrily A. Kuhn, RNC, PhD

CHAPTER OUTLINE

BOX

KEY TERMS

Kinins   Monoamines
Lysosomal enzymes   Prostaglandins

LEARNING OBJECTIVES

After reading this chapter, the student will be able to:

1. Identify those drugs commonly used as anti-inflammatory medications.
2. Differentiate among the anti-inflammatory medications as to mechanism of action, route of administration, pharmacokinetics, adverse effects, contraindications and precautions, and interactions.
3. Identify specific areas to assess in the patient requiring anti-inflammatory medications to formulate appropriate patient outcomes.
4. Plan the nursing interventions necessary to administer anti-inflammatory medications and choose appropriate teaching strategies to gain patient compliance.
5. Evaluate the patient at various stages of treatment to measure the effectiveness of nursing interventions.

The *prostaglandins*, first discovered in the 1930s, have been detected in almost every tissue and body fluid and take part in almost every biologic function. They are not stored in the body, but are produced and released under certain conditions, such as cell damage (injury, inflammation, or tumor).

Several groups of prostaglandins, synthesized from essential fatty acids through the arachidonic acid cascade, have been recognized and are referred to by the letters A, B, C, D, E, F, H, I, and non-PG (thromboxane). A numerical subscript (1, 2, or 3) may be added, indicating the prostaglandin series (e.g., PGI_2). The prostaglandins PGE and PGF are currently best known. PGE and PGF are stable in blood, but are rapidly metabolized (80% to 90%) on a single pass through either the kidneys or the liver. Once synthesized, prostaglandins are released locally, where they may act as local mediators of cellular action leading to a wide variety of functional changes followed by a local metabolism or secondary "overflow" release into the ve-

nous circulation for eventual metabolism. The prostaglandins have been described as having an "awesome and bewildering" diversity of actions, which include the following:

1. vasodilation
2. increased cardiac output
3. increased capillary permeability
4. stimulation of uterine contractions
5. either vasodilation or constriction of bronchioles (PGE_1 and PGE_2 dilate, PGF_2 constricts)
6. possible pain production
7. interruption of early pregnancy, causing abortion
8. stimulation of adrenal and pituitary secretion
9. release of lysosomal enzymes
10. inhibition of platelet aggregation
11. stimulation of erythropoietin production
12. suppression of the immune response by inhibiting both T and B lymphocyte activity

13. inhibition of gastric acid secretion and stabilization of the gastric mucosa
14. prevention of release of histamine from sensitized leukocytes
15. elevation of body temperature
16. vascular dilatation in kidney to help regulate renal vascular resistance

KININS, MONOAMINES, AND LYSOSOMAL ENZYMES

Along with prostaglandins, other substances play a role in inflammation, including kinins, monoamines, and lysosomal enzymes. *Kinins*, including bradykinin, are biologically active polypeptides formed as a result of injury or inflammation and are powerful vasodilators. Vasodilation is also accompanied by increased permeability of the vessels, resulting in local redness, edema, burning, and throbbing pain. In the lung, bradykinin causes bronchospasm and bronchoconstriction when it is released following a stimulus.

The *monoamines* (substances that contain one amine radical), including histamine and serotonin, are stored in the mast cell in the lung and other body cells and are released as a result of body injury. Both bradykinin and histamine encourage the phagocytic cells to migrate from the bloodstream to the place of injury. The lysosomal membrane surrounding the cell is damaged when phagocytic cells are broken down as they attempt to engulf foreign particles. As a result of lysosomal breakdown, several *lysosomal enzymes*, including proteases and hydrolases, are released. These begin to clean up the damaged phagocytes and their original prey (for example, uric acid crystals), but also begin to break down the collagenous connective tissue within the arthritic joint. This leads to the development of more prostaglandins, bradykinin, and histamine, causing the inflammation to worsen, as shown in Figure 57–1.

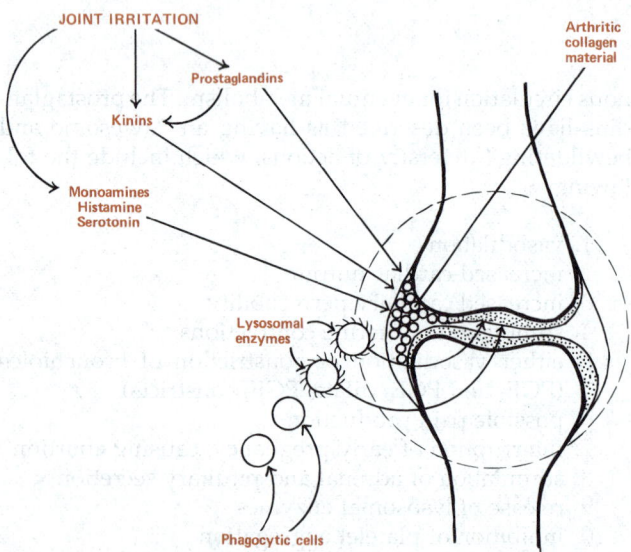

Figure 57–1. As part of the inflammatory process, prostaglandins, kinins, and monoamines are released, along with lysosomal enzymes released by the damaged phagocytic cell, resulting in more inflammation and pain.

ANTI-INFLAMMATORY DRUGS

Inflammatory diseases range from rheumatoid arthritis and degenerative joint disease to connective tissue disorders such as lupus erythematosus and scleroderma, as presented in Table 57–1. Therapeutic agents for treating anti-inflammatory diseases include prostaglandins, acetaminophen, salicylates, nonsteroidal anti-inflammatory drugs (NSAIDs), salicylate-like medications, gold products, antimalarials, cytotoxic medications, and antigout drugs, classified in Table 57–2. Salicylates, NSAIDs, and salicylate-like medications provide symptomatic relief of the disease, but it is unknown whether they actively alter the course of disease. Gold products and antigout products suppress the destructive course of the disease whereas antimalarials and cytotoxic drugs may or may not have this effect. Research is ongoing.

The choice of drug depends on the acuteness and severity of the disease. Patients often have remissions and exacerbation of symptoms. During early treatment, conservative therapy is used such as rest, exercise, physical therapy, avoidance of activities that activate discomfort, maintenance of normal weight and emotional stability. Salicylates are often the first drugs used as they are inexpensive and often produce rapid results.

ACTION

Anti-inflammatory agents, at least in part, act by inhibiting prostaglandin synthesis. In addition, most are thought to have an analgesic effect either by acting peripherally or by displacing certain peptides from their protein-binding sites to exert a protective effect on the tissues. Some agents such as salicylates also have an antipyretic effect that may aid in decreasing warmth of the affected area as well as in decreasing swelling.

USES

Anti-inflammatory drugs are used primarily to treat autoimmune diseases, including arthritis. The anti-inflammatory drugs are used for both short- and long-term therapy. The medications used for short-term therapy are normally used for 1 to 4 weeks, owing to their severe adverse effects. When the long-term medications are prescribed, the patient is evaluated by the physician in 1 to 2 weeks to ascertain if the medication is effective. Anti-inflammatory agents are also used to manage acute postoperative pain and cancer pain.

PROSTAGLANDINS

Research has demonstrated that nonsteroidal anti-inflammatory agents inhibit prostaglandin synthesis and thereby help to relieve pain. There is great promise for the potential use of currently known prostaglandins (and their derivatives) and for drugs that work through prostaglandin inhibition. Prostaglandins are currently used to

Table 57–1. INFLAMMATORY DISEASES

Arthritis

DEFINITION: A group of conditions or disorders resulting from the body's own antigen-antibody reaction.

CLASSIFICATION OF ARTHRITIS BY THE AMERICAN RHEUMATIC ASSOCIATION AND ARTHRITIS FOUNDATION:

- I. Polyarthritis of unknown origin (includes rheumatoid arthritis)
- II. Connective tissue disorders (includes lupus erythematosus)
- III. Rheumatic fever
- IV. Degenerative joint diseases (includes osteoarthritis)
- V. Nonarticular rheumatism
- VI. Diseases with which arthritis is frequently associated
- VII. Associated with known infectious agents
- VIII. Traumatic and/or neurogenic disorders
- IX. Associated with known biochemical or endocrine disorders (includes gout)
- X. Tumor and tumorlike conditions
- XI. Allergy and drug reactions

Condition	Pathologic Process	Sex Preference/ Onset Age (yr)	Symptoms
Rheumatoid arthritis	Chronic, systemic, inflammatory	F, 20–40	Joints swollen, painful, and inflamed, leading to calcification, immobility, and deformity (Fig. 56–1)
Osteoarthritis	Chronic, localized, degenerative	F, 45–55	Slow degeneration of spine and weight-bearing joints
Gouty arthritis	Acute, familial, metabolic disorder of purine metabolism	M, 35+	Joint or joints swollen, painful, and inflamed; can lead to chronic deformity (may be precipitated by certain medications)
Juvenile arthritis	Systemic inflammatory disease affecting one or more joints	Undetermined	Joint swollen, painful, and inflamed; 75% have remission without joint damage

Connective Tissue Diseases

DEFINITION: Conditions that affect and destroy connective tissue.

TYPES: Lupus erythematosus
        Polyarteritis nodosa
        Scleroderma

Condition	Pathologic Process	Sex Preference/ Onset Age (yr)	Symptoms
Lupus erythematosus	Chronic, systemic; produces antibodies that attack own nucleoproteins	F, 15+	Swollen joints, skin rash, multiple organ damage, generalized alopecia, photosensitivity
Polyarteritis nodosa	Chronic, diffuse, inflammatory; necrosis of small arteries	F, 25+	Damage to small to medium-sized arteries in major organs of body leading to organ damage
Scleroderma	Chronic, diffuse	M, 35+	Skin thickens and has pigmentation changes; respiratory impairment

TREATMENTS INCLUDE:

Medications, including salicylates and nonsteroidal anti-inflammatory drugs, gold compounds, steroids, cytotoxic agents, and antigout preparations.

Minimization of functional limitation, discomfort, infection, and deformity.

Education regarding self-help devices (Self-Help Devices Office, Institute of Physical Medicine and Rehabilitation, 400 East 34th Street, New York, NY 10016).

Helping patient develop support system to maintain independence as long as possible.

Establishment of realistic goals.

Maintenance of prescribed exercise and/or rest program to improve circulation, promote relaxation, relieve pain, improve range of motion, including heat and cold application.

Maintenance of routine schedule of sleep (firm mattress is recommended).

---

treat rheumatoid arthritis, fever, headache, patent ductus arteriosus, midtrimester abortion and induction of labor (Chapter 48), and peripheral vascular disease. Possible future uses include the following: hypertension, heart failure, bronchial asthma, burns, glaucoma, coronary, and deep-vein thrombosis.

○ **Misoprostol** (Cytotec), a synthetic prostaglandin E_1 analog, inhibits gastric acid secretion and has mucosal protective properties. Patients who take NSAIDs are at increased risk of upper gastrointestinal (GI) tract bleeding, which may be prevented with prophylactic use of misoprostol.

Table 57–2. ANTI-INFLAMMATORY CLASSES

Agent	OTC	Rx
Group I Agents: Salicylates and Nonsteroidal Anti-inflammatory Agents		
A. Salicylates		
Aspirin	X	
Choline salicylate (Arthropan)	X	
Choline magnesium trisalicylate (Trilisate)	X	X
Diflunisal (Dolobid)		X
B. Propionic Acid Derivatives		
Fenoprofen (Nalfon)		X
Flurbiprofen (Ansaid)		X
Ibuprofen (Motrin, Rufen)	X	X
Naproxen (Naprosyn, Anaprox, Aleve)	X	
Ketoprofen (Orudis)	X	X
Oxaprozin (Daypro)		X
C. Indoles (Acetic Acids)		X
Indomethacin (Indocin)		X
Sulindac (Clinoril)		X
Ketorolac (Toradol)		X
Tolmetin (Tolectin)		X
Etodolac (Lodine)		X
Nabumetone (Relafen)		X
Diclofenac (Voltaren)		X
D. Pyrazolones		
Phenylbutazone (Butazolidin)		X
Oxyphenbutazone (Tandearil)		X
E. Fenamates		
Mefenamic acid (Ponstel)		X
Meclofenamate sodium (Meclomen)		X
F. Oxicams		
Piroxicam (Feldene)		X
Group II Agents		
A. Gold Products		
Gold sodium thiomalate (Myochrisine)		X
Aurothioglucose (Solganal)		X
Auranofin (Ridaura)		X
B. D-penicillamine (Cuprimine)		X
C. Hydroxychloroquine (Plaquenil)		X
Group III Agents		
(Oral and intersynovial; see Chapter 44).		
Group IV Agents: Cytotoxic agents (last-ditch effort; unapproved use at this time; see Chapter 55)		
Cyclophosphamide (Cytoxan)		X
Azathioprine (Imuran)		X
Methotrexate (Rheumatrex)		X

ACTION Misoprostol can increase bicarbonate and mucus production in the stomach, which is inhibited by the NSAIDs. Misoprostol also inhibits basal and nocturnal gastric acid secretion and acid secretion in response to a variety of stimuli including meals, histamine, pentagastrin, and coffee.

USES Misoprostol is used to prevent both aspirin- and NSAID-induced gastric ulcers in persons at high risk for ulcer formation (which includes those with a past history of ulcer disease and the elderly) and in patients with concomitant debilitating diseases. Misoprostol is taken for the duration of aspirin or NSAID therapy. Misoprostol does not prevent duodenal ulcers in patients on NSAIDs.

Misoprostol is also used to reduce the incidence of kidney rejection and improves renal function in renal transplant patients who are being treated with cyclosporine (Sandimmune) and prednisone. Recent research indicates that misoprostol may improve fat absorption in patients with cystic fibrosis. Research is continuing in this area.

because of its abortifacient properties it is being studied to enhance abortions.

Pharmacokinetics, dosages, and nursing implications for misoprostol are presented in Table 57–3.

CONTRAINDICATIONS AND PRECAUTIONS Misoprostol is contraindicated in patients with prior allergy to the prostaglandins.

▼ CLINICAL ALERT

Misoprostol is contraindicated in pregnancy as it has abortifacient properties and actually produces uterine contractions that may endanger pregnancy. It should be administered only to women who are capable of complying with effective contraceptive measures. It is suggested that pregnant nurses handle misoprostol with gloves not their bare hand.

Misoprostol is used cautiously in persons with renal impairment as misoprostol is excreted 80% in the urine. Dosage may need to be decreased. Safety has not been established in children under age 18. Misoprostol should not be administered to nursing mothers because it is excreted in milk and could cause significant diarrhea in nursing infants.

ADVERSE EFFECTS The most common adverse effect is diarrhea, which occurs in 13% to 40% of patients. The diarrhea is generally self-limiting and resolves within 8 days. If diarrhea continues, it may necessitate discontinuation of misoprostol. Diarrhea and other GI symptoms such as abdominal pain, nausea, flatulence, dyspepsia, and vomiting can be reduced by administering misoprostol after meals and at bedtime and by avoiding coadministration with magnesium-containing antacids.

Additional adverse effects can occur in females and include spotting, cramps, hypermenorrhea, menstrual disorders, and dysmenorrhea.

INTERACTIONS Antacids, particularly magnesium-containing antacids, reduce the total availability of misoprostol. This does not appear to be clinically important as misoprostol acts locally in the stomach. Plasma concentrations are also diminished when misoprostol is taken with food.

ACETAMINOPHEN

○ **Acetaminophen** (Tylenol and many others) is the first-line treatment for osteoarthritis pain in the hip and knee, according to a guideline published by the American College of Rheumatology (1996). Acetaminophen is discussed in Chapter 18.

SALICYLATES

Salicylates are the most extensively employed analgesic, antipyretic, and anti-inflammatory chemical group used today. Although the potential of these drugs to alleviate pain is much lower than that of the narcotic analgesics,

Table 57–3. ANTI-INFLAMMATORY MEDICATIONS: PROSTAGLANDINS AND SALICYLATES

DRUG NAME/ROUTE AND DOSAGE	PHARMACOKINETICS/ DYNAMICS	NURSING IMPLICATIONS
PROSTAGLANDINS		
misoprostol (Cytotec)		
Adults: 100–200 μg PO 4 times daily	**Onset:** rapid **Peak:** 9–15 min **Duration:** 3 hr **½L:** 20–40 min **PB:** 80–90% **B:** liver **E:** 80% urine	**ASSESSMENT:** Pregnancy test (pregnancy category X). **INTERVENTION:** Therapy is begun after a negative pregnancy test 2 wk before. It is then started on 2nd or 3rd day of next menstrual period. **Patient Teaching**—Instruct patient to take after meals and at bedtime. Warn patient *not* to take magnesium-containing antacids concurrently. Teach patient not to give this medicine to anyone else. **EVALUATION:** Evaluate for diarrhea and gynecologic disorders. Report these to physician.
SALICYLATES		
acetylsalicylic acid (aspirin)		
Adults: 325–650 PO, rectal q 4–6 hr, or 500 mg q 3 hr, or 1000 mg q 6 hr (extended release) as needed (not to exceed 6 g/day) **Children 2–11 yr:** 60–110 mg/kg per day PO, rectal in 4–6 divided doses **anti-inflammatory** **Adults:** 2.6–5.2 g PO, rectal in divided doses **Children:** 90–130 mg/kg/day PO, rectal in divided doses **prevention of transient ischemic attacks** **Adults:** 325 mg–1.3 g PO, rectal daily in 2–4 divided doses **prevention of myocardial infarction** **Adults:** 81–325 mg/day PO, rectal	**Onset:** PO, 15–30 min; rectal, 1–2 hr **Peak:** PO, 1–3 hr; rectal, 4–5 hr **Duration:** PO, 3–6 hr; rectal, 7 hr **½L:** 2–3 hr (low doses); up to 15–39 hr (aspirin in high doses) **PB:** concentration dependent: 90%–100% at low dose, 25%–60% at high dose, 33% (pure aspirin) **B:** liver **E:** kidneys	**ASSESSMENT:** Assess pain and limitation of movement; note type, location, and intensity of pain before and 30–60 min following administration. Assess fever and associated symptoms. Assess for pregnancy (category D). **INTERVENTION:** Food will decrease absorption rate, but will not alter total amount absorbed. Crushing tablets increases absorption rate. **Patient Teaching**—Advise patient not to crush or chew enteric-coated tablets. Tell patient that tablets with acetic odor should be discarded. Warn patients on long-term therapy to contact physician before undergoing surgery. (Drug may need to be withheld for at least 1 wk before surgery). Advise parents that Centers for Disease Control and Prevention warn against giving aspirin to children or adolescents with varicella (chicken pox) or influenza-like or viral illnesses because of possible association with Reye's syndrome. Advise patient to avoid concurrent use of alcohol with medication to minimize possible gastric irritation. **EVALUATION:** Evaluate if pain is not relieved and notify physician. Pain should be relieved without significant alteration in level of consciousness, respiratory status, or blood pressure. Contact physician if tinnitus, unusual bleeding of gums, bruising, or black, tarry stools or if fever returns or lasts longer than 3 days.

aspirin-like drugs are often preferred because they do not lead to addiction and have fewer side effects. The two main groups of salicylate derivatives include acetylsalicylic acid (aspirin) and salicylic acid–based drugs (choline salicylate, choline magnesium trisalicylate, and diflunisal).

ACTION

The salicylates inhibit prostaglandin synthesis, resulting in a decrease in the development of pain and deformity in the person with arthritis. Salicylates are thought to stabilize the lysosomal membrane, thereby preventing it from releasing substances that cause inflammation. Also, salicylates inhibit formation of excessive amounts of prostaglandins in the brain, which may possibly account for their effectiveness in treatment of headaches. Some re-

searchers believe that salicylates have their site of action centrally within the brain.

○ **Acetylsalicylic acid** (aspirin) reduces pain and fever. Aspirin is generally more effective than salicylic acid–based drugs, but may cause greater GI side effects.

Pharmacokinetics for aspirin, as well as dosages and nursing implications, are presented in Table 57–3.

CONTRAINDICATIONS AND PRECAUTIONS Aspirin is contraindicated in patients with salicylate sensitivity, in patients with GI disease such as ulcers or bleeding, and in those with glucose-6-phosphate dehydrogenase (G6PD) deficiency because these conditions are worsened. Aspirin is used with caution in hypoprothrombinemia, bleeding disorders, and Hodgkin's disease. Caution is used in situations in which there is risk of bleeding, because aspirin decreases platelet aggregation (decreasing clot formation) and prolongs bleeding time, causing the patient to bleed excessively. The use of aspirin and other salicylates in children with varicella infections or influenza-like viruses has been reported to increase the risk of developing Reye's syndrome; therefore aspirin is contraindicated in children. The mechanism is unknown.

ADVERSE EFFECTS   The most common adverse effect of aspirin and the other salicylates is their tendency to cause GI upset and ulcer formation.

 CLINICAL ALERT

Aspirin causes local gastric mucosal irritation by increasing the entry of acid into the mucosa. In toxic doses, salicylates may cause tinnitus (ringing in the ears) or a whole spectrum of adverse effects called "salicylism" including changes in mentation and perception; changes in GI, liver, kidney, and respiratory function; and increased uric acid production.

INTERACTIONS   Aspirin interacts with several drug types and chemical substances. Because it increases the amount of active drug in the blood by displacing other drugs from plasma proteins, aspirin increases anticoagulant effect, raises methotrexate levels, and enhances hypoglycemic response to sulfonylurea antidiabetic agents. When used with alcohol and corticosteroids, aspirin increases the risk of GI bleeding and ulceration through its irritant action. Drugs that acidify the urine such as ascorbic acid or ammonium chloride may increase the plasma concentration of the salicylates. Products that contain large amounts of alkali and sodium, such as Alka-Seltzer, are not suitable for long-term use as larger dosages of aspirin may be needed to compensate for increased excretion caused by the resulting alkalosis. Aspirin decreases the uricosuric effect of probenecid and pyrazolones.

NONSTEROIDAL ANTI-INFLAMMATORY DRUGS

The nonsteroidal anti-inflammatory drugs (NSAIDs) are classified into several groups, as follows:

1. propionic acid derivatives, including ibuprofen, fenoprofen, naproxen, flurbiprofen, ketoprofen, and oxaprozin
2. indole analogs or acetic acid drugs such as indomethacin, sulindac, tolmetin, nabumetone, ketorolac tromethamine, etodolac, and diclofenac sodium
3. oxicam drugs such as piroxicam
4. pyrazolone derivatives, including phenylbutazone
5. fenamates such as meclofenamate sodium and mefanamic acid

ACTION

Most of the NSAIDs presumably act by inhibiting the enzyme cyclooxygenase, thus blocking the synthesis of prostaglandins E_2 which, owing to their potent vasodilator effect, increase vascular permeability and increase the inflammatory process. In addition, NSAIDs may also af-

fect T-cell function, stabilize lysosomal membranes, inhibit chemotaxis of inflamed cells, and decrease release of superoxide radicals (which also contribute to inflammation). These agents do not produce tolerance or physical or psychologic dependence. NSAIDs do not alter the course of the underlying disease.

USES

Most of the nonsteroidal anti-inflammatory drugs are effective in alleviating symptoms of rheumatoid arthritis and osteoarthritis, such as swelling, pain, stiffness, and tenderness. They are also effective in relieving mild to moderate pain of dental extractions, postsurgical pain, cancer pain, primary dysmenorrhea, and soft tissue athletic injuries. NSAIDs are especially effective for bone pain due to tumor metastasis. However, caution is used when administering NSAIDs to oncology patients because the antipyretic effect that these drugs have may mask infection. In addition, because of their effect on platelet function, they may promote hemorrhage.

Pharmacokinetics, dosage, and nursing implications are featured in Table 57–4.

CONTRAINDICATIONS AND PRECAUTIONS

The NSAIDs are contraindicated in patients with GI lesions, in patients sensitive to these or similar drugs, or who are allergic to aspirin or iodides, or who have induced symptoms of asthma, rhinitis, urticaria, angioedema, or bronchospasm. These conditions may be exacerbated by NSAIDs. NSAIDs are given cautiously to persons with a previous history of GI ulceration as bleeding may occur, in renal or hepatic disease as serum levels may be elevated increasing the possibility of toxicity, or in cardiac disease as fluid retention may occur compromising cardiac function. Because the NSAIDs impair platelet aggregation and prolong bleeding time, they are given cautiously to persons with bleeding disorders. These medications are generally stopped 24 to 48 hours before surgery. The nonsteroidal and anti-inflammatory drugs cross the placental barrier and are found in breast milk. They are given to pregnant (either category B or C) or lactating women with caution, because their effects on the fetus are unknown.

ADVERSE EFFECTS

Many adverse effects may result from NSAIDs; these include GI irritation leading to nausea, vomiting, heartburn, GI bleeding, and ulceration.

 CLINICAL ALERT

NSAIDs are responsible for one-fifth of all admissions to hospitals with bleeding or perforated peptic ulcers and thousands of deaths worldwide. Gastrointestinal bleeding is a significant problem in the elderly. The gastric ulcer may be a silent condition, detectable only on visual examination. Intestinal inflammation is also found in about two-thirds of long-time (more than 6 months) users.

Table 57–4. NONSTEROIDAL ANTI-INFLAMMATORY DRUGS (NSAIDs)

NSAID	Selected Trade Names	Available Generically	Time to Peak Levels (hr)[a]	Half-life (hr)	Antiheumatic Action		Max. Recommended Daily Dose (mg)
					Onset (days)	Peak (wks)	
Indole Analogs (acetic acids)							
Diclofenac potassium	Cataflam	No	0.33–2	Approx. 2	ND	ND	200
Diclofenac sodium	Voltaren	No	2–3	1–2	ND	ND	200
Etodolac	Lodine	No	1–2	7.3	ND	ND	1200
Indomethacin	Indocin	Yes	1–2	4.5	Within 7	1–2	200
Indomethacin (sustained release)	Indocin E-R Indocin SR	Yes	2–4	4.5–6	Within 7	1–2	150
Ketorolac	Toradol	No	0.5–1	2.4–8.6	ND	ND	IM: 120[b] Oral: 40
Nabumetone[c]	Relafen	No	2.5–4	22.5–30[d]	ND	ND	2000
Sulindac	Clinoril	Yes	2–4	7.8 (16.4)[d]	Within 7	2–3	400
Tolmetin	Tolectin Tolectin DS	Yes	0.5–1	1–1.5	Within 7	1–2	2000
Fenamates							
Meclofenamate	Meclomen	Yes	0.5–1	2 (3.3)[e]	Few days	2–3	400
Mefenamic Acid	Ponstel	No	2–4	2–4	ND	ND	1000
Propionic Acid Derivatives							
Fenoprofen	Nalfon	Yes	1–2	2–3	2	2–3	3200
Flurbiprofen	Ansaid	No	1.5	5.7	ND	ND	300
Ibuprofen OTC	Aches-N-Pain Advil Bayer Select Pain Relief Formula Excedrin IB Ibu-Tab Medipren Midol IB Motrin IB Nuprin Trendar	Yes	1–2	1.8–2.5	Within 7	1–2	1200
Rx	Childrens Advil or Motrin Ibu-Tab Motrin Rufen						3200
Ketoprofen	Orudis (OTC)	Yes (some forms)	1.2	2.1	ND	ND	300
	Oruvail	No	0.5–2	2–4	ND	ND	300
Naproxen	Naprosyn Naprelan	Yes	2–4 30 min	12–15 15–20 hr	Within 14	2–4	1500
Naproxen sodium	Aleve (OTC) Anaprox Anaprox DS	No Yes	1–2	12–13	Within 14	2–4	600 1375
Oxaprozin	Daypro	No	3–5	42–50	Within 7	ND	1800
Oxicam							
Piroxicam	Feldene	Yes	3–5	30–86	7–12	2–3	20

Source: Adapted from Facts and Comparisons Drug Newsletter. 13(4):29, 1994.
[a]Food decreases absorption rate; may delay time to peak levels.
[b]150 mg on first day.
[c]Active metabolite of nabumetone is acetic acid.
[d]Half-life of active metabolite.
[e]Half-life with multiple doses.
ND = no data.

The relative GI toxicity of selected NSAIDs in descending order is as follows: phenylbutazone, indomethacin, mefanamic acid, sulindac, tolmetin sodium, naproxen, fenoprofen, and ibuprofen. Many medications are best administered with food or milk to avoid GI irritation. Other adverse effects include bone marrow depression effects such as anemia and decreased white blood count (WBC); renal effects such as decreased glomerular filtration rate and decreased renal blood flow mediated by inhibition of prostaglandin synthesis; hepatitis-like syndrome (rare), which is reversible and often accompanied by abnormal liver function tests; skin eruptions; central nervous system (CNS) symptoms such as tinnitus, headache, dizziness, and blurred vision; and allergic reactions manifested as hives, anaphylaxis, and asthmatic broncho-spasm. There is often a cross-sensitivity to other NSAIDs and yellow food dye.

Frequent complete blood counts (CBCs) are performed when taking the drugs such as phenylbutazone and in-domethacin. If changes occur, the medication is discon-tinued and other therapies instituted. These agents inhibit platelet aggregation, and therefore bleeding may occur.

INTERACTIONS

Interactions include an increase in the ulcerogenic effects when nonsteroidal anti-inflammatory drugs are given concurrently with corticosteroids or salicylates. They are given cautiously with anticoagulants, as they increase the incidence of bleeding. Also, concurrent aspirin adminis-tration may decrease anti-inflammatory effects. The anti-hypertensive effects of beta-adrenergic blockers and an-giotension-converting enzyme (ACE) inhibitors may be decreased if NSAIDs are taken concurrently. Probenecid may increase the plasma level and the half-life of most of the agents. Hydantoins and other highly bound drugs may be displaced and cause toxicity; therefore, close mon-itoring must be done.

PROPIONIC ACID DERIVATIVES

The propionic acid derivatives include **ibuprofen** *(Motrin, Rufen)*, **fenoprofen** *(Nalfon)*, **naproxen** *(Naprosyn, Ana-prox, Aleve)*, **flurbiprofen** *(Ansaid)*, **ketoprofen** *(Orudis, Oruval)*, and **oxaprozin** *(Daypro)*. Ibuprofen, naproxen, and ketoprofen are featured in Table 57-5.

○ **Ibuprofen** (Motrin, Rufen) is administered to treat all types of arthritis, tendonitis, bursitis, primary dys-menorrhea, and mild to moderate pain. A therapeutic ef-fect may occur after one tablet or it may take as long as 2 weeks. Ibuprofen is also available over-the-counter (OTC) in doses of 200 mg and is safe for long-term therapy.

○ **Naproxen** (Naprosyn, Naprelan) is used for vari-ous types of arthritis, tendonitis, bursitis, acute gout, mild to moderate pain, and primary dysmenorrhea. Naproxen is safe for acute and long-term therapy.

Table 57–5. NONSTEROIDAL ANTI-INFLAMMATORY DRUGS: PROPIONIC ACID DERIVATIVES

DRUG NAME/ROUTE AND DOSAGE	PHARMACOKINETICS/ DYNAMICS	NURSING IMPLICATIONS
all proprionic acid derivatives		
		ASSESSMENT: Obtain baseline blood studies and thor-ough GI history. Assess for pregnancy (category B). **INTERVENTION: Patient Teaching**—Caution patient to avoid aspirin and alcoholic beverages while taking medication and, if GI upset occurs, to take drug with food, milk, or antacids. Advise patient to use caution when driving or operating heavy equipment. **EVALUATION:** Notify physician if persistent rash, itching, black stools, edema, or weight gain occurs.
ibuprofen (Motrin) (Rufen) and many others		
Adults: 200–800 mg PO 3–4 times daily; maximum daily dose 3200 mg	**Onset:** 30–60 min **Peak:** 1–2 hr **Duration:** 2–4 hr **½L:** 1.8–2.5 hr **PB:** 90%–99% **B:** liver **E:** urine (5%–10% unchanged), liver	Same as for all plus: **ASSESSMENT:** Assess for pregnancy (category un-known). **INTERVENTION:** Give lowest possible dose to decrease side effects. OTC product should be taken for no more than 3 days for fever and 10 days for pain before con-sulting a physician.
naproxen (Naprosyn)		
Adults: 250–750 mg PO 2 times daily; maximum daily dose 1500 mg *Children:* total dose 10 mg/kg PO in 2 doses	**Onset:** 1–2 hr **Peak:** 2–4 hr **Duration:** 7–12 hr **½L:** 12–15 hr **PB:** 99% **B:** liver **E:** urine (70% unchanged)	Same as for all plus: **INTERVENTION:** Symptomatic relief may not occur for 2 wk.
ketoprofen (Orudis)		
Adults: 150–300 mg/day PO, single or divided daily dose; maximum dose 300 mg/day	**Onset:** 0.5 hr **Peak:** 0.5–2 hr **Duration:** 4–8 hr **½L:** 2–4 hr **PB:** 99% **B:** liver **E:** urine	Same as for all plus: **INTERVENTION:** Reduce dose in renal disease.

○ **Ketoprofen** (Orudis, Oruval) is used to treat all types of arthritis, mild to moderate pain, and primary dysmenorrhea. Dosages are reduced in the elderly or those with renal dysfunction. It is safe for both acute and long-term therapy.

○ **Fenoprofen** (Nalfon) is safe for acute and long-term therapy for all types of arthritis and mild to moderate pain. It is administered orally in doses of 200 to 600 mg three to four times daily (30 minutes before meals or 2 hours after meals is best).

○ **Flurbiprofen** (Ansaid) is used for both acute and long-term treatment of all types of arthritis. The dosage is 50 to 100 mg orally two to four times a day.

○ **Oxaprozin** (Daypro) is used for the management of osteo and rheumatoid arthritis. Dosing is 600 mg two times daily or 1200 mg once daily.

INDOLE ANALOGS

Indole analogs include **indomethacin (Indocin)**, **sulindac (Clinoril)**, **tolmetin (Tolectin)**, **nabumetone (Relafen)**, **ketorolac tromethamine (Toradol)**, **etodolac (Lodine)**, and **diclofenac sodium (Voltaren, Voltaren SR)**. Selected drugs are featured in Table 57–6.

○ **Indomethacin** (Indocin) is a potent anti-inflammatory analgesic with antipyretic properties and a potent prostaglandin inhibitor. Indomethacin is considered for use only in acute active disease processes owing to its potential for adverse effects. Indomethacin is used to treat all types of arthritis, ankylosing spondylitis, tendonitis, bursitis, acute painful shoulder, and acute gout. Indomethacin in suppository form may decrease the risk and severity of recurrent colic secondary to ureteral calculi. Topical eye drops are used to treat cystoid macular edema. Indomethacin in an IV form is also indicated for closure of persistent patent ductus arteriosus.

Indomethacin shares the same adverse effects as the other NSAIDs but increases frequency and severity. Also, because of these adverse effects, it is given cautiously to patients with impaired renal and hepatic function and to the elderly. Indomethacin is administered cautiously to patients with epilepsy or Parkinson's disease as these conditions may be exacerbated. Laboratory studies are done routinely when patients are on indomethacin to assess for abnormalities. It is titrated to the lowest possible effective dosage to prevent these major complications.

○ **Ketorolac tromethamine** (Toradol) exhibits anti-inflammatory, analgesic, antipyretic activity and inhibits synthesis of prostaglandins. It was the first NSAID approved for acute post-operative pain control. Pain relief occurs as early as 10 minutes after a dose of 30 to 60 mg IM or IV. It is administered immediately after surgery before pain occurs and then every 6 hours, either IM or PO, until it is no longer needed or a maximum of 5 days is reached. Administration of ketorolac tromethamine can reduce the need of narcotics for pain control. Peak plasma levels occur within 45 to 90 minutes.

▼ CLINICAL ALERT

Ketorolac tromethamine and its metabolites are primarily excreted in the kidneys, so reduced creatinine clearance (Cr Cl) results in increased plasma levels, which may lead to impaired clearance of the drug. The most serious risks associated with ketorolac are GI ulcerations, bleeding, and perforation; renal events ranging from interstitial nephritis to acute renal failure, especially in patients with preexisting kidney problems; hemorrhage; and anaphylactic reactions.

The concurrent administration of ketorolac and probenecid is contraindicated. Concomitant use of these agents decreases ketorolac clearance and increases serum concentrations as well as the half-life of ketorolac. These effects on the pharmacokinetics of ketorolac may increase the risk of toxicity (Tatro, 1995).

○ **Sulindac** (Clinoril) is safe for both acute and long-term therapy treatment for all arthritis, ankylosing spondylitis, acute painful shoulder (tendonitis/bursitis), mild to moderate pain, and acute gouty arthritis. It is a pro-drug that is converted to an active drug by the liver.

○ **Tolmetin** (Tolectin) is similar to the others in its action; however, it differs chemically. It shares the same uses as the other anti-inflammatory agents and is used in both short- and long-term management of adult and juvenile rheumatoid arthritis and osteoarthritis. The adult dosage is initially 200 to 400 mg PO three to four times daily. The maintenance dose is 600 to 1800 mg PO daily in divided doses. For children 2 years and older the dose is initially 20 mg/kg per day PO in three to four divided doses. The maintenance dose is 15 to 30 mg/kg per day PO in three to four divided doses.

○ **Nabumetone** (Relafen) is available to treat rheumatoid arthritis and osteoarthritis. Nabumetone is a pro-drug that is converted to an active drug in the liver. It is said to be as effective as other NSAIDs and causes a relatively low incidence of peptic ulcers. The usual dosage is 1000 to 2000 mg/day orally in a single dose.

○ **Etodolac** (Lodine) is available to treat rheumatoid arthritis and osteoarthritis and as a general purpose analgesic. Etodolac has no benefits over acetaminophen for pain and has more adverse GI effects. Dosage for osteoarthritis administration is 600 to 1200 mg PO in two to four divided doses, for acute pain 200 to 400 mg PO every 6 to 8 hours to a maximum dose of 1200 mg.

○ **Diclofenac sodium** (Voltaren, Voltaren SR) (Table 57–6) is indicated for the management of both acute and chronic rheumatoid and osteoarthritis and ankylosing spondylitis. Diclofenac is a phenylacetic acid derivative with both analgesic and antipyretic activity. Its exact mechanism of action is unknown; however, it is thought to decrease synthesis of prostaglandins, prostacyclin, and thromboxane. Adverse effects are similar to the other NSAIDs, with the most frequent side effect being GI complaints.

OXICAM DRUGS

○ **Piroxicam** (Feldene) is used for long-term treatment of osteoarthritis and rheumatoid arthritis. The therapeutic effects are evident early in the treatment of both diseases and progress over 8 to 12 weeks. The usual adult dose is 10 to 20 mg PO daily or in divided doses. It may

Table 57–6. NONSTEROIDAL ANTI-INFLAMMATORY DRUGS: INDOLE ANALOGS

DRUG NAME/ROUTE AND DOSAGE	PHARMACOKINETICS/ DYNAMICS	NURSING IMPLICATIONS
all indole analogs		**ASSESSMENT:** Obtain baseline blood studies and thorough GI history. **INTERVENTION: Patient Teaching**—Caution patient to avoid aspirin and alcoholic beverages while taking medication and, if GI upset occurs, to take drug with food, milk, or antacids. Advise patient to use caution when driving or operating heavy equipment. **EVALUATION:** Notify physician if persistent rash, itching, black stools, edema, or weight gain occurs.
indomethacin (Indocin) and many others **Adults:** 25–50 mg PO 2–4 times daily, maximum dose 200 mg/day; 75 mg sustained-release (SR) capsules PO qid or bid (do not crush SR capsules); or 50 mg rectally 2–4 times/day	**Onset:** 0.5–2 hr **Peak:** 1–2 hr **Duration:** PO, 4–6 hr; rectal, 8–12 hr **½L:** 4.5 hr **PB:** 99% **B:** liver **E:** urine (10%–20% unchanged), feces	Same as for all plus: **ASSESSMENT:** Obtain complete eye exam at onset of therapy and periodically. Assess for pregnancy (category unknown). **INTERVENTION:** With twice-daily dosing, medication is best taken on arising in morning and at bedtime. If stomach distress arises, give with food, milk, or antacid. Complete physical examination and laboratory studies are recommended before and during therapy. Monitor stool for bleeding, and monitor intake and output. Older patient may need lower dose. Do not crush SR form.
ketorolac tromethamine (Toradol) **Adults:** 10 mg PO q 4–6 hr for limited duration (max. 2 wk); not to exceed combined doses of 120 mg/day **Maximum Daily Dosage:** Patients over 65—60 mg/day IM; Patients under 65—120 mg/day IM; Patients with Cr Cl < 50 mL/min—60 mg/day IM	**Onset:** 5–10 min **Peak:** 30–90 min **Duration:** 4–8 hr **½L:** 2.4–8.6 hr **PB:** 99% **B:** liver **E:** urine	Same as for all plus: **ASSESSMENT:** Assess for pregnancy (category C). **INTERVENTION:** Monitor serum creatinine daily while receiving ketorolac. Discontinue drug if Cr Cl increases >0.5 mg/dL. Max. duration: 48 hr (with an automatic stop order for 48 hr—varies per institutional policy). Convert to oral therapy when patient can tolerate. Protect from light.
sulindac (Clinoril) **Adults:** 150–200 mg PO 2 times daily, maximum dose 400 mg/day	**Onset:** 1 hr **Peak:** 2–4 hr **Duration:** 7–16 hr **½L:** 7–8 hr (16 hr metabolite) **PB:** 93%–98% **B:** liver **E:** urine	Same as for all plus: **ASSESSMENT:** Assess for pregnancy (category unknown). **INTERVENTION:** Administer with food. Therapy for 7–14 days is usually sufficient.
diclofenac sodium (Voltaren) **Adults:** 100–200 mg/day PO in 2–4 divided doses	**Onset:** 1 hr **Peak:** 2–3 hr **Duration:** 4–6 hr **½L:** 1.2–1.8 hr **PB:** 99% **B:** liver (high first-pass effect) **E:** urine, feces	Same as for all plus: **ASSESSMENT:** Assess for pregnancy (category B).

be administered concurrently with fixed doses of gold salts and corticosteroids.

PYRAZOLONE DERIVATIVE

○ **Phenylbutazone** (Butazolidin) has anti-inflammatory, antipyretic, analgesic, and mild uricosuric properties.

 CLINICAL ALERT

Pyrazolone derivatives have serious side effects—agranulocytosis and aplastic anemia—and are therefore only recommended when other NSAIDs have not been successful. These drugs are best used for 1 week only, particularly in the elderly.

The exact mechanism of its effect is unknown, but it is thought to inhibit prostaglandins synthesis, leukocyte migration, and lysosomal enzymes.

USES Phenylbutazone is used more effectively for bursitis, traumatic tenosynovitis, ankylosing spondylitis, acute gout, and acute rheumatoid arthritis.

CONTRAINDICATIONS AND PRECAUTIONS Phenylbutazone is contraindicated in persons with hypersensitivity, senile patients, and in children under 14. It is given cautiously to patients with GI disease as ulceration and bleeding may occur and in those with hepatic disease as liver abnormalities may progress. Safety in pregnant and lactating women has not been established.

ADVERSE EFFECTS The most serious adverse effects of phenylbutazone are aplastic anemia and agranulocytosis, whereas the most common adverse effects are abdominal discomfort and edema (3% to 9%), nausea, dyspepsia, and rash. Because of these side effects, patients are assessed frequently during therapy. If improvement does not occur in 2 to 3 days, phenylbutazone therapy is stopped.

INTERACTIONS Phenylbutazone can enhance oral anticoagulants, so concurrent use with anticoagulants may increase the incidence of bleeding.

DOSAGE Phenylbutazone is administered orally in doses of 100 mg three to four times daily, with a maximum dose of 400 mg/day. It is administered for 7 days only.

FENAMATE DRUGS

The fenamate drugs, salicylate-like medications and prostaglandin inhibitors, include **mefenamic acid (Ponstel)** and **meclofenamate sodium (Meclomen)**, featured in Table 57–7. Both have antipyretic, analgesic, and anti-inflammatory effects and are indicated for mild to moderate pain relief for short-term use. Adverse effects are similar to all other anti-inflammatories.

Contraindications and Precautions

The fenamate drugs are contraindicated in patients sensitive to aspirin, in active peptic ulcer disease, during pregnancy (category C), and in children under 14 because a significant amount of research has not been done in this population. They are given cautiously to persons with previous history of GI ulceration or renal, hepatic, or cardiac disease as all conditions may be worsened.

Interactions

Several interactions can occur with fenamate products. They are by themselves ulcerogenic, but the ulcerogenic effects are potentiated when they are given concurrently with corticosteroids, phenylbutazone, and salicylates. As-

Table 57–7. NONSTEROIDAL ANTI-INFLAMMATORY DRUGS: FENAMATES

DRUG NAME/ROUTE AND DOSAGE	PHARMACOKINETICS/ DYNAMICS	NURSING IMPLICATIONS
all fenamates		**ASSESSMENT:** Obtain baseline blood studies and thorough GI history. **INTERVENTION: Patient Teaching**—Caution patient to avoid aspirin and alcoholic beverages while taking medication and, if GI upset occurs, to take drug with food, milk, or antacids. Advise patient to use caution when driving or operating heavy equipment. **EVALUATION:** Notify physician if persistent rash, itching, black stools, edema, or weight gain occurs.
mefenamic acid (Ponstel) ***Adults:*** 500 mg PO followed by 250 mg 3–4 times daily; maximum dose 1000 mg/day; therapy should not exceed 5–7 days.	**Onset:** 1–2 hr **Peak:** 2–4 hr **Duration:** 6 hr **½L:** 2–4 hr **PB:** 9% **B:** liver **E:** urine, feces	Same as for all plus: **ASSESSMENT:** Assess GI system, obtain baseline blood work. Assess for pregnancy (category C). **INTERVENTION:** Administer with food or antacid to reduce GI complications. After acute flare-up is over, medication should be reduced and discontinued. Patients should be placed on these medications for 1 wk only. **EVALUATION:** If rash or diarrhea occurs, notify physician.
meclofenamate sodium (Meclomen) ***Adults:*** 200–400 mg/day PO in 3–4 divided doses; maximum dose 400 mg/day.	**Onset:** 0.5–1 hr **Peak:** 0.5–2 hr **Duration:** 6 hr **½L:** 1–4 hr **PB:** 99% **B:** liver **E:** urine	Same as for all plus: **ASSESSMENT:** Assess for pregnancy (category unknown). **INTERVENTION:** Not recommended as initial drug because of GI side effects. If diarrhea becomes severe, may need to discontinue drug.

pirin may decrease the plasma level of these drugs. When anticoagulants are given concurrently, the dose of warfarin may need to be reduced to prevent bleeding.

○ **Mefenamic acid** (Ponstel) is indicated for short-term pain relief and primary dysmenorrhea, for which it generally should be used no longer than 1 week.

○ **Meclofenamate sodium** (Meclomen) is used in the management of acute and chronic rheumatoid arthritis, osteoarthritis, and relief of mild to moderate pain. It appears to be as effective as aspirin in relieving the symptoms of arthritis. Although it is less likely than aspirin to cause tinnitus, it causes more GI side effects, especially diarrhea. Some patients have developed peptic ulcer while taking meclofenamate sodium, especially those with a history of ulcer disease or those taking other anti-inflammatory drugs concurrently.

CHOICE OF NONSTEROIDAL ANTI-INFLAMMATORY DRUGS

There is little difference between the NSAIDs as far as efficacy is concerned. Some patients may respond better and with fewer side effects to one over another. Therefore, a trial period is necessary to determine the optimum drug. Cost (ranges from $20 to $170/month) and frequency of dosing is also important; once-a-day dosing enhances patient compliance. Patient response is monitored closely as the therapeutic dose may vary from patient to patient. Treatment is initiated with one drug, and the dose is gradually increased to optimal or maximal tolerated dose. If the patient has an inadequate therapeutic response, the first drug is replaced with another NSAID. Optimal therapeutic dosage is continued for at least 2 weeks before changing drugs. When rheumatoid arthritis does not respond to an NSAID, clinicians add hydroxychloroquine for patients with mild arthritis or methotrexate if the disease is more severe.

Some studies have found that ibuprofen (Motrin and others) and naproxen (Naprosyn and others) have a lower risk of serious GI complications than other NSAIDs. Nabumetone (Relafen) may cause less gastric irritation than other NSAIDs. Meclofenamate (Meclomen and others) may cause a high incidence of diarrhea, which is sometimes severe. Piroxicam (Feldene and others), which has a longer half-life and may cause a higher incidence of GI bleeding than other NSAIDs, should be avoided in elderly patients.

REMISSION-INDUCING DRUGS

The remission-inducing drugs—gold preparations (gold sodium thiomalate, aurothioglucose, auranofin), chelating agents (penacillamine), cytotoxic drugs (cyclophosphamide, azathioprine, methotrexate), and antimalarials (chloroquine, quinacrine, hydroxychloroquine)—may produce partial or complete remission. These drugs are all slow acting and require 6 weeks to 6 months of treatment before benefits can be recognized.

GOLD PREPARATIONS

Rheumatoid arthritis has been treated with parenteral gold salts for more than 50 years. (An oral preparation is also available.) Studies seem to suggest that about 50% of patients will have a positive clinical response to gold therapy. The gold preparations, which include **gold sodium thiomalate** *(GST, Myochrisine)*, **aurothioglucose** *(Soganal)*, and **auranofin** *(Ridaura)*, are featured in Table 57–8.

Action

The exact mechanism of action of gold preparations has not yet been determined. It is thought that they may inhibit the formation of abnormal proteins (such as bradykinin) by retarding the formation of disulfide bonds, or they may stabilize the collagen fibers, making them less susceptible to inflammation. Gold seems to alter the progression of the disease by suppressing synovial inflammation and inhibiting the activity of lysosomal enzymes, reducing lymphocyte proliferation, and lessening phagocytic activity within the joint. However, therapy is often necessary for 3 to 4 months before any response can be noted. Gold therapy is the most costly of all therapies; however, it is beneficial and cost effective in some patients. Gold products have beneficial effects in approximately 80% to 90% of the patients when a cumulative dosage of 200 to 400 mg has been reached.

Contraindications and Precautions

The contraindications of gold products are toxicity to heavy metals, renal or hepatic disease, congestive heart failure, hypertension, uncontrolled diabetes, and acute hepatitis as all of these conditions can be worsened from gold deposits in tissues. Oral gold is also contraindicated in persons with bone marrow aplasia, pulmonary fibrosis, and exfoliative dermatitis. Safety in pregnancy (category C), lactating women, and children has not been established.

Adverse Effects

The most common adverse effects occur secondary to the deposits of gold in the tissues and include pruritus, dermatitis, alopecia, skin pigment changes (gray to blue coloration), metallic taste, stomatitis, nephrotic syndrome and proteinuria, allergic reactions, and thrombocytopenia. Adverse effects most generally appear when the cumulative dose of gold is 400 to 800 mg of parenteral gold. These adverse effects are experienced by about 40% of the population receiving gold compounds. Less commonly, anemias, hepatitis, and gold deposits in eyes are experienced.

○ **Gold sodium thiomalate** (GST, Myochrysine) is 50% gold and is administered by IM injection. In most cases, clinical improvement does not occur until 1 g has been administered. With clinical improvement, the dosage is decreased.

○ **Aurothioglucose** (Solganal), like gold sodium thiomalate, contains approximately 50% gold. It is admin-

Table 57–8. REMISSION-INDUCING DRUGS: GOLD PRODUCTS AND CHELATING AGENTS

DRUG NAME/ROUTE AND DOSAGE	PHARMACOKINETICS/ DYNAMICS	NURSING IMPLICATIONS
GOLD PRODUCTS		
gold sodium thiomalate (Myochrisine) (contains 50% gold)		
Dosage highly individualized. *Initial Dose*–10 mg IM; *Second Injection*–25 mg; *Third Injection and Thereafter*–25–50 mg weekly until response occurs or an upper limit of 1 g administered, or until toxicity occurs.	**Onset:** slow **Peak:** 2–6 hr (blood levels); 1–2 mo (therapeutic effect) **Duration:** 6 mo **½L:** 14–168 days: single dose; 14–40 days by third dose; up to 168 days after 11th dose **PB:** 95%–99% **B:** none **E:** urine, feces	For all: **ASSESSMENT:** Baseline CBC, blood urea nitrogen, and creatinine are obtained before start of therapy and at regular intervals thereafter. Assess for pregnancy (category C). **INTERVENTION:** Exposure to sun may aggravate dermatitis, so patient should wear hats and long-sleeved clothing for protection. Therapeutic effects may not be seen for 6–8 wk. May continue to improve for as long as 1 yr. When administering, agitate bottle before medication is withdrawn into syringe to ensure uniform suspension. Use 20 or 21-gauge needle. Then inject medication deep intragluteally with patient in recumbent position. It is best if patient can remain recumbent for 30 min. (Transient side effects, such as dizziness, facial flushing, and vertigo may be experienced). Medication should be preserved in tightly closed light-resistant container and should not be used if darker than pale yellow. **EVALUATION:** Notify physician for continued rash, sore mouth, indigestion, and diarrhea.
aurothioglucose (Solganal) (contains 50% gold)		
1st Dose–10 mg/wk IM; *2nd and 3rd Dose*–25 mg/wk; *4th and Other Doses*–50 mg/wk; continue until 0.8–1.0 g has been given and evaluate; if improvement, give 25 mg q 3–4 wk.	**Onset:** slow **Peak:** 4–6 hr (levels); 1–2 mo (effect) **Duration:** 6 hr **½L:** 3–27 days **PB:** 85%–95% **B:** none **E:** urine, feces	Same as for all plus: **INTERVENTION:** Use an 18-gauge needle. Keep patient lying flat for 15 min.
auranofin (Ridaura) (contains 29% gold)		
Adults: 6 mg/day PO; if no response in 6 mo, increase to 9 mg/day; if no response in another 3 mo, discontinue.	**Onset:** rapid **Peak:** 1–2 hr (levels); 8–16 wk (effect) **Duration:** 6 mo **½L:** 26 days **PB:** 60% **B:** NA **E:** urine (85% unchanged), feces	Same as for all.
CHELATING AGENTS		
D-penicillamine (Cuprimine)		
Adults: 125–250 mg PO daily; up to 1 g/day, with increases every 1–3 mo. *Children:* 5 mg/kg per day PO; up to 10–15 mg/kg per day.	**Onset:** 1–3 mo **Peak:** 130 min **Duration:** 1–3 mo **½L:** 60 min **PB:** NA **B:** liver **E:** urine, feces	**ASSESSMENT:** Assess patient before and during therapy for skin, blood, renal, and hepatic problems. Assess temperature daily (may be first sign of allergy). Routine CBC and renal studies are done q 2 wk for 6 mo, then monthly. **INTERVENTION:** Administer on empty stomach (30–60 min before, or 2 hr after meals). Separate other medications by 1 hr. Capsules may be opened and mixed with juice. Patient may need supplemental vitamin B6. If patient has remission for 6 mo, gradually reduce dose of drug. Continue with other drug therapy while administering penicillamine. **EVALUATION:** Notify physician if skin rash, unusual bruising, bleeding, sore throat, exertional dyspnea, fever, or chills occurs.

NA = not available.

istered only intramuscularly in the gluteal muscle. If there is no improvement when large doses have been administered, aurothioglucose is discontinued.

○ **Auranofin** (Ridaura) is an oral gold product for adult rheumatoid arthritis. This drug is indicated for patients who have not responded or cannot tolerate the NSAIDs.

In controlled studies, fewer patients dropped out of therapy because of side effects due to auranofin than because of those due to injectable gold. Therapeutic effects may start in 3 to 4 months but also may not be seen for 6 months. If response is inadequate after 6 months, dosage can be increased. If there is still inadequate response in 3 months, auranofin should be discontinued.

CHELATING AGENTS

○ **D-Penicillamine** (Cuprimine) is a chelating agent recommended for the removal of excess copper in patients with Wilson's disease (Table 57–8). In numerous studies in England, it has been shown to be effective in suppressing disease activity in rheumatoid arthritis. Its direct action in rheumatoid arthritis is still under investigation; but it does reduce serum immunoglobulins (IgM and IgG) and, with prolonged use, also reduces titers of the rheumatoid factor and decreases erythrocyte sedimentation rate (ESR). D-Penicillamine helps to control the symptoms of rheumatoid arthritis, but complete remissions are rare. As with gold, it may take 2 to 3 months before any effects, such as reduction in pain, swelling, and tenderness, are recognized. The duration of action may be months or years after the medication is discontinued.

CONTRAINDICATIONS AND PRECAUTIONS D-Penicillamine is contraindicated in pregnancy, blood dyscrasias, and renal insufficiency. If fever develops, the drug is discontinued. It is given cautiously to individuals who are allergic to penicillin because of the possibility of hypersensitivity and to patients who are currently using or have taken gold salts within the past 4 months.

ADVERSE EFFECTS D-Penicillamine has many dangerous adverse effects, so the patient must continue under medical supervision during therapy. These include GI complaints, allergic reactions, bone marrow depression, alopecia, and increased skin friability. This drug should not be given concurrently with salicylates, NSAIDs, or corticosteroids because of the increased incidence of serious GI side effects.

CYTOTOXIC MEDICATIONS

Three very potent cytotoxic medications that are commonly used to treat cancer, **cyclophosphamide *(Cytoxan)*, azathioprine *(Imuran)*,** and **methotrexate *(Rheumatrex)*,** can also be used as anti-inflammatory agents. These medications depress lymphocyte activity. The lymphocytes are primarily responsible for the damage to the connective tissue. Methotrexate is often considered a first-line drug by many rheumatologists. A single weekly dose is usually used. See Chapter 54 for more information on these drugs.

ANTIMALARIAL MEDICATIONS

The antimalarials—**chloroquine *(Aralen)*, quinacrine *(Atabrine)*,** and **hydroxychloroquine *(Plaquenil)*—**can be used as anti-inflammatory agents in both rheumatoid arthritis and lupus erythematosus (see Chapter 58). These preparations are rapidly absorbed from the GI tract. A patient receiving these preparations for long-term therapy should have his or her eyes evaluated frequently for macular degeneration, a common complication.

OTHER AGENTS FOR RHEUMATOID ARTHRITIS

Other agents used to treat rheumatoid arthritis include **sulfasalazine *(Azulfidine)*** and investigational agents from several drug classifications. These include cyclosporine, amiprilose, and monoclonal anti-CD4 antibodies. In addition, various combinations of second-line drugs are being evaluated.

○ **Sulfasalazine** (Azulfidine), used to treat inflammatory bowel disease for many years, is now used to treat rheumatoid arthritis. Several studies have found sulfasalazine as effective as gold and penicillamine (and less toxic) and more effective than hydroxychloroquine in preventing progression of the joint disease.

ANTIGOUT AGENTS

Gout, a metabolic disorder of purine metabolism resulting in hyperuricemia, is classified as primary or secondary. Primary hyperuricemia results from either overproduction or decreased renal excretion of uric acid. Secondary hyperuricemia develops during the course of another disease or secondary to chemotherapy.

The symptoms of gout appear when the serum uric acid level is above 6 mg/dL. Urate crystals are deposited in synovial fluid, which eventually precipitates an acute attack. Before therapy is started, it is important to clearly diagnose acute gout as the symptoms may resemble several other types of arthritis.

The primary agents used in the treatment of gout are **colchicine,** featured in Table 57–9; the uricosurics **probenecid *(Benemid)*** and **sulfinpyrazone *(Anturane)*;** and **allopurinol *(Lopurin, Zyloprim)*.** Colchicine is effective in about 90% of all cases provided it is started immediately after the attack begins. If started later, it is less effective. The uricosurics, probenecid (Benemid) and sulfinpyrazone (Anturane), inhibit the tubular reabsorption of uric acid in the kidney. Consequently, uric acid is excreted and serum levels are decreased. Allopurinol (Lopurin, Zyloprim) inhibits the conversion of xanthine to uric acid by the inhibition of the enzyme xanthine oxidase. Ultimately, there is a reduced serum uric acid level, which begins in about 24 to 48 hours. See Figure 57–2 for site of action of each of these agents.

Table 57–9. ANTIGOUT DRUGS

DRUG NAME/ROUTE AND DOSAGE	PHARMACOKINETICS/ DYNAMICS	NURSING IMPLICATIONS
colchicine		
acute gout 0.5–1.2 mg/hr PO × 10 doses or until GI side effects occur; maximum dose 4–8 mg **chronic gout** 0.5–1.2 mg/day PO **iv use** *Adults:* 1–3 mg over 2–5 min IV to start, then 0.5 mg q 6 hr; max. dose 4 mg in 24 hr or one course of therapy	**Onset:** 20 min **Peak:** 0.5–2 hr **Duration:** 9 days **½L:** 20 min (plasma) **PB:** NA **B:** liver **E:** urine (10%–20% unchanged), bile	For all: **ASSESSMENT:** Baseline uric acid levels and CBC are obtained and periodically checked during therapy. Assess for pregnancy: colchicine (category C—oral; D—parenteral); probenecid, sulfinpyrazone (unknown); and allopurinol (C). **INTERVENTION:** Administer immediately before, during, or after meal to limit gastric irritation. Increase fluid intake to at least 3000 mL/day (assuming there are no contraindications to increased fluid intake) to prevent formation of uric acid stones by kidney. Activity of affected joint is limited during acute attack. May begin exercise, warmth, and physical therapy when pain and swelling subside, generally about 24–72 hr from onset of therapy. Understand and follow diet limitations. Patients may be encouraged to test their urinary pH with nitrazine paper. A highly acidic urine tends to occur during gout attack. If urinary pH is decreasing, patients should notify physician and begin their medication immediately. **Patient Teaching**—Lifelong therapy may be required to control symptoms. The patient should not take aspirin or aspirin-containing medications without consulting physician. If analgesic is required, acetaminophen is recommended. Patient should not experiment with drug dosage but should take prescribed dose. Limit alcohol intake. **EVALUATION:** Notify physician if rash, sore throat, fever, or unusual bleeding, bruising, or weakness occurs. Discontinue as soon as gout pain is relieved.
probenecid (Benemid)		
Adults: 250 mg PO 2 times daily; increased to 1 g/day over many weeks to control symptoms	**Onset:** 30 min **Peak:** 2–4 hr **Duration:** 5–8 hr **½L:** 4–9 hr **PB:** 85%–95% **B:** liver **E:** urine	Same as for all plus: **INTERVENTION:** Take with food or antacid. Do not start drug until acute gouty attack has subsided. Try to alkalize urine. Drink at least 6–8 glasses of water to prevent development of kidney stones.
sulfinpyrazone (Anturane)		
Adults: Initial Dose—100–200 mg PO 2 times daily; up to 200–400 mg 2 times daily *Maintenance Dose*—200–800 mg/day	**Onset:** 30 min **Peak:** 1–2 hr **Duration:** 4–6 hr **½L:** 2.2–3 hr **PB:** 98%–99% **B:** liver **E:** urine (50% unchanged)	Same as for all plus: **INTERVENTION:** Give with meals. Drink at least 10–12 glasses of fluid per day.
allopurinol (Zyloprim)		
Adults: 200–800 mg PO 1–2 times daily; maximum dose 800 mg/day	**Onset:** 30–60 min (blood levels); 24–48 hr (therapeutic effect) **Peak:** 1.5–4.5 hr (levels); 1–3 wk (effect) **Duration:** 18–30 hr (levels); 1–2 wk (effect) **½L:** 1–2 hr (metabolite, 18–30 hr) **PB:** NA **B:** liver **E:** urine, feces (20%)	Same as for all plus: **INTERVENTION:** Take with meals. Do not take excessive vitamin C as there is increased risk of kidney stone formation. Drink at least 10–12 glasses of fluids per day. **EVALUATION:** Observe caution when performing tasks requiring alertness. Notify physician of skin rash.

NA = not available.

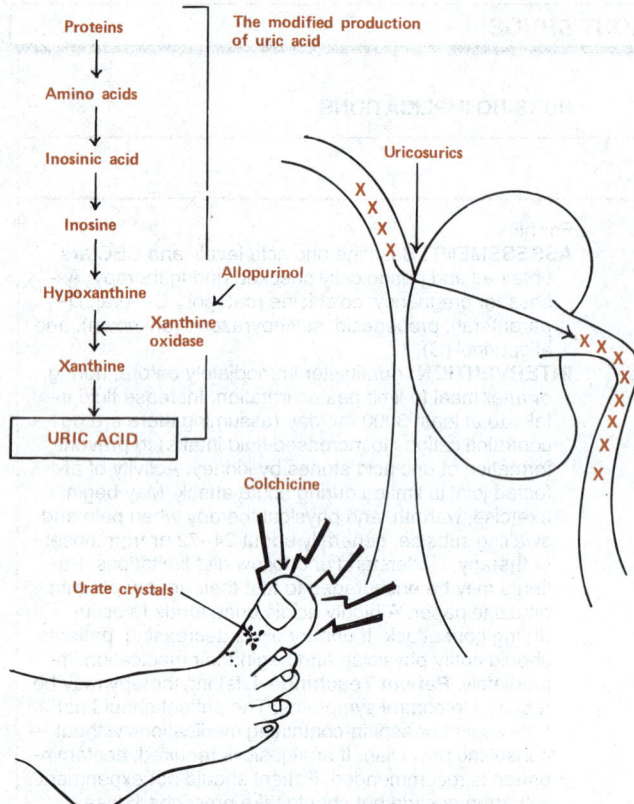

Figure 57–2. Three mechanisms of action of antigout medications. Colchicine opposes leukocyte phagocytosis, which inhibits further deposits; uricosurics interfere with tubular reabsorption of uric acid; and allopurinol interferes with xanthine oxidase, an enzyme necessary for uric acid production.

CONTRAINDICATIONS AND PRECAUTIONS

All antigout medications are contraindicated in patients with hypersensitivity, GI or hepatic disease, or blood dyscrasias as these conditions may be aggravated or worsened. It is given cautiously to the elderly or to debilitated patients as adverse effects are worsened. Use in pregnancy (allopurinol—category C), lactating women, and children has not been established.

ADVERSE EFFECTS

The most common adverse effects of the antigout drugs include bone marrow depression and blood dyscrasias. GI symptoms, especially diarrhea, are also common, particularly with maximal doses.

○ **Colchicine** may inhibit leukocyte activity in the joint, diminish phagocytosis, and reduce inflammation. Colchicine can relieve pain, but it is not an analgesic. Colchicine is not a uricosuric and does not prevent the progression of gout to chronic gouty arthritis. Colchicine's suppressive effects reduce the incidence of acute attacks only.

○ **Probenecid** (Benemid) is started only after the initial attack of gout has subsided, as its administration may make the acute symptoms worse. As well as being used

as an antigout medication, probenecid is also used as an adjunct to therapy with penicillin or other short-acting penicillin preparations and zidovudine (AZT). It inhibits the tubular secretion of penicillin, and zidovudine increases plasma levels two to four times. It is frequently given to prolong the effectiveness of penicillin when treating gonorrhea or gonococcal infections in both men and women.

INTERACTIONS Probenecid inhibits the renal excretion and therefore may increase the plasma levels of NSAIDs, acyclovir, sulfonylureas, dapsone, methotrexate, clofibrate, and penicillamine. Concurrent use with ketorolac decreases the clearance of ketorolac and increases the half-life; therefore, this combination is contraindicated. Concurrent therapy with salicylates inhibits its uricosuric effects. Probenecid interferes with laboratory test results such as urinary 17-ketosteroids and bromsulphalein (BSP), inhibiting excretion of the steroid compounds and the dye BSP.

○ **Sulfinpyrazone** (Anturane) has little anti-inflammatory effect and is not recommended for acute gout attacks but only for chronic prophylaxis or for intermittent gout attacks. It also inhibits platelet aggregation.

○ **Allopurinol** (Zyloprim) inhibits xanthine oxidase, thus reducing the production of uric acid. It is the preferred drug in the treatment of tophaceous gout. It is also used in patients receiving cytotoxic agents that break down cellular nucleic acid and leads to acute uric acid nephropathy. If allopurinol is given during acute attacks, colchicine or another NSAID is also given to treat the attack. A fall in both serum and urinary uric acid begins in 2 to 3 days. However, 1 week or more of therapy may be required before the full effects of the drug are achieved.

Allopurinol is also being used in the management of patients with leukemia; lymphoma; and malignancies with acute, urate-induced, obstructive uropathy; and also for treatment of urinary tract stones. Several potential uses for allopurinol have recently surfaced. Because of its antioxidant properties, allopurinol may prove beneficial in preventing superoxide-induced tissue damage, such as inflammatory joint disease, myocardial ischemia, alcoholic liver disease, and organ survival before and during transplantation.

Several studies have examined the role of allopurinol in decreasing mortality of patients undergoing coronary artery bypass surgery. These studies have shown that allopurinol reduces the incidence of postoperative dysrhythmias; in one study, the need for postoperative inotropic support was decreased and the rate of peripheral warming was increased.

USING THE NURSING PROCESS

ASSESSMENT

- Obtain a thorough nursing history to develop the database, as summarized in Table 57–10. All the information is used later when preparing the nursing-care plan. The patient requiring anti-inflammatory

Assessment

Assess past history/presence of inflammatory disease, e.g., rheumatoid arthritis, gout.
Assess level of activity and ability to maintain activities of daily living.
Assess nutritional status.
Assess laboratory studies, e.g., CBC, sedimentation rate, uric acid, immunoglobulin, or rheumatoid factor levels.
Assess psychologic state and determine how illness has affected life.

Nursing Diagnosis Pain

RELATED TO: Distention of tissues by accumulation of fluid/inflammatory process.

Desired Outcomes/Evaluation Criteria

Reports pain is relieved/controlled. Appears relaxed, able to sleep/rest and participate in activities appropriately. Incorporates relaxation skills and diversional activities into pain-control program.

Nursing Actions	Rationale
Investigate complaints of pain, noting location and intensity (scale of 1–10). Note precipitating factors and nonverbal pain cues.	Helpful in determining pain management needs and effectiveness of therapy.
Have patient assume position of comfort while in bed or sitting in chair.	In severe disease/acute exacerbation, total bedrest may be necessary to limit pain/injury to joints.
Maintain neutral position of affected joints with pillows, sandbags, trochanter rolls, splints, braces.	Rests painful joints.
Encourage frequent changes of position. Assist as needed.	Prevents general fatigue and joint stiffness.
Encourage use of stress management techniques, e.g., progressive relaxation, Therapeutic Touch, biofeedback, visualization, guided imagery, self-hypnosis, and controlled breathing.	Promotes relaxation, provides sense of control, and may enhance coping abilities.
Administer medications as indicated, e.g., acetylsalicylates (ASA) nonsteroidal anti-inflammatory drugs (ibuprofen, naproxen, misoprostol).	ASA exerts an anti-inflammatory and mild analgesic effect, decreasing stiffness and increasing mobility. Used when patient does not respond to aspirin or to enhance effects of aspirin. Given to decrease or prevent the incidence of gastric irritation and ulceration when NSAIDs are administered concurrently. (Contraindicated in pregnant women/nursing mothers).
Discuss taking drugs with food, milk, or antacids.	Minimizes gastric upset and irritation.

Nursing Diagnosis: Impaired Physical Mobility

RELATED TO: Skeletal deformity, pain/discomfort, intolerance to activity.

AS EVIDENCED BY: Reluctance to attempt movement/inability to purposefully move, limited range of motion, decreased muscle strength.

Desired Outcomes/Evaluation Criteria

Maintains position of function and absence of contractures. Displays increased strength and function of affected and/or compensatory body part. Demonstrates techniques/behaviors that enable resumption/continuation of activities.

Nursing Actions	Rationale
Evaluate/continuously monitor degree of joint inflammation/pain.	Level of activity/exercise is dependent on progression/resolution of inflammatory process.
Maintain bed/chair rest when indicated.	Systemic rest is mandatory during acute exacerbations and throughout course of disease.
Assist with active/passive ROM as well as resistive exercises and isometrics when patient is able.	Maintains/improves joint function, muscle strength, and general stamina.
Demonstrate use of pillows, sandbags, trochanter rolls, splints, and braces for positioning.	Promotes joint stability and maintains proper joint position and body alignment, minimizing contractures.
Provide safe environment, e.g., raised chairs/toilet seat, use of handrails in tub/shower and toilet, proper use of mobility aids, wheelchair safety.	Avoids accidental injuries/falls.
Consult with physical/occupational therapists.	Helpful in formulating exercise/activity program based on individual needs and in identifying mobility devices/adjuncts.
Administer medications as indicated, e.g., antirheumatic agents (gold, Myochrisine, or auranofin) or steroids.	Chrysotherapy (gold salts) may produce dramatic/sustained remission but may result in rebound inflammation if discontinued or if serious side effects occur, e.g., nitritoid crisis with dizziness, blurred vision, flushing, progressing to anaphylactic shock. May be necessary to suppress acute systemic inflammation.

Continued on the following page

Table 57–10. NURSING PROCESS FOR PATIENT RECEIVING PROSTAGLANDINS AND ANTI-INFLAMMATORIES, *Continued*	
Nursing Diagnosis: Body Image Disturbance/Role Performance **RELATED TO:** Disfigurement, changes in ability to perform usual tasks, increased energy expenditure. **AS EVIDENCED BY:** Change in structure/function of affected parts, negative self-talk, feelings of helplessness or hopelessness.	**Desired Outcomes/Evaluation Criteria** Verbalizes increased confidence in ability to deal with illness, changes in lifestyle, and possible limitations. Makes realistic goals/plans for future.

Nursing Actions	**Rationale**
Encourage verbalization about concerns of disease process, future expectations.	Provides opportunity to identify fears/misconceptions and deal with directly.
Discuss meaning of loss/change to patient/significant other (SO). Ascertain how patient views self as man/woman in usual lifestyle functioning, including sexual aspects. Discuss patient's perception of how SO perceives limitations.	Identifying how illness affects perception of self and interactions with others will determine need for further intervention/counseling. Verbal/nonverbal cues from SO may have major impact on how patient views self.
Acknowledge and accept feelings of grief, hostility, dependency.	Constant pain is wearing, and feelings of anger and hostility are common. Acceptance provides feedback that feelings are normal.
Involve patient in planning care and scheduling activities.	Enhances feelings of competency/self-worth, encourages independence and participation in therapy.

Other Suggested Nursing Diagnosis: Knowledge Deficit.

drugs may be acutely ill in a hospital or relatively healthy, with the condition being treated on an outpatient basis. The course of most of these conditions is variable. A group of patients may have one acute attack and then completely remit; another group may have repeated remissions and exacerbations; and another group may have inexorable progression of the disease, which is unresponsive to therapeutic modalities.

- Assess the activity level of the patient and identify what assistance is needed with activities of daily living. Both the patient and family should understand that fatigue or malaise present with these diseases is not laziness but a disease symptom that could disappear as therapy progresses. Assessment of ability to do household work, to accomplish on-the-job and specific activities such as climbing stairs and personal hygiene is made. It is often useful to ask the patient which specific activities are most impaired by the disease and to follow this as an indicator of improvement.
- Assess dietary intake. Recent research indicates that there is a connection between nutrition and arthritis. Most of these research findings still need to be replicated in larger groups of patients. Currently, eliminating milk, cheese, and yogurt can reduce joint stiffness, pain, and swelling in certain patients. Cereal grains (wheat, oat, rye), shrimp, and sodium nitrate (food preservative) can trigger joint problems in some arthritics. Patients should eliminate one food at a time from their diets. If symptoms improve, the food is eliminated permanently. One food substance, eicosapentaenoic acid—a fatty acid found in fish such as salmon, mackerel, tuna, rainbow trout, and sardines—when included in the diet, may alleviate symptoms of arthritis.

- Obtain laboratory tests such as CBC, sedimentation rate, uric acid levels, immunoglobulin or rheumatoid factor levels, and radiographs to develop the baseline data and periodically to monitor treatment and assess for adverse effects of medication.
- Assess psychologic status. The diagnosis of anti-inflammatory disease may cause great anxiety in both the patient and family. During the intervention phase, teaching emphasis is placed on the broad spectrum of disease manifestations and multiple options for therapy.

NURSING DIAGNOSIS

- Typical nursing diagnoses for a patient requiring anti-inflammatory medications include Pain, Impaired Mobility, Knowledge Deficit, and Body Image Disturbance.

PLANNING AND INTERVENTION

- Develop the goals of nursing intervention. Typical goals of nursing intervention when caring for the patient requiring anti-inflammatory drugs are included in Table 57–10. These include reducing pain and inflammation, maintaining joint mobility, and preventing deformity.

Juvenile arthritis varies from adult disease in that children frequently have more joint deformity. The prognosis for most children is good if treatment is begun immediately.

- Involve families in the patient's education. The more they know, the more likely that the patient and family are to be compliant with the treatment program.

- When patients taking NSAIDs, need elective surgery, discontinue the drugs at least 5 half-lives before to decrease the likelihood of postoperative GI bleeding and hypotension.

Patient Teaching

- Teach the patient important points about the anti-inflammatory drugs. This information is summarized in the Nursing Implications column of the drug tables and in Table 57–11.
- Monitor patients taking NSAIDs for GI side effects, including irritation and bleeding. To reduce the risk of bleeding, the drugs are administered with food or milk. Enteric-coated aspirin may be helpful. Misoprostol may be administered concurrently with NSAIDs or aspirin to prevent gastric ulcer formation. The best way to monitor GI bleeding is to have a baseline CBC done before therapy begins, with follow-up testing every 4 to 6 months.

When NSAIDs do cause upper GI bleeding, the blood that reaches the colon is usually digested and is, therefore, unlikely to react with the hemoccult reagent. For this reason, a positive hemoccult test in a NSAID-treated patient should not be attributed to upper GI bleeding. This patient needs to have a thorough colorectal workup.

- Monitor and attempt to obtain relief of pain. NSAIDs may not adequately control pain with active disease. If additional pain medications are needed, codeine or propoxyphene may be justified. Patients need to be taught not to take alcohol, tranquilizers, sedatives, or other CNS depressants along with their pain medication. Non-drug alternatives to pain medication may also be tried, such as relaxation techniques, biofeedback, or transcutaneous electrical nerve stimulation (TENS). Acute exacerbation may also be treated with low-dose, short-term steroids. Patients with acute joint flare-up may receive the corticosteroids directly into the joint. This injection usually brings relief in 24 to 48 hours. Adjunctive therapies such as splints and physical therapy may also be helpful.
- Alcohol may increase the risk of hepatic injury caused by acetaminophen or GI bleeding due to NSAIDs, but the relative risk of OTC doses of these drugs in patients who drink small amounts of alcohol is unknown. Regular use of any analgesic should be discouraged in alcohol drinkers, and those who do use them should be encouraged to use the lowest possible doses.
- Teach the patient about dietary limitations when he or she is diagnosed as having gout. The diet usually includes placing the patient on a purine-limited diet, increasing fluid volume daily, and limiting beer, ale, or wine, as they may precipitate a gout attack. The patient should not take aspirin or aspirin-containing medications without consulting the physician. If an analgesic is required, acetaminophen is recommended.
- Teach the patients not to experiment with their drug dosages, but to take the prescribed dose. For example, taking a subtherapeutic dose of sulfinpyrazone can precipitate an acute gout attack.

The therapeutic choices of drugs available to treat inflammatory diseases is great. At this time, no one can predict which drug will be best for an individual patient, but the vast majority of patients do respond to therapy. Besides pharmacologic therapy, the nurse must stress occupational therapy, counseling, and exercise to achieve the goal of a creative, functional person who has achieved some freedom from disease.

EVALUATION

- Evaluate the effectiveness of anti-inflammatory drugs on a predetermined list of outcome evaluation criteria (see Table 57–10).
- Work with the patient and family to ensure their complete assistance and support. The primary reasons for noncompliance are forgetting the medication, stopping it because all the symptoms have been eliminated, and stopping it because of side effects. Education for the patient with arthritis must stress that stopping the medication for any period of time only causes a flare-up of the symptoms, possibly with more damage resulting. With gout, the average patient may have only four or five attacks in a lifetime, even if he or she is on no medication.
- Determine whether or not the patient can open the medication bottles. Childproof tops may be impossible for the individual with arthritic hands to open. Upon request, the pharmacist can put a regular cap on the prescription. The patient can also ask for a

---

Table 57–11. PATIENT TEACHING INFORMATION—ANTI-INFLAMMATORY AGENTS

Dear Patient:
This drug has been ordered for you. This is what you should know about your drug to get the most from your therapy. Anti-inflammatory drugs are used to decrease redness and soreness in diseases such as arthritis and bursitis.

☐ 1. Drugs will be taken (until your symptoms disappear for _____ days; for several months until your symptoms are controlled; for the rest of your life).
☐ 2. Drugs should be taken (with meals; between meals—see Drug Tables for specific information).
☐ 3. Interactions with other drugs are possible with your medication. Do not take any drug without first checking with your physician or pharmacist.
☐ 4. If you forget your drug until your next dose time, forget it. Do not try to catch up.
☐ 5. Do not stop your drug without talking to your physician first.
☐ 6. Side effects can occur from your drug. They might include upset stomach and headache. Additional side effects include (_____). If any of these occurs, tell your doctor.
☐ 7. Weigh yourself every week. Call your physician if you have a change of more than 5 lb in a week.
☐ 8. Check your stool for presence of blood. Stools may appear black or have actual blood in them.
☐ 9. Keep all drugs out of the reach of small children.
☐ 10. Store your medication in a tight, moisture-resistant container.

large bottle with a regular cap to store aspirin or related OTC preparations. The nurse stresses the importance of properly labeling and storing these medications out of the reach of children as they do not have childproof caps.

- Evaluate for the adverse effects of medications. If an unusual symptom is noted, the patient is encouraged to call the physician or nurse.
- Evaluate the patient for any unusual weight gain or edema. All medications are discontinued promptly if the patient complains of diarrhea, skin rash, or bleeding from any body area.
- Obtain and evaluate patient and family compliance. The nurse stresses the importance of continued medical care. During a remission, the dosages are likely to be reduced; during an exacerbation, they are increased. The nurse is always alert for possible drug interactions. In addition, all other evaluation criteria are evaluated before the patient leaves the nurse's care. All previously taught material is reviewed and updated, if necessary, to ensure that the patient's knowledge base remains accurate.

As long as there is no cure for arthritis, new drugs will continually be developed to treat the symptoms. As they are released, the media will herald them as the latest miracle cure, often raising false hopes for the millions of arthritis sufferers. These patients need continued education that nurses can provide concerning the benefits of these new therapies.

The bibliography for this chapter can be found in Appendix B, which begins on page 1054.

CHAPTER REVIEW QUESTIONS*

1. The prostaglandins have a diversity of action, which includes:
   a. Vasoconstriction.
   b. Decreased cardiac output.
   c. Increased capillary permeability.
   d. Platelet aggregation.

2. Misoprostol (Cytotec) is contraindicated in the following patient condition:
   a. Pregnancy.
   b. Gastric ulcers.
   c. Glaucoma.
   d. Diabetes mellitus.

3. Short-term anti-inflammatory medications are used for:
   a. One to two months only.
   b. A temporary cure.
   c. Pain relief.
   d. Minimal side effects.

4. Salicylates are thought to relieve arthritic pain by:
   a. Enhancing platelet aggregation.
   b. Releasing neurologic blockers.
   c. Stimulating bradykinin synthesis.
   d. Inhibiting prostaglandin synthesis.

5. The nonsteroidal anti-inflammatory drugs:
   a. Are administered cautiously to patients with renal disease.
   b. Do not cross the placental barrier and are safe for pregnant women.
   c. Are used as a substitute for patients allergic to aspirin.
   d. Are primarily used as a cure for clinically significant hangover.

6. Antigout agents, known as the uricosurics, include probenecid and sulfinpyrazone. These agents act by:
   a. Increasing the activity of leukocytes and synovial cells.
   b. Stimulating the breakdown of purine in the liver.
   c. Inhibiting the tubular reabsorption of uric acid.
   d. Inhibiting the conversion of xanthine to uric acid.

*See Appendix A, which begins on page 1051, for answers.

BUILDING YOUR CRITICAL THINKING SKILLS

CONSTIPATION

Case Study 2: Constipation

A 65-year-old woman comes to the clinic with reports of fatigue, chronic constipation, and red stools. She is suspected of having a GI bleed. Stool samples for occult blood are negative, and her hemoglobin and hematocrit are normal for her age. She states she has been taking Feen-A-Mint and Pepto-Bismol for several months.

1. What effect could the combination of these two over-the-counter drugs be for this patient?
2. How should the nurse address this patient's problem?

CHAPTER 58

Anti-Infectives

Sandra L. Preston, PharmD
Laurie L. Briceland, PharmD

CHAPTER OUTLINE

TABLES

BOX

KEY TERMS

Acetylation
Aerobic organisms
Anaerobic organisms
Antibiotic-associated colitis
Bacterial resistance
Bactericidal
Bacteriostatic
Beta-lactam
Beta-lactamase
Beta-lactamase inhibitors
Broad-spectrum agents
Chromosomal mutation
Crystalluria
Disulfiram-like reaction
DNA gyrase
DNA polymerase
Enterohepatic recirculation
Eosinophilia
Glucose-6-phosphate
　dehydrogenase deficiency
Gray baby syndrome
Host defenses
Interstitial nephritis
Narrow-spectrum agents
Normal flora
Nosocomial
Para-aminobenzoic acid
Pathogen
Penicillinase
Peptidoglycan
Plasmids
Pseudotumor cerebri
RNA polymerase
Sterols (ergosterol)
Superinfection
Synergy
Tetrahydrofolic acid
　reductase
Thymidine kinase
Translocation

LEARNING OBJECTIVES

After reading this chapter, the student will be able to:

1. Formulate a specific plan to assess the teaching needs of a patient requiring an anti-infective agent.
2. Develop the nursing diagnoses relative to the teaching needs of a patient requiring anti-infective agents.
3. Plan the nursing intervention necessary to teach the patient requiring anti-infective agents.
4. Develop teaching and evaluation tools or techniques specific to the learning needs of the patient requiring medication.
5. Evaluate the effectiveness of nursing intervention to promote patient compliance with the treatment regimen.

Anti-infective agents are commonly used in clinical practice to treat infection due to a *pathogen*, an organism which causes disease. The term "anti-infective" can be used to describe antibacterial, antiviral, antifungal, antiparasitic, antiprotozoal, antileprotic, and antituberculous agents. The desired therapeutic outcome with anti-infective agents is to eradicate infection while avoiding drug-induced toxicity.

INTRODUCTION TO PATHOGENS AND ANTIMICROBIAL THERAPY

The population of microorganisms inhabiting internal and external surfaces of healthy human beings is often referred to as the *normal flora*. Important anatomic locations populated by various bacteria, fungi, and protozoa include the oropharynx, upper and lower intestine, lower genitourinary tract, conjunctiva, and skin. Other locations in the body such as the blood and cerebrospinal fluid are sterile, meaning that the presence of microbes is abnormal and indicates infection.

Normal bacterial flora functions to prevent pathogens from causing infection by suppressing their growth through competition. When the normal flora is altered, pathogenic organisms can cause infection. The most dramatic alterations of the normal flora come about as a result of administering antibiotics. A common example is the occurrence of vaginal yeast infections in patients taking *broad-spectrum* antibiotics (e.g., tetracyclines, cephalosporins). By elimination of the normal vaginal flora by the broad-spectrum antibiotic, there is a subsequent overgrowth of yeast, causing clinical vaginitis. This is an example of *superinfection*.

Another example of the protective role of normal flora is seen in patients who experience *antibiotic-associated colitis* (AAC). The colitis is due to a toxin that is produced by the bacterium *Clostridium difficile*. Under antibiotic-free conditions, the intestinal growth of this organism is limited by the presence of normal flora. When patients receive antibiotics that suppress the normal intestinal flora (e.g., ampicillin, cephalosporins, and clindamycin), *C. difficile* begins to multiply and produce toxin. Fever, abdominal cramping, watery diarrhea, mucus in the stool are present. The stool may also contain blood. AAC may be life threatening. The offending antibiotic is stopped and either oral metronidazole 250–500 mg every 6–8 hours or oral Vancomycin 125 mg every 6 hours is administered.

The administration of potent, broad-spectrum antibiotics to hospitalized patients can result in colonization and infection with organisms resistant to numerous antibiotics including the antibiotic being prescribed. Colonization and infection with multidrug-resistant bacteria is most often seen in patients who have received prolonged courses of antibiotics (e.g., burn patients). For this reason, narrow-spectrum antibiotic therapy is prescribed as often as possible and for only the appropriate duration of treatment.

Finally, other infections can increase risk of a secondary infection. Patients who experience viral respiratory tract infections often develop secondary bacterial infections. In this situation, the initial viral infection is believed to alter the epithelial cells lining the oropharynx, thus allowing pathogenic bacteria to colonize the area. These pathogenic bacteria can invade the host and cause a secondary bacterial infection.

ANTIMICROBIAL SPECTRUM

Antibiotic agents may be broad spectrum or *narrow spectrum* (effective against only a few types of organisms). The organisms themselves are usually classified by whether they absorb the Gram laboratory stain (gram-positive or gram-negative) and/or whether they require the presence of oxygen (*aerobic* or *anaerobic*) to live and grow. However, many organisms elude classification in this way and it is increasingly common for specific organisms to be directly named and associated with the spectrum of activity of individual antibiotics and other anti-infectives.

HOW ANTIMICROBIAL AGENTS EXERT THEIR EFFECT

Antibiotic agents exert their effect on bacteria in one of two ways. *Bacteriostatic* agents inhibit bacterial growth. Subsequent bacterial death therefore depends on the *host defenses*. The immune system acts as the host defense system and is made up of leukocytes, complement, and immunoglobulins that act to subsequently destroy the pathogen. Erythromycin and clindamycin are examples of such agents.

Some antibiotics are *bactericidal*, meaning that the bacteria are killed after exposure. Examples of drugs acting in this manner include the penicillins, cephalosporins, imipenem, and the quinolones. These agents are preferable in patients who are immunocompromised or if the site of infection is in an area with limited host defenses (e.g., meningitis, endocarditis).

BACTERIAL RESISTANCE TO ANTIBIOTICS

Bacterial resistance is said to occur when a bacterium is not susceptible to the effects of a certain anti-infective agent. Bacteria become resistant to antibiotics by altering genetic material that codes for biochemical changes within their cells. The mechanisms by which bacteria alter their genetic material include *chromosomal mutation*, recombination of DNA, and transfer of *plasmids* (small pieces of DNA containing genetic information).

Chromosomal mutation occurs spontaneously among a given population of bacteria. Suppression of the nonmutant bacteria by antibiotics allows the mutant organisms to multiply. Chromosomal mutation usually increases bacterial resistance by causing the bacteria to produce an enzyme that inactivates the antibiotic. Mutation may also induce changes in bacterial membranes, preventing antibiotic penetration, and may alter the target site of the antibiotic, thus preventing attachment.

Transfer of plasmids may be achieved by numerous mechanisms from one bacteria to another. Plasmids contain instructions for the bacteria. These genetic instructions give the bacterial cell the ability to synthesize enzymes that inactivate antibiotics or to alter membrane permeability, preventing antibiotic entry into the cell. The most common example of plasmid-mediated resistance is the elaboration of *beta-lactamase* enzymes (e.g., penicillinase, cephalosporinase) by various bacteria.

Bacterial resistance is increasingly becoming a problem in the clinical setting. Organisms such as *Staphylococcus aureus* and *Staphylococcus epidermidis* can be resistant to many antibiotics, including methicillin owing to alterations in the penicillin-binding proteins in the bacteria that the drug must bind to exert its effect. These organisms are termed methicillin-resistant *S. aureus* (MRSA), methicillin-resistant *S. epidermidis* (MRSE). Vancomycin must be used to treat an infection caused by these organisms, and careful infection control measures must be taken to avoid transmission to other patients.

Other organisms for which bacterial resistance is increasing in certain geographic areas includes *Enterococcus species* and *Streptococcus pneumoniae*. Resistant gram-negative organisms may be a particular problem in the intensive care units. It is important that these resistant organisms be identified and be treated with appropriate anti-infective agents.

GENERAL PRINCIPLES OF ANTI-INFECTIVE THERAPY

Frequently, the selection of appropriate antibiotic therapy is made without the results of culture and sensitivity data. The following factors are considered when selecting an antibiotic regimen:

1. infecting organism (suspected or confirmed)
2. antibiotic sensitivity of the organism
3. site of infection
4. status of host defenses and organ function
5. antibiotic pharmacokinetics
6. monitoring of therapy

Infecting Organism   In most clinical situations in which infection is suspected, the pathogen is not identified within the first 24 to 48 hours. This lag period requires that initial treatment be directed against the most likely bacteria responsible for the infectious process. For this reason, knowledge of the normal flora, the status of host defenses, and underlying disease is important. If an organism is subsequently identified or documented, antimicrobial therapy may then be directed against the specific pathogen(s).

Antibiotic Sensitivity Testing   Collecting various body fluids or tissues for routine culture and antibiotic sensitivity testing is very important when infection is suspected. Initial or empiric broad-spectrum coverage may then be narrowed or streamlined based on test results.

Site of Infection   Although an organism may be identified, it is important to consider the site of infection. Antibiotics may not reach the necessary body compartment in sufficient concentrations (e.g., aminoglycosides in bacterial meningitis) to eradicate the infecting organism; therefore, alternative dosing regimens or routes of administration must be considered.

Host Defenses and Organ Function   An awareness of the patient's host defenses is important. Patients may be immunocompromised because of underlying diseases (e.g., cancer, AIDS) or drug therapy (e.g., corticosteroids). In these cases, the infecting organism may not be the usual bacterial pathogen, but instead may be a fungus (e.g., *Candida albicans*), a virus (e.g., cytomegalovirus), or a parasite (e.g., *Pneumocystis carinii*). In addition, these patients may require broader-spectrum antibiotics and more aggressive management because of their decreased ability to fight infection.

The primary organ of elimination for most antibiotics is the kidney and/or the liver. In patients with impaired renal or hepatic function, the dose of most antibiotics is reduced or the interval of drug administration increased. Antimicrobial agents for which no reduction in dose is necessary in patients with renal insufficiency are chloramphenicol, nafcillin, oxacillin, cloxacillin, dicloxacillin, clindamycin, cefoperazone, ceftriaxone, erythromycin, and metronidazole. In addition, hemodialysis and peritoneal dialysis can have a major impact on antibiotic removal from the body.

Antibiotic Pharmacokinetics   Antibiotics are absorbed, distributed, metabolized, and excreted in a variety of ways. Knowledge of the severity of infection, the site of infection, and so on, help guide in the selection of appropriate antibiotics.

Monitoring of Therapy   Clinical evaluation of antibiotic effectiveness is discussed in later sections. Several antibiotics (e.g., aminoglycosides, chloramphenicol, vancomycin) are monitored by measuring drug concentrations in blood. Knowledge of the desired antibiotic concentration minimizes both underdosing and potential toxicity associated with overdosing. Selected laboratory values (as discussed in each antibiotic section) are followed during therapy.

COMBINATION THERAPY AND PROPHYLACTIC USE

Combination anti-infective therapy is often indicated to achieve adequate broad-spectrum coverage. For empiric therapy for infections due to an unknown pathogen, it is desirable to obtain antimicrobial coverage for all potentially infecting organisms. In some instances, a combination of two agents can enhance the antibacterial activity, with more than a simple additive effect. When the activity of the combination is greater than the activity of either agent alone, *synergy* is said to occur. An example is the combination of an aminoglycoside and a penicillin for infections due to *Pseudomonas aeruginosa* or *Enterococcus faecalis*. Enhanced antibacterial activity is achieved with combination.

Combination therapy is used for treatment of active tuberculosis to prevent emergence of resistance, which can occur when only one drug is used. Because of the high numbers of organisms in patients with active tuberculosis, there is most likely a subpopulation resistant to a drug. If only that drug is used as treatment, the patient responds to the drug at first; however, the resistant subpopulation continues to grow and the patient relapses.

Prophylactic use of anti-infective agents is often indicated when there is potential risk for infection. When deciding whether or not to use anti-infective prophylaxis for a patient, the efficacy of prophylaxis must outweigh the toxicity associated with its use. Cost considerations are also evaluated. For instance, if the cost of an infection due to a pathogen outweighs the cost associated with the prophylaxis, it may be appropriate to use prophylaxis. One must also take into account which patient population is at risk for the infection. The HIV-positive population and the neutropenic patient population are often given anti-infective prophylaxis. These patient are at increased risk of development of certain infections due to their immunosuppression. In the HIV-positive population, prophylaxis is the standard of care for infections such as *P. carinii* pneumonia. Other patients who receive prophylaxis include patients undergoing certain surgical procedures or patients predisposed to bacterial endocarditis who are undergoing dental procedures.

PENICILLINS

Penicillins are natural or synthetic beta-lactam antimicrobial agents produced by or derived from species of the mold *Penicillium* and other fungi. Natural penicillins are produced by the process of fermentation. Synthetic penicillins are produced by chemical modification of the natural penicillin structure. Members of the penicillin family are classified into the following categories:

1. natural penicillins—penicillin G (Pfizerpen, Pentids, others) and penicillin V (Pen Vee K, V-Cillin K, Veetids, others)
2. penicillinase-resistant (antistaphylococcal) penicillins—methicillin (Staphcillin), nafcillin (Nafcil, Unipen), oxacillin (Prostaphlin), cloxacillin (Tegopen), and dicloxacillin (Dynapen, Pathocil)
3. broad-spectrum penicillins—ampicillin (Amcill, Omnipen, Polycillin), ampicillin/sulbactam (Unasyn), amoxicillin (Amoxil, Polymox, Trimox), amoxicillin/clavulanic acid (Augmentin), and bacampicillin (Spectrobid)
4. extended-spectrum (antipseudomonal) penicillins—oral carbenicillin (Geocillin), ticarcillin (Ticar), ticarcillin/clavulanic acid (Timentin), mezlocillin (Mezlin), piperacillin (Pipracil), and piperacillin/tazobactam (Zosyn)

Selected penicillins are featured in Table 58–1.

ACTION

Antimicrobial agents possessing a four-membered beta-lactam ring structure are able to bind bacterial cell wall components, preventing cross-linking of *peptidoglycan*, which is essential for cell wall synthesis. *Beta-lactam* agents may also bind to other enzymes regulating various aspects of bacterial cell division. Ultimately, defective cell wall synthesis leads to cell lysis and destruction of the organism. Beta-lactam agents are often referred to as cell wall active agents.

SPECTRUM OF ACTIVITY

In general, the penicillins are active against gram-positive cocci and bacilli (rods), and some gram-negative cocci. Certain derivatives (e.g., ampicillin, mezlocillin) are active against gram-negative bacilli.

Natural Penicillins Penicillin G and penicillin V are active against a wide range of aerobic, gram-positive organisms, including various species of streptococci, enterococci, and non-penicillinase-producing staphylococci. (*Penicillinases* are enzymes produced by bacteria that destroy the beta-lactam nucleus and render the penicillin molecule microbiologically inactive). The natural penicillins are also active against some gram-negative cocci, including non-penicillinase-producing strains of *Neisseria gonorrhoeae* and *Neisseria meningitidis* and certain mouth flora anaerobic organisms. In addition, *Actinomyces israelii*, *Pasteurella multocida*, *Listeria monocytogenes*, and *Treponema pallidum* are highly sensitive to penicillin.

Penicillinase-Resistant Penicillins Antistaphylococcal penicillins have been structurally modified to prevent or resist penicillinase inactivation and are indicated for the treatment of staphylococcal infections, including *S. aureus* and coagulase-negative staphylococci (*S. epidermidis*). These drugs are less active than penicillin G against other penicillin G–sensitive organisms and are not effective in treatment of infection with MRSA or MRSE.

Broad-Spectrum Penicillins These agents are active against most organisms sensitive to penicillin G and are also active against some gram-negative bacilli. The advantage of this category is enhanced activity against *E. faecalis* and common gram-negative urinary tract pathogens (e.g., *Escherichia coli*, *Proteus mirabilis*). Only non-penicillinase-producing strains of *Haemophilus influenzae* type B are susceptible to the ampicillins, as this class is not stable to beta-lactamase inactivation. However, the addition of *beta-lactamase inhibitors* such as clavulanic acid or sulbactam to ampicillin derivatives (e.g., amoxicillin/clavulanic acid [Augmentin] and ampicillin/sulbactam [Unasyn]) has broadened the spectrum of these agents to include coverage of penicillinase-producing microorganisms (e.g., *S. aureus*, *H. influenzae*).

Extended-Spectrum Penicillins Further modification of the basic penicillin structure has lead to enhanced activity against gram-negative bacilli (especially *P. aeruginosa*), while retaining activity similar to that of the broad-spectrum penicillins. The combination agents, ticarcillin/clavulanic acid (Timentin) and piperacillin/tazobactam (Zosyn) are useful against beta-lactamase–producing strains of organisms, to which other members of the class are not stable. These agents are often used to treat *nosocomial* (originating in the hospital) gram-negative infections, either as single-agent therapy, or combined with an aminoglycoside to enhance bactericidal activity.

PHARMACOKINETICS

Oral Absorption Penicillin G is rapidly inactivated within the acidic environment of the stomach, particularly when food is present, resulting in variable and inconsistent absorption. Penicillin VK (the K stands for the

Table 58–1. PENICILLINS

DRUG NAME/ROUTE AND DOSAGE	PHARMACOKINETICS/ DYNAMICS	NURSING IMPLICATIONS
amoxicillin (Amoxil) ***Adults over 20 kg:*** 250–500 mg q 8 hr ***Children:*** 20–40 mg/kg per day PO in divided doses q hr	**Peak:** 1–2 hr **A:** 80% **PB:** 20% **½L:** 1–1.3 hr **E:** renal, hepatic	**ASSESSMENT:** Obtain a history before administering drug to determine previous use of and allergic reactions to penicillins or cephalosporins. Obtain specimens for culture and sensitivity prior to initiating therapy. Assess patient for infection; check vital signs and appearance of wound, sputum, urine, and stool; determine WBC. Assess for pregnancy (category C). **INTERVENTION:** Observe patients for signs of anaphylaxis; if these occur, discontinue drug and notify physician. **Patient Teaching**—Advise patient to report signs of superinfection and allergy. **EVALUATION:** Check to see if fever and symptoms have resolved. WBC should return to normal. Report adverse effects.
amoxicillin/clavulanic acid (Augmentin) ***Adults:*** 250–500 mg PO q 8 hr ***Children:*** 20–40 mg/kg per day in 3 divided doses	Same as for amoxicillin	Same as for amoxicillin.
ampicillin (Principen and others) ***Patients >40 kg:*** 250–500 mg IV or IM q 4–6 hr (1–12 gm per day) ***Patients <40 kg:*** 25–50 mg/kg per day IV or IM in 4 equally divided doses (100–400 mg/kg per day)	**Peak:** PO 1–2 hr, IV immediate **A:** 50% **PB:** 20% **½L:** 1–1.3 hr **E:** renal, hepatic	Same as for amoxicillin.
ampicillin/sulbactam (Unasyn) ***Adults:*** 1.5–3.0 g IV q 6 hr	Same as for ampicillin	Same as for amoxicillin.
penicillin G (Pfizerpen) ***Adults:*** 4–24 million units IV or IM daily ***Children:*** 50,000–250,000 U/kg per day IV or IM in 4–6 divided doses	**Peak:** 1–2 hr **A:** 15%–30% **PB:** 60% **½L:** 0.7 hr **E:** renal, hepatic	Same as for amoxicillin.
penicillin VK (V-Cillin K and others) ***Adults and Children >12 yr:*** 125–500 mg PO q 6 hr ***Children <12 yr:*** 15–50 mg/kg per day PO in 4–6 divided doses	**Peak:** 0.5–1 hr **A:** 60% **PB:** 80% **½L:** 0.5 hr **E:** renal, hepatic	Same as for amoxicillin.
piperacillin (Pipracil) ***Adult:*** 3–4 g IV or IM q 4–6 hr ***Children:*** 50–300 mg/kg per day IV or IM q 8 hr (200–500 mg/kg per day) ***Neonates:*** 100 mg/kg/dose q 12 hr	**Peak:** 0.5–1 hr (IM) **A:** 0% **PB:** 19% **½L:** 0.5–1.2 hr **E:** renal 70%, biliary 30%	Same as for amoxicillin.
ticarcillin (Ticar) ***Adults and Children >40 kg:*** 150–300 mg/kg per day IV in 4–6 divided doses ***Children <40 kg:*** 50–300 mg/kg per day IV q 4–6 hr ***Neonates:*** 1–7 days, <2000 g: 75 mg/kg IV q 12 hr; 1–7 days, >2000 g: 75 mg/kg IV q 8 hr	**Peak:** 0.5–1 hr **A:** 0% **PB:** 50% **½L:** 1.0–1.3 hr **E:** renal, hepatic	Same as for amoxicillin. **ASSESSMENT:** Assess for pregnancy (category UK)

potassium salt), a phenoxymethyl derivative, overcomes this gastric inactivation problem. Penicillin V is resistant to acid hydrolysis and is able to pass through the stomach to the upper portion of the small intestine, where absorption occurs. Food intake has minimal effect on the breakdown of penicillin VK. Oxacillin, cloxacillin, and dicloxacillin are rapidly but incompletely absorbed following oral administration. Absorption is less variable when they are taken on an empty stomach.

Ampicillin is well absorbed following oral administration, but food intake may result in altered absorption. Amoxicillin is absorbed more rapidly and to a greater extent than ampicillin, and absorption is unaffected by food intake. Of the extended-spectrum penicillins, only carbenicillin is available orally; it must be taken as the indanyl ester formulation. Following absorption, the ester is removed by hydrolysis, delivering free carbenicillin to the systemic circulation.

Intramuscular Absorption Intramuscular (IM) penicillins are designed for deep injection. Intramuscular administration results in lower peak serum concentrations than that found with penicillins given intravenously and can be uncomfortable. In many clinical situations (e.g., meningitis, endocarditis) in which high serum penicillin concentrations are desired, the intravenous route is preferred. The primary indication for IM administration is when compliance with an oral regimen is inconvenient or the patient's compliance behavior is in question. Long-acting preparations of penicillin G (aqueous procaine and benzathine) are available for these situations. Benzathine penicillin G is very slowly absorbed following IM injection and provides the longest antibiotic effect of all long-acting penicillin preparations (average 26 days). Aqueous procaine penicillin G provides a source of penicillin for up to 24 hours. Procaine has local anesthetic properties, which make injections less painful. Patients with a history of hypersensitivity reactions to procaine should receive an intradermal skin test (0.1 mL of a 1% procaine solution) prior to administration of aqueous procaine penicillin G.

Distribution Following administration, all penicillins distribute out of blood vessels and into interstitial fluids. Penicillins do not penetrate cell membranes easily, however, when inflammation is present, membrane permeability increases and a greater amount of penicillin can cross physiologic membranes. For example, penicillin penetration is enhanced during meningitis (meningeal inflammation) but progressively decreases as the inflammatory process subsides.

Metabolism and Excretion Natural and broad-spectrum penicillins are predominantly excreted by the kidney via glomerular filtration and proximal tubular secretion in the unchanged form. When tubular secretion is blocked by another compound (e.g., probenecid), the serum concentration of penicillin is maintained for a longer period. In patients with reduced renal function (decreased creatinine clearance), the dosage of penicillins may need to be reduced to prevent toxicity.

Penicillinase-resistant penicillins and selected extended-spectrum penicillins (e.g., mezlocillin) are secreted in the bile (40% to 50%) and do not require extensive dosage alterations in patients with renal failure.

CONTRAINDICATIONS AND PRECAUTIONS

These drugs are avoided in patients with a history of penicillin or other beta-lactam (cephalosporin, imipenem) allergy. Doses of many penicillins are adjusted in patients with renal insufficiency. Safe use during pregnancy has not been established.

ADVERSE EFFECTS

Hypersensitivity Reactions Penicillin hypersensitivity may present as anaphylactic reactions, serum sickness, contact dermatitis, or local injection reactions. Anaphylactic reactions occur in previously sensitized patients and are rare, but can be life threatening. Immediate treatment includes epinephrine, corticosteroids, saline or plasma expanders, and other resuscitative measures. Serum sickness usually occurs 7 to 10 days after treatment is initiated. The clinical presentation may include fever, arthritis, urticaria, lymphadenopathy, and generalized edema.

Neurotoxicity High doses of penicillins may induce convulsions or coma secondary to direct central nervous system (CNS) irritation. Neurotoxicity is more likely to occur in patients receiving large doses, having renal impairment, and/or having an underlying CNS disease.

Nephropathy *Interstitial nephritis* (inflammation of renal tissue) may occur in patients receiving parenteral penicillin therapy. The onset is usually within 2 to 4 weeks after initiating therapy. A rising serum creatinine level and blood urea nitrogen (BUN) may indicate decreased renal function, whereas increases in blood and urinary eosinophils (*eosinophilia* and *eosinophiluria*, respectively) suggest a possible drug-induced reaction has occurred. Fever and rash may also occur. This reaction usually subsides when the penicillin is discontinued; however, in some cases corticosteroids may be administered in an attempt to correct the deterioration in renal function.

Hematologic Effects A fall in hemoglobin concentration and laboratory evidence of hemolysis in a patient receiving high-dose intravenous penicillin may indicate the presence of penicillin-induced immune hemolytic anemia. This adverse effect can be life threatening if the penicillin is continued. Withdrawal of penicillin usually results in a return of the hemoglobin to a normal value. Similarly, a dose-related bone marrow suppressive effect may decrease the white blood cell count (WBC). The onset is approximately 3 weeks after the initiation of therapy and is reversible upon penicillin withdrawal. Penicillins (primarily carbenicillin and ticarcillin) may induce platelet dysfunction (inhibit platelet aggregation), resulting in a prolonged bleeding time. The effects may be exaggerated in patients with preexisting coagulation abnormalities (such as uremia or hepatic disease). Platelet function returns to baseline after the drug is discontinued.

Electrolyte Disturbances Extended-spectrum penicillins (carbenicillin and ticarcillin) are administered as disodium salts. Patients with underlying renal or cardiac disease may not tolerate the excess sodium load. Newer members of this class (e.g., mezlocillin, piperacillin, azlocillin) are monosodium salts and may be useful alternatives in these patients. All penicillins, if given in high doses, may induce hypokalemia. In clinical situations in which high doses of penicillins are indicated, supplemental potassium may be required.

Hepatotoxicity   Certain penicillins (e.g., oxacillin, carbenicillin) have been associated with an elevation in serum enzymes that are of hepatic origin (e.g., serum aspartate aminotransferase [AST]). The onset of this particular adverse effect is approximately 3 weeks after therapy is initiated; however, serum enzyme elevations return to normal on withdrawal of the offending agent.

INTERACTIONS

Penicillins are bactericidal agents active against dividing bacterial cells. When penicillins are administered concurrently with bacteriostatic (inhibiting bacterial growth) antibiotics (e.g., chloramphenicol, erythromycin, tetracyclines), the activity of the penicillin may be decreased.

Patients who are receiving anticoagulants (e.g., warfarin, heparin) may be at risk for bleeding when high doses of carbenicillin and ticarcillin are prescribed concurrently. High concentrations of penicillins (200 μg/mL) may microbiologically inactivate aminoglycoside antibiotics. Because of this interaction, penicillins and aminoglycosides are not admixed in the same intravenous fluid. From a clinical standpoint, this interaction is relevant in patients with poor renal function in whom elevated serum concentrations of both agents may be present.

Salicylates may compete with penicillin G for renal excretion and consequently prolong the serum half-life of penicillin G.

Probenecid inhibits the renal tubular secretion of penicillins, resulting in elevated penicillin concentrations. This interaction is used therapeutically to sustain penicillin concentrations in patients with gonorrhea.

CEPHALOSPORINS

The cephalosporins were first isolated from *Cephalosporium acremonium*. The basic structure for cephalosporins can be modified chemically to provide a large number of derivatives that have activity against many microorganisms. Although not an absolute classification system, the following nomenclature may be a convenient method for recalling the large number of cephalosporins. Some selected cephalosporins are featured in Table 58–2:

1. first generation—cephalothin (Keflin, Seffin), cefazolin (Ancef, Kefzol), cephapirin (Cefadyl), cephalexin (Keflex), cephradine (Velosef, Anspor), cefadroxil (Duricef, Ultracef)
2. second generation—cefamandole (Mandol), cefmetazole (Zefazone), cefoxitin (Mefoxin), cefaclor (Ceclor), cefuroxime (Zinacef, Ceftin), cefonocid (Monocid), cefotetan (Cefotan), cefprozil (Cefzil).
3. third generation—cefotaxime (Claforan), moxalactam (Moxam), cefoperazone (Cefobid), ceftizoxime (Cefizox), ceftriaxone (Rocephin), ceftazidime (For-

taz, Tazicef, Tazidime), cefixime (Suprax), cefpodoxime (Vantin), ceftibuten (Cedax).
4. fourth generation—cefepime (Maxipime)

ACTION

The mechanism of action of cephalosporins is similar to that of penicillins (see Action in penicillin section) and includes inhibition of cell wall synthesis, resulting in cell death.

SPECTRUM OF ACTIVITY

First Generation   The first-generation cephalosporins inhibit the growth of most gram-positive cocci including penicillinase-producing staphylococci and streptococci, but excluding enterococci. These cephalosporins are effective against certain gram-negative bacilli, including *E. coli, Klebsiella pneumoniae, mirabilis, Salmonella* species, and *Shigella* species.

Second Generation   The second-generation cephalosporins offer a broadened gram-negative antimicrobial spectrum in comparison with first-generation agents. In general, these cephalosporins are more active against both the gram-negative bacilli mentioned previously and strains of indole-positive *Proteus* species, *Enterobacter cloacae, Enterobacter aerogenes,* and *H. influenzae.* Cefoxitin, although less active against *H. influenzae* than cefamandole and cefuroxime, has greater activity against anaerobic bacteria, including *Bacteroides fragilis.* Cefotetan and cefmetazole are comparable to cefoxitin in anaerobic activity.

Third Generation   Third-generation cephalosporins broaden the gram-negative spectrum farther to include activity against *Serratia marcescens* and *P. aeruginosa.* These agents are more potent against selected gram-negative organisms and anaerobic pathogens than other cephalosporin classes. Ceftazidime and cefoperazone are the most active against *P. aeruginosa.* Against *B. fragilis,* ceftizoxime demonstrates the greatest activity as compared with the other third-generation agents but has less activity than cefoxitin and cefotetan. In general, as the gram-negative activity of cephalosporins has been enhanced, their activity against gram-positive cocci has decreased. As a result, patients receiving third-generation cephalosporins with minimal gram-positive activity may be at increased risk of developing gram-positive coccal infections. The orally available agents, (cefpodoxime, ceftibuten, cefixime) however, do not have antipseudomonal coverage.

Fourth Generation   The prototype drug for this generation, cefepime, has a broader spectrum of activity than third-generation cephalosporins. There is increased gram-positive coverage for staphylococcal infections; however, its anaerobic coverage is decreased. Cefepime is stable to hydrolysis by many beta-lactamases and thus may be useful for treatment of infections resistant to other cephalosporins.

PHARMACOKINETICS

Absorption   Food may affect absorption and the time to peak plasma level. Consult the individual drug litera-

Table 58–2. CEPHALOSPORINS

DRUG NAME/ROUTE AND DOSAGE	PHARMACOKINETICS/ DYNAMICS	NURSING IMPLICATIONS
cefadroxil (Duricef) ***Adults:*** 500 mg-1–2 g/day PO in 1 or 2 divided doses ***Children:*** 15 mg/kg PO q 12 hr	**A:** >90% **PB:** 15%–20% **½L:** 1.1–2 hr **E:** renal	**ASSESSMENT:** Obtain a history before administering drug to determine previous use of and allergic reactions to cephalosporins or penicillins (possible cross-sensitivity). Obtain specimens for culture and sensitivity prior to initiating therapy. Assess patient for infection; check vital signs and appearance of wound, sputum, urine, and stool; determine WBC; check for earache. Assess for pregnancy (category B). **INTERVENTION:** Observe patient for signs of anaphylaxis; if these occur, discontinue drug and notify physician. **Patient Teaching**—Advise patient to report signs of superinfection and allergy. Tell patient to notify physician if fever and diarrhea develop, especially if stool contains blood, pus, or mucus. Advise patient not to treat diarrhea without consulting physician or pharmacist. **EVALUATION:** Check to see if fever and symptoms have disappeared. Check WBC. Report adverse effects.
cefazolin (Ancef, Kefzol) ***Adults:*** 0.5–2 g IV or IM q 6–8 hr ***Children and Infants >1 mo:*** 25–50 mg/kg per day IV or IM in 3–4 divided doses	**PB:** 84% **½L:** 1.8 hr **E:** renal	Same as for cefadroxil.
cefixime (Suprax) ***Adults and Children >12 yr:*** 400 mg PO qd or 200 mg PO q 12 hr ***Children Under >12 yr, <50 kg:*** 8 mg/kg per day PO in 1–2 divided doses	**A:** 30%–50% **PB:** 65% **½L:** 3–4 hr **E:** renal	Same as for cefadroxil. Food delays absorption and peak plasma level by 1 hr.
cefotaxime (Claforan) ***Adults and Children >49 kg:*** 1–2 g IV or IM q 6–12 hr ***Neonates:*** 50 mg/kg IV or IM q 8–12 hr ***Infants and Children <13 yr, <50 kg:*** 25–200 mg/kg per day IV or IM in 4–6 divided doses	**PB:** 38% **½L:** 0.9–1.7 hr **E:** renal, liver (active metabolites)	Same as for cefadroxil.
cefoxitin (Mefoxin) ***Adults:*** 1–2 g IV or IM q 6–8 hr ***Children >3 mo:*** 80–160 mg/kg per day IV or IM in equally divided doses q 4–6 hr	**PB:** 73% **½L:** 0.7–1.1 hr **E:** renal	Same as for cefadroxil.
ceftazidime (Fortaz, Tazidime) ***Adults and Children >12 yr:*** 1–2 g IV or IM q 8–12 hr ***Infants and Children 1 mo–12 yr:*** 25–50 mg/kg IV q 8 hr ***Neonates <1 mo:*** 30–50 mg/kg IV q 12 hr	**PB:** 5%–24% **½L:** 1.4–2 hr **E:** renal	Same as for cefadroxil.
ceftizoxime (Cefizox) ***Adults:*** 1–2 g IV or IM q 8–12 hr ***Children >6 mo:*** 33–50 mg/kg IV/IM q 6–8 hr	**PB:** 30% **½L:** 1.7 hr **E:** renal	Same as for cefadroxil plus: **EVALUATION:** Monitor patient for signs of bleeding.

Continued on the following page

Table 58–2. CEPHALOSPORINS, Continued

DRUG NAME/ROUTE AND DOSAGE	PHARMACOKINETICS/ DYNAMICS	NURSING IMPLICATIONS
ceftriaxone (Rocephin)		
Adults: 0.5–2 g IV or IM q 12–24 hr **Children:** 50–100 mg/kg per day IV or IM in divided doses q 12 hr	**PB:** 95% **½L:** 5.8–10.9 hr **E:** renal and biliary	Same as for cefadroxil.
cefuroxime sodium (Zinacef)		
Adults: 750–1.5 g IV or IM q 6–8 hr **Infants and Children >3 mo:** 50–240 mg/kg per day IV or IM in equally divided doses q 6–8 hr	**PB:** 33%–50% **½L:** 1–2 hr **E:** renal	Same as for cefadroxil.
cephalexin (Keflex)		
Adults: 250 mg 1 qm PO q 6 hr **Children:** 25–50 mg/kg per day PO in 4 equally divided doses	**A:** 90% **PB:** 14% **½L:** 0.5–1.2 hr **E:** renal	**INTERVENTION:** Patient should avoid taking with food.

ture to determine which products can and cannot be taken with food. Cephalosporins can be administered intramuscularly and are well absorbed from the site of injection. Large volumes (more than 2 mL) may be painful when injected.

Distribution All cephalosporins (oral and parenteral) distribute throughout the body fluids, but do not penetrate cells to a great extent. The first generation cephalosporins do not penetrate the cerebrospinal fluid (CSF) and are not to be used for the treatment of bacterial meningitis. However, cefuroxime and third-generation agents do penetrate the CSF and achieve even higher concentrations in the CSF in the presence of meningitis.

Metabolism and Excretion The first-generation cephalosporins, with the exception of cephalothin and cephapirin (both of which are deacetylated in the liver), are primarily eliminated from the body by the kidneys. Second-generation cephalosporins are mainly excreted by the kidneys and to a lesser extent in the bile. Sixty percent or more of an administered dose of cefotaxime, moxalactam, ceftizoxime, and ceftazidime are excreted by the kidneys. Cefoperazone and ceftriaxone are 40% or more metabolized by the liver and excreted in the bile. With the exception of cefoperazone and ceftriaxone, major dosage modifications are necessary in the presence of renal insufficiency. Cefepime is primarily renally eliminated, and doses must be adjusted in patients with renal impairment.

CONTRAINDICATIONS AND PRECAUTIONS

Avoid use in patients with a history of penicillin or related compound (beta-lactam) allergy. Doses of many agents should be adjusted in renal insufficiency. Use cautiously in pregnant or lactating women.

ADVERSE EFFECTS

Hypersensitivity Reactions As with penicillins, hypersensitivity reactions are the most common adverse reaction of cephalosporins. A small percentage of patients with penicillin allergy are cross-sensitive to the cephalosporins, probably because of their structural similarities (see penicillin toxicity).

Coagulation Disorders When high doses are given, cephalosporins may alter the coagulation mechanism and expose patients to a risk of bleeding. Cephalosporins (cefamandole, cefoperazone, cefotetan, and cefmetazole) may inhibit normal platelet function and depress the hepatic synthesis of the vitamin K–dependent clotting factor, prothrombin, leading to prolongation of the prothrombin time (PT). Patients at risk for this adverse effect are those with malnutrition or renal insufficiency, patients receiving prolonged antibiotic therapy, and patients receiving relatively high-dose therapy with one of the previously mentioned agents. It is recommended that patients at risk and receiving any of these agents be given prophylactic vitamin K to prevent PT prolongation. Platelet effects do not influence the PT but rather prolong the bleeding time. Patients with preexisting platelet dysfunction, such as is seen in renal failure, are probably at increased risk.

Gastrointestinal System Patients receiving oral cephalosporins may experience diarrhea, nausea, or vomiting. In some, these side effects may be alleviated by taking the drug with food. AAC or pseudomembranous colitis (PMC), due to the overgrowth of C. difficile, is another complication of the cephalosporins seen after therapy has been initiated or following a course of therapy.

Neurotoxicity High doses of cephalosporins administered to patients with impaired kidney function may induce seizures. For this reason, cephalosporins primarily excreted by the kidneys should have their dosage adjusted when renal failure is present.

Nephrotoxicity In patients with preexisting renal disease, cephalosporins and aminoglycosides may have additive toxicity on the kidneys. This direct toxicity is relatively rare; however, these agents may induce interstitial nephritis like that seen with penicillins.

INTERACTIONS

Patients receiving cefamandole, moxalactam, or cefoperazone may experience a disulfiram-like reaction if they ingest ethanol. Patients may experience headache, flushing, dizziness, nausea, and vomiting within 30 minutes of ethanol ingestion.

MONOBACTAMS

Aztreonam (Azactam) is structurally a synthetic monocyclic antimicrobial agent, or monobactam, and is currently the only one in its class. Table 58–3 features pharmacokinetics and dosage.

○ **Aztreonam** (Azactam) disrupts bacterial cell wall synthesis like the penicillins and the cephalosporins. The spectrum of activity of aztreonam is limited to aerobic gram-negative rods (e.g., *E. coli*, *K. pneumoniae*, *Proteus* species, *Enterobacter* species, and *P. aeruginosa*). In addition, it is active against *N. gonorrhoeae* and *H. influenzae*. It has no activity against gram-positive organisms or against anaerobic microorganisms.

CONTRAINDICATIONS AND PRECAUTIONS Use with caution in patients with an aztreonam allergy. Doses may need adjustment in renal insufficiency. Safe use in pregnancy and lactation and in children has not been established.

ADVERSE EFFECTS Aztreonam has the same toxicity profile as many of the penicillin and cephalosporin antibiotics. However, cross-sensitivity with other beta-lactam drugs is minimal to nonexistent.

CARBAPENEMS

Imipenem/cilastatin (Primaxin) and **meropenem (Merrem)** are the carbapenems currently available. Dosage and pharmacokinetics are in Table 58–3.

○ **Imipenem/cilastastin** (Primaxin) contains two drugs. Imipenem interferes with bacterial cell wall synthesis, which results in elongation and subsequent lysis of the microorganism. Cilastatin inhibits the enzymatic breakdown of imipenem in the kidneys, making it effective against organisms that infect the urinary tract. This anti-infective has the broadest antibacterial spectrum of any beta-lactam antibiotic currently on the market. It is extremely potent against staphylococci and streptococci, with variable activity against the enterococci. It has no activity against methicillin-resistant staphylococci. Imi-

---

Table 58–3. MONOBACTAMS AND CARBAPENEMS

DRUG NAME/ROUTE AND DOSAGE	PHARMACOKINETICS/ DYNAMICS	NURSING IMPLICATIONS
MONOBACTAMS		
aztreonam (Azactam) **Adults:** 500 mg–2 g IV q 6–12 hr **Children:** 30–50 mg/kg IV q 6–12 hr	**PB:** 60–70% **½L:** 1.7 hr **E:** renal, liver	**ASSESSMENT:** Obtain specimens for culture and sensitivity prior to initiating therapy. Assess patient for infection; check vital signs and appearance of wound, sputum, urine, stool; determine WBC. Assess for pregnancy (category B). **INTERVENTION:** None. **EVALUATION:** Evaluate for fever and symptom resolution. Check WBC. Report adverse reactions.
CARBAPENEMS		
imipenem-cilastatin (Primaxin) **Adults:** 250–500 mg IV q 6–8 hr; rarely, up to 4 g/day may be used. **Children:** 15–25 mg/kg IV q 6 hr	**PB:** 20% **½L:** 1–1.3 hr **E:** renal 75%, nonrenal 25%	Same as for aztreonam plus: **ASSESSMENT:** Obtain a history before administering drug to determine previous use of and allergic reactions to penicillins or related compounds (possible cross-sensitivity). Assess for pregnancy (category C).
meropenem (Merrem) **Adults:** 0.5–1 g IV q 8 hr	**PB:** minimal **½L:** 0.8–1 hr **E:** renal, biliary	Same as for imipenem.

penem is active against Enterobacteriaceae (e.g., *E. coli*, *Klebsiella* species, *Enterobacter* species, *P. mirabilis*) and *P. aeruginosa*. In addition, it maintains activity against *H. influenzae*, *N. meningitidis*, and *N. gonorrhoeae*. Its anaerobic activity is also very broad and includes *B. fragilis*, *Peptostreptococcus* and *Peptococcus*, and *Fusobacterium*.

CONTRAINDICATIONS AND PRECAUTIONS Use with caution in patients with a history of penicillin or other beta-lactam allergy. Safe use in pregnancy and lactation has not been established. Use with caution in patients with underlying CNS disorders.

ADVERSE EFFECTS Patients allergic to penicillin antibiotics are considered allergic to imipenem. Infrequent reactions have been drug fever, urticaria, pruritis, and other rashes. Phlebitis, thrombophlebitis, and erythema (redness) have been reported following the intravenous administration of imipenem. Severe nausea and vomiting (which may or may not occur with episodes of hypotension, dizziness, and sweating) have been attributed to infusions of imipenem. This effect is unpredictable and may occur inconsistently in the same patient. Slowing the infusion may be the only intervention necessary; however, the drug may need to be discontinued in selected situations.

Seizures have been reported in up to 1.5% of patients receiving imipenem. This adverse effect appears to be more common in elderly patients with renal insufficiency and other predisposing factors such as head injury, intracranial neoplasm, and/or a history of seizures or alcohol abuse. The dose of imipenem in such high-risk patients should not exceed 2 grams per day.

INTERACTIONS Concomitant administration of probenecid with imipenem results in increased serum concentrations (and possible toxicity) of imipenem. Concomitant administration of ganciclovir with imipenem has been reported to result in an increased likelihood of seizures.

○ **Meropenem's** (Merrem), spectrum of activity are similar to imipenem. Meropenem has slightly better activity against *P. aeruginosa* and *P. cepacia*, but activity against Enterococci species may be reduced.

CONTRAINDICATIONS AND PRECAUTIONS Avoid use in patients with a hypersensitivity to penicillins or related compounds.

ADVERSE EFFECTS Meropenem has less propensity to induce seizures than imipenem. Its usefulness in meningitis may therefore be increased.

CARBACEPHEMS

Loracarbef (Lorabid), is a carbacephem and is available for oral administration at an adult dose of 200–400 mg twice daily.

○ **Loracarbef** (Lorabid) is a cell wall active agent (see penicillins) with greater chemical stability than the cephalosporins. This stability enhances serum and tissue drug concentrations and enables an oral suspension dosage form to be stored unrefrigerated without degradation.

SPECTRUM OF ACTIVITY Loracarbef is active against gram-positive organisms such as *S. aureus*, *S. pneumoniae*,

and *S. pyogenes*. It is also active against aerobic gram-negative organisms including *E. coli*, *Moraxella catarrhalis*, and *H. influenzae*. Loracarbef is stable to beta-lactamase inactivation and thus is useful against beta-lactamase–producing strains of the above organisms.

CONTRAINDICATIONS AND PRECAUTIONS Use with caution in patients with a history of penicillin or other beta-lactam allergy.

ADVERSE EFFECTS Diarrhea and vomiting were the most common side effects found with loracarbef. As with all beta-lactam agents, hypersensitivity reactions (rash, urticaria, pruritus) occur in a small percentage of patients.

INTERACTIONS Probenecid inhibits the renal excretion of loracarbef and may prolong the half-life from 1 hour to 1.5 hours.

AMINOGLYCOSIDES

In 1944, streptomycin, a product of *Streptomyces griseus*, was discovered. The emergence of resistance has limited its usefulness to select clinical situations. Subsequently, neomycin (Mycifradin) and kanamycin (Kantrex) were introduced, but their usefulness was limited by toxicity and the development of resistance. Currently, **gentamicin (Garamycin)**, **tobramycin (Nebcin)**, **amikacin (Amikin)**, and **netilmicin (Netromycin)** are the aminoglycosides used for the treatment of gram-negative bacillary infections; they are featured in Table 58–4. Paromomycin is an orally available nonabsorbable aminoglycoside that has use in the treatment of intraintestinal amebic infection.

ACTION

After transport across cell membranes, aminoglycosides act at the 30S bacterial ribosome to interrupt protein synthesis. Although other antibiotics that alter protein synthesis may be bacteriostatic, the effects of aminoglycosides are bactericidal. Bacterial resistance to aminoglycosides may be related to failure to cross or penetrate the cell membrane, altered binding to ribosomes, or inactivation by microbial enzymes. When penicillin is added to aminoglycoside therapy, the cell wall is altered (by the penicillin), thus allowing the aminoglycoside to more easily penetrate the cell. This is an excellent example of antibiotic synergy.

SPECTRUM OF ACTIVITY

The primary indication for the aminoglycosides is for the treatment of infection caused by aerobic gram-negative bacilli (e.g., enterobacteriaceae). In general, certain strains of *P. aeruginosa* are more sensitive to tobramycin than to gentamicin, whereas strains of *S. marcescens* are more sensitive to gentamicin than to tobramycin. Bacteria resistant to gentamicin, tobramycin, and netilmicin are usually sensitive to amikacin. The aminoglycosides possess activity against staphylococci and are used in combination with beta-lactam agents or vancomycin to treat enterococcal or viridan streptococcal infections. Anaerobic bacteria are resistant to aminoglycosides.

Table 58–4. AMINOGLYCOSIDES

DRUG NAME/ROUTE AND DOSAGE	PHARMACOKINETICS/ DYNAMICS	DRUG CONCENTRATION	NURSING ASSESSMENT
amikacin (Amikin) **Adults and Children:** 15–20 mg/kg per day in 2 divided doses **Infants <1 wk old:** 7.5– 10 mg/kg, IV/IM q 12 h **> 1 wk old:** 10–12.5 mg/kg IV/IM q 8–12 hr	**PB:** 4% **½L:** 2–3 hr **E:** renal	**Peak:** 20–35 μg/mL **Trough:** <10 μg/mL	**ASSESSMENT:** Obtain specimens for culture and sensitivity prior to initiating therapy. Assess patient for infection; check vital signs; appearance of wound, sputum, urine, and stool; WBC. Assess for pregnancy (category D). **INTERVENTION:** none **EVALUATION:** Monitor serum concentrations. Monitor serum creatinine and BUN. Check hearing and balance. Check for resolution of fever and symptoms, WBC.
gentamicin (Garamycin) **Adults:** Loading Dose—2 mg/kg IV/IM Maintenance Dose—1–1.5 mg/kg IV/IM q 8 hr **Children:** 2–2.5 mg/kg IV/IM q 8 hr **Infants:** 2.5 mg/kg IV/IM q 8 hr **Neonates <1 wk:** 2.5 mg/ kg IV/IM q 12 hr	**PB:** <10% **½L:** 2–3 hr **E:** renal	**Peak:** 6–10 μg/mL **Trough:** <2 μg/mL	Same as for amikacin. **ASSESSMENT:** Assess for pregnancy (category C).
tobramycin (Nebcin) **Adults:** Loading Dose—2 mg/kg Maintenance Dose—1–1.5 mg/kg IV/IM q 8 hr **Children:** 2–2.5 mg/kg IV/ IM q 8 hr **Premature or Full-Term Infants <4 wk:** 2.5 mg/ kg IV/IM q 12 hr	**PB:** <10% **½L:** 2–3 hr **E:** renal	Same as for gentamicin	Same as for amikacin. **ASSESSMENT:** Assess for pregnancy (category D).

PHARMACOKINETICS

Absorption Aminoglycosides are poorly absorbed after oral administration. This property is employed clinically when neomycin is prescribed to sterilize the bowel prior to surgery. Neomycin is also used to eliminate urease-producing bacteria in patients with hepatic encephalopathy and thus prevent the absorption of ammonia (the product of urease activity on intestinal urea). Aminoglycosides are absorbed rapidly after intramuscular injection, most times the IV route is preferred.

Distribution Aminoglycosides penetrate bronchial secretions (sputum), CSF, and eye fluids poorly. Low CSF concentrations following parenteral administration may require direct injection of these antibiotics into the CSF (intrathecally or intraventricularly). Similarly, in serious eye infections, periocular injections may be indicated. Aminoglycosides do achieve sufficient concentrations in peritoneal fluid (e.g., ascites) that are useful for treating peritonitis. Aminoglycoside administration during pregnancy may result in amniotic fluid and fetal plasma exposure to these agents; therefore they should be used in pregnancy only if their potential benefit outweighs the risk.

Metabolism and Excretion Aminoglycosides are eliminated from the body almost entirely by glomerular filtration. There is little tubular secretion and no hepatic metabolism. The serum half-life of these agents is approximately 2 hours in patients with normal renal function and may be prolonged up to 50 to 60 hours in anuric patients.

CONTRAINDICATIONS AND PRECAUTIONS

Use with caution in patients allergic to aminoglycosides. Use with caution in patients with preexisting renal disease, myasthenia gravis, and/or receiving concomitant renal toxic agents (e.g., amphotericin B, vancomycin).

ADVERSE EFFECTS

Ototoxicity Auditory and vestibular symptoms may occur in patients receiving aminoglycoside therapy. Risk factors for aminoglycoside ototoxicity are impaired renal function, prolonged therapy, and/or concomitant treatment with other ototoxic drugs (e.g., furosemide [Lasix]). Patients receiving this combination are monitored by audiometry and for altered vestibular function (e.g., dizziness, light-headedness). Ototoxicity occurs uncommonly but may be irreversible.

○ **Nephrotoxicity** All aminoglycosides are potentially nephrotoxic agents; thus aminoglycoside serum concentrations and renal function are monitored closely during therapy. Although usually reversible, nephrotoxicity can substantially increase patient morbidity and costs. Risk factors for nephrotoxicity include advanced age, shock (hypotension), dehydration, preexisting renal disease, or concurrent administration of other nephrotoxic drugs (e.g., amphotericin B).

○ **Neuromuscular Blockade** This effect is secondary to inhibition of acetylcholine release. Although uncommon, this effect may be seen patients with myasthenia gravis or in patients receiving concurrent neuromuscular blocking agents (e.g., pancuronium bromide, succinylcholine), who may experience prolongation of their respiratory paralysis when these agents are used concomitantly with aminoglycosides. Treatment with calcium salts may reverse the impaired respiratory function.

MONITORING AMINOGLYCOSIDE THERAPY

The toxicity of aminoglycosides is a primary impetus for close surveillance during treatment. Renal impairment caused by these agents is usually reflected by an increase in serum creatinine 3 to 4 days into therapy, indicating that renal damage has already occurred. In many insti-

tutions, aminoglycoside serum concentrations are measured routinely to monitor for toxicity as well as efficacy. Peak and trough levels are in Table 58–4. Peak serum concentrations are obtained approximately 30 minutes after the aminoglycoside infusion has finished, and the trough serum concentration are obtained immediately before the aminoglycoside infusion is started.

INTERACTIONS

Penicillins have the potential to inactivate aminoglycosides in certain situations (see section on drug interactions of penicillins).

SULFONAMIDES

The sulfonamides were the first effective group of antibiotics used for the treatment of bacterial infections in humans in 1935. The sulfonamides are often categorized into groups based upon their rate of absorption and excretion. While not limited to the groups below, some of the more commonly used agents can be classified as follows:

1. short acting: rapid absorption, rapid excretion—sulfisoxazole (Gantrisin), sulfadiazine (Microsulfon)
2. medium acting: rapid absorption, slow excretion—sulfamethoxazole (Gantanol)
3. ultra-long acting: used in combination with pyrimethamine for the treatment of malaria—sulfadoxine (Fansidar)

The dosage and pharmacokinetics are listed in Table 58–5.

Table 58–5. SULFONAMIDES

DRUG NAME/ROUTE AND DOSAGE	PHARMACOKINETICS/ DYNAMICS	NURSING IMPLICATIONS
sulfadiazine **Adults:** 2–4 g/day PO in 3–6 divided doses **Children >2 mo:** 150 mg/kg per day PO in 4–6 divided doses **Children <2 mo:** 100–150 mg/kg per day PO in 4–6 divided doses	A: 70–100% PB: 32%–56% ½L: 13 hr E: renal	**ASSESSMENT:** Obtain a history before administering drug to determine previous use of and allergic reactions to penicillins and cephalosporins (possible cross-sensitivity). Obtain specimens for culture and sensitivity prior to initiating therapy. Assess patient for infection; check vital signs; check appearance of wound, sputum, urine, and stool; determine WBC. Assess for pregnancy (category C). **INTERVENTION: Patient Teaching**—Advise patient to avoid sunlight or ultraviolet light. **EVALUATION:** Evaluate for resolution of fever and symptoms. Check WBC.
trimethoprim/sulfamethoxazole (co-trimoxazole) (Bactrim) (Septra) **Adults:** 160 mg TMP/800 mg SMX PO q 12 hr or 8–10 mg/kg TMP/40–50 mg/kg SMX IV q 6–12 hr **Children >2 mo:** 8 mg/kg per day TMP/SMX q 12 hr	A: 70%–100% PB: TMP 50%, SMX 65% ½L: TMP 10 hr; SMX 7–12 hr E: hepatic, renal	

ACTION

Bacterial and human cells utilize folic acid derivatives to build purines, which are essential components in the synthesis of DNA. Human cells are able to use folic acid present in the diet, whereas bacteria must synthesize folate from *para-aminobenzoic acid* (PABA). The biochemical conversion of PABA to folate involves a sequence of steps, each catalyzed by the enzyme dihydrofolic acid synthetase. Because sulfonamides are structurally similar to PABA, they compete for this enzyme. The net result of this competition is a decrease in the synthesis of folic acid and suppression of purine synthesis. Without the building blocks of DNA, the bacterial cell is unable to survive and death ensues. Sulfamethoxazole has been combined with another antibiotic, trimethoprim. Trimethoprim is able to compete with another enzyme (*tetrahydrofolic acid reductase*) in the chain of events leading up to the synthesis of folic acid. This sequential inhibition of the folic acid pathway has markedly enhanced the activity of each component of the drug combination.

SPECTRUM OF ACTIVITY

The sulfonamides were originally very effective antibiotics; however, their clinical value presently is limited by the development of bacterial resistance. Trimethoprim (TMP) is more active than sulfamethoxazole (SMZ) against most bacteria, and for the most part, TMP/SMZ is aimed at aerobic gram-negative bacteria (e.g., Enterobacteriaceae); however, gram-positive organisms (e.g., *Staphylococci, Streptococci, L. monocytogenes*), *Nocardia asteroides, Xanthomonas maltophilia*, and the protozoal organism *P. carinii* are also susceptible. When present in combination, TMP and SMZ frequently inhibit organisms at much lower concentrations of each drug than would be inhibitory individually.

CONTRAINDICATIONS AND PRECAUTIONS

Use with caution in patients with a sulfonamide allergy or with previous toxicity (e.g., bone marrow toxicity, Stevens-Johnson syndrome). Avoid use in newborns and in pregnancy. Dosage may need adjustment in renal insufficiency.

ADVERSE EFFECTS

Hypersensitivity Reactions   Rashes are common during sulfonamide treatment and may be life threatening. The most common rashes are maculopapular or urticarial, but more serious reactions like erythema nodosum or exfoliative dermatitis also occur. The most serious form of cutaneous hypersensitivity is the Stevens-Johnson syndrome, consisting of erythema and ulceration of the mucous membranes (e.g., eyes, mouth, and urethra). This syndrome has been described with all sulfonamides. Serum sickness and drug fever are also noted during treatment with these agents. Patients with AIDS are more likely to develop rashes secondary to sulfonamide therapy.

Hematopoietic Disorders   Acute hemolytic anemia may occur in patients whose red blood cells are sensitized owing to a lack of a specific enzyme, *glucose-6-phosphate dehydrogenase* (G6PD deficiency). Agranulocytosis or aplastic anemia can occur during sulfonamide therapy owing to a direct toxic effect on bone marrow. Both of these reactions are uncommon; however, if they occur, prompt discontinuation of the offending drug is essential.

Urinary Tract Abnormalities   The deposition of the sulfonamide crystals (*crystalluria*) within the tissue of the urinary tract may occur. Maintenance of adequate fluid intake (more than 1000 mL/day) and in certain situations alkalinization of the urine (to increase solubility) prevent crystalluria.

Hepatitis   Rarely, focal or diffuse necrosis of the liver secondary to direct toxicity or hypersensitivity may occur. Immediate drug withdrawal is recommended.

INTERACTIONS

Patients receiving oral anticoagulants (e.g., warfarin sodium) who have trimethoprim-sulfamethoxazole added to their therapy may experience a further prolongation of the international normalized ratio (INR) and increased risk of bleeding.

The combination of sulfonamides and oral hypoglycemic agents (e.g., tolbutamide and chlorpropamide) may lead to excessive decreases in blood sugar. Patients taking these agents should be monitored closely.

Patients who are stabilized on anticonvulsant therapy with phenytoin may experience signs of phenytoin toxicity (e.g., nystagmus, ataxia) when sulfonamides are prescribed concurrently. Close observation for phenytoin toxicity is important when these agents are used together.

○ **Trimethoprim-sulfamethoxazole**   (Bactrim, Septra) is a combination of a sulfonamide (sulfamethoxazole) and a folic acid antagonist (trimethoprim). It was developed to promote the synergistic effect against certain bacteria.

MACROLIDES

The marcrolides include **erythromycin (*E-Mycin, Ilosone, Erythro, Ilotycin, Erythrocin*)**, **clarithromycin (*Biaxin*)**, **azithromycin (*Zithromax*)**, and **dirithromycin (*Dynabac*)**. Dosage and pharmacokinetics are featured in Table 58–6.

○ **Erythromycin** is available as erythromycin base (E-Mycin, ERYC), erythromycin estolate (Ilosone), erythromycin ethylsuccinate (EryPed, Erythro), erythromycin gluceptate (Ilotycin), erythromycin lactobionate (Erythrocin), and erythromycin stearate (Erythrocin).

ACTION   Erythromycin penetrates the cell wall of sensitive bacteria and reversibly binds to the 50S ribosomal subunit, thereby inhibiting *translocation*, a step in polypeptide chain formation. This ribosomal binding fails to occur in resistant bacteria. Both bacteriostatic and bactericidal activity can be seen with erythromycin; the specific activity depends on the microorganism and the drug concentration.

Table 58–6. MACROLIDES

DRUG NAME/ROUTE AND DOSAGE	PHARMACOKINETICS/ DYNAMICS	NURSING IMPLICATIONS
erythromycin base (Emycin and others) *Adults:* 250–500 mg PO q 6–12 hr (up to 4 g/day) *Children:* 30–50 mg/kg per day PO in divided doses	A: 60% PB: 65% ½L: 1.5–2 hr E: biliary, renal	**ASSESSMENT:** Obtain history to determine if prior allergic reaction occurred. Assess for pregnancy (category C). **INTERVENTION:** Avoid IM injections as they are very painful. **Patient Teaching**—Tell patient to avoid taking drug with food. **EVALUATION:** Check for resolution of fever and symptoms; check WBC. Report adverse reactions.
clarithromycin (Biaxin) *Adults:* 250–500 mg PO bid *Children:* 7.5 mg/kg PO bid	A: 55% PB: 42%–72% ½L: 4.3 hr E: 80% hepatic, 30% renal	Same as for erythromycin base except: Food does not interfere with absorption. **ASSESSMENT:** Assess for pregnancy (category C).
azithromycin (Zithromax) *Adults:* 500 mg PO day 1, then 250 mg daily for 2–5 days *Children:* 10 mg/kg PO once daily **chlamydia** *Adults:* Single 1 g dose	A: 37% PB: 7%–50% ½L: 25–68 hr E: hepatic	Same as for erythromycin base. **ASSESSMENT:** Assess for pregnancy (category C).
dirithromycin (Dynobac) *Adults:* 500 mg PO once daily	PB: 15%–30% ½L: 20–50 hr E: biliary	Same as for erythromycin base.

SPECTRUM OF ACTIVITY Erythromycin is active against most gram-positive microorganisms, with limited activity against gram-negative organisms and variable activity against anaerobic gram-negative bacteria. Staphylococci and streptococci are usually sensitive to erythromycin, but erythromycin-resistant strains have been reported. Erythromycin is very active against *Mycoplasma pneumoniae*, *Legionella pneumophila*, *T. pallidum*, *Campylobacter jejuni*, and *Chlamydia trachomatis*.

CONTRAINDICATIONS AND PRECAUTIONS Use erythromycin with caution in patients with history of allergy. Although safe use in pregnancy and lactation has not been established, it is often used in these patients.

ADVERSE EFFECTS Gastrointestinal symptoms such as nausea, vomiting, epigastric distress, and diarrhea are dose-related side effects often experienced with erythromycin. Another dose-related side effect is phlebitis and a burning sensation at the site of intravenous infusion. This adverse reaction can be prevented by diluting erythromycin in at least 100 mL of diluent (e.g., normal saline or 5% dextrose) and infusing the dose over 1 hour or more.

Side effects unrelated to the dose of erythromycin include hypersensitivity reactions (e.g., skin rash, drug fever, eosinophilia) and hepatotoxicity (e.g., cholestatic jaundice). The hepatotoxicity occurs with the estolate and the ethylsuccinate forms of the drug. It can occur in both adults and children in approximately 10 to 20 days after initial exposure and within hours after subsequent exposures to erythromycin. Clinically, abdominal pain, nausea and vomiting, jaundice, acholic (clay colored) stools, dark urine, right upper quadrant tenderness and an enlarged liver are seen. Abnormalities detected by laboratory tests include increased white blood cells; increased number of eosinophils (eosinophilia); and elevated bilirubin, alkaline phosphatase, AST, and ALT levels. These adverse effects are reversible when the drug is discontinued.

Erythromycin has been reported to cause tinnitus, vertigo, and transient hearing loss. Most cases of hearing loss have occurred following IV administration. The onset is within 36 hours to 1 week, and recovery occurs within 24 hours to 2 weeks after discontinuation of the drug. Recovery time is not dose related. All reported cases of ototoxicity secondary to erythromycin have been reversible. Patients receiving large doses, with renal and/or hepatic dysfunction, the elderly, and females seem to be at greatest risk. The concomitant administration of other ototoxic agents (e.g., furosemide, aminoglycosides) also contributes to the ototoxic potential of erythromycin.

INTERACTIONS Erythromycin inhibits the metabolism of theophylline and may precipitate signs of theophylline toxicity (e.g., tachycardia, nervousness, nausea). The common setting for the interaction between erythromycin and theophylline is in a patient with chronic lung disease receiving theophylline therapy who develops acute bronchitis or pneumonia and erythromycin is added to the drug regimen. Patients stabilized on theophylline and requiring erythromycin should be monitored clinically and with theophylline serum concentrations.

Erythromycin may also decrease the metabolism of corticosteroids, resulting in enhanced steroid effects. The dosage of the steroid may need to be reduced when erythromycin is prescribed concurrently. Erythromycin also inhibits the breakdown of phenytoin and carbamazepine, and toxicity may be precipitated by the addition of this antibiotic. Patients receiving both of these agents may experience nausea, vomiting, nystagmus, or ataxia and require dosage reduction of carbamazepine or phenytoin.

Digoxin is partially metabolized by bacteria in the GI tract, and when the normal flora is altered by erythromycin ingestion digoxin absorption may increase. When a patient who is stabilized on digoxin requires erythromycin, the patient should be observed for signs of digitalis toxicity (anorexia, nausea, vomiting, green-yellow vision, bradycardia).

Erythromycin may inhibit the hepatic metabolism of nonsedating antihistamines (terfenadine, astemizole, and cisapride), which may lead to drug accumulation and possibly serious cardiac dysrhythmias. These two drugs should not be prescribed concurrently.

○ **Clarithromycin** (Biaxin) is a macrolide antibiotic chemically similar to erythromycin. A single change in clarithromycin's ring structure has rendered the agent stable to gastric inactivation (unlike erythromycin) and has reduced the incidence of GI toxicity compared to erythromycin. Clarithromycin has the same mechanism of action as erythromycin.

SPECTRUM OF ACTIVITY Clarithromycin is more active than erythromycin against most Streptococci and Staphylococci, *L. pneumophila*, *M. catarrhalis*, and *C. trachomatis*. Clarithromycin is also active against *Mycobacterium avium complex* and *Toxoplasma gondii*, opportunistic infections commonly associated with AIDS.

ADVERSE EFFECTS Diarrhea, nausea, and abdominal pain may occur in a small percentage of patients taking clarithromycin.

INTERACTIONS Clarithromycin may inhibit the metabolism of other drugs metabolized by the liver, including theophylline and carbamazepine. Relatively few studies examining other drug-drug interactions of clarithromycin are currently available.

○ **Azithromycin** (Zithromax) has a nitrogen atom added to its structural ring, which protects the agent from gastric acid inactivation and increases its tissue penetration properties and serum half-life. Azithromycin has the same mechanism of action as erythromycin.

SPECTRUM OF ACTIVITY Azithromycin is less active than erythromycin against gram-positive organisms such as staphylococci and streptococci, but is more active than other macrolides against *H. influenzae*. Azithromycin is also active against *M. catarrhalis*, *L. pneumophila*, *M. pneumoniae*, and *C. trachomatis*.

INTERACTIONS It is not yet known whether azithromycin inhibits the metabolism of other agents hepatically cleared because relatively few studies examining drug-drug interactions of azithromycin are currently available.

○ **Dirithromycin** (Dynabac) has the same mechanism of action and spectrum of activity as erythromycin.

CONTRAINDICATIONS AND PRECAUTIONS Avoid use in a patient with a prior hypersensitivity to dirithromycin or a related compound.

INTERACTIONS The data suggest that a low likelihood of an interaction with theophylline or cyclosporine may exist. It is not known how the drug interacts with other agents.

QUINOLONES

The first quinolone synthesized in 1962 was nalidixic acid (NegGram). However, the rapid development of resistance and inadequate tissue penetration has significantly limited the overall clinical use of nalidixic acid. This agent has been largely replaced by the newer fluorinated quinolones—**norfloxacin (Noroxin)**, **ciprofloxacin (Cipro)**, **ofloxacin (Floxin)**, **lomefoxacin (Maxaquin)**, **levofloxacin (Levaquin)**; and **sparfloxacin**—which achieve far superior tissue penetration and enjoy widespread clinical utility. The dosage and pharmacokinetics are featured in Table 58–7.

CONTRAINDICATIONS AND PRECAUTIONS Avoid in patients with prior hypersensitivity reactions. Avoid during pregnancy and lactation and in children.

ADVERSE EFFECTS Norfloxacin is usually well tolerated; however, nausea, vomiting, or abdominal pain and diarrhea may occur after ingestion. Neurotoxicity, an uncommon complication of therapy with norfloxacin, may result in headache, drowsiness, dizziness, visual disturbances, and rarely seizures. Allergic reactions (itching, hives, rashes, and photosensitivity) also may occur.

INTERACTIONS The absorption of norfloxacin is reduced if administered concurrently with cation-containing agents, such as magnesium, aluminum, or calcium-containing antacids; sucralfate; or zinc or iron preparations. Therefore, these drugs should not be administered concomitantly or should be separated by at least 2 hours.

The urinary elimination of norfloxacin is decreased in the presence of probenecid; therefore, urine levels of norfloxacin may be subtherapeutic.

○ **Norfloxacin** (Noroxin) exerts its rapid bactericidal effect by interfering with bacterial *DNA gyrase*, an enzyme instrumental in the stranding of bacterial DNA synthesis.

SPECTRUM OF ACTIVITY Norfloxacin has excellent activity against most urinary tract pathogens including Enterobacteriaceae, Enterococci, *Staphylococcus saprophyticus*, and *P. aeruginosa*. It is also active against those organisms responsible for enteritis such as *Salmonella*, *Shigella*, *C. jejuni*, *Yersinia enterocolitica*, and *E. coli*.

Though widely distributed to many tissues including the prostate, norfloxacin does not achieve tissue concentrations adequate to treat systemic infections. Thus, its clinical utility is limited to the treatment of urinary tract infections (UTIs), because the drug achieves adequate urinary concentrations.

○ **Ciprofloxacin** (Cipro) has the same mechanism of action as norfloxacin.

SPECTRUM OF ACTIVITY Ciprofloxacin has broad-spectrum activity encompassing both gram-positive (e.g.

Table 58–7. QUINOLONES

DRUG NAME/ROUTE AND DOSAGE	PHARMACOKINETICS/ DYNAMICS	NURSING IMPLICATIONS
ciprofloxacin (Cipro) **Adults:** 250–750 mg PO q 12 hr 200–400 mg IV q 12 hr	**A:** 70%–80% **PB:** 20%–40% **½L:** 3–5 hr **E:** hepatic, renal	**ASSESSMENT:** Obtain specimen for culture and sensitivity prior to initiating therapy. Use is contraindicated in children <16 yr. Assess for pregnancy (category C). **INTERVENTION: Patient Teaching—**Teach patient not to administer concomitantly with antacids, iron, or calcium supplements. **EVALUATION:** Evaluate for resolution of fever and symptoms.
enoxacin (Penetrex) **Adults:** 200–400 mg PO twice daily	**A:** 90% **PB:** 40% **½L:** 3–6 hr **E:** renal	Same as for ciprofloxacin. Take 1 hour before or 2 hours after meals.
lomefloxacin (Maxaquin) **Adults:** 400 mg PO qd	**A:** 98% **PB:** 10% **½L:** 7.75 hr **E:** renal	Same as for ciprofloxacin.
norfloxacin (Noroxin) **Adults:** 400 mg PO twice daily	**A:** 30%–50% **PB:** 10%–15% **½L:** 3–4 hr **E:** hepatic, renal	Same as for ciprofloxacin. Take 1 hour before or 2 hours after meals with 8 oz H_2O. Patient should be well hydrated.
ofloxacin (Floxin) **Adults:** 200–400 mg PO/IV twice daily	**A:** 90% **PB:** 20%–32% **½L:** 5–10 hr **E:** renal	Same as for ciprofloxacin.

S. aureus, S. epidermidis, E. faecalis) and gram-negative (e.g., Enterobacteriaceae, *P. aeruginosa*) microorganisms. Ciprofloxacin is not active against anaerobic pathogens and has poor activity against *S. pneumoniae*. Resistance develops rapidly to methicillin-resistant staphylococci, limiting ciprofloxacin's use.

ADVERSE EFFECTS Additional adverse effects include bone and cartilage toxicities have been shown in immature animal models. However, this adverse effect is rarely seen in humans. Until further studies are conducted, this drug should be avoided in pediatric patients whose skeletal growth is incomplete.

INTERACTIONS Additional interactions with ciprofloxacin are that it interferes with the metabolism of theophylline, increasing serum concentrations of theophylline and resulting in theophylline toxicity. Theophylline levels are monitored closely in patients receiving these drugs concurrently. Similarly, ciprofloxacin may interfere with the metabolism of caffeine; thus, patients may wish to switch to decaffeinated beverages while taking ciprofloxacin.

○ **Ofloxacin** (Floxin) and levofloxacin (levaquin) have the same mechanism of action, spectrum of activity, and contraindications, as ciprofloxacin except that there is increased gram positive-coverage with levofloxacin.

INTERACTIONS Drug interactions seen with ciprofloxacin are likely to occur with ofloxacin and levofloxocin with the exception of the interaction with theophylline or caffeine.

○ **Lomefloxacin** (Maxaquin) is an additional quinolone that offers no apparent advantages over ciprofloxacin or ofloxacin. Sparfloxacin, like levofloxacin, has expanded gram-positive activity.

TETRACYCLINES

The tetracyclines, discovered in 1948, include **tetracycline (Achromycin, Sumycin), demeclocycline (Declomycin), doxycycline (Vibramycin),** and **minocycline (Minocin).** Selected tetracyclines are featured in Table 58–8. Although the various members of the tetracycline family possess a few specific differences, the group will be discussed as a whole.

Table 58–8. TETRACYCLINES

DRUG NAME/ROUTE AND DOSAGE	PHARMACOKINETICS/ DYNAMICS	NURSING IMPLICATIONS
doxycycline (Vibramycin) ***Adults and Children >8 yr, >45 kg:*** 200 mg PO followed by 100 mg q 12 hr, 200 mg IV followed by 100–200 mg/day in one or two infusions ***Children >8 yr, <45 kg:*** 4.4 mg/ kg followed by 2.2 mg/kg per day IV/PO	**A:** 93% **PB:** 25%–93% **½L:** 14–24 hr **E:** hepatobiliary	**ASSESSMENT:** Obtain specimens for culture and sensitivity prior to initiating therapy. Assess for pregnancy (category UK). **INTERVENTION: Patient Teaching**—Tell patient to avoid taking medication with dairy products or antacids. Protect skin from sunlight. **EVALUATION:** Evaluate for resolution of fever and symptoms. Report adverse reactions.
minocycline (Minocin) ***Adults:*** 200 mg followed by 100 mg PO/IV q 12 hr ***Children >8 yr:*** 4 mg/kg followed by 2 mg/kg q 12 hr	**A:** 90%–100% **PB:** 55%–88% **½L:** 15–20 hr **E:** hepatic	Same as for doxycycline.
tetracycline (Achromycin) ***Adults:*** 250–500 mg PO q 6–12 hr ***Children >8 yr:*** 25–50 mg/kg per day PO in 4 divided doses	**A:** 60%–80% **PB:** 20%–67% **½L:** 6–12 hr **E:** renal	Same as for doxycycline.

ACTION

The site of action of the tetracyclines is the 30S ribosome, with access depending on both a passive diffusion process and an active process that is energy dependent. Once inside the bacterial cell wall, tetracyclines inhibit protein synthesis and are bacteriostatic antibiotics. Resistance to tetracyclines appears to occur by three mechanisms: (1) alteration in the ribosome; (2) production of an inactivating enzyme; and (3) permeability changes in the organism.

SPECTRUM OF ACTIVITY

As a class, tetracyclines can be considered broad-spectrum antibiotics. They demonstrate clinical efficacy against organisms frequently resistant to other agents (e.g., *Rickettsiae, Mycoplasma, Chlamydia*). In general, tetracyclines are more active against gram-positive organisms than gram-negative organisms; however, resistance has significantly limited their usefulness. Minocycline is more active than other derivatives against *S. aureus*. *S. pyogenes* is generally sensitive; however, group B, C, and G streptococci demonstrate variable susceptibilities. *N. meningitidis* and *N. gonorrhoeae* are both inhibited although 50% of the former strains may be resistant. Against aerobic gram-negative rods (e.g., *E. coli, K. pneumoniae, E. aerogenes, P. mirabilis*), the activity of the tetracyclines is variable. Activity against *H. influenzae* is poorest with oxytetracycline and tetracycline. Indole-positive *Proteus* species (e.g., *Proteus vulgaris*) and *Pseudomonas* species are resistant. The anaerobic spectrum is most impressive with doxycycline and includes *B. fragilis*.

PHARMACOKINETICS

Absorption Oral absorption of tetracyclines is incomplete and can be enhanced by taking these agents without food or other medications. Concomitant administration of milk, milk-containing products, antacids (aluminum hydroxide), sodium bicarbonate, calcium and magnesium salts, and iron preparations impairs absorption and decreases the amount of tetracycline therapeutically available. Food appears to interfere less with the absorption of doxycycline and minocycline. Alterations in gastric pH (as after antacid administration) may also decrease absorption of tetracyclines.

Distribution Lipid solubility plays an important role in the distribution. Doxycycline and minocycline are the most lipid soluble and thus penetrate into various tissues (e.g., spinal fluid) the best. Also, minocycline demonstrates exceptionally good penetration of saliva, which makes it an ideal agent for the treatment of the meningococcal carrier state. Tetracyclines cross the placenta and umbilical cord, and fetal plasma concentrations have been reported to reach 60% of the level in the maternal circulation. These agents are also found in breast milk.

Metabolism and Excretion Tetracyclines are excreted in the urine and feces to varying degrees. Doxycycline, minocycline are primarily eliminated by nonrenal routes, whereas demeclocycline, tetracycline are mainly excreted in the urine. Doxycycline exhibits the most unusual mode of elimination, as it is secreted into the intestinal lumen, bound by the feces, and eliminated. Tetracyclines, as a class of antibiotics, are actively secreted into the bile and undergo a process known as *enterohepatic recirculation*, in which the drug is secreted into the biliary tract and is subsequently reabsorbed in the gallbladder or GI tract. Minocycline and doxycycline require minimal dosage adjustment in patients with reduced renal function. The other tetracyclines should be dosage adjusted in patients with renal disease.

CONTRAINDICATIONS AND PRECAUTIONS

Avoid use in patients with an allergy to tetracyclines. Avoid use during pregnancy and in children younger than age 10.

ADVERSE EFFECTS

Gastrointestinal Tetracyclines have the potential to cause GI irritation following oral administration. Patients may complain of epigastric burning, nausea, vomiting, or diarrhea. These problems are more common with large doses, and certain patients may require smaller doses at more frequent intervals. Taking these agents with food may help in certain cases; however, absorption is compromised.

Phototoxicity Demeclocycline and doxycycline are most commonly associated with a "sunburn" reaction. However, patients taking any tetracycline should avoid direct sunlight or sunlamps. Minocycline appears to be least likely to cause this phototoxic reaction.

Hepatotoxicity All tetracyclines have the potential to induce acute hepatic injury (fatty liver). It appears that high doses (greater than 2 g/day), intravenous administration, and pregnancy may be associated with developing a toxic hepatic reaction.

Nephrotoxicity A possible association has been suggested between tetracycline treatment and decreased kidney function, especially in patients with preexisting renal insufficiency. Demeclocycline has been reported to antagonize the effect of antidiuretic hormone (ADH), leading to a situation of drug-induced diabetes insipidus (e.g., excessive thirst and urination). Because of this side effect, demeclocycline has been used therapeutically in patients with the syndrome of inappropriate ADH (SIADH) secretion in which excess ADH is present.

Effects on Calcified Tissue Tetracyclines bind to calcium found in teeth and bones. The patients most susceptible to this effect are neonates and infants prior to their first dentition. Brown discoloration of teeth has been described in children from birth until the age of 8. These effects can also appear in the child when tetracycline is given during pregnancy from midpregnancy to delivery. Therefore, pregnant women and children should not receive tetracyclines. Skeletal deposition of tetracyclines can also occur in the fetus and young child. Bone growth can be depressed up to 40% after prolonged tetracycline exposure.

Thrombophlebitis Tetracyclines are very irritating to veins when administered intravenously. Injection sites may have to be rotated and infusion solutions diluted in some patients.

Catabolic Effects Tetracyclines may induce a catabolic effect in human cells owing to inhibition of protein synthesis. The effect is dose-related and may induce a negative nitrogen balance and elevations in BUN.

Hypersensitivity Reactions Hypersensitivity to tetracyclines is uncommon. Patients may present with various skin reactions, angioedema, anaphylaxis, or burning eyes. These reactions may last for weeks or months after the tetracycline is discontinued. When a patient displays hypersensitivity to one tetracycline, it should be assumed the patient is hypersensitive (allergic) to all members of the tetracycline family.

Hematologic Toxicity Long-term administration of tetracyclines has been associated with leukocytosis, atypical lymphocyte formation, and thrombocytopenia.

Ototoxicity Minocycline has been reported to induce vestibular toxicity. The patient may complain of dizziness, ataxia, nausea, or vomiting. This effect is dose related and subsides when minocycline is discontinued or the daily dose decreased.

Intracranial Pressure Elevations Increased intracranial pressure (*Pseudotumor cerebri*) has been described in infants primarily and in adults. The symptoms of headache and blurred vision disappear once the drug is discontinued.

Superinfections Broad-spectrum antibiotic therapy can lead to resistant organisms that may overgrow the respiratory and GI tract. Staphylococcal enterocolitis, pseudomembranous colitis, and vaginal, oral, pharyngeal yeast infections are all examples of the results of altering the normal host bacterial flora.

INTERACTIONS

Tetracycline absorption may be decreased when administered orally with various compounds containing divalent (Mg^{2+}, Ca^{2+}) or trivalent (Fe^{3+}, Al^{3+}) cations. Common examples include magnesium-, calcium-, or aluminum-containing antacids; dairy products (Ca^{2+}); and iron (Fe^{3+}) preparations. The net effect is a decrease in the antibacterial effect of tetracycline.

Tetracyclines are reported to decrease the efficacy of oral contraceptives. Synthetic estrogens (e.g., oral contraceptive agents) are excreted in the bile almost exclusively as glucuronide or sulfate conjugates. These conjugates, on reaching the gut, are hydrolyzed by enzymes present in intestinal microorganisms to liberate the unchanged drug (oral contraceptive agent), which is then reabsorbed. Treatment with tetracyclines, which undergo the same type of enterohepatic recirculation, could be expected to interfere with this oral contraceptive hydrolytic process by eliminating the gut microorganisms and thus reduce or abolish the reabsorption of the active oral contraceptive drug. The risk of pregnancy could be significant, and alternative methods of contraception should be recommended until the course of therapy is complete.

MISCELLANEOUS ANTIBIOTICS

The miscellaneous antibiotics include **clindamycin (Cleocin)**, chloramphenicol **(Chloromycetin)**, vancomycin

(Vancocin, Vancoled), and **metronidazole (Flagyl)**. Several are featured in Table 58–9.

○ **Clindamycin** (Cleocin) is a chemical modification of lincomycin, an agent no longer used clinically.

ACTION Clindamycin inhibits bacterial protein synthesis by binding to the 50S ribosomal subunit (site of action similar to erythromycin and chloramphenicol).

SPECTRUM OF ACTIVITY Clindamycin, like erythromycin, has activity against most gram-positive organisms (e.g., *S. aureus*, *S. epidermidis*, *S. pneumoniae*, *S. pyogenes*, and viridans streptococcus). Organisms resistant to erythromycin are usually resistant to clindamycin. Clindamycin is inactive against *E. faecalis* and aerobic gram-negative organisms. The anaerobic spectrum of clindamycin is its major strong point. Anaerobic microorganisms (gram-positive and -negative, cocci and rods) above (respiratory tract) and below (abdomen and pelvis) the diaphragm are usually susceptible to clindamycin. Most *Bacteroides* species (e.g., *B. fragilis*) are inhibited by clindamycin; however, resistance has been reported.

PHARMACOKINETICS Oral absorption with either dosage form is complete, with peak serum concentrations attained within 1 to 2 hours of ingestion. Food does not significantly interfere with drug absorption. Parenteral administration is usually well tolerated and peak serum concentrations following IM administration are reached in 3 hours (1 hour in children).

Clindamycin is metabolized in the liver to two major (microbiologically active) metabolites. Both metabolites and the parent drug are eliminated in bile and urine. Ten percent of an administered dose is excreted unchanged in the urine with a small percentage (less than 5%) appearing in the feces. The half-life of clindamycin is minimally prolonged in patients with renal insufficiency. Patients with liver disease have prolonged serum half-lives, and dosage reductions may be indicated for individuals with severe hepatic disease.

CONTRAINDICATIONS AND PRECAUTIONS Clindamycin is contraindicated in patients with a history of allergy. Safety in pregnancy and lactation has not been established.

ADVERSE EFFECTS Local thrombophlebitis may occur following intravenous administration, and skin rash is noted in 10% of patients receiving clindamycin.

The most notable problem associated with clindamycin therapy is antibiotic-associated diarrhea and pseudomembranous colitis. The offending antibiotic should be

Table 58–9. MISCELLANEOUS ANTIBIOTICS

DRUG NAME/ROUTE AND DOSAGE	PHARMACOKINETICS/ DYNAMICS	NURSING IMPLICATIONS
clindamycin (Cleocin) **Adults:** 150–450 mg PO q 6 hr; 300–900 mg IV/IM q 6–8 hr **Children:** 8–25 mg/kg per day PO in 3–4 divided doses; 15–40 mg/kg per day IV/IM in 3–4 divided doses	**A:** 23%–80% **PB:** 93% **½L:** 2–3 hr **E:** hepatic, biliary, renal	**ASSESSMENT:** Obtain specimens for culture and sensitivity prior to initiating therapy. Assess for severe diarrhea. Assess for pregnancy (category UK). **INTERVENTION: Patient Teaching**—Instruct patient to report first signs of severe diarrhea. Take with full glass of water or with food to avoid esophageal irritation. Absorption is not affected by food. **EVALUATION:** Evaluate for resolution of fever and symptoms. Check WBC. Report adverse reactions to physician.
metronidazole (Flagyl) **Adults:** 500 mg–1 g PO/IV q 6–8 hr **amebiasis** 750 mg PO three times daily for 10 days **thrichmoniasis** 2 g single dose or 500 mg PO twice daily for 7 days	**A:** 80%–100% **PB:** <20% **½L:** 6–8 hr **E:** hepatic	**ASSESSMENT:** Do not give as an IV bolus. Obtain specimens for culture and sensitivity prior to administration of therapy. Assess for pregnancy (category B). **INTERVENTION: Patient Teaching**—Instruct patient to take medication with food. Avoid all alcohol. Causes disulfiram effect. May cause darkening of urine. **EVALUATION:** Evaluate for resolution of fever and symptoms. Report any adverse reactions.
vancomycin (Vancocin) **Adults:** 500 mg–1 g IV q 6–12 hr, 125 mg PO q 6 hr **Children >1 mo:** 10–15 mg/kg IV over q 6 hr, 40 mg/kg per day PO in four divided doses **Neonates <1 mo:** 10 mg/kg IV q 8–12 hr, 10 mg/kg per day PO in divided doses	**A:** <1% **PB:** 52%–56% **½L:** 6 hr **E:** renal	**ASSESSMENT:** Assess for previous allergy. Assess for pregnancy (category C). **INTERVENTION:** Do not administer IM. Infuse at least 60 min. Avoid IV infiltration. **Patient Teaching**—Remind patient to report any sign of rash. **EVALUATION:** Evaluate for resolution of fever and symptoms. Check WBC. Report any adverse reactions. Monitor peak (23–35 μg/mL) and trough (8–10 μg/mL) serum concentrations.

NA = not available.

discontinued if possible, and the *C. difficile* may be treated with oral metronidazole or vancomycin.

○ **Chloramphenicol** (Chloromycetin), was discovered in 1947. Today, the clinical use of chloramphenicol is limited as a result of the development of more active and safer anti-infectives.

○ **Vancomycin** (Vancocin, Vancoled, and others) is a narrow-spectrum bactericidal glycopeptide antibiotic produced by the soil microorganism *Streptomyces orientalis*.

ACTION The primary mechanism of action of vancomycin is to inhibit cell wall synthesis at a point distinct from that of penicillins and cephalosporins. In addition, vancomycin also has been shown to inhibit ribonucleic acid (RNA) synthesis and to alter bacterial cell wall permeability.

SPECTRUM OF ACTIVITY Vancomycin is primarily active against gram-positive bacteria and is considered the drug of choice for MRSA or MRSE. However, against *E. faecalis* it is only bacteriostatic, and combination therapy with an aminoglycoside is usually necessary for treating these infections. It is inactive against gram-negative bacteria. Vancomycin administered orally is also active against *C. difficile*, the responsible organism in antibiotic-associated colitis.

PHARMACOKINETICS Vancomycin is poorly absorbed when administered orally (less than 1%), with most of the dose appearing in the feces. This is the rationale for prescribing oral vancomycin for *C. difficile* antibiotic-associated colitis, an entity confined to the GI tract. For systemic infections, vancomycin is administered intravenously. Intramuscular administration results in muscle necrosis and should be avoided.

Approximately 90% of an IV dose of vancomycin is excreted by the kidneys. It is imperative that dosage be decreased in patients with renal dysfunction to avoid toxicity. The elimination half-life of vancomycin in subjects with normal renal function is approximately 6 hours. In anuric patients, the half-life of the drug is remarkably prolonged (up to 240 hours) and once-weekly dosing may be appropriate. Hemodialysis does not remove vancomycin from the body.

CONTRAINDICATIONS AND PRECAUTIONS Use vancomycin with caution in patients with prior hypersensitivity reactions. Safe use during pregnancy has not been established.

ADVERSE EFFECTS Hearing loss may occur in patients receiving vancomycin. Deafness may be preceded by ringing in the ears and is associated with elevated serum concentrations of vancomycin. Prolonged high serum concentrations of vancomycin are usually seen in patients with decreased renal function in whom the dosage has not been reduced.

Combined use of vancomycin with other nephrotoxic agents (e.g., aminoglycosides) may result in additive nephrotoxicity.

A side effect unique to vancomycin is that related to the rapid infusion of large doses of vancomycin. It is characterized by fever, chills, paresthesias (numbness), and erythema (reddening) at the base of the neck and the upper back and may be followed by hypotension. It usually begins 10 minutes after the start of the infusion and re-

solves 15 to 20 minutes after the infusion has stopped. The reaction seems to be related to histamine release and is not a hypersensitivity (or immunologic) reaction. It may be minimized by reducing the dose, slowing the rate of infusion, or premedicating with antihistamines.

Patients receiving IV vancomycin may experience thrombophlebitis, neutropenia (decreased number of white cells), and thrombocytopenia (decreased number of platelets).

○ **Metronidazole** (Flagyl) was synthesized in 1959 and is an excellent drug for treating anaerobic infections.

ACTION Metronidazole is reduced to microbiologically active intermediary metabolites that react with bacterial DNA, disrupting transcription and replication. The end result is cell death.

SPECTRUM OF ACTIVITY Metronidazole is active against obligate (strict) anaerobes, including *B. fragilis*. It has limited activity against above-the-diaphragm mouth anaerobes, such as peptostreptococci. Metronidazole also has activity against *Trichomonas vaginalis*, *Entamoeba histolytica*, *Giardia lamblia*, *C. jejuni*, and *Gardnerella vaginalis*.

PHARMACOKINETICS Metronidazole is completely absorbed from the GI tract. An IV formulation is available for treatment of systemic infection.

This agent is extensively metabolized by the liver with less than 10% excreted unchanged in the urine. Dosage reduction is necessary only in patients with severely impaired renal function.

CONTRAINDICATIONS AND PRECAUTIONS Use of metronidazole is contraindicated during the first trimester of pregnancy. Use with caution in patients with prior hypersensitivity reactions. Avoid the concomitant use of alcohol and alcohol-containing products.

ADVERSE EFFECTS The most common GI effects of metronidazole therapy are nausea, anorexia, cramping, and diarrhea. An unpleasant metallic taste and dry mouth have also been described.

Neurologic adverse effects of metronidazole include dizziness, vertigo, and numbness or tingling in the extremities.

Darkened urine has been noted and attributed to a metabolite of metronidazole. Rashes (erythematous, maculopapular, and pruritic) and reversible neutropenia have also been described. Thrombophlebitis may be one of the most frequent effects seen with the IV form of the drug.

INTERACTIONS A *disulfiram-like reaction* may occur if patients ingest ethanol (alcohol) while taking metronidazole. Flushing, dizziness, sweating, and nausea are the clinical manifestations of this response.

Metronidazole may inhibit the hepatic metabolism of anticoagulants (warfarin), thus increasing the risk of bleeding. Clinical signs of bleeding, as well as PT prolongation are monitored closely when this combination is prescribed.

ANTITUBERCULAR AGENTS

Two important features distinguish the treatment of tuberculosis from other therapies for infections. First, effective treatment of tuberculosis requires anti-infective administration for a prolonged period—from 6 to 24 months—owing to the slow-growing nature of the organism. Second, the development of bacterial resistance to antitubercular agents occurs intrinsically. Therefore, combination therapy is indicated to minimize the emergence of resistance.

Antitubercular drugs may be thought of as either first-line or second-line agents. Drugs considered first line—**isoniazid (INH), rifampin** or **rifampicin (Rimactane), ethambutol (Myambutol),** and **pyrazinamide**—provide the most effective antituberculous activity with an acceptable degree of toxicity. Second-line agents—**ethionamide (Trecator-SC), para-aminosalicylic acid (PAS),** and **cycloserine (Seromycin)**—provide adequate antimicrobial activity but have excessive toxicities. The use of these latter agents is reemerging as multidrug-resistant strains of tuberculosis are increasing. Selected antitubucular agents are featured in Table 58–10.

FIRST-LINE ANTITUBERCULAR AGENTS

○ **Isoniazid** (INH) is the primary choice for therapy against *Mycobacterium tuberculosis.*

ACTION AND RESISTANCE Tubercle bacilli sensitive to INH possess a mechanism for transportation of the compound intracellularly. After entry into the cell, the drug interferes with the formation of an essential metabolite for the organism. INH is bactericidal against *M. tuberculosis.* Resistance to isoniazid is thought to occur because mutant organisms prevent penetration of the antibiotic into the cell.

PHARMACOKINETICS Isoniazid is rapidly absorbed from the GI tract with peak serum concentrations achieved within 1 to 2 hours after administration. Aluminum-containing antacids may interfere with absorption.

INH is extensively metabolized in the liver by a process known as *acetylation.* This metabolic pathway is catalyzed by the enzyme N-acetyl transferase. A patient's rate of acetylation (either fast or slow) is genetically determined and dependent on race. Ninety percent or more of Orientals are fast acetylators, whereas only 45% to 50% of Caucasians are considered to be fast acetylators. Thus, the serum half-life of INH is variable: 1.1 hours for a fast acetylator and 3.1 hours for a slow acetylator. The kidneys do not contribute significantly to the elimination of the parent drug (INH); however, the drug is hemodialyzable

Table 58–10. ANTITUBERCULAR AGENTS

DRUG NAME/ROUTE AND DOSAGE	PHARMACOKINETICS/ DYNAMICS	NURSING IMPLICATIONS
isoniazid (INH) *Adults:* 5–10 mg/kg PO (up to 300 mg daily) given once daily *Infants and Children:* 10–20 mg/kg PO given once daily	A: rapid PB: minimal ½L: 1.1 hr (widely variable) E: hepatic	**ASSESSMENT:** Coadminister with vitamin B₆ (pyridoxine). Compliance with medication regimen must be enforced. Assess for pregnancy (category UK). **INTERVENTION: Patient Teaching**—Instruct patient to continue medication through entire treatment course. Minimize alcohol intake due to increased risk of hepatitis. **EVALUATION:** Evaluate for resolution of fever and symptoms. Evaluate patient compliance. Report any adverse reactions.
ethambutol (Myambutol) *Adults:* 15–30 mg/kg PO once daily	A: 80% PB: 8%–22% ½L: 3–4 hr E: renal, hepatic	**ASSESSMENT:** Compliance with regimen must be enforced. Assess for pregnancy (category UK). **INTERVENTION:** Same as for isoniazid. **EVALUATION:** Same as for isoniazid.
pyrazinamide *Adults:* 15–30 mg/kg PO, maximum 2 g	A: rapid and complete PB: 50% ½L: 9 hr E: renal, hepatic	Same as for ethambutol.
rifampin (Rifadin) *Adults:* 600 mg PO once daily *Children:* 10–20 mg/kg PO once daily not to exceed 600 mg per day	A: well absorbed PB: 84%–91% ½L: 1.5–5 hr E: hepatic	**ASSESSMENT:** Same as for ethambutol. Obtain list of concurrent medications and screen for potential drug interactions. Assess for pregnancy (category C). **INTERVENTION: Patient Teaching**—Inform patient that rifampin may discolor tears, urine, and saliva and may cause discoloration of contact lenses. Stress importance of completion of therapy. **EVALUATION:** Same as for ethambutol.

and the usual dose is given following the dialysis procedure.

CONTRAINDICATIONS AND PRECAUTIONS INH administration is avoided if the patient experienced a prior hypersensitivity reaction. INH is used cautiously in patients with hepatic disease.

ADVERSE EFFECTS Nausea, vomiting, and diarrhea have been reported with INH but are not common. Hypersensitivity reactions (fever and maculopapular rash) may occur.

Hepatotoxicity is a well-known side effect of INH and most likely the result of a toxic metabolite of the drug, acetylhydrazine. It is possible that rapid acetylators are more likely to develop INH-induced hepatitis because they metabolize more INH to acetylhydrazine. Although the reaction can occur in a patient receiving only INH, it is more likely to occur in someone taking both INH and rifampin. INH frequently (10% to 20%) causes a rise in liver enzymes (e.g., ALT, AST), which occurs a week to months after the start of therapy. It may persist without progression or resolve spontaneously. In most patients it disappears once the drug is discontinued. One of the more notable side effects of INH may be an overt and sometimes fatal hepatitis, indistinguishable from viral hepatitis. The overall incidence seems to be approximately 1%; however, there is an association with age (the older the patient, the more likely this type of hepatitis). Hepatitis is rare in patients younger than 20 years of age. Although hepatitis can occur anytime during INH therapy, it is more likely during the first 2 months of treatment. Alcohol (especially daily consumption) can increase the likelihood of hepatitis, as can the concomitant administration of rifampin.

Agranulocytosis, eosinophilia, thrombocytopenia, and anemia have been reported with INH therapy. Thus, it is important to monitor CBCs when a patient receives INH.

INH interferes with the normal action of pyridoxine (vitamin B₆), an essential component in nerve function. As a result, peripheral neuritis may develop. This common toxicity (seen in 20% of patients) can be prevented by the prophylactic administration of pyridoxine (25 to 50 mg/day). Additional neurotoxicities reported are convulsions, optic neuritis, muscle twitching, dizziness, ataxia, and toxic encephalopathy. Mental status changes may appear during INH treatment, and patients may manifest euphoria, memory loss, loss of self-control, and psychoses.

INTERACTIONS INH may inhibit the metabolism of phenytoin, leading to toxicity (nystagmus, ataxia, and confusion). A reduction of phenytoin dosage may be required until the INH is discontinued. Similarly, symptoms of carbamazepine intoxication have been reported in patients who have had INH prescribed concurrently.

Corticosteroids may stimulate hepatic enzymes that metabolize INH, decreasing the antitubercular activity. This interaction may require higher doses of INH.

○ **Rifampin** (Rimactane), or rifampicin, is a semisynthetic derivative of rifamycin B, an antibiotic produced by *Streptomyces mediterranei*.

ACTION DNA-dependent RNA polymerase, a crucial enzyme in RNA synthesis, is inhibited by the presence of rifampin. These effects are limited to bacteria, and mammalian cells are unaffected. Bacterial resistance develops when a modification of the DNA-dependent *RNA polymerase* is made, enabling the enzyme to escape binding to rifampin.

SPECTRUM OF ACTIVITY Rifampin is a broad-spectrum antibacterial agent with activity against many gram-positive and gram-negative microorganisms, as well as *Mycobacterium tuberculosis*. Rifampin is very active versus *S. aureus*, *N. meningitides*, *N. gonorrhoeae*, and *H. influenzae*. The primary clinical use for rifampin is in the treatment of tuberculosis and selected staphylococcal infections. Against *M. tuberculosis* rifampin is bactericidal and is often used in combination with INH and/or streptomycin to increase the effectiveness of treatment and prevent emergence of resistance. Against staphylococci, it may be used in combination with an antistaphylococcal penicillin (e.g., nafcillin).

PHARMACOKINETICS Following oral administration, rifampin is well absorbed. Food has been shown to delay absorption and decrease peak plasma concentrations. Rifampin enters the systemic circulation and is eventually excreted in bile and into the small intestine. Reabsorption of rifampin from the GI tract occurs, and the drug returns to the systemic circulation, (enterohepatic recirculation).

Rifampin is distributed throughout body fluids, including the CSF. The extent of distribution is evident from the orange-red color change imparted to the urine, feces, saliva, sputum, tears, and sweat. Patients should be made aware of this color change so as not to be alarmed. Rifampin may also tint contact lenses orange-red. The drug has been measured in the fetal circulation and is secreted into breast milk. Rifampin also penetrates phagocytic cells and can kill intracellular organisms.

The plasma half-life of rifampin is prolonged in patients with hepatic disease. Minimal rifampin is excreted through the kidneys; therefore, dosage alteration is not required in patients with renal disease. The effects of dialysis on rifampin serum concentrations are insignificant.

CONTRAINDICATIONS AND PRECAUTIONS Rifampin is not used in patients with a prior hypersensitivity reaction or in pregnant patients. Use cautiously in patients with hepatic or renal disease.

ADVERSE EFFECTS Hypersensitivity to rifampin is rare; however, a cutaneous syndrome has been described in patients receiving daily or intermittent therapy with rifampin. Typically this reaction occurs early in the course of therapy and is manifested by flushing and pruritis (itching) with or without a rash. Areas most often involved are the face and scalp, with watering and redness of the eyes also occurring.

Rifampin-induced hepatitis is not an uncommon side effect of the drug. However, it is usually asymptomatic in nature and transient with mild elevation in transaminase enzymes (e.g., serum alanine aminotransferase [ALT]). A more serious and symptomatic form of hepatitis can occur. Patients at particular risk for this are the elderly patient, the patient with preexisting liver disease, or the alcoholic. Additive toxicity may occur when rifampin is used in combination with other antitubercular agents known to cause liver injury (e.g., INH, pyrazinamide).

Rifampin is known to induce thrombocytopenia more often when intermittent therapy, as opposed to daily therapy, is used.

INTERACTIONS Rifampin is a potent inducer of liver enzymes and has been reported to increase the metabolism of anticoagulants, oral contraceptives, methadone, quinidine, oral hypoglycemic agents, and corticosteroids. The increased metabolic capability results in a decreased pharmacologic effect of these agents, and therefore higher dosages may be required. In the case of oral contraceptive agents, patients receiving rifampin should be instructed to use an alternative method of birth control.

○ **Ethambutol** (Myambutol) probably acts as an antimetabolite and inhibits mycobacterial RNA synthesis. Its precise mechanism of action is not known.

SPECTRUM OF ACTIVITY Ethambutol is active (bacteriostatic) against *M. tuberculosis*. Against other atypical mycobacterial species (e.g., avium-intracellulare) the drug is active in vitro; however, combination therapy with other antimycobacterial agents is often necessary for effective clinical results.

PHARMACOKINETICS Ethambutol is well absorbed after oral administration and unaffected by food. It distributes to most body tissues including the lung and is localized within pulmonary alveolar macrophages. In the presence of inflammation, CSF penetration is seen. Most (80%) of an oral dose of ethambutol is excreted unchanged in the urine. Dosage alteration in patients with reduced renal function is necessary. Ethambutol is hemodialyzed, and the daily dose should be administered after the dialysis procedure.

CONTRAINDICATIONS AND PRECAUTIONS Ethambutol is not recommended in children younger than 13 years of age. Avoid use in patients with a prior hypersensitivity reaction. Use with caution in patients with renal impairment.

ADVERSE EFFECTS Ethambutol is generally well tolerated, and hypersensitivity reactions and hepatitis are rare.

Retrobulbar neuritis is considered the major toxicity of ethambutol and is clearly a dose-related phenomenon. If the dose of ethambutol is 15 mg/kg per day or less, this adverse effect is extremely uncommon. This effect is readily reversible if recognized early and the drug is discontinued; however, optic atrophy and blindness may result if therapy is continued. Symptoms include blurring of vision, central blind spots or constriction of the visual fields, and/or alterations in red/green color perception. Patients should be made aware of this toxicity and instructed to report any changes in visual function.

Because of its ability to decrease the renal clearance of uric acid, ethambutol can induce an elevation in serum uric acid concentrations (hyperuricemia). However, it seldom causes acute gouty attacks.

○ **Pyrazinamide,** a derivative of nicotinamide, was synthesized in 1952.

ACTION The manner in which pyrazinamide suppresses the growth of the tubercle bacillus is unknown. It is inactive against other bacteria and is bacteriostatic against *M. tuberculosis*. As with other antitubercular drugs, resistance may develop during prolonged treatment, particularly if the drug is used alone.

PHARMACOKINETICS Pyrazinamide is rapidly and completely absorbed following oral ingestion, with peak plasma concentrations occurring in 2 hours. The drug penetrates well into the liver, lungs, kidneys, and CSF of patients with tuberculous meningitis. Pyrazinamide enters cells that have phagocytized tubercle bacilli. Pyrazinamide is metabolized in the liver by hepatic microsomal enzymes and excreted in its original form by glomerular filtration (3%). The dosage of pyrazinamide is adjusted accordingly in patients with impaired hepatic or renal function.

CONTRAINDICATIONS AND PRECAUTIONS Pyrazinamide is contraindicated in hepatic disease and in children. Use cautiously in the presence of gout, diabetes mellitus, renal impairment, and peptic ulcer disease.

ADVERSE EFFECTS Patients may experience mild degrees of anorexia and nausea. Vomiting is much less common.

The incidence of hepatotoxicity secondary to pyrazinamide is variable and ranges from 2% to 20% of patients. Patients should be monitored closely for signs of hepatic injury (jaundice or altered liver function tests) while on pyrazinamide.

One of the metabolites of pyrazinamide inhibits the tubular secretion of uric acid, causing hyperuricemia. Early studies reported certain patients who developed clinical gout secondary to elevations of serum uric acid; thus, patients with prior abnormalities of uric acid metabolism should be monitored during pyrazinamide treatment.

Arthralgias can occur, which may be the result of elevated serum uric acid levels. Unlike gout, the joint pain usually involves both large and small joints (most commonly the shoulders, knees, and fingers) and often involves more than one type of joint. The onset is usually during the first two months after treatment has been initiated, is usually self-limiting, and responds readily to symptomatic therapy (e.g., aspirin).

SECOND-LINE ANTITUBERCULAR AGENTS

○ **Ethionamide** (Trecator-SC), a derivative of isonicotinic acid, was discovered in France in 1956 and was subsequently shown to be an effective antitubercular drug. Its mechanism of action is unknown.

CONTRAINDICATIONS AND PRECAUTIONS Use ethionamide cautiously in patients with diabetes mellitus, in pregnant patients, and in children.

ADVERSE EFFECTS Gastrointestinal complaints are the major adverse effects of ethionamide, which limits its use. Patients receiving the drug may complain of excessive salivation, nausea, vomiting, anorexia, diarrhea, abdominal pain, or a metallic taste. In some patients, these effects are severe enough to require discontinuation of therapy. Gastrointestinal side effects may be more common in women than men.

Liver damage is uncommon with this agent. However, it has been reported and patients should be monitored for hepatic dysfunction.

In the clinical setting, patients ingesting ethionamide

may experience mental status changes. Giddiness and headache are common. In addition, depression, acute psychoses, and dizziness may be reported. Patients may experience visual alterations or peripheral nerve abnormalities (tingling fingers).

Ethionamide is teratogenic in animals and should be avoided during pregnancy.

○ **Para-aminosalicylic acid (PAS),** in 1946, was found to have tuberculostatic effect. Clinical usage of this agent has decreased with newer, less toxic antitubercular agents on the market.

○ **Cycloserine** (Seromycin) is a broad-spectrum antibiotic produced by *Streptomyces orchidaceus* and *Streptomyces garyphalus*. Although cycloserine is active against other microorganisms, its primary clinical indication is as a second-line antituberculous agent.

ACTION Cycloserine is a cell wall–active antibiotic; however, it appears to work at a site different from that of other cell wall–active agents (e.g., the penicillins).

PHARMACOKINETICS Cycloserine is well absorbed when given orally, and peak serum concentrations are reached in 3 to 4 hours. The drug is not appreciably bound to serum protein and thus it has a large volume of distribution throughout the body. The CSF is extremely accessible to cycloserine, with concentrations comparable to serum concentrations. Cycloserine is primarily eliminated by the kidneys (about 65%) by glomerular filtration. Approximately 35% is metabolized. The dosage of cycloserine is decreased in patients with reduced renal function.

CONTRAINDICATIONS AND PRECAUTIONS Avoid use in patients with a prior hypersensitivity reaction. Use cautiously in patients with CNS disorders or renal impairment and during pregnancy. Use cautiously in children.

ADVERSE EFFECTS The most common reactions to cycloserine are related to the CNS. The excellent penetration of cycloserine into the CFS may result in psychosis, somnolence, headache, tremor, vertigo, confusion and depression, aggression, visual disturbances, slurred speech, insomnia, seizures, and hyperreflexia. All these reactions appear to be dose related and are less likely to occur with lower daily doses (e.g., 0.5 g/day). The drug is avoided in patients with a history of epilepsy or psychiatric illness. Hypersensitivity reactions and hepatitis are rare.

ANTILEPROTIC AGENTS

Agents classified as antileprotics—**dapsone (DDS)** and **clofazamine *(Lamprene)***—are used to treat leprosy and are also being used to treat some AIDS-related opportunistic infections. These drugs pharmacokinetics and dosage are featured in Table 58–11.

○ **Dapsone** (DDS) is a sulfone that is bacteriostatic and probably acts by interfering with folate synthesis, similar to the sulfonamides. It has activity against *Mycobacterium leprae* and *P. carinii*.

CONTRAINDICATIONS AND PRECAUTIONS Avoid use of drug in patients with a prior hypersensitivity to dapsone and possibly sulfonamides. Administer with caution to patients with G6PD deficiency.

ADVERSE EFFECTS A dose-related hemolysis is seen in most patients, as manifested by a decreased hemoglobin and increased reticulocyte count. In patients with G6PD deficiency, this response may be exaggerated. Dapsone has an increased oxidative potential; therefore, methemoglobinemia may also occur, leading to fatigue, difficulty breathing, and cyanosis. Dapsone may also cause phototoxic reactions.

INTERACTIONS Rifampin decreases dapsone serum concentrations owing to induction of the hepatic microenzymes and subsequent increased clearance of dapsone. Concurrent administration of trimethoprim and dapsone may increase the serum concentrations of both drugs, which may lead to increased frequency of adverse effects of both drugs.

○ **Clofazimine** (Lamprene) is believed to bind to mycobacterial DNA and inhibit its growth. The exact mechanism of action is unknown. Clofazimine has activity against *M. leprae* and *M. avium* complex.

CONTRAINDICATIONS AND PRECAUTIONS Safe use in pregnancy or lactation has not been established. Use with

Table 58–11. ANTILEPROTIC AGENTS		
DRUG NAME/ROUTE AND DOSAGE	**PHARMACOKINETICS/ DYNAMICS**	**NURSING IMPLICATIONS**
clofazimine (Lamprene) *Adults:* 100 mg PO once daily	A: 50% ½L: 70 days E: biliary	**ASSESSMENT:** Assess for pregnancy (category C). **INTERVENTION: Patient Teaching**—Instruct patient to take drug with meals. Warn patient that skin discoloration may occur. **EVALUATION:** Evaluate for resolution of symptoms.
dapsone (DDS) *Adults:* 50–300 mg PO daily	A: nearly 100% PB: 70%–90% ½L: 10–50 hrs E: hepatic	**ASSESSMENT:** Assess history to determine if the patient has a known G6PD deficiency. **INTERVENTION:** Monitor patient for development of hemolytic anemia (monitor hemoglobin). **EVALUATION:** Evaluate for resolution of symptoms.

caution in patients with hepatic disease or with a prior sensitivity to clofazimine.

ADVERSE EFFECTS Skin pigmentation changes (pink to brownish-black) can occur in up to 75% to 100% of patients receiving clofazimine for several weeks. This effect is reversible, but may require several months or years to disappear completely. Skin dryness can also occur, which can be treated with oils or emollients. Abdominal pain, nausea, vomiting, and diarrhea occur in about half of patients receiving clofazimine.

ANTIFUNGAL AGENTS

Commonly prescribed antifungal agents include **amphotericin B** *(Fungizone)*, **flucytosine** *(Ancobon)*, **miconazole** *(Monistat IV)*, **ketoconazole** *(Nizoral)*, **nystatin** *(Mycostatin)*, **clotrimazole** *(Lotrimin, Mycelex)*, **fluconazole** *(Diflucan)*, and **itraconazole** *(Sporanox)*. Selected antifungal agents their dosage and pharmacokinetics are featured in Table 58–12.

Table 58–12. ANTIFUNGAL AGENTS

DRUG NAME/ROUTE AND DOSAGE	PHARMACOKINETICS/ DYNAMICS	NURSING IMPLICATIONS
amphotericin B (Fungizone) **Adults:** Test dose 1 mg; if tolerated 0.25–1 mg/kg per day IV. Not to exceed a total daily dose of 1.5 mg/kg	**PB:** 95% **½L:** 24 hr **E:** nonrenal	**ASSESSMENT:** Assess for pregnancy (category B). **INTERVENTION:** Infuse over 4–6 hr. Monitor phlebitis. Premedicate with diphenhydramine, acetaminophen, and meperidine. **Patient Teaching**—Instruct patient to report any fever, chills, shaking, dizziness, or flushing during infusion. **EVALUATION:** Evaluate for resolution of fever and symptoms. Report any adverse reactions.
fluconazole (Diflucan) **Adults:** 50–400 mg PO/IV daily in one or two doses	**A:** 90% **PB:** 11% **½L:** 31 hr **E:** renal	**ASSESSMENT:** Assess patient for concurrent medications that may interact with fluconazole. Assess for pregnancy (category C). **INTERVENTION: Patient Teaching**—Tell patient that fluconazole may be taken without regard to meals. **EVALUATION:** Evaluate patient for resolution of fever and symptoms.
flucytosine (Ancobon) **Adults:** 50–150 mg/kg per day PO in four divided doses	**A:** 75%–90% **PB:** 2%–4% **½L:** 2.5–6 hr **E:** renal	**ASSESSMENT:** Assess for pregnancy (category C). **INTERVENTION:** Assess initial doses may decrease GI upset. **Patient Teaching**—Tell patient to report any nausea. **EVALUATION:** Monitor patient renal function and serum concentrations (desired concentrations 50–100 μg/mL).
itraconazole (Sporanox) **Adults:** 200 mg PO once or twice daily	**PB:** 99.8% **½L:** 13–30 hr **E:** hepatic	**ASSESSMENT:** Assess patient for any concurrent medications that may interact with itraconazole. Assess for pregnancy (category C). **INTERVENTION: Patient Teaching**—Inform patient that itraconazole should be taken with food to ensure maximal absorption. **EVALUATION:** Evaluate patient for resolution of fever and symptoms.
ketoconazole (Nizoral) **Adults:** 200–400 mg PO once daily **Children >2 yr:** 3.3–6.6 mg/kg PO. Single daily dose.	**A:** variable **PB:** 84%–99% **½L:** 8 hr **E:** renal, hepatic	**ASSESSMENT:** Assess patient for any concurrent medications that may interact with ketoconazole. Assess for pregnancy (category C). **INTERVENTION: Patient Teaching**—Instruct patient not to take drug with antacids or histamine H_2 blockers. **EVALUATION:** Evaluate for resolution of fever and symptoms.

CONTRAINDICATIONS As a group, safe use during pregnancy has not been established. They are not used in patients with a known prior hypersensitivity.

○ **Amphotericin B** (Fungizone) is a product of a soil organism, *Streptomyces nodesus*, and was discovered in 1956.

ACTION The antifungal activity of amphotericin B is related to its ability to bind to *ergosterol*, which is the principal *sterol* on the fungal cell membrane. As a result of this binding phenomenon, pores appear in the cell membrane and life-sustaining cellular materials "leak" out of the organism, ultimately causing fungal death. Amphotericin B has a greater affinity for components of fungal membranes than for human membranes. However, toxicity of this agent is thought to be caused by altered membrane permeability of human cells.

SPECTRUM OF ACTIVITY Amphotericin B is either fungistatic (inhibits fungal growth) or fungicidal (kills fungi), depending on the concentration attained and the sensitivity of the fungus. It is active against many of the fungi seen commonly in hospitalized patients such as *Candida* species, *Cryptococcus neoformans*, and *Aspergillus fumigatus*. The antifungal activity of amphotericin B is enhanced (synergy) when administered together with tetracyclines, rifampin, or 5-flucytosine. The alteration in the membrane permeability induced by amphotericin B makes it easier for the other agent (e.g., 5-flucytosine) to penetrate the fungal cell wall.

ADVERSE EFFECTS Patients may experience thrombophlebitis, fever, chills, headache, anorexia, nausea, and vomiting during and after intravenous administration. These adverse effects may represent drug toxicity or patient hypersensitivity. A 1-mg test dose of amphotericin B can be administered to determine patient hypersensitivity. The addition of heparin or hydrocortisone and a prolonged duration of infusion (4 to 6 hours) may overcome these reactions. Premedication with diphenhydramine (Benadryl) and acetaminophen (Tylenol) can decrease the fever and chills associated with the drug's administration.

Most patients experience a decrease in renal function during amphotericin B therapy, which is monitored clinically by changes in the serum creatinine concentration. When the serum creatinine level reaches 2.5 mg/dL, the drug is usually discontinued and then resumed again after 2 to 3 days or an every-other-day administration regimen is followed. Normal saline infusion both before and after amphotericin B infusion may minimize nephrotoxicity.

With amphotericin B–induced renal dysfunction, the kidneys may excrete excess potassium, leading to severe hypokalemia. Patients are monitored closely and given potassium supplements when indicated. Hypomagnesemia may also occur and requires magnesium supplementation. Metabolic acidosis due to altered renal acidifying mechanisms can also occur during amphotericin B administration.

Patients receiving amphotericin B usually develop mild anemia owing to suppression of red blood cell production in the bone marrow. This effect is reversible when the drug is discontinued.

INTERACTIONS Concurrent administration of amphotericin B with other nephrotoxic agents (e.g., aminoglycosides, cisplatinum, furosemide) may have additive toxic effects on the kidneys.

There are currently several other types of amphotericin B formulations on the market. These include **liposomal amphotericin B** and **amphotericin B lipid complex (ABLC)**. To potentially decrease amphotericin B toxicity, lipid formulations of amphotericin B have been developed. These preparations appear to accumulate preferentially in organs of the reticuloendothelial system rather than the kidneys. These drugs, however are very expensive. They are therefore recommended to be used in patients with a life-threatening mycoses for whom conventional therapy has failed or who are intolerant to conventional amphotericin B therapy.

○ **Flucytosine** (Ancobon), also known as 5-flucytosine or 5-FC, is a synthetic antimetabolite of the fluoropyrimidine series.

ACTION 5-FC penetrates fungal cells with the help of an enzyme known as cytosine permease. Once inside the cell, 5-FC is converted by cytosine deaminase to 5-FU (5-fluorouracil), which is then incorporated into RNA, disrupting protein synthesis and resulting in cell death. Part of the selective action of 5-FC is the fact that human cells do not contain the enzyme cytosine deaminase. Fungi may develop resistance to 5-FC as a result of a deficiency of permease activity; resistance to 5-FC develops rapidly when it is prescribed alone.

SPECTRUM OF ACTIVITY 5-FC has been prescribed in combination with other antifungals for the treatment of infections caused by *C. albicans*, *C. neoformans*, *Torulopsis glabrata*, and *Aspergillus* species.

ADVERSE EFFECTS Patients receiving 5-FC may develop nausea, vomiting, or diarrhea and may require a dosage reduction. 5-FC induces bone marrow suppression, which may lead to neutropenia, thrombocytopenia, or anemia. Patients at risk for this particular side effect appear to be individuals with decreased renal function.

○ **Miconazole** (Monistat IV) is an imidazole antifungal agent. In addition to its use as a topical antifungal (available over-the-counter [OTC] for treatment of vaginal yeast infections), it is also available for IV administration, though it is rarely used in this form due to an association with cardiotoxicity.

Miconazole has a similar mechanism of action to clotrimazole.

SPECTRUM OF ACTIVITY Miconazole inhibits the growth of *C. albicans*, *C. neoformans*, *Blastomyces dermatitidis*, *Histoplasma capsulatum*, *Coccidioides immitis*, and *Aspergillus*, *Trichophyton*, and *Epidermophyton* species.

ADVERSE EFFECTS Miconazole appears to suppress red blood cell production. This effect is dose related and disappears when miconazole is discontinued. Intravenous dosing may result in symptoms such as nausea, vomiting, or diarrhea. Intravenous infusions of miconazole may cause thrombophlebitis when given through peripheral veins. This problem is avoided by administering the drug via larger central veins.

INTERACTIONS Miconazole and anticoagulants administered concurrently may result in prolongation of the PT and an increased risk of bleeding. Concurrent administration with hypoglycemic agents may result in hypoglycemia.

○ **Ketoconazole** (Nizoral) is an imidazole antifungal agent similar in structure and spectrum of activity to miconazole.

ACTION The mechanism of antifungal action is impairment of ergosterol biosynthesis and alteration in the cell membrane, which leads to cell death. In addition, ketoconazole may affect oxidative and peroxidative systems within fungal organisms, resulting in the intracellular accumulation of toxic endoperoxides.

ADVERSE EFFECTS Following oral doses of 400 to 600 mg per day of ketoconazole, patients may complain of mild nausea and occasional vomiting. These symptoms may be alleviated by taking the drug with meals. Asymptomatic elevations in transaminase enzymes has been reported in 2% to 5% of patients, but symptomatic hepatic disease is rare. High doses or prolonged therapy may result in sexual impotence, hair loss, and gynecomastia due to ketoconazole's ability to inhibit testosterone and adrenocorticotropic hormone synthesis.

INTERACTIONS The solubility of ketoconazole and subsequent absorption of the drug depends on an acid environment. Agents that increase the pH of the stomach, including antacids and H_2 antagonists, affect the absorption of ketoconazole and thus should be avoided or properly spaced. The plasma half-life of cyclosporine is reported to be prolonged by ketoconazole. Rifampin is a known enzyme stimulator and can increase the metabolism of ketoconazole, resulting in a decrease in clinical effect of the antifungal agent. Prolonged INR has been reported with the concomitant administration of ketoconazole and oral anticoagulants (e.g., warfarin sodium). Patients receiving both agents should be monitored for potential bleeding episodes.

▼ **CLINICAL ALERT**

Ketoconazole may inhibit the hepatic metabolism of terfenadine, astemizole, and cisapride, leading to an increase in drug serum levels and possible development of life-threatening cardiac dysrhythmias. These drugs are administered concurrently to patients.

○ **Nystatin** (Mycostatin) is used primarily for topical therapy of superficial fungal infections. Nystatin is administered orally (swish and swallow) and vaginally, but is not absorbed systemically.

ACTION Nystatin binds to fungal cell membranes (specifically sterols) and induces an alteration in cell permeability, which results in cell death.

SPECTRUM OF ACTIVITY Nystatin inhibits the growth of various fungi including *Candida albicans*, *C. neoformans*, *H. capsulatum*, *B. dermatitidis*, *C. immitis*, and *Aspergillus*.

ADVERSE EFFECTS Minimal toxicity is associated with topical administration of nystatin; however, following oral ingestion of large doses, nausea and diarrhea may occur.

○ **Clotrimazole** (Lotrimin, Mycelex) was synthesized in Germany in 1967; however, GI toxicity has limited its clinical application to topical treatment of superficial fungal infections. It is available OTC for the treatment of vaginal yeast infection. Like other imidazole antifungal agents (e.g., miconazole, ketoconazole), clotrimazole appears to effect the fungal cell wall, which leads to "leakage" of vital cellular elements and ultimately to cell death. It has the same spectrum of activity as nystatin. Systemic absorption is minimal and thus side effects are rare.

○ **Fluconazole** (Diflucan), approved in 1990, was the first member of a new class of antifungal agents known as triazoles. Fluconazole is available for oral and IV administration.

ACTION Like ketoconazole, this drug impairs ergosterol biosynthesis. Unlike ketoconazole, it is specific for fungal enzyme systems and spares many of the enzyme systems found in humans.

SPECTRUM OF ACTIVITY Fluconazole is primarily active against *Candida* species, *C. neoformans*, *C. immitis*, and *H. capsulatum*.

ADVERSE EFFECTS Mild nausea, vomiting, and abdominal cramps may be associated with the oral use of fluconazole. Asymptomatic and transient elevations in AST and ALT have been reported, and a much less commonly reported adverse effect has been hepatic necrosis. This unusual adverse effect has been fatal. A relatively benign rash following the administration of fluconazole has been reported, as well as a more serious form of erythema multiforme, Stevens-Johnson syndrome, which can be life threatening.

INTERACTIONS An interaction between fluconazole and cyclosporine can result in elevated plasma levels of cyclosporine. Patients receiving both drugs should be monitored for cyclosporine-induced nephrotoxocity. Concomitant use of fluconazole and warfarin sodium (Coumadin) can lead to an enhanced anticoagulant effect because of the inhibition of warfarin sodium metabolism. Patients receiving oral hypoglycemic agents (e.g., tolbutamide, glipizide, and glyburide) and fluconazole concomitantly may be more susceptible to the hypoglycemic effects of these drugs. Administration of fluconazole to a patient receiving therapeutic doses of phenytoin (Dilantin) may lead to elevated phenytoin levels and clinical signs of toxicity (nystagmus, ataxia, and lethargy). Coadministration of fluconazole and rifampin may result in subtherapeutic fluconazole plasma concentrations. Careful monitoring of patients for response to therapy is important when these two agents are given together.

○ **Itraconazole** (Sporanox), like fluconazole, impairs ergosterol biosynthesis. In addition to acting against the same microorganisms as those affected by fluconazole, itraconazole has activity against *Aspergillus* species, *H. capsulatum*, and *B. dermatiditis*.

CONTRAINDICATIONS AND PRECAUTIONS Because of decreased absorption, itraconazole may by inappropriate in patients with achlorhydria. Adverse effects for itraconazole are the same of those for fluconazole.

INTERACTIONS Antacids can increase the pH of the stomach and can decrease itraconazole's absorption. Didanosine contains an antacid buffer and can exert the same effect. Itraconazole can inhibit hepatic metabolism of astemizole and terfenadine and can increase risk of cardiac dysrhythmias and cardiac arrest. Itraconazole can increase serum concentrations of oral hypoglycemics, potentially leading to hypoglycemia.

ANTIVIRAL AGENTS

Important antiviral agents are **acyclovir (Zovirax)**, **ganciclovir (Cytovene)**, **famciclovir (Famvir)**, **valacyclovir (Valtrex)**, **foscarnet (Foscavir)**, **ribavirin (Virazole)**, **amantadine (Symmetrel)**, and **rimantadine (Flumadine)**, and their dosage and pharmacokinetics are featured in Table 58–13. Antiretroviral agents are discussed in Chapter 61.

CONTRAINDICATIONS AND PRECAUTIONS For all antivirals, avoid use in patients with a prior hypersensitivity reaction. Use cautiously in patients with renal impairment, in pregnant patients, and in children.

○ **Acyclovir** (Zovirax), a acyclic nucleoside analog of guanosine, is the first antiviral compound that requires a viral enzyme for activation.

ACTION Acyclovir requires viral enzymatic activation by *thymidine kinase* before it becomes virustatic. Acyclovir binds much more avidly to viral thymidine kinase than to host (human) cell thymidine kinase. This enzyme phosphorylates acyclovir to its active form, acyclovir triphosphate, which inhibits viral *DNA polymerase*, an enzyme necessary for viral DNA synthesis. Three mechanisms of resistance to acyclovir have been documented: (1) The resistant virus lacks adequate thymidine kinase activity, (2) there is a decrease in DNA polymerase sensitivity to acyclovir, and (3) the enzyme thymidine kinase has a decreased specificity for acyclovir.

SPECTRUM OF ACTIVITY Acyclovir is active against herpes viruses, including herpes simplex type 1 (HSV 1), herpes simplex type 2 (HSV 2) and varicella-zoster virus (VZV). Other herpes viruses (e.g., cytomegalovirus and Epstein-Barr virus) are less susceptible.

Most of the drug is eliminated unchanged by both glomerular filtration and tubular secretion. The half-life of acyclovir is markedly prolonged (about 20 hours) in the presence of renal impairment, such that dosage reductions are required.

ADVERSE EFFECTS With high doses administered intravenously, a poor solubility may cause acyclovir to crystallize within the kidney tubules, causing renal damage. This toxicity is avoided by infusing acyclovir slowly over at least 1 hour and keeping the patient well hydrated. Injection site reactions (irritation, inflammation) may also occur. These effects may be alleviated by infusing acyclovir slowly and rotating injection sites. CNS toxicity reactions, such as lethargy, delirium, tremulousness, or seizures, have also been reported in patients receiving acyclovir.

○ **Ganciclovir** (Cytovene), was the first effective antiviral agent for the treatment of cytomegalovirus (CMV) retinitis. An oral form of the drug was approved in 1995 for maintenance therapy of CMV retinitis.

ACTION Ganciclovir requires enzymatic conversion to a triphosphorylated compound (ganciclovir triphos-

phate) for its antiviral activity. Ganciclovir is markedly more active than acyclovir, probably the result of the infected cell generating higher concentrations of ganciclovir triphosphate than of acyclovir triphosphate.

SPECTRUM OF ACTIVITY AND RESISTANCE Ganciclovir is active against herpes viruses and is comparable to acyclovir against HSV and VZV, more active against Epstein-Barr Virus (EBV), and markedly more active than acyclovir against CMV. Resistance to ganciclovir has been identified; the mechanism appears to be a reduction in the capacity of the virally infected cell to phosphorylate (activate) ganciclovir.

PHARMACOKINETICS The bioavailability of oral ganciclovir is 6% to 9% when administered with food. It appears that absorption increases with an increasing number of calories but is not affected by fat content of the food. Serum concentrations attained by oral ganciclovir are lower then that of IV ganciclovir, so oral ganciclovir is approved only for use as maintenance therapy in patients with non-sight-threatening CMV retinitis.

ADVERSE EFFECTS Significant neutropenia (absolute neutrophil count less than 1000 cells/mm^3) is the major dose-limiting side effect of ganciclovir. Its onset is about 14 days after the start of therapy with recovery taking up to 3 weeks following discontinuance of therapy. Bone marrow transplant recipients appear to be at increased risk of neutropenia. Other adverse effects include elevated liver function tests (AST and ALT), thrombocytopenia (20% incidence), eosinophilia (10% incidence), mental status changes, and phlebitis.

INTERACTIONS Concomitant administration of zidovudine and ganciclovir may have additive bone marrow toxicity, and the incidence of neutropenia may be higher than when either agent is used alone. Generalized seizures have been reported in patients receiving imipenem-cilastatin concomitantly with ganciclovir. Concurrent administration of oral ganciclovir and didanosine increases serum concentrations of didanosine by up to 400%, increasing risk of didanosine toxicity (peripheral neuropathy).

○ **Famciclovir** (Famvir) has a mechanism of action and spectrum of activity that are similar to that of acyclovir.

ADVERSE EFFECTS Headache and dizziness may occur in patients. Nausea, vomiting, and diarrhea were reported in clinical trials of famciclovir.

○ **Valacyclovir** (Valtrex) has a mechanism of action and adverse effects similar to famciclovir and acyclovir. This compound is the prodrug of acyclovir, meaning that the oral form of the drug is rapidly absorbed and metabolized to acyclovir. The drug is approved for treatment of herpes zoster, but is most effective when initiated within 48 hours of the onset of the zoster rash.

CONTRAINDICATIONS AND PRECAUTIONS Avoid use in immunocompromised patients because of potential development of thrombotic thrombocytopenia purpura/hemolytic uremic syndrome.

○ **Foscarnet** (Foscavir), also known as trisodium phosphonoformate, is used for the treatment of CMV retinitis.

ACTION Foscarnet reversibly inhibits herpesvirus-induced DNA polymerase activity, a necessary enzyme

Table 58–13. ANTIVIRAL AGENTS

DRUG NAME/ROUTE AND DOSAGE	PHARMACOKINETICS/ DYNAMICS	NURSING IMPLICATIONS
acyclovir (Zovirax) **Adults:** 5 mg/kg IV every 8 hr; 200 mg PO 3–5 times daily **Children <2 yr:** 250 mg/m² IV every 8 hr; also available as ointment, applied to lesion every 3 hr	**A:** 20% **PB:** 9%–33% **½L:** 2–3 hr **E:** renal	**ASSESSMENT:** Monitor for phlebitis. Infuse over 1 hr. Use finger cot or gloves to apply ointment. Assess for pregnancy (category C). **INTERVENTION: Patient Teaching**—Instruct patient to use gloves or finger cot when applying ointment to lesions. **EVALUATIONS:** Evaluate for resolution of fever and symptoms. Report any adverse reactions.
amantadine (Symmetrel) **Adults:** 200 mg PO daily in 1–2 doses **Children 1–9 yr:** 4.4–8.8 mg/kg once daily or in 2 divided doses	**A:** 100% **PB:** NA **½L:** 24 hr **E:** renal	**ASSESSMENT:** Assess for pregnancy (category C). **INTERVENTION: Patient Teaching**—Instruct patient to complete course of therapy. **EVALUATION:** Evaluate for resolution of fever and symptoms. Monitor for and report adverse reactions.
famciclovir (Famvir) **Adults:** 500 mg PO every 8 hr for 7 days	**A:** 77% **PB:** <20% (penciclovir) **½L:** 2.3 hrs **B:** hepatic **E:** renal	**EVALUATION:** Evaluate for resolution of fever and symptoms.
foscarnet (Foscavir) **Adults:** Induction—60 mg/kg IV every 8 hr Maintenance—90–120 mg/kg IV daily	**PB:** 14%–17% **½L:** 3–7 hr **E:** renal	**ASSESSMENT:** Assess patient for renal impairment prior to initiating dose. Maintain adequate hydration. Assess for pregnancy (category C). **INTERVENTION: Patient Teaching**—Instruct patients to report any tingling in perioral area, numbness in extremities, or paresthesias during or after infusion. **EVALUATION:** Report any adverse reactions.
ganciclovir (Cytovene) **Adults:** Induction—5 mg/kg IV q 12 hr for 14–21 days Maintenance—5 mg/kg IV daily or 6 mg/kg IV 5 days per wk, or 1000 mg PO 3 times daily or 500 mg PO 6 times daily every 3 hr	**A:** PO 6%–9% **PB:** 1%–2% **½L:** 4 hr **E:** renal	**ASSESSMENT:** Assess patient for impaired renal function prior to beginning therapy. Assess for pregnancy (category C). **INTERVENTION: Patient Teaching**—Instruct patient to take capsules with food to increase absorption. **EVALUATION:** Monitor WBC. Monitor renal function.
rimantadine (Flumadine) **Adults:** 100 mg PO twice daily for 7 days	**A:** well absorbed **PB:** NA **½L:** 25–32 hr **E:** hepatic	Same as for amantadine.
valacyclovir (Valtrex) **Adults:** 1 g PO bid for 7 days	**A:** 54% **½L:** 2.5–3.3 hr **PB:** 13.5%–17.9% **E:** renal	**EVALUATION:** Evaluate for resolution of symptoms.

NA = not available.

in viral replication. In addition, foscarnet inhibits reverse transcriptase, an enzyme necessary for viral replication of the human immunodeficiency virus (HIV).

SPECTRUM OF ACTIVITY Foscarnet is active against herpes viruses, particularly CMV and acyclovir-resistant HSV. Foscarnet has also demonstrated activity against human immunodeficiency virus (HIV).

ADVERSE EFFECTS A twofold to threefold increase in serum creatinine may occur in up to 45% of patients, representing the major dose-limiting adverse effect of foscarnet. The effect is usually reversible and may be minimized by dosage reduction, use of intermittent rather than continuous infusions, provision of adequate prehydration, and avoidance of concurrent nephrotoxic agents, such as aminoglycosides.

Transient elevations in serum calcium and phosphate levels occur commonly during foscarnet therapy, perhaps because of foscarnet replacing phosphate in bone or foscarnet chelation with ionized calcium. These effects usually cause no symptoms in patients receiving foscarnet.

Patients may experience a decrease in hemoglobin. However, foscarnet does not appear to induce neutropenia.

INTERACTIONS Concurrent administration of potentially nephrotoxic agents (pentamidine, acyclovir, aminoglycosides) may result in additive nephrotoxicity with foscarnet. Avoidance of such combinations is recommended.

○ **Ribavirin** (Virazole) is a purine nucleoside analog approved for aerosolized administration the treatment of respiratory syncytial virus (RSV).

ACTION Ribavirin must be activated to the triphosphorylated form (ribavirin triphosphate) for virustatic activity. Ribavirin interferes with viral RNA production, resulting in inhibition of viral replication.

SPECTRUM OF ACTIVITY Ribavirin is a broad-spectrum virustatic antiviral compound with activity against a number of RNA and DNA viruses. Its major indication is for the treatment of severe lower respiratory tract infections secondary to RSV, commonly found in infants.

ADVERSE EFFECTS Worsening of the patient's respiratory status and the development of bacterial pneumonia and/or pneumothorax have been reported. Cardiac arrest, hypotension, and digitalis intoxication have also been reported. With the aerosol form, rash and conjunctivitis can occur. Ribavirin has been shown to be teratogenic in small animals. Thus, a major concern is the risk of toxicity to health-care workers of childbearing potential who may inhale ribavirin while caring for a patient receiving aerosolized ribavirin. Data suggest that health-care personnel should minimize their exposure to ribavirin, particularly if the drug is administered by oxygen tent.

○ **Amantadine** (Symmetrel), a chemically synthesized compound, is approved for prevention of influenza A viral infections or as an adjunctive therapy to immunization.

ACTION After viral attachment to host cell membranes, amantadine prevents uncoating of the virus, which results in inhibition of viral replication. Resistance to amantadine appears to be a genetically determined property, and amantadine-resistant strains of influenza viruses can be selected.

SPECTRUM OF ACTIVITY Amantadine is a narrow-spectrum antiviral agent, primarily active against influenza A viruses.

CONTRAINDICATIONS AND PRECAUTIONS Use cautiously in patients with renal impairment or congestive heart failure, during pregnancy or lactation, or in children.

ADVERSE EFFECTS Amantadine is well tolerated in the dosage range of 200 to 300 mg per day. Most adverse effects are transient and rapidly reversible on discontinuation. Patients may experience nervousness, difficulty in concentration, dizziness, light-headedness, slurred speech, ataxia, drowsiness, and insomnia. In addition, blurred vision, dry mouth, and palpitations have been reported. Livedo reticularis, a diffuse, rose-colored mottling of the skin usually confined to the lower extremities, has been described with amantadine. Mild ankle edema is usually present and most noticeable when the patient is standing or is exposed to cold. It is reversible in 2 to 6 weeks on discontinuation and is relatively benign even when the drug is continued.

○ **Rimantadine** (Flumadine) is an approved antiviral agent with a profile similar to amantadine. The major difference is that whereas amantadine is almost completely renally eliminated, rimantadine undergoes partial hepatic metabolism. There has also been a decrease in reported adverse affects (particularly CNS effects) with rimantadine as compared to amantadine.

ANTIPROTOZOAL AGENTS

Antiprotozoal agents include **pentamidine isethionate (NebuPent, Pentam 300)** and **atovaquone (Mepron)**.

○ **Pentamidine isethionate** (NebuPent, Pentam 300) is effective in the treatment of leishmaniasis and trypanosomal protozoal infections, diseases rarely encountered in the United States. However, pentamidine's major use is in the treatment and prophylaxis of *P. carinii* pneumonia, a frequent opportunistic infection found in patients with AIDS.

ACTION Pentamidine interferes with oxidative phosphorylation and synthesis of nucleic acids and alters the ability of *P. carinii* organisms to utilize extracellular nutritional constituents and metabolize glucose.

PHARMACOKINETICS Because of its poor absorption from the GI tract, pentamidine is not available for oral administration. Following IM administration, the drug is well absorbed with peak plasma concentrations reached in approximately 1 hour. The drug is usually administered by IV infusion.

The drug is widely distributed in the body with tissue concentrations highest in the kidneys, followed by the liver, and then other tissues (e.g., lungs). Very little of the drug is found in the brain.

Pentamidine undergoes no biotransformation and is slowly released from tissue stores and eliminated unchanged by the kidney. The half-life of the drug in patients with normal renal function is approximately 6 hours. Dosing alterations need to be made in the patient with decreased kidney function as drug accumulation does occur. Hemodialysis and peritoneal dialysis apparently have no effect on the removal of pentamidine from the plasma.

ADVERSE EFFECTS Adverse effects that occur following IV administration of pentamidine include (in order of occurrence) hypotension, followed by tachycardia, nausea and/or vomiting, facial flushing, pruritis, unpleasant taste, hallucinations, and syncope (fainting). These reactions may be minimized if pentamidine is infused over at least 60 minutes.

Following IM administration moderate-to-severe pain at the injection site, sterile abscess formation, or dermal necrosis of the overlying skin have been reported. Following IV infusions of pentamidine, urticaria occurring at the infusion site, phlebitis, and thrombosis have been seen.

Mild and reversible nephrotoxicity is the most frequent adverse systemic reaction to pentamidine. In addition, leukopenia (decrease in white blood cells) or neutropenia (decrease in polymorphonuclear leukocytes), anemia, and thrombocytopenia are also seen. Abnormalities in glucose metabolism with resultant hypoglycemia has been described, and up to 5% of patients receiving pentamidine may develop hyperglycemia. Pancreatitis is another reported adverse effect. Liver function test abnormalities (e.g., transaminase enzyme elevations) have been reported. Other less frequent systemic adverse reactions include skin rashes, alopecia, hypocalcemia, hyperkalemia, decreased folic acid levels, and fever.

▼ CLINICAL ALERT

The daily dose of the drug is based on total body weight of the patient and renal function. In general, patients with normal renal function should receive 3 to 4 mg/kg per day of pentamidine. If the IM route is used, the site of injection should be rotated daily. Intravenous doses of pentamidine should be diluted in 50 to 100 mL of diluent and infused over at least 60 minutes so as to minimize immediate adverse effects. For patients with renal insufficiency, the dose of pentamidine may be reduced and/or the interval of administration extended. This is recommended for patients with a creatinine clearance of less than 35 mL/min.

Aerosolized pentamidine is used to deliver greater concentrations of drug to the site of the infection (lungs) and to decrease systemic adverse reactions. By this route of administration, doses of 300 mg over 30 to 45 minutes have been given once monthly as prophylaxis. Bronchospasm and a metallic taste in the mouth have been reported as an adverse reaction to aerosolized pentamidine.

○ **Atovaquone** (Mepron) may inhibit synthesis of nucleic acid and adrenosine triphosphate (ATP) in susceptible organisms. Its exact mechanism of action is not understood. Atovaquone has activity against *P. carinii* and *T. gondii*.

PHARMACOKINETICS   Atovaquone is administered orally, but its bioavailability is low. To increase absorption, it is recommended that the drug be administered with a high-fat meal (more than 23 g). Atovaquone is highly lipophilic, but penetration into the CNS is poor. It is primarily (94%) eliminated unchanged in the feces.

CONTRAINDICATIONS AND PRECAUTIONS   Avoid use in patients with an allergy to atovaquone. Safety in pregnancy and lactation has not been established.

ADVERSE EFFECTS   There are relatively few adverse reactions to atovaquone. The main reactions include rash, nausea, vomiting, cough, and insomnia.

ANTIPARASITIC AGENTS

Antiparasitic agents include amebicides (agents that kill amebae), anthelmintics (agents that destroy parasitic intestinal worms), and antimalarials (agents that prevent or relieve malaria). The dosage and pharmacokinetics of these agents are featured in Table 58–14.

AMEBICIDES

The amebicides include **iodoquinol (diiodohydroxyquin) (Diodoquin)** and **paromomycin (Humatin)**. Metronidazole, discussed previously, is also classified as an amebicide.

○ **Iodoquinol** (Diodoquin) produces a local amebicidal effect. The exact mechanism of action is unknown. Iodoquinol has activity against *E. histolytica* and *Balantidium coli*.

PHARMACOKINETICS   Iodoquinol is not systemically absorbed and thus is effective only against intestinal amebic infection.

CONTRAINDICATIONS AND PRECAUTIONS   Use with caution in patients with a prior hypersensitivity to iodine, iodoquinol, or primaquine.

ADVERSE EFFECTS   Because iodoquinol has very little systemic absorption, adverse effects are minimal. Fever and hypersensitivity reactions may occur. Thyroid gland enlargement may occur if there is systemic absorption.

ANTHELMINTICS

Pyrantel pamoate (Antiminth), **mebendazole (Vermox)**, and **thiabendazole (Mintezol)** are drugs belonging to the anthelmintics classification. Dosages and pharmacokinetics for these agents are found in Table 58–14.

CONTRAINDICATIONS AND PRECAUTIONS   All the antihelmintics are avoided in known hypersensitivity. Safety during pregnancy and lactation has not been established.

ADVERSE EFFECTS   Common to all antihelmintics include nausea, vomiting, and rash.

○ **Pyrantel pamoate** acts as a depolarizing neuromuscular blocking agent that paralyzes the helminth. The parasite is then expelled from the body. The drug has activity against *Ascaris lumbricoides, Enterobius vermicularis* (pinworm), *Ancylostoma duodenale* (hookworm), *Necator americanus*, and *Trichostrongylus* species.

ADVERSE EFFECTS   Common adverse reactions include dizziness, and drowsiness.

INTERACTIONS   Concurrent administration of piperazine may antagonize the effects of pyrantel.

○ **Mebendazole** (Vermox) blocks uptake of glucose in helminths, depleting energy stores and killing the parasite. Mebendazole is active against *A. lumbricoides, E. vermicularis, A. duodenale, N. americanus, Trichuris trichiura, Capillaria philippinensis, Gnathostoma spinigerum, Echinococcus multilocularis*, and *Trichinella spiralis*.

Table 58–14. ANTIPARASITIC AGENTS: AMEBICIDES, ANTHELMINTICS, AND ANTIMALARIALS

DRUG NAME/ROUTE AND DOSAGE	PHARMACOKINETICS/ DYNAMICS	NURSING IMPLICATIONS
AMEBICIDES		
iodoquinol (diiodohydroxyquin) (Diodoquin) ***Adults:*** 650 mg PO 3 times daily for 20 days ***Children:*** 30–40 mg/kg per day PO in 3 divided doses for 20 days. Do not exceed 1.95 gm in 24 hr for 20 days.	**A:** minimal **PB:** NA **½L:** 11–14 hr **E:** NA	**ASSESSMENT:** Assess for pregnancy. **INTERVENTION: Patient Teaching**—Instruct patient to complete course of therapy. **EVALUATION:** Evaluate patient for resolution of symptoms. Report any adverse reactions.
paromomycin (Humatin) ***Adults:*** 25–35 mg/kg per day PO in 3 divided doses for 5–10 days.	**A:** none **E:** gastrointestinal	**ASSESSMENT:** Assess patient for evidence of intestinal obstruction (contraindication). **INTERVENTION: Patient Teaching**—Instruct patient to take drug with meals. **EVALUATION:** Evaluate for resolution of symptoms. Report any adverse reactions.
ANTIHELMINTICS		
mebendazole (Vermox) ***Adults and Children:*** 100 mg PO twice daily for 3 days	**A:** 2%–10% **PB:** highly **½L:** 2.8–9 hr **E:** hepatic, gastrointestinal	**ASSESSMENT:** Assess for pregnancy (category C). **INTERVENTION:** Drug may be chewed, swallowed, crushed, or mixed with food. **EVALUATION:** Evaluate for resolution of symptoms. Report any adverse reactions.
pyrantel pamoate (Antiminth) ***Adults and Children:*** 11 mg/kg PO once (maximum 1 g)	**A:** poor **PB:** NA **½L:** NA **E:** gastrointestinal, liver	**INTERVENTION: Patient Teaching**—Instruct patient to complete course of therapy. Drug may be taken with meals. **EVALUATION:** Evaluate for resolution of symptoms. Report any adverse reactions.
thiabendazole (Mintezol) ***Adults and Children:*** 25 mg/kg PO twice daily for 2–5 days, maximum 3 g/day	**A:** rapid **PB:** NA **½L:** NA **E:** renal	**INTERVENTION: Patient Teaching**—Tell patient urine drug may cause urine to have unusual odor. Instruct patient to take drug after meals. **EVALUATION:** Evaluate for resolution of symptoms. Report any adverse reactions.
ANTIMALARIALS		
chloroquine (Aralen) **initial treatment—Amebicides** ***Adults:*** 600 mg of base (1000 mg of phosphate tablet) PO daily for 2 days followed by 300 mg of base in 6 hr and again on days 2 and 3. 2.5 mg/kg of base IM every 4 hr, not to exceed 25 mg/kg **prophylaxis—Amebicides** ***Adults:*** 300 mg of base (500 mg of phosphate tablet) PO per wk; begin 1 wk prior to exposure; continue during vacation and for 6 wk after vacation ***Children:*** 5 mg/kg of base PO per week; up to 300 mg of base; follow previous regimen	**A:** rapid and complete **PB:** 50%–65% **½L:** 3–5 days **E:** nonrenal	**ASSESSMENT:** Assess for previous allergy. **INTERVENTION: Patient Teaching**—Instruct patient to complete full course of therapy. **EVALUATION:** Evaluate for resolution of symptoms. Report any adverse reactions.

Continued on the following page

Table 58–14. ANTIPARASITIC AGENTS: AMEBICIDES, ANTHELMINTICS, AND ANTIMALARIALS, *Continued*

DRUG NAME/ROUTE AND DOSAGE	PHARMACOKINETICS/ DYNAMICS	NURSING IMPLICATIONS
quinine sulfate (Quinamm, Q-vel)		
Adults: 300 mg salt (250 mg base) PO 3 times daily for 3–10 days	**A:** almost complete **PB:** 70% **½L:** 4–5 hr **E:** hepatic	**ASSESSMENT:** Assess female patients for possibility of pregnancy (contraindication). **EVALUATION:** Evaluate for resolution of symptoms. Report any adverse reactions.

NA = not available.

CONTRAINDICATIONS AND PRECAUTIONS Use with caution in patients with hepatic impairment.

ADVERSE EFFECTS Hypersensitivity reactions may occur, along with a dose-associated neutropenia, which is reversible.

○ **Thiabendazole** (Mintezol) may inhibit the enzyme functions in parasites. Its exact mechanism of action is unclear. Thiabendazile has vermicidal activity against *A. lumbricoides, Strongloides stercoralis, N. americanus, A. duodenale, T. trichiura, Ancylostoma braziliense,* and *E. vermicularis.*

ADVERSE EFFECTS Anorexia and diarrhea may occur. Other adverse effects include a urinary odor due to renal elimination of the drug.

ANTIMALARIALS

Antimalarial agents include **chloroquine *(Aralen)*** and **quinine sulfate *(Quinamm, Q-vel)*.**

○ **Chloroquine** (Aralen) may bind to and alter the properties of DNA in susceptible parasites. The exact antimalarial action is unknown.

SPECTRUM OF ACTIVITY Chloroquine has activity against *Plasmodium ovale, Plasmodium malariae, Plasmodium vivax,* and some strains of *Plasmodium falciparum.* Because chloroquine resistance has increasingly become a problem in many geographic areas, a patient who has acquired malaria, particularly *P. falciparum* malaria, from an area with known chloroquine resistance should be treated with a different agent (e.g., quinine).

CONTRAINDICATIONS AND PRECAUTIONS Use of chloroquine is not recommended during pregnancy.

ADVERSE EFFECTS Chloroquine may cause corneal opacities, mainfested as blurred vision or other change in vision. Agranulocytosis, aplastic anemia, neutropenia, and thrombocytopenia are rare reactions to chloroquine. Symptoms may include sore throat, fever, weakness, fatigue, and bleeding.

○ **Quinine sulfate** (Quinamm, Q-vel) is thought to produce its effect by disrupting intracellular transport in the parasite. Quinine has activity against *P. vivax, P. ovale, P. malariae,* and *P. falciparum* (including chloroquine-resistant strains).

CONTRAINDICATIONS AND PRECAUTIONS Quinine has been shown to cause congenital malformations in fetuses, particularly in large doses. The drug has also been associated with stillbirths. Benefit of use of the drug must be weighed against risk to the fetus.

ADVERSE EFFECTS In overdose, ventricular dysrhythmias and myocardial depression may occur.

INTERACTIONS Concurrent use of quinine and mefloquine should be avoided as the combination may increase risk of development of seizures and electrocardiogram (ECG) abnormalities, predisposing patients to dysrhythmias.

USING THE NURSING PROCESS

ASSESSMENT

The nurse plays an important role in the management of patients with infection. The therapeutic goal in patients being treated for an infection is to maximize the efficacy of the antimicrobial agent while minimizing toxicity associated with the therapy. Because of the frequency of patient contact, the nurse is invaluable in assessing whether this goal is being achieved.

• Obtain a history of the illness, as essential clues to the nature of the infection may be identified. Table 58–15 summarizes the nursing process for administration of anti-infectives. In addition, a knowledge of prior drug allergies is important when antibiotics are to be prescribed. A detailed description of the type of allergic reaction the patient experienced is imperative as many patients may have experienced a side effect (such as nausea or vomiting) and mistakenly labeled the response a drug allergy. An awareness of the patient's current disease states and drug therapy is important because many antibiotics may interact with other medications the patient is receiving (see drug interaction sections under each anti-infective agent).

• Determine vital signs (temperature, blood pressure, pulse, respiratory rate). An elevated body temperature (fever) is a cardinal sign of the presence of inflammation and/or infection. The cardiovascular response to infection may present as a rapid heart rate or as a drop in blood pressure. For every degree Farenheit of elevation in temperature, there is an increase in heart rate of approximately eight to ten beats per minute. Metabolic acidosis secondary to infection often elicits a compensatory increase in respiratory rate, and sweating may lead to fluid imbalance.

• Assess for clinical signs and symptoms related to in-

Table 58–15. NURSING PROCESS FOR ADMINISTRATION OF ANTI-INFECTIVES

Assessment

Assess previous/current use of prescription drugs (especially antibiotics, glucocorticoids), history of drug sensitivity/allergic reactions. Assess nutritional status.
Assess for presence/history of liver, kidney, or gastrointestinal disorders, pregnancy/nursing.
Assess infection site; associated signs and symptoms, e.g. presence of temperature elevation, tachycardia, malaise, arthralgias, myalgias.

Nursing Diagnosis: Knowledge Deficit

RELATED TO: Lack of information/misinterpretation, unfamiliarity with resources.
AS EVIDENCED BY: Questions, statement of concern, inaccurate follow-through of instructions/development of preventable complications.

Desired Outcomes/Evaluation Criteria

Identifies relationship of signs/symptoms to the disease process and correlates symptoms with causative factors. Correctly performs necessary procedures and explains reasons for actions.

Nursing Actions	Rationale
Provide information about disease process and future expectations.	Understanding allows patient to make informed choices and participate in treatment regimen.
Demonstrate correct administration of prescribed drug.	Ensures safe administration and desired therapeutic effect; IV, IM, oral (tablet and liquid) may be used.
Discuss foods to avoid while on antibiotics.	Certain foods can interfere with optimal therapeutic level of drug.
Determine financial circumstances of patient/family.	Patient may not be able to afford drug but be afraid to ask for assistance or know what resources are available.
Identify signs/symptoms that require physician notification, e.g. continued fever, chills, diaphoresis, rash.	Provides for prompt evaluation and intervention to alter treatment.
Encourage intake of nutritionally balanced diet, adequate rest periods.	Promotes healing and general wellness.
Review necessity of personal hygiene and environmental cleanliness.	Helps to control environmental exposure by diminishing number of pathogens present.

Nursing Diagnosis: Risk for Infection

RELATED TO: Absence of or inadequate/inappropriate drug therapy.

Desired Outcomes/Evaluation Criteria

Achieves timely wound healing, is free of purulent drainage or erythema, is afebrile.

Nursing Actions	Rationale
Obtain culture/sensitivities from site of infection.	Identifies organism and determines most appropriate drug.
Administer anti-infective agents.	Specific choice usually determined by results of culture and sensitivities. Prompt treatment of infection can prevent progression to life-threatening situations (e.g., septicemia).
Emphasize importance of taking drug exactly as prescribed and completing course of treatment.	Patient may think that he or she is well when symptoms abate and believe the drug is no longer needed.
Monitor signs/symptoms of infection, noting reduction of temperature, decreased WBC, reduced pain and swelling, redness.	Should subside within 48 hr and be resolved within 7–10 days.
Stress proper handwashing techniques.	First-line defense against infection.
Maintain aseptic technique when inserting invasive lines, administering IV fluids/medications, changing IV bottles.	Prevents cross-contamination, introduction of bacteria.
Cleanse incisions/insertion sites daily/PRN with appropriate solutions.	Prevents introduction of bacteria/contamination of site.
Monitor appropriate laboratory studies (e.g., CBC, liver/renal function).	Tests can monitor for adverse drug reactions for certain drugs.
Demonstrate proper handling/disposal of infective or soiled material (e.g., dressings, tissues).	Reduces risk of contamination, limits spread of airborne organisms.
Recommend avoidance of crowds, contact with infected persons.	Reduces risk of secondary infection.

fection that may be present when the patient is examined. General signs and symptoms may be malaise, arthralgias, myalgias, or drowsiness. In other situations, clinical findings may be more specific to the site of infection. For example, a patient may describe a productive cough and shortness of breath (pneumonia); burning on urination, frequency, urgency (UTI); or a stiff neck (meningitis).

• Assess patient laboratory reports. A CBC with differential count is an important diagnostic tool when infection is suspected. An increase in the number of leukocytes including an increased number of immature neutrophils (bands) (shift to the left) is a common finding in bacterial infections. Analysis of body fluids that are thought to be infected is also an important diagnostic aid. In addition, body fluids (urine, sputum, peritoneal fluid, CSF, joint fluid) are examined for the presence of cells (leukocytes, RBCs, and so on), changes in pH, glucose, and protein. Body fluids suspected of being infected should be Gram stained and cultured in the laboratory to determine the presence of bacteria. Accurate sample collection and rapid transportation to the laboratory are important aspects of this process. If an organism is grown from a body fluid, it is tested against a battery of antibiotics to determine sensitivity patterns.

- Assess for radiographic confirmation of infection, if appropriate. A common example is the use of a chest radiograph to document pneumonia. More complex testing may be done, depending on the site of infection (bone scan, computerized tomography, magnetic resonance imaging).

NURSING DIAGNOSIS

- Typical nursing diagnoses for a patient requiring anti-infective therapy include the following: Knowledge Deficit, Risk for Infection, Ineffective Thermoregulation, Diarrhea, Fatigue, and Risk for Altered Body Temperature (see Table 58–15).

PLANNING AND INTERVENTION

The nursing diagnoses are used by the nurse as the goals of intervention are established. The goals of nursing intervention are included in Table 58–15.

- Constant observation of the patient allows the nurse to follow the outcome of anti-infective therapy. Normalization of body temperature and laboratory tests, as well as sterilization of body fluids, often provides evidence of antibiotic efficacy. However, the nurse must be keenly aware of signs and symptoms of treatment failure or drug toxicity. Also, accurate timing of sample collections is extremely important when antibiotic concentrations are measured in blood.
- Maintain appropriate handwashing technique, which will prevent the spread of microorganisms among patients. Be aware of both infected patients and those at risk of infection.

Nursing Responsibilities when Administering Anti-infectives

The nurse in the hospital situation has several nursing responsibilities when administering anti-infective agents. These are featured in the Nursing Implications column in each of the drug tables.

- Administer antibiotics at the proper time. Consideration must be given to the effect that food or antacids may have on the rate and extent of antibiotic absorption. In certain cases (e.g., tetracyclines, quinolones) the patient may have to avoid the use of aluminum-containing or magnesium-containing antacids and schedule antibiotic administration around other maintenance medications. Meals can effect the absorption of many anti-infective agents; therefore, patients may have to be instructed on the appropriate timing of their antibiotics in relationship to meals.

Frequently, IV antibiotics must be administered because of the severity of the infection and/or because of a nonfunctioning GI tract. Intravenous anti-infectives are administered over a 30 to 60 minute period using intravenous equipment—partial fills, burettes, or piggybacks. Phlebitis may frequently be a problem associated with the route of administration, and the nurse must evaluate the IV site daily for complications.

- When the nurse administers IM anti-infectives, the sites are always rotated to enhance absorption. The site is massaged by either the nurse or the patient for a full 2 minutes after each injection to improve circulation. Intramuscular injections should be avoided in patients with small muscle mass, decreased circulation, or sepsis because absorption is erratic and unreliable.

Patient Teaching

During the intervention phase, the nurse is responsible for patient teaching, featured in Table 58–16.

Table 58–16. PATIENT TEACHING INFORMATION—ANTI-INFECTIVES

Dear Patient:
   This drug has been prescribed for you. This is what you should know about your drug to get the most from your therapy.

- ☐ 1. Anti-infectives are taken until all symptoms have gone away to prevent reinfection.
- ☐ 2. Do not stop taking your anti-infective without consulting with your physician. Take the medication until all is gone.
- ☐ 3. All anti-infectives should be taken as prescribed. Do not save any medication until next time.
- ☐ 4. Take your anti-infective 1 hour before, with, or 1 to 2 hours after meals, as you have been taught by your nurse, pharmacist, or physician.
- ☐ 5. Always check with your physician or pharmacist before taking other medications, as interactions may occur.
- ☐ 6. If you forget to take your anti-infective for a period of time, do not take the dose. *Do not* try to catch up by taking two doses at the same time. Take all medication as prescribed.
- ☐ 7. If you have any side effects from your anti-infectives, consult your physician or pharmacist. Common side effects include the following: (a list of side effects specific for each drug the patient is on should be included).
- ☐ 8. Store your medication in a tight and moisture-resistant container to prevent deterioration.
- ☐ 9. Anti-infectives may also be taken prophylactically (to prevent infection) for tooth extractions and other minor surgical procedures as prescribed by your physician. Again, take all these medications as ordered.

- Teach the patient that a full course of therapy is extremely important to adequately treat the underlying infection. Often the patient is treated as an outpatient or released from the hospital before therapy is concluded. Therefore, educate the patient to continue treatment and take all of the medication prescribed. Caution patients about the dangers of saving a few tablets until next time.

- Educate the patient in the use of handwashing techniques, proper food preparation (washing hands before and after preparation), and proper disposal of waste products (sputum, urine, stool) to limit the further spread of infection.

- Teach the importance of proper nutrition with adequate protein, vitamins, and minerals and of getting enough rest during the acute and recovery phases of infection.

EVALUATION

During the evaluation phase, the effectiveness of treatment through outcome evaluation criteria is assessed, and is included in Table 58–15.

- Evaluate the patient's response to therapy. A successful therapy is indicated by a reduction in the severity or a complete loss of symptomatology. In most cases, an effective treatment begins to reduce symptoms within 2 days. However, several infections, such as tuberculosis or fungal infections, may take weeks to months to resolve. The infection should be brought under control with the patient experiencing no adverse drug reactions. The most common adverse reaction is GI complaints (e.g., nausea, vomiting, and diarrhea). Nausea and vomiting can be minimized by decreasing the dose of the anti-infective agent or scheduling the doses to coincide with meals, assuming meals do not interfere with drug absorption. Diarrhea is generally self-limited and subsides when the anti-infective agent is discontinued. When diarrhea occurs, increasing the bulk in the diet and taking *Lactobacillus* cultures (yogurt, buttermilk, or Lactinex tablets) helps to restore the normal intestinal flora and reduce diarrhea. The possibility of pseudomembranous colitis must always be considered in the setting of broad-spectrum antibiotic therapy and profuse diarrhea. Females may experience vaginitis secondary to antibiotic therapy, requiring specific treatment.

- Evaluate the site of drug administration when the patient is receiving IV or IM antibiotics for inflammation, phlebitis, and sterile abscess formation. Rotation of the IV site every 48 hours may help to reduce these side effects.

- Review and update all previously taught material before the patient's discharge to ensure that the patient's knowledge base remains accurate.

The bibliography for this chapter can be found in Appendix B, which begins on page 1054.

CHAPTER REVIEW QUESTIONS*

1. Mr. Smith is a 45-year-old male who has recently undergone intensive cancer chemotherapy and is presently being treated for a *Candida albicans* line sepsis with amphotericin B. All of the following adverse reactions are associated with amphotericin B and should be monitored for by the nurse, *except*:
   a. Anemia.
   b. Hypokalemia.
   c. Nephrotoxicity.
   d. Ototoxicity.

2. Mrs. Jones has been receiving isoniazid, rifampin, and pyrazinamide for treatment of active pulmonary tuberculosis. Which of the following drugs interacts with rifampin?
   a. Acetaminophen.
   b. Oral contraceptive.
   c. Aluminum-containing antacid.
   d. Pyrazinamide.

3. Which of the following drugs is the most useful for treatment of a *Pseudomonas aeruginosa* pneumonia?
   a. Cefazolin.
   b. Ceftriaxone.
   c. Ceftazidime.
   d. Azithromycin.

4. Mrs. Miller has a history of hives and difficulty breathing when she took penicillin several years ago. Which of the following drugs can be safely administered to the patient?
   a. Erythromycin.
   b. Imipenem.
   c. Cefazolin.
   d. Amoxicillin.

5. Routine monitoring of serum concentrations occurs with which of the following drugs?
   a. Tobramycin.
   b. Gentamicin.
   c. Vancomycin.
   d. All of the above.

6. Your patient recently underwent surgery and is being treated with antibiotics for a wound infection. You notice that the patient is developing reddening at the base of the neck and in the upper back along with hypotension. This reaction could be attributed to:
   a. Rapid infusion of vancomycin.
   b. Rapid infusion of gentamicin.
   c. Too slow an infusion of vancomycin.
   d. None of the above.

*See Appendix A, which begins on page 1051, for answers.

BUILDING YOUR CRITICAL THINKING SKILLS

INFECTION

Case Study 1: Fever in Immunocompromised Client

A 36-year-old female has recently completed a round of chemotherapy for breast cancer. She currently has a temperature of 102.4 °F. Emperic antibiotic therapy coverage with piperacillin, tobramycin, and oxacillin is started. Blood cultures remain negative. However, the client's temperature remains elevated after 5 days of antibiotic therapy.

1. What else could be causing the elevated temperature?
2. What additional therapy could be instituted for this client?

Case Study 2: Urinary Tract Infection

A 65-year-old man with a history of peptic ulcer disease, has had four relapses of urinary tract infections and receives a diagnosis of chronic prostatitis. He is started on ciproflaxacin. However, after 2 weeks of therapy, the symptoms continue.

1. Why aren't the client's symptoms being alleviated?
2. Are there other data regarding the client's history the nurse should collect?

CHAPTER 59

Immunity and Immunizations

Merrily A. Kuhn, RNC, PhD

CHAPTER OUTLINE

Infectious Diseases and Immunity
Immunizations
Using the Nursing Process

TABLES

Drug Tables

Nursing Process

Patient Teaching

KEY TERMS

Active immunity
Antibodies
Attenuated organisms
Immunity
Immunization

Passive immunity
Serum
Toxoid
Vaccine

LEARNING OBJECTIVES

After reading this chapter, the student will be able to:

1. Identify medications commonly used as vaccines and immunizations.
2. Differentiate vaccines, serums, and toxoids.
3. Differentiate among the immunizations as to mechanism of action, route of administration, pharmacokinetics, adverse effects, contraindications and precautions, and interactions.
4. Identify specific areas to assess in the patient requiring immunizations to formulate appropriate patient outcomes.
5. Plan the nursing interventions necessary to administer immunizations and choose appropriate teaching strategies to gain patient compliance.
6. Evaluate the patient at various stages of treatment to measure the effectiveness of nursing interventions.

Vaccination or *immunization* is a deliberate attempt to protect humans against disease through the administration of antigens, antibodies, or infectious agents. Immunization has made a major impact on mortality reduction and population growth. Immunization has a long history, but only in the twentieth century has this practice become routine. Immunization has controlled nine major diseases in parts of the world: diphtheria, tetanus, yellow fever, pertussis, poliomyelitis, measles, mumps, rubella, and smallpox, which has been completely eradicated. Immunization against influenza, hepatitis B, pneumococci, and *Haemophilus influenza* has made major headways against these infections. But, much still remains to be done, even in developed countries.

The history of immunization dates to the sixth century in China. Edward Jenner's work with cowpox vaccination in 1810 was the first scientific attempt to control an infectious disease by means of a deliberate systematic inoculation. Later, in the 1880s, Louis Pasteur developed the rabies vaccine. By the end of the 1890s, vaccines were available against typhoid, plague, cholera, and diphtheria.

After World War II, numerous immunizations were developed such as polio, measles, mumps, rubella, and adenovirus, all composed of attenuates (to be described later); polio and rabies composed of killed virus; and pneumococcus, meningococcus, *H. influenza*, and hepatitis B composed of purified protein. In the final years of the twentieth century, new technologies are available, and the new wave of vaccine development continues.

INFECTIOUS DISEASES AND IMMUNITY

An infectious disease is any disease caused by the growth of pathogenic organisms in the body. Infectious diseases are a major health problem in developing countries. Also, because many people from developed countries like the United States travel abroad, there is increased interest in preventing these diseases. Table 59–1 features a brief review of infectious diseases and how they can be treated.

Immunity, which can be either innate (natural) or acquired, is the ability of the body to develop relative resistance to disease after exposure to the agent responsible for causing the disease. Figure 59–1 and Table 59–2 illustrate and compare innate and acquired immunity. Immunity based on the development of *antibodies* (immunoglobulin; serum protein that combines with and destroys antigens) is probably the most efficient type of immunity. This type of immunity is subdivided into that which is actively acquired and that which is passively acquired, as follows:

1. innate or natural immunity (natural, artificial)
2. acquired immunity (natural, artificial)
   a. actively acquired
   b. passively acquired

ACTIVE VERSUS PASSIVE IMMUNITY

Acquired immunity can be active or passive. The term *active immunity* refers to those antibodies produced by the body in response to an antigen (the immune system is discussed in detail in Chapter 54) that functions to destroy the offending pathogen that has entered the body. Actively acquired immunity is obtained when an antigenic substance—one that has lost its ability to produce illness but is able to stimulate antibody formation—is injected into the body. Active acquired immunization can be obtained with live *attenuated organisms* (microorganisms or cells that have been rendered less capable of producing disease), dead organisms, or toxins. Attenuated vaccines contain viable but weakened organisms that produce a mild infection of little danger to the host. It has the advantage, however, of producing a much more permanent form of immunity than killed vaccines. Several vaccines are available as both killed (e.g., Salk polio vaccine) and attenuated (e.g., Sabin polio vaccine). *Toxoids* are detoxified but still antigenically active poisons excreted by certain bacteria. Antibodies formed against toxoids are fully reactive with the natural toxin and provide an excellent immunity against diseases caused by toxigenic bacteria such as tetanus and diphtheria.

Passive immunity is immunity that is achieved by the introduction of antibodies produced by someone other than the patient. Passive immunity can be achieved through antibody transfer from mother to infant via the placenta or breast milk (naturally acquired) and through immunization with antibodies from another human or animal (artificially acquired). Injections of hyperimmune serum, antiserum, or globulins are examples of artificially acquired immunizations.

Both active immunity and passive immunity are used for prophylactic treatment of disease. Active immunization is generally given far in advance of the exposure to the infectious agent. When the incubation time of the disease is longer than the time required for antibody formation, such as with rabies or smallpox, it is possible for the individual to be immunized after exposure. Passive immunity can also be administered prior to or immediately after exposure.

Active immunity requires 5 to 14 days to develop after the primary immunization. This is the time it takes for the protective antibodies to appear in the serum. Once active immunity is obtained, it persists for relatively long periods, usually years. This occurs because once the plasma cells are activated to produce antibodies, they continue to do so for the lifetime of the cell. The half-life of a human antibody is about 25 days. Active immunity can be restored easily through booster injections.

Passive immunity provides immediate but only moderately effective protection. Because the body is not actively producing antibodies against the disease, passive immunity persists only for several days or hours. The body does, however, make antibodies against the administered foreign antibody, which hastens its removal. The half-life of injected antibodies is about 7 days (without internal replacement).

IMMUNIZATIONS

Immunizations, often referred to as vaccinations, are classified as serums, vaccines, or toxoids, as presented in Table 59–3.

SERUMS

Serums are obtained from humans or animals in which antibodies have been formed against a pathogenic organism. Serum derived from a human source is likely to cause fewer allergic reactions than one obtained from an animal source. Serums are purified and standardized for injection. Dosages, adverse effects, and nursing implications for selected serums are featured in Table 59–4.

Serums provide temporary immunity against disease. They can also prevent formation of active antibodies in an Rh-negative mother carrying or delivering an Rh-positive infant.

There are currently three types of serums available, as follows:

1. immune globulin for general use
2. immune globulin with known antibodies against certain antigens
3. animal antitoxins and serums

Immune globulin preparations are prepared from serum using ethanol fractionation, a process that separates the protein and lipoprotein components. The use of ethanol fractionation inactivates the live human immunodeficiency virus (HIV). However, HIV antibodies are passively transmitted.

Table 59–1. SELECTED INFECTIOUS DISEASES AND THEIR MANAGEMENT

	Infectious Sources	Entry Site	Infective Organism	Incubation Period	Method of Spread	Therapy*	Prophylaxis
Chickenpox (varicella)	Human cases	Probably nasopharynx	Varicella-zoster (V-Z) virus	12–17 days	Probably respiratory droplets	Acyclovir (?)	Varicella-zoster globulin (VZIG) primarily for immunocompromised children and certain neonates exposed in utero
Diphtheria	Human cases and carriers; fomites; raw milk	Nasopharynx	*Corynebacterium diphtheriae*	2–5 days	Nasal and oral secretions; respiratory droplets	Diphtheria antitoxin; penicillin	Active immunization with diphtheria toxoid
Influenza	Human cases	Respiratory tract	Virus	24–72 hr	Respiratory	Amantadine; rimantadine	Influenza virus vaccine
Measles	Human cases	Respiratory mucosa	Virus	8–13 days	Nasopharyngeal secretions	None	Measles vaccine
Meningococcal meningitis	Human cases and carriers	Nasopharynx; tonsils	*Neisseria meningitidis*	2–10 days	Respiratory droplets	Penicillin; ampicillin; chloramphenicol	Meningococcal polysaccharide vaccine for persons at risk; rifampin/sulfadiazine for carriers or contacts
Mumps	Human cases (early)	Upper respiratory tract	Virus	2–3 wk (avg. 18 days)	Respiratory droplets	None	Live mumps vaccine
Pneumococcal pneumonia	Human carriers	Respiratory mucosa	*Streptococcus pneumoniae*	Variable	Respiratory droplets	Penicillin G; erythromycin	Polyvalent pneumococcal vaccine; control of upper respiratory infections; avoidance of alcoholic intoxication
Poliomyelitis	Human cases and carriers	Gastrointestinal tract	Polioviruses (types I, II, III)	7–14 days	Pharyngeal secretions; fecal-oral	None	Oral polio vaccine (OPV), the live attenuated vaccine containing all 3 strains of poliovirus—produces long-lasting immunity in most recipients
Rubella (German measles)	Human cases	Respiratory mucosa	Virus	14–23 days	Nasopharyngeal secretions	None	Rubella virus vaccine; immune globulin (human) given to contacts of rubella; rubella in early stages of pregnancy legally recognized as indication for abortion
Tetanus	Contaminated soil; infected wounds	Penetrating and crush wounds	*Clostridium tetani*	4–21 days (avg. 10 days)	Horse and cattle feces	Tetanus immune globulin (human—TIG) and tetanus toxoid; penicillin	Wound debridement; toxoid booster injections for patients previously immunized; tetanus toxoid and tetanus immune globulin (separate sites and separate syringes) for nonimmune persons

Table 59–1. SELECTED INFECTIOUS DISEASES AND THEIR MANAGEMENT, *Continued*

	Infectious Sources	Entry Site	Infective Organism	Incubation Period	Method of Spread	Therapy*	Prophylaxis
Tuberculosis	Sputum from human cases; milk from infected cows (rare in U.S.)	Respiratory mucosa	*Mycobacterium tuberculosis*	Variable	Sputum; respiratory droplets	Isoniazid; ethambutol; rifampin; streptomycin; pyrazinamide	Early discovery and adequate treatment of active cases; milk pasteurization, BCG vaccine
Whooping cough (pertussis)	Human cases	Respiratory tract	*Bordetella pertussis*	Commonly 7 days	Infected bronchial secretions	Erythromycin; ampicillin	Active immunization with vaccine; case isolation

*Please refer to guides and package inserts for specific current dosages and uses.

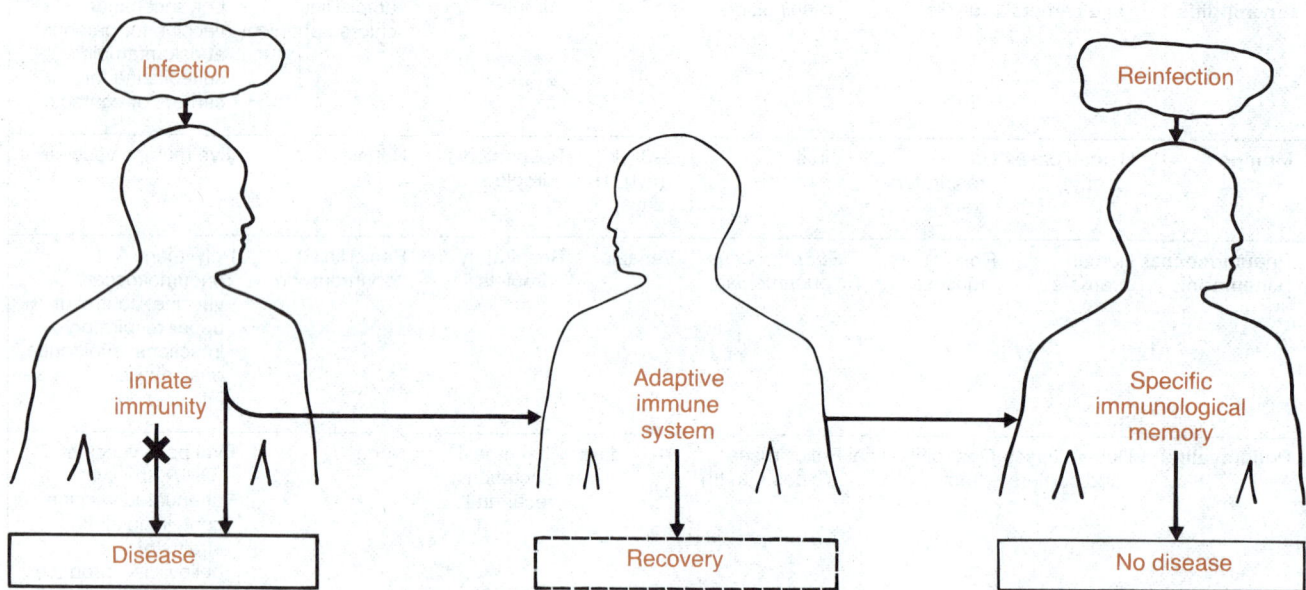

Figure 59–1. Adaptive and innate immunity. When an infectious agent enters the body, it first encounters elements of the innate immune system. These may be sufficient to prevent disease, but if not, a disease results and the adaptive immune system is activated. The adaptive immune system produces recovery from the disease, and a specific immunologic memory is established so that following reinfection with the same agent no disease results; the individual has acquired immunity to the infectious agent.

Table 59–2. IMMUNITY

Type	How Obtained	Response Triggered	Comments
Natural	• Born with • Acquired from mother • Exposure to disease	Nonspecific	Natural mechanisms—intact skin, lysozyme in tears, cilia in respiratory tract, GI juices/enzymes, pH in vagina/semen, interferon
Acquired	• Developing disease • Immunization	Antibody dependent	May be active or passive (see text for further discussion)

Table 59–3. IMMUNIZATION TYPES

Type	Source	Use	Examples
Serum	Serum from animal or human used for injection	• Prevention • Relieves symptoms • Provides long-term active immunity	Serum globulin Rabies immune globulin BCG Hepatitis vaccines Tetanus Diphtheria
Vaccine	Suspension of live or killed or attenuated microorganisms		
Toxin	Poison substance secreted by microorganism treated to reduce toxicity	• Creates active immunity	
Antitoxin	Obtained from horses	• Provides passive immunities after exposure to microorganism	Tetanus antitoxin Rabies antitoxin Diphtheria antitoxin
Antivenin	Obtained from insect, snake, or spider, and made less toxic	• Passive immunity after exposure to insect, spider, or snake bites	Black widow antivenin Crotalidae antivenin
Attenuate	Made directly from microorganism, but virulance reduced to protect host	• Provides more permanent immunity	Measles

Table 59–4. IMMUNIZATIONS: SERUMS

DRUG NAME/ROUTE AND DOSAGE	ADVERSE EFFECTS	NURSING IMPLICATIONS
immune globulin intravenous (IGIV) (Gamimune N) (Gammagard S/D) (Gammar-IV) (Sandoglobulin) (Venoglobulin-I) **immune globulin intramuscular** (IGIM) (Gamastan) (Gammar)		

DRUG NAME/ROUTE AND DOSAGE	ADVERSE EFFECTS	NURSING IMPLICATIONS
hepatitis a exposure *Adults and Children:* 0.02–0.06 mL/kg IM. **igg deficiency** *Adults:* 1.3 mL/kg IM followed by 0.66 mg/kg every 3–4 wk, not to exceed 3 mL. **measles (rubeola)** *Adults and Children:* 0.25 mL/kg IM within 6 days of exposure. **rubella** *Adults:* 0.55 mL/kg IM within 72 hr of exposure. **immunodeficiency syndrome** *Adults and Children:* 100–400 mg/kg IV q 3 wk or monthly, depending on product. **idiopathic thrombocytopenic purpura** *Adults and Children:* 400–2000 mg/kg IV, depending on product brand, for 2–7 days. **prevention of bacterial infections in hiv-infected children** *Children:* 400 mg/kg IV q 28 days. **prevention of bacterial infections in b-cell chronic lymphocytic leukemia** *Adults:* 400 mg/kg IV q 21–28 days.	**Most Common:** Local tenderness **Life Threatening:** Anaphylaxis (IV), angioedema **Other:** Chest tightness, dyspnea, faintness, fever chills, headache, myalgia, nausea and vomiting, stiffness at injection site, urticaria, hypersensitivity reactions	**ASSESSMENT:** Assess for recent immunoglobulin administration, as these antibodies interfere with immune response. Assess for particles or color change in vial. Assess baseline vital signs and temperature. **INTERVENTION:** Do not mix with other medications. Inject IM or SC in either the anterolateral aspect of upper thigh or deltoid of arm. Store at 2–8°C. Mix in 5% dextrose in water only. Swirl gently to mix. Administer IV at a flow rate of 0.5–1 mL/min; after 15 min may increase to 1.5–2.5 mL/min. **EVALUATION:** If chest pain or chills occur, stop IV infusion and notify physician.

Continued on the following page

Table 59–4. IMMUNIZATIONS: SERUMS, *Continued*

DRUG NAME/ROUTE AND DOSAGE	ADVERSE EFFECTS	NURSING IMPLICATIONS
cytomegalovirus immune globulin iv, human (CMV-IGIV)		
Administer within 72 hours of transplant. **Adults:** Start at 15 mg/kg per hr; if no adverse effect, increase to 30 mg/kg per hr until full dose of 150 mg/kg is administered. At weeks 2, 4, 6, and 8 post-transplant, give 100 mg/kg; at weeks 12 and 16 posttransplant, give 50 mg/kg.	Same as for immune globulin plus: **Other:** Hypotension, muscle cramps	**INTERVENTION:** If nausea, back pain, or flushing occur, slow down infusion rate. Mix powder with 50 mL of sterile water, then release the residual vacuum, which will hasten dissolution. Do not shake, and avoid foaming to prevent protein degradation. Allow to dissolve for 30 min. Administer at correct dosage. Use within 6 hr of mixing.
hepatitis b immune globulin (HBIG) (HyperHep) (Hep-B-Gammagee)		
Adults: 0.06 mL/kg IM within 7 days of exposure and 2nd injection 28–30 days later. *After sexual exposure*–0.6 mL/kg IM within 14 days. **Children and Newborns:** 0.5 mL IM within 24 hr of birth; repeat at 3 and 6 mo.	Same as for immune globulin plus: **Other:** Dizziness, headache	Very expensive. Use only in persons at high risk for developing hepatitis B. **ASSESSMENT:** Assess baseline vital signs and temperature. **INTERVENTION:** Administer adult dose in deltoid and pediatric dose in vastus lateralis. Aspirate carefully before injecting solution. Store at 2–8°C. **Patient Teaching**—Teach patient importance of receiving 2 or 3 injections.
tetanus immune globulin (TIG) (Hyper-Tet)		
Prophylaxis: 250–500 units IM. **Treatment:** 3000–6000 units IM.	Same as for immune globulin plus: **Other:** Nephrotic syndrome	**INTERVENTION:** store at 2–6°C; do not freeze.
rho (d) immune globulin (Gamulin Rh) (RhoGAM) (HypRho-D) **rho (d) immune globulin microdose** (Mini-Gamulin Rh) (MICRhoGAM) (HypRho-D Mini-Dose) **rho (d) immune globulin iv**		
Lab determines fetal packed red blood cell volume: 1 vial if fetal RBC is 15 mL; if more than 15 mL, administer more than 1 vial. 1 vial standard dose = 300 μg; 1 vial of microdose = 50 μg. **Antepartum:** Administer 1 vial standard dose IM or 1500 IU IV at 28th wk of gestation. **Postpartum:** Administer 1 vial standard dose IM or 600 IU IV within 72 hr. **After Abortion, Miscarriage, or Ectopic Pregnancy:** 1 microdose vial administered within 72 hr.	Same as for immune globulin plus: **Other:** Fever, splenomegaly	**INTERVENTION:** IM—Administer at 28th wk of gestation or within 72 hr of delivery of ectopic pregnancy, trauma, amniocentesis, or abortion. If 1 vial is needed, inject entire vial IM. If more than 1 vial is needed, inject at different injection sites but all within 72 hours. Reinforce patient education regarding temporary protection. Inform that subsequent pregnancies will require treatment. IV—Infuse over 3–5 min. Do not mix with other drugs.

People receiving immune globulins may develop transient, positive HIV antibody tests. Passively transmitted antibodies clear from the body within 6 months of the time immune globulin is received. Thus, patients testing positive to either the enzyme-linked immunosorbent assay (ELISA) or Western blot confirmation tests for HIV, but who have no identifiable risk factors, should have repeat antibody testing. By the end of 6 months the test results become negative if the antibodies were, indeed, passively received from the immune globulin injection.

Pharmacokinetics

Serums are absorbed well after either intramuscular or intravenous administration. Immunity is obtained almost immediately but it is short term, lasting only 1 to 12 weeks.

Contraindications and Precautions

A contraindication to all serums is a known hypersensitivity or previous anaphylactic reaction. They are all contraindicated in patients with isolated immunoglobulin A (IgA) deficiency, as circulating IgE antibodies may react with IgA in the product and induce anaphylactoid reactions. Patients with coagulation disorders and thrombocytopenia may be relative contraindications because these products are administered IM.

Serums are considered safe in children and the elderly. They are not used during pregnancy (category C) unless clearly indicated. Safety during lactation is unknown.

Adverse Effects

The agents used for passive immunity may cause reactions that range from mild local discomfort to severe anaphylaxis, although this is rare. A few patients may experience fever and general malaise, chills, and headache.

Interactions

As a general rule, live virus vaccines are administered 14 to 30 days before or 6 to 12 weeks after serums to prevent interference with the development of immunity.

○ **Immune globulin intravenous** *(IGIV, Gamimune N, Gammagard S/D, Gammar-IV, Sandoglobulin, Venoglobulin-I)* and *immune globulin intramuscular (IGIM, Gamastan, Gammar)* are obtained from pooled plasma of approximately 1000 human donors and contain standardized antibodies to diphtheria, poliomyelitis, measles, and hepatitis A. They are used in patients with immunodeficiency syndromes, idiopathic thrombocytopenia purpura, measles, varicella, rubella, B-cell chronic lymphocytic leukemia, and thrombocytopenia, and in patients exposed to hepatitis A. The protection obtained from immune globulin varies from 6 weeks to several months depending on the dosage. Immune globulin is also used today to treat IgG deficiency.

○ **Cytomegalovirus immune globulin IV, human** *(CMV-IGIV, CytoGam)* contains IqG antibodies and a relatively high concentration of antibodies directed against CMV. This serum can raise the antibody level to a sufficient level to reduce the incidence of CMV-IGIV. CMV-IGIV is administered to persons following renal transplant. Seronegative persons receiving a seropositive kidney develop CMV at a rate of 75%. After receiving CMV-IGIV, the incidence of CMV is reduced by 50%.

○ **Hepatitis B immune globulin** *(HBIG, HyperHep, Hep-B-Gammagee)* is obtained from the pooled plasma of donors with a high titer of antibodies to hepatitis B surface antigen (HBsAg) and then concentrated by cold alcohol fractionation. HBIG is indicated only for the postexposure prophylaxis of hepatitis following needle sticks or exposure to blood or other body fluids from patients known to be positive for hepatitis B surface antigen.

○ **Tetanus immune globulin** *(TIG, Hyper-Tet)*, obtained from human plasma, is effective in producing passive immunity in patients whose wounds may be contaminated with *Clostridium tetani* and in treating tetanus.

○ **Rho (D) immune globulin** *(Gamulin Rh, RhoGAM)* is administered to nonsensitized (negative indirect Coombs, negative antibody titer) Rh-negative women who are pregnant or who give birth to Rh-positive infants. Rho (D) immune globulin effectively suppresses the immune response in nonsensitized Rho (D)–negative women who have received Rh-positive blood during fetal-maternal transfer.

▼ **CLINICAL ALERT**

At the time of delivery, Rho (D) immune globulin is administered to prevent hemolytic disease of the newborn (erythroblastosis fetalis) in subsequent pregnancies.

Rho (D) immune globulin is also administered to nonsensitized Rh-negative women after spontaneous or induced abortions, ectopic pregnancies, aminocentesis, abdominal trauma, and any other occurence of transplacental hemorrhage. Rho (D) immune globulin is not indicated for infants or the elderly.

Other Serums

○ **Varicella-zoster immune globulin** (VZIG), obtained from human plasma with high titers of varicella-zoster antibodies, is used to prevent or ameliorate varicella. There are limited supplies of VZIG, so patients should meet the following criteria to receive this immunization. The patient has one or more of the following conditions—neoplastic disease, immunodeficiency, immunosuppression, or prematurity—or is a newborn whose mother develops chickenpox within 48 hours after delivery or 5 days before delivery.

ADVERSE REACTIONS The most frequent adverse reaction is pain at the injection site. Less frequent reactions include GI symptoms, headache, rash, and respiratory symptoms.

○ **Lymphocyte-immune globulin, antithymocyte globulin (equine)** (Atgam) is a lymphocyte suppressant that reduces the number of circulating thymus-dependent lymphocytes. Suppressing T-cell function reduces humoral reactions associated with renal transplant rejection. Lymphocyte-immune globulin is also indicated in the treatment of moderate to severe aplastic anemia unsuited for bone marrow transplant.

ADVERSE REACTIONS Patients frequently experience fever, chills, leukopenia, thrombocytopenia, and dermatologic reactions.

RABIES PROPHYLAXIS PRODUCTS

Although there are few cases of rabies in the United States, each year approximately 25,000 persons receive rabies prophylaxis. Rabies is endemic throughout the world in animal populations except in the United Kingdom, Japan, and Antarctica. It is a viral infection that can be transmitted to domestic animals as well as people. Once the virus enters the body it incubates for 10 to 60 days. The virus travels along afferent sensory nerve pathways to the spinal cord and then on to the brain where it multiplies. The virus then travels down efferent motor nerve pathways to all areas of the body, particularly the salivary glands.

Immediate and thorough washing of all bite wounds

and scratches with soap and water is perhaps the most effective measure for preventing rabies. The two types of immunizing products for rabies are vaccines and globulins. The vaccines include **human diploid cell rabies vaccine (HDCV)** and **rabies vaccine adsorbed (RVA).** Vaccines induce active immunity within 7 to 10 days and last for up to 1 year. The globulins, which include only **rabies immune globulin, human (RIG),** provide rapid passive immunity that lasts a short time (half-life is 21 days).

Before prophylaxis treatment is begun, it is important to consider the type of animal and the type of exposure. The animal in most likely to be carnivorous (skunk, fox, coyote, raccoon, dog, or cat) or a bat. An unprovoked attack is more likely to mean that the animal is rabid. The rabies virus is transmitted through a break in the skin, so a bite with puncture wounds or a scratch or open wound that is contaminated with saliva is considered dangerous. Dosages, adverse effects, and nursing implications for the rabies prophylaxis products are presented in Table 59–5.

VACCINES

Vaccines provide active immunity for a prolonged period of time. The vaccines, unlike immune serum or antitoxin, which contain exogenous antibodies, include specific antigens that induce endogenous production of antibodies. Vaccines are featured in Table 59–6. There are two general types of vaccines, as follows:

1. bacterial vaccines prepared from whole or purified capsular polysaccharides of killed bacteria, including **bacillus Calmette-Guérin (BCG) vaccine; pneumococcal vaccine, polyvalent (Pneumovax 23, Pnu-Immune 23); hemophilus B conjugate vaccine (HibTITER, PedvaxHIB, ProHIBiT);** and others
2. viral vaccines containing live attenuated or inactive non-living viruses, including **hepatitis B vaccine (Energix-B, Recombivax HB); hepatitis A vaccine (HAV, Havrix); poliovirus vaccine, live, oral, trivalent (Sabin); poliovirus vaccine, inactivated (IPV); influenza virus vaccine (Fluogen, Fluzone, Fluviron);** and others

Pharmacokinetics

Vaccines provide long-term or permanent immunity against disease. The onset of action begins in several days to several weeks. The peak action time varies as does the duration of action. Immunity can vary from 1 year with influenza vaccine to 10 years with tetanus toxoid.

Contraindications and Precautions

Vaccines are contraindicated in persons with a history of hypersensitivity or serious adverse reactions and in the immunocompromised patient. Safety in the elderly and children varies with the type of vaccine. Safety in pregnancy (category C) and lactation is unknown.

Table 59–5. RABIES PROPHYLAXIS PRODUCTS

DRUG NAME/ROUTE AND DOSAGE	ADVERSE EFFECTS	NURSING IMPLICATIONS
all rabies prophylaxis products		
	Less Common: Serum sickness, erythema and urticaria, local pain	**ASSESSMENT:** Assess type of animal and type of exposure. Assess for previous allergic reaction and current febrile infection, both contraindications. **INTERVENTION: Patient Teaching**—Teach patient importance of receiving all injections to develop immunity.
human diploid cell rabies vaccine (HDCV) (IMOVAX Rabies Vaccine)		
Preexposure Prophylaxis: 1 mL IM on days 0, 7, and 21 or 28 days (total 3 doses) **Postexposure Prophylaxis:** 1 mL IM on days 0, 3, 7, 14, and 28 (total 5 doses) **Postexposure Prophylaxis in Previously Immunized Person:** 1 mL IM on days 0 and 3 (total 2 doses)	Same as for all plus: **Less Common:** Nausea, abdominal pain	Same as for all.
rabies vaccine adsorbed (RVA)		
Same as above	Same as for all	Same as for all.
rabies immune globulin, human (RIG) (Hyperab) (Imogam)		
20 IU/kg, half administered into the wound and half IM	Same as for all plus: **Less Common:** Nephrotic syndrome **Life Threatening:** Anaphylactic shock, angioedema	Same as for all plus: **INTERVENTION:** Administer IM into lateralis in children. Store at 2–8°C, do not freeze. Administer rabies vaccine concurrently.

Table 59–6. BACTERIAL AND VIRAL VACCINES

DRUG NAME/ROUTE AND DOSAGE	ADVERSE EFFECTS	NURSING IMPLICATIONS
BACTERIAL VACCINES		For all products: **INTERVENTION:** Administer SC or IM preferably in the deltoid or lateral midthigh. See manufacturer's directions accompanying vaccine for specific information.
bacillus Calmette-Guérin (BCG) vaccine (TheraCys) (TICE BCG)		
scarification *Adults and Children:* 0.2–0.3 mL on skin followed by multiple-puncture gun. Allow to dry for 24 hr. Repeat in 2–3 mo if still TB negative. **bladder cancer** *Adults:* TheraCys–1 mL injected deep into bladder for 6 wk, then 1 dose at 3, 6, 12, 18, and 24 mo. *TICE BCG*–2 mL for 6 wk then monthly follow-ups.	**Common:** Local pain **Life Threatening:** Lymphadenitis, death **Less Common:** Mild arthralgia, swelling	**ASSESSMENT:** Assess for presence of TB. Assess immunocompetence. Assess for pregnancy (category C). **INTERVENTION:** Store at 2°–8°C. Do not expose to light. Add 1 mL sterile water to each ampule. Allow to stand for 1 min. Do not shake. Withdrawal of solution will yield homogenous suspension. Drop 0.2–0.3 mL onto cleansed surface of skin and administer percutaneously using a sterile multiple-puncture disk (scarification). Keep vaccine site clean until local reaction has disappeared. Do not administer IV, SC, or interdermally. Keep away from persons with active TB for 6–12 weeks. **EVALUATION:** Conduct postvaccine TB test in 2–3 mo. If not positive, revaccinate.
pneumococcal vaccine polyvalent (Pneumovax 23) (Pnu-Immune 23)		
Adults: 0.5 mL SC or IM.	**Common:** Local erythema, induration, soreness, low-grade fever. **Life Threatening:** Guillain-Barre syndrome, anaphylaxis **Less Common:** arthralgia, paresthesia, rash	**ASSESSMENT:** Assess for acute infection and previous history of pneumococcal pneumonia. **INTERVENTION:** Refrigerate at 2°–8°C. Do not administer IV or intradermal. May need a booster in 6 yr. **EVALUATION:** Evaluate for local reactions.
hemophilus B polysaccharide complex (PedvaxHIB) (ProHIBiT) **hemophilus B oligosaccharide complex** (HibTITER)		
ProHIBiT *Age 15 mo–5 yr:* 0.5 mL IM single dose. Booster at 15 mo. **HibTITER** *Age 2–6 mo:* 0.5 mL IM 3 times at 2-mo intervals. Booster at 15 mo. *Age 7–11 mo:* 0.5 mL IM 2 times at 2-mo intervals. Booster at 15 mo. *Age 12–14 mo:* 0.5 mL IM single dose. Booster at 15 mo. **PedvaxHIB** *Age 2–14 mo:* 0.5 mL IM 2 times at 2-mo intervals. *Age ≥15 mo:* 0.5 mL IM single dose.	**Common:** Fever, local erythema, induration, tenderness **Less Common:** Anorexia, diarrhea, irritability, vomiting, seizures	**INTERVENTION:** Administer IM in outer aspect of vastus lateralis or deltoid; do not administer IV. With PedvaxHIB, use only diluent provided.
VIRAL VACCINES		
hepatitis B vaccine (Engerix-B) (Recombivax HB)		
Infants Born to HBsAg-Positive Mothers: Recombivax HB–5 μg within 7 days of birth and 1 and 6 mo later (or at 1, 2, and 12 mo).		

Continued on the following page

Table 59–6. BACTERIAL AND VIRAL VACCINES, *Continued*

DRUG NAME/ROUTE AND DOSAGE	ADVERSE EFFECTS	NURSING IMPLICATIONS
VIRAL VACCINES, Continued		
hepatitis B vaccine (Engerix-B) (Recombivax HB), *Continued*		
Energix-B –10 μg within 7 days of birth and 1 and 6 mo later (or at 1, 2, and 12 mo). **Recombivax HB** (10 μg = 1 mL) **Children 11–19 yr:** 0.5 mL IM at 0, 1, 6 mo. **Adults ≥20 yr:** 1 mL IM at 0, 1, 6 mo. **Engerix-B** (20 μg = 1 mL) **Children 11–19 yr:** 1 mL IM at 0, 1, 6 mo. **Adults ≥20 yr:** 1 mL IM at 0, 1, 6 mo. **routine infant immunization** **Birth–10 yr:** 0.5 mL IM at 0, 1, 6 mo old with 1st dose within 12 hr of birth. **postexposure prophylaxis** **Adults:** Initial 1 mL within 7 days of exposure, 2nd dose in 1 mo, 3rd dose in 6 mo.	**Common:** Headache, soreness, pain, induration, tenderness **Life Threatening:** Guillain-Barre syndrome **Less Common:** Light headedness, vertigo, dizziness, insomnia, fatigue, weakness, arthralgia, myalgia, upper respiratory infection, nausea, vomiting, diarrhea, abdominal pain, cramps, thrombocytopenia	**ASSESSMENT:** Assess for acute infection. **INTERVENTION:** Administer IM in deltoid in adults or anterolateral thigh in infants and children. **EVALUATION:** Evaluate for local and systemic reactions.
hepatitis A vaccine, inactivated (HAV) (Havrix)		
Adults: 1440 ELU IM on day 0. 1-mL booster 6–12 mo later. **Children:** 360 ELU IM on day 0 and 30. A booster 6–12 months later.	Same as above	**INTERVENTION:** Inject into deltoid. Do not use gluteal region. **Patient Teaching—**Teach patient to still maintain water and food precautions to avoid infection.
poliovirus vaccine, live, oral, trivalent (Sabin) (OPV) (Orimune)		
0.5 mL PO 3 times at 6–12 wk of age, 6–8 wk later, then 8–12 mo later.	**Life Threatening:** Paralysis	**ASSESSMENT:** Assess for acute infection. **INTERVENTION:** For oral use only. Keep frozen. If defrosted during transport, 10 freeze-thaw cycles allowed. Once defrosted, vaccine should be used with 30 days. Once opened, vaccine should be used within 7 days.
poliovirus vaccine, inactivated (IPV) (IPOL) (Poliovax)		
Adults: 0.5 mL SC × 2 at 1- to 2-mo intervals, and 0.5 mL 6–12 mo later (total 3 doses). **Children:** 0.5 mL SC at 2 mo, 4 mo, and 6–12 mo later.	**Common:** Fever, tenderness **Less Common:** Rashes, pruritis	**ASSESSMENT:** Assess for acute infection. **INTERVENTION:** For SC use only.
influenza virus vaccine (Fluogen) (Fluzone) (Fluviron)		
Children 6–35 mo: 0.25 mL IM × 1 or 2 doses. **Children 3–8 yr:** 0.5 mL IM × 1 or 2 doses. **Children 9 yr and Over:** 0.5 mL IM, 1 dose.	**Common:** Local soreness **Less Common:** Erythema, fever, malaise, myalgia	**ASSESSMENT:** Assess for acute infection. **INTERVENTION:** Do not administer IV. Administer IM in deltoid in adults and anterolateral aspect of thigh in children. Store in refrigerator. Do not freeze as potency is destroyed.

Adverse Effects

Adverse effects from immunizations are similar to those experienced from agents that produce passive immunity. Local symptoms at the injection site are most common. Mild systemic symptoms can include mild arthralgia, anorexia, and drowsiness.

Bacterial Vaccines

○ **Bacillus Calmette-Guérin (BCG) vaccine** provides active immunity for persons who are at high risk of contracting tuberculosis (TB). BCG vaccine is recommended for infants and children with risk of intimate and prolonged exposure to persons with untreated TB, who cannot be placed on long-term preventative therapy. Health-care workers continually exposed to persons with active TB should be followed by tuberculin skin testing surveillance and receive isoniazid prophylaxis in case of TB skin test conversion. This vaccine is also appropriate for persons who will be residing in countries where there is an increased incidence of tuberculosis.

There has been an upsurge in tuberculosis in the United States in the last several years. The biggest increases are among Hispanic, African-Americans, and Asian-Americans. It is estimated that 10 to 15 million persons in the United States carry TB, but only 10% become ill. There is also an increase in the number of patients who are presenting with a drug-resistant strain.

BCG is also used for intravesical treatment of primary or relapsed carcinoma in situ of the bladder. The exact mechanism of action is unknown, but live BCG provokes an inflammatory response that includes activation of macrophages, a delayed hypersensitivity reaction, and stimulation of T and B lymphocytes and natural killer T cells. BCG injected into the bladder can lead to prolonged remission and a 45% chance of remaining free of disease 5 years later.

○ **Pneumococcal vaccine polyvalent** (Pneumovax 23, Pnu-Immune 23) contains 23 of the most common prevalent or invasive pneumococcal sero types, which account for 85% to 90% of all pneumococcal pneumonias. It is useful in adults and children over age 2 with all chronic illnesses, particularly cardiovascular and pulmonary diseases for which there is increased morbidity associated with respiratory infections. The pneumococcal vaccine is also useful in persons over age 65 who are otherwise healthy.

○ **Hemophilus B conjugate vaccine** (ProHIBiT, HibTITER, and PedvaxHIB) is indicated for immunization against invasive diseases caused by *H. influenzae* type B (Hib), such as meningitis, epiglottitis, and pericarditis. Hemophilus B conjugated vaccine is prepared from purified capsular polysaccharide covalently bound to diphtheria toxoid (ProHIBiT) or meningococcal protein (PedvaxHIB); or from capsular oligosaccharide convalently bound to diphtheria CRM$_{197}$ protein (HibTITER)

▼ CLINICAL ALERT

The largest group at risk for contracting Hib diseases are children under age 5 years, with approximately 12% of the cases occurring in children 18 to 24 months of age. The primary Hib diseases seen in children are epiglottitis, septic arthritis, sepsis, pneumonia, and meningitis. Even with advances in antimicrobial therapy, there remains a 5% mortality rate from *H. influenzae* and a high incidence of mental retardation in those who survive meningitis.

The initial vaccination is given at age 24 months (HibTITER, PedvaxHIB) or 15 months (ProHIBiT). Children who were not vaccinated at 24 months can be given the vaccine up to age 5 years. A physician may decide a child aged 18 to 23 months should be vaccinated if the child is in a high-risk group such as being asplenic or

immunosuppressed, having sickle cell anemia or a malignancy, or attending a day-care center. The Hib vaccine can be given at the same time as the DPT vaccine, but a different injection site is used to prevent possible interaction.

Other Bacterial Vaccines

○ **Cholera vaccine** is available in the United States for cholera prophylaxis in persons traveling to or residing in cholera-infested areas. Immunity is brief, lasting only 3 to 6 months. Use of the cholera vaccine does not prevent transmission of infection. A booster is recommended after 6 months if exposure is to be continued. However, the traveler's best protection from cholera is to avoid food and water that may be contaminated.

○ **Meningococcal vaccine** is effective against meningitis caused by a variety of microorganisms, but not meningitis associated with *Neisseria meningitidis*. Meningitis vaccine is recommended for persons above age 2 years who are at risk in epidemic areas, for laboratory personnel who are at risk of exposure, for travelers going to highly endemic areas, and for persons who are asplenic and who have a terminal complement component deficiency.

○ **Typhoid vaccine,** produced from killed *Salmonella typhi*, is about 70% to 90% effective in preventing typhoid fever. Protection lasts about 3 years, but can be extended by increasing the number of injected organisms. Typhoid vaccine is recommended for persons traveling to areas where typhoid fever is endemic.

○ **Staphphage lysate** (SPL), a bacterial antigen from *Staphylococcus aureus,* is used to treat either staphylococcal infections or polymicrobial infections with a staphylococcus component. SPL is recommended for all patients who have had a spleenectomy. This vaccine is rated pregnancy category B. It can be administered subcutaneously, intranasally, or topically.

Viral Vaccines

Viral vaccines provide immunity for viral infections such as hepatitis B, measles, mumps, rubella, polio, and influenza. Viral vaccines are featured in Table 59–6.

○ **Hepatitis B vaccine** (Engerix, Recombivax HB), available to individuals who are at risk of contracting the hepatitis B virus (HBV), are derived from HBsAg in yeast cells. The recombinant products produce immunity in 93% to 99% of subjects. Boosters of either product may be required in 5 years if titers fall below 10 U/mL.

HBV causes approximately 5000 deaths per year from cirrhosis or hepatocellular cancer. The serious sequelae of HBV occur mostly in chronic carriers; acquiring the disease at birth leads to an 80% to 90% risk of becoming a carrier, compared to a 5% to 10% risk when the disease is acquired after age 5.

▼ CLINICAL ALERT

Hepatitis B vaccine is highly recommended for all infants at birth and may protect against HBV infection for at least

9 years. The first hepatitis B injection is administered within the first 12 hours of life, with the remaining injections administered at 4 and 6 to 18 months. The vaccine is also recommended for all health-care workers working with blood and blood products; persons at risk because of their sexual practices; and infants born to HBsAg-positive mothers.

Hepatitis B vaccine is greatly underused. It is suggested that only 40% of health-care workers at risk for developing hepatitis have been immunized. If an individual does not have HBV acquired immunity or has not been immunized with Heptavax-B and is exposed to HBV, hepatitis B immune globulin (HBIG) is given, which offers passive immunity.

Hepatitis B vaccine also protects against Hepatitis D. Hepatitis D can infect and cause illness only in persons infected with hepatitis B.

○ **Hepatitis A vaccine** (HAV, Havrix) is recommended for persons traveling to areas where hepatitis A is endemic (e.g., Africa, Mexico, Middle East), persons engaging in high-risk sexual activity, users of illicit IV drugs, and persons with chronic liver disease.

○ **Poliovirus vaccine, live, oral, trivalent** (OPV, TOPV, Sabin, Orimune) is a live attenuated vaccine that produces active immunity in about 90% of persons. The live virus is preferred to inactivated preparations as it multiplies in the host and provokes the production of serum antibodies. Live poliovirus is then shed by the host for about 3 weeks.

The poliovirus vaccine is used for prophylaxis against poliomyelitis, primarily in childhood. The child receives 2 or 3 oral doses with 6 to 12-week intervals between doses. Simultaneous administration of two or more live virus vaccines should be avoided.

○ **Poliovirus vaccine, inactivated (IPV)** (Salk, IPOL, Poliovax) is prepared from three different inactivated polioviruses and provides active immunity against poliomyelitis. The viruses are grown in monkey kidney cells (IPOL) or in human diploid cells (Poliovax). These production techniques provide a very consistent immunogenic vaccine. Poliovirus vaccine is recommended for persons over age 18 who are at risk, including travelers to countries where polio is endemic and health-care workers. The vaccine is administered subcutaneously in the deltoid muscle. Three doses at 4-week intervals followed by a booster dose 6 to 12 months later is recommended. Boosters are given after 3 to 5 years.

○ **Influenza virus vaccine** (Fluogen, Fluzone, Fluvirin) is made from inactivated viruses grown in eggs. It is available in the United States as a split-virus (Fluogen), as a whole-virus (Fluzone), and as a purified-surface-antigen vaccine (Fluviron). Split and purified-surface-antigen formulas are less likely to cause adverse reactions.

Influenza is one of the most common viral respiratory infections, affecting several hundred million people yearly. In previous years influenza has been both endemic and pandemic and caused millions of deaths. Each year the United States Public Health Services Committee on Immunizations Practice recommends which influenza vaccine is to be used because the antigen components of the influenza strain change.

The influenza virus vaccine is recommended for persons 6 months or older who would be at risk if they developed influenza. This group includes persons with chronic cardiovascular or pulmonary disorders and all residents (regardless of age) of nursing homes or chronic care facilities. It is also desirable for persons over age 45 and for all health-care workers. Health-care workers are immunized because they are capable of transmitting nosocomial infections. About 2 weeks after the vaccine, antibody levels are usually sufficient to prevent disease. The best time for the injection is in November.

Persons recently vaccinated with the flu vaccine may test positive to HIV-1, hepatitis C, and human-T-lymphotropic virus type 1, despite having no infection. No one who has had the flu vaccine is at risk for infection from any of these diseases.

Other Viral Vaccines

○ **Mixed respiratory vaccine** (MRV) is prepared from many strains of bacterial organisms commonly found in the respiratory tract including two general classes of streptococci, several strains of *S. aureus*, four different pneumococci, *Moraxella catarrhalis*, *Klebsiella pneumoniae*, and *H. influenzae*. More research is needed on this vaccine before it is determined to be fully effective for the labeled indications.

Measles, Mumps, and Rubella Vaccines

Measles, mumps, and rubella vaccines are available individually or in combination.

○ **Measles vaccine** (Attenuvax) is available as a live, attenuated vaccine, developed on chicken embryos, that produces a modified infection in susceptible individuals. The vaccine is effective for about 8 years. Measles vaccine is primarily used in children 15 months or older and also in adults in epidemic situations.

During the years 1963 through 1967, the vaccine consisted of a killed virus, but was later found to be ineffective. Persons immunized between 1963 and 1967 are at risk for contracting the disease unless they have been revaccinated. In 1967, the measles vaccine was changed to an attenuate. The attenuated form has been very successful in providing immunity if it is administered after 15 months of age. Prior to age 15 months, the child has passive immunity to the disease in the form of maternal antibodies. If immunized with a live vaccine before age 15 months, the maternal antibodies destroy the microorganism before antibody production (active immunity) is stimulated. Occasionally, a younger child who has been exposed to the disease is immunized early. If this happens, the immunization is generally repeated at age 15 months to ensure immunity.

○ **Rubella virus vaccine, live** (Meruvax II) is a live, attenuated vaccine that gives protection against rubella for about 6 years. It is recommended for children 12 months to puberty, leukemia patients in remission, and nonpregnant females with negative serologic tests. Immunity is indicated by a rubella antibody titer of 1:8 or greater. In the past, if a female received rubella vaccine and became pregnant, termination of pregnancy was recommended. The U.S. Public Health Service still suggests that pregnancy should be a contraindication, but if pregnancy should occur there is no reason to terminate, as the risk of congenital deformities is so rare.

○ **Mumps virus vaccine** (Mumpsvax) is a live vaccine that induces an effective antibody response in 97% of children and 93% of adults. Immunity persists for about 10 years. The mumps virus vaccine is recommended for children 12 months or older.

Investigational Vaccines

Many vaccines are currently under development and investigation. These include *Escherichia coli* vaccine, cytomegalovirus vaccine, hepatitis C vaccine, hepatitis E vaccine, herpes simplex 2 vaccine, HIV vaccine (see discussion that follows), Klebsiella vaccine, melanoma vaccine, Lyme disease vaccine, *Pseudomonas* vaccine, and respiratory syncytial virus vaccine. Vaccines must progress through the FDA approval process just as drugs must.

Human Immunodeficiency Virus The acquired immune deficiency syndrome (AIDS) was described in 1981, and the etiological agent, human immunodeficiency virus (HIV) was identified in 1983–1984. Currently there are two well-characterized subtypes of the virus—HIV-1 and HIV-2—which are both spreading throughout the world. HIV has already become the leading cause of death in the United States of young adult males and females.

HIV is a member of the lentivirus subfamily of cytopathic retroviruses. These viruses are characterized by slow, progressive infections in which the virus escapes host immune defenses. The viruses are contained within an envelope glycoprotein that contains reverse transcriptase enzyme and RNA. A potential problem in the development of an HIV vaccine is the geographically divergent envelope glycoprotein. A proposed explanation for this divergence is a high rate of mutation.

Although much is known about the pathogenesis of HIV infection, there are still many questions that must be addressed in the development of an HIV vaccine. If current technologies are capable of developing a vaccine, studies lasting a minimum of several years and involving thousands of individuals probably are necessary to assess its safety and efficacy. An effective vaccine appears to be many years away.

TOXOIDS

Toxoids are used for active immunization against tetanus, diphtheria, and pertussis (whooping cough). These agents are reviewed in detail in Table 59–7.

○ **Tetanus toxoid** is used for active immunization against tetanus in both adults and children. The toxin, produced by the virulent tetanus bacillus, has been treated with formaldehyde to reduce its toxicity. Tetanus immunization is recommended for all persons beginning at age 2 months. It is particularly important for adults to maintain their immunization if there is an increased risk of lacerations and abrasions such as with firemen, military personnel, farm and utility workers, and people

working with horses. It is recommended that elderly nursing home residents be routinely vaccinated for tetanus because of their vulnerability to pressure ulcers. In the last 10 years, approximately 20% of tetanus cases have been associated with chronic wounds.

Immunization is generally started in infants by using adsorbed diphtheria, tetanus toxoid, and pertussis vaccine (DTP) or adsorbed diphtheria and tetanus toxoids. The tetanus and diphtheria toxoid is recommended to protect persons over age 6.

○ **Diphtheria toxoid, adsorbed** is used for active immunization against diphtheria in infants and children under 6. It is not used in the treatment of actual diphtheria infections.

○ **Diphtheria, tetanus toxoids and pertussis vaccine, adsorbed** (DTP) contains diphtheria and tetanus toxoid, which have been detoxified by formaldehyde, with pertussis vaccine. In the past, this was the agent of choice for routine immunization of children less than 6 years of age. It is not recommended for persons over age 7. DTP confers protection for at least 10 years.

Today, a new diphtheria and tetanus toxoid and acellular pertussis vaccine (DTaP, ACEL-IMUNE, Tripedia) is suggested for the fourth or fifth doses of DTP, usually given at 15 or 18 months and before school entry. The DTaP vaccine causes fewer side effects locally and systemically.

Pertussis contains killed *Bordetella pertussis* organisms, which provides protection against whooping cough. Only bacteria that possess a capsule are selected for this vaccine, as the capsule presence correlates highly with virulence.

Because of the decline in pertussis-related mortality prior to the institution of widespread immunization, some researchers argue that pertussis vaccine is currently superfluous and that it should be abandoned except for certain high-risk groups. In addition, pertussis vaccine may be associated with encephalopathy, infantile spasms, and sudden infant death syndrome.

In spite of these difficulties and uncertainties, it is the consensus of most authorities that the benefits of the vaccine to the individual and to the public far outweigh the risks, even with the current impossibility of providing a precise mathematical estimate of the benefit-risk ratio.

○ **Diphtheria and tetanus toxoid, combined** (DT, Td) has both the diphtheria and tetanus toxoids, which are inactivated by formaldehyde. This vaccine is used when the triple vaccine DTP is contraindicated and in children above 7 years of age and adults.

USING THE NURSING PROCESS

ASSESSMENT

- Determine if the individual has had immunizations before and if there has been an allergic reaction. For certain immunizations, it is all-important to assess for allergies to animal products, sulfites, and thimerosal. Also, many vaccines are not given to a patient with an acute infection or to anyone who is immunosup-

Table 59–7. TOXOIDS		
DRUG NAME/ROUTE AND DOSAGE	**ADVERSE EFFECTS**	**NURSING IMPLICATIONS**
tetanus toxoid, fluid **tetanus toxoid, adsorbed**		
Fluid (0.5 mL contains 4 or 5 Lf of tetanus toxoid): 0.5 mL IM or SC × 3 doses at 4 to 8 wk intervals, 4th dose 6–12 mo later, booster 0.5 mL q 10 yr. Adsorbed (0.5 mL contains 5 or 10 Lf of tetanus toxoid): 0.5 mL IM × 2 doses at 4 to 8 week intervals, 3rd dose 6–12 mo later, booster 0.5 mL q 10 yr.	**Common:** Local erythema and induration, nodule pruritis **Life Threatening:** Hypersensitivity reactions **Less Common:** Tachycardia, hypotension, low grade fever, chills, malaise, generalized aches and pains, flushing	**ASSESSMENT:** Assess for active acute infection. **INTERVENTION:** Administer in deltoid or vastus lateralis. **EVALUATION:** Report any severe adverse reaction.
diphtheria and tetanus toxoid and pertussis vaccine, adsorbed (DTP)		
0.5 ml IM × 3 doses at 4 to 8 wk intervals.	**Common:** Erythema, induration, pain, swelling, and nodules at injection site; fretfulness, drowsiness **Life Threatening:** Sudden infant death syndrome **Less Common:** Anorexia, vomiting	Same as above.
diphtheria and tetanus toxoid combined (DT—Pediatric) (Td—Adults)		
pediatric adsorbed toxoid **Infants:** 0.5 mL × 3 doses at 4-wk intervals and another dose 6–12 mo later. **Children 1–6 yr:** 0.5 mL IM × 2 doses at 4-week intervals and another dose 6–12 mo later; 0.5 mL IM booster at 4–6 yr. **adult adsorbed toxoid** **Adults and Children 7 yr:** 0.5 mL IM × 2 doses at 4 to 6-week intervals and 3rd dose 6–12 mo later.	Same as above	Same as above.

pressed. Therefore, an adequate history is obtained from the patient and family. Typical nursing assessments for patient receiving immunizations are included in Table 59–8.

Most immunizations are received during childhood. Table 59–9 presents the recommended immunization schedules. Six vaccines are recommended for routine use in adults living in the United States: tetanus-diphtheria toxoid every 10 years; influenza vaccine yearly for persons with chronic disease; pneumococcal vaccine every 5 years for high-risk individuals and those more than 65 years of age; hepatitis B vaccine for everyone with boosters as needed every 5 years; measles to appropriate people; and rubella for unimmunized young women and health-care workers. Children and adults at risk of contracting infectious diseases who were not vaccinated in childhood may require further immunization. These risk groups include persons traveling to foreign countries,

health-care workers, immigrants to this country, the elderly, and the chronically ill.

Vaccines are intended for use by healthy individuals, and the manufacturer usually indicates precautions or contraindications. Minor nonfebrile illnesses in children are not contraindications for inoculation. A vaccine is given at a later date to a child who has a febrile illness.

It is important for the nurse to understand what type of immunizations can be administered together. Immune globulin is not given for 3 months before or at least 2 weeks after a live viral vaccine, although it does not appear to interfere with the immune response to oral poliovirus vaccine or to yellow fever vaccine.

NURSING DIAGNOSIS

- Typical nursing diagnoses for a patient receiving immunizations include Knowledge Deficit, Risk for Infection, and Altered Protection.

Table 59–8. NURSING PROCESS FOR PATIENT REQUIRING IMMUNIZATIONS

Assessment

Assess previous immunization history and reactions that may have occurred.
Assess allergies to animal products and thimerosal.
Assess presence of acute infection and/or immunosuppression; pregnancy.

Nursing Diagnosis: Knowledge Deficit	Desired Outcomes/Evaluation Criteria
RELATED TO: Lack of exposure/recall, information misinterpretation/unfamiliarity with resources. **AS EVIDENCED BY:** Questions, statement of concern, inaccurate follow-through of instruction/development of preventable complications.	Verbalizes understanding of disease process and need for immunizations. Participates in treatment regimen.

Nursing Actions	Rationale
Provide information about diseases and need for protection.	Provides knowledge base for patient to make informed choices. May enhance cooperation with regimen.
Review expected side effects and potential adverse reactions that need to be reported.	Preparation for normalcy of reaction helps patient cope with minor discomforts and recognize more serious problems.
Discuss correct regimen for booster shots.	Full course of immunization promotes optimal protection.
Instruct in proper aftercare, e.g., do not apply heat or cold to local reaction, use antipyretics to relieve fever.	Improper care can increase reactions.

Nursing Diagnosis: Risk for Infection	Desired Outcomes/Evaluation Criteria
RELATED TO: Inadequate acquired immunity.	Verbalizes understanding of individual causative risk factor(s). Achieves immunity.

Nursing Actions	Rationale
Administer serum (e.g., immune globulin, Hyper-Tet); vaccine (e.g., Mumpsvax, Fluogen); or toxoid (e.g., DTP), according to individual need.	Although some people are born with innate immunity to certain diseases, most people have to acquire immunity in some way.
Discuss need to contact physician/public health department before traveling out of country.	Determines need for additional immunizations related to specific area individual is visiting.
Instruct patient to maintain record of vaccination/booster shots.	Proof of immunization for certain diseases is required by schools and health departments in effort to control outbreaks of disease and for determining future health-care needs.

Other Suggested Nursing Diagnosis: Altered Protection.

PLANNING AND INTERVENTION

- Prepare the immunization. Vaccines are stored according to manufacturers instructions. Follow their specific recommendations for temperature and light as listed in Tables 59–4, 59–5, and 59–6. Most vaccines are stored in the refrigerator (not on the door), as the temperature is higher on the door. If vaccines are to be transported, ice packs are used to protect vaccines, and they are transported in styrofoam containers. Polio vaccines are transported with dry ice only.
- Administer the vaccine into the correct injection site. Most vaccines are mixed just prior to administration.
- Provide the patient with information about potential adverse reactions, home treatment for these reactions, and when to call the physician. If additional injections or boosters are necessary, teach the patient about when to return to the clinic or doctor's office. A patient teaching table, presented in Table 59–10, is included with additional information that should be taught to the patient. Many fact sheets are available from the Centers for Disease Control in Atlanta.

Persons who are traveling abroad must have current immunizations. Table 59–11 reviews some tips for persons traveling abroad.

EVALUATION

- Evaluate for side effects and/or complications. Immunizations are, for the most part, very safe and effective drugs. Localized redness and swelling at the injection site and fever are common reactions. Minor symptoms that mimic the disease itself are also common. For example, mild rashes may follow the injection of the measles and rubella vaccine, and minor swelling of the salivary glands may follow the administration of the mumps vaccine. About 5% of the children who get the rubella vaccine complain of some aching and swelling of the joints. Common side

Table 59–9. IMMUNIZATION SCHEDULES FOR CHILDREN

Recommended Schedule for Childhood Immunizations

Age	Immunization
0–first 12 hr	HBV
2 mo	DPT, OPV, Hib
4 mo	DPT, OPV, HBV, Hib
6 mo	DPT, Hib, HBV
12 mo	TB Test*
15 mo	DTaP, OPV, MMR, HBV, Hib
4–6 yr	DTaP, OPV, MMR
10–14 yr	MMR
14–16 yr	DT, Td†, DTaP

Recommended Immunization Schedules for Infants and Children Not Initially Immunized at Usual Recommended Times in Early Infancy

Time of Visit	Immunization
1st visit	DPT, OPV, TB test, HBV
1 mo after 1st visit	MMR (not given before age 15 mo), Hib (for children aged 18–60 mo)
2 mo after 1st visit	DPT, OPV, HBV, Hib
4 mo after 1st visit	DPT, OPV
10–16 mo after last dose	DTaP, HBV, Hib, OPV
Preschool	DTaP, OPV (may not be necessary if last DPT and OPV given after age 4 yr.)

HBV = (Engerix-B or Recombivax B) Hepatitis B vaccine; DPT = Diphtheria and tetanus toxoids with pertussis vaccine; OPV = Oral, attenuated poliovirus vaccine contains types 1, 2, and 3; Hib = Conjugate *Haemophilus influenza* type B vaccine; DTaP = diphtheria, tetanus, acellular pertussis vaccine; MMR = Live measles, mumps, and rubella viruses in combined vaccine; DT, Td = Adult tetanus toxoid (full dose) and diphtheria (reduced dose) in combination.
*May be repeated every 2 yr.
†Repeat every 10 yr.

effects are explained to the client and family before an immunization is administered so that they are not surprised or alarmed when they occur. Any unusual reaction is reported immediately to a physician, who will forward this information to the Centers for Disease Control. To prevent possible complications, any woman who is pregnant or planning to become pregnant in the immediate future should consult her physician before receiving any immunization.

Table 59–10. PATIENT TEACHING INFORMATION—IMMUNIZATIONS

Dear Patient:
This drug has been prescribed for you. This is what you should know about your drug to get the most from your therapy.

☐ 1. This immunization will protect you from . . . (disease) . . . for approximately . . . (time period) . . . It may then be necessary to receive a booster.

☐ 2. Typical side effects from your immunization include redness and soreness and also _____ . Call your doctor if severe side effects occur.

Table 59–11. INTERNATIONAL TRAVEL IMMUNIZATION GUIDELINES

Immunization	Comment
Cholera	Not usually recommended (only 50% effective and lasts only 3–6 mo). Travelers to high-risk areas (South America) should be warned not to drink untreated water and not to eat raw fish or uncooked or unpeeled fruits and vegetables.
Hepatitis A	IgG 2 mL administered close to departure date. For trips over 3 mo: 5 mL, then repeat q 5 mo. For endemic areas only.
Hepatitis B	Recommended only for health professionals and for people who expect to have sexual contacts in Southeast Asia or Africa or stay longer than 6 mo. Inject into deltoid in series of 3 doses over minimum periods of 2 mo.
Measles	People born after 1956 who have not received 2 doses of measles vaccine or had the disease should receive a booster, but not at the same time as IgG.
Meningococcal Disease	Only if traveling to areas where epidemics are occurring: Kenya and Tanzania and sub-Saharan African countries, Middle East, India, Nepal. Administer in single dose.
Polio	Primary vaccination or a booster is recommended.
Tetanus, Diphtheria	Booster q 10 yr.
Typhoid	Oral vaccine; 1 capsule qid or 4 capsules starting 2 wk before departure when traveling to endemic areas.
Yellow Fever	Only if traveling to Africa, South America, or Asia. Boosters are given every 10 yr.
Malaria	No drug guarantees immunity. If symptoms occur, take mefloquine. In all malarious areas, use room sprays, mosquito nets for beds, window screens, clothing with long sleeves, long pants, and insect repellents containing 15% to 20% diethyltoluamide (deet), especially during the evening and night hours.

• Administer if febrile reactions occur. Antipyretics can be used to relieve symptoms. If local reaction occurs, the patient is told not to apply heat or cold because both are likely to increase the local reaction. To reduce local subcutaneous skin reactions, the needle can be changed after the liquid is withdrawn from the vial. This is particularly helpful to decrease the irritation of DPT.

The bibliography for this chapter can be found in Appendix B, which begins on page 1054.

CHAPTER REVIEW QUESTIONS*

1. An advantage of passive immunity is that it:
   a. Stimulates the body to produce antibodies.
   b. Provides immediate protection.
   c. Persists for an extended period.
   d. Treats diseases effectively.

2. Children should not receive the attenuated measles vaccine before 15 months because:
   a. Maternal antibodies destroy the attenuated virus before antibody production occurs.
   b. The child's immune system is too young to respond with antibody production.
   c. The attenuated virus is too strong and will produce an active form of the disease.
   d. Antibodies which are produced by a child less than 15 months are immature.

3. A nursing intervention associated with immunization is to:
   a. Teach patients that unusual side effects are to be expected.
   b. Mix vaccines at least 6 hours before administration.

*See Appendix A, which begins on page 1051, for answers.

   c. Change the needle before injecting the vaccine.
   d. Keep vaccines in a warm place for storage.

4. What is the time required for development of active immunity in response to vaccine?
   a. 6 months
   b. 6 hours
   c. 5 to 14 days
   d. 25 to 75 days

5. A possible serious adverse effect associated with pneumococcal vaccine (Polyvalent) is:
   a. Lymphadenitis.
   b. Serum sickness.
   c. Sudden Infant Death Syndrome
   d. Guillain-Barre Syndrome

6. Which of the following statements is *correct* regarding rabies immune globulin (RIG)?
   a. It is obtained from the plasma of hyperimmunized chicken donors.
   b. RIB should be administered 6 days after the rabies vaccine.
   c. Half of the dose is administered into the wound, the other half intramuscularly.
   d. There are no known adverse effects associated with RIB.

CHAPTER 60

Medications Used in Organ Transplantation

Brenda K. Shelton, MS, RN, CCRN, OCN

KEY TERMS

Allograft
Antilymphocyte globulins
Autograft
Cytokines
Donor
Graft
Histocompatibility leukus antigens (HLA)
HLA tissue typing
Immunosuppressant agents
Isografts
Monoclonal antibodies
Polypeptide antibiotics
Recipient
Rejection
Syngeneic
T-3 complex

LEARNING OBJECTIVES

After reading this chapter, the student will be able to:

1. Describe the immunology of transplantation and graft rejection.
2. Differentiate between the immunosuppressive agents in relation to action, indications, adverse reactions, contraindications and precautions, and interactions.
3. Design an assessment plan for patients receiving immunosuppressive agents.
4. Plan nursing interventions appropriate to the administration and teaching of patients receiving immunosuppressive agents.

Organ transplantation as a specialized area of clinical practice has expanded considerably with advanced surgical techniques and improved ability to prevent rejection of transplanted organs. The nurse caring for patients who have received organ transplants needs to become familiar with *immunosuppressant agents*, or antirejection drugs. This chapter outlines the immunologic aspects of organ transplantation and rejection and the clinical application of the five categories of immunosuppressant agents.

ORGAN TRANSPLANT IMMUNOLOGY

The growth of organ transplantation as a therapy for individuals with end-organ failure has paralleled advances in immunology that have helped health-care providers identify the method by which self is recognized and foreign is rejected. Organ transplantation has become successful because of perfection of genetic tissue typing and the development of effective immunosuppressive drugs that block the body's natural rejection of foreign proteins. In every transplant, there is a *donor* that provides the organ for transplant and a human *recipient* of the donated organ. Donors of the organ to be transplanted may be other persons or animals. The transplanted tissue is called a *graft*, and person to person transplant is called an *allograft*. Transplant survival ranges from one year to complete cures. Types of organ transplants are listed with their key characteristics in Table 60–1.

Transplanted tissue is accepted or rejected by the recipient based on the activity of a specific inherited block of genetic antigens found on chromosome 6 called *histocom-*

Table 60–1. ORGANS TRANSPLANTED

Organ	Example of Clinical Indication	5-yr Graft Success Rates	Donor Type	Complications
Skin	Burns	>95%	Autograft Allograft Xenograft	Rejection, infection
Bone marrow	Hematologic malignancies, immune deficiencies, aplastic anemia, solid tumors, genetic disorders	40%–80%	Autograft Allograft	Rejection, graft-versus-host disease, infection, organ failure
Kidney	End-stage renal disease	85%	Allograft	Toxicities rejection, infection
Heart	Congenital heart disease, cardiomyopathies	40%	Allograft	Rejection or dysrhythmias
Liver	Congenital biliary atresia, end-stage liver failure	40%–60%	Allograft	Rejection, bleeding
Lungs	Chronic obstructive pulmonary disease, pulmonary hypertension, pulmonary fibrosis	40%–60%	Allograft	Rejection, respiratory failure, infection
Pancreas	Diabetes, chronic pancreatitis	60%–80%	Allograft	Rejection
Cornea	Cataracts	>95%	Allograft	Opacification

patibility leukocyte antigens (HLA). These antigens are proteins on cell surface markers that identify the cell as different from self. The immune system mounts a response against HLA antigens that it perceives are foreign (such as those in the transplanted organ), characterizing *rejection.* There are more than 100 different encoding genes that have been identified by site and named A, B, C, and D. Each coding site carries the gene from the individual's father and mother. As a consequence, siblings are most likely to share common genetic codons and are often used to donate organs for transplantation for each other.

HLA antigens also have been functionally separated into class I (A, B, and C) antigens or class II (D) antigens. Class II antigens are thought to be responsible for the initial response in graft rejection. Class II antigens stimulate the production of antigen-reactive T-helper lymphocytes, which then stimulate B lymphocytes to produce antibodies against the class I antigens on the foreign tissue. A region on the T-helper cell, known as the antigen recognition structure or *T-3 complex,* is responsible for recognizing foreign antigens and sending a signal to the interior of the T cell telling it to make cytokines. *Cytokines* are cell-killing substances produced by T cells to destroy foreign proteins. The closer the HLA match between donor and recipient, the less likely the host's immune system will reject it, and the more likely the graft will thrive.

Individual HLA typing is accomplished by tissue typing for class I antigens and mixed lymphocyte culture (MLC) for class II antigens. *HLA tissue typing* is performed by adding sensitized sera to a culture of recipient and donor lymphocytes, and a cross-matching procedure ascertains the degree of reactivity the cells have against each other. Recipient cells that proliferate and are activated signal a high potential for rejection.

ABO (blood typing) compatibility is also important for the success of engraftment. Although not essential, transplanted organs without ABO compatibility are at risk for graft ischemia and cell hemolysis by recipient immunologic cells. Other more relevant criteria for eligibility for transplantation may include absence of metastasizing malignancies, absence of active infection, and healthy organ function in the rest of the body.

IMMUNOLOGY OF REJECTION

Despite close HLA matching of donor and recipient, incompatibility of tissue proteins may still result in graft rejection by the host. Rejection is not present in *autografts* because the tissue is self; it is limited in *syngeneic* (identical twin donor) transplants due to identical HLA matching. Rejection is an immunologic response involving both B lymphocytes and T lymphocytes. The three types of rejection are hyperacute, acute, and chronic. The major immunologic and clinical characteristics of these types of rejection are outlined in Table 60–2. Rejection is the most common reason for unsuccessful transplant survival; hence, pharmacologic agents are given in an attempt to suppress this immunologic response by the body.

Table 60–2. TYPES OF TRANSPLANT REJECTION

Rejection Type	Immunologic Characteristics	Agents Used
Hyperacute	Recipient has preformed anti-ABO or anti-HLA class I antibodies. Recipient's antibodies bind to vascular endothelium of transplanted organ, triggering clotting.	Preventive agents—antimetabolites, anti-inflammatory agents
Acute	Macrophages and B lymphocytes of the transplant recipient encounter HLA antigens of the transplanted organ and stimulate the T-lymphocyte cytotoxic response, and B lymphocytes target antibody to the graft.	Cyclosporine, antibodies
Chronic	Minor histocompatibility antigens not involved to the HLA complex cause low-level chronic stimulation of T lymphocytes and vascular clotting.	Anti-inflammatory agents

PRINCIPLES OF PHARMACOLOGIC IMMUNOSUPPRESSIVE THERAPY

The major principles of pharmacologic therapy in the prevention and treatment of transplant rejection involve immune suppression and modulation. The choice of agents may depend on the type of organ transplant, characteristics of the donor, type of rejection, and personal preference. Combinations of drugs are often preferred for their broader spectrum of immunosuppression and the possible limitation of single-organ toxicity. All transplants except *isografts* (transplant tissue from one part of the body to another) require intensive posttransplant immune suppression.

When rejection is suspected, immediate diagnosis via organ biopsy is necessary to plan interventions. Other causes, especially infections, can render similar symptoms. Immediate, aggressive treatment is essential to prevent dangerous ischemia and necrosis of the graft. Once rejection is controlled, immunosuppressive therapy is tapered, and the patient is observed for recurrence of rejection symptoms. Immunosuppressive therapy is categorized into several main groups according to the therapy's primary mode of action: (1) anti-inflammatory agents, (2) antimetabolites, (3) cytotoxic agents, (4) antibodies, and (5) polypeptide antibiotics. Of the five, the first three are most common. These categorizations are based on a variety of sources that are not standard drug classifications at this time. Antibodies are further subdivided into those agents that destroy lymphoid cells (*antilymphocyte globulins*) and those agents that block lymphoid cell activity (*monoclonal antibodies*). Selected drugs from several of these categories are featured in Table 60–3.

Table 60–3. ORGAN TRANSPLANTATION DRUGS: ANTIMETABOLITES, ANTIBODIES, AND POLYPEPTIDE ANTIBIOTICS		
DRUG NAME/ROUTE AND DOSAGE	**PHARMACOKINETICS/ DYNAMICS**	**NURSING IMPLICATIONS**
ANTIMETABOLITES		
azathioprine (Imuran)		
Oral and intravenous doses are the same. **transplantation (dose defined by renal transplant data)** *Initial dose*–3–5 mg/kg per day 1–3 days prior to transplant. *Maintenance dose*–1–3 mg/dg per day beginning 3–6 weeks after transplant and continuing for variable time periods. **rheumatoid arthritis** 1 mg/kg per day for 6–8 wk, increased by 0.5 mg/kg per day at 4-wk intervals up to 12–14 wk, doses are tapered in increments of 0.5 mg/kg per day.	**Onset:** PO, 6–8 wk; IV, days to weeks **Peak:** PO, 12 wk **Duration:** PO, NA; IV, days to weeks **½L:** 5 hr **PB:** 30% **B:** liver **E:** renal (as metabolites)	**ASSESSMENT:** Gastrointestinal (GI) irritation is common, but severe oral and esophageal ulceration is an indication of GI hypersensitivity. Assess oral cavity, voice, and ability to swallow every day; mild hepatic enzyme elevation may occur, but assessment for symptoms of hepatic failure, encephalopathy, or veno-occlusive disease should be made at least weekly— check hepatic enzymes; observe for jaundice, unexplained weight gain, right upper quadrant abdominal tenderness, ascites. Assess neurologic status for signs of hepatic encephalopathy; frequent complete blood counts and coagulation tests will be performed. Inspect intravenous tubing for cloudiness to detect precipitates that may occur in incompatible solutions or solutions mixed longer than 24 hours. Assess for pregnancy (category unknown). **INTERVENTION:** Azathioprine is converted to 6-mercaptopurine over time, and IV solutions and tubing should be managed as hazardous. Azathioprine administration should be planned around mealtime to reduce GI toxic effects. Give oral form with food or milk to reduce GI side effects. Store tablets protected from light and heat. Administer reconstituted doses within 24 hr; dilute in at least 50 mL normal saline (NS) or dextrose 5% and administer over 30–60 min. Provide soothing oral anesthetics in presence of irritation. **Patient Teaching—** Provide patient oral care instruction for management of stomatitis, and teach infection prevention strategies. **EVALUATION:** Observe for signs/symptoms of graft rejection throughout therapy. Evaluate for nursing problems and response to interventions as outlined in nursing plan.
ANTIBODIES		
equine antithymocyte globulin (Atgam)		
Prevention and treatment of rejection uses same doses.	**Onset:** variable **Peak:** variable	**ASSESSMENT:** Assess patient's history for evidence of previous bone marrow suppression or hepatic or renal

Continued on the following page

Table 60–3. ORGAN TRANSPLANTATION DRUGS: ANTIMETABOLITES, ANTIBODIES, AND POLYPEPTIDE ANTIBIOTICS, *Continued*

DRUG NAME/ROUTE AND DOSAGE	PHARMACOKINETICS/ DYNAMICS	NURSING IMPLICATIONS

ANTIBODIES, *Continued*

equine antithymocyte globulin (Atgam), *Continued*

delay onset rejection

Adults: 15 mg/kg per day for 14 days with additional alternate day doses up to 21 doses (routinely about 7 additional doses).

rejection

Adults: 10–30 mg/kg per day for 14 days with additional alternate day doses up to 21 doses (routinely about 7 additional doses).

Children: 5–25 mg/kg per day for 14 days with additional alternate day doses up to 21 doses. Dose is administered over 4–8 hr.

Duration: NA
½L: NA
PB: NA
B: NA
E: natural degradation; renal 1%

dysfunction. Assess baseline volume status and heart's function (blood pressure, heart rate, central venous pressure (CVP), edema, jugular venous pulsations (JVP); check results of recent chest x-ray films or arterial blood gases (ABGs). Assess skin response to test dose (0.1 mL of a 1:1000 dilution NS)—10-mm wheal and flare reaction indicates possible hypersensitivity. Assess for pregnancy (category C).

INTERVENTION: Plan for skin test dose to identify hypersensitivity before IV administration; have emergency equipment readily available. Provide cardiac monitoring for frequent pulse checks for rate and rhythm during first dose. Limit other fluids during infusion. Determine that no evident active infections are present prior to therapy. Dilute medication in 250–1000 mL 0.45% or 0.9% NS; avoid medication contact with air (protein is denatured); If mixing, add to inverted bottle of diluent; keep refrigerated. Use an in-line 0.2 to 1.0-micron filter and administer by slow IV infusion (4–8 hr) within 12 hours of reconstitution. Monitor IV catheter site for erythema, pain, warmth. Premedicate patient with tylenol and/or benadryl as ordered by physician. Do not administer concomitantly with blood products or amphotericin B. Assess vital signs during first infusion q 15 min × 4, q 30 min × 4, q 60 min × 4, then routinely. Monitor dextrostix (at least bid); perform intake and output measurements (report intake > output) and weigh patient daily. *Patient Teaching*—Teach patient symptoms to report that may signal hypersensitivity (dyspnea, itching, chest discomfort) and infection prevention strategies.

EVALUATION: Carefully observe and evaluate patient during first infusion for signs/symptoms of hypersensitivity or anaphylaxis (can occur even after negative skin test); auscultate heart and lung sounds throughout therapy to detect cardiopulmonary complications; provide oxygen saturation monitoring or obtain ABGs as ordered if patient subjectively reports dyspnea or has high risk for hypoxemia or pulmonary edema; monitor CVP and/or JVP for hypervolemia and heart failure; report alterations in mental status or agitation; manage serum sickness symptoms with tylenol, warm blankets, and supportive measures; provide antiemetic therapy.

muromonab-CD3 (Orthoclone OKT3)

Adults: 5 mg daily over approximately 1 min for 10–14 days (15 min is reported as acceptable).

Onset: minutes
Peak: NA
Duration: few days (?)
½L: NA
PB: No
B: NA
E: natural degradation

ASSESSMENT: Assess patient history for previous hypersensitivity to proteins, particularly of murine origin. Assess baseline cardiopulmonary status for signs of hypervolemia, heart failure, hypoxemia; check results of recent chest x-ray films and ABGs.

INTERVENTION: Determine patient's dry weight prior to therapy and attempt to achieve this weight prior to start of OKT3. Determine physician's preference for premedication: tylenol, nonsteroidal anti-inflammatory agents, benadryl, or hydrocortisone may be ordered prior to administration. Determine that no infection is present prior to therapy; be certain patient is afebrile prior to all doses of drug (variable according to physician preference); discuss plans of whether to reduce dose of concomitant immunosuppressive medications (usually are reduced). Withdraw drug from vial using a

Continued on the following page

Table 60–3. ORGAN TRANSPLANTATION DRUGS: ANTIMETABOLITES, ANTIBODIES, AND POLYPEPTIDE ANTIBIOTICS, *Continued*

DRUG NAME/ROUTE AND DOSAGE	PHARMACOKINETICS/ DYNAMICS	NURSING IMPLICATIONS
ANTIBODIES, *Continued*		
muromonab-CD3 (Orthoclone OKT3), *Continued*		low protein-binding 0.2 or 0.22 micron filter and discard filter needle. Administer through needle or needleless system (no filter); administer with dextrose solution flushing line. Cardiac monitor or rhythm checks throughout the first and second infusions or if during a second cycle of treatment. Assess vital signs during first and second doses—q 15 min × 4, q 30 min × 2; q 60 min × 3, then routinely; subsequent dose vital signs, temperature, and blood pressure q 1 hr × 4. Measure intake and output throughout therapy and weigh patient daily. **Patient Teaching**—Teach patient symptoms of hypersensitivity reactions and infection prevention strategies. **EVALUATION:** Have emergency equipment and supplemental oxygen readily available during therapy. Administer antipyretics for several hr after infusion as ordered for fever. Auscultate heart and lung sounds throughout therapy to detect cardiopulmonary complications; provide oxygen saturation monitoring or obtain ABGs as ordered if patient subjectively reports dyspnea or has high risk for hypoxemia or pulmonary edema; monitor CVP and/or JVP for hypervolemia and heart failure. Monitor CD3 antibody levels during therapy.
POLYPEPTIDE ANTIBIOTICS		
cyclosporine (Neoral) (Sandimmune)		
Induction: *Oral*–14–25 mg/kg per day liquid-filled capsule given with food or milk (is ⅓ of IV dose). *Intravenous*–5–6 mg/kg per day infused over 2–6 hr. **Maintenance:** *Oral*–5–10 mg/kg per day.	**Peak:** variable **Duration:** 3–5 hr **½L:** biphasic—initial: 1.2 hr; terminal: 19–27 hr **PB:** 90% **B:** NA **E:** Bile (primarily), renal 6%	**ASSESSMENT:** Assess patient history for drugs likely to interact with cyclosporine. Identify renal insufficiency through BUN, creatinine, creatinine clearance. Determine existence and therapeutic status of hypertension; ascertain history of seizure disorder, psychiatric disease, and pancreatitis—last episode, precipitators, characteristics, therapeutics at present. Determine baseline oral health, and check baseline cholesterol and triglycerides. Assess for pregnancy (category C). **INTERVENTION:** Identify patient-specific risk factors for enhanced or reduced cyclosporine effects or levels. Plan for preventive oral health care to reduce complications related to gum hyperplasia. Plan for routine blood monitoring of cyclosporine levels, chemistry (especially BUN and creatinine), and liver function tests. Consider need to discontinue or reduce dose of other immunosuppressive agents. Dilute dose in 20–100 mL NS or dextrose 5%; use glass infusion bottle or mix oral solution in plastic cup (may leach polyvinylchloride [PVC]). Administer IV dose over 2–6 hr; mix oral form in corn oil and food or milk diluent; *do not* give oral doses with meals—will alter absorption; protect diluted oral or IV solutions from light. Measure intake and output throughout therapy and weigh patient daily. Institute seizure precautions and perform dextrostix checks at least bid. **Patient Teaching**—Teach patient oral hygiene measures to prevent complications related to gum hyperplasia; symptoms of seizures (altered sensory perceptions, muscle twitching, memory loss); reportable symptoms of hypertension (headache, visual disturbances, lethargy, fullness of head); symptoms of hyperglycemia (lethargy, thirst, polyuria); and to take oral form with milk or food.

Continued on the following page

Table 60–3. ORGAN TRANSPLANTATION DRUGS: ANTIMETABOLITES, ANTIBODIES, AND POLYPEPTIDE ANTIBIOTICS, *Continued*

DRUG NAME/ROUTE AND DOSAGE	PHARMACOKINETICS/ DYNAMICS	NURSING IMPLICATIONS
POLYPEPTIDE ANTIBIOTICS, *Continued*		
cyclosporine (Neoral) (Sandimmune),*Continued*		**EVALUATION:** Monitor blood pressure throughout therapy—administer antihypertensives as ordered; monitor cholesterol and triglycerides and report abdominal pain (especially right upper quadrant); constantly evaluate fluid volume status and need for medications that may alter cyclosporine effects or enhance renal dysfunction; follow up any neurologic changes with physician evaluation and cyclosporine level; administer antiemetics as ordered for nausea and vomiting.
tacrolimus (Prograf) **Adults:** 0.15–0.3 mg/kg per day PO in bid dosing; 0.05–0.1 mg/kg per day IV as continuous infusion. **Children:** Administered the same doses as adults, but the upper end of this dose range is usually required and tolerated by children.	**Onset:** immediate **Peak:** 1.5–3.5 hr **Duration:** NA **½L:** 11.7 hr in liver transplant patients; 21.2 hr in normal volunteers **PB:** 75%–99% **B:** liver **E:** renal 1% (most metabolized before excretion)	**ASSESSMENT:** Assess for hypersensitivity first 30 min of infusion. Assess for pregnancy (category C). **INTERVENTION:** Must be diluted with NS or dextrose to a concentration of 4–20 μg; Do not use PVC because it alters stability of solution and leaches phthalates from PVC containers. Have emergency equipment available for possible anaphylaxis; anaphylaxis to IV form does not necessarily preclude oral use; start oral dose 8–12 hr after IV dose discontinued. Food decreases absorption up to 27%. **Patient Teaching**—Teach patient reportable symptoms of hypertension (headache, visual disturbances, lethargy, fullness of head), and hyperglycemia (lethargy, thirst, polyuria). Instruct patient to take oral form with milk or food. **EVALUATION:** Blood trough concentrations 9.8–19.4 ng/mL 10–13 hr postdose are useful in regulating dose, but fixed relationships between blood concentrations and effective immune suppression are not established.

NA = not available.

ANTI-INFLAMMATORY AGENTS

Anti-inflammatory agents prevent rejection of a graft by providing nonspecific suppression of the inflammatory and immune responses. The adrenocortical steroids such as prednisone and methylprednisilone act by stabilizing cell membranes, suppressing monocytic activity, diminishing sensitivity of host to antigens, and reducing the sensitization and lymphokine production by T lymphocytes. Chronic and high-dose steroids are used for immune suppression, causing increased risk of infection and cushingoid symptoms in these patients. These medications are covered in depth in Chapter 57.

ANTIMETABOLITES

ACTION

Antimetabolite medications interfere with cell nutrition (e.g., nucleic acid synthesis) or enzymatic activity by replacing a substance needed by the cell, which leads to cell death. Because antimetabolites participate in cell activities, there is little free drug circulating. Specific dosages, pharmacokinetics, adverse effects, and interactions for antimetabolites are presented in Chapter 55 because antimetabolites are more often used as antineoplastic medications, but a review of the prototype drug **azathioprine** *(Imuran)* is included in Table 60–3.

USES

Agents in this category used as immunosuppressive therapy include methotrexate and azathioprine. Because these antimetabolites suppress T-cell reaction to an antigen, they are not believed to be effective once a rejection process has been initiated. As a consequence, antimetabolites are used to prevent graft rejection, but they are not initiated when rejection occurs; they are usually discontinued when there is immunologic confirmation of rejection.

CONTRAINDICATIONS AND PRECAUTIONS

Antimetabolites have many potential toxicities, which vary with specific patient characteristics. When given with other immunosuppressive agents or with renal or hepatic insufficiency, these toxic effects may be exacerbated, requiring careful observation for infection, bone marrow suppression, renal failure, and hepatic injury. This is a particular concern when used for patients receiving kidney or liver transplants. Renal disease warrants reduced dosing and careful monitoring for an increased incidence of drug side effects or toxicities. The risks associated with infectious complications must be constantly balanced against the risk of rejection symptoms if the antimetabolite were to be discontinued. It is preferred to try to treat infections while maintaining the patient on therapy, so that rejection symptoms do not occur and necessitate change in the immunosuppressive regimen.

A concern in long-term use of antimetabolites is the potential for death and mutation of normal cells. The body's rapidly dividing cells such as skin, mucosa, and bone marrow are affected most. Patients with existing conditions such as skin lesions, gastrointestinal bleeding, or bone marrow suppression may have worsening of their problem if given antimetabolites. Secondary malignancies common in long-term treatment with antimetabolites are due to normal cell mutation and may occur during treatment or years later. Lymphoproliferative malignancies are the most common. Antimetabolite medications are also considered hazardous to the person administering the agent, so precautions recommended for handling of chemical hazards should be observed during administration. These guidelines usually are available through hospital safety officers and in oncology nursing references.

Hypersensitivity, although uncommon, is an absolute contraindication to further therapy. Because the agents resemble naturally occurring substances, the body may reject them as foreign protein. Hypersensitivity reactions are characterized by a combination of symptoms often mimicking serum sickness: fever, rigors, myalgias, arthralgia, maculopapular rash, and rarely, dyspnea or hypotension.

ADVERSE EFFECTS

The adverse effects noted with antimetabolites used as cancer chemotherapeutic agents are less evident in the doses used for immunosuppression. Side effects that do occur relate to the destruction of the body's rapidly dividing cells and include the following: alopecia, anemia, leukopenia, thrombocytopenia, oral lesions, anorexia, nausea, vomiting, and diarrhea.

○ **Azathioprine** (Imuran) is an analog of the chemotherapeutic agent mercaptopurine. The precise mechanism of action for this agent is unknown; however, it is known for suppression of inflammation and T-cell reactivity to antigens. This agent is used in conjunction with other immunosuppressive agents in renal and cardiac transplantation and in management of exacerbations of rheumatoid arthritis. Other uses for azathioprine have included alleviation of nephrotic conditions, immune thrombocytopenia, and autoimmune hemolytic anemia.

ADVERSE EFFECTS Unique effects noted with azathioprine include fever, jaundice, pancreatitis, skin rash, and arthralgias. Fever and skin rash occur during or shortly after administration and are thought to be a type of hypersensitivity reaction. It is unknown why arthralgias occur. This agent is toxic to the liver and pancreas, causing an inflammatory response with cholestasis and accompanying jaundice and pancreatitis.

▼ **CLINICAL ALERT**

An unusual but life-threatening adverse effect of azathioprine is veno-occlusive disease (VOD) of the liver. The usual presenting symptoms include weight gain, right upper quadrant tenderness, and hyperbilirubinemia. Permanent discontinuation of the drug is necessary when VOD is suspected.

INTERACTIONS Allopurinol interferes with metabolism of azathioprine, increasing the risks of toxicities, particularly bone marrow suppression. Dose reduction of azathioprine (25% to 35% of usual dose) is recommended to moderate these affects, although specific patient monitoring will determine the precise dose to administer.

CYTOTOXIC AGENTS

ACTION

Cytotoxic immunosuppressants, such as cyclophosphamide and chlorambucil, act by inhibiting DNA synthesis and T-cell cytokine release, which control both T-cell and B-cell responses against foreign proteins. The sensitivity of lymphoid elements to cytotoxicity is greater than the other bone marrow elements, making these agents effective as immunosuppressive therapy. The therapeutic index between immune-suppressing activity and general cytotoxicity is narrow as reflected in their more common use as anticancer agents. Lower dose, continuous therapy with agents such as cyclophosphamide, chlorambucil, and thioguanine is characteristic of their application in immune suppression after organ transplantation. Pharmacokinetics, adverse effects, and interactions for specific agents are presented in Chapter 55, where these drugs are discussed in detail.

USES

Cytotoxic agents are used as a preventive and therapeutic treatment against graft rejection for all types of organ transplant. The broad-spectrum immune-suppressing effects make them good baseline agents after organ transplantation. Cytotoxic agents are particularly used in bone marrow transplantation because of their additional anticancer effects.

CONTRAINDICATIONS AND PRECAUTIONS

Nonspecific suppression such as occurs in cytotoxic therapy incurs an increased risk for various infectious pathogens requiring careful monitoring of blood counts and observation for symptoms of infection. Long-term bone marrow suppression may occur with large doses of these drugs. Supression of the immune system also increases the incidence of lymphoproliferative malignancies. Cytotoxic agents, like antimetabolites, are also considered health hazards to caregivers and require special protective techniques when being administered.

ANTIBODIES

A number of antibody preparations have been used as immunosuppressive therapy. Some antibodies are directed toward destruction of lymphoid cells (antilymphocyte globulins), whereas others block the immunologic function of lymphocytes (monoclonal antibodies). Antilymphocyte globulins currently in use are **equine antithymocyte globulin (ATG, Atgam)**, **antilymphocyte globulin (ALG)**, and **antilymphocyte serum (ALS)**. The only monoclonal antibody currently used for immunosuppressive therapy is **muromonab-CD3 (Orthoclone OKT3).** Dosages, pharmacokinetics, and nursing implications for ATG and muromonab-CD3 are presented in Table 60–3.

ACTION

Antithymocyte or antilymphocyte sera lower the number of circulating T lymphocytes and reduce the body's reactivity to T cells and their cytokines. These antibodies are all derived from nonhuman sources and as such may cause the production of atypical antibodies. The most common source is the horse (equine); however, rabbit-derived ATG (RATG) are also promising in renal, pancreatic, and cardiac transplants. The antilymphocyte globulins are polyclonal antibodies because they are derived after animals are injected with human thymocytes (thymus gland is the source of T cells in humans) and red blood cells, which stimulate the animal to produce nonspecific IgG antibodies. These polyclonal antibodies are so named because they react to more than one antigen. Even though not specific, the primary action of lymphocytotoxicity is directed at T lymphocytes. These agents are administered to the graft recipient, and the foreign antibodies directly attack the host's T cells and reduce their circulating number. This causes specific T-cell suppression by reduced number of T cells without reducing immune activity of other cells. The various antilymphocyte preparations differ qualitatively and quantitatively because of differences in source (e.g., horse versus rabbit) and method of producing the antiserum. Certain of these formulations are used in different types of transplant; for example, ATG is used most often in bone marrow transplant, but ALG may be used in cardiac transplant. These differences are currently based on individual preferences, not sound clinical research findings.

Monoclonal antibodies provide selective immunosuppression and allow for administration of a purer protein fraction. These agents (e.g., muromonab-CD3) are developed through a hybridization technique that involves in-

jecting a mouse with human T cells. The mouse creates B-cell specific antibodies against human T cells that are harvested and fused with human myeloma cells, allowing for rapid and massive reproduction. The hybrid cells are reimplanted into the mouse where they become activated and rapidly multiply. They are then recollected in large enough quantities to be purified and administered to humans. When given to humans, the monoclonal antibody complex recognizes the T-3 complex on the human T cell and acts against it in three ways: (1) It coats the T cells, which aids their removal by reticuloendothelial cells; (2) it destroys the T-3 structure, and (3) it directly blocks T-cell killer activity. The activation and therapeutic effects of antibodies are widely variable in relation to the potency of the antibody preparation, the type of graft, and the host's immunologic reactivity. The absorption and serum concentration of these drugs are not important to their therapeutic effects. The drugs' effects are related to their direct activity on T cells, which may be immediate or delayed. Immediate anti–T cell effects are seen when monoclonal antibodies are given.

USES

Antibodies have been used to both prevent graft-versus-host reactions in bone marrow transplantation and treat graft rejection in other organ transplants. They are most often used in conjunction with other nonspecific agents such as corticosteroids or antimetabolites to delay or diminish the severity of rejection, but prolonged graft survival has not been demonstrated. Used mostly to treat rejection, these agents have facilitated important advances in the management of acute episodes of rejection in all types of allotransplantation and reversal of aplastic anemia without transplantation.

CONTRAINDICATIONS AND PRECAUTIONS

Hypersensitivity reactions and serum sickness occur more frequently with these agents because the antibodies are foreign proteins created by nonhuman sources. Immediate hypersensitivity is monitored for very closely. The incidence of anaphylaxis varies from 1% to 4% in patients receiving antibody therapy. Hypersensitivity is most commonly found during or immediately after the first dose of antibody substance and declines in severity with subsequent doses. To accurately identify these reactions relating to the antibody substance, antibodies should not be administered concomitantly with blood products, plasma protein derivatives, or amphotericin B.

▼ CLINICAL ALERT

Patients with altered left ventricular function are given these agents cautiously because pulmonary edema has been noted, particularly during the first dose. Fluid overload is a problem throughout therapy, as it relates to the limited anti-inflammatory response generated by administration of foreign proteins.

Serious infections also are of grave concern during anti-body immunosuppressive therapy. Increased incidence of viral and opportunistic infections (e.g., *Pneumocystis carinii*) have been noted during therapy. Patients developing life-threatening infections may have antibody therapy discontinued; however, this is not done without careful thought of the consequences. Therapy discontinuation eliminates the rejection suppression and enhances the development of antibodies against the antibody agent. Thus, when these agents are used in patients who develop such antibodies, the therapeutic effects are negligible.

ADVERSE EFFECTS

Most adverse effects related to antibodies relate to the body's recognition of the antibody as a foreign protein and subsequent hypersensitivity reactions. Symptoms that relate to hypersensitivity include skin rash, respiratory difficulty, nasal stuffiness, fever, chills, myalgias, and arthralgias. Serum sickness may occur in the polyclonal antibody preparations such as ATG, but not with monoclonal antibodies.

INTERACTIONS

General interactions with other medications are not known. The specificity of immune suppression with monoclonal antibodies allows for administration without discontinuation of other immunosuppressive therapy. Polyclonal preparations have a broader spectrum and may or may not be used with other agents. Antibodies do exert additive immunosuppressive effects, and some argue that this is the desired response, whereas others advocate lowering the doses of the concomitant agents. There are few drugs that are compatible when given concomitantly.

○ **Equine antithymocyte globulin** (ATG, Atgam) or lymphocyte immune globulin is primarily IgG antibody from horses injected with human thymus lymphocytes. ATG is lymphocyte-selective and reduces the number of circulating thymus-dependent lymphocytes (T cells), leading to a functional immune suppression. ATG has been used with all types of organ transplantation but is used more often as primary therapy when the risk of rejection may be higher, such as with heart-lung transplantation or unrelated bone marrow transplants. In less risky transplants, ATG may be reserved as alternative therapy when rejection symptoms occur. ATG is also used as primary treatment of aplastic anemia.

CONTRAINDICATIONS AND PRECAUTIONS Secondary to the polyclonal and general nature of the antibody infused as ATG, the incidence of anaphylaxis is about 1%, and serum sickness is 5% (renal allograft transplant with other immunosuppressives) to 85% (aplastic anemia). The manufacturer strongly recommends an intradermal skin test for reactivity before the first dose of the drug; however, the sensitivity of the test to predict systemic reactions is unconfirmed, and reactions may occur even with a negative skin test.

The use of ATG in children is limited. Although it has been used for renal transplants in patients aged 3 months to 19 years, its efficacy and side-effect profile is not well established. The safety of this agent in pregnant women has not been established and should be avoided. It is unknown whether this agent affects fertility. Mutagenicity studies are inconclusive. Although increased incidence of lymphoproliferative disorders have occurred in some patients suppressed with a regimen containing ATG, it is uncertain which immunosuppressive agent was the precursor.

ATG is compatible only with normal saline, and it will precipitate with other substances. Even without the presence of incompatible substances, ATG proteins may clump and form a precipitate in the intravenous tubing. In-line filters and frequent observation for cloudiness in the intravenous tubing are recommended.

ADVERSE EFFECTS Reduction of white blood cells (leukopenia) occurs with this agent the same as with others, but lymphopenia does not occur, which preserves some natural protection against viral infection. ATG is diluted in a large amount (1 to 2 L) of fluid, and hence has been reported as causing hypervolemia and pulmonary edema in susceptible patients. Other effects for which the mechanisms are unknown include thrombocytopenia, diarrhea, headache, and stomatitis.

○ **Muromonab-CD3** (Orthoclone OKT3) is a murine monoclonal antibody to the T-3 complex of the T lymphocytes. Studies on combination immunosuppressive therapy have shown that muromonab-CD3 may both delay and reduce severity of graft rejection as well as reverse the rejection process. Because of this lymphocyte-selective immunosuppressive action, muromonab-CD3 is used in immune-mediated diseases such as aplastic anemia, leukemia, lymphoma, multiple sclerosis, and transplantation. Most clinical experience in transplantation has been with renal allografts; however, there is growing interest in the use of muromonab-CD3 in cardiac, hepatic, and bone marrow transplant. Its primary use is as an adjunct to conventional therapy in the setting of graft rejection. An additional benefit of this agent is its lack of renal and hepatic toxicities, permitting immunosuppressive therapy to continue when other agents must be discontinued owing to organ toxicity.

CONTRAINDICATIONS AND PRECAUTIONS Muromonab-CD3 is usually reserved for patients who have failed conventional therapy because its benefit as a preventative is unproved, and repeated therapy with it has resulted in the development of antibodies to the drug, rendering it ineffective. Patients on other immunosuppressive therapy were less likely to develop these anti-OKT3 antibodies. Retreatment after the development of anti-OKT3 antibodies has been successful but requires close monitoring of antibody titers in the patient's blood.

ADVERSE EFFECTS Severe hypersensitivity and serum sickness is unusual because of the purity of this protein product; however, flulike and inflammatory symptoms are the hallmark of OKT3 treatment. The increased incidence of pulmonary edema and viral infection potentially occurring with the antibody agents is also significant with muromonab-CD3. Precautions and monitoring are the same with this agent as with others.

POLYPEPTIDE ANTIBIOTICS

ACTION

Polypeptide antibiotics, or cyclic peptides, are agents derived from bacteria or fungi that target specific proteins found on lymphoid cells called cyclophilins. They are similar to antibiotics in structure and gross function; however, their T-cell specificity is little understood. These agents have become the mainstay of immunosuppressive therapy because of their ability to block activation and mediator release by T cells without the usual myelosuppression. The only polypeptide antibiotics currently available for use are **cyclosporine *(Sandimmune)*** and **tacrolimus *(Prograf)*** (see Table 60–3). Oral and intravenous formulations are available and are equally bioavailable. The liver fully metabolizes these drugs into both active and inactive metabolites, primarily excreted in bile. Lipoprotein binding is present, although it does not appear to affect drug distribution in body fluids and tissues. No accurate method of measuring and interpreting drug levels has been established with these agents, hence making it difficult to define therapeutic levels.

USES

Polypeptide antibiotics are used to prevent graft rejection in all types of organ transplant except pancreatic and corneal, but their major limiting factor is the high incidence of rejection as soon as the agent is discontinued. Many clinicians recommend using corticosteroids concomitantly with polypeptides to provide a more comprehensive antirejection regimen. In addition to their use in transplant patients, these agents may also be used to manage disorders such as systemic lupus erythematosis, insulin-dependent diabetes mellitus, and rheumatoid arthritis.

CONTRAINDICATIONS AND PRECAUTIONS

Because of the risk of severe hypersensitivity and anaphylaxis (0.1% to 2%), close monitoring during the first one or two infusions of polypeptide antibiotics is essential.

ADVERSE EFFECTS

Polypeptide antibiotics act on cyclophilins in the body, producing the variety of adverse effects seen. Specific adverse effects are addressed within the agent-specific data.

INTERACTIONS

Polypeptide antibiotics have relatively strong immunosuppressing qualities, and other agents may be discontinued when these are employed. This side-effect profile is also significant, precluding therapy with other agents causing additive toxicities.

○ **Cyclosporine** (Neoral, Sandimmune) is a potent immunosuppressive agent that acts by inhibiting primary immune responses of T cells and humoral activity of B cells. The exact mechanism of action has not been determined, but it appears to involve a reversible inhibition of lymphocytic growth and cytotoxic activity. The primary benefit of this agent is its lack of myelosuppression. Cyclosporine is used in all types of allografts; however, it has been studied most in the renal and bone marrow transplant populations. Cyclosporine is an effective immunosuppressing rejection-preventive agent, but it is not viewed as effective for management of acute rejection.

CONTRAINDICATIONS AND PRECAUTIONS Oral absorption in prolonged therapy is reported as erratic, and frequent laboratory blood studies may be required. A microemulsion formulation with the trade name Neoral is better absorbed. High doses of drug also have been reported to contribute to hepatic dysfunction, and therapy should be monitored carefully when the patient has hepatic disease.

▼ **CLINICAL ALERT**

Immunosuppression using cyclosporine is undertaken with extreme caution in patients with existing or high risk for renal insufficiency. The drug is nephrotoxic (25% to 37% of patients) and excreted through the kidneys, necessitating therapeutic monitoring and dose reduction for these patients. Renal toxicity may be difficult to differentiate from graft rejection in the renal transplant patient.

Because of the unusual but potential risk of anaphylaxis associated with the intravenous form of this drug, oral formulations are used whenever possible. Children have safely received cyclosporine, but an increased propensity for seizures is noted. Currently cyclosporine is not viewed as mutagenic, but it can influence fetal growth and cause premature birth.

▼ **CLINICAL ALERT**

Cyclosporine is administered with caution to patients who have persistent unresolved hypertension. Hypertension can be exacerbated by cyclosporine therapy and tends to be unresponsive to standard interventions. If left untreated, hypertension can lead to stroke or seizures. This may be particularly risky if the patient is thrombocytopenic from other immunosuppressive therapy or has received a bone marrow transplant.

ADVERSE EFFECTS The most common adverse effects of cyclosporine therapy include transient gum hyperplasia, hirsutism, and fine tremors of the hands. Cyclosporine causes hypertension in 40% to 50% of recipients, dictating caution when given to patients with known heart disease or to patients with refractory hypertension (American Hospital Formulary Service, 1994). Hypertensive seizures have been reported in a small number of patients (American Hospital Formulary Service, 1994). Tremors and at times life-threatening seizures have occurred in patients receiving cyclosporine; however, the relationship is unclear. Some researchers speculate that elevated serum cyclosporine levels may predict this complication, whereas others correlate its incidence to variables such as concomitant use of corticosteroids, existence of hypertension, or coexisting hypomagnesemia.

Rare reactions (fewer than 2%) include anemia, thrombocytopenia, anorexia, gastritis or peptic ulcer, hiccups, muscle pain, hyperglycemia, tinnitus, hearing loss, fever, and brittle fingernails. Moderate elevations in hepatic transaminases have been noted in some patients; however, the levels usually return to normal after dose reduction or discontinuation of the drug. The mechanism of this effect is unknown.

INTERACTIONS   Because nephrotoxicity of cyclosporine may be additive, it is recommended that other nephrotoxic drugs are avoided whenever possible. Short-term omission of doses while monitoring drug levels may be first attempted to prevent the emergence of rejection symptoms likely to occur if the drug is discontinued. Other medications that enhance cyclosporine levels include erythromycin, diltiazem, rifampin, corticosteroids, phenytoin, phenobarbital, and intravenous sulfamethazine and trimethoprim. Monitoring cyclosporine levels while the patient is on these medications ensures maximization of the effective dose.

O **Tacrolimus**   (Prograf) is a polypeptide antibiotic derived from *Streptomyces tsukubaenis* (a strain of soil fungus). It is similar in composition to rifamycin and erythromycin. Tacrolimus acts by inhibiting T-lymphocyte activation and the production of interleukin-2, but the exact mechanism is unknown. It is FDA approved for use in combination with corticosteroids for prophylaxis of rejection in liver and pancreas transplants.

CONTRAINDICATIONS AND PRECAUTIONS   Because tacrolimus is a nephrotoxin, it is administered cautiously to patients with renal or hepatic insufficiency. Tacrolimus causes decreased renin and aldosterone levels, resulting in potentially dangerous concomitant increased serum potassium levels; it is withheld if the patient has hyperkalemia. The oral form of the drug is poorly absorbed, requiring frequent therapeutic monitoring during treatment; however, the high incidence of hypersensitivity reactions associated with the intravenous form of the drug necessitates oral administration whenever possible (see Table 60–3).

ADVERSE EFFECTS   The most frequent adverse effects of tacrolimus therapy are constipation or diarrhea, insomnia, headache, tremors, nausea, abdominal pain, fever, and itching. Many of these effects subside with long-term therapy. Mild hypertension occurs in one-third to one-half of patients. Some patients experience fewer adverse effects with tacrolimus than with cyclosporine.

USING THE NURSING PROCESS

Immunosuppressive agents prevent the host's recognition of transplanted tissue (by preventing T-cell activity) and thus prevent graft rejection. Nurses caring for patients taking drugs in this classification must constantly assess for signs and symptoms of rejection phenomena that signal that pharmacologic therapy must be readjusted. Symptoms of rejection vary with each type of organ transplant, but are generally reflective of systemic infection or organ failure. The challenge to balance adequate immune suppression with the risk of infection requires complex assessment and communication with other health-team members. An overview of the most important nursing problems and interventions for these patients is included in Table 60–4.

ASSESSMENT

- Know the specific signs and symptoms of graft rejection with each type of transplant and develop a plan to monitor for them.
- Signs of graft rejection often necessitate graft biopsy followed by a change in the immunosuppressive medications. Assess the patient's and family's understanding of the rejection process, the risk of rejection in each unique patient situation, and how immunosuppressive medications affect this process.
- Assess vigilantly for signs and symptoms of infection. All transplant patients are at risk for infectious complications, especially with fungal, viral, and opportunistic organisms, and display few of the usual signs and symptoms of infection. Because most patients have had herpes simplex virus, one of the most common infectious complications is reactivation of herpetic infection.
- When infection is suspected, the patient's social and activity history is elicited to determine if there have been exposures to communicable diseases.
- Each immunosuppressive medication has varying immunosuppressing qualities and must be considered in formulating a plan.

NURSING DIAGNOSIS

The most common nursing diagnoses for the patient receiving immunosuppressants are found in Table 60–4. Additional nursing diagnoses may center around the patient's specific symptoms of rejection, which are monitored to assess for response to changes in the immunosuppressive therapy.

PLANNING AND INTERVENTION

- Provide meticulous hygiene and protection against infection. Although no specific infection prevention guidelines for immunosuppressed patients have been provided by the Centers for Disease Control and Prevention (CDC), most routine patient care is performed more frequently and thoroughly in these patients (e.g., daily bathing, daily clothing and linen change, frequent oral care). Antibiotic ointments are usually used on dressing sites, and dressings are changed daily. Beyond universal precautions, some clinicians continue to wear masks and/or gloves

Table 60–4. NURSING PROCESS FOR PATIENT REQUIRING IMMUNOSUPPRESSIVE THERAPY

Assessment:

Assess type of tranplant.
Assess indication for immunosuppressive therapy—rejection prevention or treatment?
Assess medication profile—antibiotics, number and type of immunosuppressives.
Assess current active infections.
Assess risk factors for infection—altered barriers (e.g., skin breakdown), invasive devices, WBC, nutritional status.
Assess fluid volume status—hypervolemia, hypovolemia, edema?
Assess cardiopulmonary function.
Assess hepatorenal function.
Assess bone marrow reserve.

Nursing Diagnosis: Risk for Infection

RELATED TO: Immunosuppression

Desired Outcomes/Evaluation Criteria

Nursing Actions	Rationale
Monitor temperature every 4 hr while patient is awake.	Provides earliest symptom of infection—immunocompromised patients show few overt symptoms of infection.
Fever work-up to include physical assessment, blood cultures from two sites, urine cultures, sputum cultures, wound cultures, and chest x-ray films. Send cultures for bacteria, fungus, virus, and key opportunistic organisms.	The best time for culture results to be positive is at time of fever spike. Total body evaluation is essential in these patients.
Check lines and orifices for potential infections daily.	Sites most likely to become infected.
Perform routine surveillance body, excrement, or blood cultures as ordered.	Cultures will reveal colonizations and early infection with pathogens.
Provide environment free of pathogens— no fresh flowers, limited fresh fruits or vegetables, limit public exposure to communicable diseases, good handwashing, aseptic technique for all dressing changes, hepafiltered room if possible, no room proximity to patients infected with resistant organisms.	Infections acquired from the environment and caregivers can be avoided with good infection control technique.
Provide conservative infection control practices for these patients—daily dressing changes, IV tubing changes every 48 hr.	Centers for Disease Control and Prevention do not dictate clear guidelines for routine care of these patients, but guidelines err on conservative side.

Nursing Diagnosis: Fluid Volume Overload

RELATED TO: Renal dysfunction

Desired Outcomes/Evaluation Criteria

Desired Outcomes/Evaluation Criteria
Intake equal to output within 250 mL
Absence of heart failure symptoms.
Absence of edema.

Nursing Actions	Rationale
Measure intake and output during therapy.	Most accurate reflection of total body fluid.
Use existing measurements of vascular volume status—orthostasis, CVP, JVP.	Assists in demonstrating body's tolerance of additional fluids.
Daily weights.	Reflects total body fluid, but not location.
Daily assessment of edema, ascites, and so on.	Identifies amount of extravascular volume.
Frequent assessment of breath and heart sounds for signs of pulmonary edema—crackles in lungs, gallop heart sounds.	Assists in early identification of cardiopulmonary compromise from volume overload.

Nursing Diagnosis: Impaired Gas Exchange

RELATED TO: Drug-related anemia or hypersensitivity reactions.

Desired Outcomes/Evaluation Criteria

Normal breath sounds.
Oxygen saturation >90% and PaO_2 >60.
Patient verbalizes improvement of respiratory symptoms with oxygen or other therapeutic interventions.

Table 60–4. NURSING PROCESS FOR PATIENT REQUIRING IMMUNOSUPPRESSIVE THERAPY, *Continued*	
Nursing Actions	**Rationale**
Assess repiratory status throughout: immunosuppressive therapy—respiratory rate and depth, dyspnea, adventitious sounds, dull percussion (pleural effusions).	Identify early signs of altered oxygenation.
Evaluate oxygen saturation through noninvasive pulse oximetry.	Oxygen saturation is good measure of tissue perfusion with oxygen.
Obtain arterial blood gases as ordered.	Arterial blood gases are definitive measure of ventilation and gas exchange.
Position in high Fowlers with arms supported or elevated or in reverse Trendelenburg.	Best positions for ventilation.
Administer sedatives cautiously in the presence of respiratory difficulty.	Sedation reduces ventilation—may worsen oxygenation or ventilation disorder.
Administer diuretics as ordered.	Oxygenation problems in these patients are often due to fluid overload.
Administer blood products as ordered.	RBCs will increase oxygen-carrying capacity.
Administer oxygen as ordered—evaluate subjective response to oxygen and check oxygen saturation or arterial blood gas for objective response.	Oxygen therapy is medication/treatment—should always be evaluated for subjective and objective improvement.
Have patient cough, deep breathe, and turn every 2–4 hr.	Enhances oxygenation, prevents atelectasis and pneumonia.

Other Suggested Nursing Diagnoses: Altered Cardiac Output; Altered Nutrition; Altered Mucous Membranes; Altered Urinary Elimination; Hyperthermia; and Pain.

when caring for these patients; however, literature does not support this practice.

- To safeguard against infection, patients who are receiving immunosuppressive therapy should eat public food cautiously, wash fruits and vegetables before eating them, avoid fresh flowers, and limit public exposure to communicable diseases.
- Additional measures to prevent infection in the hospitalized patient include avoidance of invasive procedures, injections, and rectal procedures.

Patient Teaching

A patient education tool to be used for patients prescribed immunosuppressive agents is included in Table 60–5.

- Ascertain the patient's and family's understanding of the expected and adverse effects of immune suppression and teach them infection prevention techniques. It is essential to observe patient or family performance of these practices to determine their understanding of aseptic technique and the importance of early intervention for potential infection.

EVALUATION

- Evaluation of the effectiveness of therapy is a shared responsibility of all team members. Evaluate patient responses to drug therapy. The nurse understands the signs and symptoms of graft rejection for any patient receiving immunosuppressive therapy and constantly monitors for their occurrence. Because some agents are used to prevent graft rejection and others are implemented to treat graft rejection symptoms, a

clear plan for identifying desirable and undesirable patient responses is necessary.

- Evaluate effectiveness of therapy. In the absence of symptoms of rejection, the tapering and discontinuation of immunosuppressive therapy varies widely from one type of transplant to another. Therapy may range from 8 weeks to years. In patients with evidence of rejection, immunosuppressive treatment may be for life.
- Evaluate patient for signs and symptoms of infection. When multiple immunosuppressive therapies are used, immune suppression may be additive, placing the patient at even greater risk for infection. Symptoms of infection in these patients will be subtle because of their lack of inflammatory response. Many transplant patients receive routine cultures of blood and orifices (mouth, nose, anus, vagina) to monitor for organism colonization and early infection.
- Evaluate patient for fever. Because fever is the only presenting symptom in immune-suppressed patients, a temperature of 38.5°C requires a full fever work-up, which includes two sets of blood cultures, line cultures, urine culture, stool culture, chest radiograph, and sputum culture.
- Evaluate patient for drug adverse effects and toxicity. Each immunosuppressive agent has a side-effect and toxicity profile that must be considered when evaluating patients. However, renal, hepatic, and bone marrow (hematologic) functions are monitored frequently; just after the transplant this may be daily and later may be only monthly, depending on drugs used, dosage, and personal risks for certain effects.

The bibliography for this chapter can be found in Appendix B, which begins on page 1054.

Table 60–5. PATIENT TEACHING INFORMATION—IMMUNOSUPPRESSIVE THERAPY

Dear Patient:

You have been prescribed a drug to help prevent/treat rejection of your transplanted _____. These drugs are called immuno-suppressive drugs because they block your body's immune reaction to kill the _____ that has been transplanted into your body. This drug is called _____. Some information that will assist you in caring for yourself while taking this medication is listed below:

- ☐ 1. Immunosuppressive drugs block the immune system.
- ☐ 2. You will be more prone to infections while taking this drug.
- ☐ 3. The signs of an infection will not be the same while you are taking this drug—they will be milder, but this does not mean that the infection is less.
- ☐ 4. The most common sign of infection is a fever. Take your temperature at least every day and when you feel sick, warm, chilly, or not right. If you have a fever of 101.3°F (38.5°C) or more, you should call your doctor or his or her answering service *right away*.
- ☐ 5. Any delay in calling the doctor or getting the proper antibiotic (medicine to fight infection) can be dangerous and lead to severe infection.
- ☐ 6. To prevent infections, you should take a bath and change clothes every day. If you have any cuts, scrapes, or special dressings, these should be changed every day.
- ☐ 7. You should be careful about eating at restaurants. Certain foods may cause infections for you. The foods to avoid include fish, mayonaise, eggs, and rare meat.
- ☐ 8. Avoid crowds and places where people with colds and flu may give you their illness.
- ☐ 9. Wash all fresh fruits and vegetables thoroughly before eating them.
- ☐ 10. Avoid fresh flowers, gardening, and stagnant water. These spread infection.
- ☐ 11. Your pets may give you infection, so have them checked by the veterinarian and wash after you have had contact with them.
- ☐ 12. Protect your skin from injury and burns by wearing gloves, testing bath water for excessive heat, wearing shoes with cotton socks, and wearing cotton underwear.

If you have further questions about your medicine or its effects, please feel free to contact the doctor/nurse at _____.

CHAPTER REVIEW QUESTIONS*

1. Patricia Hightower is a 64-year-old woman who has undergone successful heart transplant surgery. She is being cared for in the surgical intensive care unit and receiving cyclosporine (Sandimmune) intravenously. Which of the following data should be noted before therapy with this agent?
   a. Serum amylase.
   b. Creatinine and BUN.
   c. LDH and CPK.
   d. T_3, T_4 levels.

2. Which of the following findings would the nurse report promptly after assessing the patient receiving cyclosporine?
   a. Evidence of hair loss.
   b. Heart rate of 100 bpm.
   c. Urine output of 40 mL/hr.
   d. Drainage from incision.

3. After 3 days of intravenous therapy with cyclosporine, a patient is to be converted to an oral dosage of cyclosporine. The nurse will administer oral cyclosporine:
   a. On an empty stomach.
   b. With meals.
   c. With an antacid.
   d. Before bedtime.

4. When planning specific nursing care for a patient receiving cyclosporine therapy, the nurse will include:
   a. Weighing patient once a week.
   b. Limiting mobility.
   c. Maintaining isolation.
   d. Performing oral care.

5. The nurse will monitor patients receiving cyclosporine therapy for:
   a. Nausea.
   b. Alopecia.
   c. Tremors.
   d. Palpitations.

*See Appendix A, which begins on page 1051, for answers.

Agents Used in the Management of HIV Infection and Acquired Immunodeficiency Syndrome (AIDS)

Brenda K. Shelton, MS, RN, CCRN, OCN

CHAPTER OUTLINE

KEY TERMS

Acquired immunodeficiency
    syndrome (AIDS)
AIDS dementia complex
    (ADC)
Antiretroviral agents
Enzyme-linked
    immunosorbent assay
    (ELISA)
HIV culture
HIV seroconversion
Human immunodeficiency
    virus (HIV)

Kaposi's sarcoma (KS)
Opportunistic infection (OI)
Protease inhibitors
Retrovirus
Reverse transcriptase
Reverse transcriptase
    inhibitors
T4 Helper or CD4
    lymphocyte
Western blot test

LEARNING OBJECTIVES

After reading this chapter, the student will be able to:

1. Describe the immune deficits that occur with HIV
   infection.
2. Outline the mechanism of action and key characteristics
   of antiretroviral agents.
3. Design an assessment plan for patients receiving antiretroviral agents.
4. Plan nursing interventions appropriate to the administration and teaching of patients receiving antiretroviral
   agents.

---

*A*cquired immunodeficiency syndrome (AIDS) is the severe end-disorder of an immune deficit caused by viral destruction of cells with CD4 receptor sites on their surfaces. AIDS was first described in 1981 when previously healthy individuals with no risk factors for immunodeficiency presented with opportunistic infections and unusual cancers such as *Kaposi's sarcoma (KS)*. The *human immunode-*

ficiency virus (HIV), identified in 1983, is the causative agent for AIDS.

HIV survives only in body tissues, blood, and secretions such as semen and breast milk. The primary source of infection is through blood transmission. Blood may cross directly from one individual to another via shared needles among intravenous drug users, traumatic sexual encounters, blood transfusion, placental blood sharing between mother and fetus, or open wound contact with infected blood. Currently, the highest risk group are those having unprotected sexual encounters with HIV-positive persons. Universal blood donor testing has reduced the incidence of HIV in transfused patients, but those receiving multiple transfusions and multidonor products such as cryoprecipitate carry a slight risk of contracting the disease. Although isolated from many body fluids, HIV infection is not believed to be transmitted by tears, emesis, or urine.

World Health Organization statistics and subsequent mortality and household survey statistics estimate that 630,000 to 897,000 cases of AIDS have occurred within the United States alone. AIDS has been a problem in densely populated and impoverished areas with intravenous drug usage and prostitution.

PATHOPHYSIOLOGY

HIV is a *retrovirus* known for its ability to incorporate itself into the normal cell's ribonucleic acid (RNA), causing replication of virus cells, not normal cells. HIV cells are protected by an "envelope," or protective coating that deters destruction. HIV preferentially binds to the human CD4 molecule found on *T4 (helper) lymphocytes* and monocytes, causing destruction and compromised cellular immune function. T4 lymphocytes are responsible for battling intracellular infections; assisting in production of immunoglobulin; and recognizing malignant cell transformation, allograft rejection, and delayed-type hypersensitivity (DTH). In HIV infection, immunoglobulins may be produced in excessive quantity but are ineffectual in function. The consequence is hyperallergy but inability to recognize and destroy invading pathogens. HIV's effects on the monocyte/macrophage lead to tissue infection and liberation of inflammatory mediators such as tumor necrosis factor. It is postulated that the wasting syndrome associated with AIDS is related to these mediators (Fan et al., 1994). Infections are often due to encapsulated or protected organisms that notoriously pass the neutrophil and are destroyed by the monocytes. Examples of infections of this variety are tuberculosis, *mycobacterium avium-intracellulare* (MAI), and *Pneumocystis carinii*.

Within 3 to 6 weeks of viral exposure, an infected person may present with transient flu or mononucleosis symptoms. Within 8 to 12 weeks after exposure, 95% of all affected persons have *HIV seroconversion* as evidenced by the presence of serum HIV antibodies. The average time from seroconversion to symptomatic disease is 7 to 12 years, with longer periods for younger persons. (Bartlett, J, 1996).

Numerous tests are used to diagnose exposure to HIV. The most common tests employed include *enzyme-linked immunosorbent assay (ELISA)*, *Western blot test*, gp 24 core protein, *HIV culture*, and polymerase chain reaction (PCR). In addition, home tests using saliva are now available. The first test to be done in suspected HIV infection is the ELISA, a blood test for the presence of antibodies to HIV. The ELISA is used by blood banks to detect infected blood products. ELISA has a false-positive rate of about 5%, so all positive ELISAs are followed by another test, usually the Western blot test. The Western blot test detects antibodies specific to viral proteins. This test is nonspecific when used alone but considered 99.9% diagnostic when accompanied by a positive ELISA. Other tests that are acceptable for confirmation of HIV infection as defined by the Centers for Disease Control and Prevention (CDC) include (1) antigen assays for p24, gp41, or gp 120/160; (2) viral DNA polymerase chain reaction (PCR); and (3) HIV genetic material on viral culture. The p24 antigen test is used most in diagnosis of the acute retroviral syndrome that precedes seroconversion (Bartlett, J, 1996). Once the diagnosis of HIV infection has been made, the CD4 count is most helpful in predicting patient symptoms and clinical problems.

The absolute CD4 count, which normally ranges from 600 to 1200 cells per mm^3, is the best measure of the severity of HIV disease. When the CD4 count is below 500 cells per mm^3, immune compromise and potential opportunistic infection or cancer begins; and when the count falls below 200 cells per mm^3, mortality related to infection and cancer is significant. Recent changes require CDC case-reporting criteria based on these CD4 counts, as presented in Table 61–1. Nevertheless, true AIDS (seroconversion and reduced CD4 helper count) is known to present as one or more of three major clinical manifestations: neurologic disease, opportunistic infection, or cancers.

Neurologic Disease

AIDS-related neurologic disease occurs in 60% to 80% of all patients and is related to opportunistic infection in 80% of those cases. Other types of neurologic disease include lymphoma, cerebral vascular accident, aseptic meningitis, and HIV infestation of neurologic cells. HIV invasion of the brain causes patients to exhibit personality changes, memory deficits, muscle atrophy, and polyneuropathies. An encephalitis-type syndrome known as *AIDS dementia complex (ADC)*, or AIDS dementia is thought to affect at least two-thirds of persons in the terminal phase of HIV infection. Approximately one-fourth of these patients may not have obvious symptoms but reveal abnormalities such as slowed thought processes, poor balance and coordination, apathy, dysphoria, difficulty concentrating, or regression when neurologically tested. There is no known cure for this syndrome, although symptoms improve with antiretroviral treatment.

Opportunistic Infections

Opportunistic infections (OIs) are those infections that do not usually occur in an immunocompetent host. Organisms considered opportunistic may encompass those not normally pathogenic, unusually severe infections, or unusual presentations for certain organisms. Many OIs are the consequence of reactivation of a latent infection within the host that has lain dormant but becomes active when cell-mediated immunity fails. The prevalence of specific opportunistic infections is constantly changing as antimicrobial prophylaxis regimens are established and patients survive previously fatal infectious complications.

Table 61–1. CDC CASE DEFINITIONS FOR AIDS

	Clinical Categories		
CD4 Cell Categories	**A** **Asymptomatic, or PGL or Acute HIV Infection**	**B** **Symptomatic[†]** **(not A or C)**	**C*** **AIDS Indicator Condition (1987)**
1. >500/mm³ (≥29%)	A1	B1	C1
2. 200–499/mm³ (14–28%)	A2	B2	C2
3. <200/mm³ (<14%)	A3	B3	C3

Indicator Conditions

Candidiasis, of esophagus, trachea, bronchi, or lungs
Cervical cancer, invasive[‡]
Coccidioidomycosis, extrapulmonary[‡]
Cryptococcosis, extrapulmonary
Cryptosporidiosis with diarrhea >1 month
Cytomegalovirus of any organ other than liver, spleen, or lymph nodes
Herpes simplex with mucocutaneous ulcer >1 month or bronchitis, pneumonitis, esophagitis
Histoplasmosis, extrapulmonary[‡]
HIV-associated dementia[‡]: Disabling cognitive and/or motor dysfunction interfering with occupation or activities of daily living
HIV-associated wasting[‡]: Involuntary weight loss >10% of baseline plus chronic diarrhea (≥2 loose stools/day ≥30 days) or chronic weakness and documented enigmatic fever ≥30 days
Isosporosis with diarrhea >1 mo[‡]
Kaposi's sarcoma in patient under 60 yr (or over 60 yr[‡])
Lymphoma of brain in patient under 60 yr (or over 60 yr[‡])
Lymphoma, non-Hodgkins of B-cell or unknown immunologic phenotype and histology showing small, noncleaved lymphoma or immunoblastic sarcoma
Mycobacterium avium or *M. kansaii*, disseminated
Mycobacterium tuberculosis, disseminated[‡]
Mycobacterium tuberculosis, pulmonary[‡§]
Nocardiosis[‡]
Pneumocystis carinni pneumonia
Pneumonia, recurrent-bacterial (≥2 episodes in 12 mo)[‡§]
Progressive multifocal leukoencephalopathy
Salmonella septicemia (nontyphoid), recurrent[‡]
Strongyloidosis, extraintestinal
Toxoplasmosis of internal organ
Wasting syndrome due to HIV (as defined above—HIV-associated wasting)

*All cases in categories A3, B3, and C1–3 are reported as AIDS, based on the AIDS-indicator conditions and/or a CD4 cell count <200/mm³. AIDS indicator conditions include three new entries: recurrent bacterial pneumonia, invasive cervical cancer, and pulmonary tuberculosis.
[†]Symptomatic conditions not included in category C that are (a) attributed to HIV infection or indicative of a defect in cell-mediated immunity, or (b) considered to have a clinical course or management that is complicated by HIV infection. Examples of B conditions include but are not limited to bacillary angiomatosis; thrush; vulvovaginal candidiasis that is persistent, frequent, or poorly responsive to therapy; cervical dysplasia (moderate or severe); cervical carcinoma in situ; constitutional symptoms such as fever (38.5° C) or diarrhea >1 month; oral hairy leukoplakia; herpes zoster involving two episodes or >1 dermatome; ITP; listeriosis; PID (especially if complicated by a tubo-ovarian abscess); and peripheral neuropathy.
[‡]Requires positive HIV serology.
[§]Added in the revised case definition 1993. Modified from CDC definitions.

However, cytomegalovirus of the colon, retina, or lungs remains the most lethal opportunistic infection associated with AIDS. The antimicrobial treatment of these infections is overviewed within the discussion of antimicrobial therapy in Chapter 58. Common prophylaxis regimens used in patients with HIV infection are noted in Table 61–2.

Cancers in AIDS

Malignant disease in AIDS comprises approximately 12% of all cases. Cancers that have been strongly correlated with HIV infection include Kaposi's sarcoma and non-Hodgkins lymphomas. Kaposi's sarcoma (KS) when associated with AIDS is an aggressive, invasive soft-tissue sarcoma usually occurring with CD4 counts between 200 and 500 cells per mm³ and in strong association with herpes simplex virus 8 (HSV8) (Bartlett, JG, 1996). Kaposi's sarcoma is manifested by uncontrolled proliferation of raised reddish-purple nodules on the skin and mucous membranes of the mouth, gastrointestinal (GI) tract, lymph nodes, lungs, and liver. Lesion invasion into the GI tract often may cause bowel obstruction or GI bleeding, and pulmonary lesions cause airway obstruction or respiratory failure. KS treatment is moderately successful and may include local radiation therapy, biotherapy, and chemotherapy. *Antiretroviral agents* have been shown to slow or halt the spread of KS and are therefore the preferred first treatment. Other agents with limited efficacy against this tumor include vincristine, vinblastine, etoposide, adriamycin, and alpha interferon.

Lymphoma is another significant malignancy associ-

Table 61–2. PROPHYLACTIC ANTIMICROBIAL THERAPY BASED ON CD4 COUNT

		CD4 <200/mm³			CD4 <100/mm³	
	Cost	Agent	Cost/Yr	Agents		Cost/Yr
All patients: **Pneumococcal vaccine**	$10.60	**PCP prophylaxis:**		**Deep fungal prophylaxis:**		
PPD positive or anergy + high risk:		TMP-SMX—1 DS/d*	$ 25	Fluconazole—100 mg/d,		$2500
INH 300 mg/d		Alternatives:		200 mg/d*		$5000
(Influenza vaccine)	$14.60	Dapsone—50 mg/d,	$ 65			
(Hepatitis B vaccine)	$5/yr	—100 mg/d*	$ 65	*M. avium* **prophylaxis:**		
	$160	Aerosolized pentamidine—		Rifabutin—300 mg/d*		$2390
		300 mg/mo*	$1200	Clarithromycin—500 mg/d,		$1004
				1 g/d		$2008
				Toxoplasmosis prophylaxis:		
				Positive serology +		
				contraindication to TMP-SMX		
				Dapsone 50 mg/d +		
				pyrimethamine 50 mg/wk +		
				folinic acid 25 mg/wk*		$ 818

*Efficacy for prevention of infection by stated pathogen documented in controlled trial with HIV-infected patients; the only regimen with documented benefit in prolonging survival is TMP-SMX (JAMA 259:1185, 1988).
†CD4 cell strata for initiating prophylaxis for deep fungal infections and toxoplasmosis is arbitrary; for *M. avium* prophylaxis, the PHS recommendation is <100/mm³.

ated with HIV infection. Most AIDS-related lymphomas are B-cell lymphomas, and brain metastases may be present at the time of diagnosis (normally rare in lymphoma). These lymphomas have proven resistant to conventional treatment, but the usual and investigational chemotherapeutic agents are used.

TREATMENT OF HIV INFECTION

There are four goals of medical treatment for HIV infection. The first goal is to enhance early detection of HIV infection. Early treatment with antiretroviral agents or antimicrobial therapy can reduce the progression of HIV infection and its opportunistic infections. The second goal is to support and encourage research and development of antiretroviral agents. These medications offer the most realistic hope of halting disease progression. The Food and Drug Administration (FDA) has licensed five *reverse transcriptase inhibitors* and three *protease inhibitors*, which will be discussed in this chapter. The third goal is to continue exploration of therapies to restore immunologic function. The fourth goal is to expand our capability for early identification and treatment of opportunistic infections, cancer, and HIV-related clinical syndromes.

Treatment of HIV virus and the related complications will encompass all types of antimicrobial therapy. Antimicrobial therapy is directed toward the suspected pathogens based on clinical presentation, previous infections, and CD4 count. A program of prophylactic antimicrobial therapy based on the CD4 count is shown in Table 61–2.

Treatment of symptomatic HIV-positive individuals or those with CD4 counts below 500 per mm³ include administration of an antiretroviral agent. Due to cumulative toxicities that occur with long-term use, many patients receive combination or alternating therapy that reduces the adverse effects of each inividual agent. Combination therapy is also implemented when the patient's CD4 count continues to decrease despite what is perceived as

adequate therapy. Agents for the treatment of infectious and malignant HIV-related syndromes can be found in Chapters 55, 56, and 58. Specific information on antiretroviral agents as used in the management of the HIV infected patient is included in Tables 61–3 and 61–4.

REVERSE TRANSCRIPTASE INHIBITORS

The reverse transcriptase inhibitors include **zidovudine (Azidothymidine, AZT, Compound S, Retrovir), didanosine (ddI, Videx), zalcitabine (Hivid), stavudine (d4T, Zerit),** and **lamivudine (3TC, Epivir).**

ACTION

Because *reverse transcriptase* replacement is the mechanism by which HIV destroys normal CD4 cells, drugs such as those in this category, which have a blocking effect on viral reverse transcriptase, can halt the replication and growth of HIV in humans. There is minor variability in the action of these agents.

USES

Reverse transcriptase inhibitor antiretroviral medications are indicated for all symptomatic, HIV-seroconverted patients with a CD4 count less than 500 per mm³ (National Institute of Allergy and Infectious Diseases, NIH, and U.S. Public Health Service, 1993). Some patients may opt for therapy if their CD4 count is below 500 cells per mm³, and yet they remain asymptomatic; and in rare cases, asymptomatic patients with CD4 counts greater than 500 cells per mm³ will receive antiretroviral therapy. "Symptomatic" is defined as having acute retroviral syndrome, diffuse lymphadenopathy, or one of the AIDS indicator diseases. When opportunistic infections or cancer (other than KS) are the primary presenting problem, treatment

Table 61–3. REVERSE TRANSCRIPTASE INHIBITORS

DRUG NAME/ROUTE AND DOSAGE	PHARMACOKINETICS/ DYNAMICS	NURSING IMPLICATIONS
zidovudine (Retrovir) Dosage regimen varies depending on protocols and concurrent drug administration. *Adults:* 200 mg (two capsules) PO tid for a 4-wk induction period, then 100 mg every 4 hr; or 200 mg PO tid when given with zalcitabine.	**Onset:** NA **Peak:** 0.5–1.5 hr **Duration:** NA **½L:** 1 hr **PB:** NA **B:** 75% **E:** metabolism to a glucuronide in liver and renally excreted (15%–20% unchanged)	**ASSESSMENT:** Assess patient history for bone marrow disease or medications that deplete bone marrow reserve; important to note and increase frequency of hematologic assessment parameters. Assess medication history to identify bone marrow suppressants (e.g., cancer chemotherapy, allopurinol), neurotoxic agents (e.g., vinca alkaloids, neuromuscular agents), or medications metabolized by glucuronidation (e.g., tylenol, aspirin). Assess baseline neurologic examination findings (especially depression, orientation, cognitive ability, and peripheral neuropathies) to help identify risk of toxicity and to assist in monitoring response to intervention in AIDS dementia; assess ability to perform fine motor activities (e.g., buttoning shirt) to assess for developing peripheral neuropathies. Assess for renal or hepatic dysfunction or bone marrow suppression. Assess for pregnancy (category C). **INTERVENTION:** Store medication protected from light. Institute infection prevention precautions. Administer erythropoietin and leukocyte growth factors as ordered to counteract bone marrow suppression. Treat discomfort such as headache and myalgias cautiously owing to analgesic interference with metabolism. Refer for obtainment of a wig or use of scarves if alopecia occurs. Institute seizure precautions as indicated by history and risk factors. Administer RBC transfusions as ordered. Encourage use of sleep medications if insomnia is problematic. Monitor time, amount, consistency of stools; identify existing food intolerances that exacerbate diarrhea; encourage foods that may cause constipation in others (e.g., cheese, starch); administer antidiarrheal medications as ordered. **Patient Teaching**—Teach patient importance of not missing doses. Teach safety precautions to patient with altered peripheral sensations (from peripheral neuropathy). Instruct patient to report abdominal pain or fatty food intolerance. **EVALUATION:** Monitor hematologic counts (CBC, HgB, HCT, platelets) routinely—they may begin to drop as early as 2 wk (usually drop after 6–12 wk of therapy). Monitor antiseizure drug levels carefully during zidovudine treatment. Check neurologic status at least biweekly; while patient is on therapy check for orientation changes, altered sensation, discomfort, disrupted fine motor skills.
didanosine (ddl) (Videx) Dosage is reduced in renal or hepatic impairment. Dose is determined based on weight. *Adults:* Available as 25-mg, 50-mg, 100-mg, or 150-mg buffered tablets; or buffered powder for oral solution (100-mg, 167-mg, 250-mg, or 375-mg single-dose packets) to ensure adequate buffering to prevent degradation of drug: >75 kg—300 mg bid (tablets), 375 mg bid (powder); 50–74 kg—200 mg bid (tablets), 250 mg bid (powder); 35–49 kg—125 mg bid (tablets), 167 mg bid (powder).	**Onset:** 2 min **Peak:** 0.6–1 hr **Duration:** NA **½L:** Adults—1.3–1.6 hr; children—0.8 hr **PB:** <5% **B:** Metabolized into several metabolites **E:** renal (about 50%)	Same as for zidovudine plus: **ASSESSMENT:** Assess for existing hypertension, GI disorders or intolerances. Assess history of constipation, dermatologic disorder, arthritis, pancreatitis, and cholecystitis. Assess medication history for agents known to have altered activity when given concomitantly. Assess GI/abdominal at least weekly. Assess for pregnancy (category B). **INTERVENTION:** Store in normal room temperature—avoid heat and cold. Give in prescribed dose to ensure adequate absorption. *Do not* give with meals or other medications; administer with antacids to enhance absorption—if patient finds unpalatable, add flavoring. Institute seizure precautions as indicated by history and risk factors. Develop bowel regimen to prevent constipation—encourage fluids, excercise. Encourage meticulous skin care cleansing, moisturizers, and antipruri-

Continued on the following page

Table 61–3. REVERSE TRANSCRIPTASE INHIBITORS, *Continued*

DRUG NAME/ROUTE AND DOSAGE	PHARMACOKINETICS/ DYNAMICS	NURSING IMPLICATIONS
didanosine (ddI) (Videx), *Continued*		
Pediatric: Following specific instructions, reconstitute 2-g or 4-g bottle of pediatric powder for oral solution for a final admixture of 10 mg/mL BSA 1.1–1.4 m^2—100 mg bid (tablets), 125 mg bid (powder); BSA 0.8–1 m^2—75 mg bid (tablets), 94 mg bid (powder); BSA 0.5–0.7 m^2—50 mg bid (tablets), 62 mg bid (powder); BSA <0.4 m^{2}2—25 mg bid (tablets), 31 mg bid (powder).		tics (as ordered) for rash or irritation; frequent oral care with saliva substitutes as needed; soft food and cold liquids to reduce oral discomfort; antimicrobial oral rinses if stomatitis is severe; oral anesthetics as needed. Monitor intake and output with cardiac function—report signs/symptoms of heart failure. Apply warm compresses or clothing to aching joints. **Patient Teaching**—Encourage patient to identify food likes and aversions; discuss these to determine if patient is consuming adequate amounts and a well-balanced diet. **EVALUATION:** Determine efficacy or drug levels of important drugs that may be given concomitantly (e.g., dapsone, zidovudine, ribavarin). Check neurologic status at least biweekly; while patient is on therapy check for orientation changes, altered sensation, discomfort, disrupted fine motor skills. Check amylase, lipase as ordered. Assess for hair loss and provide referrals for wigs as appropriate. Monitor uric acid as ordered.
zalcitabine (Hivid)		
Adults and Children: 0.750 mg (one tablet) PO concomitantly with zidovudine 200 mg every 8 hr. *Adults and Children with Peripheral Neuropathies:* After therapy break, 0.375 mg PO with zidovudine 200 mg every 8 hr. *Patients <30 kg:* No dose reduction is required.	**Onset:** NA **Peak:** 0.8–1.6 hr **Duration:** NA **½L:** 1.2 hr **PB:** <4% **B:** hepatic **E:** renal (at least 70%)	Same as for zidovudine plus: **ASSESSMENT:** Assess GI disorders or intolerances. Assess history of pancreatitis or cholecystitis. Assess oral health at baseline and intermittently throughout therapy. Assess GI/abdominal at least weekly. Assess oral cavity including swallowing ability at least weekly; assess airway patency if oropharyngeal ulceration exists. **INTERVENTION:** Given only in conjunction with zidovudine. *Do not* take with food, as absorption is reduced. Store tablets at room temperature—extremes of heat alter effectiveness. Encourage frequent oral care and special mouth rinses and topical anesthetics with stomatitis. Institute seizure precautions as indicated by history and risk factors. **EVALUATION:** Check neurologic status at least biweekly; while on therapy check for orientation changes, altered sensation, discomfort, disrupted fine motor skills. Check amylase, lipase as ordered. Monitor intake and output with cardiac function—report signs/symptoms of heart failure.
stavudine (d4T) (Zerit)		
Dose is determined based on weight: <60 kg—30 mg PO bid; >60 kg—40 mg PO bid.	**Onset:** NA **Peak:** >1 hr **Duration:** NA **½L:** 1 hr **PB:** NA **B:** unclear **E:** renal (50% unchanged)	Same as for zidovudine.
lamivudine (3TC) (Epivir)		
Adults: 150 mg PO bid alone or with zidovudine. *Adults with Severe Peripheral Neuropathies:* Give a therapy break until pain resolves and resume at 50% original dose.	**Onset:** NA **Peak:** 1–1.5 hr **Duration:** NA **½L:** 2–4 hr **PB:** <36% **B:** liver (small %) **E:** renal (70%)	Same as for zidovudine.

NA = not available.

Table 61–4. ANTIRETROVIRAL PROTEASE INHIBITORS

DRUG NAME/ROUTE AND DOSAGE	PHARMACOKINETICS/ DYNAMICS	NURSING IMPLICATIONS
saquinavir (SQV) (Invirase) *Adults:* 600 mg PO tid with reverse transcriptase inhibitors.	**Onset:** NA **Peak:** NA **Duration:** NA **½L:** 1–2 hr **PB:** NA **B:** liver (90%) **E:** biliary (P450 cytochrome)	**ASSESSMENT:** Assess history of pancreatitis. Assess nutritional status. Assess abdomen periodically. Assess for pregnancy (category B). **INTERVENTION:** Give small frequent feedings; avoid aromatic foods if nauseated; and serve food on cardboard trays to reduce odors. Monitor time, amount, and consistency of stools; identify existing food intolerances that exacerbate diarrhea; encourage foods that may cause constipation in others (e.g., cheese, starch). Administer antidiarrheal medications as ordered, within 2 hr of a high-fat meal for best absorption. **Patient Teaching**—Instruct patient to report intractable nausea and vomiting or diarrhea and to not miss medication doses as development of resistance is rapid. **EVALUATION:** Evaluate manifestations of AIDS and patient regression or progression while on medication, monitor CD4 counts.
ritonavir (Norvir) *Adults:* 600 mg PO bid alone or with reverse transcriptase inhibitors. To enhance GI tolerance, give 300 mg bid for 1 day, 400 mg bid for 2 days, 500 mg bid for 1 day, then 600 mg bid thereafter.	**Onset:** NA **Peak:** 2–4 hr **Duration:** NA **½L:** 3.5 hr **PB:** 98%–99% **B:** liver **E:** urine, feces (85%)	Same as for saquinavir plus: **ASSESSMENT:** Check baseline and monitor cholesterol and triglyceride levels; assess history of cholecystic disease. **INTERVENTION:** assess for abdominal pain, rebound tenderness; administer medication with food if possible. **Patient Teaching**—Advise patient that taste aversions (especially to liquids) may occur. Instruct patient to report severe and intractable abdominal discomfort and numbness or tingling of the extremities.
indinavir (Crixivan) *Adults:* 800 mg PO tid with reverse transcriptase inhibitors.	**Onset:** NA **Peak:** NA **Duration:** NA **½L:** 1.5–2 hr **PB:** NA **B:** 60%–70% **E:** biliary (P450 cytochrome)	Same as for saquinavir plus: **ASSESSMENT:** Monitor bilirubin levels as ordered. **INTERVENTION:** Ensure fluid intake of at least 48 oz daily to prevent nephrolithiasis, provide hard candies for alleviation of metallic taste, monitor platelet count for thrombocytopenia. **Patient Teaching**—Instruct patient to report skin or scleral yellow discoloration or blood in urine. Tell patient to maintain adequate fluid intake.

NA = not available.

with antiretroviral agents may be delayed until those complications have been stabilized. These agents may be used as a possible prophylaxis for known occupational HIV exposure.

CONTRAINDICATIONS AND PRECAUTIONS

▼ CLINICAL ALERT

All available reverse transcriptase inhibitors must be given cautiously to individuals with renal insufficiency as these agents are metabolized and excreted renally.

Drugs that interfere with renal clearance of this drug may also be important to recognize, because toxicity is worsened when the drug's metabolism and clearance are hindered.

Concomitant use of medications causing peripheral neuropathy may increase the incidence of this side effect and hence is not recommended. Medications in this group include chloramphenicol, vinca alkaloids, cisplatin, dapsone, hydralazine, isoniazid, metronidazole, nitrofurantoin, phenytoin, and ribavirin. Patients exhibiting signs of neuropathy should have a therapy break or discontinuation of the drug until symptoms resolve. Because other neurotoxicities are also common, patients with neurologic impairment should be monitored carefully throughout administration. These agents are used to treat AIDS dementia, so neurologic disease is not a contraindication to therapy.

ADVERSE EFFECTS

Reverse transcriptase inhibitors, although having similar therapeutic activity, have some variation in side effects. The most typical adverse effects expected are neurologic in nature. Symptoms may be as mild as insomnia in some but will cause confusion, peripheral neuropathies, and seizures in others. All patients with a history of neuropsychiatric problems should have frequent monitoring for these nontherapeutic responses.

▼ CLINICAL ALERT

Another unique adverse effect associated with these agents is the risk of producing pancreatitis. In treatment with zidovudine, its incidence is rare; however, didanosine and zalcitabine have reported incidence rates between 1% and 4% with associated morbidity and mortality. As a consequence, patients' amylase level, cholesterol level, and liver function tests are monitored at least bimonthly during therapy.

Although most prevalent in zidovudine, all reverse transcriptase inhibitors have some bone marrow suppression. It is often the dose-limiting side effect of zidovudine, the first-line therapy for HIV infection. Anemia and leukopenia are common; thrombocytopenia is more unusual. Zalcitabine is the least toxic to marrow, producing anemia only rarely.

INTERACTIONS

Reverse transcriptase inhibitors have few interactions clearly identified at this time. It is speculated that at least some agents interact with other medications. It is prudent to evaluate all concurrent medications the patient is taking and attempt to discontinue any that are not essential. This is particularly important if other medication the patient is taking produces bone marrow suppression or pancreatitis.

○ **Zidovudine** (Azidothymidine, AZT, Compound S, Retrovir) was used, then abandoned as an anticancer drug in 1964, only to become the most significant agent currently available to treat HIV infection. It is a thymidine analog that specifically reduces reverse transcriptase activity of HIV-1 (AIDS virus). Because reverse transcriptase replacement is the mechanism by which HIV destroys normal CD4 cells, this blocking effect can halt the replication and growth of HIV in humans. Zidovudine is approved for use in patients with symptomatic HIV infection with a confirmed positive *Pneumocystis* culture or an absolute CD4 lymphocyte count of less than 500/mm³. In studies with HIV-seropositive mothers, the use of zidovudine therapy reduced fetal transmission of HIV infection from 25% to 5.4%.

CONTRAINDICATIONS AND PRECAUTIONS Zidovudine should be used cautiously in patients with granulocyto-

penia (granulocyte count less than 1000/mm³) or anemia (Hgb less than 9.5 mg/dL).

ADVERSE EFFECTS Most adverse effects associated with zidovudine have been the hematologic toxicities of anemia and granulocytopenia. Forty-five percent are reported to have had one of these signs. Other side effects may include fingernail discoloration, myalgias, liver function abnormalities, skin rash, altered taste sensation, numbness and tingling of extremities, dizziness, anxiety, and tremors when given in large doses. Rarely, seizures or encephalitis occur. Patients receiving zidovudine for more than 1 year may develop myopathy, which manifests as extremity weakness and tenderness, muscle atrophy, increased lactic dehydrogenase (LDH), and increased creatine phosphokinase (CPK).

INTERACTIONS The antiviral effects of this medication can be enhanced by acyclovir, interferon, didanosine (ddI), and granulocyte-macrophage colony-stimulating factor (GM-CSF). Its effects are antagonized by thymidine and ribavirin. The concurrent use of acetaminophen, aspirin, indomethacin, or probenecid may increase the toxic effects of zidovudine. Patients should consult with their physician before taking any of these medications while on zidovudine.

○ **Didanosine** (ddI, Videx) is a reverse transcriptase inhibitor licensed for the treatment of HIV-infected patients. The exact mechanism of antiretroviral activity for didanosine is unknown. It appears to inhibit the production of viral reverse transcriptase, leading to inability for the virus to replicate. Didanosine is indicated for treatment of HIV infection in adults and children 6 months or older who are intolerant to zidovudine or who have demonstrated clinical or immunologic deterioration during zidovudine therapy. Examples of patients who may qualify are those with significant bone marrow suppression on zidovudine or those who develop worsening KS when on zidovudine.

CONTRAINDICATIONS AND PRECAUTIONS The magnesium load of these tablets will also worsen any hypermagnesemia present (this is more prevalent in renal failure). This high magnesium may also induce diarrhea. Prescribing information for didanosine has been obtained from clinical trials, and many concerns about safety of administration in pregnancy, less obvious contraindications, and potential long-term effects are not available.

ADVERSE EFFECTS The major dose-limiting adverse effects are peripheral neuropathy and pancreatitis. Peripheral neuropathies occurring in 34% of patients are thought to be dose and duration related. Symptoms such as tingling and shooting "electrical" pain tend to occur most often in the soles of the feet and at night. Other neurologic effects reported less often include restlessness, irritability, anxiety, depression, insomnia, and dizziness. Rare instances of ataxia, speech disorders, and seizures have been reported.

One of the most serious adverse effects reported is pancreatitis. Occurring in up to 20% of patients receiving this drug, pancreatitis has been fatal in about 1% of the cases (American Hospital Formulary Service, 1996). In patients receiving didanosine for an average of 8.5 months, abdominal pain and amylasemia have occurred in 7% to

18% of patients, but therapy of less than five months reduces this incidence slightly (American Hospital Formulary Service, 1996).

Other side effects with an occurrence rate less than 15% include diarrhea, nausea, vomiting, asymptomatic hyperuricemia, rash, pruritis, elevated transaminases, myalgias, arthralgias, and alopecia.

INTERACTIONS The most important interactions related to this medication are those that alter gastric absorption rate. Acid or fasting stomachs reduce absorption, whereas milk-based products and antacids enhance absorption of didanosine.

○ **Zalcitabine** (Hivid) is an RNA reverse transcriptase inhibitor indicated only in combination with zidovudine for treatment of adults with advanced HIV infection (CD4 count less than 300/mm³) who have demonstrated significant clinical or immunologic deterioration). Patients who have had progressive symptoms of HIV disease despite adequate therapy may benefit from a combination of zidovudine and zalcitabine.

CONTRAINDICATIONS AND PRECAUTIONS Information regarding the safety of combined Hivid and zidovudine is limited by the number of patients who have been treated, the diversity of patients treated, and the potential combined toxicities, which have not yet been defined. This drug's use in children less than 13 years old, asymptomatic individuals, and pregnant women has not been established. The use of zalcitabine in patients with hepatic impairment, preexisting liver disease, or alcohol abuse has been shown to worsen hepatic impairment in 12% of patients treated. Monitoring and dose reduction as needed is recommended for these patients. Patients with existing peripheral neuropathies were excluded from all studies evaluating efficacy of this therapy and thus should be treated cautiously with zalcitabine.

ADVERSE EFFECTS The major clinical toxicity observed with zalcitabine therapy is peripheral neuropathy, occurring in 17% to 31% of patients receiving zalcitabine alone. These effects were noted in patients receiving monotherapy with zalcitabine and may be enhanced when given in combination with zidovudine. Other serious toxicities that have occurred in clinical trials evaluating zalcitabine include oral or esophageal ulceration, cardiomyopathy heart failure, and anaphylactoid reactions. Other minor reactions (occurring in 10% to 20% of patients) include headache and fatigue.

INTERACTIONS If intravenous pentamidine is used to treat *Pneumocystis carinii* pneumonia, zalcitabine treatment is interrupted owing to potential inactivation of pentamidine. Other possible interactions with specific medications have not been investigated.

○ **Stavudine** (d4T, Zerit) is a reverse transcriptase inhibitor that requires intracellular activation for its antiretroviral activity. It is indicated in advanced HIV disease when patients have become resistant or profoundly toxic with prolonged zidovudine exposure.

CONTRAINDICATIONS AND PRECAUTIONS Because bone marrow suppression is more common with this agent than others, it is administered cautiously to patients who have experienced profound bone marrow suppression from other antiretroviral therapies.

ADVERSE EFFECTS The most common adverse effects are headache, insomnia, nausea, diarrhea, granulocytopenia, fever, and rash.

INTERACTIONS No interactions are known at this time.

○ **Lamivudine** (3TC, Epivir) is a reverse transcriptase inhibitor that has a more specific action on reverse transcriptase codons. Lamivudine is only the second drug (after AZT) to be approved for initial therapy. This specificity enhances the risk of resistance if used as monotherapy, but makes it an ideal agent when used concomitantly with a more generally active agent such as zidovudine. Lamuvudine has the same contraindications and precautions as other reverse transcriptase inhibitors. Its major adverse effect is peripheral neuropathy, but it does not appear to enhance toxicity when administered with zidovudine. Other clinical information regarding adverse effects and interactions is not available at this time.

NONNUCLEOSIDE REVERSE TRANSCRIPTASE INHIBITORS (NNRTI)

These chemically distinct compounds directly bind to the functional enzyme complex of reverse transcriptase and act to inhibit polymerization and replacement of normal cell RNA. These agents have activity only against HIV-1, leading to development of viral mutants of the HIV-2 variety. Although extensive evaluation of nevirapine and delavirdine have been underway, no medications in this category have yet been licensed by the Food and Drug Administration.

PROTEASE INHIBITORS

Protease inhibitors used to manage HIV include **Saquinavir (SQV, Invirase)**, ritonavir **(Norvir)**, and **indinavir (Crixivan)**.

ACTION

After HIV initially incorporates itself into the cell's DNA, it remains dormant until the infected cell is activated. The initialized viral DNA becomes transcribed into messenger RNA and creates viral specific proteases that create viral proteins. The antiretroviral protease inhibitors block the formation of viral protein, stopping the viral replication process. These chemically distinct compounds are extraordinarily specific for HIV-1, but not HIV-2.

USES

Because these drugs are specific protease inhibitors that theoretically increase the risk of resistant viral mutants, these agents are best for patients with advanced disease who are heavily pretreated with reverse transcriptase inhibitors. These drugs can reduce the viral load to a point where it is undetectable in the blood.

CONTRAINDICATIONS AND PRECAUTIONS

There are no identified contraindications or precautions at this time, but these agents are not recommended for use with children or pregnant or lactating women. Cross-resistance between protease inhibitors has been noted, encouraging the use of combination therapy with reverse transcriptase agents.

ADVERSE EFFECTS

Gastrointestinal discomfort in the form of nausea, vomiting, diarrhea, or abdominal cramping are the primary adverse effects of these agents. Elevated hepatic transaminases and asymptomatic hyperbilirubinemia have also been reported.

INTERACTIONS

Rifampin and rifabutin decrease blood levels of all protease inhibitors. *Mycobacterium* prophylaxis is changed from rifabutin to clarithromycin when patients are receiving protease inhibitors.

○ **Saquinavir** (SQV, Invirase) has been used as either monotherapy in patients with CD4 counts less than 100 cells per mm^3 and in combination with zidovudine. It is licensed for treatment of advanced HIV disease in combination with a reverse transcriptase agent. Precautions, adverse effects, and interactions are as defined in the general drug category.

INTERACTIONS Saquinavir blood levels may be reduced if given with phenobarbital, phenytoin, dexamethasone, or carbamazepine. Saquinavir levels are increased by ketoconazole and itraconazole. When given with terfenadine, astemizole, cisapride, calcium channel blockers, and quinidine, these drug levels may be increased and enhance their arrythmogenicity or sedation properties. Levels of clindamycin, dapsone, and triazolam are also increased when given with saquinavir.

○ **Ritonavir** (Norvir) has been used both alone and in combination with reverse transcriptase inhibitors for treatment of advanced HIV disease. In patients with fewer than 100 CD4 cells per mm^3, there is demonstrated prolongation of life and delayed disease progression (Hirsch, 1996).

INTERACTIONS Significant increases in plasma concentrations of the following medications prohibit concurrent administration: amiodarone, alprazolam, astemizole, bepridil, bupropion, cisapride, clorazepate, clozapine, diazepam, encainide, estazolam, flurazepam, flecainide, meperidine, midazolam, propoxyphene, propafenone, quinidine, piroxicam, rifabutin, terfenadine, triazolam, and zolpidem.

○ **Indinavir** (Crixivan) has been used both alone and in combination with reverse transcriptase inhibitors for treatment of advanced HIV disease. In patients with fewer than 100 CD4 cells per mm^3, delayed disease progression and prolonged survival have been demonstrated (Hirsch, 1996).

INTERACTIONS Indinavir coadministered with ketoconazole may result in indinavir level increased 70% or more. When given with astemizole, cisapride, midazolam, terfenadine, or triazolam, these drug levels may be increased and enhance their arrythmogenicity or sedation properties.

IMMUNE MODULATORS

A number of lymphokines known to enhance T-lymphocyte activity or replication have been used to boost immune function, particularly in asymptomatic individuals. Passive transfer of HIV-specific antibody preparations is also under study (Hirsch, 1996). Biologic agents currently under investigation for this purpose include interleukin-2 (IL-2), gamma interferon, thymopentin, thalidomide, and pentoxyfylline (Hirsch, 1996). Initial reports of IL-2 studies demonstrate increased peripheral blood CD4 cell counts.

USING THE NURSING PROCESS

ASSESSMENT

Assessment of patients receiving antiretroviral therapy involves constant assessment for HIV disease response or progression as well as toxicities of therapy. Table 61–5 suggests assessment data that must be collected and shows how to apply other steps of the nursing process for these patients.

- Provide emotional support for patients undergoing therapy; responses often take weeks. Responses may be seen as reduction in the patient's symptoms (e.g., Kaposi's lesions) or an improvement in an opportunistic infection. Patients who are unresponsive to one agent are changed to another or a combination of agents.
- Assess patients for complications of HIV infection (neurologic disease, opportunistic infection, cancers) throughout antiretroviral therapy.
- Ongoing assessment includes frequent neurologic, respiratory, GI, and integumentary assessments.
  - Because of the high incidence of AIDS-related neurologic disease as well as defined neurotoxicities of antiretroviral agents, neurologic assessment includes parameters that will detect brain stem dysfunction as well as cognitive impairment. Components of the neurologic exam include response to voice and painful stimuli, alertness and orientation, motor strength and appropriateness of activity, short-term memory, ability to follow complex commands, reasoning ability, calculation ability, and peripheral sensation.

    Enlist the assistance of family members who are good sources for knowledge of the patient's personality. They can detect subtle changes that may

Table 61–5. NURSING PROCESS FOR PATIENT REQUIRING ANTIRETROVIRAL MEDICATIONS

Assessment

Assess AIDS classification—current presentation, existence of AIDS dementia.
Assess CD4 lymphocyte count.
Assess history of bone marrow suppression, pancreatitis, and gallbladder disease.
Assess current medications.
Assess history of mental illness, AIDS dementia, depression, anxiety; how patient resolved distress.
Assess baseline neurologic, GI, and hematologic status.
Assess renal and hepatic function.

Nursing Diagnosis: Sensory-Perceptual Alterations (Peripheral Neuropathies)

Desired Outcomes/Evaluation Criteria

Does not have complaints of pain. Exercises safety precautions appropriate to decreased peripheral sensation in performing ADl.

Nursing Actions	**Rationale**
Discuss safety precautions for patients with decreased peripheral sensation.	Patients can injure themselves without being aware of it.
Assist with walking as needed.	Peripheral neuropathies alter ability to walk with a normal gait.
Encourage zippers or snaps rather than buttons.	Zippers and snaps are easier for the patient to manage independently.
Provide pain medications as needed.	Numbness, tingling, and shooting pains from peripheral neuropathies may be severe enough to require medication.
Keep covers off of feet if sensitive.	Feet are often sensitive to touch.

Nursing Diagnosis: Risk for Infection

Desired Outcomes/Evaluation Criteria

Is afebrile. Reports no symptoms of infection.

Nursing Actions	**Rationale**
Monitor temperature often.	Provides early symptom of infection.
Observe skin, mucous membranes, orifices for signs and symptoms infection.	Infection is most likely to occur in orifices and at breaks in barrier integrity.
Identify specific times at risk for infection through WBC counts.	Patient risks of infection depend in part on severity of neutropenia; awareness of patient's CBC assists in nursing actions and patient education to protect against infection.
Avoid exposure to infectious diseases when leukopenic.	Prevents acquisition of community infectious illnesses.

Nursing Diagnosis: Altered Nutrition, less than body requirements

Desired Outcomes/Evaluation Criteria

Calculated nutritional needs are met by meals and planned supplementation. Denies nausea, vomiting, abdominal pain, distention, diarrhea. Normal amylase and lipase levels.

Nursing Actions	**Rationale**
Assess abdomen often for tenderness, distention.	Helps to detect pancreatitis or bowel infections.
Monitor amylase, lipase as ordered.	Detects laboratory evidence of pancreatitis.
Administer antiemetics as ordered.	Helps to counteract potential nausea, vomiting.
Encourage small, frequent feedings.	Helps to enhance nutrition and counteract nausea/vomiting.
Reduce aromatic meals.	Helps to reduce nausea/vomiting.
Encourage diversional activities.	Helps to decrease awareness of GI distress.
Supplement nutrient intake with vitamins, special high protein and high calorie supplements.	Enhance nutritional balance.
Administer antidiarrheal agents as ordered.	Diarrhea causes fluid and electrolyte depletion that can lead to malnutrition.
Weigh patient periodically.	Body weight reflects overall nutritional status.

Other Suggested Nursing Diagnoses: Altered Thought Processes; Impaired Gas Exchange; Decreased Cardiac Output; Pain; Altered Oral Mucous Membranes; Diarrhea; Activity Intolerance; Fatigue; Dysfunctional Grieving

DELIVERING HOME HEALTH CARE

Antiretroviral Therapy

Most patients with HIV infection will receive antiretroviral drugs sometime within the course of their illness, and many will take them for almost the entire duration of their 3- to 10-year illness. Because the disease process and other concomitant medications display similar clinical findings, careful nursing evaluation during therapy is essential. Each medication has specific considerations and common as well as unique adverse effects.

Once started, patients receive antiretroviral therapy for the duration of their illness. Prescription plans, Medicaid, and Medicare usually provide coverage for these medications; however, patients without a prescription plan may obtain free medications through clinical trial participation or via special support services with the pharmaceutical company. Most antiretroviral therapy is initiated in the ambulatory setting, but ongoing monitoring, drug changes, and dose adjustments may be directed by phone and require home-care follow-up. Key nursing implications include the following guidelines.

GENERAL GUIDELINES IN CARING FOR PATIENTS TAKING ANTIRETROVIRAL AGENTS:

- It is essential for the patient to take all doses to prevent the HIV virus from entering the white blood cells.
- Each medication has special recommendations for administration that will affect absorption. Provide patient and family education on how to take as directed.

GUIDELINES FOR ADVERSE EFFECT MONITORING:

- Antiretroviral agents can cause bone marrow suppression. Assess the patient for the following:
  - Anemia—tachycardia, hypotension, full and bounding pulses, hypothermia, cold intolerance, pallor, palmar erythema
    - Bleeding—petichiae, ecchymoses, bleeding or oozing mucous membranes, gums that bleed easily with toothbrushing, dark or tarry stools
  - Infection—fever, subnormal temperature, chills or rigors, pain or erythema of a localized area, cloudy urine, diarrhea, foul odor to stool, crackles on breath sound auscultation, low diastolic blood pressure
- Pancreatitis is a rare but life-threatening complication of several antiretroviral agents. Report epigastric or abdominal pain, especially if it is worst after eating fatty foods.
- Peripheral neuropathies are common with some antiretroviral agents. Patients will have limited peripheral sensation and be at risk for injury. With each home visit:
  - Assess the safety of the home—be certain small or sharp objects are not on the floor, remove throw rugs without a rubber backing, look for sharp edges or projecting objects in the household.
  - Teach strategies to prevent injury—wearing slippers for walking, always using a potholder for stovetop cooking, using an elbow to check the temperature of bath water, purchasing clothes that do not require small buttoning (use zippers or Velcro closures).
  - Assess for the presence of significant symptoms—difficulty with fine motor movements like buttoning shirts, reduced sensation of the feet or fingers.

indicate neurologic impairment before health-care providers.
  - Perform respiratory assessment to detect clues of the presence of respiratory infection or drug-related congestive heart failure.
  - Perform GI assessment for diarrhea, abdominal pain, abdominal distension that may indicate infection, tumor-induced bowel obstruction, and drug intolerances.
  - Assess nutrient intake and tolerance, presence of nausea or vomiting (thalidomide is being studied to improve appetite and weight gain), characteristics of stool elimination patterns, and the status of bowel sounds. These are important parameters that reflect nutritional adequacy.
  - Frequently assess the skin and mucous membranes for infection, adverse drug reactions, and dermatologic presentation of Kaposi's sarcoma and lymphoma. Have all rashes and skin lesions further evaluated by expert clinicians to determine if a skin biopsy is indicated.
- Assist in monitoring of essential laboratory tests reflecting disease or drug toxicity. Laboratory tests for hepatic dysfunction (bilirubin, transaminase levels);

bowel inflammation (amylase or lipase level); electrolyte (blood chemistries) balance; and stool cultures are ordered first.
- Measure intake and output and weigh patient frequently to monitor for renal dysfunction; antiretroviral metabolites are cleared through the kidneys.
- Perform blood urea nitrogen and creatinine at least every 1 to 2 months to monitor for renal compromise.
- Monitor for concomitant administration of other agents known to cause peripheral neuropathies, which may increase the occurrence of this adverse effect. Particular care should be taken if the patient is also receiving aminoglycosides, amphotericin-B, chloramphenicol, cisplatin, dapsone, disulfiram, ethionamide, foscarnet, metronidazole, nitrofurantoin, phenytoin, ribavirin, and vinca alkaloid chemotherapy agents.
- Monitor for concomitant administration of other agents with bone marrow–suppressing qualities such as the following: allopurinol, amphotericin-B, cancer chemotherapeutic agents, dapsone, flucytosine, gancyclovir, histamine blockers, nonsteroidal anti-inflammatory agents (NSAIDs), pentamidine, salicylates, and steroids.

NURSING DIAGNOSIS

Nursing diagnoses for patients receiving antiretroviral agents are similar to those for patients with HIV who are not receiving antiretrovirals; however, some specific nursing problems associated with the pharmacologic agents exist.

▼ **CLINICAL ALERT**

The side effects of these medications are similar to manifestations of the disease itself.

The most common nursing diagnoses are as follows: Sensory-Perceptual Alterations; Risk for infection; and Altered Nutrition, Less than Body Requirements (see Table 61–5).

PLANNING AND INTERVENTION

Nurses caring for the patient receiving antiretroviral agents should be well aware of the patient's personal history and health status. Patient teaching information is provided in Table 61–6.

- Review recent laboratory tests and all medications with the patient on every office visit or weekly when hospitalized.
- Review new symptoms and concerns at every visit to identify potential interactions and nonessential medications that can be discontinued. Patients receiving antiretroviral therapy should have all other nonessential medications discontinued to reduce potential interactions or cumulative side effects.
- Protect the patient against infectious complications regardless of therapy status. Implement institutional standards for care of the immunocompromised patient. Encourage meticulous hygiene measures.
- Plan nursing care or assist the patient to stagger activity to conserve energy and reduce oxygena-

tion demands when antiretroviral treatment causes anemia.
- Anti-HIV agents do not reduce the infectiousness of the patient; hence universal precautions and safe sexual practices should be reinforced with patients, families, and friends.
- Use a variety of teaching methods with written reinforcement to educate the patient and family about antiretroviral therapy.
- An abdominal flat-plate x-ray film can show bowel obstruction, paralytic ileus, bowel perforation, or shifting of abdominal contents. Because tumors of the bowel are an additional risk factor for these patients, a computerized tomography (CT) scan of the abdomen may also be obtained.
- Routine blood work throughout therapy includes complete blood counts (CBCs) at least every 1 to 2 months. Patients with toxicity or marginal bone marrow reserve are likely to have CBCs performed weekly or biweekly.

EVALUATION

Evaluation of the effectiveness of therapy is an ongoing responsibility of all members of the health-care team. A patient is usually provided initial treatment of approximately 8 to 12 weeks to ascertain a response to an agent. If the patient demonstrates disease stabilization, he or she continues antiretroviral therapy for as long as the condition is stable, which could be anywhere from 5 months to 5 or more years. If no clinical or immunologic response is evident, another agent is used. Patients are most likely to become resistant to therapy in the late stages of the illness, when generally all antiretroviral agents fail to halt the destruction of CD4 cells.

- Develop established routines for evaluating toxicities of anti-HIV agents on an individual basis. Single-agent therapy reflects the toxicities associated with that agent. Alternating regimens using zidovudine and didanosine cause different effects than using zidovudine in combination with zalcitabine. A history

---

Table 61–6. PATIENT TEACHING INFORMATION—ANTIRETROVIRAL THERAPY

Dear Patient:
  Your doctor has prescribed a drug to stop the AIDS virus from killing a valuable immune cell in the body called a CD4 cell. This drug prevents the AIDS virus from infecting more cells in your body but does not reverse the infection that has occurred. The name of your drug is _____. Some information that will assist you in caring for yourself while taking this medication is listed below:

☐ 1. Anti-HIV drugs block the virus from infecting more immune cells in your body.
☐ 2. These drugs must be taken exactly on time.
☐ 3. The drug you are taking must be taken at least 2 hours before or after eating.
☐ 4. You may be more prone to infections or bleeding while taking this drug. Regular doctor's visits and blood tests will check for this problem and help the doctor decide when to change the medicine or give you special instructions to prevent problems.
☐ 5. You will still be prone to infections because of the HIV infection; continue all you are presently doing to prevent infection.
☐ 6. Report to your doctor any stomach pain, sick feelings, or trouble eating.
☐ 7. Report to your doctor any trouble feeling with your fingers or toes or pain in the hands or feet.
☐ 8. Practice only protected sex, and/or use only sterile needles, as this medication does not make the virus go away, and you can still pass it to other people.
☐ 9. Other side effects special to this medicine are:
  _____
  _____

  If you have further questions about your medicine or its effects, please feel free to contact the doctor/nurse at _____.

of pancreatitis and peripheral neuropathies is partic-ularly important to note, as these are significant tox-icities of antiretroviral therapy.

- Monitor CD4 counts to detect response to therapy. Reduction in the CD4 count may result in the addi-tion of another agent or changing to a different agent.
- Evaluation of key laboratory tests such as complete blood count, blood chemistry (including blood urea nitrogen and creatinine), and hepatic transaminases provide information about organ dysfunction, re-quiring alteration in the treatment plan.

- Evaluate baseline data, which will assist in defining the nature and frequency of monitoring for adverse reactions. Recognizing the patient's individual risk for adverse and toxic effects is also used to prioritize patient teaching.
- Evaluate the patient's disease status and prescribed medications. These can affect assessment of neuro-logic, GI, and hematologic systems.

The bibliography for this chapter can be found in Ap-pendix B, which begins on page 1054.

CHAPTER REVIEW QUESTIONS*

1. A patient with HIV infection is treated with which category of drugs?
   a. Antifungal.
   b. Antibiotic.
   c. Antiviral.
   d. Antiretroviral.

2. The most common side effect of zidovudine is:
   a. Pancreatitis.
   b. Leukopenia.
   c. Peripheral neuropathies.
   d. Alopecia.

3. A patient taking didanosine for treatment of HIV infection should be taught to:
   a. Take it with antacids.
   b. Take it only with meals.

   c. Take it on an empty stomach.
   d. Mix the medication in solution before taking it.

4. Ms. Smith has recently tested positive for HIV antibodies from probable blood exposure. She is asymptomatic, and her CD4 count is 800 cells per mm^3. The most appropriate treatment at this time is:
   a. Zidovudine.
   b. Zidovudine and zalcitabine.
   c. Observation only.
   d. Didanosine.

5. A contraindication for treatment with reverse transcriptase in-hibitors or protease inhibitors is:
   a. HIV neurologic disease.
   b. Pancreatitis.
   c. Thrombocytopenia.
   d. Active GI infection.

*See Appendix A, which begins on page 1051, for answers.

UNIT 15

DRUGS AFFECTING THE VISUAL, AUDITORY, AND INTEGUMENTARY SYSTEMS

UNIT OUTLINE

CHAPTER 62

Overview of the Anatomy and Physiology of the Eye and Ear

Merrily A. Kuhn, RNC, PhD

CHAPTER OUTLINE

The Eye
The Ear

KEY TERMS

Accommodation reflex
Aqueous humor
Cerumen
Cornea

Sclera
Trabecular meshwork
Tympanic membrane

LEARNING OBJECTIVES

After reading this chapter, the student will be able to:

1. Identify major anatomic structures of the eyes.
2. Explain the function of the refractory media and how vision occurs.
3. Identify major anatomic structures of the ear.
4. Explain the mechanisms of hearing and equilibrium.

This chapter reviews the function of the refractory media, the mechanisms of vision, and the mechanisms of hearing and equilibrium. For a complete review of the anatomy and physiology of the eye and ear, refer to an anatomy and physiology or nursing text.

THE EYE

STRUCTURE OF THE EYE

The eyes, located in the bony cavities or orbits in the anterior cranium, function as the body's organs of vision. The eye is composed of three layers: the outer, middle, and inner, as shown in Figure 62–1. The outer layer consists of the *cornea*, or anterior covering, which is clear and colorless, and the *sclera*, or posterior covering, which is thick and opaque. The highly vascular middle layer is composed of the ciliary body and processes, the iris anteriorly, the lens, and the choroid posteriorly. The ciliary muscles, which form the main part of the ciliary body, are the muscles that increase the visual acuity of the eye by

changing the shape of the lens. The iris (the colored portion of the eye) is a diaphragm with a circular center opening, the pupil, which regulates the amount of light admitted. When a person faces strong light or focuses on a nearby object, the pupil constricts; when the person faces dim light or focuses on a distant object, the pupil dilates to allow more light to enter.

The inner layer of the eyes, the retina, has only a posterior portion. It is composed of several layers of nerve cells that translate the light waves to neural impulses; these are then transmitted via the optic nerve to the brain, which interprets them as sight. The retina contains photoreceptive nerve cells of two types: cones (about 100 million) for daylight and color vision, and rods (about 6 million) for vision at low levels of illumination. Cones are most densely concentrated in the fovea centralis central depression (a small depression in the center of the macula near the center of the retina). The fovea is the portion of the retina where visual acuity is the greatest. The macula is a region located almost exactly at the posterior pole of the eye; it is slightly yellow in appearance. Rods are entirely absent from the fovea and macula, and their num-

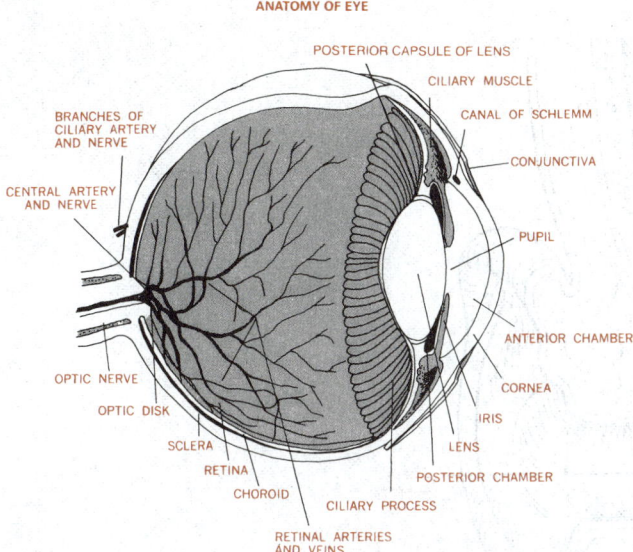

ANATOMY OF EYE

POSTERIOR CAPSULE OF LENS
CILIARY MUSCLE
CANAL OF SCHLEMM
CONJUNCTIVA
PUPIL
ANTERIOR CHAMBER
CORNEA
IRIS
LENS
POSTERIOR CHAMBER
CILIARY PROCESS
RETINAL ARTERIES AND VEINS
CHOROID
RETINA
SCLERA
OPTIC DISK
OPTIC NERVE
CENTRAL ARTERY AND NERVE
BRANCHES OF CILIARY ARTERY AND NERVE

Figure 62–1. Anatomy of eye. (From Thomas, CL [ed]: Taber's Cyclopedic Medical Dictionary, ed 17. FA Davis, Philadelphia, 1993, with permission.)

ber increases in density toward the periphery of the retina. The rods also function as motion detectors.

The anterior chamber of the eye is filled with a watery-clear substance called *aqueous humor*, which is continuously produced by the ciliary body and associated structures at a rate of 2 to 5 mL/min. Figure 62–2 depicts the normal flow of aqueous humor, which transports nutrients to the eye tissues and carries away cellular debris. Aqueous humor enters the anterior chamber to maintain the shape and intraocular pressure within the chamber (normally 12 to 25 mm Hg). Aqueous humor is formed by the ciliary processes in much the same manner as cerebrospinal fluid is formed by the choroid plexus. The ciliary epithelium actively secretes sodium chloride and bicarbonate ions, which, in the presence of carbonic anhydrase (an enzyme that catalyzes the formation of carbonic acid from carbon dioxide and water), promote the osmosis of a large amount of water into the eye.

Aqueous humor furnishes nutritional support to the crystalline (or avascular) lens and cornea. Normally, the same amount of aqueous humor enters the eye as exits it. The aqueous humor flows into the anterior chamber and then enters the *trabecular meshwork*—filtering tissue located in the anterior chamber angle between the periphery of the iris and the cornea—and then the canal of

Schlemm. A thin-walled vein that encircles the eye, the canal of Schlemm conveys the aqueous humor into the venous system.

An increase in the rate of aqueous secretion or resistance to humoral outflow can cause intraocular pressure to increase to 60 mm Hg or more. This leads to the development of glaucoma, permanent atrophy of the optic nerve, and blindness.

MECHANISMS OF VISION

The image enters the eye through the cornea and passes through the aqueous humor in the anterior chamber. The image is then transmitted through the crystalline lens, which is suspended in the eye by suspensory ligaments. The lens is 65% water and 35% protein and changes shape to allow proper focusing of the image. Light rays converge on the lens, are bent, and move into the posterior cavity. In the posterior cavity, the light rays pass through the vitreous humor and are transmitted to the retina.

The eye has several reflexes, some to protect and others to assist in sight. The *accommodation reflex* allows the pupil to become smaller when the gaze shifts from a distant to a closer object. The ciliary muscles controlled by the nervous system also function in accommodation by changing the size of the lens: as a near object is viewed, the ciliary muscles contract, causing the lens to bulge and become more convex; to view a distant object, the ciliary muscle relaxes, allowing the lens to flatten and become less convex. Because the lens can narrow, the refractory power of the eye allows us to see printed matter and other small subject as well as large or distant objects. There is a direct and consensual reflex of both eyes, allowing both eyes to see the same object.

VISION TESTING

Several tests are available to test visual acuity such as the Snellen test and perimetry to examine the extent of the visual field. Eyedrops (mydriatics and cycloplegics) may be instilled into the eye to assist with further examination of the retina. More information on eye testing can be found in medical-surgical texts.

THE EAR

The ears are the organs of hearing and assist with maintaining equilibrium (balance). Each ear is composed of three major divisions: the external, middle, and inner, shown in Figure 62–3.

The external ear has two parts, the auricle (pinna) and the external auditory canal (meatus). The auricle, composed of cartilage and skin, is the protrusion on the side of the head that funnels the sound into the external auditory canal. The external auditory canal is about 1.25 inches long and travels inward, forward, and downward. Modified sweat glands within the canal secrete *cerumen* (earwax), which lubricates the canal lining and traps foreign material. Cerumen also helps to prevent bacterial overgrowth. The canal ends at the *tympanic membrane*

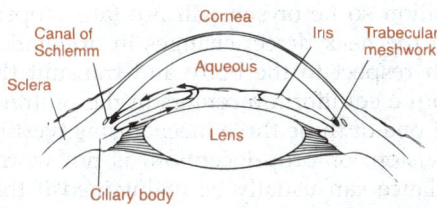

Cornea
Canal of Schlemm
Iris
Trabecular meshwork
Aqueous
Sclera
Lens
Ciliary body

Figure 62–2. Normal flow of aqueous humor. Aqueous humor is produced in the ciliary body and flows through anterior chamber and out the canal of Schlemm.

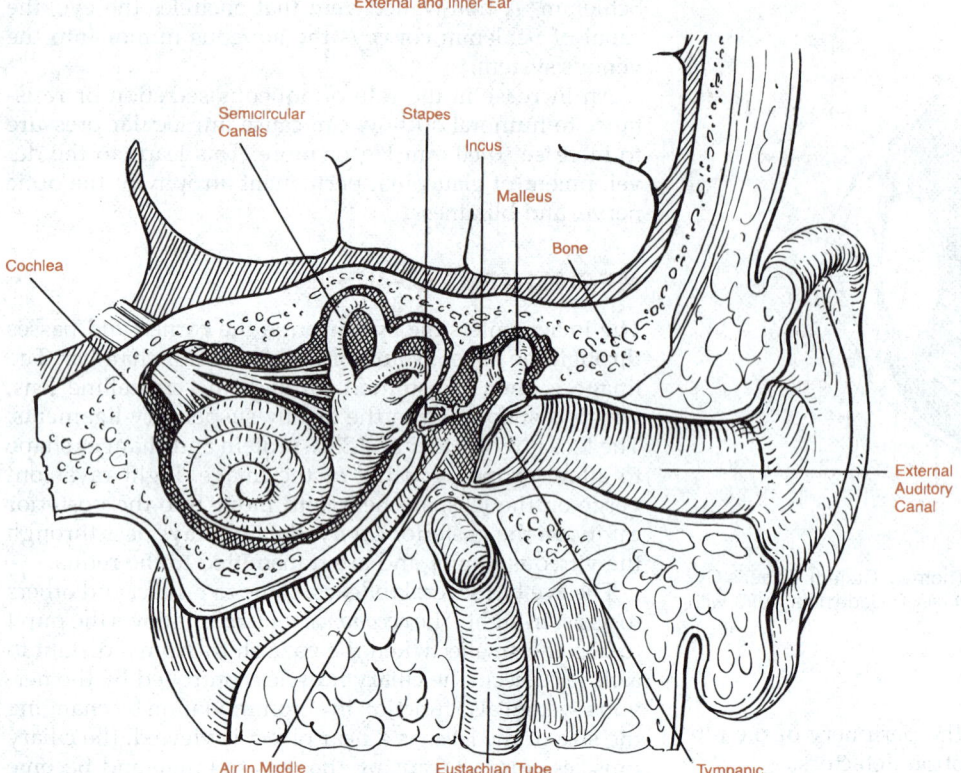

External and Inner Ear

Semicircular Canals

Stapes

Incus

Malleus

Bone

Cochlea

External Auditory Canal

Air in Middle Ear Area

Eustachian Tube (Leading to Pharynx)

Tympanic Membrane

Figure 62–3. External and inner ear. (From Thomas, CL [ed]: Taber's Cyclopedic Medical Dictionary, ed 16. FA Davis, Philadelphia, 1989, with permission.)

(eardrum), which separates the external ear from the middle ear.

The middle ear, or tympanic cavity, is a hollowed-out area of the temporal bone that contains auditory ossicles (bones): malleus (hammer), incus (anvil), and stapes (stirrup). The malleus is attached to the tympanic membrane and to the incus. The incus is connected to the stapes, which, in turn, fits through the oval window and attaches to a small area in the cochlea. The eustachian tube connects the middle ear area with the nasopharynx and serves to equalize air pressure and provide drainage. The round window, below the oval window, permits the cochlea to bulge slightly into the middle ear area as the stapes vibrates the cochlear membrane.

The inner ear consists of the cochlea, the semicircular canals, and the vestibule. The vestibule contains the suspended utricle and saccule separated by perilymphatic fluid. It opens into the oval and round windows, the cochlea, and the semicircular canals.

The cochlea contains the organ of Corti, the hearing sense organ. The cells of this organ have tiny hairlike strands (cilia) that protrude into the fluid of the cochlea. The three bony semicircular canals house the membranous semicircular canals and are separated from them by perilymphatic fluid.

The eighth cranial nerve travels to the temporal lobe of the cerebral cortex from the ear in two branches. The cochlear division, originating in the cochlea (in the organ of Corti), is responsible for hearing impulses. The vestibular division, originating in the vestibule and the semicircular canals, transmits messages to the brain that assist with postural adjustments (maintain balance).

Hearing is accomplished by sound waves moving through the air in the auditory canal, causing the tympanic membrane and auditory ossicles to vibrate. The cochlea is stimulated by the vibration. The cilia of the organ of Corti send the impulse to the brain along the acoustic nerve to the temporal lobes of the cerebral cortex for interpretation.

MECHANISMS OF EQUILIBRIUM

Equilibrium is maintained by automatic shifts of tone in the muscles from one side of the body to the other, or forward and backward, in accordance with various signals arriving from the vestibular apparatus, the eyes, and the proprioceptors. Visual images help the person to maintain equilibrium by simple visual detection of the upright stance. Any slight linear or angular movement of the body instantaneously shifts the visual images to the retina, which then relays impulses to the equilibrium center. Therefore, optic information is similar to that processed by the semicircular canals and can help equilibrium centers predict that the person will need to correct body position so he or she will not fall. Proprioceptive centers in the neck detect changes in orientation of the head with respect to the body and transmit this information to the equilibrium centers in the central nervous system. If one of these three mechanisms (vestibular apparatus, vision, or proprioception) is not working correctly, balance can usually be maintained if the person performs all movements slowly.

The bibliography for this chapter can be found in Appendix B, which begins on page 1054.

CHAPTER REVIEW QUESTIONS*

1. The refractory mechanism occurs through which *correct* sequence to focus light rays on the retina?
   a. Lens, cornea, vitreous humor, aqueous humor.
   b. Aqueous humor, cornea, vitreous humor, lens.
   c. Cornea, aqueous humor, lens, vitreous humor.
   d. Cornea, vitreous humor, lens, aqueous humor.

2. Normal intraocular pressure is:
   a. 12 to 25 mm Hg.
   b. 50 to 60 mm Hg.
   c. 2 to 10 mm Hg.
   d. 30 to 46 mm Hg.

*See Appendix A, which begins on page 1051, for answers.

3. Which of the following statements is *correct* regarding the aqueous humor?
   a. It is found in the posterior chamber of the eye.
   b. Aqueous humor is continually produced by the choroid plexus.
   c. It furnishes nutritional support to the iris and retina.
   d. Aqueous humor maintains intraocular pressure in the eye.

4. The function of the eustachian tube is to:
   a. Direct sound waves into the inner ear.
   b. Equalize air pressure in the middle ear.
   c. Secrete lubrication for the auditory canal.
   d. Vibrate against the tympanic membrane.

CHAPTER 63

Medications Used in Eye Disorders

Merrily A. Kuhn, RNC, PhD

CHAPTER OUTLINE

KEY TERMS

Cycloplegics
Esotropia
Iontophoresis
Miosis
Miotic
Mydriasis

Mydriatic
Retrobulbar injection
Strabismus
Trabeculoplasty
Vagotonia

LEARNING OBJECTIVES

After reading this chapter, the student will be able to:

1. Identify those medications commonly used for eye disorders.
2. Differentiate among the medications used for eye disorders as to mechanism of action, route of administration, pharmacokinetics, adverse effects, contraindications, and interactions.
3. Identify specific areas to assess in the patient requiring medications for eye disorders to formulate appropriate patient outcomes.
4. Plan the nursing interventions necessary to administer medications for eye disorders and choose appropriate teaching strategies to gain patient compliance.
5. Evaluate the patient at various stages of treatment to measure the effectiveness of nursing interventions.

More than half of the world's population has eye problems. Although many conditions are correctable with eyeglasses or contact lenses, others require medication to control or treat. Antibacterial, anti-inflammatory, antifungal, and antiviral agents are often used to treat inflammatory eye disorders. Topical anesthetics are used either to allow examination of the eye or to enable surgical operations to be performed on the eye. *Mydriatics* are used to dilate the pupil during eye examinations and *cycloplegics* to paralyze the ciliary muscle of the eye and prevent accommodation. Lubricants are sometimes needed to replace tears or to prevent damage to the cornea when blinking is absent. *Miotics* (drugs that constrict the pupil with cholinergic action), sympathomimetic medications, carbonic anhydrase inhibitors, and osmotic agents are used to treat and control glaucoma, which is featured in Table 63–1. Ocular medications are most often administered topically as sterile solutions, ointments, or conjunc-

Table 63–1. COMPARISON OF GLAUCOMAS		
	Open-Angle Glaucoma	**Narrow-Angle Glaucoma**
Incidence	Most common.	Least common.
Etiology	Diabetes, severe myopia.	Trauma, inflammation, papillary dilatation.
Pathophysiology	Clogging of trabecular meshwork with tissue debris.	Anterior chamber is too tight for aqueous humor to flow freely through it.
Progression	Slowly, usually in both eyes simultaneously.	Quickly, often a medical emergency, occurs in one eye only.
Vision loss	Peripheral is lost first, followed by precise central vision. Blindness develops in months or years.	Blindness can occur in 3 to 5 days.
Treatment	Medications: miotics, beta-blockers, diuretics, mydriatics. Surgery.	Medications: diuretics. Surgery: cryosurgery, laser surgery.

tival inserts and are easy to instill into the eye. Although ointments remain in contact with the eye longer than solutions, they leave a film over the eye that may interfere with vision. On the other hand, solutions may be responsible for a higher incidence of contact dermatitis than ointments, as they are more likely to contain preservatives and other common sensitizers. Less frequently, ocular medications may be administered through the application of packs; administered by *iontophoresis* (administration of drugs via an electrical current); subconjunctival or *retrobulbar injection* (injection of drugs behind the eyeball); or injection directly into either eye chamber.

Most eye medications are discussed in other chapters of this book and are reviewed only briefly with their usual ophthalmic dosages. This chapter discusses in detail the diagnostic aids, miotics, mydriatics, cycloplegics, lubricants, and topical anesthetics.

DIAGNOSTIC AIDS

Several preparations—**fluorescein sodium (AK-Fluor, Fluorescite), fluorexon (Fluoresoft), rose bengal (Rosets),** and **tear test strips (Sno-Strips)**—are available for diagnostic purposes. Other groups of medications are also used in diagnosing problems of the eye, including mydriatics and cycloplegics.

○ **Fluorescein sodium** (AK-Fluor, Fluorescite, and others), a nontoxic water-soluble dye, can be applied to the cornea of the eye. The dye stains denuded areas of epithelium such as scratches a bright green color, whereas foreign bodies in the eye are surrounded by a green ring. Areas having a loss of conjunctiva are stained yellow. The staining of the eye disappears in about 30 minutes. If the nasolacrimal drainage system is patent, the dye that has been instilled in the eye appears in the nasal secretions. Fluorescein sodium is also used to fit hard contact lenses, to test lacrimal patency, and to identify defects in retinal pigment epithelium in retinal photography.

Solutions of fluorescein are easily contaminated with *Pseudomonas aeruginosa*, so the dye is impregnated onto strips of dry filter paper (Fluor-I-Strip—9 mg; Flu-Glo—0.6 mg; Fluoret—1 mg). The filter paper is moistened with a sterile solution and is then gently brought into contact with the conjunctiva, allowing the dye to disperse.

Other diagnostic products are Fluress and Fluoracaine, which combine fluorescein and a local anesthetic. One drop of a 0.25% solution can facilitate removal of foreign bodies from the eye.

○ **Fluorexon** (Fluoresoft) is a fluourescent solution (0.35%) used to fit soft (hydrogel) contact lenses because it has less than a 55% water content and does not stain soft lenses. The lens should be washed with saline after fluorexon use.

○ **Rose bengal** (Rosets) is a dye that stains dead or degenerated epithelial cells (1 to 3 mg strips). It is used for routine ocular exams or when superficial corneal or conjunctival tissue change is suspected.

○ **Tear test strips** (Sno-Strips) are used in the eye before any topical medication (especially an anesthetic) is administered or other procedures are carried out, particularly manipulation of the eyelids.

When any of these staining agents are used topically, the patient is told that these agents may be irritating and cause discomfort and staining of the eye and skin around the eye for a short time. The skin staining can be washed off with mild soap and water.

ANTI-INFECTIVE DRUGS

Anti-infective agents may be administered systemically or locally in the form of drops, ointments, packs, corneal baths, or even injections into the anterior chamber. Eye infections require prompt treatment to prevent the spread of infection and damage to the eye, which can result in impaired vision.

The causative organisms are identified when possible, but treatment should not be withheld while awaiting results of a culture or smear. Table 63–2 features a selection of the commonly used antibacterial (effective against most gram-positive and gram-negative organisms), antifungal, and antiviral agents used in treating eye disorders. Many anti-infectives are also available in combination with each other or with other groups of medications, such as steroids and decongestants. The table identifies the general indications and usual doses for topical conjunctival, parenteral, and intravenous dosages when applicable, as well as nursing implications. Although most anti-infectives do not penetrate the eye when given systemically, a few anti-infectives are capable of penetration when the blood–aqueous humor barrier is weakened by inflammation or injury.

Table 63–2. OPHTHALMIC ANTIBACTERIAL, ANTIFUNGAL, AND ANTIVIRAL AGENTS

ORGANISMS COVERED	STRENGTH/DOSAGE	NURSING IMPLICATIONS
ANTIBACTERIAL AGENTS		
all antibacterial agents		
	No more than 20 mL should be prescribed initially, and prescription should not be refilled without consultation with physician.	**ASSESSMENT:** Assess for prior hypersensitivity. Assess history of symptoms, previous drug hypersensitivity. Carefully assess local (contact dermatitis) and other systemic reactions. **INTERVENTION:** Tilt head back, place medication in conjunctival sac, and close eye. Apply light finger pressure on the lacrimal sac for 1 min following instillation. Keep medications sterile. Avoid touching application tip to reduce contamination. Administer only as directed. Administer correct vehicle—ointment or liquid. **EVALUATION:** Notify physician if stinging, burning, or itching becomes pronounced or if redness, irritation, swelling, or pain persists.
bacitracin (Bacitracin Ophthalmic)		
Gram-positive; gonorrheal	500 units bacitracing/g. **Subconjunctival:** ¼″ ointment 1–3 times daily.	
gentamicin sulfate (Gentacidin) (Gentamicin) (Gent-AK)		
Gram-positive; gram-negative	**Topical:** 1 gtt 0.3% solution q 1–4 hr; ointment q 3–4 hr. **Subconjunctival:** 10–30 mg in 0.5 mL aqueous solution.	Same as for all.
neomycin sulfate (Myciguent)		
Gram-positive; gram-negative	**Topical:** ointment 3–4 times/day. **Subconjunctival:** 100–500 mg in 0.5 mL isotonic NaCl.	Same as for all plus: **INTERVENTION:** May be absorbed through eyes following topical application.
sulfacetamide sodium (Sulamyd) (AK-Sulf)		
Gram-positive; gram-negative	**Topical:** 1–2 gtt 10%, 15%, or 30% solution q 2–3 hr.	**ASSESSMENT:** Assess for prior hypersensitivity. **INTERVENTION:** May cause sensitivity to bright lights; minimized by wearing sunglasses. **EVALUATION:** Do not discontinue without consulting physician. Notify physician if no improvement in 7–8 days or if condition worsens.
tobramycin (Tobrex)		
Gram-positive; gram-negative	**Topical:** 0.3% solution 3–4 times/day; ointment hs.	Same as for all plus: **INTERVENTION:** May be absorbed through eyes following topical application.
ANTIFUNGAL AGENTS		
natamycin (Natacyn)		
Fungi (*Candida, Asperigillus, Cephalosporium, Fusarium,* and *Penicillium* species)	**Topical:** 1 gtt of 5% solution q 1–2 hr.	**ASSESSMENT:** Carefully note local (contact dermatitis) and systemic reaction. **INTERVENTION:** Keep medications sterile. Administer only as directed. Avoid exposure of medication to excessive light and heat. Shake well before use. **EVALUATION:** If not effective after 7–10 days, the infection is likely not sensitive to this agent.

Continued on the following page

Table 63–2. OPHTHALMIC ANTIBACTERIAL, ANTIFUNGAL, AND ANTIVIRAL AGENTS, *Continued*

ORGANISMS COVERED	STRENGTH/DOSAGE	NURSING IMPLICATIONS
ANTIVIRAL AGENTS		
idoxuridine (IDU) (Herplex) (Stoxil)		
Herpes simplex keratoconjunctivitis (some strains of herpes simplex are resistant to idoxuridine)	**Topical:** ointment 0.5% q 4 hr; solution 1 gtt 0.1% q 1–2 hr daily and q 2–4 hr nightly.	For all antiviral medications: **ASSESSMENT:** Assess for prior hypersensitivity and pregnancy. Use cautiously. **INTERVENTION:** Carefully note local (contact dermatitis) and systemic reactions. Keep medications sterile. Administer only as directed. Administer correct vehicle— ointment or liquid. Do not mix with other medication. To prevent recurrence of herpes, medication should be administered for 5–7 days after healing has occurred. Improvement usually occurs in 7–8 days and may continue up to 21 days. **Patient Teaching**—Warn patient to wear dark glasses because idoxuridine may cause photosensitivity. **EVALUATION:** If no improvement in 7 days or if pain, burning, or irritation occurs, notify physician.
vidarabine (Adenine arabinoside) (Ara-A) (Vira-A)		
Herpes simplex types 1 and 2, idoxuridine-resistant herpes, varicella and varicella zoster.	**Topical:** solution 3%, 2–4 qtt q 1–2 hr.	Same as for all.
trifluridine (Viroptic)		
Herpes simplex I and II, keratoconjunctivitis, idoxuridine-resistant herpes.	**Topical:** solution 1%, 1 gtt 2–4 hr (maximum daily dose 9 gtt).	Same as for all plus: **INTERVENTION:** Drop medicine on lower lid while looking up. Release lower lid. Keep eye open and do not blink for at least 30 sec. Wait 5 min before using other drops. Do not blink more than usual.

Topical application is often the route of choice for ophthalmic drugs. This route is selected to decrease the risk of systemic side effects and toxicities or because the medication used is rarely or never administered systemically.

▼ CLINICAL ALERT

Topical application of ophthalmic drugs is more likely to result in local inflammation than other routes and can sensitize the patient to that particular preparation.

CONTRAINDICATIONS AND PRECAUTIONS

Antibiotics are contraindicated in persons hypersensitive to a component of the product. Antibiotics are contraindicated in epithelial herpes simplex keratitis, vaccinia, and varicella as these conditions may worsen.

ADVERSE EFFECTS

In general, side effects experienced by patients receiving topical anti-infective drugs include local skin and eye irritation and conjunctivitis.

ANTI-INFLAMMATORY DRUGS

The eye structures, because they are delicate, may develop functional damage such as scarring and impaired vision occurring secondarily to inflammation. Anti-inflammatory medications—including the nonsteroidal anti-inflammatory drugs and the adrenal corticosteroids in particular—are indicated in certain nonpyogenic inflammatory conditions of the eye to control inflammation and ultimately reduce the amount of permanent scarring and visual loss.

Corticosteroids are most commonly used in acute ocular disorders caused by hypersensitivity or allergic reactions. The most commonly used preparations are **dexamethasone** *(Decadron, Maxidex)*, **fluorometholone** *(FML)*, **prednisolone** *(Econopred, Metreton, Pred-Forte)*, and **rimaxolone** *(Vexol)*, featured in Table 63–3. Corticosteroids used in eye disorders may be administered topically, injected into the eye itself, or used systemically.

▼ CLINICAL ALERT

The eyes are monitored closely for signs of infection because corticosteroids decrease defense mechanisms and

Table 63–3. ANTI-INFLAMMATORY AGENTS USED IN EYE DISORDERS

CORTICOSTEROIDS

TOPICAL DOSAGE	NURSING IMPLICATIONS
dexamethasone (Decadron) and others **0.1% suspension:** 1–2 gtt into conjunctival sac q 1 hr day, q 2 hr night.	For all corticosteroids: **ASSESSMENT:** Carefully assess local (contact dermatitis) fungal infection, acute infections, viral disease, tuberculosis, ocular herpes simplex, all of which are contraindicated, and systemic reactions. **INTERVENTION:** Keep medications sterile. Administer correct vehicle—ointment or liquid. Use only for short periods under close medical supervision. Do not rub eyes because steroids increase bruisability of delicate eye tissue. Administer only as directed. **Patient Teaching**—Advise patient the corticosteroids may cause sensitivity to bright light and to wear dark glasses for protection. **EVALUATION:** Do not discontinue before physician has ordered discontinuation. If no improvement in 7–8 days, or if pain, itching, or swelling occurs, notify physician.
fluorometholone (FML Forte) **0.25% or 0.1% suspension:** 1–2 gtt into conjunctival sac q 1 hr day, q 2 hr night. **0.1% ointment:** Apply thin coat to lower conjuctival sac 3–4 times/day.	Same as for all.
prednisolone acetate (Pred-forte) (Encopred Plus) **1% suspension:** 1–2 gtt into conjunctival sac q 1 hr day, q 2 hr night.	Same as for all.

NONSTEROIDAL ANTI-INFLAMMATORY AGENTS (NSAIDs)

TOPICAL DOSAGE	NURSING IMPLICATIONS
flurbiprofen sodium (Ocufen) **0.03% solution:** 1 gtt q 30 min beginning 2 hr before surgery.	For all nonsteroidal anti-inflammatory agents: **ASSESSMENT:** Assess for abnormal bleeding; systemic absorption may interfere with platelet aggregaton. Assess for hypersensitivity and epithelial herpes, both contraindicated. **INTERVENTION:** Keep medication sterile. **EVALUATION:** Do not discontinue before physician has ordered discontinuation. If no improvement in 7–8 days, or if pain, itching, or swelling occurs, notify physician.
suprofen (Profenal) **1% solution:** 2 gtt 3, 2, and 1 hr before surgery.	Same as for all NSAIDs.
diclofenac sodium (Voltaren) **0.1% solution:** 1 gtt q 4 hr beginning 24 hr after surgery for 2 wk.	Same as for all NSAIDs.
ketorolac tromethamine (Acular) **0.5% solution:** 1 gtt qid. May be used long term without major complication.	Same as for all NSAIDs plus: **INTERVENTION:** One of the most expensive NSAIDs for opthalmic use.

thus reduce resistance to pathogen invasion. Corticosteroids applied topically increase the potential for fungal infections, are related to an increased incidence of glaucoma and cataracts, and may delay wound healing. Because of these complications, they are used for short-term therapy only.

Additional information on corticosteroids can be found in Chapter 44.

The ophthalmic nonsteroidal anti-inflammatory drugs (NSAIDs)—**flurbiprofen sodium (Ocufen), suprofen (Profenal), diclofenac sodium (Voltaren),** and **ketorolac tromethamine (Acular)**—decrease prostaglandin concentrations in the eye, which theoretically might contribute to decreased itching and inflammation. Flurbiprofen sodium (Ocufen) and suprofen (Profenal) are administered from 2 to 3 hours before surgery and are used to decrease intraoperative miosis. Diclofenac sodium (Voltaren) is used postoperatively to decrease inflammation following cataract extraction. Ketorolac (Acular) relieves itching in seasonal allergic conjunctivitis. These drugs have analgesic, antipyretic, and anti-inflammatory properties.

CONTRAINDICATIONS

Anti-inflammatory drugs are contraindicated in patients with hypersensitivity. They are also contraindicated in patients with fungal or viral infections, acute infections, tuberculosis, or ocular herpes simplex because these conditions will worsen.

ADVERSE EFFECTS

Posterior subcapsular cataracts (usually irreversible) may develop. In addition, there may be an increase in intraocular pressure, glaucoma, impaired healing, masked symptoms of infection, and eye irritation. Systemic side effects may occur with prolonged use.

LOCAL ANESTHETICS

Local anesthetics, featured in Table 63–4, inhibit pain sensation, so the eye can be examined, foreign bodies removed, or superficial surgery performed. All of the commonly used topical anesthetics—**tetracaine hydrochloride** *(Pontocaine)* and **proparacaine hydrochloride** *(Ophthaine, Ophthetic)*—produce adequate corneal anesthesia within 13 to 36 seconds and generally have a duration of approximately 15 to 20 minutes. If longer anesthesia is needed, the application can be repeated. Local anesthetics stabilize the neuron so it is less permeable to ions, thus preventing the transmission of nerve impulses.

CONTRAINDICATIONS AND PRECAUTIONS

Local anesthetics are contraindicated in persons with known hypersensitivity. They are administered cautiously to persons with heart disease because they cause sweating, hypotension, dysrhythmia, and even cardiac arrest. They are also administered cautiously to persons with hyperthyroidism as they can cause restlessness, excitement, nausea and vomiting, twitching, convulsions, and therefore exacerbations of hyperthyroidism.

ADVERSE EFFECTS

Patients may complain of temporary stinging, burning, tearing, conjunctival redness, and photophobia due to local irritation.

 CLINICAL ALERT

Local anesthetics can also delay wound healing. Permanent corneal opacification and scarring have been reported with prolonged use.

Central nervous system (CNS) disturbances occasionally occur and are related to systemic absorption of the topical agent.

Table 63–4. ANESTHETICS FOR EYE DISORDERS

TOPICAL DOSAGE	NURSING IMPLICATIONS
proparacaine hydrochloride (Ophthaine) (Ophthetic)	
0.5% solution: 1–2 gtt into conjunctival sac q 1 hr day, q 2 hr night.	For all: **ASSESSMENT:** Carefully assess local (contact dermatitis) and systemic reactions. Assess for hyperthyroidism, cardiac disease, open lesions of eye as these may be contraindicated. **INTERVENTION:** Keep medications sterile. Administer only as directed. Try not to blink more than usual. Warm ointment in hand several min before use. Administration is short term. Generally not given to patient for home use. Place eye patch over eye to protect it from injury. Corneal reflexes return within 1 hr. Before use of other eye drops wait 5 min. Before use of other ointment, wait 10 min. **EVALUATION:** Evaluate for temporary stinging, burning, conjunctival erythema, photophobia, epithelial damage, retardation of healing. Report to physician.
tetracaine hydrochloride (Pontacaine)	
0.5% solution: 1–2 gtt into conjunctival sac q 1 hr day, q 2 hr night. **0.5% ointment:** Apply thin coat to lower conjunctival sac 3–4 times/day.	Same as for all.

LUBRICANTS

Lubricants may be needed by healthy individuals to replace tears or to moisten contact lenses or artificial eyes; by ill individuals with keratitis or neuroparalytic keratitis occurring during unconsciousness; or to protect the eye during surgical or diagnostic procedures. Individuals may lose their blink reflex owing either to anesthesia or to acute or chronic CNS disorders. Lubricants or artificial tears contain balanced amounts of salts to maintain ocular tonicity (0.9% sodium chloride); buffers like boric acid to adjust the pH; viscosity agents like hydroxpropyl methylcellulose or polyvinyl alcohol to prolong eye contact time; and preservatives like benzalkonium chloride, chlorobutanol, and thimerosal to maintain sterility.

○ **Hydroxyropyl methylcellulose products** (Lacril, Isopto Plain, Tears Naturale, and others) are nonirritating and can be used for prolonged periods of time to lubricate the eye. Excessive use may cause the lubricant to dry on the eyes and form sandlike granules. These particles can be washed out with a sterile eye-irrigating solution.

A hydroxypropyl cellulose insert that is placed into the inferior cul-de-sac of the eye is available under the trade name Lacrisert. This insert, which may be inserted once or twice daily, stabilizes and thickens the precorneal tear film and prolongs tear film breakup time. Patients may demonstrate allergies to these products, usually to the preservatives (e.g., thimerosal), such as redness of the eyes, and should refrain from using them. Caution soft contact lens wearers to read labels carefully as some of the products should not be used with soft lenses.

○ **Petrolatum-based ointments** (Artificial tears, Hypotears, Liquifilm tears, and others) are often applied to hard contact lenses to lubricate them before insertion. These lubricating ointments also are added to other eye products to prolong the contact time of topically applied preparations. Many of these lubricants are available over-the-counter (OTC) as drops or ointments.

DECONGESTANTS

Products containing adrenergic drugs such as **naphazoline** (0.01% to 0.03%), **phenylephrine** (0.08% to 0.2%), and **tetrahydrozoline** (0.01% to 0.05%), featured in Table 63–5, may be used to cause constriction of the conjunctival blood vessels. These products may temporarily relieve itching and minor irritation caused by chemical or mechanical irritants or by immediate-type allergic reactions. They are not effective in treating delayed hypersensitivity reaction. The percent following each product is the concentration found to be safe and effective by the FDA Advisory Review Panel on OTC ophthalmic drug products.

▼ CLINICAL ALERT

In the concentration present in OTC products, adrenergic drugs rarely cause serious side effects. However, prolonged or indiscriminate use of this product is avoided, as this can lead to neglect of symptoms of serious eye disease or to rebound vasodilation with increased redness.

Vasoconstrictors are applied topically to the eye (1 to 2 drops every 3 to 4 hours or as needed) until symptoms subside. Local application of decongestant adrenergic drugs may cause browache, headache, blurred vision, irritation, lacrimation, allergic conjunctivitis, and local dermatitis. In patients predisposed to narrow-angle glaucoma, these products may precipitate an acute attack of angle-closure glaucoma.

○ **Naphazoline** (Allerest, Clear Eyes, Opcon), available in OTC and prescription solutions, is used as a topical ocular vasoconstrictor to soothe, refresh, moisturize, and remove redness due to minor eye irritation.

○ **Tetrahydrozoline hydrochloride** (Murine Plus,

Table 63–5. OPHTHALMIC VASOCONSTRICTORS

DRUG NAME/ROUTE AND DOSAGE	PHARMACOKINETICS/ DYNAMICS	NURSING IMPLICATIONS
naphazoline (Clear Eyes) (Nafazair)		
0.012%–0.05% solution (OTC) or 0.025%–0.1% solution (Rx): 1–2 gtt q 3–4 hr	**Onset:** minutes **Duration:** 2–3 hr	For all ophthalmic vasoconstrictors: **ASSESSMENT:** Assess for contact dermatitis. Assess for cause of irritation. Assess for long-standing diabetes, advanced arteriosclerotic heart disease, debilitated or elderly patient with intraocular lens implant (contraindications). **INTERVENTION:** Keep medication sterile.
tetrahydrozoline (Murine Plus) (Visine)		
0.05% solution: 1–2 gtt 2–4 times daily	**Onset:** minutes **Duration:** 2–3 hr	Same as for all.

Visine, Optigene 3), available in OTC products, is used as a topical eye decongestant.

MIOTICS

There are two distinct types of miotics: direct-acting cholinergics and cholinesterase inhibitors. They produce the same effect but differ in their pharmacologic mechanisms. Table 63–6 contains dosages, pharmacokinetics, and nursing implications of selected miotics.

ACTION

Both types of miotics are capable of penetrating the cornea rapidly and completely. Both groups of drugs induce constriction of the pupil *(miosis)*, contraction of the ciliary muscle controlling accommodation, widening of the spaces within the trabecular meshwork, and ultimately cause a fall in intraocular pressure that is associated with decreased resistance to the outflow of aqueous humor.

The direct-acting cholinergic medications—**pilocarpine hydrochloride *(Isopto Carpine, Akarpine, Pilocar)*, pilocarpine nitrate *(Pilagan)*, pilocarpine ocular system *(Ocusert Pilo)*,** and **carbachol *(Miostat)*** —are chemically related to acetylcholine, the chemical mediator of nerve impulse transmission. They are used primarily in the treatment of open-angle glaucoma.

The cholinesterase inhibitors, **isoflurophate *(Floropryl)*, physostigmine *(Eserine)*, demecarium *(Humorsol)*,** and **echothiophate *(Phospholine)*,** are also used in the treatment of open-angle glaucoma and are effective in treating *strabismus* (eye disorder in which optic axes cannot be directed to the same object). The cholinesterase-inhibitor miotics inhibit cholinesterase, an enzyme that destroys acetylcholine, thereby leaving acetylcholine free to act on the ciliary muscle and iris sphincter, causing pupil constriction and spasm of accommodation. When cholinesterase is inhibited, the destruction of acetylcholine depends on the synthesis of new enzyme or eventual diffusion away from the action site. The cholinesterase inhibitors cause more ciliary spasm with discomfort and blurred vision than do the cholinergic miotics. The cholinesterase inhibitors may be short-acting (and reversible) or long-acting (and irreversible). However, even the "irreversible" products eventually wear off.

USES

Miotics are used primarily to lower intraocular pressure in open-angle glaucoma (see Table 63–1). Unless the elevated intraocular pressure in glaucoma is lowered, blood flow to the retina is reduced, resulting in retinal damage and visual field loss.

CONTRAINDICATIONS AND PRECAUTIONS

Both types of miotics are contraindicated in hypersensitivity, secondary forms of glaucoma, and in acute inflammation of the eye. Safety in pregnancy (category C), lactation, and children has not been established. Both types of miotics are administered cautiously to persons with narrow-angle glaucoma because these drugs may precipitate acute-angle closure. It is suggested that cholinesterase-inhibitor miotics be discontinued prior to surgery, as their action can interfere with the breakdown of succinylcholine (a commonly used muscle relaxant), resulting in prolonged muscle paralysis and apnea.

ADVERSE EFFECTS

The miotics cause many local side effects including burning, itching, smarting, and ciliary spasm. There is reduced visual acuity in bright light due to papillary dilation. Systemic side effects can also occur. These include hypertension, tachycardia, pulmonary edema, salivation, nausea, vomiting, diarrhea, lacrimation, and muscle tremor, which are related to the direct cholinergic effect on body tissues.

DIRECT-ACTING CHOLINERGICS

○ **Pilocarpine hydrochloride** (Isopto-Carpine, Akarpine, Pilocar) or **pilocarpine nitrate** (Pilagan) is definitely the preferred miotic for both emergency, initial, and maintenance therapy for open-angle glaucoma. In most persons, particularly those over age 50 who do not have cataracts, pilocarpine is relatively free of undesirable side effects and is better tolerated than other miotics.

ADVERSE EFFECTS In addition to the general miotic side effects, pilocarpine causes side effects in about 80% of all patients. Additional symptoms of conjunctival and ciliary congestion and ocular and periorbital pain rarely persist for more than 2 weeks.

○ **Pilocarpine ocular system** (Ocusert Pilo) is a form of pilocarpine currently available as a clear, flexible, elliptical, waferlike object slightly larger than a hard contact lens, with a white edge for easier visualization. It is inserted into the conjunctival sac for the continuous treatment of open-angle glaucoma. It is available as Ocusert Pilo-20 and Ocusert Pilo-40, releasing pilocarpine at rates of 20 and 40 μg/hour for 1 week, respectively. The nurse may instruct patients to initially insert the Ocusert at bedtime. First it is gently rinsed with tap water to prevent massive initial release of pilocarpine, which results in severe miosis and ciliary body spasm. The initial releasing dose is approximately equal to one drop of a 1%, 2%, or 3% pilocarpine solution depending on the dosage being administered. The Ocusert may be moved digitally from the upper to the lower conjunctival sac if irritation occurs. It continues to release pilocarpine for about 1 week, freeing the patient from frequent medication administration and increasing compliance.

○ **Carbachol** (Isopto Carbachol) is a potent synthetic choline ester, similar to acetylcholine, used to treat open-angle and narrow-angle glaucoma and to produce miosis during surgery. It is effective in lowering intraocular pressure in glaucoma patients who have become refractory or allergic to pilocarpine, or when pilocarpine

Table 63–6. MIOTICS: DIRECT-ACTING CHOLINERGICS AND CHOLINESTERASE INHIBITORS

DRUG NAME/ROUTE AND DOSAGE	PHARMACOKINETICS/ DYNAMICS	NURSING IMPLICATIONS
DIRECT-ACTING CHOLINERGICS		
pilocarpine hydrochloride (Isopto Carpine) (Pilocar) (Akarpine) and others **pilocarpine nitrate** (Pilagan) *0.25%–10% solution:* 1–2 gtt any solution up to 6 times daily. *Gel:* Apply 0.5″ ribbon to lower conjunctival sac.	**Onset:** 10–30 min (miosis); within 60 min (IOP) **Peak:** 30 min (miosis); 75 min (IOP) **Duration:** 4–8 hr (miosis); 4–14 hr (IOP)	For all direct-acting cholinergics: **ASSESSMENT:** Carefully assess local (contact dermatitis) and systemic reactions. Assess for previous hypersensitivity. **INTERVENTION:** Keep medications sterile. Administer only as directed. Administer correct vehicle—ointment or liquid. Apply gentle pressure to the nasolacrimal canal for 102 min after administration to prevent drainage of solution from intended area. Avoid hazardous activities such as driving car or operating heavy equipment because some blurring of vision will occur. Miosis that occurs causes difficulty in dark adaption. May be instilled in both eyes. Patient should not rub or squeeze lids together after administration of medication. Store in tight, light-resistant container away from excessive heat. Patients should wear identification noting they have glaucoma and medications being taken. **EVALUATION:** If stinging and blurring continue, notify physician.
pilocarpine ocular system (Ocusert Pilo-20) (Ocusert Pilo-40) *Adults:* 20 μg/hr for 1 wk or 40 μg/hr for 1 wk.	**Onset:** 1.5–2 hr **Peak:** 6 hr **Duration:** 1 wk	Same as for all. **PATIENT TEACHING:** Always check placement before going to bed and on rising.
carbachol (Miostat) (Isopto Carbachol) *0.75%–3% topical solution:* 1–2 gtt q 6–8 hr. **intraocular surgery** *0.01% solution for injection:* 0.5 mL into anterior chamber before or after securing sutures.	**Onset:** 10–20 min (IOP) **Peak:** 4 hr (IOP) **Duration:** 4–8 hr (miosis); 4 hr (IOP) **Onset:** immediate (miosis) **Peak:** 2–5 min (miosis)	Same as for all.
CHOLINESTERASE INHIBITORS		
physostigmine salicylate (Isopto Eserine) *0.25% ointment or 0.25%–0.5% solution:* 1–2 gtt 4 times daily.	**Onset:** 20–30 min **Peak:** 2–6 hr **Duration:** 12–48 hr	For all cholinesterase inhibitors: **ASSESSMENT:** Assess for local irritation, previous hypersensitivity, glaucoma, and other inflammatory diseases (contraindications). **INTERVENTION:** First dose should be administered by physician and tonometer readings taken at least hourly for 3–4 hr to observe for transient, paradoxic increase in intraocular pressure. Avoid prolonged contact with skin. Bedtime administration may minimize visual side effects. Patients need constant medical supervision while on medication. Ointment is inactivated by water, so tube should be tightly capped between uses. **EVALUATION:** Notify physician if nausea, vomiting, cramps, or prolonged diarrhea occurs.
demecarium bromide (Humorsol) *0.125%–0.25% solution:* 1 gtt q 12–48 hr.	**Onset:** 10 min–1 hr (miosis) **Peak:** 2–4 hr (miosis); 24 hr (IOP) **Duration:** 3–10 days (miosis); 9 days (IOP)	Same as for all.

Continued on the following page

Table 63–6. MIOTICS: DIRECT-ACTING CHOLINERGICS AND CHOLINESTERASE INHIBITORS, *Continued*

DRUG NAME/ROUTE AND DOSAGE	PHARMACOKINETICS/ DYNAMICS	NURSING IMPLICATIONS
CHOLINESTERASE INHIBITORS		
echothiophate iodide (Phospholine Iodide)		
0.03%–0.25% solution: 1 gtt q 12 hr	**Onset:** 10–30 min (miosis) **Peak:** 0.5 hr (miosis); 24 hr (IOP) **Duration:** 1–4 wk (miosis); days–weeks (IOP)	Same as for all.
isoflurophate (Floropryl)		
0.025% ointment: ¼" strip or less q 8–72 hr.	**Onset:** 10–30 min (miosis) **Peak:** 0.5 hr (miosis); 24 hr (IOP) **Duration:** 1–4 wk (miosis); 1 wk (IOP)	Same as for all.

cannot be used. It is more potent and longer acting than pilocarpine because of its slower inactivation by cholinesterase.

Carbachol is also used for single intraocular administration by an ophthalmologist during eye surgery. No more than 0.5 mL is instilled into the anterior chamber of the eye before or after securing sutures. Miosis is usually maximal 2 to 5 minutes after application.

CHOLINESTERASE INHIBITORS

The cholinesterase inhibitors inhibit the enzyme cholinesterase and thus enhance the effects of endogenous acetylcholine. The increased cholinergic activity in the eye leads to intense miosis and contraction of the ciliary muscle and loss of accommodation.

The cholinesterase inhibitors are used to treat open-angle glaucoma, following iridectomy, and in convergent strabismus. Dosages, pharmacokinetics, and nursing implications for the ophthalmic cholinesterase inhibitors are found in Table 63–6.

Contraindications and Precautions

The cholinesterase inhibitors are contraindicated in narrow-angle glaucoma (prior to iridectomy) owing to the possibility of increasing the angle blockage. The cholinesterase inhibitors are administered cautiously to persons who must drive at night as accommodation is lost and vision is poor. They are administered cautiously to persons with marked *vagotonia* (hyperirritability of the parasympathetic nervous system), bronchial asthma, spastic gastrointestinal (GI) disturbances, peptic ulcer, and pronounced bradycardia and hypotension as all these conditions are worsened owing to the increased activity of acetylcholine.

Adverse Effects

Ocular side effects are most common and include burning and stinging, allergic follicular conjunctivitis, lid muscle twitching, conjunctival and ciliary redness, browache,

headache, and myopia with blurred vision. Prolonged use may cause conjunctival thickening.

Interactions

Succinylcholine given concurrently with cholinesterase inhibitors during surgery may cause respiratory or cardiovascular collapse. Systemic anticholinesterases for myasthenia gravis may cause an additive effect.

❍ **Physostigmine** (Eserine) is available as an ointment or solution and is administered into the conjunctival sac.

❍ **Demecarium** (Humorsol) is a potent, long-acting quaternary ammonium compound and the most toxic of this group. It is used when patients have become refractory to the less toxic drugs. Besides its use in open-angle glaucoma, it is also used in accommodative *esotropia* (convergent strabismus). Demecarium causes contraction of ciliary muscle. Carbonic anhydrase inhibitors are used frequently in conjunction with demecarium to enhance its action.

❍ **Isoflurophate** (Floropryl) is a potent, long-acting organophosphorus cholinesterase inhibitor. Isoflurophate is available as a 0.025% ointment, which is usually applied in a strip of ¼ inch or less every 8 to 72 hours to the conjunctival sac.

❍ **Echothiophate** (Phospholine) is an extremely potent, long-acting quaternary organophosphorus compound, similar in almost all ways to demecarium. Unlike demecarium, however, the cholinesterase inhibition produced by echothiophate is irreversible until new enzyme is produced. Echothiophate is available in many combinations.

BETA-ADRENERGIC BLOCKERS

Another approach in treating chronic open-angle glaucoma is the use of the beta-adrenergic blocking (sympatholytic) agents: **timolol (Timoptic, Betimol), betaxolol (Betoptic), levobunolol (Betagan Liquifilm), metipranolol (Optipranolol)**, and **carteolol (Ocupress)**. Refer to Table 63–7 for dosages, pharmacokinetics, and nursing implications.

Action

Beta receptors, besides being located in the heart, skeletal muscles, and bronchioles, have been identified in ocular tissue, primarily in the ciliary muscle and in the sphincter muscle of the iris. Beta-blockers combine reversibly with these receptors to block the response to sympathetic nerve stimulation or circulating catecholamine. (More detailed information on beta-receptor sites is presented in Chapter 17).

Timolol, levobunolol, carteolol, and metipranolol are noncardioselective beta 1– and beta 2–blockers, whereas betaxolol is a cardioselective beta 1–blocker. Intraocular pressure is lowered, although the exact mechanism is unknown; however, it appears to be by decreasing production of aqueous humor. There is a reduction in intraocular pressure (IOP) with little or no effect on pupil size or accommodation. All beta-blockers except betaxolol have approximately equivalent potency. The choice is generally based on local or systemic side effects.

CONTRAINDICATIONS AND PRECAUTIONS

Patients with signs of cerebrovascular insufficiency may have a worsening of their symptoms related to the decreased blood pressure and pulse. Because betaxolol is a cardioselective beta-blocker, these effects are minimal. There are no well-controlled studies in pregnant women, so these products are used only if the benefits outweigh

---

Table 63–7. OPHTHALMIC BETA-ADRENERGIC BLOCKING MEDICATIONS		
DRUG NAME/ROUTE AND DOSAGE	**PHARMACOKINETICS/ DYNAMICS**	**NURSING IMPLICATIONS**
timolol maleate (Timoptic) (Betimol) *0.25%–0.5% soluton:* 1–2 times daily	**Onset:** 30 min **Peak:** 1–2 hr **Duration:** 12–24 hr	For all: **ASSESSMENT:** Assess for hypersensitivity, bronchospasm, COPD, congestive heart failure, bradycardia, and heart block, which are all contraindications. Assess for local (contact dermatitis) and systemic reactions. Keep medications sterile. Administer only as directed. All other antiglaucoma eye medications should be discontinued on 2nd day of timolol therapy. Frequently monitor vital signs and blood pressure during initial therapy for side effects. **EVALUATION:** Tolerance has been noted, so follow-up appointment must be kept. Notify physician of severe stinging or discomfort.
betaxolol (Betoptic) *0.25%–0.5% solution:* 1 gtt 2 times daily	**Onset:** 10–30 min **Peak:** 2 hr **Duration:** 12 hr	Same as for all.
levobunolol (Betagan Liquifilm) *0.25%–0.5% solution:* 1 gtt 1–2 times daily	**Onset:** <60 min **Peak:** 2–6 hr **Duration:** 12–24 hr	Same as for all.
metipranolol hydrochloride (Optipranolol) *0.3% solution:* 1 gtt 1–2 times daily	**Onset:** <30 min **Peak:** 2 hr **Duration:** 12–24 hr	Same as for all.
carteolol (Ocupress) *1% solution:* 1 gtt bid	**Onset:** NA **Peak:** NA **Duration:** 12 hr	Same as for all.

NA = not available.

the risk. Caution is advised when administering to nursing mothers as these products are excreted in milk. Safety in children has not been established.

▼ CLINICAL ALERT

Ophthalmic beta-adrenergic blockers produce systemic effects; therefore, patients with bronchial asthma, severe chronic obstructive pulmonary disease (COPD), bradycardia, and heart block should not receive them as these conditions are worsened. Patients with diabetes may experience spontaneous hypoglycemia, and the signs of hypoglycemia may be masked by beta-blockers.

ADVERSE EFFECTS

Many side effects can occur from these drugs, including headache, dysrhythmias, nausea, and depression, all secondary to the systemic beta effect of these drugs. All beta-blockers may cause transient but brief eye discomfort, including ocular irritation and visual disturbances.

INTERACTIONS

Concurrent quinidine, oral beta-blockers, and calcium antagonists have an additive slowing effect on the conduction system.

○ **Timolol maleate**   (Timoptic, Betimol) does not alter papillary diameter or reactivity to light, but it enhances the mydriatic effect of epinephrine. Timolol is better tolerated than most miotics in young adults and in older patients with cataracts because it does not cause spasm of accommodation or miosis. If it becomes necessary to change from one ophthalmic beta-blocker to timolol, the first agent is discontinued after proper dosing on one day and timolol is started on the following day with one drop of 0.25% solution. The dosage can be increased if needed. If it is necessary to change from another antiglaucoma agent to timolol, on the first day continue with the agent being used and add one drop of 0.25% timolol twice daily. The next day discontinue the first agent completely. The dosage of timolol can be increased if needed.

ADVERSE EFFECTS   Reported adverse effects include ocular irritation, hypersensitivity, and visual disturbances. Recently, sexual dysfunction (impotence, decreased libido, and decreased ejaculation volume) has been identified as an adverse effect; in most cases, symptoms reversed when timolol was stopped.

○ **Betaxolol**   (Betoptic) is as effective as timolol and may be safer in asthmatics and patients with COPD.

○ **Levobunolol hydrochloride**   (Betagon) is a long-acting nonselective beta-blocker for topical treatment of chronic open-angle glaucoma. It is as effective as timolol.

○ **Metipranolol hydrochloride**   (Optipranolol), is used to lower IOP in patients without ocular hypertension and patients with open-angle glaucoma.

○ **Carteolol**   (Ocupress) can be used alone or in combination with other intraocular pressure-lowering drugs.

CARBONIC ANHYDRASE INHIBITORS

For the ciliary body to produce aqueous humor, it must have the enzyme carbonic anhydrase present. Carbonic anhydrase inhibitors—**acetazolamide (Diamox)**, **methazolamide (Neptazane)**, **dorzolamide hydrochloride (Trusopt)**, and **dichlorphenamide (Daranide)**—interfere with the production of carbonic acid, which leads to a reduced level of bicarbonate ions and a systemic acidosis. This is associated with reduced aqueous humor formation and decreased intraocular pressure. The systemic acidosis also adds to the ocular hypotensive effect. These drugs were first developed as diuretics but are now used almost solely for the treatment of glaucoma, particularly when adequate control cannot be achieved with miotics alone. Carbonic anhydrase inhibitors are used in conjunction with miotics and osmotic agents to treat both open-angle and narrow-angle glaucoma as well as angle-closure attacks.

The most common adverse effects, although usually not severe, include lethargy, anorexia, drowsiness, depression, malaise, diuresis, and numbness and tingling of the face and extremities. The frequency and intensity of these side effects are dose related, and some are associated with systemic acidosis. These side effects are often the cause of patient intolerance to these products. When diuresis is produced, potassium depletion can occur. Carbonic anhydrase inhibitors frequently cause gastric distress, nausea, vomiting, and diarrhea. All of these effects are due to a local irritant action that may be alleviated by taking the drug with food. For more information on carbonic anhydrase inhibitors, see Table 63–8 and Chapter 38.

OSMOTIC AGENTS

Osmotic diuretics are administered intravenously or orally for short-term reduction of intraocular pressure and vitreous volume. By increasing the plasma osmolarity, fluid is drawn from the eyeball and pressure is reduced. The most commonly used osmotic agents include **glycerin topical (Ophthalgan)**, **glycerin oral (Osmoglyn)**, **urea (Ureaphil)**, **isosorbide (Ismotic)**, **hypertonic sodium chloride (Adsorbonac)**, and **glucose (Glucose 40)**, featured in Table 63–9. Osmotic agents are generally effective in patients who do not respond to miotics or carbonic anhydrase inhibitors. They are generally given preoperatively and postoperatively for this reason.

In general, the side effects include temporary burning and irritation upon installation. All osmotic agents are given cautiously to persons with cardiac conditions because of the possible development of pulmonary edema and congestive heart failure due to the pulling of fluid from the tissues. The weakened heart is unable to pump

Table 63–8. OPHTHALMIC CARBONIC ANHYDRASE INHIBITORS

DRUG NAME/ROUTE AND DOSAGE	PHARMACOKINETICS/ DYNAMICS	NURSING IMPLICATIONS
acetazolamide sodium (Diamox)		
Adults: 250 mg PO 1–4 times/ day; or 500 mg timed-release (TR) capsule PO once or twice daily **Children:** 8–30 mg/kg per day PO divided in 3 equal doses	**Onset:** PO, 1 hr; TR, 2 hr **Peak:** PO 2–4 hr; TR, 3–6 hr **Duration:** PO, 8–12 hr; TR, 18–24 hr **½L:** 5 hr **PB:** 93% **B:** NA **E:** urine (unchanged)	For all ophthalmic carbonic anhydrase inhibitors: **ASSESSMENT:** Assess for sensitivity, renal or hepatic dysfunction. Assess for dehydration, potassium balance, and vital signs. Assess for pregnancy (acetazolamide and dorzolamide—category C; methazolamide—category D). **INTERVENTION:** Do not change brands. Take early in day, as it will increase urination. May cause GI upset; take with meals. May increase blood sugar in diabetes; monitor carefully. **EVALUATION:** Evaluate effectiveness of therapy (decrease in IOP in glaucoma); if patient cannot tolerate one carbonic anhydrase inhibitor or if therapy is not effective, switching to another may be more effective or tolerable.
methazolamide (Neptazane)		
Adults: 25–100 mg PO q 6–8 hr	**Onset:** 2–4 hr **Peak:** 6–8 hr **Duration:** 10–18 hr **½L:** NA **PB:** 55% **B:** NA **E:** urine (55% unchanged)	Same as for all.
dorzolamide hydrochloride (Trusopt)		
2% solution: 1 gtt tid	**½L:** 4 mo **PB:** 33% **E:** urine	Same as for all plus: **ASSESSMENT:** Assess for sulfonamide sensitivity.

the added volume, and the kidneys are unable to excrete the volume rapidly enough. Osmotic agents are given cautiously to the elderly because of the possible development of dehydration. Glycerin, because it is a carbohydrate, may cause the diabetic patient to develop hyperglycemia and glycosuria. Isosorbide may be useful in the diabetic as it does not cause hyperglycemia.

MYDRIATICS AND CYCLOPLEGICS

Mydriatics are used to dilate the pupil, and cycloplegics paralyze accommodation. Mydriatics and cycloplegics are featured in (Table 63–10). Two groups of drugs, anticholinergics and alpha adrenergics, acting by different mechanisms, cause *mydriasis* (dilation of the pupil).

ACTION

Anticholinergics, the muscarinic antagonists, inhibit the parasympathetic nervous system, whereas alpha adrenergics mimic the sympathetic nervous system. At times, both types of medications can be combined to achieve marked mydriasis. However, the anticholinergics alone are capable of producing cycloplegia.

Anticholinergics paralyze the ciliary muscle and the dilator muscle of the iris, causing both dilation of the pupil and the paralysis of accommodation. This action is achieved through the blockage of acetylcholine. As the anticholinergics relax the ciliary muscle, the lens becomes less convex, and therefore accommodation for close vision becomes more difficult. Alpha-adrenergics, on the other hand, contract the dilator muscle of the iris, causing dilation of the pupil; but they have only a slight effect on the ciliary muscle, so that accommodation is not affected.

The adrenergics, besides producing mydriasis and slight relaxation of the ciliary muscle, constrict conjunctival blood vessels. They probably also decrease formation of aqueous humor, thereby causing a drop in intraocular pressure. This vasodilation may be the mechanism by which the rate of aqueous humor production is decreased.

USES

The anticholinergic mydriatics and cycloplegics, such as **atropine sulfate (Atopisol)**, **cyclopentolate (Cyclogyl)**, **homatropine hydrobromide (Isopto Homatropine)**, **scopolamine hydrobromide (Isopto Hyoscine)**, and **tropicamide (Mydriacyl)**, are used in eye examinations for accurate measurement of refractory errors and preoper-

Table 63–9. OSMOTIC AGENTS USED IN EYE DISORDERS

DRUG NAME/ROUTE AND DOSAGE	PHARMACOKINETICS/ DYNAMICS	NURSING IMPLICATIONS
glycerin topical (Ophthalgan) **glycerin oral** (Osmoglyn) **50% solution:** 1–1.8 g/kg PO 1–1.5 hr prior to surgery. **Solution:** 1–2 gtt into eye before examination.	**Onset:** PO and topical, 10–30 min **Peak:** PO and topical, 1–1.5 hr **Duration:** PO, 4–8 hr; topical, 4–5 hr **½L:** 30–45 min **PB:** NA **B:** liver (80%), kidneys (20%) **E:** NA	For all: **ASSESSMENT:** Carefully assess fluid and electrolyte balance, urinary output, and vital signs. Assess for previous hypersensitivity. Assess for pregnancy—category C. **INTERVENTION:** Headache may be relieved by having patient lie down during and after oral administration. Flavoring with lemon or lime juice and serving it over cracked ice may reduce nausea and vomiting.
isosorbide (Ismotic) **45% solution:** Initial dose–1.5 g/kg PO; Dosage range–1–3 g/kg 2–4 times daily.	**Onset:** 10–20 min **Peak:** 1–1.5 hr **Duration:** 5–6 hr **½L:** 5–9.5 hr **PB:** **B:** NA **E:** NA	Same as for all plus: **INTERVENTION:** May be useful in diabetics as it does not affect blood sugar. Pregnancy—category B.
urea (Ureaphil) **Adults:** 30% solution—0.5–2g/kg IV at 60 gtt/min, not to exceed 4 mL/min. **Children:** 30% solution—0.1–1.5 g/kg IV over 30 min.	**Onset:** 30–45 min **Peak:** 1 hr **Duration:** 5–6 hr **½L:** NA **PB:** **B:** in GI tract **E:** kidney	**ASSESSMENT:** Assess for severe renal impairment, active cerebral bleeding, marked dehydration, liver failure, as all are contraindications. **INTERVENTION:** Unstable; must be prepared before each administration. Urea is irritating to tissues and causes pain on injection.
hypertonic sodium chloride (Adsorbonac) **2%–5% solution:** Instill 1–2 gtt into eye q 3–4 hr **5% ointment:** Apply ¼" strip qid.	**Onset:** 10–30 min **Peak:** 1–1.5 hr **Duration:** 4–5 hr **½L:** 30–45 min	Same as for urea.

atively and postoperatively to cause pupillary dilation.

When a short-acting anticholinergic such as cyclopentolate, homatropine, or tropicamide is used to produce mydriasis and cyclopegia for eye examinations or refractions, pilocarpine (a cholinergic miotic) may be used to counteract both the mydriasis and cycloplegia.

The strong alpha vasoconstriction preparations—**phenylephrine 2.5%** and **10% (Neo-Synephrine)** and **hydroxyamphetamine 10% (Paredrine)**—are used to cause vasoconstriction and pupillary dilation for eye examinations and during surgery. The intermediate strength **epinephrine** 0.5% and 2% **(Epitrate)** are used to manage open-angle glaucoma, alone or in combination with other drugs.

CONTRAINDICATIONS AND PRECAUTIONS

The mydriatics are contraindicated in patients who have had previous hypersensitivity to the preparation and for patients who have certain cardiac problems, such as tachycardia. They are also contraindicated in patients with glaucoma, as they may precipitate an attack of narrow-angle glaucoma because of their action of dilation of the pupil and narrowing of the iridocorneal angle where the canal of Schlemm is located. They are also administered cautiously to elderly and debilitated patients because of their local and systemic side effects. Safe use in pregnancy (atropine and homatropine category C) has not been established.

ADVERSE EFFECTS

The mydriatics are generally not absorbed systemically after ocular instillation. But if absorption does occur, the anticholinergic drugs can cause side effects, the most commonly observed including dryness of the mouth, flushing, and, rarely, tachycardia, fever, delirium, inhibition of sweating, and coma. In addition, pupillary dilation from either local or systemic administration can precipitate acute glaucoma (angle-closure attack) in those with narrow-angle glaucoma. Although serious systemic

Table 63–10. MYDRIATICS AND CYCLOPLEGICS

DRUG NAME/ROUTE AND DOSAGE	PHARMACOKINETICS/ DYNAMICS	NURSING IMPLICATIONS
ANTICHOLINERGIC MYDRIATICS AND CYCLOPLEGICS		
atropine suflate (Atropisol) *Adults:* 1–2 gtt 0.5%–3% solution 1–4 times daily; or small amount of 0.5%–1% ointment in conjunctival sac 1–3 times daily *Children:* 1–2 gtt 0.5% solution 1–3 times daily before examination	**Mydriasis:** Onset—30–40 min; Duration—7–12 days **Cycloplegia:** Peak—1–3 hr; Duration—6–14 days	For all: **ASSESSMENT:** Carefully assess local (contact dermatitis) and systemic reactions. Physician should assess intraocular tension before and during use. Narrow-angle glaucoma is contraindication. Assess cardiac condition. **INTERVENTION:** Keep medications sterile. Administer only as directed. Administer correct vehicle—ointment or liquid. Blurred vision may occur. Wear dark glasses in bright light if photophobia occurs. To avoid systemic absorption, compress lacrimal sac by digital pressure for 1–3 min after instillation. Heavily pigmented eyes may require larger doses. If epinephrine is being administered concurrently with miotics, miotic is instilled 2–10 min before epinephrine. **Patient Teaching—** Caution patient about driving and performing tasks requiring alertness, as these medications may cause drowsiness. **EVALUATION:** If severe eye pain, headache, spots before eyes, or acute eye redness occurs, discontinue use and consult physician.
cyclopentolate (Cyclogyl) (Used only as mydriatic.) 0.5%, 1%, and 2% solution *Adults:* 1–2 gtt, repeated in 5–10 min if needed *Children:* 1 gtt, followed in 5–10 min with another application of 0.5% or 0.1% solution	**Mydriasis:** Onset—30–60 min; Duration—1 day	Same as for all.
homatropine hydrobromide (Isopto-Homatropine) 2% solution—mydriasis; 5% solution—cycloplegia *Adults:* 1–2 gtt 2%–5% solution q 3–4 hr *Children:* 1 gtt 2% solution	**Mydriasis:** Peak—10–30 min; Duration—6 hr–3 days **Cycloplegia:** Peak—30–60 min; Duration—10–48 hr	Same as for all.
scopolamine hydrobromide (Isopto Hyoscine) *0.25% solution:* 1–2 gtt	**Mydriasis:** Peak—20–30 min; Duration—3–7 days **Cycloplegia:** Peak—30–60 min; Duration—3–7 days	Same as for all.
tropicamide (Mydriacyl) (Tropicacyl) *0.5% and 1% solution:* 1–2 gtt	**Mydriasis:** Onset—20–40 min; Duration—6–7 hr **Cycloplegia:** Peak—20–35 min; Duration—1–6 hr	Same as for all.
ALPHA-ADRENERGIC MYDRIATICS		
epinephrine hydrochloride (Epifrin) *0.25%, 0.5%, 0.1%, and 2% solution:* 1–2 qtt up to 1–4 times daily	Ocular pressure drop: **Onset:** 1 hr **Peak:** 4 hr **Duration:** 24 hr	Same as for all plus: **INTERVENTION:** Do not use while wearing soft contact lenses. Tell patient to immediately report any decrease in visual acuity.

Continued on the following page

Table 63–10. MYDRIATICS AND CYCLOPLEGICS, *Continued*		
DRUG NAME/ROUTE AND DOSAGE	**PHARMACOKINETICS/ DYNAMICS**	**NURSING IMPLICATIONS**
ALPHA-ADRENERGIC MYDRIATICS		
phenylephrine (Neo-Synephrine)		
0.12 %, 2.5%, or 10% solution *Adults:* 1 gtt 2.5% or 10% solution	**Mydriasis:** Onset—0–1 hr; Peak—3 hr **Cycloplegia:** Onset—15–60 min; Peak—0–90 min **Duration:** 3–7 hr (10%)	Same as for all plus: **INTERVENTION:** When a 10% solution is used, prevent systemic absorption by pressing gently on nasolacrimal canal for 1–2 min after administration.
apraclonidine hydrochloride (Iopidine)		
Adults: 1 gtt 0.1% solution in operative eye 1 hr before surgery	**Onset:** 1 hr **Peak:** 3–5 hr **Duration:** 12 hr	Same as for all.

side effects are rare with the adrenergic drugs, patients with underlying heart disease are monitored closely for increases in blood pressure and pulse.

ANTICHOLINERGIC MYDRIATICS AND CYCLOPLEGICS

Both local and systemic side effects are similar to those of other anticholinergic preparations. The local effects include photophobia, loss of accommodation, contact dermatitis, edema around the eye, and conjunctivitis. Patients must report any of these symptoms as soon as they become evident. If the patient is experiencing systemic side effects at the time of the next scheduled dose, he or she is instructed to omit that dose. These drugs are always stored in a safe place out of the reach of children because of their toxicity.

○ **Atropine sulfate** (Atropisol, Atropine), the most potent of all cycloplegic drugs, is a tertiary amine derived from *Atropea belladonna*. It is commonly used as a mydriatic and cycloplegic when administered locally as an ointment or gel and has many other uses when administered systemically. (See other chapters.) It is frequently used to dilate the pupil in acute inflammations such as anterior uveitis and iritis. In addition, it is used for the initial examination of patients with convergent strabismus and, because of the long duration of action, is the preferred drug for refraction of children with accommodative esotropia.

○ **Homatropine hydrobromide** (Isopto-Homatropine) is a synthetic alkaloid with action, contraindications, precautions, and side effects similar to those of atropine. It may be preferred over atropine for certain ophthalmic purposes, as its duration of action is shorter. It is useful in producing mydriasis and cycloplegia for diagnostic purposes (See Table 63–10).

○ **Cyclopentolate** (Cyclogyl) is more potent and has a shorter duration of action than homatropine. It is used only as a mydriatic.

○ **Scopolamine hydrobromide** (Isopto-Hyoscine) is a belladonna alkaloid similar in most ways to atropine sulfate, but is more rapid acting and has a shorter duration of action. Scopolamine can be used with no side effects in patients who have demonstrated a sensitivity to atropine sulfate.

○ **Tropicamide** (Mydriacyl, Tropicacyl) is a derivative of tropic acid, with all pharmacologic properties being similar to atropine. It is useful for diagnostic purposes but ineffective for treating inflammatory conditions. It is a rapid-acting, short-duration mydriatic and cycloplegic. Eye examinations must be completed within 35 minutes of the first administration, or another dose of medication is needed.

ALPHA-ADRENERGIC MYDRIATICS

Several of the alpha-adrenergic mydriatics—**epinephrine hydrochloride** *(Epifrin)*, **phenylephrine** *(Neo-Synephrine)*, and **apracloridine hydrochloride** *(Iopidine)*—are featured in Table 63–10.

○ **Epinephrine hydrochloride** (Adrenal Chloride, Epifrin, Glaucon) is a naturally occurring or synthetically prepared catecholamine. It lowers IOP by decreasing aqueous humor production; it therefore is useful in treating glaucoma. During initial therapy for open-angle glaucoma, however, pilocarpine or other miotics may be used along with epinephrine to effect control. Epinephrine prevents the rapid absorption of local ophthalmic anesthetics.

○ **Phenylephrine** (Neo-Synephrine) is a potent, non-catecholamine, direct-acting sympathomimetic, similar in most aspects to epinephrine. It is frequently used as a mydriatic and as an aid to produce cycloplegia. It is also used as a decongestant and vasoconstrictor and for pupil dilatation in uveitis, wide-angle glaucoma, and surgery. It also provides temporary relief of minor eye irritation caused by hayfever, dust, wind, sun, smog, and hard contact lenses.

○ **Apraclonidine hydrochloride** (Iopidine) is a relatively selective alpha-adrenergic agonist that does not have local anesthetic properties. It is instilled into the eye to control and reduce IOP that can occur in patients after argon laser *trabeculoplasty* (surgical manipulation of the trabecular meshwork of the eye to treat glaucoma) and iridotomy. Increases in IOP can lead to visual field loss and optic nerve damage.

CONTRAINDICATIONS AND PRECAUTIONS Apraclonidine is contraindicated in persons hypersensitive to its components or to clonidine (antihypertensive), which is chemically related.

ADVERSE EFFECTS When apraclonidine was used during laser surgery adverse effects reported included upper lid elevation (in 1.3% of patients), conjunctival blanching, and mydriasis.

USING THE NURSING PROCESS

ASSESSMENT

- Obtain a thorough nursing history to develop the database. The patient requiring eye medications may be acutely ill and hospitalized or may be relatively healthy with a condition such as glaucoma being discovered on a routine physical or eye examination. See Table 63–11 for information when preparing the nursing care plan.
- Assess for the presence of similar symptoms like "pink eye" among close friends or relatives.
- Assess for pupil size and the presence of redness or edema in or around the eye. Visual acuity, peripheral vision, and optic fundi are assessed.
- Determine if there has been a change in visual acuity during the past several months.
- Obtain laboratory data, such as eye culture results as ordered. Cultures may be helpful in determining the organisms that cause inflammation and infection.
- Assess medication history. Many eye problems may be precipitated by both prescription and OTC medications. Table 63–12 features commonly used prescription and OTC medications; identifies the way they are likely to affect the eye, and indicates the frequency that eye examinations are administered to the patient while the medication is being taken. Some of these medications can cause temporary or permanent damage to the eye. If the patient has been on, or is currently taking, eye medications, it is important to identify specific medications and dosage, the reason they were chosen or prescribed, and how long the patient has been taking them. It is also important to know whether the patient has experienced any allergic reaction to eye medications in the past including OTC drugs and contact lens products. The nurse also must assess the activity level of the patient. Does the patient operate heavy equipment or drive a car? Does the patient do many activities at night and therefore need good night vision? Can the patient administer his or her own eye drops or ointments?

NURSING DIAGNOSIS

- Typical nursing diagnoses for the patient with an eye disorder include the following: Knowledge Deficit, Physical Imobility, Infection, Visual Sensory Perceptual Alteration, and Anticipatory Grieving (see Table 63–11).

PLANNING AND INTERVENTION

- Develop the goals of nursing intervention from the nursing diagnoses. Typical nursing goals when caring for the patient requiring medications for eye disorders are included in Table 63–11.

Administration Guidelines

- Always wash the hands thoroughly before administering any eye medication.
- Never touch the tip of the eye dropper or the tube of ointment to any surface.
- Close container immediately after use.
- Do not store eye medications where there is the possibility of extremes of heat such as in a car.
- Teach patient that eye medications may cause temporary stinging or blurred vision.
- Use only medications marked for ophthalmic use. Antibiotics or steroids for otic or dermatologic use are not to be used in the eye.
- The normal eye can hold about 10 μL of fluid. Because the average dropper delivers 25 to 50 μL per drop, generally more than one drop is not useful. Owing to rapid lacrimal drainage (16% per minute) and limited eye capacity, if multiple-drop therapy is needed, the best interval between drops is 5 minutes. This ensures that the first drop is not flushed away by the second and that the second drop is not diluted by the first. Do not use drops that have changed color.
- Minimize systemic absorption of ophthalmic drops by compressing the lacrimal sac for 1 to 2 minutes during and following instillation of drops. This retards passage of drops via the nasolacrimal duct into areas of potential absorption such as nasal and pharyngeal mucosa.
- Certain factors may increase the absorption of ophthalmic dosage forms, including lax eyelids of some patients (usually the elderly), which creates a greater reservoir for retention of drops; and hyperemic or diseased eyes. Topical anesthesia also increases the bioavailability of ophthalmic agents by decreasing the blink reflex and the production and turnover of tears.
- Discourage the use of eyecups because of potential contamination and risk of spreading disease.
- It is important for ophthalmic medications to remain uncontaminated after opening. Use solutions and drops within 4 weeks and ointments within 3 months. Monitor expiration dates closely. Do *not* use outdated medication.
- Suspensions and solutions remain in the eye longer than other fluids. Ophthalmic suspensions mix with

Table 63–11. NURSING PROCESS FOR PATIENT WITH EYE DISORDERS

Assessment

Assess pupil size, acuity, peripheral vision, and optic fundi; presence of discharge; redness, edema in or around the eye.
Assess laboratory data, e.g., eye culture.
Assess current medication history.

Nursing Diagnosis: Knowledge Deficit

RELATED TO: Lack of exposure/recall, unfamiliarity with information resources/misinterpretation, cognitive limitation.
AS EVIDENCED BY: Questions, statement of concern, inaccurate follow-through of instructions/development of preventable complications.

Desired Outcomes/Evaluation Criteria

Verbalizes understanding of condition/disease process and treatment. Currently performs necessary procedures and explains reasons for the actions.

Nursing Actions	Rationale
Review information about individual condition, prognosis, type of procedures.	Enhances understanding and promotes cooperation with treatment regimen.
Discuss possible effects/interactions between eye medications and patient's medical problems.	Use of topical eye medications (e.g., sympathomimetic agents, β-blockers, anticholinergic agents) can cause BP to rise in hypertensive patients, precipitate dyspnea in patients with COPD, mask the symptoms of a hypoglycemic crisis in insulin-dependent diabetics.
Instruct in proper method of instilling eye drops, counting drops as indicated.	Correction application can limit absorption into systemic circulation, minimizing problems such as drug interactions and unwanted/untoward systemic effects.
Suggest use of dark glasses/reduced room lighting as indicated.	Can reduce discomfort associated with photophobia.
Recommended wearing medical identification bracelet if appropriate.	Reduces risk that person with glaucoma will receive contraindicated drugs in emergency situation.
Identify signs/symptoms requiring prompt evaluation, e.g., sharp/sudden pain, decreased/blurred vision, increased photophobia, flashes of light/floating particles in visual field, lid swelling, purulent discharge, redness, watering of eyes, photophobia.	Early intervention can prevent development of serious complications, possible loss of vision.
Stress importance of routine follow-up care, as indicated.	Periodic monitoring reduces risk of serious complications.

Nursing Diagnosis: High Risk for Spread Infection

RELATED TO: Inadequate primary defenses.

Desired Outcomes/Evaluation Criteria

Verbalizes understanding of individual causative/risk factor(s). Identifies interventions to prevent/reduce risk of spread of infection. Demonstrates proper technique for instillation of eye drops.

Nursing Actions	Rationale
Administer antibacterial, antifungal, or antiviral agent as appropriate.	Used to treat existing infection.
Discuss reasons for infection, how it can be spread, and treatment needs.	Understanding of how infection is transmitted promotes accurate care and cooperation with treatment regimen.
Stress importance of washing hands before and after instilling eye drops.	Prevents possible introduction of other pathogens/spread of infection.
Encourage rest and limit eye activity.	Promotes healing.
Discuss ways to prevent reinfection. Recommend abstaining from use of eye makeup during acute infection and routinely discard/replace eye makeup.	Reduces risk of recurrence and spreading infection.

Nursing Diagnosis: Visual Sensory-Perceptual Alteration

RELATED TO: Altered sensory reception, altered status of sense organ
AS EVIDENCED BY: Progressive loss of visual field.

Desired Outcomes/Evaluation Criteria

Maintains current visual field/acuity without further loss.

Nursing Actions	Rationale
Administer appropriate drug, e.g., Diamox, Osmitrol, timolol.	Controls intraocular pressure preventing further loss of vision.
Demonstrate administration of eye drops, e.g., counting drops.	Helps patient to follow proper procedure. Medication regimen is vital to prevent progression of disease. Some drugs cause pupil dilation, increasing IOP and potentiating additional loss of vision.
Discuss importance of maintaining drug schedule/not missing doses.	Glaucoma can be controlled, not cured, and maintaining consistent medication regimen is vital to prevent progression of disease.

Continued on the following page

Table 63–11. NURSING PROCESS FOR PATIENT WITH EYE DISORDERS, *Continued*

Nursing Actions	Rationale
Discuss medications that should be avoided, e.g., mydriatic drops, overuse of topical steroids.	Some drugs cause pupil dilation, increasing IOP and potentiating additional loss of vision.
Monitor vital signs during initial therapy.	Blood pressure may drop and pulse may slow with β-adrenergic blocking medications.
Reduce environmental clutter, clear travel paths as needed.	Reduces safety hazards related to changes in visual fields.
Encourage expression of feelings about actual/possible loss of vision.	While early intervention may prevent blindness, the patient faces the possibility or may already have experienced partial or complete loss of vision.

Other Suggested Nursing Diagnoses: Impaired Physical Mobility, Anticipatory Grieving, and Risk of injury.

Table 63–12. OCULAR TOXICITY OF VARIOUS DRUGS

Medications	Ptosis	Miosis	Vision Changes	Mydriasis	Oculogyric Crisis	Optic Neuritis	Nystagmus	Diplopia	Ocular Palsies	Conjunctivitis	Papilledema	Frequency* of Follow-up	Comments
Central Nervous System Drugs													
Chlorpromazine (Thorazine)			x	x								2	Increased pigmentation on all parts of eyes, degeneration of retina
Phenytoin (Dilantin)	x		x				x	x		x		3	
Haloperidol (Haldol)			x	x	x							1	
Levodopa (L-Dopa)				x								1	
Morphine		x	x									1, 3	Myopia
Tricyclic antidepressants (e.g., Elavil)				x								2	Cycloplegia, aggravation of narrow-angle glaucoma
Diazepam (Valium)			x				x	x				1	Acute glaucoma
Nasal decongestants			x	x									
Anti-Infectives													
Tetracycline			x								x	2	
Sulfonamides							x						
Medications to Treat Tuberculosis													
Ethambutol (Myambutol)			x			x						2	Green vision lost
Isoniazid (INH)						x						2	Keratitis
Cardiovascular Medications													
Digitalis preparations								x	x			3	Color vision disturbances especially xanthopsia (yellow vision), halos
Quinidine			x			x						3	
Amiodarone												1	Ocular deposits occur
Diuretics													
Thiazide (Diuril)												3	Myopia, xanthopsia (yellow vision)
Furosemide (Lasix)			x									3	
Antirheumatoid Medications													
Gold salts						x				x		3	Gold deposits in eye
Ibuprofen (Motrin)			x									1	Color vision disturbances, changes in tear quality
Indomethacin (Indocin)					x			x				3	Cause corneal deposits
Salicylates				x	x	x				x		3	Retinal hemorrhages
Hormonal Agents													
Corticosteroids	x			x							x		Cataracts, retinopathy, myopia, exophthalmia
Oral contraceptives					x	x					x	1, 2	Alterations in corneal curvature

*1: should be seen if symptoms arise; 2, 3–6 months; 3, 6–12 months.

tears less rapidly and remain in the cul de sac longer than solutions. The clearance rate of ophthalmic ointments from the eye is approximately 0.5% per minute; ophthalmic ointments provide maximum contact between drug and ophthalmic tissues and structures. Ophthalmic ointments may impede delivery of other ophthalmic drugs to the affected site by serving as a barrier to contact. If more than one kind of ointment is needed, wait about 10 minutes before applying the second drug. Ointments may blur vision during the waking hours. Use with caution in conditions where visual clarity is critical (e.g., operating motor equipment, reading).

- If the ophthalmic disorder persists or worsens, contact the physician.

Proper Use of Ophthalmic Solutions

1. Tilt the head backward or have the patient lie down and gaze upward. Gently pull down lower eyelid to form a pouch. Hold the dropper above the eye and place the prescribed volume of drops inside the lower lid. Avoid contact of the dropper with the eye, finger, or any surface. Release the lid slowly. The patient should try to keep the eye open (not blink) for 30 seconds after administration.

2. Apply gentle pressure with fingers to the bridge of the nose (inside corner of eye) for 1 to 2 minutes. This retards drainage of solution from the intended area.

3. Do not rub the eye. Minimize blinking. Do not close the eyes tightly after instillation; this may express medication from the cul de sac.

4. In situations where the instillation of eye drops is difficult (e.g., pediatric patients, adults with particularly strong blink reflex) the close-eye method may be used. This involves the patient lying down, placing the prescribed number of drops on the eyelid in the inner corner of the eye, then opening the eye so that drops will fall into it by gravity.

Proper Use of Ophthalmic Ointments

1. When opening the ointment tube for the first time, squeeze out and discard the first 0.25 inch of ointment—it may be too dry. Hold the ointment tube in the hand for a few minutes to warm the ointment, which will facilitate flow. Gently pull down the lower lid to form a pouch and place 0.25 to 0.5 inch of ointment inside the lower lid. Have the patient close the eye for 1 to 2 minutes and roll the eyeball in all directions. Temporary blurring may occur.

2. Remove excessive ointment around the eye or ointment tube tip with tissue.

Patient Teaching

The patient will often be self-administering eye medications at home. Make sure the patient knows and understands several basic measures to administer eye medication safely, the reasons for the use of the eye medication, and the correct way to administer them. Figure 63–1 depicts the proper administration of eye drops and eye oint-

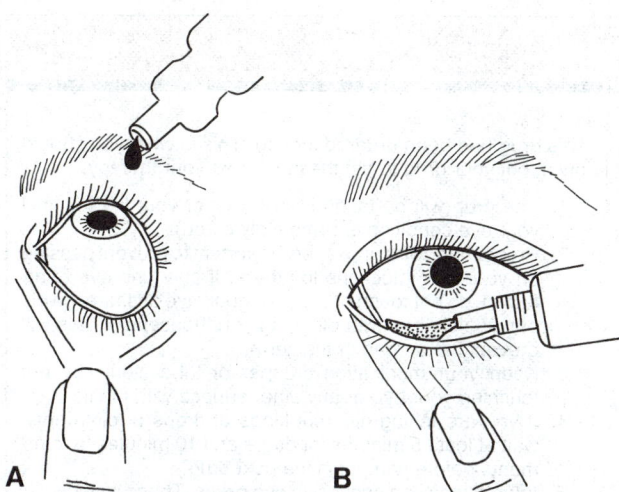

Figure 63–1. **(A)** Eye drops are administered onto the lower lid, which has been pulled down with the forefinger. The eye is then closed for 30 seconds to allow the medication to flow over the entire eye. The medication applicator approaches the eye from below and outside the patient's field of vision. Do not let dropper tip touch any surface, including eyelashes. **(B)** Eye ointment is administered onto the lower lid, which is pulled down with the forefinger. Only a small amount (¼ inch) of ointment need be used. The eye is then closed to allow the medication to flow over the entire eye.

ments. Sterile technique must be maintained to prevent contamination of the dropper. Patient teaching information is found in Table 63–13.

For safe administration of these drugs, refer to the information found in each drug table in the Nursing Implications column. Directions may need to be repeated several times to ensure patient understanding and continued compliance. Eye conditions (particularly glaucoma) associated with possible blindness frequently cause high anxiety levels in patients. Anxious patients may be unable to comprehend simple instructions. Written instructions for reference are helpful to ensure compliance once the patient returns home.

- Teach the patient signs and symptoms that would indicate a worsening of the condition or an acute exacerbation of the disease. Give the patient specific and individualized instructions, appropriate to the particular situation, on what to do and whom to contact when these symptoms occur.
- Teach the patient specifics about his or her medication (see appropriate drug tables).

Cataracts

Cataracts develop most often in the elderly when the crystalline lens develops a greater percentage of protein. Recent research indicates that there are drugs that can increase or decrease the risk of developing cataracts. Drugs known to increase the risk of cataract development include steroids and nifedipine (Procardia). Drugs taken regularly that may reduce the risk of developing cataracts by 50% or more include aspirin, acetaminophen, and ibuprofen (Motrin, Advil). Researchers suspect that analgesics protect against cataracts by lowering levels of plasma glucose, a possible contributor to cataract formation.

Table 63–13. PATIENT TEACHING INFORMATION—EYE MEDICATIONS

Dear Patient:

This drug has been ordered for you. This is what you should know about your drug to get the most from your therapy.

- ☐ 1. The drug will be taken for the rest of your life (or until your eye condition is completely cured).
- ☐ 2. Proper handwashing is very important to prevent passing on your eye infections to others. If only one eye is affected, do not touch or rub your good eye or share towels or wash clothes with others in your household. This will prevent the spread of the germs.
- ☐ 3. Keep your medication dropper or tube sterile by not touching your eye or any other surface with the tip.
- ☐ 4. If you are taking different kinds of drops or ointments, wait at least 5 minutes for drops and 10 minutes for ointments before you put in the next drug.
- ☐ 5. Interactions can occur with eye drugs. These include . . . [include specific information from drug tables].
- ☐ 6. If you forget your drug until it is almost time for your next dose, forget the dose; *do not* try to catch up.
- ☐ 7. Do not stop your drug without your doctor's knowledge.
- ☐ 8. Sometimes side effects may occur from eye drugs. The most usual is irritation and redness around the eye. If redness, itching, or swelling occurs, contact your doctor. Other side effects include . . . [fill in specific information from drug tables].
- ☐ 9. The safety precautions for your particular drug include . . . [fill in information found in drug tables].
- ☐ 10. Store your drugs away from direct heat and freezing and cap them tightly. Do not touch the tip of the applicator. Discard old, discolored, or cloudy solutions.

GUIDELINES FOR PROPER USE OF OPHTHALMIC SOLUTIONS

- ☐ 1. Tilt the head backward or lie down and gaze upward.
- ☐ 2. Gently pull down lower eyelid to form a pouch.
- ☐ 3. Hold the dropper above the eye and place the prescribed volume of drops inside the lower lid.
- ☐ 4. Avoid touching the dropper to the eye, finger, or any other surface.
- ☐ 5. Release the lid slowly.
- ☐ 6. You should try to keep the eye open (not blink) for 30 seconds after putting the drug in.
- ☐ 7. Press gently with fingers to the bridge of the nose (inside corner of eye) for 1–2 minutes. This keeps the drug in the eye and doesn't let it drain out.
- ☐ 8. Do not rub the eye. Do not blink too much. Do not close the eyes tightly after putting the drug in; this may squeeze the medication from the eyelid pouch.
- ☐ 9. Do not rinse the dropper.

GUIDELINES FOR PROPER USE OF OPHTHALMIC OINTMENTS

- ☐ 1. When opening the ointment tube for the first time, squeeze out and throw away the first 0.25 inch of ointment as it may be too dry.
- ☐ 2. Holding the ointment tube in the hand for a few minutes will warm the ointment and help it flow better.
- ☐ 3. Gently pull down the lower lid to form a pouch.
- ☐ 4. Place 0.25–0.5 inch of ointment inside the lower lid by squeezing the tube gently.
- ☐ 5. Close the eye for 1–2 min and roll the eyeball in all directions.
- ☐ 6. Your eyesight may be blurred for a little while. Do not do things for which you need to see clearly, such as driving, until blurring clears.
- ☐ 7. Remove extra ointment around the eye or ointment tube tip with tissue.

Contact Lenses

Several forms of contact lenses are marketed today—hard and soft with the soft available as daily wear or extended-wear lenses. All contact lenses float on a film of tears and do not actually come in contact with the cornea.

Many products are available OTC for the contact lens wearer: storage and soaking solutions, wetting solutions, wetting and cleaning solutions, rewetting solutions, cleaning solutions and gels, rinsing and storage solutions, surfactant cleaning solutions, enzymatic cleaners, and chemical disinfectants. It is important to choose the correct product for the contact lens being used.

Patients using OTC or prescription antihistamines or anticholinergics should not be fitted for contact lenses while using these products as tear quality may be compromised. Such patients should be advised to discontinue contact lens wear until they have stopped using the drugs.

Various drugs (e.g., the anti-inflammatory drug sulfasalazine) stain soft contact lenses a deep yellow color. Routine cleaning removes the stain from daily-wear lenses; however, extended-wear lenses are stained permanently. Therefore, patients wearing extended-wear lenses must remove their lenses during therapy.

EVALUATION

- Evaluate the effectiveness of the medications used for eye disorders as well as other nursing and medical goals. This evaluation is based on a list of outcome evaluation criteria developed in relation to the goals determined by the nurse, patient, and family (see Table 63–11).
- Work with the patient and family to ensure their complete assistance and support. A patient who understands the importance of continued medical treatment is usually compliant. A person does not wish to lose his or her sight; consequently, the person is usually most willing to comply with the treatment regimens. The primary reasons for noncompliance are forgetting to take the medication, discontinuing the medication because of feeling well, or deliberately stopping it because of the uncomfortable side effects. A patient with a chronic disease, such as glaucoma, must understand that the medication controls disease but does not cure it; therefore, lifelong therapy is required. The patient must also be made aware of the importance of continued follow-up for his or her eye condition.
- Evaluate for adverse effects. If the patient experiences headache, eye pain, vision changes, continued redness, or irritation, or the condition worsens for more than 3 days, the physician should be notified. The offending product is usually discontinued.

Teach the patient about potential side effects so that a patient taking medication at home reports any unusual symptoms to the physician or nurse.

The bibliography for this chapter can be found in Appendix B, which begins on page 1054.

CHAPTER REVIEW QUESTIONS*

1. Fluorescein sodium can be used in the eye to:
   a. Fit soft contacts.
   b. Test lacrimal patency.
   c. Remove foreign bodies from the eye.
   d. Stain the eye for 60 minutes.

2. The antiviral medication idoxuridine (IDU) is administered:
   a. For 5 to 7 days after healing has occurred.
   b. Concurrently with boric acid solution.
   c. In a liquid form only.
   d. Systemically to treat herpes simplex virus.

3. Anti-inflammatory eye medications, such as dexamethasone, are used primarily for:
   a. Treatment of fungal infections.
   b. Management of acute infections.
   c. Long-term treatment of glaucoma.
   d. Reduction of permanent scarring.

*See Appendix A, which begins on page 1051, for answers.

4. Which of the following agents is a cholinesterase inhibitor used to treat open-angle glaucoma?
   a. Methazolamide (Neptazane).
   b. Carbachol (Isopto Carbachol).
   c. Physostigmine (Eserine).
   d. Betaxolol (Betopic).

5. Caution is advised when administering beta-adrenergic blockers, such as timolol maleate (Timoptic), with the following medication:
   a. Potassium chloride.
   b. Digoxin.
   c. Aspirin.
   d. Iodine.

6. Acetazolamide (Diamox) is useful in treating glaucomas because of which of the following actions?
   a. Production of systemic alkalosis.
   b. Interference with production of carbonic acid.
   c. Production of osmotic diuresis.
   d. Direct contraction of ciliary muscles.

BUILDING YOUR CRITICAL THINKING SKILLS

ADDITIVE EFFECTS/TOXIC EFFECTS

Patient 1

Doug, age 73, is admitted to the emergency department after falling to the floor. His pulse on admission is 38 beats/minute. He has had hypertension for 12 years and has recently been diagnosed with glaucoma.

Focus of Inquiry: 12-lead ECG is obtained and shows a sinus bradycardia.

Analysis and Synthesis: Recall that antihypertensive medications may slow the heart. Examine the patient's current drug regimen. Doug has been taking labetalol (Lopresser) for his blood pressure for 10 years. His blood pressure has been well controlled. His new glaucoma medicine is metipranolol hydrochloride (Optic Pranolol).

New Supposition: The bradycardia, causing the fall, is most likely relative to the administration of two beta-blockers. The beta-blocker eye medication was most likely absorbed systemically and caused excessive slowing of the heart rate.

Resolution: The beta-blocker glaucoma drug is changed to another type of drug such as a miotic (e.g., pilocarpine) to lower intraocular pressure.

Patient 2

Jane, age 36, was diagnosed with a severe inflammatory condition in her eye about 8 weeks ago. She was seen by a doctor at that time but moved to another city about 4 weeks ago. Since then, the eye condition has worsened.

Focus of Inquiry: Currently her left eye has thick yellow-green drainage and her vision is cloudy. A fungal infection is diagnosed.

Analysis and Synthesis: Recall that medications used for acute inflammation, such as steroids, are used for short-term use only. Determine what medication was originally prescribed and how long it was used.

New Supposition: Jane shows the eye drops that were prescribed—rimaxolone (Vexol). Rimaxolone is a steroid that should have been used for only 10–14 days, and she has now used it daily for 8 weeks. The fungal infection is most likely a consequence of long-term use of the steroid.

Resolution: The steroid is discontinued. An antifungal eye drop is ordered, and she is told to return to the clinic in 1 week. The importance of a return visit is stressed.

CHAPTER 64

Medications Used in Ear Disorders

Merrily A. Kuhn, RNC, PhD

CHAPTER OUTLINE

Anti-Infectives
Antihistamine-Decongestants
Local Anesthetics
Combination Products
Cerumenolytic Medications
Using the Nursing Process

TABLES
Drug Tables
Selected Otic Anti-Infectives, 980
Nursing Process
Nursing Process for Patient Receiving Ear Medications, 982
Patient Teaching
Patient Teaching Information—Ear Medications, 983

KEY TERMS

Cerumen
Conductive hearing loss
Myringitis

Tinnitus
Vertigo

LEARNING OBJECTIVES

After reading this chapter, the student will be able to:

1. Identify those medications commonly used for ear disorders.
2. Differentiate among the medications used for ear disorders as to mechanism of action, route of administration, pharmacokinetics, adverse effects, contraindications, and interactions.
3. Identify specific areas to assess in the patient requiring medications for ear disorders to formulate appropriate patient outcomes.
4. Plan the nursing interventions necessary to administer medications for ear disorders and choose appropriate teaching strategies to gain patient compliance.
5. Evaluate the patient at various stages of treatment to measure the effectiveness of nursing interventions.

Otic medications are administered locally to prevent or treat conditions of the external ear and are generally dissolved or suspended in a liquid vehicle for easier administration in the external ear canal. A few creams or ointments are available to be used on dry, crusted lesions. Generally, the medications used to treat ear conditions, which are featured in Table 64–1, are the same preparations commonly used to treat problems in other areas of the body. Examples include anti-infectives; local anesthetics; and combination products containing anti-infectives, adrenal corticosteroids, and/or local anesthetics. Cerumenolytic preparations are used to remove or loosen wax accumulations. It may be necessary to administer systemic medications when there are severe external infections, when the pain associated with the ear problem cannot be managed with the application of heat or topically applied medications, or when it is preferable or nec-

essary to reach the middle ear via the circulatory system. Because all of the medications used in otic disorders are discussed in other parts of this text, there is only a brief discussion of the specific action of these preparations.

ANTI-INFECTIVES

EXTERNAL EAR PROBLEMS

The anti-infectives, featured in Table 64–2, employed most commonly as otic medications for external use include **polymyxin B** and **neomycin** alone, or in combinations with hydrocortisone. The addition of the hydrocortisone reduces redness, itching, and edema within the ear. **Tetracycline, sulfonamides, chloramphenicol, gentami-**

Table 64–1. EAR DISEASE	
External Ear	
Types	External otitis: acute localized; acute diffuse; chronic diffuse; progressive, necrotizing
Age	Most common in infants and young children but can affect all age groups
Causative Organism	Staphylococcus, Pseudomonas, Proteus, fungi
Management	(1) Cleansing of the external canal to remove desquamated material, purulent secretions, cerumen (wax), and previously instilled topical medications, often done by irrigation; (2) application of appropriate medications; and (3) alteration of the pH to restore normal bacterial flora, the ear canal being normally acidic
Middle Ear	
Types	Otitis media; acute, chronic
Etiology	Often follows viral infections of the upper respiratory tract
Causative Organism	Streptococcus, pneumococcus, *Haemophilus influenzae*
Symptoms	Earache, feeling of fullness and pressure in the ear, loss of hearing, and accumulation of debris behind tympanic membrane may cause it to perforate or rupture owing to increased pressure.
Management	Systemic antibiotics, systemic analgesics, or surgical opening of tympanic membrane (myringotomy) to relieve pressure and promote drainage
Mastoiditis	
Definition	Inflammation of the mastoid antrum and cells
Etiology	May follow middle ear infection, sore throat, or respiratory infection
Symptoms	Earache, ringing in the ears, and painful, swollen mastoid process
Management	Anti-infectives; if ineffective, surgery

cin, **nitrofurazone, neomycin, ampicillin, penicillin G,** and **nystatin** are also used, orally or parenterally, when necessary (see Chapter 58 for more information on anti-infectives).

▼ CLINICAL ALERT

Topical therapy should be discontinued after 10 days to prevent overgrowth of fungal organisms or if the infection spreads. Oral products are then used, if necessary.

Another antimicrobial preparation used in external otic diseases is **acetic acid** as a 2% solution. It is often the drug of choice because of (1) a broad spectrum of antimicrobial activity that includes both fungi and *Pseudomonas* species; (2) a lack of bacterial resistance, and therefore, there is no chance of the patient developing resistant strains; (3) an absence of toxic or allergic actions; (4) an absence of cross-sensitivity with other medications; (5) low cost; and (6) stability with a long shelf-life, and thus it can be used many times.

INNER EAR PROBLEMS

Amoxicillin *(Amoxil)* and **ampicillin *(Polycillin)*** are currently first-line drugs effective for otitis media. **Erythromycin *(E-Mycin),* sulfamethoxazole/trimethoprim *(co-trimoxazole, Bactrim),*** and **amoxicillin/clavulanate potassium *(Augmentin)*** are second-line drugs that are used if the first-line drugs are ineffective, usually after 48 to 72 hours. The third-line drugs are of the cephalosporin group, particularly **cefaclor *(Ceclor).*** Pneumococcal and streptococcal infections are often treated with a 10-day course of oral penicillin G or penicillin V or with a single

injection of penicillin V. Parenteral administration may be ordered when the patient is noncompliant with oral therapy. If patients are allergic to the penicillins, erythromycin (for gram-positive organisms) or sulfonamides (for gram-negative organisms) are usually effective.

ANTIHISTAMINE-DECONGESTANTS

Orally administered antihistamine-decongestant products are used as an adjunct, along with anti-infectives, in treating patients with acute otitis media. Research demonstrates that antihistamine-decongestants reduce nasal congestion and middle ear effusion. Antihistamine-decongestants are believed to improve eustachian tube patency and to promote resolution of the underlying pathology. As edema around the eustachian tube orifice is reduced, drainage from the middle ear is enhanced.

The side effects experienced from the antihistamine-decongestants include dry mouth, somnolence, and blurred vision.

Several antihistamine-decongestant combination products are available, many of them over the counter (OTC). These include the following: Actifed—60 mg pseudoephedrine HCl and 2.5 mg triprolidine (OTC); Dimetane Decongestant—10 mg phenylephrine HCl and 4 mg brompheniramine maleate (OTC); Dimetapp—25 mg phenylpropanolamine HCl and 4 mg brompheniramine maleate (OTC); Drixoral Plus—60 mg pseudoephedrine sulfate, 3 mg dexbrompheniramine maleate, and 500 mg acetaminophen (OTC); Ornade—75 mg phenylpropanolamine HCl and 12 mg chlorpheniramine maleate (Rx); and Triminic Allergy Tablets—25 mg phenylpropanolamine HCl and 4 mg chlorpheniramine maleate (OTC).

Table 64–2. SELECTED OTIC ANTI-INFECTIVES*

DRUG NAME	MODE OF ADMINISTRATION	DOSE	ADVERSE EFFECTS*
acetic acid (Acetic acid otic solution 2% and other irritating solutions)			
	Topical	4–6 gtt q 2–3 hr	Local irritation and sensitivity reactions
ampicillin (Polycillin, Omnipen, Amcill)			
	PO, IM, IV	*Adults:* 1,000–12,000 mg/ day in divided doses of 4–6 hr *Children:* 50–200 mg/kg per day in divided doses q 4–6 hr	GI upset, increased SGOT, superinfection, hypersensitivity, BLOOD DYSCRASIAS, NEUROTOXICITY, ANAPHYLAXIS, INTERSTITIAL NEPHRITIS
penicillin (Penicillin G, Pentids, V-Cillin, Pen-Vee)			
	IM	*Pen G:* *Adults:* 600,000–1.2 million units/day *Children:* 500,000–1 million units/day *Pen V: Adults:* 125–250 mg q 6–8 hr *Pen V, PO, Children over 12 yr:* 15–50 mg/kg per day in 3–6 divided doses	Hypersensitivity reactions, GI upset, blood dyscrasias, neuropathy, superinfections
amoxicillin (Amoxil, Larotid, Polymox)			
	PO	*Adults:* 250–500 mg tid *Children under 20 kg:* 20–40 mg/kg per day in divided doses q 8 hr	Same as above
cefaclor (Ceclor)			
	PO	*Adults:* 250–500 mg tid *Children:* 20 mg/kg per day in doses q 8 hr	Same as above
amoxicillin, clavulanate (Augmentin)			
	PO	*Adults:* 250 mg q 8 hr *Children over 40 kg:* 40 mg/kg per day in divided doses q 8 hr	Diarrhea common

*CAPITALS indicate life-threatening effects. Also, prolonged use may lead to superinfection (herpes simplex, vaccinia, and so on). All drugs are contraindicated during pregnancy and lactation if previous sensitivity and safety have not been established.

LOCAL ANESTHETICS

To control the pain associated with ear infections, local anesthetics are often used topically. They may be used alone or in combination with either anti-infective or anti-inflammatory agents or both. Local anesthetic preparations include **Americaine otic drops, Auralgan otic solution, Otodyne otic solution, Otolgesis otic solution,** and **Tympagesis ear drops.** The usual dosage is 1 to 6 drops in each ear as ordered.

Pain relief for ear disorders may best be accomplished by using systemic analgesics such as Tylenol or other drugs rather than local agents. Tylenol is recommended, as most ear infections occur in children.

COMBINATION PRODUCTS

The combination products contain anti-infectives and either local anesthetics or anti-inflammatory agents or both. In general, these combination products are frowned upon by much of the medical community, which believes that only the single ingredient that is really needed should be used. A corticosteroid, when combined with an anti-infective, may decrease the ultimate effectiveness of the anti-infective. Commonly used combination otic medications include the following: **Cortisporin Otic** (solution) or **Otocort** (solution)—5 mg neomycin sulfate, 10,000 units polymyxin B sulfate, and 1% hydrocortisone; **VoSol Otic**—1% hydrocortisone, 2% acetic acid in isopropyl alcohol, 3% propylene glycol diacetate, 0.02% benzethonium chloride, and 0.015% sodium acetate; **Swimear, Dri/Ear, Ear-Dry,** or **Aurocaine 2**—2.75% boric acid in isopropyl alcohol.

CERUMENOLYTIC MEDICATIONS

Cerumen (ear wax) is produced by glands in the outer one-third of the external canal and has bacteriostatic and fungistatic properties. Normally, cerumen slowly moves toward the external opening of the ear where it is washed out and does not cause obstruction or a loss of hearing. However, this mechanism may break down if the individual frequently attempts to remove the cerumen deposits manually.

The type of wax is genetically determined. Persons living in western countries produce moist cerumen, whereas persons living in eastern countries produce dry cerumen. The ear canal is less effective in clearing dry cerumen than moist cerumen. If the ear canal becomes blocked by cerumen, a significant *conductive hearing loss* (hearing loss resulting from the mechanical inability of sound waves to be transmitted to the auditory nerves) may occur and the obstruction may predispose to the development of external otitis.

Gentle irrigation with hypertonic sodium chloride or hydrogen peroxide solutions may be necessary to soften, loosen, and flush out dried cerumen deposits. If the individual has chronic difficulty, the periodic instillation of one or two drops of olive oil, sweet almond oil, mineral oil, glycerin, or hydrogen peroxide softens the deposits and promotes normal removal. The cerumenolytics on the market, triethanolamine polypeptide oleate-condensate (Cerumenex) and carbamide peroxide (Debrox), are expensive and work no better than the agents just named. Cerumenex causes more local irritation than does Debrox.

USING THE NURSING PROCESS

ASSESSMENT

- Obtain a thorough nursing history to develop the database. The nursing process is summarized in Table 64–3. The patient requiring otic medications is generally relatively healthy and is often treated as an outpatient.
- Assess for *tinnitus* (ringing in the ear) or hearing loss. At times, medications given for other purposes may cause ear symptoms. During the initial assessment,

all medications the patient is taking, both prescription and OTC, are identified. Medications that commonly cause ear symptoms are listed in Table 64–4. At this time, drug regulatory agencies are not required to test new drugs for ototoxic effects. Adverse otologic effects must, therefore, await recognition during general clinical trials. The risk of ototoxicity is greatly increased in patients with impaired renal function and, in general, is more likely in the elderly. Most drugs causing ototoxicity also cause nephrotoxicity (e.g., aminoglycoside antibiotics).

▼ **CLINICAL ALERT**

Some drugs, particularly the aminoglycoside antibiotics, have the capacity to damage the eighth cranial nerve, sometimes irreversibly. The onset of hearing loss may not occur until sometime after treatment is discontinued or may continue to progress even when treatment is stopped. Eighth cranial nerve damage may occur to the vestibular portion, causing the patient to complain of *vertigo* (disturbed equilibrium characterized by dizziness and light-headedness) and tinnitus; or to the auditory portion, which often leads to temporary or permanent loss of high-frequency sound perception. Auditory toxicity is particularly common with kanamycin, neomycin, and streptomycin.

- Assess predrug, postdrug, and with biweekly testing when appropriate in a patient taking ototoxic drugs. Intratherapeutic monitoring is most appropriate for those over 50 years old or those who may be prone to exceeding therapeutic concentrations of a potential ototoxic antibiotic.
- Assess how the individual normally cares for his or her ears, as improper hygiene practices may be the source of the problem. Inform the patient of proper ear care procedures if needed.

NURSING DIAGNOSIS

- Typical nursing diagnoses for a patient with ear problems include Knowledge Deficit, Pain, Anxiety, and Risk for Trauma (see Table 64–3).

PLANNING AND INTERVENTION

- Develop the goals of nursing intervention from the nursing diagnoses during the planning phase. Typical nursing actions are included in Table 64–3.

Patient Teaching

- Make certain that the patient knows and understands the information presented in Table 64–5 and Figure 64–1 to ensure the safe administration of medications and the prevention of further ear problems.
- Teach the patient how to do ear irrigations. Irrigations must be done very gently to prevent damaging

Table 64–3. NURSING PROCESS FOR PATIENT RECEIVING EAR MEDICATIONS

Assessment

Assess history of current illness/condition, previous occurrence (and frequency) of infection.
Assess routine care, how often and how ears are cleaned, whether patient is swimmer.
Assess medication use (prescription and OTC drugs).
Assess dizziness.

Nursing Diagnosis: Knowledge Deficit	**Desired Outcomes/Evaluation Criteria**
RELATED TO: Lack of exposure/recall, unfamiliarity with information resources/misinterpretation. **AS EVIDENCED BY:** Questions, statement of concern, inaccurate follow-through of instruction/development of preventable complications.	Verbalizes understanding of individual condition/disease process and treatment. Correctly performs necessary procedures and explains reasons for the actions.

Nursing Actions	**Rationale**
Provide information about individual condition, treatment rationale, and expected outcomes.	Understanding of reasons for ear problems helps patient to make informed choices and cooperate with treatment regimen.
Review drug dosage, administration schedule, need to continue for specified number of days.	Promotes correct procedure and enhances potential for positive outcome.
Instruct in administration of ear drops/ medications or irrigations. Have individual return demonstration of procedure.	Provides optimal benefit from medication.
Identify possible detrimental side effects (e.g., hypersensitivity) or signs of inadequate treatment (e.g., continuing pain, drainage) and importance of seeking medical attention.	Early identification allows for prompt intervention and prevention of further problems.
Demonstrate correct procedure for ear care.	Reduces risk of recurrence.
Discuss reasons for infection related to swimming, use of diving hoods or ear phones.	Swimmer's ear is common summer malady, usually due to *Pseudomonas aeruginosa* or other gram-negative organism.
Suggest use of ear plugs, limiting time in water, and drying ear thoroughly after swimming or showering/shampooing.	Use of barrier/proper care can reduce recurrence of these infections.

Nursing Diagnosis: Risk for Trauma	**Desired Outcomes/Evaluation Criteria**
RELATED TO: Balancing difficulties.	Identifies and corrects potential risk factors in environment. Demonstrates appropriate actions to reduce risk of injury.

Nursing Actions	**Rationale**
Monitor complaints of dizziness, swaying gait.	Indicators of vestibular disturbances.
Note hazards in environment and take measures to correct.	Can prevent injury from falls related to impaired balance.
Assist patient as necessary when walking	May need help until vertigo is resolved.
Determine origin of symptoms and refer for medical evaluation.	Vertigo may be side effect of drugs such as acetylsalicylic acid or aminoglycosides or result of infection.

Other Suggested Nursing Diagnoses: Pain and Anxiety.

Table 64–4. MEDICATIONS ADVERSELY AFFECTING THE EAR

Drug	Tinnitus	Vertigo	Hearing Loss
Gentamicin, tobramycin, kanamycin, neomycin	x	x	x (mild to moderate, high frequency)
Streptomycin	x	x	x (moderate to severe)
Loop diuretics (e.g., ethacrynic acid, furosemide, bumex)	—	—	x (mild to moderate)
Salicylates and other nonsteroidal anti-inflammatory agents	x	x	—
Chloroquine	x	x	—
Platinol	—	—	x (high frequency)
Minocycline	—	x	—

Important to monitor hearing ability when doses are increased, when there is increased duration of treatment, or with decreased renal function.

Table 64–5. PATIENT TEACHING INFORMATION—EAR MEDICATIONS

Dear Patient:

This drug has been ordered for you. This is what you should know about your drug to get the most from its use.

☐ 1. You must take ear drugs until your ear problem is resolved.

☐ 2. To give ear medications correctly, you must straighten the ear canal. Tip your head slightly to the opposite side, grasp the top of the ear (auricle) firmly and pull it upward, back, and slightly out. Press gently on the skin flap over the opening (tragus) after putting on the medicine or use an ear wick to move the medication down into the canal. (Cotton plugs do not help the medication move.) (Figure 64–1 shows ear medication instillation.) If you are administering a topical ear medication to a young child, the child is held securely to prevent hurting the ear. A child's ear is pulled down by the ear lobe to open the ear canal.

☐ 3. The interactions that may occur with your drugs include: ―――――.

☐ 4. If you forget your ear drug until almost when the next dose is due, forget the dose; do *not* try to catch up.

☐ 5. Typical side effects for your ear medications include: ―――――

☐ 6. If you usually get earaches during the warm weather or after swimming, you should try to keep your ear canals dry. After swimming, you can put a few drops of either ethyl or isopropyl alcohol (70% to 95%) or isopropyl alcohol mixed with vinegar into the ear to help dry the canal and prevent a ready source of infection.

☐ 7. Do not put or poke any foreign objects, such as hairpins, cotton-tipped swabs, match sticks, fingernails, or other small objects into your ear canal for any purpose.

☐ 8. Take all of your drugs as ordered by your physician.

☐ 9. Store your drug in a dry, light-resistant container.

the tympanic membrane and therefore are best performed by direct visualization. The most frequently used irrigating solutions include aluminum acetate solution (Burow's solution), dilute (10% to 20%) ethyl alcohol solution, hydrogen peroxide (3% mixed 1:1 with water), hypertonic (3%) sodium chloride solution, and 1% acetic acid solution.

Swimmer's Ear

A common malady, particularly during the summer, is swimmer's ear. It is usually due to *Pseudomonas aeruginosa*

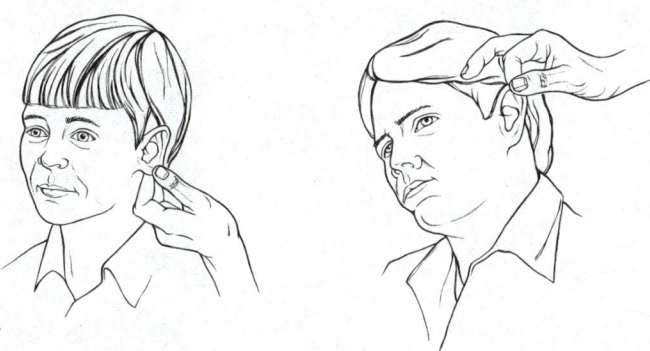

Figure 64–1. To instill ear drops in a child, pull down on the ear lobe to straighten the external canal. To instill ear drops in an adult, pull up and back on the auricle to straighten the external canal.

or other gram-negative organism. Rarely is the infection fungal. Swimmer's ear may occur when a person's ears have been exposed to prolonged heat or moisture as from swimming or the use of diving hoods or ear phones.

In the earliest, mildest form of swimmer's ear, which is sometimes called the pre-inflammatory stage, itching and a feeling that the ear is plugged are the most typical complaints. If the canal has been kept dry and free from trauma, the condition rarely needs medication attention. However, if there has been trauma to the skin of the canal from scratching, infection occurs. The canal is red, swollen, and tender. In all but the mildest cases, pushing on the tragus, pulling the auricle up and back, or exerting gentle outward pressure in the canal with an otoscope speculum causes discomfort. As the infection progresses, the canal fills with varying amounts of cheesy green-blue-gray discharge composed of bacteria, leukocytes, desquamated epithelial cells, and serous fluid. This external otitis is often accompanied by *myringitis* (inflammation of the eardrum, usually because of infection).

The best approach to swimmer's ear is prevention. When teaching the patient, recommend that he or she limit time in the water. The time is determined by trial and error but is generally less than 1 hour. Shake the head to loosen water and dry the ear with the corner of a towel. The ear is allowed to dry completely for an hour or two before going back in the water.

In addition, a solution of equal parts of water and vinegar or vinegar and rubbing alcohol can be prepared. A few drops are put in each ear on arising in the morning, after each swim, and at bedtime. The solution should remain in the ear for at least 5 minutes. Nothing is inserted into the ear canal that could cause injury to the delicate epithelial lining.

If these measures are not effective, medical treatment is obtained. After treatment begins, the individual should stay out of the water for at least 7 days. It is permissible to shower or bathe each day and shampoo the hair every other day if the ear is dried immediately afterwards and ear medications put in. Typical ear medications that are ordered include local antibiotics, systemic antipruritics, and analgesics. Medications are generally continued for several days after all signs and symptoms have resolved.

Evaluation

• Evaluate the effectiveness of the medications used for ear disorders, based on a list of outcome evaluation criteria that has been developed in relation to the goals determined by the nurse, patient, and family (see Table 64–3).

• Evaluate for potential side effects of the medications, and instruct patients to report any unusual symptoms to the physician or nurse. In general, medications applied topically to the ear have few side effects. The most frequent complaint is contact dermatitis. Any local redness or itching is reported at once and the medication discontinued.

• Evaluate for patient compliance with the treatment regimen. Work with the patient and family to ensure their complete assistance and support, and stress the importance of continued medical care. Many of the patients with ear disorders are children, so assistance from the school or camp nurse in administering the medication may need to be elicited. The primary reason for noncompliance is forgetting medication. Develop a method that the patient and family can use to help them remember the medication schedule and to evaluate its effectiveness.

The bibliography for this chapter can be found in Appendix B, which begins on page 1054.

CHAPTER REVIEW QUESTIONS*

1. A solution that can be used to irrigate the ears is:
   a. 10% acetic acid.
   b. Full-strength hydrogen peroxide.
   c. 50% ethyl alcohol.
   d. Burow's solution.

2. When performing a nursing assessment on the patient requiring ear medications, the nurse is aware that:
   a. Over-the-counter medications are free of ototoxic effects.
   b. Patients with renal dysfunction are less prone to ototoxicity.
   c. Aminoglycoside antibiotics may damage the eighth cranial nerve.
   d. Vestibular damage causes loss of high-frequency sound perception.

3. The nurse instructs patients and families on proper administration of ear medications, which includes:
   a. Pulling the auricle downward and slightly in for the adult.

   b. Inserting cotton plugs after administration.
   c. Tipping the head toward the affected side before instillation.
   d. Applying gentle pressure on the tragus after instillation.

4. Swimmer's ear is usually due to:
   a. Gram-positive organisms.
   b. Gram-negative organisms.
   c. Viral infections.
   d. Fungal infections.

5. Which of the following agents can be used to soften and remove cerumen deposits?
   a. Augmentin.
   b. Ornade.
   c. Debrox.
   d. Aerosporin.

*See Appendix A, which begins on page 1051, for answers.

CHAPTER 65

Medications for Common Skin Disorders

Merrily A. Kuhn, RNC, PhD

CHAPTER OUTLINE

TABLES

KEY TERMS

Collodions
Comedones
Creams
Emollients
Keratolytics

Lichenified lesions
Lotions
Ointment
Protectives

LEARNING OBJECTIVES

After reading this chapter, the student will be able to:

1. Identify those medications commonly used in skin disorders.
2. Differentiate among the skin disorder medications as to mechanism of action, route of administration, pharmacokinetics, adverse effects, contraindications, and interactions.
3. Identify specific areas to assess in the patient requiring skin disorder medications to formulate appropriate patient outcomes.
4. Plan the nursing interventions necessary to administer skin disorder medications and choose appropriate teaching strategies to gain patient compliance.
5. Evaluate the patient at various stages of treatment to measure the effectiveness of nursing interventions.

The skin, the largest single organ in the body, acts as a barrier between the environment and the body. It protects the body from external conditions such as heat and cold and from harmful agents such as organisms and chemicals. The skin is also actively involved with temperature control and in regulation of fluid balance. It produces pigment, giving itself color, and synthesizes vitamin D.

The skin is composed of three main layers: the epidermis, the dermis, and the hypodermis, as shown in Figure 65–1. It is a living tissue and requires a supply of oxygen and nutrients. The skin also has appendages, including hair follicles, sebaceous glands, sweat glands, and the nails.

Diseases of the skin can be classified by the location of their causative agent. These classifications include diseases of the appendages, diseases caused by parasites and insects, bacterial diseases, viral diseases, fungal diseases, eczema and dermatitis, skin conditions caused by sunlight, and malignant tumors of the skin. Table 65–1 identifies the common dermatologic conditions, their assessable characteristics, and their management.

Dermatologic agents are so vast in number that it would be difficult to cover them all in this chapter. Many of these preparations are also used to treat other conditions and have been discussed elsewhere in this text. Only a brief review will be given for those groups of products.

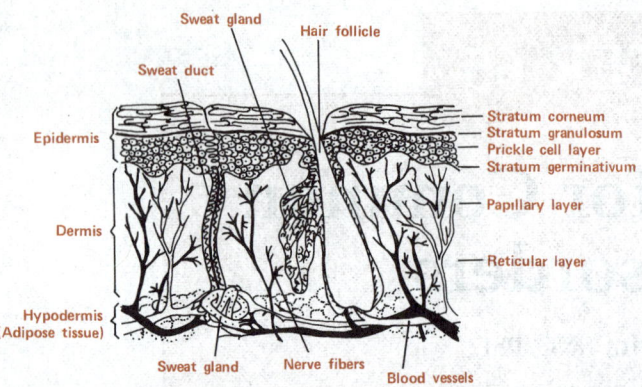

Figure 65–1. The three layers of the skin are the epidermis, the dermis, and the hypodermis. The horny, or keratinized, layer is the uppermost layer. Hair, glandular structures, and other organs associated with the skin are found within the dermis.

Dermatologic preparations include emollients to soften or soothe irritated skin; anti-infectives, such as antiseptic, antibacterial, antifungal, antiviral, or antiparasitic agents; counterirritants to produce mild irritation of the skin to produce healing; keratolytics to soften scales and loosen the horny layer of skin; antipruritics to allay itching; protectives to protect the skin from the outside environment; and cleansers such as soaps and shampoos to clean the skin.

CREAMS, OINTMENTS, EMULSIONS, AND LOTIONS

Emollients, found as creams or ointments, are oily or fatty substances that soften or soothe irritated skin by allowing

Table 65–1. COMMON SKIN CONDITIONS WITH NURSING INTERVENTIONS

Condition	Assessable Characteristics	Intervention Pharmacologic	Nonpharmacologic
Diseases of the Appendages Seborrheic dermatitis	Chronic, common, recurrent lesions, which are dry or greasy, scaly red patches over upper body.	Detergent shampoos, astringents, drying agents, emollients.	Frequent baths and shampooing; well-balanced diet, avoidance of excessive stress.
Acne rosacea	Chronic; common in females in the fourth and fifth decades. Lesions are in middle third of face and appear as areas of vasodilation with papules and pustules.	Tetracycline.	Avoid facial hyperemia by eliminating alcohol, spicy foods, excessive sun exposure.
Acne vulgaris	Found in 90% of teenagers. Lesions are inflammation of pilosebaceous follicles with formation of cysts.	Frequent washing (2–3 times a day) of affected skin with soap; drying agents, keratolytics, irritants, or abrasives. Tetracyclines and other antibiotics (topical and systemic).	Frequent exposure to sunlight when medicine is not used, well-balanced diet.
Parasites and Insects Scabies	Irritation of skin in folds—wrist, between fingers, genitals, buttock, waist. Pruritus varies.	1% lindane (Kwell, Gamene) cream/lotion. Lotion should be left in place 24 hr. Benzyl benzoate (10%) lotion.	All clothes and bedding thoroughly washed or dry cleaned; good hygiene; education.
Pediculosis	Minute, red, noninflamed areas over skin in affected area.	Lindane shampoo.	Same as above.
Bacterial Diseases Impetigo	Facial lesions, generally in children. Circular lesions, starting as vesicles and progressing to pustules.	Benzathine penicillin G IM single dose 600,000 units in children ≤6 yr, 1.2 million units in patients >7 yr of age. Or 10 days' therapy with erythromycin 250 mg PO qid or penicillin VK 250 mg PO qid. For staphylococcal impetigo, dicloxacillin 250 mg PO qid.	Washing with mild soaps, warm tap water, saline soaks; washing with bactericidal or bacteriostatic soaps.

Continued on the following page

Table 65–1. COMMON SKIN CONDITIONS WITH NURSING INTERVENTIONS, *Continued*

Condition	Assessable Characteristics	Intervention	
		Pharmacologic	*Nonpharmacologic*
Viral Diseases **Herpes simplex**	Lesions are one time only or recurrent at same site. Begin as local burning and tingling followed by multiple, grouped, tiny vesicles on an erythematous base.	Drying agents. Acyclovir topically or IV.	Avoid contact with infected individual.
Warts (verrucae)	Papillary growths anywhere on the skin surface.	Cryotherapy; drying agents; caustics.	Contagious; avoid direct contact with others.
Fungal Infections **Ringworm of the foot** (tinea pedis)	Lesions between toes characterized by cracking and blisters containing a watery liquid.	Topical antibacterial and antifungal agents; antifungal powder.	Keep area clean and dry; wear clogs in any public shower; educate on prevention.
Eczema and Dermatitis **Contact dermatitis**	Lesions occur anywhere on body and appear as reddened, edematous vesicles and bullae; itching usually present.	Wet dressing. Medications to control and relieve itching.	Identify causative agent and prevent further contact.
Atopic dermatitis (allergic eczema)	Lesions most commonly occur on face, neck, scalp, and diaper area shortly after birth. Areas are dry, excoriated, and edematous; and they itch.	Antipruritic, anti-inflammatory agents and lubricants control pruritus. Wet dressings (Burrow's solution). Topical steroids.	Mild soaps. Dry climate. Avoid irritants.
Pityriasis rosea	Fawn-colored, scaly lesions that appear on trunk and extremities; pruritus.	Most patients require no treatment; however, antihistamines and emollients can be used to control pruritus. Tepid baths (Aveeno oatmeal) 10–15 min daily.	Noninfectious. Limit ultraviolet exposure.
Psoriasis	Lesions are thick, scaly plaques characterized by sharply demarcated deep red covered lesions by thick overlying silver scales. Emotional stress and anxiety cause exacerbations. Often occurs on elbows, hands, knees, feet, and in genital areas.	Anti-inflammatory agents (potent fluorinated steroids). Antineoplastic drugs (methotrexate). Keratolytics. Coal tar therapy in combination or alternating with corticosteroids. Photoactive drugs (psoralens) in combination with ultraviolet light. Retinoic acid. Anthralin (Dithranol) Calcipotriene (Emersal) Etretinate (Tegison)	Frequent exposure to sunlight. Control stress and anxiety. Avoid cold climates.

the skin to retain water. *Creams* are emulsions of oil in water or water in oil. Water-in-oil emulsions have a more hydrating effect and provide more lubrication and occlusion, but oil-in-water emulsions are less greasy and more easily removed. When the amount of oil exceeds that of water by a certain proportion, the emulsion changes from a pourable cream to a semisolid *ointment*. Ointments are greasier than creams, and unmedicated ointments are not irritating to the skin. Ointments and creams are used as effective vehicles to dissolve active ingredients or medications so that they may be applied to the skin. Creams and ointments are particularly suitable for the chronic inflammatory stage of skin diseases. Dry, scaling, thickened, pruritic, and *lichenified lesions* (a general term applied to a variety of skin reactions that are characterized by the presence of papules or circumscribed red elevations) respond to their softening and lubricating properties.

Emollients may have as a base preparation fixed oils, such as olive, flaxseed, or cottonseed. Glycerin is usually mixed with water or rose water (oil-in-oil emulsion), and often is useful in treating cracked, irritated lips and skin. Petrolatum (petroleum jelly—water-repellent ointment) is a purified, semisolid mixture of hydrocarbons derived from petroleum. Lanolin (water-in-oil emulsion), a purified hydrous sheep wool fat that can absorb water, is mixed with 25% to 30% water. Cold cream (water-in-oil emulsion) is a combination of spermaceti, white wax, and mineral oil. Hydrogenated vegetable oil (Crisco) can also be used as an emollient. Most other emollients are prepared from these bases. Yellow ointment (yellow wax) and petroleum is a water-repellent ointment, and zinc ointment (petroleum white ointment and 20% zinc oxide) is a water-absorbent ointment.

Lotions are usually liquid suspensions (require shaking before application) or dispersions that can be prepared by mixing solid ingredients that have been made into a paste consistency with a liquid in which they are insoluble. Medicated lotions (Calamine lotion, Caladryl lotion) are often used as anti-inflammatory agents because they provide a drying, protective, and cooling effect. Lotions (aluminum acetate solution [Burow's solution], potassium permanganate solution, and zinc stearate), are used for subacute inflammatory lesions after the severe exudate phase has ceased. Lotions can also be used as a wash for the skin, soaks, or wet dressings on ulcers or burns. Although lotions are predominantly water, they have a "drying" effect on the skin when the water evaporates. Lotions are generally not a good vehicle for delivering medications.

In general, the more chronic and scaly the lesions, the more likely highly hydrating products, such as ointments with oil emulsions, are used.

RUBS AND LINIMENTS

Rubs and liniments are used for the temporary relief of muscular aches, rheumatism, arthritis, sprains, and neuralgia. Common products sold over the counter (OTC) include Aspercreame, Myoflex, Hot Cream/Balm/Stick, Ben Gay, Deep-down Rub, and many others. These products contain combinations of antiseptics, local anesthetics, analgesics, and counterirritants. A heating pad is not used with these products as irritation or burning of the skin may occur. Some of these products contain salicylates, and if used over a large area of the skin may cause salicylate side effects such as tinnitus, nausea, or vomiting.

ANTI-INFECTIVE AGENTS

Anti-infective agents include antiseptic, antibacterial, antifungal, antiviral, and antiparasitic drugs. All the anti-infectives are discussed in detail in Chapter 58. Topical antibiotics are safe and effective in certain conditions, primarily acne, rosacea, and nasal carriage of *Staphylococcus*

aureus. In general, antibiotics are safe, but extensive use may encourage the emergence of resistant bacteria.

ANTISEPTICS

Several antiseptic solutions are available, including **sodium hypochlorite *(Dakin's)*, chlorhexidine gluconate *(Hibiclens)*, acetic acid, hydrogen peroxide,** and **hexachlorophene *(pHisoHex)*.** It is important to use the antiseptic solution that best suits the patient's condition.

○ **Sodium hypochlorite** (Dakin's) is a chloride solution which loosens, dissolves, and deodorizes necrotic tissue and blood clots. It kills most common bacteria, spores, amebas, fungi, protozoa, viruses, and yeasts. It is used for irrigating and cleaning necrotic or purulent wounds, or for packing necrotic, not purulent, wounds since it is inactivated by copious pus.

▼ **CLINICAL ALERT**

Sodium hypochlorite burns, so it should not be in contact with healing or normal tissue. Recent studies demonstrate that sodium hypochlorite interferes with the body's natural wound-healing process.

Sodium hypochlorite loses its potency during storage, so fresh solution is prepared frequently.

○ **Chlorhexidine gluconate** (Hibiclens) is effective for cleansing wounds caused by staphylococci, reptococci, and other gram-positive bacteria. It is used for irrigating and cleansing wounds but not for packing because it may cause contact dermatitis.

○ **Acetic acid** as a 0.25% solution is effective for irrigating, cleansing, and packing wounds infected by *Pseudomonas aeruginosa*. Healthy skin surrounding the wound must be protected with a petrolatum barrier because it excoriates the skin.

○ **Hydrogen peroxide** as a 3% solution has effervescent action that releases gas and breaks up necrotic tissue. It is used to irrigate and clean necrotic tissue and pus from open wounds. It is not used to pack wounds because it decomposes too rapidly. When epithelial tissue begins to form, hydrogen peroxide is discontinued because it inhibits tissue formation.

○ **Hexachlorophene** (pHisoHex, Soy-Dome Cleanser, Pre-op) is a combination of hexachlorophene, a bacteriostatic agent with activity against staphylococci and other gram-positive bacteria, and alcohol. Alcohol dries and irritates tissues and forms a film that can actually promote infection; it is not a very effective germicide. All hexachlorophene products are well rinsed from the skin after their use to prevent systemic absorption.

▼ **CLINICAL ALERT**

Hexachlorophene is heavily absorbed through broken skin and can cause neurotoxicity. It should not be used on any type of wound.

ANTIBACTERIALS

When antibacterial drugs are needed, the less absorbable antibiotics such as bacitracin, neomycin, and polymyxin B are generally used. Common combinations of all three products include Mity-mycin, Mycitracin Triple Antibiotic, and Triple Antibiotic. In addition, Neo-Polycin Ointment is a combination of zinc, bacitracin, neomycin, and polymyxin B. Topical application of these preparations is not effective for acute, superficial, and relatively localized infections. Systemic antibiotics are preferred for more severe, chronic, deep, or generalized infections. These products are applied one to five times daily to the infected area and covered if needed.

○ **Mupirocin** (Bactroban) is a topical antibacterial active against impetigo caused by *Stapholococcus* or *Streptococcus* species. It is applied three times daily. If improvement is not observed within 3 to 5 days, it is discontinued.

ANTIFUNGALS

When antifungal agents are used, the skin is washed at least daily with soap and water and patted dry. Antifungal agents applied to the skin may cause erythema, stinging, blistering, peeling, pruritis, urticaria, and general skin irritation. Treatment is often protracted, but if no results are obtained after 4 weeks of treatment, the patient is reevaluated. Table 65–2 features the most common antifungal dermatologic agents, their general uses, and specific comments concerning use.

ANTIVIRALS

The primary topical antiviral agent used today is acyclovir (Zovirax). Acyclovir, which inhibits DNA replication in the virus, is a synthetic acyclic purine necleoside analog that has activity against herpes simplex types 1 and 2, varicella-zoster, Epstein-Barr, and cytomegalovirus. The major adverse effects include mild pain and transient burning and stinging. Acyclovir is available as a 5% ointment that is applied (completely covering the lesion) every 3 hours six times daily for 1 week. A rubber glove is used to apply the ointment to prevent the spread of infection.

ANTIPARASITICS

Antiparasitic agents are used to kill parasitic arthropods including the causative agents for scabies (mange) and pediculosis (lice). The object of treatment of scabies and pediculosis is elimination of the offending organisms and prevention or treatment of secondary infections. These products are available as shampoos, creams, spray, or lotions. The drugs are well absorbed through intact skin and thus may be harmful during pregnancy and in young children because of their thinner skin.

Antiparasitic preparations may irritate the skin, eyes, and mucous membranes, and may even cause allergic reactions. When signs of severe intolerance develop, the medications are discontinued and the inflammation allowed to subside before alternative therapy is substituted.

Common antiparasitic agents are listed in Table 65–3 with additional information.

STIMULANTS AND IRRITANTS

Stimulants and irritants produce a mild irritation to the surface of the skin, causing hyperemia and inflammation, which promote healing. Coal tar, obtained from the destructive distillation of coal, is most widely used and is soluble in most ointment bases, oils, pastes, and alcohols, but not in plain water. Tars are sometimes used in treating psoriasis, seborrheic dermatitis, and atopic dermatitis. They can also act as antiseptics.

▼ **CLINICAL ALERT**

Tars in general have an unpleasant odor, frequently stain the skin and hair, and cause phototoxicity.

Coal tar is available as a cream, emulsion, lotion, ointment, soap, and shampoo and is also available in combination with steroids.

○ **Compound benzoin tincture,** available as a spray-on solution, is a demulcent and stimulant. It is used to protect the skin when the patient has bedsores, ulcers, cracked nipples, and fissures of any orifice such as the lips or anus. The mild irritation that is caused produces increased blood flow and healing.

KERATOLYTICS

Keratolytics—preparations that dissolve keratin—include **salicylic acid (Wart-Off, Freezone, Compound W)**, resorcinol **(Fostex Medicated Bar, Meted 2, Sebulex)**, podophyllum resin **(Pod-Ben-25)**, podofilox **(Condylox)**, cantharidin **(Cantharone)**, and masoprocol **(Actinex)**. These medications soften scales and loosen the horny layer of skin, resulting in minimal peeling or extensive desquamation. Keratolytic preparations are of use in treating superficial fungal infections, seborrheic dermatitis, psoriasis, and localized dermatitis. Keratolytics are available as gels, ointments, creams, plasters, or *collodions* (liquid compounds containing pyroxylin dissolved in ether or alcohol, which dry to a tenacious film).

○ **Salicylic acid** (Wart-off, Freezone, Compound W, and many others) is used to treat seborrheic dermatitis, acne, psoriasis, and to thin and remove calluses.

▼ **CLINICAL ALERT**

Salicylic acid can be absorbed systemically, even from small open lesions. In high enough concentrations, it is slowly excreted in the urine and can cause salicylism, characterized by dizziness and tinnitus. Therefore, salicylic acid is not applied to large surface areas or open wounds.

Table 65–2. TOPICAL ANTIFUNGAL AGENTS*

Generic Name/Trade Name	General Use											Comments/Dosage
	SFI‡	Tinea pedis	Tinea cruris	Tinea corporis	Tinea manuum	Tinea versicolor	Candidiasis‡	Athlete's Foot	Ringworm	Diaper Rash	Jock Itch	
												For all: Rub gently into the skin. Avoid friction or wearing tight clothing over infected area.
Haloprogin (Halotex)	X	X	X	X	X							Apply twice daily for 2–3 wk.
Miconazole nitrate (Micatin, Monistat-Derm, and others)		X	X			X	X					Apply sparingly twice daily (once a day for tinea versicolor).
Clotrimazole (Lotrimin, Mycelex)		X	X	X		X	X					Rub into area twice daily; improvement seen in 1 wk.
Ketoconazole (Nizoral)			X	X		X						Two times daily. May need treatment for 2–3 wk.
Undecylenic acid and derivatives (Desenex, Kool Foot, many others)								X	X	X	X	Cleanse and dry area, then apply product.
Econazole nitrate (Spectazole)		X	X	X		X	X					For tinea pedis, cruris, corporis, cutaneous candiasis, apply two times daily; for tinea versicolor, apply once daily.
Ciclopirox olamine (Loprox)		X	X	X		X	X					Gently massage into affected area twice daily. Reevaluate after 4 wk.
Triacetin (Fungoid)	X	X										Apply two times daily. Continue 1 wk after symptoms disappear.
Oxiconazole nitrate (Oxistat)		X	X									Apply daily for 2 wk or 1 mo for tinea pedis.
Sulconazole nitrate (Exelderm)			X	X		X						Gently massage small amount into affected area and surrounding skin 1 or 2 times a day. Improvement occurs within 1 wk, but continue therapy for 3–4 wk.
Naftifine HCl (Naftin)			X	X								Gently massage into affected area and surrounding skin. Use cream once a day, and gel twice a day. Wash hands after application.
Clioquinol (Vioform)							X					Apply 2–3 times daily, (can also be used for eczema).

*Many antifungal combination products are also available.
†SFI = superficial fungal infections.
‡Nystatin (Mycostatin and others) and amphotericin B (Fungizone) are also used for candidiasis.

Table 65–3. TOPICAL ANTIPARASITIC AGENTS

Name	General Use	Specific Directions and Comments*
Lindane† (gamma benzene hexachloride) (Kwell, Scabene, G-Well)	Scabies, pediculosis	**Cream, lotion:** Apply for 8–12 min and then remove by thorough washing. **Shampoo:** Apply for 4 min and then rinse thoroughly. Second application may be necessary 4–7 days later. Treat sexual contacts concurrently.
Crotamiton (Eurax)	Scabies	**Cream, lotion:** Thoroughly massage into skin of whole body. Reapply 24 hr later. Change clothing and bed linen next morning. Take cleansing bath 48 hr after 2nd application. Stains clothes, is cosmetically unattractive.
Permethrin (Nix, Elimite)	Pediculosis capitis	**Liquid, cream:** Wash, rinse, and towel-dry hair. Apply sufficient volume to saturate hair and scalp. Allow to remain on hair 10 min. Rinse with water.
Malathion (Ovide)	Head lice	**Lotion:** Sprinkle lotion on dry hair and rub gently until scalp is moistened. Allow to dry naturally. After 8–12 hr wash hair with nonmedicated shampoo. Rinse, use a fine-toothed comb to remove lice. Repeat in 7–9 days if needed.
Nit Removal System (Step 2)	Lice	**Cream rinse:** Shake well. Apply to wet hair and allow to remain 10 min. Rinse with warm water and dry hair with hair dryer. Used to loosen and remove lice after other pediculosis treatments.

*Clean clothing and bedding also as patient is treated: Dryclean, put in hot cycle of washing machine, or place in sealed bag 30–35 days, which surpasses life span of arthropods.
†Resistance is beginning to develop.

Salicylic acid is also available in combination with benzoic acid, marketed as Whitfield's ointment.

○ **Podophyllum resin** (Pod-Ben-25) is used for various types of skin cancer. Podophyllum resin causes direct degeneration of embryonic or tumor cells. Podophyllum resin is applied daily to the skin. The lesion sloughs off leaving a superficial ulcer and moderate dermatitis. After the therapy is discontinued, the lesions are dressed with a mild antiseptic ointment. The lesions generally heal within a few days.

○ **Cantharidin** (Cantharone) is used in treating warts and molluscum contagiosum. Cantharidin has an exfoliation effect only on epidermal cells. The site of application may experience tingling, itching, and burning and may be extremely tender for 2 to 6 days.

○ **Masoprocol** (Actinex) has antiproliferative activity against keratinocytes and is used to treat actinic keratoses. It is administered daily for 28 days, and the hands are washed thoroughly after spreading cream. Occlusive dressings are not to be used. Transient burning may be experienced after administration.

ANTIPRURITICS

Antipruritics are medications that allay itching of both the skin and mucous membranes. These preparations are applied as wet dressings, pastes, lotions, creams, or ointments. Itching is one of the most frequent complaints of patients with dermatologic conditions and is the one most poorly tolerated. Cornstarch or oatmeal baths; lotions of calamine or phenol applied to the site; or dressings moistened with solutions of potassium permanganate, aluminum subacetate, boric acid, or normal saline are all used to allay itching. See Table 65–4 for commonly used antipruritic medications.

Baths may be used to cleanse or medicate the skin or reduce the temperature. Persons with dry skin should bathe less frequently. Soothing baths have 1 to 2 ounces per gallon of bran, starch, or gelatin added. Antipruritic baths have 1 ounce per gallon of oilated oatmeal, Alpha-Keri, or Lubath added.

Systemic medication such as antihistamines, diphenhydramine (Benadryl), or some phenothiazine derivatives, in particular trimeprazine (Temaril), may also be administered to reduce itching. Trimeprazine is believed to have an antipruritic activity largely because of its antihistamine effect, reducing the pruritic action of histamine. Cyproheptadine (Periactin), a drug that blocks both histamine and serotonin (also an itch mediator), is also a very effective antipruritic. Dry skin is a common cause for itching. Emollients may help to rehydrate the skin and prevent further difficulties.

PROTECTIVES

Protectives are either films or preparations that form a film on the skin to protect it from irritations such as light, moisture, air, and dust. This action promotes natural healing without the usual formation of a dry crust over the wound. Preparations used as protectives include transparent films applied to the skin, such as flexible collodion (Second Skin and many others); bandages impregnated

Table 65–4. ANTIPRURITICS

Preparation	Action
LOTIONS/PASTES	
Phenol 0.5–2%	Local anesthetic
Menthol 0.1–2%	Cooling effect
Camphor 1–3%	Cooling effect
Calamine lotion	Astringent and cooling effect
BATHS (per gallon tub water)	
Cornstarch (1 cup cornstarch with 1 cup baking soda)	Cools and soothes
Oatmeal (1 cup)	Cools and soothes
Aveeno (colloidal oatmeal—1 cup)	Cools and soothes
WET DRESSING	
Potassium permanganate (dilute to 1:4,000–1:16,000)	Cools and soothes
Aluminum acetate (Burow's solution, dilute 1:10–1:40)	Moderate germicidal activity
Boric acid (1 tbsp in 1 liter of water)	Mild germicidal activity; cools and soothes
Sodium chloride 0.9% (2 tsp in 1 liter of water)	Cools and soothes
Magnesium sulfate (Epsom salt—8 tsp in 1 liter of water)	Cools and soothes
Silver nitrate 0.25% solution	Good germicidal action

with special medications, such as zinc oxide paste in an Unna's boot (Dome-Paste, Gelocast); or preparations that act as sunscreens to protect the skin from ultraviolet light. Protectives are featured in Table 65–5.

The dressings vary in porosity and absorbency, but all hydrate the wound surface, and many fend off environmental bacteria as well as reduce the pain and cost of treatment. Some act as nonabsorbent "second skins," allowing exudate to collect beneath the dressing, forming an artificial blister. Most products are waterproof, reduce friction with other surfaces, have a long life, and reduce pain as the drugs protect sensitive areas such as donor skin graft sites. Others form a gel-like coating over the wound surface. Occlusion can hasten the separation of necrotic tissue by keeping the wound fluid in intimate contact with the wound surface. Wound fluid contains enzymes that lyse dead tissue, a process called autolytic debridement.

In some instances protectives may reduce offensive odors. The odor that may accumulate under a dressing is pronounced when the dressing is removed or when leakage occurs. The odor normally disappears when the wound is cleansed.

Research (Hoffman, 1992) indicates that polyurethane film dressings, which have been used over IV sites for many years, actually allow more fluid to collect under the dressing, which may support the growth of bacteria. Hoffman found "a 53% higher risk of catheter bacterial infections for peripheral catheters using transparent versus gauze dressings. With central venous catheters, there was a 78% risk."

There is no single product that is ideal for all wound types. The choice of dressing depends on the wound size, location, exudate, depth, presence of infection, and necrosis. The dressing type needs to change as the wound heals or worsens. For example, an absorptive paste or powder is a good choice for a craterlike ulcer and yellow necrotic slough and moderate drainage. As the slough is replaced by granulation tissue that fills the wound space and drainage decreases, a less hydrophilic wafer or sheet dressing would be appropriate.

Preparations such as Dome-Paste or Gelocast are specially marketed products that are commonly used to improve healing in stasis ulcers. These semihard casts are impregnated with zinc oxide, zinc stearate, and aluminum silicate product and give mechanical support, which improves healing by preventing further trauma and providing a coating action on the skin.

SUNSCREENS

The skin must often be protected from the ultraviolet rays of the sun, which can cause acute or chronic injury to the skin. The acute injury is sunburn; the chronic effects include degenerative changes such as wrinkling and pigment alterations, premalignant actinic keratoses, basal and squamous cell carcinoma, and possibly malignant melanoma. Ultraviolet exposure is composed of UVB (mid-range ultraviolet) and UVA (long-range ultraviolet). UVB, the major cause of sunburn, peaks in temperate latitudes between 10 AM and 3 PM, while UVA is fairly constant throughout the day. Both contribute to chronic skin injury, including aging and skin cancer. After 60 minutes of continuous exposure to UVA, sunburn can also occur.

Chemical sunscreens act by absorbing ultraviolet rays in the medium wavelength range (UVB range), which are primarily absorbed in the epidermis. Long wavelength UV light (UVA range) can cause tanning and is responsible for most photosensitivity reactions that occur with many drugs and cosmetics. UVA deeply penetrates the dermis and causes serious skin damage. Ultimate sunscreen effectiveness depends on UV absorption spectrum, concentration, and vehicle.

The best sunscreens contain PABA (para-aminobenzoic acid) or its derivatives. Many commercial products are available containing various percentages of these agents.

▼ CLINICAL ALERT

These products are beneficial only if they are applied before sun exposure to prevent burning. Most suntan lotions

Table 65–5. PROTECTIVES

Preparation	Ingredients	Uses
Flexible Collodion	Collodion with 2% camphor and 3% castor oil	Transparent protective film
Styptic Collodion	20% tannic acid	Astringent
Tegaderm	Self-adhering transparent polyurethane dressing, permeable to air and water vapor	Seals in body's normal defenses against invasion, promotes natural healing without crust formation. To cover pressure sores, skin donor sites, minor abrasions.
Duo-Derm	Hydroactive particles embedded in a polymer base, which are softened by wound moisture and act as a protective gel over healing tissue	Hastens wound healing and prevents contamination of leg ulcers, pressure sores, or other open wounds. Can be left in place up to 7 days.
PolySkin	Self-adhering transparent polyurethane dressing, gas and oxygen permeable	To cover central and peripheral IV sites; change at least every 2–3 days.
Ensure-It (Deseret)	Self-adhering transparent polyurethane dressing, vapor and gas permeable, that does not stick to itself	To cover central and peripheral IV sites, pressure sores, and superficial wounds; change every 48 hr.
Op-Site	Self-adhering transparent polyurethane dressing, vapor and gas permeable	Can be used as an incision drape and sutured through. As backing for split-thickness grafts (change after 10 days), as covering for donor sites, superficial burns, and ostomies, change at least every 7–10 days.
Tegasorb	Self-adhering, hypoallergenic, hydrocolloid adhesive	Partial- and full-thickness pressure ulcers.
Uniflex	Self-adhering transparent polyurethane dressing, vapor and gas permeable; hypoallergenic	To cover central or peripheral IV sites and pressure sores; change every 2–5 days.
Mediskin and Silver	Silver ions with porcine xenograft (stored at freezer temperatures; must be thawed for 2–3 hr before use)	Used to cover full- or partial-thickness burns, skin donor sites, and pressure sores for aggressive antibacterial action and pain relief. Change every 2–7 days depending on use.
Zinc oxide paste (Unna's boot) Dome-Paste Gelocast	Zinc oxide Zinc stearate	Mechanical support; prevent crusting and trauma; stimulate healing

now contain a numbering system (sun protection factor or SPF) of 1 to 50. Preparations with the numeral 1 have minimal protection, whereas those numbered 50 have maximal protection from the sun's rays. The FDA has recommended that SPFs above 30 no longer be allowed as they offer no real additional protection.

Table 65–6 describes skin characteristics and type and the suggested SPF protection.

Sunscreens are most effective when applied about 30 minutes to 1 hour before exposure to the sun so that they can penetrate the skin. All sunscreens should be reapplied after swimming or sweating. The term "waterproof" has been removed from suntan products. Environment con-

Table 65–6. SUGGESTED SPF BASED ON PATIENT CHARACTERISTICS

Skin Characteristics	Skin Type	Suggested Product SPF
Never burns; deeply pigmented (insensitive)	VI	None indicated
Rarely burns; tans profusely (dark brown; insensitive)	V	2–4
Burns minimally; always tans well (moderate brown; normal)	IV	4–8
Burns moderately; tans gradually (light brown; normal)	III	8–12
Always burns easily; tans minimally (sensitive)	II	12–20
Always burns easily; never tans (sensitive)	I	20–30

ditions such as altitude, snow, sand, and water all affect erythema-producing ultraviolet light. The intensity of sunlight at 5000 feet is about 20% greater than at sea level. Fresh snow and white sand are effective reflectors. Water is a variable reflector, depending on the angle of the sun and the presence or absence of waves. Reflected light from any of these sources can cause an additive effect and can strike the skin in previously unexposed areas.

▼ CLINICAL ALERT

Researchers currently suggest that by preventing sunburn and by regularly using sunscreens (SPF 15) for the first 18 years of life, it is possible to decrease the incidence of basal and squamous cell carcinoma of the skin by 78%. Even this approach will not totally prevent degenerative skin changes.

Sunscreens are all capable of causing contact dermatitis and photosensitivity reactions. If any of these occur, the product should be discontinued at once.

Sunblocks containing titanium dioxide, red petrolatum, or zinc oxide are also available today in many colors. These products prevent all solar radiation from reaching the skin. Sun blocks are particularly useful for the nose, lips, cheeks, and tips of the ears.

GROWTH FACTORS

One of the most exciting new developments in wound healing is the isolation and development of growth factors. Growth factors are normally released by platelets, macrophages, and other cells as the inflammatory stage of cell repair begins. These factors stimulate cells to divide and migrate, resulting in wound healing formation of granulation tissue and new epidermis. Over 30 growth factors have been identified. One product developed from platelet-derived growth factors is Procuren solution.

○ **Procuren solution** is an autologous product made from a small amount of each patient's blood, processed in a specially equipped laboratory. Procuren promotes faster healing by actively stimulating growth of granulation tissue, capillaries, and epithelium. Procuren is derived from platelets derived from growth factors. All neurotic tissue is removed, and infection is treated. A thin layer of Procuren is applied to the wound, and it is covered with petrolatum—impregnated gauze. The material is left in place for 12 hours and then washed off with tap water irrigation. During the remaining 12 hours of the day, the wound is covered with sulfadiazine (Silvadene). Procuren is available from CuraTech, Inc., Minneapolis, MN (612-942-8181).

CLEANSERS

Cleansers, including soaps and shampoos, are used to clean the surface of the skin. Cleansers are featured in Table 65–7.

Table 65–7. CLEANSERS AND SOAPS

Soaps, Neutral Soaps, or Soap Substitutes	
Acne Aide Detergent Soap	Dove
Alpha-Keri	pHisoDerm
Aveenobar	Vel
Caress	

Superfatted Soaps	
Basis	Dermalab Soap
Camay	Nivea Creme Soap
Coast	Shield

Soap-Free Products	
Ancet	Lowila cake
Ceta	Neutrogena
Green soap	

Bacteriostatic Agents and Deodorant Soaps	
Betadine Skin Cleanser	Jergens Clear Complexion Bar
Dial	Lifebuoy
Fostex Cake	Phase III
Ionax	Safeguard
Ionax Scrub	Sulfur Soap
Irish Spring	Zest

SOAPS

The belief that soap is bad for the complexion is incorrect. Clean skin helps promote healthy skin. Soaps used, particularly on the face, should be mild and contain a minimum amount of irritating substances. Ordinary soaps are sodium or potassium salts of fatty acids having an alkaline pH. Many different sources of fatty acids can be used—for example, olive oil, coconut oil, and glycerin. Because an alkaline pH can be irritating to injured skin, several soap or soaplike products have a pH of less than 7.5, which is less irritating. Other soaps are superfatted (have large quantities of fat) to reduce their alkalinity. Therapeutic cleansers are "soap free" and are less irritating to sensitive skin. "Modified" soap products contain emollient components or are adjusted to neutral or slightly acidic pH. Some soaps also contain bacteriostatic agents, providing a deodorant effect. Numerous controlled studies have suggested that bacteriostatic soaps have value in the prophylaxis of cutaneous bacterial infections.

SHAMPOOS

Shampoos are liquid soaps or detergents used to wash the hair and scalp and to relieve pruritus. Several shampoos are effective in the temporary treatment of dandruff but are usually not curative. Dandruff is now generally thought to be caused by an inflammatory reaction to a commensal yeast, *Pityrosporon ovale*. In general, one to two teaspoonfuls is lathered into the hair and allowed to remain there for 2 to 3 minutes, then rinsed and repeated.

○ **Selenium sulfide shampoos** (ExSel, Selsun Blue) are temporarily effective for the treatment of dandruff and tinea versicolor. These products are not used when there is an acute inflammation present, as increased absorption may occur. The 2.5% suspension is available only by prescription (ExSel), whereas the less potent products can be bought without prescription (Selsun Blue).

○ **Zinc pyrithione shampoos** (Danex, Sebulon, Therapy Z, Head and Shoulders) are widely available nonprescription formulas used for the temporary treatment of dandruff. These products may be used twice weekly if needed.

○ **Tar derivative shampoos** (Tegrin, Pentrax, Denorex, Zetar, and Polytar) help to correct abnormalities of keratenization by decreasing epidermal proliferation and dermal filtration. They also have antipruritic and antibacterial activity. Tar derivative shampoos are used for treatment of scalp psoriasis, eczemas, seborrheic dermatitis, dandruff, cradle cap, and other oil or itchy scalp conditions.

○ **Ketoconazole** (Nicoral), an antifungal agent, is available as a prescription-only shampoo for the treatment of seborrheic dandruff.

ENZYMES

Dermatologic conditions are often treated with topical enzyme preparations, although some physicians question their use. Enzyme preparations help to digest necrotic tissue through their proteolytic action (sutilains, fibrolysin, and desoxyribonuclease) or to digest collagenous tissue debriding dermal ulcers or burns (collagenase). Refer to Chapter 66 for more information.

CORTICOSTEROIDS

The corticosteroids (discussed in detail in Chapter 44), when used topically, possess anti-inflammatory, antipruritic, and vasoconstrictive actions. The relative strength of the topical steroid is determined more by its base or vehicle and the type of lesion treated rather than by the percentage strength. The vehicle (available as gels, lotions, sprays, ointments, and creams) alters the vasoconstrictor property and the therapeutic efficacy. Table 65–8 lists examples of corticosteroids available by potency. Group I is the most potent; group VII is the least potent. No significant differences exist among agents within groups II to IV. Most topical corticosteroids are in suspension, and the addition of a solvent (propylene glycol) enhances dissolution and may improve absorption.

Topical steroids are contraindicated in patients demonstrating previous sensitivity to steroids; in those with current systemic fungal, viral, or bacterial infections; and in those with current complications related to steroid therapy. Use for long periods during pregnancy (category C) is contraindicated owing to the increased risk to the fetus.

Adverse effects of steroids include hypopigmentation; acneform eruptions; allergic contact dermatitis; burning; dryness; folliculitis; irritation; itching; overgrowth of bacteria, fungi, and viruses; and skin atrophy. Skin atrophy is common and may become clinically significant in 3 to 4 weeks when using a potent topical corticosteroid. Atrophy occurs more readily at sites where percutaneous absorption is high. Systemic effects occur rarely but can cause adrenal suppression, Cushing's syndrome, striae, skin atrophy, and ocular effects (glaucoma and cataracts). These effects occur more frequently when occlusive dressings are used.

▼ **CLINICAL ALERT**

Children are particularly at risk for developing adverse effects from topical corticosteroids, so they are monitored closely.

IMMUNOSUPPRESSIVE AGENTS

○ **Cyclosporine** (Sandimmune), described in detail in Chapter 60, is one of the major drugs used to reduce the incidence of organ rejection after transplant. Multiple trials have confirmed its usefulness in psoriasis at steadily decreasing dosages. Cyclosporine acts principally via its interference with the function of the helper T-cell lymphocytes.

ACNE PRODUCTS

Acne, primarily affecting adolescents and young adults, is due to an exaggerated response to androgenic steroids such as testosterone and 17-hydroxyprogesterone. Patients with mild acne have oily skin and closed and open *comedones* (blackheads; discolored dried sebum plugging an excretory duct of the skin). Patients with moderate acne have papules, pustules, and inflammation. These lesions may lead to pitting and hypertrophic scars.

Acne is associated with development of keratin plugs at the base of the sebaceous follicle. Treatment is aimed at removing the keratin plug; reducing the amount of free fatty acid formation on the skin, which, in turn, reduces inflammation; decreasing sebum production; and reducing bacteria that lead to inflammation. By modifying the cause of the acne, the patient's appearance is also improved.

Treatment for acne includes nondrug and drug therapies. Nondrug therapies are aimed at reducing effects of irritating chemicals or drugs such as corticosteroids, androgens, and oral contraceptives with a high amount of androgens; humid environments; and heavy occlusive cosmetics. Comedone extraction, dermabrasion, or collagen injection may be useful in a select group of patients.

Drug therapy includes two major groups: (1) cleansers (Aconomel, Bravisol, Clearasil Medicated Cleanser, Fostex, Oxy-Wash, pHisoDerm, and Stri-Dex) and drying agents (Aconomel, Dry and Clear, Ionax, Listerex, Oxy-5/10, Stri-Dex) and (2) antibiotics. These products generally contain a combination of benzoyl peroxide, an antiseptic, drying, and keratolytic agent; sulfur, an antiseptic agent; resorcinol or salicylic acid, keratolytic agents; hexachlorophene, an antiseptic and cleanser; alcohol, a drying agent and antiseptic; and other ingredients to dry, color,

Table 65–8. TOPICAL STEROIDS

STEROID %	STEROID PRODUCT NAME	VEHICLE*	NURSING IMPLICATIONS
group I (super-high potency)			For all products:
0.05%	diflorasone diacetate (Psorcon)	C, O	**ASSESSMENT:** Assess type and location of lesion to determine best product: lotions for hair areas; creams and ointments for dry scaly areas; sprays, lotions, and gels for scalp or hair; sprays for weeping lesions.
	halobestasol propionate (Ultravate)	C, O	**INTERVENTION:** Monitor plasma cortisol levels if prolonged therapy is necessary. **Patient Teaching**—Apply products sparingly in light film, rubbing gently. Avoid prolonged contact with eyes, genital and rectal areas, face, and in skin creases. Wash area with soap just prior to application to increase drug penetration. May apply to skin alone or with dry occlusive dressing.
			EVALUATION: Monitor for toxic reactions, liver dysfunction, worsening of condition. Report burning, irritation, and infection to physician.
group II (high potency)			Same as for all.
0.1%	amcinonide (Cyclocort)	C, O, L	
0.05%	betamethasone dipropionate (Diprosone)	C, O	
0.25%		C, O, G	
0.01%	desoximetasone (Topicort)	C	
	betamethasone valerate (Valisone)		
group III (medium potency)			Same as for all.
0.05%	desoximetasone (Topicort LP)	C	
0.2%	hydrocortisone (Westcort)	C, O	
0.5%	triamcinolone acetonide	C, O, L	
group IV (low potency)			Same as for all.
0.05%	desonide (DesOwen, Tridesilon)	C	
0.05%	flurandrenolide (Cordran, Cordran SP)	L, O, C	
group V (lowest potency) (May be ineffective for some indications)			Same as for all.
0.1%	dexamethasone (Decadron Phosphate)	C	
1.0%	hydrocortisone (Cort-Dome)	C, O	

*O = ointment; C = cream; G = gel; L = lotion.

and scent the product. Most of these products are available in several forms—lotions, gels, creams, or ointments.

Based on recommendations of an advisory panel on OTC antimicrobial (II) drug products, the FDA has published a monograph on topical acne drug products. Benzoyl peroxide, sulfur, and resorcinol with sulfur are considered to be safe and effective for the treatment of acne. Salicylic acid 0.5% to 2% is also safe and effective, but data are insufficient to determine the safety of concentrations above 2%. Astringents (aluminum and zinc salts), which promote drying, are classified as ineffective. Antiseptics, which are present in many formulations, are classified as unsafe and/or ineffective. The antimicrobial, povidone iodine, is considered safe, but data are insufficient to permit its final classification as effective.

Mild acne can be treated with bar soaps, soap-free cakes, liquid cleansers, lotions, gels, and creams. Abrasives remove surface debris, and alcohol or acetone promotes drying. For moderate acne, topical anti-inflammatory drugs such as **benzoyl peroxide, tretinoin (Retin-A), isotretinoin (Accutane), azelaic acid (Azelex), adapaline (Differin),** and antibiotics are useful.

The side effects of acne products can include excessive redness; extreme dryness of the skin, leading to blistering and crusting; temporary pigmentation changes; and peeling of the skin. Patients are cautioned about not overusing these products. The same product is used each day for a period of time. If another products is to be tried, the first is discontinued or used only as indicated by the physician. All products are kept away from the eyes, inside the nose, mucous membranes, hair, and colored fabric.

○ **Benzoyl peroxide** (Benzac, Fostex, Dryox, and many more), is a keratolytic agent which is bacteriostatic and may decrease the production of irritant-free fatty acids in the follicle. Benzoyl peroxide is not applied under an occlusive dressing because of a high incidence of local irritation.

○ **Tretinoin** (Retin-A) and **adapaline** (Differin) are acids of vitamin A acid that are used to treat acne vulgaris, skin cancer, and aging of the skin. Tretinoin decreases cohesiveness of the epithelial cells, increasing cell mitosis and turnover.

Tretinoin is contraindicated in patients hypersensitive to any component. Tretinoin is potentially irritating, particularly when used correctly. Within 48 hours, the skin generally becomes red and begins to peel. Temporary hyperpigmentation and hypopigmentation can also occur with tretinoin. Adapaline does not carry the hypopigmentation warning. Patients using tretinoin should avoid sun exposure as photosensitivity may occur.

Tretinoin is applied liberally to the skin. The hands are washed thoroughly immediately after applying. Therapeutic results should be seen after 2 to 3 weeks but may not be optimal until after 6 weeks. Patients may use cosmetics, but the skin needs to be cleansed thoroughly before applying tretinoin.

○ **Isotretinoin** (Accutane) is also a metabolite of vitamin A. Its use is reserved for persons who have not responded to other therapies including systemic antibiotics. It is used to treat severe recalcitrant cystic acne.

Isotretinoin has many adverse effects including xerosis and facial desquamation, palmoplantar desquamation, pruritis, brittle nails, and hair loss. Corneal opacities have been reported. Approximately 25% of patients have an elevated triglyceride level, 15% develop a decrease in high density lipoprotein (HDL), and about 7% have an increase in cholesterol. Use during pregnancy or in women who could become pregnant is contraindicated owing to the increased risk of fetal abnormalities.

Isotretinoin is administered with meals two times daily for 15 to 20 weeks. If another course of therapy is needed, an 8-week lapse of time should occur. Photosensitivity may occur, so the patient needs to decrease sun and sunlamp exposure. Alcohol consumption should be eliminated during therapy as alcohol may potentiate the serum triglyceride elevation.

ANTIBIOTICS

Local antibiotics are also used to treat acne, the most common being clindamycin (Cleocin-T), erythromycin (many products), tetracycline (Topicycline), and meclocycline (Meclan). When inflammation is severe, systemic tetracycline is warranted. Therapeutic response generally requires 6 to 12 weeks of therapy. The major side effects of the antibiotics include acute contact dermatitis, transient stinging or burning, staining of the skin, erythema, and skin tenderness.

POISON IVY TREATMENT PRODUCTS

Poison ivy treatment products are used topically to relieve itching, pain, and discomfort associated with ivy, oak, or sumac poisoning. These products (calamine, Calomox, Rhuli Cream/Spray/Gel, Ivy-Rid, Ivy-Chex) may contain antiseptics, astringents, counterirritants, local anesthetics, antipruritics, and antimicrobials in any combination. If rash develops, these products are discontinued.

BURN PRODUCTS

Products available to treat burns include **nitrofurazone (Furacin)**, **mafenide (Sulfamylon)**, **silver sulfadiazine (Flint SSD, Silvadene)**, and **silver nitrate**, all featured in Table 65–9.

○ **Nitrofurazone** (Furacin) is applied topically to the burn as a solution, ointment, or cream. It is a synthetic nitrofuran and has a broad spectrum of antibacterial activity. Nitrofurazone is used in second- or third-degree burns where bacterial resistance to other agents is a real or potential problem.

○ **Mafenide** (Sulfamylon) is a water-soluble cream that is bacteriostatic for both gram-negative and gram-positive organisms. Mafenide is used to treat second- and third-degree burns to reduce the bacteria present in avascular tissues.

Mafenide diffuses through devascularized areas of the

Table 65–9. BURN PRODUCTS

DRUG NAME/ROUTE AND DOSAGE	ADVERSE EFFECTS	NURSING IMPLICATIONS
nitrofurazone (Furacin) *Topical:* Apply ¹⁄₁₆″ film directly to burn.	**Common:** Contact dermatitis, rash **Less Common:** pruritis, local edema	For all: **ASSESSMENT:** Assess degree of burn depth, vital signs, temperature, urinary output, and renal function. Assess for pregnancy (category C). **INTERVENTION:** Apply directly to burn with sterile gloved hand. Wash burn daily. Whirlpool baths daily assist with wound debridement. **Patient Teaching**—Caution patient to avoid exposure of skin undergoing treatment to sun. **EVALUATION:** Notify physician of fever, rash, or worsening of burn.
mafenide (Sulfamylon) *Topical:* Apply ¹⁄₁₆″ film 1–2 times daily.	**Common:** Local pain, rash **Life-threatening:** Bone marrow depression, hemolytic anemia **Less Common:** Hyperventilation, metabolic acidosis, itching, hives, blisters	Same as for nitrofurazone plus: **ASSESSMENT:** Assess burn frequently for development of super infections. **INTERVENTION:** Keep burn covered with mafenide at all times. **Patient Teaching**—Teach patient that drug may cause local discomfort and burning. **EVALUATION:** Notify physician if hyperventilation occurs. If acidosis develops, mafenide is washed off skin.
silver sulfadiazine (Silvadene) (Flint SSD) *Topical:* Apply ¹⁄₁₆″ film 1–2 times daily (keep burn covered at all times with silver sulfadiazine).	**Common:** Rash, itching **Less Common:** Leukopenia, interstitial nephritis	Same as for nitrofurazone plus: **ASSESSMENT:** Monitor CBCs, particularly WBCs, frequently. If leukopenia develops, discontinue drug.
silver nitrate (ointment: 10%; solution: 10%, 25%, 50% in 30 mL) *Topical:* *Ointment*—Apply to dressing for 5 days PRN; do not apply to wounds, cuts, or broken skin. *Solution*—Apply cotton applicator dipped in solution to affected area 2–3 times a week for 2–3 wk PRN.	Same as for nitrofurazone	Same as for nitrofurazone plus: **ASSESSMENT:** Assess levels of sodium and potassium in serum electrolytes.

CBC = complete blood count; WBC = white blood count.

skin and is absorbed, rapidly metabolized, and excreted through the kidneys. Both mafenide and its metabolites are strong carbonic anhydrase inhibitors and, therefore, may precipitate metabolic acidosis usually compensated by hyperventilation.

○ **Silver sulfadiazine** (Flint SSD, Silvadene) has a broad spectrum of activity against gram-negative bacteria, gram-positive bacteria, and yeasts. Silver sulfadiazine is released slowly from the cream, which is selectively toxic to bacteria. Silver sulfadiazine is used primarily to prevent sepsis in patients with second- and third-degree burns. Silver sulfadiazine is not a carbonic anhydrase inhibitor and, therefore, does not cause acidosis. Rash and itching do occur from topical application.

○ **Silver nitrate** is an aqueous, antiseptic solution active against gram-negative bacteria. Patients have dressings applied to their burns, which are then kept moist with silver nitrate. Silver nitrate stains anything that it comes in contact with brown or black. This discoloration is usually not permanent. Silver nitrate used for long periods or on extensive burns may precipitate fluid and electrolyte imbalances.

Biologic dressings, including skin obtained from humans (homografts), from other animals (xenographs or heterographs), or amnion from human placentas, are being used today on large burns. These coverings are featured in Table 65–10. They provide a temporary wound closure until autographing is complete and are also used to debride dirty wounds after eschar separation. They decrease evaporative fluid and protein loss, protect new nerve endings, and provide a bacterial barrier enhancing reepithelialization. When the biologic dressing appears to be taking, or adheres to the granulating wound surface with a minimum of underlying exudate, the patient is ready for permanent placement of an autograft. Because of the cost of biologic dressings, synthetic substitutes have also become available, such as Biobrane and artificial skin (Integra).

Table 65–10. BURN COVERINGS

Type of Dressing	Indications	Source and Description	Nursing Considerations
Allograft Homograft	Debride untidy wounds. Protect granulation tissues after escharotomy. Cover excised wounds immediately. Serve as test graft before autograft.	Human cadaver skin, about 0.015 inch thick	Observe for exudate; also watch for local and systemic signs of infection and rejection. Change: Varies greatly.
Xenograft Heterograft	Same as for homograft. Cover meshed autografts. Protect exposed tendons. Cover partial-thickness burns that are eschar free and clean or only slightly contaminated.	Pigskin similar to human skin, harvested after slaughter, then cryopreserved or lyophilized for long-term storage	Observe for signs of infection. Change: 2–5 days.
Amnion	Protect partial-thickness burns. Temporary cover granulation tissue awaiting autograft.	Amnionic and chorionic membranes collected from human placentas under sterile conditions	Apply to clean wounds. Change: 48 hr.
Biobrane	Cover donor graft sites. Protect clean, superficial, partial-thickness burns and excised wounds awaiting autografts. Cover meshed autografts.	Nylon fabric bonded to silicon rubber membrane, containing collagenous porcine peptides Elastic and durable; adheres to wound surface until removed or sloughed by spontaneous reepithelialization	Useful for wounds awaiting autograft. It is permeable to antimicrobiais, which can be applied over it. Change: 3–14 days.
Artificial Skin (Integra)	Temporary cover for partial- and full-thickness burns.	Mixture of protein from cowhide and complex CHO derived from shark cartilage	As early as 10 days after the graft, postage stamp patches of plastic are peeled away and replaced by slivers of patient's own epidermal tissue. Use only once.
Duo-Derm	Cover small partial-thickness burns. Prevent bacterial contamination.	Hydroactive dressing that interacts with moisture on skin, creating bond that makes it adhere Interacts with wound exudate to produce soft moist gel, facilitating removal	Use size that allows dressing to extend beyond wound onto healthy skin. Be careful to distinguish pus from liquefied material that normally remains in wound. Change: daily.
Op-Site	Cover clean partial-thickness burns and clean donor sites to reduce pain from these wounds. Provide moist environment for reepithelialization.	Thin, transparent elastic film that adheres to dry surfaces, conforms to body contours, and stretches with movement Occlusive and waterproof; permeable to moisture, vapor, and air	Maintain closed dressing; if exudate forms, drain aseptically with needle and syringe, seal hole with OP-Site patch Check for pooling of exudate in dependent areas. Change: 2–5 days.
N-Terface	Cover partial thickness burns and newly applied autografts. Eliminate shearing of epithelium and protect healing tissue.	Surface material used between burn and outer dressing Translucent, nonabsorbent, and nonreactive; permeable to air and fluid	Shortens time it normally takes to change dressing, eliminating soaking and other steps required with conventional gauze dressing. Change: 2–5 days.
Vigilon	Clean small partial-thickness burns.	Colloidal suspension on a polyethylene mesh support Permeable to gases and water vapor; provides moist environment Compatible with topical preparations	For occlusive use, remove one polyethylene film backing and place uncovered side on wound; for nonocclusive use, remove both backings and secure over wound with gauze or tape. Change: daily.

USING THE NURSING PROCESS

The patient requiring medications for skin disorders may be acutely ill in the hospital or relatively healthy and self-treating a dermatologic problem with OTC preparations. High standards of skin maintenance must be maintained, especially in debilitated and aged patients.

ASSESSMENT

- Obtain a thorough nursing history to develop the database. Include a family history of any serious systemic disease in the assessment. Other data to obtain from the patient are included in Table 65–11.
- Obtain laboratory tests, such as wound cultures or blood counts as ordered.
- Assess all skin conditions. Wearing gloves during the exam may help protect against transmission. However, scabies and lice mites can penetrate cloth and paper isolation gowns. Often scabies and lice can be confused with other less serious conditions. Scabies can be mistaken for eczema, poison ivy, or a scratch, while pediculosis, or lice infestations, look like dandruff. There are two species of lice—head lice (*Pediculus capitis*) and body lice (*Pediculus corporis*). Both types feed by sucking blood. When they bite, the affected area itches. Because adult lice feed five times a day, each meal lasting 35 to 40 minutes, they can cause a lot of itching. Lice are very difficult to get rid of. They sometimes fall off injured, but leave voluntarily only if their host becomes too hot, because of fever, or too cold, because of death.
- Inspect patient's shoulders, armpits, buttocks, waist, or abdomen, as these are areas where clothing or bed linen comes in close contact with the body. If lice are present, there are small bites, scratch marks, and sometimes patchy discolorations, crusted areas, or infection. Lymph nodes may also be enlarged as a result of inflammation and infection. If lice are suspected, inspect the patient's undergarments, especially the seams, for lice and eggs. If lice or eggs are found, the infection control department of the hospital is notified. Itching can persist even after lice are dead, especially if the skin is already irritated from scratching. A soothing lotion or solution of baking soda and water may help.
- Assess the quality of the skin in ill patients and prevent its breakdown, which can lead to infection. Some of the factors that put a patient at risk for skin breakdown include the following: incontinence, poor nutritional status, anemia, hypoxia, stress, limited mobility, limited or decreased sensation, or redness over a bony prominence that lasts over 15 minutes. The Agency for Health Care Policy and Research has developed and released guidelines that assist the nurse to identify patients at risk for pressure ulcers and to define early interventions and treatments. Several types of mattresses are available to prevent patients at risk from having skin breakdown.
- Monitor oxygenation. Oxygen is critical for healing. It also supports phagocytic defense, angiogenesis, and collagen synthesis and stabilizes cell structure. Thus, hypoxia impairs all wound healing. Anemia is an enemy to healing when it is severe (hematocrit below 20 g/dL). Stress triggers the release of catecholamines, which constrict blood vessels and reduce blood flow. Therefore, any interventions that can reduce stress may improve wound healing.
- Monitor for side effects of medications, which include skin reactions ranging from photosensitivity to skin eruptions. Medications suspected of causing the skin

---

Table 65–11. NURSING PROCESS FOR PATIENT REQUIRING MEDICATIONS FOR THE SKIN

Assessment

Assess current illness/condition, note debilitation, incontinence, presence of allergies.
Inspect skin for reddened areas, decreased sensation, lesions, bites, scratches, patchy excoriations, crusted areas, infection, and/or presence of scabies, lice.
Assess source of current infestation.
Assess family history of systemic disease.
Assess current medication use, including prescribed, OTC, and street drugs.
Review laboratory tests (e.g., wound cultures or blood counts).

Nursing Diagnosis: Impaired Skin Integrity	Desired Outcomes/Evaluation Criteria
RELATED TO: External factors (e.g., chemical substance, physical immobilization), mechanical factors (e.g., pressure, trauma), and internal factors (e.g., medication, altered circulation, nutritional state, excretions/secretions, edema, skeletal prominence). **AS EVIDENCED BY:** Complaints of itching, pain, disruption of skin surface, destruction of skin layers, invasion of body structures.	Verbalizes understanding of condition and causative factors. Identifies interventions appropriate for specific condition. Verbalizes relief of discomfort/itching. Displays timely healing.

Continued on the following page

Table 65–11. NURSING PROCESS FOR PATIENT REQUIRING MEDICATIONS FOR THE SKIN, *Continued*

Nursing Actions	Rationale
Administer/apply therapeutic agent (e.g., use of topical sprays, creams, ointment, or soaks).	Promotes healing/alleviates condition.
Instruct in aseptic/clean technique for dressing changes and proper disposal of soiled dressings.	Prevents spread of bacteria and promotes healing.
Maintain strict skin hygiene, using mild, nondetergent soap (if any), drying gently and thoroughly and lubricating with lotion or emollient.	Cleansing skin and using lubricants can keep it soft/pliable and can protect skin, which is susceptible to breakdown.
Examine feet and nails routinely and provide foot/nail care as indicated.	Jagged, rough nails can cause tissue infection by scratching adjacent skin areas.
Provide balanced diet (e.g., adequate protein, vitamins A and E).	A positive nitrogen balance and improved nutritional state can prevent skin breakdown and promote healing.

Nursing Diagnosis: Pain	Desired Outcomes/Evaluation Criteria
RELATED TO: Injuring agents (biologic, chemical, physical, and psychologic). **AS EVIDENCED BY:** Complaints, self-focusing, restlessness, autonomic responses.	Reports pain reduced/controlled. Follows prescribed pharmacologic regimen. Verbalizes methods that provide relief. Sleeps/rests appropriately.

Nursing Actions	Rationale
Administer analgesics as indicated.	Reduces pain and itching.
Keep area clean, dress wounds carefully.	Assists body's natural process of repair and prevents infection.
Promotes use of progressive relaxation, breathing exercises, visualization.	Refocuses attention, relieves muscle tension, enhances sense of control, and helps to reduce pain and discomfort.
Encourage tub baths with Burow's solution, soda.	Soothes skin and promotes relief of itching.
Be available to patient for listening and discussion of condition and expected outcome.	Presence of pain/itching can stress individual coping abilities.

Nursing Diagnosis: Knowledge Deficit	Desired Outcomes/Evaluation Criteria
RELATED TO: Lack of exposure/recall, information misinterpretation/unfamiliarity with resources. **AS EVIDENCED BY:** Questions, statement of concern, inaccurate follow-through of instructions/development of preventable complications.	Verbalizes understanding of condition/disease process and treatment. Identifies relationship of signs/symptoms to the disease process and correlates symptoms with causative factors. Correctly performs necessary procedures and explains reasons for actions.

Nursing Actions	Rationale
Review physiologic importance of skin and measures to maintain skin functioning.	Understanding promotes proper care and helps patient to feel in control of situation.
Identify expected actions, side effects, and possible interactions with other drugs.	Helps patient to know what to anticipate and to be able to differentiate between expected and potentially dangerous symptoms.
Demonstrate appropriate amount of therapeutic agent for application, duration of treatment.	Correct usage reduces likelihood of untoward effects (e.g., inflammation, dermatitis). Condition may be slow to resolve, and patient may be tempted to discontinue therapy.
Discuss necessity of inspecting skin on a regular basis.	Provides opportunity for early intervention/prevention of recurrence/complications.
Stress importance of adequate fluid intake.	Helps to maintain skin turgor.
Review modes of transmission of infectious conditions or infestations as appropriate.	Can prevent spread/recurrence.
Encourage open discussion of patient's attitude toward condition/skin manifestations and expected results.	Some diseases/conditions can be temporarily or permanently disfiguring and may have a negative emotional effect.

Other Suggested Nursing Diagnoses: Impaired Social Interaction, Risk for Injury, and Impaired Adjustment.

reaction are discontinued. These reactions can be mild to very severe. Table 65–12 features selected medications that are known to cause dermatologic side effects, and Table 65–13 features selected medications that can cause life-threatening skin eruptions.

Other reactions secondary to medication include skin eruptions, which may be nonspecific and generalized in nature or may occur in the same site each time the medication is given. Eruptions may appear as either contact dermatitis or exfoliative dermatitis, with either wet or dry lesions. When a rash is observed, it is best to discontinue all topical and systemic medications that might be causing the rash, if possible, until the rash disappears. Medications are then added to the patient's daily regimen one at a time to determine the offending agent. At times, the causative agent may not be determined. One of the most serious dermatologic reactions to medications is the Stevens-Johnson (S-J) syndrome. The S-J syndrome is a severe form of erythema multiforme in which lesions may involve both the oral and anogenital mucosa. Systemic symptoms may also occur such as general malaise, fever,

Table 65–12. CHARACTERISTIC CLINICAL CUTANEOUS ERUPTIONS AND SELECTED CAUSATIVE AGENTS

Acneiform and Pustular

ACTH	Phenobarbital
Corticosteroids	Isoniazid (INH)
Iodides	Oral contraceptives
Lithium	Ethambutol
Phenytoin	

Alopecia

Antithyroid drugs	Colchicine
Oral contraceptives	Propranolol
Anticoagulants	Levodopa
Allopurinol	Indomethacin
Cytotoxic agents	Testosterone (in women)
Thallium	Valproate

Lichenoid and Lichen Planus–like

Gold salts	Methyldopa
Quinidine	Penicillamine
Thiazides	Sulfonylureas
Hydroxychloroquine	Chlorothiazide and related
Eurosemide	drugs

Eczematous

Chlorpromazine	Sulfonamides
Chlorothiazide	Thiamine
Meprobamate	Iodides
Penicillin	Tolbutamide
Procaine (and other local anesthetics)	Chlorpropamide
	Aminophylline
Aminoglycoside antibiotics	

Erythema Multiforme

Chlorpropamide	Sulfonamides
Penicillin	Thiazine derivatives
Phenothiazines	

Erythema Nodosum

Iodides	Oral contraceptives
Sulfonamides	Salicylates
Penicillin	Antibiotics

Table 65–12. CHARACTERISTIC CLINICAL CUTANEOUS ERUPTIONS AND SELECTED CAUSATIVE AGENTS, *Continued*

Exanthematic (Scarlatiniform, Morbilliform)

Anticonvulsants	Meprobamate
Antihistaminics	Penicillin
Barbiturates	Phenothiazines
Gold salts	Phenylbutazone
Griseofulvin	Streptomycin
Insulin	Sulfonamides

Pigmentary Changes

Chlorpromazine	Cytoxan
Fluorouracil	Gold salts
Estrogens	Phenytoin
Doxorubicin	

Porphyria (Exacerbation)

Barbiturates	Oral contraceptives
Androgens	Sulfonamides
Estrogens	Sulfonylureas

Purpuric

Barbiturates	Quinidine
Chlorothiazide	Sulfonamides
Chlorpromazine	(chemotherapeutics,
Gold salts	antidiabetics, and diuretics)
Griseofulvin	Phenylbutazone
Iodides	

Urticarial

Chloramphenicol	Penicillin
Enzymes	Phenothiazines
Griseofulvin	Salicylates
Insulin	Streptomycin
Opiates	Sulfonamides
Indomethacin	Tetracyclines

Source: Adapted from Moschella, SL. et al: Dermatology, vol 1. Drugs and the Skin. WB Saunders, Philadelphia, 1985, p 1040, with permission. Modified in 1996.

headache, arthralgia, and conjunctivitis. The development of the S-J syndrome may be either an allergic or an idiosyncratic reaction. The true mechanism for its development is unknown.

Photosensitivity occurs when patients are exposed to sunlight or ultraviolet light during or after receiving certain drugs. This photosensitivity can either be a phototoxic reaction, often associated with a nonimmunologic reaction, or a photoallergic reaction, which is associated with an immunologic reaction. Because these reactions can occur up to a year after discontinuing certain medications, it is important to obtain a past medication history. See Table 65–14 for selected drugs that can cause photosensitivity.

Dermatitis is a complaint of many patients and has various causes. Contact dermatitis can occur following contact with poison oak and ivy, some antibiotics, some OTC analgesics, and certain metals such as gold. Irritant dermatitis is associated with eruptions from direct contact with cosmetics, chemicals, dyes, or detergents. Seborrheic dermatitis is a yellowish-pinkish scaling of the scalp, face, and trunk. Atopic dermatitis has a characteristic distribution in persons with a family history of allergic diseases.

Table 65–13. LIFE-THREATENING DRUG-INDUCED SKIN ERUPTIONS & SELECTED DRUGS INVOLVED

Exfoliative Dermatitis

Barbiturates	Measles virus vaccine
Carbamazepine (Tegretol)	Nitroglycerin
Demeclocycline (Declomycin)	Oral antidiabetic agents
Diphtheria, tetanus toxoids,	Penicillin
and pertussis vaccine;	Phenothiazines
absorbed and Salk	Phenylbutazone (Butazolidin)
poliomyelitis vaccine	Phenytoin (Dilantin)
Furosemide (Lasix)	Streptomycin
Gold salts	Sulfasalazine (Azulfidine)
Griseofulvin (Grifulvin)	Sulfonamides
Isoniazid	Tetracyclines

Stevens-Johnson Syndrome
(erythema multiforme)

Ampicillin	Pentazocine (Talwin)
Barbiturates	Phenobarbital
Carbamazepine (Tegretol)	Phenylbutazone (Butazolidin)
Chloramphenicol	Phenytoin (Dilantin)
Clindamycin	Procaine penicillin, aqueous
Codeine	injection and oral mixed
Mephenytoin (Mesantoin)	sulfonamide preparation
Oxyphenbutazone	Sulfathiazole
(Tandearil)	Sulfonamides
Penicillin	Tetracycline

Toxic Epidermal Necrosis
(Lyell's syndrome)

Antihistamines	Pentazocine (Talwin)
Barbiturates	Phenobarbital
Gold salts	Phenylbutazone (Butazolidin)
Ipecac	Phenytoin (Dilantin)
Neomycin sulfate	Procaine penicillin, aqueous
Nitrofurantoin (Furadantin)	injection and oral mixed
Oxyphenbutazone	sulfonamide preparation
(Tandearil)	Sulfonamides
Penicillin	Tetracycline

Lupus Erythematosus

Gold compounds (long term)	Phenytoin (Dilantin)
Griseofulvin (Fulvicin)	Primidone (Mysoline)
Hydantoin anticonvulsants	Propylthiouracil
Hydralazine (Apresoline)	Reserpine (long term)
Isoniazid (INH)	Rifampin (Rifadin,
Methyldopa (Aldomet)	Rimactane, Rifampicin)
Penicillin	Streptomycin
Phenobarbital (long term)	Tetracycline
Phenothiazines	Thiazides (long term)
Phenylbutazone (Butazolidin)	

Source: Martin, EW: Hazards of Medication, ed 2. Provest, Fayetteville, NC, 1978, with permission. Modified in 1996.

When dermatitis is the problem, skin testing may be able to diagnose the allergen. Emotional stress and food allergies may also be causative agents and may need to be modified during the intervention phase. The reaction can be as mild as a slight reddening or as severe as open blisters. Because it is often hard to pin down the source of an allergy, the dermatologist often gets rid of the symptoms without knowing the cause. This can condemn the patient to a life of recurring, frustrating skin problems. Every attempt should be made during the initial assessment to determine the causative agent.

NURSING DIAGNOSIS

- Typical nursing diagnoses for a patient with dermatologic conditions include Pain, Knowledge Deficit, and Impaired Skin Integrity (see Table 65–11).

PLANNING AND INTERVENTION

- Develop the goals of nursing intervention from the nursing diagnoses. Typical nursing goals for the patient requiring medications that affect the skin are included in Table 65–11.

Patient Teaching

- Educate the patient about his or her medications. Table 65–15 presents patient teaching information.

Patients administering their own medication have a tendency to apply topical preparations more freely and for longer periods than prescribed. Very careful directions are given to patients to prevent the inflammation and dermatitis that can result from overuse of topical agents.

Table 65–14. SELECTED AGENTS THAT MAY CAUSE PHOTOSENSITIVITY REACTIONS

Anticancer Drugs
Fluorouracil (Fluoroplex and others)
Methotrexate (Folex and others)
Vinblastine (Velban and others)

Antidepressants
Amitriptyline (Elavil and others)
Phenelzine (Nardil)

Antidiabetics
Glipizide (Glucotrol and others)
Glyburide (DiaBeta and others)
Tolbutamide (Orinase and others)*

Antihypertensives
Captopril (Capoten)
Diltiazem (Cardizem and others)
Methyldopa (Aldomet and others)
Nifedipine (Procardia and others)

Antimicrobials
Ciprofloxacin (Cipro)
Demeclocycline (Declomycin and others)*
Doxycycline (Vibramycin and others)*
Sulfonamides
Tetracycline (Achromycin and others)

Antipsychotic Drugs
Haloperidol (Haldol and others)
Prochlorperazine (Compazine and others)*
Trifluromazine (Vesprin)

Diuretics
Most thiazides*
Furosemide (Lasix and others)*

Nonsteroidal Anti-inflammatory Drugs
Most drugs in group

*Reactions occur more frequently.

Table 65–15. PATIENT TEACHING INFORMATION—DERMATOLOGIC AGENTS

Dear Patient:

This drug has been prescribed for you. This is what you should know about your drug to get the most from your therapy.

- ☐ 1. You will take your drug until your current condition is cleared up.
- ☐ 2. Whenever topical agents are used to treat a skin disorder, the skin is washed daily before each dose of drug with mild soaps and patted dry before the next dose of drug is applied. If you have a moist lesion, a small amount of medication is gently rubbed into the area. If the lesion is dry or scaly, a thin film is applied over the area. A tongue blade may be helpful in applying the drug. When the lesion is under a hairy area, the hair may have to be parted to ensure the drug is rubbed into the skin.
- ☐ 3. There are several reactions that can occur with your drug. They include: _____ . If any of these occur, consult your doctor.
- ☐ 4. Typical side effects from dermatologic agents include staining of the skin, clothes, and nails; local allergic reactions; photosensitivity; and a drying effect. Often, staining of the clothes, photosensitivity, and excessive drying can be eliminated on small areas of the body by placing an occlusive dressing over the area. Check with your doctor to see if this technique is permissible.
- ☐ 5. Occlusive dressing may sometimes be ordered by your doctor to enhance the treatment of psoriasis and for persistent inflammatory dermatoses. The area is cleaned and shaved (if necessary) before the treatment begins. Any scales or crusts are removed. The drug is applied and is then covered with a plastic wrap (Saran Wrap, Handi-Wrap). A moist gauze may be applied over the skin under the plastic wrap if additional moisture is desired. The edges of the plastic wrap are sealed with tape. It is left in place anywhere from 7 or 8 hours to 12–24 hours. (If the dressing is to be worn only part of the day, you may choose to apply it only during the night.) The therapy is continued for several days after the lesion has cleared to prevent a relapse.
- ☐ 6. All tight and constricting clothing is avoided over the affected area. Clothing is washed daily to prevent recontamination. The clothing should also be dry and aerated so that undue moisture does not develop.

When patients have acquired infectious dermatologic conditions, the nurse is often responsible for educating the patient and the family about transmission and further prevention of the condition.

Patients with parasitic infections are treated as a family group, with all members of the family group treated at once. All persons having had sexual contact with the patient are also treated simultaneously when patients have pediculosis pubis. All clothing and bed linen are cleaned at the same time.

Many skin lesions are chronic and may lead to psychologic problems, feelings of rejection, and poor body image, which may then further aggravate the symptoms. Much of today's advertising indicates that a smooth, blemish-free skin is a necessity. A patient with a chronic disorder may become overly embarrassed about his or her condition. Patients and family may need additional counseling to successfully cope with the condition. The nurse is always careful to avoid showing any sign of rejection to a patient with a skin condition. Offering helpful suggestions such as the use of cosmetic cover-ups like Erase and Covermark or growing a beard may be helpful in camouflaging facial lesions or scarring. However, these may not be appropriate in the patient with active acne. In addition, the nurse educates the consumer to evaluate product advertising intelligently.

EVALUATION

- Evaluate the effectiveness of the medications for dermatologic conditions. This evaluation is based on a predetermined list of evaluation criteria previously developed in relation to the goals of treatment, as determined by the nurse, patient, and family. Typical outcome evaluation criteria are included in Table 65–11.
- Evaluate skin lesions daily while the patient is in the hospital or on each subsequent visit to the clinic or office. Acute conditions generally subside in 3 to 4 weeks. Chronic conditions may have periods of remission. Lesions that do not show improvement after 4 weeks of therapy must be reevaluated.
- Work with the patient and family to ensure their complete assistance, support, and compliance. Patients who understand the importance of their continued medical treatment are usually more compliant. The primary reason for noncompliance usually is forgetting to take the medication or not liking the unpleasant side effects. Teach the patient taking medications at home what potential side effects or unusual symptoms need to be reported to the physician, nurse, or pharmacist.
- Evaluate the patient's knowledge. All previously taught material is reviewed and updated, if necessary, to ensure that the patient's knowledge base remains accurate.

The bibliography for this chapter can be found in Appendix B, which begins on page 1054.

CHAPTER REVIEW QUESTIONS*

1. Which of the following is correct regarding emollients?
   a. The suspension requires shaking before application.
   b. They have a drying effect on the skin when the water evaporates.
   c. Emollients have fixed oils as a base preparation.
   d. They are predominantly water in base.

2. A common side effect of acyclovir (Zovirax) is:
   a. Photosensitivity.
   b. Hives.
   c. Mild pain.
   d. Pigment changes.

3. When a patient who is receiving medications for a skin disorder develops a reaction, the nurse will plan to:
   a. Discontinue medications one at a time.

*See Appendix A, which begins on page 1051, for answers.

b. Obtain a complete medication history.

c. Assume the rash is due to the current medication(s).

d. Continue all medications and document all nursing care.

4. When treating and assessing patients with pediculus (lice), the nurse is aware that:

a. They are easy to treat.

b. Cloth and paper gowns provide adequate protection.

c. Lymph nodes may be enlarged as a result of inflammation.

d. Itching should ease as soon as lice are removed.

5. A common adverse effect of topical steroids is:

a. Skin atrophy.

b. Moist, weeping skin.

c. Striae.

d. Hyperpigmentation.

SELECTED ISSUES IN PHARMACO-THERAPEUTICS

CHAPTER 66

Enzymes as Therapeutic Agents

Merrily A. Kuhn, RNC, PhD

CHAPTER OUTLINE

KEY TERMS

Depolymerization   Hypodermoclysis
Enzymes   Proteolytic
Fibrinolytic   Spondylolisthesis
Flocculation

LEARNING OBJECTIVES

After reading this chapter, the student will be able to:

1. Identify medications commonly used as enzymes.
2. Differentiate among the enzymes as to mechanism of action, route of administration, pharmacokinetics, adverse effects, contraindications and precautions, and interactions.
3. Identify specific areas to assess in the patient requiring enzymes to formulate appropriate patient outcomes.
4. Plan the nursing interventions necessary to administer enzymes and choose appropriate teaching strategies to gain patient compliance.
5. Evaluate the patient at various stages of treatment to measure the effectiveness of nursing interventions.

Enzymes are proteins needed by the body to act as catalysts in chemical reactions. Enzymes mediate reactions but are not altered or consumed by the reaction. Nearly every step in the metabolism of nutrients, as well as subsequent growth and repair of body parts, depends on enzymes. Most subcellular particles such as mitochondria, microsomes, and lysosomes also need enzymes to function properly. Many enzymes function only in the presence of cofactors such as ions of calcium (Ca^{2+}), choride (Cl^-), or nonprotein organic compounds. If these cofactors are missing, the enzymatic reaction does not occur.

ENZYMES

Enzymes can be divided into two primary groups: *proteolytic*—those that digest protein; and *fibrinolytic*—those

that dissolve fibrin. The name of most enzymes contains two parts: the name of the substrate that is acted on and the suffix "ase." For example, collagenase is an enzyme that breaks down collagen.

USES

Enzymes have many therapeutic uses: to promote healing of wounds, to debride skin ulcers, to replace deficient digestive enzymes (see Chapter 50), to dissolve clots (see Chapter 35), and to liquefy tracheobronchial secretions (see Chapter 40). Most enzymes are applied topically as creams or ointments. Only a few enzymes (e.g., replacement enzymes or digestants) are available for systemic use. Because enzymes are proteins, they are destroyed by the proteolytic enzymes of the intestinal tract when administered orally. Table 66–1 lists selected enzymes and

Table 66–1. ENZYMES

DRUG NAME/ROUTE AND DOSAGE	SOURCE	NURSING IMPLICATIONS
ENZYMES TO PROMOTE WOUND HEALING		
papain (Panafil) (Panafil White)		
Topical: 10% ointment once or twice daily	Papaya	**all enzymes** **ASSESSMENT:** Assess for skin reactions and for wound healing. Assess within first 24 hr of treatment; a febrile state often occurs due to accumulation of leukocytes at wound site. This may be avoided by frequent aspiration of exudate from wound. Assess vision when ophthalmic products are used. **INTERVENTION:** All powders are stored in cool, dry place and reconstituted just before use. Do not store reconstituted product for more than 24 hr. When mixing, medications are rolled or turned gently, not agitated. This prevents excessive flocculation. Medications are discontinued at first sign of sensitivity. Enzymes must be in immediate contact with purulent wound material to be most effective. Wounds are cleansed with prescribed irrigating solution between doses. Wounds are irrigated or cleansed gently to prevent damage to healthy tissue. Itching and stinging often occur after topical application, but they should subside. If symptoms persist, notify physician. Light dressings and cellophane wrap may be used over wound to prevent soiling of clothing. Change all dressings frequently to prevent contamination and to remove necrotic debris. Body cavities are drained at least every 6–10 hr and enzyme solution replaced. Store at 8–15°C. **EVALUATION:** Evaluate for hypersensitivity reactions. Report stinging and burning to physician.
hyaluronidase (Wydase)		
Clysis **Adults:** 150 units in 1000 mL solution **Children under 3 yr:** limit to 200 mL **Premature infants:** should not exceed 25 mL/kg daily **Subcutaneous Urography** **Adults:** 75 units	Bovine	Same as for all enzymes plus: **INTERVENTION:** For hypodermoclysis, dose of hyaluronidase is injected into rubber tubing close to needle of running clysis solution. Alternatively, dose of hyaluronidase may be injected under skin prior to clysis. Amount of fluid administered and flow rate are no faster than if fluid were administered IV. When administering fluid to children via this route, the nurse is particularly cautious about overhydration.
ENZYMES FOR SKIN ULCERS		
sutilains (Travase)		
Topical: apply 82,000 units/g ointment 3–4 times/day	Bacteria	Same as for all enzymes plus: **INTERVENTION:** Thoroughly cleanse wound of heavy metal, antibacterials, or antiseptics, which may denature enzyme activity. Thoroughly moisten wound with sodium chloride or water and apply loose thin dressing after applying thin film extending ¼ to ½ inch beyond area to be debrided. Refrigerate ointment at 2–8°C.

Continued on the following page

Table 66–1. ENZYMES, *Continued*		
DRUG NAME/ROUTE AND DOSAGE	**SOURCE**	**NURSING IMPLICATIONS**
ENZYMES FOR SKIN ULCERS		
collagenase (Santyl)		
Topical: *Ointment*–250 units/g once or more daily	Bacteria	Same as for all enzymes plus: **INTERVENTION:** Apply at least daily with tongue depressor blade directly to deep wound. Prior to application, cleanse wound of debris by gently rubbing with a gauze pad with water or Dakin's solution, followed by sterile saline. Remove all excess ointment each time dressing is changed. Terminate use when necrotic tissue is gone. Applied only to injured area. Causes erythema in healthy tissues. Protect healthy tissue with zinc oxide paste.
fibrinolysin and desoxyribonuclease (Elase)		
Topical: *Ointment*–1 unit fibrinolysin, 666 units desoxyribonuclease g 1–3 times daily. *Dry powder*–25 units fibrinolysin, 15,000 units desoxyribonuclease 1–3 times daily ***Intravaginal:*** 5 g ointment deep vaginal at bedtime × 5 applications.	Bovine	Same as for all enzymes plus: **INTERVENTION:** Clean wound with water, pat dry. Apply thin layer and cover with petrolatum gauze. Flush away necrotic debris with saline. For deep wounds, clean and replace medication q 6–10 hr. For best effect, mix solution just prior to use.

their dosages, sources (bovine, porcine, plant, or bacterial), and nursing implications.

CONTRAINDICATIONS AND PRECAUTIONS

In general, enzyme preparations are contraindicated in patients sensitive to the original source, such as beef, pork, pineapple, or papaya. Cross-sensitivity also must be assessed in patients before starting therapy. These products are not given to pregnant women or children under age 12.

▼ CLINICAL ALERT

Because many of the enzymes are fibrinolytic agents, they are contraindicated in patients with bleeding disorders, those currently receiving anticoagulants, or those who have current hemorrhages, as they further increase the anticoagulant effect by dissolving fibrin.

ADVERSE EFFECTS

The major adverse effect produced by the enzymes is hypersensitivity. Because these agents are foreign proteins that are applied topically or taken orally, immunologic reactions may result. When applied topically, these reactions may result in localized itching, stinging, or tingling. When taken internally, the reactions lead to nausea, vomiting, pruritus, and rash. The patient is told to notify the physician immediately if these reactions occur, and the enzyme preparation is discontinued.

ENZYMES TO PROMOTE WOUND HEALING

Enzymes may aid in wound healing. Medications such as **papain** *(Papase, Panafil, Panafil White)*, **hyaluronidase** *(Wydase)*, and **chymopapain** *(Chymodiactin)* reduce inflammation resulting from trauma and infections. These enzymes also dissolve fibrin clots, which helps to reduce the size of surface hematomas. They may also be used surgically to dissolve fibrin clots in episiotomies.

In general, enzyme administration is only adjunctive therapy. For example, when enzymes are used to debride a large stasis ulcer, other drugs such as periphjeral vasodilators and systemic or local antibiotics are also employed. To be effective, the enzyme must be in contact with the affected tissue in adequate concentrations for a sufficient length of time. If necessary, the wound is first surgically debrided. Once the treatment of the wound is completed, enzymes are discontinued because their function is complete. If enzymes are not administered to a clean, debrided wound, healing may be delayed. See Table 66–1 for additional information.

○ **Papain** (Papase, Panafil), a combination of proteolytic enzymes extracted from the papaya plant, is used topically for enzymatic debridement, promotion of normal healing, and when combined with chlorophyll derivatives, deodorization of surface lesions. Papain does not injure or affect healthy tissue or cells. Hydrogen peroxide cannot be used to irrigate the wound, because it inactivates the papain.

○ **Hyaluronidase** (Wydase), a mucolytic enzyme of bovine origin, facilitates the absorption of fluids given by subcutaneous *hypodermoclysis* (the introduction of large quantities of fluids into the subcutaneous tissues). By increasing the rate of fluid absorption in the subcutaneous tissue, the pain and tissue tension caused by the fluid injection are reduced. Another use for hyaluronidase is to inject it subcutaneously into an infiltrated IV site where a potent vasoconstrictor, such as norepinephrine (Levophed) or metaraminol (Aramine), has infiltrated. This reduces the sloughing of tissue likely to occur secondary to infiltration. It is also used to perform subcutaneous urography.

Hyaluronidase is used in ophthalmic surgery to increase the reabsorption of transudates and edema to prevent damage to the eye.

○ **Chymopapain** (Chymodiactin), a proteolytic enzyme derived from papaya, is used in the treatment of patients with herniated lumbar intervertebral disc who have not responded to an adequate trial of conservative therapy. Although the exact mechanism of action of chymopapain has not been established, the herniated portion of the intervertebral disc is usually absent from its former site following administration directly into the herniated disc. About 75% of patients respond favorably to this drug.

CONTRAINDICATIONS AND PRECAUTIONS Chymopapain is contraindicated in patients who have previously been injected with any form of chymopapain due to the high likelihood of allergic reaction, and in patients with severe *spondylolisthesis* (spinal cord tumor) or cauda equina lesion as these conditions do not improve with chymopapain.

ADVERSE EFFECTS Frequent adverse effects of chymopapain include back pain, stiffness, and soreness. Patients are instructed that they may experience back pain or involuntary muscle spasm in the lower area of the back for several days after drug administration.

▼ **CLINICAL ALERT**

Anaphylaxis, which can be immediate or delayed up to 1 hour after drug administration, is the most serious adverse effect of chymopapain, occurring in about 1% of patients. Other serious adverse effects include paraplegia or paraparesis and central nervous system hemorrhage. Chymopapain is extremely toxic when injected intrathecally; therefore, great care is taken to ensure that the dura is not penetrated during injection. Because of these adverse effects and complications, chymopapain is used only in a hospital setting by physicians experienced in its use.

DOSAGE For intradiscal administration, 5 mL of sterile water for injection is added to a vial containing 10,000 units of chymopapain, which provides a final solution containing 2,000 units/mL. The usual adult dose of chymopapain is 2,000 to 4,000 units per disc as a single injection. Bacteriostatic water for injection must not be used for reconstitution as it may inactivate the enzyme. Before needles are inserted into the vial of drug, the stopper is cleansed with alcohol; the alcohol is allowed to completely evaporate prior to insertion of the needle as it may inactivate the chymopapain.

ENZYMES TO PROMOTE SURGICAL HEALING

An enzyme, **chymotrypsin** *(Catarase)*, which is both proteolytic and fibrinolytic, promotes rapid healing in certain surgical applications. It is administered both preoperatively and postoperatively to prevent infection and to promote a more rapid and less painful recovery, such as in cataract surgery. It is instilled into the eye prior to surgery to soften the lens so it can be removed more easily. After surgery, chymotrypsin promotes rapid healing of both the eye or ear. It is believed that postsurgical inflammation, pain, and edema are due to accumulation of fibrin that occludes capillaries and lymph vessels. Proteolytic and fibrinolytic enzymes dissolve the fibrin clot, thus allowing greater blood flow to the area for increased healing. Chymotrypsin is derived from bovine tissues and administered four times daily.

ENZYMES TO REMOVE EXUDATES

Enzymes are also used to remove exudates, although their use is controversial. Several preparations, including **sutilains** *(Travase)*, **collagenase** *(Santyl)*, and **fibrinolysin** and **desoxyribonuclease** *(Elase)*, are used to aid in wound debridement. Primarily, these products promote the *depolymerization* (conversion of compounds into smaller molecules) of desoxyribonucleic acid. In addition, because injured tissue cells are protected from further damage by desoxyribonucleic acid, enzymes alter the previously thick, purulent drainage to a thin liquid material that can easily be wiped or irrigated off the wound, which promotes wound healing.

To ensure that these products are used properly, the wound is prepared before their application. The wound is cleaned and cross-hatching of eschar on burns is performed to allow adequate enzyme contact with the wound. Products that interfere with the action of these enzymes, such as cleansers, heavy metals, and antiseptics, are not used concurrently. These enzyme preparations are adjuncts to surgical debridement and not a replacement for surgery.

○ **Sutilains** (Travase), a proteolytic enzyme derived from bacteria, is particularly useful in removing nonviable or necrotic tissues and purulent exudates from second- or third-degree burns, decubitus ulcers, traumatic injuries, and peripheral vascular disease wounds. This enzyme is virtually inactive on viable tissue. See Table 66–1 for specific application instructions. Sutilains functions best in a pH range of 6.0 to 6.8. If the wound is not affected after 24 to 48 hours of use, the medication is discontinued.

Drug interactions are known to occur with sutilains. Concomitant use of metallic ion-containing compounds such as thimerosal (Merthiolate) interferes with its activity. The use of detergents and antiseptics like iodine and nitrofurazone also decreases its effectiveness.

○ **Collagenase** (Santyl, Biozyme-C), a proteolytic enzyme derived from bacteria, is used as a topical debriding agent. It not only acts on the desoxyribonucleic acid, but also on both denatured (changed protein) and undenatured (unchanged) collagen. By acting on both types of collagen, collagenase produces an effective debridement of the collagen tissue at the wound edges where the necrotic tissue is anchored. This encourages the formation of granulation tissue at the edges and quicker epithelialization of wounds. The best pH range for its proteolytic activity is 6 to 8.

○ **Fibrinolysin and desoxyribonuclease** (Elase), a proteolytic and fibrinolytic enzyme product derived from bovine plasma and pancreas, acts on both deoxyribonucleic acid and fibrin to debride wounds, including burns, decubitus ulcers, and inflamed or infected lesions.

OTHER ENZYMES TO REMOVE EXUDATES

○ **Dextranomer** (Debrisan) is a cross-linked polymer of dextran chains available as beads 0.1 to 0.3 mm in diameter or as a paste. It is not a debriding agent but is a cleansing agent that actually absorbs peptides and pro-

---

Table 66–2. NURSING PROCESS FOR PATIENT RECEIVING TOPICAL ENZYMES

Assessment

Assess illness/condition requiring enzyme treatment.
Assess history of allergies to products from which enzymes are produced, e.g., beef, pork, papaya, pineapple, or bacteria.
Assess current medication use, especially anticoagulants.
Assess presence of bleeding disorders, current hemorrhage.

Nursing Diagnosis: Impaired Skin Integrity	**Desired Outcomes/Evaluation Criteria**
RELATED TO: External (hyperthermia/hypothermia, physical immobilization, trauma, internal altered circulation/nutritional state) excretions/secretions and edema. AS EVIDENCED BY: Complaints of itching, pain, numbness, pressure, disruption of skin surfaces.	Verbalizes understanding of condition and causative factors. Identifies interventions appropriate for specific condition. Observed improvement in wound/lesion healing.

Nursing Actions	**Rationale**
Perform skin testing as indicated.	Determines sensitivity to enzyme medication.
Review importance of skin and measures to maintain proper skin functioning.	Helps patient to understand individual situation and enhances cooperation with treatment regimen.
Discuss factors necessary to improve general health/well-being, e.g., nutrition, cleanliness.	Improves body's own ability to heal.
Monitor vital signs and evaluate open wound.	Elevation of temperature and pulse may be indicators of infection.
Cleanse open area, assist with debridement as indicated, apply enzymes (e.g., Papase, Travase) to wound; or apply proteolytic and fibrinolytic agents (e.g., Catarase) preoperatively and postoperatively as appropriate.	Useful for debridement of large stasis ulcers, burns; reduces opportunity for bacterial contamination and enhances healing.

Nursing Diagnosis: Knowledge Deficit	**Desired Outcomes/Evaluation Criteria**
RELATED TO: Lack of exposure/recall, information misinterpretation, unfamiliarity with information resources. AS EVIDENCED BY: Questions, statement of concern, inaccurate follow-through of instruction/development of preventable complications.	Verbalizes understanding of condition/disease process and treatment. Correctly performs necessary procedures and explains reasons for the actions.

Nursing Actions	**Rationale**
Provide information about pathophysiology of condition, treatment regimen, and expected outcomes.	Understanding of own condition helps patient to make informed decisions and participate fully in treatment regimen.
Instruct in proper application/use of enzyme medications.	Promotes optimal healing.
Discuss probability of burning sensation at site and measures to take to minimize discomfort.	Common side effect may impair cooperation with treatment regimen. Knowing what to expect can help patient to cope with situation and achieve desired effects.
Discuss possible interactions with other drugs.	Can prevent negative result from accidental combination(s).
Review indications for medical evaluation.	Persistent symptoms, indications of infection may indicate need for change in or further treatment.

Other Suggested Nursing Diagnosis: Risk for Infection.

teins. Dextranomer is effective in wet wounds only. Do not pack dextranomer into wounds tightly because maceration of surrounding tissue may result.

USING THE NURSING PROCESS

ASSESSMENT

The patient requiring enzymes may be acutely ill in the hospital or relatively healthy, with his or her condition being treated on an outpatient basis. The patient may have a decubitus ulcer needing care, a necrotic wound after surgery or trauma, or a burn; or may be receiving enzymes to assist with wound healing. Because enzymes are used to treat such a wide variety of conditions, the nursing assessments must be specific for the individual patient's condition.

- Obtain a thorough nursing history to develop the database. Typical information obtained from the patient and family is included in Table 66–2.
- Assess the wound daily either in the hospital or at home to determine if therapeutic effects are occurring. When the wound is completely debrided, enzymes are discontinued as they may retard healing.
- Assess the patient for a history of allergies to the products from which enzymes are produced, such as beef, pork, bacteria, papaya, or pineapple. Skin testing (discussed later) may be performed if allergies are suspected.

NURSING DIAGNOSIS

- Typical nursing diagnoses for a patient receiving enzymes include Impaired Skin Integrity, Knowledge Deficit, and Risk for Infection (see Table 66–2).

PLANNING AND INTERVENTION

- Develop the goals of nursing intervention from the nursing diagnoses. The goals of planning and intervention for a patient requiring enzymes are included in Table 66–2.

Nursing Responsibilities

As the nurse administers these medications, certain basic information should be understood.

- Store all powders in a cool, dry place, and reconstitute just before use. Enzymes are not stored for more than 24 hours after reconstitution.
- Roll or turn medication gently when mixing; do not agitate. This prevents excessive *flocculation* (the formation of thin translucent fibers) in the preparation.
- Skin test patients before administering enzymes. Administer a small amount of medication subcutaneously to assess sensitivity. If a wheal and localized itching occur within 5 minutes and last for 20 to 30 minutes, the medication is not used and the patient is informed about the positive allergic reaction. Enzymes are discontinued at the first sign of sensitiv-

---

Table 66–3. PATIENT TEACHING INFORMATION—ENZYMES

Dear Patient:
This drug has been prescribed for you. This is what you should know about your drug to get the most from your therapy.

- ☐ 1. Your drug must be taken until your current medical problem is cleared up.
- ☐ 2. Drug interactions can occur with your drug. Check with your pharmacist or physician before taking any other drug.
- ☐ 3. Do not stop your drug until told to do so by your physician.
- ☐ 4. Typical side effects of your drug include _____. If these occur, contact your physician.
- ☐ 5. If you are applying enzymes to your wound, follow the specific directions taught to you by your nurse, including _____. Do not use other solutions to wash your wound.
- ☐ 6. Store your drug tightly capped, in a cool dry place.

---

ity—redness, extreme itching, or other unusual local or systemic reactions.

- Cleanse or irrigate wounds gently to prevent damage to healthy tissue. Itching and stinging often occur after topical application, but generally subside. If symptoms persist, the physician is notified. Enzymes must be in direct contact with purulent material on the wound to be effective. Light dressings and cellophane wrap may be used over the wound to enhance drug effect and prevent soiling of clothing. Skin surfaces are kept clean and moist with saline solution to ensure enzymatic activity.
- Change dressings frequently to prevent contamination and to remove necrotic debris. Transparent, occlusive, synthetic films such as Op Site, Bioclusive, and Tegaderm may be indicated to minimize bacterial contamination, drying, and pain. Skin grafting may need to be performed in lesions larger than 3 cm. Antiseptics containing heavy metals such as silver (e.g., siver nitrate) or mercury are not applied to the affected area because these substances and other detergent antiseptics may inactivate the enzymes.
- Drain enzymes used within body cavities at least every 6 to 10 hours and replace enzyme solution. Within the first 24 hours of treatment, a febrile state often occurs due to the accumulation of leukocytes at the wound site. This may be avoided by frequent aspiration of exudate from the wound.

Patient Teaching

- Ensure the patient can administer his or her medication safely, and that he or she knows and understands all patient teaching materials found in Table 66–1 in the Nursing Implications column. If this is not possible, a home health referral is considered. A teaching guide for enzymes is featured in Table 66–3.

EVALUATION

- Develop evaluation criteria on an individual basis through discussion among the nurse, patient, and family. The information from the database, obtained in the original assessment, is used to formulate the criteria for evaluation (see Table 66–2).

- Work with the patient and family to ensure their complete assistance and support. Once they understand the importance of their continued medical treatment, most patients are usually compliant. The primary reason for noncompliance is usually forgetting the medication or not using it because of the local burning or irritation that may occur.
- Evaluate the patient's knowledge of side effects to which he or she may have to become accustomed as

well as major side effects, which must be reported to the physician. The presence of side effects is continually evaluated. The dose of the enzyme may be lowered, or the medication changed or stopped completely, depending on the reaction.

- Review and update all previously taught material, if necessary, to ensure that the patient's knowledge base remains accurate.

The bibliography for this chapter can be found in Appendix B, which begins on page 1054.

CHAPTER REVIEW QUESTIONS*

1. As a class of drugs, enzymes are:
   a. Given intravenously to aid digestion.
   b. Synthesized proteins from plants or animals.
   c. Known to be immunologically neutral.
   d. Altered by the reactions that they mediate.

2. To prepare the skin for sutilains (Travase) therapy, the following should be used:
   a. Soap and water.
   b. Isotonic sodium chloride solution.
   c. Hexachlorophene.
   d. Iodine.

3. The nurse will include the following information when teaching the patient about enzyme replacement therapy:

*See Appendix A, which begins on page 1051, for answers.

   a. Enteric-coated tablets are to be chewed, then followed by water.
   b. Mild stinging may occur when tablets are absorbed buccally.
   c. Bowel movements should increase while on digestive enzymes.
   d. Store enzyme tablets in the refrigerator.

4. A side effect for which the nurse would monitor with regard to chymopapain intradiscal administration is:
   a. Photosensitivity.
   b. Difficulty voiding.
   c. Back pain.
   d. Drowsiness.

CHAPTER 67

Using the Nursing Process with Patients Who Abuse Drugs, Alcohol, and Other Substances

Ellen O'Donnell, RN, CRNA

CHAPTER OUTLINE

Etiology and Progression of Substance Disorders
Concepts Basic to the Nursing Approach
Health Consequences of Substance Abuse
Treatment of Substance Disorders
Attitudes of Health Professionals About Drug Abuse
Using the Nursing Process
Impaired Practice Among Nurses and Other Health
   Professionals

TABLES

Drug Tables

Classes of Abused Drugs and Their Actions, 1016
Smoking Deterrents, 1020
Drugs Used in Treating Substance Dependence, 1023

Nursing Process

Nursing Process by Drug Class Being Abused, 1024

KEY TERMS

Addiction
Anhedonia
Dual diagnosis
Early remission
Enabling behaviors
Impaired practice
Polysubstance abuse/
   dependence

Progression
Substance abuse
Substance dependence
Sustained remission
Tolerance
Withdrawal

LEARNING OBJECTIVES

After reading this chapter, the student will be able to:

1. Define terms related to drug abuse.
2. Identify drugs of frequent abuse.
3. Describe psychologic and physical dependency states.
4. List components of a nursing assessment.
5. List nursing diagnoses relevant to a patient who abuses drugs.
6. Formulate the nursing-care plan for the patient with problems related to drug abuse.
7. Describe outcomes to evaluate interventions with patients who abuse drugs.
8. Formulate patient teaching on the health consequences of drug use.
9. List implications of impaired nursing practice.

The abuse of alcohol and other drugs is widely acknowledged as a major health problem in American society. Abuse of and dependence on a variety of drugs are so common that one in four individuals is estimated to have personal experience with a family member or friend who is, or was, substance dependent. Furthermore, at any given time, 20% to 35% of all persons hospitalized in non-psychiatric settings suffer from some degree of substance abuse. The prevalence of substance abuse and related medical problems ensures that students and practitioners of nursing will care for large numbers of individuals for whom alcohol and/or drug use has been an important life issue. This number has been increased by the growth of HIV-AIDS among intravenous drug users and their partners. Lastly, nurses need to remember they are not

The publisher gratefully acknowledges the contribution of Madeline A. Naegle to the third edition.

immune. Dependence on prescription and illicit drugs is an ongoing concern for health professionals themselves.

The public has various ways of classifying drugs. They differentiate between "social" drugs (alcohol, nicotine, caffeine), prescription drugs (narcotic analgesics, sedatives, amphetamines), over-the-counter (OTC) drugs, and illicit drugs (marijuana, heroin, hallucinogens, inhalants, cocaine). Health professionals, however, classify drugs by their psychoactive effect, which is determined largely by their action on the central nervous system, as presented in Table 67–1. Table 67–2 lists some common street names of drugs by classification.

Table 67–1. CLASSES OF ABUSED DRUGS AND THEIR ACTIONS

ACTION	SITE OF ACTION	LENGTH OF EFFECT	POTENTIAL FOR ADDICTION
PSYCHEDELIC DRUGS			
LSD, psilocybin, mescaline, MDA (Ecstasy), **DOM, DMT, STP**			
Euphoria; altered perceptions; somatic effects (dizziness, tremors, weakness, nausea); psychotic-like symptoms; flashbacks **Objective signs:** Dilated pupils, emotional swings, suspiciousness, paranoia, bizarre behavior	CNS (modify neurotransmitters) Taken orally	**O:** 30–45 min **D:** 8–12 hr; STP 6–9 hr, mescaline 12–14 hr; LSD 10–12 hr	Psychologic dependence only.
CANNABINOIDS			
marijuana, hashish (THC) (*Cannabis sativa*) (*Cannabis indica*)			
Failure in judgment/memory; mild intoxication; euphoria; relaxation; sexual arousal; panic states and psychosis in high doses **Objective signs:** Reddened eyes; heart rate to 140; pulse, respirations, BP increase	CNS Cardiovascular system Smoked	**Admin/dose:** dependent **O:** immediate **D:** 3–7 hr	Moderate. Psychologic dependence and long-term effects occur.
OPIOIDS (NARCOTICS, SYNTHETIC NARCOTICS)			
codeine, morphine, heroin, hydromorphone (Dilaudid), **methadone, meperidine** (Demerol)			
Analgesia, euphoria; escape; reduction in sexual and aggressive drives; sedation, sleepiness **Objective signs:** respiratory depression; constipation; impaired intellectual function, constricted pupils, scratching	Bind in receptor sites, CNS, GI tract Taken orally and injected, inhaled	**O:** depends on route of admin **D:** 4–24 hr	High tolerance and withdrawal occur.
SEDATIVE HYPNOTICS			
barbiturates: secobarbital (Seconal), **pentobarbital** (Nembutal), **amobarbital** (Amytal), **amobarbital/secobarbital** (Tuinal) **barbiturate-like:** (Quaaludes), **benzodiazapines, minor tranquilizers** (Librium) (Valium) (Clonopin)			
Drowsiness/sedation/sleep; euphoria, escape/loss of inhibition, reduction of aggressive and sexual drives; emotional instability; poor judgment	CNS (ascending reticular activating system) Taken orally and injected	**O:** 30–45 min **D:** 4–5 hr	High tolerance and life-threatening withdrawal occur. Cross-tolerance to all CNS depressants occurs.

Continued on the following page

Table 67–1. CLASSES OF ABUSED DRUGS AND THEIR ACTIONS, *Continued*

ACTION	SITE OF ACTION	LENGTH OF EFFECT	POTENTIAL FOR ADDICTION
STIMULANTS			
amphetamine (Methaphetamine) (Dexedrine), **cocaine, crack** (free base), **caffeine**			
Euphoria/grandiosity; energy; excitation; relief of fatigue; depression; wakefulness; suppression of appetite; aggressive feelings; paranoia; reproductive dysfunction in women **Objective signs:** Sweating; dilated pupils; weight loss; vital signs elevated; tremors; seizures; restlessness; psychomotor agitation	CNS (synapses)	**D:** 2–6 hr	High: Tolerance and withdrawal occur.
PHENCYCLIDINES			
PCP (Angel Dust)			
Detachment from surroundings; decreased sensory awareness; illusions of superhuman strength; acute intoxication **Objective signs:** Flushing; fear; sweating; coma; agitation; incoherent speech; aggression	CNS Inhaled	**O:** 2–3 min up to 45 min Prolonged effects	Psychologic only.
INHALANTS			
benzene (paint thinner) (cleaning fluid) (glue), **nitrites, freons, nitrous oxide**			
Euphoria; giddiness; headache; fatigue **Objective signs:** Increase in vital signs; damage to kidneys, liver; disorientation	Cardiac effects CNS Inhaled	Rapid absorption	Psychologic only.
BEVERAGE/ALCOHOL			
beer, wine, liquor			
Relaxation; sedation; release of inhibition **Objective signs:** incoordination; nausea; ataxia; vomiting; impaired cognitive function; slurred speech	CNS Respiratory system Taken orally	**O:** 20 min–1 hr Dose related	High: Tolerance and life-threatening withdrawal occur.

Source: Naegle, MA. Psychiatric Mental Health Nursing: A Client-Centered Approach. JB Lippincott, Philadelphia, 1989, with permission.
O = onset; D = duration; BP = blood pressure.

ETIOLOGY AND PROGRESSION OF SUBSTANCE DISORDERS

The development of drug dependence is complex, and theories about etiology abound with a minimum of evidence. It has been shown that substance disorders are common in some families, which suggests a genetic influence may be operant in some individuals. Opponents of this theory argue that no gene has been identified as causing addiction. These opponents point out that the familial predisposition could be a result of behaviors learned in

Table 67–2. COMMON STREET NAMES FOR ABUSED DRUGS BY CLASSIFICATION	
Classification/Drug	**Street Names**
CNS Depressants	
Chlordiazepoxide (Librium)	Green-and-whites, libs, roaches
Secobarbital (Seconal)	Red birds, red devils
Pentobarbital (Nembutol)	Yellow jackets, nembies, yellowbirds
Amobarbital (Amytal)	Bluebirds, blue angels, blue devils
Glutethimide (Doriden)	Gorilla pills, GBs, Cibas, D
Cannabinoids	
Marijuana, hashish	Pot, grass, reefer, weed, Panama red, Acapulco gold, joint, Mary Jane, MJ, hemp, jive, loco weed, sativa, Texas tea, Sweet Lucy, many others
CNS Stimulants	
Cocaine	Coke, snow, gold dust, girl, flake, C, Carrie, Cecil, dream, happy dust, heaven dust, joy powder, nose candy, crystal
Hydrochloride cocaine	Rock, crack
Amphetamine sulfate (Benzedrine)	Bennies, footballs, greenies, uppers, co-pilots, crossroads, roses, truck drivers, wake ups, whites, black beauties, jolly beans
Dextroamphetamine (Dexedrine)	Dexies, oranges, hearts, Christmas trees, wedges, spots
Methamphetamine (Desoxyn)	Chris, Christine, crystal, meth, speed, crack
Hallucinogens	
Lysergic acid diethylamide (LSD)	Acid, cube, big D, California sunshine, blue dots, barrels, black magic, blue acid, blue heaven, chocolate chips, cupcakes, domes, Hawaiian sunshine, micro dots, peace tablets, squirrels, strawberry field, purple haze, purple ozone
Mescaline	Peyote, cactus buttons, mescal, half moon, big chief
Dimethyltryptamine	DMT, businessman's trip
Phencyclidine	Angel dust, dummy dust, PCP, hog, peace pill, rocket fuel, sheets
Opiates/Narcotics	
Heroin	H, horse, junk, noise, pee, scag, shit, skid, smack, boy, doojee, hairy, Harry, TNT
Opium	Black stuff, poppy, tar, hop, pin, yen, skee, wen shee, big O
Morphine	M, morph, morphie, morpho, white stuff, cube juice, emsel, hocus, Miss Emma, unkie, white merchandise
Codeine	Schoolboy, robo, romo, syrup
Designer Drugs	
Fentanyl analog	China White
Meperidine analogs	MPPP, synthetic heroin
3,4-methylene-dioxymethamphetamine	MDMA, MDA, Adam, Ectasy, XTC

the family. It is possible that both genetics and learned behavior affect the development of substance dependence.

The concept of access certainly influences at least the type of drug used. In neighborhoods where heroin and crack cocaine are readily available, we see high rates of dependence on these drugs. Medical professionals often become dependent on prescription opiates and sedatives with anesthesiologists and nurse anesthetists generally selecting fentanyl as their drug of choice.

Peer pressure is frequently cited as the reason many people experiment with drugs and alcohol. In some social sets peer pressure may result in continued abusive use but may not explain the development of dependence. For example, one hundred young men may join a college fraternity in which the excessive use and abuse of alcohol is engaged in for the 4 years of college. However, statistically, only ten to twelve of these men continue to drink alcoholically once they leave college and enter another social climate.

Personality factors may influence the development of substance dependence. Borderline and antisocial personality disorders are both associated with high rates of alcohol and drug abuse. Most substance abusers, however, are neither borderline nor antisocial. The so-called addictive personality is probably a myth. Professionals in the treatment of addicts and alcoholics find a wide range of personality types among their patients. A substance abuser may be aggressive or meek, extroverted or introverted, intelligent or slow-witted, optimistic or pessimistic. A substance abuser may be a priest, doctor, nurse, firefighter, or a police officer along with career thieves, prostitutes, and murderers.

Pharmacologic factors may contribute to the development of dependence. Individuals may use sedatives to help them cope with the death of a loved one or opiates to relieve the pain of a back injury and find that the withdrawal states produced by these drugs cause them to continue using the drugs long after the grief or physical pain have eased. Most people who use drugs for these reasons, however, do not develop a dependence on them.

These factors may all contribute to the beginning of a substance dependence problem, but why some people with the same influences develop drug or alcohol problems and others do not, we cannot adequately explain. People at high risk for this disorder include those with a family history of substance abuse/dependence, a history of multiple losses and traumatic life events, unresolved psychologic conflicts, and extensive emotional or economic deprivation. Psychoactive drug use is only one method of coping with such issues, and why some people choose this method over others is difficult to say.

Although the reasons why people develop these disorders are various and unclear, the *progression* of substance disorders is remarkably consistent. This progression was first described in regard to alcoholics, but has been found to apply quite well to drug users also.

Initial experimental use progresses to social use and to "relief" use. Relief use occurs, for example, after a difficult day, an anxiety-producing event, or even as a necessary means for celebration. This may then become heavy social use with daily ingestion. This stage can continue for a number of years without significant symptoms of dependence before progressing to a stage of heavy daily use with multiple social, occupational, medical, and legal complications. If the disease is not arrested, it may progress to a late chronic phase of continuous substance binging in which virtually all other interests (work, family, social, recreational, and spiritual) are abandoned and which ends in complete incapacitation and death if recovery is not instituted.

The rate of progression varies widely. Some people move from experimentation to late-stage disease in a few years, and others take several decades to reach the same point. It is important for the nurse to keep in mind that recovery may occur at any point in the progression. The timely intervention of a perceptive and knowledgeable professional may spare the patient from much damage incurred during later stages of dependence.

CONCEPTS BASIC TO THE NURSING APPROACH

The term *addiction* refers to a compulsive physiologic need for a habit-forming drug. However, not all drugs of abuse cause physiologic dependence, and the range of behaviors and patterns of use in people with drug problems cannot be described by such a narrow definition. Therefore, health professionals currently speak of addictive behaviors in terms of abuse and dependence.

Substance abuse refers to a pattern of substance use that causes impairment of the user's ability to meet normal obligations at work, school, or home; use in situations that create physical danger (e.g., driving a car); recurrent legal problems from substance use; or continued use of the substance despite persistent social or interpersonal problems stemming from such use.

The individual suffering from *substance dependence* generally has many of the symptoms of abuse as well as signs of a more advanced problem. These may include the development of tolerance and withdrawal. When *tolerance* is present the user must markedly increase the amount of the drug used to achieve the same effect. In *withdrawal* the user experiences a distressing syndrome of physiologic symptoms when he or she decreases or tries to stop using a substance. However, tolerance and withdrawal are not absolutely necessary for a diagnosis of dependence. Other signs of dependence include taking the substance in larger amounts or over a longer period of time than the user intended, persistent desire or unsuccessful attempts to decrease or control substance use, spending a great deal of time in obtaining the substance or recovering from its effects (e.g., the alcoholic hangover), giving up important social or occupational activities because of substance

use, and continued substance use despite knowledge of a physical or psychologic problem that is caused or exacerbated by such use.

It is common for people to use more than one drug. For example, someone may be dependent on heroin and cocaine while also abusing alcohol and sedatives. This is called *polysubstance abuse/dependence.*

Substance abusers are famous for using the psychologic defense of denial. They deny that their drinking or drug use is a problem, and they minimize the consequences they suffer as a result of that use. Some addicts forced to admit, for example, that shooting heroin in their veins several times a day is a problem will then deny that it is possible to recover. They believe they are incurable. In either case, denial serves an important function. If one denies that substance use is a problem or denies that recovery is possible, then one does not have to change and can continue in the comfortable, if painful, cycle of dependence.

The term *dual diagnosis* was coined to describe people with a major psychiatric disorder as well as a substance disorder. For instance, a patient with bipolar disorder may drink large amounts of alcohol during a manic episode to control his or her symptoms. This may eventually result in the development of alcohol dependence in addition to the bipolar disorder. The nurse must be diligent in addressing both disorders. Patients whose psychiatric problems can be adequately controlled with treatment are unlikely to adhere to the treatment if their substance use continues unabated. By the same token, substance users who achieve abstinence through treatment are unlikely to maintain that abstinence while distressed by an untreated psychiatric disorder.

When patients manage to recover from the substance abuse/dependence for more than one month they are considered to be in *early remission*. When that recovery has continued for more than 12 months they enter *sustained remission*. There is considerable disagreement about when, if ever, a patient can be considered cured or recovered.

HEALTH CONSEQUENCES OF SUBSTANCE ABUSE

The most commonly abused substances—nicotine, alcohol, opioids, stimulants, sedatives, volatile inhalants, hallucinogens, and phencyclidine—have health consequences ranging from medically benign to life threatening or fatal, depending on the substance.

Nicotine The medical consequences of nicotine dependence are encountered often as this is the most commonly abused drug in our culture. These consequences include cardiovascular disease; emphysema; and lung, oral, head and neck, and gastrointestinal (GI) cancers. Table 67–3 features products available to assist with nicotine withdrawal.

Alcohol The myriad medical problems arising from alcohol dependence are often seen and treated without anyone addressing the primary cause. These problems include oral and GI cancers, esophagitis, alcoholic gastritis,

Table 67–3. SMOKING DETERRENTS

DRUG NAME/ROUTE AND DOSAGE	PHARMACOKINETICS/ DYNAMICS	NURSING IMPLICATIONS
nicotine transdermal system (Habitrol) (Nicoderm) (Nicotrol) (ProStep)		
Habitrol–21 mg/day first 6 wk; 14 mg/day next 2 wk; 7 mg/day last 2 wk. Entire therapy 8–12 wk. Wear 24 hr. *Nicoderm*–21 mg/day first 6 wk; 14 mg/day next 2 wk; 7 mg/day last 2 wk. Entire therapy 8–12 wk. Wear 24 hr. *Nicotrol*–15 mg/day first 12 wk; 10 mg/day next 2 wk; 5 mg/day last 2 wk. Entire therapy 14–20 wk. Apply in AM remove hs. *ProStep*–22 mg/day 4–8 wk; 11 mg/day 2–4 wk. Entire therapy 6–12 wk. Wear 24 hr.	**Onset:** 2–4 hr **½L:** 1–2 hr **B:** liver **E:** urine 10%	**ASSESSMENT:** Assess patient's desire to stop smoking. Patient should stop smoking immediately. Drugs replace nicotine in receptor sites to overcome withdrawal symptoms. Assess for pregnancy (category X). Patient should not breast-feed. **INTERVENTION:** Apply system as soon as removed from protective pouch. Use only if pouch is intact. Apply only once a day to nonhairy, clean, dry skin site on upper body or upper outer arm. Skin sites should not be reused for 1 wk. Upon removal, place in protective pouch and dispose. **EVALUATION:** If severe GI symptoms occur, call physician.
nicotine polacrilex (Nicorette, Nicorette DS)		
2 mg—9–30 pieces/day. 4 mg—9–20 pieces/day.	Same as above.	Same as above plus: **ASSESSMENT:** Assess teeth and jaw for pain. Assess for furosemide use; may reverse effects of propranolol and theophylline. Assess diabetics as Nicorette may decrease requirements for insulin. **INTERVENTION:** Chew slowly to minimize side effects. Chew each piece for 30 min. Chew a piece q 1–2 hr. Avoid eating or drinking for 15 min before and after chewing gum. Gradually decrease pieces chewed by 1/day. **EVALUATION:** Evaluate for nausea, vomiting, nonspecific GI complaints, CNS, and insomnia.
lobeline (Bantron)		
1 tablet PO after meals with half glass of water; do not use longer than 6 wk.	**Onset:** NA **½L:** NA **B:** NA **E:** NA	**ASSESSMENT:** Assess desire to stop smoking. Assist patient to enter an antismoking program. Monitor for epigastric pain, nausea, vomiting, and heartburn. **INTERVENTION:** If GI symptoms occur, they may be lessened by an antacid. **EVALUATION:** Notify physician of nausea, vomiting, palpitations, or convulsion.

NA = not available.

---

pancreatitis, alcoholic liver disease (fatty liver, alcoholic hepatitis, and cirrhosis), nutritional deficiencies, macrocytic anemia, pancytopenia from alcoholic bone marrow depression, alcohol poisoning (overdose), traumatic injuries (incurred while intoxicated), withdrawal seizures, alcoholic brain damage (e.g., Wernicke-Korsakoff syndromes, alcoholic dementia), alcoholic myopathy, and mental health problems (e.g., depression, suicidal thoughts and behavior). A patient being treated for any of these problems should be assessed for the possibility that alcohol dependence is causing or contributing to that problem. If alcohol dependence is found, the patient must be informed of the connection between drinking and the medical disorder and should be offered specific treatment for alcoholism. Another concern is the development of fetal alcohol syndrome in the babies of women who drink during pregnancy. This syndrome is characterized by prenatal and postnatal growth deficiencies, microcephaly,

various facial malformations, central nervous system (CNS) dysfunction, and varying degrees of organ system malformations in affected children. Mental retardation is fairly common, but even in children less affected we see behavioral difficulties including hyperactivity, attention deficits, impulsivity, and poor motor control. Also, any nurse dealing with a suspected case of child abuse/neglect should investigate the possibility that alcohol or other drug abuse is a contributing factor.

Opioids Opioids are fairly medically benign. Other than the constant danger of overdosing and hemorrhoids caused by chronic constipation, these drugs do not cause significant organ damage. However, opioid users suffer many consequences caused by the lifestyle associated with illicit drug use (e.g., violent injuries) and the route of administration. Addicts who inject opioids rarely have easy access to sterile equipment, and this exposes them to the risks of bacterial endocarditis, abscesses, infectious hepatitis, and AIDS. Also, accidental overdoses are not uncommon.

Stimulants Users of cocaine and amphetamines are constantly overstimulating their cardiovascular and central nervous systems, resulting in myocardial infarctions, cerebrovascular accidents, and psychotic episodes. Evidence also shows that prolonged or high-dose stimulant abuse may result in a permanent mood disorder characterized by *anhedonia* (loss of the ability to experience pleasure) or constant low-level depression. Babies born to women who abuse stimulants during pregnancy are often born with significant CNS and other organ damage. There are even reports of babies suffering prenatal strokes as a result of their mother's stimulant use.

Sedatives Barbiturates and minor tranquilizers do not cause significant organ damage; however, they are often associated with accidental overdose. This may be related to the memory impairment typically incurred during sedative intoxication causing users to forget how many pills they have already taken. Also, once tolerance develops, users suffer severe mood swings as their blood levels of the drug rise and fall. This often precipitates suicidal behavior and psychiatric admissions. Abusers of sedatives are also prone to accidental injuries incurred while intoxicated.

Marijuana Although there are many controversial studies on the long-term effects of marijuana smoking, there is very little reliable data about suspected problems (e.g., the amotivational syndrome). However, one well-confirmed danger of marijuana smoking is its effect on the lungs. Heavy marijuana smokers are subject to the same risks as tobacco smokers. These risks include bronchitis, emphysema, and lung cancer. In fact, marijuana smoke contains higher concentrations of the same carcinogens found in tobacco smoke.

Volatile Inhalants The medical problems of most concern from the use of petroleum distillates, solvents, glue, and so on, are those of the nervous system. These include acute and chronic encephalopathy, peripheral neuropathy, Parkinsonism, visual loss, and cerebellar ataxia. Depending on the particular substance inhaled, other problems include renal, hepatic, pulmonary, cardiac, and hematologic toxicity.

Hallucinogens The consequences of hallucinogen abuse are generally related to psychiatric problems of varying duration. These may include psychoses, depressive reactions, flashbacks, anxiety, and paranoid states.

Phencyclidine Phencyclidine users are exposed to the same risks as users of other hallucinogens. However, other medical consequences peculiar to phencyclidine include hyperthermia, atropine-like toxicity, hypertensive crisis, and rhabdomyolysis with resultant renal failure.

TREATMENT OF SUBSTANCE DISORDERS

Although spontaneous remission or stabilization of substance disorders occasionally occurs, it is by no means the norm. Once dependence has developed the user requires help to achieve and maintain comfortable abstinence. Some attempts at maintaining a pattern of controlled substance use rather than abstinence have been tried, but the relapse rate to addictive use and all its problems tends to be unacceptably high; such programs have not flourished. Most treatment programs aim for complete abstinence from all mood-altering substances. There are several treatment modalities available.

DETOXIFICATION

Some patients require medical detoxification before rehabilitation can begin. Although many people feel this is the only treatment needed, studies show that over 95% of addicts and alcoholics relapse after detoxification alone. Detoxification may be done on an outpatient basis, in an inpatient detoxification unit, or in a medical unit while the patient is concurrently being treated for one of the medical complications of substance use. Referral for further rehabilitative treatment is always appropriate following successful completion of detoxification.

TWELVE-STEP PROGRAMS

The twelve-step programs of organizations such as Alcoholics Anonymous (AA) or Narcotics Anonymous (NA) are by far the most successful treatment approaches in the United States to date. These programs are based on the premise that dependence is a physical, mental, and spiritual disorder. It is addressed by attendance at self-help meetings, working the steps of recovery (which address denial, atonement for guilt-producing actions, and spiritual growth), acquiring sober sponsors to assist in recovery, and helping others afflicted with the disorder to achieve sobriety. There are usually ancillary programs (e.g., Al-Anon) to assist family and friends of the dependent person.

Most professional treatment programs are based on the twelve-step philosophy and encourage intensive involvement with self-help groups as part of the treatment. Some treatment centers offer inpatient rehabilitation components that typically last 2 to 4 weeks and offer intensive education about the disease, group therapy, and individual counseling. Most centers offer a variety of outpatient programs, which vary in their intensity and duration. Halfway houses where the recovering person may live while working or attending school are also available.

RATIONAL RECOVERY

Rational Recovery, another self-help program, is based on the philosophy of rational emotive therapy developed by Albert Ellis. It is often proposed as an alternative to the twelve-step programs for people who are alienated by the spiritual component of those programs. The availability of these meetings varies according to geographic location but is considerably lower than the twelve-step programs.

THERAPEUTIC COMMUNITIES

Therapeutic communities are long-term inpatient programs (often up to 2 years) that offer behavioral modification, group therapy, and education about the disease. Assistance with general education and vocational training may also be offered, which may be especially useful for the addict who dropped out of school and has no useful work skills. Most therapeutic communities also offer outpatient programs. It is not uncommon for these programs to recommend twelve-step involvement to their clients, especially during the reentry phase of treatment.

RELIGIOUS TREATMENT CENTERS

Some religions have set up substance disorder treatment centers based on the teachings and principles of the particular religion. Christian treatment centers are particularly plentiful, and many have been helped by this approach.

PSYCHIATRIC TREATMENT CENTERS

Many psychiatric hospitals have substance disorder treatment units. They usually offer a variety of inpatient and outpatient options. These are especially useful for the dual diagnosis patient who suffers from another psychiatric disorder in addition to substance abuse/dependence. In dual diagnosis units the importance of complying with treatment for the psychiatric disorder is stressed along with maintaining abstinence from drugs of abuse. Most psychiatric treatment centers also recommend involvement in twelve-step programs to their patients.

NEUROBIOLOGIC TREATMENT APPROACHES

Because of the relationship between neurochemistry and its disturbance in substance abuse, many professionals are researching medications to restore neurochemical balance. Although this research is in its infancy, it may hold great promise for the treatment of substance disorders.

METHADONE MAINTENANCE PROGRAMS

Methadone maintenance treatment programs (MMTPs) were developed to help heroin addicts who have failed repeatedly at abstinence treatments or those who are not willing to attempt abstinence. These are programs of agonist therapy where the opioid addict is started on a dose of methadone that is equivalent to their opioid tolerance. That dose is then gradually increased to a much higher level where the patient is maintained. The purpose is to increase the addict's tolerance to a level where the use of heroin (or other opioids) would have no noticeable effect. Because methadone can be given orally once a day, this spares the addict from the infectious dangers of intravenous drug use, constant struggles with withdrawal symptoms, and the legal and social problems associated with illicit drug use. It is a good example of the "harm reduction" philosophy of substance disorder treatment. MMTPs are not without problems. The person is still dependent on an opioid, many continue to abuse other classes of drugs (alcohol, cocaine, sedatives, and/or marijuana) while on an MMTP, and it is difficult to detoxify

from such a high dose of opioids if the patient wishes to attempt abstinence. However, for some patients MMTPs are a tremendous help. They can function normally in society, hold a job, avoid disease (AIDS, hepatitis, endocarditis), and avoid arrest for drug-related crimes while not having to give up the use of opioids.

ADJUNCTIVE PHARMACOTHERAPY

Some patients are helped by the use of antagonists or other medications while recovering. Disulfiram (Antabuse) is a medication for recovering alcoholics that produces immediate and severely distressing symptoms (facial flushing, palpitations, difficulty breathing, dizziness, nausea, and vomiting) if they ingest even a minute quantity of alcohol. The patient takes the medication daily and, although it does not affect craving for alcohol, it is hoped that fear of a reaction will prevent the person from drinking. Naltrexone (ReVia) is an opioid antagonist that blocks the effect of opioids. It is sometimes used for heroin addicts to help them maintain abstinence. Recent research suggests that naltrexone may decrease the craving for alcohol and decrease relapse rates in recovering alcoholics. Indeed, this medication has become far more popular with alcoholics than heroin addicts. See Table 67–4 for more information on disulfiram and naltrexone.

ATTITUDES OF HEALTH PROFESSIONALS ABOUT DRUG ABUSE

Health professionals with a negative or pessimistic attitude toward substance abusers are unlikely to engage in helpful interactions with them. These attitudes are influenced by education, personal experience, experiences with addicted patients, and experiences with family members and friends who are substance dependent. Association with a substance abuser in the nurse's personal life may have produced feelings of frustration, anger, and pain. By the time patients are hospitalized with the medical complications of dependence, they are often in the late stages of the disorder and have a relatively poor prognosis. Such patients tend to be difficult. They lie about their problem, are demanding or manipulative in an attempt to obtain psychoactive medication, and tend to be noncompliant with medical treatment regimens. These are powerful reinforcement for negative attitudes. The education received by most professionals is woefully inadequate to overcome such negativism. Professionals need to be exposed to recovering individuals to achieve an optimistic outlook for dealing with substance abusers. It is no accident that many professionals who work in the field are recovering themselves. Recovering people know from their own experience that the problem is not incurable. They also tend to develop acquaintances and friendships among recovering people. Other professionals could overcome their negativism in similar ways. Student professionals could do rotations in substance abuse treatment centers, and all professionals are welcome to attend

Table 67–4. DRUGS USED IN TREATING SUBSTANCE DEPENDENCE

DRUG NAME/ROUTE AND DOSAGE	PHARMACOKINETICS/DYNAMICS	NURSING IMPLICATIONS
ALCOHOL ANTAGONIST		
disulfiram (Antabuse) 200–500 mg PO daily	**Onset:** 0.5–3 hr **Peak:** 3–12 hr **Duration:** 1–2 wk **½L:** NA **PB:** NA **B:** liver **E:** urine, lungs	**ASSESSMENT:** Assess for intoxication. Never administer while patient is intoxicated or without patient's knowledge. Recent use of metronidazole paraldehyde, alcohol, or alcohol-containing preparations; severe myocardial disease; coronary occlusion; hypersensitivity to disulfiram or other thiuram derivatives are all contraindicated. **INTERVENTION:** Observation, documentation. Monitor for flushing, nausea, vomiting, headache, weakness, dizziness, skin eruptions, impotence. **Patient Teaching**—Teach patient to read all OTC product labels closely to assess for alcohol. **EVALUATION:** Evaluate for severe nausea, vomiting, or hypotension; notify physician.
OPIOID ANTAGONIST		
naltrexone (Revia) 50 mg PO daily or 100–150 mg 2–3 times weekly	**Onset:** 15–30 min **Peak:** 1 hr **Duration:** 24–72 hr **½L:** 3.9–12.9 hr **PB:** 21% **B:** liver **E:** urine	**ASSESSMENT:** Assess for acute hepatitis or liver failure. **Patient Teaching**—Warn patient that attempts to overcome the blockade with large amounts of heroin may result in life-threatening circumstances. **EVALUATE:** Evaluate for severe anxiety, insomnia, headache, or rash; notify physician.

open meetings of Alcoholics Anonymous and Narcotics Anonymous.

Occasionally health professionals engage in *enabling behaviors*. These are behaviors that support the patient's continuing use of the drug by failure to confront the addicts with the consequences of their illness or shielding them from experiencing these consequences. Families do this by participating in denial of the problem; making excuses for the addict, covering up their drug use to keep employers and others unaware; and supplying money, housing, food, and so on when the addict is not able to fulfill his or her obligations. Professionals engage in enabling behaviors by omitting drug and alcohol use histories, providing care for the medical consequences of addiction (e.g., cirrhosis, endocarditis, AIDS) without exploring the underlying causes, and failing to make appropriate referrals for substance disorder treatment. Professionals may do this to avoid alienating the patient or because of their own discomfort with the problem or with therapeutic confrontation.

USING THE NURSING PROCESS

ASSESSMENT

- Obtain a comprehensive nursing assessment using both history taking and observational skills. In a routine history and physical a short-form drug history is used as a screening mechanism. On admission to a drug/alcohol treatment unit or when the short-form screening indicates a significant substance problem, an extensive substance evaluation is indicated. Assessment data is found in Table 67–5.
- Establish rapport by asking for other nonthreatening information (e.g., general medical history and social history) before asking about substance use. Substance users are reluctant to be truthful about their problem for a number of reasons. Some fear the professional will be judgmental. They often have high levels of guilt and have no reason to believe you will judge them any less harshly than they judge themselves. They may minimize their use to hide the extent of their problem or exaggerate the amount used for fear the hospital will give them an inadequate dose of detoxification medication and cause them to suffer withdrawal. Even if they intend to be truthful, it is difficult. Once intoxicated they may not really remember how much they used. Because they rarely use the same amount each day, they will try to estimate usual usage. These estimations are often laughably inaccurate. When street drugs are used, it is important to keep in mind that drug dealers never indicate the number of milligrams of pure drug in a package. One addict's three bag a day heroin habit may be worse than another's six bag a day habit be-

Table 67–5. NURSING PROCESS BY DRUG CLASS BEING ABUSED

HALLUCINOGEN INTOXICATION/WITHDRAWAL (LSD, CANNABIS)

Assessment

Assess mental status, noting degree of agitation and psychomotor activity, presence of emotional swings, suspiciousness, paranoia, bizarre behavior.
Assess baseline vital signs, noting hypertension, tachycardia, tachypnea.

Nursing Diagnosis: Risk for Injury

RELATED TO: Clouded sensorium.
AS EVIDENCED BY: Impaired judgment, poor coordination, and diminished perception of pain.

Desired Outcomes/Evaluation Criteria

Maintains physiologic stability and injury does not occur.

Nursing Actions

Have someone known to the patient accompany him or her and provide support, comfort, and close observation. Provide nonthreatening environment with subdued, pleasant stimuli.
Avoid use of phenothiazines.

Administer Valium as indicated.

Rationale

Patient is disoriented, experiencing perceptual distortions and hallucinations that can increase likelihood of injury.

Antipsychotic drugs may increase anticholinergic effects of ingested drug, causing hypotension.
Acts as a tranquilizer with calming effect to reduce risk of injury.

Nursing Diagnosis Altered Thought Processes

RELATED TO: Physiologic changes, impaired judgment with loss of memory.
AS EVIDENCED BY: Inaccurate interpretation of environment, bizarre thinking, disorientation.

Desired Outcomes/Evaluation Criteria

Demonstrates return of memory and ability to function with absence of visual/auditory disturbances.

Nursing Actions

Provide safe, nonthreatening environment with close observation and diversion from disturbing internal experiences.
Anticipate some form of unpredictable behavior.
Tell patient that current thoughts and feelings are a result of drug effect.
Administer medications, e.g., Valium, as indicated.

Rationale

Alteration in thinking leads to inability to process information correctly, affecting patient's response to environment.

Being prepared for the unexpected allows opportunity to manage situation effectively.

Provides reassurance about body integrity and safety.

May provide tranquilizing effect.

PHENCYCLIDINE INTOXICATION/WITHDRAWAL (PCP)

Assessment

Assess baseline vital signs, presence of flushing, fever, sweating. Observe for increasing anxiety, fear, irritability, and agitation. Note changes in behavior pattern and exaggerated emotional responses.
Assess signs of neurologic irritation, hyperactivity, incoherent speech, level of consciousness.
Assess degree of sensory awareness, presence of delusions, detachment from surrounds.

Nursing Diagnosis: Risk for Violence: Self-directed or directed at others

RELATED TO: Toxic reactions to drugs, exogenous chemical alteration.
AS EVIDENCED BY: Abnormal behavior.

Desired Outcomes/Evaluation Criteria

Acknowledges reality of situation and understanding of the relationship of behavior to drug use.

Nursing Actions

Place in a darkened, quiet, nonthreatening environment with a nonintrusive observer.
Speak in a soft nonthreatening voice. Avoid use of "talk-down" techniques.
Observe behavior without administering drugs before a decision about use of other drugs is made.
Administer Valium as indicated.

Rationale

Lowers stimulation, decreasing the likelihood of confusion and fear and lessening the chance of violent response.

May have a calming effect, but "talk-downs" may increase agitation level.

Allows for a clear clinical picture to develop.

Provides calming effect to help control behavior.

Continued on the following page

Table 67–5. NURSING PROCESS BY DRUG CLASS BEING ABUSED *Continued*

PHENCYCLIDINE INTOXICATION/WITHDRAWAL (PCP)

Nursing Diagnosis: Altered Tissue Perfusion, Cardiopulmonary/cerebral

RELATED TO: Alterations in blood flow (hypertensive crisis).
AS EVIDENCED BY: Decreased level of consciousness, hypotension/hypertension

Desired Outcomes/Evaluation Criteria

Maintains/achieves physiologic stability evidenced by patent airway and adequate respiratory/cardiac function. Regains/maintains usual level of consciousness free of adverse neurologic symptoms/complications.

Nursing Actions	**Rationale**
Elevate head of bed, keep head in midline position.	Enhances venous drainage, reducing risk of vascular congestion and increased intracranial pressure and possibility of hemorrhage.
Observe for pupillary or vital sign changes, decreased level of consciousness.	Provides for early detection and intervention to minimize increased intracranial pressure/injury.
Administer antihypertensive medications as indicated.	Effective in lowering blood pressure to prevent hypertensive crisis.

DEPRESSANT INTOXICATION/WITHDRAWAL (BARBITURATES, SEDATIVES, OPIOIDS)

Assessment

Assess baseline vital signs, noting hypertension, respiratory depression.
Assess mental/emotional state (e.g., lability, belligerence, lethargy, agitation, anxiety, presence of confusion or delirium) and degree of impairment, duration of problems.
Assess concurrent alcohol and other drug use.

Nursing Diagnosis: Risk for Injury

RELATED TO: Depression/agitation, psychologic stress, IV drug-use techniques.
AS EVIDENCED BY: hyperactive behavior, seizure activity.

Desired Outcomes/Evaluation Criteria

Verbalizes understanding of risk factors of taking drugs.
Completes withdrawal without injury to self, development of complications.

Nursing Actions	**Rationale**
Provide quiet, lighted room with close observation.	Reduces stimuli that may potentiate agitation/seizure activity and possibility of injury.
Restrict activity/assist as necessary.	Presence of orthostatic hypotension, hyperreflexion, and muscle cramping increases risk of traumatic injury.
Maintain frequent contact, reorient as needed. Provide seizure precautions.	Provides reassurance/reduces anxiety. May prevent injury if seizures occur during withdrawal.
Evaluate changes in behavior/emotional state.	Drug intoxication can precipitate alterations in perceptions/psychotic behavior and may result in hallucinations and precipitate suicidal/homicidal behavior.
Administer emetics, assist with gastric lavage if indicated.	Emptying stomach may be effective when drug has been recently ingested.
Administer activated charcoal per protocol. Administer phenobarbital or methadone, Trexan as indicated by drug used.	Reduces intestinal absorption of ingested drugs. Phenobarbital's prolonged effect provides smoother sedation, while methadone/Trexan replace heroin or other narcotic effects.
Observe for dehydration, record I/O, monitor temperature.	Hyperpyrexia may occur with withdrawal or occur with infectious process, requiring additional fluid replacement to promote clearance of drug.
Maintain IV line as appropriate.	Provides avenue for emergency drugs/fluid replacement.

ALCOHOL INTOXICATION/WITHDRAWAL

Assessment

Assess respiratory rate, depth, rhythm, and breath sounds.
Assess level of consciousness, behavioral responses, presence of hallucinations/impaired cognitive function, slurred speech.
Assess degree of fear and reality of threat perceived by the patient.
Assess coordination, note ataxia.
Assess information as soon as possible on drug/alcohol ingestion.

Nursing Diagnosis: Ineffective Breathing Pattern

RELATED TO: Direct effect of alcohol toxicity on respiratory center, decreased energy, presence of chronic respiratory inflammatory processes, and sedative effects of drugs given to decrease alcohol withdrawal symptoms.
AS EVIDENCED BY: Hypoventilation.

Desired Outcomes/Evaluation Criteria

Displays normal breathing pattern free of symptoms of respiratory distress and cyanosis.

Nursing Actions	**Rationale**
Establish patient airway. Elevate head of bed and position on side as indicated.	Respiratory depression can lead to hypoxia and eventually cardiovascular collapse.
Encourage cough and deep breathing. Suction as needed.	Facilitates lung expansion and clearance of secretions, reducing risk of atelectasis.

Continued on the following page

Table 67–5. NURSING PROCESS BY DRUG CLASS BEING ABUSED, *Continued*

ALCOHOL INTOXICATION/WITHDRAWAL

Nursing Actions	**Rationale**
Monitor level of consciousness and vital signs closely.	Treatment and medication are administered in accordance with level of consciousness.
Initiate resuscitation efforts as necessary.	
Administer supplemental oxygen as indicated.	Helpful in preventing/reducing hypoxia associated with CNS/respiratory depression.

Nursing Diagnosis: Sensory-Perceptual Alteration (Specify)	**Desired Outcomes/Evaluation Criteria**
RELATED TO: Exogenous chemical alteration (alcohol use/sudden cessation) and endogenous (electrolyte imbalance, elevated ammonia and blood urea nitrogen), sleep deprivation, psychologic stress.	Reports absence of auditory/visual hallucinations. Maintains optimal level of consciousness.
AS EVIDENCED BY: Disorientation, bizarre thinking, exaggerated responses.	

Nursing Actions	**Rationale**
Provide safe, quiet environment and regulate lighting as indicated. Speak in calm voice.	Promotes rest and limits hyperactive responses to aid in control of hallucinations and reduce risk of personal injury.
Provide supervision and interpersonal support. Refrain from judgmental comments.	Patient is disoriented, frightened, guilty, and needs assistance to avoid additional complications.
Administer Valium cautiously as indicated.	Decreases CNS stimulation but may potentiate respiratory depression.
Administer Antabuse as indicated.	Produces a highly sensitive reaction to alcohol with unpleasant side effects, promoting abstinence.
Refer to substance abuse treatment program upon resolution of acute intoxication.	Patient is unable to respond to health-oriented referral during acute state.

STIMULANT INTOXICATION/WITHDRAWAL (AMPHETAMINES, COCAINE/CRACK)

Assessment

Assess information on type and kind of drugs ingested.
Assess perceptions; behavioral responses; and presence of hallucinations, paranoia, aggressive feelings.
Assess extent of fatigue and excitation/psychomotor acceleration (e.g., sweating, dilated pupils, tremors, seizures).
Assess degree of fear and reality of threat perceived by the patient.
Assess vital signs, noting presence of tachycardia, hypertension, tachypnea, hyperpyrexia.
Assess suppression of appetite, weight loss.

Nursing Diagnosis: Decreased Cardiac Output	**Desired Outcomes/Evaluation Criteria**
RELATED TO: Drug effect on myocardium/electrical conduction, and preexisting myocardiomyopathy.	Demonstrates adequate cardiac output and normalization of vital signs and cardiac rhythm.
AS EVIDENCED BY: Hypotension.	

Nursing Actions	**Rationale**
Monitor cardiac activity, anticipate cardiac arrest, and implement resuscitative measures as necessary.	Tachycardia and arrhythmias are common and may be life threatening.
Administer medications, e.g., propranolol (Inderal) and lidocaine.	β-adrenergic blockers reduce cardiac oxygen demand. Lidocaine may be used in emergency situation to control/prevent ventricular arrythmias.

Nursing Diagnosis: Fear	**Desired Outcomes/Evaluation Criteria**
RELATED TO: Paranoid delusions.	Discusses reality base of persecutory fears. Demonstrates appropriate range of feelings and lessened fear.
AS EVIDENCED BY: Suspiciousness and concerns about actions of others.	

Nursing Actions	**Rationale**
Be concrete, clear in communication.	Promotes accurate understanding and helps to lessen fear.
Acknowledge awareness of patient's feelings. Encourage verbalization of fear.	Ventilation can lessen intensity of fearfulness.
Assist patient in reality-checking fears.	Patient can further reduce fear by understanding difference between reality and delusions.

cause he or she is getting a purer product. You may increase the accuracy of the history by pointing out inconsistencies to the patient, using repeat histories by different professionals in other disciplines, correlating the information in the history with physical signs or laboratory findings, and using collateral histories. Collateral histories are histories obtained from other people close to the substance user. A woman may tell you that she takes 5 milligrams of diazepam three times a day "just like my doctor ordered." Her husband may reveal that he has found bills from several doctors and empty pill bottles hidden all over the house.

- Obtain the following information in a comprehensive substance history:
  - Alcohol use (Do you ever drink alcohol? How often? How much? When was your last drink? How old were you when you had your first real drink? When did you start daily drinking?)
  - Drug use (What other drugs have you used? How much? How often? When was the last use for each substance mentioned? Do you take pain pills or sedatives from a doctor? When did you first try each substance mentioned?)
  - Family substance history (In your opinion, does anyone else in your family have a drinking or drug problem?)
  - Social problems from drug use (Have any of your family or friends complained about your drinking or drug use? Has your spouse threatened to leave you? Have your parents threatened to kick you out?)
  - Employment problems (Are you in trouble at work for lateness? Absences? Poor performance? Trouble getting along with co-workers?)
  - Medical problems from drug use (Have you ever had a seizure? Memory blackout? Accidental overdose? Hepatitis? Pancreatitis? Endocarditis? AIDS test? Has a doctor ever told you that your liver was enlarged or that your liver tests were abnormal?)
  - Psychiatric history (Have you ever been treated by a psychiatrist? Psychiatric admissions? Therapy for depression, marriage counseling, personal problems? Have you ever tried to kill yourself? Do you feel suicidal now? Have you ever seen or heard things that weren't really there?)
  - Legal problems (Have you ever been arrested? What for? Have you done time in prison? How much? Are you on parole or probation now?)
  - Treatment history (Have you ever been treated for a drinking or drug problem in the past? What type of treatment? How often? When was your last treatment?)
  - Abstinence history (What is the longest time you were ever able to remain sober and drug free? How did you do that?)
- Correlate the information from the history with careful observation of physical signs and a review of the patient's laboratory data. Important observations include the following:
  - Mental status (Is patient alert, lethargic, somnolent, agitated, hyperkinetic, intoxicated? Does patient appear depressed, cheerful, anxious, hostile, paranoid, grandiose? Is patient's affect appropriate to the situation and his or her mood?)
  - Activity (Is patient restless? Unable to sit still? Falling asleep between questions? Repeatedly scratching as if itching? Note repeated yawning or sneezing. Are tremors noticed when patient is sitting still or when asked to extend the arms?)
  - Eyes (Does patient maintain good eye contact? Pupil size should be recorded in millimeters or described—dilated, larger than midsize, midsize, smaller than midsize, constricted, pinpoint. Note signs of redness or tearing.) Eye signs are especially important in patients abusing opiates such as heroin. These patients often claim they have not used heroin for at least a day prior to admission and need medication immediately because they feel sick. If that is true their pupils should be dilated to midsize or larger, indicating opiate withdrawal. Commonly, though, their pupils are constricted to pinpoint, indicating recent ingestion of a significant dose of opiates. A nurse who does not notice this risks overmedicating the patient into an overdose.
  - Skin (Note any needle track marks or scarring over veins, multiple bruises on extremities, rashes, burns, lacerations or scars on wrists, spider angiomata, poor skin turgor, diaphoresis, palmar erythema, abscesses, edema, facial flushing, pallor, gooseflesh, or rhinorrhea.)
- Assess the patient's general state of hygiene, odors on the breath (e.g., alcohol), slurred speech, ataxia, and nutritional status.
- Assess laboratory data. Urine toxicology results should be consistent with the drugs the patient reports using. If the toxicology results are to be reported to the patient's employer or parole officer or are critical for their medical care, the nurse must supervise the specimen collection to prevent the patient from substituting another urine sample or diluting the sample with water to decrease the drug concentration below a detectable level. Blood alcohol levels and Breathalyzers are more reliable indicators of recent drinking than urine toxicology. Liver function tests are usually abnormal in alcoholics and sometimes abnormal in intravenous drug users who have been exposed to hepatitis. Alcoholics with more advanced liver disease also have prolonged clotting times and elevated bilirubin. Macrocytic anemia consistent with folate deficiency is common in alcoholics. They also may reveal a pancytopenia consistent with alcoholic bone marrow depression. Intravenous drug users may have elevated white cell counts from infections or low white cell counts, which may be an ominous sign of advanced HIV infection. It is not unusual for alcoholics to have electrolyte disturbances and hypomagnesemia as a result of poor nutrition combined with frequent diarrhea, nausea, and vomiting.

Alcohol and drug users are often interested in the results of their laboratory tests. It is very helpful to review their laboratory results with them and explain any abnormalities that are connected with alcohol or drug abuse. It is interesting to note that most intravenous drug users believe they have been tested for HIV any time blood is drawn. They then assume they are HIV-negative if nobody tells them they have AIDS. It is important to make it a point to inform them if HIV testing was not done and either offer counseling and testing at your facility or refer them to a public health center for anonymous testing.

NURSING DIAGNOSIS

- Examples of nursing diagnoses relating to substance abuse include the following: Risk for Injury; Altered Thought Processes; Risk for Violence, Self-directed or directed at others; Altered Tissue Perfusion; Ineffective Breathing Pattern; Ineffective Individual Coping; Sensory-Perceptual Alteration; Sleep Pattern Disturbance; and Altered Nutrition, Less than body requirements.

NURSING INTERVENTIONS

- It is essential that nurses be educated about substance abuse/dependence to recognize signs that interventions for the problem would be appropriate. Whenever confronted with a patient suffering medical consequences of substance abuse, the professional should include interventions for the drug problem in the patient's care plan. Nurses also have opportunities to intervene at earlier stages of the disease if they are vigilant. Occupational nurses may become aware of workers who suffer repeated small injuries on the job or have a suspicious pattern of absences (e.g., frequently call in sick on Mondays). These things should precipitate a complete substance abuse evaluation. The school nurse should be aware that children from families with a substance problem often manifest behavioral or learning difficulties at school. By speaking with teachers and family members as well as the child, the teacher may uncover the problem and initiate recovery for the whole family. Nurses in mental health clinics and private practice should be sure to elicit a comprehensive drug/alcohol history on every client who comes to the intake process. Some methods of early intervention include the following:
  - refusal to accept the client's excuses, rationalizations, and continuing dysfunctional behavior
  - expressing sincere concern about the client's health as a result of drug-using behavior
  - giving truthful feedback and interpretations of the results of laboratory tests, screening histories, and evaluative tools
  - referring family members (who are often distressed by the addict's behavior long before the addict is) to appropriate treatment or self-help groups
  - advising the primary caregiver (e.g., patient's family physician) about signs and symptoms of a substance problem you have observed
  - promoting communication among all caregivers involved with the client

The purpose of such early interventions is to overcome the denial of the addict and those closely involved with him or her. To be successful they must be carried out with a respectful attitude of caring concern for the individuals involved. The nurse must take care to avoid inducing guilt and shame, which only lead to further estrangement. Many people believe that the substance-dependent individual must admit the problem and ask for help before interventions can succeed. This is absolutely untrue. Most are aware of the problem on some level, but all are ambivalent about seeking treatment. This is because successful treatment means they will have to give up the drugs or alcohol, which have become necessary for their comfort and pleasure. The idea of the intervention is to point out the terrible price they pay for this mode of relief and offer assistance toward developing a better style of coping. Some people seek treatment because they have been threatened with loss of a job, family, or legal freedom. These are powerful inducements to change and make it much easier for treatment professionals to accomplish their goals.

Withdrawal Syndromes

Some drugs have a characteristic withdrawal syndrome of unpleasant physiologic and psychologic symptoms. The appearance of such withdrawal symptoms is one of the criteria on which a diagnosis of dependence may be based. General principles of withdrawal include the following:

- The acute discomfort involved typically causes dependent persons to seek immediate relief by taking whatever drug they need to relieve that discomfort.
- Withdrawal symptoms tend to be opposite in nature from the direct effects of the drug.
- Withdrawal from all classes of substances produces symptoms of acute anxiety and protracted depression.
- Polysubstance use is increasingly the norm; any withdrawal syndrome may be accompanied by a second set of symptoms or may be masked by intoxication from another substance.
- Because the substance abuser may be self-medicating for a major psychiatric disorder or a personality disorder that predates the drug use, the withdrawal syndrome can evoke evidence of a previously masked set of psychiatric symptoms such as phobias, anxiety disorders, mood disorders, or borderline personality.
- Although an uncomplicated detoxification may be safely carried out on an outpatient basis by a knowledgeable physician, this will often be unsuccessful because the patient requires a controlled environment in order to abstain from illicit drug use during the detoxification process.
- When caring for a patient in withdrawal it is important to remember that neither the history nor the patient's subjective complaints are accurate means to determine the amount of detoxification medication required. An alcoholic may well swear that he or she feels fine and does not need more medication while you notice the patient's hands are tremulous and vital signs are elevated. A heroin addict may complain of severe withdrawal discomfort while objectively you

note pinpoint pupils, nose scratching, and constipation—all signs that the patient is more than adequately medicated. The patient's complaints should instigate an evaluation by the nurse, but when the objective signs do not agree with the subjective complaints (or lack of them), the nurse must treat according to the objective signs.

Not all classes of substances provoke significant withdrawal. Psychedelic drugs, cannabinoids, phencylidines, and inhalants have not been documented to produce withdrawal syndromes requiring treatment. Significant withdrawal often occurs in those dependent on alcohol, sedatives, opioids, and stimulants.

Withdrawal from Sedatives and Alcohol

Untreated withdrawal from sedatives and alcohol can be life threatening. Depending on the extent of dependence, hospitalization and close supervision is optimal. Although the symptoms for withdrawal from alcohol are similar to those from sedatives, the time frame for their occurrence differs. Early symptoms such as tremors, sweating, diarrhea, increased heart rate, increased blood pressure, anxiety, and insomnia begin a few hours after the last drink of alcohol but do not develop until the third day after the last use of benzodiazepines.

Later symptoms of seizures, hallucinations, delirium, and hyperpyrexia also have a varying onset dependent on the drug used. Seizures in the alcoholic usually occur 7 to 38 hours after cessation of drinking, and delirium tremens appears 2 to 3 days after the last drink and usually starts to subside in 1 to 5 days if the patient survives. With some barbiturates and hypnotics, withdrawal symptoms typically begin 12 to 24 hours after the last use and peak in 24 to 72 hours. For many benzodiazepines and phenobarbital, the withdrawal symptoms do not peak until the fifth to the eighth day after the last dose.

A protracted withdrawal syndrome of anxiety and sleep disturbances may persist in the alcoholic long after acute withdrawal has resolved. In the sedative user the protracted withdrawal often includes severe anxiety, mood swings, insomnia, nightmares, difficulty concentrating, parasthesias, and forgetfulness. These symptoms

may persist for several months. Many recovering people have reported that it was very helpful to be warned of these protracted symptoms during their initial detoxification. The knowledge that these difficulties were to be expected and would eventually resolve was very comforting to them in the early months of recovery.

The major syndromes associated with alcohol withdrawal are reviewed in Table 67–6.

Treatment for sedative or alcohol withdrawal is carried out with a sedative taper accompanied by stabilization of fluid and electrolyte balance. The most commonly used drugs are Librium, Valium, and phenobarbital (Chapter 25) although any sedative, theoretically, could be used.

Withdrawal from Opioids

Withdrawal from opioids is rarely life threatening but causes a range of discomforts in the user. The dose, length of use, frequency of use, and expectations of the user are important factors in determining the severity of withdrawal symptoms. Early signs and symptoms of opioid withdrawal include craving for the drug, lacrimation, piloerection, rhinorrhea, anxiety, irritability, dilated pupils, yawning, sneezing, depression, muscle or bone aches, and insomnia. These symptoms begin 6 to 12 hours after the last dose for short-acting opioids (e.g., heroin, morphine) and 24 to 48 hours after the last dose of methadone, which has a long duration of action. Later signs and symptoms developed by those with severe dependency include nausea, vomiting, diarrhea, abdominal cramps, and dehydration. The withdrawal symptoms tend to peak at 48 to 72 hours and subside over 5 to 7 days for short-acting opioids. For methadone (Chapter 18) the syndrome tends to be milder in intensity but more protracted, with peak intensity reached in 4 to 8 days and a total duration of more than 14 days.

Treatment for opioid withdrawal consists of an opioid taper (preferably using methadone) carried out over several days. Recently, clonidine (Chapter 30) has been used to treat opioid withdrawal with benzodiazepines (Chapter 25) sometimes used to augment the treatment. This method is somewhat less comfortable than an opioid taper and is therefore less acceptable to many addicts.

See Table 67–4 for information on drugs used to treat opioid withdrawal and overdose.

Table 67–6. SYNDROMES ASSOCIATED WITH ALCOHOL WITHDRAWAL

State	Peak Time of Onset and Duration	Signs and Symptoms
Alcohol withdrawal	P: 24 hr D: 3 days–2 wk	Tremulousness, irritability, nausea, vomiting, autonomic hyperactivity; increased vital signs, sleep disturbance
Alcohol seizures	P: 7–38 hr following cessation of alcohol	Grand mal seizures that occur in bursts; 2–6 seizures
Alcohol withdrawal delirium	P: Gradual; 2–3 days after cessation of alcohol D: 4–5 days	Marked variations in levels of consciousness, e.g., confusion, disorientation, perceptual disturbance, autonomic hyperactivity; life threatening
Alcohol hallucinosis	P: Within 48 hr or less after last drink D: 3 days–2 wk	Clear sensorium but vivid auditory hallucinations of a persecutory nature Agitation, fearfulness, increased suicide potential

Withdrawal from Stimulants

There is controversy surrounding the concept of withdrawal from stimulants. It is agreed that there are no dangerous symptoms requiring medical treatment. However, there are three phases of abstinence easily recognized by stimulant users that may contribute to relapse to stimulant use. The first phase is the "crash." This follows a stimulant binge of a few days duration. The crash starts soon after the binge ends, and the early phase is characterized by a depressed mood with anxiety and stimulation from the drug continuing. Within a few hours this progresses to symptoms of hypersomnolence and hyperphagia (increased appetite). For the next 1 to 4 days the user just wants to sleep and eats heartily during brief periods of waking. After waking from the crash the user's sleep is normalized but he or she commonly suffers from anhedonia, dysphoria, anergia, anxiety, and a high craving for stimulants. This withdrawal phase lasts 1 to 10 weeks. This is followed by the extinction phase in which the mood normalizes and the drug craving becomes more episodic in nature.

Treatment for stimulant withdrawal consists mainly of preventing relapse, sometimes by inpatient rehabilitation. Various drugs, including antidepressants and bromocriptine, have been used to relieve dysphoria and prevent relapse, but their value is debated.

Nursing Interventions Directed toward Recovery

- Once the patient has acknowledged the disease and entered treatment, the nursing interventions are more straightforward and include the following:
  - Denial is a continuing issue that should be repeatedly confronted.
  - Education about the disease is vital and often alleviates guilt the patient has about being an alcoholic or drug addict.
  - The education given by the nurse about the process of recovery depends partly on the philosophy of the particular treatment center, but ethical practitioners do not withhold information about other modalities of treatment available that might be appropriate for the patient.
  - Involvement of the family and significant others in treatment should be strongly encouraged. It greatly improves the prognosis for recovery.
  - Spiritual counseling should be made available to the patient who wishes it.
  - The patient should be assisted in identifying changes he or she may need to make to stay comfortably sober. Examples of such changes include separation from relationships with active alcoholics or drug users, changing a particularly inappropriate job (e.g., bartender), or changing the work schedule to decrease stress and make participation in ongoing treatment or self-help groups easier.
  - Relapse prevention techniques such as identifying substance-use triggers and ways to avoid or deal with them should be stressed.
  - Self-esteem can be improved by helping the patient identify personal assets and giving positive feedback about his or her efforts toward recovery.
  - The patient needs to be encouraged to form relationships with other recovering people and become comfortable in turning to them for support when the professional treatment is concluded.
- Maintain appropriate boundaries when dealing with substance-dependent patients. Although the professional may help someone locate self-help programs, he or she should never offer to accompany the patient to meetings when off duty. Giving the patient money or other concrete assistance demeans them and robs them of the satisfaction gained by solving their own problems. It is unethical and unhealthy for a nurse to have a social relationship with the patient outside of treatment or in any way imply that this might be possible when treatment ends. This advice may seem self-evident, but substance abuse patients are often quite skilled at drawing others into their problems and creating enabling relationships however unconsciously. In the final analysis, the patient recovers through his or her own efforts. The nurse can best assist by maintaining a nonjudgmental attitude and showing respect for the patient and confidence in his or her ability to recover.

EVALUATION

- Evaluate the results of the nursing interventions.

It is easy to deem the interventions successful when patients acknowledge their disease, participate fully in treatment, and remain sober and drug free. However, the nurse who considers the interventions a failure if this does not occur is making a mistake. Recovery is a long process, and progress must be measured in degrees. Sometimes the most that can be ensured is a safe detoxification. A heroin addict may not give up drugs, but may stop sharing needles as a result of the teaching and thus be saved from contracting AIDS or hepatitis. If the patient refuses treatment but the nurse has assisted the spouse and children to enter a family self-help program, the intervention may relieve a tremendous amount of human distress. Not infrequently the alcoholic or addict recovers only after the rest of the family learns a healthier mode of interaction. Keep in mind that many recovering people report they acted on information about their problem and available treatment many months or even years after they received it. Sometimes they need to hear the same thing from many people before they can accept it. Your actions may give individuals hope that a better life is possible for them even if you never get the satisfaction of seeing them recover while they are your patients. Do not fall into the trap of thinking you know which patients will recover and which are hopeless cases. Professionals who work in the field are often dismayed when a person who they were sure would recover is readmitted in relapse, and they are often pleasantly surprised when a patient who appeared to reject all their help recovers very nicely. The nurse must offer the best care and advice possible to all substance abusing patients and have faith that some peoples' lives will be better for it.

IMPAIRED PRACTICE AMONG NURSES AND OTHER HEALTH PROFESSIONALS

Studies to determine the number of health professionals with substance disorders have been unable to provide reliable data. Even when studies are conducted by anonymous questionnaires, significant underreporting is found when concurrent urine toxicologies are obtained. Health professionals' vulnerability to substance disorders is increased by accessibility and attitude. It is estimated that nurses and physicians suffer a rate of narcotics addiction 30 to 100 times that of the general population. Doctors, nurses, dentists, and pharmacists routinely handle and administer psychoactive drugs and observe positive effects from them. The professional's knowledge of pharmacology often supports the illusion that he or she knows enough about drugs not to become addicted. Once caught in the cycle of dependence, the professional's guilt and shame inhibit him or her from seeking help. There is a tendency to attempt self-treatment long after it has been proven fruitless. This shame is also responsible for an unusually high likelihood of suicide among health professionals who develop substance disorders. These deaths are particularly poignant because health professionals who receive treatment for the disorder have extremely high rates of recovery. Consequently many professional organizations have implemented programs to assist peers who are experiencing problems and help them to accept treatment.

Impaired practice is defined as the inability to meet standards of practice because cognitive, interpersonal, and psychomotor skills are compromised by the use of drugs, alcohol, or by psychiatric illness. Impaired practice is most readily identified by changes in job performance and the deteriorating quality of the professional's work. Typical patterns include high absenteeism, many excuses for poor job performance, problems with documentation of narcotic administration, interpersonal problems with patients and co-workers, decreased productivity, and withdrawal from communities and professional activities.

The practitioner whose professional judgment is impaired by drugs or alcohol poses a threat to the patient, his or her own well-being, and professional standards. Impaired practice is in violation of the ethical Code for Nurses and places the nurse at risk for legal action, loss of license, and possible criminal conviction. It is important to recognize that the nurse who practices while impaired has lost control of drug or alcohol use and continues to use drugs compulsively with little rational consideration of the consequences.

Constructive intervention takes two primary forms: (1) supervisory intervention, including objective assessment of the quality of job performance and referral of the nurse to an employee assistance program and treatment; and (2) peer assistance intervention by trained volunteers who contact the nurse and attempt to motivate him or her to seek treatment. Employing institutions are encouraged to treat rather than fire impaired nurses and to develop policies that make available sick time, employee healthcare benefits, and, when necessary, disability insurance for the nurse. Recognition that addiction is a treatable disease is central to the management of impaired practice and the key to changing negative attitudes and providing opportunities for recovery and a return to practice.

Recovering nurses who return to practice may submit to a period of urine toxicology monitoring, a change of position to one in which narcotics are not handled, a stable shift assignment to facilitate continuing treatment, or self-help participation and follow-up by the employee assistance program or professional peer association. These are methods of assisting the nurse in early recovery to stay sober and assure the employing institution and the public that the nurse's practice is no longer impaired.

All nurses should be aware that it is the *self-administration* of mood-altering drugs that leads to dependence and that they should be very cautious about self-treatment of any problem. Nurses with a substance problem would do well to realize that they will be much better off seeking treatment *now* rather than waiting to be "caught" and suffering possible professional and legal catastrophe.

Federal law protects the confidentiality of all those who enter treatment for substance disorders. The treatment center is not allowed to inform your employer or anyone else about your disorder or treatment unless you give them written permission to do so.

The bibliography for this chapter can be found in Appendix B, which begins on page 1054.

CHAPTER REVIEW QUESTIONS*

1. Which statement is *not* correct regarding the definition of terms related to drug abuse?
   a. Dependency refers to a state in which the person needs a specific drug to maintain abilities to function.
   b. Drug abuse is the use of drugs that create legal, emotional, social, and health problems for the individual.
   c. Tolerance develops when a person requires the drug to experience positive feelings and a sense of self-esteem.
   d. Physical dependence develops when the person experiences physical withdrawal symptoms when the drug wears off.

2. Which statement is correct regarding etiologic factors of drug and alcohol dependency?
   a. Physical dependency always has a genetic etiology or causative factor.
   b. Current theories adequately explain the causes of drug and alcohol dependency.
   c. Drug and alcohol dependency can be viewed as involving a single factor.
   d. Scientific understanding of dependency is at an early point in development.

3. In the assessment of the patient who abuses drugs, the nurse should:
   a. Use the street names for drugs during the information-gathering phase.
   b. Begin the interview with discussion of sensitive information about drug use.
   c. Note only verbal responses to questions designed to elicit information on drug and alcohol usage.
   d. Use direct questioning to make the patient feel more comfortable.

4. All of the following statements are correct regarding the impaired nurse *except:*
   a. Nurses develop addictive illness at the same rate as people in the general population.

*See Appendix A, which begins on page 1051, for answers.

b. Recognition that addiction is treatable is central to the management of impaired practice.
c. The trend in employing institutions is to treat the impaired nurse before firing him or her.
d. Impaired practice is most rapidly identified by changes in job performance.

5. A therapeutic reaction of the nurse to the individual drug abuser includes all of the following *except:*
   a. Developing knowledge related to drug treatment.
   b. Shielding the patient from painful realizations.
   c. Including a drug history in comprehensive assessment.
   d. Making appropriate referrals for substance abuse.

6. When administering nicotine transdermal patches, patient teaching includes which of the following?
   a. Apply patch to any area of the body once every 3 days.
   b. Do not reuse skin site for 1 week.
   c. Therapy can be used for 9 to 10 months.
   d. Patches are worn for only 6 hours each day.

CHAPTER 68

Emergency Situations, Hypotension, and Shock

Merrily A. Kuhn, RNC, PhD

CHAPTER OUTLINE

KEY TERMS

Antigenicity	Dromotropic effect
Colloidal osmotic pressure	Plasma expanders
Colloids	Pulmonary artery pressure

LEARNING OBJECTIVES

After reading this chapter, the student will be able to:

1. Identify those medications commonly used in emergency situations, hypotension, and shock.
2. Identify specific areas of assessment in the patient requiring medications in emergency situations, hypotension, and shock to formulate appropriate patient outcomes.
3. Identify the sympathomimetics and colloids commonly administered in hypotension and shock.
4. Plan nursing interventions necessary to administer medications in emergency situations and choose appropriate teaching strategies to gain patient compliance.
5. Evaluate the patient at various stages of treatment to measure the effectiveness of nursing interventions.

The nurse working in an intensive care area, emergency room, or operating room is frequently confronted with emergency situations. However, the nurse working in hospital clinics, industrial locations, nursing homes, public health facilities, schools, or homes of clients can also be confronted with emergencies. Regardless of where it occurs, the nurse is expected to function calmly and efficiently in any emergency situation.

This chapter briefly summarizes the emergency situations previously discussed in this text in an easy-to-use table. Table 68–1 features the emergency condition along with its most common assessable findings and the drug of choice with its primary reason for administration. This table can serve as a fast reference source in an emergency situation. Most of these are potent, dangerous medications with many adverse effects, interactions, and contraindications. The nurse must know how these might act and interact within the body before administering them.

This chapter also discusses nursing considerations for administering drugs to acutely ill patients and includes altered drug pharmacokinetic behaviors in patients with various organ diseases and drug interactions that are likely to occur. This chapter also discusses the care of a patient who develops hypotension and shock and reviews colloid solutions and adrenergic drugs and their nursing implications.

CONSIDERATIONS FOR DRUG THERAPY IN THE ACUTE-CARE SETTING

Patients admitted to an intensive care unit (ICU) are often those who are the most likely to receive multiple-drug therapy or frequently changing drug orders, experience drug-drug interactions, display altered pharmacokinetic behavior, and incur drug-induced toxicity. In addition, these patients commonly have multiple disease processes and require supplemental intravenous or enteral nutritional support. The situation is often intimidating to many

Table 68–1. SUMMARY OF EMERGENCY SITUATIONS AND DRUG MANAGEMENT

Condition	Assessment Findings	Drug of Choice	Uses	Chapter
Acute adrenal insufficiency	Dehydration, hypotension, weakness, fever, lethargy, nausea, vomiting, abdominal pain. Check the following laboratory data: serum sodium, serum glucose, and serum potassium.	Hydrocortisone sodium phosphate (Hydrocortone Phosphate) or hydrocortisone sodium succinate (Solu-Cortef). Note: Fluid replacement is also critical and is usually carried out with isotonic sodium chloride or glucose in saline.	Replacement of glucocorticoids.	44
Acute pulmonary edema	Intense dyspnea, tachycardia, hypotension, crackles, intense anxiety, pink frothy sputum. Laboratory data: ECG changes, chest radiograph changes, acid-base changes.	Digoxin (Lanoxin)	Strengthen and slow cardiac rate.	29
		Aminophylline	Bronchial dilatation.	40
		Furosemide (Lasix)	Reduce fluid overload.	37
		Morphine sulfate	Reduce anxiety and tachypnea. Reduce preload.	18
Cardiac dysrhythmias	Irregular pulse with changes in blood pressure and neurologic status. Laboratory data: ECG changes.	Atropine	Sinus bradycardia, first-degree atrioventricular block.	16
		Lidocaine (Xylocaine)	Ventricular dysrhythmias; premature ventricular contractions (PVCs), ventricular tachycardia.	31
		Phenytoin (Dilantin)	Paroxysmal atrial tachycardia (PAT) especially due to digitalis toxicity, ventricular arrhythmias; PVCs, ventricular tachycardia.	31
		Procainamide (Pronestyl) Propranolol (Inderal)	Atrial dysrhythmias; premature atrial contractions (PACs), atrial fibrillation. PAT.	31
		Quinidine	Ventricular dysrhythmias; PVCs, ventricular tachycardia.	31
		Verapamil (Calan) Dilitiazem (Cardizem)	Supraventricular tachycardia, PAT, atrial flutter, atrial fibrillation.	31
Cardiac or respiratory arrest	Absence of pulse and respirations. No response to external stimuli. Brain death develops in 4 min if untreated.	Epinephrine (Adrenalin)	Initiate cardiac rhythm in standstill.	17
Cardiogenic shock	Hypotension, tachycardia, and tachypnea, increasing fatigue, increasing restlessness, lethargy, cool clammy skin.	Digitalis products	Improve cardiac performance.	29
		Vasopressors: Dopamine (Intropin)	Improve renal perfusion.	68
		Norepinephrine (Levophed)	Same as above.	68
		Inotropics: Dobutamine (Dobutrex)	Improves cardiac performance, improves cardiac output.	68
		Vasodilators: Isoproterenol (Isuprel)	Counteracts vasoconstriction, increases cardiac output, facilitates AV conduction.	68
		Nitroglycerin	Reduces preload, dilates venous capacitance vessels.	32
Cholinergic crisis	Diplopia, dysarthria, difficulty chewing, dyspnea, generalized weakness, restlessness, anxiety, irritability, salivation, anorexia, nausea, burping, vomiting, abdominal cramps, diarrhea, increased bronchial secretions, lacrimation, perspiration, blurred vision, miosis.	Atropine sulfate	Produces an anticholinergic response to modify cholinergic crises and improve condition.	16

Table 68–1. SUMMARY OF EMERGENCY SITUATIONS AND DRUG MANAGEMENT, *Continued*

Condition	Assessment Findings	Drug of Choice	Uses	
Diabetic ketoacidosis	Kussmaul respirations, flushed dry skin, acetone odor to breath, dehydration, hypotension, shock, coma, or stupor. Laboratory data: elevated blood sugar (over 300 mg/100 mL), acidosis, glycosuria.	Regular insulin	Lowers blood glucose level.	45
Hemorrhagic shock	Increased anxiety, lethargy, coma, hypotension, cool clammy skin, anorexia, increasing fatigue, tachypnea. Laboratory data: decreased hemoglobin and hematocrit.	Ringer's lactate	Replaces volume	11
		Whole blood and components	Replaces volume	34
		Dopamine (Intropin)	Elevates blood pressure (correct hypovolemia first).	68
		Norepinephrine (Levophed)		68
Hypertensive crisis	Sustained blood pressure over 120 diastolic, severe retinopathy, renal impairment, headache, hypertensive encephalopathy.	Diazoxide (Hyperstat IV)	Causes vasodilation of peripheral arterioles.	30
		Sodium nitroprusside (Nipride)	Potent-acting vasodilator	30
		Propranolol (Inderal)	Causes arteriolar vasodilation, thereby reducing vascular resistance.	30
		Furosemide (Lasix)	Reduce fluid volume.	17
		Calcium channel blockers	Reduce SVR.	32
Hypotensive crisis	Blood pressure less than 80 mm Hg systolic, cool clammy skin, tachycardia, tachypnea, lethargy.	Dopamine (Intropin)	Elevates blood pressure (correct hypovolemia first).	68
		Norepinephrine (Levophed)	Same as above.	68
		Dobutamine (Dobutrex)	Improves cardiac performance, improves cardiac output.	68
Insulin shock	Diaphoresis, weakness, nervousness, shakiness, irritability, impaired vision, headache, unconsciousness, convulsions. Laboratory data: blood glucose decreases below 50 mg/100 mL.	Glucagon	Elevates blood glucose level.	45
Myasthenic crisis	Ptosis, diplopia, dysarthria, dysphagia, difficulty chewing, dyspnea, generalized weakness, restlessness, anxiety, irritability.	Edrophonium chloride (Tensilon)	To distinguish between myasthenic and cholinergic crises.	23
		Pyridostigmine (Mestinon)	To improve myasthenic condition.	
Narcotic overdosage (including codeine, hydromorphone, morphine, and meperidine)	Respiratory depression, which may progress to apnea, coma, possible seizures, cardiac arrest, circulatory collapse, miosis with morphine derivatives, mydriasis with meperidine derivatives, cold clammy skin, hypothermia, muscular flaccidity.	Naloxone (Narcan)	Narcotic antagonist.	18
Overdosage of propoxyphene hydrochloride (Darvon)	Stupor, coma, convulsions, ECG abnormalities, circulatory collapse, miosis, diabetes insipidus, respiratory depression.	Naloxone (Narcan)	Antidote.	18
Status asthmaticus	Prolonged expiratory time, tachypnea, tachycardia, labored breathing, diaphoresis, wheezing (in severe cases, chest may be silent).	Epinephrine. If no response after second dose of epinephrine, then:	Bronchial dilation.	17
		Aminophylline		40

Table 68–1. SUMMARY OF EMERGENCY SITUATIONS AND DRUG MANAGEMENT, *Continued*

Condition	Assessment Findings	Drug of Choice	Uses	
Status epilepticus	Rapid recurrence of seizure activity, generally tonic-clonic in nature; respiratory depression, respiratory acidosis, hyperthermia, cardiac decompensation.	Diazepam (Valium) Phenytoin (Dilantin) Phenobarbital (Luminal)	Control seizure activity.	25 20 20
Thyrotoxic crisis or thyroid storm	Fever above 100°F, tachycardia, congestive heart failure, restlessness, diaphoresis, tremor, CNS dysfunction, somnolence, coma, psychosis, diarrhea, abdominal pain. Laboratory data: hyperglycemia; elevated T_3, T_4, and T_7 values.	Propranolol (Inderal)	Decreases manifestations of crisis; also blocks conversion of thyroxine to triiodothyroinine.	17
		Acetaminophen (avoid aspirin)	Antipyretic.	18
		Propylthiouracil	Blocks synthesis of thyroid hormone.	46
		Iodide (Lugol's solution; sodium iodide)	Inhibits release of thyroid hormone.	46
		Hydrocortisone sodium succinate (Solu-Cortef)	To prevent adrenal insufficiency.	44

health-care professionals; however, a sound understanding of pathophysiology and therapeutics often allows one to see past the intravenous lines and various life-support systems and provide appropriate drug therapy.

ALTERED DRUG PHARMACOKINETIC BEHAVIOR

When administering medications to the critically ill, the goal is to attain a therapeutic effect while minimizing toxicity. It is important for the nurse to have an understanding of normal pharmacokinetics so that he or she is able to identify differences in the critically ill.

Absorption

In the acute-care setting, the usual route of drug administration—oral ingestion—is inappropriate for various reasons. Patients who are comatose, experiencing gastrointestinal (GI) bleeding, or recovering from surgery may not be able to receive medicine orally. In addition, many new medications are not available as oral preparations and so require parenteral (IV or IM) administration.

The IV route creates four major concerns: storage, solution, compatibility, and delivery. The nurse must understand how the drug is diluted, used, and stored. For example, nitroprusside sodium spontaneously degrades in about 24 hours and may require special IV tubing. Amphotericin B easily precipitates in sodium chloride, so it is mixed only with dextrose.

Optimally, each drug is administered separately to avoid interactions and incompatibilities; however, this is rarely possible in critical care. Current drug compatibility charts should be readily available on each unit for reference.

The intravenous route is generally preferred in acute situations because the onset of action is more rapid—often within minutes. The nurse must be knowledgeable about the mixing and administration of these medica-

tions. For example, a bolus of digoxin (Lanoxin) or furosemide (Lasix) is given undiluted over at least 10 minutes; phenytoin (Dilantin) is given at 50 mg/min and no faster; and protamine sulfate is given over 10 to 15 minutes. Administering medications faster than recommended may increase the incidence of adverse effects, including hypotension and dysrhythmia.

Intramuscular or subcutaneous administration is not appropriate in patients who are hypotensive, such as those with septic shock or severe cardiac failure. When the blood pressure is lower than normal, blood is shunted away from the peripheral areas of the body. This usually leads to underperfusion of skeletal muscle and thus to erratic drug absorption.

When oral administration is possible, certain factors affecting absorption are considered. Patients with severe edema (heart failure, nephrotic syndrome, cirrhosis, hypoproteinemia) often have fluid accumulation within the intestinal mucosa, leading to decreased absorption. Also, many patients in the ICU receive continuous antacid administration to prevent stress-related ulceration of the GI tract. In this situation, the patient's drug therapy is reviewed to identify any medication in which absorption may be altered by concurrent antacid administration (e.g., oral digitalis drugs, tetracyclines, quinidine, and salicylates).

Distribution

The factors controlling drug distribution are complex and often altered in critically ill patients. Drug distribution to the tissues depends on protein binding. In certain disease states (cirrhosis, nephrotic syndrome, malnutrition, and others), the serum albumin concentration may be lower than normal and drugs may display altered distribution characteristics. Highly bound drugs like penicillins, cephalosporins, sulfonamides, anticoagulants, nonsteroidal anti-inflammatory drugs, and propranolol (to name just a few) are not bound; therefore, drug effect is increased.

The increased free drug is also available for elimination. Digoxin, although not highly bound, can have clinically relevant changes in drug distribution. In patients with end-stage renal disease, a reduced maintenance dose is required because the kidney has a decreased ability to eliminate digoxin, and the drug is distributed into a smaller volume. Patients with severe cirrhosis or porto-systemic shunts do not distribute drugs to the liver well. Because many drugs are metabolized in the liver, this decreased distribution and metabolism can lead to toxic effects.

Biotransformation (Metabolism)

The major site of drug metabolism is the liver. Patients with underlying hepatic disease may be admitted to the ICU for treatment of another medical problem requiring drug therapy with agents that are metabolized by the liver.

The liver has a variety of pathways by which it can metabolize drugs: the microsomal enzyme system; the cytochrome P-450 system; and others. The microsomal enzyme system can be induced with drugs like phenobarbital or phenytoin, or the microsomal enzyme system may be decreased by using cimetidine (Tagamet) for ulcers or chloramphenicol (Chloromycetin) for infection. Cimetidine and chloramphenicol have been reported to potentiate the effects of drugs such as warfarin (Coumadin), beta-blockers, lidocaine, phenytoin, theophylline, benzodiazepines, and narcotic analgesics. The cytochrome P-450 system regulates activity of steroid hormones, facilitates drug excretion, and detoxifies external poisons.

Half-life may also be affected in the critically ill. The most important use of half-life is to predict how long it takes a dosing regimen to achieve steady state concentration in the blood. When therapy is instituted, if a loading dose is not administered, then it will take four to five half-lives for the drug to reach steady state. Serum levels of drugs must be drawn appropriately to determine steady state. As an example, digoxin has a half-life of approximately 36 hours. Steady state is achieved in a patient with normal kidneys in about 1 week. If a serum level to determine steady state is drawn in 2 days, little insight into the patient's therapeutic drug level is obtained. Changing the dosage before the patient has reached steady state can prove confusing and be potentially hazardous for the patient.

In emergency situations, loading doses are usually administered intravenously. They should always be given over 3 to 5 minutes or longer (depending on the drug) to prevent unnecessary complications.

Excretion

Drugs are primarily excreted from the body via the kidneys. Many critically ill patients may either underperfuse their kidneys, have preexisting renal disease, or develop acute renal failure while in the hospital. Renal function markers (creatinine, creatinine clearance) are followed closely, and doses of drugs excreted by the kidneys are adjusted accordingly. Aminoglycosides are drugs excreted by the kidney and therefore may need their dose adjusted.

Aging also has an effect on renal function. The aging patient in a critical-care unit may also need dosage adjustments.

Most pharmacokinetic information is obtained from studies on healthy, young volunteers. This information can hardly apply to the elderly cachectic patient with myocardial infarction, heart failure, or renal failure. All pharmacokinetic phases need to be considered, but more important, so do the characteristics of the patient.

Finally, many medications administered to acutely ill patients may be nephrotoxic (e.g., aminoglycosides and amphotericin B). All drugs prescribed in this setting are reviewed for their potential to injure the kidneys. When nephrotoxic drugs are prescribed, they are carefully monitored and renal function indicators are followed closely.

PHARMACOKINETIC ALTERATIONS WITH DISEASE

Respiratory Disease

The diseased lung in critical-care patients may have an important effect on drug requirements through two mechanisms: (1) direct alteration of lung uptake, distribution, metabolism, or clearance of drugs; and (2) an indirect alteration of pharmacokinetics or drug-receptor response.

The patient with overt or impending pulmonary failure rarely has an isolated disease. There are often other associated organ dysfunctions or infections present. Important drug problems often relate to the secondary effect of hemodynamic changes or other organ alterations involved in drug metabolism. Several examples are cited, but for more detailed information see appropriate chapters in this text.

When beta-adrenergic agents, theophylline drugs, or vasodilators are administered, they may diminish hypoxic pulmonary vasoconstriction, particularly in patients with ventilation-perfusion defects. Consequently, the patient who receives nitroglycerin and other nitrates for the treatment of angina may become hypoxemic because of this or other effects on pulmonary function.

Parenteral nutrition is often used in patients with acute respiratory conditions to help maintain respiratory muscles and to decrease the possibility of sepsis. Overfeeding or feeding the patient formulas high in carbohydrates increases carbon dioxide production by elevating the respiratory quotient. This could contribute to respiratory acidosis. Nutritional therapy needs to be specifically tailored to meet the needs of the acutely ill respiratory and ventilated patient.

Respiratory patients often have fluid retention associated with other concurrent diseases. Diuretic therapy along with fluid restriction can precipitate hypokalemia, hypochloremia, or dehydration alkalosis. Progressive carbon dioxide retention and pulmonary decompensation may complicate the already marginal status of the acutely ill patient. Close monitoring of electrolyte and acid-base balance during diuresis prevents or controls this situation.

Heart Disease

Heart failure can lead to alterations in pharmacokinetics and pharmacodynamics. When it is necessary to administer drugs to a patient with heart failure, the IV route is preferable. Titratable drugs with short half-lives, which are rapidly metabolized and excreted, are drugs of choice. Monitoring kidney and liver function and acid-base balance is essential. Using drugs that have known blood levels and monitoring those levels can help prevent problems.

Liver Disease

The liver is the primary organ of metabolism and excretion for many drugs. When the patient has liver disease, the enzyme systems are less effective, blood flow is depressed, protein production is decreased, and many of the hemostatic and metabolic functions are compromised. All have a negative effect on drug utilization.

There are risks associated with all drugs, but there are three groups of drugs that should be used with extreme caution or better yet not at all in patients with liver disease. Group I drugs are those capable of causing hepatic damage even in a person with a healthy liver. Drugs in this group include acetaminophen, acetylsalicylic acid, chlorpromazine, erythromycine estolate, methotrexate, and methyldopa. Group II drugs are those that are capable of compromising liver function, such as anabolic steroids and contraceptive, prednisone, and tetracyclines. Group III drugs are those that may make the complications of liver disease worse, such as indomethacin, diuretics, meperidine, and other central nervous system (CNS) depressants.

Whenever drug therapy is required in patients with liver disease, it is preferable to use drugs whose disposition is least affected by liver dysfunction. Numerous references are available that review dosage adjustments for the patient with liver disease. These tables can easily be obtained from the pharmacy department.

Renal Disease

Patients with acute renal disease may experience acid-base imbalances, fluid derangements, and alterations in blood pressure, all of which can affect drug effectiveness and elimination. When administering drugs to patients with renal disease, either the dose should be reduced or the dosing interval prolonged to adjust for impaired elimination. Whenever possible, serum drug levels—peaks and troughs—are used to monitor drug therapy. Many commonly used drugs will have to have their dose adjusted, including penicillins, cephalosporins, aminoglycosides, many other antibiotics, sedatives and analgesics, cardiovascular and antihypertensive drugs, and diuretics.

Patients with acute renal failure may need to be dialyzed. For a drug to be dialyzable, it must be water soluble. Drugs that are generally removed by the kidneys are removed through dialysis, although at different rates of removal. Drugs removed through dialysis need to be "reloaded" following dialysis.

DRUG-DRUG INTERACTIONS

Patients in critical care are particularly susceptible to drug interactions. Patients frequently receive multiple drugs that have narrow therapeutic indices and/or are frequently implicated in drug interactions. To compound the potential problems, the patient's primary disease can have a great influence on drug disposition and response.

Patients in ICUs often require drug therapy to support the cardiovascular and pulmonary systems and to fight infection. In addition, certain patients may require anticoagulants, anticonvulsants, or some form of chemotherapy. These patients may also have multiple organ system failure or senescent organ dysfunction and require mechanical ventilation or other aggressive interventions. Critical-care patients are often so ill that adverse drug effects or interactions can easily be misinterpreted as manifestations of the patient's underlying condition, resulting in greater potential for drug toxicity and interactions. The risk increases when patients are unable to verbalize such effects owing to, for example, tracheal intubation and CNS dysfunction.

Drug-drug interactions can occur for various reasons. These include alteration in pharmacokinetics as with absorption, distribution (protein binding), metabolism, and elimination, or alteration in pharmacodynamics. Refer to Chapter 5 for more specific information.

With the increasing numbers of new drugs that are available and the use of multiple drugs in any given patient, the potential for drug interaction is limitless. The patient must be monitored closely and have drug dosages altered individually, considering age and disease states.

HYPOTENSION AND SHOCK

Patients on any unit of the hospital may experience a hypotensive and/or shock state. As hypotension and/or shock develop, the primary treatment is to restore intravascular volume, maintain blood pressure, and supply adequate oxygen to the tissues. Intravascular volume can be restored and maintained by using crystalloids (saline or dextrose solutions, discussed in Chapter 11) or colloids. The colloids in current use include albumin, dextran, and hetastarch.

▼ CLINICAL ALERT

Volume deficits develop when there is a loss of fluid volume, secondary to blood loss from hemorrhage, burns, surgery, sepsis, or other trauma. An individual can tolerate the gradual loss of up to approximately 25% (1.5 liters of total body blood volume of 5 to 6 liters) of total blood volume. However, if the loss is sudden, only approximately 10% loss is tolerated before symptoms develop. To support vital functions, blood volume must be replaced. This can be done with plasma expanders, blood, or artificial blood (see Chapter 34 for detailed information).

COLLOIDS

Colloids, or *plasma expanders,* are substances obtained from sources other than blood that have the ability to expand a depleted blood volume. Colloids are featured in Table 68–2. These substances are not artificial blood, but exert a *colloidal osmotic pressure* (oncotic pressure) similar to plasma proteins that balances the distribution of water between the intravascular and interstitial space. Thus, by increasing the pressure in the vascular bed, fluid is pulled from the interstitial compartment, and total blood volume is increased.

▼ CLINICAL ALERT

Colloids do not have oxygen-carrying capacity or contain plasma proteins or clotting factors. They are not meant to be a substitute for blood or plasma. Patients who have suffered a large blood loss still need the replacement of blood and blood components.

Colloids are readily available and inexpensive. They can be administered immediately, and the patient does

Table 68–2. COLLOIDS

DRUG NAME/ROUTE AND DOSAGE	PHARMOKINETICS/DYNAMICS	NURSING IMPLICATIONS
LOW-MOLECULAR-WEIGHT DEXTRAN		
dextran 40 (LMD 10%) (Rheomacrodex 40,000) (Gentran 40)		
Adults: 10% solution mixed with 5% dextrose (170 cal/L) or 0.9% sodium chloride 10 mL/kg rapidly, not to exceed 20 mL/kg in first 24 hr. Therapy should not continue for more than 5 days in shock state.	**Onset:** within min **Peak:** NA **Duration:** 4–6 hr **½L:** 2–6 hr **PB:** 4–6 hr **B:** urine **E:** urine	**ASSESSMENT:** Obtain baseline lab data (hemoglobin, hematocrit, serum osmolality) prior to infusion. Monitor these parameters throughout course of therapy. Monitor vital signs, urine output, specific gravity, and CVP (if available) hourly throughout infusion. Notify physician promptly if urine output decreases or CVP increases >15 cm H$_2$O. Always do type and cross-match before administration. Assess patient for signs of heart failure and for signs and symptoms of hypersensitivity. **INTERVENTION:** Initial 500 mL may be administered over 15–30 min. Distribute remainder of daily dose over 8–24 hr depending on use. Crystallization can occur at low temperatures. Submerge in warm water and dissolve all crystals before administration and then use an IV filter. Use only clear solutions. **Patient Teaching**—Instruct patient to report any discomfort or dyspnea promptly throughout course of therapy. **EVALUATION:** Signs of shock should decrease. Report severe nausea, vomiting, or urticaria to physician.
HIGH-MOLECULAR-WEIGHT DEXTRAN		
dextran 70 (Macrodex) **dextran 75** (Gentran 75)		
Adults: 6% solution mixed with 0.9% sodium chloride or 500 mL Dextrose 5% at 20–40 mL/min (usual dose). **Pediatric:** not to exceed 20 mL/kg.	**Onset:** 1 hr **Peak:** NA **Duration:** 12 hr **½L:** 12 hr **PB:** not protein bound **B:** degraded to glucose **E:** urine	Same as above plus: **ASSESSMENT:** Plasma protein levels, PT or INR, PTT when large volumes are administered. **INTERVENTION:** Monitor infusion site carefully. **EVALUATION:** For signs of pulmonary congestion and allergic reactions.
OTHER COLLOIDS		
hetastarch (Hespan)		
Adults: 500–1000 mL 6% solution in 0.9% sodium chloride not to exceed 1500 mL/day or 20 mg/kg.	**Onset:** immediate **Peak:** NA **Duration:** 24–36 hr **½L:** 17–48 days **PB:** not protein bound **B:** urine **E:** urine, liver	**ASSESSMENT:** Obtain PT or INR, PTT, clotting time, and hematocrit at baseline and then frequently. **INTERVENTION:** IV filter is not needed, but if one is used, use 5-micron filter. Do not use solution if it is cloudy, deep brown, or contains crystals. **EVALUATION:** Same as for dextran 40.

NA = not available; CVP = central venous pressure; INR = international ratio.

not have to wait for blood typing and matching. Specific uses of colloids are featured in Table 68–3. These products do not transmit hepatitis virus or human immunodeficiency virus (HIV), but they are capable of causing an anaphylactic reaction. Therefore, patients need to be monitored carefully.

Dextran and **hetastarch** *(Hespan)* are the two types of colloids available today (Table 68–2). Dextran, a polysaccharide, is prepared from sucrose and is available as either low- or high-molecular-weight. Hetastarch (Hespan) is a preparation made from cornstarch and sodium chloride.

Contraindications and Precautions

Colloids are contraindicated in patients with hypersensitivity. Colloids are not administered to patients with renal failure and severe heart failure because they increase the fluid volume, which will worsen these conditions. Colloids are administered cautiously during pregnancy (category unknown) and lactation.

Adverse Effects

Adverse effects of colloids are related to hypersensitivity (nausea, vomiting, hypotension, urticaria), hemodilation, and antiplatelet activity. Administration of large volumes of any of these products may alter coagulation and result in transient prolongation of prothrombin time (PT) or international ratio (INR), partial thromboplastin time (PTT), and bleeding and clotting times; decreased hematocrit; and may cause excessive dilation of plasma protein. Before administering any colloids, renal function is assessed. Fluid overload may occur from lack of elimination of the newly reabsorbed fluid.

Interactions

Colloids may interfere with blood typing and crossmatching; therefore, blood is drawn before colloid administration.

○ **Dextran 40,** or low-molecular-weight dextran (Gentran 40, Rheomacrodex LMD, Dextran 40), is a branched polysaccharide colloid with an average molecular weight of 40,000 daltons. It is shorter acting and more rapidly excreted than other dextrans. A 2.5% solution of dextran 40 is used as adjunctive therapy in shock as it enhances blood flow, particularly in the microcirculation, by increasing blood volume, venous return, and cardiac output; decreasing blood viscosity and peripheral vascular resistance; and reducing red blood cell (RBC) aggregation. It is sometimes used as a hemodiluent in the heart-lung machine because of its low viscosity and ability to keep blood cells from sludging in small blood vessels. Dextran 40 is also used to decrease the incidence of deep-vein thrombosis in patients recovering from orthopedic surgery as it minimizes sludging of blood in the microcirculation and decreases platelet aggregation. Seventy percent of dextran 40 is excreted within 24 hours.

Antigenicity (ability to produce an immune response to an antibody) of the dextrans is related to the degree of branching in the chemical formulation. Dextran 40 has minimal branching and consequently is relatively free of antigenic effects. However, hypersensitivity reaction can occur.

○ **Dextran 70 or 75,** or high-molecular-weight dextran (Gentran 75, Macrodex, Dextran 75), is a synthetic polysaccharide that approximates the colloid properties of albumin. Dextran 70 has a molecular weight of 70,000 daltons, whereas dextran 75 has a molecular weight of 75,000 daltons. Because of its high molecular weight, it does not leak out of blood vessels. Therefore, it has the ability to increase osmotic pressure and pull fluid back into the circulatory system for longer periods than does dextran 40. It can be used when a large volume of blood has been lost; however, because it does not have oxygen-carrying capacity, RBCs are also given as needed. Dextran 70 is primarily indicated for the management of impending shock due to trauma, surgery, hemorrhage, or burns. Fifty percent of dextran 70 or 75 is excreted within 24 hours. This expansion of plasma volume improves the hemodynamic status for 24 hours or longer.

Dextran 70 has more branching in its chemical structure, and there is a greater risk of anaphylactoid reactions. These reactions generally occur early in the infusion period in patients not previously exposed to IV dextran.

Table 68–3. SPECIFIC USES OF COLLOIDS

Uses	5% Albumin	25% Albumin	5% Plasma Protein Fraction	Dextran 40	Dextran 70	6% Hetastarch
Shock	x	x 1st	x	x	x	x
Burns	x 1st	x after 24 hr	x	—	x	x
Hypoproteinemia	x	x	x	—	—	—
Cardiopulmonary (CP) bypass	—	x	—	—	—	—
Acute liver failure	x	x	—	—	—	—
Acute nephrosis	—	x	—	—	—	—
Renal dialysis	—	x	—	—	—	—
Hyperbilirubinemia	—	x	—	—	—	—
Hemodiluent for CP bypass	—	—	—	x	—	—
Decrease incidence deep vein thrombosis	—	—	—	x	—	—

○ **Hetastarch** (Hespan) 6%, has a molecular weight of 450,000 daltons and colloidal properties similar to those of 5% human albumin. It can be used in the treatment of shock due to hemorrhage, burns, trauma, surgery, or sepsis. It can also be used to assist with the harvesting of granulocytes through the process of leukapheresis. Hetastarch is marketed as nonantigenic; however, the patient still needs to be assessed for allergic or sensitivity reactions.

The effects of hetastarch last approximately 24 to 36 hours. Forty percent of hetastarch is eliminated in 24 hours, 64% in 8 days, and 90% in 42 days. The elimination half-life is 17 days. The large molecules are removed and stored in the liver and spleen and are slowly degraded by amylase.

Other Colloids

○ **Dextran 1** (Promit), a monovalent hapten with a low molecular weight of 1000 daltons, is administered before Dextran 40, 70, or 75 to impede the occurrence of anaphylaxis. Dextran 1 binds with one of the available dextran-reacting antibodies and thus does not allow the other dextran to bind to these sites and elicit a reaction. After infusion of dextran 1, hypotension and bradycardia have been reported.

ADRENERGIC DRUGS

The adrenergic drugs, or sympathomimetics, increase blood pressure by causing vasoconstriction (increasing afterload) in the peripheral vessels; they are featured in Table 68–4. These drugs, also referred to as pressors, are given only after circulatory volume has been returned to normal or near normal.

The adrenergic drugs—**epinephrine, norepinephrine, isoproterenol (Isuprel), dopamine hydrochloride (Intropin),** and **dobutamine (Dobutrex)**—mimic the sympathetic nervous system and act in one of two ways. Epinephrine, norepinephrine, isoproterenol, and dopamine hydrochloride interact directly on the adrenergic alpha or beta receptors. Dobutamine (Dobutrex) acts by first releasing catecholamines from their storage sites, which in turn activates the alpha and beta sites.

Action Dopamine, norepinephrine, isoproterenol, and epinephrine have many physiologic responses, including a marked positive chronotropic effect to increase cardiac rate; a positive *dromotropic effect* (an effect related to conductivity of a nerve—a drug with a positive dromotropic effect on the heart increases cardiac condition) to increase conduction through the heart; a stimulatory effect on the Purkinje fibers and a decrease in ventricular refractory time, possibly resulting in ventricular dysrhythmias; and some drugs may elevate blood pressure due to increased peripheral resistance. Vasoconstriction in the peripheral vessels occurs, resulting in a rise in blood pressure and cold, clammy skin as the $alpha_1$ receptors are stimulated. The adrenergics increase forward flow back to the heart and decrease backward flow as in failure.

Adrenergic drugs can increase anxiety, increase alertness, and cause respiratory stimulation. The adrenergics also exert an effect on all nonvascular smooth muscle, in most cases leading to relaxation and less peristalsis in the GI tract. The urinary bladder relaxes, delaying the need to void. In the eye, the radial and sphincter muscles of the iris contract (dilating the pupil), giving the patient a wide-staring appearance.

Some adrenergenics, particularly isoproterenol (Isuprel) (discussed in detail in Chapter 39) and epinephrine, have a pronounced effect on the bronchial smooth muscle, which results in bronchodilation through $beta_2$ agonist stimulation. Epinephrine also constricts the bronchial vessels and inhibits bronchial secretions, which makes it effective in the management of bronchial asthma.

The adrenergenics inhibit or stimulate metabolic activity, such as insulin secretion, depending on the sympathetic nervous system receptors stimulated. However, in a stress situation, they are responsible for making more energy available to the body; so they stimulate glycogen release from the liver and skeletal muscles and fatty acid release as a result of lipolysis in the adipose tissue.

Contraindications and Precautions The adrenergic medications are contraindicated in patients with severe dysrhythmia and in those with organic brain disease as the vasoconstriction that occurs may worsen these conditions. Adrenergic drugs are administered cautiously to debilitated patients, patients with peripheral vascular disease, and those with previous hypertension, as all these conditions could be exacerbated. They are used during pregnancy only if the benefit justifies the risk to the fetus.

Adverse Effects The adverse effects of adrenergic drugs include increased anxiety and headache, dizziness, sweating, dysrhythmia, and anginal pain all related to the increased activity on alpha and beta receptors. Patients may also complain of nausea and vomiting. If any of these symptoms are severe, they are reported to the physician.

Interactions The adrenergic drugs can potentiate any positive inotropic agent (Digoxin, calcium) and enhance activity of all thyroid products. Adrenergic drugs antagonize the effects of all antihypertensives, including beta-blockers. Sodium bicarbonate neutralizes many adrenergics if injected into the same line.

○ **Epinephrine** (Adrenalin), a naturally occurring adrenergic, acts on both alpha and beta receptors and is a powerful alpha-receptor stimulator. It may be administered parenterally or as a nasal spray or ophthalmic solution. See other chapters in this text for more specific information.

○ **Norepinephrine** (Levophed) is the bitartrate salt of the body's catecholamine norepinephrine. It acts primarily on $alpha_1$, $alpha_2$, and $beta_1$ receptors to cause vasoconstriction and cardiac stimulation. The blood pressure is elevated because of norepinephrine's powerful constrictor action on both resistance and capacitance blood vessels. Because of its dual action to increase preload and afterload, norepinephrine increases arterial pressure more reliably than other available adrenergics. Because alpha-adrenergic receptors appear to be reduced in number in cerebral and coronary vessels, norepinephrine tends to increase blood flow to these areas.

Table 68–4. ADRENERGIC STIMULANTS

DRUG NAME/ROUTE AND DOSAGE	PHARMACOKINETICS/DYNAMICS	NURSING IMPLICATIONS

dopamine hydrochloride (Intropin)

common actions/uses: **AA BB CC DD EE FF GG HH II JJ KK LL**
inc inc 0 — inc dec dec — + — HF β_1, dopaminergic, α

0.5–2.0 μg/kg per min IV (renal use); 2–5 μg/kg per min may be increased to 10 μg/kg per min (blood pressure uses); increase q 10 min until desired effect.	**Onset:** 5 min **Duration:** 10 min **½L:** short, several min **PB:** UK **B:** liver, neuron **E:** urine	**ASSESSMENT:** Check vital signs closely. Assess for pregnancy (category C). **INTERVENTION:** Use microdrip tubing and infusion pumps. Maintain fluid volume. Mix 400 mg in 250 mL; concentration 1600 μg/mL. Administer through central line. Discard solutions that are discolored. Use only freshly prepared solution. Wean when discontinuing medication. **EVALUATION:** Monitor closely for infiltration. If it occurs, 5 to 10 mg of phentolamine (Regitine) should be administered to infusion site. Evaluate for headache, dysrhythmia, nausea and vomiting.

norepinephrine (Levophed)

common actions/uses: **AA BB CC DD EE FF GG HH II JJ KK LL**
inc inc inc D C dec inc — + — — α_1, α_2, β_1

Adults: Mix 2–4 mg in 500–1000 mL IV. *Initial dose*–8–12 μg/min. *Maintenance dose*–2–12 μg/min per patient response. **Children:** 2 μg/min IV or 2 μg/m² per min maintenance.	**Onset:** 1–2 min **Peak:** rapid **Duration:** 1–2 min after infusion stops **½L:** 2–2.5 min **B:** neuron **E:** urine	**ASSESSMENT:** Assess for extravasation. Monitor vital signs closely. Assess for pregnancy (category C). **INTERVENTION:** Dilute in dextrose solutions to protect from significant oxidation. During time when dosage is being increased or decreased, blood pressure is recorded at least every 2–3 min. Do not use if solution is brown. Slowly taper infusion when stopping. Maintain fluid volume. **EVALUATION:** Same as for dopamine. If infiltration occurs, stop infusion and immediately infiltrate area with phenotolamine hydrochloride (Regitine).

dobutamine hydrochloride (Dobutrex)

common actions/uses: **AA BB CC DD EE FF GG HH II JJ KK LL**
inc dec 0 — inc dec dec — — — * β_1, inc

Adults: 2.5–20 μg/kg per min IV. Increase 2.5 μg/kg per min q 10 min until desired effect. **Children:** Not recommended for use in children.	**Onset:** within 2 min **Peak:** 8–10 min **Duration:** 5–10 min **½L:** 2–3 min **PB:** UK **B:** liver **E:** urine	**ASSESSMENT:** Check vital signs closely. Assess ECG closely. Monitor ST segment. Assess for pregnancy (category UK). **INTERVENTION:** Use microdrip tubing and infusion pumps. 500 mg in 250 mL = concentration 2000 μg/mL. **ADMINISTRATION:** Maintain fluid volume. Discard solutions that are discolored. Use only freshly prepared solution. Wean when discontinuing medication. **EVALUATION:** If blood pressure and pulse exceed pre-established levels, notify physician.

AA = myocardium (heart rate); **BB** = total peripheral resistance; **CC** = blood pressure; **DD** = bronchi; **EE** = kidneys; **FF** = GI tract; **GG** = metabolic; **HH** = bronchoconstriction; **II** = hypertension; **JJ** = allergic states; **KK** = other; **LL** = receptor activated; inc = increased; dec = decreased; 0 = no effect; D = dilates; C = constricts; HF = heart failure; + = used, — = not used, * = cardiac arrest (MI and HF without profound failure).

▼ **CLINICAL ALERT**

Norepinephrine does, however, decrease blood flow to the skin, skeletal muscle, and kidney, and ischemia may result.

For this reason, norepinephrine is used only in those patients in whom an immediate increase in arterial pressure is required to maintain life or in whom an infusion of dopamine cannot maintain perfusion pressure. Recent research indicates the norepinephrine may help to reverse refractory septic shock and may improve renal function in these patients. Weaning patients off norepinephrine may be difficult because continued doses of norepinephrine block the synthesis of new norepinephrine in the sympathetic synapse, as shown in Figure 68–1; therefore, when the infusion is stopped, there is minimal norepinephrine in the body to effect changes in blood pressure. Norepinephrine causes less CNS stimulation and has less effect on metabolism than does epinephrine.

○ **Dopamine hydrochloride** (Intropin), considered to be a precursor to norepinephrine, is administered to patients with poor renal perfusion and lowered blood pressure related to shock or other diseases. Like norepinephrine, it increases blood pressure and pulse rate and acts as a vasopressor, increasing pulmonary artery obstructed pressure (PAOP), and cardiac output in larger doses. It also has a positive inotropic effect on the heart and therefore may increase myocardial ischemia. In low doses (0.5 to 2 μg/kg per minute), unlike norepinephrine, it increases mesenteric blood flow, which improves renal perfusion. In large doses (above 5 μg/kg per minute) mesenteric blood flow is reduced. Dopamine has several metabolic effects: It decreases aldosterone secretions; it inhibits thyroid-stimulation hormone and prolactin release; and it inhibits insulin secretion.

USES Dopamine is used to increase cardiac output without decreasing afterload and filling pressure. It has been used successfully for cardiocirculatory support in cases of heart failure (HF) with hypotension, or reduction in urinary flow, or both; for cardiogenic shock; and for other conditions that occur with critically ill patients. Dopamine is preferred in the patient who requires both a pressor effect and an increase in cardiac output, and who does not have marked tachycardia or ventricular irritability. Low-dose dopamine is especially beneficial when renal blood flow is impaired as in severe HF. Low doses are also used to achieve acute diuresis in patients in whom administration of diuretic agents is not desired or is ineffective. Dopamine is frequently used after coronary artery bypass grafting to support the circulation. Dopamine is the first-line adrenergic used clinically today.

CONTRAINDICATIONS AND PRECAUTIONS In addition to others, contraindications to the use of dopamine hydrochloride include pheochromocytoma because it may be worsened.

DOSAGE At lowest infusion rates of 0.5 to 2 μg/kg per minute, both DA-1 and DA-2 receptors are stimulated, which dilates mesenteric and renal beds. This rate of infusion is often used to initiate diuresis in the oliguric patient. Because the renal artery is dilated, there is increased renal blood flow, which improves urinary output, sodium excretion, and creatinine clearance. Blood pressure may decrease slightly. Higher infusion rates are generally used in the treatment of shock. When infusion rates are increased to 2 to 5 μg/kg per minute, beta$_1$ receptors are activated, which improves cardiac contractility and cardiac output. Myocardial oxygen consumption (MVO$_2$) is increased, but this does not provoke an ischemic risk. Dopamine may even increase blood flow to ischemic areas. Heart rate may increase, decrease, or remain unchanged. At infusion rates of 5 to 10 μg/kg per minute, contractility, cardiac output, and heart rate all improve. After about 10 minutes of this infusion rate, cardiac output may improve by 20% to 30%. At rates of above 10 μg/kg per minute, dopamine resembles norepinephrine and alpha activity begins, which increases the blood pressure. Weaning the patient from dopamine hydrochloride is often difficult. Several preliminary studies suggest that oral levodopa (250 to 2000 mg 4 times a day) used to treat Parkinson's disease, which is converted to dopamine, may be helpful during weaning.

○ **Dobutamine hydrochloride** (Dobutrex), a form of synthetic isoproterenol, has relatively cardioselective action on beta$_1$-adrenergic receptor sites and relatively weak action on beta$_2$ and alpha$_1$ receptors. Unlike dopamine, it does not cause the release of endogenous norepinephrine from adrenergic nerve fibers; therefore, dobutamine is relatively selective in its ability to increase myocardial contractile force. It increases the force of cardiac contraction and cardiac output by 30% to 70%, reduces the pulmonary artery occlusive pressure, increases coronary blood flow, increases stroke-work index, and improves ejection fraction, with few vascular or cardioacceleratory effects. Dobutamine increases the blood pressure but reduces systemic vascular resistance through vasodilation. Dobutamine pulls fluid back into the vascular bed, thus increasing cardiac output. Generally, in low doses, there is little increase in heart rate; but at higher doses, these changes may become significant. These ac-

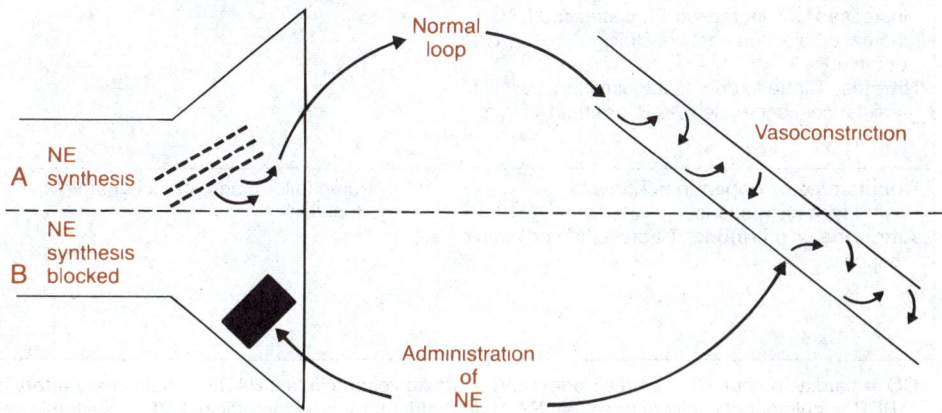

Figure 68–1. Administration of norepinephrine causes vasoconstriction in the peripheral system but also in a negative feedback loop, blocking the production of new norepinephrine in the sympathetic synapse.

tions make dobutamine hydrochloride a particularly good drug for patients with decreased blood pressure or shock resulting from depressed myocardial function. However, if vasoconstriction is required to increase blood pressure, dobutamine hydrochloride is not appropriate.

▼ **CLINICAL ALERT**

Dobutamine hydrochloride may cause cardiac ischemia, so it is important to frequently assess for ST depression. Dobutamine hydrochloride does not affect renal or mesenteric blood flow. Any effects that occur are most likely secondary to an increase in cardiac output.

USES Dobutamine hydrochloride is useful in the short-term management of patients with myocardial infarction, cardiovascular decompensation, cardiogenic shock, or acute HF, and for intermittent therapy for HF. Dobutamine infusions for only 4 hr/wk may produce a conditioning effect, which enhances exercise tolerance and increases functional classification. Another strategy is to use a 3-day infusion of dobutamine, which may improve beta-receptor activity as HF improves and downgrading (decreasing effectiveness) of beta receptors is avoided.

Research indicates that dobutamine may increase oxygen extraction by skeletal muscles and may, therefore, augment the aerobic enzyme activity of human skeletal muscles. For these reasons, dobutamine is being studied in critically ill, long-term, bedridden patients for its physical conditioning effect, thus decreasing the deconditioning effects of immobility and assisting in the rehabilitation of critical-care patients.

CONTRAINDICATIONS AND PRECAUTIONS In addition to others already listed, dobutamine hydrochloride is specifically contraindicated in persons with any obstruction to cardiac outflow, such as idiopathic hypertrophic subaortic stenosis (IHSS), because it may increase the likelihood of sudden ouflow obstruction.

DOSAGE Dobutamine hydrochloride is administered by intravenous infusion at a rate of 2.5 to 20 μg/kg per minute. Dosage is titrated by monitoring the effects on the pulmonary artery obstructive pressure rather than blood pressure. In low doses, dobutamine hydrochloride has primarily an $alpha_1$ effect, causing mild vasoconstriction. As the dosage reaches 15 μg/kg per minute, vasodilation effect occurs, which causes a reduction in afterload. In addition, infusion rates in excess of 15 μg/kg per min are likely to be accompanied by dysrhythmia because of the increased MVO_2. Dobutamine has a duration of action of 3 to 4 minutes after the infusion is terminated.

Table 68–5. COMBINATION DIRECT ADRENERGIC THERAPY AND OTHER DRUGS

Drug Combinations	Uses	Comments
Dobutamine: Titrate to hemodynamic response to increased CO, increased CI, decreased PAOP, increased ejection fraction. Dosage 5–15 μg/kg per min. **Dopamine:** Titrate not higher than required for renal dilation and increased renal output. Dosage: 0.5–5.0 μg/kg per min.	Pump failure, pulmonary congestion, poor hemodynamic function.	Superior to higher doses of either drug alone. Improves CO, CI, SVI, and mean arterial pressure and dilates renal arteries without increasing afterload.
Dopamine: Titrate to increase CO, increase CI, decrease HR. **Nitrates:** Titrate to decrease pulmonary vascular resistance, decrease PAOP less than 17 min Hg.	Congestive heart failure, hypotension, to increase peripheral vascular resistances, poor hemodynamic function	Improves CO while reducing afterload.
Dobutamine: Titrate to hemodynamic response to increased CO, increased CI, decreased PAOP, increased ejection fraction. Dosage: 5–15 μg/kg per min. **Nitroprusside:** Initially start at 16 μg/min.	Shock, congestive heart failure	Superior to either drug alone to increase CO and reduce PAOP.
Dobutamine: Titrate to hemodynamic response to increased CO, increased CI, decreased PAOP, increased ejection fraction. Dosage: 5–15 μg/kg per min. **Nitrates:** Titrate to decrease pulmonary vascular resistances, decrease PAOP less than 17 mm Hg.	Severe congestive heart failure	Improves CI while markedly decreasing left ventricular filling pressure and relieving congestion.
Dobutamine or dopamine: Titrate to hemodynamic response. **Amrinone or milrinone:** Titrate to hemodynamic response.	Pump failure, poor hemodynamic function	Improves CO and decreases PCP and RA pressure. Monitor platelets carefully with amrinone. Monitor for dysrhythmias. Decreased LV filling pressure and SVR may also decrease MVO_2.

CO = cardiac output; CI = cardiac index; SVI = stroke volume index; PAOP = pulmonary artery occlusive pressure; HR = heart rate; PCP = pulmonary capillary pressure; RA = right atrium; LV = left ventricle; SVR = systemic vascular resistance; MVO_2 = myocardial oxygen consumption.

Infusions of up to 72 hours have demonstrated no adverse effects. Infusions for more than 72 hours may be accompanied by the development of tolerance, which may possibly be due to down-regulation of beta-adrenoreceptors.

Combination of Agents

In seriously ill patients, it is often necessary to combine several adrenergics to produce a more beneficial effect. Combination is rarely started first; it usually evolves because of poor patient response to a single drug. Table 68–5 describes several drug combinations that produce a beneficial effect, that is, produce the least amount of vasoconstriction while maintaining an adequate perfusion pressure. The endpoints of therapy are reevaluated as clinical improvement occurs.

USING THE NURSING PROCESS

ASSESSMENT

- Obtain a brief but thorough physical assessment of the patient's symptoms—neurologic, cardiac, renal, respiratory, gastrointestinal, musculoskeletal, immunologic, and hematopoietic. The system with the most presenting symptoms receives the first and most thorough assessment.
- Assess for the objective signs and symptoms such as presence of extreme restlessness, orthopnea, or dyspnea; the nature of secretions—color, consistency, odor, and location; lung, cardiovascular, and GI sounds; level of anxiety; hemodynamic status; electrocardiogram results; urinary output; and muscle strength.
- Obtain laboratory data including electrocardiogram (if needed), blood and urine studies, radiographic studies, and drug levels if poisoning is suspected. Chapter 6 reviews commonly overdosed drugs and toxic agents along with their most common symptoms and management.
- Elicit subjective symptoms from the patient whenever possible, for example, pain, paresthesia, and numbness anywhere in the body; dizziness; headache; fatigue; dyspnea; change in appetite; urinary frequency; and diarrhea.

If a past medical history can be obtained for either the patient or the family, it is important to learn if the present occurrence is similar to any occurrence the patient has had before. For example, when a diabetic child presents in a semicomatose condition, the nurse questions the family about the patient's diabetic control. Is the child insulin dependent? Did he or she receive insulin this morning? Did the child eat adequate food to balance the insulin that was received? Did he or she have any GI symptoms? And, has this happened before? Often, by obtaining a thorough history of the present situation from the family or significant other, the nurse can determine the specific etiology of the situation.

- Determine if the patient has any allergies to drugs or food. Cross-sensitivity to medications is common. For example, a patient who is allergic to penicillin may also experience allergy to the cephalosporin group of antibiotics.
- Question the patient, family, or significant others about drug ingestion. Does the patient take medications on a daily basis? If so, what are they? Are they prescription, nonprescription, or drugs of abuse including street drugs such as heroin, cocaine, and marijuana, and legitimate drugs such as amphetamines and barbiturates? If the patient is suspected of having taken a drug overdose, it is important to determine the specific drug taken, as the treatment varies.
- Assessment of the patient requiring plasma expanders requires that laboratory tests be done before administration, such as hematocrit and hemoglobin levels and typing and cross-matching for blood or blood products. Plasma expanders lower hematocrit by increasing plasma volume. Other tests are performed based on the patient's diagnosis.
- Assess fluid needs carefully. The most important rule to follow in any patient is to restore vascular volume and RBC mass. Table 68–6 compares the colloid and crystalloid products.

The volume and rate of fluid administration is initially guided by arterial pressure, central venous pressure (CVP), heart rate, hematocrit, and cardiac output. The volume and rate of fluid replacement is limited by the patient's cardiac competency, especially in older patients with hypertension or ischemic heart disease. The major risk of volume expansion with any IV fluid is pulmonary edema. Therefore, a thorough and continuous respiratory assessment is performed.

When the primary circulatory problem is hypovolemia, therapy is directed toward restoration of blood volume. Because colloid solutions expand vascular volume with far less fluid infusion than crystalloid solution, hemodynamic resuscitation is likely to be accomplished more rapidly with colloids. Table 68–7 compares various IV products as to the amount of fluid returned to the vascular system. Crystalloids equilibrate across the vascular membrane such that only $\frac{1}{10}$ to $\frac{1}{4}$ of the solution remains in the plasma at the end of infusion. Crystalloids also dilute plasma proteins and consequently reduce colloidal osmotic pressure. Decreases in blood colloid osmotic pressure allows for filtration of fluid from the vascular space into the interstitial space, further potentiating the volume deficit. Also as colloidal osmotic pressure is reduced, the patient is at increased risk for developing pulmonary edema. When colloids are used, colloidal osmotic pressure is maintained, requiring less fluid for resuscitation. The possibility of pulmonary edema is also reduced.

Volume loading, in the form of fluid challenges, is often performed in acutely volume-depleted patients to compensate for sequestration or pooling of blood in the splanchnic organs and maldistribution of blood flow. As a fluid challenge is administered (50 to 200 mL of fluid over 10 minutes and repeated as necessary), the nurse carefully assesses CVP and pulmonary artery obstructive or wedge pressure (PAOP/PAWP). Disproportionate in-

Table 68–6. COMPARISON OF COLLOIDS AND CRYSTALLOIDS

Molecular Weight	Albumin 5%	Albumin 25%	Hetastarch 6%	Normal Saline	Dextran 40	Dextran 70
PV expansion (per 500 mL)	69,000	NA	69,000	—	30,000–40,000	70,000
Percent	100–150	200–300+	100–172	—	100–200	100–156
Volume	500–750	1700	500–850	100	500–1000	500–750
COP (mm Hg)	20	100	30	–30	60	45
Tonicity	Iso-oncotic	Markedly hyperoncotic	Hyperoncotic	Isotonic	Hyperoncotic	Hyperoncotic
Duration of expansion	<24 hr	<24 hr	<36 hr	Few hr	4–6 hr	12 hr
Half-life	21 days	21 days	<2 mo (17–48 days)	—	2–6 hr	12 hr
Cautions	Pulmonary edema, CHF, active bleeding, decreased platelets	See albumin 5%, give with diuretic	See albumin 5%, greater effect on coagulation	—	May cause obstructive renal failure as molecules get caught in nephron; may interfere with blood clotting	May cause obstructive renal failure as molecules get caught in nephron; may interfere with blood clotting
Allergy incidence	0.5%	0.5%	0.085%	—	>5%	>5%
Cost to the hospital per dose (approximately)	$16.40	$26.00	$52.00	$3.00	$16.50	$11.00

PV = plasma volume; COP = colloid oncotic pressure; NA = not available; CHF = congestive heart failure.

creases in CVP indicate right ventricle failure, whereas disproportionate increases in PAOP indicate left ventricle failure.

- Share with the patient and family the reason for the purpose of the therapy and help them recognize and allay their fears. IV therapy is a routine part of nursing. However, it may be a traumatic event for the patient and family. Often, to the patient and family, the administration of blood may erroneously indicate serious illness or impending death.

NURSING DIAGNOSIS

- Typical nursing diagnoses for the patient in an emergency situation include Altered Cardiac Output, Fluid Volume Deficit, Altered Nutrition, and Pain. Table 68–8 includes other suggested nursing diagnoses and goals for patient management in emergency situations.

INTERVENTION

- The patient in an emergency situation must be treated immediately, as speed may be the determining factor in averting death. Goals vary depending on the causative condition.
- Transport the patient as quickly as possible to an acute-care facility. Intravenous lines are secured, a urinary catheter inserted, and an airway maintained.
- Return intravascular volume to normal as quickly as possible. Fluids that are administered include crystalloids, colloids, or blood products.
- Monitor vital signs, cardiac respiratory, and renal function as fluid resuscitation is performed. Therapy is dictated by the results of the physical assessment and laboratory and radiography data. Therapy may include the administration of emergency medications to manage the situation.
- Administer emergency medications such as vaso-

Table 68–7. DISTRIBUTION OF COLLOIDS AND CRYSTALLOIDS

Fluid Compartment:	5% Glucose	Isotonic NaCl	Hypertonic NaCl	Iso oncotic (5%) Albumin	Hyperoncotic (25%) Albumin
Intravascular	↑ 10%	↑ 25%	↑ 25%	↑ 100%	↑ 200%–300%
Interstitial	↑ 90%	↑ 75%	↑ 75%	—	↓ Reduce fluid levels
Intracellular	↑ 90%	—	↓ Decrease cell edema	—	↓ Reduce fluid levels
To increase plasma volume by 1 liter, administer:	10 liters	4 liters	4 liters	1 liter	0.5 liters

Source: Adapted from Shoemaker, W, et al: Textbook of Critical Care Medicine. WB Saunders, Philadelphia, 1984.

Table 68–8. NURSING DIAGNOSES AND GOALS FOR PATIENT MANAGEMENT IN EMERGENCY SITUATIONS

Possible Nursing Diagnosis	Nursing Goal	Evaluation Criteria
Cardiac Output, altered, related to current disease process	Promote and maintain hemodynamic stability	Evidence of hemodynamic stability
Airway Clearance, ineffective, related to status asthmaticus	Maintenance and support of respiratory function	Evidence of respiratory stability
Coping, ineffective, individual, related to drug overdose	Maintenance and support of neurologic function	Evidence of neurologic stability
Fluid Volume Deficit (Regulatory Failure), risk for, related to insulin shock and possible increased risk of infection related to disease process	Return to and maintenance of electrolyte and acid-base balance	Evidence of electrolyte and acid-base balance stability
Fluid Volume Deficit, risk for, related to current gunshot wound	Maintenance of fluid balance	Evidence of fluid-balance stability
Nutrition altered, less than body requirements, related to massive injury	Provide nutritional support	Evidence of stable nutrition balance
Pain related to multiple fractures from automobile accident	Provide psychologic support of patient and family to reduce anxiety levels	Evidence of patient recovery and return to full function

pressors to maintain blood pressure, insulin to correct diabetic ketoacidosis, bronchodilators to reduce bronchospasms, corticosteroids to reverse symptoms in adrenal crisis, cholinergic drugs to counteract myasthenic crisis, and vasodilators to treat heart disease. The nurse is responsible for knowing the symptoms of these conditions as well as knowing about the drugs being used. The nurse probably is the individual who will be mixing and administering these emergency medications.

- Restore both cardiac and pulmonary function and maintain vital organ function. During an emergency situation, intravenous drugs are generally administered through a central line. However, if a central line is not in place, its placement may be time consuming and requires discontinuation of compressions and ventilations. To alleviate this problem, large catheters are generally inserted through the brachial vein. To enhance delivery to the central circulation, each peripheral venous injection is followed by a bolus of 50 mL of normal saline.

If a central line has not been inserted, certain drugs may be administered endotracheally. Drugs that can be used for endotracheal administration include lidocaine, epinephrine, atropine, naloxone, and diazepam. Time to attain a therapeutic blood concentration is 5 minutes for endotracheal lidocaine, 30 seconds for atropine, and 60 seconds for epinephrine.

Emergency medications are often administered by an IV infusion at a rate of a certain number of micrograms per minute. Many tables are available to assist with drug administration.

During administration, the contact time of drug solutions is minimized by using stopcocks, Y-connectors, or piggyback systems. Extension tubing is avoided. Regulation of IV infusions by drops is inaccurate as the drop size varies 50% with the solution constituents, orifice characteristics, flow rate, orifice angle, and duration of infusion. Rotary or piston pumps have a much more accurate range (±3% to 5%).

It is important to remember that there may be a delay in drug effect that is caused by slow filling of the void volume of IV catheters. Void volume of a 17 French pulmonary artery catheter to the distal lumen is 0.9 mL, a 33-inch extension tubing is 3.2 mL, and a 70-inch solution administration set is 8.9 mL.

- Assist with the placement and aftercare of hemodynamic monitor lines, such as pulmonary artery lines to measure *pulmonary artery pressure* (pressure as measured directly within the pulmonary artery that reflects the function of the right side of the heart) and cardiac output (CO); arterial lines to monitor blood pressure; and central venous lines to measure volume. Hemodynamic results are often used to determine proper dosing of vasopressor, vasodilating, or inotropic drugs.

Patients may also be placed and maintained on ventilators. The nurse inserts a Foley catheter to monitor urinary output, which, in turn, indirectly monitors cardiac output. Fluids are regulated to elicit adequate urinary output of at least 30 mL/hr as well as by blood pressure levels.

- Protect patients from developing stress ulcers and upper GI bleeds. H_2 inhibitors, antacids, and sucralfate (Carafate) are generally administered to critically ill patients to stop gastric acid secretion and to raise the gastric pH. By increasing the pH in the upper GI system, the environment becomes more favorable for the growth of gram-negative bacilli. This proliferation of these bacteria increases the incidence of gram-negative aspiration pneumonias.
- When administering colloids, check the bottle carefully. If crystals appear in the dextran bottle, they may be dissolved by placing the bottle in warm water for several minutes. The flow rate of the plasma expander is ordered by the physician. Monitor the patient throughout the infusion for signs of fluid overload and allergic reactions. Transient or prolonged

bleeding may also occur, because platelets are rendered less sticky and decrease their ability to function. Monitoring of CVP or PAOP is recommended during administration to monitor fluid levels. Any extreme hemodynamic changes may necessitate slowing or halting the infusion.

During an acute bleed, therapy is aimed at maintaining the following:

1. blood volume at 100% normal
2. hemoglobin at least 8 g/dL and hematocrit 24%
3. total serum protein at least 60% of normal
4. plasma coagulant factors above 35% of normal (except VIII—50% of normal)
5. platelets over 25% (50,000) of normal

The techniques for maintaining these criteria in an acute bleed are featured in Table 68–9. The nurse and physician work closely together in these cases to improve the patient's chance for survival.

- Check vital signs closely when administering any of the adrenergics. Hemodynamic measures, including CVP, PAOP, and CO, are monitored closely, particularly when vasopressors are administered. Table 68–10 reviews the expected hemodynamic changes that occur when vasopressors and adrenergics specifically designed to elevate blood pressure, such as norepinephrine and dopamine hydrochloride, are administered. When any vasopressor is administered, continually monitor blood volume and correct it by appropriate fluid and electrolyte replacement to maintain tissue perfusion and to avoid recurrences of hypotension when products are discontinued. The concentrations of the medications are prepared carefully using microdrip tubing and an infusion pump to control the drip rate. Also, the exact blood pressure ranges for each patient must be known. The medication is titrated to maintain the blood pressure within the given ranges. Continually monitor mentation, skin temperature, and color of the extremities to determine the effectiveness of the therapy.

When administering adrenergics, the infusion is begun at a low level and increased as necessary. Effects are seen within seconds. Infusions are tapered slowly to avoid sudden decreases in ventricular function. If marked increases in blood pressure, heart rate, or the appearance of dysrhythmia occur, the infusion is slowed. These effects are generally reversed promptly by reduction in dosage.

- Take care to prevent drug extravasation at the infusion site. If extravasation does occur, 5 to 10 mg of phentolamine in 10 to 15 mL normal saline is infil-

Table 68–9. ACUTE BLEED MANAGEMENT

Blood Loss	Fluids
20% or less (slowly)	Crystalloids (e.g., balanced solutions)
20–50%	Nonprotein plasma expanders, red cells
Over 50% (slowly) or over 20% (acutely)	Whole blood and fresh or frozen plasma
80% or more	As above. For every 5 units of blood give 1–2 units fresh frozen plasma, 1–2 units platelets to prevent hemodilution of clotting factors and bleeding

Table 68–10. VASOPRESSOR AGENTS—HEMODYNAMIC CHANGES

	Cardiac Output	PCOP	SVR	Mean Blood Pressure	Heart Rate	CVP	PVR
Norepinephrine (Levophed)	↑ slight	↑	↑	↑	↑ ↓	↑	↑
Phenylephrine (Neo-Synephrine)	↓	↑	↑	↑	↓	↑	↑
Epinephrine	↑	↑	↑	↑	↑	↑	↑
Dobutamine (Dobutrex)	↑	↓	↓	↑ with increased CO	↑ slight	↓	↓
Dopamine (Intropin)	↑	↑	↑ slight	↑	↑	↑	↔
<6 μg/kg per min	—	—	—	↑ ↓	—	—	↓
>6 μg/kg per min	↑	↑ ↑	↑ ↑	↑ ↑	↑	↑ ↑	↑
isoproterenol (Isuprel)	↑	↓	↓	↓	↑	↓	↓

↑ = increase; ↑ ↑ = greater increase; ↓ = decrease; ↔ = no change; PCOP = pulmonary capillary occlusive pressure; SVR = systemic vascular resistance; CVP = central venous pressure; PVR = pulmonary vascular resistance.

trated throughout the affected area as soon as possible to prevent tissue sloughing. If therapy is to be prolonged, it is advisable to change infusion sites at intervals to allow local vasoconstriction effects to subside. Monitor the patient's complaints of headache, vomiting, palpitation, dysrhythmia, chest pain, photophobia, and bradycardia because these may indicate overdose. A reflex bradycardia may occur as a result of a rise in blood pressure. When therapy is to be discontinued, the infusion rate is slowed gradually. Abrupt withdrawal should be avoided.

- Monitor for cold extremities. If the extremities become very cold, a 2-inch strip of nitroglycerin ointment is applied to the warmest areas of the chest or abdomen. This may be effective in increasing peripheral blood flow without affecting blood pressure.
- Fluid administration is continued until either the clinical and hemodynamic signs of hypovolemia are reversed or until the safe limit of volume expansion has been reached. Restoration of mental alertness, warm skin, urine flow greater than ½ mL/kg per hour, normal blood pressure, and hemodynamic stability are appropriate findings indicating effective volume expansion.
- Ensure that laboratory and radiographic studies are performed on time and results obtained. Patients may need large amounts of fluids, including blood or blood components, so typing and cross-matching of blood is performed.

- Emphasize health teaching to prevent further incidents.

EVALUATION

- Evaluate the nursing actions and the patient's response against the goals of nursing care. Possible evaluation criteria for the patient in an emergency situation are included in Table 68–8. Assuming that the patient recovers, actual recovery may take from 1 day to several years.
- Prevent further injury to the patient and prevent complications. Complications of immobility—thrombophlebitis, embolism, kidney stones, and muscle wasting—are examples of complications that need preventive measures.
- Evaluate the patient for the regular complications of IV therapy. The IV site and drip rate are evaluated hourly or more often, if necessary.
- Evaluate the effectiveness of treatment by a return to normal homeostatis. This is evaluated through qualitative, quantitative, and laboratory findings.
- Encourage patients to keep future appointments for follow-up visits to evaluate their progress. As the patient and family leave the acute-care situation, it is important to evaluate all previously taught material to ensure that the patient's and family's knowledge base still remains accurate.

The bibliography for this chapter can be found in Appendix B, which begins on page 1054.

CHAPTER REVIEW QUESTIONS*

1. Drugs that may be given endotracheally in an emergency situation include:
   a. Epinephrine.
   b. Bretylium.
   c. Sodium bicarbonate.
   d. Dopamine.

2. The following agent may be ordered for the patient in cardiogenic shock:
   a. Propranolol.
   b. Dobutamine.
   c. Atropine.
   d. Sodium bicarbonate.

3. The physician orders a renal dose dopamine infusion for the patient in cardiogenic shock. Which of the following ranges is appropriate?
   a. 15 to 20 μg/kg per minute.
   b. 0.5 to 2.0 μg/kg per minute.
   c. 2 to 5 μg/kg per minute.
   d. 10 to 15 μg/kg per minute.

4. An assessable clinical symptom to observe in the patient experiencing a fluid volume deficit is:
   a. Pulmonary hypertension.
   b. Increased urine output.

*See Appendix A, which begins on page 1051, for answers.

   c. Profuse sweating.
   d. Concentrated urine.

5. Which state is correct regarding drugs acting as adrenergic stimulants?
   a. Levarterenol bitartrate (Levophed) increases blood flow to the kidney and skeletal muscles.
   b. Isoproterenol hydrochloride (Isuprel) produces bronchial constriction and peripheral vasodilation.
   c. Dobutamine hydrochloride (Dobutrex) causes the release of endogenous norepinephrine from adrenergic fibers.
   d. Epinephrine (Adrenalin) causes vasodilation in the blood vessels of muscle fibers with mostly beta$_2$ receptors.

6. Which of the following statements is correct with regard to the pharmacokinetics of adrenergics?
   a. Most of these drugs are metabolized by cholinesterase in the liver and kidney.
   b. Catecholamines are concentrated only at selected tissue and organ sites.
   c. CNS effects of catecholamines are due to passage across the blood-brain barrier.
   d. Catecholamine drugs are inactivated through uptake at sympathetic nerve endings.

BUILDING YOUR CRITICAL THINKING SKILLS

HYPERTENSION, HYPOTENSION, AND DRUG TITRATION

A 47-year-old male with a long history of hypertension is brought to the emergency department with a blood pressure of 200/120 mmHg. He is admitted to the ICU and started on Nitroprusside (Nipride). The medical order is to titrate the blood pressure to 140/85. As the Nipride dose is increased, and the blood pressure brought under con-

trol, the nurse notes the client becomes increasingly restless and confused. His urine output has decreased to 15 ml in the last hour. His blood pressure is now 160/90.

1. What do the client's symptoms indicate?
2. How are these symptoms related to the client's current drug therapy?
3. What medical orders should the nurse anticipate?

APPENDIX A

Answers to Chapter Review Questions

CHAPTER 1
1. (b)
2. (b)
3. (d)
4. (c)

CHAPTER 2
1. (c)
2. (d)
3. (b)
4. (d)

CHAPTER 3
1. (c)
2. (b)
3. (a)
4. (b)
5. (a)

CHAPTER 4
1. (c)
2. (c)
3. (d)
4. (a)
5. (c)

CHAPTER 5
1. (d)
2. (c)
3. (b)
4. (b)
5. (a)
6. (b)

CHAPTER 6
1. (d)
2. (b)
3. (d)
4. (c)
5. (a)
6. (d)

CHAPTER 7
1. (c)
2. (d)
3. (a)
4. (b)
5. (a)
6. (c)

CHAPTER 8
1. (a)
2. (a)
3. (d)
4. (b)
5. (d)

CHAPTER 9
1. (c)
2. (b)
3. (d)
4. (b)

CHAPTER 10
1. (c)
2. (a)
3. (b)
4. (a)
5. (d)

CHAPTER 11
1. (a)
2. (b)
3. (d)
4. (a)
5. (c)
6. (d)

CHAPTER 12
1. (b)
2. (c)
3. (d)
4. (c)
5. (a)

CHAPTER 13
1. (c)
2. (b)
3. (b)
4. (b)
5. (a)
6. (a)

CHAPTER 14
1. (c)
2. (c)
3. (a)
4. (c)
5. (b)
6. (d)

CHAPTER 15
1. (d)
2. (a)

3. (b)
4. (a)

CHAPTER 16
1. (d)
2. (b)
3. (a)
4. (c)
5. (b)

CHAPTER 17
1. (c)
2. (d)
3. (b)
4. (d)
5. (b)

CHAPTER 18
1. (c)
2. (a)
3. (a)
4. (d)
5. (d)

CHAPTER 19
1. (d)
2. (d)
3. (a)
4. (a)
5. (c)

CHAPTER 20
1. (d)
2. (b)

3. (b)
4. (d)

CHAPTER 21

1. (b)
2. (c)
3. (c)
4. (c)
5. (a)
6. (d)
7. (b)
8. (a)

CHAPTER 22

1. (d)
2. (c)
3. (a)
4. (b)
5. (b)

CHAPTER 23

1. (b)
2. (a)
3. (d)
4. (d)
5. (a)

CHAPTER 24

1. (c)
2. (b)
3. (b)
4. (b)
5. (d)

CHAPTER 25

1. (a)
2. (c)
3. (d)
4. (d)
5. (b)

CHAPTER 26

1. (c)
2. (b)
3. (d)
4. (c)

5. (a)
6. (b)

CHAPTER 27

1. (a)
2. (b)
3. (b)
4. (a)
5. (d)
6. (c)

CHAPTER 27

1. (c)
2. (c)
3. (b)
4. (b)
5. (d)

CHAPTER 28

1. (d)
2. (b)
3. (a)
4. (d)
5. (a)
6. (d)

CHAPTER 29

1. (c)
2. (c)
3. (a)
4. (b)
5. (c)
6. (a)

CHAPTER 31

1. (c)
2. (b)
3. (a)
4. (c)
5. (c)
6. (a)

CHAPTER 32

1. (b)
2. (d)

3. (d)
4. (d)
5. (a)

CHAPTER 33

1. (c)
2. (a)
3. (c)
4. (d)
5. (b)

CHAPTER 34

1. (a)
2. (d)
3. (d)
4. (a)
5. (b)

CHAPTER 35

1. (d)
2. (c)
3. (d)
4. (b)
5. (d)
6. (d)

CHAPTER 36

1. (a)
2. (d)
3. (b)
4. (b)

CHAPTER 37

1. (d)
2. (c)
3. (a)
4. (d)
5. (b)

CHAPTER 38

1. (b)
2. (a)
3. (c)
4. (c)
5. (a)

CHAPTER 39

1. (d)
2. (b)
3. (a)
4. (a)
5. (a)

CHAPTER 40

1. (b)
2. (c)
3. (c)
4. (d)
5. (c)
6. (b)
7. (c)

CHAPTER 41

1. (a)
2. (c)
3. (b)
4. (b)

CHAPTER 42

1. (c)
2. (c)
3. (d)
4. (a)
5. (d)

CHAPTER 43

1. (c)
2. (d)
3. (c)
4. (d)
5. (c)

CHAPTER 44

1. (a)
2. (d)
3. (b)
4. (a)
5. (c)

CHAPTER 45

1. (a)
2. (b)

3. (a)
4. (d)
5. (a)

CHAPTER 46

1. (b)
2. (c)
3. (c)
4. (c)
5. (a)
6. (c)

CHAPTER 47

1. (c)
2. (a)
3. (d)
4. (b)
5. (a)
6. (a)

CHAPTER 48

1. (c)
2. (a)
3. (c)
4. (a)
5. (a)

CHAPTER 49

1. (a)
2. (c)
3. (b)
4. (c)
5. (a)

CHAPTER 50

1. (d)
2. (b)
3. (b)
4. (c)
5. (b)
6. (c)
7. (a)

CHAPTER 51

1. (b)
2. (a)
3. (c)
4. (b)
5. (a)

CHAPTER 52

1. (c)
2. (a)
3. (d)
4. (d)
5. (b)
6. (b)

CHAPTER 53

1. (d)
2. (a)
3. (c)
4. (c)

CHAPTER 54

1. (b)
2. (d)
3. (c)
4. (d)

CHAPTER 55

1. (a)
2. (c)
3. (d)
4. (b)
5. (d)

CHAPTER 56

1. (c)
2. (a)
3. (c)
4. (d)
5. (b)

CHAPTER 57

1. (a)
2. (a)
3. (c)
4. (d)
5. (a)
6. (c)

CHAPTER 58

1. (d)
2. (b)
3. (c)
4. (a)
5. (d)
6. (a)

CHAPTER 59

1. (b)
2. (a)
3. (c)
4. (c)
5. (d)
6. (c)

CHAPTER 60

1. (b)
2. (c)
3. (b)
4. (d)
5. (c)

CHAPTER 61

1. (d)
2. (c)
3. (a)
4. (c)
5. (b)

CHAPTER 62

1. (c)
2. (a)
3. (d)
4. (b)

CHAPTER 63

1. (b)
2. (a)
3. (d)
4. (c)
5. (b)
6. (b)

CHAPTER 64

1. (d)
2. (c)
3. (d)
4. (b)
5. (c)

CHAPTER 65

1. (c)
2. (c)
3. (b)
4. (c)
5. (a)

CHAPTER 66

1. (b)
2. (b)
3. (b)
4. (c)

CHAPTER 67

1. (c)
2. (d)
3. (a)
4. (a)
5. (b)
6. (b)

CHAPTER 68

1. (a)
2. (b)
3. (b)
4. (d)
5. (d)
6. (d)

APPENDIX B

Bibliography

CHAPTER 1

American Nurses Association: Guideline for Implementing the Code for Nurses. The Association, Kansas City, MO, 1990.

Doenges, ME, and Moorhouse, MF: Nurse's Pocket Guide: Nursing Diagnoses with Interventions, ed 4. FA Davis, Philadelphia, 1993.

Doenges, ME, et al: Nursing Care Plans: Nursing Diagnoses in Planning Patient Care, ed 3. FA Davis, Philadelphia, 1993.

Kozier, B, et al: Concepts and Issues in Nursing Practice. Addision-Wesley Nursing, Menlo Park, CA, 1992.

Sparks, S, and Taylor, C: Nursing Diagnosis Reference Manual, ed 2. Springhouse Corporation, Springhouse, PA, 1995.

CHAPTER 2

American Nurses Association: Guideline for Implementing the Code for Nurses. The Association, Kansas City, MO, 1990.

Carpenito, LJ: Nursing Diagnosis—Application to Clinical Practice, ed 4. JB Lippincott, Philadelphia, 1992.

Doenges, ME, and Moorhouse, MF: Application of the Nursing Process and Nursing Diagnosis: An Interactive Text for Diagnostic Reasoning, ed 2. FA Davis, Philadelphia, 1995.

Olin, BR: Facts & Comparisons. JB Lippincott, Philadelphia, 1996.

Schank, MJ: Wanted: Nurses with critical thinking skills. The Journal of Continuing Education in Nursing 21(2):87, 1990.

CHAPTER 3

American Nurses Association: Code for Nurses. The Association, Kansas City, M.O., 1985.

Carpenito, LJ: Nursing Diagnosis: Application to Clinical Practice, ed 4. JB Lippincott, Philadelphia, 1992.

Olin, BR: Facts & Comparisons. JB Lippincott, Philadelphia, 1996.

CHAPTER 4

Gillman, AG, Goodman, L, and Gilman, A (eds): Goodman and Gilman's The Pharmacological Basis of Therapeutics, ed 9. Macmillan, New York, 1995.

Staff College, Center for Drug Evaluation and Research: MedWatch Continuing Education: Drug Induced Disease. Food and Drug Administration, Washington, D.C., June 1995.

Reinberg, AC: Concepts of circadian chronopharmacology. Ann NY Acad Sci 10:102–115, 1991.

CHAPTER 5

American Society of Hospital Pharmacists: Medication Teaching Manual. American Society of Hospital Pharmacists, Washington, D.C., 1996.

Cerrato, PL: Vitamins and minerals. RN 56(6):28–32, 1993.

Gilman, AG, Goodman, LS, and Gilman, A: Goodman and Gilman's The Pharmacological Basis of Therapeutics, ed 9. Macmillan, New York, 1995.

Hansten, PD: Drug Interactions: Decision Support Tables. In Applied Therapeutics: Clinical Use of Drugs. Applied Therapeutics for Clinical Pharmacist Service, St Louis, 1994.

Kuhn, M: Drug interactions and their nursing implications. Journal of the New York Nurses Association 24(2):10–16, 1993.

Miayagawa, CI: Drug-nutrient interactions in critically ill patients. Crit Care Nurs 93(10):69–90, 1993.

Rizack, M: The Medical Letter Handbook of Adverse Drug Interactions. The Medical Letter, New Rochelle, N.Y., 1995.

Wells, P, et al: Interactions of warfarin with drugs and food. Ann Intern Med 121:676–683, Nov. 1, 1994.

CHAPTER 6

Ekins, B: The treatment of poisoning. Facts and Comparison Newsletter 14(3):17–18, 1995.

Gillman, AG, Goodman, LS, and Gilman, A (eds): Goodman and Gilman's The Pharmacological Basis of Therapeutics, ed 9. Macmillan, New York, 1995.

Kuhn, M: Anaphylaxis vs anaphylactoid reactions: Nursing interventions. Crit Care Nurs 10(50):121–137, 1990.

CHAPTER 7

Chameides, L, and Hazinski, MF (eds): Textbook of Pediatric Advance Life Support. American Heart Association, Dallas, 1994.

Cornwell, C: The Ommaya reservoir: Implications for pediatric oncology. J Pediatr Nurs 16(3):249–251, 1990.

Goodarzi, M, et al: Epidural versus patient-controlled analgesia with morphine for postoperative pain after orthopedic procedures in children. Pediatr Orthop 13:663–667, 1993.

Hazinski, MF: Nursing Care and the Critically Ill Child, ed 2. CV Mosby, St Louis, 1992.

Wong, D: Whaley and Wong's Nursing Care of Infants and Children, ed 5. Mosby Yearbook, St Louis, 1995.

CHAPTER 8

Age discrimination: Patient choice or physician bias? Clinical Oncology Alert 10(2):9–10, 1995.

Department of Health and Human Services, Office of the Inspector General: Medication Regimens: Causes of Non-compliance. DHHS, Washington D.C., June 1990.

Lee, M: Drugs and the elderly do you know the risks? AJN 96(7):25–32, 1996.

Merkatz, R, and Couig, MP: Patient education: Helping America take its medicine. AJN 92(6):56–62, 1992.

Drugwatch: Unraveling drug problems in the elderly. AJN 95(4):53, 1995.

CHAPTER 9

Andrews, M, and Boyle, J: Transcultural Concepts in Nursing Care, ed 2. JB Lippincott, Philadelphia, 1995.

Antai-Otong, D: Psychiatric Nursing: Biological and Behavioral Concepts. WB Saunders, Philadelphia, 1995.

Avery, C: Native American medicine: Traditional healing. JAMA 265(17), 1994.

Giger, JN, and Davidhizar, RE: Transcultural Nursing: Assessment and Intervention. Mosby-Year Book, St Louis, 1991.

Harwood, MA: The hot-cold theory of disease: Implication for treatment of Puerto Rican patients. JAMA 216(7):1155, 1991.

Hautman, MA: Folk health and illness beliefs. The Nurse Practitioner 4(4):27, 1979.

Kudzma, E: Drug response: All bodies are not created equal. AJN (12), 1992.

Leininger, MM: Transcultural Nursing: Concepts, Theories, and Practices. John Wiley and Sons, New York, 1978.

Moser, M: Relative efficacy of, and some adverse reactions to different antihypertensive regimes. American Journal of Cardiology 63(4):654–660, 1989.

Spector, R: Cultural Diversity in Health and Illness, ed 3. Appleton & Lange, Norwalk, Conn., 1991.

Wilson, H, and Kneisel, C: Psychiatric Nursing. Addison-Wesley, Reading, Mass., 1993.

CHAPTER 10

American Hospital Formulary Services: Drug Information 95. American Society of Hospital Pharmacists, Bethesda, Md, 1995.

Fishback, F: A Manual of Laboratory Diagnostic Tests, ed 5. JB Lippincott, St Louis, 1996.

Olin, B (ed): Facts & Comparisons. JB Lippincott, St Louis, 1997.

CHAPTER 11

Gilman, AG, et al (eds): Goodman and Gilman's The Pharmacological Basis of Therapeutics, ed 9. Macmillan, New York, 1996.

Olin, B (ed): Facts & Comparisons. JB Lippincott, St Louis, 1997.

CHAPTER 12

Gilman, AG, et al (eds): Goodman and Gilman's The Pharmacological Basis of Therapeutics, ed 9. Macmillan, New York, 1996.

McLean, R: Magnesium and it's therapeutic uses: A review. Am J of Med 96(2):363–375, 1994.

Olin, B (ed): Facts & Comparisons, JB Lippincott, St Louis, 1997.

Owens, MW, and Daniel, JL: IV magnesium sulfate in the treatment of ventricular tachycardia and acute myocardial infarction. Crit Care Nurs 13(12):83–86, 1993.

CHAPTER 13

American Pharmaceutical Association: Handbook of Nonprescription Drugs, ed 10. The Association, Washington, D.C., 1995.

Long, P: Vitamin E: Here's all you need to know. Health 14(9):94–97, 1996.

Olin, B (ed): Facts & Comparisons, JB Lippincott, St Louis, 1997.

Perez, A: Restoring electrolyte balance: Hypokalemia. RN 95(12):33–35, 1995.

Perez, A: Electrolytes. Restoring the balance: Hyperkalemia. RN 95(11):33–36, 1995.

Terry, K: Vitamin checkup. Health Jan/Feb:81–84, 1996.

CHAPTER 14

Estoup, M: Approaches and limitations of medication delivery in patients with enteral feeding tubes. Crit Care Nurs 94(2):68–80, 1994.

Gianino, S, et al: The ABCs of TPN. RN 96(2):42–47, 1996.

Miller, D, and Miller, HW: Giving meds through the tube. RN 95(1):44–47, 1995.

Miyagawa, CI: Drug-nutrient interactions in critically ill patients. Crit Care Nurs 93(10):69–90, 1993.

Olin, B (ed): Facts & Comparisons. JB Lippincott, St Louis, 1997.

Phillips, MC, and Olson, LR: The immunologic role of the gastrointestinal tract. Crit Care Nurs Clin North Am 5(1):107–120, 1993.

CHAPTER 15

Gilman, AG, et al (eds): Goodman and Gilman's The Pharmacologic Basis of Therapeutics, ed 8. Macmillan, New York, 1994.

Guyton, AC: Textbook of Medical Physiology, ed 6. WB Saunders, Philadelphia, 1996.

Price, SA, and Wilson, LM: Pathophysiology: Clinical Concepts of Disease Processes, ed 4. McGraw-Hill, New York, 1993.

CHAPTER 16

American Hospital Formulary Service: Drug Information. American Society of Hospital Pharmacists, Bethesda, Md, 1996.

Kastrup, EK (ed): Drug Facts and Comparisons, JB Lippincott, St Louis, 1997.

USP Dispensing Information: Drug Information for the Health Care Provider, United States Pharmacopeial Convention, Rockville, Md, 1996.

CHAPTER 17

AMA Drug Evaluations, ed 7. PSG Publishing, Littleton, Mass, 1994.

Dunnington, CS: Sotalol hydrochloride (Betapace): A new antiarrhythmic drug. Am J Crit Care 2(5):397–406, 1993.

Fitzgerald, JD, and Singh, B: Cardiovascular Pharmacology and Therapeutics, Churchill Livingstone, New York, 1994.

Gilman, AG, et al (eds): Goodman and Gilman's The Pharmacological Basis of Therapeutics, ed 8. Macmillan, New York, 1994.

Moser, DK: Pharmacologic management of heart failure: Neurohormonal agents. Crit Care Nurs Clin North Am 5(4):599–606, 1993.

Olin, B (ed): Facts and Comparisons, JB Lippincott, St Louis, 1997.

Paul, SC: New pharmacologic agents for emergency management of supraventricular tachydysrhythmias. Crit Care Nurs Q 16(2):35–45, 1993.

Solomon, J: Hypertension: New drug therapies. RN Magazine 94(1):26–32, 1994.

CHAPTER 18

American Pain Society: Principles of Analgesic Use in the Treatment of Acute Pain and Cancer Pain, ed 3. The Society, Skokie, Ill, 1992.

Beard, J: IM injections aren't the best. Am J Nurs 94(8):22, 1994.

Drugs for migraine. Med Lett 37(943):17–20, 1995.

Duggleby, W, and Lander, J: Cognitive status and postoperative pain: Older adults. Pain Symptom Manage 9(1):19–27, 1994.

Gibbons, K, et al: Lumbar discectomy: Use of an epidural morphine sponge for postoperative pain control. Department of Neurosurgery, School of Medicine and Biomedical Sciences, State University of New York at Buffalo, Buffalo. Unpublished paper, 1994.

Jacox, A, et al: Facts about pain control. Am J Nurs, May 1992:53.

Maxam-Moore, VA, et al: Analgesics for cardiac surgery patients in critical care: Describing current practices. Am J Crit Care 3(1):31–39, 1994.

Pasero, C, and McCaffery, M: Avoiding opioid-induced respiratory depression. Am J Nurs 94(4):28–31, 1994.

Vallerand, A: Gender differences in pain. Image 27(3):7–10, 1995.

CHAPTER 19

American Hospital Formulary Service: Drug Information. American Society of Hospital Pharmacists, Bethesda, Md, 1994.

Goodman, LS, et al: Goodman and Gilman's The Pharmacological Basis of Therapeutics, ed 8. Macmillan, New York, 1994.

CHAPTER 20

Olin, B (ed): Facts and Comparisons, JB Lippincott, St Louis, 1997.

Hopkins, S: Epilepsy: Advantages in anticonvulsant drugs. Nursing Standard 8(15):24–25, 1995.

Kelly, M: Status epilepticus. Am J Nurs 95(8):50, 1995.

Med Lett Drug Ther: Drugs for epilepsy. 37(947):37–40, April 1995.

Reinisch, JM, et al: In utero exposure to phenobarbital and intelligence deficits in adult men. JAMA 274(19):1518–1525, 1995.

Steiner, JF: Pharmacologic treatment of epilepsy. J Am Acad Physician Assistants 7(7):508–515, 1994.

CHAPTER 21

Gilman, AG, et al: Goodman and Gilman's The Pharmacological Basis of Therapeutics, ed 8. Macmillan, New York, 1994.

Healy, TEJ, and Cohen, PJ: A Practice of Anesthesia, ed 6. Edward Arnold, London. Distributed in America by Little, Brown, Boston, 1995.

Watson, DS, and James, DS: Intravenous conscious sedation, AORN J, 51(6):1512–1522, June 1990.

CHAPTER 22

Gilman, AG, et al (eds): Goodman and Gilman's The Pharmacological Basis of Therapeutics, ed 9. Macmillan, New York, 1996.

Jarpe, MB: Nursing care of patients receiving long-term infusion of neuromuscular blocking agents. Crit Care Nurs 12(10):58–61, 1992.

Rocuronium: A new neuromuscular blocker. Med Lett Drugs Ther 36(928)71–72, Aug 1994.

Olin, B (ed): Facts & Comparisons. JB Lippincott, St Louis, 1996.

Schell, HM: Neuromuscular blockage in the ICU: Looking for answers. AJN 94(11):36–41, 1994.

Snider, BS: Use of muscle relaxants in the ICU: Nursing implications. Crit Care Nurs 13(12):55–60, 1993.

Somerson, SJ, et al: Insights into conscious sedation. Am J Nurs 95(6):26–32, 1995.

CHAPTER 23

Anonymous. Tacrine (Cognex). RN 56(12):49–50, Dec 1993.

Olin, B (ed): Facts & Comparisons. JB Lippincott, St Louis, 1996.

Goodman, LS, and Gilman, AG: The Pharmaceutical Basis of Therapeutics, ed 8. New York, Macmillan, 1995.

Keltner, NL. Tacrine: A pharmacological approach to Alzheimer's disease. J Psychosoc Nur Ment Health Serv 32(3):37–39, 1994.

Surgical treatment of Parkinson's disease. Med Lett Drugs Ther 35(909):103–106, 1993.

Interferon beta-1B for multiple sclerosis. Med Lett Drugs Ther 35(900):61–64, 1993.

Dietary help for people with Parkinson's disease. Tufts Univ Diet Nutr Lett 12(10):7–8, 1994.

CHAPTER 24

Gilman, S, and Newman, SW: Essentials of Clinical Neuroanatomy and Neurophysiology. FA Davis, Philadelphia, 1992.

Hardman, JG, et al: Goodman and Gilman's The Pharmacological Basis of Therapeutics, ed 9. McGraw-Hill, New York, 1996.

Scanlon, VC, and Sanders, T: Essentials of Anatomy and Physiology, ed 2. FA Davis, Philadelphia, 1995.

Walker, E, and Neumann, C: Neurodevelopmental origins of schizophrenia. NARSAD Research Newsletter, 14–16, Spring 1994.

CHAPTER 25

Alprazolam for panic disorder. Med Lett 33:30, 1991.

Baldessarini, RJ: Drugs and the treatment of psychiatric disorders. In Gilman, AG, et al (eds): The Pharmacological Basis of Therapeutics, Pergamon, New York, 1990.

Ballinger, BR: Hypnotics and anxiolytics. Br Med J 300:446, 1990.

Drugs for Psychiatric Disorders. Med Lett 36(993):89–96, 1994.

Farnsworth, MG: Benzodiazepine abuse and dependence: Misconceptions and facts. J Fam Prac 31(4):393, 1990.

Livingston, MG: Benzodiazepine dependence. Br J Hosp Med 51(6):281–286, 1994.

Nofzinger, EA and Reynolds III, CF: Insomnia. In Conn's Current Therapy, Philadelphia, Saunders, 1996.

Rall, TW: Hypnotics and sedatives. In Gilman, AG, et al (eds): The Pharmacological Basis of Therapeutics, Pergamon, New York, 1990.

Wise, MG and Griffies, WS: A combined treatment approach to anxiety in the medically ill. J Clin Psychiatry 56(2):14–19, 1995.

Woods, JR, et al: Benzodiazepines: Use, abuse, and consequences. Pharmacol Rev 44:151–347, 1992.

CHAPTER 26

American Psychiatric Association: The Diagnostic and Statistical Manual: IV. The Association, Washington, D.C., 1994.

Drugs for Psychiatric Disorders. Med Lett 36(993):89–96, 1994.

Jefferson, JW: Lithium: The present and the future. J Clin Psychiatry 56(1):41–48, 1995.

McElroy, SL, et al: Minimizing and managing antidepressant side effects. J Clin Psychiatry (suppl 2)56:49–55, 1995.

Zanecka, JM, and Ross, JS: Management of comorbid anxiety and depression. J Clin Psychiatry (suppl 2)56:10–13, 1995.

CHAPTER 27

American Psychiatric Association: Diagnostic and Statistical Manual of Mental Disorders: IV. The Association, Washington, D.C., 1994.

Barnes, TR, and Curson, DA: Long-term depot antipsychotics: A risk-benefit assessment. Drug Safety 10(6):464–479, 1994.

Drugs for Psychiatric Disorders. Med Lett 36(993):89–96, 1994.

Meltzer, HY: An overview of the mechanism of action of clozapine. J Clin Psychiatry (9 suppl B)55:47–52, 1994.

Sigmundson, HK: Pharmacology of schizophrenia: A review. Can J Psychiatry (9 suppl 2)39:S70–75, 1994.

CHAPTER 28

Guyton, A: A Textbook of Medical Physiology, ed 9. WB Saunders, Philadelphia, 1995.

Netter, F: The Ciba Collection of Medical Illustrations, Vol 5, Heart. Ciba Pharmaceuticals, New York, 1969.

Wellens, H, and Conover, M: The ECG in Emergency Decision Making. WB Saunders, Philadelphia, 1992.

CHAPTER 29

Olin, B (ed): Facts & Comparisons. JB Lippincott, St Louis, 1997.

Redeker, NS: Aging and CV drugs. Am J Nurs 95(9):35–40, 1995.

Steiner J, et al: Incidence of digoxin toxicity in outpatients. West J Med 161(11):474–478, 1994.

Wallace, C: When digoxin harms instead of helps. RN 58(9):26–29, 1995.

Walthall, S, et al: Routine withholding of digitalis for heart rate below 60 beats per minute: Widespread nursing misconception. Heart Lung. Nov/Dec, 472–476, 1993.

CHAPTER 30

Foy, S, et al: Comparison of enalapril versus captopril on left ventricular function and survival three months after acute myocardia infarction (The "practical" study). Am J Cardiol 73(6):1180–1186, 1994.

Grossman, E, et al: Should a moratorium be placed on sublingial nifedipine capsules given for hypertensive emergencies and pseudoemergencies? JAMA Act 23/30(276):1328–1331, 1996.

Moyle, LA, et al: Uniformity of captopril benefit in the SAVE study: Subgroup analysis. Eur Soc Card (Suppl B)15:2–8, 1994.

Olin, B (ed): Facts & Comparisons. JB Lippincott, St Louis, 1997.

Redeker, N: Aging and cardiovascular pharmacology. Am J Nurs 95(9):35–40, 1995.

Solomon, J: Hypertension: New drug therapies. RN 94(1):26–32, 1994.

Drugs for hypertension. Med Lett 37(949):45–50, 1995.

CHAPTER 31

Dunnington, C: Sotalol hydrochloride. Am J Crit Care 2(5):397–405, 1993.

Norton, M: Amiodarone pulmonary toxicity: The nursing challenge. Dimensions Crit Care Nurs 13(6):302–307, 1997.

Olin, B (ed): Facts & Comparisons. JB Lippincott, St Louis, 1997.

Paul, S: New pharmacologic agents for emergency management of supraventricular tachydysrhythmias. Crit Care Nurs Q 16(2):35–45, 1993.

Thompson, E: Adenosine thallium imaging: Pharmacodynamics and patient monitoring. Dimensions Crit Care Nurs 13(4):184–192, 1994.

Yacone-Morton, LA: Antiarrhythmics. RN 95(4):26–36, 1995.

CHAPTER 32

Nisoldipine: A new calcium channel blocker for hypertension. Med Lett 38(968):13–16, Feb 1996.

Olin, B (ed): Facts & Comparisons. JB Lippincott, St Louis, 1997.

CHAPTER 33

Brown, G, et al: Regression of coronary artery disease as a result of intensive lipid-lowering therapy in men with high levels of apolipoprotein B. N Engl J Med 323:1289–1298, 1990.

Gotto, AM: Lipid lowering, regression, and coronary events: A review of the interdisciplinary council on lipids and cardiovascular risk intervention, seventh Council meeting. Circulation 92(3):646–656, 1995.

Hadley, SA, and Saarmann, L: Lipid physiology and nutritional considerations in coronary heart disease. Crit Care Nurs 11(10):28–38, 1995.

National Cholesterol Education Program: Second report of the expert panel on detection, evaluation, and treatment of high blood cholesterol in adults (Adult Treatment Panel II). Circulation 89(3):1329–1445, 1994.

Scandinavian Simvastatin Survival Study Group: Randomised trial of cholesterol lowering in 4444 patients with coronary heart disease: The Scandinavian Simvastatin Survival Study (4S). The Lancet 344:1383–1389, 1994.

Waters, D, et al: Effects of monotherapy with an HMG-CoA reductase inhibitor on the progression of coronary atherosclerosis as assessed by serial quantitative arteriography: The Canadian coronary atherosclerosis intervention trial. Circulation 89:959–968, 1994.

CHAPTER 34

Gilman, AG, et al (eds): Goodman and Gilman's The Pharmacological Basis of Therapeutics, ed 9. Macmillan, New York, 1996.

Jorgensen-Huston, C: Hemolytic transfusion reaction. Am J Nurs 96(3):47, 1996.

Olin, B (ed): Facts & Comparisons. JB Lippincott, St Louis, 1997.

CHAPTER 35

American Association of Critical Care Nurses: Quality of care: Evaluation of the effects of heparinized and nonheparinized slush solutions on the patency of arterial pressure monitoring lines: The AACN thunder project. Am J Crit Care 2(1):3–13, 1993.

Apple, S: New trends in thrombolytic therapy. RN 96(1):30–34, 1996.

Bowlby, H, et al: Heparin as adjunctive therapy to coronary thrombolysis in acute myocardial infarction. Heart Lung 24(4):292–305, July/Aug, 1995.

Catania, U-M: Monitoring Coumadin therapy. RN 94(2):29–34, 1994.

Gilman, AG, et al (eds): Goodman and Gilman's The Pharmacological Basis of Therapeutics, ed 8. Macmillan, New York, 1994.

Habib, GB: Current status on thrombolytics in acute MI. Chest 107:225–232, 1995.

Kuc, J: When heparin causes clots. RN Magazine 93(3):34–37, 1993.

Lemmon, PN, et al: Tissue plasminogen activator: The nurse's role. Crit Care Nurs 14(12):22–31, 1994.

Marchiondo, K: Pharmacologic stress testing: An alternative to exercise. Crit Care Nurs 41–45, December 1994.

National Institute of Neurological Disorders and Stroke rt-PA Stroke Study Group: Tissue plasminogen activator for acute ischemic stroke. N Engl J Med 333:1581–1587, Dec 14, 1995.

Singh, B, et al: CV Pharmacology and Therapeutics. Churchill Livingstone, New York, 1994.

Sparks, K: Are you up to date on weight-based heparin dosing? Am J Nurs 96(4):33–36, April 1996.

CHAPTER 36

McCance, K, and Huether, S: Pathophysiology. CV Mosby, St Louis, 1994.

CHAPTER 37

Olin, B (ed): Facts & Comparisons: JB Lippincott, St Louis 1997.

Materson, BJ, et al: Treatment of hypertension in the elderly. I. Blood pressure and clinical changes: Results of a Department of Veterans Affairs and Cooperative Study. Hypertension 15(4):348–360, 1990.

Singh, B, et al: Cardiovascular Pharmacology and Therapeutics. Churchill Livingstone, New York, 1994.

CHAPTER 38

Dunn, S: How to care for the dialysis patient. Am J Nurs 93(6):26–33, 1993.

Olin, B (ed): Facts & Comparisons: JB Lippincott, St Louis, 1997.

Boggs, RL, and Woolbridge-King, M: AACN Procedure Manual for Critical Care, ed 3. WB Saunders, Philadelphia, 1993.

CHAPTER 39

Mathews, LR: Cardiopulmonary Anatomy and Physiology. JB Lippincott, Philadelphia, 1996.

Des Jardins, T: Cardiopulmonary Anatomy and Physiology, ed. 2. Delmar, Albany, N.Y., 1993.

Scanlan, C, et al: Egan's Fundamentals of Respiratory Care, ed 6. Mosby, St Louis, 1995.

CHAPTER 40

Borkgren, MW, and Gronkiewicz, CA: Update your asthma care from hospital to home. Am J Nurs 95(1):26, 1995.

Chapman, S: Choosing asthma drugs. Community Nurse 1(3):5, 1995.

Eisenbeis, C: Full partner in care: Teaching your patient how to manage her asthma. Nursing 96 26(1):48, 1996.

FDA Approved New Drug Bulletin: Salmeterol xinofoate. RN 57(8):51, 1994.

Ladner, A: Asthma: New insights in the management of older adults. Geriatrics 49(11):20, 1994.

McConnell, EA: What's wrong with this patient? Investigating shortness of breath. Nursing 95 25(3):74, 1995.

Poe, RH, et al: Theophylline: Still a reasonable choice? J Respir Dis 15(1):19, 1994.

Weixier, D: Correcting metered-dose inhaler misuse. Nursing 94 24(7):62, 1994.

CHAPTER 41

Burns, SM: Respiratory pharmacology. AACN Clin Issues Adv Pract Acute Crit Care 6(2):269, 1995.

Cottrell, GP, and Surkin, HB: Pharmacology for Respiratory Care Practitioners, FA Davis, Philadelphia, 1995.

FDA Approved New Drug Bulletin: Dornase alfa (Pulmozyme). RN 57(4):41, 1994.

Howard, BA: Guiding allergy sufferers through the medication maze. RN 57(4):26, 1994.

Howder, CL: Pharmacology, ed 2. Williams & Wilkins, Baltimore, 1996.

CHAPTER 42

Goodman, AG, et al (eds): Goodman and Gilman's The Pharmacological Basis of Therapeutics, ed 8. Macmillan, New York, 1995.

Guyton, A: Textbook of Medical Physiology. WB Saunders, Philadelphia, 1990.

Price, SA, and Wilson, LM: Pathophysiology: Clinical Concepts of Disease Process, ed 2. McGraw-Hill, New York, 1994.

Wilson, J, and Foster, D: Textbook of Endocrinology. WB Saunders, Philadelphia, 1991.

CHAPTER 43

American Medical Association Department of Drugs: AMA Drug Evaluations, ed 5. PSG Publishing, Littleton, Mass, 1996.

Gilman, AG, et al: Goodman and Gilman's The Pharmacological Basis of Therapeutics, ed 8. Macmillan, New York, 1994.

Olin, B (ed): Facts & Comparisons. JB Lippincott, St Louis, 1997.

CHAPTER 44

American Medical Association Department of Drugs, Division of Drugs and Technology: Drug Evaluation, ed 7. WB Saunders, Philadelphia, 1995.

Olin, B (ed): Facts and Comparisons: Glucocorticoid Equivalencies. St Louis, June 1997.

Gilman, AG, et al: Goodman and Gilman's The Pharmacological Basis of Therapeutics, ed 8. Macmillan, New York, 1995.

Growth hormone comes up short. Health 95(5):14, 1995.

Howser, RL. What you need to know about corticosteroid therapy. Am J Nurs 95(8):44–49, 1995.

CHAPTER 45

Baily, C: Biguanides and NIDDM. Diabetes Care 15(6):755–772, 1995.

Clinical Practice Recommendations: American Diabetes Association. Diabetes Care (suppl)19:1, 1996.

Olin, B (ed): Facts & Comparisons: Drug Information. JB Lippincott, St Louis, 1997.

Gilman, AG, et al (eds): Goodman and Gilman's The Pharmacological Basis of Therapeutics, ed 8. Macmillan, New York, 1994.

Nathan, et al: The effect of intensive treatment of diabetes on the development and progression of long-term complications in insulin dependent diabetes mellitus. New Engl J Med 329:997–986, 1993.

USP Drug Information for the Health Care Professional, ed 15, vols 1 and 2. United States Pharmacopedial Convention, Rockville, Md, 1995.

White, J, and Campbell, RK: Drug; drug and drug: Disease interactions and diabetes. Diabetes Educator 21(4):283–286.

CHAPTER 46

American Medical Association, Division of Drugs: AMA Drug Evaluations, ed 7. John Wiley & Sons, New York, 1995.

American Society of Hospital Pharmacists: Hospital Formulary Service. The Society, New York, 1995.

Gilman, AG, et al: Goodman and Gilman's The Pharmacological Basis of Therapeutics, ed 8. Macmillan, New York, 1994.

Mathewson (Kuhn), M: Thyroid disorder. Crit Care Nurs 7(1):74–85, 1987.

CHAPTER 47

Bonnier, P, et al: Clinical and biologic prognostic factors in breast cancer diagnosed during post-menopausal hormone replacement therapy. Obstet Gynecol 85:11–17, Jan 1995.

Gilman, AG, et al: Goodman and Gilman's The Pharmacological Basis of Therapeutics, ed 8. Macmillan, New York, 1994.

Felson DT, et al: The effect of postmenopausal estrogen therapy on bone density in elderly women. N Engl J Med 330(10):715–16, 1994.

Hospital Formulary. American Society of Hospital Pharmacists, Washington, D.C., 1996.

Lafferty, FW, and Fiske, ME: Postmenopausal estrogen replacement: A long-term cohort study. Am J Med 97:66–77, July 1994.

Choice of contraceptives. Med Lett Drugs Ther 37(941):9–12, 1995.

Rookus, MA, and Leeuwen, FE. Oral contraceptives and the risk of breast cancer in women aged 20–54. The Lancet 344:844–51, Sept 24, 1994.

Sanchez-Guerrero, J, et al: Postmenopausal estrogen therapy and the risk for developing systemic lupus erythematosus. Ann Intern Med 122(6):430–433, 1995.

Whipple, B. Common questions about osteoporosis and menopause. Am J Nurs 95(1):69–70, 1995.

CHAPTER 48

Appleton, M et al: Magnesium sulfate versus phenytoin for seizure prophylaxis in pregnancy-induced hypertension. Am J Obstet Gynecol 165:907–913, 1991.

Briggs, G et al: Drugs in Pregnancy and Lactation, ed 4. Williams & Wilkins, Baltimore, 1994.

Gleicher, N: Principles and Practice of Medical Therapy in Pregnancy, ed 2. Appleton and Lange, Norwalk, Conn, 1992.

Mandeville, L, and Troiano, N: NAACOG High Risk Intrapartum Nursing. JB Lippincott, Philadelphia, 1992.

Rayburn, W, and Zuspan, F: Drug Therapy in Obstetrics and Gynecology, ed 3. Mosby, St Louis, 1992.

Simpson, KR, and Creehan, PA: Perinatal Nursing. JB Lippincott, Philadelphia, 1996.

Torgersen, K.L. (1996) Ask the experts: Prostaglandin E2 preparations used to ripen the cervix in preparation for induction. *AWHONN Voice.* 4(3), 4.

CHAPTER 49

Guyton, A: Medical Physiology, ed 9. WB Saunders, Philadelphia, 1995.

Price, S, and Wilson, L: Pathophysiology: Clinical Concepts of Disease Process. McGraw-Hill, New York, 1995.

CHAPTER 50

American Medical Association Department of Drugs: AMA Drug Evaluations, ed 7. PSG Publishing, Littleton, Mass, 1994.

Gilman, AG, et al: Goodman and Gilman's The Pharmacological Basis of Therapeutics, ed 9. Macmillan, New York, 1995.

Med Lett: Lansoprazole. 37(953):63–66, 1995.

Med Lett: Cisapride for nocturnal heartburn. 36(927):65–68, 1994.

Olin, B (ed): Facts & Comparisons, JB Lippincott, St Louis, 1997.

Phillips, MC, and Olson, LR: The immunologic role of the gastrointestinal tract. Crit Care Nurs Clin North Am 5(1):107–120, 1993.

Tryba, M: Sucralfate versus antacids, H_2 antagonists for stress ulcer prophylaxis: A meta analyses. Crit Care Med 19:942–949, 1991.

CHAPTER 51

American Medical Association Drug Department: AMA Drug Evaluations, ed 7. PSG Publishing, Littleton, Mass, 1994.

DiStasio, SA: Zofran makes chemo bearable. RN Magazine 93(5):56–59, 1993.

Gilman, AG, et al (eds): Goodman and Gilman's The Pharmacological Basis of Therapeutics, ed 8. Macmillan, New York, 1994.

Hogan, CM: Advances in the management of nausea and vomiting. Nurs Clin North Am 25(2):475–497, 1990.

Olin, B (ed): Facts & Comparisons. JB Lippincott, St Louis, 1996.

CHAPTER 52

American Medical Association Department of Drugs: AMA Drug Evaluations Annual, New York, 1995. The Association, 1995.

Gilman, AG, et al (eds): Goodman and Gilman's The Pharmacological Basis of Therapeutics, ed 9. McGraw-Hill, 1995.

Olin, B (ed): Facts & Comparisons. JB Lippincott, St Louis, 1996.

CHAPTER 53

American Medical Association Department of Drugs: AMA Drug Evaluations Annual 1995. The Association, 1995.

Gilman, AG, et al (eds): Goodman and Gilman's The Pharmacological Basis of Therapeutics, ed 8. McGraw-Hill Health Profession Division, 1994.

Olin, B (ed): Facts & Comparisons. JB Lippincott, St Louis, 1997.

CHAPTER 54

Allen, MA: Hematologic system. In Wright, J, and Shelton, BK (eds): Desk Reference for Certified Critical Care Nursing Practice. Jones and Bartlett Publishers, Boston, 1993.

Mandell, GL, et al (eds): Principles and Practices of Infectious Diseases, ed 4. Churchill Livingstone, New York, 1993.

Styrt, B: Infection associated with asplenia: Risks, mechanisms and preventions. Am J Med 88:33N–42N, 1990.

Tramont, EC: General or nonspecific host defense mechanisms. In Mandell, GL, et al (eds): Principles and Practices of Infectious Diseases, ed 4. Churchill Livingstone, New York, 1993.

Williams, WJ, et al (eds): Hematology, ed 5. McGraw-Hill, New York, 1994.

CHAPTER 55

Baird, SB, et al: Cancer Nursing: A Comprehensive Textbook. WB Saunders, Philadelphia, 1991.

Foley, JF, et al: Current Therapy in Cancer. WB Saunders, Philadelphia, 1994.

Horwich, A (ed): Combined Radiotherapy and Chemotherapy in Clinical Oncology. Edward Arnold, Division of Hodder & Stoughton, London, 1992.

Muggia, FM, and Speyer, JL (eds): New drug therapy. Hematol Oncol Clin North Am, April 1994.

New drugs for colon cancer. Clin Oncol Alert 5(1):2, 1990.

Skidmore-Roth, L. Mosby's 1991 Nursing Drug Reference. CV Mosby, St Louis, 1991.

Taxol Information Line, Bristol Myers Squibb, New Brunswick, NJ. Personal communication, January 1992. (Hotline 1-800-829-6587.)

Update on tamoxifen for prevention of breast cancer. Clin Oncol Alert 5(11):42, 1990. What do you do with lobular carcinoma in situ? Clin Oncol Alert 6(10):37–38, 1991.

Wickham, RS: Advances in venous access devices and nursing management strategies. Nurs Clin North Am 25(2):345–362, 1990.

Wollner, DI: New agents for the elderly with advanced cancer. Pharmacol Toxicol 17(11):1697–1708, 1992.

CHAPTER 56

Bach, JF, et al: Safety and efficacy of therapeutic monoclonal antibodies in clinical therapy. Immunol Today 14:421–425, 1993.

Creekmore, S, et al: Principles of the clinical evaluation of biologic agents. In DeVita, V, et al (eds): Biologic Therapy of Cancer. JB Lippincott, Philadelphia, 1991.

Croghan, TW: Advances in gene therapy. Hosp Formulary 26(11):880–885, 1991.

Dujulio, JE, and Liles, TM: Monoclonal antibiotics. In Reiger, PT (ed): Biotherapy: A Comprehensive Overview. Jones and Bartlett Publishers, Boston, 1995, pp 135–160.

Hidemann, W, et al: Recombinant human granulocyte-macrophage colony stimulating factor after chemotherapy in patients with myeloid leukemia at higher age or after relapse. Blood 78(5):1190–1197, 1991.

INF-b Multiple Sclerosis Study Group: Interferon beta 1b is effective in relapsing-remitting multiple sclerosis. I. Clinical results of a multicenter, randomized double-blind, placebo-controlled trial. Neurology 43:655–661, 1993.

Jassak, P: An overview of biotherapy. In Reiger, PT (ed): Biotherapy: A Comprehensive Overview. Jones and Bartlett Publishers, Boston, 1995.

Milich, E, and Fefer, A (eds): National Cancer Institute monograph, 63. U.S. Department of Health and Human Services, Public Health Service, National Institutes of Health, NIH Publication No. 83 2606, 1993.

Mitchell, M: Chemotherapy in combination with biomodulations: A 5 year experience with cyclophosphamide and interleukin-2. Semin Oncol (suppl 4)19(2):80–87, 1992.

Moldawer, NP, and Figlin, RA: The interferons. In Reiger, PT (ed): Biotherapy: A Comprehensive Overview. Jones and Bartlett Publishers, Boston, 1995, pp 67–92.

Oncology Nursing Society: Biotherapy: Recommendations for Nursing Course Content and Clinical Practicum. Oncology Nursing Press, Pittsburgh, 1995.

Pardoll, DM: Cancer vaccines. Immunol Today 14:310–316, 1993.

Smith, BR: Use of erythropoietin in AIDS and hematologic disorders. Hosp Formulary 26(8):655–661, 1991.

Wheeler, V: The future of biotherapy. In Reiger, PT (ed): Biotherapy: A Comprehensive Overview. Jones and Bartlett Publishers, Boston, 1995, pp 303–315.

CHAPTER 57

Allison, MC: Gastrointestinal damage associated with the use of nonsteroidal antiinflammatory drugs. N Engl J Med 327:749–754, Sept 1992.

AMA Drug Evaluations. PSG Publishing, Littleton, Mass, 1996.

Gilman, AG, et al (eds): Goodman and Gilman's The Pharmacological Basis of Therapeutics, ed 7. Macmillan, New York, 1995.

Drugs for rheumatoid arthritis. Med Lett Drugs Ther 36(935):101–106, Nov 1994.

Tatro, DS (ed): Drug interactions facts. Facts and Comparisons May 1995.

CHAPTER 58

Ad Hoc Committee of the Scientific Assembly on Microbiology, Tuberculosis, and Pulmonary Infection. Treatment of tuberculosis and tuberculosis infection in adults and children. Clin Infect Dis 21:9–27, 1995.

Nathwani D, Wood MJ: Penicillins. A current review of their clinical pharmacology and therapeutic use. Drugs 45:866–894, 1993.

Piddock LJV: New quinolones and gram-positive bacteria. Antimicrob Agents Chemother 38:163–169, 1994.

Rapp RP, McCraney SA, Goodman NL, Shaddick DJ: New macrolide antibiotics: usefulness in infections caused by mycobacteria other than *Mycobacterium tuberculosis*. Ann Pharmacother 28:1225–1263, 1994.

Von Rosenstiel N, Adam D: Quinolone antibacterials. An update of their pharmacology and therapeutic use. Drugs 47:872–901, 1994.

CHAPTER 59

Olin, B (ed): Facts & Comparisons. JB Lippincott, St Louis, 1997.

CHAPTER 60

American Hospital Formulary Service: AHFS drug information 94. American Society of Hospital Pharmacists, Bethesda, Md, 1994.

Department of Drugs, Division of Drugs and Toxicology: Drug evaluations 1991. American Medical Association, Bethesda, Md, 1991.

Gahart, BL: Intravenous medications, ed 11. CV Mosby, St Louis, 1994.

CHAPTER 61

Allen, MA: Human immunodeficiency virus (HIV). In Wright, J, and Shelton, BK (eds): Desk Reference for Critical Care Nursing. Jones & Bartlett Publishers, Boston, 1993.

American Hospital Formulary Service: AHFS drug information 96. American Society of Hospital Pharmacists, Bethesda, Md, 1996.

Anastasi, JK, and Rivera, JL: AIDS drug update: ddl and ddC. RN 11:41–43, 1991.

Bartlett J: Medical Management of HIV infection. Physicians and Scientists Publishing, Glenview, Ill, 1996.

Bartlett, JG: Pocketbook of infectious disease therapy. Williams & Wilkins, Baltimore, 1996.

Burroughs Wellcome: Zidovudine drug information sheet, 1992.

Centers for Disease Control: HIV/AIDS surveillance report. MMWR 39(9):1–18, 1990.

Connor, EM, et al: Reduction of maternal-infant transmission of human immunodeficiency virus type 1 with zidovudine treatment, N Engl J Med 331:1173–1180, 1994.

Davey, RT, and Lane, HC: Laboratory methods in the diagnosis and prognostic staging of infection with human immunodeficiency virus type I. Rev Infect Dis 12(5):912–930, 1990.

Fan, H, Connor, RF, and Villarreal, LP: The biology of AIDS. Jones & Bartlett Publishers, Boston, 1994.

Fauci, AS: Combination therapy for HIV infection: Getting closer. Ann Intern Med 116(1):85–86, 1992.

Hirsch, M: Treatment of HIV infection, Johns Hopkins AIDS Conference, March 21–22, 1996.

Lederman, MM: Host-directed and immuno-based therapies for human immunodeficiency virus infection, Ann Int Med 122:218–222, 1995.

Levine, AM: Therapeutic approaches to neoplasms in AIDS. Rev Infect Dis 12(5):938–943, 1990.

Meng, T, Fischl, MA, Boota, AM, et al: Combination therapy with zidivudine and dideox-ycytidine in patients with advanced human immunodeficiency virus infection. Ann Intern Med 116:13–20, 1992.

National Institute of Allergy and Infectious Diseases, NIH, and U.S. Public Health Service: State of the ART Conference on Antiretroviral therapy for adult HIV-infected patients. JAMA 270:2583, 1993.

Roche Laboratories: HIVID (zalcitabine) (package insert). Nutley, NJ, Hoffman-La Roche, 1992.

Threlkeld, S, and Hirsch, MS: Antiviral therapy: medical clinics of North America. In press, September 1996.

Valenti, WM: Early intervention in the management of HIV: A handbook for the managed healthcare professional. Burroughs Wellcome, St Louis, 1992.

CHAPTER 62

Guyton, A: Textbook of Medical Physiology. WB Saunders, Philadelphia, 1995.

Luckmann, J, and Sorensen, K: Medical-Surgical Nursing. WB Saunders, Philadelphia, 1996.

Thomas, CL (ed): Taber's Cyclopedic Medical Dictionary, ed 16. FA Davis, Philadelphia, 1989.

CHAPTER 63

AMA Department of Drugs: AMA Drug Evaluations, ed 7. PSG Publishing, Littleton, Mass, 1995.

Daroff, RB, et al: Beta-blockers: Beyond cardiology. Patient Care 13(6):47–70, June 1993.

Gilman, AG, et al (eds): Goodman and Gilman's The Pharmacological Basis of Therapeutics, ed 8. Macmillan, New York, 1994.

Topical Carbonic Anhydrase Inhibitor for Glaucoma. Med Lett 37(956):Sept 1995.

CHAPTER 64

AMA Department of Drugs: AMA Drug Evaluations, ed 6. PSG Publishing, Littleton, Mass, 1996.

Gilman, AG, et al (eds): Goodman and Gilman's The Pharmacological Basis of Therapeutics, ed 8. Macmillan, New York, 1994.

Olin, B (ed): Facts & Comparisons. JB Lippincott, St Louis, 1997.

CHAPTER 65

AMA Department of Drugs: AMA Drug Evaluations. PSG Publishing, Littleton, Mass, 1995.

American Pharmaceutical Association: Handbook of Nonprescription Drugs, ed 8. American Pharmaceutical Association, Washington, DC, 1994.

Carroll, P: Bed selection helps patients rest easy. RN 95(5):44–50, 1995.

Gilman, AG, et al (eds): Goodman and Gilman's The Pharmacological Basis of Therapeutics, ed 9. Macmillan, New York, 1995.

Hoffman, K, Weber, D, and Samsa G: Transparent polyurethane film as an IV catheter dressing. JAMA 267(15):2072–2076, 1992.

CHAPTER 66

AMA Department of Drugs: AMA Drug Evaluations, ed 7. PSG Publishing, Littleton, Mass, 1996.

Gilman, AG, et al (eds): Goodman and Gilman's The Pharmacological Basis of Therapeutics, ed 8. Macmillan, New York, 1994.

Olin, B (ed): Facts & Comparisons. JB Lippincott, St Louis, 1997.

CHAPTER 67

AMA Department of Drugs: AMA Drug Evaluations, ed 8. PSG Publishing, Littleton, Mass, 1995.

Olin, B (ed): Facts and Comparisons. JB Lippincott, St Louis, 1993.

CHAPTER 68

Gilman, AG, et al (eds): Goodman and Gilman's The Pharmacological Basis of Therapeutics, ed 8. Macmillan, New York, 1994.

Hall H: Dobutamine therapy in the home. J Home Health Care Prac 7(1):6–15, 1994.

Kuhn, M: Colloids vs. crystalloids. Crit Care Nurs 11(5):37–51, 1991.

Madsen K: Converting cardiac surgery patients from dopamine to dobutamine. Crit Care Nurs 14(2):103–108, Feb 1994.

Vermeulen, LC, Ratko, TA, Erstad, BL, et al: A paradigm for consensus: The university hospital consortium guidelines for the use of albumin, nonprotein colloid, and crystalloid solutions. Arch Intern Med 155:373–379, Feb 1995.

APPENDIX C

Resolutions to Critical Thinking Skills

CHAPTER 6

Case Study 1: Isoniazid Isoniazid (INH) is commonly used in the United States for TB prophylaxis, and it is a common cause of seizures because one side effect of the drug is pyridoxine (B$_6$) deficiency. As a result, pyridoxine should be administered concurrently with isoniazid. This patient complained of numbness and tingling in her extremities prior to her seizure activity, a significant symptom of pyridoxine deficiency. The treatment of choice is administration of intravenous pyridoxine. The nurse should also be aware that isoniazid interferes with diazepam metabolism via enzyme inhibition. Thus, diazepam doses should be reduced to prevent toxicity. When the patient is stable, the nurse should perform a nutritional assessment as pyridoxine deficiency generally is exacerbated by poor nutritional status. Teaching should include reviewing the necessity of eating foods high in B$_6$ (red meat, poultry, fish, potatoes, tomatoes, spinach, sweet potatoes) and the need of taking supplemental B$_6$ as long as the child is taking isoniazid.

Case Study 2: Lead Poisoning Because (1) the patient's symptoms do not abate with standard peptic ulcer therapy and (2) in light of the increased pain, reduced hemoglobin and hematocrit, and development of extremity weakness, the patient's diagnosis is not correct. Additional information important to this case is that he works on cars and inhales toxic fumes frequently. Lead poisoning should be suspected because of the worsening abdominal pain, anorexia, anemia, and neuropathy. Laboratory tests would reveal elevated lead content in the blood; edetate calcium disodium (calcium EDTA) should be administered for 5 days, and, after a 2-day rest period, the dosing regimen should be repeated. The patient should be advised to use a mask during working hours.

CHAPTER 17

The patient's psychosocial history has two implications for this case study: (1) Anxiety can increase catecholamine release, thus increasing myocardial oxygen demands; and (2) he has a loss of income, which may have prevented him from filling his prescriptions. The nurse should inquire as to the last time the patient took his medication. A 12-lead ECG and cardiac enzymes should be drawn to rule out preinfarction angina or myocardial infarction.

Teaching should emphasize that the medication should be taken as prescribed and never be discontinued. The social service department should be contacted to obtain financial assistance for the patient so he may buy his medication until he can return to work.

CHAPTER 18

The nurse's priority concern for this patient is her low respiratory rate. It is possible that the increased morphine dose could cause the respiratory depression. However, it could also be possible that either the medication pump or the epidural catheter has malfunctioned. Naloxone (Narcan) is the drug of choice for opiate overdose. The nurse should continue to monitor the patient's respiratory status and pain control after Narcan administration, as well as evaluate the medication pump. The patient may have received a bolus of medication when she was repositioned if the catheter was kinked. The epidural catheter should be examined for kinking or migration. Care should be taken to ensure the catheter is not kinked after any repositioning.

CHAPTER 20

The most likely causes of seizure in this patient are hyperglycemia or hypoglycemia, acidosis (diabetic ketoacidosis), electrolyte imbalance, and/or abrupt drug or alcohol withdrawal. The patient should have glucose, electrolytes, arterial blood gases, liver enzymes, and toxicology screens drawn, including Dilantin levels. Because the patient did not take his Dilantin for 3 days, it is likely that his levels are low (normal range: 10–20 μg). If the Dilantin is subtherapeutic, the patient will be given a loading dose of 1000 mg of Dilantin. The nurse should ensure the drug is given in an IV line with only normal saline running, and no faster than 50 mg/min. Cardiac rhythm should be monitored as well. The patient should be taught to take his medication as prescribed and to call his primary health-care provider if he is unable to take the medication orally for more than 1 day.

CHAPTER 26

Case Study 1: Tricyclic Antidepressants The nurse should try to ascertain the type and amount of drug that was taken. The type of drug could be obtained from the patient's physician. The amount of drug could be obtained by searching the patient's house for the bottle and determining the number of doses missing. The patient is found to be taking Imipramine, a tricyclic antidepressant. The nurse should realize that depressed patients sometimes attempt suicide by using their medication. The nurse should institute appropriate suicide precautions and contact the patient's mental health care provider. Treatment is aimed at aggressively managing the tricyclic overdose.

Case Study 2: Lithium   It is common for patients with bipolar disorders to have relapses and quit taking their medication. The nurse should assess the last time the patient took her medication. The patient's mental health–care provider should be contacted. It is likely the patient will require admission to an inpatient mental health facility, where her lithium would be restarted and adjusted. She will be discharged when her mood has stabilized and her serum lithium levels are therapeutic.

CHAPTER 27

Case Study 1: Chlorpromazine (Thorazine)   Chlorpromazine, a phenothiazine, can cause a variety of neurologic syndromes termed *extrapyramidal reactions*. The nurse should question the patient and his family about the time of onset of these symptoms and when they are the most severe. Generally, extrapyramidal reactions increase after a dose of the medication. However, the nurse should also rule out the possibility of reoccurrence of the psychosis by careful questioning about delusions, hallucinations, and so on. This patient is probably experiencing akathesia, an extrapyramidal reaction characterized by restlessness, agitation, facial tics, fine hand tremors, insomnia, and a compulsion to walk. The time of maximal risk for these symptoms is 5 to 60 days after initiating therapy with chlorpromazine. The appropriate course of action is to administer an antiparkinsonian drug, such as Cogentin, along with the Thorazine. The nurse should tell the patient to take the medications together and to call his mental health–care provider if the symptoms return. Hospitalization is not necessary.

Case Study 2: Haloperidol (Haldol)   Chronic treatment with haloperidol can lead to an extrapyramidal reaction of tardive dyskinesia (TD), which is characterized by the symptoms displayed by this patient. TD is more frequent among older female patients who have been given high doses of medications. The symptoms are most likely due to changes in the concentration of dopamine in the brain due to years of haloperidol use. TD is a chronic and irreversible condition that will worsen if the medication is withdrawn. However, patients can be assisted to live more comfortably with this condition. The nurse should provide education about the disorder and make arrangements for the patient to move into a group home for older schizophrenic adults.

CHAPTER 33

Case Study 1: Hypertriglyceridemia in Males   This patient's case provides an excellent example of the interplay

of underlying diseases on serum lipids. Diabetes is one example of a disease that causes hyperlipidemia, thus increasing the triglyceride level as well. The nurse should collect additional data relating to the patient's weight, activity level, and diet. It would not be surprising to find the patient to be overweight and sedentary. Because the hypertriglyeridemia is most likely related to poor control of his diabetes, the patient should start taking an oral hypoglycemic. The patient's plan of care should include teaching for the oral hypoglycemic agent; review of a low-fat, low-sodium, and low-cholesterol diet; and suggestions for weight loss and increasing his activity.

Case Study 2: Hypertriglyceridemia in Females   This patient has a relatively low risk for the development of hyperlipidemia at this time. However, the nurse should emphasize the need for the patient to lose weight and exercise. A goal of a 5- to 10-pound weight loss should be set; the patient's understanding of a low-fat, low-cholesterol diet should be reinforced; and the need to increase activity level should be explained.

CHAPTER 35

Coumadin is highly protein bound, predisposing it to displacement reactions by many other drugs. Further, the use of alcohol could inhibit enzymes that normally biotransform Coumadin. The nurse should ask the patient if she has been taking any additional medications, including over-the-counter drugs, and assess her alcohol intake. The patient should be taught to refrain from taking *any* medication without prior approval of her health-care provider. Further, she should be taught to limit alcohol intake to no more than one glass of wine or beer per day. Hard liquor should be avoided.

CHAPTER 37

Loop diuretics (especially when given IV in large doses) can result in ototoxicity. The lack of interest in surroundings and misinterpretation of questions could indicate a loss of hearing. The nurse needs to determine the other types of antibiotics the patient is taking and his serum potassium level. Aminoglycoside antibiotics are also ototoxic and could result in an additive effect when combined with loop diuretics. The ototoxic effect is heightened with hypokalemia. If the patient is taking an aminoglycoside, the appropriate course of action would be to change his antibiotic to something less ototoxic, such as erythromycin. Hearing acuity should be assessed frequently over the next week to 10 days.

CHAPTER 38

Recall that nonsteroidal anti-inflammatory drugs (NSAIDs) reduce renal perfusion by blocking the dilatory effects of prostaglandins. Thus, the rising creatinine could be related to the use of Motrin. The Motrin should be discontinued and the patient taught to call her health-care provider prior to taking any medication, including over-the-counter drugs. The patient's serum creatinine should be observed over the next week. If the creatinine returns to previously acceptable levels, an increased frequency of peritoneal dialysis is not necessary.

CHAPTER 40

Case Study 1: Atrovent vs. Albuterol   Bronchospasm may be caused from adrenergic blockade or by excessive cholinergic activity. Overuse of MDIs can diminish their therapeutic response. Albuterol, an adrenergic agent, is unable to reverse the bronchospasm. Thus, it may be assumed that there is excessive cholinergic activity. Atrovent (ipratropium bromide) may be a more suitable drug to administer at this time. The nurse should assist the patient to high-Fowler's position, instruct him on pursed-lip breathing, and ensure that he is not left alone until the bronchospasm improves.

Case Study 2: Alupent   Nonepisodic wheezing in a patient with asthma may be caused by low-grade persistent airway inflammation. Thus, bronchodilating agents are ineffective against this problem. Simple pulmonary function tests could be performed to assess airflow resistance at rest before and after a dose of Alupent. Even though the patient reports feeling fairly comfortable, if there is little change postadministration, another cause for the airway resistance could possibly be chronic airway inflammation. The patient's history increases the likelihood of this possibility. Thus, anti-inflammatory agents, such as beclomethasone (Vanceril) and cromalyn sodium (Intal) could be prescribed. After one month, pulmonary function testing should be repeated to see if there is any improvement.

CHAPTER 41

Case Study 1: Diphenhydramine (Benylin)   Severe coughing can stand in the way of the patient's recovery. Recall that a hyperexcitable cough reflex must be subdued thoroughly to avoid the pain and sleep deprivation it can cause. Antihistamine antitussives may be insufficient to control these harsh coughs, and their drying effects may exacerbate the problem. Thus, a nonantihistamine antitussive containing codeine, such as Robitussin-AC, may be more effective for this patient.

Case Study 2: Pseudoephedrine   Pseudoephedrine decreases nasal congestion by stimulating alpha-adrenergic receptors and causing vasoconstriction. This can cause an elevation of blood pressure. Thus, the pseudoephedrine decreases the effectiveness of the propranolol. The patient's rhinitis needs to be controlled, as does his hypertension. Because the patient's rhinitis is allergy related, an antihistamine such as clemastine is more appropriate to control these symptoms. The patient should be evaluated for effectiveness of this drug and for side effects. The patient needs to be taught to avoid nonprescription medications without prior consultation with his health-care provider.

CHAPTER 44

Exacerbations of MS are usually treated with large doses of corticosteroids. The nurse should ascertain the amount of drug the patient was taking. The nurse should also ask the patient if he has been compliant in taking the medication. Abrupt withdrawal from corticosteroids could result in an Addisonian crisis, which is manifested by symptoms similar to this patient (i.e., loss of sodium and water, potassium retention, and hypoglycemia). If the patient has discontinued his drug therapy, the drug needs to be restarted He should be retaught the vital importance of not discontinuing the drug without appropriate tapering of dose so his adrenal glands may function at normal levels.

CHAPTER 45

Insulin reactions may occur when an individual skips a meal or has an increase in activity. The nurse should assess when physical education fits into the daily school schedule. Also, the nurse should assess when the afternoon snack is taken. Developmentally, adolescent children do not want to be different from their peers. The child may not be testing her glucose prior to physical activity or consuming snacks during the afternoon because she does not want to be different. She may also be trying to deny her blood glucose is low, because she would have to eat in class. Or, with school ending at 3:00 PM, she may be trying to wait until class is over to treat the reaction. Reviewing the diabetic regimen with the child should include assessing her self-blood glucose monitoring and her ability to recognize and treat hypoglycemic reactions. Explore what makes the current regimen difficult for this child. Incorporate the child's teacher into the plan to make glucose testing and eating in class easier for the child. Referral to adolescent diabetic support groups and summer camps for children with diabetes may be helpful.

CHAPTER 48

Magnesium sulfate would cause CNS depression, including respiratory depression. Further, clearance of magnesium occurs through the kidneys, and renal function may be impaired with pregnancy-induced hypertension. Further data regarding urine output, specific gravity, and proteinuria should be assessed, as well as serum magnesium level and deep-tendon reflexes. Maternal oxygen saturation, via pulse oximetry, should be instituted. The effect of respiratory depression on fetal heart rate should also be evaluated. The nurse should notify the physician, discontinue the magnesium sulfate infusion, and prepare to administer calcium.

CHAPTER 50

The nurse should ascertain the exact amounts of medication the patient is taking. In this case, the patient was taking 100 mg of Tagamet at bedtime, and a 16-oz bottle of antacid lasted her about 1 week. Thus, she was undermedicating herself. She needs a prescription of 800 mg

Tagamet at bedtime and antacids 3 times a day, 1 hour before meals and before bedtime. Caution the patient to separate administration of antacids and Tagamet by 1 hour, and stress the importance of measuring the amount of antacid precisely. The patient may be given a supply of medication cups for home or taught household equivalents.

CHAPTER 52

Case Study 1: Diarrhea   This patient's diarrhea is most likely caused from the use of the antibiotics. The patient is experiencing antibiotic-associated colitis. He should be assessed for signs of fluid volume deficits and electrolyte imbalances. The current antibiotic should be stopped, and metronidazole (Flagyl) started to assist in healing the bowel. In addition, a bland diet and adequate fluid replacement should be prescribed. The patient should be reassessed in about 3 days to see if the diarrhea has subsided.

CHAPTER 56

Patient 1   The adverse effects of biotherapy are agent specific, dose and schedule related, and may vary with individual health variables such as disease sites and pre-existing health problems. Biotherapeutic agents augment the body's own immune response against tumor and demonstrate exacerbated symptoms in sites where the tumor is present. Therefore, hepatic insufficiency is expected as evidenced by the elevated AST, as is the bone pain. IL-2 may also cause a flulike syndrome, as well as cardiac, respiratory, hepatic, renal, and integumentary symptoms. These adverse affects and the patient's medical history suggest the nurse should evaluate respiratory effort, skin reactions, and joint pain. Patient education is very important when biotherapy is used and should include thorough review of possible side effects of medications and common interventions to alleviate these. For elevated AST, the health-care provider may elect to reduce the dose and observe the AST level; meticulous skin care and the administration of allopurinol will assist with the worsened eczema and gout.

Patient 2   Infections are most common about 2 weeks after therapy, when the neutrophils fall below 500 cells/ mm^3. Hematopoietic growth factors are often administered to shorten this neutropenic period and reduce the incidence and/or severity of infections. This may reduce hospital admissions, resulting in a cost savings to the patient, as well as enhancing her quality of life. Because of her short neutropenic period, the physician orders the G-CSF to begin 12 days after therapy. If this medication is effective, the patient should receive it during each cycle of chemotherapy.

CHAPTER 57

Case Study 2: Constipation   Feen-A-Mint contains phenolphthalein, which, if the feces are alkaline, turns the stools pink-red. The combination of Pepto-Bismol (an antidiarrheal) and Feen-A-Mint (a laxative) could be aggravating each other. Suggest she stop both medications, add bulk to her diet, and increase her daily exercise level. These changes in daily activities might improve her chronic constipation.

CHAPTER 58

Case Study 1: Fever in Immunocompromised Client In an immunocompromised client, any number of pathogens could be causing an infection and elevated temperature. Since blood cultures are negative for bacteria, and reviewing the client's drug regimen indicates there is no coverage for fungal infections, treatment for fungal infection may be indicated. Amphotericin B could be prescribed and the client's temperature monitored closely for 5–7 days.

Case Study 2: Urinary Tract Infection   The nurse should review the client's history and determine if he is taking other medications. Given his history of PUD, there may be a reaction occurring between aluminum-magnesium containing antacids and the ciproflaxacin. Recall that these types of antacids chelate with ciproflaxacin and prevent its absorption when administered concurrently. The antacid should be discontinued. Histamine blocking agents may be substituted. The client should be reassessed in 7 to 10 days.

CHAPTER 68

Restlessness, confusion, and low urine output are all characteristic signs of hypotension. Although the blood pressure of 160/90 is not low, the body perceives this large fall in BP as such. Organ perfusion has been maintained at a chronically higher level for a long time. Thus, the ordered blood pressure is too low to maintain cerebral and renal perfusion. The nurse should call the physician and obtain an order for a higher base blood pressure.

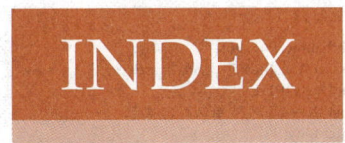

Boldface type indicates broad classifications of drugs; color indicates generic drugs; f indicates a figure; t indicates a table.

Vasodilation, 485, 485f
Vasodilators
  arterial, 432–435, 432t, 433t, 442t
  coronary, 470–474, 471t–472t, 476t–477t, 480–484, 481t–482t
  mixed arterial and venous, 432, 433t, 434–435, 442t
  peripheral, 432–435, 432t–433t, 484–485, 484f, 485t, 486t, 487
Vasopressin, 626, 628
Vasopressors, 1048, 1048t
Vasospasm, 470
Vasotec, 419, 436, 437t, 439, 440t, 559
Vasotec IV, 436, 437t, 439
Vazepam, 358t
V-Cillin, 980t
V-Cillin K, 871t
VCR, 813t
Vecuronium bromide, 304, 320, 321t, 322
Velban, 92, 812, 813t
Velosulin BR, 647, 648t
Velosulin R, 653
Velsar, 812
Venlafaxine hydrochloride, 377, 378
Venoglobulin-I, 511, 909t, 911
Venography, 117
Venous access catheters, 32, 32f
Venous access port (VAP), 32, 32f
Venous/arterial vasodilators, 432, 433t, 434–435, 442t
Ventilation, 582
Ventolin, 589, 590t
Ventricular fibrillation (VF), 407t, 465t
Ventricular tachycardia (VT), 465t
Verapamil, 56t, 435, 451t, 463, 476t, 478–479, 1034t
Verapamil controlled-release, 435, 478
Verapamil sustained-release, 435, 476t, 478
Verelan, 435, 476t
Vermox, 898, 899t
Versed, 302, 304, 305, 359
Vertigo, 981
Very low density lipoproteins (VLDL), 490
Vesicant drugs, 89
Vesiculation, 120
Vexol, 959
VF. See Ventricular fibrillation
Vibramycin, 883, 884t
Vidarabine, 959t
Videx, 939, 940t–941t, 943
Vinblastine, 92, 812, 813t
Vinca alkaloids, 812–814, 813t, 814t
Vincasar PFS, 812
Vincrex, 812
Vincristine, 89, 92, 812–813, 813t
Vindesine sulfate, 812, 813, 813t
Vinorelbine, 812, 813–814, 813t
Vioform, 990t
Viokase, 767t
Vira-A, 959t
Viral vaccines, 913t–914t, 915–917
Virazole, 895, 897

Viroptic, 959t
Visceral proteins, 182, 182t
Visine, 962t, 963
Vision, 953
Visken, 222t, 223, 232, 431, 460
Vistaril, 364, 366
Vitamin A, 156–159, 157t
Vitamin B$_1$, 161, 162t
Vitamin B$_2$, 161, 162t
Vitamin B$_3$, 164t, 491, 497, 497t
Vitamin B$_5$, 163t, 166
Vitamin B$_6$, 161, 162t, 165
Vitamin B$_9$, 163t, 165–166
Vitamin B$_{12}$, 163t, 165
Vitamin C, 59, 164t, 167
Vitamin D, 59, 157t, 159–160, 544
Vitamin D analogue, 157t
Vitamin D$_2$, 157t
Vitamin D$_3$, 157t
Vitamin E, 158t, 160
Vitamin G, 162t
Vitamin H protective factor x, 164t
Vitamin K, 158t, 160–161
Vitamin K$_1$, 160, 521t, 524
Vitamin K$_2$, 160
Vitamin K$_3$, 160
Vitamins, 155–167, 156t, 186, 190–191
  antioxidant, 167
  fat-soluble, 156–161, 157t–158t
  nursing process for, 173–177, 173t
  water-soluble, 161–167, 162t–164t
  See also specific vitamins
Vivactil, 371
Vivelle, 707
VLB, 813t
VLDL. See Very low density lipoproteins
Volatile anesthetics, 301
Voltaren, 855, 856t, 960, 960t, 961
Voltaren SR, 855
Volume of distribution, 42
Vomiting, 754, 755f, 763
  See also **Antiemetics; Emetics**
Vontrol, 758t, 760
VoSol Otic, 981
VT. See Ventricular tachycardia
VZIG, 911

W

Warfarin, 54t, 55
Warfarin sodium, 521t, 522, 523
Wart-Off, 989
Warts, 987t
Water balance, 124–125, 126f, 127–131
Water-soluble vitamins, 161–167, 162t–164t
Wax. See Cerumen
WBCs. See White blood cells
Weight, 49, 272
Wellbutrin, 377
Wellcovorin, 163t

Wellferon, 834t, 840
Westcort, 996t
Western blot test, 910, 937
White blood cells (WBCs), 504, 506t, 509, 795–796
Whole blood, 506t, 508
Whooping cough, 908t
Wingel, 741t
Winstrol, 693
Withdrawal, 1019
  from alcohol, 1029, 1029t
  from opioids, 1029
  from sedatives, 1029
  from stimulants, 1030
  syndromes, 361, 1028–1030, 1029t
Wolff-Parkinson-White (WPW) syndrome, 455, 465t
Wound healing, 1009t, 1010–1011
WPW. See Wolff-Parkinson-White (WPW) syndrome
Wydase, 1009t, 1010, 1011
Wytensin, 426, 429

X

Xamaterol, 224t
Xanax, 359, 359t, 362
Xylocaine, 306, 307t, 456–457, 458t, 721, 1034t

Y

Yutopar, 722, 723t

Z

Zalcitabine, 939, 941t, 944
Zanosar R, 806, 808t
Zantac, 743, 744t, 746
Zarontin, 282t, 289, 290t
Zaroxolyn, 549t, 550, 552
Zebeta, 222t, 223, 233
Zemuron, 304, 320, 321t, 322
Zerit, 939, 941t, 944
Zestril, 437t, 439
Zetar, 995
Zetran, 358t
Zidovudine, 939, 940t, 943
Zinacef, 875t
Zinc, 171–172, 182–183
Zinc 15, 172
Zinc gluconate, 172
Zinc oxide paste, 993t
Zinc pyrithione shampoos, 995
Zinc sulfate, 172
Zinecard, 804, 814
Zithromax, 880, 881t, 882
Zocor, 494, 495t
Zofran, 758t, 760
Zoloft, 373
Zolpidem tartrate, 364, 365–366, 365t
Zovirax, 895, 896t, 989
Zyloprim, 860, 861t, 862
Zyrtec, 603

NURSING CARE PLANS

Plans of care for the patient on . . .

DELIVERING HOME HEALTH CARE